ORTHOPEDIC PHYSICAL ASSESSMENT

SIXTH EDITION

David J. Magee, PhD, BPT, C.M.
Professor
Department of Physical Therapy
Faculty of Rehabilitation Medicine
University of Alberta
Edmonton, Alberta, Canada

ELSEVIER

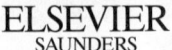

ELSEVIER
SAUNDERS

3251 Riverport Lane
St. Louis, Missouri 63043

ORTHOPEDIC PHYSICAL ASSESSMENT, ED 6   978-1-4557-0977-9

Notices

Knowledge and best practice in this field are constantly changing. As new research and experience
broaden our understanding, changes in research methods, professional practices, or medical
treatment may become necessary.

Practitioners and researchers must always rely on their own experience and knowledge in
evaluating and using any information, methods, compounds, or experiments described herein. In
using such information or methods they should be mindful of their own safety and the safety of
others, including parties for whom they have a professional responsibility.

With respect to any drug or pharmaceutical products identified, readers are advised to check the
most current information provided (i) on procedures featured or (ii) by the manufacturer of each
product to be administered, to verify the recommended dose or formula, the method and duration
of administration, and contraindications. It is the responsibility of practitioners, relying on their
own experience and knowledge of their patients, to make diagnoses, to determine dosages and the
best treatment for each individual patient, and to take all appropriate safety precautions.

To the fullest extent of the law, neither the Publisher nor the authors, contributors, or editors,
assume any liability for any injury and/or damage to persons or property as a matter of products
liability, negligence or otherwise, or from any use or operation of any methods, products,
instructions, or ideas contained in the material herein.

Previous editions copyrighted 1987, 1992, 1997, 2006, 2008.

Library of Congress Cataloging-in-Publication Data

Magee, David J., author.
   Orthopedic physical assessment / David J. Magee.—6th edition.
      p. ; cm.
   Includes bibliographical references and index.
   ISBN 978-1-4557-0977-9 (hardcover : alk. paper)
   I. Title.
   [DNLM: 1. Bone Diseases—diagnosis.   2. Orthopedic Procedures—methods.   3. Joint Diseases—
diagnosis.   4. Physical Examination—methods. WE 168]
   RD734
   616.7′075—dc23

                                                                    2013041753

Content Strategist: Jolynn Gower
Senior Developmental Editor: Christie Hart
Publishing Services Manager: Deborah Vogel
Project Manager: Brandi Flagg
Designer: Amy Buxton

Printed in Canada

Last digit is the print number: 9 8 7 6 5 4 3 2 1

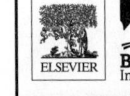

Working together
to grow libraries in
developing countries

www.elsevier.com • www.bookaid.org

To my parents,
Who taught me to pick a goal in life
and to take it seriously

To my family,
Bernice, Wendy, Shawn,
Dolly, Theo, Harry, Tommy, and Henry
My reason for being

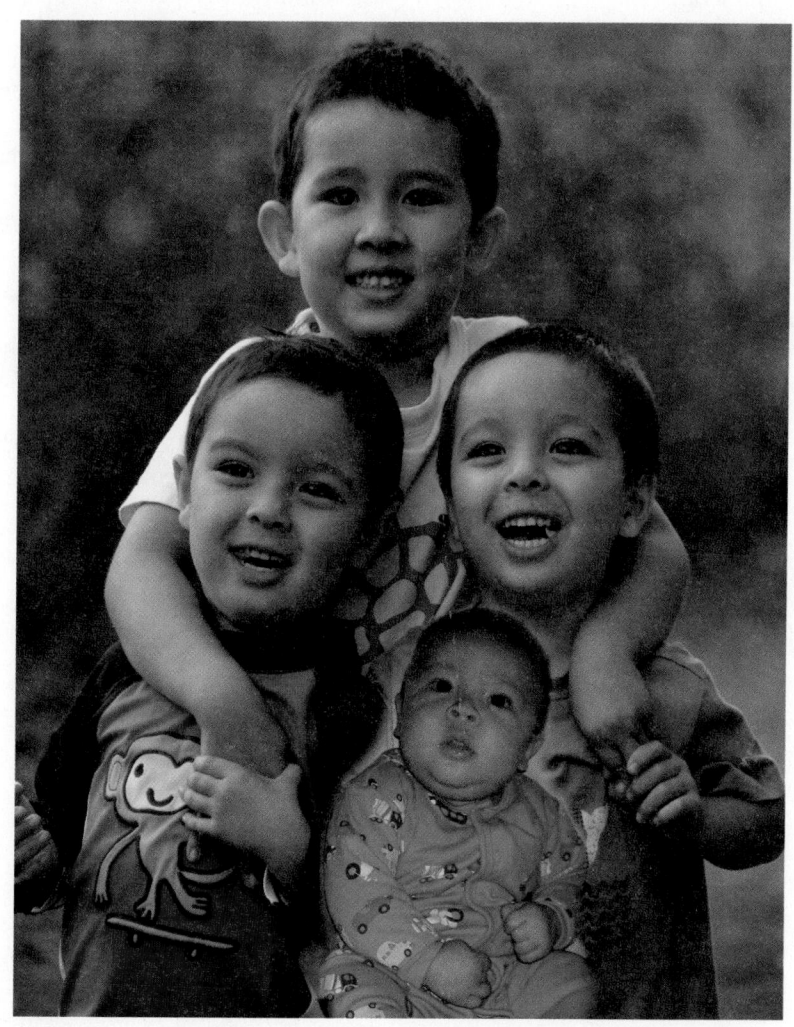

"Grandpa's Boys"

Preface to the Sixth Edition

This sixth edition is a culmination of a dream I have had for many years. When the first edition was published in 1987, I hoped at that time that I would be able to develop a series of books that would meet the needs of rehabilitation clinicians in the area of musculoskeletal conditions. With the assistance of the other editors, James Zachazewski, Sandy Quillen, and Rob Manske, and with a number of experts in their respective fields, my dream has become a reality with the **Musculoskeletal Rehabilitation Series**, with *Orthopedic Physical Assessment* being one of the four books in the series.

In this edition of *Orthopedic Physical Assessment*, information has been updated in all of the chapters as it has been previously in other editions. In addition, and in response to a number of requests, I have put the references back into the book and moved the tables on the reliability and validity of many of the special tests to the Evolve website, where they are available for those who want them. Reliability studies for testing show variability in their outcomes, so I decided to highlight key tests using different icons because the value of the tests have been demonstrated clinically and/or statistically that they contribute to determining what the problem is. Hopefully this will help students and clinicians determine which tests could be effective depending on the pathology being presented.

This book, as the title suggests, is about assessing for musculoskeletal pathology. It is not a pathology textbook. As part of the Musculoskeletal Rehabilitation Series, the companion book to *Orthopedic Physical Assessment* is *Pathology and Interventions in Musculoskeletal Rehabilitation,* which goes into much greater detail on pathological conditions and their treatment. As "bookends" to these two books, *Scientific Foundations and Principles of Practice in Musculoskeletal Rehabilitation* provides information on healing of different tissue types, pain and aging, and the principles of different types of practice to treat different musculoskeletal tissue types; and *Athletic and Sport Issues in Musculoskeletal Rehabilitation* deals with more acute injuries and issues related to the more active individual, specific groups, and specific activities as they relate to sport.

Thanks to Elsevier, this edition is in full color. Although some black and white photographs still remain because of their value in demonstrating certain pathologies, I believe these colored additions greatly enhance the book. Not only have several new color photographs and line drawings been added to this edition, access to video clips on assessment and special tests are available on the Evolve website. These videos are identified throughout the book by a video icon.

I am grateful to the people who have provided input and constructive criticism to make the book better. The support of these people, my students, and family are greatly appreciated. The book is what it is because of their help and involvement.

David J. Magee
2014

Contents

Acknowledgments

The writing of a book such as this, although undertaken by one person, is in reality the bringing together of ideas, concepts, and teachings developed and put forward by colleagues, friends, clinicians, and experts in the field of musculoskeletal assessment. When the book was first published in 1987, I had no idea of how successful it would be. It has succeeded in becoming more than I could have ever imagined in seven languages.

In particular, for this edition, I would like to thank the following people:

My family, for putting up with my moods and idiosyncrasies, especially at 4 a.m.!

Bev Evjen, my irreplaceable developmental editor and friend. Without her help, encouragement, persistence, and eye for detail, this edition, as with the four previous editions and in fact the whole musculoskeletal rehabilitation series, would not be what it is.

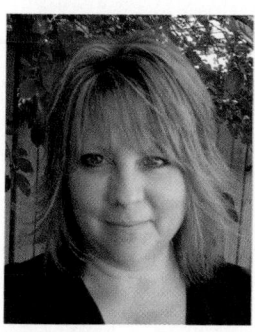

My undergraduate, graduate, and postgraduate students from Canada, the United States, Brazil, Chile, and Japan who provided me with many ideas for revisions, who collected many of the articles used as references, and helped me with many of the tables, especially the reliability and validity tables.

The many authors and publishers who were kind enough to allow me to use their photographs, drawings, and tables in the text so that explanations could be clearer and more easily understood. Without these additions, the book would not be what I hoped for.

Ted Huff, my medical illustrator, whose skills and attention to detail have made a significant contribution to the success of *Orthopedic Physical Assessment* through four editions.

My photographers, Brian Gavriloff and James Tennant, whose photographic talents add immeasurably to the book.

Dr. Andrew Porter for many of the radiographic images he provided for the diagnostic imaging portions of the book.

Dr. Rob Manske for his support and ideas in making the book better and his involvement in the accompanying videos along with Dr. Judy Chepeha. They are true professionals and I am honored to call them friends.

My models, Tanya Beasley, Judy Chepeha, Paul Caines, Lee-Anne Clayholt, Carolyn Crowell, Michelle Cuthbert, Vanessa de Oliveira Furino, Devon Fraser, Ian Hallworth, Nathaniel Hay, Sarah Kazmir, Tysen LeBlanc, Dolly Magee, Shawn Magee, Theo Magee, Tommy Magee, Harry Magee, Judy Sara, Paula Shoemaker, Holly Stevens, Brandon Thome, Joan Matthews-White, and Yung Yung Wong. Your patience and agreement to be models for the many explanatory photographs and videos is very much appreciated.

My colleagues who contributed ideas, suggestions, radiographs, and photographs, and who typed and reviewed the manuscripts.

The people at WB Saunders (Elsevier), especially Jolynn Gower, Christie Hart, Rachel McMullen, and Brandi Flagg for their ideas, suggestions, assistance, and patience.

My teachers, colleagues, and mentors who encouraged me to pursue my chosen career.

To these people and many others – thank you for your help, ideas and encouragement. Your support played a large part in the success and completion of this book.

David J. Magee
2014

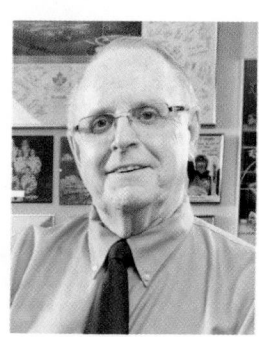

v

CHAPTER 1

Principles and Concepts

A musculoskeletal assessment requires a proper and thorough systematic examination of the patient. A correct diagnosis depends on a knowledge of functional anatomy, an accurate patient history, diligent observation, and a thorough examination. The differential diagnosis process involves the use of clinical signs and symptoms, physical examination, a knowledge of pathology and mechanisms of injury, provocative and palpation (motion) tests, and laboratory and diagnostic imaging techniques. It is only through a complete and systematic assessment that an accurate diagnosis can be made. The purpose of the assessment should be to fully and clearly understand the patient's problems, from the patient's perspective as well as the clinician's, and the physical basis for the symptoms that have caused the patient to complain. As James Cyriax stated, "Diagnosis is only a matter of applying one's anatomy."[1]

One of the more common assessment recording techniques is the problem-oriented medical records method, which uses "SOAP" notes.[2] SOAP stands for the four parts of the assessment: Subjective, Objective, Assessment, and Plan. This method is especially useful in helping the examiner to solve a problem. In this book, the subjective portion of the assessment is covered under the heading Patient History, objective under Observation, and assessment under Examination.

Although the text deals primarily with musculoskeletal physical assessment on an outpatient basis, it can easily be adapted to evaluate inpatients. The primary difference is in adapting the assessment to the needs of a bedridden patient. Often, an inpatient's diagnosis has been made previously, and any continuing assessment is modified to determine how the patient's condition is responding to treatment. Likewise, an outpatient is assessed continually during treatment, and the assessment is modified to reflect the patient's response to treatment.

Regardless of which system is selected for assessment, the examiner should establish a **sequential method** to ensure that nothing is overlooked. The assessment must be organized, comprehensive, and reproducible. In general, the examiner compares one side of the body, which is assumed to be normal, with the other side of the body, which is abnormal or injured. For this reason, the examiner must come to understand and know the wide variability in what is considered normal. In addition, the

examiner should focus attention on only one aspect of the assessment at a time, for example, ensuring a thorough history is taken before completing the examination component. When assessing an individual joint, the examiner must look at the joint and injury in the context of how the injury may affect other joints in the kinetic chain. These other joints may demonstrate changes as they try to compensate for the injured joint.

Total Musculoskeletal Assessment

- Patient history
- Observation
- Examination of movement
- Special tests
- Reflexes and cutaneous distribution
- Joint play movements
- Palpation
- Diagnostic imaging

Each chapter ends with a summary, or précis, of the assessment procedures identified in that chapter. This section enables the examiner to quickly review the pertinent steps of assessment for the joint or structure being assessed. For further information, the examiner can refer to the more detailed sections of the chapter.

PATIENT HISTORY

A complete medical and injury history should be taken and written to ensure reliability. This requires effective and efficient communication on the part of the examiner and the ability to develop a good rapport with the patient and, in some cases, family members and other members of the health care team. This includes speaking at a level and using terms the patient will understand; taking the time to listen; and being empathic, interested, caring, and professional.[3] Naturally, emphasis in taking the history should be placed on the portion of the assessment that has the greatest clinical relevance. Often the examiner can make the diagnosis by simply *listening to the patient.* No subject areas should be skipped. Repetition helps the examiner to become familiar with the characteristic history of the patient's complaints so that unusual deviation, which often indicates problems, is noticed immediately. Even if the diagnosis is obvious, the history provides valuable information about the disorder, its present state, its prognosis, and the appropriate treatment. The history also enables the examiner to determine the type of person the patient is, his or her language and cognitive ability, the patient's ability to articulate, any treatment the patient has received, and the behavior of the injury. In addition to the history of the present illness or injury, the examiner should note relevant past history, treatment, and results. Past medical history should include any major illnesses, surgery, accidents, or allergies. In some cases, it may be necessary to delve into the social and family histories of the patient if they appear relevant. Lifestyle habit patterns, including sleep patterns, stress, workload, and recreational pursuits, should also be noted.

It is important that the examiner politely but firmly keeps the patient focused and discourages irrelevant information. Questions and answers should provide practical information about the problem. At the same time, to obtain optimum results in the assessment, it is important for the examiner to establish a good rapport with the patient. In addition, the examiner should listen for any potential **red flag** signs and symptoms (Table 1-1) that would indicate the problem is not a musculoskeletal one or a more serious problem that should be referred to the appropriate health care professional.[4,5] **Yellow flag** signs and symptoms are also important for the examiner to note as they denote problems that may be more severe or may involve more than one area requiring a more extensive examination, or they may relate to cautions and contraindications to treatment that the examiner might have to consider, or they may indicate overlying psychosocial issues that may affect treatment.[6]

The patient's history is usually taken in an orderly sequence. It offers the patient an opportunity to describe the problem and the limitations caused by the problem as he or she perceives them. To achieve a good functional outcome, it is essential that the clinician heed to the patient's concerns and expectations for treatment. After all, the history is the patient's report of his or her own condition. The clinician should ask questions that are easy to understand and should not lead the patient. For example, the examiner should not say, "Does this increase your pain?" It would be better to say, "Does this alter your pain in any way?" The examiner should ask one question at a time and receive an answer to each question before proceeding with another question. Open-ended questions ask for narrative information; closed or direct questions ask for specific information. Direct questions are often used to fill in details of information given in open-ended questions, and they frequently require only a one-word answer, such as yes or no. In any musculoskeletal assessment, the examiner should seek answers to the following pertinent questions.

▼ TABLE **1-1**

Red Flag Findings in Patient History That Indicate Need for Referral to Physician

Cancer	Persistent pain at night
	Constant pain anywhere in the body
	Unexplained weight loss (e.g., 4.5 to 6.8 kg [10 to 15 lbs] in 2 weeks or less)
	Loss of appetite
	Unusual lumps or growths
	Unwarranted fatigue
Cardiovascular	Shortness of breath
	Dizziness
	Pain or a feeling of heaviness in the chest
	Pulsating pain anywhere in the body
	Constant and severe pain in lower leg (calf) or arm
	Discolored or painful feet
	Swelling (no history of injury)
Gastrointestinal/ Genitourinary	Frequent or severe abdominal pain
	Frequent heartburn or indigestion
	Frequent nausea or vomiting
	Change in or problems with bowel and/or bladder function (e.g., urinary tract infection)
	Unusual menstrual irregularities
Miscellaneous	Fever or night sweats
	Recent severe emotional disturbances
	Swelling or redness in any joint with no history of injury
	Pregnancy
Neurological	Changes in hearing
	Frequent or severe headaches with no history of injury
	Problems with swallowing or changes in speech
	Changes in vision (e.g., blurriness or loss of sight)
	Problems with balance, coordination, or falling
	Faint spells (drop attacks)
	Sudden weakness

Data from Stith JS, Sahrmann SA, Dixon KK, et al: Curriculum to prepare diagnosticians in physical therapy. J Phys Ther Educ 9:50, 1995.

1. *What is the patient's age and sex?* Many conditions occur within certain age ranges. For example, various growth disorders, such as Legg-Perthes disease or Scheuermann disease, are seen in adolescents or teenagers. Degenerative conditions, such as osteoarthritis and osteoporosis, are more likely to be seen in an older population. Shoulder impingement in young people (15 to 35 years) is more likely to result from muscle weakness, primarily in the muscles controlling

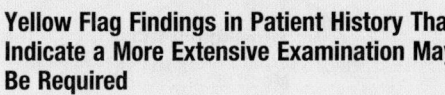

Yellow Flag Findings in Patient History That Indicate a More Extensive Examination May Be Required

- Abnormal signs and symptoms (unusual patterns of complaint)
- Bilateral symptoms
- Symptoms peripheralizing
- Neurological symptoms (nerve root or peripheral nerve)
- Multiple nerve root involvement
- Abnormal sensation patterns (do not follow dermatome or peripheral nerve patterns)
- Saddle anesthesia
- Upper motor neuron symptoms (spinal cord) signs
- Fainting
- Drop attacks
- Vertigo
- Autonomic nervous system symptoms
- Progressive weakness
- Progressive gait disturbances
- Multiple inflamed joints
- Psychosocial stresses
- Circulatory or skin changes

the scapula, whereas the condition in older people (40+ years) is more likely to be the result of degenerative changes in the shoulder complex. Some conditions show sex and even race differences. For example, some cancers are more prevalent in men (e.g., prostrate, bladder), whereas others occur more frequently in women (e.g., cervical, breast), yet still others are more common in white people.

2. *What is the patient's occupation?* What does the patient do at work? What is the working environment like? What are the demands and postures assumed?[7] For example, a laborer probably has stronger muscles than a sedentary worker and may be less likely to suffer a muscle strain. However, laborers are more susceptible to injury because of the types of jobs they have. Because sedentary workers usually have no need for high levels of muscle strength, they may overstress their muscles or joints on weekends because of overactivity or participation in activity that they are not used to. Habitual postures and repetitive strain caused by some occupations may indicate the location or source of the problem.

3. *Why has the patient come for help?* This is often referred to as the **history of the present illness** or **chief complaint.** This part of the history provides an opportunity for patients to describe in their own words what is bothering them and the extent to which it bothers them. It is important for the clinician to determine what the patient wants to be able to do functionally and what the patient is unable to do functionally. It is

also essential to ensure that the clinician knows what is important to the patient in terms of outcome, whether the patient's expectations for the following treatment are realistic, and what direction functional treatment should take to ensure the patient can, if at all possible, return to his or her previous level of activity or realize his or her expected outcome.[8]

4. *Was there any inciting trauma (macrotrauma) or repetitive activity (microtrauma)?* In other words, what was the **mechanism of injury,** and were there any predisposing factors? If the patient was in a motor vehicle accident, for example, was the patient the driver or the passenger? Was he or she the cause of the accident? What part of the car was hit? How fast were the cars going? Was the patient wearing a seat belt? When asking questions about the mechanism(s) of injury, the examiner must try to determine the direction and magnitude of the injuring force and how the force was applied. By carefully listening to the patient, the examiner can often determine which structures were injured and how severely by knowing the force and mechanism of injury. For example, anterior dislocations of the shoulder usually occur when the arm is abducted and laterally rotated beyond the normal range of motion (ROM), and the "terrible triad" injury to the knee (i.e., medial collateral ligament, anterior cruciate ligament, and medial meniscus injury) usually results from a blow to the lateral side of the knee while the knee is flexed, the full weight of the patient is on the knee, and the foot is fixed. Likewise, the examiner should determine whether there were any predisposing, unusual, or new factors (such as, sustained postures or repetitive activities, general health, or familial or genetic problems) that may have led to the problem.[9]

5. *Was the onset of the problem slow or sudden?* Did the condition start as an insidious, mild ache and then progress to continuous pain, or was there a specific episode in which the body part was injured? If inciting trauma has occurred, it is often relatively easy to determine the location of the problem. Does the pain get worse as the day progresses? Was the sudden onset caused by trauma, or was it sudden with locking because of muscle spasm (spasm lock) or pain? Is there anything that relieves the symptoms? Knowledge of these facts helps the examiner make a differential diagnosis.

6. *Where are the symptoms that bother the patient?* If possible, have the patient point to the area. Does the patient point to a specific structure or a more general area? The latter may indicate a more severe condition or referral of symptoms **(yellow flag).** The way in which the patient describes the symptoms often helps to delineate problems. Has the dominant or nondominant side been injured? Injury to the dominant side may lead to greater functional limitations.

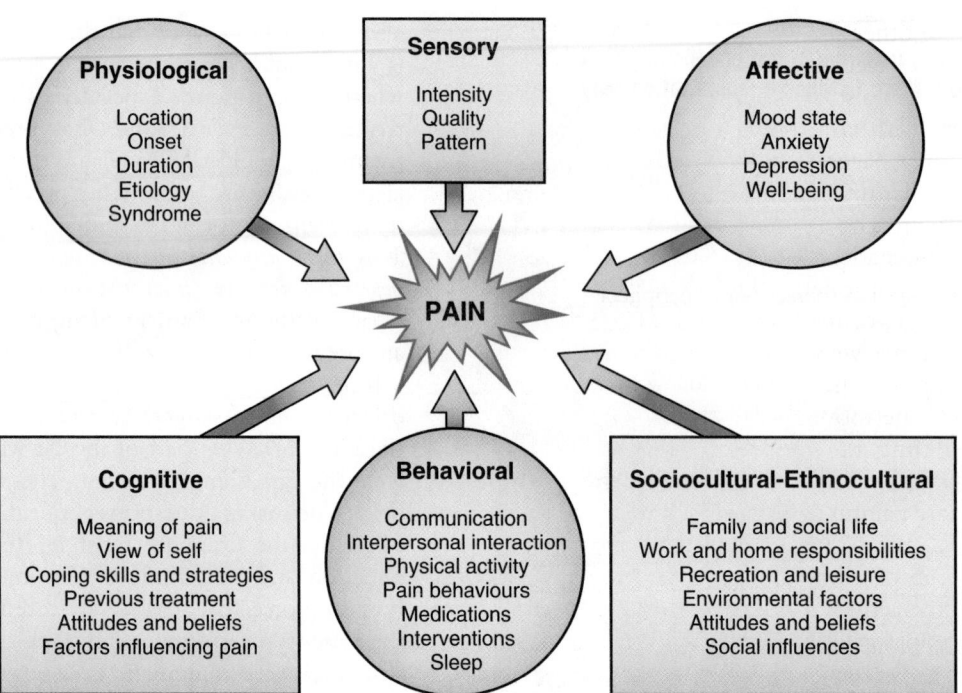

Figure 1-1 The dimensions of pain. (Redrawn from Petty NJ, Moore AP: Neuromusculoskeletal examination and assessment: a handbook for therapists, London, 1998, Churchill-Livingstone, p. 8.)

7. *Where was the pain or other symptoms when the patient first had the complaint?* Pain is subjective, and its manifestations are unique to each individual. It is a complex experience involving several dimensions (Figure 1-1).[10] If the intensity of the pain or symptoms is such that the patient is unable to move in a certain direction or hold a particular posture because of the symptoms, the symptoms are said to be severe. If the symptoms or pain become progressively worse with movement or the longer a position is held, the symptoms are said to be irritable.[11,12] **Acute pain** is new pain that is often severe, continuous, and perhaps disabling and is of sufficient quality or duration that the patient seeks help. Acute injuries tend to be more irritable resulting in pain earlier in the movement, or minimal activity will bring on symptoms, and often the pain will remain after movement has stopped.[3] **Chronic pain** is more aggravating, is not as intense, has been experienced before, and in many cases, the patient knows how to deal with it. Acute pain is more often accompanied by anxiety, whereas chronic pain is associated with depression.[13] When tissue has been damaged, substances are released leading to inflammation and **peripheral sensitization** of the nociceptors (also called **primary hyperalgesia**) resulting in localized pain. If the injury does not follow a normal healing pathway and becomes chronic, **central sensitization** (also called **secondary hyperalgesia**) may occur. Peripheral sensitization is a local phenomenon whereas central sensitization is a more central process involving the spinal cord and brain. Central

sensitization manifests itself as widespread hypersensitivity to such physical, mental, and emotional stressors as touch, mechanical pressure, noise, bright light, temperature, and medication.[14,15]

Has the pain moved or spread? The location and spread of pain may be marked on a body chart, which is part of the assessment sheet (see Appendix 1-1). The examiner should ask the patient to point to exactly where the pain was and where it is now. Are trigger points present? **Trigger points** are localized areas of hyperirritability within the tissues; they are tender to compression, are often accompanied by tight bands of tissue, and, if sufficiently hypersensitive, may give rise to referred pain that is steady, deep, and aching. These trigger points can lead to a diagnosis, because pressure on them reproduces the patient's symptoms. Trigger points are not found in normal muscles.[16]

In general, the area of pain enlarges or becomes more distal as the lesion worsens and becomes smaller or more localized as it improves. Some examiners call the former **peripheralization of symptoms** and the latter, **centralization of symptoms**.[17–19] The more distal and superficial the problem, the more accurately the patient can determine the location of the pain. In the case of referred pain, the patient usually points out a general area; with a localized lesion, the patient points to a specific location. **Referred pain** tends to be felt deeply; its boundaries are indistinct, and it radiates segmentally without crossing the midline. The term, referred pain, means that the pain is felt at a site other than the injured tissue because the same or adjacent neural segments supply the referred site. Pain also may shift as the lesion shifts. For example, with an internal derangement of the knee, pain may occur in flexion one time and in extension another time if it is caused by a loose body within the joint. The examiner must clearly understand where the patient feels the pain. For example, does the pain occur only at the end of the ROM, in part of the range, or throughout the ROM?[9]

8. *What are the exact movements or activities that cause pain?* At this stage, the examiner should not ask the patient to do the movements or activities; this will take place during the examination. However, the examiner should remember which movements the patient says are painful so that when the examination is carried out, the patient can do these movements last to avoid an overflow of painful symptoms. With cessation of the activity, does the pain stay the same, or how long does it take for the pain to return to its previous level? Are there any other factors that aggravate or help to relieve the pain? Do these activities alter the intensity of the pain? The answers to these questions give the examiner some idea of the irritability of the joint. They also help the examiner to differentiate between musculoskeletal or mechanical pain and systemic pain, which is pain arising from one of the body's systems other than the musculoskeletal system (Table 1-2).[18] Functionally, pain can be divided into different levels, especially for repetitive stress conditions.

TABLE 1-2

Differentiation of Systemic and Musculoskeletal Pain

Systemic	Musculoskeletal
• Disturbs sleep • Deep aching or throbbing • Reduced by pressure • Constant or waves of pain and spasm • Is not aggravated by mechanical stress • Associated with the following: 　○ Jaundice 　○ Migratory arthralgias 　○ Skin rash 　○ Fatigue 　○ Weight loss 　○ Low-grade fever 　○ Generalized weakness 　○ Cyclic and progressive symptoms 　○ Tumors 　○ History of infection	• Generally lessens at night • Sharp or superficial ache • Usually decreases with cessation of activity • Usually continuous or intermittent • Is aggravated by mechanical stress

From Meadows JT: Orthopedic differential diagnosis in physical therapy—a case study approach, New York, 1999, McGraw Hill, p. 100. Reproduced with permission of the McGraw-Hill Companies.

Pain and Its Relation to Severity of Repetitive Stress Activity

- Level 1: Pain after specific activity
- Level 2: Pain at start of activity resolving with warm-up
- Level 3: Pain during and after specific activity that does not affect performance
- Level 4: Pain during and after specific activity that does affect performance
- Level 5: Pain with activities of daily living (ADLs)
- Level 6: Constant dull aching pain at rest that does not disturb sleep
- Level 7: Dull aching pain that does disturb sleep

NOTE: Level 7 indicates highest level of severity.

---

9. *How long has the problem existed?* What are the duration and frequency of the symptoms? Answers to these questions help the examiner to determine whether the condition is acute, subacute, chronic, or acute on chronic and to develop some understanding of the patient's tolerance to pain. Generally, **acute conditions** are those that have been present for 7 to 10 days,

subacute conditions have been present for 10 days to 7 weeks, and **chronic conditions** or symptoms have been present for longer than 7 weeks. In **acute on chronic** cases, the injured tissues usually have been reinjured. This knowledge is also beneficial in terms of how vigorously the patient can be examined. For example, the more acute the condition, the less stress the examiner is able to apply to the joints and tissues during the assessment. A full examination may not be possible in very acute conditions. In that case, the examiner must select those procedures of assessment that will give the greatest amount of information with the least stress to the patient. Does the patient protect or support the injured part? If so, this behavior signifies discomfort and fear of pain if the part moves, usually indicating a more acute condition.

10. *Has the condition occurred before?* If so, what was the onset like the first time? Where was the site of the original condition, and has there been any radiation (spread) of the symptoms? If the patient is feeling better, how long did the recovery take? Did any treatment relieve symptoms? Does the current problem appear to be the same as the previous problem, or is it different? If it is different, how is it different? Answers to these questions help the examiner to determine the location and severity of the injury.

11. *Has there been an injury to another part of the kinetic chain as well?* For example, foot problems can lead

to knee, hip, pelvic, and/or spinal problems; elbow problems may contribute to shoulder problems; and hip problems can contribute to knee problems.

12. *Are the intensity, duration, or frequency of pain or other symptoms increasing?* These changes usually mean the condition is getting worse. A decrease in pain or other symptoms usually means the condition is improving. Is the pain static? If so, how long has it been that way? This question may help the examiner to determine the present state of the problem. These factors may become important in treatment and may help to determine whether a treatment is helping. Are pain or other symptoms associated with other physiological functions? For example, is the pain worse with menstruation? If so, when did the patient last have a pelvic examination? Questions such as these may give the examiner an indication of what is causing the problem or what factors may affect the problem. It is often worthwhile to give the patient a pain questionnaire, visual analog scale (VAS), numerical rating scale, box scale, or verbal rating scale that can be completed while the patient is waiting to be assessed.[20,21] The McGill-Melzack pain questionnaire and its short form (Figures 1-2

McGill-Melzack
PAIN QUESTIONNAIRE

Patient's name __________ Age ______
File No. ______ Date ______
Clinical category (e.g., cardiac, neurological, etc.):
Diagnosis: ______

Analgesic (if already administered):
1. Type ______
2. Dosage ______
3. Time given in relation to this test ______

Patient's intelligence: circle number that represents best estimate
1 (low) 2 3 4 5 (high)

****

This questionnaire has been designed to tell us more about your pain. Four major questions we ask are:

1. Where is your pain?
2. What does it feel like?
3. How does it change with time?
4. How strong is it?

It is important that you tell us how your pain feels now. Please follow the instructions at the beginning of each part.

© R. Melzack, Oct. 1970

Part 1. Where Is Your Pain?

Please mark, on the drawings below, the areas where you feel pain. Put E if external, or I if internal, near the areas which you mark. Put EI if both external and internal.

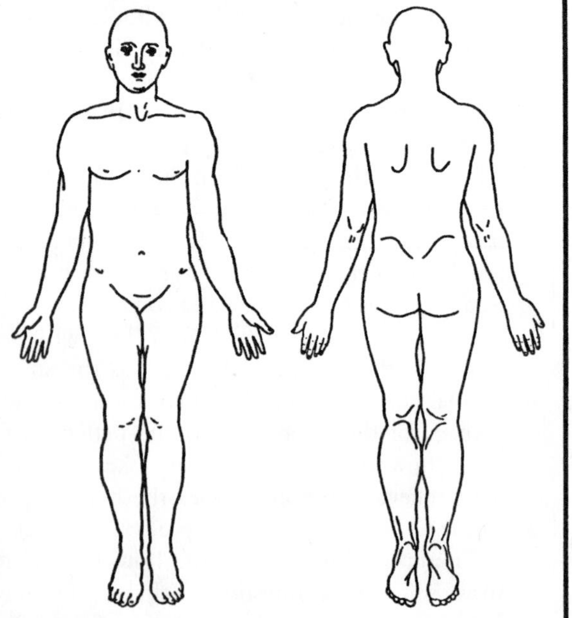

Part 2. What Does Your Pain Feel Like?

Some of the words below describe your present pain. Circle ONLY those words that best describe it. Leave out any category that is not suitable. Use only a single word in each appropriate category—the one that applies best.

1	2	3	4
Flickering Quivering Pulsing Throbbing Beating Pounding	Jumping Flashing Shooting	Pricking Boring Drilling Stabbing Lancinating	Sharp Cutting Lacerating
5	**6**	**7**	**8**
Pinching Pressing Gnawing Cramping Crushing	Tugging Pulling Wrenching	Hot Burning Scalding Searing	Tingling Itchy Smarting Stinging
9	**10**	**11**	**12**
Dull Sore Hurting Aching Heavy	Tender Taut Rasping Splitting	Tiring Exhausting	Sickening Suffocating
13	**14**	**15**	**16**
Fearful Frightful Terrifying	Punishing Gruelling Cruel Vicious Killing	Wretched Blinding	Annoying Troublesome Miserable Intense Unbearable
17	**18**	**19**	**20**
Spreading Radiating Penetrating Piercing	Tight Numb Drawing Squeezing Tearing	Cool Cold Freezing	Nagging Nauseating Agonizing Dreadful Torturing

Part 3. How Does Your Pain Change With Time?

1. Which word or words would you use to describe the pattern of your pain?

1	2	3
Continuous	Rhythmic	Brief
Steady	Periodic	Momentary
Constant	Intermittent	Transient

2. What kind of things relieve your pain?

3. What kind of things increase your pain?

Part 4. How Strong Is Your Pain?

People agree that the following 5 words represent pain of increasing intensity. They are:

1	2	3	4	5
Mild	Discomforting	Distressing	Horrible	Excruciating

To answer each question below, write the number of the most appropriate word in the space beside the question.

1. Which word describes your pain right now? ______
2. Which word describes it at its worst? ______
3. Which word describes it when it is least? ______
4. Which word describes the worst toothache you ever had? ______
5. Which word describes the worst headache you ever had? ______
6. Which word describes the worst stomach-ache you ever had? ______

Figure 1-2 McGill-Melzack pain questionnaire. (From Melzack R: The McGill pain questionnaire: major properties and scoring methods. Pain 1:280–281, 1975.)

SHORT-FORM McGILL PAIN QUESTIONNAIRE
RONALD MELZACK

PATIENT'S NAME:_____   DATE:_____

	NONE	MILD	MODERATE	SEVERE
1. THROBBING	0) ____	1) ____	2) ____	3) ____
2. SHOOTING	0) ____	1) ____	2) ____	3) ____
3. STABBING	0) ____	1) ____	2) ____	3) ____
4. SHARP	0) ____	1) ____	2) ____	3) ____
5. CRAMPING	0) ____	1) ____	2) ____	3) ____
6. GNAWING	0) ____	1) ____	2) ____	3) ____
7. HOT-BURNING	0) ____	1) ____	2) ____	3) ____
8. ACHING	0) ____	1) ____	2) ____	3) ____
9. HEAVY	0) ____	1) ____	2) ____	3) ____
10. TENDER	0) ____	1) ____	2) ____	3) ____
11. SPLITTING	0) ____	1) ____	2) ____	3) ____
12. TIRING-EXHAUSTING	0) ____	1) ____	2) ____	3) ____
13. SICKENING	0) ____	1) ____	2) ____	3) ____
14. FEARFUL	0) ____	1) ____	2) ____	3) ____
15. PUNISHING-CRUEL	0) ____	1) ____	2) ____	3) ____

|—————————————————————————|

0
NO
PAIN

10
WORST
POSSIBLE
PAIN

P P I

0 NO PAIN	____
1 MILD	____
2 DISCOMFORTING	____
3 DISTRESSING	____
4 HORRIBLE	____
5 EXCRUCIATING	____

Figure 1-3 The short-form McGill pain questionnaire. Descriptors 1 to 11 represent the sensory dimension of pain experience, and descriptors 12 to 15 represent the affective dimension. Each descriptor is ranked on an intensity scale of 0 = none, 1 = mild, 2 = moderate, 3 = severe. The present pain intensity (PPI) of the standard long-form McGill pain questionnaire and the visual analogue scale (VAS) are also included to provide overall intensity scores. For actual examination, line would be 10 cm long. (Modified from Melzack R: The short-form McGill pain questionnaire. Pain 30:193, 1987.)

and 1-3)[22–24] provide the patient with three major classes of word descriptors—sensory, affective, and evaluative—to describe their pain experience. These designations are used to differentiate patients who have a true sensory pain experience from those who think they have experienced pain (affective pain state). Other pain-rating scales allow the patient to visually gauge the amount of pain along a solid 10-cm line (visual analogue scale) (Figure 1-4) or on a thermometer-type scale (Figure 1-5).[25] It has been shown that an examiner should consistently use the same pain scales when assessing or reassessing patients to increase consistent results.[26–29] The examiner can use the completed questionnaire or scale as an indication of the pain as described or perceived by the patient. Alternatively, a self-report pain drawing (see Appendix 1-1), which (with the training and

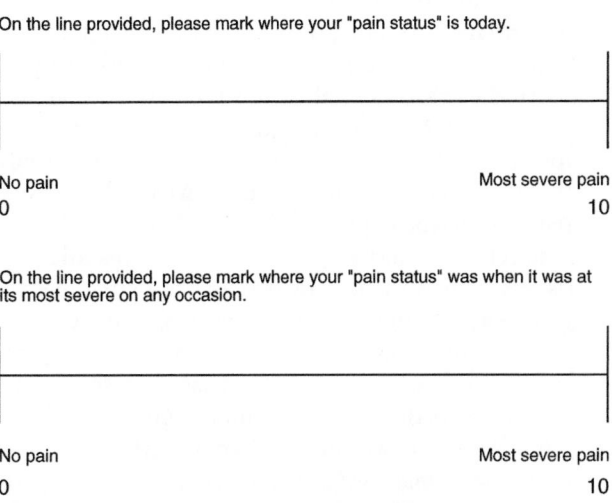

On the line provided, please mark where your "pain status" is today.

No pain
0

Most severe pain
10

On the line provided, please mark where your "pain status" was when it was at its most severe on any occasion.

No pain
0

Most severe pain
10

Figure 1-4 Visual analog scales (VASs) for pain. Example only. Note: For an actual examination, the lines would be 10 cm long.

Pain Rating Scale

Instructions:
  Below is a thermometer with various grades of pain on it from "No pain at all" to "The pain is almost unbearable." Put an X by the words that describe your pain best. Mark how bad your pain is **at this moment in time.**

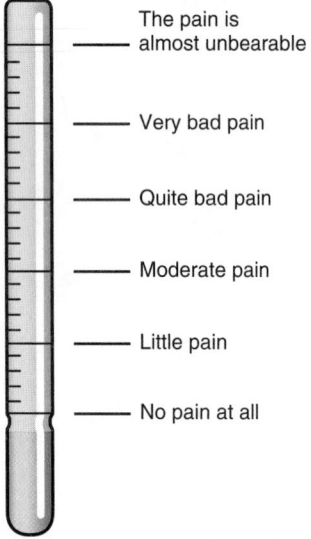

— The pain is almost unbearable

— Very bad pain

— Quite bad pain

— Moderate pain

— Little pain

— No pain at all

Figure 1-5 "Thermometer" pain rating scale. (Redrawn from Brodie DJ, Burnett JV, Walker JM, et al: Evaluation of low back pain by patient questionnaires and therapist assessment. J Orthop Sports Phys Ther 11[11]:528, 1990.)

guidelines of the raters) has been shown to have reliability, can be used for the same purpose.[30]

13. *Is the pain constant, periodic, episodic (occurring with certain activities), or occasional?* Does the condition bother the patient at that exact moment? If the patient is not bothered at that exact moment, the pain is not constant. **Constant pain** suggests chemical irritation, tumors, or possibly visceral lesions.[18] It is always there, although its intensity may vary. If **periodic** or **occasional pain** is present, the examiner should try to determine the activity, position, or posture that irritates or brings on the symptoms, because this may help determine what tissues are at fault. This type of pain is more likely to be mechanical and related to movement and stress.[18] **Episodic pain** is related to specific activities. At the same time, the examiner should be observing the patient. Does the patient appear to be in constant pain? Does the patient appear to be lacking sleep because of pain? Does the patient move around a great deal in an attempt to find a comfortable position?

14. *Is the pain associated with rest? Activity? Certain postures? Visceral function? Time of day?* Pain on activity that decreases with rest usually indicates a mechanical problem interfering with movement, such as adhesions. Morning pain with stiffness that improves with activity usually indicates chronic inflammation and edema, which decrease with motion. Pain or aching as the day progresses usually indicates increased congestion in a joint. Pain at rest and pain that is worse at the beginning of activity than at the end implies acute inflammation. Pain that is not affected by rest or activity usually indicates bone pain or could be related to organic or systemic disorders, such as cancer or diseases of the viscera. Chronic pain is often associated with multiple factors, such as fatigue or certain postures or activities. If the pain occurs at night, how does the patient lie in bed: supine, on the side, or prone? Does sleeping alter the pain, or does the patient wake when he or she changes position? Intractable pain at night may indicate serious pathology (e.g., a tumor). Movement seldom affects visceral pain unless the movement compresses or stretches the structure.[11] Symptoms of peripheral nerve entrapment (e.g., carpal tunnel syndrome) and thoracic outlet syndromes tend to be worse at night. Pain and cramping with prolonged walking may indicate lumbar spinal stenosis (neurogenic intermittent claudication) or vascular problems (circulatory or vascular intermittent claudication). Intervertebral disc pain is aggravated by sitting and bending forward. Facet joint pain is often relieved by sitting and bending forward and is aggravated by extension and rotation. What type of mattress and pillow does the patient use? Foam pillows often cause more problems for persons with cervical disorders because these pillows have more "bounce" to them than do feather or buckwheat pillows. Too many pillows, pillows improperly positioned, or too soft a mattress may also cause problems.

15. *What type or quality of pain is exhibited?* **Nerve pain** tends to be sharp (lancinating), bright, and burning and also tends to run in the distribution of specific nerves. Thus, the examiner must have detailed knowledge of the sensory distribution of nerve roots (dermatomes) and peripheral nerves as the different distributions may tell where the pathology or problem is if the nerve is involved. **Bone pain** tends to be deep, boring, and localized. **Vascular pain** tends to be diffuse, aching, and poorly localized and may be referred to other areas of the body. **Muscle pain** is usually hard to localize, is dull and aching, is often aggravated by injury, and may be referred to other areas (Table 1-3). If a muscle is injured, when the muscle contracts or is stretched, the pain will increase. Inert tissue, such as ligaments, joint capsules, and bursa, tend to exhibit pain similar to muscle pain and may be indistinguishable from muscle pain in the resting state (e.g., when the examiner is taking the history); however, pain in inert tissue is increased

when the structures are stretched or pinched. Each of these specific tissue pains is sometimes grouped as **neuropathic pain** and follows specific anatomical pathways and affect specific anatomical structures.[18] The Leeds Assessment of Neuropathic Symptoms and Signs (LANSS) Pain Scale (Figure 1-6) has been

TABLE 1-3

Pain Descriptions and Related Structures

Type of Pain	Structure
Cramping, dull, aching	Muscle
Dull, aching	Ligament, joint capsule
Sharp, shooting	Nerve root
Sharp, bright, lightning-like	Nerve
Burning, pressure-like, stinging, aching	Sympathetic nerve
Deep, nagging, dull	Bone
Sharp, severe, intolerable	Fracture
Throbbing, diffuse	Vasculature

developed to determine if neuropathic causes dominate the pain experience.[31] **Somatic pain,** on the other hand, is a severe chronic or aching pain that is inconsistent with injury or pathology to specific anatomical structures and cannot be explained by any physical cause because the sensory input can come from so many different structures supplied by the same nerve root.[12] Superficial somatic pain may be localized, but deep somatic pain is more diffuse and may be referred.[32] On examination, somatic pain may be reproduced, but visceral pain is not reproduced by movement.[32]

16. *What types of sensations does the patient feel, and where are these abnormal sensations?* If the problem is in bone, there usually is very little radiation of pain. If pressure is applied to a nerve root, radicular pain (radiating pain) results from pressure on the dura mater, which is the outermost covering of the spinal cord. If there is pressure on the nerve trunk, no pain occurs, but there is paresthesia, or an abnormal sensation, such as a "pins and needles" feeling or tingling.

THE LANSS PAIN SCALE
Leeds Assessment of Neuropathic Symptoms and Signs

NAME_____ DATE _____

This pain scale can help to determine whether the nerves that are carrying your pain signals are working normally or not. It is important to find this out in case different treatments are needed to control your pain.

A. PAIN QUESTIONNAIRE

*   Think about how your pain has felt over the last week.
*   Please say whether any of the descriptions match your pain exactly.

1) **Does your pain feel like strange, unpleasant sensations in your skin? Words like pricking, tingling, pins and needles might describe these sensations.**

   a) NO - My pain doesn't really feel like this .... (0)

   b) YES - I get these sensations quite a lot .... (5)

2) **Does your pain make the skin in the painful area look different from normal? Words like mottled or looking more red or pink might describe the appearance.**

   a) NO - My pain doesn't affect the colour of my skin .... (0)

   b) YES - I've noticed that the pain does make my skin look different from normal ..... (5)

3) **Does your pain make the affected skin abnormally sensitive to touch? Getting unpleasant sensations when lightly stroking the skin, or getting pain when wearing tight clothes might describe the abnormal sensitivity.**

   a) NO - My pain doesn't make my skin abnormally sensitive in that area .... (0)

   b) YES - My skin seems abnormally sensitive to touch in that area .... (3)

4) **Does your pain come on suddenly and in bursts for no apparent reason when you're still. Words like electric shocks, jumping, and bursting describe these sensations.**

   a) NO - My pain doesn't really feel like this .... (0)

   b) YES - I get these sensations quite a lot .... (2)

5) **Does your pain feel as if the skin temperature in the painful area has changed abnormally? Words like hot and burning describe these sensations**

   a) NO - I don't really get these sensations .... (0)

   b) YES - I get these sensations quite a lot .... (1)

B. SENSORY TESTING

Skin sensitivity can be examined by comparing the painful area with a contralateral or adjacent non-painful area for the presence of allodynia and an altered pin-prick threshold (PPT).

1) **ALLODYNIA (Pain caused by something that normally would not cause pain)**
     Examine the response to lightly stroking cotton wool across the non-painful area and then the painful area. If normal sensations are experienced in the non-painful site, but pain or unpleasant sensations (e.g., tingling, nausea) are experienced in the painful area when stroking, allodynia is present.

   a) NO, normal sensation in both areas .... (0)

   b) YES, allodynia in painful area only .... (5)

2) **ALTERED PIN-PRICK THRESHOLD**
     Determine the pin-prick threshold by comparing the response to a 23 gauge (blue) needle mounted inside a 2 ml syringe barrel placed gently on to the skin in a non-painful and then painful areas.

     If a sharp pin prick is felt in the non-painful area, but a different sensation is experienced in the painful area (e.g., none/blunt only [raised PPT] or a very painful sensation [lowered PPT]), an altered PPT is present.

     If a pinprick is not felt in either area, mount the syringe onto the needle to increase the weight and repeat.

   a) NO, equal sensation in both areas .... (0)

   b) YES, altered PPT in painful area .... (3)

SCORING:

Add values in parentheses for sensory description and examination findings to obtain overall score.

TOTAL SCORE (maximum 24) ....

If score <12, neuropathic mechanisms are **unlikely** to be contribution to the patient's pain.

If score ≥12, neuropathic mechanisms are **likely** to be contribution to the patient's pain.

Figure 1-6 The Leeds Assessment of Neuropathic Symptoms and Signs (LANSS) Pain Scale. (Modified from Bennett M: The LANSS Pain Scale: the Leeds assessment of neuropathic symptoms and signs, Pain 92:156–157, 2001.)

Paresthesia is an unpleasant sensation that occurs without an apparent stimulus or cause (to the patient). Autonomic pain is more likely to be a burning type of pain. If the nerve itself is affected, regardless of where the irritation occurs along the nerve, the brain perceives the pain as coming from the periphery. This is an example of **referred pain.**

17. *Does a joint exhibit locking, unlocking, twinges, instability, or giving way?* Seldom does locking mean that the joint will not move at all. **Locking** may mean that the joint cannot be fully extended, as is the case with a meniscal tear in the knee, or it may mean that it does not extend one time and does not flex the next time (**pseudolocking**), as in the case of a loose body moving within the joint. Locking may mean that the joint cannot be put through a full ROM because of muscle spasm or because the movement was too fast; this is sometimes referred to as **spasm locking.** **Giving way** is often caused by reflex inhibition or weakness of the muscles, and so the patient feels that the limb will buckle if weight is placed on it or the pain will be too great. Inhibition may be caused by anticipated pain or instability.

In nonpathological states, excessive ROM in a joint is called **laxity** or **hypermobility.** Laxity implies the patient has excessive ROM but can control movement in that range and no pathology is present. It is a function of the ligaments and joint capsule resistance.[33] This differs from flexibility, which is the ROM available in one or more joints and is a function of contractile tissue resistance primarily as well as ligament and joint capsule resistance.[33] Gleim and McHugh[33] describe flexibility in two parts: static and dynamic. Static flexibility is related to the ROM available in one or more joints; dynamic flexibility is related to stiffness and ease of movement. Laxity may be caused by familial factors or may be job or activity (e.g., sports) related. In any case, laxity, when found, should be considered normal (Figure 1-7). If symptoms occur, then laxity is considered to be hypermobility and has a pathological component, which commonly indicates the patient's inability to control the joint during movement, especially at end range, which implies instability of the joint. Instability can cover a wide range of pathological hypermobility from a loss of control of arthrokinematic joint movements to anatomical instability where subluxation or dislocation is imminent or has occurred. For assessment purposes, instability can be divided into translational (loss of arthrokinematic control) and anatomical (dislocation or subluxation) instability.[34] **Translational instability** (also called *pathological* or *mechanical instability*) refers to loss of control of the small, arthrokinematic joint movements (e.g., spin, slide, roll, translation) that occur when the patient attempts to stabilize (statically or dynamically) the

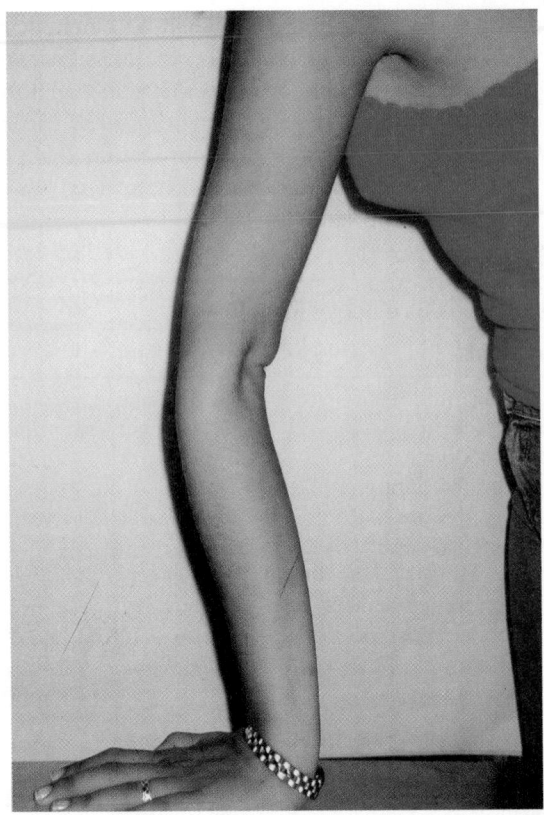

Figure 1-7 Congenital laxity at the elbow leading to hyperextension. This may also be called *nonpathological hypermobility.*

joint during movement. **Anatomical instability** (also called *clinical* or *gross instability,* or *pathological hypermobility*) refers to excessive or gross physiological movement in a joint where the patient becomes apprehensive at the end of the ROM because a subluxation or dislocation is imminent. It should be noted that there is confusion in the application of the terms used to describe the two types of instability. For example, mechanical instability is sometimes used to mean anatomical instability because of anatomical or pathological dysfunction. **Functional instability** may mean either or both types of instability and implies an inability to control either arthrokinematic or osteokinematic movement in the available ROM either consciously or unconsciously during functional movement. These instabilities are more likely to be evident during high-speed or loaded movements. Both types of instability can cause symptoms, and treatment centers on teaching the patient to develop muscular control of the joint and to improve reaction time and proprioceptive control. Both types of instability may be voluntary or involuntary. **Voluntary instability** is initiated by muscle contraction, and **involuntary instability** is the result of positioning. Another concept worth remembering during assessment for instability is the **circle concept of instability,** which was originally developed from shoulder studies[35,36] but is equally applicable to other joints. This concept states that injury to structures on one side of a joint leading to instability can, at the same time, cause injury to structures on the other side or other parts of the joint. Thus, an anterior shoulder dislocation can lead to injury of the posterior capsule. Similarly, anterolateral rotary instability of the knee leads to injury to posterior structures (e.g., arcuate-popliteus complex, posterior capsule) as well as anterior (e.g., anterior cruciate ligament) and lateral (e.g., lateral collateral ligament) structures. Thus, the examiner must be aware of potential injuries on the opposite side of the joint even if symptoms are predominantly on one side, especially when the mechanism of injury is trauma.

18. *Has the patient experienced any bilateral spinal cord symptoms, fainting, or drop attacks? Is bladder function normal? Is there any "saddle" involvement (abnormal sensation in the perianal region, buttocks, and superior aspect of the posterior thighs) or vertigo?* "Vertigo" and "dizziness" are terms often used synonymously, although vertigo usually indicates more severe symptoms. The terms describe a swaying, spinning sensation accompanied by feelings of unsteadiness and loss of balance. These symptoms indicate severe neurological problems, such as cervical myelopathy, which must be dealt with carefully and can (e.g., in cases of altered bladder function) be emergency conditions potentially requiring surgery. Drop attacks occur when the patient suddenly falls without warning or provocation but remains conscious.[18] It is caused by neurological dysfunction especially in the brain.

19. *Are there any changes in the color of the limb?* Ischemic changes resulting from circulatory problems may include white, brittle skin; loss of hair; and abnormal nails on the foot or hand. Conditions such as reflex sympathetic dystrophy, which is an autonomic nerve response to trauma, however minor, can cause these symptoms, as can circulatory problems such as Raynaud's disease.

20. *Has the patient been experiencing any life or economic stresses?* These psychological stressors are sometimes considered to be **yellow flags** that alter both the assessment and subsequent treatment.[37,38] Divorce, marital problems, financial problems, or job stress or insecurity can contribute to increasing the pain or symptoms because of psychological stress. What support systems and resources are available? Are there any cultural issues one should be aware of? Does the patient have an easily accessible living environment? Each of these issues may increase stress to the patient. Pain is often accentuated in patients with anxiety, depression, or hysteria, or patients may exaggerate their symptoms (symptom magnification) in the absence of objective signs, which may be called

psychogenic pain.[3,39,40] Thus, psychosocial aspects can play a significant role with injury.[41-44] Because of the importance of these psychosocial aspects related to movement, questionnaires such as the Fear-Avoidance Beliefs Questionnaire (FABQ)[45] (Figure 1-8) and the Tampa Scale for Kinesiophobia[46-49] have been developed. Most of the studies related to the psychosocial aspects of injury have been related to the low back but could be used for other joints. The focus of these questionnaires is on the patient's beliefs about how physical activity and work affect his or her injury and pain.[42,50,51] Table 1-4 outlines some of the psychological processes affecting pain.[42] These processes have been divided into different colored "flags" (Table 1-5), but it is important to note that these psychological flags, other than the red flag, are different from pathological "flags" previously mentioned.[44] Waddell and Main[37] consider illness behavior normal with patients who are exhibiting both a physical problem and varying degrees of illness behavior (Table 1-6). In these cases, it may be beneficial to determine the level of psychological stress or to refer the patient to another appropriate health care professional.[38] When symptoms (such as, pain) appear to be exaggerated, the examiner must also consider the possibility that the patient is malingering. Malingering implies trying to obtain a particular gain by a conscious effort to deceive.[52]

Reactions to Stress

- Aches and pains
- Anxiety
- Changed appetite
- Chronic fatigue
- Difficulty concentrating
- Difficulty sleeping
- Irritability and impatience
- Loss of interest and enjoyment in life
- Muscle tension (headaches)
- Sweaty hands
- Trembling
- Withdrawal

---

21. *Does the patient have any chronic or serious systemic illnesses or adverse social habits (e.g., smoking, drinking) that may influence the course of the pathology or the treatment?* In some cases, the examiner may use a medical history screening form (Figure 1-9) to determine the presence of conditions that may affect treatment or require referral to another health care professional.

22. *Is there anything in the family or developmental history that may be related, such as tumors, arthritis, heart*

Fear-Avoidance Beliefs Questionnaire (FABQ)

Here are some of the things which other patients have told us about their pain. For each statement please circle any number from 0 to 6 to say how much physical activities such as bending, lifting, walking, or driving affect or would affect *your* back pain.

	Completely disagree			Unsure			Completely agree
1. My pain was caused by physical activity	0	1	2	3	4	5	6
2. Physical activity makes my pain worse	0	1	2	3	4	5	6
3. Physical activity might harm my back	0	1	2	3	4	5	6
4. I should not do physical activities which (might) make my pain worse	0	1	2	3	4	5	6
5. I cannot do physical activities which (might) make my pain worse	0	1	2	3	4	5	6

The following statements are about how your normal work affects or would affect your back pain

	Completely disagree			Unsure			Completely agree
6. My pain was caused by my work or by an accident at work	0	1	2	3	4	5	6
7. My work aggravated my pain	0	1	2	3	4	5	6
8. I have a claim for compensation for my pain	0	1	2	3	4	5	6
9. My work is too heavy for me	0	1	2	3	4	5	6
10. My work makes or would make my pain worse	0	1	2	3	4	5	6
11. My work might harm my back	0	1	2	3	4	5	6
12. I should not do my normal work with my present pain	0	1	2	3	4	5	6
13. I cannot do my normal work with my present pain	0	1	2	3	4	5	6
14. I cannot do my normal work till my pain is treated	0	1	2	3	4	5	6
15. I do not think that I will be back to my normal work within 3 months.	0	1	2	3	4	5	6
16. I do not think that I will ever be able to go back to that work	0	1	2	3	4	5	6

Scoring:

fear-avoidance beliefs about work (scale 1) = (points for item 6) + (points for item 7) + (points for item 9) + (points for item 10) + (points for item 11) + (points for item 12) + (points for item 15)

fear-avoidance beliefs about physical activity (scale 2) = (points for item 2) + (points for item 3) + (points for item 4) + (points for item 5)

Items not in scale 1 or 2: 1 8 13 14 16

Interpretation:

• Minimal scale scores: 0

• Maximum scale 1 score: 42 (7 items)

• Maximum scale 2 score: 24 (4 items)

• The higher the scale scores the greater the degree of fear and avoidance beliefs shown by the patient.

Figure 1-8 Fear-Avoidance Beliefs Questionnaire (FABQ). (Modified from Waddell G, Newton M, Henderson I, et al: A fear-avoidance beliefs questionnaire [FABQ] and the role of fear-avoidance beliefs in chronic low back pain and disability. Pain 52:166, 1993.)

TABLE **1-4**

Summary of Psychological Processes

Factor	Description	Possible Effect on Pain and Disability	Example of Treatment Strategy
Attention	Pain demands our attention	• Vigilance may increase pain intensity • Distraction may decrease its pain intensity	• Distraction techniques • Interceptive exposure
Cognitions	How we think about our pain may influence it	• Interpretations and beliefs may increase pain and disability • Catastrophizing (irrational thoughts that something is far worse than it is) may increase pain • Negative thoughts and beliefs may increase pain and disability • Expectations may influence pain and disability • Cognitive sets may reduce flexibility in dealing with pain and disability	• Cognitive restructuring • Behavioral experiments designed, for example, to disconfirm unrealistic expectations and catastrophizing
Emotions and emotion regulation	Pain often generates negative feelings; these negative feelings may influence the pain as well as fuel cognitions, attention, and overt behaviors	• Fear may increase avoidance behavior and disability • Anxiety may increase pain disability • Depression may increase pain disability • Distress, in general, fuels negative cognitions and pain disability • Positive emotions might decrease pain	• Cognitive-behavioral therapy programs for anxiety and depression • Activation (to increase positive emotion) • Relaxation • Positive psychology techniques that promote well-being and positive emotions
Overt behavior	What we do to cope with our pain influences our perception of pain	• Avoidance behavior may increase disability • Unlimited activity (overactivity) may provoke pain • Pain behaviors communicate pain	• Operant, graded activity training • Exposure in vivo • Coping strategies training

Modified from Linton SJ, Shaw WS: Impact of psychological factors in the experience of pain. Phys Ther 91:703, 2011.

TABLE **1-5**

Summary of Different Types of Psychological Flags

Flag	Nature	Examples
Red	Signs of serious pathology	• Cauda equina syndrome, fracture, tumor
Orange	Psychiatric symptoms	• Clinical depression, personality disorder
Yellow	Beliefs, appraisals, and judgments	• Unhelpful beliefs about pain; indication of injury as uncontrollable or likely to worsen • Expectations of poor treatment outcome, delayed return to work
	Emotional responses	• Distress not meeting criteria for diagnosis of mental disorder • Worry, fears, anxiety
	Pain behavior (including pain coping strategies)	• Avoidance of activities due to expectations of pain and possible reinjury • Over-reliance on passive treatments (e.g., hot packs, cold packs, analgesics)
Blue	Perceptions about the relationship between work and health	• Belief that work is too onerous and likely to cause further injury • Belief that workplace supervisor and workmates are unsupportive
Black	System or contextual obstacles	• Legislation restricting options for return to work • Conflict with insurance staff over injury claim • Overly solicitous family and health care providers • Heavy work, with little opportunity to modify duties

From Nicholas MK, Linton SJ, Watson PJ, et al: Early identification and management of psychological risk factors (yellow flags) in patients with low back pain: a reappraisal, Phys Ther 91:739, 2011.

TABLE **1-6**

Spectrum of Clinical Symptoms and Signs

	Physical Disease	Illness Behavior
Pain		
Pain drawing	Localized	Nonanatomic
	Anatomic	Regional
		Magnified
Pain adjectives	Sensory	Emotional
Symptoms		
Pain	Musculoskeletal or neurologic distribution	Whole leg pain
		Pain at the tip of the tailbone
Numbness	Dermatomal	Whole leg numbness
Weakness	Myotomal	Whole leg giving way
Time pattern	Varies with time and activity	Never free of pain
Response to treatment	Variable benefit	Intolerance of treatments
		Emergency hospitalization
Signs		
Tenderness	Musculoskeletal distribution	Superficial
		Nonanatomic
Axial loading	Neck pain	Low back pain
Simulated rotation	Nerve root pain	Low back pain
Straight leg raising	Limited on formal examination	Marked improvement with distraction
	No improvement on distraction	
Motor	Myotomal	Regional, jerky, giving way
Sensory	Dermatomal	Regional

From Waddell G, Main CJ: Illness behavior. In Waddell G, editor: The back pain revolution, Edinburgh, 1998, Churchill Livingstone, p. 162.

disease, diabetes, allergies, and congenital anomalies? Some disease processes and pathologies have a familial incidence.

23. *Has the patient undergone an x-ray examination or other imaging techniques?* If so, x-ray overexposure must be considered; if not, an x-ray examination may help yield a diagnosis.

24. *Has the patient been receiving analgesic, steroid, or any other medication? If so, for how long?* High dosages of steroids taken for long periods may lead to problems, such as osteoporosis. Has the patient been taking any other medication that is pertinent? Anticoagulants (such as, aspirin or anticoagulant therapy) increase the chance of bruising or hemarthrosis because the clotting mechanism is altered. Patients may not regard over-the-counter formulations, birth control pills, and so on as medications. If such medications have been taken for a long period, their use may not seem pertinent to the patient. How long has the patient been taking the medication? When did he or she last take the medication? Did the medication help?[53] It is also important to determine whether medication is being taken for the condition under review. If analgesics or anti-inflammatories were taken just before the patient's visit for the assessment, some symptoms may be masked.

25. *Does the patient have a history of surgery or past/present illness?* If so, when was the surgery performed, what was the site of operation, and what condition was being treated? Sometimes, the condition the examiner is asked to treat is the result of the surgery. Has the patient ever been hospitalized? If so, why? Health conditions such as high blood pressure, heart and circulatory problems, and systemic diseases (e.g., diabetes) should be noted because of their effect on healing, exercise prescription, and functional activities.[3]

Taking an accurate, detailed history is very important. *Listen to the patient—he or she is telling you what is wrong!* With experience, the examiner should be able to make a **preliminary "working" diagnosis** from the history alone. The observation and examination phases of the assessment are then used to confirm, alter, or refute the possible diagnoses. What an examiner looks for in observation and tests for in examination is often related to what she or he has found when taking a history.

Date:		
Patient's Name:	DOB:	Age:
Diagnosis:	Date of Onset:	
Physician:	Therapist:	Precautions:

Medical History			Do Not Complete, For Clinician		
Have you or any immediate family member ever been told you have:	Circle one:		Relation to Patient	Date of Onset	Current Status
Cancer	Yes	No			
Diabetes	Yes	No			
Hypoglycemia	Yes	No			
Hypertension or high blood pressure	Yes	No			
Heart disease	Yes	No			
Angina or chest pain	Yes	No			
Shortness of breath	Yes	No			
Stroke	Yes	No			
Kidney disease/stones	Yes	No			
Urinary tract infection	Yes	No			
Allergies	Yes	No			
Asthma, hay fever	Yes	No			
Rheumatic/scarlet fever	Yes	No			
Hepatitis/jaundice	Yes	No			
Cirrhosis/liver disease	Yes	No			
Polio	Yes	No			
Chronic bronchitis	Yes	No			
Pneumonia	Yes	No			
Emphysema	Yes	No			
Migraine headaches	Yes	No			
Anemia	Yes	No			
Ulcers/stomach problems	Yes	No			
Arthritis/gout	Yes	No			
Other	Yes	No			

Medical Testing

1. Are you taking any prescription or over-the-counter medications?   Yes   No
   If yes, please list:
2. Have you had any x-rays, sonograms, computed tomography (CT)   Yes   No
   scans, or magnetic resonance imaging (MRI) done recently?
   If yes, when?   Where?   Results?
3. Have you had any laboratory work done recently (urinalysis or blood tests)?   Yes   No
   If yes, when?   Where?   Results?
4. Please list any operations that you have ever had and the date(s) of surgery.
   Surgery/Date:

General Health

1. Have you had any recent illnesses within the last 3 weeks (e.g., colds,   Yes   No
   influenza, bladder or kidney infection)?

Figure 1-9 Medical history screening card. (From Goodman CC, Snyder TK: Differential diagnosis in physical therapy, Philadelphia, 1990, WB Saunders.)

Continued

2. Have you noticed any lumps or thickening of skin or muscle anywhere on your body?	Yes	No
3. Do you have any sores that have not healed or any changes in size, shape, or color of a wart or mole?	Yes	No
4. Have you had any unexplained weight loss in the last month?	Yes	No
5. Do you smoke or chew tobacco?	Yes	No
If yes, how many packs/day?		
For how many months or years?		
6. How much alcohol do you drink in the course of a week?		
7. How much caffeine to you consume daily (including soft drinks, coffee, tea, or chocolate)?		
8. Are you on any special diet prescribed by a physician?	Yes	No

Special Questions for Women

1. Last Pap smear:		
2. Last breast examination:		
3. Do you perform a monthly self-breast examination?	Yes	No
4. Do you take birth control pills or do you use an intrauterine device (IUD)?	Yes	No

Special Questions for Men

1. Do you ever have difficulty with urination (e.g., difficulty in starting or continuing flow or a very slow flow or urine)?	Yes	No
2. Do you ever have blood in your urine?	Yes	No
3. Do you ever have pain on urination?	Yes	No

Work Environment

1. Occupation:		
2. Does your job involve:		
prolonged sitting (e.g., desk, computer, driving)	Yes	No
prolonged standing (e.g., equipment operator, sales clerk)	Yes	No
prolonged walking (e.g., mill worker, delivery service)	Yes	No
use of large or small equipment (e.g., telephone, fork lift, typewriter, drill press, cash register)	Yes	No
lifting, bending, twisting, climbing, turning	Yes	No
exposure to chemicals or gases	Yes	No
other: please describe		
3. Do you use any special supports:		
back cushion, neck cushion	Yes	No
back brace, corset	Yes	No
other kind of brace or support for any body part	Yes	No

For Clinician

Vital signs:

Resting pulse rate:

Oral temperature:

Blood pressure: 1st reading: 2nd reading:

Position: Extremity:

Figure 1-9, cont'd

OBSERVATION

In an assessment, observation is the "looking" or inspection phase. Its purpose is to gain information on visible defects, functional deficits, and abnormalities of alignment. Much of the observation phase involves assessment of **normal standing posture** (see Chapter 15). Normal posture covers a wide range, and asymmetric findings are common. The key is to determine whether these findings are related to the pathology being presented. The examiner should note the patient's way of moving as well as the general posture, manner, attitude, willingness to cooperate, and any signs of overt pain behavior.[54] Observation may begin in the waiting room or as the patient is being taken to the assessment area. Often the patient is unaware that observation is occurring at this stage and may present a different picture. The patient must be adequately undressed in a private assessment area to be observed properly. Male patients should wear only shorts, and female patients should wear a bra or halter top and shorts. Because the patient is in a state of undress, it is essential for the examiner to explain that observation and detailed looking at the patient are integral parts of the assessment. This explanation may prevent a potentially embarrassing situation that can have legal ramifications.

Overt Pain Behavior[54]

- *Guarding*—Abnormally stiff, interrupted or rigid movement while moving the joint or body from one position to an other
- *Bracing*—A stationary position in which a fully extended limb supports and maintains an abnormal distribution of weight
- *Rubbing*—Any contact between hand and injured area (i.e., touching, rubbing, or holding the painful area)
- *Grimacing*—Obvious facial expression of pain that may include furrowed brow, narrowed eyes, tightened lips, corners of mouth pulled back and clenched teeth
- *Sighing*—Obvious exaggerated exhalation of air usually accompanied by the shoulders first rising and then falling; patients may expand their cheeks first

---

As the patient enters the assessment area, the examiner should observe his or her gait (see Chapter 14). This initial gait assessment is only a cursory one; however, problems, such as Trendelenburg sign or drop foot, are easily noticed. If there appears to be an abnormality, the gait may be checked in greater detail after the patient has undressed.

The examiner should be positioned so that the dominant eye is used, and both sides of the patient should be compared simultaneously. During the observation stage, the examiner is only looking at the patient and does not ask the patient to move; the examiner usually does not palpate, except possibly to learn whether an area is warm or hot or to find specific landmarks.

After the patient has undressed, the examiner should observe the posture, looking for asymmetries and determining whether the asymmetries are significant or applicable to the problem being assessed. In doing so, the examiner should attempt to answer the following questions often by comparing both sides:

1. What is the normal body alignment? Anteriorly, the nose, xiphisternum, and umbilicus should be in a straight line. From the side, the tip of the ear, the tip of the acromion, the high point of the iliac crest, and the lateral malleolus (anterior aspect) should be in a straight line.
2. Is there any obvious deformity? Deformities may take the form of restricted ROM (e.g., flexion deformity), malalignment (e.g., genu varum), alteration in the shape of a bone (e.g., fracture), or alteration in the relationship of two articulating structures (e.g., subluxation, dislocation). **Structural deformities** are present even at rest; examples include torticollis, fractures, scoliosis, and kyphosis. **Functional deformities** are the result of assumed postures and disappear when posture is changed. For example, a scoliosis due to a short leg seen in an upright posture disappears on forward flexion. A pes planus (flatfoot) on weight bearing may disappear on non-weight-bearing. **Dynamic deformities** are caused by muscle action and are present when muscles contract or joints move. Therefore, they are not usually evident when the muscles are relaxed. Dynamic deformities are more likely to be seen during the examination phase.
3. Are the bony contours of the body normal and symmetric, or is there an obvious deviation? The body is not perfectly symmetric, and deviation may have no clinical implications. For example, many people have a lower shoulder on the dominant side or demonstrate a slight scoliosis of the spine adjacent to the heart. However, any deviation should be noted, because it may contribute to a more accurate diagnosis.
4. Are the soft-tissue contours (e.g., muscle, skin, fat) normal and symmetric? Is there any obvious muscle wasting?
5. Are the limb positions equal and symmetric? The examiner should compare limb size, shape, position, any atrophy, color, and temperature.
6. Because pelvic position plays such an important role in correct posture of the whole body, the examiner should determine if the patient can position the pelvis in the **"neutral pelvis" position.** This dynamic position is such that the anterior superior iliac spines are one-to-two finger widths lower than the posterior superior iliac spines on the same side in normal standing. When looking for the "neutral pelvis" position, the examiner must be able to answer three questions in the affirmative. If not, there are

probably hypomobile and/or hypermobile structures affecting the pelvic position. The three questions are:

1) Can the patient get into the "neutral pelvis" position? (If not, why not?)
2) Can the patient hold the "neutral pelvis" position while doing distal dynamic movement? (If not, why not?)
3) Can the patient control the dynamic "neutral pelvis" while doing dynamic movement (e.g., walking, running, jumping)?

If the answer to any of these questions is "no," the examiner should consider adding pelvic "core muscle" control activities to any treatment protocol.

7. Are the color and texture of the skin normal? Does the appearance of the skin differ in the area of pain or symptoms, compared with other areas of the body? Ecchymosis or bruising indicates bleeding under the skin from injury to tissues (Figure 1-10). In some cases, this ecchymosis may track away from the injury site because of gravity. Trophic changes in the skin resulting from peripheral nerve lesions include loss of skin elasticity, shiny skin, hair loss on the skin, and skin that breaks down easily and heals slowly. The nails may become brittle and ridged. Skin disorders (such as, psoriasis) may affect joints (psoriatic arthritis). Cyanosis, or a bluish color to the skin, is usually an indication of poor blood perfusion. Redness indicates increased blood flow or inflammation.

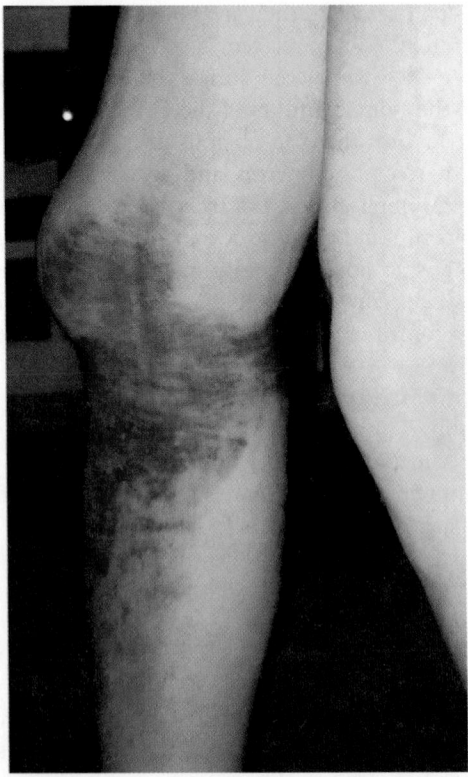

Figure 1-10 Ecchymosis around the knee following rupture of the quadriceps and dislocation of the patella. Note how the ecchymosis is tracking distally toward the foot because of gravity from the leg hanging dependent.

8. Are there any scars that indicate recent injury or surgery? Recent scars are red because they are still healing and contain capillaries; older scars are white and primarily avascular. Fibers of the dermis (skin) tend to run in one direction, along so-called cleavage or tension lines. Lacerations or surgical cuts along these lines produce less scarring. Cuts across joint flexion lines frequently produce excessive (hypertrophic) scarring. Some individuals are also prone to keloid (excessive) or hypertrophic scarring. Hypertrophic scars are scars that have excessive scar tissue but stay within the margins of the wound. Keloid scars expand beyond the margins of the wound. Are there any callosities, blisters, or inflamed bursae, indicative of excessive pressure or friction to the skin? Are there any sinuses that may indicate infection? If so, are the sinuses draining or dry?

9. Is there any crepitus, snapping, or abnormal sound in the joints when the patient moves them? Sounds, by themselves, do not necessarily indicate pathology. Sounds on movement only become significant when they are related to the patient's symptoms. Crepitus may vary from a loud grinding noise to a squeaking noise. Snapping, especially if not painful, may be caused by a tendon moving over a bony protuberance. Clicking is sometimes heard in the temporomandibular joint and may be an indication of early nonsymptomatic pathology.

10. Is there any heat, swelling, or redness in the area being observed? All of these signs along with pain and loss of function are indications of inflammation or an active inflammatory condition.

11. What attitude does the patient appear to have toward the condition or toward the examiner? Is the patient apprehensive, restless, resentful, or depressed? These questions give the examiner some indication of the patient's psychological state and how he or she will respond to the examination and treatment.

12. What is the patient's facial expression? Does the patient appear to be apprehensive, in discomfort, or lacking sleep?

13. Is the patient willing to move? Are patterns of movement normal? If not, how are they abnormal? Any alteration should be noted and included in the observation portion of the assessment.

On completion of the observation phase of the assessment, the examiner should return to the original preliminary working diagnosis made at the end of the history to see if any alteration in the diagnosis should be made with the additional information found in this phase.

EXAMINATION

Principles

Because the examination portion of the assessment involves touching the patient and may, in some cases, cause the patient discomfort, the examiner must obtain a valid consent to perform the examination before it begins. A valid consent must be voluntary, must cover the procedures to be done (informed consent), and the patient must be legally competent to give the consent (Appendix 1-2).[55,56]

The examination is used to confirm or refute the suspected diagnosis, which is based on the history and observation. The examination must be performed systematically with the examiner looking for a consistent pattern of signs and symptoms that leads to a differential diagnosis. Special care must be taken if the condition of the joint is irritable or acute. This is especially true if the area is in severe spasm or if the patient complains of severe unremitting pain that is not affected by position or medication, severe night pain, severe pain with no history of injury, or nonmechanical behavior of the joint.

Red Flags in Examination Indicating the Need for Medical Consultation[57]

- Severe unremitting pain
- Pain unaffected by medication or position
- Severe night pain
- Severe pain with no history of injury
- Severe spasm
- Inability to urinate or hold urine
- Elevated temperature (especially if prolonged)
- Psychological overlay

In the examination portion of the assessment, a number of principles must be followed.

1. Unless bilateral movement is required, the normal side is tested first. Testing the normal side first allows the examiner to establish a baseline for normal movement for the joint being tested[58] and shows the patient what to expect, resulting in increased patient confidence and less patient apprehension when the injured side is tested.

2. The patient does active movements before the examiner does passive movements. Passive movements are followed by resisted isometric movements (see later discussion). In this way, the examiner has a better idea of what the patient thinks he or she can do before the structures are fully tested.

3. Any movements that are painful are done last, if possible, to prevent an overflow of painful symptoms to the next movement that, in reality, may be symptom free.

4. If active range of motion (AROM) is not full, overpressure is applied only with extreme care to prevent the exacerbation of symptoms.

5. During AROM, if the ROM is full, overpressure may be carefully applied to determine the end feel of the joint. This often negates the need to do passive movements.

6. Each active, passive, or resisted isometric movement may be repeated several times or held (sustained) for a certain amount of time to see whether symptoms increase or decrease, whether a different pattern of movement results, whether there is increased weakness, or whether there is possible vascular insufficiency. This repetitive or sustained activity is especially important if the patient has complained that repetitive movement or sustained postures alter symptoms.

7. Resisted isometric movements are done with the joint in a neutral or resting position so that stress on the inert tissues is minimal. Any symptoms produced by the movement are then more likely to be caused by problems with contractile tissue.

8. For passive range of motion (PROM) or ligamentous tests, it is not only the degree (i.e., the amount) of the opening but also the quality (i.e., the end feel) of the opening that is important.

9. When the examiner is testing the ligaments, the appropriate stress is applied gently and repeated several times. The stress is increased up to but not beyond the point of pain, thereby demonstrating maximum instability without causing muscle spasm.

10. When testing **myotomes** (groups of muscles supplied by a single nerve root), each contraction is held for a minimum of **5 seconds** to see whether weakness becomes evident. Myotomal weakness takes time to develop.

11. At the completion of an assessment, because a good examination commonly involves stressing different tissues, the examiner must warn the patient that symptoms may exacerbate as a result of the assessment. This will prevent the patient from thinking any initial treatment may have made the patient worse and thus be hesitant to return for further treatments.

12. If, at the conclusion of the examination, the examiner has found that the patient has shown unusual signs and symptoms or if the condition appears to be beyond his or her scope of practice, the examiner should not hesitate to refer the patient to another appropriate health care professional.

Vital Signs

In some cases, the examiner may want to begin the examination by taking the patient's vital signs to establish the patient's baseline physiological parameters and vital signs (Table 1-7) and review the medical history screening card (see Figure 1-9). These include the pulse (most commonly the radial pulse at the wrist is used), blood

TABLE **1-7**

Vital Sign Normal Ranges

Age Group	Respiratory Rate	Heart Rate	Diastolic Blood Pressure	Systolic Blood Pressure	Temperature	Weight (kg)	Weight (lbs)
Newborn	30–50	120–160	Varies	50–70	97.7°F (36.5°C)	2–3	4.5–7
Infant (1–12 months)	20–30	80–140	Varies	70–100	98.6°F (37.0°C)*	4–10	9–22
Toddler (1–3 years)	20–30	80–130	48–80	80–110	98.6°F (37.0°C)*	10–14	22–31
Preschooler (3–5 years)	20–30	80–120	48–80	80–110	98.6°F (37.0°C)*	14–18	31–40
School Age (6–12 years)	20–30	70–110	50–90	80–120	98.6°F (37.0°C)*	20–42	41–92
Adolescent (13–17 years)	12–20	55–105	60–92	110–120	98.6°F (37.0°C)*	>50	>110
Adults (18+ years)	18–20	60–100	<85	<130	98.6°F (37.0°C)*	Varies	Depends on body size

*Ranges from 97.8°F to 99.1°F (36.5°C to 37.3°C).

Remember these points:
- The patient's normal range should always be taken into consideration.
- Heart rate, blood pressure, and respiratory rate are expected to increase during times of fever or stress.
- Respiratory rate for infants should be counted for a full 60 seconds.

Principles of Examination

- Tell the patient what you are doing
- Test the normal (uninvolved) side first
- Do active movements first, then passive movements, and then resisted isometric movements
- Do painful movements last
- Apply overpressure with care to test end feel
- Repeat movements or sustain certain postures or positions if history indicates
- Do resisted isometric movements in a resting position
- Remember that with passive movements and ligamentous testing, both the degree and quality (end feel) of opening are important
- With ligamentous testing, repeat with increasing stress
- With myotome testing, make sure that contractions are held for 5 seconds
- Warn the patient of possible exacerbations
- Maintain the patient's dignity
- Refer if necessary

pressure, respiratory rate, temperature (98.4°F or 37°C is normal, but it may range from 96.5°F [35.8°C] to 99.4°F [37.4°C]), and weight. Table 1-8 outlines guidelines for blood pressure measurement. High blood pressure values should be checked several times at 15- to 30-minute intervals with the patient resting in between to determine whether a high reading is accurate or is being caused by anxiety ("white coat syndrome") or some similar reason. If three consecutive readings are high, the patient is said to have high blood pressure (hypertension) (Table 1-9). If the readings remain high, further investigation may be warranted.[59-61]

Scanning Examination

The examination described in this book emphasizes the joints of the body, their movement and stability. It is necessary to examine all appropriate tissues to delineate the affected area, which can then be examined in detail. Application of tension, stretch, or isometric contraction to specific tissues produces either a normal or an appropriate abnormal response. This action enables the examiner to determine the nature and site of the present symptoms and the patient's response to these symptoms. The examination shows whether certain activities provoke or change the patient's pain; in this way, the examiner can focus on the subjective response (i.e., the patient's feelings or opinions) as well as the test findings. The patient must be clear about his or her side of the examination. For instance, the patient must not confuse questions about movement-associated pain ("Does the movement make any difference to the pain?" "Does the movement bring on or change the pain?") with questions about already existing pain. In addition, the examiner attempts to see whether patient responses are measurably abnormal. Do the movements cause any abnormalities in function? A loss of movement or weakness in muscles can be measured and therefore is an objective response. Throughout the assessment, the examiner looks for two sets of data: (1) what the patient feels (subjective) and (2) responses that can be measured or are found by the examiner (objective).

TABLE **1-8**

Guidelines for Measurement of Blood Pressure

Posture	Blood pressure obtained in the sitting position is recommended. The subject should sit quietly for 5 minutes, with the back supported and the arm supported at the level of the heart, before blood pressure is recorded.
Circumstances	No caffeine during the hour preceding the reading. No smoking during the 30 minutes preceding the reading. A quiet, warm setting.
Equipment	**Cuff size:** The bladder should encircle and cover two thirds of the length of the arm; if it does not, place the bladder over the brachial artery. If bladder is too short, misleading high readings may result. Manometer: Aneroid gauges should be calibrated every 6 months against a mercury manometer.
Technique	**Number of readings:** • On each occasion, take at least two readings, separated by as much time as is practical. If readings vary by more than 5 mm Hg, take additional readings until two consecutive readings are close. • If the initial values are elevated, obtain two other sets of readings at least 1 week apart. • Initially, take pressure in both arms; if the pressures differ, use the arm with the higher pressure. • If the arm pressure is elevated, take the pressure in one leg (particularly in patients younger than 30 years of age). **Performance:** • Inflate the bladder quickly to a pressure 20 mm Hg above the systolic pressure, as recognized by disappearance of the radial pulse. • Deflate the bladder by 3 mm Hg every second. • Record the Korotkoff phase V (disappearance), except in children, in whom use of phase IV (muffling) may be preferable if disappearance of the sounds is not perceived. • If the Korotkoff sounds are weak, have the patient raise the arm and open and close the hand 5 to 10 times, and then reinflate the bladder quickly.
Recordings	Blood pressure, patient position, arm and cuff size.

From Kaplan NM, Deveraux RB, Miller HS: Systemic hyperextension. Med Sci Sports Exerc 26:S269, 1994.

TABLE **1-9**

Classification of Hypertension by Age

	MAGNITUDE OF HYPERTENSION				
	Normal	Mild, Stage 1	Moderate, Stage 2	Severe, Stage 3	Very Severe, Stage 4
Child (6–9 years)					
Systolic	80–120	120–124	125–129	130–139	≥140
Diastolic	50–75	75–79	80–84	85–89	≥90
Child (10–12 years)					
Systolic	80–120	125–129	130–134	135–144	≥145
Diastolic	50–80	80–84	85–89	90–94	≥95
Adolescent (13–15 years)					
Systolic	110–120	135–139	140–149	150–159	≥160
Diastolic	60–85	85–89	90–94	95–99	≥100
Adolescent (16–18 years)					
Systolic	110–120	140–149	150–159	160–179	≥180
Diastolic	60–90	90–94	95–99	100–109	≥110
Adult (>18 years)					
Systolic	110–130	140–159	160–179	180–209	≥210
Diastolic	80–90	90–99	100–109	110–119	≥120

Reprinted, by permission, from McGrew CA: Clinical implications of the AHA preparticipation cardiovascular screening guidelines. Athletic Ther Today 5(4):55, 2000.

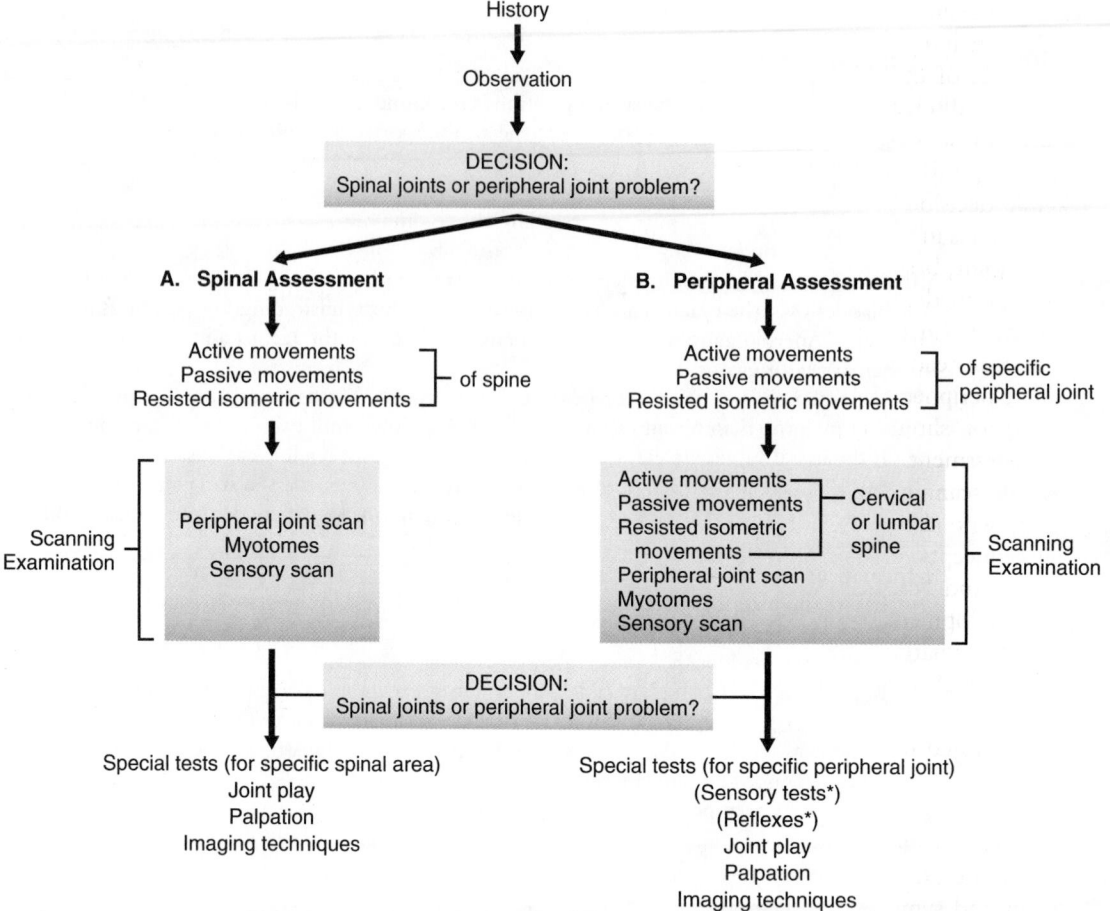

Figure 1-11 The scanning examination used to rule out referral of symptoms from the spine. **A,** Spinal assessment (i.e., based on the history, the clinician feels the problem is in the spine). **B,** Peripheral joint assessment (i.e., based on the history, the clinician feels the problem is in a peripheral joint). (*These are done if scanning examination is not done.)

When to Use the Scanning Examination

- There is no history of trauma
- There are radicular signs
- There is trauma with radicular signs
- There is altered sensation in the limb
- There are spinal cord ("long track") signs
- The patient presents with abnormal patterns
- There is suspected psychogenic pain

To ensure that all possible sources of pathology are assessed, the examination must be extensive. This is especially true if there are symptoms when no history of trauma is present. In this case, a scanning or screening examination is performed to rule out the possibility of referral of symptoms, especially from the spine. Similarly, if there is any doubt about where the pathology is located, the scanning examination is essential to ensure a correct diagnosis. The scanning examination is a "quick look" or scan of a part of the body involving the spine and extremities. It is used to rule out symptoms, which may be referred from one part of the body to another. It is divided into two scans: the upper limb scan and the lower limb scan. It is part of the examination that is used, where necessary, along with a detailed and focused examination of one or more of the joints.

As with all assessments, the use of a scanning examination depends on what the examiner found in the history and observation. For assessment of the spine, the scanning examination is integrated into the examination as a regular part of the cervical or lumbar assessment (Figure 1-11, *A*) and includes a peripheral joint scan, myotome testing, and a sensory scan. If, when assessing the peripheral joints, the examiner suspects a problem is being referred from the spine, the scanning examination is "inserted" into the examination of that joint (Figure 1-11, *B*). For the scanning examination, the peripheral joints are "scanned," with the patient doing only a few key movements at each joint. The movements should include those that may be expected to exacerbate symptoms that are derived from the history. The examiner then tests the upper or lower limb myotomes (key muscles representing a specific nerve root). After these tests, a sensory scanning examination (sensory scan) can be performed that may include the appropriate reflexes, the sensory distributions of the dermatomes and peripheral nerve distribution, and selected neurodynamic tests (e.g., upper limb tension test, slump test) if the examiner suspects some neurological involvement. At this point, the examiner makes a decision or an "educated guess" as to whether the problem is in the cervical spine, lumbar spine, or the peripheral joint, based on the information gained. Once the decision is made, the examiner either completes the spinal assessment (in the case of a suspected spinal problem) or turns instead to completing the assessment of the appropriate peripheral joint (see Figure 1-11). The scanning examination should add no more than 5 or 10 minutes to the assessment.

The idea of the scanning examination was developed by James Cyriax,[1] who also, more than any other author, originated the concepts of "contractile" and "inert" tissue, "end feel," and "capsular patterns" and contributed greatly to development of a comprehensive and systematic physical examination of the moving parts of the body. Although several of his constructs and paradigms have been questioned,[62-64] the basic principles of ensuring that all tissues are tested remains sound.

Spinal Cord and Nerve Roots

To further comprehend and ensure the value of the scanning examination, the examiner must have a clear understanding of signs and symptoms arising from the spinal

cord and nerve roots of the body and those arising from peripheral nerves. The scanning examination helps to determine whether the pathology is caused by tissues innervated by a nerve root or peripheral nerve that is referring symptoms distally.

The nerve root is that portion of a peripheral nerve that "connects" the nerve to the spinal cord. Nerve roots arise from each level of the spinal cord (e.g., C3, C4), and many, but not all, intermingle in a plexus (brachial, lumbar, or lumbosacral) to form different peripheral nerves (Figure 1-12). This arrangement can result in a single nerve root supplying more than one peripheral nerve. For example, the median nerve is derived from the C6, C7, C8, and T1 nerve roots, whereas the ulnar nerve is derived from C7, C8, and T1 (Table 1-10). For this reason, if pressure is applied to the nerve root, the distribution of the sensation or motor function is often felt or exhibited in more than one peripheral nerve distribution (Table 1-11). Therefore, although the symptoms seen in a nerve root lesion (e.g., paresthesia, pain, muscle weakness) may be similar to those seen in peripheral nerves, the signs (e.g., area of paresthesia, where pain occurs, which muscles are weak) are commonly different. The examiner must be able to differentiate a dermatome (nerve root) from the sensory distribution of a peripheral nerve, and a myotome (nerve root) from muscles supplied by a specific peripheral nerve. In addition, neurological signs and symptoms, such as paresthesia and pain, may result from inflammation or irritation of tissues, such as

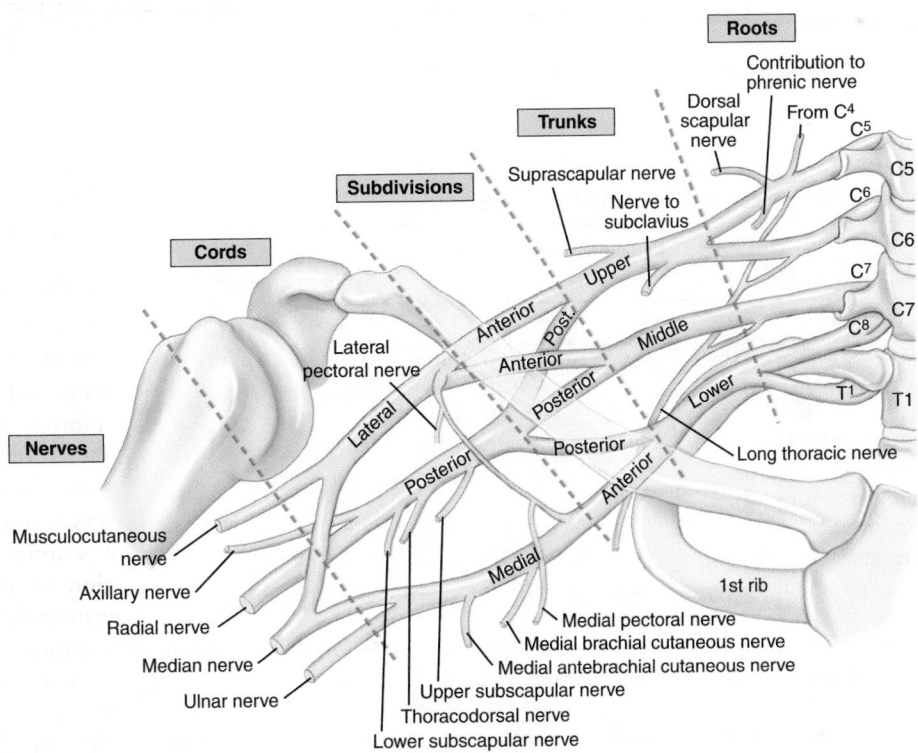

Figure 1-12 The brachial plexus. (From Neuman DA: Kinesiology of the musculoskeletal system—foundations for rehabilitation, St Louis, 2010, Mosby Elsevier, p. 150.)

TABLE 1-10

Common Peripheral Nerves and Their Nerve Root Derivation

Peripheral Nerve	Nerve Root Derivation
Axillary	C5,6
Supraclavicular	C3,4
Suprascapular	C5,6
Subscapular	C5,6
Long thoracic	C5,6,7
Musculocutaneous	C5,6,7
Medial cutaneous nerve of forearm	C8,T1
Lateral cutaneous nerve of forearm	C5,6
Posterior cutaneous nerve of forearm	C5,6,7,8
Radial	C5,6,7,8,T1
Median	C6,7,8,T1
Ulnar	C(7)8,T1
Pudendal	S2,3,4
Lateral cutaneous nerve of thigh	L2,3
Medial cutaneous nerve of thigh	L2,3
Intermediate cutaneous nerve of thigh	L2,3
Posterior cutaneous nerve of thigh	S1,2,3
Femoral	L2,3,4
Obturator	L2,3,4
Sciatic	L4,5,S1,2,3
Tibial	L4,5,S1,2,3
Common peroneal	L4,5,S1,2
Superficial peroneal	L4,5,S1
Deep peroneal	L4,5,S1,2
Lateral cutaneous nerve of leg (calf)	L4,5,S1,2
Saphenous	L3,4
Sural	S1,2
Medial plantar	L4,5
Lateral plantar	S1,2

facet joints and interspinous ligaments or other tissues supplied by the nerve roots, and they may be demonstrated in the dermatome, myotome, or sclerotome supplied by that nerve root. This irritation can contribute to the referred pain (see later discussion).

Examples of Autonomic Nervous System Involvement (Yellow Flags)

- Ringing in the ears
- Dizziness
- Blurred vision
- Photophobia (sensitivity to light)
- Rhinorrhea (runny nose)
- Sweating
- Lacrimation (tearing)
- Generalized loss of muscle strength
- Increase in heart rate
- Flushing (vasodilatation)

Nerve roots are made up of anterior (ventral) and posterior (dorsal) portions that unite near or in the intervertebral foramen to form a single **nerve root** or **spinal nerve** (Figure 1-13). They are the most proximal parts of the peripheral nervous system.

The human body has 31 nerve root pairs: 8 cervical, 12 thoracic, 5 lumbar, 5 sacral, and 1 coccygeal. Each nerve root has two components: a **somatic** portion, which innervates the skeletal muscles and provides sensory input from the skin, fascia, muscles, and joints, and a **visceral** component, which is part of the autonomic nervous system.[65] The autonomic system supplies the blood

TABLE 1-11

Nerve Root Dermatomes, Myotomes, Reflexes, and Paresthetic Areas

Nerve Root	Dermatome*	Muscle Weakness (Myotome)	Reflexes Affected	Paresthesias
C1	Vertex of skull	None	None	None
C2	Temple, forehead, occiput	Longus colli, sternocleidomastoid, rectus capitis	None	None
C3	Entire neck, posterior cheek, temporal area, prolongation forward under mandible	Trapezius, splenius capitis	None	Cheek, side of neck
C4	Shoulder area, clavicular area, upper scapular area	Trapezius, levator scapulae	None	Horizontal band along clavicle and upper scapula
C5	Deltoid area, anterior aspect of entire arm to base of thumb	Supraspinatus, infraspinatus, deltoid, biceps	Biceps, brachioradialis	None
C6	Anterior arm, radial side of hand to thumb and index finger	Biceps, supinator, wrist extensors	Biceps, brachioradialis	Thumb and index finger

TABLE **1-11**

Nerve Root Dermatomes, Myotomes, Reflexes, and Paresthetic Areas—cont'd

Nerve Root	Dermatome*	Muscle Weakness (Myotome)	Reflexes Affected	Paresthesias
C7	Lateral arm and forearm to index, long, and ring fingers	Triceps, wrist flexors (rarely, wrist extensors)	Triceps	Index, long, and ring fingers
C8	Medial arm and forearm to long, ring, and little fingers	Ulnar deviators, thumb extensors, thumb adductors (rarely, triceps)	Triceps	Little finger alone or with two adjacent fingers; *not* ring or long fingers, alone or together (C7)
T1	Medial side of forearm to base of little finger	Disc lesions at upper two thoracic levels do not appear to give rise to root weakness. Weakness of intrinsic muscles of the hand is due to other pathology (e.g., thoracic outlet pressure, neoplasm of lung, and ulnar nerve lesion). Dural and nerve root stress has T1 elbow flexion with arm horizontal. T1 and T2 scapulae forward and backward on chest wall. Neck flexion at any thoracic level.		
T2	Medial side of upper arm to medial elbow, pectoral and midscapular areas			
T3–T12	T3–T6, upper thorax; T5–T7, costal margin; T8–T12, abdomen and lumbar region	Articular and dural signs and root pain are common. Root signs (cutaneous analgesia) are rare and have such indefinite area that they have little localizing value. Weakness is not detectable.		
L1	Back, over trochanter and groin	None	None	Groin; after holding posture, which causes pain
L2	Back, front of thigh to knee	Psoas, hip adductors	None	Occasionally anterior thigh
L3	Back, upper buttock, anterior thigh and knee, medial lower leg	Psoas, quadriceps, thigh atrophy	Knee jerk sluggish, PKB positive, pain on full SLR	Medial knee, anterior lower leg
L4	Medial buttock, lateral thigh, medial leg, dorsum of foot, big toe	Tibialis anterior, extensor hallucis	SLR limited, neck flexion pain, weak or absent knee jerk, side flexion limited	Medial aspect of calf and ankle
L5	Buttock, posterior and lateral thigh, lateral aspect of leg, dorsum of foot, medial half of sole, first, second, and third toes	Extensor hallucis, peroneals, gluteus medius, dorsiflexors, hamstring and calf atrophy	SLR limited one side, neck flexion painful, ankle decreased, cross-leg raising—pain	Lateral aspect of leg, medial three toes
S1	Buttock, thigh, and leg posterior	Calf and hamstring, wasting of gluteals, peroneals, plantar flexors	SLR limited, Achilles reflex weak or absent	Lateral two toes, lateral foot, lateral leg to knee, plantar aspect of foot
S2	Same as S1	Same as S1 except peroneals	Same as S1	Lateral leg, knee, and heel
S3	Groin, medial thigh to knee	None	None	None
S4	Perineum, genitals, lower sacrum	Bladder, rectum	None	Saddle area, genitals, anus, impotence, massive posterior herniation

PKB, Prone knee bending; *SLR*, straight leg raising.
*In any part of which pain may be felt.

vessels, dura mater, periosteum, ligaments, and intervertebral discs, among many other structures.

The sensory distribution of each nerve root is called the **dermatome.** A dermatome is defined as the area of skin supplied by a single nerve root. The area innervated by a nerve root is larger than that innervated by a peripheral nerve.[66] The descriptions of dermatomes in the following chapters should be considered as examples only, because slight differences and variabilities occur with each patient, and dermatomes also exhibit a great deal of overlap.[67,68] The variability in dermatomes was aptly demonstrated by Keegan and Garrett in 1948 (Figure 1-14).[69] The overlap may be demonstrated by the fact that, in the thoracic spine, the loss of one dermatome often goes unnoticed because of the overlap of the adjacent dermatomes.

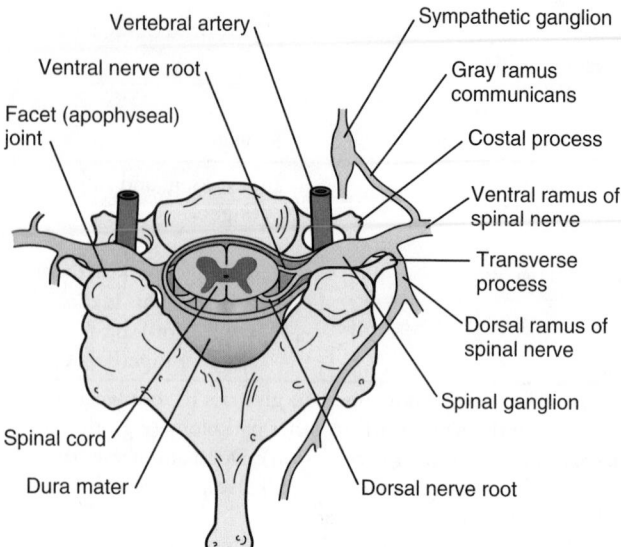

Figure 1-13 Spinal cord, nerve root portions, and spinal nerve in the cervical spine and their relation to the vertebra and vertebral artery.

Spinal nerve roots have a poorly developed epineurium and lack a perineurium. This development makes the nerve root more susceptible to compressive forces, tensile deformation, chemical irritants (e.g., alcohol, lead, arsenic), and metabolic abnormalities. For example, compression of the nerve root could occur with a posterolateral intervertebral disc herniation, a "burner" or stretching of the nerve roots or the brachial plexus in a football player or alcoholic neuritis in an alcoholic. Pressure on nerve roots leads to loss of muscle tone and mass, but the loss is often not as obvious as when pressure is applied to a peripheral nerve. Because the peripheral nerve that innervates the muscle is usually supplied by more than one nerve root, more muscle fibers are likely to be affected and wasting or atrophy is more evident if the peripheral nerve itself is damaged. In addition, the pattern of weakness (i.e., which muscles are affected) is different for an injury to a nerve root and to a peripheral nerve, because a nerve root supplies more than one peripheral nerve. Pressure on a peripheral nerve resulting in a neuropraxia leads to temporary nonfunction of the nerve. With this type of injury, there is primarily motor involvement, with little sensory or autonomic involvement, and although weakness may be demonstrated, muscle atrophy may not be evident. With more severe peripheral nerve lesions (e.g., axonotmesis and neurotmesis), atrophy is evident.

Myotomes are defined as groups of muscles supplied by a single nerve root. A lesion of a single nerve root is usually associated with paresis (incomplete paralysis) of the myotome (muscles) supplied by that nerve root. It therefore takes time for any weakness to become evident on resisted isometric or myotome testing, and for this reason, the isometric testing of myotomes is held for *at least 5 seconds.* On the other hand, a lesion of a peripheral nerve leads to complete paralysis of the muscles supplied by that nerve, especially if the injury results in an axonotmesis or neurotmesis, and the weakness therefore is evident right away. Differences in the amount of resulting paralysis arise from the fact that more than one myotome contributes to the formation of a muscle embryologically.

A **sclerotome** is an area of bone or fascia supplied by a single nerve root (Figure 1-15). As with dermatomes, sclerotomes can show a great deal of variability among individuals.

It is the complex nature of the dermatomes, myotomes, and sclerotomes supplied by the nerve root that can lead to referred pain, which is pain felt in a part of the body that is usually a considerable distance from the tissues that have caused it. Referred pain is explained as an error in perception on the part of the brain. Usually, pain can be referred into the appropriate myotome, dermatome, or sclerotome from any somatic or visceral tissue innervated by a nerve root, but, confusingly, it sometimes is not referred according to a specific pattern.[70] It is not understood why this occurs, but clinically it has been found to be so.

Many theories of the mechanism of referred pain have been developed, but none has been proven conclusively. Generally, referred pain may involve one or more of the following mechanisms:

1. Misinterpretation by the brain as to the source of the painful impulses
2. Inability of the brain to interpret a summation of noxious stimuli from various sources
3. Disturbance of the internuncial pool by afferent nerve impulses.

Referral of pain is a common occurrence in problems associated with the musculoskeletal system. Pain is often felt at points remote from the site of the lesion. The site to which pain is referred is an indicator of the segment that is at fault: it indicates that one of the structures innervated by a specific nerve root is causing signs and symptoms in other tissues supplied by that same nerve root. For example, pain in the L5 dermatome could arise from irritation around the L5 nerve root, from an L5 disc causing pressure on the L5 nerve root, from facet joint involvement at L4–L5 causing irritation of the L5 nerve root, from any muscle supplied by the L5 nerve root, or from any visceral structures having L5 innervation. Referred pain tends to be felt deeply; its boundaries are indistinct, and it radiates segmentally without crossing the midline. **Radicular** or **radiating pain,** a form of referred pain, is a sharp, shooting pain felt in a dermatome, myotome, or sclerotome because of direct involvement of or damage to a spinal nerve or nerve root.[53] A **radiculopathy** refers to radiating paresthesia, numbness or weakness but not pain.[71] A **myelopathy** is a neurogenic disorder involving the spinal cord or brain and resulting in an upper motor neuron lesion; the patterns

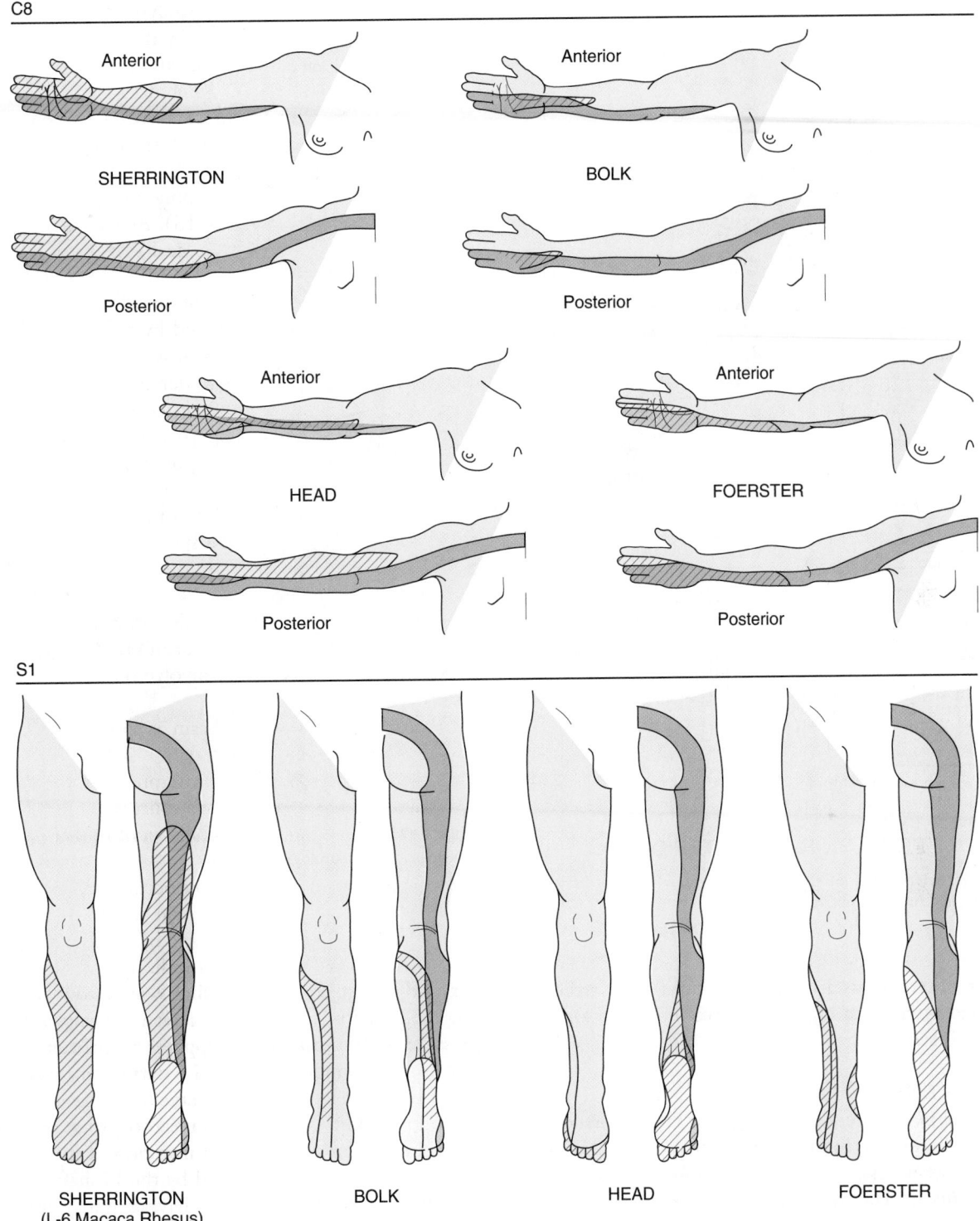

Figure 1-14 The variability of dermatomes at C8 and S1 as found by four researchers. Similar variability is demonstrated in most cervical, lumbar, and sacral vertebrae. (Redrawn from Keegan JJ, Garrett FD: The segmental distribution of the cutaneous nerves in the limbs of man, Anat Rec 101:430, 433, 1948. Copyright © 1948. This material is used by permission of Wiley-Liss, a subsidiary of John Wiley & Sons.)

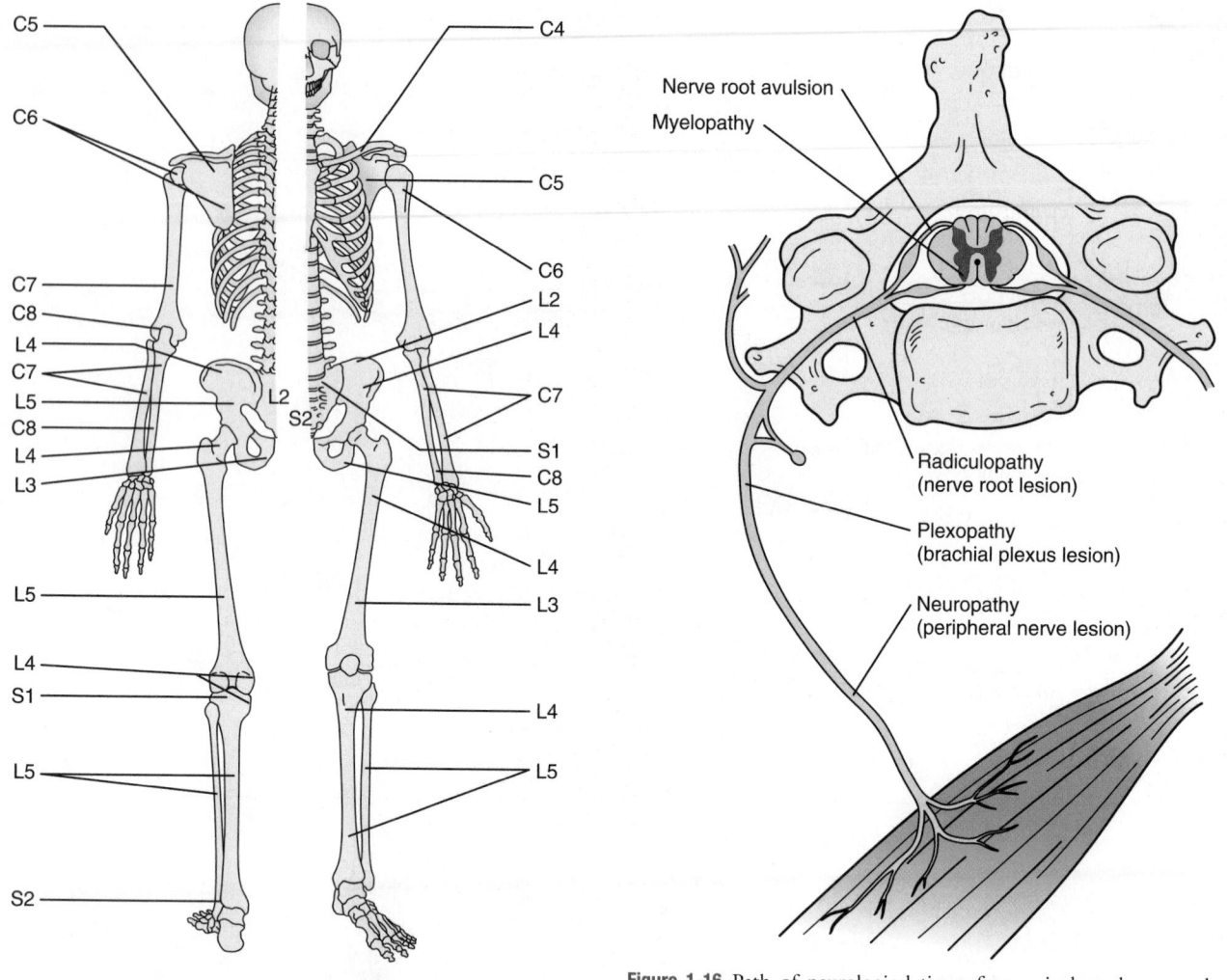

Figure 1-15 Sclerotomes of the body. Lines show areas of bone and fascia supplied by individual nerve roots.

POSTERIOR   ANTERIOR

Figure 1-16 Path of neurological tissue from spinal cord to muscles, showing sites of neurological lesions.

of pain or symptoms are different from that of radicular pain, and often both upper and lower limbs are affected (Figure 1-16).

Peripheral Nerves

Peripheral nerves are a unique type of "inert" tissue (see the later discussion) in that they are not contractile tissue, but they are necessary for the normal functioning of voluntary muscle. The examiner must be aware of potential injury to nervous tissue when examining both contractile and inert tissue. Table 1-12 shows some of the tissue changes that result when a peripheral nerve lesion occurs.

In peripheral nerves, the epineurium consists of a loose areolar connective tissue matrix surrounding the nerve fiber. It allows changes in growth length of the bundled nerve fibers (funiculi) without allowing the bundles to be strained. The perineurium protects the nerve bundles by acting as a diffusion barrier to irritants and provides tensile strength and elasticity to the nerve. Peripheral

nerves therefore are most commonly affected by pressure, traction, friction, anoxia, or cutting. Examples include pressure on the median nerve in the carpal tunnel, traction to the common peroneal nerve at the head of the fibula during a lateral ankle sprain, friction to the ulnar nerve in the cubital tunnel, anoxia of the anterior tibial nerve in a compartment syndrome, and cutting of the radial nerve with a fracture of the humeral shaft. Cooling, freezing, and thermal or electrical injury may also affect peripheral nerves.

Nerve injuries are usually classified by the systems of Seddon[72] or Sunderland.[73] Seddon, whose system is most commonly used, classified nerve injuries into neuropraxia (most common), axonotmesis, and neurotmesis (Table 1-13). Sunderland followed a similar system but divided axonotmesis and neurotmesis into different levels or degrees (Table 1-14). Any examination of a joint must include a thorough peripheral nerve examination, especially if there are neurological signs and symptoms. The

TABLE **1-12**

Signs and Symptoms of Mixed Peripheral Nerve (Lower Motor Neuron) Lesions*

Motor	Sensory	Sympathetic
• Flaccid paralysis • Loss of reflexes • Muscle wasting and atrophy • Lost synergic action of muscles • Fibrosis, contractures, and adhesions • Joint weakness and instability • Decreased range of motion and stiffness • Disuse osteoporosis of bone • Growth affected	• Loss of or abnormal sensation • Loss of vasomotor tone: warm flushed (early); cold, white (later) • Skin may be scaly (early); thin, smooth, and shiny (later) • Shallower skin creases • Nail changes (striations, ridges, dry, brittle, abnormal curving, luster lost) • Ulceration	• Loss of sweat glands (dryness) • Loss of pilomotor response

*Primarily axonotmesis and neurotmesis.

TABLE **1-13**

Classification of Nerve Injuries According to Seddon

Grade of Injury	Definition	Signs and Symptoms
Neuropraxia (Sunderland 1°)	A transient physiological block caused by ischemia from pressure or stretch of the nerve with no wallerian degeneration	• Pain • No or minimal muscle wasting • Muscle weakness • Numbness • Proprioception affected • Recovery time: minutes to days
Axonotmesis (Sunderland 2° and 3°)	Internal architecture of nerve preserved, but axons are so badly damaged that wallerian degeneration occurs	• Pain • Muscle wasting evident • Complete motor, sensory and sympathetic functions lost (see Table 1-12) • Recovery time: months (axon regenerates at rate of 1 inch/month, or 1 mm/day) • Sensation is restored before motor function
Neurotmesis (Sunderland 3°, 4°, and 5°)	Structure of nerve is destroyed by cutting, severe scarring, or prolonged severe compression	• No pain (anesthesia) • Muscle wasting • Complete motor, sensory and sympathetic functions lost (see Table 1-12) • Recovery time: months and only with surgery

Data from Seddon HJ: Three types of nerve injury. Brain 66:17–28, 1943.

TABLE **1-14**

Correlation of Seddon and Sunderland Classification of Nerve Injuries

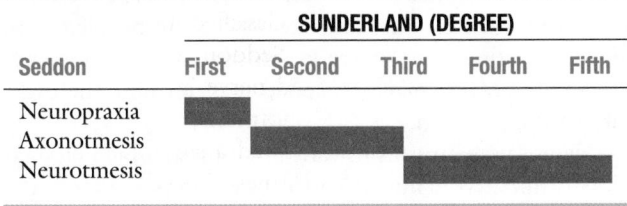

From Morrey BF, editor: The elbow and its disorders, ed 2, Philadelphia, 1993, WB Saunders, p. 814.
Shaded areas indicate equivalent terms.

examiner must be able not only to differentiate inert tissue lesions from contractile tissue lesions but also to determine whether a contractile tissue malfunction is the result of the contractile tissue itself or a peripheral nerve lesion or a nerve root lesion.

Sensory loss combined with motor loss should alert the examiner to lesions of nervous tissue.[74–76] Injury to a single peripheral nerve (e.g., the median nerve) is referred to as a **mononeuropathy.** Systemic diseases (e.g., diabetes) may affect more than one peripheral nerve. In this case, the pathology is referred to as a **polyneuropathy.** Careful mapping of the area of sensory loss and testing of the muscles affected by the motor loss allow

TABLE **1-15**

Comparison of Signs and Symptoms for C7 Nerve Root Lesion and Median Nerve Lesion at Elbow

	C7 Nerve Root	Median Nerve
Sensory alteration	Lateral arm and forearm to index, long, and ring fingers on palmar and dorsal aspect	Palmar aspect of thumb, index, middle, and half of ring finger Dorsal aspect of index, middle, and possibly half of ring finger
Motor alteration	Triceps Wrist flexors Wrist extensors (rarely)	Pronator teres Wrist flexors (lateral half of flexor digitorum profundus) Palmaris longus Pronator quadratus Flexor pollicis longus and brevis Abductor pollicis brevis Opponens pollicis Lateral two lumbricals
Reflex alteration	Triceps may be affected	None*
Paresthesia	Index, long and ring fingers on palmar and dorsal aspect	Same as sensory alternation

*No "common" reflexes are affected; if the examiner tested the tendon reflexes of the muscles listed, they would be affected.

the examiner to differentiate between a peripheral nerve lesion and a nerve root lesion. (An example is shown in Table 1-15.) If electromyographic studies are to be used to determine the grade of nerve injury, denervation cannot be evaluated for at least 3 weeks after injury to allow wallerian degeneration to occur and to allow regeneration (if any) to begin.[77–79] Muscle wasting usually becomes obvious after 4 to 6 weeks and progresses to reach its maximum by about 12 weeks following injury. Circulatory changes after nerve injury vary with time. In the initial or early stages, the skin is warm, but after about 3 weeks, the skin becomes cooler as a result of decreased circulation. Because of the decreased circulation and altered cell metabolism, trophic changes occur to the skin and nails.

When assessing a patient, the examiner must also be aware of what has been called the **double-crush syndrome** or double-entrapment neuropathy.[80–83] The theory of this lesion (which has not yet been proved but has clinical supporting evidence) is that, whereas compression or pathology at one point along a peripheral nerve or nerve root may not be sufficient to cause signs and symptoms, compression or pathology at two or more points may lead to a cumulative effect that results in apparent signs and symptoms.[84] Because of this cumulative effect, signs and symptoms may indicate one area of involvement (e.g., the carpal tunnel), whereas other areas (e.g., cervical spine, brachial plexus, thoracic outlet) may be contributing to the problem. Similarly, cervical lesions may be involved in tennis elbow (lateral epicondylitis) syndromes. Upton and McComas[80] believed that compression proximally on the nerve trunk could increase the vulnerability of the peripheral nerves or nerve roots at distal points along their paths because axonal transport

would be disrupted. In addition, diseased nerves are more susceptible to injury; thus, the presence of systemic disease (e.g., diabetes, thyroid dysfunction) may make the nerve more susceptible to compression somewhere along its path.[75] Finally, the signs and symptoms could potentially be arising from both a nerve root lesion and a peripheral nerve lesion. Only with meticulous assessment can the clinician delineate where the true problems lie, which may be due to trauma, degeneration, or anatomical anomalies.

Similarly, the loss of extensibility of the nervous tissue at one site may produce increasing tensile loads when the peripheral nerve or nerve root is stretched, leading to mechanical dysfunction.[85] This is the principle behind the **neural tension** or **neurodynamic tests**, such as the straight leg raise, slump test, and upper limb tension test,[85–87] and may provide a partial explanation for lesions, such as cervical spine lesions mimicking tennis elbow and carpal tunnel syndrome. These tests put neural tissue (e.g., neuraxis of the central nervous system [CNS], meninges, nerve roots, peripheral nerves) under tension when they are performed and may duplicate symptoms that result during functional activity.[85,87,88] For example, sitting in a car is closely mimicked by the action of the slump test and straight leg raising. However, they often do not, by themselves, indicate where the problem lies. Further testing (e.g., nerve conduction tests, electromyography [EMG]) may be needed to determine the exact site of the problem.

Neural tissue moves toward the joint at which elongation is initiated. Thus, if cervical flexion is initiated, the nerve roots, even those in the lumbar spine, move toward the cervical spine. Likewise, flexion of the whole spine causes movement toward the lumbar spine, and extension of the knee or dorsiflexion of the foot causes neural movement toward the knee or ankle.[85,87,88] These "tension points" can potentially help determine where the restriction to movement is occurring. Normally, tension tests are not painful, although the patient is often aware of increased tension or discomfort in the spine or the limb. As tension tests indicate neural mobility and sensitivity to mechanical stresses, they are considered positive only if they reproduce the patient's symptoms, or if the patient's response is altered by movement of a body part distal to where the symptoms are felt (e.g., foot dorsiflexion causing symptoms in the lumbar spine), or if there is asymmetry in the response.[85] When doing tension tests, the examiner should note the angle or position at which the restriction occurs and what the resistance feels like. With irritable conditions, only those parts of the test that are needed to cause positive results should be performed. For example, in the slump test, if neck flexion and slumping cause positive signs, there is no need to cause further discomfort to the patient by doing knee extension and foot dorsiflexion.

In the examination, testing of neurological tissue occurs during active, passive, and resisted isometric movement, as well as during functional testing, specific tests, reflexes, and cutaneous distribution and palpation.

Examination of Specific Joints

The examiner should use an unchanging, systematic approach to the examination that varies only slightly to elaborate certain clues given by the history or by asymmetric responses. For example, if the history is characteristic of a disc lesion, the examination should be a detailed one of all the tissues that may be affected by the disc and a brief one of all the other joints to exclude contradictory signs. If the history suggests arthritis of the hip, the examination should be a detailed one of the hip and a brief one of the other joints—again, to exclude contradictory signs. As the movements are tested, the examiner is looking sometimes for the patient's subjective responses and sometimes for clinical objective findings. For example, if examination of the cervical spine shows clear signs of a disc problem, as the examination is continued down the arm, the examiner looks more for muscle weakness (objective) rather than for elicitation of pain (subjective). In contrast, if the history suggests a muscle lesion, pain will probably be provoked when the arm is examined. In either case, the structures expected to be normal are not omitted from the examination. There are only a few situations in which deviation from this systematic routine should occur: when there is uncertainty about where the pathology lies (in which case, a scanning examination must be performed with combined assessment of the spine and one or more peripheral joints); when there is no history of trauma or indication of pathology in a specific joint yet the patient complains of pain in that joint

(again, a scanning examination is performed); or when the joint to be assessed is too acutely injured or irritable to do the total systematic examination.

If there is an organic lesion, some active, passive, or resisted isometric movements will be abnormal or painful, and others will not. Negative findings must balance positive ones, and the examination must be extensive enough to allow characteristic patterns to emerge. Determination of the problem is not made on the strength of the first positive finding; it is made only after it is clear that there are no other contradictory signs. Movements may be repeated several times quickly to rule out any problem, such as vascular insufficiency, or if the patient has indicated in the history that repetitive movements increase the symptoms. Likewise, sustained postures may be held for several seconds or combined movements may be performed if the history indicates increased symptoms with those postures or movements.

Contractile tissues may have tension placed on them by stretching or contraction.[1] These structures include the muscles, their tendons, and their attachments into the bone. **Nervous tissues** and their associated sheaths also have tension put on them by stretching and pinching, as do **inert tissues.** Inert tissues include all structures that would not be considered contractile or neurological, such as joint capsules, ligaments, bursae, blood vessels, cartilage, and dura mater. Table 1-16 demonstrates differential diagnosis of injuries to contractile tissue (strains and paratenonitis) and inert tissue (sprains). Some examiners separate vascular tissues from the other inert tissues; however, for the most part, when doing a musculoskeletal examination, they can be grouped with the other inert tissues with the understanding that they do present their own unique signs and symptoms.

When doing movement testing, the examiner should note whether pain or restriction predominate. If pain predominates, the condition is more acute, and gentler assessment and treatment are required. If restriction predominates, the condition is subacute, or chronic, and more vigorous assessment and treatment can be performed.

Active Movements

Active movements (AROM) are "actively" performed by the patient's voluntary muscles and have their own special value in that they combine tests of joint range, control, muscle power, and the patient's willingness to perform the movement. These movements are sometimes referred to as **physiological movements.** The end of active movement is sometimes referred to as the **physiological barrier.** Contractile, nervous, and inert tissues are involved or moved during active movements. When active movements occur, one or more rigid structures (bones) move, and such movement results in movement of all structures that attach to or are in close proximity to that bone. Although active movements are usually the first

TABLE **1-16**

Differential Diagnosis of Muscle Strains, Tendon Injury, and Ligament Sprains

	1° Strain	2° Strain	3° Strain (rupture)	Paratenonitis[a] Tendinosis[b]	1° Sprain	2° Sprain	3° Sprain
Definition	Few fibers of muscle torn	About half of muscle fibers torn	All muscle fibers torn (rupture)	[a]Inflammation of tendon [b]Intratendinous degeneration	Few fibers of ligament torn	About half of ligament torn	All fibers of ligament torn
Mechanism of Injury	Overstretch Overload	Overstretch Overload Crushing	Overstretch Overload	Overuse Overstretch Overload [b]Aging	Overload Overstretch	Overload Overstretch	Overload Overstretch
Onset	Acute	Acute	Acute	Chronic Acute	Acute	Acute	Acute
Weakness	Minor	Moderate to major (reflex inhibition)	Moderate to major	Minor to moderate	Minor	Minor to moderate	Minor to moderate
Disability	Minor	Moderate	Major	Minor to major	Minor	Moderate	Moderate to major
Muscle Spasm	Minor	Moderate to major	Moderate	Minor	Minor	Minor	Minor
Swelling	Minor	Moderate to major	Moderate to major	[a]Minor to major (thickening) [b]No	Minor	Moderate	Moderate to major
Loss of Function	Minor	Moderate to major	Major (reflex inhibition)	Minor to major	Minor	Moderate to major	Moderate to major (instability)
Pain on Isometric Contraction	Minor	Moderate to major	No to minor	Minor to major	No	No	No
Pain on Stretch	Yes	Yes	No*	Yes	Yes	Yes	No*
Joint Play	Normal	Normal	Normal	Normal	Normal	Normal	Normal to excessive
Palpable Defect	No	No	Yes (if early)	[b]May have palpable module	No	No	Yes (if early)
Crepitus	No	No	No	Possible	No	No	No
ROM	Decreased	Decreased	May increase or decrease depending on swelling	Decreased	Decreased	Decreased	May increase or decrease depending on swelling Dislocation or subluxation possible

ROM, Range of motion.
*Not if it is the only tissue injured; however, often with 3° injuries, other structures will suffer 1° or 2° injuries and be painful.

movements done, they either are not performed at all or are performed with caution during fracture healing or if the movement could put stress on newly repaired soft tissues. The examiner should note which movements, if any, cause pain or other symptoms and the amount and quality of pain that results. For example, small, unguarded movements causing intense pain indicate an acute, irritable joint. If the condition is very irritable or acute, it may not be possible to elicit all the movements desired.

In this case, only those movements that provide the most useful information should be performed. The examiner should note the rhythm of movement along with any pain, limitation, or unusual (e.g., instability jog) or trick movements that occur. Trick movements are modified movements that the patient consciously or unconsciously uses to accomplish what the examiner has asked the patient to do. For example, in the presence of deltoid paralysis, if the examiner asks the patient to abduct the arm, the patient can accomplish this movement by laterally rotating the shoulder and using the biceps muscle to abduct the arm.

Active movement may be abnormal for several reasons, and the examiner must try to differentiate the cause. Pain is a common cause for abnormal movement as is muscle weakness, paralysis, or spasm. Other causes include tight or shortened tissues, altered length-tension relationships, modified neuromuscular factors, and joint-muscle interaction. In some cases, the patient may not be able to actively move the joint through the available ROM because of weakness, pain, or tight structures. This inability to move through the available ROM is sometimes called a **lag.** The most common example of this is a quadriceps lag in which the quadriceps is not able to actively take the knee into full extension even if full passive extension is possible. (This is commonly seen after surgery.) It is important to remember that a lag may also be caused by tightness of tissues acting in the opposite direction (e.g., in the knee, tight posterior capsule, tight hamstrings, or scarring).

The active movement component of the examination is a functional test of the anatomical and dynamical aspects of the body and joints while demonstrating correct or incorrect motor function, which is the ability to demonstrate skillful and efficient movement patterns while maintaining control of voluntary postures.[7,89] The examiner should ensure the movement is performed at a smooth constant speed in the desired direction using the most efficient pathway through full ROM.[90,91] This will involve the integration and synchronization of prime movers and synergists through the whole or part of the kinetic chain involved in the movement.

When testing active movements, the examiner should note where in the arc of movement the symptoms occur. For example, pain occurs during abduction of the shoulder between 60° and 120° if there is impingement under the acromion process or coracoacromial ligament. Any increase in intensity and quality of pain should also be noted. This information helps the examiner determine the particular tissue at fault. For example, bone pain, except in the case of a fracture or tumor, often is not altered with movement. By observing the patient's reaction to pain, the examiner can get some idea of how much the condition is affecting the patient and the patient's pain threshold. By noting the pattern of movement, the quality and rhythm of the movement, the movements in other joints, and the observable restriction, the examiner can tell if the patient is "cheating" (using accessory muscles or muscle substitution) to do the movement and what tissues are affected. For example, "shoulder hiking" may indicate a capsular pattern of the shoulder or incorrect sequential firing of different muscles.

Generally, active movements are performed once or twice in each desired direction while the examiner notes the pattern of movement and any discrepancies or cheating/substitution movements. If the patient has noted pain or difficulty with any particular movements,

---

Examiner Observations During Active Movement

- When and where during each of the movements the onset of pain occurs
- Whether the movement increases the intensity and quality of the pain
- The reaction of the patient to pain
- The amount of observable restriction and its nature
- The pattern of movement
- The rhythm and quality of movement
- The movement of associated joints
- The willingness of the patient to move the part

---

these movements should be done last to ensure no overflow of symptoms to other movements. If the patient has complained that certain repetitive movements or sustained postures are the problem, the examiner should ensure that the movements are repeated (5 to 10 times) or sustained (usually 5 to 20 seconds but may depend on history) until the symptoms are demonstrated.

There are standard movements for each joint, and these movements tend to follow cardinal planes (i.e., they are single plane movements). However, if the patient complains of problems outside these standard movements or if symptoms are more likely to be elicited by combined movements (i.e., movements in multiple planes or around combined axes), repeated movements, movements with speed, or movements under compression, then these should be performed.[92-94] McKenzie has reported that repeated movements increase symptoms in irritable acute tissues or in internal derangements,[17] whereas postural dysfunctions change little with repeated movements.

In some cases, especially if the joints are not too reactive or irritable, overpressure may carefully be applied at the end of the AROM. If the overpressure does not produce symptoms and the end feel is normal, the movement is considered normal and the examiner may decide that passive movements are unnecessary.

Passive Movements

Passive movements (PROM) are primarily performed to determine the available anatomical ROM and end feel. The PROM may be within normal limits, hypermobile (see the Patient History section) or hypomobile. Palpation of measurement points can play a major role when using palpable landmarks for goniometry.[95] With passive movement, the examiner puts the joint through its ROM while the patient is relaxed. These movements may also be referred to as **anatomical movements.** The end of passive movement is sometimes referred to as the **anatomical barrier.** Normally, the physiological barrier (active movement) occurs before the anatomical barrier (passive movement) so that passive movement is always slightly greater than active movement. The movement must proceed through as full of a range as possible and should, if possible, involve the same motions as were performed actively. Positioning the patient (e.g., sitting, lying supine) may have an effect on active and passive ROM, so the examiner must consider positioning. Differences in ROM between active and passive movements may be caused by muscle contraction or spasm, muscle deficiency, neurological deficit, contractures, or pain. Active and passive ROM may be measured by goniometer, inclinometer, examiner estimation ("eyeballing"), or a similar measure.[96,97] With most of these methods, it is difficult to show consistent differences of less than 5°.[98,99] Goniometry is especially useful for measuring and recording joint or fracture deformities and has been shown to have a satisfactory level of intratester reliability,[99–101] although this may depend on the motion measured.[101] Measurements at different times show progression or regression of the deformity. Although there are sources that describe ROMs for various joints, the values given are averages and do not necessarily constitute the ROM needed to do specific activities or the ROM that is present in a specific patient. Normal mobility is relative. For example, gymnasts tend to be classed as lax (nonpathological hypermobility) in most joints, whereas elderly persons tend to be classed as hypomobile. For these individual populations, however, the available ROM may be considered normal. In reality, the important question is, does the patient have the ROM available to do what he or she wants to do functionally? Certain pathological states, such as Ehlers-Danlos syndrome, may also affect ROM. For example, if several joints demonstrate excessive ROM, a condition referred to as **benign joint hypermobility syndrome** may exist.[102] The **Beighton Hypermobility Index** for this condition is a modification of the Carter and Wilkinson Scoring Criteria (see Chapter 17). This index used in isolation, if positive, means the individual has widespread joint hypermobility. Generalized joint hypermobility is said to be present when a score of 4 or more is found on the Beighton test.[103–105]

Likewise, the **Brighton Diagnostic Criteria,** which is not widely used in orthopedics, measures joint mobility and skin abnormalities.[102,105] Using this criteria, the patient must have two major criteria, one major and two minor criteria, or four minor criteria to be diagnosed with benign joint hypermobility syndrome.

Each movement must be compared with the same movement in the opposite joint or, secondarily, with

---

Beighton Hypermobility Index Scoring Criteria[106,107]

- Patient can bend and place hands flat on floor without bending knees (1 point)
- Knee(s) can hyperextend past 0° (1 point for each knee)
- Elbow(s) can hyperextend past 0° (1 point for each elbow)
- Thumb can be bent backward to touch forearm (1 point for each thumb)
- Little finger can be bent backward beyond 90° (1 point for each little finger)

NOTE: Maximum score = 9.

Brighton Diagnostic Criteria for Benign Joint Hypermobility Syndrome

MAJOR CRITERIA
- A Beighton score of 4/9 or greater (either currently or historically)
- Arthralgia (joint pain) for longer than 3 months in four or more joints

MINOR CRITERIA
- A Beighton score of 1, 2 or 3/9 (0, 1, 2 or 3 if aged 50+)
- Arthralgia (more than 3 months) in one to three joints or back pain (more than 3 months), spondylosis, spondylolysis/spondylolisthesis
- Dislocation/subluxation in more than one joint, or in one joint on more than one occasion
- Soft tissue rheumatism (inflammatory conditions) more than three lesions (e.g., epicondylitis, tenosynovitis, bursitis)
- Marfanoid habitus (Marfan-like appearance) (tall, slim, span/height ratio more than 1.03, upper: lower segment ratio less than 0.89, arachnodactyly [long, thin, spider-like fingers] [positive Steinberg/wrist signs])
- Abnormal skin: striae, hyperextensibility, thin skin, papyraceous (paper-like) scarring
- Eye signs: drooping eyelids or myopia or antimongoloid slant
- Varicose veins or hernia or uterine/rectal prolapse

From Grahame R, Bird HA, Child A, et al: The revised (Brighton 1998) criteria for the diagnosis of benign joint hypermobility syndrome (BJHS). J Rheumatol 27:1778, 2000.

Examiner Observations During Passive Movement

- When and where during each of the movements the pain begins
- Whether the movement increases the intensity and quality of pain
- The pattern of limitation of movement
- The end feel of movement
- The movement of associated joints
- The range of motion available

---

accepted norms. Although passive movement must be gentle, the examiner must determine whether there is any limitation of range (**hypomobility**) or excess of range (**hypermobility** or **laxity**) and, if so, whether it is painful. Hypermobile joints tend to be more susceptible to ligament sprains, joint effusion, chronic pain, recurrent injury, paratenonitis resulting from lack of control (instability), and early osteoarthritis. Hypomobile joints are more susceptible to muscle strains, pinched nerve syndromes, and paratenonitis resulting from overstress.[108,109] **Myofascial hypomobility** results from adaptive shortening or hypertonicity of the muscles or from posttraumatic adhesions or scarring. **Pericapsular hypomobility** has a capsular or ligamentous origin and may result from adhesions, scarring, arthritis, arthrosis, fibrosis, or tissue adaptation. Restriction may be in all directions but not the same amount in each direction (e.g., capsular pattern). **Pathomechanical hypomobility** occurs as a result of joint trauma (micro or macro) leading to restriction in one or more directions.[18] Hypermobility is not the same as instability. Instability covers a wide range of pathological hypermobility. Although there are tests to demonstrate general hypermobility, these tests should be interpreted with caution because patients demonstrate a wide range of variability between joints and within joints.[110,111] With careful assessment, one often finds that a joint may be hypermobile in one direction and hypomobile in another direction. It must also be remembered that evidence of hypomobility or hypermobility does not necessarily indicate a pathological state in the person being assessed. The examiner should attempt to determine the cause of the limitation (e.g., pain, spasm, adhesions, compression) or hypermobility (e.g., injury, occupational, genetic, disease) and the quality of the movement (e.g., lead pipe, cogwheel).

End Feel.[1] When assessing passive movement, the examiner should apply overpressure at the end of the ROM to determine the quality of end feel (the sensation the examiner "feels" in the joint as it reaches the end of the ROM) of each passive movement (Table 1-17). Care must be taken when testing end feel, however, to be sure that severe symptoms are not provoked. If the patient is able to hold a position at the end of the physiological ROM (end range of active movement) without provoking symptoms or if the symptoms ease quickly after returning to the resting position, then the end feel can be tested. Pain with pathological end feels is common.[63] If, however, the patient has severe pain at end range, end feel should only be tested with extreme care. A proper evaluation of end feel can help the examiner to assess the type of pathology present, determine a prognosis for the condition, and learn the severity or stage of the problem. By determining if pain or restriction is the main problem, the examiner can determine if a more gentle treatment should be given (pain predominating) or a more vigorous treatment (restriction predominantly). The end feel sensations that the examiner experiences are subjective, so intrarater reliability tends to be good, whereas interrater reliability is poor.[62] Many clinicians develop their own classification with the most common ones used[63] developed by Cyriax,[1] Kaltenborn,[92] and Paris.[112]

Cyriax described three classic **normal end feels:**[1]

- *Bone-to-Bone.* This is a "hard," unyielding sensation that is painless. An example of normal bone-to-bone end feel is elbow extension.
- *Soft-Tissue Approximation.* With this type of end feel, there is a yielding compression (mushy feel) that stops further movement. Examples are elbow and knee flexion, in which movement is stopped by compression of the soft tissues, primarily the muscles. In a particularly slim person with little muscle bulk, the end feel of elbow flexion may be bone-to-bone.
- *Tissue Stretch.* There is a hard or firm (springy) type of movement with a slight give. Toward the end of ROM, there is a feeling of springy or elastic resistance. The normal tissue stretch end feel has a feeling of "rising tension or stiffness." This changing tension has led to this end feel sometimes being divided into two types: **elastic (soft)** and **capsular (hard).** This feeling depends on the thickness and type of tissue being stretched, and it may be very elastic, as in the Achilles tendon stretch, or slightly elastic, as in wrist flexion (tissue stretch), or hard as in knee extension. A hard end feel is firm with a definite stopping point, whereas soft end feel implies a softer end feel without a definite stopping place.[113] Tissue stretch is the most common type of normal end feel; it is found when the capsule and ligaments are the primary restraints to movement. Examples are lateral rotation of the shoulder, and knee and metacarpophalangeal joint extension.

In addition to the three normal types of end feel, Cyriax described five classic **abnormal end feels,** several of which have subdivisions and each of which is commonly associated with some degree of pain or restricted movement.[1,114]

- *Muscle Spasm.* This end feel is invoked by movement, with a sudden dramatic arrest of movement often accompanied by pain. The end feel is sudden and hard. Cyriax called this a "vibrant twang."[1] Some examiners divide muscle spasm into different parts. **Early muscle spasm** occurs early in the ROM, almost as soon as movement starts; this type of muscle spasm is associated with inflammation and is seen in more acute conditions. **Late muscle spasm** occurs at or near the

TABLE 1-17

Normal and Abnormal End Feels

End Feel	Example
Normal	
Bone to bone	Elbow extension
Soft tissue approximation	Knee flexion
Tissue stretch	Ankle dorsiflexion, shoulder lateral rotation, finger extension
Abnormal	
Early muscle spasm	Protective spasm following injury
Late muscle spasm	Spasm due to instability or pain
"Mushy" tissue stretch	Tight muscle
Spasticity	Upper motor neuron lesion
Hard capsular	Frozen shoulder
Soft capsular	Synovitis, soft tissue edema
Bone to bone	Osteophyte formation
Empty	Acute subacromial bursitis
Springy block	Meniscus tear

end of the ROM. It is usually caused by instability and the resulting irritability caused by movement. An example is muscle spasm occurring during the apprehension test for anterior dislocation of the shoulder. Both types of muscle spasm are the result of the subconscious efforts of the body to protect the injured joint or structure, and their occurrence may be related to how quickly the examiner does the movement. **Spasticity** is slightly different and is seen with upper motor neuron lesions. It is a form of muscle hypertonicity that offers increased resistance to stretch involving primarily the flexors in the upper limb and extensors in the lower limb and may be associated with muscle weakness. The Ashworth scale is sometimes used to measure spasticity and resistance to passive movement, but its reliability has been questioned.[115,116] A **tight muscle** may give its own unique end feel. This is similar to normal tissue stretch, but it does not have as great an elastic feel.

- *Capsular.* Although this end feel is similar to tissue stretch, it does not occur where one would expect (i.e., it occurs earlier in the ROM), and it tends to have a thicker feel to it. ROM is obviously reduced, and the capsule can be postulated to be at fault. Muscle spasm usually does not occur in conjunction with the capsular type of end feel except if the movement is fast and the joint acute. Some examiners divide this end feel into **hard capsular,** in which the end feel has a thicker stretching quality to it, and **soft capsular** (boggy), which is similar to normal tissue stretch end feel but with a restricted ROM. The hard capsular end feel is seen in more chronic conditions or in full-blown capsular patterns. The limitation comes on rather abruptly after a smooth, friction-free movement. The soft capsular end feel is more often seen in acute conditions with stiffness occurring early in the range and increasing until the end of range is reached. Maitland calls this "resistance through range."[117] Some authors interpret this soft, boggy end feel as being the result of synovitis, soft-tissue edema, or hemarthrosis.[118] Major injury to ligaments and the capsule often causes a **soft end feel** until the tension is taken up by other structures.[119]
- *Bone-to-Bone.* This abnormal end feel is similar to the normal bone-to-bone type, but the restriction occurs before the end of ROM would normally occur or where a bone-to-bone end feel would not be expected. An example is a bone-to-bone end feel in the cervical spine resulting from osteophyte formation.
- *Empty.* The empty end feel is detected when movement produces considerable pain. The movement cannot be performed or stops because of the pain, although no real mechanical resistance is being detected. Examples include an acute subacromial bursitis or a tumor. Patients often have difficulty describing the empty end feel, and there is no muscle spasm involved.
- *Springy Block.* Similar to a tissue stretch, this occurs where one would not expect it to occur; it tends to be

found in joints with menisci. There is a rebound effect with a thick stretching feel although it is not as stretchy as a hard capsular end feel, and it usually indicates an internal derangement within the joint. A springy block end feel may be found with a torn meniscus of a knee when it is locked or unable to go into full extension.

Capsular Patterns.[1] With passive movement, a full ROM must be carried out in several directions. A short, too-soft movement in the midrange does not achieve the proper results or elicit potential findings. In addition to evaluating the end feel, the examiner must look at the **pattern of limitation or restriction**. If the capsule of the joint is affected, the pattern of limitation is the feature that indicates the presence of a **capsular pattern** in the joint. This pattern is the result of a total joint reaction, with muscle spasm, capsular contraction (the most common cause), and generalized osteophyte formation being possible mechanisms at fault. Each joint has a characteristic pattern of limitation. The presence of this capsular pattern does not indicate the type of joint involvement; only an analysis of the end feel can do that. Only joints that are controlled by muscles have a capsular pattern; joints, such as the sacroiliac and distal tibiofibular joints, do not exhibit a capsular pattern. Dutton pointed out that capsular patterns are based on empirical findings rather than research, and this may be the reason capsular patterns may be different or inconsistent.[3] In fact, Hayes et al.[62] felt the pattern of limitation was useful but the proportional limitation concept should not be used. Table 1-18 illustrates some of the common capsular patterns seen in joints.

Noncapsular Patterns.[1] The examiner must also be aware of **noncapsular patterns,** for example, a limitation that exists but does not correspond to the classic capsular pattern for that joint. In the shoulder, abduction may be restricted but with very little rotational restriction (e.g., subacromial bursitis). Although a total capsular reaction is absent, there are other possibilities, such as ligamentous adhesions, in which only part of a capsule or the accessory ligaments are involved. There may be a local restriction in one direction, often accompanied by pain, and full, pain-free ROM in all other directions. A second possibility is **internal derangement,** which commonly affects only certain joints, such as the knee, ankle, and elbow. Intracapsular fragments may interfere with the normal sequence of motion. Movements causing impingement of the fragments will be limited, whereas other motions will be free. In the knee, for example, a torn meniscus may cause a blocking of extension, but flexion is usually free. Loose bodies cause limitation when they are caught between articular surfaces. A third possibility is **extra-articular lesions.** These lesions are revealed by disproportionate limitation, extra-articular adhesions, or an acutely inflamed structure limiting movement in a particular direction. For example, limited straight leg raising in the lumbar disc syndrome is referred to as a **constant length phenomenon.** This phenomenon results when the limitation of movement in one joint depends on the position in which

TABLE **1-18**

Common Capsular Patterns of Joints

Joint	Restriction*
Temporomandibular	Limitation of mouth opening
Atlanto-occipital	Extension, side flexion equally limited
Cervical spine	Side flexion and rotation equally limited, extension
Glenohumeral	Lateral rotation, abduction, medial rotation
Sternoclavicular	Pain at extreme of range of movement, especially horizontal adduction and full elevation
Acromioclavicular	Pain at extreme of range of movement, especially horizontal adduction and full elevation
Ulnohumeral (elbow)	Flexion, extension
Radiohumeral	Flexion, extension, supination, pronation
Proximal (superior) radioulnar	Supination, pronation equally limited
Distal radioulnar	Full range of movement, pain at extremes of rotation
Radiocarpal (wrist)	Flexion and extension equally limited
Intercarpal	None
Midcarpal	Equal limitation of flexion and extension
Carpometacarpal (thumb)	Abduction, extension
Carpometacarpal (fingers)	Equal limitation in all directions
Trapeziometacarpal	Abduction, extension
Metacarpophalangeal and interphalangeal	Flexion, extension
Thoracic spine	Side flexion and rotation equally limited, extension
Lumbar spine	Side flexion and rotation equally limited, extension
Sacroiliac, symphysis pubis, and sacrococcygeal	Pain when joints are stressed
Hip†	Flexion, abduction, medial rotation (but in some cases medial rotation is most limited)
Knee (tibiofemoral)	Flexion, extension
Distal tibiofibular	Pain when joint stressed
Talocrural	Plantar flexion, dorsiflexion
Talocalcaneal (subtalar)	Limitation of range of movement (varus, valgus)
Midtarsal	Dorsiflexion, plantar flexion, adduction, medial rotation
Tarsometatarsal	None
First metatarsophalangeal (big toe)	Extension, flexion
Second to fifth metatarsophalangeal	Variable
Interphalangeal	Flexion, extension

*Movements are listed in order of restriction.
†For the hip, flexion, abduction, and medial rotation are always the movements most limited in a capsular pattern. However, the order of restriction may vary.

another joint is held. The restricted tissue (in this case, the sciatic nerve) must lie outside the joint or joints (in this case, hip and knee) being tested. The constant length phenomenon may also result from muscle adhesions that cause restriction of motion.

Inert Tissue.[1] After the active and passive movements are completed, the examiner should be able to determine whether there are problems with any of the **inert tissues.** The examiner makes such a determination by judging the degree of pain and the limitation of movement within the joint. For lesions of inert tissue, the examiner may find that active and passive movements are painful in the same direction. Usually pain occurs as the limitation of motion approaches. Resisted isometric movements (discussed later) are not usually painful unless some compression is occurring. During the examination, inert tissues are tested or stressed during active and passive movements,

functional testing, selected special tests, joint play testing, and palpation.

Inert tissue refers to all tissue that is not considered contractile or neurological. Four classic patterns may be seen in lesions of inert issue, according to the ROM available (or restriction present) and the amount of pain produced.[1]

1. If the *range of movement is full and there is no pain,* there is no lesion of the inert tissues being tested by that passive movement; however, there may be lesions of inert tissue in other directions or around other joints.

2. The next possible pattern is one of *pain and limitation of movement in every direction.* In this pattern, the entire joint is affected, indicating arthritis or capsulitis. Each joint has its own capsular pattern (see Table 1-18), and the amount of limitation is not

usually the same in each direction; however, although there is a set pattern for each joint, other directions may also be affected. All movements of the joint may be affected, but the motions described for the capsular pattern usually occur in the particular order listed. For example, the capsular pattern of the shoulder is lateral rotation most limited, followed by abduction and medial rotation. In early capsular patterns, only one movement may be restricted; this movement is usually the one that has the potential for the greatest restriction. For example, in an early capsular pattern of the shoulder, only lateral rotation may be limited, and the limitation may be slight.

3. A patient with a lesion of inert tissue may experience *pain and limitation or excessive movement in some directions but not in others,* as in a ligament sprain or local capsular adhesion. In other words, a noncapsular pattern is presented. Movements that stretch, pinch, or move the affected structure cause the pain. Internal derangement that results in the blocking of a joint is another example of a lesion of inert tissue that produces a variable pattern. Extra-articular limitation occurs when a lesion outside the joint affects the movement of that joint. Because these movements pinch or stretch the involved structure (e.g., bursitis in the buttock, acute subacromial bursitis), pain and limitation of movement occur on stretch or compression of these structures. If a structure such as a ligament has been torn, the ROM may increase if swelling is minimal, especially right after injury, indicating instability (pathological hypermobility) of the joint and can be seen in spinal or peripheral joints. Swelling often masks instability because it puts the tissues under tension. Pathological hypermobility, if present, results in greater than normal movement at the joint, causes pain, puts neurogenic structures at risk, and can result in progressive deformity and degeneration.[120]

4. The final inert tissue pattern is *limited movement that is pain free.* The end feel for this type of condition is often of the abnormal bone-to-bone type, and it usually indicates a symptomless osteoarthritis—that is, osteophytes are present and restrict movement, but they are not pinching or compressing any sensitive structures. If this situation is encountered, it should be left alone because it is not causing the patient any problem other than restricted ROM and attempts at treatment could lead to further problems.

Patterns of Inert Tissue Lesions

- Pain-free, full range of motion (ROM)
- Pain and limited ROM in every direction
- Pain and excessive or limited ROM in some directions
- Pain-free, limited ROM

Resisted Isometric Movements

Resisted isometric movements are the movements tested last in the examination of the joints. This type of movement consists of a strong, static (isometric), voluntary muscle contraction, and it is used primarily to determine whether the contractile tissue is the tissue at fault, although the nerve supplying the muscle is also tested. If the muscle, its tendon, or the bone into which they insert is at fault, pain and weakness result; the amount of pain and weakness is related to the degree of injury and the patient's pain threshold. If movement is allowed to occur at the joint, inert tissue around the joint will also move, and it will not be clear whether any resulting pain arises from contractile or inert tissues. The joint, therefore, is put in a neutral or resting position (see Table 1-35 later) so that minimal tension is placed on the inert tissue. The patient is asked to contract the muscle as strongly as possible while the examiner resists to prevent any movement from occurring and to ensure that the patient is using maximum effort. To keep movement to a minimum, it is best for the examiner to position the joint properly in the resting position and then to say to the patient, "Don't let me move you." In this way, the examiner can ensure that the contraction is isometric and can control the amount of force exerted. Movement cannot be completely eliminated, but this method minimizes it. Some compression of the inert tissues (e.g., cartilage) occurs with the contraction, and there may be some joint shear as well, but it will be minimal if done as described.

If, as advocated, this isometric hold method is used, then movement against this resistance would require muscle strength of grade 3 to 5 on the muscle test grading scale (Table 1-19).[121] If the muscle strength is less than grade 3, then the methods advocated in muscle testing manuals must be used.[117,122] If the examiner is having difficulty differentiating between grade 4 and grade 5, an eccentric break method of muscle testing may be used. This method starts as an isometric contraction, but then the examiner applies sufficient force to cause an eccentric contraction or a "break" in the patient's isometric contraction. This method provides a more recognizable threshold for maximum isometric contraction.[121] It must be recognized, however, that all three methods are subjective for normal and good values. When a muscle is tested in the resting position, it is usually being tested in its position of optimum length so that maximum force, if necessary, can be elicited. In some cases, however, a muscle, because of pathology, may become lengthened or shortened leading to weakness when tested in the normal resting position. Testing a muscle in the fully lengthened position tightens the inert components of muscle and puts more stress on the contractile tissues, whereas testing it in a shortened position puts it in its weakest position. Kendall et al.,[123] for example, called muscle weakness that results from muscle lengthening **stretch weakness** or **positional weakness.** Thus, if the examiner has found ROM to be

TABLE **1-19**

Muscle Test Grading

Grade	Value	Movement Grade
5+	Normal (100%)	Complete ROM against gravity with maximal resistance
4	Good (75%)	Complete ROM against gravity with some (moderate) resistance
3+	Fair +	Complete ROM against gravity with minimal resistance
3	Fair (50%)	Complete ROM against gravity
3−	Fair −	Some but not complete ROM against gravity
2+	Poor +	Initiates motion against gravity
2	Poor (25%)	Complete ROM with gravity eliminated
2−	Poor −	Initiates motion if gravity is eliminated
1	Trace	Evidence of slight contractility but no joint motion
0	Zero	No contraction palpated

ROM, Range of motion.

limited or excessive during passive movement testing, consideration should be given to performing the isometric tests in different positions of the ROM to see if the problem is not one of strength but of muscle length. This action will also help differentiate between weakness throughout the ROM (**pathological weakness**) from weakness only in certain positions (**positional weakness**). If, in the history, the patient has complained of symptoms in a different position than those commonly tested, the examiner may modify the isometric test position to try to elicit the symptoms. If the patient has complained that a concentric, eccentric, or econcentric contraction has caused the problem, the examiner may include these movements, with or without load, in the examination, but only after the isometric tests have been completed. Econcentric or pseudo-isometric contraction involves two-joint muscles in which the muscle is acting concentrically at one joint and eccentrically at the other joint, the result being minimal or no change in muscle length. Two-joint muscles are among the most frequently injured muscles (e.g., hamstrings, biceps, gastrocnemius) often because of the different actions occurring over the two joints at the same time.

In some cases, machines may be used to measure muscle strength, but care should be taken, because these tests are often not isometric, and they are often not performed in functional positions nor at functional speeds. They do, however, provide a comparison or ratio between right and left and between different movements.

Muscle weakness, if elicited, may be caused by an upper motor neuron lesion, injury to a peripheral nerve, pathology at the neuromuscular junction, a nerve root

Examiner Observations During Resisted Isometric Movement

- Whether the contraction causes pain and, if it does, the pain's intensity and quality
- Strength of the contraction
- Type of contraction causing problem (e.g., concentric, isometric, eccentric, econcentric)

lesion, or a lesion or disease (myopathy) of the muscle, its tendons, or the bony insertions themselves. For the first four of these causes, the system of muscle test grading may be used. For nerve root lesions, myotome testing is the method of choice. When testing for muscle lesions, it is more appropriate to test the resisted movements isometrically first, to determine which movements are painful, then perform individual muscle tests, as advocated in texts such as that of Daniels and Worthingham,[122] to determine exactly which muscle is at fault.

Signs and Symptoms of Myopathy (Muscle Disease)[66]

- Difficulty lifting
- Difficulty walking
- Myotonia (inability of muscle to relax)
- Cramps
- Pain (myalgia)
- Progressive weakness
- Myoglobinuria

If the contraction appears weak, the examiner must make sure that the weakness is not caused by pain or by the patient's fear, unwillingness, or malingering. The examiner can often resolve such a finding by having the patient make a contraction on the good side first, which normally will not cause pain. Weakness that is not associated with pain or disuse is a positive neurological sign indicating that a nerve root, peripheral nerve, or upper motor neuron lesion is at least part of the problem.

Causes of Muscle Weakness

- Muscle strain
- Pain/reflex inhibition
- Peripheral nerve injury
- Nerve root lesion (myotome)
- Upper motor neuron lesion (even when muscle shows increased tone)
- Tendon pathology
- Avulsion
- Psychological overlay

Contractile Tissue.[1] With resisted isometric testing, the examiner is looking for problems of **contractile tissue,** which consists of muscles, their tendons, attachments (e.g., bone), and the nervous tissue supplying the contractile tissue. Both active movements and resisted isometric testing demonstrate symptoms if contractile tissue is affected. Other parts of the examination, which will test contractile tissue, include passive movement, functional testing, specific special tests, and palpation. Usually, passive movements are normal—that is, passive movements are full and pain free, although pain may be exhibited at the end of the ROM when the contractile or nervous tissue is stretched. If contractile tissue has been injured, active movement is painful in one direction (contraction) and passive movement, if painful, is painful in the opposite direction (stretch). Resisted isometric testing is painful in the same direction as active movement. If the muscles are tested as previously described, not all movements will be found to be affected, except in patients with psychogenic pain and sometimes in patients with an acute joint lesion, in which even a small amount of tension on the muscles around the joint provokes pain. However, if the joint lesion is acutely severe, passive movements (when tested) will be markedly affected, and there will be no confusion as to where the lesion lies. As with inert tissue, four classic patterns have been identified with lesions of contractile and nervous tissue.[1] (In this case, however, one is dealing with pain and strength rather than pain and altered ROM.)

1. Movement that is *strong and pain free* indicates that there is no lesion of the contractile unit being tested or the nervous tissue supplying that contractile unit, regardless of how tender the muscles may be when touched. The muscles and nerves function painlessly and are not the source of the patient's discomfort.

2. Movement that is *strong and painful* indicates a local lesion of the muscle or tendon. Such a lesion could be a first- or second-degree muscle strain. The amount of strength is usually determined by the amount of pain the patient feels on contraction, which results from reflex inhibition that leads to weakness or cogwheel contractions. A second-degree strain produces greater weakness and more pain than a first-degree strain. Similarly, tendinosis, tendinitis, paratenonitis, or paratenonitis with tendinosis (Table 1-20) all may lead to contractions that are strong (relative) and painful, but one that is not usually as strong as on the good side; and the pain is in or around the tendon, not the muscle.[124,125] If there is a partial avulsion fracture, again, the movement will be strong and painful. However, if the avulsion is complete, the movement will be weak and painful (see later discussion). Typically, there is no primary limitation of passive movement when contractile tissue is injured although end range may be painful (stretch), except, for example, in the case of a gross muscle tear with hematoma where the muscle, which is often in spasm, is being stretched. In this case, the patient may develop joint stiffness secondary to disuse. This is often caused by protective muscle spasm of adjacent muscles that allow, for example, some joint contracture to be superimposed on the muscle lesion. This stiffness then takes

TABLE **1-20**

Bonar's Modification of Clancy's Classification of Tendinopathies

Pathological Diagnosis	Concept (Macroscopic Pathology)	Histological Appearance
Tendinosis	Intratendinous degeneration (commonly caused by aging, microtrauma, and vascular compromise)	Collagen disorientation, disorganization, and fiber separation with an increase in mucoid ground substance, increased prominence of cells and vascular spaces with or without neovascularization, and focal necrosis or calcification
Tendinitis/partial rupture	Symptomatic degeneration of the tendon with vascular disruption and inflammatory repair response	Degenerative changes as noted above with superimposed evidence of tear, including fibroblastic and myofibroblastic proliferation, hemorrhage and organizing granulation tissue
Paratenonitis	Inflammation of the outer layer of the tendon (paratenon) alone, regardless of whether the paratenon is lined by synovium	Mucoid degeneration in the areolar tissue is seen. A scattered mild mononuclear infiltrate with or without focal fibrin deposition and fibrinous exudate is also seen
Paratenonitis with tendinosis	Paratenonitis associated with intratendinous degeneration	Degenerative changes as noted for tendinosis with mucoid degeneration with or without fibrosis and scattered inflammatory cells in the paratenon alveolar tissue

From Khan KM, Cook JL, Bonar F, et al: Histopathology of common tendinopathies—update and implications for clinical management. Sports Med 27:399, 1999.

precedence in the treatment. One should always remember that it is easier to maintain physiological function than it is to restore it.

3. Movement that is *weak and painful* indicates a severe lesion around that joint, such as a fracture. The weakness that results is usually caused by reflex inhibition of the muscles around the joint, secondary to pain.

4. Movement that is *weak and pain free* indicates a rupture of a muscle (third-degree strain) or its tendon or involvement of the peripheral nerve or nerve root supplying that muscle. If the movement is weak and pain free, neurological involvement or a tendon rupture should be suspected first. With neurological involvement, the examiner must be able to differentiate between the muscle innervation of a nerve root (myotome) and the muscle innervation of a peripheral nerve (see Table 1-15 as an example). Also, the examiner should be able to differentiate between upper and lower motor neuron lesions (see Table 1-12). Third-degree strains are sometimes masked, because if the force is great enough to cause a complete tear of a muscle, the surrounding muscles, which assisted the movement, may also be injured (first- or second-degree strain). The pain from these secondary muscles can mask the third-degree strain to the primary mover. The tested weakness, however, would be greater with the third-degree strain (and its lack of pain). Although significant pain can occur at the time of the third-degree injury, this pain usually quickly subsides to a dull ache, even when the muscle is contracting, because there is no tension on the muscle, which no longer has two attachment (origin and insertion) points. For this reason, a gap or hole in the muscle may be palpated. When the third-degree injured muscle does contract, the muscle may bunch up or bulge, giving an obvious deformity (Figure 1-17).

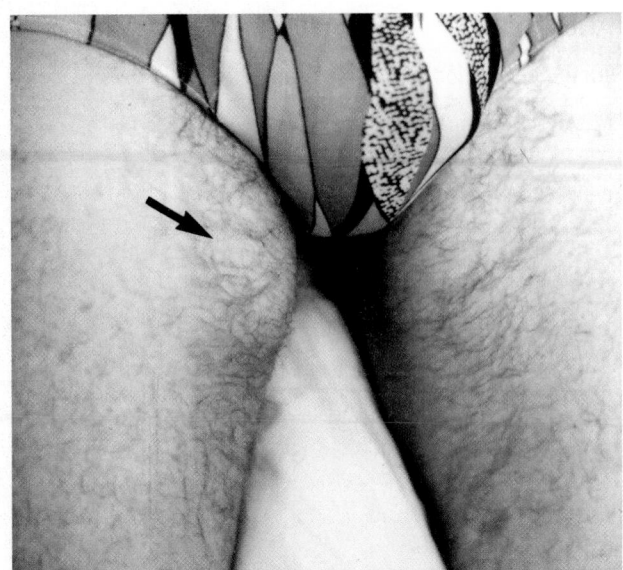

Figure 1-17 Rupture (3° strain) of right adductor muscle. Note the bulge in the muscle caused when the patient is asked to contract the muscle.

Patterns of Contractile Tissue and Nervous Tissue Lesions

- No pain, and movement is strong
- Pain, and movement is relatively strong (but not as strong as it should be)
- Pain, and movement is weak
- No pain, and movement is weak

Signs and Symptoms of Upper Motor Neuron Lesions

- Spasticity
- Hypertonicity
- Hyperreflexia (deep tendon reflexes)
- Positive pathological reflexes (e.g., Babinski, Hoffman)
- Absent or reduced superficial reflexes
- Extensor plantar response (bilateral)

If all movements around a joint appear painful, the pain is often a result of fatigue, emotional hypersensitivity, or emotional problems. Patients may equate effort with discomfort, and they must be told that they are not necessarily the same.

Janda put forth an interesting concept by dividing muscles into two groups: postural and phasic.[126] He believed that **postural** or **tonic muscles,** which are the muscles responsible for maintaining upright posture, have a tendency to become tight and hypertonic with pathology and to develop contractures but are less likely to atrophy, whereas **phasic muscles,** which include almost all other muscles, tend to become weak and inhibited with pathology. The examiner must be careful to note the type of muscle affected and the ROM available (active movements) as well as the strength and production of pain (resisted isometric movements) when testing contractile tissue. Table 1-21 shows the muscles that are postural and prone to tightness and those that are phasic and prone to weakness. Table 1-22 shows the characteristics of postural and phasic muscles. If a muscle imbalance is present, the tight muscles must first be stretched to their normal length and tone before strength can be equalized.[127,128]

Janda and his associates further expanded this concept with the "upper crossed syndrome" and "pelvic crossed syndrome," which show muscles (primarily postural) on one diagonal at a joint to be tight and hypertonic, whereas muscles on the other diagonal are weak and lengthened (Figure 1-18).[128,129] This concept of tight and hypertonic muscles in one aspect of a joint with weak lengthened muscles in the opposite aspect is one that examiners should remember for all joints, especially when looking

TABLE **1-21**

Functional Division of Muscle Groups*

Muscles Prone to Tightness (Postural Muscles)	Muscles Prone to Weakness (Phasic Muscles)
• Gastrocnemius and soleus • Tibialis posterior • Short hip adductors • Hamstrings • Rectus femoris • Iliopsoas • Tensor fasciae latae • Piriformis • Erector spinae (especially lumbar, thoracolumbar, and cervical portions) • Quadratus lumborum • Pectoralis major • Upper portion of trapezius • Levator scapulae • Sternocleidomastoid • Scalenes • Flexors of the upper limb	• Peronei • Tibialis anterior • Vastus medialis and lateralis • Gluteus maximus, medius, and minimus • Rectus abdominis • External oblique • Serratus anterior • Rhomboids • Lower portion of trapezius • Short cervical flexors • Extensors of upper limb

Modified from Jull G, Janda V: Muscles and motor control in low back pain. In Twomey LT, Taylor JR, editors: Physical therapy for the low back: clinics in physical therapy, New York, 1987, Churchill Livingstone, p. 258.
*Janda considers all other muscles neutral.

TABLE **1-22**

Characteristics of Postural and Phasic Muscle Groups

Muscles Prone to Tightness (Postural Muscles)	Muscles Prone to Weakness (Phasic Muscles)
Predominantly postural function	Primarily phasic function
Associated with flexor reflexes	Associated with extensor reflexes
Primarily two-joint muscles	Primarily one-joint muscles
Readily activated with movement (shorter chronaxie)	Not readily activated with movement (longer chronaxie)
Tendency to tightness, hypertonia, shortening, or contractures	Tendency to hypotonia, inhibition, or weakness
Resistance to atrophy	Atrophy occurs easily

Modified from Jull G, Janda V: Muscles and motor control in low back pain. In Twomey LT, Taylor JR, editors: Physical therapy for the low back: clinics in physical therapy, New York, 1987, Churchill Livingstone.

at chronic joint injuries as both types of muscles tend to be present and require different treatment approaches.

In addition, the examiner should always consider the action of **force couples** surrounding a joint. Force couples are counteracting groups of muscles functioning

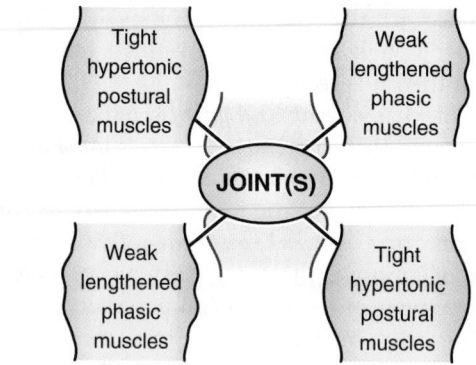

Figure 1-18 Postural and phasic muscle response to pathology producing "crossed syndromes."

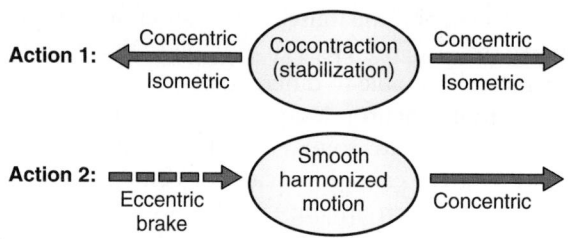

Figure 1-19 Force couple action.

either by co-contraction to stabilize a joint, or by one group acting concentrically and the opposing group acting eccentrically to cause a controlled joint motion that is smooth and harmonized (Figure 1-19).[130] Pathology to one of the force couple muscles or to one of the force couples acting about a joint can lead to muscle imbalance, instability, and loss of smooth coordinated movement.

Other Findings During Movement Testing

When carrying out the examination of the joints, the examiner must be aware of other findings that may become evident and may help to determine the nature and location of the problem. For example, it should be noted whether there is excessive ROM (hypermobility or laxity) within the joints. Comparison of the normal side with the involved side of the body gives some indication as to whether the findings on the affected side would be considered normal. For example, an apparently excessive range (laxity) may just be the normal ROM for that patient. It must also be remembered that joints on the nondominant side tend to be more flexible than those on the dominant side.

It is also important to note whether a **painful arc** is present; this finding indicates that an internal structure is being squeezed or pinched in part of the ROM. Sounds (such as, crepitus, clicking, or snapping) should be noted. To be pathologically significant however, these sounds must be related to the patient's symptoms. They may be caused by structures slipping over one another (e.g., tendons slipping over bone), loose bodies or arthritic changes in the joint, abnormal movement of structures (e.g., meniscus click on opening or closing of the temporomandibular joint), or a tear in a structure (e.g., a tear in the triangular cartilaginous disc of the wrist). **Pain at the extreme of ROM** may be caused by squeezing or stretching of structures around the joint or even in the joint, especially if the movement takes the joint into its close packed position.

Functional Assessment

Functional assessment plays an important role in the evaluation of the patient.[131] It is different from the analysis of specific movement patterns of active, passive, and resisted isometric movements used to differentiate between inert, neurological, and contractile tissue. Functional assessment may involve task analysis, observation of certain patient activities, or a detailed evaluation of the effect of the injury or disability on the patient's ability to function in everyday life. Reiman and Manske[132] have organized functional tests into different levels of difficulty for assessment purposes (Table 1-23). Determining what the patient hopes is an appropriate functional outcome, and determining what the patient can and cannot do functionally can be extremely important in the choice of

TABLE **1-23**

Levels That Can Be Used for Assessment of Function in an Individual

Levels for the Assessment of Function	Assessment Examples
Level I Assessment primarily at the level of subjective report (patient and clinician)	• Self-report measures most indicative of dysfunction • Biopsychosocial measures relevant to dysfunction • Self-report of activity rating scales (patient interpretation on specific requirements of his/her necessary activity level to return to previous level of function) • Clinician analysis of specific sport/occupation/ADLs with respect to requirements (e.g., specific type of movements, energy system involvement)
Level II Assessment primarily at the level of impairment	• Anthropometric measurements (e.g., body mass index, girth and height measurements) • Muscle length • Manual muscle testing • ROM • Sensation • Joint play
Level III Assessment primarily at the level of static observation/posture/balance	• Static posture • Static balance (bilateral and single-leg balance static assessment)
Level IV Assessment primarily at the level of dynamic posture, general movement patterns, and single plane dynamic balance	• Dynamic posture (i.e., posture of individual as he or she performs movements required) • General movement patterns (e.g., walking, transfer movements) • Dynamic balance predominantly in one plane of movement without quality assessment (e.g., functional reach test, tandem walking)
Level V Assessment primarily at the level of movement patterns encountered during higher level tasks and/or multi-planar dynamic balance	• Assessment of movement patterns the individual performs with his or her primary tasks (e.g., specific sport, occupational, and other tasks) • Four square step
Level VI Assessment primarily at the level of specific movement patterns	• Functional movement screen • Movement impairment syndrome assessment

Continued

TABLE **1-23**

Levels That Can Be Used for Assessment of Function in an Individual—cont'd

Levels for the Assessment of Function	Assessment Examples
Level VII Assessment of the individual primarily at the level of PPM occurring predominantly in one plane of movement	• 1RM testing • Trunk endurance • Sit-up endurance • Supine bridge • Loaded forward reach • Lunge • Flexed arm hang • Step-down • Single-leg squat • Single-leg inclined squat on total gym

Level VIII
 	
Assessment primarily at the level of PPM occurring predominantly in one plane of movement, but requiring one or more of the following:
• Limited base of support
• Multiple joint involvement
• Multiple muscle group involvement
• Explosive movement
	• Aerobic endurance testing one or more of the following:
	  ○ 1-mile walk
	  ○ Rockport walk
	  ○ 1- to 5-mile run
	  ○ 12-minute run
	  ○ 20-meter shuttle run
	• Wingate anaerobic power
	• Star excursion balance test
	• Knee bending in 30 seconds
	• Single jump and hop testing in one plane of movement for one or more of the following:
	  ○ Standing long jump
	  ○ Single-hop for distance
	  ○ Vertical jump
	• Seated chest pass
	• Seated shot-put throw

Level IX
 	
Assessment primarily at the level of PPM occurring predominantly in multiple planes of movement and/or requiring explosive movement
	• Jump and hop testing in multiple planes of movement or requiring multiple jumps or hops for one or more of the following:
	  ○ Side-hop
	  ○ One-legged cyclic hop
	  ○ Hexagon jump
	  ○ Modified hexagon hop
	  ○ Figure-eight hop
	  ○ Carioca drill
	  ○ 6-meter timed hop
	  ○ Triple jump for distance
	  ○ Triple hop for distance
	  ○ Single-leg crossover hop for distance
	  ○ Hop testing after fatigue
	• 300 shuttle run
	• Bosco test
	• Running-based anaerobic sprint test
	• Lower extremity functional test
	• Speed and agility testing for one or more of the following:
	  ○ Edgren side-step
	  ○ Illinois agility
	  ○ Pro agility (5-10-5)
	  ○ Three-cone drill
	  ○ T-test
	  ○ Zigzag run
	• Sidearm medicine ball throw
	• Underkoffler softball throw for distance

TABLE **1-23**

Levels That Can Be Used for Assessment of Function in an Individual—cont'd

Levels for the Assessment of Function	Assessment Examples
Level X	
Assessment primarily at the level of PPM in multiple planes and/or explosive type of movement with the quality of the performance also assessed	• Balance error scoring system • Functional throwing performance index • Multiple single-leg hop stabilization • Tinetti assessment tool
Level XI	
Assessment primarily at the level of replication of the specific tasks performed during the individual's sport/occupation/daily activity and/or clustering of PPM that replicate component(s) of the sport/occupation/daily activity	• Functional capacity evaluation • Firefighting "ability test" • BEAST90 • Functional abilities test
Level XII	
Cumulative assessment (FPT) including performance assessment (quantitative and qualitative) with self-report and biopsychosocial measures	Assessment forward and backward along the functional continuum utilizing each parameter of function (i.e., impairment, performance measures, and self-report measures) as necessary

Modified from Reiman MP, Manske RC: The assessment of function: how is it measured? A clinical perspective. J Man Manip Ther 19:95–97, 2011.
1RM, One repetition maximum; *ADL*, activity of daily living; *BEAST90*, ball-sport endurance and sprint test; *FPT*, functional performance testing; *PPM*, performance-based measures; *ROM*, range of motion.

treatments that will be successful. Primarily, functional assessment helps the examiner establish what is important to the patient and the patient's expectations. It commonly represents a measurement of a **whole-body task performance ability,** as opposed to isolated examination of a joint. That being said, Preston et al.[133] recommend that functional assessment should involve joint-specific questions and activity level questions along with general health questions. These may be in one questionnaire or in several instruments. Because it is part of each individual joint assessed, the functional testing should demonstrate whether an isolated impairment affects the patient's ability to perform everyday activities.

The examiner should attempt to establish what functional factors are important to the patient. For example, functional testing may include movements under different loads to determine the patient's ability to work or play. Likewise, repeated movements and sustained postures may be necessary for work, recreational, or social activities. In some cases, movements at different speeds or under different loads may be necessary to determine pathology.[94] A traumatic shoulder instability, for example, may not be evident in a swimmer except when he or she is actually doing the activity at the speed and load at which the activity is done in the water.

Because functional testing relates to the effect of the injury on the patient's life, those activities that cause symptoms, those that are restricted by symptoms, and the factors (e.g., strength, power, flexibility) that are needed to perform the activities must be considered. For example, if the patient is seated normally while a history is taken, the examiner knows the patient has the functional ROM (agility) for sitting with 90° of hip and knee flexion. Table 1-24 lists some functional outcome measures that should be considered. The activities should be simple, patient-oriented, and based on coordinated functional movement of the joints, and they should be activities the patient wants to do. Although most functional outcomes or tests are subjective, this does not make them any less effective.[134]

The functional assessment is important to determine the effect of the condition or injury on the patient's daily life, including his or her sex life. Functional impairment may be slightly annoying or completely disabling for the patient. Functional activities that should be tested, if appropriate, include self-care activities, such as walking, dressing, daily hygiene (e.g., washing, bathing, shaving, combing hair), eating, and going to the bathroom; recreational activities, such as reading, sewing, watching television, gardening, and playing a musical instrument; and other activities, such as driving, dialing a telephone, getting groceries, preparing meals, and hanging clothes. Goldstein nicely divided activities of human function into four broad areas, which are then broken down into more discrete levels (Table 1-25).[135] The examiner should consider which of these are important to the patient and ensure that they are considered in the assessment. Figure

TABLE **1-24**

Examples of Functional and Clinical Outcomes

Clinical Outcomes	Functional Outcomes
• Strength • Range of motion • Proprioception • Endurance (muscular) • Swelling • Pain • Psychological overlay	• Power • Agility • Kinesthetic awareness • Endurance (muscular and cardiovascular) • Speed • Activity specificity • Pain • Skill level required for activity • Psychological preparedness • Daily living skills

1-20 shows some of the daily living skills and mobility questions that may be of concern to both the examiner and the patient. The short musculoskeletal function assessment (SMFA) helps to determine how much the patient is bothered by functional problems (Figure 1-21).[136] Other functional assessment tool examples that are available include the functional capacity evaluation (FCE),[135] the functional independence measure (FIM),[137] the physical performance test,[138] the functional status test,[139] the arthritis impact measurement scale (AIMS 2),[140] the functional assessment tool (FAT),[141] the SF-36 Health Status Survey,[142,143] the Sickness Impact Profile,[144] the SMFA Questionnaire,[145] and the Sock Test.[146] The particular tool used depends on the needs of the patient and the presenting pathological problem.

TABLE **1-25**

Goldstein's Divisions of Human Function

FUNCTION: BASIC OR PERSONAL ACTIVITIES OF DAILY LIVING (ADLS)			
Activity	**Examples**	**Activity**	**Examples**
Bed activities	Moving in bed Managing pillows and blankets Reaching for objects Sitting up	Dressing activities	Putting on clothes Tying laces
		Transfer activities	Putting on socks and shoes Bed to chair Sit to stand
Hygiene activities	Brushing teeth Bathing and showering Washing Toileting Combing hair Shaving Putting on makeup	Walking activities	Getting into car Level and uneven surfaces Curbs and stairs Opening doors Walking and carrying items Distance and velocity Assistive devices Gait deviations
Eating activities	Using utensils Cutting meat Managing glass and cup		

FUNCTION: INSTRUMENTAL (ADVANCED) ACTIVITIES OF DAILY LIVING (IADLS)			
Activity	**Examples**	**Activity**	**Examples**
Meal preparation	Cutting vegetables Turning on oven	Having sex	Manipulating clothing Changing positions
Light housework	Measuring ingredients Dusting Washing dishes Mopping floors	Driving car	Getting in and out Turning wheel Adjusting pedals, mirrors
Check writing	Manipulating pen Adding and subtracting	Gardening	Kneeling Raking Digging Watering
Shopping	Pushing cart Carrying groceries Reaching Getting money out of pocket	Communicating	Using writing tools Using telephone

TABLE **1-25**

Goldstein's Divisions of Human Function—cont'd

FUNCTION: WORK ACTIVITIES			
Activity	Examples	Activity	Examples
Lifting	From table and from floor	Kneeling	On all fours and just knees
Carrying	Small and large objects	Manipulating objects	Pen, salt shaker
Stooping	Wiping floor	Climbing	Stairs and ladder
Pushing	Broom	Standing	
Pulling	Drawer and door	Walking	Slow and fast
Reaching	Into cupboard		

FUNCTION: SPORT AND RECREATIONAL ACTIVITIES			
Activity	Examples	Activity	Examples
Walking	Forward and backward Sideways Level and uneven surfaces	Hitting	Baseball bat Tennis racquet Golf club
Jogging and sprinting	Different surfaces In water	Swimming	Different strokes Different kicks
Cutting	Circles Figure-eights Crossover and sidestep	Agility	Specific drills
		Open and closed kinetic chain	Throwing and pushing
Jumping and hopping	Vertical and distance Forward and backward Level and uneven surfaces	Speed and power	Moving different sized objects at different speeds
Throwing	Underhand and overhand Two-handed Different objects	Endurance	Aerobic and anaerobic Cardiovascular and muscle
		Reaction time and proprioception	Blinking lights
Catching	One- and two-handed Different sizes and weights		

Data from Goldstein TS: Functional Rehabilitation in Orthopedics, Gaithersburg, MD, 1995, Aspen Pub. Inc., pp. 19–23.

Part of this functional assessment occurs during the history when the examiner asks the patient which activities can be done easily, which can be done with some difficulty, and which cannot be done at all. During the observation, the examiner notes what the patient can and cannot do within the confines of the assessment area. Finally, during the examination, functional testing or a work analysis may be performed. For example, when examining the hand, the examiner notes the power and dexterity exhibited during performance of fundamental maneuvers, such as gripping and pinching. Below is an example of a work activity analysis, which may be evaluated if the patient is hoping to return to that activity and to do it successfully.[147] Regardless of which functional test is used, the examiner must understand the purpose of the test. A functional test should not be done just because it is available. It should not be used in isolation but rather in conjunction with the overall assessment so that a complete assessment picture of the patient can be developed.

Example of an Analysis of Work Activity

Job title: *Packer*
Essential function: *Packing individual cobbler cups for shipping*

STEPS
1. Select a box
2. Place the box on the conveyor side rack
3. Pick up one cobbler cup in each hand
4. Place the cups into the packing box
5. Repeat steps 3 and 4 until 36 cups are in a box
6. Place the filled box on the "sealing table"
7. Fold the short flaps of the box lid
8. Fold the longer flaps of the box lid
9. Tape down the long flaps of the box using the manual taping machine
10. Place the sealed box on the pallet

From Ellexson MT: Analyzing an industry: job analysis for treatment, prevention, and placement. Orthop Phys Ther Clin 1:17, 1992.

Numerical scoring systems are often used as part of the functional assessment and often play a role in **clinical prediction rules** (also called **clinical decision rules** or **risk scores**) that quantify different parts of the history, physical examination, and laboratory results in making a diagnosis or prognosis.[148–152] By combining the different findings, it is felt that a clinician's diagnostic accuracy is increased.[5,131,148,153–155] The Ottawa Ankle and Foot Rules and the Pittsburgh Knee Rules are examples of clinical prediction rules.[95,156]

The numerical scoring systems are often more related to function as it applies to a specific joint and often a specific activity rather than to the whole body (Figure 1-22),[157] and for many, functional assessment plays only a small part. With these numerical systems, the clinician must ensure that the scoring systems really measure what they say they measure. To be effective, a numerical scoring system must demonstrate universality, practicality, reliability, reproducibility, effectiveness, and inclusiveness, and it must have been validated.[158] The terminology and methods must be described precisely; the criteria should be related to functional outcome (what the patient desires) rather than clinical outcome (what the clinician desires), and the measures must be sensitive enough to show a difference.[159] Figure 1-23 shows a functional assessment involving the entire upper limb.[160] Table 1-26 demonstrates tests that could be used in an examination of simulated activities of daily living (ADLs).[161] Similar charts can and have been developed for almost all joints of the body. However, many of these numerical scoring systems have been developed from the clinician's perspective rather than from what the patient thinks is important.

Functional tests may also be used as provocative tests to bring on the symptoms the patient has complained of or to determine how the patient is progressing or whether he or she is ready to return to activity. Examples of these tests include the hop test and disco test for the knee. These tests, in reality, could be used for all the weight-bearing (lower limb) joints. However, it must be remembered that many of these provocative or stress tests are designed for very active persons and are not suitable for all populations.

Special (Diagnostic) Tests

After the examiner has completed the history, observation, and evaluation of movement, special tests may be performed for the involved joint. Many special tests are available for each joint to determine whether a particular type of disease, condition, or injury is present. They are

Text continued on p. 53

Daily Living Skill and Mobility Questions for Functional Assessment

Daily Living Skills	Mobility
Feeding	**Supine to Sit**
(7) Are you able to feed yourself from a tray or table using ordinary utensils? Can you cut meat? Can you pour liquids from open containers?	(7) When you are lying on your back, can you sit up without using your arms or without rolling to the side? Can you do this smoothly and easily?
(4) If you use a spork or rocker knife or other helpful aid, are you able to feed yourself in a reasonable length of time?	(4) Do you use your arms to help you sit up, or do you roll to the side before sitting up? Do you have to try several times before sitting up?
(2) Are you able to feed yourself with some help from another person, for example, to help you raise a cup to your mouth or to cut meat?	(2) Does someone help you to sit up?
(0) Do you depend on another person to feed you?	(0) Are you unable to sit up?
	Sitting to Standing
Dress Upper Body	(7) Are you able to stand up from a regular chair without using your arms?
(7) Are you able to get clothes out of your closets and drawers and put them on and remove them from your upper body by yourself, including bra, slip, pullovers, and front opening shirts and blouses, as well as managing zippers, buttons, and snaps?	(4) Do you need to use your arms to help you stand up, or do you need to try several times?
	(2) Does someone need to help you stand up out of a chair?
(4) If someone lays your clothes out for you or hands them to you, are you able to dress your upper body by yourself even if it takes a little more time, or do you need some help with closures, such as buttons, zippers, snaps, or hooks? Do you use aids such as reachers, dressing hooks, button hooks, or zipper pulls?	(0) Do you depend on someone else entirely to get you out of a chair?
	Transfer—Toilet
	(7) Are you able to get on and off the toilet easily and without using your hands?
(2) Does someone help you put on your blouse or shirt or sweater because you are limited by pain, lack of strength, or limited range of motion?	(4) Do you need to use your arms to help you get on and off the toilet, or do you require assistive devices such as elevated toilet seats or grab bars?
	(2) Does someone need to help you get on and off the toilet?
(0) Do you depend on another person to dress your upper body?	(0) Are you unable to use the toilet?

Figure 1-20 **Daily living skill and mobility questions for function assessment.** (Modified from Convery FR, Minteer MA, Amiel D, et al: Polyarticular disability: a functional assessment. Arch Phys Med Rehab 58[11]:498, 1977.)

Daily Living Skills	Mobility

Dress Lower Body

(7) Are you able to put on undergarments, slacks, socks, nylons, and shoes by yourself? Can you tie shoelaces?

(4) Are you able to put on undergarments, slacks, socks, nylons, and shoes by yourself if they are laid out for you or handed to you? Do you use dressing aids such as long handled reachers? Do you avoid shoes that have laces or buckles, or do you use elastic laces or Velcro shoe closures by yourself?

(2) Does someone help you to put on undergarments, slacks, nylons, or shoes?

(0) Do you depend on another person to dress your lower body?

Grooming

(7) Are you able to comb and brush and shampoo your hair, shave, apply makeup, clean your teeth or dentures, and manage nail care by yourself without adaptations or modifications?

(4) Do you use assistive devices or adapted methods for grooming: If someone places what you need within reach, are you then able to complete grooming activities unaided? Do you use long-handled combs or brushes, suction brushes for cleaning nails or dentures, adapted shaving equipment or adapted key for rolling toothpaste tubes?

(2) Does someone actually help you shampoo or brush your hair, shave, apply makeup, clean your teeth or dentures, or manicure your nails?

(0) Do you depend on someone else entirely for your grooming needs?

Care of Perineum/Clothing at Toilet

(7) Are you able to go to the bathroom by yourself including managing your clothes, wiping yourself (and placing sanitary napkins or tampons)?

(4) Are you able to manage your clothing at the toilet and wipe yourself independently although it may be difficult, or do you use aids such as an extended reacher for wiping yourself or clothing aids?

(2) Does someone help you with your clothing at the toilet or assist you with wiping yourself (or in placement of sanitary napkins or tampons)?

(0) Do you depend on someone else to manage your clothes at the toilet for you or to wipe you (or to place sanitary napkins or tampons)?

Wash or Bathe

(7) Are you able to wash and dry your entire body by yourself, including your back and feet? Are you able to turn water faucets?

(4) Do you use bathing aids such as long handled bath brushes or sponges? Are you unable to reach some parts of your body for bathing or drying thoroughly but can still manage without help?

(2) Are you able to bathe and dry most parts of your body and have someone help you with the rest?

(0) Does someone else bathe you?

Vocational

(2) Are you employed full-time in your usual occupation? Are you a full-time homemaker and require no assistance? Are you retired for other than medical reasons?

(0) Not able to do the above

Transfer—Tub or Shower

(7) Are you able to get in and out of a tub or shower safely?

(4) Can you get in and out of a tub or shower using aids such as grab bars or special seat or lift?

(2) Does someone need to help you to get in and out of the tub or shower?

(0) Are you unable to get in and out of the tub or shower?

Transfer—Automobile

(7) Can you get in and out of a car easily, including opening and closing the door?

(4) Can you get in and out of a car by yourself if you use aids such as grab bars or if someone opens the door for you?

(2) Does someone help you get in and out of a car?

(0) Are you unable to get in and out of a car even with assistance?

Walk on Level

(7) Are you able to walk two blocks at an even pace without using a cane, crutches, walker, or adapted shoes?

(4) Do you need a cane, crutches, or walker to walk two blocks?

(2) Can you walk one block with assistance?

(0) Are you unable to walk one block even with assistance?

Walk Outdoors

(7) Are you able to walk outdoors at least two blocks without avoiding rough terrain such as grass, sand, gravel, curbs, ramps, or hills?

(4) Do you try to avoid uneven terrain? Do you use a crutch or cane for safety or balance purposes only when outside?

(2) Must you use a cane or crutches to walk at least two blocks on uneven terrain?

(0) Are you unable to walk on uneven terrain?

Up and Down Stairs

(7) Can you go up and down at least five steps safely, step over step without using the hand rail or other support?

(4) Are you able to go up and down at least five steps if you use a hand rail, cane, or crutches or if you go one step at a time?

(2) Do you need someone to help you go up and down at least five steps?

(0) Are you unable to go up and down at least five steps even with help?

Wheelchair/10 Yards

(7) Are you able to push your wheelchair without help for 10 yards? Can you turn corners and get close to bed, table, and toilet?

(4) Do you use a motorized wheelchair?

(2) Do you need someone to help you maneuver your wheelchair around corners or to help you position it?

(0) Are you unable to push your wheelchair 10 yards?

Figure 1-20, cont'd

Short Musculoskeletal Function Assessment (SMFA)

Instructions

We are interested in finding out how you are managing with your injury or arthritis this week. We would like to know about any problems you may be having with your daily activities because of your injury or arthritis.

Please answer each question by putting a check in the box corresponding to the choice that best describes you.

These questions are about how much difficulty you may be having <u>this week</u> with your daily activities because of your injury or arthritis.

	Not at All Difficult	A Little Difficult	Moderately Difficult	Very Difficult	Unable To Do
1. How difficult is it for you to get in or out of a low chair?	☐	☐	☐	☐	☐
2. How difficult is it for you to open medicine bottles or jars?	☐	☐	☐	☐	☐
3. How difficult is it for you to shop for groceries or other things?	☐	☐	☐	☐	☐
4. How difficult is it for you to climb stairs?	☐	☐	☐	☐	☐
5. How difficult is it for you to make a tight fist?	☐	☐	☐	☐	☐
6. How difficult is it for you to get in or out of the bathtub or shower?	☐	☐	☐	☐	☐
7. How difficult is it for you to get comfortable to sleep?	☐	☐	☐	☐	☐
8. How difficult is it for you to bend or kneel down?	☐	☐	☐	☐	☐
9. How difficult is it for you to use buttons, snaps, hooks, or zippers?	☐	☐	☐	☐	☐
10. How difficult is it for you to cut your own fingernails?	☐	☐	☐	☐	☐
11. How difficult is it for you to dress yourself?	☐	☐	☐	☐	☐
12. How difficult is it for you to walk?	☐	☐	☐	☐	☐
13. How difficult is it for you to get moving after you have been sitting or lying down?	☐	☐	☐	☐	☐
14. How difficult is it for you to go out by yourself?	☐	☐	☐	☐	☐
15. How difficult is it for you to drive?	☐	☐	☐	☐	☐
16. How difficult is it for you to clean yourself after going to the bathroom?	☐	☐	☐	☐	☐
17. How difficult is it for you to turn knobs or levers (for example, to open doors or to roll down car windows)?	☐	☐	☐	☐	☐
18. How difficult is it for you to write or type?	☐	☐	☐	☐	☐
19. How difficult is it for you to pivot?	☐	☐	☐	☐	☐
20. How difficult is it for you to do your usual physical recreational activities, such as bicycling, jogging, or walking?	☐	☐	☐	☐	☐
21. How difficult is it for you to do your usual leisure activities, such as hobbies, crafts, gardening, card-playing, or going out with friends?	☐	☐	☐	☐	☐
22. How much difficulty are you having with sexual activity?	☐	☐	☐	☐	☐
23. How difficult is it for you to do <u>light</u> housework <u>or</u> yard work, such as dusting, washing dishes, or watering plants?	☐	☐	☐	☐	☐
24. How difficult is it for you to do <u>heavy</u> housework <u>or</u> yard work, such as washing floors, vacuuming, or mowing lawns?	☐	☐	☐	☐	☐
25. How difficult is it for you to do your usual work, such as a paid job, housework, or volunteer activities?	☐	☐	☐	☐	☐

Figure 1-21 Short Musculoskeletal Function Assessment (SMFA). (From Swiontkowski MF, Engelberg R, Martin DP, et al: Short musculoskeletal function assessment questionnaire: the validity, reliability, and responsiveness. J Bone Joint Surg Am 81[9]: 1256–1258, 1999.)

These next questions ask how often you are experiencing problems <u>this week</u> because of your injury or arthritis.

	None of the Time	A Little of the Time	Some of the Time	Most of the Time	All of the Time
26. How often do you walk with a limp?	☐	☐	☐	☐	☐
27. How often do you avoid using your painful limb(s) or back?	☐	☐	☐	☐	☐
28. How often does your leg lock or give-way?	☐	☐	☐	☐	☐
29. How often do you have problems with concentration?	☐	☐	☐	☐	☐
30. How often does doing too much in one day affect what you do the next day?	☐	☐	☐	☐	☐
31. How often do you act irritable toward those around you (for example, snap at people, give sharp answers, or criticize easily)?	☐	☐	☐	☐	☐
32. How often are you tired?	☐	☐	☐	☐	☐
33. How often do you feel disabled?	☐	☐	☐	☐	☐
34. How often do you feel angry or frustrated that you have this injury or arthritis?	☐	☐	☐	☐	☐

These questions are about how much you are bothered by problems you are having <u>this week</u> because of your injury or arthritis.

	Not at All Bothered	A Little Bothered	Moderately Bothered	Very Bothered	Extremely Bothered
35. How much are you bothered by problems using your hands, arms, or legs?	☐	☐	☐	☐	☐
36. How much are you bothered by problems using your back?	☐	☐	☐	☐	☐
37. How much are you bothered by problems doing work around your home?	☐	☐	☐	☐	☐
38. How much are you bothered by problems with bathing, dressing, toileting, or other personal care?	☐	☐	☐	☐	☐
39. How much are you bothered by problems with sleep and rest?	☐	☐	☐	☐	☐
40. How much are you bothered by problems with leisure or recreational activities?	☐	☐	☐	☐	☐
41. How much are you bothered by problems with your friends, family or other important people in your life?	☐	☐	☐	☐	☐
42. How much are you bothered by problems with thinking, concentrating, or remembering?	☐	☐	☐	☐	☐
43. How much are you bothered by problems adjusting or coping with your injury or arthritis?	☐	☐	☐	☐	☐
44. How much are you bothered by problems doing your usual work?	☐	☐	☐	☐	☐
45. How much are you bothered by problems with feeling dependent on others?	☐	☐	☐	☐	☐
46. How much are you bothered by problems with stiffness and pain?	☐	☐	☐	☐	☐

Figure 1-21, cont'd

Shoulder Evaluation Form

Diagnosis:
Aim of Procedure:
Operation:
Shoulder: right: left:
Arm Dominance: right: left:

The rating in each category can be adjusted
according to the AIM of the procedure.

Patient's Name:
Hospital Unit #:
Date of Operation:
Date of Follow-up:
Surgeon:
Preoperative rating:
Postoperative rating:
Patient's Evaluation (circle):
Exc.   Good   Fair   Poor

Unit Rating
(circle one in
each category)

Unit Rating
(circle one in
each category)

I. PAIN (15)

1.	None	15
2.	Slight during activity	12
3.	Increased pain during activities	6
4.	Moderate/severe pain in activity	3
5.	Severe pain, dependent on medication	0 ___

II. STABILITY (25)

1.	Normal. Shoulder stable and strong in all positions	25
2.	Mild apprehension in normal use of arm. No subluxation or dislocation	20
3.	Avoids elevation and external rotation. Rare subluxation	10
4.	Recurrent subluxations ("Dead arm syndrome"). Positive apprehension test or recurrent dislocation	5
5.	Recurrent dislocation	0 ___

III. FUNCTION (25)

1.	Normal function. All activities of daily living. Performs all work, sport/recreation prior to injury. Lifting 30+ lb. Swimming, tennis, throwing. **Combat**	25
2.	Mild limitation in sports and work. Can throw, but limited in baseball. Strong in tennis, football, swimming, lifting (15–20 lb) and combat. Performs all personal care.	20
3.	Moderate limitation in overhead work and lifting (10 lb) and athletics. Unable to throw or serve in tennis. Swims sidestroke. Difficulty with body care (perineal care, back pocket, combing hair, reaching back). Aid necessary at times.	10
4.	Severe limitations. Unable to perform usual work or lifting. No athletics. Sedentary occupation. Unable to perform body care without aid. Can feed self and comb hair.	5
5.	Complete disability of extremity	0 ___

IV. MOTION (25)

Abduction and forward flexion

151 to 170°	15
121 to 150°	12
91 to 120°	10
61 to 90°	7
31 to 60°	5
Less than 30°	0 ___

IR   Thumb to scapula — 5
     Thumb to sacrum — 3
     Thumb to trochanter — 2
     Less than trochanter — 0 ___

ER   (with arm at side)
     80° — 5
     60° — 3
     30° — 2
     Less than 30° — 0 ___

V. STRENGTH (10) (compared to opposite shoulder)

(specify method = manual, spring gauge, Cybex)

Normal	10
Good	6
Fair	4
Poor	0 ___

TOTAL UNITS

Excellent	(100–85 units) ___
Good	(84–70 units)
Fair	(69–50 units)
Poor	(49 units or less)

Figure 1-22 Shoulder evaluation form. (Modified from Rowe CR: The shoulder, Edinburgh, 1988, Churchill Livingstone, p. 632.)

TABLE **1-26**

Summary Description of Tests in Simulated Activities of Daily Living Examination (SADLE)

Test	Measure	Units	Instrumentation
Two leg standing, eyes open	Maximum time of three 30-second trials	Seconds	Stopwatch
One leg standing, eyes open	Maximum time of three 30-second trials	Seconds	Stopwatch
Two leg standing, eyes closed	Maximum time of three 30-second trials	Seconds	Stopwatch
One leg standing, eyes closed	Maximum time of three 30-second trials	Seconds	Stopwatch
Tandem walking with supports	Time to take 10 heel-to-toe steps	Steps/sec	Stopwatch and parallel bars
Tandem walking without supports	Time to take 10 heel-to-toe steps	Steps/sec	Stopwatch and parallel bars
Putting on a shirt	Average time of two trials	Seconds	Stopwatch and shirt
Managing three visible buttons	Average time of two trials	Seconds	Stopwatch and cloth with three buttons mounted on a board
Zipping a garment	Average time of two trials	Seconds	Stopwatch and cloth with zipper mounted on a board
Putting on gloves	Average time of two trials	Seconds	Stopwatch and two garden gloves
Dialing a telephone	Average time of two trials	Seconds	Stopwatch and telephone
Tying a bow	Average time of two trials	Seconds	Stopwatch and large shoelaces mounted on a board
Manipulating safety pins	Average time of two trials	Seconds	Stopwatch and two safety pins
Picking up coins	Average time of two trials	Seconds	Stopwatch and four coins placed on a plastic sheet
Threading a needle	Average time of two trials	Seconds	Stopwatch, thread, and large-eyed needle
Unwrapping a Band-Aid	Time for one trial	Seconds	Stopwatch and one Band-Aid
Squeezing toothpaste	Average time of two trials	Seconds	Stopwatch, tube of toothpaste, and a board
Cutting with a knife	Average time of two trials	Seconds	Stopwatch, plate, fork, knife, and Permoplast
Using a fork	Average time of two trials	Seconds	Stopwatch, plate, fork, and Permoplast

Modified from Potvin AR, Tourtellotte WW, Dailey JS, et al: Simulated activities of daily living examination. Arch Phys Med Rehab 53:478, 1972.

sometimes called *clinical accessory, provocative, motion, palpation,* or *structural tests.* These tests, although strongly suggestive of a particular disease or condition when they yield positive results, do not necessarily rule out the disease or condition when they yield negative results. This will depend on the sensitivity and specificity of each test as well as the skill and experience of the clinician.

Special tests should seldom be used in isolation or as "stand alone" tests. They should only be considered as part of an overall clinical assessment that includes history, observation, and the rest of the examination.[162,163] One of the problems with special tests is that many clinicians, especially those with less experience, hope that any special tests they use will give them a definitive answer as to what is wrong. Although a special test may give a definitive answer, more commonly it does not, but combined with the other information from the assessment, a clearer picture of the problem arises. No physical test is 100%

reliable, valid, sensitive, or specific. In this book, the author has highlighted key tests that the clinician should practice, become comfortable with, and become confident in their use because the value of these tests has been demonstrated clinically (via examiner experience) and/or statistically to show that they contribute to determining what the problem is. It is better to learn one or two tests well and to be confident and proficient in their use rather than learning all the possible tests used to confirm a certain pathology. The following key ("Key to Classifying Special Tests") has been developed to give an indication whether the author feels it is worthwhile to learn to do the test based on present evidence and the clinician's experience. That being said, even the tests with a ✓ icon will or can be ineffective if the conditions outlined in the following green box are not met. Without these conditions being met, even the best test may fail to confirm the diagnosis regardless of its utility score, QUADUS

Upper Extremity Function Test

Basic Function	*Date* _____	
	Right	**Left**

Grasp
1. Block 4 in. (Item 1)
2. Block 3 in. (Item 2)
3. Block 2 in. (Item 3)
4. Block 1 in. (Item 4)

Grip
5. Pipe 1¾ in. (Item 5)
6. Pipe ¾ in. (Item 6)

Lateral Prehension
7. Slate 1 × ⅝ × 4 in. (Item 7)

Pinch
8. Ball 3 in. (Item 8)
    Marble ⅝ in. (Item 9)
9. Index finger and thumb
10. Middle finger and thumb
11. Ring finger and thumb
12. Small finger and thumb
    Ball-bearing ⁷⁄₁₆ in. (Item 10)
13. Index finger and thumb
14. Middle finger and thumb
15. Ring finger and thumb
16. Small finger and thumb
    Ball-bearing ¼ in. (Item 11)
17. Index finger and thumb
18. Middle finger and thumb
19. Ring finger and thumb
20. Small finger and thumb
    Ball-bearing ⁵⁄₃₂ in. (Item 12)
21. Index finger and thumb
22. Middle finger and thumb
23. Ring finger and thumb
24. Small finger and thumb

Placing
25. Washer over nail (Item 13)
26. Iron to shelf (Item 14)

Supination and Pronation
27. Pour water from pitcher to glass
28. Pour water from glass to glass (pronation)
29. Pour water back to first glass (supination)
30. Place hand behind head
31. Place hand on top of head
32. Hand to mouth

33. Write name _____

TOTAL _____

Smedly Dynamometer Reading:
Does pain interfere with function?

Scoring:	3—Performs test normally
	2—Completes test, but takes abnormally long time or has great difficulty
	1—Performs test partially
	0—Can perform no part of test

Score:	0–25:	Trace
	26–50:	Very poor
	51–75:	Poor
	76–89:	Partial
	90–98:	Functional
	99–100:	Maximal (dominant hand) (96-nondominant hand)

Figure 1-23 Upper extremity function test. (Modified by permission of the publisher from Carroll D: A quantitative test of upper extremity function. J Chron Dis 18:482, 1965. Copyright © 1965 by Elsevier Science.)

score, or reliability or validity value. The research on the tests is important, but so is the experience of the clinician and the "state" of the patient. The ☑ icon does not imply the tests are infallible. It means they are useful along with the history and the rest of the examination in making a diagnosis.

Key for Classifying Special Tests

The following is based on the author's clinical experience and review of the literature:

☑ Implies that the test has moderate to strong statistical (research) and clinical (examiner experience) support, or the author has found the test useful along with the history and examination in making a clinical diagnosis

⚠ Implies that the test has minimal statistical (research) and some clinical (examiner experience) support, or the author has found the test helpful along with the history and examination in making a clinical diagnosis

❓ Implies that the test has insufficient statistical (research) evidence, but it may demonstrate clinical support for its use in the hands of an experienced examiner along with the history and examination in making a clinical diagnosis

Special Test Considerations

Any special test, regardless of its classification, can be positively or negatively affected by the:

- Patient's ability to relax
- Presence of pain and the patient's perception of the pain
- Presence of patient apprehension
- Skill of the clinician
- Ability and confidence of the clinician

When deciding to use these diagnostic tests or grouping or clustering them in clinical prediction rules, the examiner must determine if the test will give reliable and useful information that will help in the diagnosis and subsequent treatment.[164,165] To be useful, a diagnostic test must give reliable data (i.e., consistent results regardless of who does the test), must be valid (i.e., test what it says it tests), and must be accurate to maximize patient outcomes.[164,166] As previously stated, care must be taken considering the usefulness of a special test, because the test is influenced by both the patient and the clinician. One single study reporting on the reliability, validity, or other measures of test usefulness gives a good indication that the test can be useful in certain circumstances (in this case, those circumstances used to test the test), but research studies always involve compromises in terms of what is controlled and what is not controlled when doing the study. For example, many tests are confirmed

TABLE 1-27

Benchmark Intraclass Correlation Coefficient Values

Value	Description
<0.75	Poor to moderate agreement
>0.75	Good agreement
>90	Reasonable agreement for clinical measurements

Data from Portney LG, Walkins MP: Foundations of clinical research—applications to practice. Upper Saddle River, NJ, 2000, Prentice-Hall, p. 565.

during surgery when the patient is unconscious. Looking at the analysis of one test by different authors shows the wide variability in outcomes.[167,168] Given all these factors, it is easy to see that special tests, although they have an important role to play, should not be used in isolation, nor should they be the single deciding factor in making a diagnosis.

Reliability may be affected by cooperation of the patient, which may be influenced by the patient's ability to relax, tolerate pain, describe apprehension, and show sincerity; it may be affected by the skill of the clinician, which may be influenced by experience, his or her ability to relax, and to confidently do the test; and it may be affected by the calibration of equipment.[164] Several methods are used to determine reliability, but the intraclass correlation coefficient (ICC) is the preferred index because it reflects both agreement and correlation among ratings.[169] It is calculated through analysis of variance (ANOVA) using variance estimates.[169] Table 1-27 shows ICC agreement values that are illustrative for diagnostic tests. With nominal data, the kappa statistic (κ) is applied after the percentage agreement between testers has been determined.[169]

When performing a test, it is also useful, in terms of reliability, to know the standard error of measurement (SEM).[169] The SEM reflects the reliability of the response when the test is performed many times. It is an indication of how much change there might be when a test is repeated. If the SEM is small, then the test is stable with minimal variability between tests.[169]

Diagnostic tests should be evaluated on their diagnostic accuracy or ability to determine which people have the condition or disease and those who do not as this will have an impact on subsequent treatment and patient outcomes.[170] The most useful methods of determining whether a test is a good test for the pathology under consideration are sensitivity, specificity, and likelihood ratios.[164–166,169–178] Sensitivity implies the ability of a test to identify people who have a particular condition, dysfunction, or disease when they do (i.e., a true positive).[164,166,169,174,178] Specificity, on the other hand, is used to determine which people do not have a particular condition, dysfunction, or disease (i.e., a true negative).[164,166,169,174,178] Sensitivity and specificity values for tests are usually based on a gold standard, or reference test (e.g., diagnostic imaging, what was found at surgery).[178,179] If the clinician is unsure that the patient has a particular condition, dysfunction or disease, then the examiner would want to use a test of exclusion or discovery that has a high sensitivity as it will rule out those people who do not have the problem, provided the test's specificity is equal to or higher than another test testing for the same thing.[173] On the other hand, if the examiner has a high level of suspicion (based on the preceding history, observation, and examination) that the problem is present and wants to confirm that decision (confirmation test), then the examiner would want a test with higher specificity to "rule in" those people who do have the problem, provided the test's sensitivity is equal to or higher than another test testing for the same thing.[166,173] This is especially true if further evaluation or treatment is expensive or dangerous. To prevent healthy people from receiving unnecessary expensive or dangerous treatment, high specificity is desired.[174] In an ideal world, one would want a test that has both high sensitivity and high specificity. To try to solve these differences in levels of sensitivity and specificity, likelihood ratios are often recommended as determinants of the usefulness of a test.[164,166,170,173,175,180] Likelihood ratios are based on determining the odds that a condition, dysfunction, or disease is present by combining sensitivity and specificity to indicate whether the test will raise or lower the probability of the patient having the condition, dysfunction, or disease.[164,175] The higher the likelihood ratio, the greater is the likelihood that the patient has the problem.

There are two other issues that the clinician should be aware of when considering special or diagnostic tests. Although beyond the scope of this book, clinicians should also consider responsiveness, which is the ability of a test to detect a clinically important change, and the minimal clinical important difference (MCID), which is the smallest difference in the result of a test that the clinician perceives as beneficial or significant in the context that it may result in a particular treatment or change in treatment.[171,172,181]

Tests can be more accurately performed right after injury (during the period of tissue shock—5 to 10 minutes after injury), under anesthesia, or in chronic conditions where pain may be less of a factor. Each examiner tends to use those tests he or she has found to be clinically effective. Under no circumstances should special tests be used in isolation, nor is it necessary to learn all of the special tests. They should be viewed as an integral part of a total examination.[182] They should be considered as tests to confirm a tentative diagnosis, to make a differential diagnosis, to differentiate between structures, to understand unusual signs, or to unravel difficult signs and symptoms.[93]

Special Test Uses[93]

- To confirm a tentative diagnosis
- To make a differential diagnosis
- To differentiate between structures
- To understand unusual signs
- To unravel difficult signs and symptoms

For each joint examination described in this book, specific tests are mentioned for specific conditions. The tests can be used to differentiate contractile, inert, and neurological pathology.

Today, most clinicians want to use only tests that are highly reliable and have good sensitivity and specificity. Although this goal is highly desirable, it is not always possible. Several books have quantified the value of some of these tests, and in reviewing these books it will be seen that for many of the tests their utility is questioned.[167,168] Thus, as previously mentioned, these tests should not be used in isolation but as part of a much larger assessment. In this book, the author has included many special tests— more like an encyclopedia of tests, rather than only the ones that have shown good reliability, sensitivity, or specificity. This has been done for three reasons (1) to provide a source for different tests, (2) to provide test examples for individuals who may want to test the reliability, specificity, and sensitivity of the tests where this has not been done before, and (3) to show that test results depend on the state of the patient and the ability and experience of the clinician. Tests that the author has found to be particularly effective and have provided useful and reliable information have been highlighted in boxes, and the author recommends that the students learn *these* tests. Many of the tests are similar and show similar results; the choice of which ones to use depends on which ones give the best results for the individual examiner and which tests provide the most useful and reliable information to the examiner.[183] For example, both the Lachman test and anterior drawer test may be used to test the anterior cruciate ligament although the literature indicates the Lachman test is more sensitive.[184,185]

If desired, the examiner can design his or her own special tests or modify the described tests. Sometimes, the examiner can reproduce the same movement that the patient described as the mechanism of injury, which may provoke the symptoms. However, the addition of too many special tests only makes the picture more confusing and the diagnosis more difficult. Also, care should be taken when performing these tests, because they are usually provocative tests and will provoke signs and symptoms, including pain and apprehension. Thus, special tests should be done with caution and may be contraindicated in the presence of severe pain, acute and irritable conditions of the joints, instability, osteoporosis, pathological bone diseases, active disease processes, unusual signs and symptoms, major neurological signs, and patient apprehension.

In addition to the special tests, the examiner may also make use of **laboratory tests** ordered by a physician for specific conditions. With osteomyelitis, for example, a positive blood culture is likely to be obtained, the white blood cell count will be elevated, and the erythrocyte sedimentation rate will be increased. If a physician is the examiner, he or she may decide to draw fluid out of a joint (aspirate) with a hypodermic needle to view the synovial fluid. Tables 1-28 to 1-30 present normal laboratory values, laboratory findings in some bone diseases, and a classification of synovial fluid as examples of laboratory tests and values.

Reflexes and Cutaneous Distribution

After the special tests, the examiner can test the superficial, deep tendon, or pathological reflexes to obtain an indication of the state of the nerve or nerve roots supplying the reflex. If the neurological system is thought to be normal, there is no need to test the reflexes or cutaneous distribution. However, if the examiner is unsure whether there is neurological involvement, both reflexes and sensation should be tested to clarify the problem and where the problem actually is.

Most often, the deep tendon reflexes (sometimes referred to as *muscle stretch reflexes*)[32] are tested with a reflex hammer. A deep tendon reflex can be elicited from almost any tendon with practice. The more common deep tendon reflexes tested are shown in Table 1-31. Tables 1-32 and 1-33 demonstrate superficial and pathological reflexes. Superficial reflexes are provoked by superficial stroking, usually with a sharp object. A pathological reflex is not normally present, except in the very young (less than 5 to 7 months) in whom the cerebrum is not developed enough to suppress this reflex.[32] If it is present in adults and children, it often signals a pathological condition.

With a loss or abnormality of nerve conduction, there is a diminution (hyporeflexia) or loss (areflexia) of the stretch reflex. Aging also causes a decreased response. Upper motor neuron lesions produce findings of spasticity, hyperreflexia, hypertonicity, extensor plantar responses, reduced or absent superficial reflexes, and weakness of muscles distal to the lesion. Lower motor neuron lesions involving nerve roots or peripheral nerves produce findings of flaccidity, hyporeflexia or areflexia, hypotonicity, fasciculation, fibrillations, and weakness and atrophy of the involved muscles (see Table 1-12).[186]

Deep tendon reflexes are performed to test the integrity of the spinal reflex, which has a sensory (afferent) and motor (efferent) component.[11] Abnormal deep tendon reflexes are not clinically relevant unless they are found with sensory or motor abnormalities. To properly test the

TABLE 1-28

Normal Laboratory Values Used in Orthopedic Medicine*

Laboratory Test	Normal Range
White blood cell (WBC) count	$4–9 \times 10^9$/L
Red blood cell (RBC) count	$4.3–5.4 \times 10^{12}$/L (male) $3.8–5.2 \times 10^{12}$/L (female)
Hematocrit (HCT)	38–50% (male) 34–46% (female)
Hemoglobin (Hgb)	130–170 g/L (male) 115–160 g/L (female)
Erythrocyte sedimentation rate (ESR)	0–10 mm/hr (male) 0–15 mm/hr (female) 0–10 mm/hr (children)
Myoglobin (Mb)	30–90 ng/mL
Ferritin	25–465 µg/mL (male) 15–200 µg/mL (female)
Platelet count	140,000–350,000/mm³
Calcium	8.5–10.5 mg/dl
Ionized calcium	4.2–5.4 mg/dl
Alkaline phosphatase	25–92 U/L
Antinuclear antibodies screen	Negative
Uric acid	3.5–7.2 mg/dl (male) 2.6–6.0 mg/dl (female)
Rheumatoid arthritis factor	<1.20

*Values may vary slightly depending on equipment used.

deep tendon reflexes, the patient must be relaxed and the examiner must ensure that the muscle of the tendon to be tested is relaxed. The tendon to be tested is put on slight stretch, and an adequate stimulus is applied by dropping the reflex hammer onto the tendon. The examiner should tap the tendon five or six times to uncover any fading reflex response, indicative of developing nerve root signs. If the deep tendon reflexes are difficult to elicit, the reflexes often can be enhanced by having the patient clench the teeth or squeeze the hands together (**Jendrassik maneuver**) when testing the lower limb or squeeze the legs together when testing the upper limb. These activities increase the facilitative activity of the spinal cord and thereby accentuate minimally active reflexes.[187]

Superficial reflexes are tested by stroking the skin with a moderately sharp object that does not break the skin. The expected responses are shown in Table 1-32. A great deal of practice is needed to become proficient in testing the superficial reflexes.

Pathological reflexes, which are not usually evident because they are suppressed by the cerebrum at the brain stem or spinal cord level (see Table 1-33), may indicate upper motor neuron lesions if present on both sides or lower motor neuron lesions if present on only one side.[32] Improper stimulation (e.g., too much pressure) may lead to voluntary withdrawal in normal subjects, and the

TABLE **1-29**

Laboratory Findings in Bone Disease

Condition	Calcium	Inorganic Phosphorus	Alkaline Phosphatase	Calcium	Phosphorus
Hyperparathyroidism, primary	↑	↓	↑	↑	↑
Hyperparathyroidism, secondary	N-↓	↑	R↑	↑	↑
Hyperthyroidism, marked	N	N	↑	↑	↑
Hypothyroidism	N	N	N	N	N
Senile osteoporosis	N	N-O↓	N	N	N
Rickets (child)	↓	↓	↑	N	N
Osteomalacia (adult)	N-↓	↓	↑	N	N
Paget disease	R↑	R↓	↑	N	N
Multiple myeloma	↑	N-↑	R↑	↑	↑

Adapted from Quinn J: Introduction to the musculoskeletal system. In Meschan I: Synopsis of analysis of roentgen signs in general radiology, Philadelphia, 1976, W.B. Saunders Co., p. 27.
N, Normal; *O*, occasionally; *R*, rarely; ↑, increased; ↓, decreased.

TABLE **1-30**

Classification of Synovial Fluid

Type	Appearance	Significance
Group 1	Clear yellow	Noninflammatory states, trauma
Group 2*	Cloudy	Inflammatory arthritis; excludes most patients with osteoarthritis
Group 3	Thick exudate, brownish	Septic arthritis; occasionally seen in gout
Group 4	Hemorrhagic	Trauma, bleeding disorders, tumors, fractures

From Curran JF, Ellman MH, Brown NL: Rheumatologic aspects of painful conditions affecting the shoulder. Clin Orthop Relat Res 173:28, 1983.
*Inflammatory fluids will clot and should be collected in heparin-containing tubes. All group 2 or 3 fluids should be cultured if the diagnosis is uncertain.

TABLE **1-31**

Common Deep Tendon Reflexes

Reflex	Site of Stimulus	Normal Response	Pertinent Central Nervous System Segment
Jaw	Mandible	Mouth closes	Cranial nerve V
Biceps	Biceps tendon	Biceps contraction	C5–C6
Brachioradialis	Brachioradialis tendon or just distal to the musculotendinous junction	Flexion of elbow and/or pronation of forearm	C5–C6
Triceps	Distal triceps tendon above the olecranon process	Elbow extension/muscle contraction	C7–C8
Patella	Patellar tendon	Leg extension	L3–L4
Medial hamstrings	Semimembranosus tendon	Knee flexion/muscle contraction	L5, S1
Lateral hamstrings	Biceps femoris tendon	Knee flexion/muscle contraction	S1–S2
Tibialis posterior	Tibialis posterior tendon behind medial malleolus	Plantar flexion of foot with inversion	L4–L5
Achilles	Achilles tendon	Plantar flexion of foot	S1–S2

examiner must take care not to confuse this reaction with the pathological response. The two most commonly tested pathological reflexes are the Babinski reflex (lower limb) and the Hoffman reflex (upper limb).

To be of clinical significance, findings must show asymmetry between bilateral reflexes unless there is a central lesion. The eliciting of reflexes often depends on the skill of the examiner. The examiner should not be overly concerned if the reflexes are absent, diminished, or excessive on both sides, especially in young people, unless a central lesion is suspected. Exercise just before testing or patient anxiety or tenseness may lead to accentuated tendon reflexes.[87] Hyporeflexia or areflexia indicates a lesion of a peripheral nerve or spinal nerve root as a result of impingement, entrapment, or injury. Examples would be nerve root compression, cauda equina syndrome, or peripheral neuropathy. Hyporeflexia or areflexia may be seen in the absence of muscle weakness or atrophy because of the involvement of the efferent loop of the reflex arc in the reflex. Hyperactive or exaggerated reflexes (hyperreflexia) indicate upper motor neuron lesions as seen in neurological disease and cerebral or brain stem impairment. If a disc herniation and compression occur above the cervical enlargement in the cervical spine, the reflexes of the upper extremity are exaggerated. If the cervical enlargement is involved (which is more commonly the case), then some reflexes are exaggerated and some are decreased.[188]

TABLE 1-32

Superficial Reflexes

Reflex	Normal Response	Pertinent Central Nervous System Segment
Upper abdominal	Umbilicus moves up and toward area being stroked	T7–T9
Lower abdominal	Umbilicus moves down and toward area being stroked	T11–T12
Cremasteric	Scrotum elevates	T12, L1
Plantar	Flexion of toes	S1–S2
Gluteal	Skin tenses in gluteal area	L4–L5, S1–S3
Anal	Contraction of anal sphincter muscles	S2–S4

Deep Tendon Reflex Grading

0—Absent (areflexia)
1—Diminished (hyporeflexia)
2—Average (normal)
3—Exaggerated (brisk)
4—Clonus, very brisk (hyperreflexia)

TABLE 1-33

Pathological Reflexes*

Reflex	Elicitation	Positive Response	Pathology
Babinski[†]	Stroking of lateral aspect of sole of foot	Extension of big toe and fanning of four small toes Normal reaction in newborns	Pyramidal tract lesion Organic hemiplegia
Chaddock's	Stroking of lateral side of foot beneath lateral malleolus	Same response as above	Pyramidal tract lesion
Oppenheim's	Stroking of anteromedial tibial surface	Same response as above	Pyramidal tract lesion
Gordon's	Squeezing of calf muscles firmly	Same response as above	Pyramidal tract lesion
Piotrowski's	Percussion of tibialis anterior muscle	Dorsiflexion and supination of foot	Organic disease of central nervous system
Brudzinski	Passive flexion of one lower limb	Similar movement occurs in opposite limb	Meningitis
Hoffman (Digital)[‡]	"Flicking" of terminal phalanx of index, middle, or ring finger	Reflex flexion of distal phalanx of thumb and of distal phalanx of index or middle finger (whichever one was not "flicked")	Increased irritability of sensory nerves in tetany Pyramidal tract lesion
Rossolimo's	Tapping of the plantar surface of toes	Plantar flexion of toes	Pyramidal tract lesion
Schaeffer's	Pinching of Achilles tendon in middle third	Flexion of foot and toes	Organic hemiplegia

*Bilateral positive response indicates an upper motor neuron lesion. Unilateral positive response may indicate a lower motor neuron lesion.
[†]Test most commonly performed in lower limb.
[‡]Test most commonly performed in upper limb.

At the same time, the examiner can perform a **sensory scanning examination** by checking the cutaneous distribution of the various peripheral nerves and the dermatomes around the joint being examined. The sensory examination is performed for several reasons. First, it is used to determine the extent of sensory loss, whether that loss is caused by nerve root lesions, peripheral nerve lesions, or compressive tunnel syndromes. Second, because function is often tied to sensation, it is used to determine the degree of functional impairment. Third, because sensory function returns before motor function, it can be used to determine nerve recovery after injury or repair as well as when reeducation can commence. Also, if sensory function remains after injury to the spinal cord, it is a good indication that some motor function, at least, will be restored.[189] Finally, it is part of the total assessment and is often necessary for medicolegal reasons. Although the sensory distribution of peripheral nerves may vary from person to person, they tend to be more consistent than dermatomes.[69,190] The examiner must be able to differentiate between sensory loss involving a nerve root (dermatome) and that involving a peripheral nerve (see Table 1-15 for an example).

The sensory examination begins with a quick scan of sensation. To do this, the examiner runs his or her relaxed hands relatively firmly over the skin to be tested bilaterally and asks the patient whether there are any differences in sensation. The patient's eyes may be open for the scan. If the patient notes any differences in sensation between the affected and unaffected sides, then a more detailed sensory assessment is performed. The examiner should note the patient's ability to perceive the sensation being tested and the difference, if any, between the two sides of the body. In addition, distal and proximal sensitivities should be compared for each form of sensation tested. During the detailed sensory testing, the patient should keep his or her eyes closed so that the results will indicate the patient's perception and interpretation of the stimuli, not what the patient sees happening. With the detailed sensory testing, the examiner marks out, or delineates, the specific area of altered sensation and then correlates the area with the known dermatome and peripheral nerve distribution. The examiner must be aware, however, that the abnormal sensation does not necessarily come from the indicated nerve root or peripheral nerve; because of referred pain, it may come from any structure supplied by that nerve root. In some cases, the paresthesia may involve no specific pattern, or it may involve the entire circumference of a limb. This "opera glove" or "stocking" paresthesia or anesthesia may result from vascular insufficiency or systemic disease.

Superficial tactile (light touch) sensation, which is commonly the first sensation affected, can be tested with a wisp of cotton, soft hairbrush, or small paint or makeup brush. Superficial pain can be tested with a flagged pin (holding a piece of tape attached to a pin), pinwheel, or

TABLE **1-34**

Nerve Fiber Classification

Sensory Axons	Axon Diameter (μm)	Conduction Velocity (m/sec)	Innervation
Ia (Aα)	12–22	65–130	Muscle spindles (annulospiral endings)
Ib (Aα)	12–22	65–130	Golgi tendon organs
II (Aβ)	5–15	20–90	Pressure, touch, vibration (flower spray endings)
III (Aδ)	2–10	6–45	Temperature, fast pain
IV (C)	0.2–1.5	0.2–2.0	Slow pain, visceral, temperature, crude touch

other sharp object. Only light tapping should be used. About 2 seconds should elapse between each stimulus to avoid summation. It is the group II afferent fibers (Table 1-34) that are being tested. Perception to pin prick may range from absence of awareness, through pressure sensation, hyperanalgesia with or without radiation, localization, and sensation of sharpness, to normal perception.

If desired, the examiner may also test other sensations. Two test tubes (one with hot water, one with cold) are used to assess sensitivity to temperature (lateral spinothalamic tract and group III fibers), one containing hot water and one containing cold water. A normal response to this test does not necessarily mean that the patient has normal temperature sensation. Rather, the patient can distinguish between hot and cold, each at one level in the range, but not necessarily between different degrees of hot and cold. Sensitivity to vibration (i.e., how long until vibration stops) may be tested by holding a tuning fork (usually 30- or 256-cps tuning forks are used) against bony prominences; this tests the integrity of group II fibers and the dorsal column and medial lemniscal systems. Deep pressure pain (group II Aβ fibers) can be tested by squeezing the Achilles tendon, the trapezius muscle, or the web space between the thumb and index finger or by applying a knuckle to the sternum. To test proprioception and motion (i.e., the skin and joint receptors, muscle spindles, dorsal column and medial lemniscal systems, and group I and II fibers), the patient's fingers or toes are passively moved, and the patient is asked to indicate the direction of movement and final position while keeping the eyes closed. To ensure that pressure on the patient's skin cannot be used as a clue to direction of movement, the test digit should be grasped between the examiner's thumb and index finger.

Cortical and discriminatory sensations may be tested by two-point discrimination, point localization, texture discrimination, stereognostic function (i.e., identification of familiar objects held in the hand), and graphesthesia (i.e., recognition of letters or numbers written with a blunt object on the patient's palms or other body parts). These techniques also test the integrity of the dorsal column and lemniscal systems.

Joint Play Movements

All synovial and secondary cartilaginous joints, to some extent, are capable of an active ROM, termed "voluntary movement" (also called *active physiological movement*) through the action of muscles crossing over the joint. In addition, there is a small ROM that can be obtained only passively by the examiner; this movement is called **joint play** or **accessory movement.** These accessory movements are not under voluntary control; they are necessary, however, for full painless function of the joint and full ROM of the joint. **Joint dysfunction** signifies a loss of joint play movement.

The existence of joint play movement is necessary for full, pain-free voluntary movement to occur. An essential part of the detailed assessment of any joint includes an examination of its joint play movements. If any joint play movement is found to be absent or decreased, this movement must be restored before the patient can regain functional voluntary movement. In most joints, this movement is normally less than 4 mm in any one direction.

In some cases, joint play movements may be similar to or the same as movements tested during passive movements or ligamentous testing. This is most obvious in joints that have minimal movement and in joints that do not have muscles acting directly on them, such as the sacroiliac joints and superior tibiofibular joints.

Mennell's Rules for Joint Play Testing[191]

- The patient should be relaxed and fully supported
- The examiner should be relaxed and should use a firm but comfortable grasp
- One joint should be examined at a time
- One movement should be examined at a time
- The unaffected side should be tested first
- One articular surface is stabilized, while the other surface is moved
- Movements must be normal and not forced
- Movements should not cause undue discomfort

Loose Packed (Resting) Position

To test joint play movement, the examiner places the joint in its resting position, which is the position in its ROM at which the joint is under the least amount of stress; it is also the position in which the joint capsule has its greatest capacity.[192] The resting position (sometimes called the *loose packed* or *maximum loose packed position*) is one of minimal congruency between the articular surfaces and the joint capsule with the ligaments being in the position of greatest laxity and passive separation of the joint surfaces being the greatest. This position may be the anatomical resting position, which is usually considered in the midrange, or it may be just outside the range of pain and spasm. The advantage of the loose packed position is that the joint surface contact areas are reduced and are always changing to decrease friction and erosion in the joints. The position also provides proper joint lubrication and allows the arthrokinematic movements of spin, slide, and roll. It is therefore the most common position used for treatment using joint play mobilizations. Examples of resting positions are shown in Table 1-35.

Close Packed (Synarthrodial) Position

The close packed position should be avoided as much as possible during an assessment except to stabilize an adjacent joint, because in this position, the majority of joint structures are under maximum tension. In this position, the two joint surfaces fit together precisely—that is, they are fully congruent. The joint surfaces are tightly compressed; the ligaments and capsule of the joint are maximally tight; and the joint surfaces cannot be separated by distractive forces. It is the position of maximum joint stability. Thus, this position is commonly used during treatment to stabilize the joint, if an adjacent joint is being treated. Ligaments, bone, or other joint structures, if injured, become more painful as the close packed position is approached. If a joint is swollen, the close packed position cannot be achieved.[119] In the close packed position, no accessory movement is possible. Examples of the close packed positions of most joints are shown in Table 1-36.

Palpation

Initially, palpation for tenderness plays no part in the assessment, because referred tenderness is real and can be misleading. Only after the tissue at fault has been identified is palpation for tenderness used to determine the exact extent of the lesion within that tissue, and then palpation is done only if the tissue lies superficially and within easy reach of the fingers. Palpation is an important assessment technique that must be practiced if it is to be used effectively.[193–196] Tenderness often does enable the examiner to name the affected ligament or the specific section or exact point of the tearing or bruising.

To palpate properly, the examiner must ensure that the area to be palpated is as relaxed as possible. For this to be done, the body part must be supported as much as possible. As the ability to perform palpation develops, the examiner should be able to accomplish the following:

1. Discriminate differences in tissue tension (e.g., effusion, spasm) and muscle tone (i.e., spasticity, rigidity,

TABLE 1-35

Resting (Loose Packed) Position of Joints

Joint	Position
Facet (cervical, thoracic and lumbar spine)	Midway between flexion and extension
Temporomandibular	Mouth slightly open (freeway space), lips together, teeth not in contact
Glenohumeral	40° to 55° abduction, 30° horizontal adduction (scapular plane)
Acromioclavicular	Arm resting by side in normal physiological position
Sternoclavicular	Arm resting by side in normal physiological position
Ulnohumeral (elbow)	70° flexion, 10° supination
Radiohumeral	Full extension, full supination
Proximal (superior) radioulnar	70° flexion, 35° supination
Distal (inferior) radioulnar	10° supination
Radiocarpal (wrist)	Neutral with slight ulnar deviation
Intercarpal	Neutral or slight flexion
Midcarpal	Neutral or slight flexion with ulnar deviation
Carpometacarpal (thumb)	Midway between abduction-adduction and flexion-extension
Carpometacarpal (fingers)	Midway between flexion and extension
Metacarpophalangeal	Slight flexion
Interphalangeal	Slight flexion
Sacroiliac (resting)	Neutral pelvis
Sacroiliac (loose pack)	Counternutation
Hip	30° flexion, 30° abduction, slight lateral rotation
Knee (tibiofemoral)	25° flexion
Distal tibiofibular	Plantar flexion
Talocrural (ankle)	10° plantar flexion, midway between maximum inversion and eversion
Subtalar (talocalcaneal)	Midway between extremes of range of movement
Midtarsal	Midway between extremes of range of movement
Tarsometatarsal	Midway between extremes of range of movement
Metatarsophalangeal	10° extension
Interphalangeal	Slight flexion

TABLE 1-36

Close Packed Position of Joints

Joint	Position
Facet (cervical, thoracic, and lumbar spine)	Full extension
Temporomandibular	Clenched teeth
Glenohumeral	Full abduction and lateral rotation
Acromioclavicular	Arm abducted to 90°
Sternoclavicular	Maximum shoulder elevation and protraction
Ulnohumeral (elbow)	Extension with supination
Radiohumeral	Elbow flexed 90°, forearm supinated 5°
Proximal radioulnar	5° supination
Distal radioulnar	5° supination
Radiocarpal (wrist)	Extension with radial deviation
Intercarpal	Extension
Midcarpal	Extension with ulnar deviation
Carpometacarpal (thumb)	Full opposition
Carpometacarpal (fingers)	Full flexion
Metacarpophalangeal (fingers)	Full flexion
Metacarpophalangeal (thumb)	Full opposition
Interphalangeal	Full extension
Sacroiliac	Nutation
Hip	Full extension, medial rotation, abduction
Knee (tibiofemoral)	Full extension, lateral rotation of tibia
Distal tibiofibular	Maximum dorsiflexion
Talocrural (ankle)	Maximum dorsiflexion
Subtalar	Supination
Midtarsal	Supination
Tarsometatarsal	Supination
Metatarsophalangeal	Full extension
Interphalangeal	Full extension

flaccidity). **Spasticity** refers to muscle tonus in which there may be a collapse of muscle tone during testing. It is the result of hypersensitivity of the reflex arc and changes in the CNS resulting in overactivity of muscles and is a component of an upper motor neuron lesion.[197] **Rigidity** refers to involuntary resistance being maintained during passive movement

and without collapse of the muscle. It is the result of hypertonia seen in extrapyramidal lesions.[197] **Flaccidity** means there is no muscle tone.

2. Distinguish differences in tissue texture. For example, the examiner can, in some cases, palpate the direction of fibers or presence of fibrous bands.
3. Identify shapes, structures, and tissue type and thereby detect abnormalities. For example, bone deformities (such as, myositis ossificans) may be palpated.
4. Determine tissue thickness and texture and determine whether it is pliable, soft, and resilient. Is there any obvious swelling? Edema is an abnormal accumulation of fluid in the intercellular spaces; swelling, on the other hand, is the abnormal enlargement of a

Examiner Observations When Palpating a Patient

- Differences in tissue tension and texture
- Differences in tissue thickness
- Abnormalities
- Tenderness
- Temperature variation
- Pulses, tremors, and fasciculations
- Pathological state of tissues
- Dryness or excessive moisture
- Abnormal sensation

Swelling

- Comes on soon after injury → blood
- Comes on after 8 to 24 hours → synovial
- Boggy, spongy feeling → synovial
- Harder, tense feeling with warmth → blood
- Tough, dry → callus
- Leathery thickening → chronic
- Soft, fluctuating → acute
- Hard → bone
- Thick, slow-moving → pitting edema

body part. It may be the result of bone thickening, synovial membrane thickening, or fluid accumulation in and around the joint. It may be intracellular or extracellular (edema), intracapsular or extracapsular. Swelling may be localized (encapsulated), which may indicate intra-articular swelling, a cyst, or a swollen bursa. Visualization of swelling depends on the depth of the tissue (a swollen olecranon bursa is more obvious than a swollen psoas bursa) and the looseness of the tissues (swelling is more evident on the dorsum of the hand than on the palmar aspect because the dorsal tissues are not "held down" to adjacent tissue). Swelling that develops immediately or within 2 to 4 hours of injury is probably caused by blood extravasation into the tissues (ecchymosis) or joint. Swelling that becomes evident after 8 to 24 hours is caused by inflammation and, in a joint, by synovial swelling. Bony or hard swelling may be caused by osteophytes or new bone formation (e.g., in myositis ossificans). Soft-tissue swelling such as edematous synovium produces a boggy, spongy feeling (like soft sponge rubber), whereas fluid swelling is a softer and more mobile, fluctuating feeling. Blood swelling is usually a harder, thick, gel-like feeling, and the overlying skin is usually warmer. Pus is thick and less fluctuant; the overlying skin is warm, and the temperature is usually elevated. Older, longstanding soft-tissue swelling (such as, a skin callus) feels like tough, dry leather. Synovial hypertrophy has a hard, thick feeling to it with little give. The more leathery the thickening feels, the more likely it is to be chronic and caused by local symptoms. Softer thickenings tend to be more acute and associated with recent symptoms.[117] Pitting edema is thick and slow moving, leaving an indentation after pressure is applied and removed. It is commonly caused by circulatory stasis and is most commonly seen in the distal extremities. Long-lasting swelling may cause reflex inhibition of the muscles around the joint, leading to atrophy and weakness. Blood swelling within a joint is usually aspirated because of the irritating and damaging effect it has on the joint cartilage.

5. Determine joint tenderness by applying firm pressure to the joint. The pressure should always be applied with care, especially in the acute phase.

Grading Tenderness When Palpating

- Grade I—Patient complains of pain
- Grade II—Patient complains of pain and winces
- Grade III—Patient winces and withdraws the joint
- Grade IV—Patient will not allow palpation of the joint

6. Feel variations in temperature. This determination is usually best done by using the back of the examiner's hand or fingers and comparing both sides. Joints tend to be warm in the acute phase, in the presence of infection, with blood swelling, after exercise, or if they have been covered (for example, with an elastic bandage).
7. Feel pulses, tremors, and fasciculations. Fasciculations result from contraction of a number of muscle cells innervated by a single motor axon. The contractions are localized, are usually subconscious, and do not involve the whole muscle. Tremors are involuntary movements in which agonist and antagonist muscle groups contract to cause rhythmic movements of a joint. Pulses indicate circulatory sufficiency and should be tested for rhythm and strength if circulatory problems are suspected. Table 1-37 indicates the more commonly palpated pulses that may be used to determine circulatory sufficiency and location.
8. Determine the pathological state of the tissues in and around the joint. The examiner should note any tenderness, tissue thickening, or other signs or symptoms that would indicate pathology. Painful scars or neuromas may be diagnosed using the **thumbnail test.** This test involves running the dorsum of the thumbnail over the scar. If this action elicits a

TABLE **1-37**

Common Circulatory Pulse Locations

Artery	Location
Carotid	Anterior to sternocleidomastoid muscle
Brachial	Medial aspect of arm midway between shoulder and elbow
Radial	At wrist, lateral to flexor carpi radialis tendon
Ulnar	At wrist, between flexor digitorum superficialis and flexor carpi ulnaris tendons
Femoral	In femoral triangle (sartorius, adductor longus, and inguinal ligament)
Popliteal	Posterior aspect of knee (deep and hard to palpate)
Posterior tibial	Posterior aspect of medial malleolus
Dorsalis pedis	Between first and second metatarsal bones on superior aspect

sharp pain, it is a possible indication of a neuroma within the scar. Diffuse sensitivity may suggest complex regional pain syndrome (reflex sympathetic dystrophy).

9. Feel dryness or excessive moisture of the skin. For example, acute gouty joints tend to be dry, whereas septic joints tend to be moist. Nervous patients usually demonstrate increased moisture (sweating) in the hands.

10. Note any abnormal sensation, such as dysesthesia (diminished sensation), hyperesthesia (increased sensation), anesthesia (absence of sensation), or crepitus. Soft, fine crepitus may indicate roughening of the articular cartilage, whereas coarse grating may indicate badly damaged articular cartilage or bone. A creaking, leathery crepitus (snowball crepitation) is sometimes felt in tendons and indicates pathology. Tendons may "snap" over one another or over a bony prominence. Loud, snapping, pain-free noises in joints are usually caused by cavitation, in which gas bubbles form suddenly and transiently owing to negative pressure in the joint.

Palpation of a joint and surrounding area must be carried out in a systematic fashion to ensure that all structures are examined. This procedure involves having a starting point and working from that point to adjacent tissues to assess their normality or the possibility of pathological involvement. The examiner must work slowly and carefully, applying light pressure initially and working into a deeper pressure of palpation, then "feeling" for pathological conditions or changes in tissue tension.[193] The uninvolved side should be palpated first so that the patient has some idea of what to expect and to enable the examiner to know what "normal" feels like. Any differences or abnormalities should be noted and contribute to the diagnosis.

Diagnostic Imaging

Although it is important, the diagnostic imaging portion of the examination is usually used only to confirm a clinical opinion and must be interpreted within the context of the whole examination.[198,199] As with special tests, diagnostic imaging should be viewed as one part of the assessment to be used when it will help confirm or establish a diagnosis.[200] In some cases, clinical decision rules have been developed (e.g., Ottawa ankle and foot rules). These rules increase the accuracy of diagnostic assessments, but the examiner should be aware that the rules apply primarily to acute, first-time injuries.[198] Although this book has examples of diagnostic imaging in each chapter, the reader is advised to consult more detailed texts on the subject for more in-depth knowledge.[201–204]

Reasons for Ordering Diagnostic Imaging

- To confirm a diagnosis
- To establish a diagnosis
- To determine the severity of injury
- To determine the progression of a disease
- To determine the stage of healing
- To enhance patient treatment
- To determine anatomical alignment

Plain Film Radiography

Conventional plain film radiography (also called *x-rays* although this term is technically incorrect; they should be called x-ray films[203]) is the primary means of diagnostic imaging for musculoskeletal problems. It offers the advantages of being readily available, being relatively cheap, and providing good anatomical resolution. On the negative side, it does expose the patient to radiation, and it offers poor differentiation of soft-tissue structures and is not sensitive to subtle pathology.[198] Radiographs are not taken indiscriminately. Because x-rays have the potential for causing cell damage, there should be a clear indication of need before a radiograph is taken, and the process should not be considered routine.[205]

Radiographs are viewed as though the patient was standing in front of the viewer in the anatomical position.[203] For example, using an anteroposterior (AP) x-ray film of a patient's right lower limb would be viewed with the fibula on the viewer's left hand side regardless of the position of the anatomical side marker.[203]

Normally, the clinician orders a minimum of two projections at a 90° orientation to each other—most

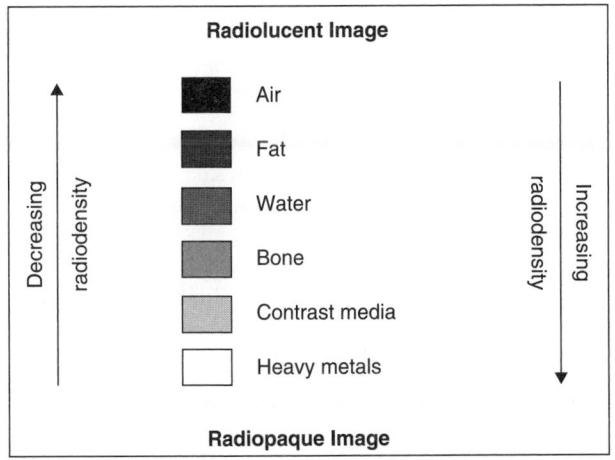

Figure 1-24 Radiographic density (shades of gray) as related to object radiodensity. Note that the shade may vary depending on thickness of tissue. (From Richardson JK, Iglarsh ZA: Clinical orthopaedic physical therapy, Philadelphia, 1995, WB Saunders, p. 630.)

Rules to Minimize Errors When Taking X-Rays[210]

1. If possible, the patient should be awake
2. The x-ray beam must be perpendicular to the anatomical region being examined
3. The x-ray source should be the farthest possible distance from the region being examined (minimal distance: 2.75 m)

Uses of Plain Film Radiography[201]

- Fractures
- Arthritis
- Bone tumors
- Skeletal dysplasia

---

commonly, AP and lateral projections. Two views are necessary because x-rays take planar images; so all structures in the path of the x-ray beam are superimposed on each other, and abnormalities may be difficult to evaluate with only one view. Two views give information concerning the dimensions of a structure, whether foreign bodies or lesions are present and their location, and to determine the alignment of fractures.[203] Other views may be obtained, depending on clinical circumstances and specific needs.[205–208] In the lumbar spine, AP, lateral, and oblique views are commonly taken.

X-rays are part of the electromagnetic spectrum and have the ability to penetrate tissue to varying degrees. X-ray imaging is based on the principle that different tissues have different densities and produce images in different shades of gray.[209] The greater the density of the tissue, the less penetration of x-rays there is, and the whiter its image appears on the film (Figure 1-24). In order of descending degree of density are the following structures: metal, bone, soft tissue, water, fat, and air. These differences give the six basic densities on the x-ray plate.

When viewing the x-rays, the examiner must identify the film, noting the name, age, date, and sex of the patient, and the examiner must identify the type of projection taken (e.g., AP, lateral, tunnel, skyline, weight-bearing, stress-type). Rules that should be kept in mind to minimize diagnostic errors when taking radiographs are outlined in the following box.

The x-ray plates that are developed after exposure to the roentgen rays enables the examiner to see any fractures, dislocations, foreign bodies, or radiopaque substances that may be present. The main function of plain x-ray examination is to rule out or exclude fractures or serious disease such as infection (osteomyelitis),

ankylosing spondylitis, or tumors and structural body abnormalities such as developmental anomalies, arthritis, and metabolic bone diseases. Thus, the main purpose of x-ray films is to determine the state of bone and its surrounding soft tissue. Bone remodelling (the taking up [osteoblastic action] and removal [osteoclastic action] of bone) goes on continuously in the body with the rate of change being the result of several factors, such as disuse, aging or disease. If removal occurs quicker than uptake, then **osteoporosis** (decrease in bone mass) results. Remodelling is related to **Wolff's law,** which states that changes in form and function of bone is followed by changes in its internal structure or that bone responds (like any tissue) to the stress and strain placed on it. For x-ray films, osteoporosis (similar to other conditions such as osteomalacia) results in an increase in radiolucency. This increased radiolucency is called **osteopenia.**

Commonly, an **ABCDs search pattern** is used when looking at radiological images (Table 1-38).[203] With soft-tissue injuries, clinical findings should take precedence over x-ray findings. It is desirable to know whether an x-ray has been taken so that the examiner can obtain the films if necessary. The examiner should be aware of obvious and unusual x-ray findings that distract attention from other tissue that is actually the cause of the pain; such x-ray abnormalities are significant only if clinical examination bears out their relevance. With experience, the examiner becomes able to detect many important soft-tissue changes on x-ray examination, such as effusion in joints, tendinous calcifications, ectopic bone in muscle, tissue displaced by tumor, and the presence of air or foreign body material in the tissues. Radiographs may also be used to indicate bone loss. For osteoporosis to be evident on x-ray, approximately 30% to 35% of the bone must be lost (Figure 1-25). **Cortical thickness** can be

TABLE **1-38**

ABCDs Search Pattern for Radiologic Image Interpretation

Division	Evaluates	LOOK FOR Normal Findings	LOOK FOR Variations/Abnormalities
A: Alignment	General skeletal architecture	Gross normal size of bones Normal number of bones	Supernumerary (extra) bones Absent bones Congenital deformities Developmental deformities Cortical fractures
	General contour of bone	Smooth and continuous cortical outlines	Avulsion fractures Impaction fractures Spurs Breaks in cortex continuity
	Alignment of bones to adjacent bones	Normal joint articulations Normal spatial relationships	Markings of past surgical sites Fracture Joint subluxation Joint dislocation
B: Bone density	General bone density	Sufficient contrast between soft-tissue shade of gray and bone shade of gray Sufficient contrast within each bone, between cortical shell and cancellous center	General loss of bone density resulting in poor contrast between soft tissues and bone Thinning or absence of cortical margins
	Texture abnormalities	Normal trabecular architecture	Appearance of trabeculae altered; may look thin, delicate, lacy, coarsened, smudged, fluffy
	Local bone density changes	Sclerosis at areas of increased stress, such as weight-bearing surfaces or sites of ligamentous, muscular, or tendinous attachments	Excessive sclerosis (increase in bone density) Reactive sclerosis that walls off a lesion (e.g., tumor) Osteophytes
C: Cartilage spaces	Joint space width	Well-preserved joint spaces imply normal cartilage or disk thickness	Decreased joint spaces imply degenerative or traumatic conditions
	Subchondral bone	Smooth surface	Excessive sclerosis as seen in degenerative joint disease Erosions as seen in the inflammatory arthritides
	Epiphyseal plates	Normal size relative to epiphysis and skeletal age	Compare contralaterally for changes in thickness that may be related to abnormal conditions or trauma
D: Soft tissues	Muscles Fat pads and fat lines	Normal size of soft-tissue image Radiolucent crescent parallel to bone Radiolucent lines parallel to length of muscle	Gross wasting Gross swelling Displacement of fat pads from bony fossae into soft tissues indicates joint effusion Elevation or blurring of fat planes indicates swelling of nearby tissues
	Joint capsules	Normally indistinct	Observe whether effusion or hemorrhage distends capsule
	Periosteum	Normally indistinct Solid periosteal reaction is normal in fracture healing	Observe periosteal reactions: solid, laminated or onionskin, spiculated or sunburst, Codman's triangle
	Miscellaneous soft-tissue findings	Soft tissues normally exhibit a water-density shade of gray	Foreign bodies evidenced by radiodensity Gas bubbles appear radiolucent Calcifications/ossification appear radiopaque

Modified from McKinnis LN: Fundamentals of musculoskeletal imaging, Philadelphia, 2005, F.A. Davis, pp. 40–41.

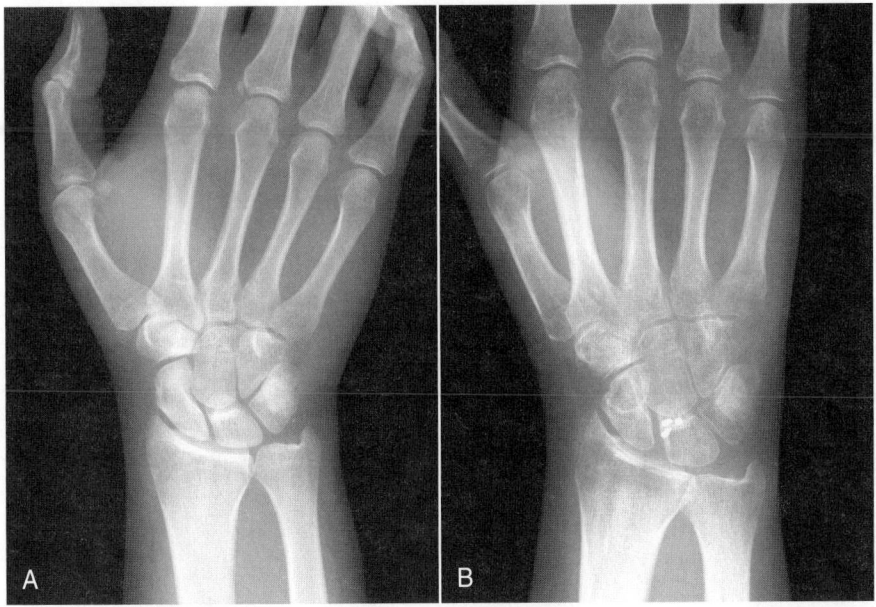

Figure 1-25 Osteoporosis of immobilization and disuse. Radiographs obtained immediately before wrist ligament reconstruction (**A**) and 2 months later (**B**) are shown. **B,** Observe the extent of the osteopenia. (From Resnick D, Kransdorf MJ: Bone and joint imaging, Philadelphia, 2005, Elsevier, p. 547.)

used to determine bone loss. The most common place for measuring cortical thickness is the midpoint of the second or third metacarpal shaft (Figure 1-26). Normally, the sum should be one-half of the total bone diameter.

Examiner Observations When Viewing an X-Ray Film

- Overall size and shape of bone
- Local size and shape of bone
- Number of bones
- Alignment of bones
- Thickness of the cortex
- Trabecular pattern of the bone
- General density of the entire bone
- Local density change
- Margins of local lesions
- Any break in continuity of the bone
- Any periosteal change
- Any soft-tissue change (e.g., gross swelling, periosteal elevation, visibility of fat pads)
- Relation among bones
- Thickness of the cartilage (cartilage space within joints)
- Width and symmetry of joint space
- Contour and density of subchondral bone

The examiner should keep in mind the maturity of the patient when viewing films. Skeletal changes occur with age,[211] and the appearance and fusion of the epiphyses, for example, may be important in interpreting the pathology of the condition seen. Soft-tissue structures as well as bone can be seen, provided there is something to outline them. For example, the joint capsule may be silhouetted by the pericapsular fat, or air in the lungs may silhouette a cardiac shadow. Anatomical variations and anomalies must be ruled out before pathology can be

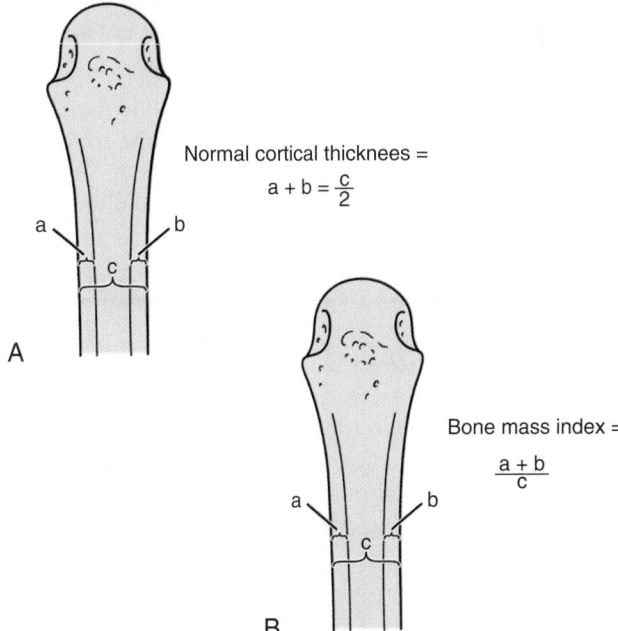

Normal cortical thicknees =
$$a + b = \frac{c}{2}$$

Bone mass index =
$$\frac{a + b}{c}$$

Figure 1-26 A, Cortical thickness measurements are usually based on the cortices at the midshaft of the second or third metacarpal. Normally, the sum of the two cortices should equal approximately one-half the overall diameter of the shaft. **B,** Cortical thickness may also be expressed as an index of bone mass, which is the sum of the cortices divided by diameter.

ruled in; for example, accessory navicular, bipartite patella, and os trigonum may be confused with fractures by the unsuspecting examiner. The fabella is often confused with a loose body in the knee in the AP projection x-ray film.

Radiographs may also be used to determine the maturity index of a patient. A special film of the wrist is taken to assess skeletal maturity (Figure 1-27). These films can be compared with established films in a bone atlas such

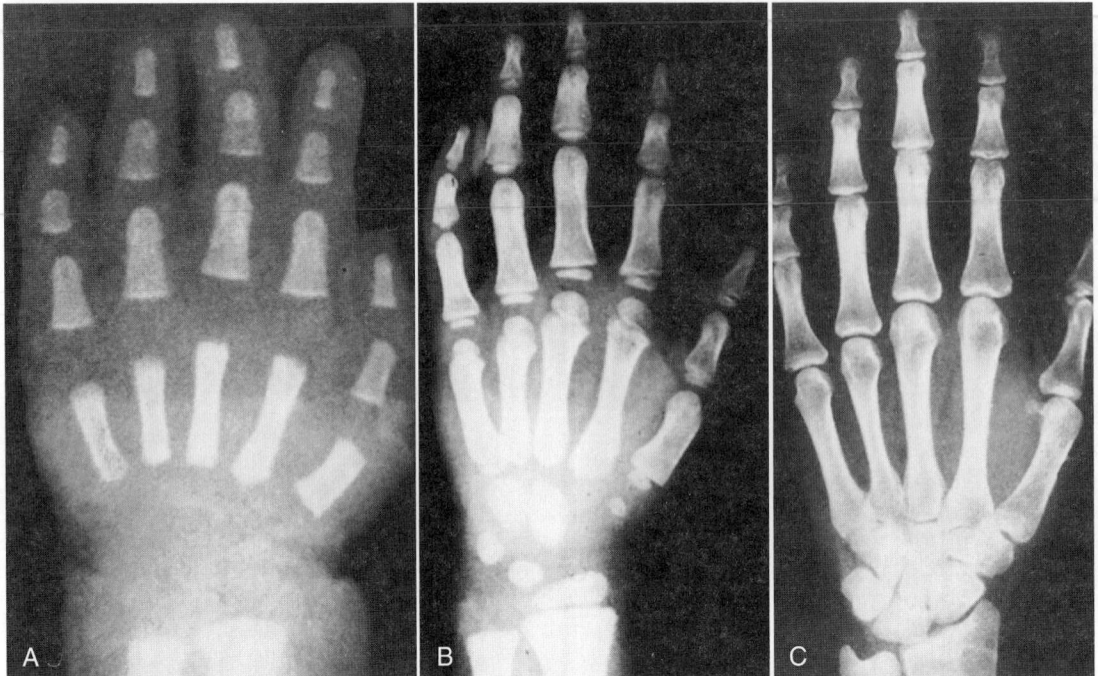

Figure 1-27 X-ray films showing skeletal maturity. **A,** Male, newborn. **B,** Male, 5-years-old. **C,** Female, 17-years-old.

as that compiled by Gruelich and Pyle.[211] For the spine, Sanders et al.[212] have advocated the use of the simplified Tanner-Whitehouse-III Skeletal Maturity Assessment (Table 1-39). This is often done before epiphysiodesis and leg-lengthening procedures to ensure that the child is of a suitable skeletal age to do the procedure.

Arthrography

Arthrography is an invasive technique in which air, a water-soluble contrast material containing iodine, or a combination of the two (double contrast) is injected into a joint space, and a radiograph is taken of the joint. The air or contrast material outlines the structures within the joint or communicating with the joint (Figure 1-28). It is especially useful in detecting abnormal joint and bursal communications, synovial abnormalities, articular cartilage lesions, and the extent of or pathology to the capsule.[203] It is used primarily in the hip, knee, ankle, shoulder, elbow, and wrist.[205]

Uses of Arthrography[201]

- Steroid injections
- Aspirations
- Joint kinematics

Computed Arthrography (Computed Tomography Arthrography)

This technique combines arthrography and computed tomography (CT) to image joints. This method provides

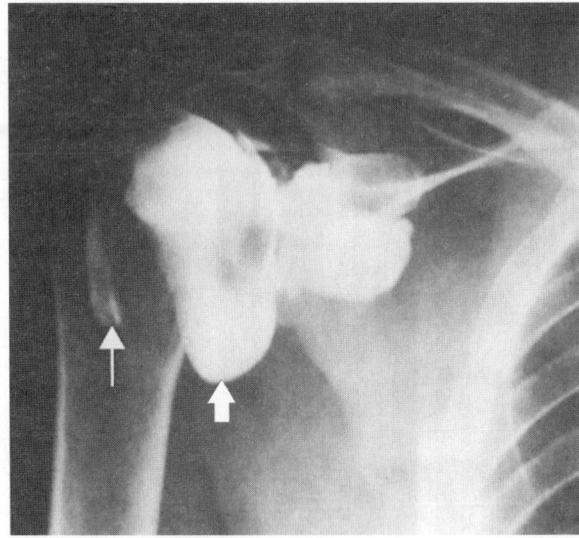

Figure 1-28 Normal arthrogram, shoulder in lateral rotation. Note the good dependent fold *(wide arrow)* and the outline of the bicipital tendon *(narrow arrow)*. (From Neviaser TJ: Arthrography of the shoulder. Orthop Clin North Am 11:209, 1980.)

a three-dimensional definition of the joint, and the dye helps to delineate articular surfaces and joint margins. It is usually reserved for those cases in which conventional CT scanning has not provided adequate anatomical detail (e.g., shoulder instability).[34,205,208]

Venogram and Arteriogram

With a venogram or an arteriogram, radiopaque dye is injected into specific vessels to outline abnormal

TABLE **1-39**

Key Findings of the Simplified Tanner-Whitehouse-III Skeletal Maturity Assessment

Stage	Key Features	Tanner-Whitehouse-III Stage	Greulich and Pyle Reference	Related Maturity Signs
1. Juvenile slow	Digital epiphyses are not covered	Some digits are at stage E or less	• Female: 8 years and 10 months • Male: 12 years and 6 months (note fifth middle phalanx)	Tanner stage 1
2. Preadolescent slow	All digital epiphyses are covered	All digits are at stage F	• Female: 10 years • Male: 13 years	Tanner stage 2, starting growth spurt
3. Adolescent rapid—early	The preponderance of digits is capped. The second through fifth metacarpal epiphyses are wider than their metaphyses	All digits are at stage G	• Female: 11 and 12 years • Male: 13 years and 6 months and 14 years	Peak height velocity, Risser stage 0, open pelvic triradiate cartilage
4. Adolescent rapid—late	Any of distal phalangeal physes are clearly beginning to close	Any distal phalanges are at stage H	• Female: 13 years (digits 2, 3, and 4) • Male: 15 years (digits 4 and 5)	Girls typically in Tanner stage 3, Risser stage 0, open triradiate cartilage
5. Adolescent steady—early	All distal phalangeal physes are closed. Others are open	All distal phalanges and thumb metacarpal are at stage I. Others remain at stage G	• Female: 13 years and 6 months • Male: 15 years and 6 months	Risser stage 0, triradiate cartilage closed: menarche only occasionally starts earlier than this
6. Adolescent steady—late	Middle or proximal phalangeal physes are closing	Middle or proximal phalanges are at stages H and I	• Female: 14 years • Male: 16 years (late)	Risser sign positive (stage 1 or more)
7. Early mature	Only distal radial physis is open. Metacarpal physeal scars may be present	All digits are at stage I. The distal radial physis is at stage G or H	• Female: 15 years • Male: 17 years	Risser stage 4
8. Mature	Distal radial physis is completed closed	All digits are at stage I	• Female: 17 years • Male: 19 years	Risser stage 5

From Sanders JO, Khoury JG, Kishan S, et al: Predicting scoliosis progression from skeletal maturity: a simplified classification during adolescence. J Bone Joint Surg Am 90(3):541, 2008.

Uses of CT Arthrograms[201]

• Loose bodies
• Joint surfaces

---

conditions (Figure 1-29). This technique may be used to diagnose arteriosclerosis, investigate tumors, and demonstrate blockage after traumatic injury.

Myelography

Myelography is an invasive imaging technique that is used to visualize the soft tissues within the spine. A water-soluble radiopaque dye is injected into the epidural space by spinal puncture and allowed to flow to different levels of the spinal cord, outlining the contour of the thecal sac, nerve roots, and spinal cord. A plain x-ray film is then taken of the spine (Figures 1-30 and 1-31). In many cases today, CT scans and magnetic resonance imaging (MRI) scans have taken the place of myelograms.[205] This technique is used to detect disc disease, disc herniation, nerve root entrapment, spinal stenosis, and tumors of the spinal cord. The clinician should be aware that myelograms can have adverse side effects. Grainger[213] reported that 20% to 30% of patients receiving myelograms complained of headache, dizziness, nausea, vomiting, and seizures.[209]

Tomography and Computed Tomography

Tomography has become a common imaging technique for musculoskeletal disorders, especially when computer enhanced (CT scan). It produces cross-sectional images of the tissues. Conventional tomography, which is also called *thin-section radiography* or *linear tomography*, tends

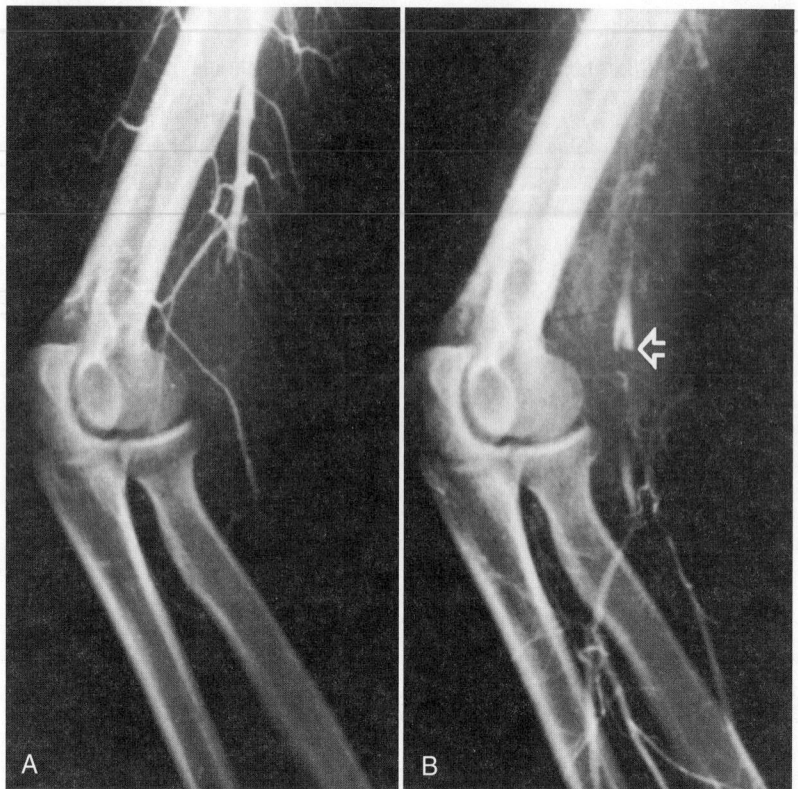

Figure 1-29 Occlusion of brachial artery. A, Arteriogram of a young man with a previously reduced elbow dislocation and an ischemic hand shows an occluded brachial artery. **B,** A later film shows fresh clot *(arrow)* in the brachial artery and reconstituted radial and ulnar arteries. Primary repair and thrombectomy treated the ischemic symptoms. (From McLean G, Frieman DB: Angiography of skeletal disease. Orthop Clin North Am 14:267, 1983.)

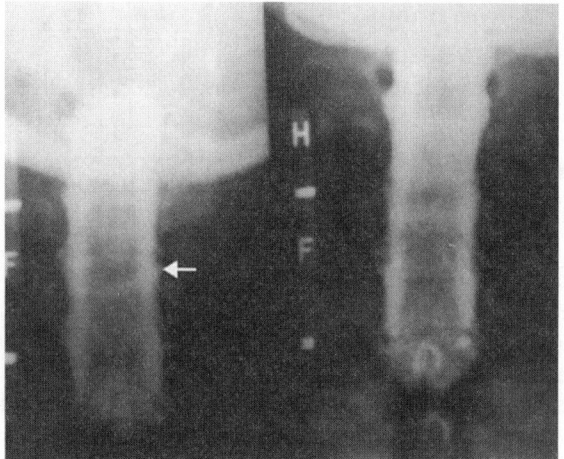

Figure 1-30 Myelogram of cervical spine. Note how radiopaque dye fills root sheaths *(arrow)*.

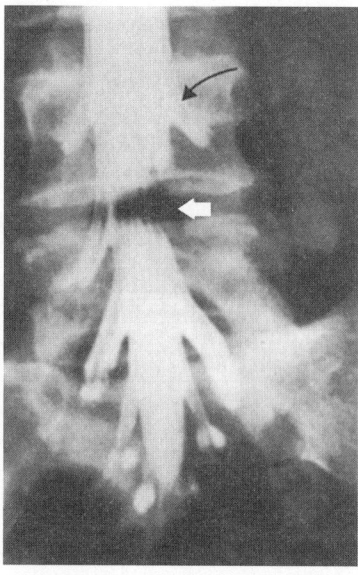

Figure 1-31 Myelogram of lumbar spine showing extrusion of nucleus pulposus of L4–L5 *(large arrow)*. Note how radiopaque dye fills dural recesses *(small arrow)*. (From Selby DK, Meril AJ, Wagner KJ, et al: Water-soluble myelography. Orthop Clin North Am 8[1]:82, 1977.)

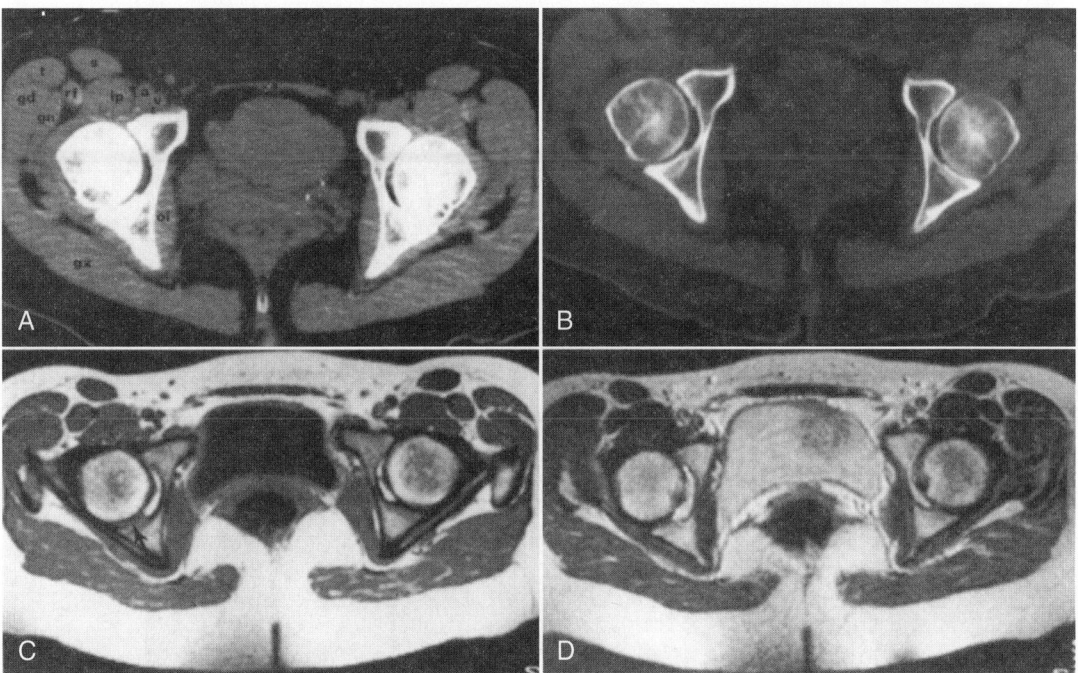

Figure 1-32 A, Normal computed tomographic (CT) image at the level of the mid acetabulum obtained with soft-tissue window settings shows the homogenous, intermediate signal of musculature. *a,* Common femoral artery; *gd,* gluteus medius; *gn,* gluteus minimus; *gx,* gluteus maximus; *ip,* iliopsoas; *oi,* obturator internus; *ra,* rectus abdominis; *rf,* rectus femoris; *s,* sartorius; *t,* tensor fascia lata; *v,* common femoral vein. **B,** Axial CT at bone window settings reveals improved delineation of cortical and medullary osseous detail. Note anterior and posterior semilunar acetabular articular surfaces and the central nonarticular acetabular fossa. **C,** Normal midacetabular T1-weighted axial 0.4-T magnetic resonance image (MRI) (*TR,* 600 msec; *TE,* 20 msec) of a different patient shows a normal, high-signal-intensity image of fatty marrow (adult pattern) and subcutaneous tissue, low-signal-intensity image of muscle, and absence of signal in the cortical bone. The thin articular hyaline cartilage is of intermediate signal intensity *(arrow).* **D,** T2-weighted MRI (*TR,* 2,000 msec; *TE,* 80 msec) shows decreasing high signal intensity in fatty marrow and subcutaneous tissue with increased signal intensity in the fluid-filled urinary bladder. (From Pitt MJ, Lund PJ, Speer DP: Imaging of the pelvis and hip. Orthop Clin North Am 21[3]:553, 1990.)

to show one small area or plane in focus with other areas or planes appearing fuzzy or blurred. The conventional tomogram is seldom used today except when subtle bone density alterations are sought.

The CT scan involves the same thin cross sections or "slices" taken at specific levels (Figure 1-32). CT scans produce cross-sectional images based on x-ray attenuation. Because of computer enhancement, CT produces superior tissue contrast resolution compared with conventional x-rays, thus enabling greater details of subtle bone pathology.[198,214] CT provides excellent bony architecture detail and has good resolution of soft-tissue structures.[204] Its disadvantages include limited scanning plane, cost, exposure to radiation (dosage similar to or greater than that of plain x-rays), alteration of the image by artifacts, and degradation of soft-tissue resolution in obese people.[34,205] The CT scan, or computed axial tomography (CAT) scan, is a radiological technique that may be used to assess for disc protrusions, facet disease, or spinal stenosis.[215] The technique may also be used to assess complex fractures, especially those involving joints, dislocations, patellofemoral alignment and tracking, osteonecrosis, tumors, and osteomyelitis. Because only a small

cross-sectional area in one plane is viewed with each scan, multiple images or scans are taken to get a complete view of the area.[34] CT arthrography may be used to enhance assessment of intra-articular structures and may be used for patients who cannot tolerate conventional MRI.

Uses of Computed Tomography Scans[201]

- Complex fractures
- Comminuted fractures
- Intra-articular fragments
- Fracture healing (e.g., non-union)
- Bone tumors

Single photon emission computed tomography (SPECT) scanning is a specialized type of CT scanning used in orthopedics primarily to detect spondylolysis.[204]

Radionuclide Scanning (Scintigraphy)[216]

With bone scans (osteoscintigraphy), chemicals labeled with radioactive isotopes (radioactive tracers) such as

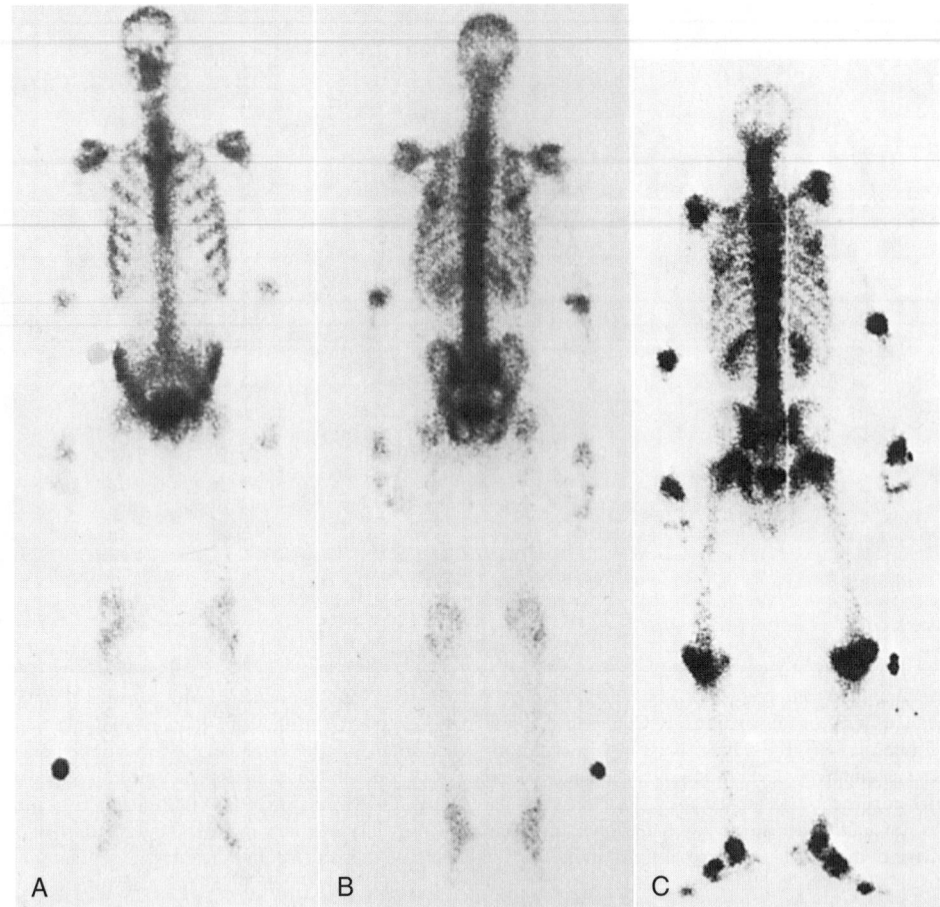

Figure 1-33 Whole body bone scans. A, Normal adult anterior scan. **B,** Normal adult posterior scan. **C,** Posterior scan showing joint involvement of rheumatoid arthritis. (From Goldstein HA: Bone scintigraphy. Orthop Clin North Am 14:244, 250, 1983.)

technetium-99m–labeled methyl diphosphonate complexes are intravenously injected several hours before the scan to localize specific organs that concentrate the particular chemical. The isotope is then localized where there is a high level of metabolic activity (e.g., bone turnover) relative to the rest of the bone. The radiograph reveals a "hot spot" (Figure 1-33) indicating areas of increased mineral turnover.[203] Although plain film radiographs do not show bone disease or stress fractures until there is 30% to 50% bone loss, bone scans show bone disease or stress fractures with as little as 4% to 7% bone loss (Figure 1-34).[215] Because the isotope is excreted by the kidneys, the kidneys and bladder are often visible in bone scans. Bone scans are used for lytic (bone-loss) diseases, infection, fractures, and tumors. They are highly sensitive to bone abnormalities but do not tell what the abnormality is (low specificity). The whole body may be imaged, and a gamma camera picks up the tracer.[205] High resolution MRI and CT scans are replacing bone scans in some cases.[217]

Discography

The technique of discography involves injecting a small amount of radiopaque dye into the nucleus pulposus of

---

Uses of Scintigraphy

- Skeletal metastases
- Stress fractures
- Osteomyelitis

---

an intervertebral disc (Figure 1-35) under radiographic guidance. It is not a commonly used technique but may be used to determine disruptions in the nucleus pulposus or the annular fibrosus and is sometimes used as a provocative test to see whether injection into the disc brings on the patient's symptoms.[205]

Magnetic Resonance Imaging

MRI is a noninvasive, painless imaging technique with high contrast resolution that uses exposure to magnetic fields, not ionizing radiation, to obtain an image of bone and soft tissue. MRI is based on the effect of a strong magnetic field on hydrogen atoms. T1 images show good anatomical detail of soft tissues (Figure 1-36), whereas T2 images are used to demonstrate soft-tissue pathology that

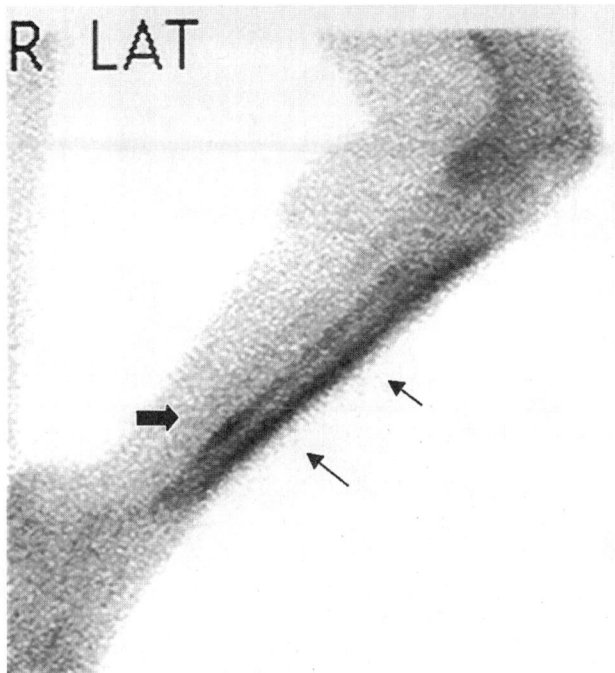

Figure 1-34 Stress fracture of the tibia and anterior shin splint. A short fusiform area of increased uptake in the posterior aspect of the distal shaft of the tibia represents a stress fracture *(large arrow)*. A long longitudinal area of increased uptake in the anterior aspect of the tibial shaft is consistent with a shin splint *(small arrow)*. (From Resnick D, Kransdorf MJ: Bone and joint imaging, Philadelphia, 2005, Elsevier, p. 103.)

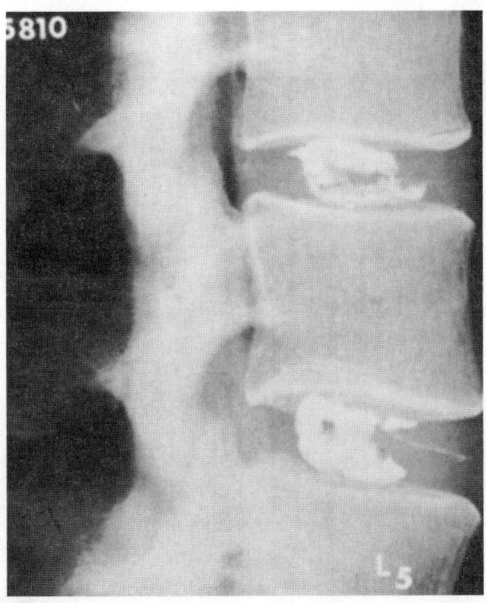

Figure 1-35 Normal discogram shown with barium paste. (From Farfan HF: Mechanical disorders of the low back, Philadelphia, 1973, Lea & Febiger, p. 96.)

alters tissue water content.[34,213] MRI offers excellent tissue contrast, is multiplanar (i.e., can image in any plane), and has no known adverse effects. In some patients, claustrophobia is a problem, and artifacts may result if the patient does not remain still.[211] For musculoskeletal conditions,

plane film radiographs are commonly taken and viewed to determine if an MRI is necessary.[199]

MRI is used to assess for spinal cord tumors, intracranial disease, and some types of CNS diseases (e.g., multiple sclerosis); it largely replaced myelography in the evaluation of disc pathology. It also aids in the diagnosis of muscle, meniscal and ligamentous tears, synovial pathology, abnormal patellofemoral tracking, joint pathology, cartilage, bone marrow pathology, osteonecrosis, stress fractures, and osteochondral lesions.[34,201,218]

Uses of Magnetic Resonance Imaging[200]

- Intra-articular structures (e.g., meniscus, loose bodies)
- Musculotendinous injury
- Joint instability
- Osteomyelitis
- Fractures
- Stress injury
- Disc disease
- Soft tissue tumors
- Skeletal malformations
- Bone bruises

On the negative side, MRI is expensive, and specificity of pathology (e.g., tendon strain versus tendinitis) may not be possible with its use, and there is a high prevalence of positive findings in asymptomatic patients.[219,220] The presence of some metallic objects (e.g., cardiac pacemakers) may make its use contraindicated because of the magnetic pull, especially if the objects are not solidly fixed to bone. It has been reported that MRI is safe with prosthetic joints and internal fixation devices, provided that they are stable.[205]

MR arthrography may enhance assessment of intra-articular structures, such as shoulder instability, ankle impingement, labral tears, wrist ligament tears and loose bodies.[201,221]

Fluoroscopy

Fluoroscopy is a technique that is used to show motion in joints through x-ray imaging; it also may be used as a guidance technique for injections (e.g., in discography). It is only rarely used because of the amount of radiation exposure. It is sometimes used to position fracture fragments and to demonstrate abnormal motion.

Diagnostic Ultrasound

Like therapeutic ultrasound, diagnostic ultrasound involves transmission of high-frequency sound waves (5 to 10 MHz) into the tissues by a transducer through a coupling agent with calculation of the time it takes for the echo to return to the transducer from different interfaces. The depth of the structure is determined, and an

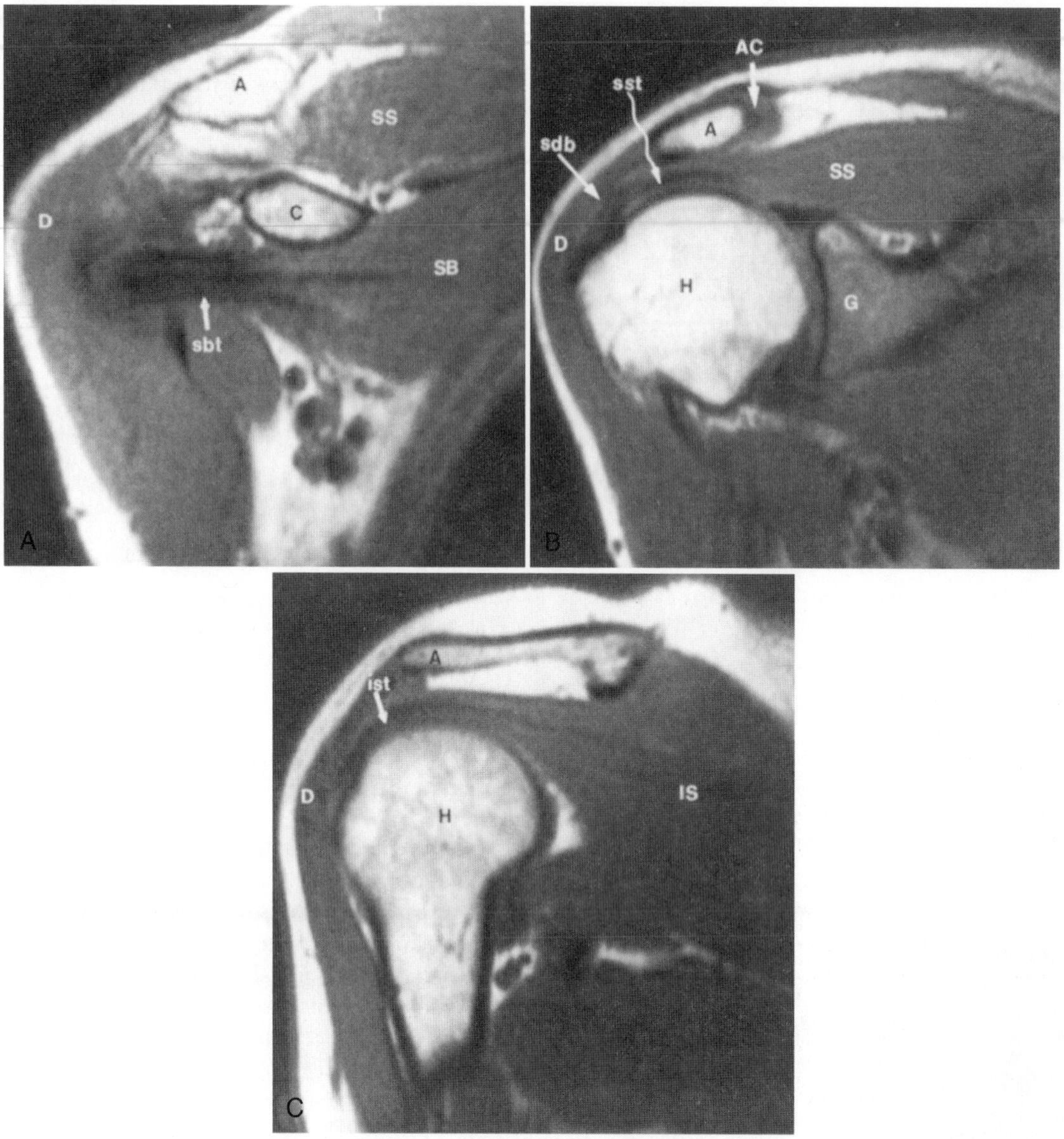

Figure 1-36 Magnetic resonance T1-weighted coronal oblique images from anterior (**A**) to posterior (**C**). *A,* Acromion; *AC,* acromioclavicular joint; *C,* coracoid; *D,* deltoid muscle; *G,* glenoid of scapula; *H,* humerus; *IS,* infraspinatus muscle; *ist,* infraspinatus tendon; *SB.* subscapularis muscle; *sbt,* subscapularis tendon; *sdb,* subdeltoid-subacromial bursa; *SS,* supraspinatus muscle; *sst,* supraspinatus tendon; *T,* trapezius muscle. (From Mayer SJ, Dalinka MK: Magnetic resonance imaging of the shoulder. Orthop Clin North Am 21:500, 1990.)

image is formed. Each tissue has a unique echo texture that relates to its internal structure (Figure 1-37).[34,222]

In the hands of an experienced operator, ultrasound can provide good image detail and cross-sectional images in different planes. No radiation is used, and no harmful biological effects have been reported. It has the advantage of providing dynamic (moving) real-time images; tissues can be visualized as they move. It also allows localization of any tenderness or palpable mass.[34,222] Therefore, it is used to assess soft-tissue injury, such as tendon, ligament, or muscle pathology, soft-tissue masses (e.g., tumor, ganglion, cyst, inflamed bursa), effusion, and congenital dislocation of the hip, and it allows dynamic visualization of muscle.[204,223] Doppler ultrasound may be used for vascular assessment.

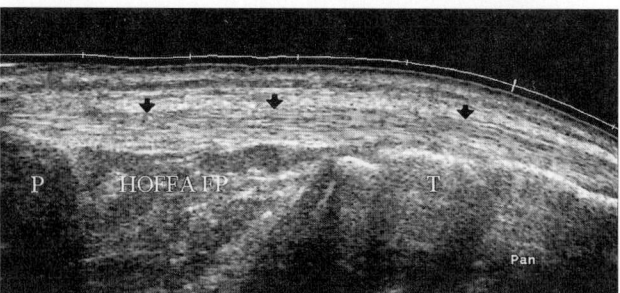

Figure 1-37 Diagnostic ultrasound—patellar tendon. A longitudinal extended field of view of a normal patellar tendon shows a well-defined hyperechoic tendon with a fine intrasubstance fibrillar pattern *(arrows).* Note the infrapatellar fat pad *(Hoffa's FP),* the inferior pole of the patella *(P),* and the tibial tubercle *(T).* (From Resnick D, Kransdorf MJ: Bone and joint imaging, Philadelphia, 2005, Elsevier, p. 81.)

Uses of Ultrasonography[200]
• Hip dysplasia in children
• Joint effusion
• Tendon pathology
• Ligament tears
• Soft tissue tumors
• Vascular disease

The disadvantages of diagnostic ultrasound include limited contrast resolution, limited depth of penetration, small viewing field, and lack of penetration of bone.[34,222] The use of diagnostic ultrasound has a difficult learning curve, and the quality and interpretation of the images depend on the operator.

Xeroradiography

Xeroradiography is a technique in which a xeroradiographic plate replaces the normal x-ray film. On the plate, there is a thin layer of a photoconductor material, which enhances the image (Figure 1-38). This technique is used when the margins between areas of different densities need to be exaggerated.[208,224]

PRÉCIS

Each chapter ends with a précis of the assessment to serve as a quick reference. The précis does not follow the text description exactly but is laid out so that each assessment involves minimal movement of the patient to decrease patient discomfort. For example, all aspects of the examination that are performed with the patient standing are done first, followed by those done with the patient sitting, and so on.

CASE STUDIES

Case studies are provided as written exercises to help the examiner develop skills in assessment. Based on the presented case study, the reader should develop a list of appropriate questions to ask in the history based on the pathology of the conditions, what should especially be noted in observation, and what part of the examination is essential to make a definitive diagnosis. Where appropriate, example diagnoses are given in parentheses at the end of each question. At the end of the case study, the reader can develop a table showing the differential diagnosis for the case described. Tables 1-40 and 1-41 illustrate such differential diagnosis charts.

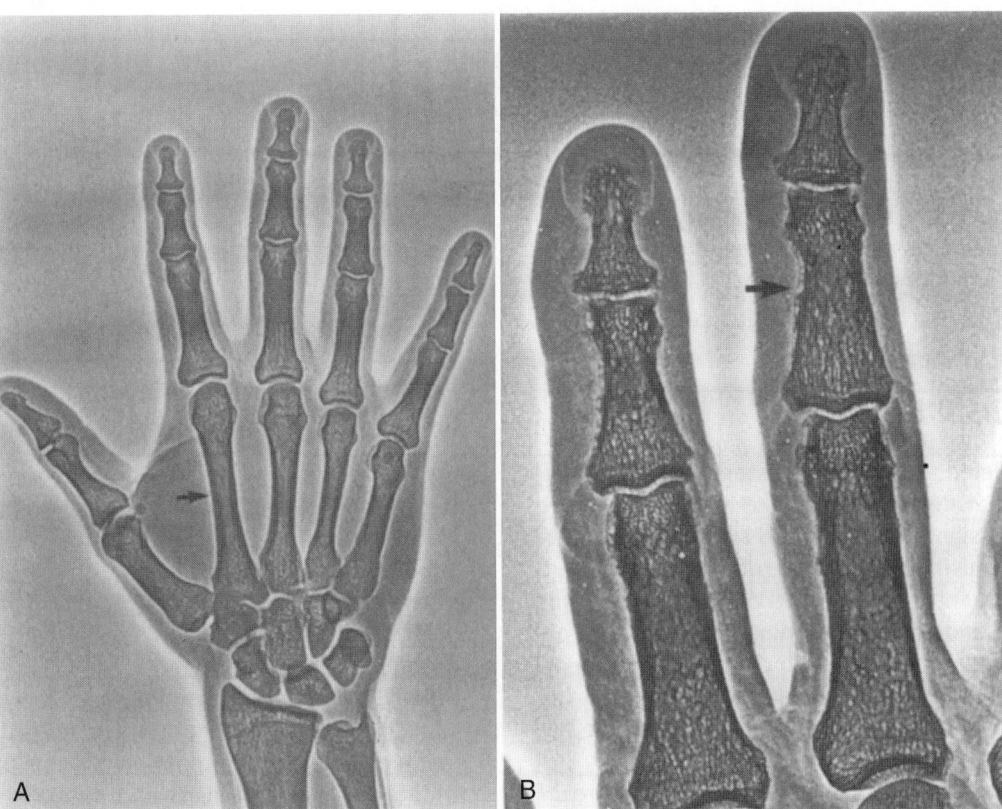

Figure 1-38 Xeroradiography. A, Normal examination. Note the ability to demonstrate both soft tissues and bony structures on a single examination. The halo effect *(arrow)* around the bony cortices is an example of edge enhancement. **B,** Hyperparathyroid bone changes shown on xeroradiography. The subperiosteal bone resorption *(arrow)* and distal tuft erosion are well shown. (**A,** From Weissman BN, Sledge CB: Orthopedic radiology, Philadelphia, 1986, WB Saunders, p. 11. **B,** From Seltzer SE, Weissman BN, Finberg HJ, et al: Improved diagnostic imaging in joint diseases. Semin Arthritis Rheum 11[3]:315, 1982.)

CONCLUSION

Having completed all parts of the assessment, the examiner can look at the pertinent objective and subjective facts, note the significant signs and symptoms to determine what is causing the patient's problems, and design a proper treatment regimen based on the findings. This is the normal and correct reasoning process.[225,226] If the assessment is not followed through completely, the treatment regimen may not be implemented properly, and this may lead to unwarranted extended care of the patient and increased health care costs.

Occasionally, patients present with a mixture of signs and symptoms that indicates two or more possible problem areas. Only by adding the positive findings and subtracting the negative findings can the examiner determine the probable cause of the problem. In many cases, the decision may be an "educated guess," because few problems are "textbook perfect." Only the examiner's knowledge, clinical experience, and diagnosis, followed by trial treatment, can conclusively delineate the problem.

Finally, when the assessment has been completed, the clinician should warn the patient about a possible exacerbation of symptoms and should not hesitate to refer the patient to another health care professional if the patient has presented with unusual signs and symptoms or if the condition appears to be beyond the scope of the examiner's practice.

TABLE **1-40**

Differential Diagnosis of Claudication and Spinal Stenosis

Vascular Claudication	Neurogenic Claudication	Spinal Stenosis
Pain* is usually bilateral	Pain is usually bilateral but may be unilateral	Usually bilateral pain
Occurs in the calf (foot, thigh, hip, or buttocks)	Occurs in back, buttocks, thighs, calves, feet	Occurs in back, buttocks, thighs, calves, and feet
Pain consistent in all spinal positions	Pain decreased in spinal flexion Pain increased in spinal extension	Pain decreased in spinal flexion Pain increased in spinal extension
Pain brought on by physical exertion (e.g., walking)	Pain increased with walking	Pain increased with walking
Pain relieved promptly by rest (1 to 5 minutes)	Pain decreased by recumbency	Pain relieved with prolonged rest (may persist hours after resting)
Pain increased by walking uphill		Pain decreased when walking uphill
No burning or dysesthesia	Burning and dysesthesia from the back to buttocks and leg or legs	Burning and numbness present in lower extremities
Decreased or absent pulses in lower extremities	Normal pulses	Normal pulses
Color and skin changes in feet—cold, numb, dry, or scaly skin, poor nail and hair growth	Good skin nutrition	Good skin nutrition
Affects ages from 40 to over 60	Affects ages from 40 to over 60	Peaks in seventh decade of life; affects men primarily

Modified from Goodman CC, Snyder TE: Differential diagnosis in physical therapy, ed 2, Philadelphia, 1995, W.B. Saunders Co., p. 539.
*"Pain" associated with vascular claudication may also be described as an "aching," "cramping," or "tired" feeling.

TABLE **1-41**

Differential Diagnosis of Contractile Tissue (Muscle) and Inert Tissue (Ligament) Pathology

	Muscle	Ligament
Mechanism of Injury	Overstretching (overload) Crushing (pinching)	Overstretching (overload)
Contributing Factors	Muscle fatigue Poor reciprocal muscle strength Inflexibility Inadequate warm-up	Muscle fatigue Hypermobility

TABLE **1-41**

Differential Diagnosis of Contractile Tissue (Muscle) and Inert Tissue (Ligament) Pathology—cont'd

	Muscle	Ligament
Active Movement	Pain on contraction (1°, 2°) Pain on stretch (1°, 2°) No pain on contraction (3°) Weakness on contraction (1°, 2°, 3°)	Pain on stretch or compression (1°, 2°) No pain on stretch (3°) ROM decreased
Passive Movement	Pain on stretch Pain on compression	Pain on stretch (1°, 2°) No pain on stretch (3°) ROM decreased
Resisted Isometric Movement	Pain on contraction (1°, 2°) No pain on contraction (3°) Weakness on contraction (1°, 2°, 3°)	No pain (1°, 2°, 3°)
Special Tests	If test isolates muscle, weakness and pain on contraction (1°, 2°) or weakness and no pain on contraction (3°)	If test isolates ligament, ROM and pain affected
Reflexes	Normal unless 3°	Normal
Cutaneous Distribution	Normal	Normal
Joint Play Movement (in Resting Position)	Normal	Increased ROM, unless restricted by swelling
Palpation	Point tenderness at site of injury Gap if palpated early Swelling (blood—ecchymosis late) Spasm	Point tenderness at site of injury Gap if palpated early Swelling (blood/synovial fluid)
Diagnostic Imaging	MRI, arthrogram, and CT scan show lesion	MRI, arthrogram, and CT scan show lesion Stress x-ray shows increased ROM

CT, Computed tomography; *MRI,* magnetic resonance imaging; *ROM,* range of motion.

REFERENCES

1. Cyriax J: Textbook of orthopaedic medicine, vol. 1: diagnosis of soft tissue lesions, ed 8, London, 1982, Balliere Tindall.
2. Weed L: Medical records that guide and teach: part I. N Engl J Med 278:593–600, 1968.
3. Dutton M: Orthopedic examination, evaluation and intervention, New York, 2004, McGraw-Hill.
4. Stith JS, Sahrmann SA, Dixon KK, et al: Curriculum to prepare diagnosticians in physical therapy. J Phys Ther Educ 9:46–53, 1995.
5. Adams ST, Leveson SH: Clinical prediction rules. BMJ 344:8312–8322, 2012.
6. Stewart J, Kempenaar L, Lanchlan D: Rethinking yellow flags. Man Ther 16:196–198, 2011.
7. American Physical Therapy Association: Guide to physical therapist practice, second edition, American Physical Therapy Association. Phys Ther 81:9–746, 2001.
8. Martin RR, Mohtadi NG, Safran MR, et al: Differences in physician and patient ratings of items used to assess hip disorders. Am J Sports Med 37:1508–1512, 2009.
9. Maitland GD: Neuro/musculoskeletal examination and recording guide, Glen Osmond, South Australia, 1992, Lauderdale Press.
10. Vranceanu AM, Barsky A, Ring D: Psychosocial aspects of disabling musculoskeletal pain. J Bone Joint Surg Am 91:2014–2018, 2009.
11. Petty NJ, Moore AP: Neuromusculoskeletal examination and assessment: a handbook for therapists, London, 1998, Churchill-Livingstone.
12. McGuire DB: The multiple dimensions of cancer pain: a framework for assessment and management. In McGuire DB, Yarbo CH, Ferrell BR, editors: Cancer pain management, ed 2, Boston, 1995, Jones & Bartlett.
13. Wiener SL: Differential diagnosis of acute pain by body region, New York, 1993, McGraw-Hill.
14. Nijs J, Van Houdenove B, Oostendorp RA: Recognition of central sensitization in patients with musculoskeletal pain: application of pain neurophysiology in manual therapy practice. Man Ther 15:135–141, 2010.
15. Smart KM, Blake C, Staines A, et al: Clinical indicators of nociceptive, peripheral neuropathic and central mechanisms of musculoskeletal pain: a Delphi survey of clinical experts. Man Ther 15:80–87, 2010.
16. Travell JG, Simons DG: Myofascial pain and dysfunction: the trigger point manual, Baltimore, 1983, Williams & Wilkins.
17. McKenzie RA: The lumbar spine: mechanical diagnosis and therapy, Waikane, New Zealand, 1982, Spinal Publications.
18. Meadows JT: Orthopedic differential diagnosis in physical therapy: a case study approach, New York, 1999, McGraw Hill.
19. Arendt-Nielsen L, Fernandez-de-las-Penas C, Graven-Nielson T: Basic aspects of musculoskeletal pain: from acute to chronic pain. J Man Manip Ther 19(4):186–193, 2011.
20. Jensen MP, Karoly P, Braver S: The measurement of clinical pain intensity: a comparison of six methods. Pain 27:117–126, 1956.
21. Strong J: Assessment of pain perception in clinical practice. Manual Ther 4:216–220, 1999.
22. Melzack R: The McGill pain questionnaire: major properties and scoring methods. Pain 1:277–299, 1975.
23. Melzack R, Torgerson WS: On the language of pain. Anesthesiology 34:50–59, 1971.
24. Melzack R: The short-form McGill pain questionnaire. Pain 30:191–197, 1987.
25. Brodie DJ, Burnett JV, Walker JM, et al: Evaluation of low back pain by patient questionnaires and therapist assessment. J Orthop Sports Phys Ther 11:519–529, 1990.
26. Scott J, Huskisson EC: Vertical or horizontal visual analogue scales. Ann Rheum Dis 38:560, 1979.
27. Langley GB, Sheppeard H: The visual analogue scale: its use in pain management. Rheumatol Int 5:145–148, 1985.
28. Carlsson AM: Assessment of chronic pain: aspects of the reliability and validity of the visual analogue scale. Pain 16:87–101, 1983.
29. Huskisson EC: Measurement of pain. Lancet 2(7889):1127–1131, 1974.
30. Lacey RJ, Lewis M, Jordan K, et al: Interrater reliability of scoring of pain drawings in a self-report health survey. Spine 30:E455–E458, 2005.

31. Bennett M: The LANSS Pain Scale: the Leeds assessment of neuropathic symptoms and signs. Pain 92:147–157, 2001.

32. Halle JS: Neuromusculoskeletal scan examination with selected related topics. In Flynn TW, editor: The thoracic spine and rib cage: musculoskeletal evaluation and treatment, Boston, 1996, Butterworth-Heinemann.

33. Gleim GW, McHugh MP: Flexibility and its effect on sports injury performance. Sports Med 24:289–299, 1997.

34. Lee M: Biomechanics of joint movements. In Refshauge K, Gass E, editors: Musculoskeletal physiotherapy, Oxford, England, 1995, Butterworth-Heinemann.

35. Bowen MK, Warren RF: Ligamentous control of shoulder stability based on selective cutting and static translation experiments. Clin Sports Med 10:757–782, 1991.

36. Terry GC, Hammon D, France P, et al: The stabilizing function of passive shoulder restraints. Am J Sports Med 19:26–34, 1991.

37. Waddell G, Main CJ: Illness behavior. In Waddell G, editor: The back pain revolution, Edinburgh, 1998, Churchill Livingstone.

38. Main CJ, Waddell G: Psychologic stress. In Waddell G, editor: The back pain revolution, Edinburgh, 1998, Churchill Livingstone.

39. Barsky AJ, Goodson JD, Lane RS, et al: The amplification of somatic symptoms. Psychosomatic Med 50:510–519, 1988.

40. Chaturvedi SK: Prevalence of chronic pain in psychiatric patients. Pain 24:231–237, 1987.

41. Main CJ, George SZ: Psychosocial influences on low back pain: why should you care? Phys Ther 91:609–613, 2011.

42. Linton SJ, Shaw WS: Impact of psychological factors in the experience of pain. Phys Ther 91:700–711, 2011.

43. Hill JC, Fritz JM: Psychosocial influences on low back pain, disability and response to treatment. Phys Ther 91:712–721, 2011.

44. Nicholas MK, Linton SJ, Watson PJ, et al: Early identification and management of psychological risk factors ("yellow flags") in patients with low back pain: a reappraisal. Phys Ther 91:737–753, 2011.

45. Waddell G, Newton M, Henderson I, et al: A fear-avoidance beliefs questionnaire (FABQ) and the role of fear-avoidance beliefs in chronic low back pain and disability. Pain 52:157–168, 1993.

46. Vlaeyen J, Kole-Snijders A, Boeren R, et al: Fear of movement/(re)injury in chronic low back pain and its relation to behavioral performance. Pain 62:363–372, 1995.

47. Miller RP, Kori SH, Todd DD: The Tampa Scale. Unpublished report, Tampa, FL, 1991.

48. Murphy DR, Hurwitz EL: The usefulness of clinical measures of psychologic factors in patients with spinal pain. J Manip Physiol Ther 34:609–613, 2011.

49. Hapidou EG, O'Brien MA, Pierrynowski MR, et al: Fear and avoidance of movement in people with chronic pain: psychometric properties of the 11 item Tampa Scale for Kinesiophobia (TSK-11). Physiother Can 64:235–241, 2012.

50. George SZ, Stryker SE: Fear-avoidance beliefs and clinical outcomes for patients seeking outpatient physical therapy for musculoskeletal pain conditions. J Orthop Sports Ther 41:249–259, 2011.

51. Gray H, Adefolarin AT, Howe TE: A systematic review of instruments for the assessment of work-related psychosocial factors (blue flags) individuals with non-specific low back pain. Man Ther 16:531–543, 2011.

52. LoPiccolo CJ, Goodkin K, Baldewicz TT: Current issues in the diagnosis and management of malingering. Ann Med 31:166–174, 1989.

53. Goodman CC, Snyder TE: Differential diagnosis in physical therapy, Philadelphia, 1995, WB Saunders.

54. Keefe FJ, Block AR: Development of an observation method for assessing pain behavior in chronic low back pain patients. Behav Ther 13:363–375, 1982.

55. Refshauge KM, Latimer J: The physical examination. In Refshauge KM, Gass E, editors: Musculoskeletal physiotherapy, Oxford, England, 1995, Butterworth-Heinemann.

56. Delany C: Should I warn the patient first? Aust J Physiother 42:249–255, 1996.

57. Ross MD, Boissonnault WG: Red flags: to screen or not to screen. J Orthop Sports Phys Ther 40:682–684, 2010.

58. Macedo LG, Magee DJ: Differences in range of motion between dominant and nondominant sides of upper and lower extremities. J Manip Physiol Ther 31:577–582, 2008.

59. Kaplan NM, Deveraux RB, Miller HS: Systemic hyperextension. Med Sci Sports Exerc 26:S268–S270, 1994.

60. Zabetakis PM: Profiling the hypertensive patient in sports. Clin Sports Med 3:137–152, 1984.

61. Sanders B, Nemeth WC: Preparticipation physical examination. J Orthop Sports Phys Ther 23:144–163, 1996.

62. Hayes KW, Petersen C, Falconer J: An examination of Cyriax's passive motion tests with patients having osteoarthritis of the knee. Phys Ther 74:697–708, 1994.

63. Peterson CM, Hayes KW: Construct validity of Cyriax's selective tension examination: association of end feels with pain in the knee and shoulder. J Orthop Sports Phys Ther 30:512–527, 2000.

64. Franklin ME, Conner-Kerr T, Chamness M, et al: Assessment of exercise-induced minor muscle lesions: the accuracy of Cyriax's diagnosis by selective tissue paradigm. J Orthop Sports Phys Ther 24:122–129, 1996.

65. Williams P, Warwick R, editors: Gray's anatomy, ed 36, Edinburgh, 1980, Churchill Livingstone.

66. Kandel ER, Schwartz JH, Jessell TM: Principles of neural science, New York, 2000, McGraw Hill.

67. Nitta H, Tajima T, Sugiyama H, et al: Study on dermatomes by means of selective lumbar spinal nerve block. Spine 18:1782–1786, 1993.

68. Downs MB, Laport E: Conflicting dermatome maps: educational and clinical implications. J Orthop Sports Phys Ther 41:427–434, 2011.

69. Keegan JJ, Garrett ED: The segmental distribution of the cutaneous nerves in the limbs of man. Anat Rec 101:409–437, 1948.

70. Grieve GP: Referred pain and other clinical features. In Boyling JD, Palastanga N, editors: Grieve's modern manual therapy: the vertebral column, ed 2, Edinburgh, 1994, Churchill Livingstone.

71. Smyth MJ, Wright V: Sciatica and the intervertebral disc: an experimental study. J Bone Joint Surg Am 40:1401–1418, 1958.

72. Seddon HJ: Three types of nerve injury. Brain 66:17–28, 1943.

73. Sunderland S: Nerve and nerve injuries, Edinburgh, 1978, Churchill Livingstone.

74. Wilgis EF: Techniques for diagnosis of peripheral nerve loss. Clin Orthop 163:8–14, 1982.

75. Tardif GS: Nerve injuries: testing and treatment tactics. Phys Sports Med 23:61–72, 1995.

76. Omer GE: Physical diagnosis of peripheral nerve injuries. Orthop Clin North Am 12:207–228, 1981.

77. Harrelson GL: Evaluation of brachial plexus injuries. Sports Med Update 4:3–8, 1989.

78. Wilbourn AJ: Electrodiagnostic testing of neurologic injuries in athletes. Clin Sports Med 9:229–245, 1990.

79. Leffert R: Clinical diagnosis, testing, and electromyographic study in brachial plexus traction injuries. Clin Orthop 237:24–31, 1988.

80. Upton AR, McComas AJ: The double crush in nerve-entrapment syndromes. Lancet 2:359–362, 1973.

81. Mackinnon SE: Double and multiple "crush" syndromes. Hand Clin 8:369–390, 1992.

82. Lee Dellon A, Mackinnon SE: Chronic nerve compression model for the double crush hypothesis. Ann Plast Surg 26:259–264, 1991.

83. Nemoto K, Matsumoto N, Tazaki K, et al: An experimental study on the "double crush" hypothesis. J Hand Surg Am 12:552–559, 1987.

84. Schmid AB, Coppieters MW: The double crush syndrome revisited—a Delphi study to reveal current expert views on mechanisms underlying dual nerve disorders. Man Ther 16:557–562, 2011.

85. Butler D: Mobilisation of the nervous system, Melbourne, 1991, Churchill Livingstone.

86. Elvey RL: Treatment of arm pain associated with abnormal brachial plexus tension. Aust J Physiother 32:225–230, 1986.

87. Shacklock M: Neurodynamics. Physiotherapy 81:9–16, 1995.

88. Shacklock M, Butler D, Slater H: The dynamic central nervous system: structure and clinical neurobiomechanics. In Boyling JD, Palastanga N, editors: Grieve's modern manual therapy: the vertebral column, ed 2, Edinburgh, 1994, Churchill Livingstone.

89. Sahrmann SA: Diagnosis and treatment of movement impairment syndromes, St Louis, 2002, Mosby.

90. Shumway-Cook A, Woollacott M: Motor control: theory and practical applications, Baltimore, 1995, Williams & Wilkins.

91. Schmidt RA, Lee TD: Motor control and learning: a behavioral emphasis, Champaign, IL, 1999, Human Kinetics.

92. Kaltenborn FM: Manual mobilization of the extremity joints, Oslo, Norway, 1980, Olaf Norlis Bokhandel.

93. Ombregt L, Bisschop P, ter Veer HJ, et al: A system of orthopedic medicine, London, 1995, WB Saunders.

94. Jull GA: Examination of the articular system. In Boyling JD, N Palastanga, editors: Grieve's modern manual therapy: the vertebral column, ed 2, Edinburgh, 1994, Churchill Livingstone.

95. Myers A, Canty K, Nelson T: Are the Ottawa ankle rules helpful in ruling out the need for x-ray examination in children? Arch Dis Child 90:1309–1311, 2005.

96. Lea RD, Gerhardt JJ: Range-of-motion measurements. J Bone Joint Surg Am 77:784–798, 1995.

97. Williams JG, Callaghan M: Comparison of visual estimation and goniometry in determination of a shoulder joint angle. Physiotherapy 76:655–657, 1990.

98. Bovens AM, van Baak MA, Vrencken JG, et al: Variability and reliability of joint measurements. Am J Sports Med 18:58–63, 1990.

99. Boone DC, Azen SP, Lin CM, et al: Reliability of goniometric measurements. Phys Ther 58(11):1355–1360, 1978.

100. Mayerson NH, Milano RA: Goniometric measurement reliability in physical medicine. Arch Phys Med Rehabil 65:92–94, 1984.

101. Riddle DL, Rothstein JM, Lamb RL: Goniometric reliability in a clinical setting: shoulder measurements. Phys Ther 67:668–673, 1987.

102. Remvig L, Jensen DV, Ward RC: Epidemiology of general joint hypermobility and basis for the proposed criteria for benign joint hypermobility syndrome: review of the literature. J Rheumatol 34(4):804–809, 2007.

103. Remvig L, Jensen DV, Ward RC: Are diagnostic criteria for general joint hypermobility and benign joint hypermobility syndrome based on reproducible and valid tests? A review of the literature. J Rheumatol 34(4):798–803, 2007.

104. Juul-Kristensen B, Rogind H, Jensen DV, et al: Inter-examiner reproducibility of tests and criteria for generalized joint hypermobility and benign joint hypermobility syndrome. Rheumatology 46:1835–1841, 2007.

105. Wolf JM, Cameron KL, Owens BD: Impact of joint laxity and hypermobility on the musculoskeletal system. J Am Acad Orthop Surg 19(8):463–471, 2011.

106. Aslan UB, Çelik E, Cavlak U, et al: Evaluation of interrater and intrarater reliability of Beighton and Horan joint mobility index. Fizyoterapi Rehabilitasyon 17(3):113–119, 2006.

107. Hirsch C, Hirsch M, John MT, et al: Reliability of the Beighton Hypermobility Index to determine the general joint laxity performed by dentists. J Orofacial Ortho 68:342–352, 2007.

108. Beighton P, Grahame R, Borde H: Hypermobility of joints, Berlin, 1983, Springer-Verlag.

109. Wynne-Davies R: Hypermobility. Proc R Soc Med 64:689–693, 1971.

110. Carter C, Wilkinson J: Persistent joint laxity and congenital dislocation of the hip. J Bone Joint Surg Br 46:40–45, 1969.

111. Nicholas JS, Grossman RB, Hershman EB: The importance of a simplified classification of motion in sports in relation to performance. Orthop Clin North Am 8:499–532, 1977.

112. Paris SV, Patla C: E1 course notes: extremity dysfunction and manipulation, Atlanta, 1988, Patris.

113. Riddle DL: Measurement of accessory motion: critical issues and related concepts. Phys Ther 72:865–874, 1992.

114. Petersen CM, Hayes KW: Construct validity of Cyriax's selective tissue examination: association of end-feels with pain at the knee and shoulder. J Orthop Sports Phys Ther 30:512–521, 2000.

115. Pandyan AD, Johnson GR, Price CI, et al: A review of the properties and limitations of the Ashworth and modified Ashworth scales as measures of spasticity. Clin Rehab 13:373–383, 1999.

116. Haas BM, Bergstrom E, Jamous A, et al: The inter rater reliability of the original and of the modified Ashworth scale for the assessment of spasticity in patients with spinal cord injury. Spinal Cord 34:560–564, 1996.

117. Maitland GD: Palpation examination of the posterior cervical spine: the ideal, average and abnormal. Aust J Physiother 28:3–11, 1982.

118. Clarkson HM, Gilewich GB: Musculoskeletal assessment: joint range of motion and manual muscle strength, Baltimore, 1989, Williams & Wilkins.

119. Evans P: Ligaments, joint surfaces, conjunct rotation and close pack. Physiotherapy 74:105–114, 1988.

120. Pope MH, Frymoyer JW, Krag MH: Diagnosing instability. Clin Orthop 279:60–67, 1992.

121. Sapega AA: Muscle performance evaluation in orthopedic practice. J Bone Joint Surg Am 72:1562–1574, 1990.

122. Hislop HJ, Montgomery J: Daniels and Worthingham's muscle testing: techniques of manual examination, Philadelphia, 1995, WB Saunders.

123. Kendall HO, Kendall FP, Boynton DA: Posture and pain, Huntington, NY, 1970, Robert E. Krieger.

124. American Academy of Orthopedic Surgeon: Athletic training and sports medicine, ed 2, Park Ridge, IL, 1991, American Academy of Orthopedic Surgeons.

125. Khan KM, Cook JL, Bonar F, et al: Histopathology of common tendinopathies: update and implications for clinical management. Sports Med 27:393–408, 1999.

126. Janda V: On the concept of postural muscles and posture in man. Aust J Physiother 29:83–85, 1983.

127. Schlink MB: Muscle imbalance patterns associated with low back syndromes. In Watkins RG, editor: The spine in sports, St Louis, 1996, Mosby.

128. Jull GA, Janda V: Muscles and motor control in low back pain: assessment and management. In Twomey LT, Taylor JR, editors: Physical therapy of the low back, New York, 1987, Churchill Livingstone.

129. Janda V: Muscles and motor control in cervicogenic disorders: assessment and management. In Grant R, editor: Physical therapy of the cervical and thoracic spine, New York, 1994, Churchill-Livingstone.

130. Watson CJ, Schenkman M: Physical therapy management of isolated serratus anterior muscle paralysis. Phys Ther 75:194–202, 1995.

131. Laupacis A, Sekar N, Stiell IG: Clinical prediction rules—a review and suggested modifications of methodological standards. JAMA 277:488–494, 1997.

132. Reiman MP, Manske RC: The assessment of function: how is it measured? A clinical perspective. J Man Manip Ther 19:91–99, 2011.

133. Paxton EW, Fithian DC, Stone ML, et al: The reliability and validity of knee-specific and general health instruments in assessing acute patellar dislocation outcomes. Am J Sports Med 31:487–492, 2003.

134. Epstein AM: The outcomes movement: will it get us where we want to go? N Engl J Med 323:266–270, 1990.

135. Goldstein TS: Functional rehabilitation in orthopedics, Gaithersburg, MD, 1995, Aspen.

136. Swiontkowski MF, Engelberg R, Martin DP, et al: Short musculoskeletal function assessment questionnaire: validity, reliability, and responsiveness. J Bone Joint Surg Am 81:1245–1260, 1999.

137. Research Foundation, State University of New York: Guide for use of the uniform data set for medical rehabilitation including the functional independence measure (FIM), Buffalo, NY, 1990, Research Foundation, State University of New York.

138. Reuben DB, Siu AL: An objective measure of physical function of elderly outpatients: the physical performance test. J Am Geriatr Soc 38:1105–1112, 1990.

139. Jette AM: Functional status index: reliability of a chronic disease evaluation instrument. Arch Phys Med Rehabil 61:395–401, 1980.

140. Meenan R, Mason JH, Anderson JJ, et al: AIMS 2: the content and properties of a revised and expanded arthritis impact measurement scales health status questionnaire. Arthritis Rheum 25:1–10, 1990.

141. Brimer MA, Shuneman G, Allen BR: Guidelines for developing a functional assessment for an acute facility. Phys Ther Forum 12:22–25, 1993.

142. Gatchel RJ, Polatin PB, Mayer TG, et al: Use of the SF-36 health status survey with a chronically disabled back pain population: strength and limitations. J Occup Rehab 8:237–245, 1998.

143. Gatchel RJ, Mayer T, Dersh J, et al: The association of the SF-36 health status survey with 1-year socioeconomic outcomes in a chronically disabled spinal disorder population. Spine 24:2162–2170, 1999.

144. Bergner M, Bobbitt RA, Pollard WE, et al: The sickness impact profile: validation of a health status measure. Medical Care 14:57–67, 1976.

145. Swiontkowski MF, Engelberg R, Martin DP, et al: Short musculoskeletal function assessment questionnaire: validity, reliability and responsiveness. J Bone Joint Surg Am 81:1245–1260, 1999.

146. Strand LI, Wie SL: The sock test for evaluating activity limitation in patients with musculoskeletal pain. Phys Ther 79:136–145, 1999.

147. Ellexson MT: Analyzing an industry: job analysis for treatment, prevention, and placement. Orthop Phys Ther Clin 1:15–21, 1992.

148. McGinn TG, Guyatt GH, Wyer PC, et al: Users' guides to medical literature: XXII: how to use articles about clinical decision rules. JAMA 284(7):79–84, 2000.

149. Backstrom KM, Whitman JM, Flynn TW: Lumbar spinal stenosis—diagnosis and management of the aging spine. Man Ther 16:308–317, 2011.

150. Haskins R, Rivett DA, Osmotherly PG: Clinical prediction rules in the physiotherapy management of low back pain: a systemic review. Man Ther 17:9–21, 2012.

151. Flynn T, Fritz J, Whitman J, et al: A clinical prediction rule for classifying patients with low back pain who demonstrate short-term improvements with spinal manipulation. Spine 27:2835–2843, 2002.

152. Glynn PE, Weisbach PC: Clinical prediction rules—a physical therapy reference manual, Sudbury, MA, 2011, Jones and Bartlett Publishers.

153. Reilly BM, Evans AT: Translating clinical research into clinical practice: impact of using prediction rules to make decisions. Ann Intern Med 144:201–209, 2006.

154. Wasson JH, Sox HC, Neff RK, et al: Clinical prediction rules—applications and methodological standards. N Eng J Med 313:793–799, 1985.

155. Toll DB, Janssen KJ, Vergouwe, Moons KG: Validation, updating and impact of clinical prediction rules: a review. J Clin Epidemiol 61:1085–1094, 2008.

156. Brehant JC, Stiell IG, Visentin L, et al: Clinical decision rules "in the real world": how a widely disseminated rule is used in everyday practice. Acad Emerg Med 12:948–957, 2005.

157. Rowe CR: The shoulder, Edinburgh, 1988, Churchill Livingstone.

158. Lippitt SB, Harryman DT, Matsen FA: A practical tool for evaluating function: the simple shoulder test. In Matsen FA, Fu FH, Hawkins RJ, editors: The shoulder: a balance of mobility and stability, Rosemont, IL, 1993, American Academy of Orthopedic Surgeons.

159. Gerber C: Integrated scoring systems for the functional assessment of the shoulder. In Matsen FA, Fu FH, Hawkins RJ, editors: The shoulder: a balance of mobility and stability, Rosemont, IL, 1993, American Academy of Orthopedic Surgeons.

160. Carroll HD: A quantitative test of upper extremity function. J Chron Dis 18:479–491, 1965.

161. Potvin AR, Tourtellotte WW, Dailey JS, et al: Simulated activities of daily living examination. Arch Phys Med Rehabil 53:476–486, 1972.

162. Cook C: The lost art of the clinical examination: an overemphasis on clinical special tests. J Man Manip Ther 18:3–4, 2010.

163. Hegedus EJ: Studies of quality and impact in clinical diagnosis and decision making. J Man Manip Ther 18:5–6, 2010.

164. Cipriani D, Noftz J: The utility of orthopedic clinical tests for diagnosis. In Magee DJ, Zachazewski JE, Quillen SW, editors: Scientific foundations and principles of practice in musculoskeletal rehabilitation, Philadelphia, 2007, Elsevier.

165. Greenhalgh T: How to read a paper: papers that report diagnostic or screening tests. Br Med J 315:540–543, 1997.

166. Fritz JM, Wainner RS: Examining diagnostic tests: an evidence-based perspective. Phys Ther 81:1546–1564, 2001.

167. Cook CE, Hegedus EJ: Orthopedic physical examination tests—an evidence based approach, Upper Saddle River, NJ, 2008, Prentice Hall Pearson.

168. Cleland J, Koppenhaver S: Orthopedic clinical examination: an evidence-based approach for physical therapists, ed 2, Philadelphia, 2011, Saunders Elsevier.

169. Portney LG, Walkins MP: Foundations of clinical research: applications to practice, Upper Saddle River, NJ, 2000, Prentice Hall.

170. Schwartz JS: Evaluating diagnostic tests: what is done—what needs to be done. J Gen Int Med 1:266–267, 1986.

171. Guyatt GH, Deyo RA, Charlson M, et al: Responsiveness and validity in health status measurement: a clarification. J Clin Epidemiol 42:403–408, 1989.

172. Jaeschke R, Singer J, Guyatt GH: Measurement of health status: ascertaining the minimally clinical important difference. Control Clin Trials 10:407–415, 1989.

173. Boyko EJ: Ruling out or ruling in disease with the most sensitive or specific diagnostic test: short cut or wrong turn? Med Decision Making 14:175–179, 1994.

174. Hagen MD: Test characteristics: how good is that test? Med Decision Making 22:213–233, 1995.

175. Jaeschke R, Guyatt GH, Sackett DL: Users' guides to the medical literature. III. How to use an article about a diagnostic test. B. What are the results and will they help me in caring for my patients? The Evidence-Based Medicine Working Group. JAMA 271:703–707, 1994.

176. Anderson MA, Forman TL: Return to competition: functional rehabilitation. In Zachazewski JE, Magee DJ, Quillen WS, editors: Athletic injuries and rehabilitation, Philadelphia, 1996, WB Saunders.

177. Lijmer JG, Mol BW, Heisterkamp S, et al: Empirical evidence of design-related bias in studies of diagnostic tests. JAMA 282:1061–1066, 1999.

178. Schulzer M: Diagnostic tests: a statistical review. Muscle Nerve 17:815–819, 1994.

179. Cook C: Challenges with diagnosis: sketchy reference standards. J Man Manip Ther 20:111–112, 2012.

180. Sackett DL: A primer on the precision and accuracy of the clinical examination. JAMA 267:2638–2644, 1992.

181. Wright A, Hannon J, Hegedus EJ, et al: Clinimetrics corner: a closer look at the minimal clinically important difference (MCID). J Man Manip Ther 20:160–166, 2012.

182. McGregor AH, Doré CJ, McCarthy ID, et al: Are subjective clinical findings and objective clinical tests related to the motion characteristics of low back pain subjects? J Orthop Sports Phys Ther 28:370–377, 1998.

183. Kuroda R, Hoshino Y, Kubo S, et al: Similarities and differences of diagnostic manual tests for anterior cruciate ligament insufficiency—a global survey and kinematics assessment. Am J Sports Med 40:91–99, 2012.

184. Jonsson T, Althoff B, Peterson L, et al: Clinical diagnosis of ruptures of the anterior cruciate ligament: a comparative study of the Lachman test and the anterior drawer sign. Am J Sports Med 10:100–102, 1982.

185. Rosenberg TD, Rasmussen GL: The function of the anterior cruciate ligament during anterior drawer and Lachman's testing. Am J Sports Med 12:318–322, 1984.

186. Cervical Spine Research Society: The cervical spine, Philadelphia, 1989, JB Lippincott.

187. Hagbarth KE, Wallen G, Burke D, et al: Effects of the Jendrassik maneuver on muscle spindle activity in man. J Neurol Neurosurg Psych 38:1143–1153, 1975.

188. Bland JH: Disorders of the cervical spine, Philadelphia, 1987, WB Saunders.

189. Poynton AR, O'Farrell DA, Shannon F, et al: Sparing of sensation to pin prick predicts recovery of a motor segment after injury to the spinal cord. J Bone Joint Surg Br 79:952–954, 1997.

190. Hockaday JM, Whitty CWM: Patterns of referred pain in the normal subject. Brain 90:481–495, 1967.

191. Mennell JM: Joint pain, Boston, 1972, Little Brown & Co.

192. Kaltenborn FM: Mobilization of the extremity joints: examination and basic treatment techniques, Oslo, Norway, 1980, Olaf Norlis Bokhandel.

193. Lewit K, Liebenson C: Palpation: Problems and implications. J Manip Physiol Ther 16:586–590, 1993.

194. Gerwin RD, Shannon S, Hong CZ, et al: Interrater reliability in myofascial trigger point examination. Pain 17:591–595, 1997.

195. Njoo KH, Van der Does E: The occurrence and interrater reliability of myofascial trigger points in the quadratus lumborum and gluteus maximus: a prospective study in non-specific low back patients and controls in general practice. Pain 58:317–321, 1994.

196. Snider KT, Snider EJ, Degenhardt BF, et al: Palpatory accuracy of lumbar spinous processes using multiple bony landmarks. J Manip Physiol Ther 34:306–313, 2011.

197. Ivanhoe CB, Reistetter TA: Spasticity: the misunderstood part of the upper motor neuron syndrome. Am J Phys Med Rehabil 83(suppl):S3–S9, 2004.

198. Deyle GD: Musculoskeletal imaging in physical therapy practice. J Orthop Sports Phys Ther 35:708–721, 2005.

199. Deyle GD: The role of MRI in musculoskeletal practice: a clinical perspective. J Man Manip Ther 19(3):152–161, 2011.

200. Khan KM, Tress BW, Hare WS, et al: Treat the patient, not the x-ray: advances in diagnostic imaging do not replace the need for clinical interpretation. Clin J Sports Med 8:1–4, 1998.

201. Johnson TR, Steinbach LS: Essentials of musculoskeletal imaging, Rosemont, IL, 2003, American Academy of Orthopedic Surgeons.

202. Resnick D, Kransdorf MJ: Bone and joint imaging, Philadelphia, 2005, Elsevier.

203. McKinnis LN: Fundamentals of musculoskeletal imaging, Philadelphia, 2005, FA Davis.

204. Coris EE, Zwygart K, Fletcher M, et al: Imaging in sports medicine: an overview. Sports Med Arthrosc Rev 17:2–12, 2009.

205. Bigg-Wither G, Kelly P: Diagnostic imaging in musculoskeletal physiotherapy. In Refshauge K, Gass E, editors: Musculoskeletal physiotherapy, Oxford, England, 1995, Butterworth-Heinemann.

206. Jones MD: Basic diagnostic radiology, St Louis, 1969, Mosby.

207. Miller WT: Introduction to clinical radiology, New York, 1982, MacMillan.

208. Gross GW: Imaging. In Stanitski CL, DeLee JC, Drez D, editors: Pediatric and adolescent sports medicine, Philadelphia, 1994, WB Saunders.

209. Fischbach F: A manual of laboratory diagnostic tests, ed 3, Philadelphia, 1988, JB Lippincott.

210. Ghanem I, El Hage S, Rachkidi R, et al: Pediatric cervical spine instability. J Child Orthop 2:71–84, 2008.

211. Gruelich WW, Pyle SU: Radiographic atlas of skeletal development of the wrist and hand, Stanford, CA, 1959, Stanford University Press.

212. Sanders JO, Khoury JG, Kishan S, et al: Predicting scoliosis progression from skeletal maturity: a simplified classification during adolescence. J Bone Joint Surg Am 90(3):540–543, 2008.

213. Grainger RG: The spinal canal. In Whitehouse GH, Worthington BS, editors: Techniques in diagnostic radiology, Oxford, England, 1983, Blackwell Scientific.

214. Buckwalter KA: Computerized tomography in sports medicine. Sports Med Arthrosc Rev 17:13–20, 2009.

215. Evans RC: Illustrated essentials in orthopedic physical assessment, St Louis, 1994, Mosby Year Book.

216. Hsu W, Hearty TM: Radionuclide imaging in the diagnosis and management of orthopedic disease. J Am Acad Orthop Surg 20(3):151–159, 2012.

217. Leffers D, Collins L: An overview of the use of bone scintigraphy in sports medicine. Sports Med Arthrosc Rev 17:21–24, 2009.

218. Black BR, Chong LR, Potter HG: Cartilage imaging in sports medicine. Sports Med Arthrosc Rev 17:68–80, 2008.

219. Silvis ML, Mosher TJ, Smetana BS, et al: High prevalence of pelvis and hip magnetic resonance imaging findings in asymptomatic collegiate and professional hockey players. Am J Sports Med 39:715–721, 2011.

220. Hurd WJ, Eby S, Kaufman KR, et al: Magnetic resonance imaging of the throwing elbow in the uninjured high school-aged baseball pitcher. Am J Sports Med 39:722–728, 2011.

221. Murray PJ, Shaffer BS: MR imaging of the shoulder. Sports Med Arthrosc Rev 17:40–48, 2008.

222. Weiss DB, Jacobson JA, Karunakar MA: The use of ultrasound in evaluating orthopedic trauma patients. J Am Acad Orthop Surg 13:525–533, 2005.

223. Nofsinger C, Konin JG: Diagnostic ultrasound in sports medicine. Sports Med Arthrosc Rev 17:25–30, 2008.

224. Weissman BNW, Sledge CB: Orthopedic radiology, Philadelphia, 1986, WB Saunders.

225. Jones MA: Clinical reasoning in manual therapy. Phys Ther 72:875–884, 1992.

226. Jones MA, Rivett DA: Clinical reasoning for manual therapists, Edinburgh, 2004, Butterworth Heinemann.

SUGGESTED READINGS

Bassett LW, Gold RH, Seeger LL: MRI of the musculoskeletal system, London, 1989, Martin Dunitz.

Boissonnault W, Goodman C: Physical therapists as diagnosticians: drawing the line on diagnosing pathology. J Orthop Sports Phys Ther 36:351–353, 2006.

Bombardier D, Tugwell P: Measuring disability: guidelines for rheumatology studies. J Rheum 10(suppl.):68–73, 1983.

Bonica JJ: The management of pain, Philadelphia, 1953, Lea & Febiger.

Burckhardt CS: The use of the McGill pain questionnaire in assessing arthritis pain. Pain 19:305–314, 1984.

Chafetz N, Genant HK: Computed tomography of the lumbar spine. Orthop Clin North Am 14:147–149, 1983.

Clark CR, Bonfiglio M: Orthopedics: essentials of diagnosis and treatment, New York, 1994, Churchill Livingstone.

Cohen J, Bonfiglio M, Campbell CJ: Orthopedic pathophysiology in diagnosis and treatment, Edinburgh, 1990, Churchill Livingstone.

Convery FR, Minteer MA, Amiel D, et al: Polyarticular disability: a functional assessment. Arch Phys Med Rehab 58:494–499, 1977.

Cox HT: The cleavage lines of the skin. J Bone Joint Surg Br 29:234–240, 1942

Curran JF, Ellman MH, Brown NL: Rheumatologic aspects of painful conditions affecting the shoulder. Clin Orthop 173:27–37, 1983.

Currey HLF: Clinical examination of the joints: an introduction to clinical rheumatology, Toronto, 1975, Pitman Medical.

Cyriax J: Examination of the spinal column. Physiotherapy 56:2–6, 1970.

Dahlin LB, Lundberg G: The neuron and its response to peripheral nerve compression. J Hand Surg Br 15:5–10, 1990.

Farfan HF: Mechanical disorders of the low back, Philadelphia, 1973, Lea & Febiger.

Forrester DM, Brown JC: The radiology of joint disease, Philadelphia, 1987, WB Saunders.

French S: History taking in physiotherapy assessment. Physiotherapy 74:158–160, 1988.

Gartland JJ: Fundamentals of orthopedics, Philadelphia, 1979, WB Saunders.

Goldstein HA: Bone scintigraphy. Orthop Clin North Am 14:243–256, 1983.

Goodman CC, Snyder TE: Differential diagnosis in physical therapy: musculoskeletal and systemic conditions, Philadelphia, 1990, WB Saunders.

Grieve GP: Common vertebral joint problems, London, 1981, Churchill Livingstone.

Groenvold M, Bjorner JB, Klee MC, et al: Test for item bias in a quality of life questionnaire. J Clin Epidemiol 48:805–816, 1995.

Hall S: The response to injury in the peripheral nervous system. J Bone Joint Surg Br 87:1306–1319, 2005.

Hammond MJ: Clinical examination and the physiotherapist. Aust J Physiother 15:47–54, 1969.

Harris ML: Flexibility. Phys Ther 49:591–601, 1969.

Hawkins RJ: Musculoskeletal examination, St Louis, 1995, Mosby Year Book.

Health JR: Problem oriented medical systems. Physiotherapy 64:269–270, 1978.

Hoppenfeld S: Physical examination of the spine and extremities, New York, 1976, Appleton-Century-Crofts.

Irwig L, Tosteson ANA, Gatsonis C, et al: Guidelines for meta-analyses evaluating diagnostic tests. Ann Int Med 120:667–676, 1994.

Jackson R: Headaches associated with disorders of the cervical spine. Headache 6:175–179, 1967.

Janda V: Muscle function testing, London, 1983, Butterworths.

Jones MA, Jones HM: Principles of the physical examination. In Boyling JD, Palastang N, editors: Grieve's modern manual therapy, ed 2, Edinburgh, 1994, Churchill Livingstone.

Judge RD, Zuidema GD, Fitzgerald FT: Clinical diagnosis: a physiologic approach, Boston, 1982, Little Brown & Co.

Kaplan RM, Bush JW, Berry CC: Health status: types of validity and the index of well-being. Health Sci Res 11:478–507, 1976.

Lee P, Jasani MK, Dick WC, et al: Evaluation of a functional index in rheumatoid arthritis. Scand J Rheum 2:71–77, 1973.

Little H: The rheumatological physical examination, Orlando, FL, 1986, Grune & Stratton.

Loomis J: Rehabilitation outcomes: the clinician's perspective. Can J Rehab 7:165–170, 1994.

MacConnaill MA, Basmajian JV: Muscles and movements: a basis for human kinesiology, Baltimore, 1977, Williams & Wilkins.

Massey EW, Riley TL, Pleet AB: Co-existent carpal tunnel syndrome and cervical radiculopathy (double crush syndrome). South Med J 74:957–959, 1981.

Mayer SJ, Dalinka MK: Magnetic resonance imaging of the shoulder. Orthop Clin North Am 21:497–513, 1990.

McLean G, Freiman DB: Angiography of skeletal disease. Orthop Clin North Am 14:257–270, 1983.

Mulrow CD, Linn WD, Gaul MK, et al: Assessing quality of a diagnostic test evaluation. J Gen Int Med 4:288–295, 1989.

Neviaser TJ: Arthrography of the shoulder. Orthop Clin North Am 11:205–217, 1980.

Nilsson N: Measuring cervical muscle tenderness: a study of reliability. J Manip Physiol Ther 18:88–90, 1995.

Noonan TJ, Garrett WG: Muscle strain injury: diagnosis and treatment. J Am Acad Orthop Surg 7:262–269, 1999.

Novey DW: Rapid access guide to the physical examination, Chicago, 1988, Year Book Medical.

Palmer ML, Epler M: Clinical assessment procedures in physical therapy, Philadelphia, 1990, JB Lippincott.

Pitt MJ, Lund PJ, Speer DP: Imaging of the pelvis and hip. Orthop Clin North Am 21:545–559, 1990.

Post M: Physical examination of the musculoskeletal system, Chicago, 1987, Year Book Medical.

Reading AE: Testing pain mechanisms in persons in pain. In Wall PD, Melzack R, editors: Textbook of pain, Edinburgh, 1984, Churchill Livingstone.

Refshauge KM, Latimer J: The history. In Refshauge K, Gass E, editors: Musculoskeletal physiotherapy, Oxford, 1995, Butterworth-Heinemann.

Robertson EA, MH Zweig, Van Steirteghem AC: Evaluating the clinical efficacy of laboratory tests. Am J Clin Pathol 79:78–86, 1983.

Sahrmann S: Are physical therapists fulfilling their responsibilities as diagnosticians? J Orthop Sports Phys Ther 35:556–558, 2005.

Saunders HD: Evaluation of a musculoskeletal disorder. In Gould JA, editor: Orthopedics and sports physical therapy, St Louis, 1990, Mosby.

Saunders HD, Saunders R: Evaluation, treatment and prevention of musculoskeletal disorders, vols 1 and 2, ed 3, Chaska, MN, 1993, HD Saunders.

Schaible HG, Grubb BD: Afferent and spinal mechanisms of joint pain. Pain 55:5–54, 1993.

Seidal HM, Ball JW, Dains JE, et al: Mosby's guide to physical examination, St Louis, 1987, Mosby.

Selby DK, Meril AJ, Wagner KJ, et al: Water-soluble myelography. Orthop Clin North Am 8:79–83, 1977.

Sheps SB, Schechter MT: The assessment of diagnostic tests: a survey of current medical research. JAMA 252:2418–2422, 1984.

Simon GE: Methodologic standards for diagnostic test assessment studies. J Gen Int Med 3:518–520, 1988.

Singer KP: A new musculoskeletal assessment in a student population. J Orthop Sports Phys Ther 8:34–41, 1986.

Smith LK: Functional tests. Phys Ther Rev 34:19–21, 1954.

Spengler DM: Low back pain: assessment and management, Orlando, FL, 1982, Grune & Stratton.

Squire LF, Colaiace WM, Strutynsky N: Exercises in diagnostic radiology, vol 3: bone, Philadelphia, 1972, WB Saunders.

Starkey C, Ryan J: Evaluation of orthopedic and athletic injuries, Philadelphia, 1996, FA Davis.

Wadsworth CT: Manual examination and treatment of the spine and extremities, Baltimore, 1988, Williams & Wilkins.

Warren MJ: Modern imaging of the spine: the use of computed tomography and magnetic resonance. In Boyling JD, Palastanga N, editors: Grieve's modern manual therapy, ed 2, Edinburgh, 1994, Churchill Livingstone.

Zimny NJ: Diagnostic classification and orthopedic physical therapy practice: what can we learn from medicine? J Orthop Sports Phys Ther 34:105–115, 2004.

APPENDIX 1-1

Example of an Assessment Form

DATE:

NAME:

AGE:

OCCUPATION:

HISTORY

Mechanism of Injury:

Aggravating/Easing Factors or Movements:

24-Hour History:

Improving/Static/Worse

New/Old Injury

Past History (include social and family history):

Diagnostic Imaging:

OBSERVATION (POSTURE)

EXAMINATION

ACTIVE MOVEMENTS   PASSIVE MOVEMENTS

EXT   EXT
L   R   L   R

FLEX   FLEX

Comments:

End Feel:

Capsular Pattern:

Mark where symptoms are:

VAS: Intensity of Pain

no   pain as bad
pain   as it could
0   possibly get
                                                            10

Pain: constant, periodic, episodic, occasional

RESISTED ISOMETRIC MOVEMENTS	**FUNCTIONAL TESTING**
Comments:	

NEUROLOGICAL TESTS

Sensory Scan:

Reflexes:

Neurological Special Tests:

SPECIAL TESTS

JOINT PLAY MOVEMENTS

PALPATION

Tenderness, Effusion

(use reverse side for other comments)

APPENDIX 1-2

Example of Informed Consent/Patient Authorization

PATIENT AUTHORIZATION

I hereby authorize and grant permission to _____,

a _____, to carry out any assessment and examination, procedures, and
         occupation

treatments as may be necessary to assess and treat my condition or injury.

The above-named _____ has agreed to provide me with understandable:
            occupation

information on:

- my diagnosis, as known
- the treatment being suggested
- significant risks, benefits of treatment, and possible alternatives to this treatment
- reasonable additional procedures which may be necessary
- the potential risks of foregoing the suggested care

I hereby authorize and grant permission to the above-named _____ to
             occupation

communicate with any health care professional that rehabilitation of my condition may indicate.

I hereby authorize and grant permission to the above-named _____ to
             occupation

release information regarding my condition and my ability to return to normal activity or work to my

insurance company/employer/lawyer or their representative.

I, _____, understand the conditions and information as
       patient's name

verbally provided and voluntarily give my consent to the above authorizations.

_____   _____   _____
    date   signature   witness

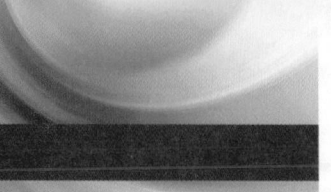

CHAPTER 2

Head and Face

Casualty officers and clinicians working in emergency care settings are often the ones who assess the head and face. In these settings, the assessment involves the bony aspects of the head and face as well as the soft tissues. The soft-tissue assessment involves primarily the sensory organs, such as the skin, eyes, nose, and ears, whereas the muscles are tested only as they relate to injury to these structures. Joints and their integrity are not the main objects of the assessment. Because the temporomandibular joints and cervical spine are discussed in Chapters 3 and 4, this chapter deals with only the head, the face, and their associated structures.

APPLIED ANATOMY

The head and face are made up of the cranial vault and facial bones. The **cranial vault,** or skull, is composed of several bones: one frontal, two sphenoid, two parietal, two temporal, and one occipital (Figure 2-1). Of these, the strongest is the occipital bone, and the weakest are the temporal bones. The frontal bone forms the forehead, and the temporal and sphenoid bones form the antero-lateral walls of the skull, or the temples of the head. The parietal bones form the top and posterolateral portions of the skull, and the occipital bones form the posterior portion of the skull. The cranial vault reaches 90% of its ultimate size by age 5.

In addition to the cranial vault bones, there are 14 **facial bones.** These bones develop more slowly than the cranial bones, reaching only 60% of their ultimate size by age 6. The facial skeleton is composed of the mandible, which forms the lower jaw; the maxilla, which forms the upper jaw on each side; the nasal bones, which form the bridge of the nose; and the palatine, lacrimal, zygomatic, and ethmoid bones, which form the remainder of the face. It is the zygomatic bone that gives the cheek its prominence. The sphenoid bones also form part of the orbital cavity. The facial skull has several cavities for the eyes (orbital), nose (nasal), and mouth (oral), as well as spaces for nerves and blood vessels to penetrate the bony structure. Weight is saved in the skull area by the addition of sinus cavities (Figure 2-2).

The muscles of the head and face are controlled primarily by the 12 **cranial nerves.** The cranial nerves and their chief functions are shown in Table 2-1. The cranial nerves generally contain both sensory and motor fibers. However, some cranial nerves are strictly sensory (olfactory and optic), whereas others are strictly motor (oculomotor, trochlear, and hypoglossal).

The **external eye** is composed of the eyelids (upper and lower), conjunctiva (a transparent membrane covering the cornea, iris, pupil, lens, and sclera), lacrimal gland, eye muscles, and bony skull orbit (Figure 2-3). Muscles of the eye, their actions, and their nerve supply are shown in Table 2-2. The muscles and movements of the eye are shown in Figure 2-4. To produce some of the actions, the various muscles of the eye must work in concert. The **eyelids** protect the eye from foreign bodies, distribute tears over the surface of the eye, and limit the amount of light entering the eye. The **conjunctiva** is a thin membrane covering the majority of the anterior surface of the eye. It helps to protect the eye from foreign bodies and desiccation (drying up). The lacrimal gland provides tears, which keep the eye moist (Figure 2-5). The eye itself is made up of the sclera, cornea, and iris as well as the lens and retina (Figure 2-6). The **sclera** is the dense white portion of the eye that physically supports the internal structures. The **cornea** is very sensitive to pain (e.g., the extreme pain that accompanies corneal abrasion) and separates the watery fluid of the anterior chamber of the eye from the external environment. It permits transmission of light through the lens to the retina. The **iris** is a circular, contractile muscular disc that controls the amount of light entering the eye and contains pigmented cells that give color to the eye. The **lens** is a crystalline structure located immediately behind the iris that permits images from varied distances to be focused on the retina. It is primarily the lens and its supporting ligaments that separate the eye into chambers: the anterior chamber (aqueous humor) and the posterior chamber (vitreous humor). Finally, the **retina** is the primary sensory structure of the eye that transforms light impulses into electrical impulses that are then transmitted by the optic nerve to the brain, which interprets the impulses as the objects seen.

The **external ear** consists of cartilage covered with skin. Its primary purpose is to direct sound and to protect the external auditory meatus, through which sound is transmitted to the eardrum. The external ear, which is sometimes called the *pinna, auricle,* or *trumpet,* consists

APPENDIX 1-2

Example of Informed Consent/Patient Authorization

PATIENT AUTHORIZATION

I hereby authorize and grant permission to _____,

a _____, to carry out any assessment and examination, procedures, and
occupation

treatments as may be necessary to assess and treat my condition or injury.

The above-named _____ has agreed to provide me with understandable:
occupation

information on:

- my diagnosis, as known
- the treatment being suggested
- significant risks, benefits of treatment, and possible alternatives to this treatment
- reasonable additional procedures which may be necessary
- the potential risks of foregoing the suggested care

I hereby authorize and grant permission to the above-named _____ to
occupation

communicate with any health care professional that rehabilitation of my condition may indicate.

I hereby authorize and grant permission to the above-named _____ to
occupation

release information regarding my condition and my ability to return to normal activity or work to my

insurance company/employer/lawyer or their representative.

I, _____, understand the conditions and information as
patient's name

verbally provided and voluntarily give my consent to the above authorizations.

_____   _____   _____
date   signature   witness

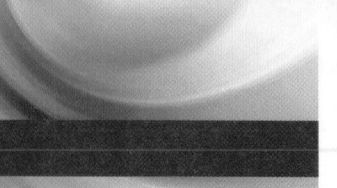

Head and Face

Casualty officers and clinicians working in emergency care settings are often the ones who assess the head and face. In these settings, the assessment involves the bony aspects of the head and face as well as the soft tissues. The soft-tissue assessment involves primarily the sensory organs, such as the skin, eyes, nose, and ears, whereas the muscles are tested only as they relate to injury to these structures. Joints and their integrity are not the main objects of the assessment. Because the temporomandibular joints and cervical spine are discussed in Chapters 3 and 4, this chapter deals with only the head, the face, and their associated structures.

APPLIED ANATOMY

The head and face are made up of the cranial vault and facial bones. The **cranial vault,** or skull, is composed of several bones: one frontal, two sphenoid, two parietal, two temporal, and one occipital (Figure 2-1). Of these, the strongest is the occipital bone, and the weakest are the temporal bones. The frontal bone forms the forehead, and the temporal and sphenoid bones form the anterolateral walls of the skull, or the temples of the head. The parietal bones form the top and posterolateral portions of the skull, and the occipital bones form the posterior portion of the skull. The cranial vault reaches 90% of its ultimate size by age 5.

In addition to the cranial vault bones, there are 14 **facial bones.** These bones develop more slowly than the cranial bones, reaching only 60% of their ultimate size by age 6. The facial skeleton is composed of the mandible, which forms the lower jaw; the maxilla, which forms the upper jaw on each side; the nasal bones, which form the bridge of the nose; and the palatine, lacrimal, zygomatic, and ethmoid bones, which form the remainder of the face. It is the zygomatic bone that gives the cheek its prominence. The sphenoid bones also form part of the orbital cavity. The facial skull has several cavities for the eyes (orbital), nose (nasal), and mouth (oral), as well as spaces for nerves and blood vessels to penetrate the bony structure. Weight is saved in the skull area by the addition of sinus cavities (Figure 2-2).

The muscles of the head and face are controlled primarily by the 12 **cranial nerves.** The cranial nerves and their chief functions are shown in Table 2-1. The cranial

nerves generally contain both sensory and motor fibers. However, some cranial nerves are strictly sensory (olfactory and optic), whereas others are strictly motor (oculomotor, trochlear, and hypoglossal).

The **external eye** is composed of the eyelids (upper and lower), conjunctiva (a transparent membrane covering the cornea, iris, pupil, lens, and sclera), lacrimal gland, eye muscles, and bony skull orbit (Figure 2-3). Muscles of the eye, their actions, and their nerve supply are shown in Table 2-2. The muscles and movements of the eye are shown in Figure 2-4. To produce some of the actions, the various muscles of the eye must work in concert. The **eyelids** protect the eye from foreign bodies, distribute tears over the surface of the eye, and limit the amount of light entering the eye. The **conjunctiva** is a thin membrane covering the majority of the anterior surface of the eye. It helps to protect the eye from foreign bodies and desiccation (drying up). The lacrimal gland provides tears, which keep the eye moist (Figure 2-5). The eye itself is made up of the sclera, cornea, and iris as well as the lens and retina (Figure 2-6). The **sclera** is the dense white portion of the eye that physically supports the internal structures. The **cornea** is very sensitive to pain (e.g., the extreme pain that accompanies corneal abrasion) and separates the watery fluid of the anterior chamber of the eye from the external environment. It permits transmission of light through the lens to the retina. The **iris** is a circular, contractile muscular disc that controls the amount of light entering the eye and contains pigmented cells that give color to the eye. The **lens** is a crystalline structure located immediately behind the iris that permits images from varied distances to be focused on the retina. It is primarily the lens and its supporting ligaments that separate the eye into chambers: the anterior chamber (aqueous humor) and the posterior chamber (vitreous humor). Finally, the **retina** is the primary sensory structure of the eye that transforms light impulses into electrical impulses that are then transmitted by the optic nerve to the brain, which interprets the impulses as the objects seen.

The **external ear** consists of cartilage covered with skin. Its primary purpose is to direct sound and to protect the external auditory meatus, through which sound is transmitted to the eardrum. The external ear, which is sometimes called the *pinna, auricle,* or *trumpet,* consists

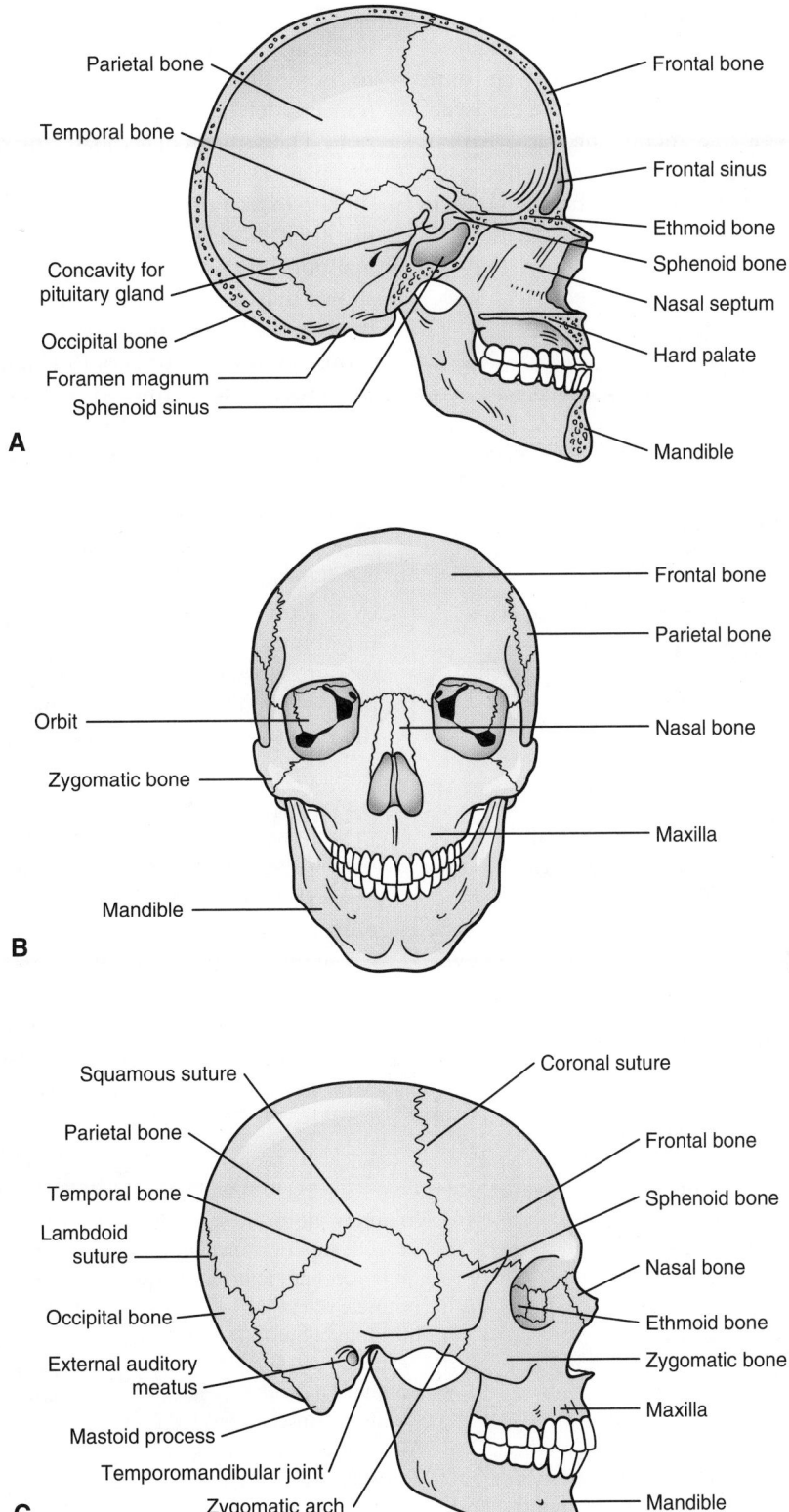

Figure 2-1 Bones of the head and face. A, Interior view. **B,** Anterior view. **C,** Lateral view. (Redrawn from Jenkins DB: Hollinshead's functional anatomy of the limbs and back, Philadelphia, 1991, WB Saunders, pp. 332–333.)

of the helix and lobule around the outside and the triangular fossa, antihelix, concha, tragus (a cartilaginous projection anterior to external auditory meatus), and antitragus on the inside (Figure 2-7). The **middle ear** structures consist of the tympanic membrane, or eardrum, which vibrates when sound hits it and sends vibrations through the ossicles—called the *malleus* (hammer), *incus* (anvil), and *stapes* (stirrup)—to the cochlea. The cochlea, which is part of the inner ear, transmits the sound waves to the vestibulocochlear nerve (cranial nerve VIII), which transmits electrical impulses to the brain for interpretation. The semicircular canals, the other part of the inner ear, play a significant role in maintaining balance.

The **external nose,** like the external ear, consists primarily of cartilage covered with skin. However, its proximal portion contains bone covered with skin. Figure 2-8 shows the bone and cartilage makeup of the nose. The floor of the nose consists of the hard and soft palates and forms the roof of the mouth (Figure 2-9). Cartilage and the nasal, frontal, ethmoid, and sphenoid bones form the roof of the nose. The frontal and maxillary bones form the nasal bridge. Three bony structures called *turbinates* (superior, middle, and inferior) form the lateral aspects of the nose, which increase the surface area of the nose and thereby warm, humidify, and filter more of the inspired air. The nose is divided into two chambers (vestibules) by a septum. These chambers are lined with a mucous membrane containing hairs that collect debris and other foreign substances from the inspired air. The cribriform plate of the ethmoid bone contains the sensory fibers of the olfactory nerve (cranial nerve I) for smell.

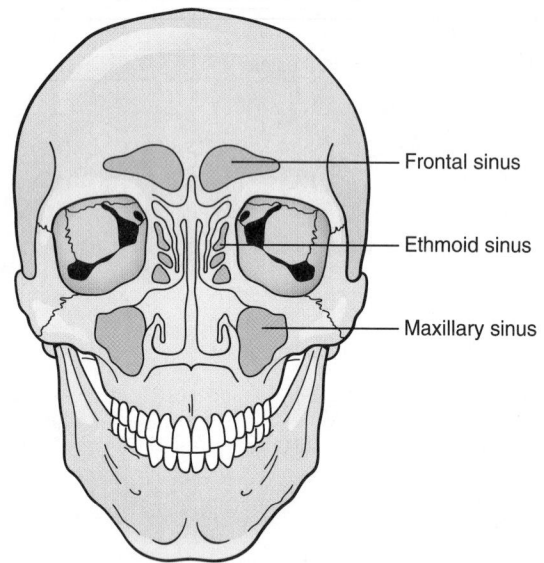

Figure 2-2 The nasal sinuses. (Modified from Swartz HM: Textbook of physical diagnosis, Philadelphia, 1989, WB Saunders, p. 166.)

- Frontal sinus
- Ethmoid sinus
- Maxillary sinus

PATIENT HISTORY

In addition to the questions listed under Patient History in Chapter 1, the examiner should obtain the following

TABLE 2-1

Cranial Nerves and Methods of Testing

Nerve	Afferent (Sensory)	Efferent (Motor)	Test
I. Olfactory	Smell: Nose	—	Identify familiar odors (e.g., chocolate, coffee)
II. Optic	Sight: Eye	—	Test visual fields
III. Oculomotor	—	Voluntary motor: Levator of eyelid; superior, medial, and inferior recti; inferior oblique muscle of eyeball Autonomic: Smooth muscle of eyeball	Upward, downward, and medial gaze Reaction to light
IV. Trochlear		Voluntary motor: Superior oblique muscle of eyeball	Downward and lateral gaze
V. Trigeminal	Touch, pain: Skin of face, mucous membranes of nose, sinuses, mouth, anterior tongue	Voluntary motor: Muscles of mastication	Corneal reflex Face sensation Clench teeth; push down on chin to separate jaws
VI. Abducens		Voluntary motor: Lateral rectus muscle of eyeball	Lateral gaze
VII. Facial	Taste: Anterior tongue	Voluntary motor: Facial muscles Autonomic: Lacrimal, submandibular, and sublingual glands	Close eyes tight Smile and show teeth Whistle and puff cheeks Identify familiar tastes (e.g., sweet, sour)

TABLE **2-1**

Cranial Nerves and Methods of Testing—cont'd

Nerve	Afferent (Sensory)	Efferent (Motor)	Test
VIII. Vestibulocochlear (acoustic nerve)	Hearing: Ear Balance: Ear	—	Hear watch ticking Hearing tests Balance and coordination test
IX. Glossopharyngeal	Touch, pain: Posterior tongue, pharynx Taste: Posterior tongue	Voluntary motor: Unimportant muscle of pharynx Autonomic: Parotid gland	Gag reflex Ability to swallow
X. Vagus	Touch, pain: Pharynx, larynx, bronchi Taste: Tongue, epiglottis	Voluntary motor: Muscles of palate, pharynx, and larynx Autonomic: Thoracic and abdominal viscera	Gag reflex Ability to swallow Say "Ah"
XI. Accessory	—	Voluntary motor: Sternocleidomastoid and trapezius muscle	Resisted shoulder shrug
XII. Hypoglossal	—	Voluntary motor: Muscles of tongue	Tongue protrusion (if injured, tongue deviates toward injured side)

Adapted from Hollinshead WH, Jenkins DB: Functional anatomy of the limbs and back, Philadelphia, 1981, WB Saunders, p. 358; and Reid DC: Sports injury assessment and rehabilitation, New York, 1992, Churchill Livingstone, p. 860.

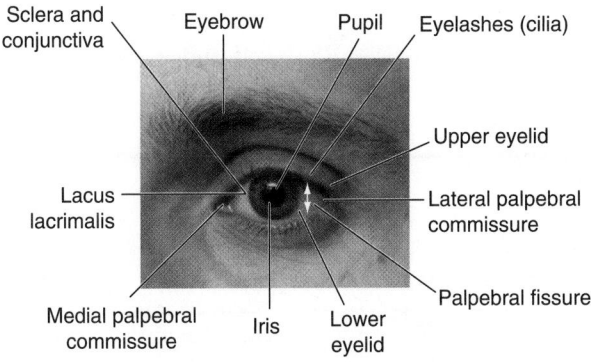

Figure 2-3 External features of the eye.

TABLE **2-2**

Muscles of the Eye: Their Actions and Nerve Supply

Action	Muscles Acting	Nerve Supply
Moves pupil upward	Superior rectus	Oculomotor (CN III)
Moves pupil downward	Inferior rectus	Oculomotor (CN III)
Moves pupil medially	Medial rectus	Oculomotor (CN III)
Moves pupil laterally	Lateral rectus	Abducens (CN VI)
Moves pupil downward and laterally	Superior oblique	Trochlear (CN IV)
Moves pupil upward and laterally	Inferior oblique	Oculomotor (CN III)
Elevates upper eyelid	Levator palpebrae superioris	Oculomotor (CN III)

CN, Cranial nerve.

information from the patient who has sustained an injury to the head or the face:

1. *What happened?* This question determines the mechanism of injury and, potentially, the area of the brain or face injured (Table 2-3). A pathological classification for acute traumatic brain injuries is shown in the box on p. 89.[1] A forceful blow to a resting, movable head usually produces maximum brain injury beneath the point of impact (Figure 2-10). This type of injury, called a **coup injury,** is usually caused by linear or translational acceleration.[2] It often causes focal ischemic lesions, especially in the cerebellum, leading to alterations in smooth, coordinated movements, equilibrium, and posture. If the head is moving and strikes an unyielding object, such as the ground, maximum brain injury is usually sustained in an area opposite the site of impact.

This **contrecoup injury** is the result of impact deceleration. The injury occurs on the side of the head opposite to that receiving the blow, because the

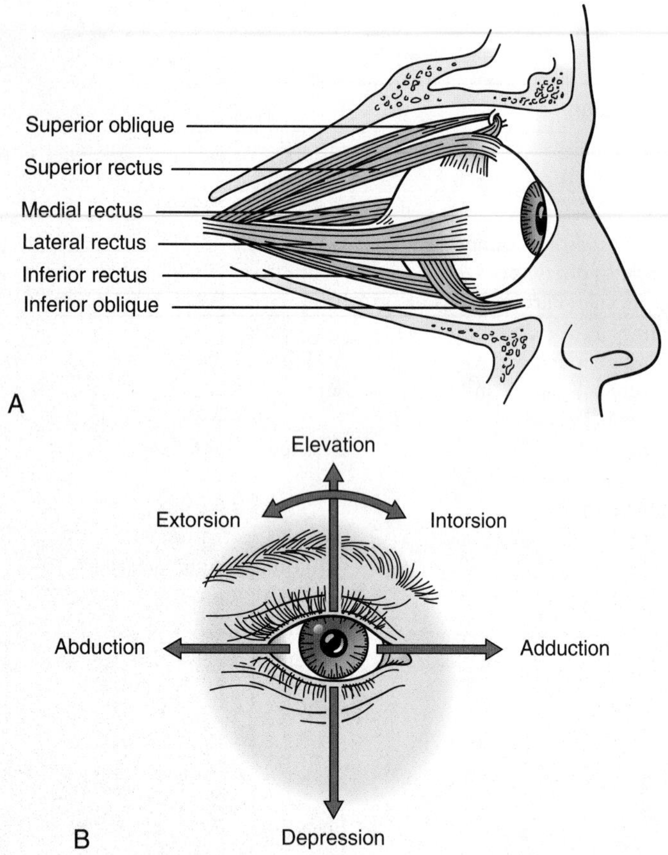

Superior oblique
Superior rectus
Medial rectus
Lateral rectus
Inferior rectus
Inferior oblique

A

Lacrimal gland

Puncta

Tear sac

Nasolacrimal duct

Canaliculi

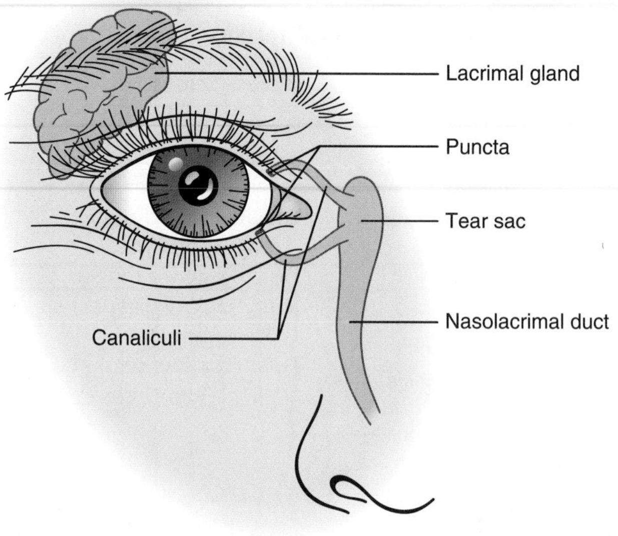

Figure 2-5 The lacrimal apparatus. (Modified from Swartz HM: Textbook of physical diagnosis, Philadelphia, 1989, WB Saunders, p. 126.)

Elevation

Extorsion   Intorsion

Abduction   Adduction

B   Depression

Figure 2-4 Muscles (**A**) and movements (**B**) of the eye. (Modified from Swartz HM: Textbook of physical diagnosis, Philadelphia, 1989, WB Saunders, pp. 125–126.)

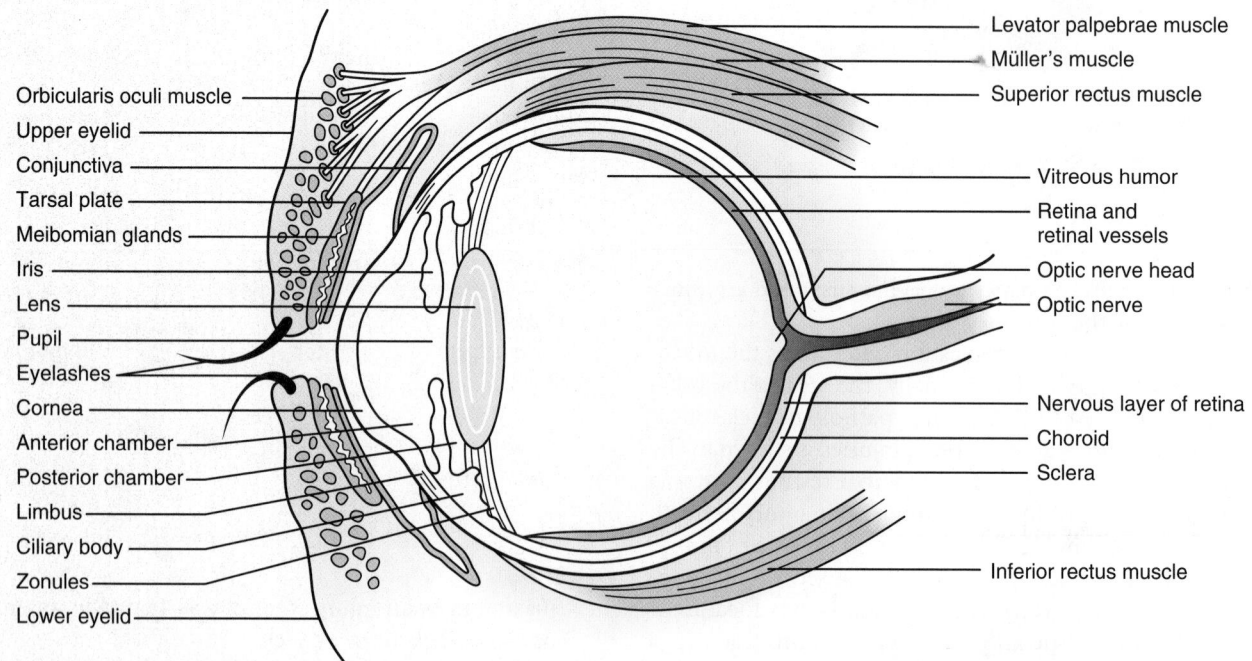

Orbicularis oculi muscle
Upper eyelid
Conjunctiva
Tarsal plate
Meibomian glands
Iris
Lens
Pupil
Eyelashes
Cornea
Anterior chamber
Posterior chamber
Limbus
Ciliary body
Zonules
Lower eyelid

Levator palpebrae muscle
Müller's muscle
Superior rectus muscle

Vitreous humor
Retina and retinal vessels
Optic nerve head
Optic nerve

Nervous layer of retina
Choroid
Sclera

Inferior rectus muscle

Figure 2-6 Cross section of the eye. (Modified from Swartz HM: Textbook of physical diagnosis, Philadelphia, 1989, WB Saunders, p. 132.)

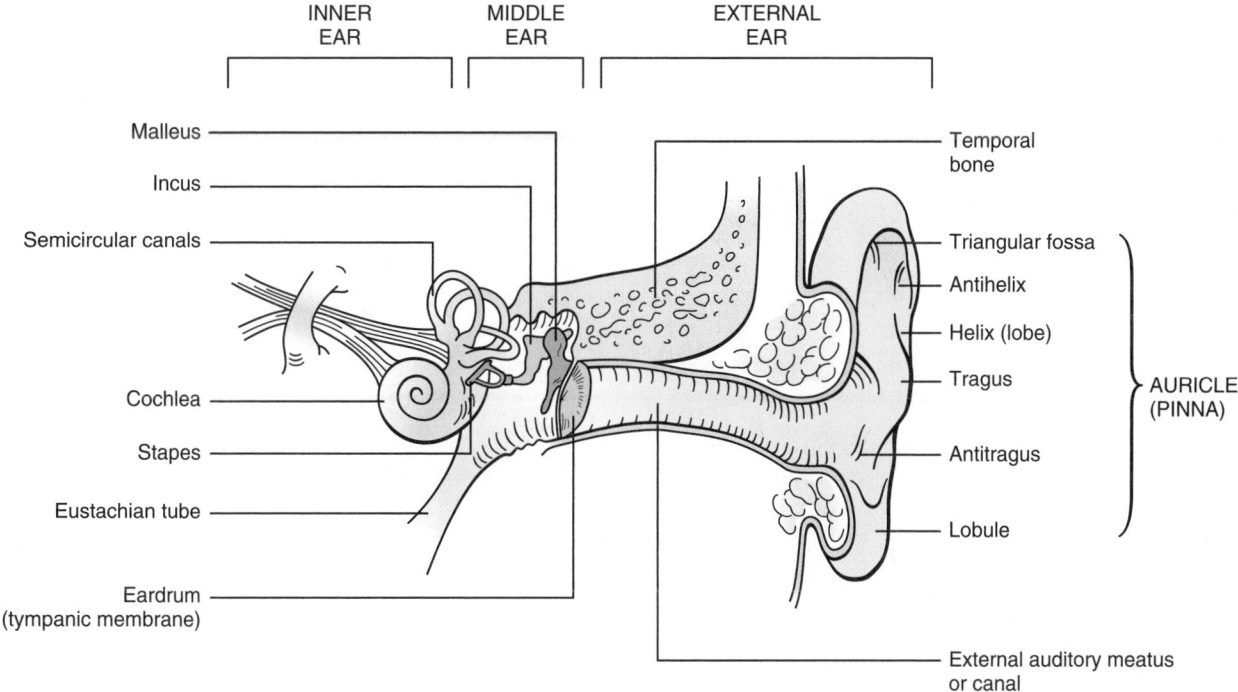

Figure 2-7 A cross-sectional view through the ear.

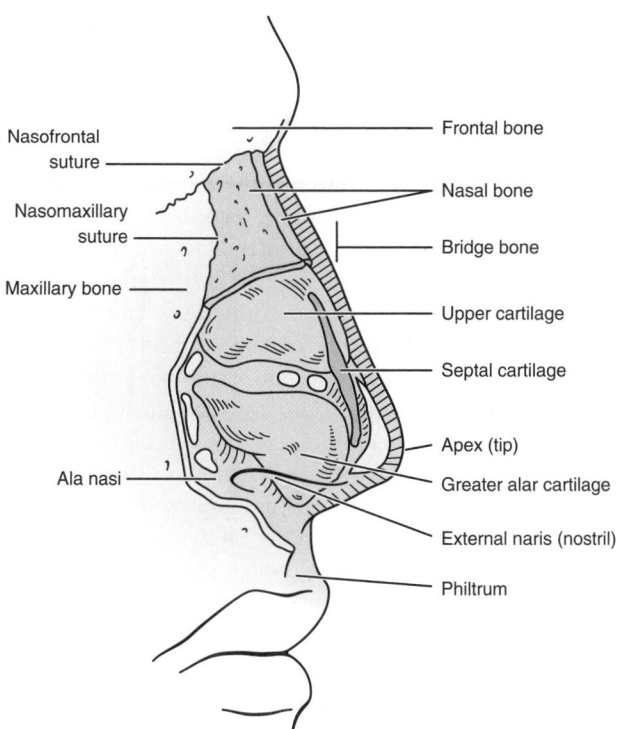

Figure 2-8 The bony and cartilaginous structures of the nose.

Pathological Classification of Acute Traumatic Brain Injury

- Diffuse brain injury
  - Cerebral concussion
  - Diffuse axonal injury
- Focal brain injury
  - Epidural hematoma
  - Subdural hematoma
  - Cerebral contusion
  - Intracerebral hemorrhage
  - Subarachnoid hemorrhage
  - Intraventricular hemorrhage
- Skull fracture
- Penetrating brain injury

Modified from Jordan BD: Brain injury in boxing. Clin Sports Med 28:561–578, 2009.

point of impact. Because of the lack of cushioning on the trailing edge, greater injury is likely to occur to the brain on the side opposite the impact. The brain may also experience a "shaking" caused by repeated reverberation within the brain after the head has been struck. This type of injury often results in the signs and symptoms of a concussion with the degree of the concussion depending on the severity of the injury (Table 2-4). Concussion severity is only determined after signs and symptoms have disappeared and any neurological and cognitive testing is normal.[3] If the cervical spine is taken beyond its normal range of

head is accelerating before impact, which squeezes the cerebrospinal fluid away from the trailing edge (the side away from the impact). The fluid moves toward the impact side, thereby thickening the cerebrospinal fluid and offering a cushioning effect at the

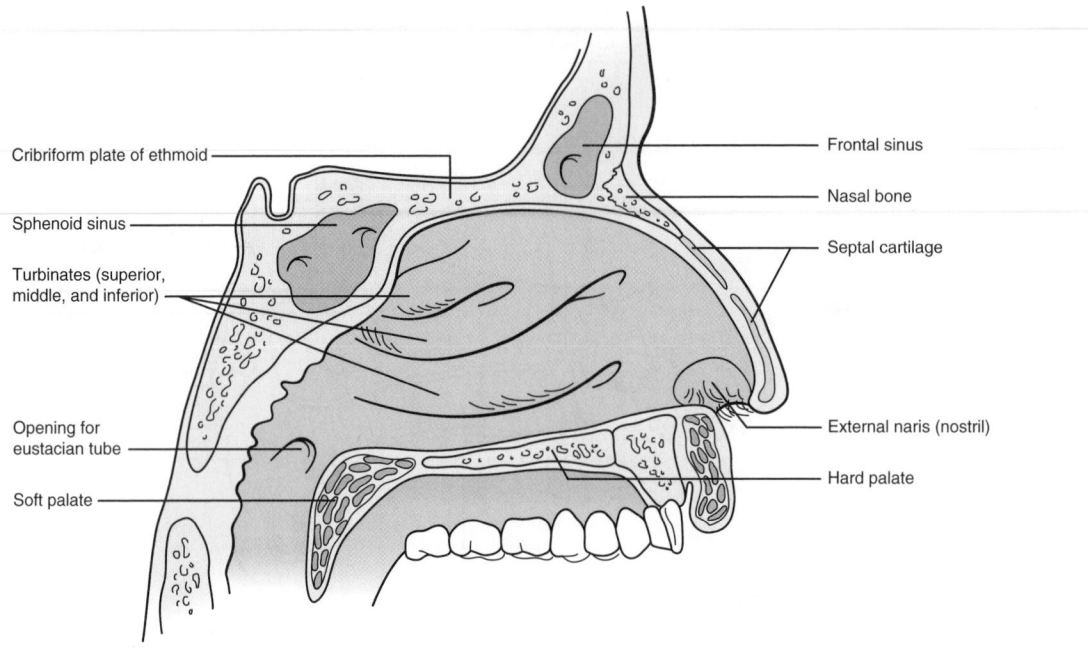

Figure 2-9 Cross section of the nose and nasopharynx.

TABLE **2-3**

Areas of the Brain and Their Function

Area of the Brain	Function
Cerebrum	Cognitive aspects of motor control Memory Sensory awareness (e.g., pain, touch) Speech Special senses (e.g., taste, vision)
Cerebellum	Coordinate and integrate motor behavior Balance Motor learning Motor control (muscle contraction and force production)
Diencephalon (thalamus)	Regulation of body temperature and water balance Control of emotions Information processing to cerebrum
Brain stem	Control of respiratory and heart rates Peripheral blood flow control

motion, especially into rotation or side flexion, there may be a twisting of the cerebral hemisphere, brain stem, carotid artery, or carotid sinus that can result in injury to these structures or ischemia to the brain. Those areas of the brain that are most susceptible to damage include the temporal lobes, anterior frontal lobe, posterior occipital lobe, and upper portion of the midbrain.[4]

2. *Did the patient lose consciousness? If so, how long was the patient unconscious? Has the patient suffered a*

concussion before? These questions are often difficult for the patient to answer or the examiner to know, because the patient may have been momentarily stunned and the time may have been so short that the patient believed there was no loss of consciousness. In other words, loss of consciousness may have been only momentary or, more traditionally, it may have lasted seconds to minutes. If the examiner is working with a sports team, accurate records are essential to record the severity (see later discussion) and the number of concussions suffered by the athlete and to ensure that proper care is instituted so that the athlete is not allowed to return to competition too soon. A **concussion** (a subset of mild traumatic brain injury) is a pathophysiological process that affects the brain and is caused by direct or indirect biomechanical forces. At present, there is no known threshold for a consussion.[5–8] Risk factors are shown in Table 2-5,[9] and stages of concussion are shown in Table 2-6.[10] Signs and symptoms of concussions are shown in Table 2-7.[11–13] Women appear to be more susceptible to concussions than men,[14] and traumatic brain injury is different in children than adults.[9,15,16] Concussions can result from a blow to the head or jaw or a fall on the buttocks from a height and can result in an inability to process information. Their effect is cumulative, and the risk of having another concussion following an initial concussion is four to six times greater than someone who has not had a concussion.[12,17] Concussions can lead to continued and severe problems (e.g., post-concussion syndrome, second-impact syndrome).[10,12,17–20] To be maximally effective, athletes should have done baseline tests in their

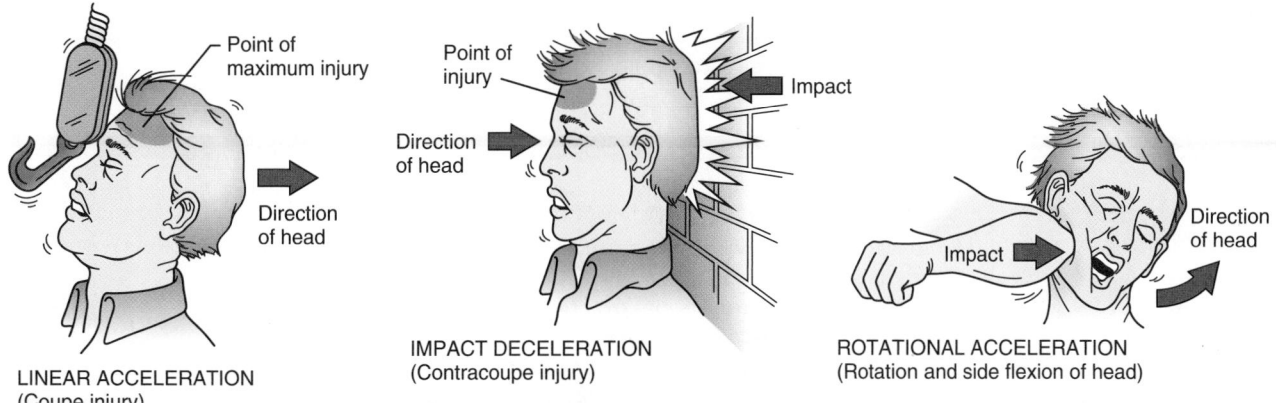

Figure 2-10 Mechanisms of injury to the brain.

TABLE **2-4**

Signs and Symptoms* of Concussion (Torg Classification)

	Grade 1	Grade 2	Grade 3	Grade 4	Grade 5
Confusion	None or momentary	Slight	Moderate	Severe	Severe
Amnesia	No	Posttraumatic amnesia <30 min	Posttraumatic amnesia <30 min Retrograde amnesia	Posttraumatic amnesia >30 min Retrograde amnesia	Posttraumatic amnesia >24 hours Retrograde anmesia
Residual symptoms	No	Perhaps	Sometimes	Yes	Yes
Loss of consciousness	No	No	No	Yes (<5 min)	Yes (>5 min)
Tinnitus	No	Mild	Moderate	Severe	Often severe
Dizziness	No	Mild	Moderate	Severe	Usually severe
Headache	No	May be present (dull)	Often	Often	Often
Disorientation and unsteadiness	None or minimal	Some	Moderate	Severe (5 to 10 min)	Often severe (>10 min)
Blurred vision	No	No	No	Not usually	Possible
Post-concussion syndrome	No	Possible	Possible	Possible	Possible
Personality changes	No	No	No	Possible	Possible

Data from Vegso JJ, Torg JS: Field evaluation and management of intracranial injuries. In Torg JS, editor: Athletic injuries to the head, neck and face, St Louis, 1991, Mosby, pp. 226–227.
*These signs and symptoms should only be used as a guide in acute situations.

pre-participation evaluation and have an extensive concussion history taken covering somatic, neurobehavioral, and cognitive symptoms (Table 2-8).[3,12,21-26] In 2012, the International Conference on Concussion in Sport updated a Sideline Concussion Assessment Tool—3rd edition (SCAT3) (Figure 2-11) and added the Sport Concussion Assessment Tool for children ages 5 to 12 years (Child-SCAT3)[8] (Figure 2-12). Kelly and Rosenberg[12,13] have developed a Standardized Assessment of Concussion (SAC) (Figure 2-13),[27,28] which provides a concise

evaluation method for concussion by including measures of orientation, immediate memory, concentration, delayed recall, and other parameters. Lovell and Burke have developed a similar form for ice hockey.[29]

These tests are often combined with computerized neurocognitive testing to try to predict how long recovery will take.[30,31] Ideally, this neurocognitive testing should be done individually at preseason evaluations to establish a baseline and should be updated every 2 years.[32,33] If pre-injury values are not available, normative data may be used.[34] An

TABLE 2-5

Risk Factors That May Prolong or Complicate Recovery from Concussion

Factors	Modifier
Symptoms	Number of concussions Duration of symptoms (>10 days) Severity (intensity and duration)
Signs	Prolonged loss of consciousness (>1 min), amnesia (anterograde and/or retrograde)
Sequelae	Concussive convulsions
Temporal	Frequency—repeated concussions over time Timing—injuries close together in time "Recency"—recent concussion or traumatic brain injury
Threshold	Repeated concussions occurring with progressively less impact force or slower recovery after each successive concussion
Age	Child and adolescent (<18-years-old) may recover slower
Co- and pre-morbidities	Migraine Depression or other mental health disorders Attention deficit hyperactivity disorder Learning disabilities Sleep disorders
Medication	Psychoactive drugs Anticoagulants
Behavior	Dangerous style of play
Sport	High risk activity Contact and collision sport High sporting level

Modified from McCrory P, Meeuwisse W, Johnston K, et al: Consensus statement on concussion in sport—The 3rd International Conference on Concussion in Sport held in Zurich, November 2008. Clin J Sport Med 19(3):189, 2009.

TABLE 2-6

Severity Stages of Concussive Injury

Acute Concussion	Post-Concussion Syndrome	Prolonged Post-Concussion Syndrome	Chronic Traumatic Encephalopathy
• **Physical (somatic) symptoms:** Headache, dizziness, hearing loss, balance difficulty, sleep disturbances, nausea/vomiting, sensitivity to light or noise, diminished athletic performance • **Cognitive deficits:** Loss of short-term memory (anterograde and/or retrograde), difficulty with focus or concentration, confusion, loss of consciousness, disorientation, inability to focus, delayed verbal and/or motor responses, excessive drowsiness, decreased attention, diminished work or school performance • **Emotional (affective) disturbances:** Irritability, anger, fear, mood swings, decreased libido	• Persistent concussion symptoms • Usually lasting 1 to 6 weeks after MTBI • Self-limiting	• Symptoms lasting over 6 months • Lowered concussion threshold • Diminished athletic performance • Diminished work or school performance	• Latency period (usually 6 to 10 years) • Personality disturbances • Emotional lability • Marriage/personal relationship failures • Depression • Alcohol/substance abuse • Suicide attempt/completion

Modified from Sedney CL, Orphanos J, Bailes JE: When to consider retiring an athlete after sports-related concussion. Clin Sports Med 30(1):189–200, 2011.
MTBI, Mild traumatic brain injury.

TABLE 2-7

Signs and Symptoms of Concussions

Acute	Late (Delayed)
• Lightheadedness • Delayed motor and/or verbal responses • Memory or cognitive dysfunction • Disorientation • Amnesia • Headache • Balance problems/incoordination • Vertigo/dizziness • Concentration difficulties • Loss of consciousness • Blurred vision • Vacant stare (befuddled facial expression) • Photophobia • Tinnitus • Nausea • Vomiting • Increased emotionality • Slurred or incoherent speech	• Persistent low grade headache • Easy fatiguability • Sleep irregularities • Inability to perform daily activities • Depression/anxiety • Lethargy • Memory dysfunction • Lightheadedness • Personality changes • Low frustration tolerance/irritability • Intolerance to bright lights, loud sounds

TABLE 2-8

Concussion Symptoms

Somatic	Neurobehavioral	Cognitive
• Headache • Nausea • Vomiting • Balance problems • Light/sound sensitivity • Numbness/tingling • Dizziness	• Sleeping more or less than usual • Drowsiness • Fatigue • Sadness • Nervousness • Trouble falling asleep	• Feeling "slowed down" • Feeling "in a fog" • Concentration difficulty • Remembering difficulty • Confusion • Amnesia (anterograde and/or retrograde) • Loss of consciousness • Inability to focus • Delayed motor and verbal responses • Excessive drowsiness

Data from Piland SG, Motl RW, Guskiewicz KM, et al: Structural validity of a self-report concussion-related symptoms scale, Med Sci Sports Exerc 38(1):27–32, 2006; Herring SA, Cantu RC, Guskiewicz KM, et al: Concussion (mild traumatic brain injury) and the team physician: a consensus statement—2011 update. Med Sci Sports Exerc 43(12): 2414, 2011.

example of such a computerized post-concussion assessment is the ImPACT test; ImPACT stands for Immediate Post-Concussion Assessment and Cognitive Testing.[31,32,35–37]

There are several different grading systems for concussions (Table 2-9). It should be pointed out, however, that the International Conference on Concussion in Sport[3] recommended that grade scales be abandoned, because concussion severity can only be determined retrospectively after all signs and symptoms have cleared, the neurological examination is normal, and cognitive function has returned to normal.[38] The conference group felt concussions should be grouped as simple or complex. Simple concussion implies that the injury resolves over 7 to 10 days without complications. Neurophysiological screening does not play a role, but mental status screening is part of the assessment. Complex concussions are those in which persistent symptoms and specific sequelae (i.e., convulsions, loss of consciousness for longer than 1 minute, prolonged cognitive impairment) occur.[3] This includes people with more than one concussion. In this case, neurophysiological testing does play a role.[13,39–42] Table 2-10 shows some neurophysiological tests that could be used for post-concussion assessment.

Grades of concussion, such as those advocated by Torg (see later discussion and Table 2-4), can play a role in the acute phase but should be used with caution if making return to activity decisions.[43] With each grade, the signs and symptoms worsen, and the sequelae are more evident. No signs and symptoms under exertion (i.e., simulating the activity the person will return to) should be evident, even with simple concussions.

With a **grade I concussion,** the patient is slightly confused and may have a dazed look. The patient is completely lucid within 5 to 15 minutes; has no amnesia, sequelae, or residual symptoms; and has had no loss of consciousness. Some people refer to the grade I concussion as the patient's having his or her "bell rung."

With a **grade II concussion,** there is slight confusion, and posttraumatic amnesia becomes evident. **Posttraumatic (anterograde) amnesia** is the loss of memory for events occurring immediately after wakening or from the moment of injury. Posttraumatic amnesia is considered to be the length of time from injury until conscious memory returns. In the acute state, it may take time for posttraumatic amnesia to become obvious. Sometimes, the patient will remember what happened immediately after the injury, but as time goes on (up to 1 to 2 hours after the injury), posttraumatic amnesia becomes evident. This is one of the reasons it is advisable to reassess acute head

Text continued on p. 102

SCAT3™

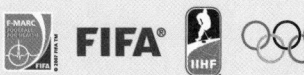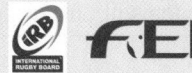

Sport Concussion Assessment Tool – 3rd Edition

For use by medical professionals only

Name	Date/Time of Injury:	Examiner:
	Date of Assessment:	

What is the SCAT3?[1]

The SCAT3 is a standardized tool for evaluating injured athletes for concussion and can be used in athletes aged from 13 years and older. It supersedes the original SCAT and the SCAT2 published in 2005 and 2009, respectively.[2] For younger persons, ages 12 and under, please use the Child SCAT3. The SCAT3 is designed for use by medical professionals. If you are not qualified, please use the Sport Concussion Recognition Tool.[1] Preseason baseline testing with the SCAT3 can be helpful for interpreting post-injury test scores.

Specific instructions for use of the SCAT3 are provided on page 3. If you are not familiar with the SCAT3, please read through these instructions carefully. This tool may be freely copied in its current form for distribution to individuals, teams, groups and organizations. Any revision or any reproduction in a digital form requires approval by the Concussion in Sport Group.
NOTE: The diagnosis of a concussion is a clinical judgment, ideally made by a medical professional. The SCAT3 should not be used solely to make, or exclude, the diagnosis of concussion in the absence of clinical judgment. An athlete may have a concussion even if their SCAT3 is "normal."

What is a concussion?

A concussion is a disturbance in brain function caused by a direct or indirect force to the head. It results in a variety of non-specific signs and/or symptoms (some examples listed below) and most often does not involve loss of consciousness. Concussion should be suspected in the presence of **any one or more** of the following:

- Symptoms (e.g., headache), or
- Physical signs (e.g., unsteadiness), or
- Impaired brain function (e.g. confusion) or
- Abnormal behavior (e.g., change in personality).

SIDELINE ASSESSMENT

Indications for Emergency Management

NOTE: A hit to the head can sometimes be associated with a more serious brain injury. Any of the following warrants consideration of activating emergency procedures and urgent transportation to the nearest hospital:

- Glasgow Coma score less than 15
- Deteriorating mental status
- Potential spinal injury
- Progressive, worsening symptoms or new neurologic signs

Potential signs of concussion?

If any of the following signs are observed after a direct or indirect blow to the head, the athlete should stop participation, be evaluated by a medical professional, and **should not be permitted to return to sport the same day** if a concussion is suspected.

Any loss of consciousness?		Y N
"If so, how long?"		
Balance or motor incoordination (stumbles, slow/labored movements, etc.)?		Y N
Disorientation or confusion (inability to respond appropriately to questions)?		Y N
Loss of memory:		Y N
"If so, how long?"		
"Before or after the injury?"		
Blank or vacant look:		Y N
Visible facial injury in combination with any of the above:		Y N

1 Glasgow Coma Scale (GCS)

Best eye response (E)

No eye opening	1
Eye opening in response to pain	2
Eye opening to speech	3
Eyes opening spontaneously	4

Best verbal response (V)

No verbal response	1
Incomprehensible sounds	2
Inappropriate words	3
Confused	4
Oriented	5

Best motor response (M)

No motor response	1
Extension to pain	2
Abnormal flexion to pain	3
Flexion/withdrawal to pain	4
Localizes to pain	5
Obeys commands	6
Glasgow Coma Score (E + V + M)	of 15

GCS should be recorded for all athletes in case of subsequent deterioration.

2 Maddocks Score[3]

"I am going to ask you a few questions. Please listen carefully and give your best effort."
Modified Maddocks questions (1 point for each correct answer)

What venue are we at today?	0	1
Which half is it now?	0	1
Who scored last in this match?	0	1
What team did you play last week/game?	0	1
Did your team win the last game?	0	1
Maddocks score		of 5

Maddocks score is validated for sideline diagnosis of concussion only and is not used for serial testing.

Notes: Mechanism of Injury ("Tell me what happened"?):

_____

_____

_____

_____

Any athlete with a suspected concussion should be REMOVED FROM PLAY, medically assessed, monitored for deterioration (i.e., should not be left alone) and should not drive a motor vehicle until cleared to do so by a medical professional. No athlete diagnosed with concussion should be returned to sports participation on the day of injury.

Figure 2-11 Sport Concussion Assessment Tool—3rd edition (SCAT3). (© 2013 Concussion in Sport Group. Br J Sports Med 47:259–262, 2013.)

BACKGROUND

Name: _____ Date: _____

Examiner: _____

Sport/team/school: _____ Date/time of injury: _____

Age: _____ Gender: ☐ M ☐ F

Years of education completed: _____

Dominant hand: ☐ right ☐ left ☐ neither

How many concussions do you think you have had in the past? _____

When was the most recent concussion? _____

How long was your recovery from the most recent concussion? _____

Have you ever been hospitalized or had medical imaging done for a head injury? ☐ Y ☐ N

Have you ever been diagnosed with headaches or migraines? ☐ Y ☐ N

Do you have a learning disability, dyslexia, ADD/ADHD? ☐ Y ☐ N

Have you ever been diagnosed with depression, anxiety or other psychiatric disorder? ☐ Y ☐ N

Has anyone in your family ever been diagnosed with any of these problems? ☐ Y ☐ N

Are you on any medications? If yes, please list: ☐ Y ☐ N

SCAT3 to be done in resting state. Best done 10 or more minutes post excercise.

SYMPTOM EVALUATION

3 How do you feel?

"You should score yourself on the following symptoms, based on how you feel now."

	none		mild		moderate		severe
Headache	0	1	2	3	4	5	6
"Pressure in head"	0	1	2	3	4	5	6
Neck pain	0	1	2	3	4	5	6
Nausea or vomiting	0	1	2	3	4	5	6
Dizziness	0	1	2	3	4	5	6
Blurred vision	0	1	2	3	4	5	6
Balance problems	0	1	2	3	4	5	6
Sensitivity to light	0	1	2	3	4	5	6
Sensitivity to noise	0	1	2	3	4	5	6
Feeling slowed down	0	1	2	3	4	5	6
Feeling like "in a fog"	0	1	2	3	4	5	6
"Don't feel right"	0	1	2	3	4	5	6
Difficulty concentrating	0	1	2	3	4	5	6
Difficulty remembering	0	1	2	3	4	5	6
Fatigue or low energy	0	1	2	3	4	5	6
Confusion	0	1	2	3	4	5	6
Drowsiness	0	1	2	3	4	5	6
Trouble falling asleep	0	1	2	3	4	5	6
More emotional	0	1	2	3	4	5	6
Irritability	0	1	2	3	4	5	6
Sadness	0	1	2	3	4	5	6
Nervous or anxious	0	1	2	3	4	5	6

Total number of symptoms (Maximum possible 22) _____

Symptom severity score (Maximum possible 132) _____

Do the symptoms get worse with physical activity? ☐ Y ☐ N

Do the symptoms get worse with mental activity? ☐ Y ☐ N

☐ self rated ☐ self rated and clinician monitored

☐ clinician interview ☐ self rated with parent input

Overall rating: If you know the athlete well prior to the injury, how different is the athlete acting compared to his/her usual self?

Please circle one response:

no different	very different	unsure	N/A

Scoring on the SCAT3 should not be used as a stand-alone method to diagnose concussion, measure recovery, or make decisions about an athlete's readiness to return to competition after concussion. Since signs and symptoms may evolve over time, it is important to consider repeat evaluation in the acute assessment of concussion.

COGNITIVE & PHYSICAL EVALUATION

4 Cognitive assessment
Standardized Assessment of Concussion (SAC) [4]

Orientation (1 point for each correct answer)

What month is it?	0	1
What is the date today?	0	1
What is the day of the week?	0	1
What year is it?	0	1
What time is it right now? (within 1 hour)	0	1
Orientation score		**of 5**

Immediate memory

List	Trial 1	Trial 2	Trial 3	Alternative word list		
elbow	0 1	0 1	0 1	candle	baby	finger
apple	0 1	0 1	0 1	paper	monkey	penny
carpet	0 1	0 1	0 1	sugar	perfume	blanket
saddle	0 1	0 1	0 1	sandwich	sunset	lemon
bubble	0 1	0 1	0 1	wagon	iron	insect
Total						

Immediate memory score total	**of 15**

Concentration: Digits Backward

List	Trial 1	Alternative digit list		
4-9-3	0 1	6-2-9	5-2-6	4-1-5
3-8-1-4	0 1	3-2-7-9	1-7-9-5	4-9-6-8
6-2-9-7-1	0 1	1-5-2-8-6	3-8-5-2-7	6-1-8-4-3
7-1-8-4-6-2	0 1	5-3-9-1-4-8	8-3-1-9-6-4	7-2-4-8-5-6
Total of 4				

Concentration: Month in Reverse Order (1 pt. for entire sequence correct)

Dec-Nov-Oct-Sept-Aug-Jul-Jun-May-Apr-Mar-Feb-Jan	0	1

Concentration score	**of 5**

5 Neck Examination:

Range of motion   Tenderness   Upper and lower limb sensation & strength

Findings: _____

6 Balance examination

Do one or both of the following tests.

Footwear (shoes, barefoot, braces, tape, etc.)

Modified Balance Error Scoring System (BESS) testing [5]

Which foot was tested (i.e., which is the **non-dominant** foot) ☐ Left ☐ Right

Testing surface (hard floor, field, etc.) _____

Condition

Double leg stance:	_____ Errors
Single leg stance (non-dominant foot):	_____ Errors
Tandem stance (non-dominant foot at back):	_____ Errors

And/Or

Tandem gait [6,7]

Time (best of 4 trials): _____ seconds

7 Coordination examination
Upper limb coordination

Which arm was tested: ☐ Left ☐ Right

Coordination score	**of 1**

8 SAC Delayed Recall [4]

Delayed recall score	**of 5**

INSTRUCTIONS

Words in *italics* throughout the SCAT3 are the instructions given to the athlete by the tester.

Symptom Scale

"You should score yourself on the following symptoms, based on how you feel now."

To be completed by the athlete. In situations where the symptom scale is being completed after exercise, it should still be done in a resting state, at least 10 minutes post exercise.

For total number of symptoms, maximum possible is 22.

For symptom severity score, add all scores in table, maximum possible is $22 \times 6 = 132$.

SAC[4]

Immediate Memory

"I am going to test your memory. I will read you a list of words and when I am done, repeat back as many words as you can remember, in any order."

Trials 2 & 3:

"I am going to repeat the same list again. Repeat back as many words as you can remember in any order, even if you said the word before."

Complete all 3 trials regardless of score on trial 1 & 2. Read the words at a rate of one per second. **Score 1 pt. for each correct response.** Total score equals sum across all 3 trials. Do not inform the athlete that delayed recall will be tested.

Concentration

Digits backward

"I am going to read you a string of numbers and when I am done, repeat them back to me backwards, in reverse order of how I read them to you. For example, if I say 7-1-9, you would say 9-1-7."

If correct, go to next string length. If incorrect, read trial 2. **One point possible for each string length.** Stop after incorrect on both trials. The digits should be read at the rate of one per second.

Months in reverse order

"Now tell me the months of the year in reverse order. Start with the last month and go backward. So you'll say December, November ... Go ahead."

1 pt. for entire sequence correct

Delayed Recall

The delayed recall should be performed after completion of the Balance and Coordination Examination.

"Do you remember that list of words I read a few times earlier? Tell me as many words from the list as you can remember in any order."

Score 1 pt. for each correct response

Balance Examination

Modified Balance Error Scoring System (BESS) testing[5]

This balance testing is based on a modified version of the Balance Error Scoring System (BESS).[5] A stopwatch or watch with a second hand is required for this testing.

"I am now going to test your balance. Please take your shoes off, roll up your pant legs above ankle (if applicable), and remove any ankle taping (if applicable). This test will consist of three twenty second tests with different stances."

(a) Double leg stance:

"The first stance is standing with your feet together with your hands on your hips and with your eyes closed. You should try to maintain stability in that position for 20 seconds. I will be counting the number of times you move out of this position. I will start timing when you are set and have closed your eyes."

(b) Single leg stance:

"If you were to kick a ball, which foot would you use? [This will be the dominant foot.] Now stand on your non-dominant foot. The dominant leg should be held in approximately 30 degrees of hip flexion and 45 degrees of knee flexion. Again, you should try to maintain stability for 20 seconds with your hands on your hips and your eyes closed. I will be counting the number of times you move out of this position. If you stumble out of this position, open your eyes and return to the start position and continue balancing. I will start timing when you are set and have closed your eyes."

(c) Tandem stance:

"Now stand heel-to-toe with your non-dominant foot in back. Your weight should be evenly distributed across both feet. Again, you should try to maintain stability for 20 seconds with your hands on your hips and your eyes closed. I will be counting the number of times you move out of this position. If you stumble out of this position, open your eyes and return to the start position and continue balancing. I will start timing when you are set and have closed your eyes."

Balance testing – types of errors

1. Hands lifted off iliac crest
2. Opening eyes
3. Step, stumble, or fall
4. Moving hip into > 30 degrees abduction
5. Lifting forefoot or heel
6. Remaining out of test position > 5 sec

Each of the 20-second trials is scored by counting the errors, or deviations from the proper stance, accumulated by the athlete. The examiner will begin counting errors only after the individual has assumed the proper start position. **The modified BESS is calculated by adding one error point for each error during the three 20-second tests. The maximum total number of errors for any single condition is 10.** If a athlete commits multiple errors simultaneously, only one error is recorded but the athlete should quickly return to the testing position, and counting should resume once subject is set. Subjects that are unable to maintain the testing procedure for a minimum of **five seconds** at the start are assigned the highest possible score, ten, for that testing condition.

OPTION: For further assessment, the same 3 stances can be performed on a surface of medium density foam (e.g., approximately 50 cm x 40 cm x 6 cm).

Tandem Gait[6,7]

Participants are instructed to stand with their feet together behind a starting line (the test is best done with footwear removed). Then, they walk in a forward direction as quickly and as accurately as possible along a 38mm wide (sports tape), 3 meter line with an alternate foot heel-to-toe gait ensuring that they approximate their heel and toe on each step. Once they cross the end of the 3m line, they turn 180 degrees and return to the starting point using the same gait. A total of 4 trials are done and the best time is retained. Athletes should complete the test in 14 seconds. Athletes fail the test if they step off the line, have a separation between their heel and toe, or if they touch or grab the examiner or an object. In this case, the time is not recorded and the trial repeated, if appropriate.

Coordination Examination

Upper limb coordination

Finger-to-nose (FTN) task:

"I am going to test your coordination now. Please sit comfortably on the chair with your eyes open and your arm (either right or left) outstretched (shoulder flexed to 90 degrees and elbow and fingers extended), pointing in front of you. When I give a start signal, I would like you to perform five successive finger to nose repetitions using your index finger to touch the tip of the nose, and then return to the starting position, as quickly and as accurately as possible."

Scoring: 5 correct repetitions in < 4 seconds = 1

Note for testers: Athletes fail the test if they do not touch their nose, do not fully extend their elbow or do not perform five repetitions. **Failure should be scored as 0.**

References & Footnotes

1. This tool has been developed by a group of international experts at the 4th International Consensus meeting on Concussion in Sport held in Zurich, Switzerland in November 2012. The full details of the conference outcomes and the authors of the tool are published in The BJSM Injury Prevention and Health Protection, 2013, Volume 47, Issue 5. The outcome paper will also be simultaneously co-published in other leading biomedical journals with the copyright held by the Concussion in Sport Group, to allow unrestricted distribution, providing no alterations are made.

2. McCrory P et al., Consensus Statement on Concussion in Sport – the 3rd International Conference on Concussion in Sport held in Zurich, November 2008. British Journal of Sports Medicine 2009; 43: i76-89.

3. Maddocks, DL; Dicker, GD; Saling, MM. The assessment of orientation following concussion in athletes. Clinical Journal of Sport Medicine. 1995; 5(1): 32–3.

4. McCrea M. Standardized mental status testing of acute concussion. Clinical Journal of Sport Medicine. 2001; 11: 176–181.

5. Guskiewicz KM. Assessment of postural stability following sport-related concussion. Current Sports Medicine Reports. 2003; 2: 24–30.

6. Schneiders, A.G., Sullivan, S.J., Gray, A., Hammond-Tooke, G. & McCrory, P. Normative values for 16-37 year old subjects for three clinical measures of motor performance used in the assessment of sports concussions. Journal of Science and Medicine in Sport. 2010; 13(2): 196–201.

7. Schneiders, A.G., Sullivan, S.J., Kvarnstrom. J.K., Olsson, M., Yden. T. & Marshall, S.W. The effect of footwear and sports-surface on dynamic neurological screening in sport-related concussion. Journal of Science and Medicine in Sport. 2010; 13(4): 382–386.

Figure 2-11, cont'd

ATHLETE INFORMATION

Any athlete suspected of having a concussion should be removed from play, and then seek medical evaluation.

Signs to watch for

Problems could arise over the first 24–48 hours. The athlete should not be left alone and must go to a hospital at once if they:

- Have a headache that gets worse
- Are very drowsy or can't be awakened
- Can't recognize people or places
- Have repeated vomiting
- Behave unusually or seem confused; are very irritable
- Have seizures (arms and legs jerk uncontrollably)
- Have weak or numb arms or legs
- Are unsteady on their feet; have slurred speech

Remember, it is better to be safe.
Consult your doctor after a suspected concussion.

Return to play

Athletes should not be returned to play the same day of injury.
When returning athletes to play, they should be **medically cleared and then follow a stepwise supervised program,** with stages of progression.

For example:

Rehabilitation stage	Functional exercise at each stage of rehabilitation	Objective of each stage
No activity	Physical and cognitive rest	Recovery
Light aerobic exercise	Walking, swimming or stationary cycling keeping intensity, 70 % maximum predicted heart rate. No resistance training	Increase heart rate
Sport-specific exercise	Skating drills in ice hockey, running drills in soccer. No head impact activities	Add movement
Non-contact training drills	Progression to more complex training drills, eg passing drills in football and ice hockey. May start progressive resistance training	Exercise, coordination, and cognitive load
Full contact practice	Following medical clearance participate in normal training activities	Restore confidence and assess functional skills by coaching staff
Return to play	Normal game play	

There should be at least 24 hours (or longer) for each stage and if symptoms recur the athlete should rest until they resolve once again and then resume the program at the previous asymptomatic stage. Resistance training should only be added in the later stages.

If the athlete is symptomatic for more than 10 days, then consultation by a medical practitioner who is expert in the management of concussion, is recommended.

Medical clearance should be given before return to play.

Scoring Summary:

Test Domain	Score		
	Date:	Date:	Date:
Number of Symptoms of 22			
Symptom Severity Score of 132			
Orientation of 5			
Immediate Memory of 15			
Concentration of 5			
Delayed Recall of 5			
SAC Total			
BESS (total errors)			
Tandem Gait (seconds)			
Coordination of 1			

Notes:

_____

_____

_____

_____

_____

_____

_____

_____

_____

_____

_____

_____

_____

_____

_____

CONCUSSION INJURY ADVICE

(To be given to the **person monitoring** the concussed athlete)

This patient has received an injury to the head. A careful medical examination has been carried out and no sign of any serious complications has been found. Recovery time is variable across individuals and the patient will need monitoring for a further period by a responsible adult. Your treating physician will provide guidance as to this timeframe.

If you notice any change in behavior, vomiting, dizziness, worsening headache, double vision or excessive drowsiness, please contact your doctor or the nearest hospital emergency department immediately.

Other important points:

- Rest (physically and mentally), including training or playing sports until symptoms resolve and you are medically cleared
- No alcohol
- No prescription or non-prescription drugs without medical supervision. Specifically:
  - No sleeping tablets
  - Do not use aspirin, anti-inflammatory medication or sedating pain killers
- Do not drive until medically cleared
- Do not train or play sport until medically cleared

Clinic phone number

Patient's name _____

Date/time of injury _____

Date/time of medical review _____

Treating physician _____

Contact details or stamp

Figure 2-11, cont'd

Child-SCAT3™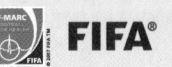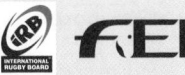

Sport Concussion Assessment Tool for children ages 5 to 12 years

For use by medical professionals only

What is childSCAT3?[1]

The ChildSCAT3 is a standardized tool for evaluating injured children for concussion and can be used in children aged from 5 to 12 years. It supersedes the original SCAT and the SCAT2 published in 2005 and 2009, respectively.[2] For older persons, ages 13 years and over, please use the SCAT3. The ChildSCAT3 is designed for use by medical professionals. If you are not qualified, please use the Sport Concussion Recognition Tool.[1] Preseason baseline testing with the ChildSCAT3 can be helpful for interpreting post-injury test scores.

Specific instructions for use of the ChildSCAT3 are provided on page 3. If you are not familiar with the ChildSCAT3, please read through these instructions carefully. This tool may be freely copied in its current form for distribution to individuals, teams, groups and organizations. Any revision and any reproduction in a digital form require approval by the Concussion in Sport Group.

NOTE: The diagnosis of a concussion is a clinical judgment, ideally made by a medical professional. The ChildSCAT3 should not be used solely to make, or exclude, the diagnosis of concussion in the absence of clinical judgment. An athlete may have a concussion even if their ChildSCAT3 is "normal."

What is a concussion?

A concussion is a disturbance in brain function caused by a direct or indirect force to the head. It results in a variety of non-specific signs and/or symptoms (like those listed below) and most often does not involve loss of consciousness. Concussion should be suspected in the presence of any one or more of the following:

-Symptoms (e.g., headache), or
-Physical signs (e.g., unsteadiness), or
-Impaired brain function (e.g. confusion) or
-Abnormal behavior (e.g., change in personality).

SIDELINE ASSESSMENT

Indications for Emergency Management

NOTE: A hit to the head can sometimes be associated with a more severe brain injury. If the concussed child displays any of the following, then do not proceed with the ChildSCAT3; instead activate emergency procedures and urgent transportation to the nearest hospital:

- Glasgow Coma score less than 15
- Deteriorating mental status
- Potential spinal injury
- Progressive, worsening symptoms or new neurologic signs
- Persistent vomiting
- Evidence of skull fracture
- Post traumatic seizures
- Coagulopathy
- History of Neurosurgery (e.g., Shunt)
- Multiple injuries

1 Glasgow Coma Scale (GCS)

Best eye response (E)

No eye opening	1
Eye opening in response to pain	2
Eye opening to speech	3
Eyes opening spontaneously	4

Best verbal response (V)

No verbal response	1
Incomprehensible sounds	2
Inappropriate words	3
Confused	4
Oriented	5

Best motor response (M)

No motor response	1
Extension to pain	2
Abnormal flexion to pain	3
Flexion/withdrawal to pain	4
Localizes to pain	5
Obeys commands	6
Glasgow Coma Score (E + V + M)	of 15

GCS should be recorded for all athletes in case of subsequent deterioration.

Potential signs of concussion?

If any of the following signs are observed after a direct or indirect blow to the head, the child should stop participation, be evaluated by a medical professional and **should not be permitted to return to sport the same day** if a concussion is suspected.

Any loss of consciousness?	Y	N
"If so, how long?"		
Balance or motor incoordination (stumbles, slow/labored movements, etc.)?	Y	N
Disorientation or confusion (inability to respond appropriately to questions)?	Y	N
Loss of memory:	Y	N
"If so, how long?"		
"Before or after the injury?"		
Blank or vacant look:	Y	N
Visible facial injury in combination with any of the above:	Y	N

2 Sideline Assessment – Child-Maddocks Score[3]

"I am going to ask you a few questions, please listen carefully and give your best effort."

Modified Maddocks questions (1 point for each correct answer)

Where are we at now?	0	1
Is it before or after lunch?	0	1
What did you have last lesson/class?	0	1
What is your teacher's name?	0	1
Child-Maddocks score		of 4

Child-Maddocks score is for sideline diagnosis of concussion only and is not used for serial testing.

Any child with a suspected concussion should be REMOVED FROM PLAY, medically assessed and monitored for deterioration (i.e., should not be left alone). No child diagnosed with concussion should be returned to sports participation on the day of injury.

BACKGROUND

Name:	Date/Time of Injury:
Examiner:	Date of Assessment:
Sport/team/school:	
Age:	Gender: M F
Current school year/grade:	
Dominant hand:	right left neither
Mechanism of Injury ("Tell me what happened"?):	

For parent/carer to complete:

How many concussions has the child had in the past?		
When was the most recent concussion?		
How long was the recovery from the most recent concussion?		
Has the child ever been hospitalized or had medical imaging done (CT or MRI) for a head injury?	Y	N
Has the child ever been diagnosed with headaches or migraines?	Y	N
Does the child have a learning disability, dyslexia, ADD/ADHD, seizure disorder?	Y	N
Has the child ever been diagnosed with depression, anxiety or other psychiatric disorder?	Y	N
Has anyone in the family ever been diagnosed with any of these problems?	Y	N
Is the child on any medications? If yes, please list:	Y	N

Figure 2-12 Sport Concussion Assessment Tool for children ages 5 to 12 years (Child-SCAT3). (© 2013 Concussion in Sport Group. Br J Sports Med 47:263–266, 2013.)

SYMPTOM EVALUATION

3 Child report

Name:

	never	rarely	sometimes	often
I have trouble paying attention	0	1	2	3
I get distracted easily	0	1	2	3
I have a hard time concentrating	0	1	2	3
I have problems remembering what people tell me	0	1	2	3
I have problems following directions	0	1	2	3
I daydream too much	0	1	2	3
I get confused	0	1	2	3
I forget things	0	1	2	3
I have problems finishing things	0	1	2	3
I have trouble figuring things out	0	1	2	3
It's hard for me to learn new things	0	1	2	3
I have headaches	0	1	2	3
I feel dizzy	0	1	2	3
I feel like the room is spinning	0	1	2	3
I feel like I'm going to faint	0	1	2	3
Things are blurry when I look at them	0	1	2	3
I see double	0	1	2	3
I feel sick to my stomach	0	1	2	3
I get tired a lot	0	1	2	3
I get tired easily	0	1	2	3

Total number of symptoms (Maximum possible 20)

Symptom severity score (Maximum possible 20 x 3 = 60)

☐ self rated   ☐ clinician interview   ☐ self rated and clinician monitored

4 Parent report

The child

	never	rarely	sometimes	often
has trouble sustaining attention	0	1	2	3
Is easily distracted	0	1	2	3
has difficulty concentrating	0	1	2	3
has problems remembering what he/she is told	0	1	2	3
has difficulty following directions	0	1	2	3
tends to daydream	0	1	2	3
gets confused	0	1	2	3
is forgetful	0	1	2	3
has difficulty completeing tasks	0	1	2	3
has poor problem solving skills	0	1	2	3
has problems learning	0	1	2	3
has headaches	0	1	2	3
feels dizzy	0	1	2	3
has a feeling that the room is spinning	0	1	2	3
feels faint	0	1	2	3
has blurred vision	0	1	2	3
has double vision	0	1	2	3
experiences nausea	0	1	2	3
gets tired a lot	0	1	2	3
gets tired easily	0	1	2	3

Total number of symptoms (Maximum possible 20)

Symptom severity score (Maximum possible 20 x 3 = 60)

Do the symptoms get worse with physical activity?   ☐ Y   ☐ N

Do the symptoms get worse with mental activity?   ☐ Y   ☐ N

☐ parent self rated   ☐ clinician interview   ☐ parent self rated and clinician monitored

Overall rating for parent/teacher/coach/carer to answer.
How different is the child acting compared to his/her usual self?
Please circle one response:

no different	very different	unsure	N/A

Name of person completing parent-report:

Relationship to child of person completing parent-report:

Scoring on the ChildSCAT3 should not be used as a stand-alone method to diagnose concussion, measure recovery or make decisions about an athlete's readiness to return to competition after concussion.

COGNITIVE & PHYSICAL EVALUATION

5 Cognitive assessment
Standardized Assessment of Concussion – Child Version (SAC-C)[4]

Orientation (1 point for each correct answer)

What month is it?	0	1
What is the date today?	0	1
What is the day of the week?	0	1
What year is it?	0	1

Orientation score — of 4

Immediate memory

List	Trial 1		Trial 2		Trial 3		Alternative word list		
elbow	0	1	0	1	0	1	candle	baby	finger
apple	0	1	0	1	0	1	paper	monkey	penny
carpet	0	1	0	1	0	1	sugar	perfume	blanket
saddle	0	1	0	1	0	1	sandwich	sunset	lemon
bubble	0	1	0	1	0	1	wagon	iron	insect
Total									

Immediate memory score total — of 15

Concentration: Digits Backward

List	Trial 1	Alternative digit list		
6-2	0 1	5-2	4-1	4-9
4-9-3	0 1	6-2-9	5-2-6	4-1-5
3-8-1-4	0 1	3-2-7-9	1-7-9-5	4-9-6-8
6-2-9-7-1	0 1	1-5-2-8-6	3-8-5-2-7	6-1-8-4-3
7-1-8-4-6-2	0 1	5-3-9-1-4-8	8-3-1-9-6-4	7-2-4-8-5-6
Total of 5				

Concentration: Days in Reverse Order (1 pt. for entire sequence correct)

Sunday-Saturday-Friday-Thursday-Wednesday-Tuesday-Monday	0	1

Concentration score — of 6

6 Neck Examination:

Range of motion   Tenderness   Upper and lower limb sensation & strength

Findings:

7 Balance examination

Do one or both of the following tests.

Footwear (shoes, barefoot, braces, tape, etc.)

Modified Balance Error Scoring System (BESS) testing[5]

Which foot was tested (i.e., which is the **non-dominant** foot)   ☐ Left   ☐ Right

Testing surface (hard floor, field, etc.)

Condition

Double leg stance: — Errors

Tandem stance (non-dominant foot at back): — Errors

Tandem gait[6,7]

Time taken to complete (best of 4 trials): _____ seconds

If child attempted, but unable to complete tandem gait, mark here.   ☐

8 Coordination examination
Upper limb coordination

Which arm was tested: ☐ Left   ☐ Right

Coordination score — of 1

9 SAC Delayed Recall[4]

Delayed recall score — of 5

Since signs and symptoms may evolve over time, it is important to consider repeat evaluation in the acute assessment of concussion.

Figure 2-12, cont'd   *Continued*

INSTRUCTIONS

Words in *italics* throughout the ChildSCAT3 are the instructions given to the child by the tester.

Sideline Assessment – child-Maddocks Score

To be completed on the sideline/in the playground, immediately following concussion. There is no requirement to repeat these questions at follow-up.

Symptom Scale[8]

In situations where the symptom scale is being completed after exercise, it should still be done in a resting state, at least 10 minutes post exercise.

On the day of injury

- the child is to complete the Child Report, according to how he/she feels now.

On all subsequent days

- the child is to complete the Child Report, according to how he/she feels today, **and**
- the parent/carer is to complete the Parent Report according to how the child has been over the previous 24 hours.

Standardized Assessment of Concussion – Child Version (SAC-C)[4]

Orientation

Ask each question on the score sheet. A correct answer for **each question scores 1 point.** If the child does not understand the question, gives an incorrect answer, or no answer, then the score for that question is 0 points.

Immediate memory

"I am going to test your memory. I will read you a list of words and when I am done, repeat back as many words as you can remember, in any order."

Trials 2 & 3:

"I am going to repeat the same list again. Repeat back as many words as you can remember in any order, even if you said the word before."

Complete all 3 trials regardless of score on trial 1 & 2. Read the words at a rate of one per second. **Score 1 pt. for each correct response.** Total score equals sum across all 3 trials. Do not inform the child that delayed recall will be tested.

Concentration
Digits Backward:

"I am going to read you a string of numbers and when I am done, you repeat them back to me backwards, in reverse order of how I read them to you. For example, if I say 7-1, you would say 1-7."

If correct, go to next string length. If incorrect, read trial 2. **One point possible for each string length.** Stop after incorrect on both trials. The digits should be read at the rate of one per second.

Days in Reverse Order:

"Now tell me the days of the week in reverse order. Start with Sunday and go backward. So you'll say Sunday, Saturday ... Go ahead."

1 pt. for entire sequence correct

Delayed recall

The delayed recall should be performed after completion of the Balance and Coordination Examination.

"Do you remember that list of words I read a few times earlier? Tell me as many words from the list as you can remember in any order."

Circle each word correctly recalled. **Total score equals number of words recalled.**

Balance examination

These instructions are to be read by the person administering the childSCAT3, and each balance task **should be demonstrated to the child.** The child should then be asked to copy what the examiner demonstrated.

Modified Balance Error Scoring System (BESS) testing[5]

This balance testing is based on a modified version of the Balance Error Scoring System (BESS).[5] A stopwatch or watch with a second hand is required for this testing.

"I am now going to test your balance. Please take your shoes off, roll up your pant legs above ankle (if applicable), and remove any ankle taping (if applicable). This test will consist of two different parts."

(a) Double leg stance:
The first stance is standing with the feet together with hands on hips and with eyes closed. The child should try to maintain stability in that position for 20 seconds. You should inform the child that you will be counting the number of times the child moves out of this position. You should start timing when the child is set and the eyes are closed.

(b) Tandem stance:
Instruct the child to stand heel-to-toe with the non-dominant foot in the back. Weight should be evenly distributed across both feet. Again, the child should try to maintain stability for 20 seconds with hands on hips and eyes closed. You should inform the child that you will be counting the number of times the child moves out of this position. If the child stumbles out of this position, instruct him/her to open the eyes and return to the start position and continue balancing. You should start timing when the child is set and the eyes are closed.

Balance testing – types of errors - Parts (a) and (b)

1. Hands lifted off iliac crest
2. Opening eyes
3. Step, stumble, or fall
4. Moving hip into > 30 degrees abduction
5. Lifting forefoot or heel
6. Remaining out of test position > 5 sec

Each of the 20-second trials is scored by counting the errors, or deviations from the proper stance, accumulated by the child. The examiner will begin counting errors only after the child has assumed the proper start position. **The modified BESS is calculated by adding one error point for each error during the two 20-second tests. The maximum total number of errors for any single condition is 10.** If a child commits multiple errors simultaneously, only one error is recorded but the child should quickly return to the testing position, and counting should resume once subject is set. Children who are unable to maintain the testing procedure for a minimum of **five seconds** at the start are assigned the highest possible score, ten, for that testing condition.

OPTION: For further assessment, the same 2 stances can be performed on a surface of medium density foam (e.g., approximately 50cm x 40cm x 6cm).

Tandem Gait[6,7]

Use a clock (with a second hand) or stopwatch to measure the time taken to complete this task. Instruction for the examiner – **Demonstrate the following to the child:**

The child is instructed to stand with their feet together behind a starting line (the test is best done with footwear removed). Then, they walk in a forward direction as quickly and as accurately as possible along a 38mm wide (sports tape), 3 meter line with an alternate foot heel-to-toe gait ensuring that they approximate their heel and toe on each step. Once they cross the end of the 3m line, they turn 180 degrees and return to the starting point using the same gait. A total of 4 trials are done and the best time is retained. Children fail the test if they step off the line, have a separation between their heel and toe, or if they touch or grab the examiner or an object. In this case, the time is not recorded and the trial repeated, if appropriate.

Explain to the child that you will time how long it takes them to walk to the end of the line and back.

Coordination examination

Upper limb coordination
Finger-to-nose (FTN) task:

The tester should **demonstrate it to the child**.

"I am going to test your coordination now. Please sit comfortably on the chair with your eyes open and your arm (either right or left) outstretched (shoulder flexed to 90 degrees and elbow and fingers extended). When I give a start signal, I would like you to perform five successive finger to nose repetitions using your index finger to touch the tip of the nose as quickly and as accurately as possible."

Scoring: 5 correct repetitions in < 4 seconds = 1
Note for testers: Children fail the test if they do not touch their nose, do not fully extend their elbow, or do not perform five repetitions. **Failure should be scored as 0.**

References & Footnotes

1. This tool has been developed by a group of international experts at the 4th International Consensus meeting on Concussion in Sport held in Zurich, Switzerland in November 2012. The full details of the conference outcomes and the authors of the tool are published in The BJSM Injury Prevention and Health Protection, 2013, Volume 47, Issue 5. The outcome paper will also be simultaneously co-published in other leading biomedical journals with the copyright held by the Concussion in Sport Group, to allow unrestricted distribution, providing no alterations are made.

2. McCrory P et al., Consensus Statement on Concussion in Sport – the 3rd International Conference on Concussion in Sport held in Zurich, November 2008. British Journal of Sports Medicine 2009; 43: i76-89.

3. Maddocks, DL; Dicker, GD; Saling, MM. The assessment of orientation following concussion in athletes. Clinical Journal of Sport Medicine. 1995; 5(1): 32–3.

4. McCrea M. Standardized mental status testing of acute concussion. Clinical Journal of Sport Medicine. 2001; 11: 176–181.

5. Guskiewicz KM. Assessment of postural stability following sport-related concussion. Current Sports Medicine Reports. 2003; 2: 24–30.

6. Schneiders, A.G., Sullivan, S.J., Gray, A., Hammond-Tooke, G. & McCrory, P. Normative values for 16-37 year old subjects for three clinical measures of motor performance used in the assessment of sports concussions. Journal of Science and Medicine in Sport. 2010; 13(2): 196–201.

7. Schneiders, A.G., Sullivan, S.J., Kvarnstrom. J.K., Olsson, M., Yden. T. & Marshall, S.W. The effect of footwear and sports-surface on dynamic neurological screening in sport-related concussion. Journal of Science and Medicine in Sport. 2010; 13(4): 382–386.

8. Ayr, L.K., Yeates, K.O., Taylor, H.G., & Brown, M. Dimensions of post-concussive symptoms in children with mild traumatic brain injuries. Journal of the International Neuropsychological Society. 2009; 15:19–30.

Figure 2-12, cont'd

CHILD ATHLETE INFORMATION

Any child suspected of having a concussion should be removed from play, and then seek medical evaluation. The child must NOT return to play or sport on the same day as the suspected concussion.

Signs to watch for

Problems could arise over the first 24–48 hours. The child should not be left alone and must go to a hospital at once if they develop any of the following:

- New headache, or headache gets worse
- Persistent or increasing neck pain
- Becomes drowsy or can't be woken up
- Can not recognize people or places
- Has nausea or vomiting
- Behaves unusually, seems confused, or is irritable
- Has any seizures (arms and/or legs jerk uncontrollably)
- Has weakness, numbness or tingling (arms, legs or face)
- Is unsteady walking or standing
- Has slurred speech
- Has difficulty understanding speech or directions

Remember, it is better to be safe.
Always consult your doctor after a suspected concussion.

Return to school

Concussion may impact on the child's cognitive ability to learn at school. This must be considered, and medical clearance is required before the child may return to school. **It is reasonable for a child to miss a day or two of school after concussion, but extended absence is uncommon.** In some children, a graduated return to school program will need to be developed for the child. The child will progress through the return to school program provided that there is no worsening of symptoms. If any particular activity worsens symptoms, the child will abstain from that activity until it no longer causes symptom worsening. Use of computers and internet should follow a similar graduated program, provided that it does not worsen symptoms. This program should include communication between the parents, teachers, and health professionals and will vary from child to child. The return to school program should consider:

- Extra time to complete assignments/tests
- Quiet room to complete assignments/tests
- Avoidance of noisy areas such as cafeterias, assembly halls, sporting events, music class, shop class, etc.
- Frequent breaks during class, homework, tests
- No more than one exam/day
- Shorter assignments
- Repetition/memory cues
- Use of peer helper/tutor
- Reassurance from teachers that student will be supported through recovery through accommodations, workload reduction, alternate forms of testing
- Later start times, half days, only certain classes

The child is not to return to play or sport until he/she has successfully returned to school/learning, without worsening of symptoms. Medical clearance should be given before return to play.

If there are any doubts, management should be referred to a qualified health practitioner, expert in the management of concussion in children.

Return to sport

There should be no return to play until the child has successfully returned to school/learning, without worsening of symptoms.
Children must not be returned to play the same day of injury.
When returning children to play, they should **medically cleared and then follow a stepwise supervised program,** with stages of progression.

For example:

Rehabilitation stage	Functional exercise at each stage of rehabilitation	Objective of each stage
No activity	Physical and cognitive rest	Recovery
Light aerobic exercise	Walking, swimming or stationary cycling keeping intensity, 70 % maximum predicted heart rate. No resistance training	Increase heart rate
Sport-specific exercise	Skating drills in ice hockey, running drills in soccer. No head impact activities	Add movement
Non-contact training drills	Progression to more complex training drills, e.g., passing drills in football and ice hockey. May start progressive resistance training	Exercise, coordination, and cognitive load
Full contact practice	Following medical clearance participate in normal training activities	Restore confidence and assess functional skills by coaching staff
Return to play	Normal game play	

There should be approximately 24 hours (or longer) for each stage and the child should drop back to the previous asymptomatic level if any post-concussive symptoms recur. Resistance training should only be added in the later stages.
If the child is symptomatic for more than 10 days, then review by a health practitioner, expert in the management of concussion, is recommended.
Medical clearance should be given before return to play.

Notes:

_____

_____

_____

_____

✂ -

CONCUSSION INJURY ADVICE FOR THE CHILD AND PARENTS/CARERS
(To be given to the **person monitoring** the concussed child)

This child has received an injury to the head. A careful medical examination has been carried out and no sign of any serious complications has been found. It is expected that recovery will be rapid, but the child will need monitoring for the next 24 hours by a responsible adult.

If you notice any change in behavior, vomiting, dizziness, worsening headache, double vision or excessive drowsiness, please call an ambulance to transport the child to hospital immediately.

Other important points:

- Following concussion, the child should rest for at least 24 hours.
- The child should avoid any computer, internet or electronic gaming activity if these activities make symptoms worse.
- The child should not be given any medications, including pain killers, unless prescribed by a medical practitioner.
- The child must not return to school until medically cleared.
- The child must not return to sport or play until medically cleared.

Clinic phone number ▭

Patient's name _____

Date/time of injury _____

Date/time of medical review _____

Treating physician _____

┌─────────────────────────────┐
│   │
│   │
│   │
│   │
│   │
│   Contact details or stamp │
└─────────────────────────────┘

Figure 2-12, cont'd

SAC: Standardized Assessment of Concussion

NAME: _____

AGE: ___ SEX: ___ EXAMINER: _____

Nature of Injury: _____

Date of Exam: _____ Time: _____ No. _____

1) ORIENTATION:

Month: _____	0	1
Date: _____	0	1
Day of Week: _____	0	1
Year: _____	0	1
Time (within 1 hour): _____	0	1

Orientation Total Score _____ /5

2) IMMEDIATE MEMORY: (all 3 trials are completed regardless of score on trials 1 & 2; score equals sum across all 3 trials)

LIST	TRIAL 1	TRIAL 2	TRIAL 3
Elbow	0 1	0 1	0 1
Apple	0 1	0 1	0 1
Carpet	0 1	0 1	0 1
Saddle	0 1	0 1	0 1
Bubble	0 1	0 1	0 1
Total			

Immediate Memory Score _____ /15

3) CONCENTRATION:

Digits Backward: (If correct, go to next string length. If incorrect, read trial 2. Stop after incorrect on both trials.)

4-9-3	6-2-9	0	1
3-8-1-4	3-2-7-9	0	1
6-2-9-7-1	1-5-2-8-6	0	1
7-1-8-4-6-2	5-3-9-1-4-8	0	1

Months in Reverse Order: (entire reverse sequence correct for 1 point)
DEC-NOV-OCT-SEP-AUG-JUL
JUN-MAY-APR-MAR-FEB-JAN   0   1

Concentration Total Score _____ /5

EXERTIONAL MANEUVERS (when appropriate):

5 jumping jacks	5 push-ups
5 sit-ups	5 knee-bends

4) DELAYED RECALL

Elbow	0	1
Apple	0	1
Carpet	0	1
Saddle	0	1
Bubble	0	1

Delayed Recall Score _____ /5

SUMMARY OF TOTAL SCORES:

Orientation	_____	/ 5
Immediate Memory	_____	/ 15
Concentration	_____	/ 5
Delayed Recall	_____	/ 5

OVERALL TOTAL SCORE _____ / 30

Figure 2-13 **Standardized Assessment of Concussion (SAC).** (Redrawn from McCrea M, Kelly JP, Kluge J, et al: Standard assessment of concussion in football players. Neurology 48[3]:586–588, 1997.)

injuries every 15 to 30 minutes. Manzi and Weaver reported that a patient who had sustained a period of posttraumatic amnesia of less than 60 minutes was considered to have sustained a mild head injury.[44] If the period of posttraumatic amnesia lasted from 1 to 24 hours, moderate head injury was considered to have occurred. If the posttraumatic amnesia lasted for more than 1 week, the patient was considered to have sustained a serious head injury. If the duration of the posttraumatic amnesia was more than 7 days, full return to neurological function was highly unlikely.[44] With a grade II concussion, the patient may experience mild tinnitus (ringing in the ears), mild dizziness, and a dull headache with some disorientation. Dizziness at the time of injury has been reported to be a sign of risk for protracted recovery.[45] The patient who experienced a grade II concussion may also develop a **post-concussion syndrome** (i.e., have continual neurological problems after the concussion), which is observed in about 10% of concussion cases. The signs and symptoms of this syndrome include persistent headaches, especially with exertion; inability to concentrate; and irritability. The symptoms may last from several weeks to several years.

TABLE **2-9**

Classification Systems for Concussions

System	Grade I (Mild)	Grade Ia	Grade II (Moderate)	Grade III (Severe)	Grade IV
Cantu	No LOC or PTA < 30 min	N/A	LOC < 5 min, PTA 30 min to 24 hrs	LOC > 5 min, PTA > 24 hrs	N/A
Torg	(Grade I to II) No LOC or amnesia (except PTA)			(Grade III–IV) LOC < few minutes, PTA or retrograde amnesia	(Grade V–VI) LOC/coma, confusion, amnesia
Colorado Consortium	Confusion without amnesia, no LOC	N/A	Confusion and amnesia, no LOC	LOC	N/A
Virginia Neurological Institute	Short LOC, PTA < 1 hr, GCS score = 15	Short LOC, PTA 1 to 24 hrs, GCS score = 15	LOC < 5 min, PTA ≥ 24 h, GCS score > 15 for < 5 min	LOC < 5 min, PTA N/A, GCS score < 15 for < 1 hr	LOC 5 to 60 min, PTA N/A, GCS score < 12 for > 5 min or < 15 for > 1 hr
American Academy of Neurology	No LOC, Symptoms < 15 min	N/A	No LOC, Symptoms > 15 min	Any LOC	N/A

From Durand P, Adamson GJ: On-the-field management of athletic head injuries, J Am Acad Orthop Surg 12:194, 2004. Adapted with permission from Macciocchi SN, Barth JT, Littlefield LM: Outcome after mild head injury. Clin Sports Med 17:27–36, 1998.
GCS, Glasgow Coma Scale; *LOC,* loss of consciousness; *PTA,* posttraumatic amnesia.

TABLE **2-10**

Examples of Neurophysiological Tests

Test	Ability Evaluated
Continuous Performance Test	Sustained attention, reaction time
Controlled Oral Word Association Test	Word fluency, word retrieval
Delayed Recall (from Hopkins Verbal Learning Test)	Delayed learning from previously learned word list
Digit Span (from Wechsler Memory Scale—revised)	Attention span
Grooved-Pegboard Test	Motor speed and coordination
Hopkins Verbal Learning Test	Verbal memory (memory for words)
Immediate Measurement of Performance and Cognitive Testing (IMPACT)	Attention span, sustained and selective attention, reaction time, memory
Number/Symbol Matching	Processing speed, visual motor speed
Orientation Questionnaire	Orientation, post traumatic amnesia
Sequential Digit Tracking	Sustained attention, reaction time
Stroop Test	Mental flexibility, attention
Symbol Digit Modalities	Visual scanning, attention
Symbol Memory	Immediate visual memory
Trail-Making Test	Visual scanning, mental flexibility
Verbal Working Memory	Word memory, working memory
Visual Span	Visual attention, immediate memory
Visual Symbol Search	Visual scanning, reaction time
Word/Colour Tracking	Focused attention, response inhibition

Data from Maroon JC, Lovell MR, Norwig J, et al: Cerebral concussion in athletes: evaluation and neurophysiological testing. Neurosurg 47:659–672, 2000.

> ### Head Injury Severity Based on Length of Posttraumatic Amnesia
>
> | | |
> |---|---|
> | Less than 60 minutes: | Mild |
> | 1 to 24 hours: | Moderate |
> | More than 1 week: | Serious (full return of neurological function unlikely) |

A patient with a **grade III concussion** has the same symptoms as someone with a grade II concussion and also experiences retrograde amnesia. **Retrograde amnesia** is loss of memory of events that occurred before the injury. It may take 5 to 10 minutes for retrograde amnesia to develop after the concussion, and amnesia may involve only a few minutes before the injury. For this reason, the patient should be questioned frequently about what happened before the injury occurred and how it occurred, to see if there is any change in the patient's memory pattern. There is always some degree of permanent retrograde amnesia with these patients.

With a **grade IV concussion,** the patient loses consciousness for 5 minutes or less. The level of consciousness may vary; the patient may be comatose, stuporous, obtunded, lethargic, confused, or fully alert. The patient goes through the following stages of recovery: unconsciousness (also called *paralytic coma*), stupor, obtundity, lethargy, confusion (with or without delirium), near lucidity with automatism, and finally full alertness. **Stupor** implies that the patient is only partially conscious and has reduced responsiveness. **Obtundity** implies the patient has reduced sensitivity to painful or unpleasant stimuli. **Lethargy** implies a state of sluggishness, dullness, or serious drowsiness. **Confusion** implies that the patient is disoriented in terms of time, place, or person. **Delirium** means that the patient may experience illusions, hallucinations, restlessness, or incoherence. **Lucidity with automatism** implies that the patient appears to be alert and fully recovered but acts only mechanically and is not really aware of what he or she is doing. With a grade IV concussion, there may be subtle changes in the patient's personality and memory function. Both retrograde and posttraumatic amnesia are evident, and the patient demonstrates mental confusion and complains of tinnitus and dizziness to a greater degree than is seen with a grade III concussion. The patient also has residual headaches and is unsteady for 5 to 10 minutes after regaining consciousness. The literature has reported that loss of consciousness, by itself, is not a good predictor of the degree of neurophysiological loss or damage with a head injury.[46] The severity of the head injury is best determined by the administration of different neurophysiological tests (e.g., GOAT test,[47]

Hopkins Verbal Learning Test,[48] Trail Making Test, Wisconsin Card Sorting Test, Digit Symbol Substitution Test [DSST],[49] and measures of decision time[49]) as well as considering all signs and symptoms the patient demonstrates.[6,8,15,50–53] To ensure adequate data, however, these tests must also have been administered before the injury (e.g., in a pre-participation evaluation in sports).[6,35]

> ### Levels of Consciousness
>
> | | |
> |---|---|
> | • **Alertness** | Is readily aroused, oriented, and fully aware of surroundings |
> | • **Confusion** | Memory is impaired
Is confused and disoriented |
> | • **Lethargy** | Sleeps when not stimulated
Is drowsy and inattentive
Responds to name
Loses train of thought
Shows decreased spontaneous movement
Has slow and fuzzy thinking |
> | • **Obtundity** | Responds to loud voice or shaking
Responds to painful stimulus (withdrawal)
Is confused when aroused
Talks in monosyllables
Mumbles and is incoherent
Needs constant stimulation to cooperate |
> | • **Stupor** (semicoma) | Responds to painful stimuli (withdrawal), shaking
Groans, mumbles
Exhibits reflex activity |
> | • **Coma** | Does not respond to painful or any other stimuli |

With a **grade V concussion,** the patient has experienced a paralytic coma or unconsciousness for 5 minutes or longer. This grade of concussion involves bruising of the brain, and there is prolonged retrograde amnesia as well as posttraumatic amnesia. The patient complains of severe tinnitus, unsteadiness for longer than 10 minutes, blurred vision, poor light accommodation, and a headache that feels "different" from most headaches. Both the autonomic and the peripheral nervous systems can be affected through their control by the brain. These patients may also experience nausea, vomiting, and sometimes convulsions. The recovery after a grade V concussion may be one of two types. In type A, the patient goes from a paralytic coma through stupor, confusion, lucidity, and full alertness, which is similar to a grade IV concussion but more severe. The individual with a type B grade V concussion experiences a paralytic coma that is associated with secondary cardiorespiratory collapse and is of much greater concern to the examiner, especially during the initial assessment, when the body's essential functions must be maintained.

More severe diffuse brain injuries are associated with more severe neurological dysfunction. With these injuries, loss of consciousness lasts for more than 24 hours, and recovery is never complete, leading to deficits in intelligence, reasoning, and memory and to changes in personality. Shearing brain injuries tend to be more severe than diffuse brain injuries and lead to abnormal brain stem signs, such as decerebrate rigidity.[43]

3. *If the patient has had an injury to the head, are there any associated symptoms in the neck or problems with breathing, altered vision, discharge from the nose or ears, or urinary or fecal incontinence?* These symptoms indicate severe brain or spinal cord injury, and the patient must be handled with extreme care.

4. *What are the sites and boundaries of pain?* This question helps the examiner determine what structures have been injured. It is important to keep in mind that the patient may be experiencing a referral of pain.

5. *What type of pain is the patient experiencing?* The type of pain indicates the type of structure injured (see Table 1-3).

6. *Is there any paresthesia, abnormal sensation, or lack of sensation?* Are smell (cranial nerve I), vision (cranial nerve II), taste (cranial nerve VII), and hearing (cranial nerve VIII) normal? These questions give the examiner some idea of whether neurological structures (especially the cranial nerves) have been injured and, if so, which ones.

Head Signs and Symptoms Requiring Specialist Care

- Presence of amnesia
- Prolonged residual symptoms
- Loss of consciousness
- Prolonged headache
- Post-concussion syndrome
- Personality changes
- More than one first- or second-degree concussion
- Prolonged disorientation, unsteadiness, or confusion (more than 2 to 3 minutes)
- Blurred vision
- Dizziness (more than 5 minutes)
- Tinnitus (more than 5 minutes)

---

7. *What activities aggravate the particular problem?*
8. *What activities ease the particular problem?*
9. *Does the patient have a **headache,** and, if so, where* (Tables 2-11 and 2-12)? Is the headache tolerable? What type of headache is it? Is it a throbbing, pounding, boring, shocklike, dull, nagging, or

---

TABLE **2-11**

Type of Headache Pain and Usual Causes

Type of Pain	Usual Causes
Acute	Trauma, acute infection, impending cerebrovascular accident, subarachnoid hemorrhage
Chronic, recurrent	Migraine (definite pattern of irregular interval); eyestrain; noise; excessive eating, drinking, or smoking; inadequate ventilation
Continuous, recurrent	Trauma
Severe, intense	Meningitis, aneurysm (ruptured), migraine, brain tumor
Intense, transient, shocklike	Neuralgia
Throbbing, pulsating (vascular)	Migraine, fever, hypertension, aortic insufficiency, neuralgia
Constant, tight (bandlike), bilateral	Muscle contraction

TABLE **2-12**

Location of Headache and Usual Causes

Location	Usual Causes
Forehead	Sinusitis, eye or nose disorder, muscle spasm of occipital or suboccipital region
Side of head	Migraine, eye or ear disorder, auriculotemporal neuralgia
Occipital	Myofascial problems, herniated disc, eyestrain, hypertension, occipital neuralgia
Parietal	Hysteria (viselike), meningitis, constipation, tumor
Face	Maxillary sinusitis, trigeminal neuralgia, dental problems, tumor

---

constant-pressure type of headache? Is the pain of the headache aggravated by movement or by rest? What is the exact location of the headache? Is the headache affected by position or time of day (Table 2-13)? Does it cover the entire head, the sinus region, or behind the eyes? Does it present a "hat band" distribution, or does it affect the neck or the occiput area? It is important for the examiner to record the location, character, duration, and frequency of the headache, as well as any factors that appear to either aggravate or relieve the pain so that a diagnosis can be made and any changes can be noted (Table 2-14). Figure 2-14 shows a headache disability questionnaire that may be used to determine the severity of headache and its effect on everyday activity.[54]

TABLE **2-13**

Effect of Position or Time of Day on Headache

Position or Time of Day When Headache Is Worst	Usual Causes
Morning	Sinusitis, migraine, hypertension, alcoholism, sleeping position
Afternoon	Eyestrain, muscle tension
Night	Intracranial disease, osteomyelitis, nephritis
Bending	Sinusitis
Lying horizontal	Migraine

10. *Is the patient dizzy, unsteady, or having problems with balance?* The examiner should also note whether the dizziness occurs when the patient suddenly stands up, turns, or bends, or whether it occurs without movement. Remember that "dizziness" is a word that patients sometimes use to indicate unsteadiness in walking. Dizziness is usually associated with problems of the middle ear, vertebrobasilar insufficiency, or problems in the upper cervical spine. Vertigo implies a rotary component; the patient's environment seems to whirl around the patient, or the patient's body seems to rotate in relation to the environment. If the patient complains of dizziness or vertigo, the time of onset and duration of these attacks should be noted. A description of the type of motion that occurs and any other associated symptoms should be included. Balance may be affected by problems within the brain or the semicircular canals in the inner ear. The examiner should also note whether the patient is talking about unsteadiness, loss of balance, or actual falling.

11. *Is the patient unduly irritated or having trouble concentrating?* The patient's state indicates the severity of the injury.

12. *Does the patient know where he or she is, who he or she is, the day, and the time of day?* Does the patient have some idea of what was happening when the injury occurred? These types of questions reveal the severity of the injury.

13. *Does the patient have any memory of past events or what occurred before or after the injury?* This type of question tests for retrograde amnesia, posttraumatic amnesia, and injury severity, which can be determined by asking the patient straightforward questions about events in the patient's own past, such as birth date or year of graduation from high school or university. The examiner may also ask questions about the injury, preceding events, and posttraumatic events. Questions such as "What day is it?" "Who is the opposition?" "Who is winning?" and "What is your telephone number and address?" test the

patient's static memory ability. The examiner must ensure that he or she or someone present at the time of the examination knows the answer to these questions. Although it is common to ask these orientation questions (e.g., time, place), it has been shown that these questions can be unreliable in sporting situations when compared with memory assessment.[55,56] The examiner can assess **recent memory** by asking the patient to remember the names for two to five persons or common objects, such as the color "red," the number "five," the name "Mr. Smith," and the word "pride," and then asking the patient to name them 5 or 10 minutes later. The patient may be asked to repeat the words two or three times when the examiner initially says them to test immediate recall or to ensure that the patient can say and recall the words. **Immediate recall,** another form of memory, is best tested by asking the patient to repeat a series of single digits. Normally, a person can repeat at least six digits, and many people can repeat eight or nine. The examiner may also ask the patient to repeat the months of the year backward in a similar type of test. Memory is generally thought to be formed and stored in certain regions of the temporal lobes. The parietal lobe of the brain is thought to enable one to appreciate the environment, to interpret visual stimuli, and to communicate.

Common Head Injury Tests

- Static memory (What day is it? Who's winning?)
- Immediate recall (repeat series of single digits)
- Recent memory (recall three common objects or names after 15 minutes)
- Short term memory (What is the game plan?)
- Processing and concentration ability (minus-7 test, multiplying)
- Abstract relationships
- Coordination (eye-hand tests)
- Balance (Romberg test)
- Myotomes
- Eye coordination
- Visual disturbance tests

14. *Can the patient solve simple problems?* Because concussions reduce one's ability to process information, it is important to determine the patient's **reasoning and processing ability.** For example, does the patient know his or her home telephone number? Is the patient able to do the "minus 7" or "serial 7" test (i.e., count backward from 100 by sevens)? This test gives the examiner some idea of the patient's calculating ability and concentration skills. Mathematic ability (the ability to add, subtract, multiply, and divide) can also be evaluated to test processing

TABLE 2-14

Headaches: A Differential Diagnosis

Disorder	Sex/Age Predominance	Nature of Pain	Frequency	Location	Duration	Prodromal Events	Precipitating Factors	Cause	Familial Predisposition	Other Possible Symptoms
Migraine	Female/20 to 40 years	Builds to throbbing and intense	Usually not more than twice a week; may be nocturnal	Usually unilateral	Several hours to days	Visual disturbances can occur contralateral to pain site	Unknown, may be physical, emotional, hormonal, dietary	Vasomotor	Yes	Nausea, vomiting, pallor, photophobia, mood disturbances, fluid retention
Cluster (histamine) headache	Male/40 to 60 years	Excruciating, stabbing, burning, pulsating	1 to 4 episodes per 24 hours; nocturnal manifestation	Unilateral, eye, temple, forehead	Minutes to hours	Sleep disturbances or personality changes can occur	Unknown, may be serotonin, histamine, hormonal blood flow	Vasomotor	Minor	Ipsilateral sweating of face, lacrimation, nasal congestion or discharge
Hypertension headache	None	Dull, throbbing, nonlocalized	Variable	Entire cranium, especially occipital region	Variable	None	Activity that increases blood pressure	High blood pressure; diastolic >120 mm Hg	Only as related to hypertension	
Trigeminal neuralgia (tic douloureux)	Female/40 to 60 years	Excruciating, spontaneous, lancinating, lightning	Can occur many (12 or more) times per day	Unilateral along trigeminal nerve area	30 seconds to 1 minute	Disagreeable tingling	Touch (cold) to affected area	Neurological	None	Reddened conjunctiva, lacrimation
Glossopharyngeal neuralgia	Male/40 to 60 years	Excruciating, spontaneous, lancinating, lightning	Can occur many (12 or more) times per day	Unilateral retrolingual area to ear	30 seconds to 1 minute	None	Movement or contact of the pharynx	Neurological	None	
Cervical neuralgia	None	Dull pain or pressure in head		Bilateral, occipital, frontal, or facial	Variable	None	Posture or head movement	Neurological, pressure on roots of spinal nerves	None	Dizziness, auditory disturbances
Eye disorders	None	Generalized discomfort in or around the eyes	Intensify with sustained visual effort	Entire cranium	During and after visual effort	None	Impairment of eye function	Cornea, iris, or intraocular pain	Possible	Diminished vision, sensitivity to light
Sinus, ear, and nasal disorders	None	Dull, persistent	Variable	Frontal, temporal, ear, nose, occipital	Variable	None	Infection, allergy, chemical, bending, straining	Blockage, inflammation, infection	None	

Modified from Esposito CJ, Grim GA, Binkley TK: Headaches: a differential diagnosis. J Craniomand Pract 4:320–321, 1986.

HEADACHE DISABILITY QUESTIONNAIRE

Name: ....   Date: ..../........./.............   Score   /90

Please read each question and circle the response that best applies to you.

1. How would you rate the usual pain of your headache on a scale from 0 to 10?

| 0 | 1 | 2 | 3 | 4 | 5 | 6 | 7 | 8 | 9 | 10 | WORST |
NO   PAIN
PAIN

2. When you have headaches, how often is in the pain severe?

NEVER 1–9% 10–19% 20–29% 30–39% 40–49% 50–59% 60–69% 70–79% 80–89% 90–100% ALWAYS
0   1   2   3   4   5   6   7   8   9   10

3. On how many days in the last month did you actually lie down for an hour or more because of your headaches?

NONE 1–3   4–6   7–9   10–12 13–15 16–18 19–21 22–24 25–27 28–31 EVERY DAY
0   1   2   3   4   5   6   7   8   9   10

4. When you have a headache, how often do you miss work or school for all or part of the day?

NEVER 1–9% 10–19% 20–29% 30–39% 40–49% 50–59% 60–69% 70–79% 80–89% 90–100% ALWAYS
0   1   2   3   4   5   6   7   8   9   10

5. When you have a headache while you work (or school), how much is your ability to work reduced?

NOT   1–9% 10–19% 20–29% 30–39% 40–49% 50–59% 60–69% 70–79% 80–89% 90–100% UNABLE
0   1   2   3   4   5   6   7   8   9   10   TO WORK
REDUCED

6. How many days in the last month have you been kept from performing housework or chores for at least half of the day because of your headaches?

NONE 1–3   4–6   7–9   10–12 13–15 16–18 19–21 22–24 25–27 28–31 EVERY DAY
0   1   2   3   4   5   6   7   8   9   10

7. When you have a headache, how much is your ability to perform housework or chores reduced?

NOT   1–9% 10–19% 20–29% 30–39% 40–49% 50–59% 60–69% 70–79% 80–89% 90–100% UNABLE
0   1   2   3   4   5   6   7   8   9   10   TO PERFORM
REDUCED

8. How many days in the last month have you been kept from non-work activities (family, social or recreational) because of your headaches?

NONE 1–3   4–6   7–9   10–12 13–15 16–18 19–21 22–24 25–27 28–31 EVERY DAY
0   1   2   3   4   5   6   7   8   9   10

9. When you have a headache, how much is your ability to engage in non-work activities (family, social or recreational) reduced?

NOT   1–9% 10–19% 20–29% 30–39% 40–49% 50–59% 60–69% 70–79% 80–89% 90–100% UNABLE
0   1   2   3   4   5   6   7   8   9   10   TO PERFORM
REDUCED

Figure 2-14 Headache Disability Questionnaire. (From Niere K, Quin A: Development of a headache-specific disability questionnaire for patients attending physiotherapy. Man Ther 14:45–51, 2009.)

ability. In addition, the examiner can ask the patient to name several important people from the present in reverse chronological order (e.g., the last three presidents of the United States) or to give the names of some familiar capital cities. Finally, the patient should be tested on his or her ability to comprehend abstract relations. For example, the examiner may quote a common proverb, such as "A bird in the hand is worth two in the bush," and then ask the patient to explain what the expression means. Patients with organic mental impairment and certain patients with schizophrenia may give a concrete answer, failing to recognize the abstract principle involved.[44] The ability to conceptualize, abstract, plan ahead, and formulate rational judgments of problems or events is largely a function of the frontal lobes.

15. *Can the patient talk normally?* Patients with lesions of the parietal lobe have difficulty communicating and understanding what is occurring around them. **Dysarthria** indicates defects in articulation, enunciation, or rhythm of speech. It usually results from extraneural problems, such as poor-fitting dentures, malformation of the oral structures, or impairment of the musculature of the tongue, palate, pharynx, or lips because of incoordination, weakness, or abnormal innervation. It is characterized by slurring, slowness of speech, indistinct speech, and breaks in normal speech rhythm. **Dysphonia** is a disorder of vocalization characterized by the abnormal production of sounds from the larynx. Dysphonia is usually caused by various abnormalities of the larynx itself or of its innervation. The principal complaint of dysphonia is hoarseness, ranging from mild roughness of the voice to an inability to produce sound. **Dysphasia** denotes the inability to use and understand written and spoken words as a result of disorders involving cortical centers of speech or their interconnections in the dominant cerebral hemisphere. With all of these conditions, the peripheral mechanisms for speech remain intact.

16. *Does the patient have any allergies, or is the patient receiving any medication?* Allergies may affect the eyes and nose, as may medications. Medications themselves may mask some symptoms.

17. *Is the patient having any problems with the eyes?* Monocular **diplopia** (blurred vision when looking with one eye) may result from hyphema, a detached lens, or other trauma to the globe of the eye.[57] Binocular diplopia (blurred vision when looking through both eyes) occurs in 10% to 40% of patients with a zygoma fracture. It may be caused by soft-tissue entrapment, neuromuscular injury (intraorbital or intramuscular), hemorrhage, or edema. It disappears when one eye is closed. Double vision, which occurs when the good eye is closed, indicates that some structure of the eye is injured. If it occurs with both eyes open,

TABLE 2-15

Common Visual Eye Symptoms and Disease States

Visual Symptom	Associated Causes
Loss of vision	Optic neuritis
	Detached retina
	Retinal hemorrhage
	Central retinal vascular occlusion
Spots	No pathological significance*
Flashes	Migraine
	Retinal detachment
	Posterior vitreous detachment
Loss of visual field or presence of shadows or curtains	Retinal detachment
	Retinal hemorrhage
Glare, photophobia	Iritis (inflammation of the iris)
	Meningitis (inflammation of the meninges)
Distortion of vision	Retinal detachment
	Macular edema
Difficulty seeing in dim light	Myopia
	Vitamin A deficiency
	Retinal degeneration
Colored haloes around lights	Acute narrow angle glaucoma
	Opacities in lens or cornea
Colored vision changes	Cataracts
	Drugs (digitalis increases yellow vision)
Double vision	Extraocular muscle paresis or paralysis

From Swartz MH: Textbook of physical diagnosis, Philadelphia, 1989, WB Saunders, p. 132.
*May precede a retinal detachment or be associated with fertility drugs.

something is affecting the free movement of the eyes (Tables 2-15 and 2-16).

18. *Does the patient wear glasses or contact lenses?* If the patient wears glasses, are the lenses treated (hardened) or made of polycarbonate? If they are hardened, how long ago were they treated? If the patient wears contact lenses, are they hard, soft, or extended-wear lenses? Did the patient wear eye protectors? If so, what type were they? Are the patient's eyes watering? Is there any pain in the eyes? Small perforating injuries may be painless. If the patient complains of flashes of bright light, "a curtain falling in front of the eye," or floating black specks, these findings may indicate retinal detachment. These questions tell the examiner whether the eyewear or eyes need to be examined in greater detail.

19. *Is the patient having any problem with hearing?* Does the patient complain of an earache? If so, when was the onset, and what is the duration of the earache? Does the patient complain of pain or a discharge from the ear? Is the earache associated with an upper

TABLE **2-16**

Common Nonvisual Eye Symptoms and Disease States

Nonvisual Symptom	Associated Causes
Itching	Dry eyes
	Eye fatigue
	Allergies
Tearing	Emotional states
	Hypersecretion of tears
	Blockage of drainage
Dryness	Sjögren syndrome
	Decreased secretion as a result of aging
Sandiness, grittiness	Conjunctivitis
Fullness of eyes	Proptosis (bulging of the eyeball)
	Aging changes in the lids
Twitching	Fibrillation of orbicularis oculi
Eyelid heaviness	Fatigue
	Lid edema
Dizziness	Refractive error
	Cerebellar disease
Blinking	Local irritation
	Facial tic
Lids sticking together	Inflammatory disease of lids or conjunctivae
Foreign body sensation	Foreign body
	Corneal abrasion
Burning	Uncorrected refractive error
	Conjunctivitis
	Sjögren syndrome
Throbbing, aching	Acute iritis (inflammation of the iris)
	Sinusitis (inflammation of the sinuses)
Tenderness	Lid inflammations
	Conjunctivitis
	Iritis
Headache	Refractive errors
	Migraine
	Sinusitis
Drawing sensation	Uncorrected refractive errors

From Swartz MH: Textbook of physical diagnosis, Philadelphia, 1989, WB Saunders, p. 133.

respiratory tract infection, swimming, or trauma? The patient should also be questioned on his or her method of cleaning the ear. If there appears to be a hearing loss, the patient should be asked whether the hearing loss came on quickly or slowly, whether the patient hears best on the telephone (amplified sound) or in a quiet or noisy environment, and whether speech is heard soft or loud. Does the patient use a hearing aid?

20. *Is the patient having any problems with the nose?* Has the patient used nose drops or spray? If so, how much, how often, and for how long? Does the patient have any nasal discharge, and if so, is its character watery, mucoid, purulent, crusty, or bloody? Does the discharge have any odor (indicative of infection), and is it unilateral or bilateral? Does the patient exhibit any associated nasal symptoms, such as sneezing, nasal congestion, itching, or mouth breathing? Does the patient complain of a nosebleed, and has the patient had many nosebleeds? If so, how frequent are the nosebleeds, what is the amount of the bleeding, and what appears to be causing the bleeding? Positive responses to any of these questions indicate that the nose must be examined in greater detail.

21. If the examiner is concerned about the mouth and teeth or the temporomandibular joints, questions related to these areas can be found in Chapter 4. It is important, however, to ensure that the patient's dental occlusion and biting alignment have not been altered. Are all the teeth present, and are they symmetrical? Is there any swelling or bleeding around the teeth? Are the teeth mobile, or is part of a tooth missing? Is the pulp exposed? Each of these questions helps determine whether the teeth have been injured. Teeth that have been avulsed, if intact, should be reimplanted as quickly as possible. If reimplanted after cleansing (rinsed in saline solution or water) within less than 30 minutes, the tooth has a 90% chance of being retained. If it is not possible to reimplant the tooth, it should be kept moist in saline, or the patient should keep it between the gum and cheek while dental care is sought.

22. Questions concerning the neck and cervical spine can be found in Chapter 3.

OBSERVATION

For proper observation[58-61] of the head and face, any hat, helmet, mouth guard, or face guard should be removed. If a neck injury is suspected or if the patient presents an emergency situation, the examiner may take the time to remove only those items that are interfering with immediate emergency care. If a neck injury is suspected, extreme caution should be observed when removing the item. When assessing the head and face, the examiner must also observe and assess the posture of the cervical spine and the temporomandibular joints; see Chapters 3 and 4 for detailed descriptions of observation of these areas.

When observing the head and face, it is essential that the examiner look at the face to note the position and shape of the eyes, nose, mouth, teeth, and ears and look for deformity, asymmetry, facial imbalance, swelling, lacerations, foreign bodies, or bleeding during rest, with movement, or with different facial expressions.[62] One should also note, as much as possible, the individual's normal facial expression. A patient's facial expression often reflects the patient's general feeling and well-being.

A dazed or vacant look often indicates problems. While talking to the patient, the examiner should watch for any asymmetry of facial motion or change in facial expression when the patient answers; slight facial asymmetry is common. In addition, small degrees of paralysis may not be obvious unless one attempts an exaggerated expression. If some facial paralysis is suspected, the examiner should ask the patient to make exaggerated facial expressions that will demonstrate the paralysis. If facial asymmetry is present, one should note whether all of the features on one side of the face are affected or only a portion of the face is affected. For example, with facial nerve (cranial nerve VII) paralysis, the entire side of the face is affected, although the most noticeable differences will occur around one eye and one side of the mouth. If only one side of the mouth is involved, then a problem with the trigeminal nerve (cranial nerve V) should be suspected. Any changes in the shape of the face or unusual features (such as, masses, edema, puffiness, coarseness, prominent eyes, amount of facial hair, excessive perspiration, or skin color) should be noted. Eye puffiness is often one of the earliest signs of edema in the face. Skin color may include cyanosis, pallor, jaundice, or pigmentation, and each may be indicative of different systemic problems.

The examiner should view the patient from the front, side, behind, and above, noting the area behind the ears, at the hairline, and around the crown of the head as well as on the face (Figure 2-15). An examiner who suspects a skull (cranial vault) injury should look behind the ears, at the hairline, and around the crown of the head for any deformity, bruising, or laceration.

Viewing from the front, the examiner should observe the patient's hairline, noting any abnormalities. The soft tissues (such as, the eyelids, eyebrows, cheeks, lips, nose, and chin) should be inspected for lacerations, bruising, or hematoma (Figures 2-16 and 2-17). The eyes should be level. For example, a zygoma fracture causes the eye on the affected side to drop (Figure 2-18). The two eyes should be compared for prominence or retraction (Figure 2-19). If there appears to be any bulging, especially unilaterally, the examiner should tilt the patient's head forward or back and, looking from above, compare each cornea with the lid below, noting whether one or both corneas bulge beyond the lid margins. If one or both eyes appear to bulge, the examiner can use a pocket ruler to roughly measure the distance from the angle of the eye to the corneal apex.

Immediate referral for further examination by a specialist is required for an embedded corneal foreign body; haze or blood in the anterior chamber (hyphema); decreased or partial vision; irregular, asymmetric, or poor pupil action; diplopia or double vision; laceration of the eyelid or impaired lid function; perforation or laceration of the globe; broken contact lens or shattered eyeglass in the eye; unexplained eye pain that is stabbing or deep and throbbing; blurred vision that does not clear with blinking; loss of all or part of the visual field; protrusion of one eye relative to the other; an injured eye that does not move as fully as the uninjured eye; or abnormal pupil size or shape. A teardrop pupil usually indicates iris entrapment in a corneal or scleral laceration. In addition, the eyes should be observed from the lateral aspect. The normal distance from the cornea to the angle of the eye is 16 mm or less. The distances between the upper and lower lids should be the same for both eyes. When the eyes open, the superior eyelid should cover a portion of the iris but not the pupil itself. If it covers more of the

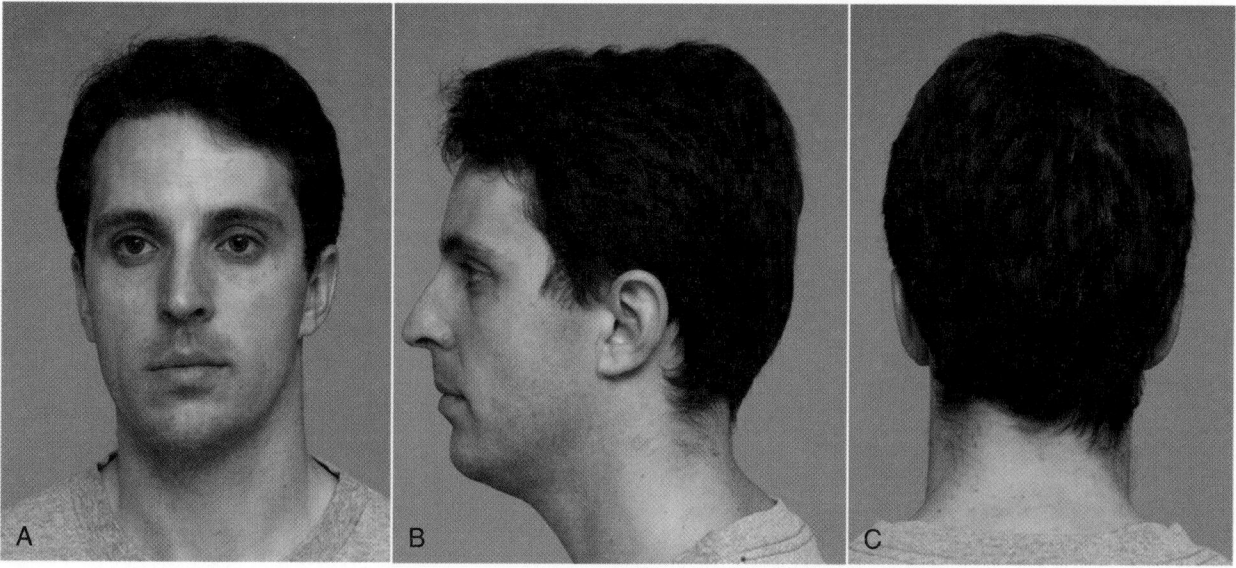

Figure 2-15 Views of the head and face. A, Anterior. **B,** Side. **C,** Posterior.

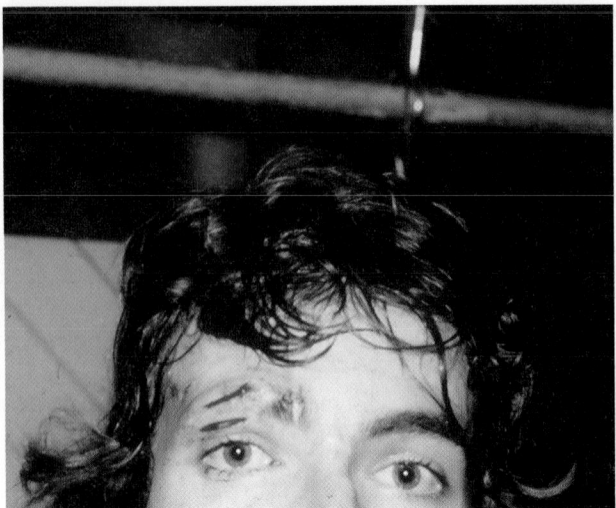

Figure 2-16 Lacerations to the upper eyelid and eyebrow.

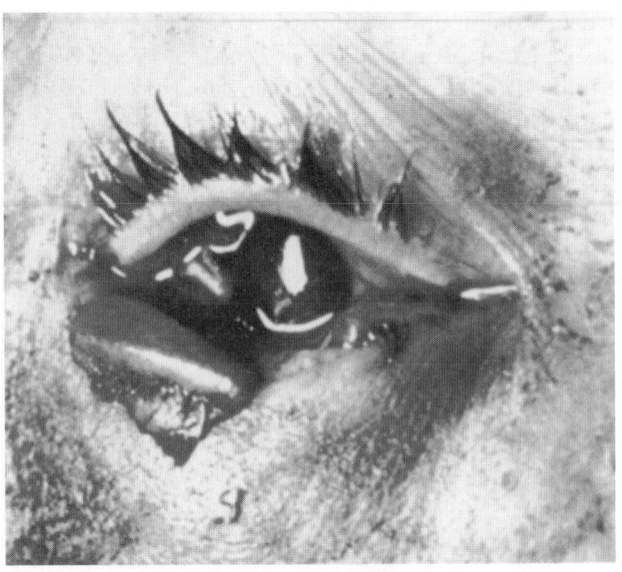

Figure 2-19 A severe glancing or direct blow to this right eye has resulted in a ruptured globe. Note the depressed eye. (From Pashby TJ, Pashby RC: Treatment of sports eye injuries. In Schneider RC, et al, editors: Sports injuries: mechanisms, prevention and treatment, Baltimore, 1985, Lippincott Williams & Wilkins p. 589.)

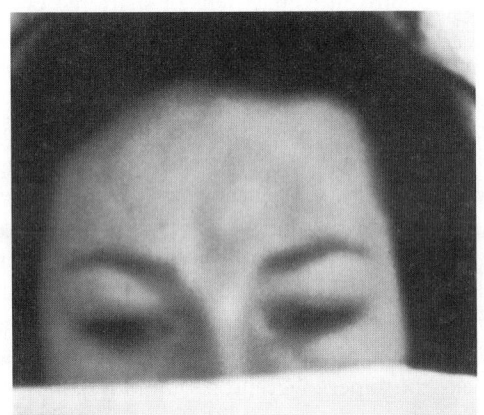

Figure 2-17 Contusion to the forehead caused by a racquetball ball.

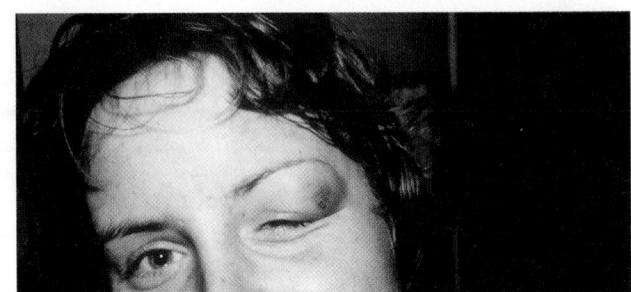

Figure 2-20 Black eye (periorbital ecchymosis).

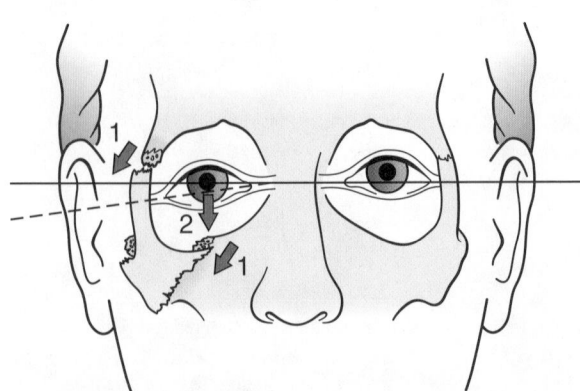

Figure 2-18 Inferior displacement of the zygoma *(1)* results in depression of the lateral canthus and pupil *(2)* because of depression of the suspensory ligaments that attach to the lateral orbital, Whitnall tubercle. (Modified from Ellis E: Fractures of the zygomatic complex and arch. In Fonseca RJ, Walker RV, editors: Oral and maxillofacial trauma, Philadelphia, 1991, WB Saunders, p. 446.)

iris than the other upper eyelid does or if it extends over the iris or pupil, ptosis or drooping of that eyelid should be suspected. If the eyelid does not cover part of the iris, retraction of the eyelid should be suspected. Are the eyelids everted or inverted? Normally, they are neither. The examiner should also note whether the patient can close both eyes completely. If an eye injury is suspected, this action should be done carefully, because closing the eyes can increase intraocular pressure. The lids should be pressed together only enough to bring the eyelashes together. Any inflammation or masses, especially on the lid margin, should be noted. If present, a "black eye," or periorbital contusion, should also be noted (Figure 2-20). The lashes should be viewed to see if there is even distribution along the lid margins. "Raccoon eyes," which are purple discolorations of the eyelids and orbital regions, may indicate orbital fractures, basilar skull fractures, or a fracture of the base of the anterior cranial fossa.[58] This sign takes several hours to develop.

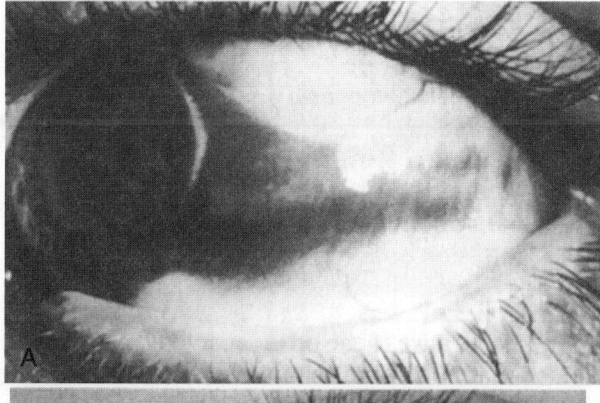
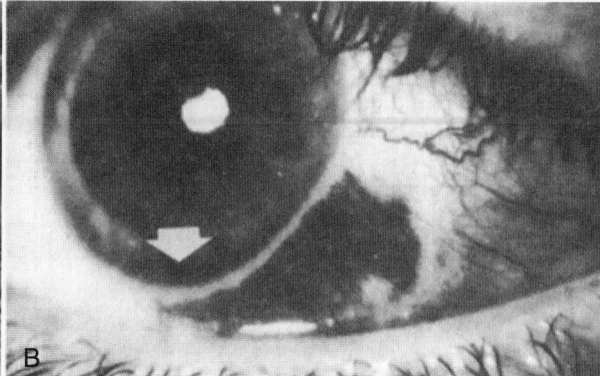
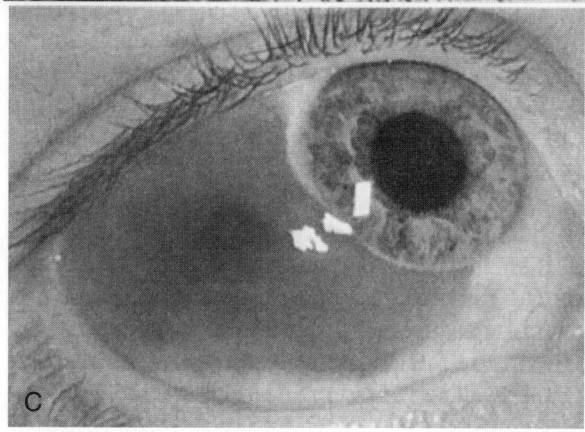

Figure 2-21 A, Posttraumatic conjunctival hemorrhage without other ocular or orbital damage. **B,** Posttraumatic conjunctival hemorrhage from blunt injury with a small hyphema *(arrow)*. In this case, the injury was significant because of the presence of blood in the anterior chamber. **C,** Subconjunctival ecchymosis with no lateral limit should suggest osseous orbital fractures. (**A** and **B,** From Paton D, Goldberg MF: Management of ocular injuries, Philadelphia, 1976, WB Saunders, p. 182. **C,** From Lew D, Sinn DP: Diagnosis and treatment of midface fractures. In Fonseca RJ, Walker RV, editors: Oral and maxillofacial trauma, Philadelphia, 1991, WB Saunders, p. 250.)

Eye Signs and Symptoms Requiring Specialist Care

- Foreign body that is not easily removed
- Eye does not move properly
- Altered pupil action
- Abnormal pupil size or shape
- Double vision
- Blurred vision
- Decreased or partial vision
- Loss of part or all of visual field
- Laceration of eye or eyelid
- Blood between cornea and iris (hyphema)
- Impaired eyelid function
- Penetration of eye or eyelid
- Eye pain
- Sharp or throbbing eye pain
- Protrusion or retraction of eye

The conjunctiva should be inspected for hemorrhage, laceration, and foreign bodies.[62] If the patient complains of "something in the eye," eversion of the upper eyelid usually reveals a foreign body that can often be easily brushed away. Displaced contact lenses are often found in this upper area of the eye. The conjunctival covering of the lower lid may be examined by having the patient look upward while the examiner draws the lower lid downward. The conjunctiva should be examined as being a continuous sheet of epithelium from the globe to the lids. The color of the sclera should also be noted. Posttraumatic conjunctival hemorrhage (Figure 2-21) and possible scleral lacerations (Figure 2-22) should be noted, if present. In dark-skinned patients, pigmented areas may show up as small dark spots or patches near the limbus. The shape and color of the cornea should be inspected. The anterior chambers of the eye should be inspected and compared for clarity and depth.[63] If present, hyphema in the form of haze or actual blood pooling (Figure 2-23) in the anterior eye chamber should be noted.[57] If there is any potential for or evidence of bleeding in the anterior chamber of the eye, the patient's activity should be curtailed, because increased activity increases the chances of secondary hemorrhage during the first week after injury. Examination of the cornea with a penlight shone obliquely on the eye should be carried out to look for foreign bodies, abrasions, or lacerations. Corneal injuries can lead to lacrimation (tearing), photophobia (intolerance to light), or blepharospasm (spasm of the eyelid orbicular muscle) as well as extreme pain from exposure of sensory nerve endings. A fluorescein strip dipped into tears that are exposed as the lower lid is pulled downward will readily outline abrasions.

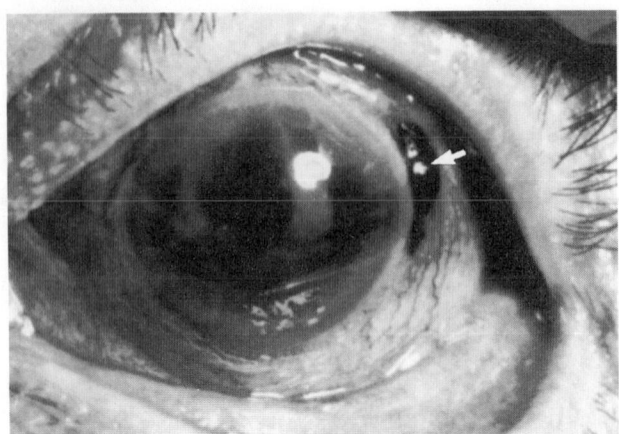

Figure 2-22 Scleral rupture *(arrow)* at the limbus after blunt trauma. The iris and ciliary body have prolapsed into the subconjunctival space. (From Paton D, Goldberg MF: Management of ocular injuries, Philadelphia, 1976, WB Saunders, p. 310.)

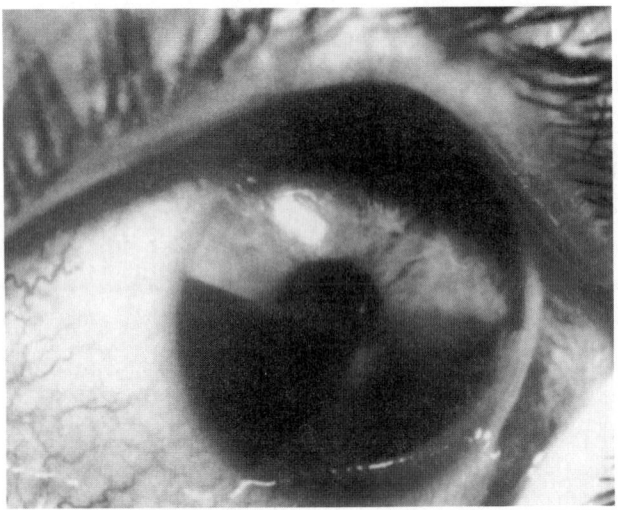

Figure 2-23 Hyphema in the anterior chamber of the eye. (From Easterbrook M, Cameron J: Injuries in racquet sports. In Schneider RC, et al, editors: Sports injuries: mechanisms, prevention and treatment, Baltimore, 1985, Lippincott Williams & Wilkins, p. 556.)

The pupillary size (diameter range, 2 to 6 mm; mean, 3.5 mm), shape (round), and symmetry should be compared with those of the other eye. Elliptical pupils often indicate a corneal laceration. The color of the irises of the eyes should be compared. When looking at the pupils, the examiner should note whether the pupils are equal. Are the pupils smaller or larger than normal? Are they round or irregularly shaped? The pupils are normally slightly unequal in 5% of the population, but inequality of pupil size should initially be viewed with suspicion. For example, unilateral dilation may be the result of a sympathetic nerve response following a blow to the face.[4] Pupils tend to be smaller in infants, the elderly, and persons with hyperopia (farsightedness), whereas they tend to be slightly dilated in persons with myopia (nearsightedness) or light-colored irises.

The nose should be inspected for any deviations in shape, size, or color.[62] The skin should be smooth without swelling and should conform to the color of the face. The airways are usually oval and symmetrically proportioned. If a discharge is present, its character (i.e., color, smell, texture) should be noted and described. Bloody discharge occurs as a result of epistaxis or trauma, such as a nasal fracture, zygoma fracture, or skull fracture. Mucoid discharge is typical of rhinitis. Bilateral purulent discharge can occur with upper respiratory tract infection. Unilateral purulent, thick, greenish, and often malodorous discharge usually indicates the presence of a foreign body.

Depression of the nasal bridge can result from a fracture of the nasal bone. Nasal flaring is associated with respiratory distress, whereas narrowing of the airways on inspiration may indicate chronic nasal obstruction and be associated with mouth breathing. The nasal mucosa should be deep pink and glistening. A film of clear discharge is often apparent on the nasal septum. The nasal septum should be close to midline and fairly straight, appearing thicker anteriorly than posteriorly. If present, a hematoma in the septal area should be noted. Asymmetric posterior nasal cavities may indicate a deviation of the nasal septum.

With the patient's mouth closed, the lips should be observed for symmetry, color, edema, and surface abnormalities. Lipstick should be removed before the assessment. The lips should be pink and have vertical and horizontal symmetry, both at rest and with movement. Dry, cracked lips may be caused by dehydration from wind or low humidity, whereas deep fissures at the corners of the mouth may indicate overclosure of the mouth or riboflavin deficiency.

Drooping of the mouth on one side, sagging of the lower eyelid, and flattening of the nasolabial fold suggest possible facial nerve (cranial nerve VII) involvement. The patient is also unable to pucker the lips to whistle.

The shape and position of the jaw and teeth should also be noted anteriorly and from the side.[62] Asymmetry may indicate a fracture of the jaw (Figure 2-24), whereas bleeding around the gums of the teeth may indicate fracture, avulsion, or loosening of the teeth (Figure 2-25). If teeth are missing, they must be accounted for. If they are not accounted for, an x-ray may be required to ensure that the teeth have not entered the abdominal or chest cavity. Pain on percussion of the teeth often indicates damage to the periodontal ligament.

From the side, the examiner should look for any asymmetry or depression, which may indicate pathology. The examiner should inspect the auricles of the ears for size, shape, symmetry, landmarks, color, and position on the head. To determine the position of the auricle, the examiner can draw an imaginary line between the outer canthus of the eye and occipital protuberance (Figure 2-26). The top of the auricle should touch or be above this line.[50] The examiner can then draw another

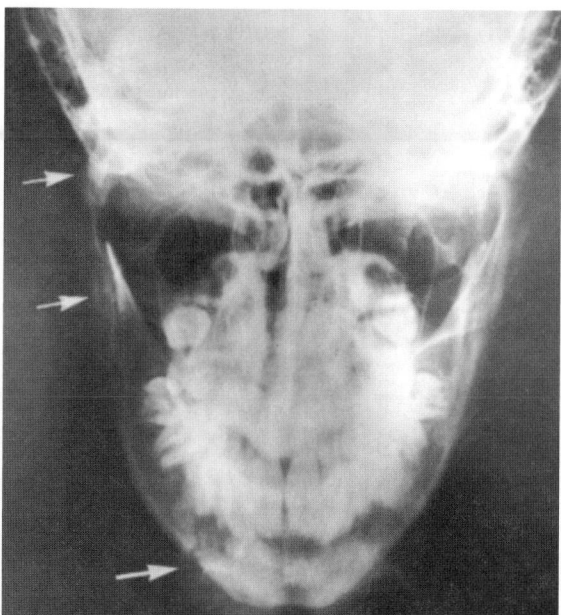

Figure 2-24 Fracture of the neck of the condyle on the right *(upper arrows)* with fracture through the mandible on the same side *(lower arrow)*. When one fracture is shown in the mandible, search carefully for the second. (From O'Donoghue DH: Treatment of injuries to athletes, Philadelphia, 1984, WB Saunders, p. 115.)

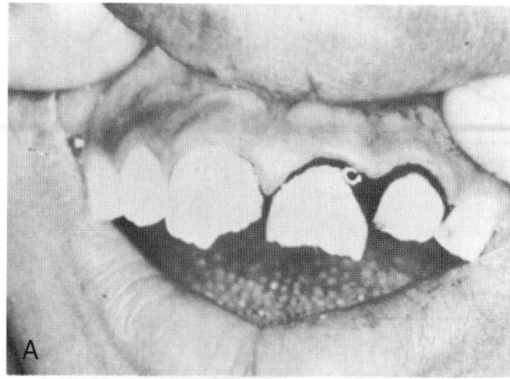

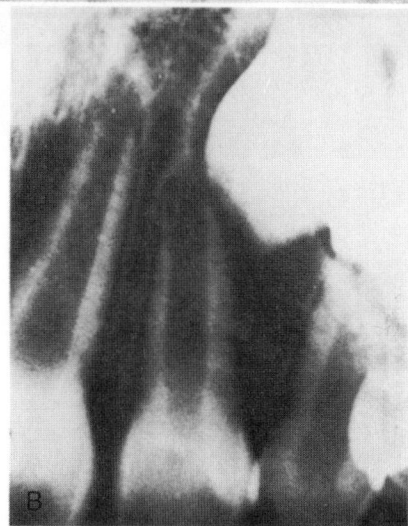

Figure 2-25 A 9-year-old boy was hit in the mouth with a ball while he was playing baseball. The right maxillary central and lateral incisors were chipped. **A,** Avulsed teeth reimplanted with finger pressure. **B,** Radiograph of root canal with wide-open apex. Reimplanted quickly, these teeth may not require root canal treatment. (From Torg JS: Athletic injuries to the head, neck and face, Philadelphia, 1982, Lea & Febiger, p. 247.)

imaginary line perpendicular to the previous line and just anterior to the auricle. The auricle's position should be almost vertical. If the angle is more than 10° posterior or anterior, it is considered abnormal. An auricle that is set low or is at an unusual angle may indicate chromosomal aberrations or renal disorders. In addition, the lateral and medial surfaces and surrounding tissues should be examined, noting any deformities, lesions, or nodules. The auricles should be the same color as the facial skin without moles, cysts, or other lesions or deformities. Athletes, especially wrestlers, may exhibit a cauliflower ear (hematoma auris), which is a keloid scar forming in the auricle because of friction to or twisting of the ear (Figure 2-27). Blueness may indicate some degree of cyanosis. Pallor or excessive redness may be the result of vasomotor instability or increased temperature. Frostbite can cause extreme pallor or blistering (Figure 2-28).

The examiner should look posteriorly for any asymmetry or depression. The positions of the ears (height, protrusion) can be compared by observing them from behind. A low hairline may indicate conditions such as Klippel-Feil syndrome. The examiner should also look for the presence of **Battle sign.** This sign, which takes as long as 24 hours to appear, is demonstrated by purple and blue discoloration of the skin in the mastoid area and may indicate a temporal bone or basilar skull fracture.

The examiner then views the patient from overhead (superior view) to note any asymmetry from above (Figure 2-29). This method is especially useful when

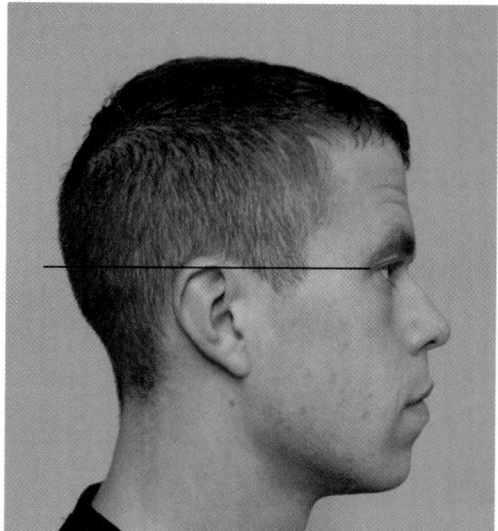

Figure 2-26 Auricle alignment. Normal position shown.

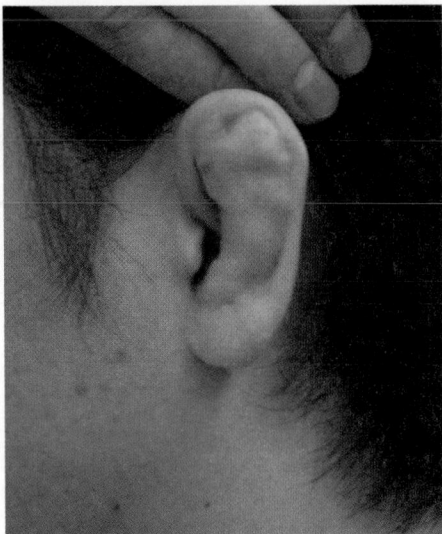

Figure 2-27 Cauliflower ear (hematoma auris).

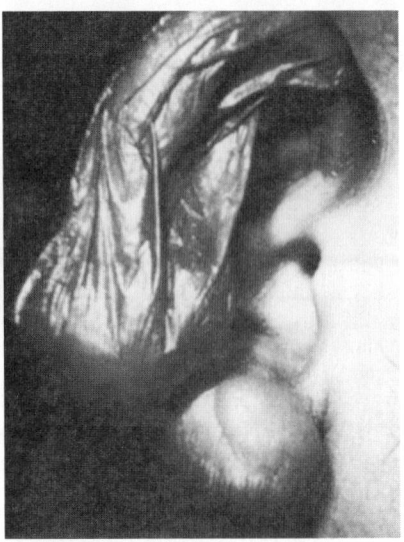

Figure 2-28 Auricular frostbite with development of massive vesicles that are beginning to resolve spontaneously. (From Schuller DE, Bruce RA: Ear, nose, throat and eye. In Strauss RH, editor: Sports medicine, ed 2, Philadelphia, 1991, WB Saunders, p. 191.)

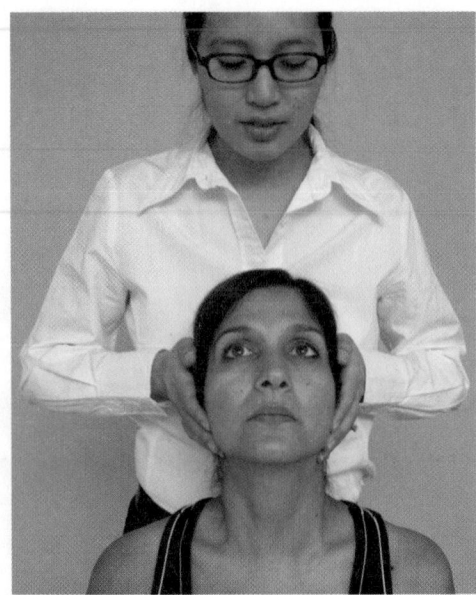

Figure 2-29 View of the patient from above to look for bilateral symmetry of the face.

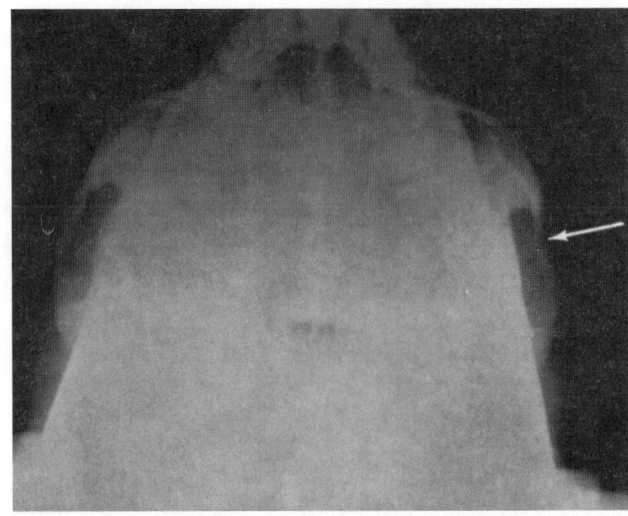

Figure 2-30 **Typical fracture of zygomatic arch** on the right *(arrow)*. Note normal arch on the left. (From O'Donoghue DH: Treatment of injuries to athletes, Philadelphia, 1984, WB Saunders, p. 114.)

looking for a possible fracture of the zygoma (Figure 2-30). The deformity is easier to detect if the examiner carefully places the index fingers below the infraorbital margins along the zygomatic bodies and then gently pushes into the edema to reduce the effect of the edema (Figure 2-31).

EXAMINATION

The examination of the head and face differs from the orthopedic assessment of other areas of the body because the assessment does not involve joints. The only joints that could be included in the assessment are the temporomandibular joints, and these joints are discussed in Chapter 4.

Examination of the Head

Many problems in the head and face may be problems referred from the cervical spine, temporomandibular joint, or teeth. However, if one suspects a head injury, it is necessary to keep a close watch on the patient, noting any changes and when these changes occur. The examiner should implement a **Neural Watch** so that any changes that occur over time can be determined easily (Table 2-17). The testing should occur at 15- or 30-minute

Signs and Symptoms of Maxillary and Zygomatic Fractures

- Facial asymmetry
- Loss of cheek prominence
- Palpable steps
  - Infraorbital rim (zygomaticomaxillary suture)
  - Lateral orbital rim (frontozygomatic suture)
  - Root of zygoma intraorally
  - Zygomatic arch between the ear and the eye (zygomaticotemporal suture)
- Hypoesthesia/anesthesia
  - Cheek, side of nose, upper lip, and teeth on the injured side
  - Compression of the infraorbital nerve as it courses along the floor of the orbit to exit into the face via the foramen beneath the orbital rim

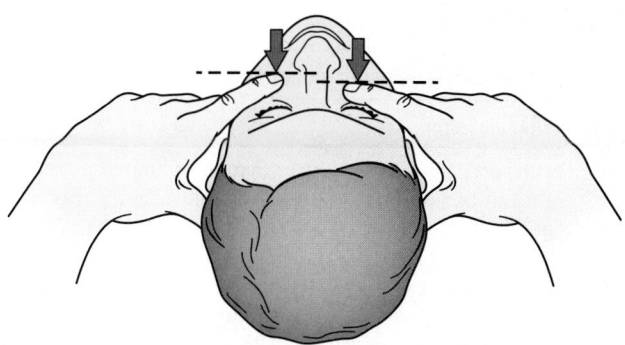

Figure 2-31 Method of assessing posterior displacement of the zygomatic complex from behind the patient. The examiner should firmly but carefully depress the fingers into the edematous soft tissues while palpating along the infraorbital areas. (Modified from Ellis E: Fractures of the zygomatic complex and arch. In Fonseca RJ, Walker RV, editors: Oral and maxillofacial trauma, Philadelphia, 1991, WB Saunders, p. 443.)

TABLE **2-17**

Neural Watch Chart

Unit		Time 1 ( )	Time 2 ( )	Time 3 ( )	Unit		Time 1 ( )	Time 2 ( )	Time 3 ( )
I Vital signs	Blood pressure Pulse Respiration Temperature				VI Pupils	Size on right Size on left Reacts on right Reacts on left			
II Conscious and	Oriented Disoriented Restless Combative				VII Ability to move	Right arm Left arm Right leg Left leg			
III Speech	Clear Rambling Garbled None				VII Sensation	Right side (normal/ abnormal) Left side (normal/ abnormal) Dermatome affected (specify) Peripheral nerve affected (specify)			
IV Will awaken to	Name Shaking Light pain Strong pain								
V Nonverbal reaction to pain	Appropriate Inappropriate "Decerebrate" None								

Modified from American Academy of Orthopedic Surgeons: Athletic training and sports medicine, Park Ridge, IL, 1984, AAOS, p. 399.

TABLE **2-18**

Graduated Return-to-Play Protocol for Returning an Individual to Sport

Rehabilitation Stage	Functional Exercise at Each Stage of Rehabilitation	Objective of Each Stage
1. No activity	Symptom limited physical and cognitive rest	Recovery
2. Light aerobic exercise	Walking, swimming or stationary cycling keeping intensity less than 70% maximum permitted heart rate; no resistance training	Increase heart rate
3. Sport-specific exercise	Skating drills in ice hockey, running drills in soccer; no head impact activities	Add movement
4. Non-contact training drills	Progression to more complex training drills (e.g., passing drills in football and ice hockey); may start progressive resistance training	Exercise, coordination, and cognitive load
5. Full-contact practice	Following medical clearance participate in normal training activities	Restore confidence and assess functional skills by coaching staff
6. Return to play	Normal game play	

Modified from McCrory P, Meeuwisse WH, Aubry M, et al: Consensus statement on concussion in sport: the 4th International Conference on Concussion in Sport held in Zurich, November 2012. Br J Sports Med 47(5):250–258, 2013.

Head Examination

- Concussion
- Headache
- Memory tests
- Neural Watch (Glasgow Coma Scale)
- Expanding intracranial lesion
- Proprioception
- Coordination
- Head injury card

---

intervals, depending on the severity of the injury and the changes recorded.

The issue of whether a patient should be allowed to return to competition or high-level activity following a concussion, and how soon, is one that has not been completely settled, although clinicians are becoming more concerned about the consequences of concussions.[11,64–70] Research has shown that the brain is vulnerable to reinjury for 3 to 5 days following concussions because of altered blood flow and metabolic dysfunction.[11] If the examiner is contemplating allowing the patient to return to activity because all symptoms have disappeared, graduated provocative stress tests (Table 2-18) should be considered before allowing the patient to return. These tests are commonly related to the sport but may include jumping jacks, sit-ups, pushups, deep knee bends, and lying supine for 1 minute with feet elevated or similar activities that may be related to what the patient will return to functionally (e.g., rapid head movements, straining or holding breath). These activities should be viewed as actions that increase intracranial pressure and can cause a different physiological response in concussed athletes,[71] which may lead to symptoms.[4,72] Although the guidelines outlined in Table 2-19 may appear excessively precautionary, they are designed to prevent **second impact syndrome,** which is potentially catastrophic injury with a mortality rate close to 50% or permanent brain injury.[18,64,73–77]

The examiner should always be looking for the possibility of an expanding intracranial lesion resulting from a leaking or torn blood vessel. Normally, the brain has a fixed volume that is enclosed in a nonexpansile structure, namely, the skull and dura mater. These lesions may be caused by epidural hemorrhage (usually tearing of one of the meningeal arteries as a result of high-speed impact), subarachnoid hemorrhage (usually as a result of an aneurysm), or subdural hemorrhage (usually as a result of tearing of bridging veins between the brain and cavernous sinus).[64] These injuries are emergency conditions that must be looked after immediately because of their high mortality rate (as much as 50%). An **expanding intracranial lesion** is indicated by an altered lucid state (state of consciousness), development of inequality of the pupils, unusual slowing of the heart rate that primarily occurs after a lucid interval, irregular eye movements, and eyes that no longer track properly. There is also a tendency for the patient to demonstrate increased body temperature and irregular respirations. Normal intracranial pressure measures from 4 to 15 mm Hg, and an intracranial pressure of more than 20 mm Hg is considered abnormal. Intracranial pressure of 40 mm Hg causes neurological dysfunction and impairment. Although in the emergency care setting there is no way of determining the intracranial pressure, the signs and symptoms mentioned indicate that the pressure is increasing. Most patients who experience an increase in intracranial pressure complain of severe headache, and this symptom is often followed

TABLE **2-19**

Return-to-Play Guidelines Following Head Injury

Grade of Concussion	On-the-Field Treatment	First Concussion	Second Concussion	Third Concussion
Simple: Loss of consciousness <1 minute; posttraumatic amnesia <30 minutes	Remove athlete from the competition	Athlete may return to play if asymptomatic for 1 week	Obtain CT scan; athlete may return in 2 weeks if asymptomatic for 1 week	Athlete sidelined a minimum of 1 month; may return then if asymptomatic for 1 week
Complex: Loss of consciousness >1 minute; posttraumatic amnesia >30 minutes	Remove athlete from the competition; transport athlete to a hospital for emergency evaluation of the player by a neurosurgeon and to obtain diagnostic neuroimaging	Obtain CT scan, remove from play for a minimum of 1 month; athlete may then return to play if asymptomatic for 1 week	Obtain CT scan; consider terminating for season	Terminate athlete for season; athlete may return next season if asymptomatic, but permanent retirement from contact sports should be considered

Modified from Warren WL, Bailes JE, Cantu RC: Guidelines for safe return to play after athletic head and neck injuries. In Cantu RC, editor: Neurologic athletic head and spine injuries, Philadelphia, 2000, WB Saunders.
CT, Computed tomography.

by vomiting (sometimes projectile vomiting). Finally, an expanding intracranial lesion causes increased weakness on the side of the body opposite that on which the lesion has occurred.

Signs and symptoms that indicate a good possibility of recovery from a head injury, especially after the patient experiences unconsciousness, include response to noxious stimuli, eye opening, pupil activity, spontaneous eye movement, intact oculovestibular reflexes, and appropriate motor function responses. Neurological signs that indicate a poor prognosis after a head injury include nonreactive pupils, absence of oculovestibular reflexes, severe extension patterns or no motor function response at all, and increased intracranial pressure.[44]

Signs and Symptoms of an Expanding Intracranial Lesion

- Altered state of consciousness
- Nystagmus
- Pupil inequality
- Irregular eye movements
- Abnormal slowing of heart
- Irregular respiration
- Severe headache
- Intractable vomiting
- Positive expanding intracranial lesion tests (lateralizing)
- Positive coordination tests
- Decreasing muscle strength
- Seizure

It is important when examining the unconscious or conscious patient for a possible head injury to determine the individual's level of consciousness, which may be determined using the **Glasgow Coma Scale** ✓ (Table 2-20). The first test relates to eye opening. Eye opening may occur spontaneously, in response to speech, or in response to pain, or there may be no response at all. Each of these responses is given a numerical value: spontaneous eye opening, *4;* response to speech, *3;* response to pain, *2;* and no response, *1.* Spontaneous opening of the eyes indicates functioning of the ascending reticular activating system. This finding does not necessarily mean that the patient is aware of the surroundings or of what is happening, but it does imply that the patient is in a state of arousal. A patient who opens his or her eyes in response to the examiner's voice is probably responding to the stimulus of sound, not necessarily to the command to open the eyes. If unsure, the examiner may use different sound-making objects (e.g., bell, horn) to elicit an appropriate response.

The second test involves motor response; the patient is given a grade of 6 if there is a response to a verbal command. Otherwise, the patient is graded on a 5-point scale depending on the motor response to a painful stimulus (see Table 2-20). When scoring motor responses, it is the ease with which the motor responses are elicited that constitutes the criterion for the best response. Commands given to the patient should be simple, such as, "Move your arm." The patient should not be asked to squeeze the examiner's hand, nor should the examiner place something in the patient's hand and then ask the patient to grasp it. This action may cause a reflex grasp, not a response to a command.[44]

TABLE **2-20**

☑ **Glasgow Coma Scale***

				Time 1 ( )	Time 2 ( )
Eyes	Open	Spontaneously	4		
		To verbal command	3		
		To pain	2		
		No response	1	___	___
Best motor response	To verbal command	Obeys	6		
	To painful stimulus†	Localizes pain	5		
		Flexion—withdrawal	4		
		Flexion—abnormal (decorticate rigidity)	3		
		Extension (decerebrate rigidity)	2		
		No response	1	___	___
Best verbal response‡		Oriented and converses	5		
		Disoriented and converses	4		
		Inappropriate words	3		
		Incomprehensible sounds	2		
		No response	1	___	___
Total			3–15	___	___

*The Glasgow Coma Scale, which is based on eye opening and verbal and motor responses, is a practical means of monitoring changes in level of consciousness. If responses on the scale are given numerical grades, the overall responsiveness of the patient can be expressed in a score that is the summation of the grades. The lowest score is 3, and the highest is 15.
†Apply knuckles to sternum; observe arms.
‡Arouse patient with painful stimulus if necessary.

If the patient does not give a motor response to a verbal command, then the examiner should attempt to elicit a motor response to a painful stimulus. It is the type and quality of the patient's reaction to the painful stimulus that constitute the scoring criteria. The stimulus should not be applied to the face, because painful stimulus in the facial area may cause the eyes to close tightly as a protective reaction. The painful stimulus may consist of applying a knuckle to the sternum, squeezing the trapezius muscle, or squeezing the soft tissue between the thumb and index finger (Figure 2-32). If the patient moves a limb when the painful stimulus is applied to more than one point or tries to remove the examiner's hand that is applying the painful stimulus, the patient is localizing, and a value of 5 is given. If the patient withdraws from the painful stimulus rapidly, a normal reflex withdrawal is being shown, and a value of 4 is given.

However, if application of a painful stimulus creates a decorticate or decerebrate posture (Figure 2-33), an abnormal response is being demonstrated, and a value of 3 is given for the decorticate posture (injury above red nucleus) or a value of 2 is given for decerebrate posture (brain stem injury). **Decorticate posturing** results from lesions of the diencephalon area, whereas decerebrate posturing results from lesions of the midbrain. With decorticate posturing, the arms, wrists, and fingers are flexed, the upper limbs are adducted, and the legs are extended, medially rotated, and plantar flexed.

Decerebrate posturing, which has a poorer prognosis, involves extension, adduction, and hyperpronation of the arms, whereas the lower limbs are the same as for decorticate posturing.[78] Decerebrate rigidity is usually bilateral. If the patient exhibits no reaction to the painful stimulus, a value of 1 is given. It is important to be sure the "no" response is caused by a head injury and not a spinal cord injury leading to lack of feeling or sensation. Any difference in reaction between limbs should be carefully noted; this finding may indicate a specific focal injury.[44]

In the third test, verbal response is graded on a 5-point scale to measure the patient's speech in response to simple questions, such as "Where are you?" or "Are you winning the game?" For verbal responses, the patient who converses appropriately and shows proper orientation, being aware of oneself and the environment, is given a grade of 5. The patient who is confused is disoriented and unable to completely interact with the environment; this patient is able to converse using the appropriate words and is given a grade of 4. The patient exhibiting inappropriate speech is unable to sustain a conversation with the examiner; this person would be given a grade of 3. A vocalizing patient only groans or makes incomprehensible sounds; this finding leads to a grade of 2. Again, the examiner should note any possible mechanical reason for the inability to verbalize. If the patient makes no sounds and thus has no verbal response, a grade of 1 is assigned.

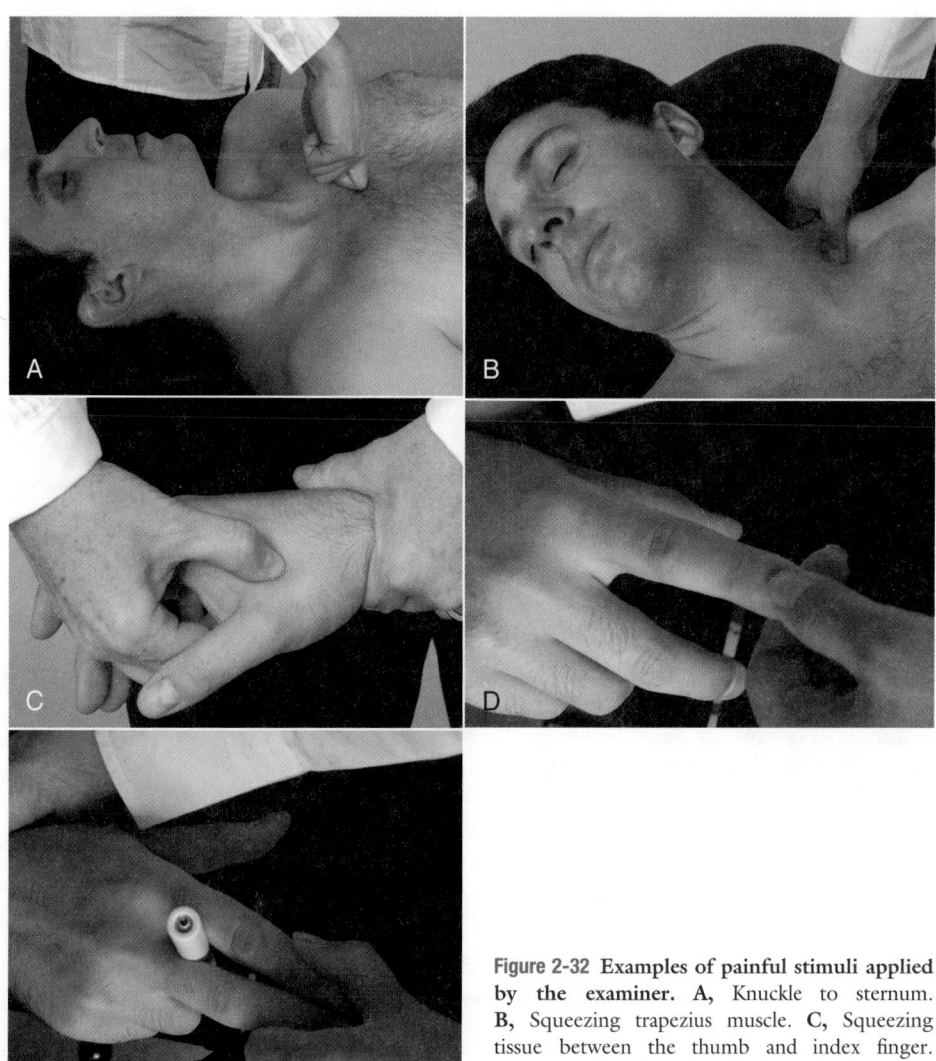

Figure 2-32 Examples of painful stimuli applied by the examiner. A, Knuckle to sternum. **B,** Squeezing trapezius muscle. **C,** Squeezing tissue between the thumb and index finger. **D,** Squeezing a fingertip. **E,** Squeezing an object between two fingers.

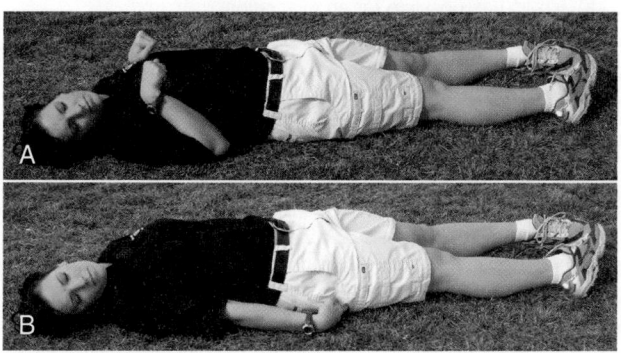

Figure 2-33 A, Decorticate rigidity. **B,** Decerebrate rigidity.

It is vital that the initial score on the **Glasgow Coma Scale** be obtained as soon as possible after the onset of the injury. The scale can then be repeated at 15- or 30-minute intervals, especially in the early stages, if changes are noted. If the score is between 3 and 8, emergency care is required. With the Glasgow Coma Scale, the initial score is used as a basis for determining the severity of the patient's head injury. Patients who maintain a score of 8 or lower on the Glasgow Coma Scale for 6 hours or longer are considered to have a serious head injury. A patient who scores between 9 and 11 is considered to have a moderate head injury, and one who scores 12 or higher is considered to have a mild head injury.[44]

Head Injury Severity Based on Score Maintained on Glasgow Coma Scale (6 or More Hours)

8 or less:	Severe head injury
9 to 11:	Moderate head injury
12 or more:	Mild head injury

TABLE **2-21**

Rancho Los Amigos Scale of Cognitive Function

Level I	No response
Level II	Generalized response
Level III	Localized response
Level IV	Confused, agitated
Level V	Confused, inappropriate
Level VI	Confused, appropriate
Level VII	Automatic, appropriate
Level VIII	Purposeful, appropriate

From Hagen C, Malkmus D, Durham P: Levels of cognitive functioning. In Rehabilitation of the brain injured adult—comprehensive management, Downey, CA, 1980, Professional Staff Association of Rancho Los Amigos.

The Rancho Los Amigos Scale of Cognitive Function may also be used to assess the patient's cognitive abilities. This scale is an eight-level progression from level I, in which the patient is nonresponsive, to level VIII, in which the patient's behavior is purposeful and appropriate (Table 2-21). The Rancho Los Amigos Scale provides an assessment of cognitive function and behavior only, not of physical functioning.[44]

If a person receives a head injury, such as a mild concussion, and is not referred to the hospital, the examiner should ensure that someone accompanies the person home and that someone at home knows what has happened so he or she can monitor the patient in case the patient's condition worsens. Appropriate written instructions should be sent home concerning the individual. The **Head Injury Card** is an example (Figure 2-34).

Levin and colleagues reported the use of the Galveston Orientation and Amnesia Test (GOAT),[47] which they believe measures orientation to person, place, and time, and the memory of events preceding and following head trauma (Figure 2-35). As the patient improves, the total GOAT score should increase.

The examiner may also wish to determine whether the patient has suffered an upper motor neuron lesion. Testing the deep tendon reflexes (see Table 1-31) or the pathological reflexes (see Table 1-33) or having the patient perform various balance and coordination tests may help to determine whether this type of lesion has occurred. However, the pathological reflexes may not be elicited owing to shock. Deep tendon reflexes are accentuated on the side of the body opposite that on which the brain injury has occurred. Balance can play an important role in the assessment of a head-injured patient. Balance involves the integration of several inputs (e.g., visual, proprioceptive, and vestibular systems) that are analyzed by the brain to allow a proper action. For example, in standing, the body is inherently unstable, and only the integration of input from various sources enables the patient to stand and to make appropriate corrections

---

Home Health Care Guidelines: Head Injury Care

The person you have been asked to watch has suffered a head injury, which at this time does not appear to be severe. However, to ensure proper care, please ensure that the following guidelines are followed for the next 24 hours.

1. Limited physical activity for at least 24 hours (rest quietly, **do not drive a vehicle**).

2. Liquid diet only for the next 8 to 24 hours (**no alcohol**).

3. Apply ice to the head for approximately 15 minutes every hour to relieve discomfort and swelling.

4. Tylenol may be given as needed but NO aspirin. No other medication for 24 hours without doctor's approval.

5. Awaken the patient every 2 hours during the next _____ hours and be aware of any symptoms in #6.

6. Appearance of any of the following signs and symptoms means that you should consult a doctor or go to an emergency room at a hospital **immediately**:

   - Nausea and/or vomiting
   - Weakness or numbness in arm, leg, or any other body part
   - Any visual difficulties or dizziness
   - Ringing in the ears
   - Mental confusion or disorientation, irritability, restlessness, forgetfulness
   - Loss of coordination
   - Unusual sleepiness or difficulty in awakening
   - Progressively worsening headache
   - Persistent intense headache after 48 hours
   - Unequal pupil size; slow or no pupil reaction to light
   - Difficulty breathing
   - Irregular heartbeat
   - Convulsions or tremors

7. Call to arrange an appointment with your doctor or the team physician/therapist* for a follow-up visit. If unable to contact your doctor, go to an emergency room as soon as possible for an evaluation.

   *Consult: _____ at _____
   phone number

   or: _____ at _____
   phone number

SPECIAL INSTRUCTIONS, APPOINTMENTS:

Figure 2-34 Home health care guidelines for patients with head injuries. (Modified from Allman FL, Crow RW: On-field evaluation of sports injuries. In Griffin LY, editor: Orthopedic knowledge update: sports medicine, Rosemont, IL, American Academy of Orthopaedic Surgeons, 1994, p. 14.)

to maintain proper standing posture. Balance and coordination can be tested in several ways. The examiner can ask the patient to stand and walk a straight line with the eyes open and then with the eyes closed while the examiner is noting any difference. He or she can then ask the

---

Galveston Orientation and Amnesia Test (GOAT)

Name _____ Date of test _____

Age _____   Sex M F   Day of the week S M T W Th F S

Date of birth _____   Time   AM   PM

Diagnosis _____ Date of injury _____

Error
points

1. What is your name? (2) _____ When were you born? (4) _____ _____

   Where do you live? (4) _____

2. Where are you now? (city) (5) _____ Location (e.g., hospital) (5) _____ _____
                                            (unnecessary to state name of hospital)

3. On what date were you admitted to this hospital? (5) _____   _____

   How did you get here? (5) _____

4. What is the first event you can remember *after* the injury? (5) _____ _____
   Can you describe in detail (e.g., date, time, companions) the first event you can recall after injury?

   (5) _____

5. Can you describe the last event you recall *before* the accident? (5) _____ _____
   Can you describe in detail (e.g., date, time, companions) the first event you can recall before injury?

   (5) _____

6. What time is it now? _____ (1 for each 1/2 hour removed from correct time, to maximum of 5)   _____

7. What day of the week is it? _____ (1 for each day removed from correct one)   _____

8. What day of the month is it? _____ (1 for each day removed from correct date, to maximum   _____
   of 5)

9. What is the month? _____ (5 for each month removed from correct one, to maximum of 15)   _____

10. What is the year? _____ (10 for each year removed from correct one, to maximum of 30)   _____

Total error points   _____

Total GOAT score (100 minus total error points)   _____

Figure 2-35 Galveston Orientation and Amnesia Test. Examiner adds up only error points, not positive responses. For example, if patient remembers the first name but not the last name, he or she would get 1 error point. (Modified from Levin HS, O'Donnell VM, Grossman RG: The Galveston Orientation and Amnesia Test: a practical scale to assess cognition after head injury. J Nerve Ment Dis 167[11]:677, 1979.)

patient to bring the finger to the nose or the heel of the foot to the opposite knee with the eyes closed (Figure 2-36). The **Balance Error Scoring System (BESS)** has been developed as an objective test for balance. The test has six parts—three on a solid floor and three on a foam surface (Figure 2-37). On each surface, three progressive stances are attempted: double leg stance, single leg stance, and heel-to-toe tandem stance. Each of the six stances is evaluated for 20 seconds with the patient closing the eyes

and hands on iliac crests. The examiner counts the number of errors for each test (Table 2-22). Provided one has a baseline score, a score of three or more errors than baseline indicates balance impairment.[25,79-82] These tests and others described under Special Tests assess balance and coordination.

Muscle tone and strength may also play a role in assessing the patient for head injury. Increased unilateral muscle tone usually implies contralateral cerebral peduncle

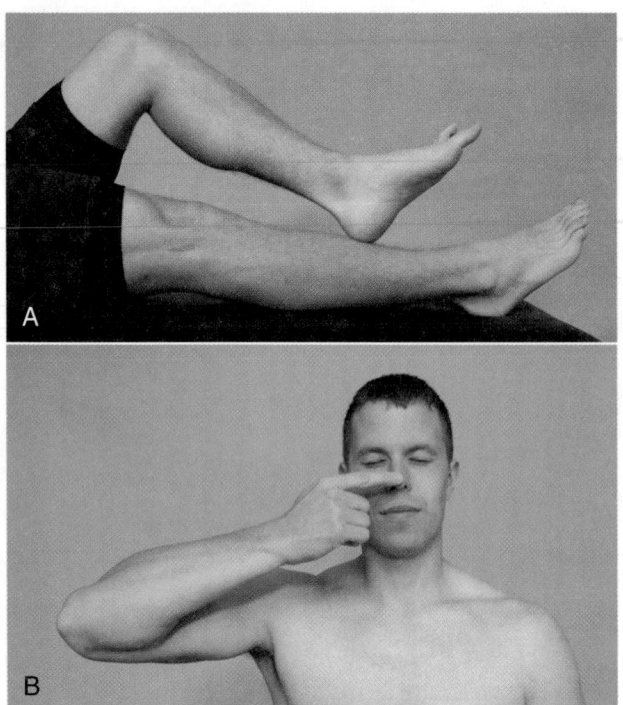

Figure 2-36 Performing coordination exercises. A, Touching knee with opposite heel. **B,** Touching nose with index finger with eyes closed.

TABLE **2-22**

Balance Error Scoring System (BESS) Countable Errors

Errors

- Hands lifted off the iliac crests
- Opening eyes
- Step, stumble, or fall
- Moving a hip into more than 30° of flexion or extension
- Lifting the forefoot or heel
- Remaining out of the testing position for more than 5 seconds

From Guskiewicz KM, Ross SE, Marshall SW: Postural stability and neuropsychological deficits after concussion in collegiate athletes. J Athl Train 36(3):265, 2001.

compression. Flaccid muscle tone implies brain stem infarction, spinal cord transection, or spinal shock. Unilateral effects, such as hemiparesis, may be seen with a stroke.

Examination of the Face[59–63,83]

Once a head injury has been ruled out or if no head injury is suspected, the examiner can inspect the face for injury. Major trauma and subsequent injury to the face should be assessed first. If major trauma has not occurred, only those areas of the face that have been affected by the trauma (e.g., eyes, nose, ears) need be assessed. The

patient may initially be tested for fractures with the use of a tongue depressor if the patient can open her or his mouth. The patient is asked to bite down as hard as possible on the tongue depressor (Figure 2-38, *A*). The examiner should note whether the patient is able to bite down strongly and hold the contraction and where any pain is elicited.

Facial Examination

- Bone and soft tissue contours
- Fractures
- Mandible
- Maxilla
- Zygoma
- Skull
- Cranial nerves
- Facial muscles

To test for a maxillary fracture, the examiner grasps the anterior aspect of the maxilla with the fingers of one hand and places the fingers of the other hand over the bridge of the patient's nose or forehead. The examiner then gently pulls the maxilla forward (Figure 2-39). If the fingers of the other hand at the nose feel movement or the examiner feels the test hand moving forward, a Le Fort II or III fracture may be present (Figure 2-40). If the maxilla moves without movement at the nose, either the maxilla is horizontally fractured, or a Le Fort I fracture is present. With a Le Fort I fracture, the palate is separated from the superior portion of the maxilla, and the upper tooth-bearing segment of the face moves alone. The nasal bones, midportion of the face, and maxilla move if a Le Fort II fracture is present. With a Le Fort III fracture, the middle third of the face separates from the upper third of the face; this is often called a *craniofacial separation.* The patient may complain of lip or cheek anesthesia and double vision (diplopia) with any of these fractures.

The examiner then asks the patient to open his or her mouth slightly. The examiner carefully applies pressure bilaterally at the angles of the mandible (Figure 2-38, *B*). Localized pain, lower lip anesthesia, and intraoral laceration may indicate a fracture of the mandible. Malocclusion of the teeth is often seen with fractures of the mandible or maxilla (Figure 2-41). Alterations in smell (cranial nerve I) are often seen with frontobasal and naso-ethmoidal fractures. Skull fractures are often associated with clear nasal discharge (spinal fluid rhinorrhea), clear ear discharge (otorrhea), or a salty taste. If blood accompanies the fluid, the examiner can use a gauze pad to collect the fluid. If cerebrospinal fluid is mixed with the blood, the examiner may observe a "halo" effect as the fluid collects on the gauze pad (Figure 2-42). If the

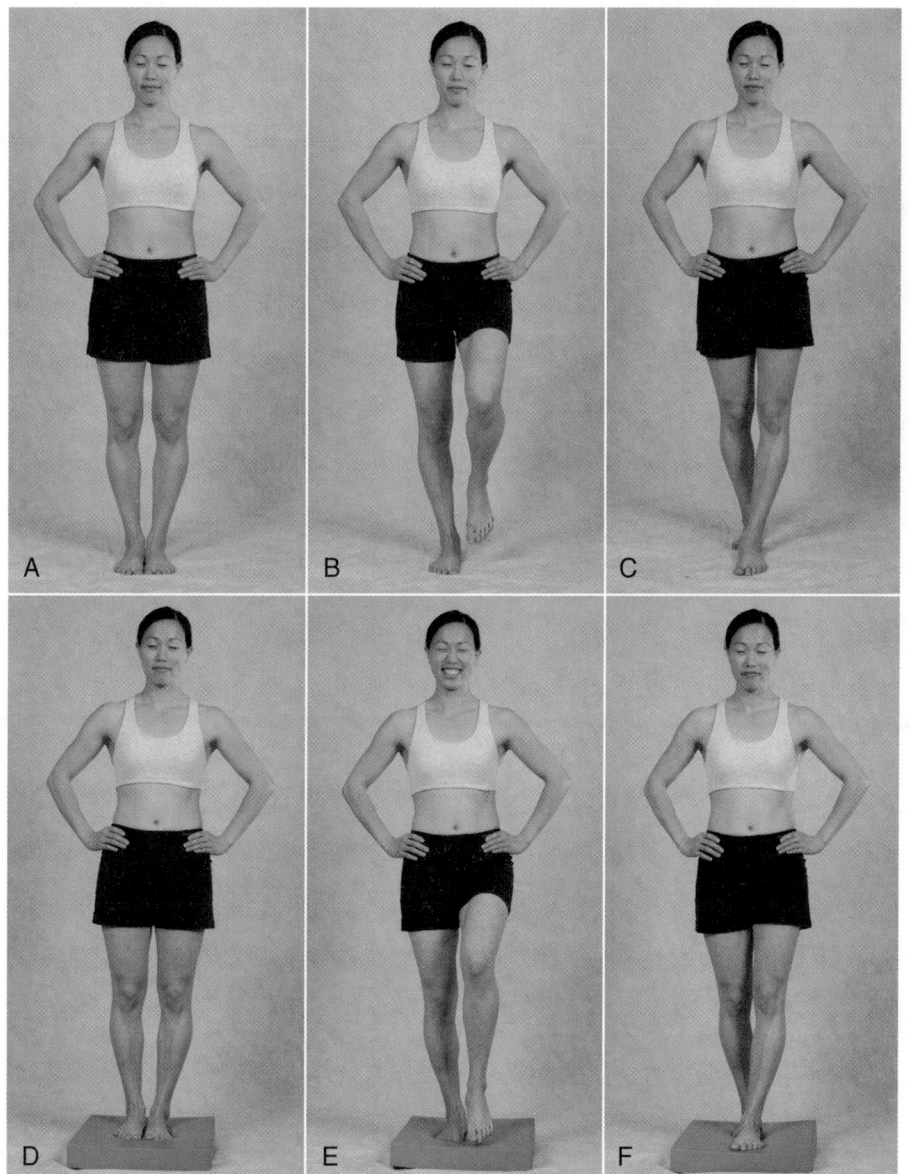

Figure 2-37 Stances for the Balance Error Scoring System (BESS). A, Double leg stance on a solid floor. **B,** Single leg stance on a solid floor. **C,** Heal to toe tandem stance on a solid floor. **D,** Double leg stance on a foam surface. **E,** Single leg stance on a foam surface. **F,** Heel to toe tandem stance on a foam surface.

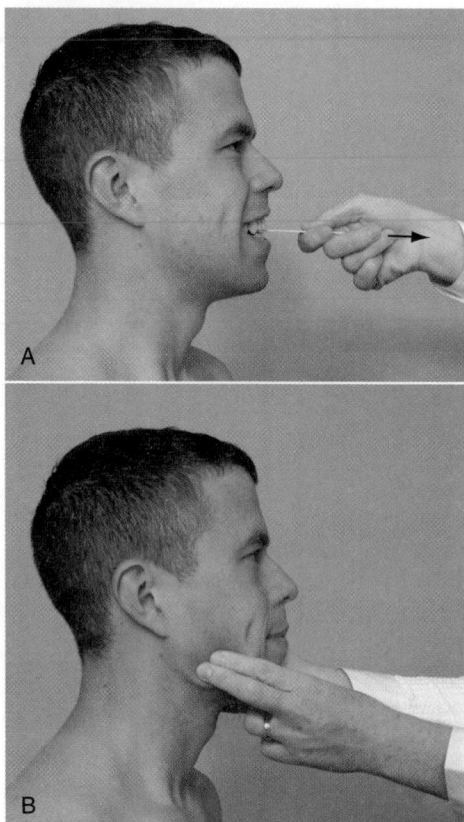

Figure 2-38 Testing for mandibular fracture. A, Patient bites down on tongue depressor while examiner tries to pull it away. **B,** Pressure at the angles of the mandible.

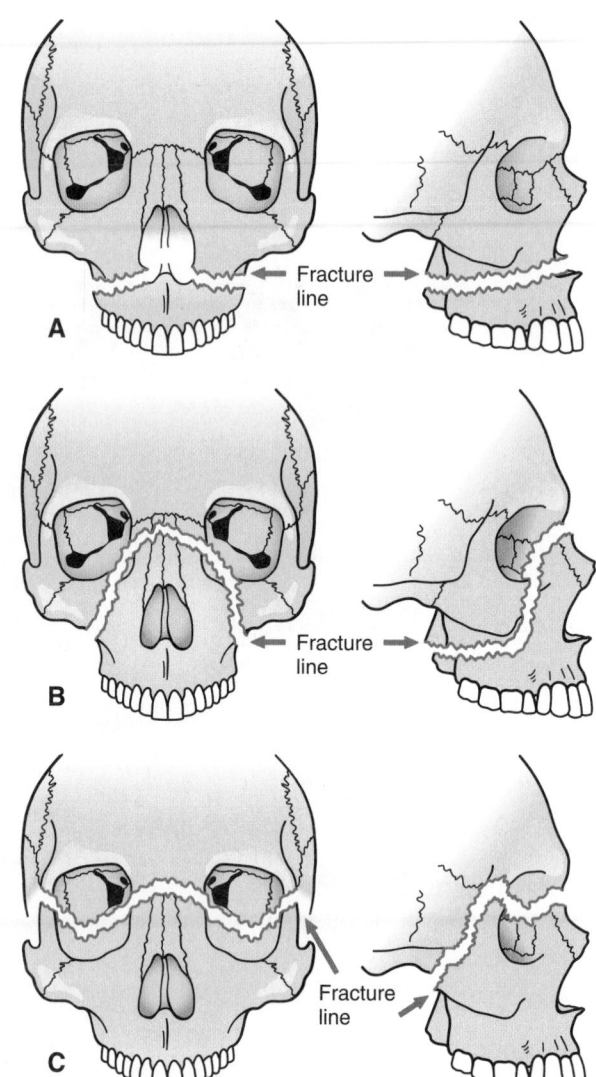

Figure 2-40 Le Fort fractures. A, Le Fort I. **B,** Le Fort II. **C,** Le Fort III.

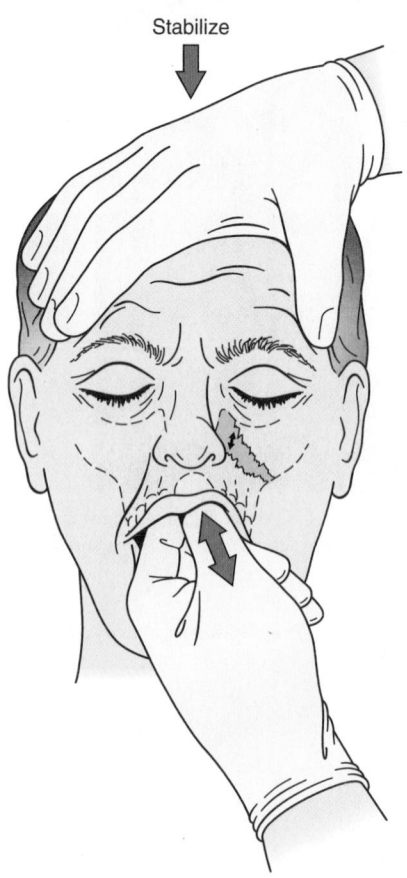

Figure 2-39 Testing for maxillary fracture.

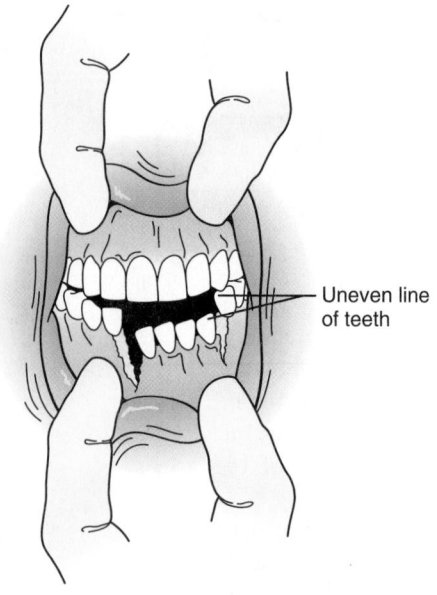

Figure 2-41 Malocclusion of teeth may be associated with fracture of mandible or maxilla.

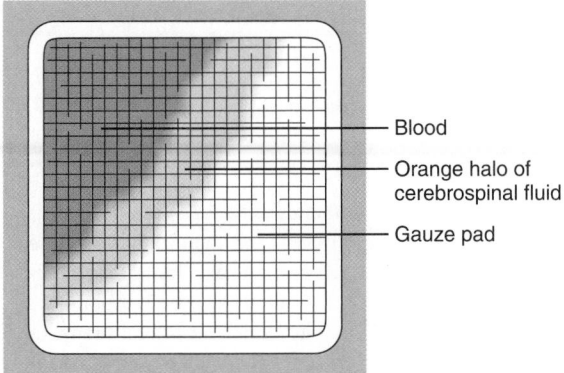
— Blood

— Orange halo of cerebrospinal fluid

— Gauze pad

Figure 2-42 An orange halo will form around the blood on a gauze pad if cerebrospinal fluid is present.

eardrum has not been perforated, blood may be visible behind it. Skull fractures may also result in blurred or double vision, loss of smell (anosmia), dizziness, tinnitus, and nausea and vomiting as well as signs and symptoms of concussion. Orbital floor fractures or dislocations are often accompanied by anesthesia of the skin in the midface or anesthesia of the cheek, lip, maxillary teeth, and gingiva.[84] Zygoma fractures are detected by observation (see Figure 2-31). They may also cause unilateral epistaxis, double vision, and anesthesia and be associated with eye injuries. Mouth opening may also be affected.

After major trauma has been ruled out, the examiner may test the muscles of the face (Table 2-23) especially if injury to these structures is suspected. Excluding the temporomandibular joint, the muscles of the face are different from most muscles in that they move the skin and soft tissues rather than joints. For example, the frontalis muscle may be weak if the eyebrows do not raise symmetrically. The corrugator muscle draws the eyebrows medially and downward (frowning). The orbicularis oris muscle approximates and compresses the lips, whereas the zygomaticus muscles raise the lateral angle of the mouth (smiling).

Examination of the Eye[59–62]

If the eyelids are swollen shut, the examiner should initially assume that the globe has been ruptured. A penetrating wound of the eyelid should be assessed carefully, because it may be associated with a globe injury. The examiner should not force the eyelid open, because intraocular pressure can force extrusion of the ocular contents if the globe has been ruptured. The patient should also be instructed not to squeeze the eyelids tight, because this action can increase the intraocular pressure from a normal value of 15 mm Hg up to approximately 70 mm Hg.

To examine the normal functioning of the eye muscles and several of the cranial nerves (II, III, IV, and VI), the examiner asks the patient to move through the six cardinal positions of gaze (Figure 2-43). The examiner holds the patient's chin steady with one hand and asks the patient to follow the examiner's other hand while the examiner traces a large "H" in the air. The examiner should hold the index finger or pencil approximately 25 cm (10 inches) from the patient's nose. From the midline, the finger or pencil is moved approximately 30 cm (12 inches) to the patient's right and held. It is then moved up approximately 20 cm (8 inches) and held, moved down 40 cm (16 inches) (20 cm relative to midline) and held, and moved slowly back to midline. The same movement is repeated on the other side. The examiner should observe movement of both eyes, noting whether the eyes follow the finger or pencil smoothly. The examiner should also observe any parallel movement of the eyes in all directions. If the eyes do not move in unison or if only one eye moves, something is affecting the action of the muscles. One of the most common causes of one eye's not moving after trauma to the eye is a blowout fracture of the orbital floor (Figure 2-44). Because the inferior muscles become "caught" in the fracture site, the affected eye demonstrates limited movement (Figure 2-45), especially upward. The patient with this type of fracture may also demonstrate depression of the eye globe, blurred vision, double vision, and conjunctival hemorrhage.

Occasionally, when looking to the extreme side, the eyes will develop a rhythmic motion called *end-point nystagmus*. **Nystagmus** is a rhythmic movement of the eyes with an abnormal slow drifting away from fixation and rapid return. With end-point nystagmus, there is a quick motion in the direction of the gaze followed by a slow return. This test differentiates end-point nystagmus from pathological nystagmus, in which there is a quick movement of the eyes in the same direction regardless of gaze. Pathological nystagmus exists in the region of full binocular vision, not just at the periphery. Cerebellar nystagmus is greater when the eyes are deviated toward the side of the lesion.

While testing the cardinal positions, the examiner should also watch for lid lag. Normally, the upper lid

TABLE **2-23**

Muscles of the Face

	Action	Cranial Nerve
Muscles of the Mouth		
Orbicularis oris	Compresses lips against anterior teeth, closes mouth, protrudes lips	VII (Zygomatic, buccal, and mandibular branches)
Depressor anguli oris	Depresses angle of mouth	VII (Buccal and mandibular branches)
Levator anguli oris	Elevates angle of mouth	VII (Zygomatic and buccal branches)
Zygomaticus major	Draws angle of mouth upward and back	VII (Zygomatic and buccal branches)
Risorius	Draws angle of mouth laterally	VII (Zygomatic and buccal branches)
Muscle of the Lips		
Levator labii superioris	Elevates upper lip, flares nostril	VII (Zygomatic and buccal branches)
Muscle of the Cheek		
Buccinator	Compresses cheeks against molar teeth; sucking and blowing	VII (Buccal branches)
Muscle of the Chin		
Mentalis	Puckers skin of chin, protrudes lower lip	VII (Mandibular branches)
Muscle of the Nose		
Nasalis	Compresses nostrils Dilates or flares nostrils	VII (Zygomatic and buccal branches)
Muscle of the Eye		
Orbicularis oculi	Closes eye forcefully Closes eye gently Squeezes lubricating tears against eyeball	VII (Temporal and zygomatic branches)
Muscles of the Forehead		
Procerus	Transverse wrinkling of bridge of nose	VII (Temporal and zygomatic branches)
Corrugator	Vertical wrinkling of bridge of nose	VII (Temporal branches)
Frontalis	Pulls scalp upward and back	VII (Temporal branches)

Adapted from Liebgott B: The anatomical basis of dentistry, St Louis, 1986, Mosby, pp. 242–243.

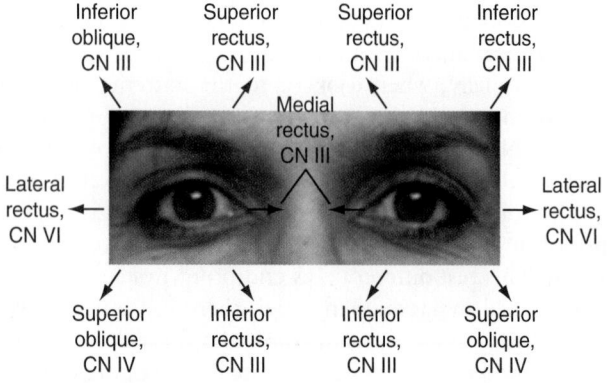

Figure 2-43 The six cardinal fields of gaze, showing eye muscles and cranial nerves involved in the movement.

covers the top of the iris, rising when the patient looks up and quickly lowering as the eye lowers. With lid lag, the upper lid delays lowering as the eye lowers.

Peripheral vision, or the visual field (peripheral limits of vision), can be tested with the confrontation test (Figure 2-46). The patient is asked to cover the right eye while the examiner covers his or her own left eye so that the open eyes of the examiner and of the patient are directly opposite each other. While the examiner and the patient look into each other's eye, the examiner fully extends his or her right arm to the side, midway between the patient and the examiner, and then moves it toward them with the fingers waving. The patient tells the examiner when he or she first sees the moving fingers. The examiner then compares the patient's response with the time or distance at which the examiner first noted the fingers. The test is then repeated to the other side.

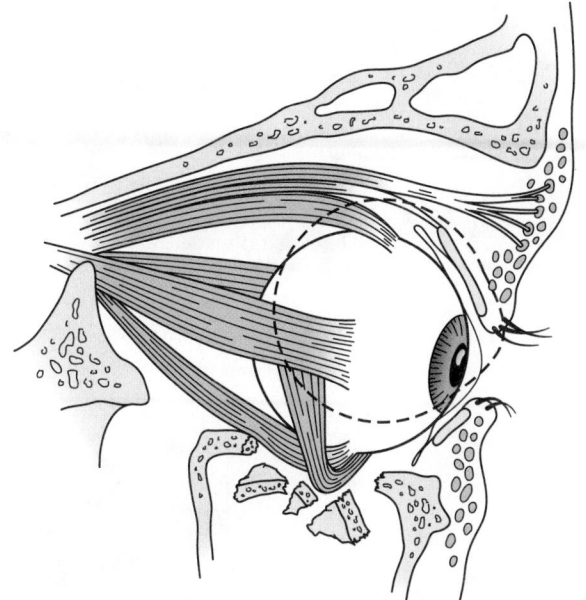

Figure 2-44 Blowout fracture of the orbital floor. The dashed line indicates normal position of the globe. The inferior oblique and inferior rectus muscles are "caught" in the fracture site, preventing the eye from returning to its normal position. (Modified from Paton D, Goldberg MF: Management of ocular injuries, Philadelphia, 1976, WB Saunders, p. 63.)

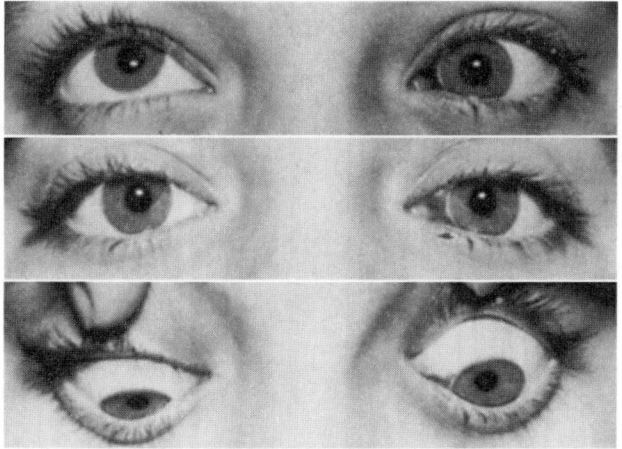

Figure 2-45 Fresh blowout fracture of left orbit with limitation of upward *(top)* and downward *(bottom)* movements of the left eye. (Modified from Paton D, Goldberg MF: Management of ocular injuries, Philadelphia, 1976, WB Saunders, p. 65.)

The nasal, temporal, superior, and inferior fields should all be tested in a similar fashion. The visual field should describe angles of 60° nasally, 90° temporally, 50° superiorly, and 70° inferiorly. Double simultaneous testing may also be performed. This method uses two stimuli (e.g., moving fingers) that are simultaneously presented in the right and left visual fields, and the patient is asked which finger is moving. Normally, the patient should say "both," without hesitation. With any loss of vision field (i.e., if the patient is unable to see in the same visual

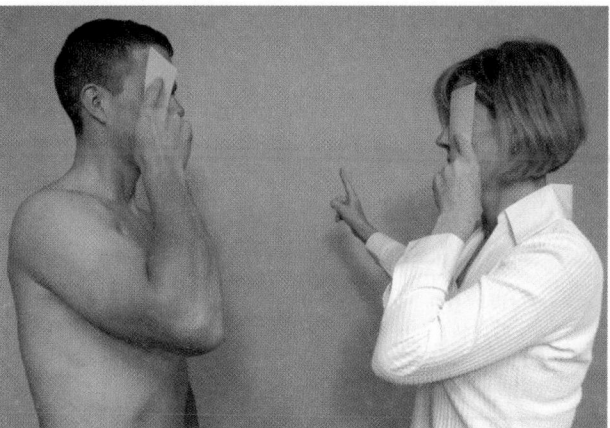

Figure 2-46 Confrontation eye test.

fields as before), the patient must be referred for further examination.

The eyelids should be everted to look at the underside of the eyelid and to give a clearer view of the globe, especially if the patient complains of a foreign body. The upper eyelid may be everted with the use of a special lid retractor or a cotton swab (Figure 2-47). The patient is asked to look down and to the right and then down and to the left while the superior aspect of the eye is examined. The examiner can check the inferior aspect of the eye and its conjunctival lining by carefully pulling the lower eyelid downward and gently holding it against the bony orbit. Next, the patient is asked to look up and to the right and then up and to the left while the inferior aspect of the eye is examined. These two techniques may also be used to look for a contact lens that has migrated away from the cornea.

Both eyelids should be checked for laceration. Lacerations in the area of the lacrimal gland are especially important to detect because, if they are not looked after properly, the tearing function of the lacrimal gland may be lost (Figure 2-48).

The reaction of the pupils to light should then be tested. First, the light in the room is dimmed. The pupils dilate in a dark environment or with a long focal distance and constrict in a light environment or with a short focal distance. The examiner shines a pen light directly into one of the patient's eyes for approximately 5 seconds (Figure 2-49). Normally, constriction of the pupil occurs, followed by slight dilation. The pupillary reaction is classified as brisk (normal), sluggish, nonreactive, or fixed. An oval or slightly oval pupil or one that is fixed and dilated indicates increased intracranial pressure. The fixation and dilation of both pupils is a terminal sign of anoxia and ischemia to the brain. If the dilation is significant, an injury to the optic nerve may be suspected. If both pupils are midsize, midposition, and nonreactive, midbrain damage is usually indicated. In a fully conscious, alert patient who has sustained a blow near the eye, a dilated,

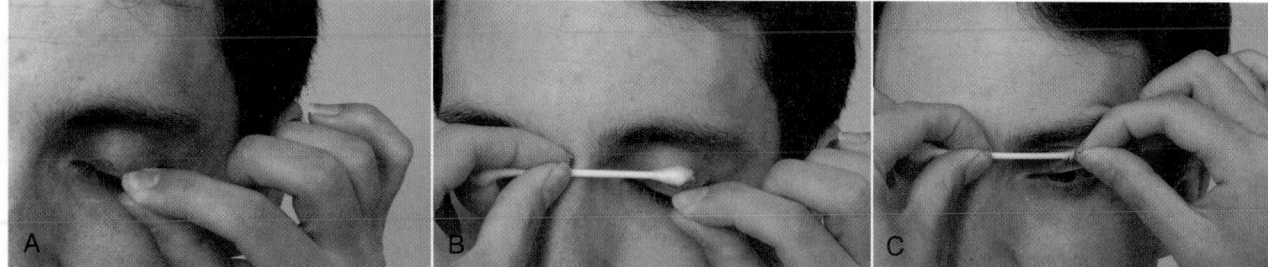

Figure 2-47 Eversion of the eyelid. A, Grasping eyelash. **B,** Putting moistened cotton-tipped applicator over eyelid. **C,** Everting eyelid over the cotton-tipped applicator.

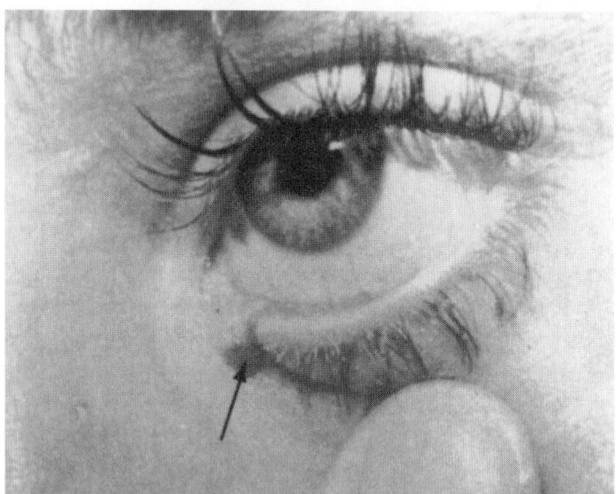

Figure 2-48 A lower lid laceration *(arrow).* (From Pashby TJ, Pashby RC: Treatment of sports eye injuries. In Schneider RC, et al, editors: *Sports injuries: mechanisms, prevention and treatment,* Baltimore, 1985, Lippincott Williams & Wilkins, p. 576.)

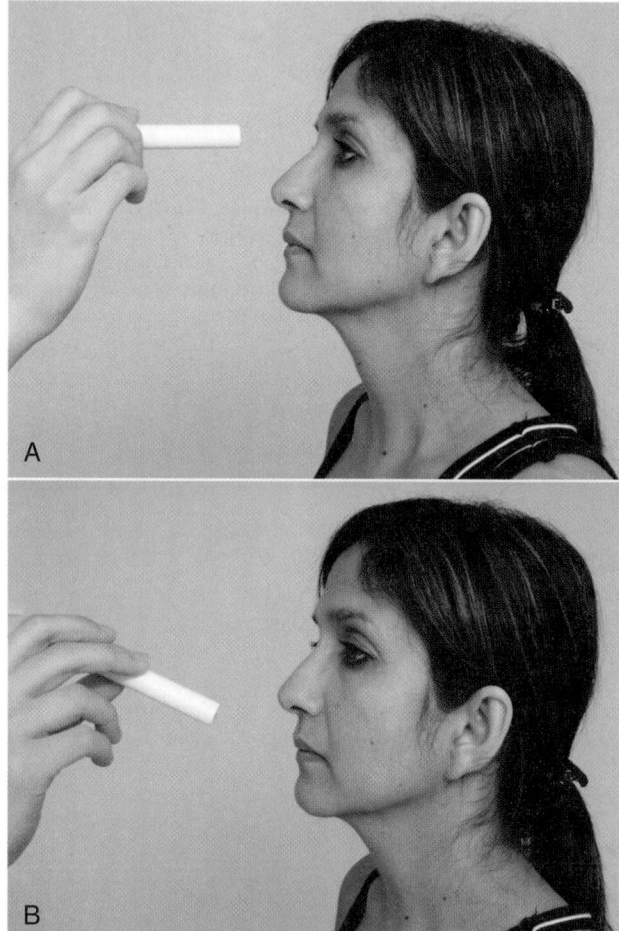

Figure 2-49 Testing the pupils for reaction to light. A, Light shining in eye. **B,** Light shining away from eye.

fixed pupil usually implies injury to the ciliary nerves of the eye rather than brain injury. The other eye is tested similarly, and the results are compared.

Normally, both pupils constrict when a light is shined in one eye. The reaction of the eye being tested is called the **direct light reflex;** the reaction of the other pupil is called the **consensual light reflex.** This reaction is brisker in the young and people with blue eyes.[63] If the optic nerve is damaged, the affected pupil constricts in response to light in the opposite eye (consensual) and dilates in response to light shined into it (direct). If the oculomotor nerve is affected, the affected pupil is fixed and dilated and does not respond to light, either directly or consensually. If the pupils do not react, it is an indication of injury to the oculomotor nerve and its connections or of injury to the head. The eye also appears laterally displaced owing to paresis of the medial rectus muscle.

The pupil is then tested for constriction to accommodation. The patient is asked to look at a distant object and then at a test object—a pencil or the examiner's finger held 10 cm (4 inches) from the bridge of the nose. The pupils dilate when the patient looks at a far object and constrict when the patient focuses on the near object. The eyes also adduct (go "cross-eyed") when the patient looks at the close object. These actions are called the **accommodation-convergence reflex.**[63] When looking at distant objects, the eyes should be parallel. Deviation or lack of parallelism is called **strabismus** and indicates weakness of one of the extraocular muscles or lack of neural coordination.[85]

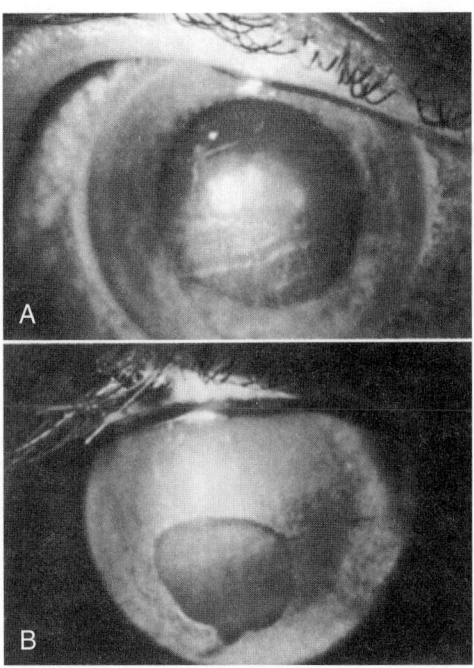

Figure 2-50 **Corneal abrasion. A,** Without fluorescein. **B,** With fluorescein. (From Torg JS: *Athletic injuries to the head, neck and face,* Philadelphia, 1982, Lea & Febiger, p. 262.)

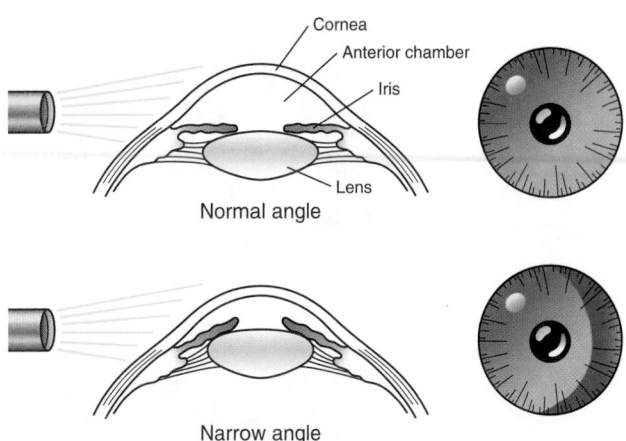

Figure 2-51 **Normal and narrow corneal angle (depth of anterior chamber).** (Modified from Swartz HM: *Textbook of physical diagnosis,* Philadelphia, 1989, WB Saunders, p. 144.)

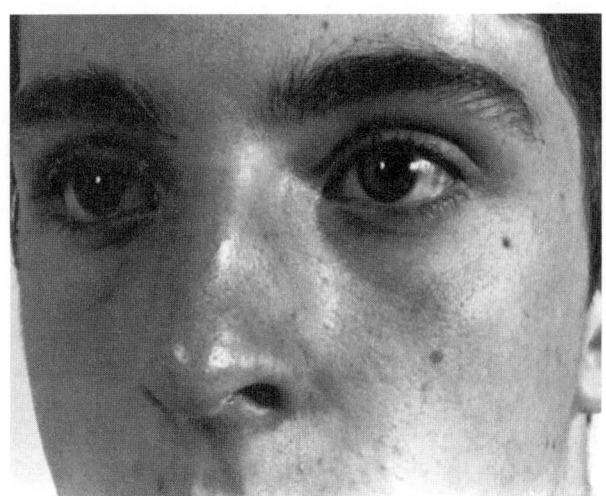

Figure 2-52 **Symmetry of gaze.** Note white "dots" of light on pupils.

When inspected under normal overhead light, the lens of the eye should be transparent. Shining a light on the lens may cause it to appear gray or yellow. The cornea should be smooth and clear. If the patient has extreme pain in the corneal area, a corneal abrasion should be suspected (Figure 2-50). An appropriate specialist may test for corneal abrasion by using a fluorescein strip and a slit lamp. The cornea should be crystal clear when it is viewed, and the iris details should match those of the other eye.

To check for depth of the anterior chamber of the eye or a narrow corneal angle, the examiner shines a light obliquely across each eye. Normally, it illuminates the entire iris. If the corneal angle is narrow because of a shallow anterior chamber, the examiner will be able to see a crescent-shaped shadow on the side of the iris away from the light (Figure 2-51). This finding indicates an anatomical predisposition to narrow-angled glaucoma.

To test for **symmetry of gaze,** the examiner aims a light source approximately 60 cm (24 inches) from the patient while standing directly in front of the patient and holding the light distant enough to prevent convergence of the patient's gaze. The patient is asked to stare at the light. The dots of reflected light on the two corneas should be in the same relative location (Figure 2-52). When one eye does not look directly at the light, the reflected dot of light moves to the side opposite the deviation. For example, if the eye deviates medially, the reflection appears more laterally placed than in the other eye. The examiner can approximate the angle of deviation by

noting the position of the reflection. Each millimeter of displacement in the reflection represents approximately 7° of ocular deviation. To bring out a mild deviation, the examiner may use a cover-uncover test (Figure 2-53). The patient looks at a specific point, such as the bridge of the examiner's nose. One of the patient's eyes is then covered with a card. Normally, the uncovered eye will not move. If it moves, it was not straight before the other eye was covered. The other eye is then tested in a similar fashion.

Visual acuity is tested using a vision chart. **Visual acuity** is the ability of the eye to perceive fine detail, for example, when reading. If a standard eye wall chart is not available, a pocket visual acuity card may be used. This pocket card is usually viewed at a distance of 35 to 36 cm (14 inches). As with the wall chart, the patient is asked to examine the smallest line possible. If neither eye chart is available, any printed material may be used. A patient

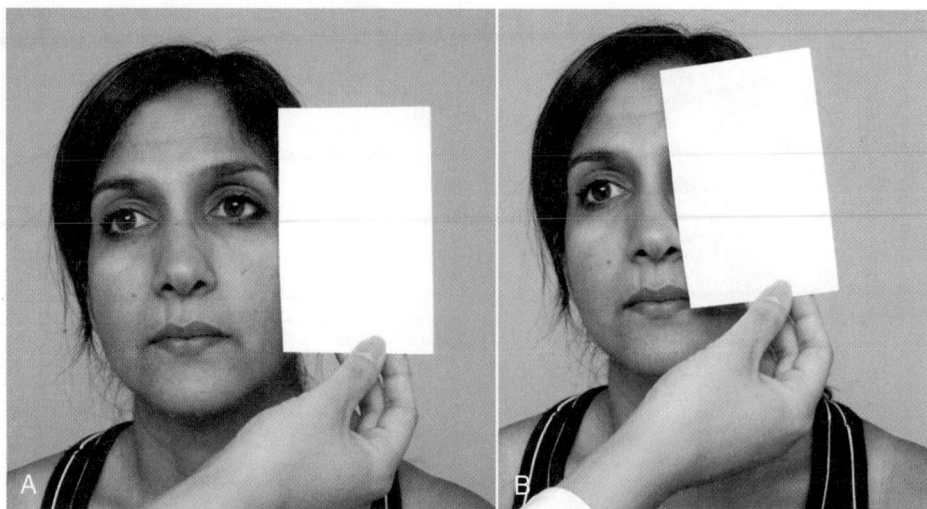

Figure 2-53 Cover-uncover test for mild ocular deviation. As patient gazes at a specific point (**A**), examiner covers one eye and looks for movement in uncovered eye (**B**).

who wears glasses or contact lenses should be tested both without and with the corrective lenses. The test is done quickly so that the patient cannot memorize the chart. Visual acuity is recorded as a fraction in which the numerator indicates the distance of the patient from the chart (e.g., 20 ft) and the denominator indicates the distance at which the normal eye can read the line. Thus, 20/100 means the patient can read at 20 ft what the average person can read at 100 ft—the smaller the fraction, the worse the myopia (nearsightedness). Patients with corrected vision of less than 20/40 should be referred to the appropriate specialist.[63] Intraocular examination with an ophthalmoscope, if available, may reveal lens, vitreous, or retinal damage.

Examination of the Nose[59–65]

Patency of the nasal passages can be determined by occluding one of the patient's nostrils by pushing a finger against the side of the nostril. The patient is then asked to breathe in and out of the opposite nostril with the mouth closed. The process is repeated on the other side. Normally, no sound is heard, and the patient can breathe easily through the open nostril.

Nasal Examination

- Patency
- Nasal cavities
- Sinuses
- Fracture
- Nasal discharge (bloody, straw-colored, clear)

If available, a nasal speculum and light may be used to inspect the nasal cavity. The nasal mucosa and turbinates can be inspected for color, foreign bodies, and abnormal masses (e.g., polyp). The nasal septum should be in midline and straight and is normally thicker anteriorly than posteriorly. If the nasal cavities are asymmetric, it may indicate a deviated septum. If the patient demonstrates a septal hematoma, it must be treated fairly quickly, because the hematoma may cause excessive pressure on the septum, making it avascular. This avascularity can result in a "saddle nose" deformity owing to necrosis and absorption of the underlying cartilage (Figure 2-54).

Illumination of the frontal and maxillary sinuses may be performed if sinus tenderness is present or infection is suspected. The examination must be performed in a completely darkened room. To illuminate the maxillary sinuses, the examiner places the light source lateral to the patient's nose just beneath the medial aspect of the eye. The examiner then looks through the patient's open mouth for illumination of the hard palate. To illuminate the frontal sinuses, the examiner places the light source against the medial aspect of each supraorbital rim. The examiner looks for a dim red glow as light is transmitted just below the eyebrow. The sinuses usually show differing degrees of illumination. The absence of a glow indicates either that the sinus is filled with secretions or that it has never developed.

Examination of the Teeth[59–65]

The examiner should observe the teeth to see if they are in normal position and whether any teeth are missing, chipped, or depressed (see Figure 2-25). Using the gloved index finger and thumb, the examiner applies mild pressure to each tooth, pressing inward toward the tongue

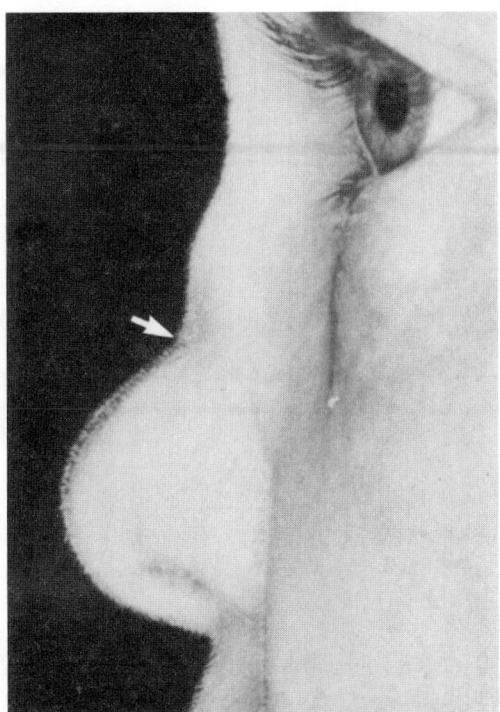

Figure 2-54 "Saddle nose" deformity *(arrow)* that occurred as a result of loss of septal cartilage support secondary to septal hematoma and abscess. (From Handler SD: Diagnosis and management of maxillofacial injuries. In Torg JS, editor: Athletic injuries to the head, neck and face, Philadelphia, 1982, Lea & Febiger, p. 232.)

and outward toward the lips. Normally, a small amount of movement is observed. If a tooth is loose, excessive movement or increased pain or numbness relative to other teeth indicates a positive test. A tooth that has been avulsed may be cleansed with warm water and reinserted into the socket. The patient is then referred to the appropriate specialist.

Tooth Examination

- Number of teeth
- Position of teeth
- Movement of teeth
- Condition of teeth
- Condition of gums

Examination of the Ear[58–62]

Examination of the ear deals primarily with whether the patient is able to hear. Several tests may be used to examine hearing.

⚠ *Rinne Test.* The Rinne test is performed by placing the base of the vibrating tuning fork against the patient's mastoid bone. The examiner counts or times the interval with a watch. The patient tells the examiner when he or

---

Ear Examination

- Tenderness (exterior and interior)
- Ear discharge (bloody, straw-colored, clear)
- Hearing
- Balance

---

she no longer hears the sound, and the examiner notes the number of seconds. The examiner then quickly positions a still-vibrating tine 1 to 2 cm (0.5 to 0.8 inch) from the auditory canal and asks patient to indicate when he or she no longer hears the sound. The examiner then compares the number of seconds the sound was heard by bone conduction and by air conduction. The counting or timing of the interval between the two sounds determines the length of time that sound is heard by air conduction (see Figure 2-56). Air-conducted sound should be heard twice as long as bone-conducted sound. For example, if bone conduction is heard for 15 seconds, the air conduction should be heard for 30 seconds.[58–60]

❓ *Schwabach Test.* This test compares the patient's and examiner's hearing by bone conduction. The examiner alternately places the vibrating tuning fork against the patient's mastoid process and against the examiner's mastoid bone until one of them no longer hears a sound. The examiner and patient should hear the sound for equal amounts of time.[58,59]

❓ *Ticking Watch Test.* The ticking watch test uses a nonelectric ticking watch to test high-frequency hearing. The examiner positions the watch approximately 15 cm (6 inches) from the ear to be tested, slowly moving it toward the ear. The patient then indicates when he or she hears the ticking sound. The distance can be measured and will give some idea of the patient's ability to hear high-frequency sound.[58,59]

❓ *Weber Test.* The examiner places the base of a vibrating tuning fork on the midline vertex of the patient's head. The patient should hear the sound equally well in both ears (Figures 2-55 and 2-56). If the patient hears better in one ear (i.e., the sound is lateralized), the patient is asked to identify which ear hears the sound better. To test the reliability of the patient's response, the examiner repeats the procedure while occluding one ear with a finger and asks the patient which ear hears the sound better. It should be heard better in the occluded ear.[58,59]

❓ *Whispered Voice Test.* The patient's response to the examiner's whispered voice can be used to determine hearing ability. The examiner masks the hearing in one of the patient's ears by placing a finger gently in the patient's ear canal. Standing approximately 30 to 60 cm (12 to 24 inches) away from the patient, the examiner whispers one- or two-syllable words and asks the patient to repeat them. If the patient has difficulty, the examiner gradually increases his or her volume until the patient

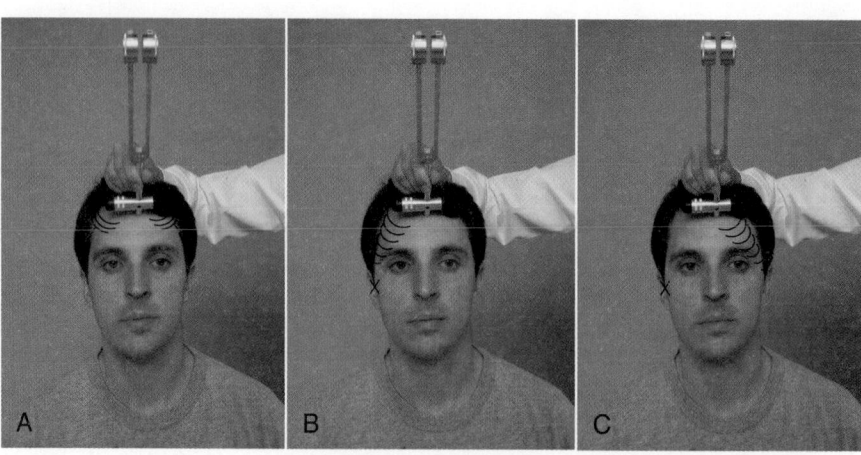

Figure 2-55 The Weber test. A, When a vibrating tuning fork is placed on the center of the forehead, the sound is heard in the center without lateralization to either side (normal response). **B,** In the presence of a conductive hearing loss, the sound is heard on the side of the conductive loss. **C,** In the presence of sensorineural loss, the sound is better heard on the opposite (unaffected) side.

responds appropriately. The procedure is repeated in the other ear. The patient should be able to hear whispered words in each ear at a distance of 30 to 60 cm (12 to 24 inches) and respond correctly at least 50% of the time.[58,59]

Conductive hearing loss implies that the patient experiences a reduction of all sounds rather than difficulty in interpreting sounds. **Sensorineural or perceptual hearing loss** indicates that the patient has difficulty interpreting the sounds.

To examine the internal structure of the ear, the examiner may use an otoscope if one is available. In this case, the examiner would observe the canal as well as the eardrum (tympanic membrane), noting any blockage, excessive wax, swelling, redness, transparency (usually pearly gray), bulging, retraction, or perforation of the eardrum.

Special Tests

Examiners perform only those special tests that they think will have value in helping to confirm a diagnosis. For example, the tests for expanding intracranial lesions would not be performed with a facial injury unless an associated injury to the brain or other neurological tissues is suspected.

For the reader who would like to review them, the reliability, validity, specificity, sensitivity, and odds ratios of some of the special tests used for the head and face are available on the Evolve website.

Tests for Expanding Intracranial Lesions

For each of these tests, the patient must be able to stand normally when the eyes are open.

❓ *Neurological Control Test—Upper Limb.* The examiner asks the patient to stand with his or her arms forward flexed 90° and eyes closed. The patient holds this position for approximately 30 seconds. If the examiner notes that one arm tends to move or drift outward and downward, the test is considered positive for an expanding intracranial lesion on the side opposite the side with the drift.

❓ *Neurological Control Test—Lower Limb.* The examiner asks the patient to sit on the edge of a table or in a chair with his or her legs extended in front and not touching the ground. The patient closes his or her eyes for approximately 20 to 30 seconds. If the examiner notes that one leg tends to move or drift, the test is considered positive for an expanding intracranial lesion on the side opposite that with the drift.

✓ *Romberg Test.* The examiner asks the patient to stand with feet together and arms by the sides with the eyes open. The examiner notes whether the patient has any problem with balance. The patient then closes his or her eyes for at least 20 seconds, and the examiner notes any differences. A positive Romberg test is elicited if the patient sways or falls to one side when the eyes are closed, and this reaction indicates an expanding intracranial lesion, possible disease of the spinal cord posterior columns, or proprioceptive problems.

⚠ *Walk or Stand in Tandem Test.* Patients with expanding intracranial lesions demonstrate increasing difficulty in walking in tandem ("walking the line") or standing in tandem (one foot in front of other). Standing in tandem is more difficult to perform than walking in tandem.

Tests for Coordination

✓ *Balance Error Scoring System.* See earlier discussion of BESS on p. 123.

⚠ *Finger Drumming Test.* The patient drums the index and middle finger of one hand up and down as quickly as possible on the back of the other hand. The test is repeated with the opposite hand. The examiner compares the two sides for coordination and speed.

❓ *Finger-Thumb Test.* The patient touches each finger with the thumb of the same hand. The normal or uninjured side is tested first, followed by the injured side. The examiner compares the two sides for coordination and timing.

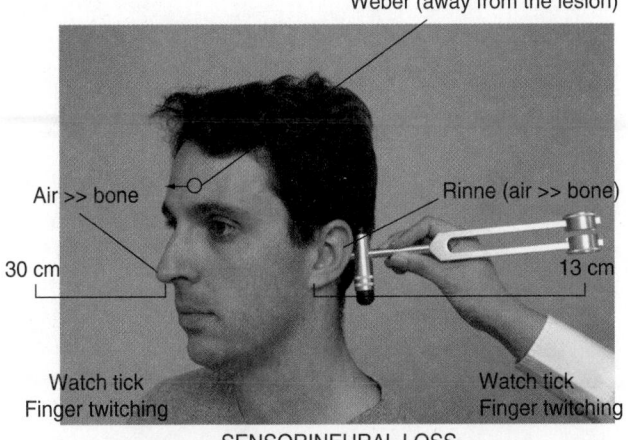

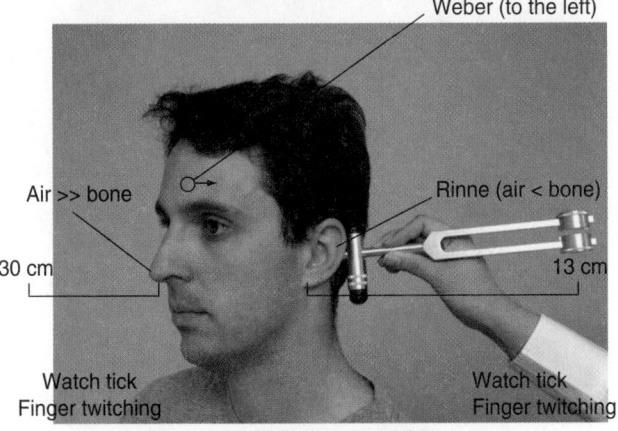

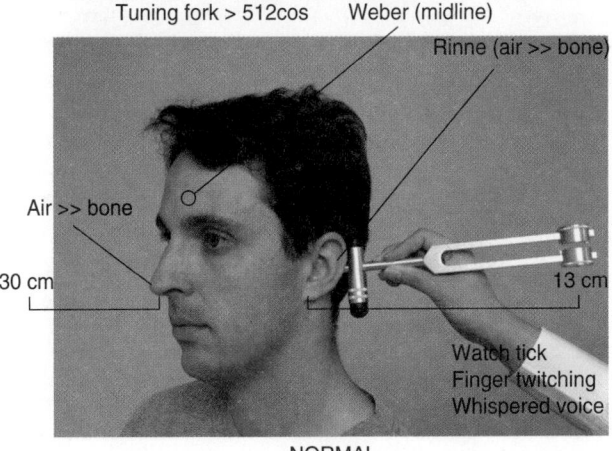

Figure 2-56 Bedside hearing tests and results with sensorineural or conductive loss in left ear and with normal hearing.

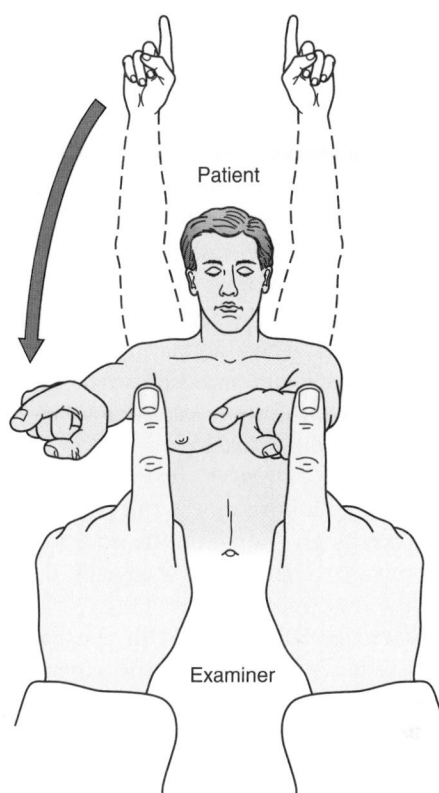

Figure 2-57 Past pointing. (Redrawn from Reilly BM: Practical strategies in outpatient medicine, Philadelphia, 1991, WB Saunders, p. 195.)

⚠ *Finger-to-Nose Test.* The patient stands or sits with the eyes open and brings the index finger to the nose. The test is repeated with the eyes closed. Both arms are tested several times with increasing speed. Normally, the tests should be accomplished easily, smoothly, and quickly with the eyes open and closed.

❓ *Hand "Flip" Test.* The patient touches the back of the opposite, stationary hand with the anterior aspect of the fingers, flips the test hand over, and touches the opposite hand with the posterior aspect of the fingers. The movement is repeated several times with both sides being tested. The examiner compares the two sides for coordination and speed.

❓ *Hand-Thigh Test.* The patient pats his or her thigh with the hand as quickly as possible. The uninjured side is tested first. The patient may be asked to supinate and pronate the hand between each hand-thigh contact to make the test more complex. The examiner watches for speed and coordination and compares the two sides.

❓ *Heel-to-Knee Test.* The patient, who is lying supine with the eyes open, takes the heel of one foot and touches the opposite knee with the heel and then slides the heel down the shin. The test is repeated with the eyes closed, and both legs are tested. The test can be repeated several times with increasing speed; the examiner notes any differences in coordination or the presence of tremor. Normally, the test should be accomplished easily, smoothly, and quickly with the eyes open and closed.

❓ *Past Pointing Test.* The patient and examiner face each other. The examiner holds up both index fingers approximately 15 cm (6 inches) apart. The patient is asked to lift the arms over the head and then bring the arms down to touch the patient's index fingers to the examiner's index fingers (Figure 2-57). The test is repeated with the patient's eyes closed. Normally, the test can be performed without difficulty. Patients with vestibular disease have problems with past pointing. The test may also be used to test proprioception.

Tests for Proprioception

❓ *Past Pointing Test.* The test is performed as described under Tests for Coordination.

⚠️ *Proprioceptive Finger-Nose Test.* The patient keeps the eyes closed. The examiner lightly touches one of the patient's fingers and asks the patient to touch the patient's nose with that finger. The examiner then touches another finger on the other hand, and the patient again touches the nose. Patients with proprioceptive loss have difficulty doing the test without visual input.

❓ *Proprioceptive Movement Test.* With the patient's eyes closed, the examiner moves the patient's finger or toe up or down by grasping it on the sides to lessen clues given by pressure. The patient then tells the examiner which way the digit moved.

❓ *Proprioceptive Space Test.* With the patient's eyes closed, the examiner places one of the patient's hands or feet in a selected position in space. The patient then imitates that position with the other limb or to find the hand or foot with the other limb. True proprioceptive loss causes the patient to be unable to properly position or to find the normal limb with the limb that has proprioceptive loss.

Reflexes and Cutaneous Distribution

With a head injury patient, deep tendon reflexes (see Table 1-31) should be tested. Accentuation of one or more of the reflexes may indicate trauma to the brain on the opposite side. Pathological reflexes (see Table 1-33) may also be altered with a head injury.

The **corneal reflex** (trigeminal nerve, cranial nerve V) is used to test for damage or dysfunction to the pons. In some cases, the patient may look to one side to avoid involuntary blinking. The examiner touches the cornea (not the eyelashes or conjunctiva) with a small, fine point of cotton (Figure 2-58). The normal response is a bilateral blink, because the reflex arc connects both facial nerve nuclei. If the reflex is absent, the test is considered positive.

The **gag reflex** may be tested using a tongue depressor that is inserted into the posterior pharynx and depressed toward the hypopharynx. The reflex tests cranial nerves IX and X, and its absence in a trauma setting may indicate caudal brain stem dysfunction.

Consensual light reflex may be tested by shining a light into one eye. This action causes the lighted pupil to constrict. If there is normal communication between the two oculomotor nerves, the nonlighted pupil also constricts.

The **jaw reflex** is usually tested only if the temporomandibular joint or cervical spine is being examined.

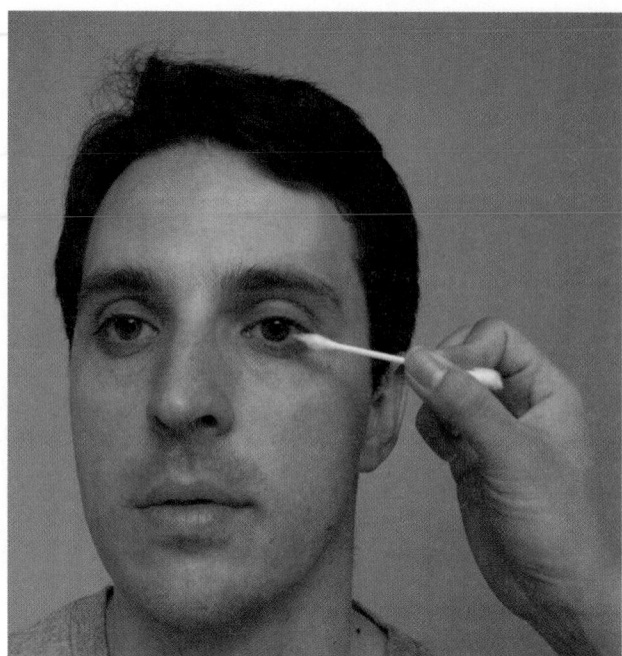

Figure 2-58 Test of corneal reflex.

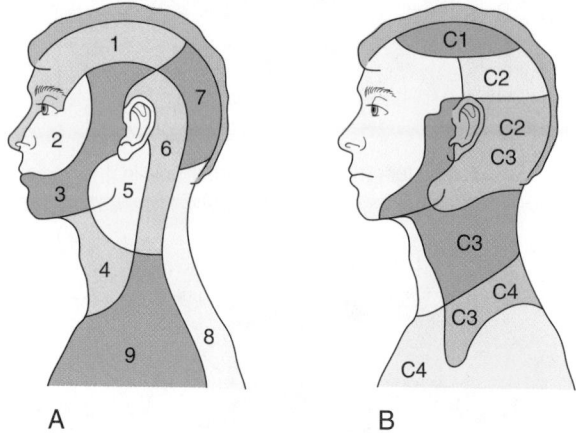

Figure 2-59 A, Sensory nerve distribution of the head, neck and face. *1,* Ophthalmic nerve; *2,* maxillary nerve; *3,* mandibular nerve; *4,* transverse cutaneous nerve of neck (C2–C3); *5,* greater auricular nerve (C2–C3); *6,* lesser auricular nerve (C2); *7,* greater occipital nerve (C2–C3); *8,* cervical dorsal rami (C3–C5); *9,* suprascapular nerve (C5–C6). **B,** Dermatome pattern of the head, neck, and face. Note the overlap of C3.

The examiner should check the sensation of the head and face, keeping in mind the differences in dermatome and sensory nerve distributions (Figure 2-59). Lip anesthesia or paresthesia is often seen in patients with mandibular fracture.

Nerve Injuries of the Head and Face

Bell's palsy involves paralysis of the facial nerve (cranial nerve VII) and usually occurs where the nerve emerges from the stylomastoid foramen. Pressure in the foramen caused by inflammation or trauma affects the nerve and, therefore, the muscles of the face (occipitofrontalis, corrugator, orbicularis oculi, and the nose and mouth muscles) on one side. The inflammation may result from a middle ear infection, viral infection, chilling of the face, or tumor. The observable result is smoothing of the face on the affected side owing to loss of muscle action, the eye on the affected side remaining open, and the lower eyelid sagging. The patient is unable to wink, whistle, purse the lips, or wrinkle the forehead. Speech sounds, especially those requiring pursing of the lips, are affected, resulting in slurred speech. The mouth droops, and it and the nose may deviate to the opposite side, especially in longstanding cases, of which there are remarkably few (90% of patients recover completely within 2 to 8 weeks). Facial sensation on the affected side is lost, and taste sensation is sometimes lost as well. The House-Brackmann Facial Nerve Grading System (Table 2-24) may be used to grade the level of facial nerve involvement.[86]

Joint Play Movements

Because no articular joints are involved in the assessment of the head and face, there are no joint play movements to test.

Palpation

During palpation of the head and face, the examiner should note any tenderness, deformity, crepitus, or other signs and symptoms that may indicate the source of pathology. The examiner should note the texture of the skin and surrounding bony and soft tissues. Normally, the patient is palpated in the sitting or supine position, beginning with the skull and moving from anterior to posterior, to the face, and finally to the lateral and posterior structures of the head.

The skull is palpated by a gentle rotary movement of the fingers, progressing systematically from front to back. Normally, the skin of the skull moves freely and has no tenderness, swelling, or depressions.

The temporal area and temporalis muscle should be laterally palpated for tenderness and deformity. The external ear or auricle and the periauricular area should also be palpated for tenderness or lacerations.

The occiput should be palpated posteriorly for tenderness. The presence of Battle sign should be noted, if observed, because this signals a possible basilar skull fracture.

The face is palpated beginning superiorly and working inferiorly in a systematic manner. Like the skull, the

---

TABLE **2-24**

House-Brackmann Facial Nerve Grading System

Parameter	Grade I	Grade II	Grade III	Grade IV	Grade V	Grade VI
Overall appearance	Normal	Slight weakness on close inspection	Obvious but not disfiguring difference between both sides	Obvious weakness and/or disfiguring asymmetry	Only barely perceptible motion	No movement
At rest	Normal symmetry	Normal symmetry	Normal symmetry	Normal symmetry	Asymmetry	Asymmetry
Forehead movement	Normal with excellent function	Moderate-to-good function	Slight-to-moderate function	None	None	None
Eyelid closure	Normal closure	Complete with minimum effort	Complete with maximal effort	Incomplete closure with maximal effort	Incomplete closure with maximal effort	No movement
Mouth	Normal and symmetric	Slight asymmetry	Slight asymmetry with maximum effort	Asymmetry with maximum effort	Slight movement	No movement
Synkinesis contracture and/or hemifacial spasm	None	May have very slight synkinesis; no contracture or hemifacial spasm	Obvious but not disfiguring synkinesis contracture and/or hemifacial spasm	Synkinesis contracture and/or asymmetrical facial spasm leading to disfiguring severe enough to interfere with function	Synkinesis contracture and/or hemifacial spasm usually absent	No movement

Modified from Dutton M: Orthopedic examination, evaluation, and intervention, New York, 2004, McGraw Hill, p. 1130. Adapted from House JW, Brackmann DE: Facial nerve grading system. Otolaryngol Head Neck Surg 93:146–147, 1985.

forehead is palpated by gentle rotary movements of the fingers, feeling the movement of the skin and the occipitofrontalis muscle underneath. Normally, the skin of the forehead moves freely and is smooth and even with no tender areas. The examiner then palpates around the eye socket or orbital rim, moving over the eyebrow and supraorbital rims, around the lateral side of the eye, and along the zygomatic arch to the infraorbital rims, looking for deformity, crepitus, tenderness, and lacerations (Figure 2-60, *A* and *B*). The orbicularis oculi muscles surround the orbit, and the medial side of the orbital rim and nose are then palpated for tenderness, deformity, and fracture. The nasal bones, including the lateral and alar cartilage, are palpated for any crepitus or deviation (Figure 2-60, *C*). The septum should be inspected to see if it has widened, possibly indicating a septal hematoma, which often occurs with a fracture. It should also be determined whether the patient can breathe through the nose or smell.

The frontal and maxillary sinuses should be inspected for swelling. To palpate the frontal sinuses, the examiner uses the thumbs to press up under the bony brow on each side of the nose (Figure 2-61, *A*). The examiner then presses under the zygomatic processes using either the thumbs or index and middle fingers to palpate the maxillary sinuses (Figure 2-61, *B*). No tenderness or swelling over the soft tissue should be present. The sinus areas may also be percussed to detect tenderness. A light tap directly over each sinus with the index finger can be used to detect tenderness.

The examiner then moves inferiorly to palpate the jaw. The examiner palpates the mandible along its entire length, noting any tenderness, crepitus, or deformity. The examiner, using a rubber glove, may also palpate along the mandible interiorly, noting any tenderness or pain (Figure 2-60, *D*). The outside hand may be used to stabilize the jaw during this procedure. The mandible may

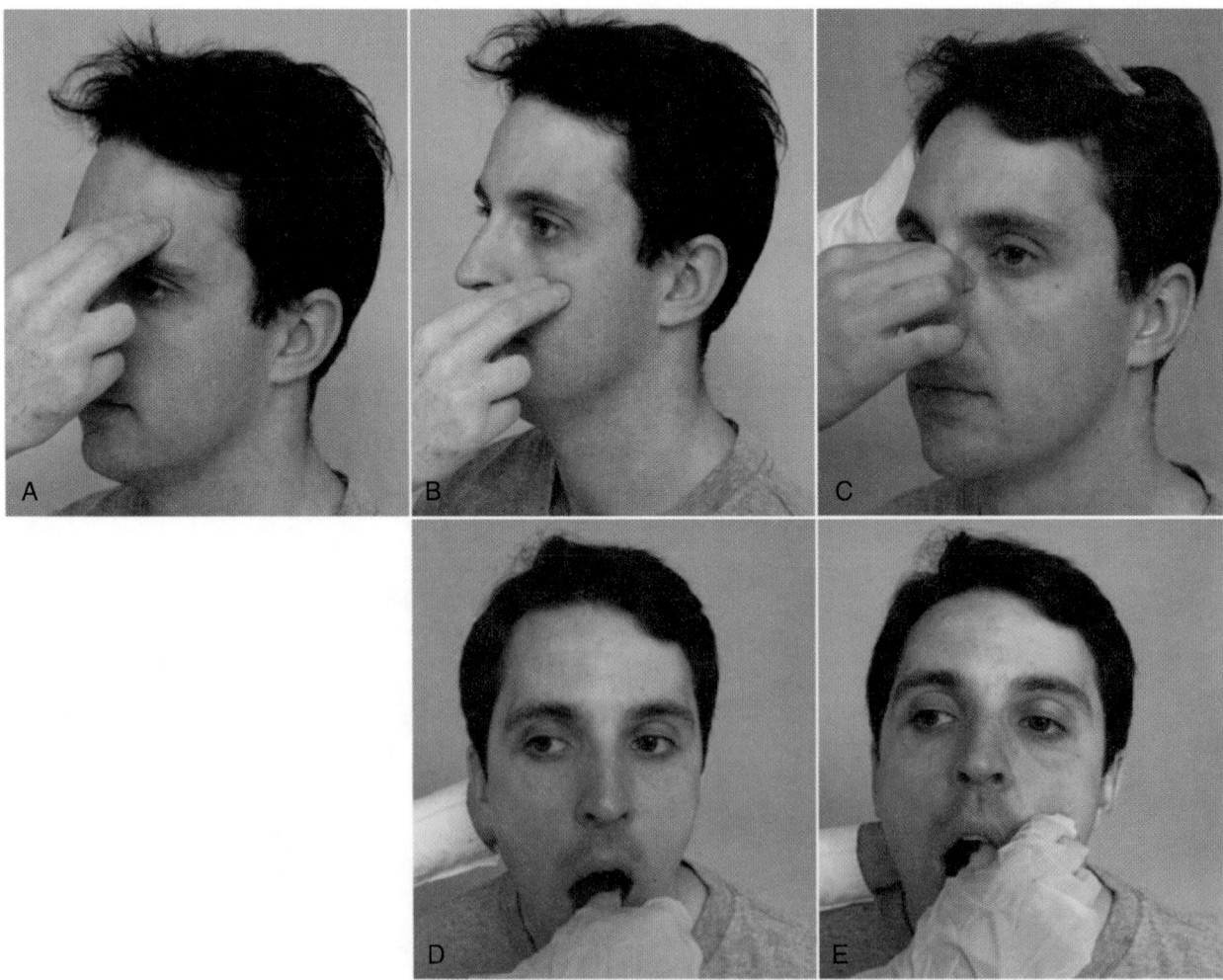

Figure 2-60 Palpation of the face. A, Upper orbital rim. **B,** Lower orbital rim. **C,** Nose. **D,** Mandible. **E,** Maxilla.

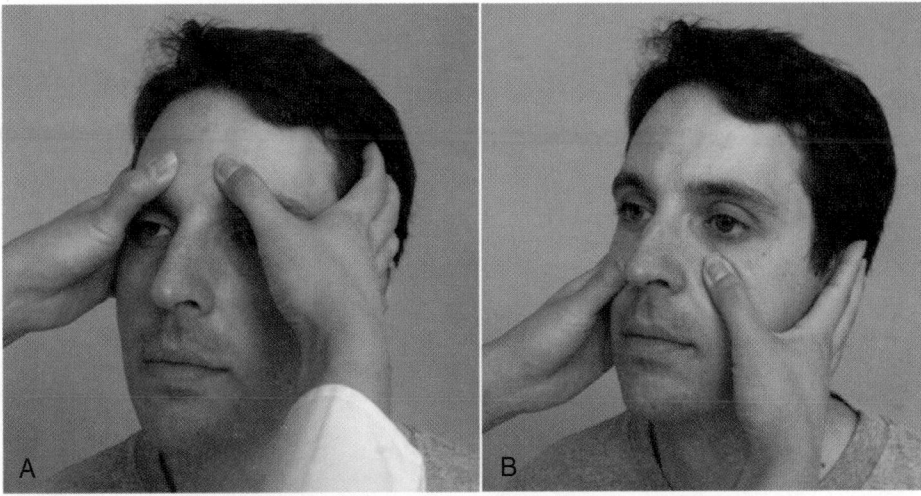

Figure 2-61 **A,** Palpation of frontal sinuses. **B,** Palpation of maxillary sinuses.

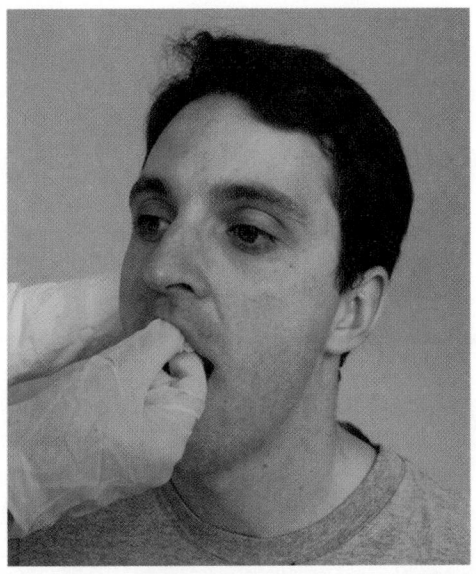

Figure 2-62 Palpation of maxillary fracture with anteroposterior rocking motion.

The trachea should be palpated for midline position. The examiner places a thumb along each side of the trachea, comparing the spaces between the trachea and the sternocleidomastoid muscle, which should be symmetric. The hyoid bone and the thyroid and cricoid cartilages should be identified. Normally, they are smooth and nontender and move when the patient swallows.

Diagnostic Imaging

Plain Film Radiography
Common x-rays taken involving the head and face are outlined in the following box.

Common X-Ray Views of the Head and Face Depending on Pathology

- Anteroposterior view (Figure 2-63)
- Lateral view (Figure 2-64)

---

also be tapped with a finger along its length to see if signs of tenderness are elicited. The muscles of the cheek (buccinator) and mouth (orbicularis oris) should be palpated at the same time.

The maxilla may be palpated in a similar fashion, both internally and externally, noting position of the teeth, tenderness, and any deformity (Figure 2-60, *E*). The examiner may grasp the teeth anteriorly to see if the teeth and mandible or maxilla move in relation to the rest of the face, which may indicate a Le Fort fracture (Figure 2-62).

Anteroposterior View. The examiner should note the normal bone contours, looking for fractures of the various bones (Figures 2-65 and 2-66; see Figure 2-63).

Lateral View. The examiner should again note bony contours, looking for the possibility of fractures (Figure 2-67).

Computed Tomography
Computed tomography scans help to differentiate between bone and soft tissue and give a more precise view of fractures (Figures 2-68 and 2-69). The Canadian

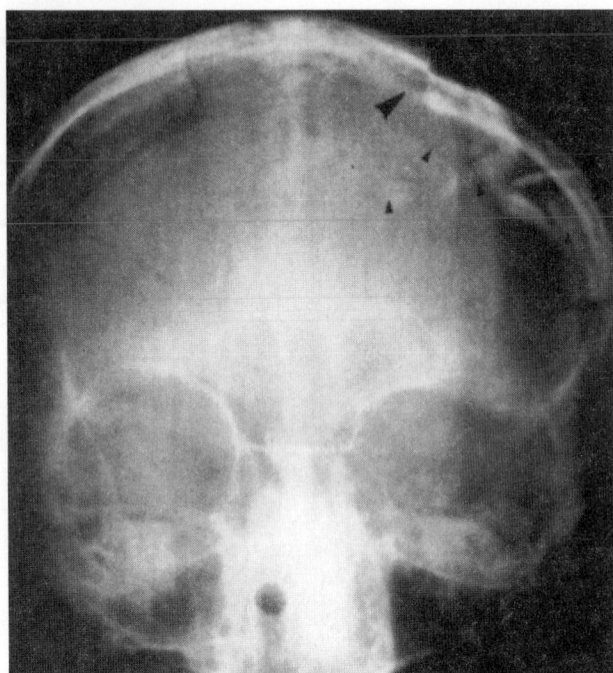

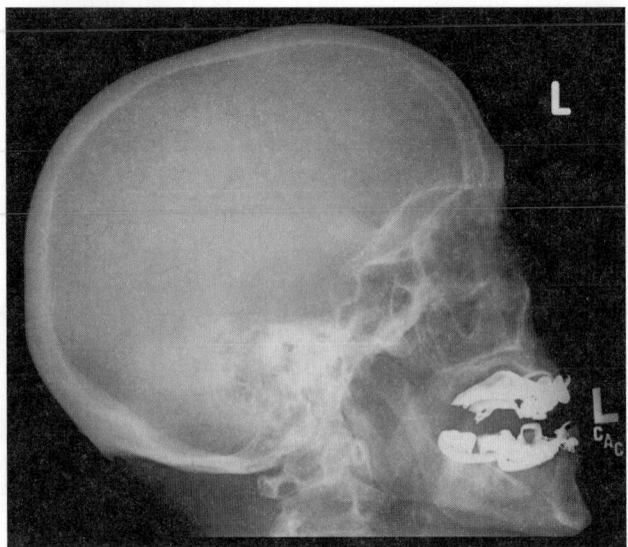

Figure 2-64 Normal lateral view of the head and face.

Figure 2-63 Normal anteroposterior view of the head and face showing a depressed parietal skull fracture *(large arrow)* with multiple bony fragments into the brain *(small arrows)*. (From Albright JP, et al: Head and neck injuries in sports. In Scott WN, et al, editors: Principles of sports medicine, Baltimore, 1984, Lippincott Williams & Wilkins, p. 53.)

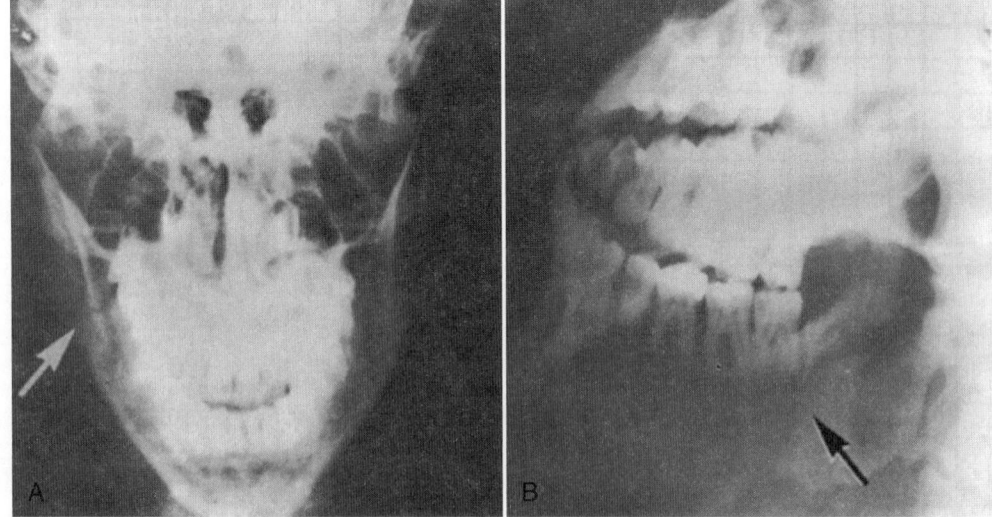

Figure 2-65 Incomplete fracture of angle of mandible on the left side *(arrows)*. **A,** Anteroposterior view. **B,** Lateral view. (From O'Donoghue DH: Treatment of injuries to athletes, Philadelphia, 1984, WB Saunders, p. 114.)

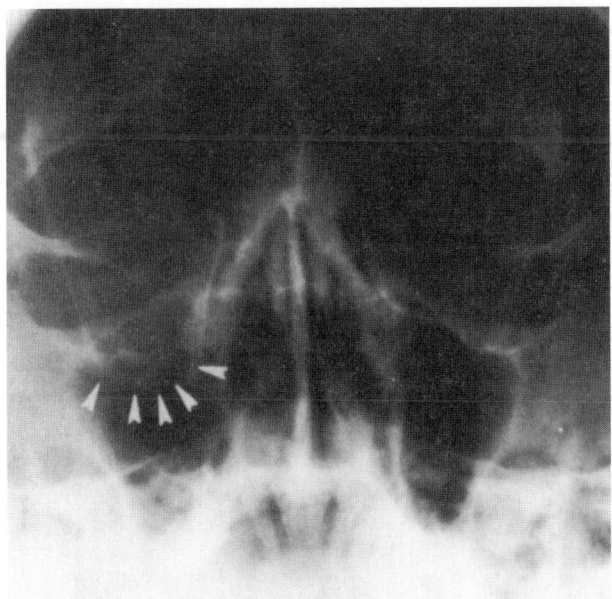

Figure 2-66 Plain posteroanterior view showing blowout fracture of the orbit *(arrows)*. (From Paton D, Goldberg MF: Management of ocular injuries, Philadelphia, 1976, WB Saunders, p. 70.)

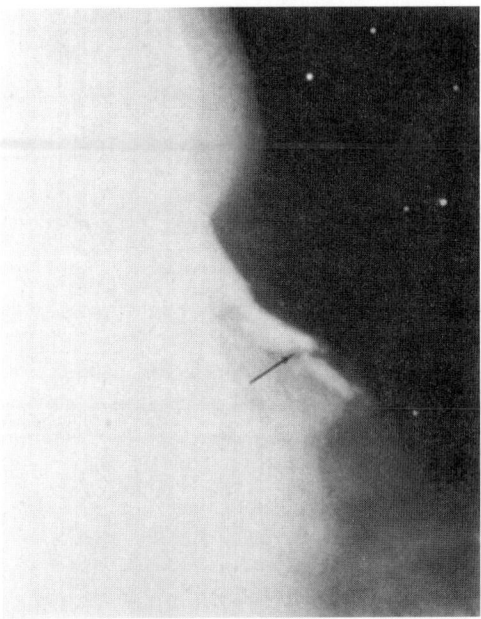

Figure 2-67 Lateral radiograph of the nasal bones demonstrating a nasal fracture *(arrow)*. (From Torg JS: Athletic injuries to the head, neck and face, Philadelphia, 1982, Lea & Febiger, p. 229.)

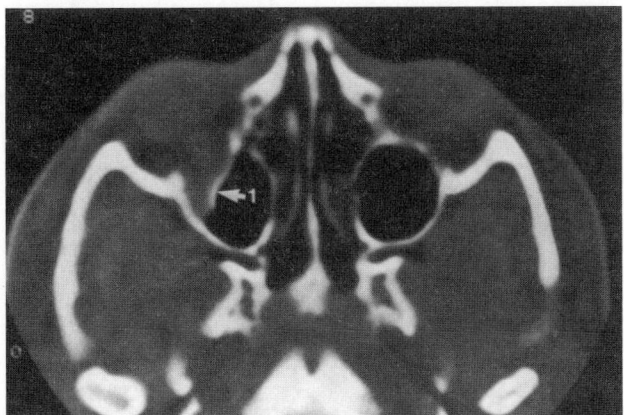

Figure 2-68 Axial computed tomogram of orbital blowout fracture showing fracture of the orbit *(1)* with orbital contents herniated into the maxillary sinus. (From Sinn DP, Karas ND: Radiographic evaluation of facial injuries. In Fonseca RJ, Walker RV, editors: Oral and maxillofacial trauma, Philadelphia, 1991, WB Saunders.)

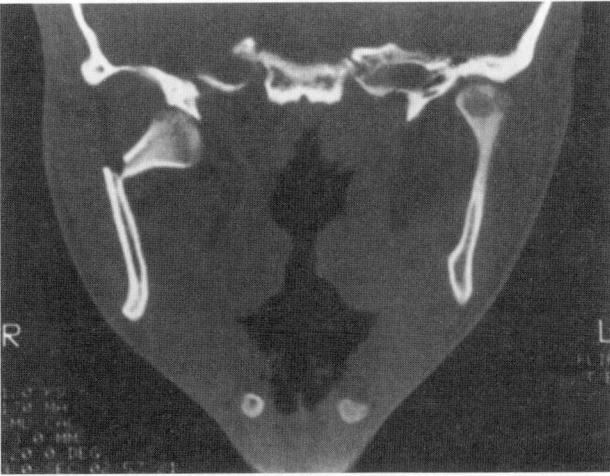

Figure 2-69 The computed tomographic scan is ideal for condylar fractures as seen in the right condyle. (From Bruce R, Fonseca RJ: Mandibular fractures. In Fonseca RJ, Walker RV, editors: Oral and maxillofacial trauma, Philadelphia, 1991, WB Saunders, p. 389.)

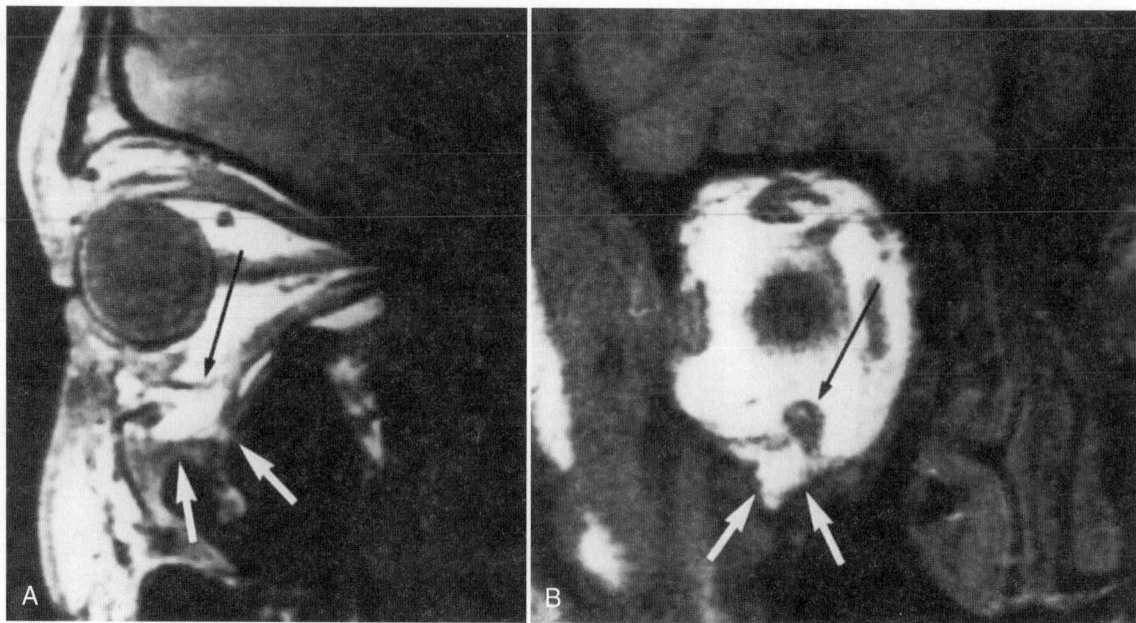

Figure 2-70 Magnetic resonance images showing blowout fracture. Sagittal (**A**) and coronal (**B**) T1-weighted scans demonstrate a blowout fracture of the right orbit with depression of the orbital floor *(white arrows)* into the superior maxillary sinus. The inferior rectus muscle *(long arrow)* is clearly identified and is not entrapped by the floor fracture. (From Harms SE: The orbit. In Edelman RR, Hesselink JR, editors: Clinical magnetic resonance imaging, Philadelphia, 1990, WB Saunders, p. 619.)

Canadian Computed Tomography Head Rule for Minor Head Injury[5]

HIGH RISK (FOR NEUROLOGICAL INTERVENTION)
- Failure to reach 15 on the Glasgow Coma Scale within 2 hours
- Suspected open skull fracture
- Any sign of basal skull fracture
- Two or more vomiting episodes
- 65-years-old or older

MEDIUM RISK (FOR BRAIN INJURY ON CT)
- Retrograde amnesia (before impact) more than 30 minutes
- Dangerous mechanism of injury

Computed Tomography (CT) Head Rule has been developed to help the clinician decide when to use CT scans in minor head injury patients.[5] The authors of the Rule have defined minor head injury as witnessed loss of consciousness, definite amnesia, or witnessed disorientation in patients with a Glasgow Coma Scale score of 13–15.

Magnetic Resonance Imaging

Magnetic resonance imaging is especially useful for demonstrating lesions of the soft tissues of the head and face and for differentiating between bone and soft tissue (Figures 2-70 and 2-71).

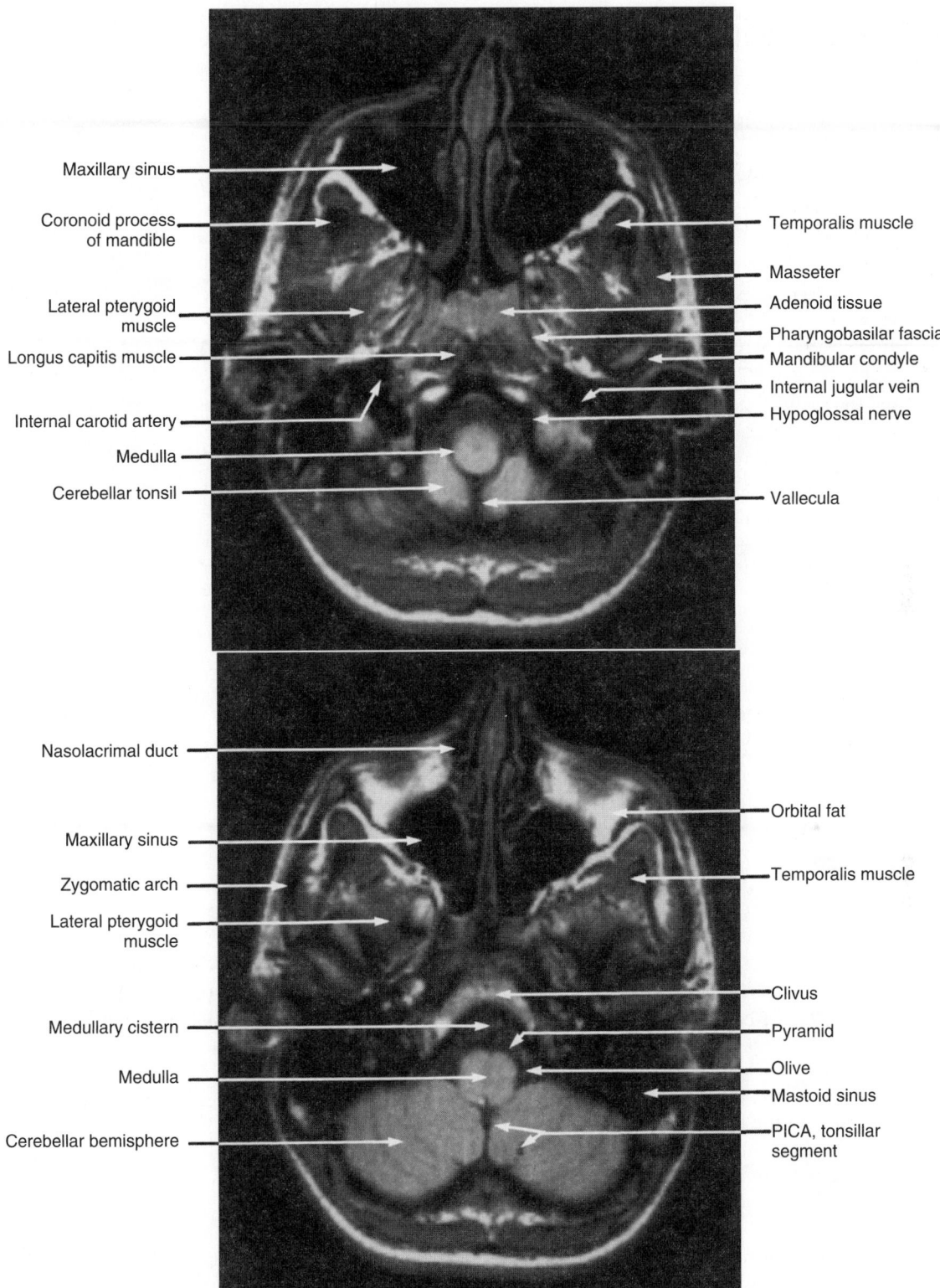

Figure 2-71 T1-weighted axial magnetic resonance images of the head and brain at two levels. *PICA,* Posterior inferior cerebellar artery. (From Greenberg JJ, et al: Brain: indications, techniques, and atlas. In Edelman RR, Hesselink JR, editors: Clinical magnetic resonance imaging, Philadelphia, 1990, WB Saunders, p. 384.)

PRÉCIS OF THE HEAD AND FACE ASSESSMENT*

History (sitting)
Observation (sitting)
Examination* (sitting)
  Head injury
    Neural Watch
    Glasgow Coma Scale
    Concussion
    Memory tests
    Headache
    Expanding intracranial lesion
    Proprioception
    Coordination
    Head injury card
  Facial injuy
    Bone and soft tissue contours
    Fractures
    Cranial nerves
    Facial muscles
  Eye injury
    Six cardinal gaze positions
    Pupils (size, equality, reactivity)
    Visual field (peripheral vision)
    Visual acuity
    Symmetry of gaze
    Hyphema
    Foreign objects, corneal abrasion

  Nystagmus
  Surrounding bone and soft tissue
Nasal injury
  Patency
  Nasal cavities
  Sinuses
  Fracture
  Nose discharge (bloody, straw-colored, clear)
Tooth injury
  Number of teeth
  Position of teeth
  Movement of teeth
  Condition of teeth
  Condition of gums
Ear injury
  Tenderness or pain
  Ear discharge (bloody, straw-colored, clear)
  Hearing tests
  Balance
Special tests
  Tests for expanding intracranial lesions
  Tests for coordination
  Tests for proprioception
Reflexes and cutaneous distribution
Palpation
Diagnostic imaging

*When examining the head and face, if only one area has been injured (e.g., the nose), then only that area needs to be examined, provided the examiner is certain that adjacent structures have not also been injured. After any examination, the patient should be warned of the possibility of exacerbation of symptoms as a result of the assessment.

CASE STUDIES

When doing these case studies, the examiner should list the appropriate questions to be asked and why they are being asked, identify what to look for and why, and specify what things should be tested and why. Depending on the patient's answers (and the examiner should consider different responses), several possible causes of the patient's problem may become evident (examples are given in parentheses). A differential diagnosis chart should be made up (see Table 2-25 as an example). The examiner can then decide how different diagnoses may affect the treatment plan.

1. A 27-year-old man was playing football. He received a "knee to the head," rendering him unconscious for approximately 3 minutes. How would you differentiate between a first-time, fourth-degree concussion and an expanding intracranial lesion?

2. A 13-year-old boy received an elbow in the nose and cheek while play-wrestling. The nose is crooked and painful and bled after the injury, and the cheek is sore. Describe your assessment plan for this patient (nasal fracture versus zygoma fracture).

3. A 23-year-old woman was in an automobile accident. She was a passenger in the front seat and was not wearing a seat belt. The car in which she was riding hit another car that had run a red light. The woman's face hit the dashboard, and she received a severe facial injury. Describe your assessment plan for this patient (Le Fort fracture versus mandibular fracture).

4. An 83-year-old man tripped in the bathroom and hit his chin against the bathtub, knocking himself unconscious. Describe your assessment plan for this patient (cervical spine lesion versus mandibular fracture).

5. An 18-year-old woman was playing squash. She was not wearing eye protectors and was hit in the eye with the ball. Describe your assessment plan for this patient (ruptured globe versus blowout fracture).

CASE STUDIES—cont'd

6. A 15-year-old boy was playing field hockey. He was not wearing a mouth guard and was hit in the mouth and jaw by the ball. There was a large amount of blood. Describe your assessment plan for this patient (tooth fracture versus mandible fracture).

7. A 16-year-old male wrestler comes to you complaining of ear pain. He has just finished a match, which he lost. Describe your assessment plan for this patient (cauliflower ear versus external otitis).

8. A 17-year-old female basketball player comes to you complaining of eye pain. She says she received a "finger in the eye" when she went up to get the ball. Describe your assessment plan for this patient (hyphema versus corneal abrasion).

TABLE **2-25**

Differential Diagnosis of 4° Concussion and Intracranial Lesion

Sign or Symptom	4° Concussion	Intracranial Lesion
Confusion	Yes, but should improve with time	Will have increased confusion with time
Amnesia	Posttraumatic, retrograde	Not usually
Loss of consciousness	Yes, but recovers	Lucid interval varies
Tinnitus	Severe	Not a factor
Dizziness	Severe, but improves	May get worse
Headache	Often	Severe
Nystagmus or irregular eye movements	Not usually	Possible
Pupil inequality	Not usually	Possible early; present later
Irregular respiration	No	Possible early; present later
Slowing of heart	No	Possible early; present later
Intractable vomiting	Not usually	Possible
Lateralization	No	Yes
Coordination affected	Yes, but improves	Yes, and gets worse
Seizure	Not usually	Possible early; probable late
Personality change	Possible	Possible

REFERENCES

1. Jordan BD: Brain injury in boxing. Clin Sports Med 28:561–578, 2009.
2. McAlindon RJ: On field evaluation and management of head and neck injured athletes. Clin Sports Med 21:1–14, 2002.
3. McCrory P, Johnston K, Meeuwisse W, et al: Summary and agreement statement of the 2nd International Conference on Concussion in Sport, Prague 2004. Clin J Sports Med 15:48–55, 2005.
4. Albright JP, Van Gilder J, El Khoury G, et al: Head and neck injuries in sports. In Scott WN, Nisonson B, Nicholas JA, editors: Principles of sports medicine, Baltimore, 1984, Williams & Wilkins.
5. Stiell IG, Wells GA, Vandemkeen K, et al: The Canadian CT Head Rule for patients with minor head injury. Lancet 357:1391–1396, 2001.
6. Harmon KG, Drezner JA, Gammons M, et al: American Medical Society for Sports Medicine position statement: concussion in sport. Br J Sports Med 47:15–26, 2013.
7. Putukian M: The acute symptoms of sport-related concussion: diagnosis and on-field management. Clin Sports Med 30:49–61, 2011.
8. McCrory P, Meeuwisse WH, Aubry M, et al: Consensus statement on concussion in sport: the 4th International Conference on Concussion in Sport held in Zurich, November 2012. Br J Sports Med 47:250–258, 2013.
9. McCrory P, Meeuwisse W, Johnston K, et al: Consensus statement on concussion in sport—3rd International Conference on Concussion in Sport, held in Zurich, November 2008. Clin J Sports Med 19:185–195, 2009.
10. Sedney CL, Orphanos J, Bailes JE: When to consider retiring an athlete after sports-related concussion. Clin Sports Med 30:189–200, 2011.
11. Wojtys EM, Hovda D, Landry G, et al: Concussion in sports. Am J Sports Med 27:676–686, 1999.
12. Kelly JP, Rosenberg JH: Diagnosis and management of concussion in sports. Neurology 48:575–580, 1997.
13. Kelly JP, Rosenberg JH: Practice parameter: the management of concussions in sports: report of the quality standards subcommittee. Neurology 48:581–585, 1997.
14. Covassin T, Elbin RJ: The female athlete: the role of gender in the assessment and management of sport related concussion. Clin Sports Med 30:125–131, 2011.
15. Meehan WP, Taylor AM, Proctor M: The pediatric athlete: younger athletes with sport-related concussion. Clin Sports Med 30:133–144, 2011.
16. Makdissi M, Davis G, Jordan B, et al: Revisiting the modifiers: how should the evaluation and management of acute concussions differ in specific groups. Br J Sports Med 47:314–320, 2013.
17. Gronwell D, Wrightson P: Cumulative effect of concussion. Lancet 2:995–997, 1975.
18. McCrory PR, Berkovic SF: Second impact syndrome. Neurology 50:677–683, 1998.
19. Evans RW: The post concussion syndrome: 130 years of controversy. Seminars in Neurology 14:32–39, 1994.
20. d'Hemecourt P: Subacute symptoms of sports-related concussion: outpatient management and return to play. Clin Sports Med 30:63–72, 2011.
21. Lovell MR, Collins MW: Neuropsychological assessment of the college football player. J Head Trauma Rehabil 13:9–26, 1998.
22. LaBotz M, Martin MR, Kimura IF, et al: A comparison of a preparticipation evaluation history form and a symptom-based concussion survey in the identification of previous head injury in collegiate athletes. Clin J Sports Med 15:73–78, 2005.
23. Piland SG, Motl RW, Guskiewicz KM, et al: Structural validity of a self-report concussion-related symptoms scale. Med Sci Sports Exerc 38:27–32, 2006.

24. Maroon JC, Lovell MR, Norwig J, et al: Cerebral concussion in athletes: evaluation and neurophysiological testing. Neurosurg 47:659–672, 2000.

25. Broglio SP, Guskiewicz KM: Concussion in sports: the sideline assessment. Sports Health 1(6):361–369, 2009.

26. Makdissi M, Darby D, Maruff P, et al: Natural history of concussion in sport-markers of severity and implications for management. Am J Sports Med 38:464–471, 2010.

27. McCrea M, Kelly JP, Kluge J, et al: Standardized assessment of concussion in football players. Neurology 48:586–588, 1997.

28. McCrea M, Kelly JP, Randolph C, et al: Standardized assessment of concussion (SAC): On-site mental status evaluation of the athlete. J Head Trauma Rehabil 13:27–35, 1998.

29. Lovell MR, Burke CJ: Concussions in ice hockey: the National Hockey League program. In Cantu RC, editor: Neurologic athletic head and spine injuries, Philadelphia, 2000, WB Saunders.

30. Lau BC, Collins MW, Lovell MR: Sensitivity and specificity of subacute computerized neurocognitive testing and symptom evaluation in predicting outcomes after sport-related concussion. Am J Sports Med 39:1209–1216, 2011.

31. Schatz P, Putz BO: Cross-validation of measures used for computer-based assessment of concussion. Appl Neuropsychol 13(3):151–159, 2006.

32. Elbin RJ, Schatz P, Covassin T: One year test-retest reliability of the online version of ImPACT in high school athletes. Am J Sports Med 39:2319–2324, 2011.

33. Moser RS, Schatz P, Neidzwski K, et al: Group vs individual administration affects baseline neurocognitive test performance. Am J Sports Med 39:2325–2330, 2011.

34. Schmidt JD, Register-Mihalik JK, Mihalik JP, et al: Identifying impairments after concussion: normative data vs individualized baselines. Med Sci Sports Exerc 44:1621–1628, 2012.

35. Lovell MR, Collins MW: Neurophysiological assessment of the college football players. J Head Trauma Rehabil 13(2):9–26, 1998.

36. Lovell MR, Iverson GL, Collins MH, et al: Measurement of symptoms following sports-related concussion: reliability and normative data for the post-concussion scale. Appl Neuropsychol 13:166–174, 2006.

37. Schatz P, Sandel N: Sensitivity and specificity of the online version of ImPACT in high school and collegiate athletes. Am J Sports Med 11:321–326, 2013.

38. Cantu RC: Concussion severity should not be determined until all post concussion symptoms have abated. Lancet 3:437–438, 2004.

39. Hinton-Bayre AD, Geffen G: Severity of sports-related concussion and neurophysiological test performance. Neurology 59:1068–1070, 2002.

40. Mrazik M, Ferrara MS, Peterson CL, et al: Injury severity and neurophysiological and balance outcomes of four college athletes. Brain Inj 14:921–931, 2000.

41. Collins MW, Grindell SH, Lovell MR, et al: Relationship between concussion and neurophysiological performance in college football players. JAMA 282:964–970, 1999.

42. Bleiberg J, Cernich A, Cameron K, et al: Duration of cognitive impairment after sports concussion. Neurosurgery 54:1073–1080, 2004.

43. Torg JS: Athletic injuries to the head, neck and face, St Louis, 1991, Mosby Year Book.

44. Manzi DB, Weaver PA: Head injury: the acute care phase, Thorofare, NJ, 1987, Slack.

45. Lau BC, Kontos AP, Collins MW, et al: Which on-field signs/symptoms predict protracted recovery from sport-related concussion among high school football players. Am J Sports Med 39:2311–2318, 2011.

46. Lovell MR, Iverson GL, Collins MW, et al: Does the level of consciousness predict neurophysiological decrements after concussion? Clin J Sports Med 9:193–198, 1999.

47. Levin HS, O'Donnell VM, Grossman RG: The Galveston orientation and amnesia test: a practical scale to assess cognition after head injury. J Nerv Ment Dis 167:675–684, 1979.

48. Brandt J: The Hopkins verbal learning test: development of a new memory test with six equivalent forms. Clin Neuropsychologist 5:125–142, 1991.

49. Maddocks D, Saling M: Neurophysiological deficits following concussion. Brain Inj 10:99–103, 1996.

50. Putukian M, Echemendia RJ: Managing successive minor head injuries: which tests guide return to play? Phys Sportsmed 24(11):25–38, 1996.

51. Johnson EW, Kegel NE, Collins MW: Neurophysiological assessment of sports-related concussion. Clin Sports Med 30:73–88, 2011.

52. Solomon GS, Dott S, Lovell MR: Long-term neurocognitive dysfunction in sports: what is the evidence? Clin Sports Med 30:165–177, 2011.

53. Echemendia RJ, Iverson GL, McCrea M, et al: Advances in neurophysiological assessment of sport-related concussion. Br J Sports Med 47:294–298, 2013.

54. Niere K, Quin A: Development of a headache-specific disability questionnaire for patients attending physiotherapy. Man Ther 14:45–51, 2009.

55. Maddocks DL, Dicker GD, Saling MM: The assessment of orientation following concussion in athletes. Clin J Sports Med 5:32–35, 1995.

56. McCrea M, Kelly JP, Kluge J, et al: Standardized assessment of concussion in football players. Neurology 48:586–588, 1997.

57. Stilger VG, Alt JM, Robinson TW: Traumatic hyphema in an intercollegiate baseball player: a case report. J Athl Train 34:25–28, 1999.

58. Seidel HM, Ball JW, Dains JE, et al: Mosby's guide to physical examination, St Louis, 1987, Mosby.

59. Swartz MH: Textbook of physical diagnosis, Philadelphia, 1989, WB Saunders.

60. Reilly BM: Practical strategies in outpatient medicine, Philadelphia, 1984, WB Saunders.

61. Novey DW: Rapid access guide to the physical examination, Chicago, 1988, Year Book Medical.

62. Kelly JP: Maxillofacial injuries. In Zachazewski JE, Magee DJ, Quillen WS, editors: Athletic injuries and rehabilitation, Philadelphia, 1996, WB Saunders.

63. Pashby TJ, Pashby RC: Treatment of sports eye injuries. In Fu FH, Stone DA, editors: Sports injuries: mechanisms, prevention, and treatment, Baltimore, 1994, Williams & Wilkins.

64. Durand P, Adamson GJ: On-the-field management of athletic head injuries. J Am Acad Orthop Surg 12:191–145, 2004.

65. Cantu RC: Guidelines for return to contact sports after cerebral concussion. Phys Sportsmed 14:75–83, 1986.

66. Robert WO: Who plays? Who sits? Managing concussions on the sidelines. Sportsmed 20:66–72, 1992.

67. Leblanc KE: Concussions in sports: guidelines for return to competition. Am Fam Phys 50:801–808, 1994.

68. Macciocchi SN, Barth JT, Alves W, et al: Neurophysiological functioning and recovery after mild head injury in collegiate athletes. Neurosurg 39:510–514, 1996.

69. Macciocchi SN, Barth JT, Littlefield LM: Outcome after sports concussion. In Cantu RC, editor: Neurologic athletic head and spine injuries, Philadelphia, 2000, WB Saunders.

70. Cantu RC: Return to play guidelines after concussion. In Cantu RC, editor: Neurologic athletic head and spine injuries, Philadelphia, 2000, WB Saunders.

71. Gall B, Parkhouse W, Goodman D: Heart rate variability of recently concussed athletes at rest and exercise. Med Sci Sports Exerc 36:1269–1274, 2004.

72. Kelly JP, Nichols JS, Filley CM, et al: Concussion in sports: guidelines for the prevention of catastrophic outcome. JAMA 266:2867–2869, 1991.

73. Macciocchi SN, Barth JT, Littlefield LM: Outcome after mild head injury. Clin Sports Med 17(1):27–36, 1998.

74. Polin RS, Alves WM, Jane JA: Sports and head injuries. In Evans RW, editor: Neurology and trauma, Philadelphia, 1996, WB Saunders.

75. Cantu RC: Return to play guidelines after a head injury. Clin Sports Med 17(1):45–60, 1998.

76. Fick DS: Management of concussion in collision sports: guidelines for the sidelines. Postgrad Med 97:53–60, 1995.

77. Cantu RC: Second-impact syndrome. Clin Sports Med 17:37–44, 1998.

78. Topel JL: Examination of the comatose patient. In Weiner WJ, Goetz CG, editors: Neurology for the non-neurologist, Philadelphia, 1989, JB Lippincott.

79. Riemann BL, Guskiewicz KM, Shields EW: Relationship between clinical and forceplate measures of postural stability. J Sports Rehab 8:71–82, 1999.

80. Valovich-McLeod TC, Barr WB, McCrea M, et al: Psychometric and measurement properties of concussion assessment tools in youth sports. J Athl Train 41:399–408, 2006.

81. McCrea M, Barr WB, Guskiewicz K, et al: Standard regression-based methods for measuring recovery from sport-related concussion. J Int Neuropsychol Soc 11:58–69, 2005.

82. Guskiewicz KM, Ross SE, Marshall SW: Postural stability and neuropsychological deficits after concussion in collegiate athletes. J Athl Train 36:263–273, 2001.

83. Fonseca RJ, Walker RV: Oral and maxillofacial trauma, Philadelphia, 1991, WB Saunders.

84. Pollock RA, Dingman RO: Management and reconstruction of athletic injuries of the face, anterior neck, and upper respiratory tract. In Schneider RC, Kennedy JC, Plant ML, editors: Sports injuries: mechanisms, treatment and prevention, Baltimore, 1985, Williams & Wilkins.

85. Simpson JF, Magee KR: Clinical evaluation of the nervous system, Boston, 1973, Little, Brown.

86. House JW, Brackmann DE: Facial nerve grading system: otolaryngol. Head Neck Surg 93:146–147, 1985.

87. Jacobson CP, Means ED: Efficacy of a monothermal warm water caloric screening test. Ann Otol Rhinol Laryngol 94:377–381, 1985.

88. Arceneaux JM: Validity and reliability of rapidly alternating movement's tests. Int J Neurosci 89:281–286, 1997.

89. Swaine BR, Sullivan SJ: Reliability of the cores for the finger to nose tests in adults with traumatic brain injury. Phys Ther 73(2):71–78, 1993.

90. Feys PG, Davies-Smith A, Jones R, et al: Intention tremor rated according to different finger-to-nose test protocols: a survey. Arch Phys Med Rehabil 84:79–82, 2003.

91. Juarez VJ, Lyons M: Interrater reliability of the Glasgow Coma Scale. J Neurosci Nurs 27(5):283–286, 1995.

92. Pettigrew LEL, Wilson JTL, Teasdale GM: Reliability of rating on the Glasgow Outcome Scales from in-person and telephone structured interviews. J Head Trauma Rehabil 18(3):252–258, 2003.

93. Rowley G, Fielding K: Reliability and accuracy of the Glasgow Coma Scale with experienced and inexperienced users. Lancet 337:535–538, 1991.
94. Fielding K, Rowley G: Reliability of assessments by skilled observers using the Glasgow Coma Scale. Aust J Adv Nurs 7(4):13–17, 1990.
95. Gill MR, Reiley DG, Green SM: Interrater reliability of Glasgow Coma Scale scores in the emergency department. Ann Emerg Med 43(2):215–223, 2004.
96. Franchignoni F, Tesio L, Martino MT, et al: Reliability of four simple, quantitative tests of balance and mobility in health elderly females. Aging Clin Exp Res 10(1):26–31, 1998.
97. Johnston DF: A new modification of the Rinne test. Clin Otolaryngol 17:322–326, 1992.
98. Thyssen HH, Brynskov J, Jansen EC, et al: Normal ranges and reproducibility for the quantitative Romberg's test. Acta Neurol Scand 66:100–104, 1982.
99. Geer F, Letz R, Green RC: Relationships between quantitative measures and neurologist's clinical rating of tremor and standing steadiness in two epidemiological studies. Neurotoxicology 21(5):753–760, 2000.

SUGGESTED READINGS

Ad Hoc Committee on Classification of Headache: Classification of headache. Arch Neurol 6:173–176, 1962.

American Academy of Orthopedic Surgeons: Athletic training and sports medicine, Chicago, 1991, AAOS.

Becser N, Borim G, Sjaastad O: Extracranial nerves in the posterior part of the head: anatomic variation and their possible clinical significant. Spine 23:1435–1441, 1988.

Booher JM, Thibodeau GA: Athletic injury assessment, St Louis, 1989, Mosby.

Boyd-Monk H: Examining the external eye. Nursing 80:58–63, 1980.

Bruce R, Fonseca RJ: Mandibular fractures. In Fonseca RJ, Walker RV, editors: Oral and maxillofacial trauma, Philadelphia, 1991, WB Saunders.

Brucker AJ, Kozart DM, Nichols CW, et al: Diagnosis and management of injuries to the eye and orbit. In Torg JS, editor: Athletic injuries to the head, neck and face, St Louis, 1991, Mosby Year Book.

Bruno LA, Gennarelli TA, Torg JS: Head injuries in athletics. In Welsh RP, Shephard RJ, editors: Current therapy in sports medicine 1985-1986, St Louis, 1985, Mosby.

Bruno LA, Gennarelli TA, Torg JS: Management guidelines for head injuries in athletics. Clin Sports Med 6:17–29, 1987.

Burde RM: Eye movements and vestibular system. In Pearlman AL, Collins RC, editors: Neurological pathophysiology, New York, 1984, Oxford University Press.

Caillet R: Head and face pain syndromes, Philadelphia, 1992, FA Davis.

Cantu RC: Guidelines for return to contact sports after a cerebral concussion. Phys Sportsmed 14:75–83, 1986.

Cantu RC, editor: Neurologic athletic head and neck injuries. Clin Sports Med 17(1):1–82, 1998.

Cox MS, Schepens CL, MacKenzie Freeman HM: Retinal detachment due to ocular contusion. Arch Ophthal 76:678–685, 1966.

Crovitz HF, Daniel WF: Length of retrograde amnesia after head injury: a revised formula. Cortex 23:695–698, 1987.

Diamond GR, Quinn GE, Pashby TJ, et al: Ophthalmologic injuries. Clin Sports Med 1:469–482, 1982.

Easterbrook M, Cameron J: Injuries in racquet sports. In Schneider RC, Kennedy JC, Plant ML, editors: Sports injuries: mechanisms, treatment and prevention, Baltimore, 1985, Williams & Wilkins.

Edelman RR, Hesselink JR: Clinical magnetic resonance imaging, Philadelphia, 1990, WB Saunders.

Ellis E: Fractures of the zygomatic complex and arch. In Fonseca RJ, Walker RV, editors: Oral and maxillofacial trauma, Philadelphia, 1991, WB Saunders.

Fahey TD: Athletic training: principles and practice, Palo Alto, CA, 1986, Mayfield.

Foreman SM, Croft AC: Whiplash injuries: the cervical acceleration/deceleration syndrome, Baltimore, 1988, Williams & Wilkins.

Frost DE, Kendall BD: Applied surgical anatomy of the head and neck. In Fonseca RJ, Walker RV, editors: Oral and maxillofacial trauma, Philadelphia, 1991, WB Saunders.

Garrison DW: Cranial nerves: a systems approach, Springfield, IL, 1986, Charles C Thomas.

Gorman BD: Ophthalmology and sports medicine. In Scott WN, Nisonson B, Nicholas JA, editors: Principles of sports medicine, Baltimore, 1984, Williams & Wilkins.

Greenberg MS, Springer PS: Diagnosis and management of oral injuries. In Torg JS, editor: Athletic injuries to the head, neck and face, St Louis, 1991, Mosby Year Book.

Halling AH: The importance of clinical signs and symptoms in the evaluation of facial fractures. Athletic Training 17:102–103, 1982.

Handler SD: Diagnosis and management of maxillofacial injuries. In Torg JS, editor: Athletic injuries to the head, neck and face, Philadelphia, 1982, Lea & Febiger.

Havener WH, Makley TA: Emergency management of ocular injuries. Ohio State Med J 71:776–779, 1975.

Hayward R: Management of acute head injuries, Oxford, 1980, Blackwell Scientific.

Hildebrandt JR: Dental and maxillofacial injuries. Clin Sports Med 1:449–468, 1982.

Hollinshead WH, Jenkins DB: Functional anatomy of the limbs and back, Philadelphia, 1981, WB Saunders.

Hugenholtz H, Richard MT: Return to athletic competition following concussion. Can Med Assoc J 127:827–829, 1982.

Jenkins DB: Hollinshead's functional anatomy of the limbs and back, Philadelphia, 1991, WB Saunders.

Jordan BD: Head injury in sports. In Jordan BD, Tsairis P, Warren RF, editors: Sports neurology, Rockville, MD, 1989, Aspen.

Kinderknecht J: Head injuries. In Zachazewski JE, Magee DJ, Quillen WS, editors: Athletic injuries and rehabilitation, Philadelphia, 1996, WB Saunders.

Kulund DN: The injured athlete, Philadelphia, 1988, JB Lippincott.

Kumamoto DP, Jacob M, Nickelsen D: Oral trauma: on field assessment. Phys Sportsmed 23:53–62, 1995.

Lampert PW, Hardman JM: Morphological changes in brains of boxers. JAMA 251:2676–2679, 1984.

Lew D, Sinn DP: Diagnosis and treatment of midface fractures. In Fonseca RJ, Walker RV, editors: Oral and maxillofacial trauma, Philadelphia, 1991, WB Saunders.

Liebgott B: The anatomical basis of dentistry, St Louis, 1986, Mosby.

Mueller FD: Catastrophic head and neck injuries. Phys Sportsmed 7:710–714, 1979.

Nasher LM: A systems approach to understanding and assessing orientation and balance disorders, Clackamas, OR, 1987, NeuroCom International.

O'Donoghue DH: Treatment of injuries to athletes, Philadelphia, 1984, WB Saunders.

Pashby RC, Pashby TJ: Ocular injuries in sports. In Welsh RP, Shephard RJ, editors: Current therapy in sports medicine 1985-1986, St Louis, 1985, Mosby.

Paton D, Goldberg MF: Management of ocular injuries, Philadelphia, 1976, WB Saunders.

Pavlov H: Radiographic evaluation of the skull and facial bones. In Torg JS, editor: Athletic injuries to the head, neck and face, St Louis, 1991, Mosby Year Book.

Powers MP: Diagnosis and management of dentoalveolar injuries. In Fonseca RJ, Walker RV, editors: Oral and maxillofacial trauma, Philadelphia, 1991, WB Saunders.

Proctor MR, Cantu RC: Head and neck injuries in young athletes. Clin Sports Med 19(4):693–715, 2000.

Reid DC: Sports injury assessment and rehabilitation, New York, 1992, Churchill Livingstone.

Rimel RW, Giordani B, Barth JT, et al: Disability caused by minor head injury. Neurosurg 9:221–228, 1981.

Root JD, Jordan BD, Zimmerman RD: Delayed presentation of subdural hematoma. Phys Sportsmed 21:61–68, 1993.

Ross RJ, Casson IR, Siegel O, et al: Boxing injuries: neurologic, radiologic and neuropsychologic evaluation. Clin Sports Med 6:41–51, 1987.

Rousseau AP: Ocular trauma in sports. In MacKenzie Freeman HM, editor: Ocular trauma in Sports, New York, 1979, Appleton-Century-Crofts.

Roy S, Irvin R: Sports medicine: prevention, evaluation, management and rehabilitation, Englewood Cliffs, NJ, 1983, Prentice-Hall.

Sandusky JC: Field evaluation of eye injuries. Athletic Training 16:254–258, 1981.

Schneider RC: Head and neck injuries in football: mechanisms, treatment and prevention, Baltimore, 1973, Williams & Wilkins.

Schneider RC, Peterson TR, Anderson RE: Football. In Schneider RC, Kennedy JC, Plant ML, editors: Sports injuries: mechanisms, prevention and treatment, Baltimore, 1985, Williams & Wilkins.

Schuller DE, Bruce RA: Ear, nose, throat, and eye. In Strauss RH, editor: Sports medicine, ed 2, Philadelphia, 1991, WB Saunders.

Schultz RC, de Camara DL: Athletic facial injuries. JAMA 252:3395–3398, 1984.

Scott WN, Nisonson B, Nicholas JA, editors: Principles of sports medicine, Baltimore, 1984, Williams & Wilkins.

Shell D, Carico GA, Patton RM: Can subdural hematoma result from repeated minor head injury? Phys Sportsmed 21:74–84, 1993.

Sinn DP, Karas ND: Radiographic evaluation of facial injuries. In Fonseca RJ, Walker V, editors: Oral and maxillofacial trauma, Philadelphia, 1991, WB Saunders.

Sitler M: Nasal septal injuries. Athletic Training 21:10–12, 1986.

Solon RC: Maxillofacial trauma. In Scott WN, Nisonson B, Nicholas JA, editors: Principles of sports medicine, Baltimore, 1984, Williams & Wilkins.

Starkey C, Ryan J: Evaluation of orthopedic and athletic injuries, Philadelphia, 1996, FA Davis.

Untevharnscheidt F: Boxing injuries. In Schneider RC, Kennedy JC, Plant ML, editors: Sports injuries: mechanisms, prevention and treatment, Baltimore, 1985, Williams & Wilkins.

Vegso JJ, Lehman RC: Field evaluation and management of head and neck injuries. Clin Sports Med 6:1–15, 1987.

Vegso JJ, Torg JS: Field evaluation and management of intracranial injuries. In Torg JS, editor: Athletic injuries to the head, neck and face, Philadelphia, 1982, Lea & Febiger.

Vinger PF: How I manage corneal abrasions and lacerations. Phys Sportsmed 14:170–179, 1986.

Wester I: Bell's palsy: the present status of electrodiagnosis and treatment. Physiother Can 23:218–221, 1971.

Zagelbaum BM, Hochman MA: A close look at a "red eye": diagnosing vision-threatening causes. Phys Sportsmed 23:85–92, 1995.

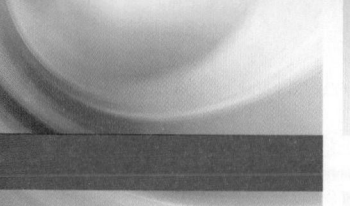

CHAPTER 3

Cervical Spine

Examination of the cervical spine involves determining whether the injury or pathology occurs in the cervical spine or in a portion of the upper limb. Cyriax[1] called this assessment the **scanning examination.** In the initial assessment of a patient who complains of pain in the neck and/or upper limb, this procedure is always carried out unless the examiner is absolutely sure of the location of the lesion. If the injury is in the neck, the scanning examination is definitely called for to rule out neurological involvement. After the lesion site has been determined, a more detailed assessment of the affected area is performed if it is outside the cervical spine.

Because many conditions affecting the cervical spine can be manifested in other parts of the body, the cervical spine is a complicated area to assess properly, and adequate time must be allowed to ensure that as many causes or problems are examined as possible.

APPLIED ANATOMY

The cervical spine consists of several pairs of joints. It is an area in which stability has been sacrificed for mobility, making the cervical spine particularly vulnerable to injury because it sits between a heavy head and a stable thoracic spine and ribs. The cervical spine is divided into two areas—the **cervicoencephalic** for the upper cervical spine and the **cervicobrachial** for the lower cervical spine. The cervicoencephalic or cervicocranial region (C0 to C2) shows the relationship between the cervical spine and the occiput, and injuries in this region have the potential of involving the brain, brainstem, and spinal cord (Figure 3-1).[2,3] Injuries in this area lead to symptoms of headache, fatigue, vertigo, poor concentration, hypertonia of sympathetic nervous system, and irritability. In addition, there may be cognitive dysfunction, cranial nerve dysfunction, and sympathetic system dysfunction.[2,3]

The **atlanto-occipital joints** (C0 to C1) are the two uppermost joints. The principal motion of these two joints is flexion-extension (15° to 20°), or nodding of the head. Side flexion is approximately 10°, whereas rotation is negligible. The **atlas** (C1) has no vertebral body as such. During development, the vertebral body of C1 evolves into the **odontoid process,** which is part of C2. The atlanto-occipital joints are ellipsoid and act in unison.

Along with the atlanto-axial joints, these joints are the most complex articulations of the axial skeleton.

There are several ligaments that stabilize the atlanto-occipital joints. Anteriorly and posteriorly are the atlanto-occipital membranes. The anterior membrane is strengthened by the anterior longitudinal ligament. The posterior membrane replaces the ligamentum flavum between the atlas and occiput. The tectorial membrane, which is a broad band covering the dens and its ligaments, is found within the vertebral canal and is a continuation of the posterior longitudinal ligament. The alar ligaments are two strong rounded cords found on each side of the upper dens passing upwards and laterally to attach on the medial sides of the occipital condyles. The alar ligaments limit flexion and rotation and play a major role in stabilizing C1 and C2, especially in rotation.[4]

The **atlanto-axial joints** (C1 to C2) constitute the most mobile articulations of the spine. Flexion-extension is approximately 10°, and side flexion is approximately 5°. Rotation, which is approximately 50°, is the primary movement of these joints. With rotation, there is a decrease in height of the cervical spine at this level as the vertebrae approximate because of the shape of the facet joints. The odontoid process of C2 acts as a pivot point for the rotation. This middle, or median, joint is classified as a **pivot (trochoidal) joint.** The lateral atlanto-axial, or facet, joints are classified as **plane joints.** Generally, if a person can talk and chew, there is probably some motion occurring at C1 to C2. At the atlanto-axial joints, the main supporting ligament is the transverse ligament of the atlas, which holds the dens of the axis against the anterior arch of the atlas. It is this ligament that weakens or ruptures in rheumatoid arthritis. As the ligament crosses the dens, there are two projections off the ligament, one going superiorly to the occiput and one inferiorly to the axis. The ligament and the projections form a cross, and the three parts taken together are called the *cruciform ligament* of the atlas (Figure 3-2).

The vertebral artery—part of the vertebrobasilar system that passes through the transverse processes of the cervical vertebrae usually starting at C6 but entering as high as C4—supplies 20% of the blood supply to the brain (primarily the hindbrain) along with the internal carotid

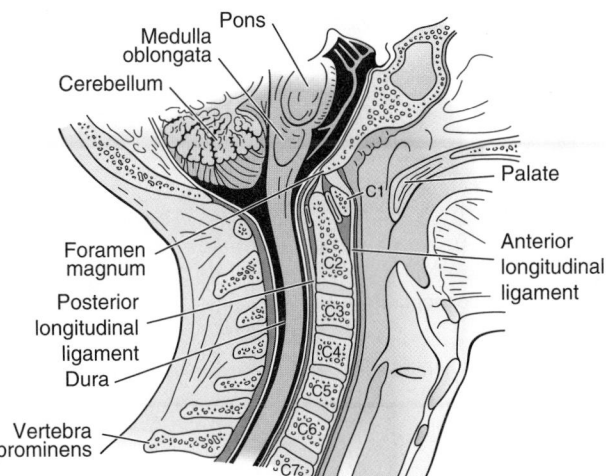

Figure 3-1 This sagittal view of the cervical spine shows the relations among the brainstem, the medulla oblongata, the foramen magnum, the spinal canal, and the cervical spine. The lower portion of the medulla is outside and below the foramen; therefore, with subluxation of the atlas on the axis, compression of the brainstem can occur through pressure of the odontoid against the upper spinal cord and the lower medulla. Note that the anterior arch of the atlas is only millimeters from the pharynx. (Redrawn from Bland JH: Disorders of the cervical spine, Philadelphia, 1994, W.B. Saunders, p. 47.)

artery (80%) (Figure 3-3).[5,6] In its path, the vertebral artery lies close to the facet joints and vertebral body where it may be compressed by osteophyte formation or injury to the facet joint. In addition, in older individuals, atherosclerotic changes and other vascular risk factors (e.g., hypertension, high fat or cholesterol levels, diabetes, smoking) may contribute to altered blood flow in the arteries.[7] The vertebral and internal carotid arteries are stressed primarily by rotation, extension, and traction movements, but other movements may also stretch the artery.[8–10] Rotation and extension of as little as 20° have been shown to significantly decrease vertebral artery blood flow.[11,12] The greatest stresses are placed on the vertebral arteries in four places: where it enters the transverse process of C6, within the bony canals of the vertebral transverse processes, between C1 and C2, and between C1 and the entry of the arteries into the skull.[13,14] These latter two areas have the greatest potential for problems (e.g., thrombosis, dissection, stroke) related to treatment and their concomitant stress on the vertebral arteries.[15] Dutton[13] reports that the most common mechanism for non-penetrating injury to the vertebral artery is neck extension, with or without side flexion or rotation.[16,17] Given the type of injury possible, symptoms may be delayed.[18,19] Symptoms related to the vertebral artery include vertigo, nausea, tinnitus, "drop attacks" (falling without fainting), visual disturbances, or, in rare cases, stroke or death.

The lower cervical spine (C3 to C7) is called the *cervicobrachial area*, since pain in this area is commonly referred into the upper extremity.[2,3] Pathology in this region leads to neck pain alone, arm pain alone, or both neck and arm pain. Thus, symptoms include neck and/or arm pain, headaches, restricted range of motion (ROM), paresthesia, altered myotomes and dermatomes, and radicular signs. Cognitive dysfunction and cranial nerve dysfunction are not commonly symptoms of injuries in this area although sympathetic dysfunction may be. Injury to both areas, if severe enough, may result in psychosocial issues.

There are 14 **facet (apophyseal) joints** in the cervical spine (C1 to C7). The upper four facet joints in the two upper thoracic vertebrae (T1 to T2) are often included in the examination of the cervical spine. The superior facets of the cervical spine face upward, backward, and medially; the inferior facets face downward, forward, and laterally (Figure 3-4). This plane facilitates flexion and extension, but it prevents simple rotation or side flexion without both occurring to some degree together. This is called a **coupled movement** with rotation and side flexion both occurring with either movement.[20] Ishii et al.[21,22] reported that between C0 and C2, as well as C7 and T1, the two movements occur in opposite directions while between C2 and C7, they occur in the same direction. These joints move primarily by gliding and are classified as **synovial (diarthrodial)** joints. The capsules are lax to allow sufficient movement. At the same time, they provide support and a check-rein type of restriction at end range. The greatest flexion-extension of the facet joints occurs between C5 and C6; however, there is almost as much movement at C4 to C5 and C6 to C7. Because of this mobility, degeneration is more likely to be seen at these levels. The neutral or resting position of the cervical spine is slightly extended. The close packed position of the facet joints is complete extension.

Cervical Spine

Resting position:	Midway between flexion and extension
Close packed position:	Full extension
Capsular pattern:	Side flexion and rotation equally limited extension

The **recurrent meningeal,** or **sinuvertebral, nerve** innervates the anterior dura sac, the posterior annulus fibrosus, and the posterior longitudinal ligament. The facet joints are innervated by the medial branch of the dorsal primary rami.[23] For C3 to C7, the main ligaments are the anterior longitudinal ligament, the posterior longitudinal ligament, the ligamentum flavum, and the supraspinal and interspinal ligaments (Figure 3-5). There are also ligaments between the transverse processes (intertransverse ligaments), but in the cervical spine, they are rudimentary.

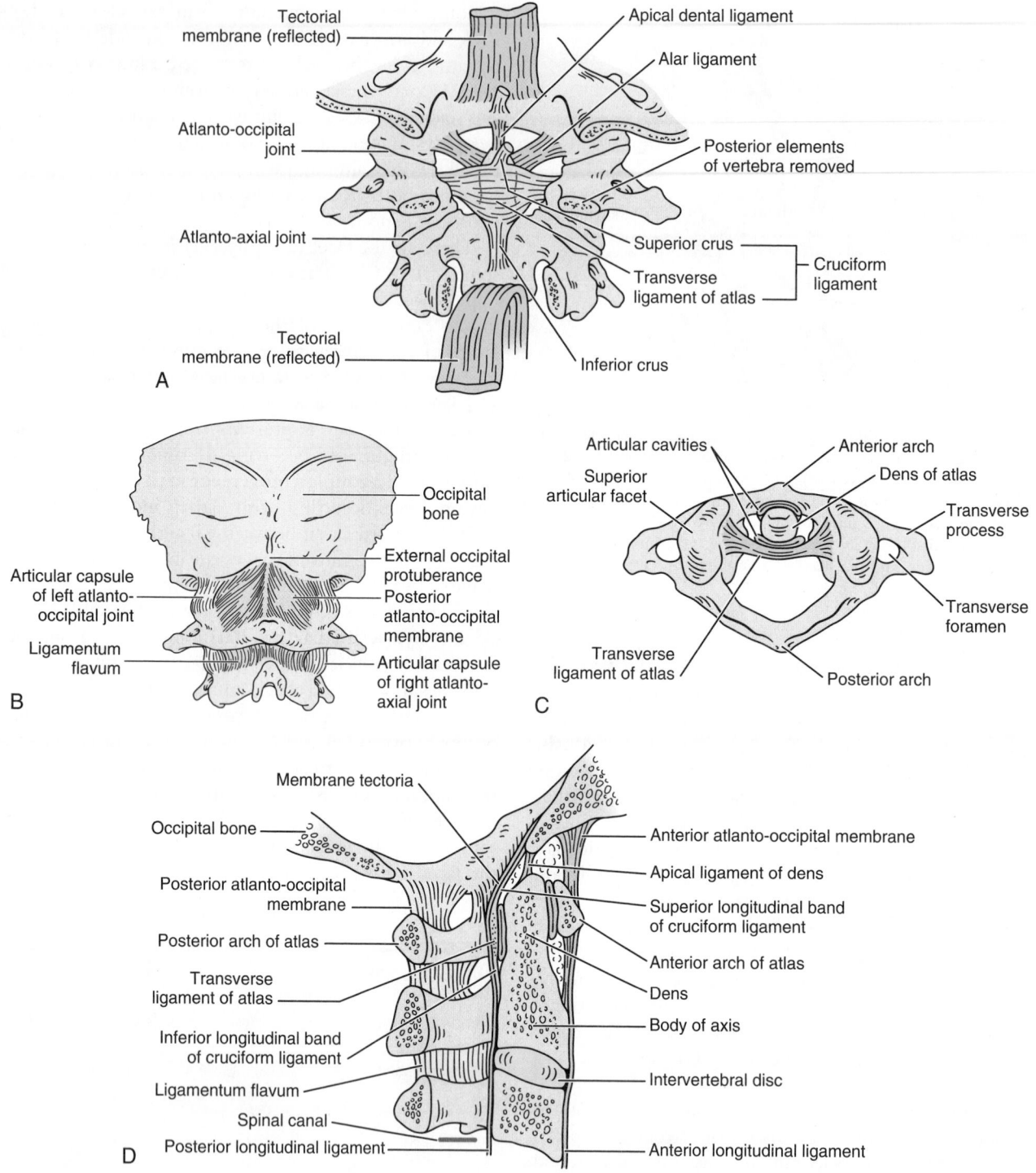

Figure 3-2 Ligaments of the upper cervical spine. A, Posterior deep view. **B,** Posterior superficial view. **C,** Superior view. **D,** Lateral view.

Some anatomists[24–27] refer to the costal or uncovertebral processes as **uncinate joints** or **joints of Luschka** (Figure 3-6). These structures were described by von Luschka in 1858. The uncus gives a "saddle" form to the upper aspect of the cervical vertebra, which is more pronounced posterolaterally; it has the effect of limiting side flexion. Extending from the uncus is a "joint" that appears to form because of a weakness in the annulus fibrosus.

The portion of the vertebra above, which "articulates" or conforms to the uncus, is called the *échancrure,* or notch. Notches are found from C3 to T1, but according to most authors,[24–27] they are not seen until age 6 to 9 years and are not fully developed until 18 years of age. There is some controversy as to whether they should be classified as real joints because some authors believe they are the result of degeneration of the intervertebral disc.

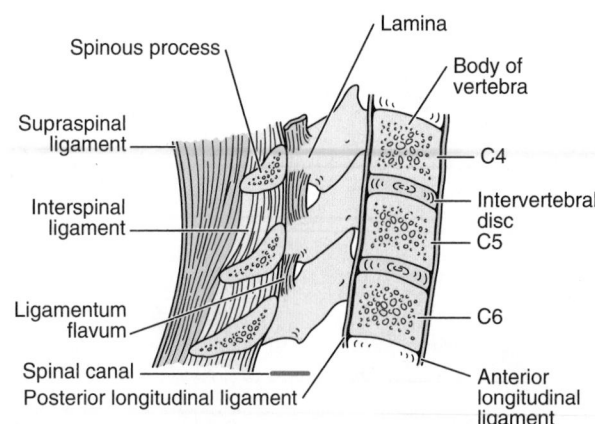

Figure 3-5 Median section of C4–C6 vertebrae to illustrate the intervertebral disc and the ligaments of the cervical spine.

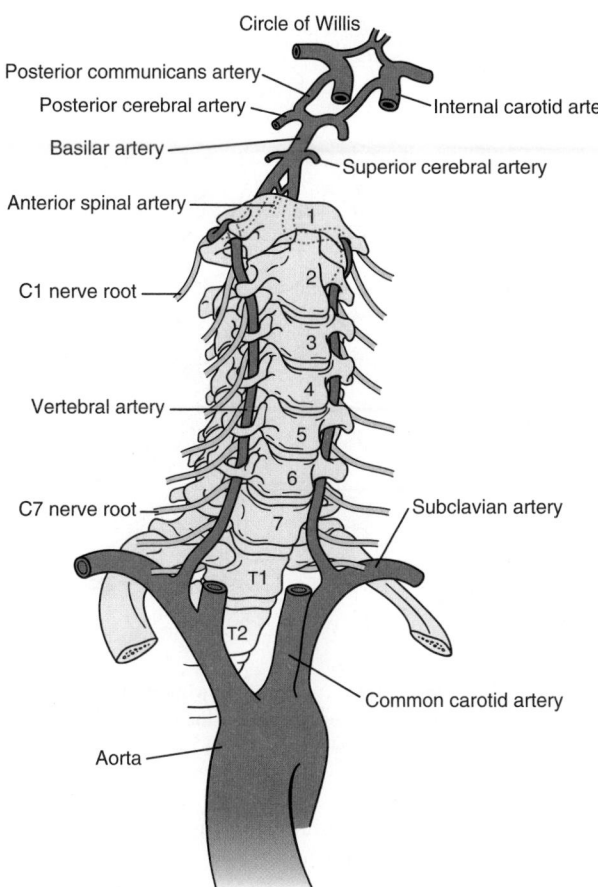

Figure 3-3 Anterolateral drawing of the course of the vertebral artery from C6 to C1 through the bony rings of the foramina transversaria. Note the double U-turn the artery makes from C2 to C1 and the posterior course around the lateral mass of the atlas. (Modified from Bland JH, Nakano KK: Neck pain. In Kelley WN, et al, editors: Textbook of rheumatology, ed 1, Philadelphia, 1981, W.B. Saunders.)

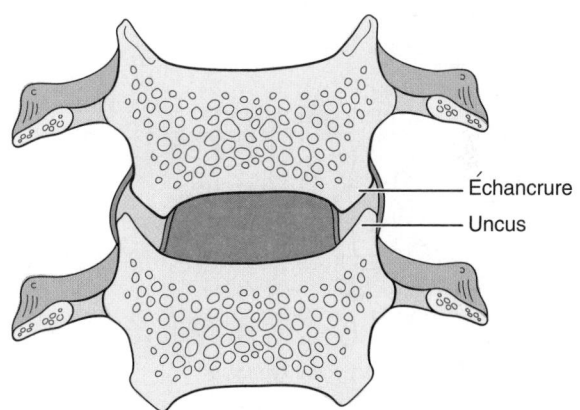

Figure 3-6 Joints of Luschka.

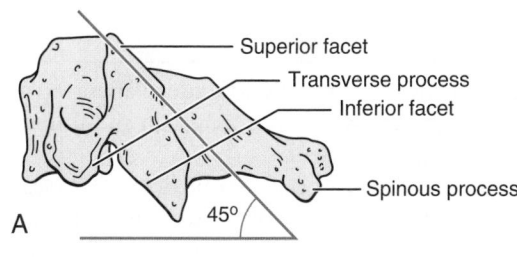

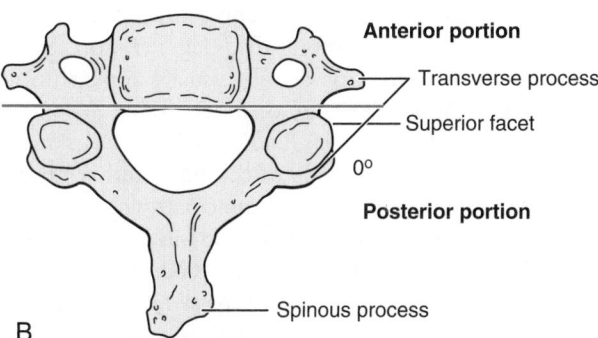

Figure 3-4 Cervical spine-plane of facet joints. A, Lateral view. **B,** Superior view.

The **intervertebral discs** make up approximately 25% of the height of the cervical spine. No disc is found between the atlas and the occiput (C0 to C1) or between the atlas and the axis (C1 to C2). It is the discs rather than the vertebrae that give the cervical spine its lordotic shape (Figure 3-7). The **nucleus pulposus** functions as a buffer to axial compression in distributing compressive forces, whereas the **annulus fibrosus** acts to withstand tension within the disc. The intervertebral disc has some innervation on the periphery of the annulus fibrosus.[28,29]

There are seven vertebrae in the cervical spine with the body of each vertebra (except C1) supporting the weight of those above it. The facet joints may bear some of the weight of the vertebrae above, but this weight is minimal if the normal lordotic posture is maintained. However, even this slight amount of weight bearing can lead to spondylitic changes in these joints. The outer ring of the vertebral body is made of cortical bone, and the inner part is made of cancellous bone covered with the cartilaginous end plate. The vertebral arch protects the spinal cord, while the spinous processes, most of which are bifid in

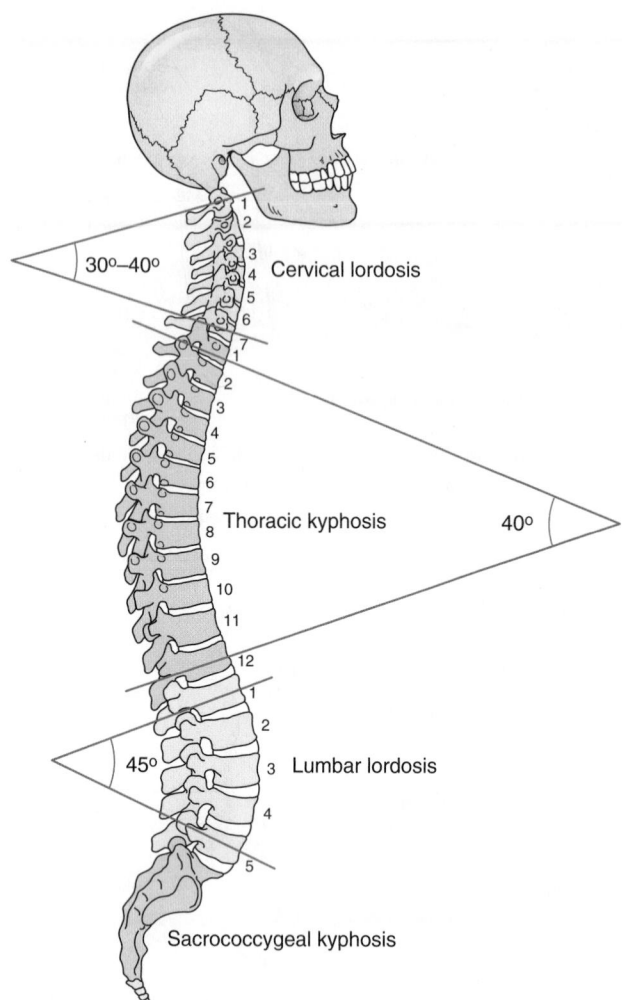

Figure 3-7 The normal sagittal plane curvatures across the regions of the vertebral column. The curvatures represent the normal resting postures of the region. (Modified from Neumann DA: Kinesiology of the musculoskeletal system—foundations for physical rehabilitation, St Louis, 2002, Mosby, p. 276.)

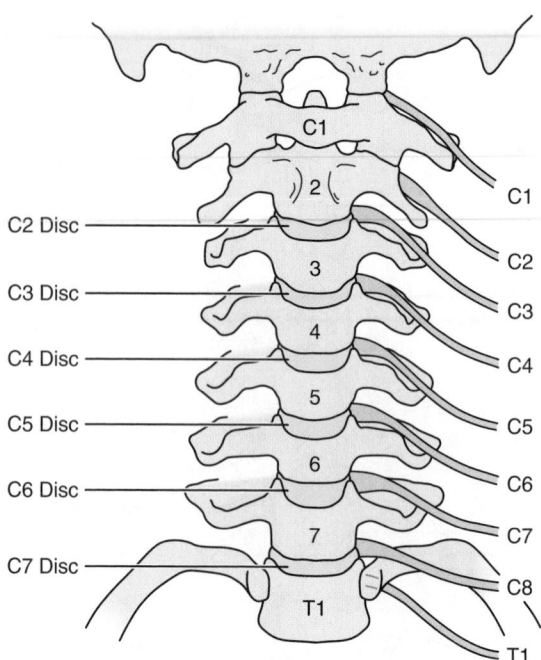

Figure 3-8 Anterior view of cervical spine showing nerve roots. Note how each cervical nerve root is numbered for the vertebra below it.

the cervical spine, provide for attachment of muscles. The transverse processes have basically the same function. In the cervical spine, the transverse processes are made up of two parts: the anterior portion that provides the foramen for the vertebral body, and the posterior portion containing the two articular facets (see Figure 3-4, *B*). In the cervical spine, the spinous processes are at the level of the facet joints of the same vertebra. Generally, the spinous process is considered to be absent or at least rudimentary on C1. This is why the first palpable vertebra descending from the external occiput protuberance is the spinous process of C2.

Although there are seven cervical vertebrae, there are eight **cervical nerve roots.** This difference occurs because there is a nerve root exiting between the occiput and C1 that is designated the C1 nerve root. In the cervical spine, each nerve root is named for the vertebra below it. As an example, C5 nerve root exists between the C4 and C5

vertebrae (Figure 3-8). In the rest of the spine, each nerve root is named for the vertebra above; the L4 nerve root, for example, exists between the L4 and L5 vertebrae. The switch in naming of the nerve roots from the one below to the one above is made between the C7 and T1 vertebrae. The nerve root between these two vertebrae is called C8, accounting for the fact that there are eight cervical nerve roots and only seven cervical vertebrae.

PATIENT HISTORY

In addition to the questions listed under Patient History in Chapter 1, the examiner should obtain the following information from the patient:

1. *What is the patient's age?* Spondylosis (also called *spondylosis deformans*) is often seen in persons 25 years of age or older, and it is present in 60% of those older than 45 years and 85% of those older than 65 years of age.[30,31] It is a generalized disease of aging initiated by intervertebral disc degeneration. Symptoms of osteoarthritis do not usually appear until a person is 60 years of age or older (Table 3-1).

2. *What are the symptoms, and which are most severe?* Table 3-2 outlines many of the signs and symptoms that may arise from cervical spine pathology.[32] Where are the symptoms most severe—in the neck, the shoulder, above or below the elbow, in the hands, and/or fingers?[33] Location of the symptoms may help determine what level of the cervical spine is involved (e.g., tingling in the middle finger may indicate a problem at C6 to C7). Are the symptoms constant,

TABLE **3-1**

Differential Diagnosis of Cervical Spondylosis, Spinal Stenosis, and Disc Herniation

	Cervical Spondylosis	Cervical Spinal Stenosis	Cervical Disc Herniation*
Pain	Unilateral	May be unilateral or bilateral	May be unilateral (most common) or bilateral
Distribution of pain	Into affected dermatomes	Usually several dermatomes affected	Into affected dermatomes
Pain on extension	Increases	Increases	May increase (most common)
Pain on flexion	Decreases	Decreases	May increase or decrease (most common)
Pain relieved by rest	No	Yes	No
Age group affected	60% of those older than 45 years 85% of those older than 65 years	11 to 70 years Most common: 30 to 60 years	17 to 60 years
Instability	Possible	No	No
Levels commonly affected	C5–C6, C6–C7	Varies	C5–C6
Onset	Slow	Slow (may be combined with spondylosis or disc herniation)	Sudden
Diagnostic imaging	Diagnostic	Diagnostic	Diagnostic (be sure clinical signs support)

*Posterolateral protrusion.

TABLE **3-2**

Signs and Symptoms Arising from Cervical Spine Pathology

Signs	Symptoms
• Anesthesia (lack of sensation) • Ataxia • Atrophy • Asymmetry • Drop attack • Dysesthesia (abnormal sensation) • Falling • Fasciculation • Hyperesthesia (increased sensitivity) • Nystagmus • Pathologic gait • Reflex changes • Spastic gait • Sweating or lack of sweating • Tender bones • Tender muscles • Tender scalp • Transient loss of hearing, consciousness, sight • Upper extremity weakness	• Arm and leg pain and ache • Auditory disturbance • Cough • Depressed mood • Diarrhea • Diplopia • Dizziness • Fatigue • Gait disturbance • Headache • Insomnia • Muscle twitch • Nausea • Pain • Paresthesia • Poor balance • "Restless arms and legs" • Sneeze • Speech disturbance • Stiff neck • Threatened faint • Tinnitus • Torticollis • Vertigo • Visual disturbance

Modified from Bland JH: Disorders of the cervical spine, Philadelphia, 1994, W.B. Saunders Co., p. 161.

TABLE **3-3**

Grading of Patients Suffering from Neck Pain

Grade	Clinical Presentation
1	No signs of major pathology Little or no interference with daily activity (ADL)
2	No signs of major pathology Interference with daily activity (ADL)
3	Pain with neurological signs of nerve compression (radiculopathy)
4	Signs of major pathology (e.g., instability, infection)

Adapted from Guzman J, Haldeman S, Carroll LJ, et al: Clinical practice implications of the Bone and Joint Decade 2000–2010 Task Force on Neck Pain and Its Associated Disorders: from concepts and findings to recommendations. J Manipulative Physiol Ther 32(2 Suppl):235, 2009.
ADL, Activity of daily living.

intermittent or variable?[33] The Bone and Joint Decade 2000–2010 Task Force on Neck Pain and its Associated Disorders recommended that neck pain sufferers be divided into four groups (Table 3-3).[34]

Watkins[35] provided a severity scale for neurological injury in football that can be used as a guideline for injury severity involving the cervical spine, especially if one is contemplating allowing the patient to return to activity (Figure 3-9). A combined score (A+B) of 4 is considered a mild episode, 4 to 7 is a moderate episode, and 8 to 10 is a severe episode. This scale

Watkins' Severity Scale for Neurological Deficit

Grade	Neurological Deficit
1	Unilateral arm numbness or dysesthesia; loss of strength
2	Bilateral upper extremity loss of motor and sensory function
3	Ipsilateral arm, leg, and trunk loss of motor and sensory function
4	Transient quadriparesis (temporary sensory loss in all 4 limbs)
5	Transient quadriplegia (temporary motor loss in all 4 limbs)

Score:_____ (A)

Grade	Time Symptoms Present
1	Less than 5 minutes
2	Less than 1 hour
3	less than 24 hours
4	Less than 1 week
5	Greater than 1 week

Score:_____ (B)

Severity Score: A + B = _____

(≤4: mild episode; 4–7: moderate episode; 8–10: severe episode)

Grade	Central Canal Diameter
1	>12 mm
2	Between 10–12
3	10 mm
4	8–10 mm
5	<8 mm

Score:_____ (C)

Return to Activity Score: A + B + C = _____

(≤6: minimum risk; 6–10: moderate risk; 10–15: severe risk)

Figure 3-9 Watkins' Severity Scale for Neurological Deficit. (Data from Watkins RG: Neck injuries in football. In Watkins RG, editor: The spine in sports, St Louis, 1996, Mosby-Year Book, p. 327.)

TABLE **3-4**

Factors That Increase Chances of Recovery from an Episode of Neck Pain

Scenario and Grade of Neck Pain	Likely Increase	Might Increase	No Effect	Not Enough Evidence to Make Determination
General population	Younger age, no previous neck pain, good physical and psychological health, good coping, good social support	Being employed	—	Gender, general exercise or fitness prior to pain episode, cervical disc changes
At work	Exercise and sports, no prior pain or prior sick leave	Changing jobs (for certain job types), white collar job, greater influence over work	Age, ergonomics/physical job demands, work-related psychosocial factors (but many such factors not studied)	Gender, compensation, litigation, obesity, smoking, cervical disc changes
After a traffic collision	No prior pain or sick leave, fewer initial symptoms, less symptom severity, Grade I WAD, good psychological health (e.g., not coping passively, no fear of movement, no post-injury anxiety), no early "overtreatment"	No prior pain problems, good prior health, non-tort insurance, no lawyer involvement, lower collision speed	Collision specific factors (such as, head position when struck, position in vehicle, direction of collision)	Age, gender, culture, prior physical fitness, cervical disc changes

From Guzman J, Haldeman S, Carroll LJ, et al: Clinical practice implications of the Bone and Joint Decade 2000–2010 Task Force on Neck Pain and Its Associated Disorders: from concepts and findings to recommendations. J Manipulative Physiol Ther 32(2 Suppl):234, 2009. *WAD*, Whiplash-associated disorder.

can be combined with radiologic information on canal size (score C) to give a general determination of the possibility of symptoms returning if the patient returns to activity. In this case, a score of 6 (A+B+C) indicates minimum risk, 6 to 10 is moderate risk, and 10 to 15 is severe risk. Watkins[35] also points out that extenuating factors (such as, age of patient, level of activity, and risk) versus benefit, also play a role and, although not included in the score, must be considered. Table 3-4 outlines some of the factors that increase the chances of recovery from neck pain. **Chronic post whiplash syndrome** can lead to anxiety, pain catastrophizing (negative or heightened orientation toward pain), and other adverse psychosocial factors over time, and it can play a major role in the symptoms felt by the patient.[36] Table 3-5 outlines yellow flags related to fear-avoidance beliefs.

3. *What was the mechanism of injury?* Was trauma, stretching, or overuse involved? Was the patient moving when the injury occurred? Table 3-6 outlines warning signs and symptoms (red flags) of serious cervical spine disorders. These questions help

determine the type and severity of injury. For example, trauma may cause a whiplash-type (acceleration) injury or whiplash associated disorder (WAD) (Table 3-7),[37] stretching may lead to "burners," overuse or sustained postures may result in thoracic outlet symptoms, and a report of an insidious onset in someone older than 55 years of age may indicate cervical spondylosis. Was the patient hit from the side, front, or behind? Did the patient see the accident coming?[38] "Burners" or "stingers" typically occur from a blow to part of the brachial plexus or from stretching or compression of the brachial plexus (Table 3-8; Figure 3-10). The answers to these questions help the examiner determine how the injury occurred, the tissues injured, and the severity of the injuries.

4. *Has the patient had neck pain before?* Table 3-9 outlines factors that decrease chances of a new episode of neck pain.[34]

5. *What is the patient's usual activity or pastime?* Do any particular activities or postures bother the patient? What type of work does the patient do? Are there any positions that the patient holds for long periods (e.g., when sewing, typing, or working at a desk)? Does the

TABLE 3-5

Clinical Yellow Flags Indicating Heightened Fear-Avoidance Beliefs

Attitudes and Beliefs	Behaviors
• Belief that pain is harmful or disabling, resulting in guarding and fear of movement • Belief that all pain must be abolished before returning to activity • Expectation of increased pain with activity or work, lack of ability to predict capabilities • Catastrophizing, expecting the worse • Belief that pain is uncontrollable • Passive attitude to rehabilitation	• Use of extended rest • Reduced activity level with significant withdrawal from daily activities • Avoidance of normal activity and progressive substitution of lifestyle away from productive activity • Reports of extremely high pain intensity • Excessive reliance on aids (braces, crutches, and so on) • Sleep quality reduced following the onset of back pain • High intake of alcohol or other substances with an increase since the onset of back pain • Smoking

From Childs JD, Fritz JM, Piva SR, et al: Proposal of a classification system for patients with neck pain. J Orthop Sports Phys Ther 34:686–700, 2004. Data from Kendall, et al: Guide to assessing psychosocial yellow flags in acute low back pain: risk factors for long-term disability and work loss, Wellington, New Zealand, 2002, Accident Rehabilitation and Compensation Insurance Corporation of New Zealand and the National Health Committee.

patient wear glasses? If so, are they bifocals or trifocals? Upper cervical symptoms may result from excessive nodding as the patient tries to focus through the correct part of the glasses. Cervicothoracic (lower cervical/upper thoracic spine) joint problems are often painful when activities that require push-and-pull motion (such as, lawn mowing, sawing, and cleaning windows) are performed. What movements bother the patient? For example, extension can aggravate symptoms in patients with radicular signs and symptoms.[39]

6. *Did the head strike anything, or did the patient lose consciousness?* If the injury was caused by a motor vehicle accident, it is important to know whether the patient was wearing a seat belt, the type of seat belt (lap or shoulder), and whether the patient saw the accident coming. These questions give some idea of the severity and mechanisms of injury. If the patient was unconscious or unsteady, the character of each episode of altered consciousness should be noted (see Chapter 2).

7. *Did the symptoms come on right away?* Bone pain usually occurs immediately, but muscle or

TABLE 3-6

Warning Signs and Symptoms of Serious Cervical Spine Disorders (Red Flags), Some of Which Will Necessitate Immediate Imaging Studies

Potential Cause	Clinical Characteristics
Fracture	Clinically relevant trauma in adolescent or adult Minor trauma in elderly patient Ankylosing spondylitis
Neoplasm	Pain worse at night Unexplained weight loss History of neoplasm Age of more than 50 or less than 20 years Previous history of cancer Constant pain, no relief with bed rest
Infection	Fever, chills, night sweats Unexplained weight loss History of recent systemic infection Recent invasive procedure Immunosuppression Intravenous drug use
Neurologic injury	Progressive neurologic deficit Upper and lower extremity symptoms Bowel or bladder dysfunction
Cervical myelopathy	Sensory disturbance of the hands Muscle wasting of hand intrinsic muscles Unsteady gait Hoffman reflex Hyperreflexia Bowel and bladder disturbances Multisegmental weakness and/or sensory changes
Upper cervical ligamentous instability	Occipital headache and numbness Severe limitation during neck active ROM in all directions Signs of cervical myelopathy
Vertebral artery insufficiency	Drop attacks Dizziness or lightheadedness related to neck movement Dysphasia Dysarthria Diplopia Positive cranial nerve signs
Inflammatory or systemic disease	Temperature more than 37° C Blood pressure more than 160/95 mm Hg Resting pulse more than 100 bpm Resting respiration more than 25 bpm Fatigue

Modified from Rao RD, Currier BL, Albert TJ, et al: Degenerative cervical spondylosis: clinical syndromes, pathogenesis, and management. J Bone Joint Surg Am 89(6):1360–1378, 2007; Childs JD, Fritz JM, Piva SR, et al: Proposal of a classification system for patients with neck pain. J Orthop Sports Phys Ther 34:688, 2004.
ROM, Range of motion.

TABLE 3-7

The Quebec Severity Classification of Whiplash Associated Disorders

Grade	Clinical Presentation
0	No neck symptoms, no physical sign(s)
1	No physical sign(s); neck pain; stiffness or tenderness only; neck complaints predominate; normal ROM; normal reflexes, dermatomes, and myotomes
2	Neck symptoms (pain, stiffness) and musculoskeletal sign(s)—such as, decreased ROM and point tenderness; soft tissue complaints (pain, stiffness) into shoulders and back; normal reflexes, dermatomes, and myotomes
3	Neck symptoms (pain, stiffness, restricted ROM) and neurological sign(s), such as decreased or absence of deep tendon reflexes, weakness (positive myotomes), and sensory (positive dermatome) deficits; x-ray shows no fracture; CT/MRI may show nerve involvement; possible disc lesion
4	Neck symptoms (pain, stiffness, restricted ROM) with fracture or dislocation and objective neurological signs, possible spinal cord signs

Modified from Spitzer WO, Skovron ML, Salmi LR, et al: Scientific monograph of the Quebec Task Force on Whiplash-Associated Disorders: redefining "whiplash" and its management. Spine 20(8 Suppl):8S–58S, 1995.
CT, Computed tomography; *MRI,* magnetic resonance imaging; *ROM,* range of motion.

ligamentous pain can either come on immediately (e.g., a tear) or occur several hours or days later (e.g., stretching caused by a motor vehicle accident). Seventy percent of whiplash patients reported immediate symptom occurrence while the rest reported delayed symptoms.[32,40-44] How long have the symptoms been present? Myofascial pain syndromes demonstrate generalized aching and at least three trigger points, which have lasted for at least 3 months with no history of trauma.[45]

8. *What are the sites and boundaries of the pain?* Have the patient point to the location or locations of the pain. Symptoms do not go down the arm for a C4 nerve root injury or for nerve roots above that level. **Cervical radiculopathy,** or injury to the nerve roots in the cervical spine, presents primarily with unilateral motor and sensory symptoms into the upper limb, with muscle weakness (myotome), sensory alteration (dermatome), reflex hypoactivity, and sometimes focal activity being the primary signs.[46-49] Acute radiculopathies are commonly associated with disc herniations, whereas chronic types are more related to spondylosis.[47] Disc herniations in the cervical spine commonly cause severe neck pain that may radiate into the shoulder, scapula and/or arm, limit ROM, and an increase in pain on coughing, sneezing, jarring, or straining.[44] **Cervical myelopathy,** or injury to the spinal cord itself, is more likely to present with spastic weakness, paresthesia, and possible incoordination in one or both lower limbs, as well as

TABLE 3-8

Differential Diagnosis of Cervical Nerve Root and Brachial Plexus Lesion

	Cervical Nerve Root Lesion	Brachial Plexus Lesion
Cause	Disc herniation Stenosis Osteophytes Swelling with trauma Spondylosis	Stretching of cervical spine Compression of cervical spine Depression of shoulder
Contributing factors	Congenital defects	Thoracic outlet syndrome
Pain	Sharp, burning in affected dermatomes	Sharp, burning in all or most of arm dermatomes, pain in trapezius
Paresthesia	Numbness, pins and needles in affected dermatomes	Numbness, pins and needles in all or most arm dermatomes (more ambiguous distribution)
Tenderness	Over affected area of posterior cervical spine	Over affected area of brachial plexus or lateral to cervical spine
Range of motion	Decreased	Decreased but usually returns rather quickly
Weakness	Transient paralysis usually Myotome may be affected	Transient muscle weakness Myotomes affected
Deep tendon reflexes	Affected nerve root may be depressed	May be depressed
Provocative test	Side flexion, rotation and extension with compression increase symptoms Cervical traction decreases symptoms Upper limb tension tests positive	Side flexion with compression (same side) or stretch (opposite side) may increase symptoms Upper limb tension tests may be positive

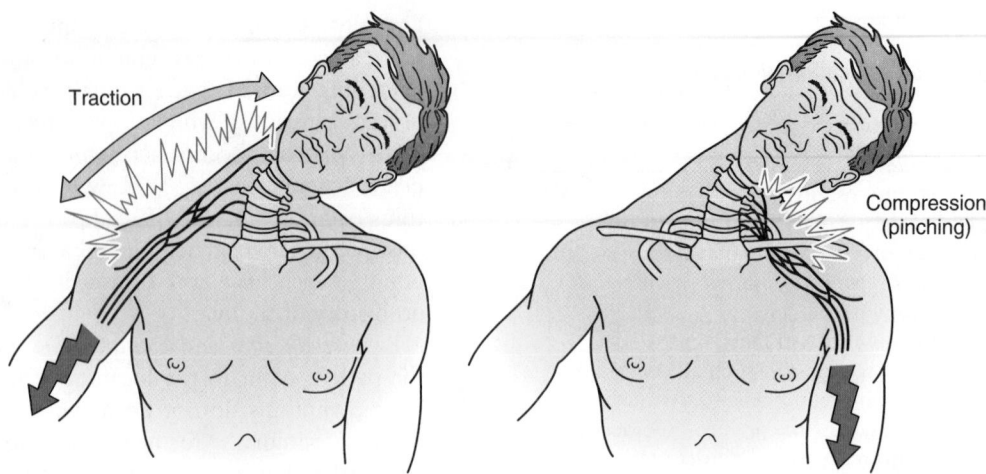

Traction

Compression (pinching)

Figure 3-10 Mechanism of injury for brachial plexus (burner or stinger) pathology.

TABLE **3-9**

Factors That Decrease Chances of Getting a New Episode of Neck Pain

Scenario and Grade of Neck Pain	Likely Decrease	Might Decrease	No Effect	Not Enough Evidence to Make Determination
General population	No previous neck pain, no other musculoskeletal problems, good psychological health	Younger age, male gender, non-smoking, changing rules in sports (like in ice hockey)	Obesity	Weight of school bags, cervical disc changes (on imaging)
At work	Younger age (peak risk in fourth and fifth decades), male gender, no previous pain in the neck, back or upper limbs, little psychological job strain, good co-worker support, active work (nonsedentary), less repetitive or precision work	Not being an immigrant or a visible minority, higher strength or endurance of the neck, not working with the neck bend for prolonged periods, non-smoking, no previous headaches, good physical health, "non-type A" personality, not working in awkward positions, light physical work, adequate keyboard position, no awkward head elbow and shoulder posture, no screen glare	Physical or sports activity during leisure, sleep quality, time spent on domestic activities, time spent on hobbies	Marital status, education, occupational class duration of employment, obesity, self-assessed health status, mental stress, job satisfaction, working with hands above the shoulder level, height of computer screen, cervical disc changes
After a traffic collision	—	Male gender, no previous neck pain, riding in back seat, side collision, no compensation for pain and suffering, specially engineered car seats and headrests	Tow bars in the car, age, type of child seat restraint	Awareness of collision, head position at time of collision, severity of collision impact, cervical disc changes (on imaging)

From Guzman J, Haldeman S, Carroll LJ, et al: Clinical practice implications of the Bone and Joint Decade 2000–2010 Task Force on Neck Pain and Its Associated Disorders: from concepts and findings to recommendations. J Manipulative Physiol Ther 32(2 Suppl):233, 2009.

TABLE **3-10**

Signs and Symptoms in Cervical Myelopathy

Motor Changes	Sensory Changes
Initial Symptoms (Predominantly Lower Limbs) • Spastic paraparesis • Stiffness and heaviness, scuffing of the toe, difficulty climbing stairs • Weakness, spasms, cramps, easy fatigability • Decreased power, especially of flexors (dorsiflexors of ankles and toes; flexors of hips) • Hyperreflexia of knee and ankle jerks, with clonus • Positive Babinski sign, extensor hypertonia • Decreased or absent superficial abdominal and cremasteric reflexes • Drop foot, crural monoplegia **Later Symptoms (In Order of Occurrence)** • Various combinations of upper and lower limb involvement • Mixed picture of upper and lower motoneuron dysfunction • Atrophy, weakness, hypotonia, hyper-reflexia to hyporeflexia, and absent deep tendon reflexes	• Headache and head pain • Neck, eye, ear, throat, or sinus pain • Sensory symptoms in the pharynx and larynx • Paroxysmal hoarseness and aphonia • Rotary vertigo • Tinnitus synchronous with pulse or continuous whistling noises • Deafness • Oculovisual changes (e.g., blurring, photophobia, scintillating scotomata, diplopia, homonymous hemianopsia, and nystagmus) • Autonomic disturbance (e.g., sweating, flushing, rhinorrhea, salivation, lacrimation, nausea, and vomiting) • Weakness in one or both legs, drop attacks with or without loss of consciousness • Numbness on one or both sides of the body • Dysphagia or dysarthria • Myoclonic jerks • Hiccups • Respiratory changes (e.g., Cheyne-Stokes respiration, Biot respiration, or ataxic respiration)

Modified from Bland JH: Disorders of the cervical spine, Philadelphia, 1994, WB Saunders, pp. 215–216.

proprioceptive and/or sphincter dysfunction (Tables 3-10 and 3-11).[50]

9. *Is there any radiation of pain?* It is helpful to correlate this answer with dermatome and sensory peripheral nerve findings when performing sensation testing and palpation later in the examination. Is the pain deep, superficial, shooting, burning, or aching? For example, when an athlete experiences a "burner," the sensation is a lightning-like, burning pain into the shoulder and arm, followed by a period of heaviness or loss of function in the arm. Figure 3-11 shows the radiation of pain with facet (apophyseal) joint pathology.[51]

10. *Is the pain affected by laughing, coughing, sneezing, or straining?* If so, an increase in intrathoracic or intra-abdominal pressure may be contributing to the problem.

11. *Does the patient have any headaches? If so, where? How frequently do they occur?* For example, do they occur every day, two times per day, two days per week, or one day per month?[52] How intense are they? How long do they last? Are they affected by medication and, if so, by how much medication, and what kind? Are there any precipitating factors (e.g., food, stress, posture)? See Tables 2-11, 2-12, and 2-13, which indicate the influence of time of day, body position, headache location, and type of pain on diagnosis of the type of headache that the patient may have. Table 2-14 outlines the salient features of some of the more

common headaches. Craniovertebral joint dysfunction commonly is accompanied by headaches. For example, C1 headaches occur at the base and top of the head, whereas C2 headaches are referred to the temporal area.

Signs of Headaches Having a Cervical Origin

• Occipital or suboccipital component to headache
• Neck movement alters headache
• Painful limitation of neck movements
• Abnormal head or neck posture
• Suboccipital or nuchal tenderness
• Abnormal mobility at C0–C1
• Sensory abnormalities in the occipital and suboccipital areas

12. *Does a position change alter the headache or pain?* If so, which positions increase or decrease the pain? The patient may state that the pain and referred symptoms are decreased or relieved by placing the hand or arm of the affected side on top of the head. This is called **Bakody's sign,** and it is usually indicative of problems in the C4 or C5 area.[53,54]

13. *Is paresthesia (a "pins and needles" feeling) present?* This sensation occurs if pressure is applied to the nerve root. It may become evident if pressure is relieved from a nerve trunk. Numbness and/or

TABLE **3-11**

Differential Diagnosis of Neurological Disorders of the Cervical Spine and Upper Limb

Cervical Radiculopathy (Nerve Root Lesion)	Cervical Myelopathy	Brachial Plexus Lesion (Plexopathy)	Burner (Transient Brachial Plexus Lesion)	Peripheral Nerve (Upper Limb)
Arm pain in dermatome distribution	Hand numbness, head pain, hoarseness, vertigo, tinnitus, deafness	Pain more localized to shoulder and neck (sometimes face)	Temporary pain in dermatome	No pain
Pain increased by extension and rotation or side flexion	Extension, rotation, and side flexion may all cause pain	Pain on compression of brachial plexus	Pain on compression or stretch of brachial plexus	No pain early; if contracture occurs (late), pain on stretching
Pain may be relieved by putting hand on head (C5, C6)	Arm positions have no effect on pain	Arm positions have no effect on pain*	Arm positions have no effect on pain*	Arm positions have no effect on pain*
Sensation (dermatome) affected	Sensation affected, abnormal pattern	Sensation (dermatome) affected	Sensation (dermatome) affected	Peripheral nerve sensation affected
Gait not affected	Wide-based gait drop attacks, ataxia; proprioception affected	Gait not affected	Gait not affected	Gait not affected
Altered hand function	Loss of hand function	Loss of arm function	Loss of function temporary	Loss of function of muscles supplied by nerve
Bowel and bladder not affected	Possible loss of bowel and bladder control	Bowel and bladder not affected	Bowel and bladder not affected	Bowel and bladder not affected
Weakness in myotome but no spasticity	Spastic paresis (especially in lower limb early, upper limb affected later)	Weakness in myotome	Temporary weakness in myotome	Weakness of muscles supplied by nerve
DTR hypoactive	Lower limb DTR hyperactive Upper limb DTR hyperactive	DTR hypoactive	DTR not affected	DTR may be decreased
Negative pathological reflex	Positive pathological reflex	Negative pathological reflex	Negative pathological reflex	Negative pathological reflex
Negative superficial reflex	Decreased superficial reflex	Negative superficial reflex	Negative superficial reflex	Negative superficial reflex
Atrophy (late sign), hard to detect early	Atrophy	Atrophy	Atrophy possible	Atrophy (not usually with neuropraxia)

DTR, Deep tendon reflexes.
*Except in neurotension test positions.

paresthesia in the hands or legs and deteriorating hand function all may relate to cervical myelopathy (see Table 3-10).

14. *Does the patient experience any tingling in the extremities?* Are the symptoms bilateral? Bilateral symptoms usually indicate either systemic disorders (e.g., diabetes, alcohol abuse) that are causing neuropathies or central space–occupying lesions.

15. *Are there any lower limb symptoms?* This finding may indicate a severe problem affecting the spinal cord (myelopathy; see Table 3-10). These symptoms may include numbness, paresthesia, stumbling, difficulty walking, and lack of balance or agility. All of these symptoms could indicate cervical myelopathy. Likewise, signs of sphincter (bowel or bladder) or sexual dysfunction may be related to cervical myelopathy.

16. *Does the patient have any difficulty walking? Does the patient have problems with balance?* Does the patient stumble when walking, have trouble walking in the dark, or walk with feet wide apart? Positive responses may indicate a cervical myelopathy. Abnormality of

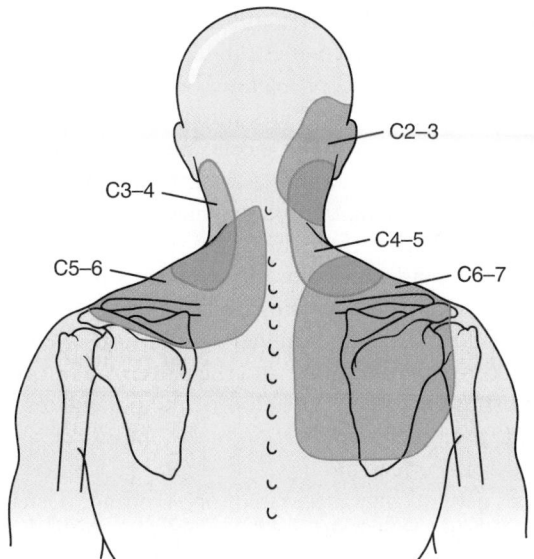

Figure 3-11 Referred pain patterns suggested with pathology of the apophyseal joints. (Redrawn from Porterfield JA, DeRosa C: Mechanical neck pain—perspective in functional anatomy, Philadelphia, 1995, W.B. Saunders, p. 104. Adapted from Dwyer A, April C, Bogduk N: Cervical zygapophyseal joint pain patterns. Spine 15:453–457, 1990.)

the cranial nerves combined with gait alterations may indicate systemic neurological dysfunction.[55]

17. *Does the patient experience dizziness, faintness, or seizures?* What is the degree, frequency, and duration of the dizziness? Is it associated with certain head positions or body positions? Semicircular canal problems or vertebral artery problems (Table 3-12) can lead to dizziness. Dizziness from a vertebral artery problem is commonly associated with other symptoms. Falling with no provocation while remaining conscious is sometimes called a **drop attack.**[56] Has the patient experienced any visual disturbances? Disturbances such as diplopia (double vision), nystagmus ("dancing eyes"), scotomas (depressed visual field), and loss of acuity may indicate severity of injury, neurological injury, and sometimes increased intracranial pressure (see Chapter 2).[53]

18. *Does the patient exhibit or complain of any sympathetic symptoms?* There may be injury to the cranial nerves or the sympathetic nervous system, which lies in the soft tissues of the neck anterior and lateral to the cervical vertebrae. The cranial nerves and their functions are shown in Table 2-1. Severe injuries (e.g., acceleration/whiplash type) can lead to hypertonia of the sympathetic nervous system.[2] Some of the sympathetic signs and symptoms the examiner may elicit are "ringing" in the ears (tinnitus), dizziness, blurred vision, photophobia, rhinorrhea, sweating, lacrimation, and loss of strength.

19. *Is the condition improving, worsening or staying the same?* The answers to these questions give the examiner some indication of the condition's progress.

TABLE 3-12

Signs and Symptoms of Vertebrobasilar Artery Insufficiency*

- Dizziness
- Giddiness
- Drop attacks
- Syncope (loss of consciousness)
- Stroke
- Diplopia, blurred vision
- Visual hallucination
- Tinnitus (ringing in the ears)
- Flushing
- Sweating
- Lacrimation (tearing)
- Rhinorrhea (runny nose)
- Scotomata (visual defect in defined area of eye[s])
- Hiccups
- Myotonic jerks
- Tremor and rigidity
- Disorientation
- Vertigo
- Photophobia (sensitivity to light)
- Numbness and tingling
- Quadriparesis (weakness in all four limbs)
- Dysphagia (difficulty swallowing)
- Dysarthria (difficulty articulating)
- Photopsia (sensation of flashing lights)
- Visual anosognosia (unawareness of visual defect)
- Nystagmus
- Ataxia (lack of voluntary muscle coordination)

Modified from Bland JH: Disorders of the cervical spine, Philadelphia, 1994, W.B. Saunders Co., p. 217.
*These paraspinal symptoms result mainly from rotation and extension of the neck, although they sometimes occur during flexion. The spectrum of neurologic symptoms and signs is as broad as that of the structures potentially involved. In a complex, bizarre, and poorly explained neurologic syndrome, vertebrobasilar artery insufficiency should be suspected.

20. *Which activities aggravate the problem? Which activities ease the problem?* Are there any head or neck positions that the patient finds particularly bothersome? These positions should be noted. For example, does reading (flexed cervical spine) bother the patient? If symptoms are not varied by a change in position, the problem is not likely to be mechanical in origin. Lesions of C3, C4, and C5 may affect the diaphragm and thereby affect breathing.

21. *Does the patient complain of any restrictions when performing movements?* If so, which movements are restricted? It is important that the patient not demonstrate the movements at this stage; the actual movements will be done during the examination.

22. *Is the patient a mouth breather?* Mouth breathing encourages forward head posture and increases activity of accessory respiratory muscles.

23. *Is there any difficulty in swallowing (dysphagia), or have there been any voice changes?* Such a change may

be caused by neurological problems, mechanical pressure, or muscle incoordination. Pain on swallowing may indicate soft- tissue swelling in the throat, vertebral subluxation, osteophyte projection, or disc protrusion into the esophagus or pharynx. In addition, swallowing becomes more difficult and the voice becomes weaker as the neck is extended.

24. *What can be learned about the patient's sleeping position?* Is there any problem sleeping? How many pillows does the patient use, and what type are they (e.g., feather, foam, buckwheat)? Foam pillows tend to retain their shape and have more "bounce;" they do not offer as much support as a good feather or buckwheat pillow. What type of mattress does the patient use (e.g., hard, soft)? Does the patient "hug" the pillow or abduct the arms when sleeping? These positions can increase the stress on the lower cervical nerve roots.

25. *Does the patient display any cognitive dysfunction?* If a possible head injury is suspected, the clinician should also consider testing for mental status (see Chapter 2).

OBSERVATION

For a proper observation, the patient must be suitably undressed. However, the examiner should also watch the patient as he or she enters the examination room, and before or while he or she undresses. The spontaneous movements of these activities can be very helpful in determining the patient's problems. For example, can the patient easily move the head when undressing? A male patient should wear only shorts, and a female patient should wear a bra and shorts for this part of the assessment. In some cases, the bra may have to be removed to determine whether there are any problems, such as thoracic outlet syndrome, thoracic symptoms being referred to the cervical spine, or functional restriction of movement of the ribs. The examiner should note the willingness of the patient to move and the patterns of movement demonstrated. Facial expression of the patient can often give the examiner an indication of the amount of pain the patient is experiencing.

The patient may be seated or standing. Usually, a standing posture is best because the posture of the whole body can be observed (see Chapter 15). Abnormalities in one area frequently affect another area. For example, excessive lumbar lordosis may cause a "poking" chin to compensate for the lumbar deformity and to maintain the body's center of gravity. In the cervical spine region, the examiner should note the following:

Head and Neck Posture. Is the head in the midline, and does the patient have a normal lordotic curvature (30° to 40°) (see Figure 3-7; Figure 3-12)? This curvature along with the other spinal curvatures in the lower spine provides a shock absorption mechanism for the spine and

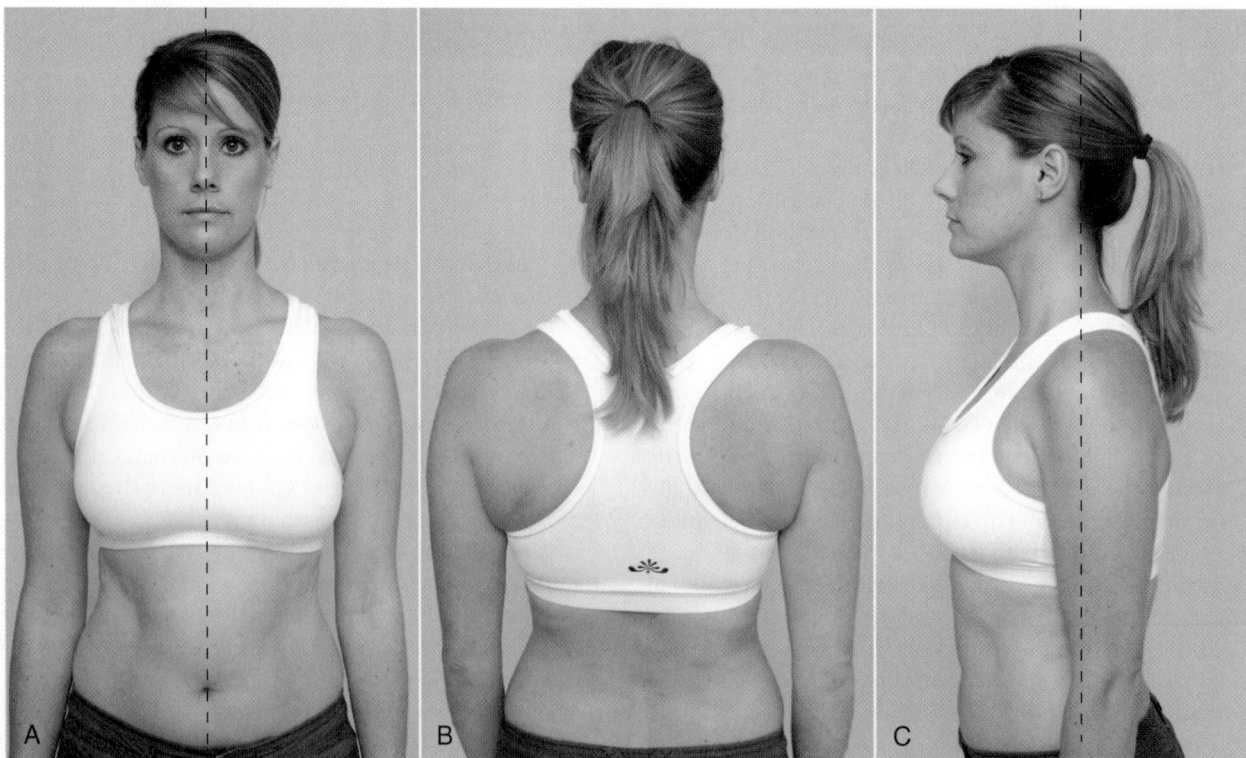

Figure 3-12 Observation views of head and neck. A, Anterior view. **B,** Posterior view. **C,** Lateral or side view. With normal posture, the ear should be in line with the shoulder and the forehead vertical. Note that this model is a "chin poker" with the head sitting anteriorly, which leads to a decrease in the lordotic curve.

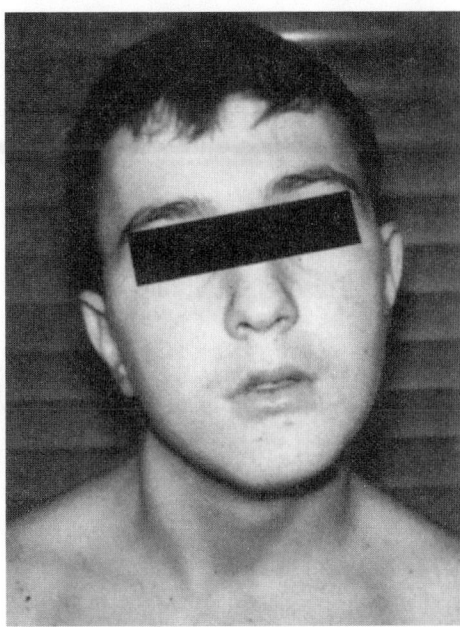

Figure 3-13 **Example of congenital torticollis** showing prominent sternocleidomastoid muscle on the right. (From Gartland JJ: Fundamentals of orthopedics, Philadelphia, 1987, WB Saunders, p. 279.)

helps the body maintain its center of gravity.[57] From the front, the chin should be in line with the sternum (manubrium) and from the side, the ears should be in line with the shoulder and the forehead vertical. Is there evidence of torticollis (congenital or acquired) (Figure 3-13), Klippel-Feil syndrome (congenital fusion of some cervical vertebra, usually C3 to C5) (Figure 3-14), or other neck deformity? Does the patient exhibit a poking chin or a "military posture?" A habitual poking chin can result in adaptive shortening of the occipital muscles. It also causes the cervical spine to change alignment resulting in increased stress of the facet joints and posterior discs and other posterior elements (Figure 3-15). The position may also lead to weaknesses of the deep neck flexors.[58] Janda[59] described a cervical **"upper crossed syndrome"** to show the effect of a "poking chin" posture on the muscles. With this syndrome, the deep neck flexors are weak, as are the rhomboids, serratus anterior, and often the lower trapezius. Opposite these weak muscles are tight pectoralis major and minor, along with upper trapezius and levator scapulae (Figure 3-16). Does the head sit in the middle of the shoulders? Is the head tilted or rotated to one side or the other, indicating possible torticollis? Does this posture appear to be habitual (in other words, does the patient always go back to this posture)? Habitual posture may result from postural compensation, weak muscles, hearing loss, temporomandibular joint problems, or wearing of bifocals or trifocals. The trapezius neck line should be equal on both sides. Head and neck posture should be checked with the patient sitting and then standing, and any differences should be noted.

Shoulder Levels. Usually the shoulder on the dominant side will be slightly lower than that on the nondominant side. With injury, the injured side may be elevated to provide protection (e.g., upper trapezius and/or levator scapulae) or because of muscle spasm. Rounded shoulders may be the result of or the cause of a poking chin. Rounding also causes the scapulae to protract, the humerus to medially rotate, and the anterior structures of the shoulder to tighten.

Muscle Spasm or Any Asymmetry. Is there any atrophy of the deltoid muscle (axillary nerve palsy) or torticollis (muscle spasm, tightness, or prominence of the sternocleidomastoid muscle) (see Figure 3-13)?

Facial Expression. The examiner should observe the patient's facial expression as the patient moves from position to position, makes different movements, and explains the problem. Such observation should give the examiner an idea of how much the patient is subjectively suffering.

Bony and Soft-Tissue Contours. If the cervical spine is injured, the head tends to be tilted and rotated away from the pain, and the face is tilted upward. If the patient is hysterical, the head tends to be tilted and rotated toward the pain, and the face is tilted down.

Evidence of Ischemia in Either Upper Limb. The examiner should note any altered coloration of the skin, ulcers, or vein distention as evidence of upper limb ischemia.

Normal Sitting Posture. The nose should be in line with the manubrium and xiphoid process of the sternum. From the side, the ear lobe should be in line with the acromion process and the high point on the iliac crest for proper postural alignment. The normal curve of the cervical spine is a lordotic type of curve. Referred pain from conditions, such as spondylosis, tends to occur in the shoulder and arm rather than the neck.

EXAMINATION

A complete examination of the cervical spine must be performed, including the neck and both upper limbs. Many of the symptoms that occur in an upper limb originate from the neck. Unless there is a history of definite trauma to a peripheral joint, an upper limb scanning examination must be performed to rule out problems within the neck.

Active Movements

The first movements that are carried out are the active movements of the cervical spine with the patient in the sitting position. The examiner is looking for differences in range of movement and in the patient's willingness to do the movement.[60] The ROM taking place in this phase is the summation of all movements of the entire cervical spine, not just at one level. This combined movement allows for greater mobility in the cervical spine while still

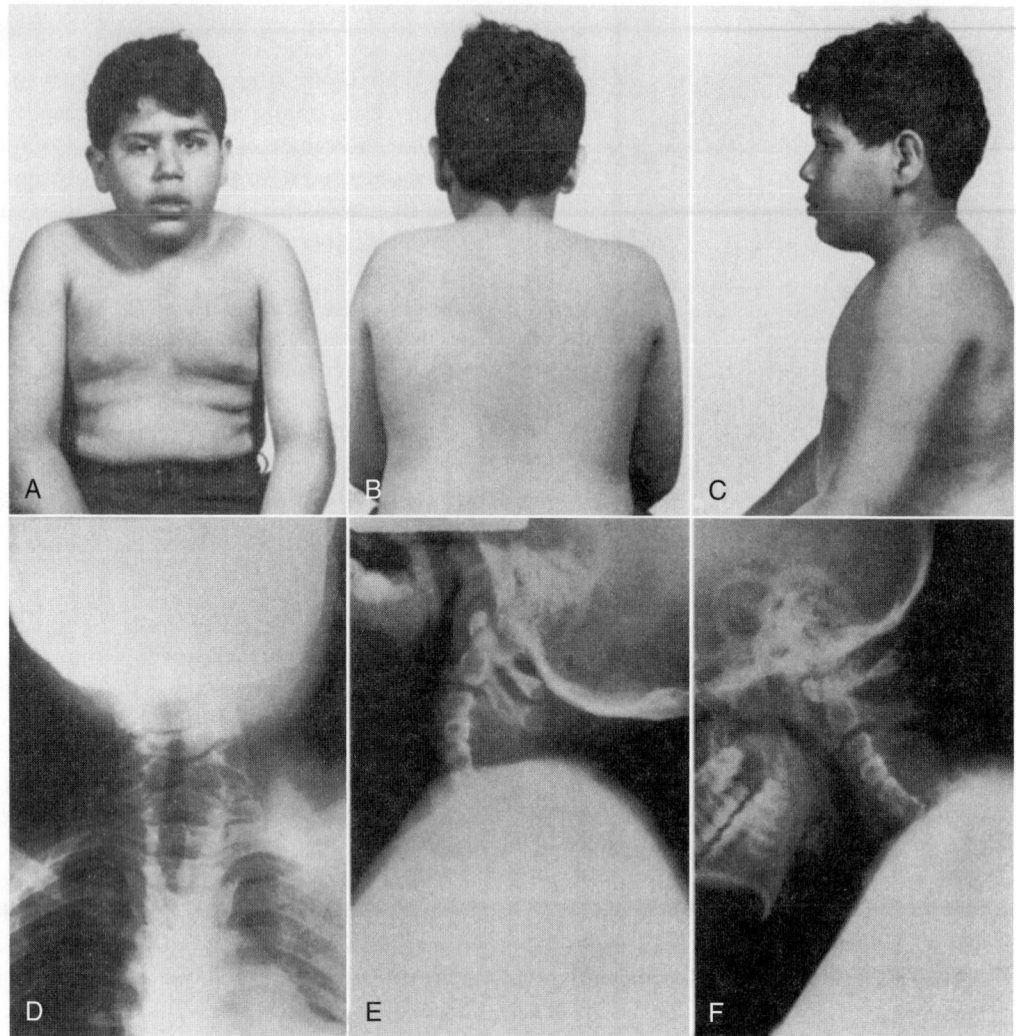

Figure 3-14 Klippel-Feil syndrome in a 12-year-old boy. Clinical appearance of the patient. **A,** Anterior view. **B,** Posterior view. **C,** Lateral view. Note the short neck with the head appearing to sit directly on the thorax. Anteroposterior **(D)** and lateral **(E,** extension; **F,** flexion) roentgenograms of the cervical spine. Note the failure of segmentation and the fusion into a homogeneous mass of bone of the four lower cervical vertebrae. (From Tachdjian MO: Pediatric orthopedics, Philadelphia, 1972, WB Saunders, p. 77.)

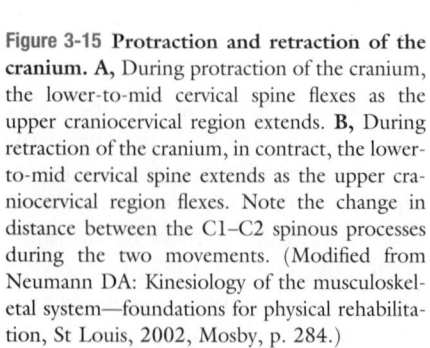

Figure 3-15 Protraction and retraction of the cranium. A, During protraction of the cranium, the lower-to-mid cervical spine flexes as the upper craniocervical region extends. **B,** During retraction of the cranium, in contract, the lower-to-mid cervical spine extends as the upper craniocervical region flexes. Note the change in distance between the C1–C2 spinous processes during the two movements. (Modified from Neumann DA: Kinesiology of the musculoskeletal system—foundations for physical rehabilitation, St Louis, 2002, Mosby, p. 284.)

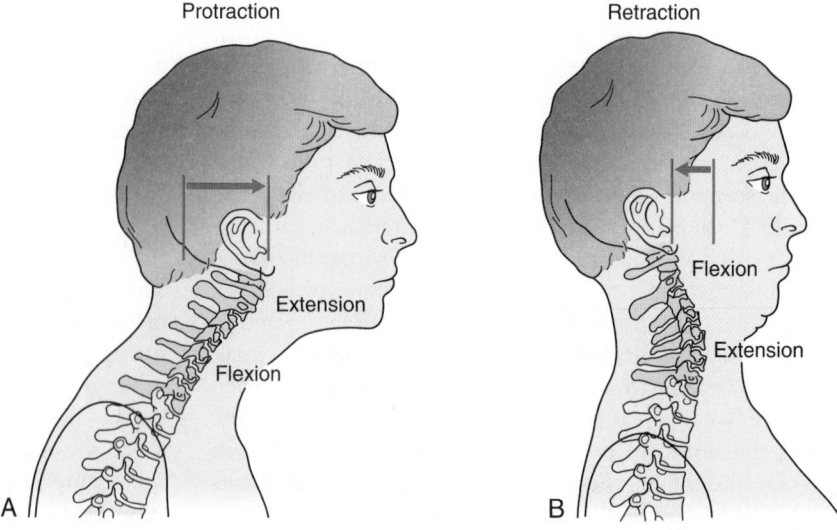

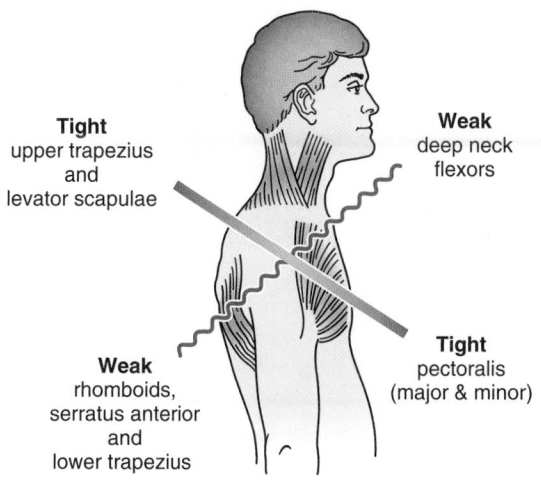

Tight
upper trapezius
and
levator scapulae

Weak
deep neck
flexors

Weak
rhomboids,
serratus anterior
and
lower trapezius

Tight
pectoralis
(major & minor)

Figure 3-16 Upper crossed syndrome.

providing a firm support for the trunk and appendages. The ROM available in the cervical spine is the result of many factors, such as the flexibility of the intervertebral discs, the shape and inclination of the articular processes of the facet joints, and the slight laxity of the ligaments and joint capsules. Female patients tend to have a greater active range of motion than males, except in flexion, but the differences are not great. The range available decreases with age, except rotation at C1 to C2, which may increase.[61,62]

The movements should be done in a particular order so that the most painful movements are done last, and no residual pain is carried over from the previous movement.[1] If the patient has complained of pain on specific movements in the history, these movements are done last. In the very acute cervical spine, only some movements—those that give the most information—are performed in order to avoid undue exacerbation of symptoms.

Active Movements of the Cervical Spine

- Flexion
- Extension
- Side flexion left and right
- Rotation left and right
- Combined movements (if necessary)
- Repetitive movements (if necessary)
- Sustained positions (if necessary)

While the patient performs the active movements, the examiner looks for limitation of movement and possible reasons for pain, spasm, stiffness, or blocking. As the patient reaches the full range of active movement, passive **overpressure** may be applied very carefully, but only if the movement appears to be full and not too painful (see passive movement in a later discussion). The overpressure

helps the examiner to test the end feel of the movement as well as differentiating between physiological (active) end range and anatomical (passive) end range. The examiner must be careful when applying overpressure to rotation or any combination of rotation, side flexion, and extension.[8] In these positions, the vertebral artery is often compressed, which can lead to a decrease in blood supply to the brain. Should this occur, the patient may complain of dizziness or feel faint. If the patient exhibits these symptoms, the examiner must use extreme care during these movements, the rest of the assessment, and treatment.

The examiner can differentiate between movement in the upper and lower cervical spine. During flexion, **nodding** occurs in the upper cervical spine, whereas **flexion** occurs in the lower cervical spine. If the nodding movement does not occur, it indicates restriction of movement in the upper cervical spine; if flexion does not occur, it indicates restriction of motion in the lower cervical spine. Movement can occur between C1 and C2 without affecting the other vertebrae, but this is not true with other cervical vertebrae. In other words, for C2 to C7, if one vertebra moves, the ones adjacent to it will also move. Thus, the active movements in the cervical spine can be divided into two parts: those testing the upper cervical spine (C0 to C2) and those involving the rest of the cervical spine (C2 to C7) (Figure 3-17). Table 3-13 gives the approximate ROMs in the different parts of the cervical spine.[63]

Flexion

To test flexion movement in the upper cervical spine, the patient is asked to nod or place the chin on the Adam's apple. Normally this movement is pain free. Positive symptoms (e.g., tingling in feet, electric shock sensation down the neck [Lhermitte sign], severe pain, nausea, cord signs) all indicate severe pathology (e.g., meningitis, tumor, dens fracture).[13] While the patient is flexing (nodding) the head, the examiner can palpate the relative movement between the mastoid and transverse process of C1 on each side comparing both sides for hypomobility or hypermobility between C0 and C1.[13] Likewise, the examiner can palpate the posterior arch of C1 and the lamina of C2 during the nodding movement to compare the relative movement.[13] For flexion, or forward bending, of the lower cervical spine, the maximum ROM is 80° to 90°. The extreme of ROM is normally found when the chin is able to reach the chest with the mouth closed; however, up to two finger widths between chin and chest is considered normal. If the deep neck flexors are weak, the sternocleidomastoid muscles will initiate the flexion movement, causing the jaw to lead the movement, not the nose, since the sternocleidomastoid muscles will cause the chin to initially elevate before flexion occurs.[52,64,65] In flexion, the intervertebral disc widens posteriorly and narrows anteriorly. The intervertebral foramen is 20% to

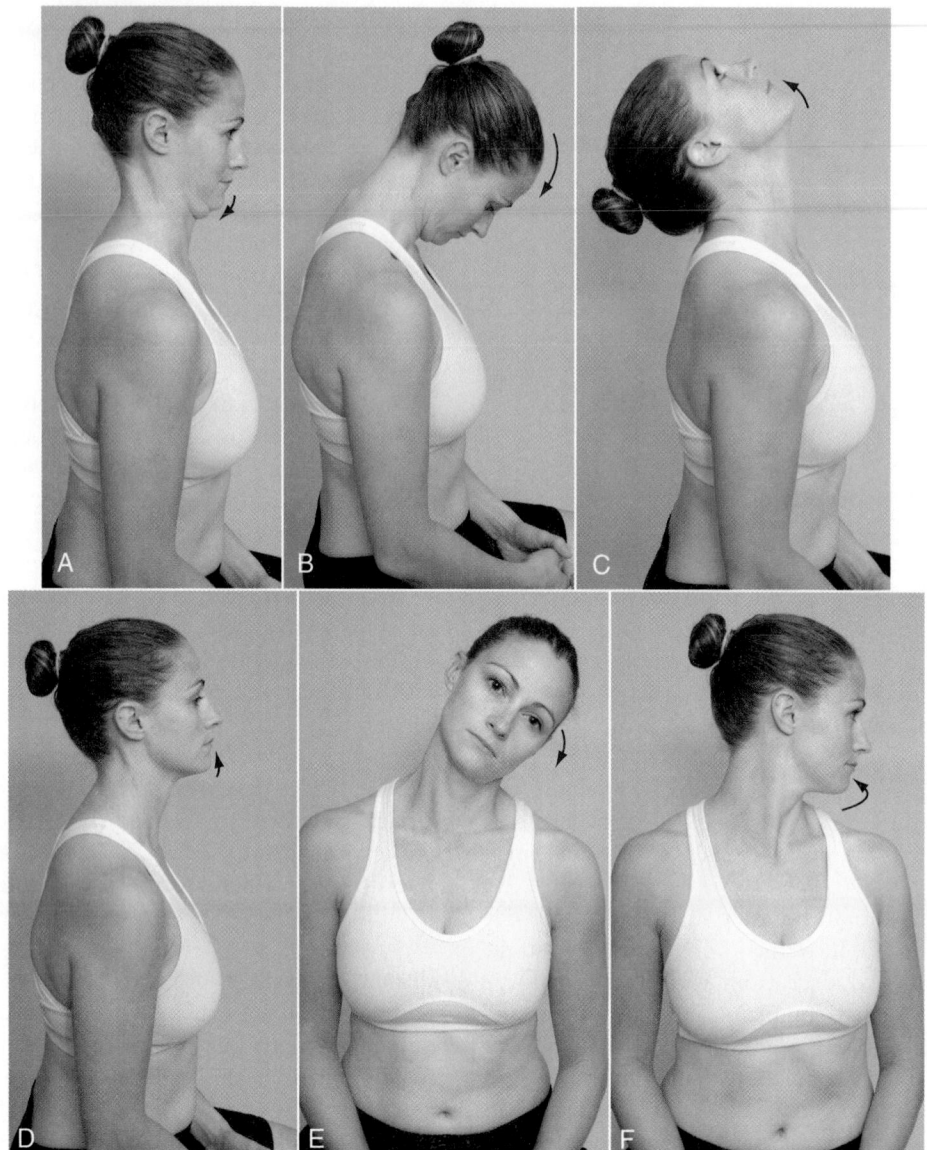

Figure 3-17 Active movements of the cervical spine. A, Anterior nodding (upper cervical spine). **B,** Flexion. **C,** Extension. **D,** Posterior nodding (upper cervical spine). **E,** Side flexion. **F,** Rotation.

30% larger on flexion than on extension. The vertebrae shift forward in flexion and backward in extension (Figures 3-18 and 3-19). Also, the mastoid process moves away from the C1 transverse process on flexion and extension. As the patient forward flexes, the examiner should look for a posterior bulging of the spinous process of the axis (C2). This bulging may result from forward subluxation of the atlas, which allows the spinous process of the axis to become more prominent. If this sign appears, the examiner should exercise extreme caution during the remainder of the cervical assessment. To verify the subluxation, the Sharp-Purser test (see under Special Tests) may be performed, but only with extreme care.

Extension

To test extension in the upper cervical spine, the patient is asked to lift the chin up without moving the neck. The examiner can lift the occiput at the same time. If serious symptoms arise (e.g., tingling in the feet, loss of balance, drop attack), it is suggestive of spinal cord compression or vertebrobasilar dysfunction.[13] Extension, or backward bending of the cervical spine, is normally limited to 70°. Because there is no anatomic block to stop movement going past this position, problems often result from whiplash or cervical strain. Normally, there is sufficient extension to allow the plane of the nose and forehead to be nearly horizontal. When the head is held in extension, the

TABLE **3-13**

Approximate Range of Motion for the Three Planes of Movement for the Joints of the Craniocervical Region*

Joint or Region	Flexion and Extension (Sagittal Plane, Degrees)	Axial Rotation (Horizontal Plane, Degrees)	Lateral Flexion (Frontal Plane, Degrees)
Atlanto-occipital joint	Flexion: 5 Extension: 10 *Total: 15*	Negligible	About 5
Atlanto-axial joint complex	Flexion: 5 Extension: 10 *Total: 15*	40–45	Negligible
Intracervical region (C2–C7)	Flexion: 35 Extension: 70 *Total: 105*	45	35
Total across craniocervical region	Flexion: 45–50 Extension: 85 *Total: 130–135*	90	About 40

From Neumann DA: Kinesiology of the musculoskeletal system—foundations for physical rehabilitation, St Louis, 2002, Mosby, p. 278.
*The horizontal and frontal plane motions are to one side only. Data are compiled from multiple sources and subject to large intersubject variations.

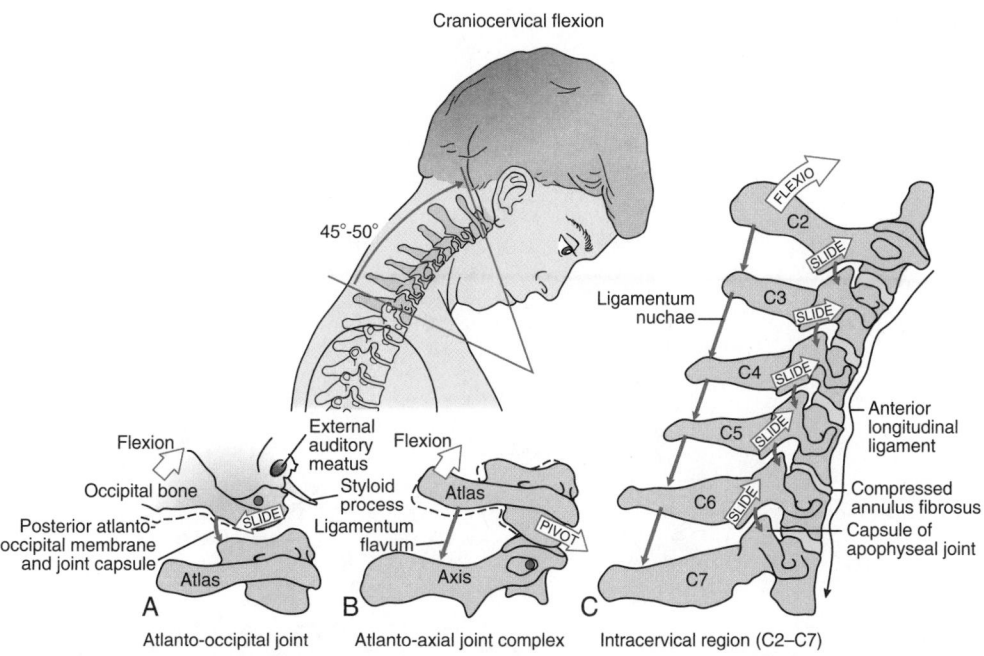

Figure 3-18 Kinematics of craniocervical flexion. A, Atlanto-occipital joint. **B,** Atlanto-axial joint complex. **C,** Intracervical region (C2–C7). Note in **C** that flexion slackens the anterior longitudinal ligament and increases the space between the adjacent laminae and spinous processes. Elongated and taut tissues are indicated by *thin black arrows;* slackened tissue is indicated by *a wavy black arrow.* (Modified from Neumann DA: Kinesiology of the musculoskeletal system—foundations for physical rehabilitation, St Louis, 2002, Mosby, p. 281.)

atlas tilts upward, resulting in posterior compression between the atlas and occiput.

Side Flexion

Side, or lateral, flexion is approximately 20° to 45° to the right and left (Figure 3-20). As the patient does the movement, the examiner can palpate adjacent transverse processes on the convex side to determine relative movement at each level. When the patient does the movement, the examiner should ensure that the ear moves toward the shoulder and not the shoulder toward the ear.

Rotation

Normally, rotation is 70° to 90° right and left, and the chin does not quite reach the plane of the shoulder (Figure 3-21). Rotation and side flexion always occur

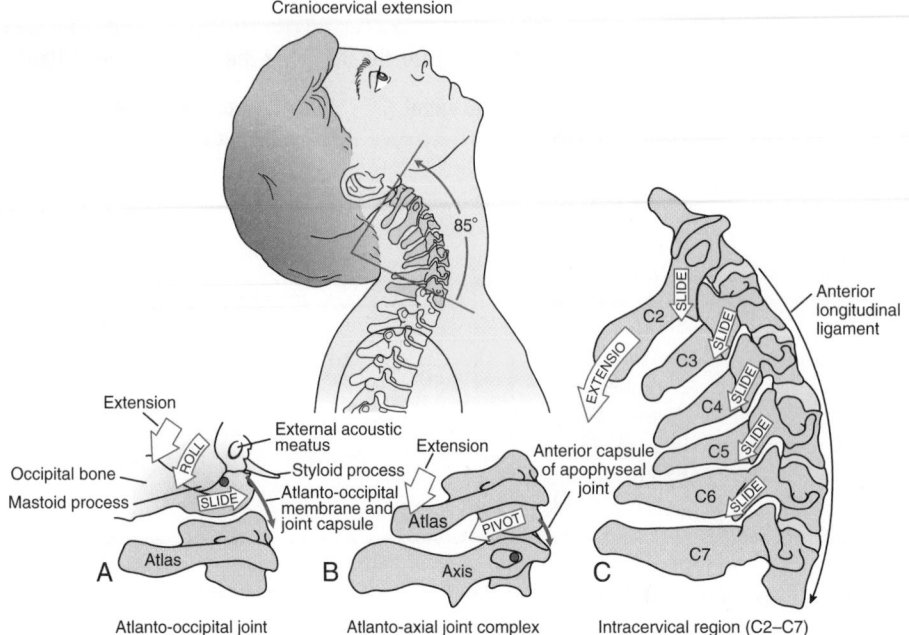

Figure 3-19 Kinematics of craniocervical extension. A, Atlanto-occipital joint. **B,** Atlanto-axial joint complex. **C,** Intracervical region (C2–C7). Elongated and taut tissues are indicated by *thin black arrows.* (Modified from Neumann DA: Kinesiology of the musculoskeletal system—foundations for physical rehabilitation, St Louis, 2002, Mosby, p. 280.)

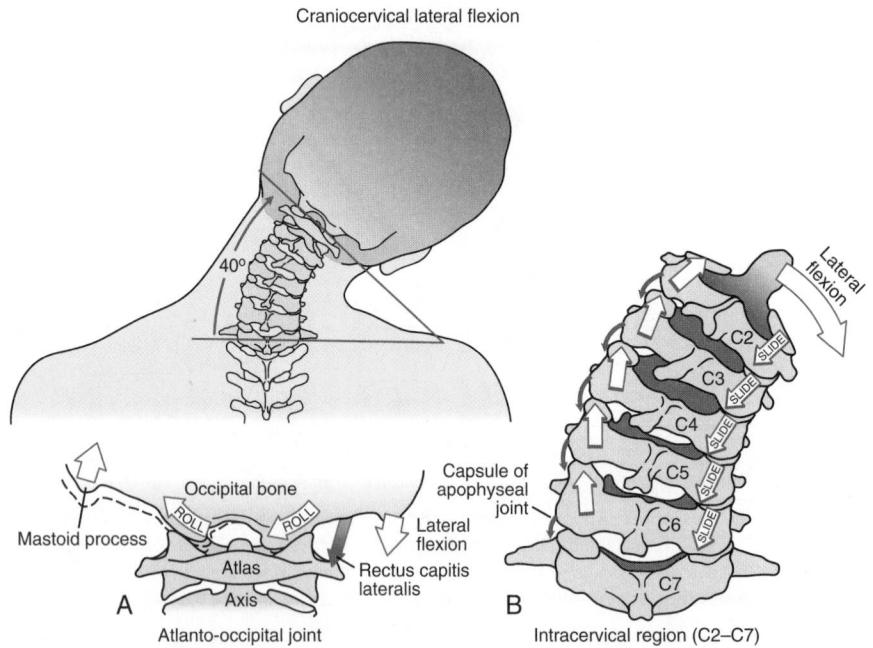

Figure 3-20 Kinematics of craniocervical lateral flexion. A, Atlanto-occipital joint. The primary function of the rectus capitis lateralis is to laterally flex this joint. Note the slight compression and distraction of the joint surfaces. **B,** Intracervical region (C2–C7). Note the ipsilateral coupling pattern between axial rotation and lateral flexion. Elongated and taut tissue is indicated by *thin black arrows.* (Modified from Neumann DA: Kinesiology of the musculoskeletal system—foundations for physical rehabilitation, St Louis, 2002, Mosby, p. 286.)

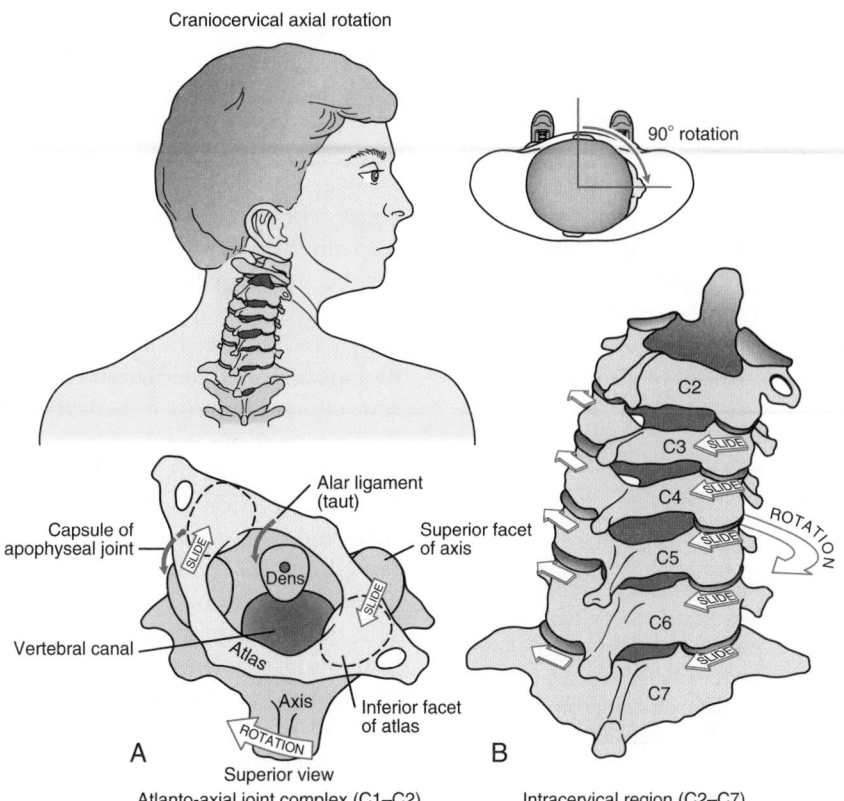

Craniocervical axial rotation

90° rotation

Alar ligament (taut)

Capsule of apophyseal joint

Superior facet of axis

Dens

Vertebral canal

Atlas

Axis

Inferior facet of atlas

ROTATION

Superior view
Atlanto-axial joint complex (C1–C2)

A

ROTATION

Intracervical region (C2–C7)

B

C2 C3 C4 C5 C6 C7

SLIDE

Figure 3-21 **Kinematics of craniocervical axial rotation. A,** Atlanto-axial joint complex. **B,** Intracervical region (C2–C7). (Modified from Neumann DA: Kinesiology of the musculoskeletal system—foundations for physical rehabilitation, St Louis, 2002, Mosby, p. 285.)

together (coupled movement) but not necessarily in the same direction.[20,21] This combined movement, which may or may not be visible in a given patient, occurs because of the shape of the articular surfaces of the facet joints; this shape is coronally oblique. Most of the rotation occurs between C1 and C2. If the patient can rotate 40° to 50°, then it is unlikely that the C1/C2 articulation is at fault.[13] If, however, side flexion occurs early to allow full motion, C1–C2 is probably involved.[13]

If, in the history, the patient has complained that **repetitive movements** or **sustained postures** have caused problems, not only should the specific movements be performed, but they should be either repeated several times or sustained to see if the symptoms are exacerbated. If a patient has complained in the history that a movement in other than a cardinal plane or a **combined movement** (e.g., side flexion, rotation, and extension combined) exacerbates the symptoms, then these movements should be performed as well. For example, the **cervical flexion-rotation test** ✓ in which the patient flexes the cervical spine to the point of pain or discomfort and then, while holding the position, rotates the head, is considered positive for pain and dysfunction arising from the C1 to C2 segment in cervicogenic headaches if pain occurs with the rotation as well.[66–68] Table 3-14 outlines examples of movement restrictions and possible causes.

Passive Movements

If the patient does not have full ROM or the examiner has not applied overpressure to determine the end feel of the movement, the patient should be asked to lie in a supine position. The examiner then passively tests flexion, extension, side flexion, and rotation, as in the active movements. The passive ROM with the patient supine is normally greater than the active and passive ROM with the patient sitting. For example, in sitting, active side flexion is about 45°, whereas in supine lying, passive side flexion is 75° to 80° with the examiner often able to take the ear to the shoulder. This increased range in the supine position results from relaxation of the muscles that, in sitting, are trying to hold the head up against gravity. For the cervical spine, therefore, passive movements with overpressure should be performed along with active movements. Active movements with overpressure at end of range do not give a true impression of end feel for the cervical spine. During passive movements, the examiner can palpate between adjacent vertebra to feel the relative amount of movement on each side. For flexion, the examiner palpates between the mastoid process and the transverse process for movement between C0 and C1 (Figure 3-22, *A*) and between the arch of C1 and spinous process of C2 for movement between C1 and

C2 (Figure 3-22, *B*). For the rest of the cervical spine and upper thoracic spine, the examiner can palpate between the spinous processes at each level while passively and progressively flexing the spine. To feel the movement, the examiner will find that as one works down the spine from C2 to C7, more flexion is required to feel the movement (Figure 3-22, *C*). Movement at each segment during side flexion and rotation may be felt by palpating the adjacent transverse processes on each side while doing the movement (Figure 3-23). To test rotation between the occiput and C1, the examiner holds the patient's head in position and palpates the transverse processes of C1 (Figure 3-24).

TABLE **3-14**

Movement Restriction and Possible Causes

Movement Restriction	Possible Causes
Extension and right side bending	Right extension hypomobility Left flexor muscle tightness Anterior capsular adhesions Right subluxation Right small disc protrusion
Flexion and right side bending	Left flexion hypomobility Left extensor muscle tightness
Extension and right side bending restriction greater than extension and left side bending	Left posterior capsular adhesions Left subluxation Left capsular pattern (arthritis, arthrosis)
Flexion and right side bending restriction equal to extension and left side flexion	Left arthrofibrosis (very hard capsular end feel)
Side bending in neutral, flexion, and extension	Uncovertebral hypomobility or anomaly

From Dutton M: Orthopedic examination, evaluation and intervention, New York, 2004, McGraw Hill, p. 1050.

The examiner must first find the mastoid process on each side and then move the fingers inferiorly and anteriorly until a hard bump (i.e., the transverse process of C1) is palpated on each side (usually below the ear lobe and just behind the jaw). Palpation in the area of the C1 transverse process is generally painful, so care must be taken. The examiner then rotates the patient's head while palpating the transverse processes; the transverse process on the side to which the head is rotated will seem to disappear (bottom one) while the other side (top one) seems to be accentuated in the normal case. If this disappearance/accentuation does not occur, there is restriction of movement between C0 and C1 on that side. To test rotation at C1–C2, the examiner stands beside the seated patient and side bends the head and neck, followed by rotation to the opposite side. As the rotation is performed, the examiner palpates the relative position of the C1 and C2 transverse processes as the head is rotated. To limit side flexion to a specific segment, as the examiner side flexes the head, the examiner applies an opposing translation force in the opposite direction to the passive movement to limit movement below that being tested.[13] With all of these movements, the end feel should be a solid tissue stretch.

Passive Movements of the Cervical Spine and Normal End Feel

- Flexion (tissue stretch)
- Extension (tissue stretch)
- Side flexion right and left (tissue stretch)
- Rotation right and left (tissue stretch)

If the passive movements with overpressure are normal and pain free, the examiner may, with great care, test other positions. For the flexion-rotation test, the patient

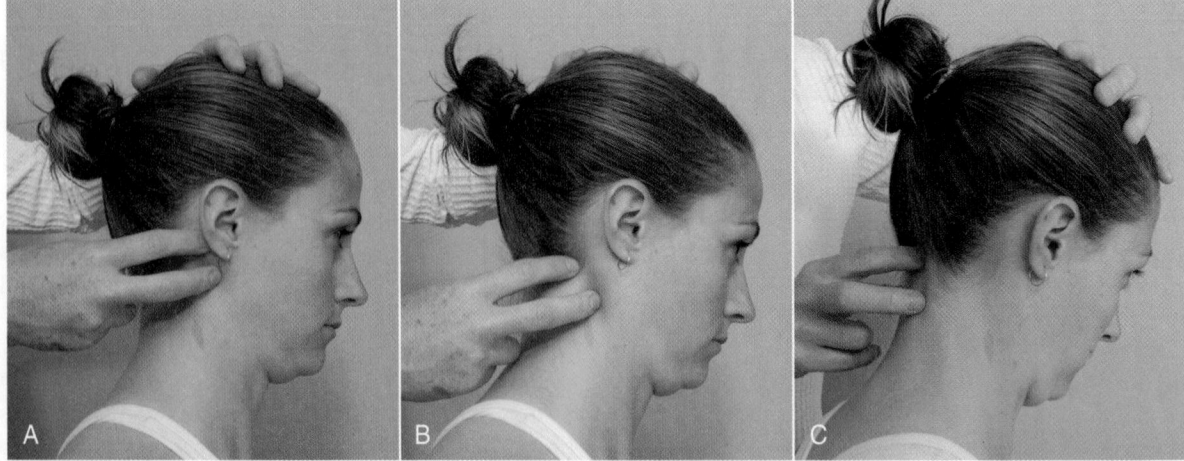

Figure 3-22 **Testing passive movement in the cervical spine. A,** Position testing for occipito-atlantal joint. **B,** Position testing for atlanto-axial joint. **C,** Flexion testing of C2–T1.

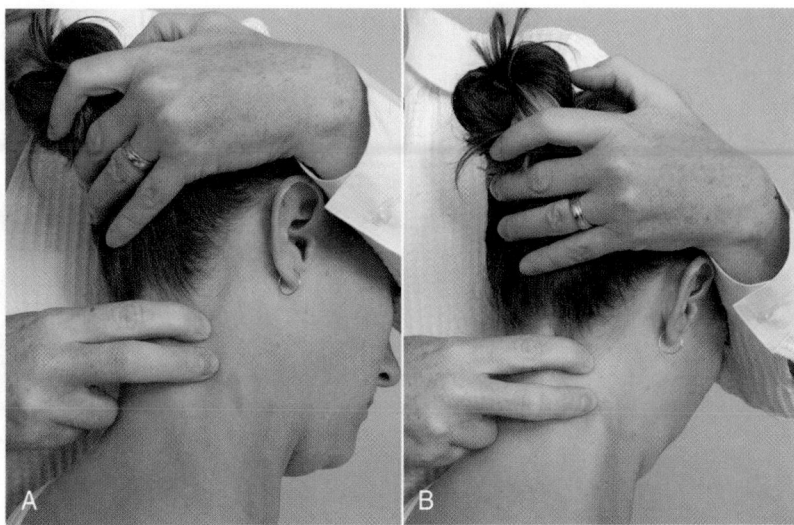

Figure 3-23 Testing passive movement in the cervical spine. A, Side flexion. **B,** Rotation.

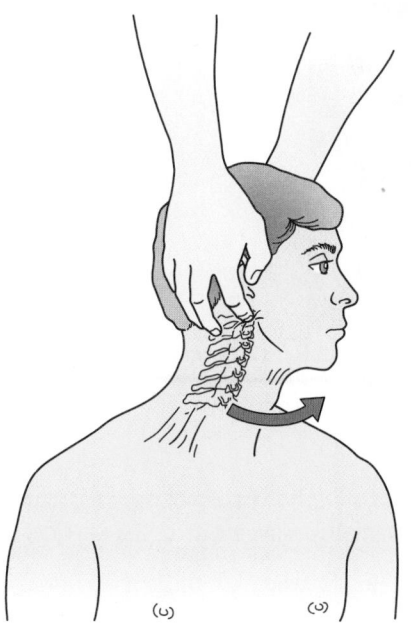

Figure 3-24 Left rotation of the occiput on C1. Note the index finger palpating the right transverse process of C1.

lies supine while the examiner flexes the neck fully and, while holding this position, passively rotates the head as far as possible within comfort limits.[69] Hall and Robinson[69] report significant restriction in rotation in patients complaining of cervicogenic headache indicating C1 to C2 segmental dysfunction. The quadrant position is end-range extension, side flexion, and rotation, a position that increases the vulnerability of anterior, posterior, and lateral tissues of the neck, including the vertebral artery.[70] If overpressure is applied in the quadrant position and symptoms result, it is highly suggestive of nerve root pathology (radicular signs), apophyseal joint involvement (localized pain), or vertebral artery involvement (dizziness, nausea).[52]

In addition to the passive movements of the whole cervical spine, physiological movements between each pair of vertebrae may be performed. These are called **passive physiological intervertebral movements (PPIVMs).** By stabilizing or blocking the movement of one vertebra (usually the distal one) and then passively moving the head through the different physiological movements (e.g., flexion, extension, side flexion, rotation), each segment can be tested. Needless to say, the amount of movement of each segment will be considerably less than the whole.[71]

Passive movements are performed to determine the end feel of each movement. This may give the examiner an idea of the pathology involved. The normal **end feels** of the cervical spine motions are tissue stretch for all four movements. As with active movements, the most painful movements are done last. The examiner should also note whether a **capsular pattern** (i.e., side flexion and rotation equally limited; extension less limited) is present. Overpressure may be used to test the entire spine (Figure 3-25, *A*) by testing it at the end of the ROM, or proper positioning may be used to test different parts of the cervical spine.[72] For example, end feel for movement of the lower cervical spine into extension is tested with minimal extension and the head pushed directly posterior (Figure 3-25, *C*), whereas the upper cervical spine is tested by "nodding" the head into extension and pushing posteriorly at an approximate 45° angle (Figure 3-25, *B*).[73]

Resisted Isometric Movements

The same movements that were done actively (flexion, extension, side flexion, and rotation) are then tested isometrically to determine relative muscle strength of each movement and to compare opposite movements.[74] It is better for the examiner to place the patient in the resting

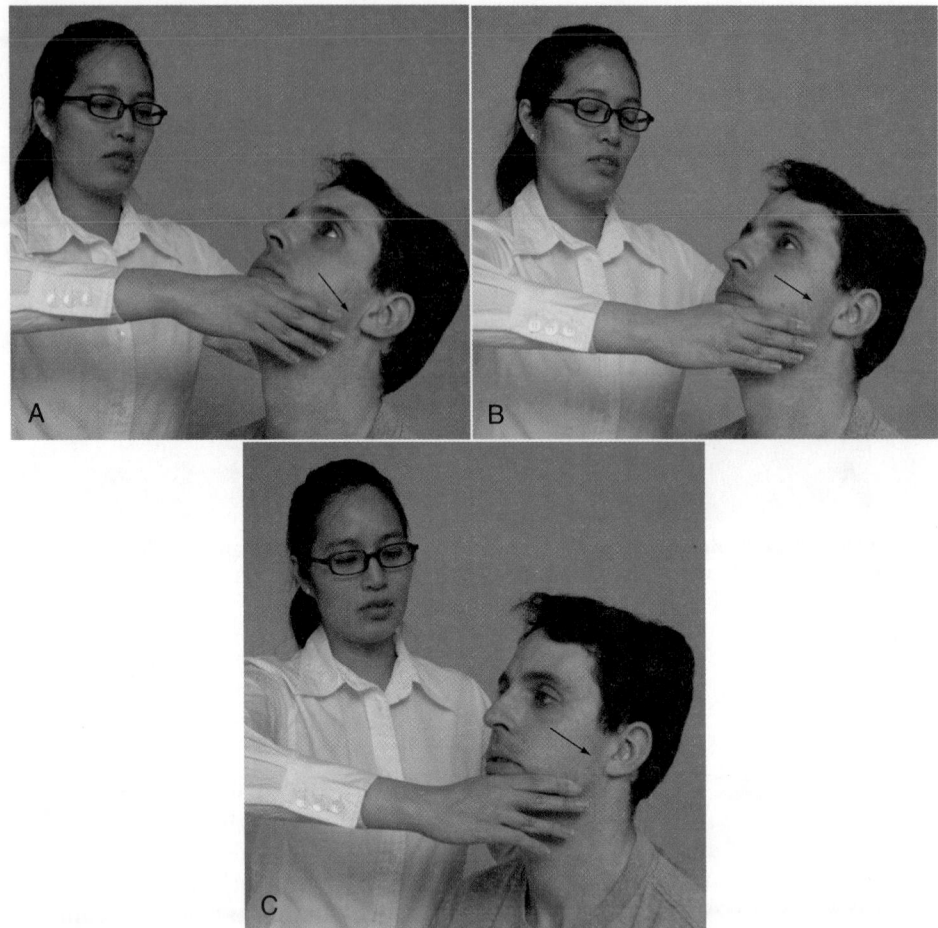

Figure 3-25 A, Overpressure to the whole cervical spine. **B,** Overpressure to the upper cervical spine. **C,** Overpressure to the low cervical spine. Clinician must differentiate between temporomandibular joint symptoms and cervical symptoms.

position and then say, "Don't let me move you," rather than to tell the patient, "Contract the muscle as hard as possible." In this way, the examiner ensures that the movement is as isometric as possible and that a minimal amount of movement occurs (Figure 3-26). The examiner should ensure that these movements are done with the cervical spine in the neutral position and that painful movements are done last. Neck flexion tests cranial nerve XI and the C1 and C2 myotomes as well as muscle strength or state. By using Table 3-15 and looking at the various combinations of muscles that cause the movement (Figure 3-27), the examiner is often able to decide which muscle is at fault. If, in the history, the patient has complained that certain loaded or combined movements (those movements giving resistance other than gravity) are painful, the examiner should not hesitate to carefully test these movements isometrically to better ascertain the problem. If a neurological injury is suspected, the examiner must carefully assess for muscle weakness to determine the structures injured. If a severe neuropraxia or axonotmesis has occurred, there may be residual weakness even though muscle atrophy may not be evident.

> **Resisted Isometric Movements of the Cervical Spine**
>
> - Flexion
> - Extension
> - Side flexion right and left
> - Rotation right and left

Scanning Examination

Peripheral Joint Scan

After the resisted isometric movements to the cervical spine have been completed, a peripheral joint scanning examination is performed to rule out obvious pathology in the extremities and to note areas that may need more detailed assessment.[1] The following joints are scanned bilaterally:

Temporomandibular Joints. The examiner checks the movement of the joints by placing the index or little fingers in the patient's ears (Figure 3-28). The pulp aspect of the finger is placed forward to feel for equality of

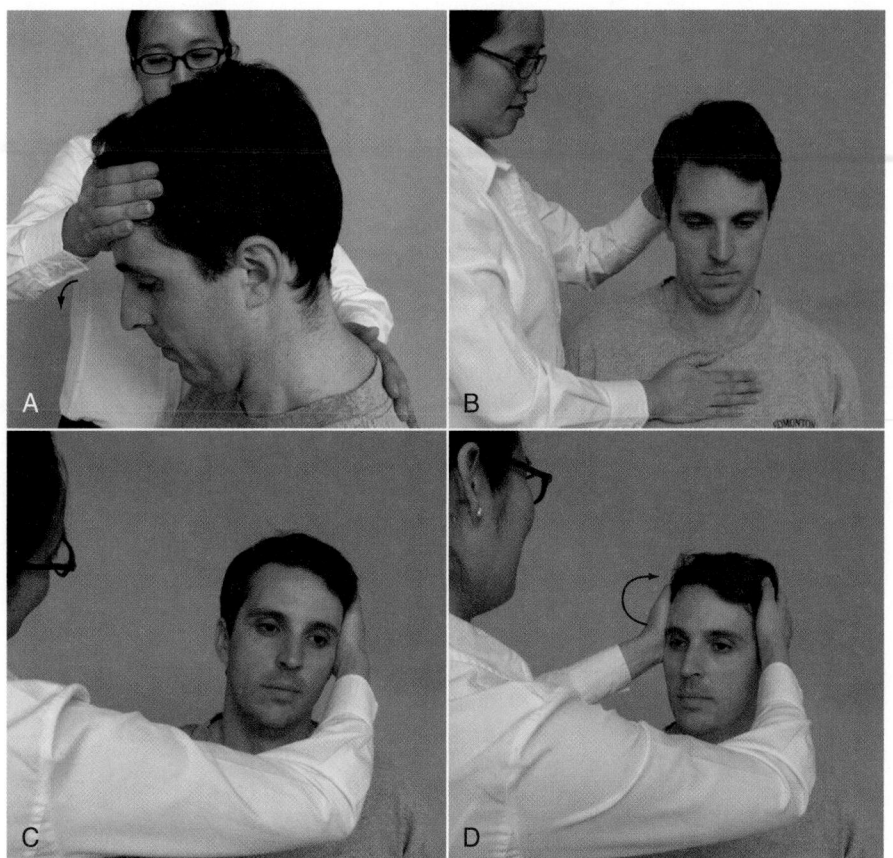

Figure 3-26 **Positioning for resisted isometric movement. A,** Flexion. Note slight flexion of neck before giving resistance. **B,** Extension. Note slight flexion of neck before giving resistance. **C,** Side flexion (left side flexion shown). **D,** Rotation (left rotation shown).

TABLE **3-15**

Muscles of the Cervical Spine: Their Actions and Nerve Supply

Action	Muscles Acting	Nerve Supply
Forward flexion of head	1. Rectus capitis anterior	C1, C2
	2. Rectus capitis lateralis	C1, C2
	3. Longus capitis	C1–C3
	4. Hyoid muscles	Inferior alveolar
		Facial
		Hypoglossal
		Ansa cervicalis
	5. Obliquus capitis superior	C1
	6. Sternocleidomastoid (if head in neutral or flexion)	Accessory, C2
Extension of head	1. Splenius capitis	C4–C6
	2. Semispinalis capitis	C1–C8
	3. Longissimus capitis	C6–C8
	4. Spinalis capitis	C6–C8
	5. Trapezius	Accessory, C3, C4
	6. Rectus capitis posterior minor	C1
	7. Rectus capitis posterior major	C1
	8. Obliquus capitis superior	C1
	9. Obliquus capitis inferior	C1
	10. Sternocleidomastoid (if head in some extension)	Accessory, C2

Continued

TABLE **3-15**

Muscles of the Cervical Spine: Their Actions and Nerve Supply—cont'd

Action	Muscles Acting	Nerve Supply
Rotation of head (muscles on one side contract)	1. Trapezius (face moves to opposite side)	Accessory, C3, C4
	2. Splenius capitis (face moves to the same side)	C4–C6
	3. Longissimus capitis (face moves to same side)	C6–C8
	4. Semispinalis capitis (face moves to same side)	C1–C8
	5. Obliquus capitis inferior (face moves to same side)	C1
	6. Sternocleidomastoid (face moves to opposite side)	Accessory, C2
Side flexion of head	1. Trapezius	Accessory, C3, C4
	2. Splenius capitis	C4–C6
	3. Longissimus capitis	C6–C8
	4. Semispinalis capitis	C1–C8
	5. Obliquus capitis inferior	C1
	6. Rectus capitis lateralis	C1, C2
	7. Longus capitis	C1–C3
	8. Sternocleidomastoid	Accessory, C2
Flexion of neck	1. Longus colli	C2–C6
	2. Scalenus anterior	C4–C6
	3. Scalenus medius	C3–C8
	4. Scalenus posterior	C6–C8
	5. Infrahyoid muscles	Ansa cervicalis
		Hypoglossal
	6. Suprahyoid muscles	Inferior alveolar
		Facial
		C1
Extension of neck	1. Splenius cervicis	C6–C8
	2. Semispinalis cervicis	C1–C8
	3. Longissimus cervicis	C6–C8
	4. Levator scapulae	C3, C4
		Dorsal scapular
	5. Iliocostalis cervicis	C6–C8
	6. Spinalis cervicis	C6–C8
	7. Multifidus	C1–C8
	8. Interspinalis cervicis	C1–C8
	9. Trapezius	Accessory
	10. Rectus capitus posterior major	C3, C4
	11. Rotatores brevis	C1
	12. Rotatores longi	C1–C8
Side flexion of neck	1. Levator scapulae	C1–C8
		Dorsal scapular
	2. Splenius cervicis	C4–C6
	3. Iliocostalis cervicis	C6–C8
	4. Longissimus cervicis	C6–C8
	5. Semispinalis cervicis	C1–C8
	6. Multifidus	C1–C8
	7. Intertransversarii	C1–C8
	8. Scaleni	C3–C8
	9. Sternocleidomastoid	Accessory, C2
	10. Obliquus capitis inferior	C1
	11. Rotatores breves	C1–C8
	12. Rotatores longi	C1–C8
	13. Longus colli	C2–C6

TABLE **3-15**

Muscles of the Cervical Spine: Their Actions and Nerve Supply—cont'd

Action	Muscles Acting	Nerve Supply
Rotation* of neck (muscles on one side contract)	1. Levator scapulae (face moves to same side)	C3, C4 Dorsal scapular
	2. Splenius cervicis (face moves to same side)	C4–C6
	3. Iliocostalis cervicis (face moves to same side)	C6–C8
	4. Longissimus cervicis (face moves to same side)	C6–C8
	5. Semispinalis cervicis (face moves to same side)	C1–C8
	6. Multifidus (face moves to opposite side)	C1–C8
	7. Intertransversarii (face moves to same side)	C1–C8
	8. Scaleni (face moves to opposite side)	C3–C8
	9. Sternocleidomastoid (face moves to opposite side)	Accessory, C2
	10. Obliquus capitis inferior (face moves to same side)	C1
	11. Rotatores brevis (face moves to same side)	C1–C8
	12. Rotatores longi (face moves to same side)	C1–C8

*Occurs in conjunction with side flexion owing to direction of facet joints.

Peripheral Joint Scanning Examination

Temporomandibular joints	Open mouth
	Closed mouth
Shoulder joints	Elevation through abduction
	Elevation through forward flexion
	Elevation through plane of scapula (SCAPTION)
	Apley's scratch test (right and left)
	Rotation in 90° abduction
Elbow joints	Flexion
	Extension
	Supination
	Pronation
Wrist and hand joints	Flexion
	Extension
	Abduction
	Adduction
	Opposition of thumb and little finger

movement of the condyles of the temporomandibular joints and for clicking or grinding as well as to ensure that the ears are clear. Pain or tenderness, especially on closing the mandible, usually indicates posterior capsulitis. As the patient opens the mouth, the condyle normally moves forward. To open the mouth fully, the condyle must rotate and translate equally bilaterally. If this does not occur, mouth opening will be limited and/or deviation of the mandible will occur (see Chapter 4). The examiner should observe the patient as he or she opens and closes the mouth and should watch for any deviation during the movement.

Shoulder Girdle. The examiner quickly scans this complex of joints (glenohumeral, acromioclavicular, sternoclavicular and "scapulothoracic" joint) by asking the patient to actively elevate each arm through abduction, followed by active elevation through forward flexion and elevation through the plane of the scapula (SCAPTION). In addition, the examiner quickly tests medial and lateral rotation of each shoulder with the arm at the side and with the arm abducted to 90°. Any pattern of restriction should be noted. If the patient is able to reach full abduction without difficulty or pain, the examiner may decide that there is no problem with the shoulder complex (see Chapter 5).

Elbow Joints. The elbow joints are actively moved through flexion, extension, supination, and pronation. Any restriction of movement or abnormal signs and symptoms should be noted, because they may be indicative of pathology (see Chapter 6).

Wrist and Hand. The patient actively performs flexion, extension, and radial and ulnar deviation of the wrist. Active movements (flexion, extension, abduction, adduction, and opposition) are performed for the fingers and thumb. These actions can be accomplished by having the patient make a fist and then spread the fingers and thumb wide. Again, any alteration in signs and symptoms or restriction of motion should be noted (see Chapter 7).

Myotomes

Having completed the peripheral joint scanning examination, the examiner should then determine muscle power and possible neurological weakness originating from the nerve roots in the cervical spine by testing the myotomes (Table 3-16 and Figure 3-29). Myotomes are tested by resisted isometric contractions with the joint at or near the resting position. As with the resisted isometric movements previously mentioned, the examiner should position the seated patient and say, "Don't let me move you," so that an isometric contraction is obtained.

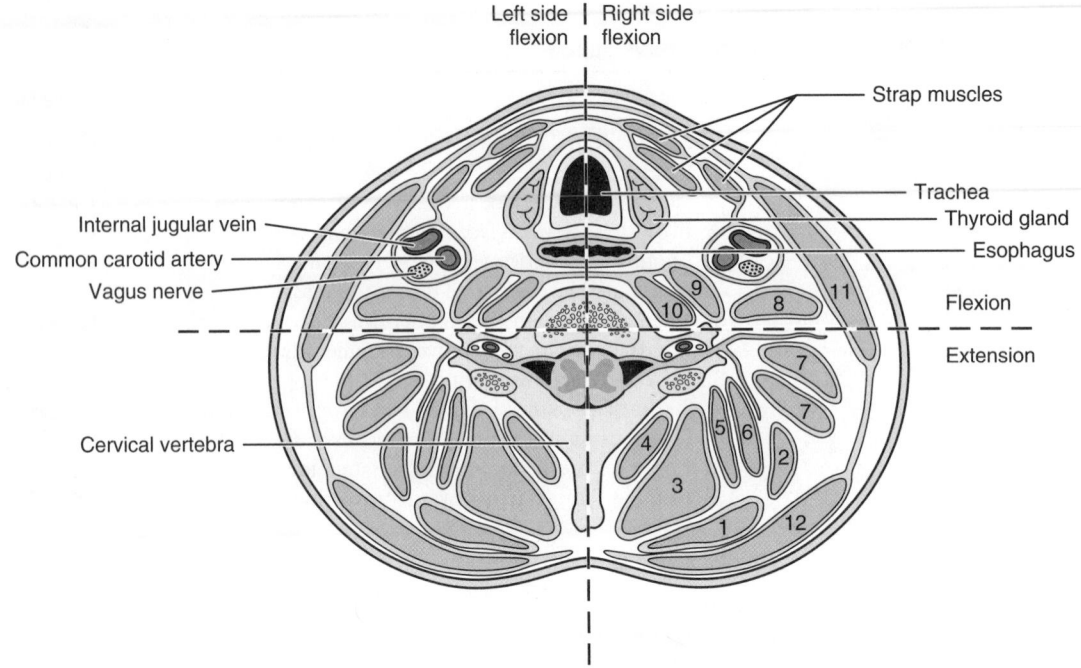

Left side | Right side
flexion | flexion

Strap muscles

Trachea

Thyroid gland

Esophagus

Flexion

Extension

Internal jugular vein

Common carotid artery

Vagus nerve

Cervical vertebra

Figure 3-27 Anatomic relations of the lower cervical spine. *1*, Splenius capitis. *2*, Splenius cervicis. *3*, Semispinalis cervicis and capitis. *4*, Multifidus and rotatores. *5*, Longissimus capitis. *6*, Longissimus cervicis. *7*, Levator scapulae. *8*, Scalenus posterior. *9*, Scalenus medius. *10*, Scalenus anterior. *11*, Sternocleidomastoid. *12*, Trapezius.

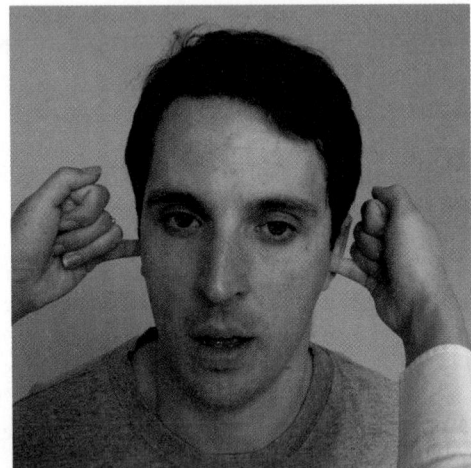

Figure 3-28 Testing temporomandibular joints.

Cervical Myotomes

- Neck flexion: C1 to C2
- Neck side flexion: C3 and cranial nerve XI
- Shoulder elevation: C4 and cranial nerve XI
- Shoulder abduction/shoulder lateral rotation: C5
- Elbow flexion and/or wrist extension: C6
- Elbow extension and/or wrist flexion: C7
- Thumb extension and/or ulnar deviation: C8
- Abduction and/or adduction of hand intrinsics: T1

The contraction should be held for *at least 5 seconds* so that weakness, if any, can be noted. Where applicable, both sides are tested at the same time to provide a comparison. If possible, the examiner must not apply pressure over the joints, because this action may mask symptoms if the joints are tender.

To test neck flexion (C1 to C2 myotome), the patient's head should be slightly flexed. The examiner applies pressure to the forehead while stabilizing the trunk with a hand between the scapulae (see Figure 3-29, *A*). The examiner should ensure the neck does not extend when applying pressure to the forehead. To test neck side flexion (C3 myotome and cranial nerve XI), the examiner places one hand above the patient's ear and applies a side flexion force while stabilizing the trunk with the other hand on the opposite shoulder (see Figure 3-29, *B*). Both right and left side flexion must be tested.

The examiner then asks the patient to elevate the shoulders (C4 myotome and cranial nerve XI) to about half of full elevation. The examiner applies a downward force on both of the patient's shoulders while the patient attempts to hold them in position (see Figure 3-29, *C*). The examiner should ensure that the patient is not "bracing" the arms against the thighs if testing is done while sitting.

To test shoulder abduction (C5 myotome), the examiner asks the patient to elevate the arms to about 75° to 80° in the scapular plane with the elbows flexed to 90° and the forearms pronated or in neutral (see Figure 3-29,

TABLE **3-16**

Myotomes of the Upper Limb

Nerve Root	Test Action	Muscles*
C1–C2	Neck flexion	Rectus lateralis, rectus capitis anterior, longus capitis, longus coli, longus cervicis, sternocleidomastoid
C3	Neck side flexion	Longus capitis, longus cervicis, trapezius, scalenus medius
C4	Shoulder elevation	Diaphragm, trapezius, levator scapulae, scalenus anterior, scalenus medius
C5	Shoulder abduction	Rhomboid major and minor, deltoid, supraspinatus, infraspinatus, teres minor, biceps, scalenus anterior and medius
C6	Elbow flexion and wrist extension	Serratus anterior, latissimus dorsi, subscapularis, teres major, pectoralis major (clavicular head), biceps, coracobrachialis, brachialis, brachioradialis, supinator, extensor carpi radialis longus, scalenus anterior, medius and posterior
C7	Elbow extension and wrist flexion	Serratus anterior, latissimus dorsi, pectoralis major (sternal head), pectoralis minor, triceps, pronator teres, flexor carpi radialis, flexor digitorum superficialis, extensor carpi radialis longus, extensor carpi radialis brevis, extensor digitorum, extensor digiti minimi, scalenus medius and posterior
C8	Thumb extension and ulnar deviation	Pectoralis major (sternal head), pectoralis minor, triceps, flexor digitorum superficialis, flexor digitorum profundus, flexor pollicis longus, pronator quadratus, flexor carpi ulnaris, abductor pollicis longus, extensor pollicis longus, extensor pollicis brevis, extensor indicis, abductor pollicis brevis, flexor pollicis brevis, opponens pollicis, scalenus medius and posterior
T1	Hand intrinsics	Flexor digitorum profundus, intrinsic muscles of the hand (except extensor pollicis brevis), flexor pollicis brevis, opponens pollicis

*Muscles listed may be supplied by additional nerve roots; only primary nerve root sources are listed.

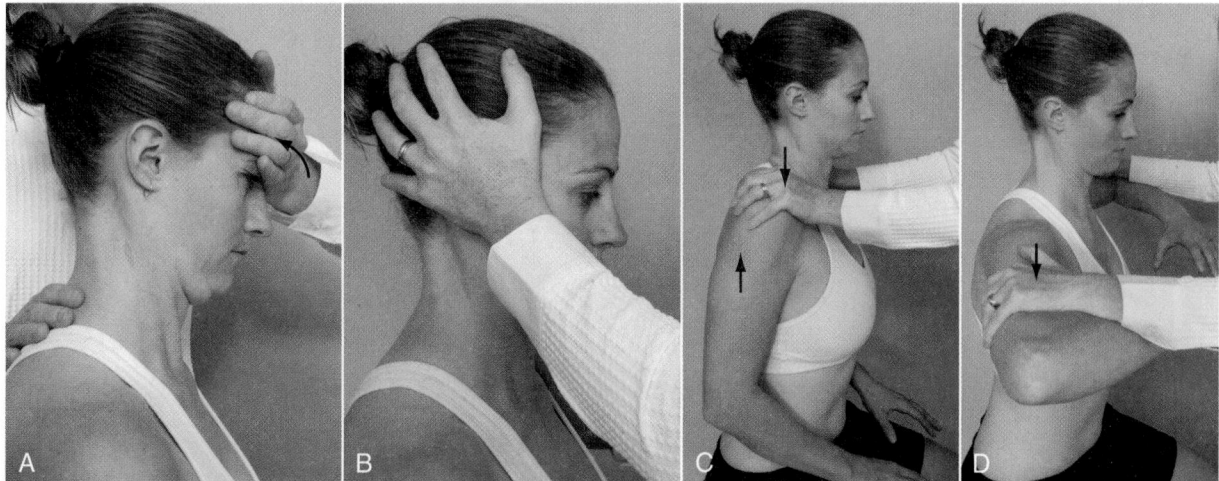

Figure 3-29 **Positioning to test myotomes. A,** Neck flexion (C1, C2). **B,** Neck side flexion to the left (C3). **C,** Shoulder elevation (C4). **D,** Shoulder abduction (C5). *Continued*

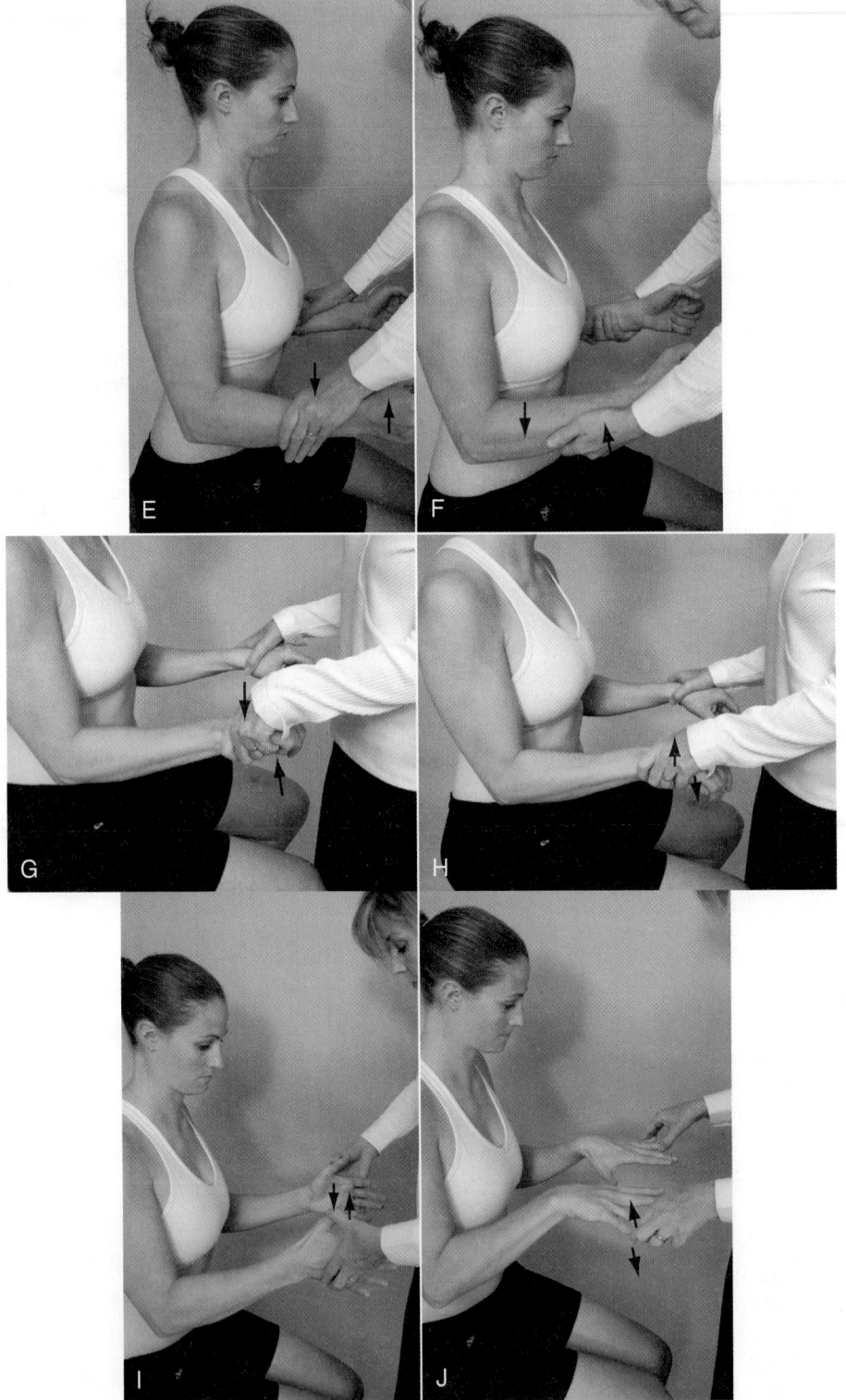

Figure 3-29, cont'd E, Elbow flexion (C6). **F,** Wrist extension (C6). **G,** Elbow extension (C7). **H,** Wrist flexion (C7). **I,** Thumb extension (C8). **J,** Finger abduction (T1).

D). The examiner applies a downward force on the humerus while the patient attempts to hold the arms in position. To prevent rotation, the examiner places his or her forearms over the patient's forearms while applying pressure to the humerus.

To test elbow flexion and extension, the examiner asks the patient to put the arms by the sides with the elbows flexed to 90° and forearms in neutral. The examiner applies a downward isometric force (see Figure 3-29, *E*) to the forearms to test the elbow flexors (C6 myotome) and an upward isometric force (see Figure 3-29, *G*) to test the elbow extensors (C7 myotome). For testing of wrist movements (extension, flexion, ulnar deviation) the patient's arms are by the side; elbows at 90°; forearms pronated; and wrists, hands, and fingers in neutral. The examiner applies a downward force (see Figure 3-29, *F*) to the hands to test wrist extension (C6 myotome), and an upward force (see Figure 3-29, *H*) to test wrist flexion (C7 myotome). To apply a lateral force (radial deviation) to test ulnar deviation (C8 myotome), the clinician stabilizes the patient's forearm with one hand and applies a radial deviation force to the side of the hand.

In the test for thumb extension (C8 myotome), the patient extends the thumb just short of full range of motion (see Figure 3-29, *I*). The examiner applies an isometric force to bring the thumbs into flexion. To test hand intrinsics (T1 myotome), the patient squeezes a piece of paper between the fingers while the examiner tries to pull it away; the patient may squeeze the examiner's fingers, or the patient may abduct the fingers slightly with the examiner isometrically adducting them (see Figure 3-29, *J*).

Sensory Scanning Examination

The examiner then tests sensation by doing a **sensory scanning examination.** This "sensory scan" is accomplished by running relaxed hands over the patient's head (sides and back); down over the shoulders, upper chest, and back; and down the arms, being sure to cover all aspects of the arm. If any difference is noted between the sides in this "sensation scan," the examiner may then use a pinwheel, pin, cotton batting, or brush (or a combination of these) to map out the exact area of sensory difference and to determine if any sensory difference is due to a nerve root (see later section on reflexes and cutaneous distribution), peripheral nerve, or some other neurological deficit. The sensory scanning examination may also include the testing of reflexes, especially the deep tendon reflexes, to test for upper and lower neuron pathology and pathological reflexes for upper motor neuron pathology, and the performance of selected neurodynamic tests (e.g., upper limb tension test, slump test) if peripheral nerve irritability is suspected.

Functional Assessment

If, in the history, the patient has complained of functional difficulties or the examiner suspects some functional impairment, a series of functional tests or movements may be performed to determine the patient's functional capacity, keeping in mind the patient's age and health. These tests may include activities of daily living (ADLs) such as the following:

Functional Assessment of the Cervical Spine

- Activities of daily living (ADLs)
- Numerical scoring table (if desired)

Breathing. Normal, unlabored breathing should be seen with the mouth closed. There should be no gulping or gasping.

Swallowing. This is a complex movement involving muscles of the lips, tongue, jaw, soft palate, pharynx, and larynx as well as the suprahyoid and infrahyoid muscles.

Looking Up at the Ceiling. At least 40° to 50° of neck extension is usually necessary for everyday activities. If this range is not available, the patient will bend the back or the knees, or both, to obtain the desired range.

Looking Down at Belt Buckle or Shoe Laces. At least 60° to 70° of neck flexion is necessary. If this range is not available, the patient will flex the back to complete the task.

Shoulder Check. At least 60° to 70° of cervical rotation is necessary. If this range is not available, the patient will rotate the trunk to accomplish this task.

Tuck Chin In. This action produces upper cervical flexion with lower cervical extension.[73]

Poke Chin Out. This action produces upper cervical extension with lower cervical flexion.[73]

Neck Strength. In athletes, neck strength should be approximately 30% of body weight to decrease chance of injury.[75]

Paresthesia. Paresthesia, especially referred to the hands, may make cooking and handling utensils particularly difficult or even dangerous.

Table 3-17 lists functional strength tests that can give the examiner some indication of the patient's functional strength capacity. For flexion, if the jaw juts forward at the beginning of the movement, it indicates an imbalance pattern of strong sternocleidomastoid and weak deep neck reflexors.[13]

Pinfold and others[76,77] developed the **Whiplash Disability Questionnaire (WDQ)** (Figure 3-30) to assess the impact of whiplash associated disorders including social and emotional problems. Vernon and Mior[78] have developed a numerical scoring functional test called the

TABLE **3-17**

Functional Strength Testing of the Cervical Spine

Starting Position	Action	Functional Test*
Supine lying	Lift head keeping chin tucked in (neck flexion)	6 to 8 repetitions: Functional 3 to 5 repetitions: Functionally fair 1 to 2 repetitions: Functionally poor 0 repetitions: Nonfunctional
Prone lying	Lift head backward (neck extension)	Hold 20 to 25 seconds: Functional Hold 10 to 19 seconds: Functionally fair Hold 1 to 9 seconds: Functionally poor Hold 0 seconds: Nonfunctional
Side lying (pillows under head so head is not side flexed)	Lift head sideways away from pillow (neck side flexion) (must be repeated for other side)	Hold 20 to 25 seconds: Functional Hold 10 to 19 seconds: Functionally fair Hold 1 to 9 seconds: Functionally poor Hold 0 seconds: Nonfunctional
Supine lying	Lift head off bed and rotate to one side keeping head off bed or pillow (neck rotation) (must be repeated both ways)	Hold 20 to 25 seconds: Functional Hold 10 to 19 seconds: Functionally fair Hold 1 to 9 seconds: Functionally poor Hold 0 seconds: Nonfunctional

Adapted from Palmer ML, Epler M: Clinical assessment procedures in physical therapy, Philadelphia, 1990, J.B. Lippincott, pp. 181–182.
*Younger patients should be able to do the most repetitions and for the longest time; with age, time and repetitions decrease.

Neck Disability Index (NDI)[79,80] (Figure 3-31), which is a modification of the Oswestry low back pain index.[81] This index and similar tests (e.g., Bournemouth Questionnaire [Figure 3-32], the Copenhagen Neck Functional Disability Scale,[82] and the Norwick Park Neck Pain Questionnaire[83,84]) can be used to detect change in patients over time.[85,86]

Special Tests

There are several special tests that may be performed if the examiner believes they are relevant and to help confirm a diagnosis. Some of these tests should always be performed (e.g., instability tests, vertebral artery tests), especially if treatment is to be given to the upper cervical spine; while others should be performed only if the examiner wants to use them as confirming tests. Some tests are provocative and should only be used if the examiner wants to cause symptoms. Other tests relieve symptoms and are used when the symptoms are present. The reliability of many of these tests commonly depends on the experience and skill of the examiner and whether the patient is sufficiently relaxed to allow the test to be performed.[87,88]

For the reader who would like to review them, the reliability, validity, specificity, sensitivity, and odds ratios of some of the special tests used in the cervical spine are available electronically on the Evolve website (see Appendix 3-1).

Tests for Cervical Muscle Strength

☑ ***Craniocervical Flexion Test.***[31,89–92] The craniocervical flexion (CCF) test is a test of the deep cervical flexor

Key Tests Performed on the Cervical Spine Depending on Suspected Pathology*

- *For cervical muscle (deep neck flexors) strength:*
  ☑ Craniocervical flexion test (CCF)
  ⚠ Deep neck flexor endurance test
- *For neurological symptoms:*
  ☑ Brachial plexus tension test
  ☑ Distraction test (if symptoms are severe)
  ☑ Foraminal compression test (three stages) (if symptoms are absent or mild)
  ☑ Upper limb neurodynamic (tension) tests (specific to particular nerve/nerve root symptoms)
- *For myelopathy:*
  ☑ Romberg test
- *For vascular signs:*†
  ❓ Hold planned mobilization/manipulation position for at least 30 seconds watching for vertebral-basilar artery signs
- *For cervical instability:*‡
  ❓ Anterior shear stress test
  ❓ Lateral flexion alar ligament stress test
  ⚠ Lateral shear test
  ❓ Rotational alar ligament stress test
  ❓ Transverse ligament stress test
- *For cervical spine mobility:*
  ☑ Cervical flexion rotation test
- *For first rib mobility:*
  ☑ First rib mobility

*The author recommends these key tests be learned by the clinician to facilitate a diagnosis. See Chapter 1, p. 55, Key for Classifying Special Tests.

†These tests should be performed if the examiner anticipates doing end-range mobilization or manipulation techniques to the cervical spine, especially the upper cervical spine. If instability of vascular signs are present, mobilization and/or manipulation should *not* be performed.

‡Before these tests are performed, the C-spine rule for radiographs should be administered, and the results should indicate that no radiographs are required.

WHIPLASH DISABILITY QUESTIONNAIRE

This questionnaire has been designed to provide information on the impact that your whiplash injury and symptoms have upon your lifestyle. Please circle a number in each section to indicate how you have been affected by the whiplash injury and symptoms. If one or more questions are not relevant to you (e.g., you don't participate in sporting activities), please leave the question blank.

NAME:..   DATE:............/............/.........

1. How much **pain** do you have today?

0	1	2	3	4	5	6	7	8	9	10
No pain										Worst pain imaginable

2. Do your whiplash symptoms interfere with your **personal care** (washing, dressing, etc.)?

0	1	2	3	4	5	6	7	8	9	10
Not at all										Unable to perform

3. Do your whiplash symptoms interfere with your **work/home/study duties**?

0	1	2	3	4	5	6	7	8	9	10
Not at all										Unable to perform

4. Do your whiplash symptoms interfere with **driving or using public transport**?

0	1	2	3	4	5	6	7	8	9	10
Not at all										Unable to travel in car/use public transport

5. Do your whiplash symptoms interfere with **sleep**?

0	1	2	3	4	5	6	7	8	9	10
Not at all										Cannot sleep

6. Do you feel more **tired/fatigued** than usual since your injury?

0	1	2	3	4	5	6	7	8	9	10
Not at all										Always

7. Do your whiplash symptoms interfere with **social activity**?

0	1	2	3	4	5	6	7	8	9	10
Not at all										Unable to socialise

8. Do your whiplash symptoms interfere with **sporting activity**?

0	1	2	3	4	5	6	7	8	9	10
Not at all										Unable to participate

Please turn the page

Figure 3-30 Whiplash Disability Questionnaire (WDQ). (From Pinfold M, Niere KR, O'Leary EF, et al: Validity and internal consistency of a whiplash-specific disability measure. Spine 29[3]:263–268, 2004.) *Continued*

Whiplash Disability Questionnaire?

9. Do your whiplash symptoms interfere with **non-sporting leisure activity**?

0	1	2	3	4	5	6	7	8	9	10
Not at all										Unable to participate

10. Do you experience **sadness/depression** as a result of your whiplash injury/symptoms?

0	1	2	3	4	5	6	7	8	9	10
Not at all										Always

11. Do you experience **anger** as a result of your whiplash injury/symptoms?

0	1	2	3	4	5	6	7	8	9	10
Not at all										Always

12. Do you experience **anxiety** as a result of your whiplash injury/symptoms?

0	1	2	3	4	5	6	7	8	9	10
Not at all										Always

13. Do you have difficulty **concentrating** as a result of your whiplash injury/symptoms?

0	1	2	3	4	5	6	7	8	9	10
Not at all										Unable to concentrate

THANK YOU FOR YOUR COOPERATION

Figure 3-30, cont'd

muscle function.[89] A pneumatic pressure device is needed for this test. The patient lies in supine with knees bent (crook lying) with head and neck in midrange, and an inflatable pressure sensor is placed under the cervical spine (Figure 3-33). Towels may be used to keep the head and neck in midrange neutral (two parallel lines: one from forehead to chin and one from tragus of ear to the line of the longitudinal neck). The pressure device is inflated to 20 mm Hg to "fill in" the lordotic curve of the cervical spine. While keeping the head/occiput stationary (no pushing down or lifting up), the patient flexes the cervical spine by nodding the head in five graded segments of increasing pressure (22, 24, 26, 28, and 30 mm Hg) and holds each for 10 seconds with 10 seconds rest between each segment. Superficial cervical muscles (e.g., sternocleidomastoid, platysma, hyoid) must remain relaxed during the test. Normally, young and middle-aged patients should be able to increase pressure to between 26 and 30 mm Hg and hold for 10 seconds without utilizing the superficial muscles. Elderly people are more likely to make greater use of the sternocleidomastoid muscle during the test.[93] A positive test is considered if the patient cannot increase pressure to at least 26 mm Hg, is unable to hold a contraction for 10 seconds, uses the superficial neck muscles, or extends the head. The performance index is calculated as the increase in pressure times the number of repetitions, while the activation score is the maximum pressure achieved and held for 10 seconds.

⚠ *Deep Neck Flexor Endurance Test.*[31,94] The patient lies supine in crook lying. The chin is maximally retracted by the patient and maintained while the patient lifts the head and neck until the head is approximately 2 to 5 cm (1 inch) above the examining table. The examiner places a hand on the table under the patient's head (occiput). The examiner watches the skin folds resulting from the chin tuck and neck flexion. As soon as the skin folds separate (due to loss of chin tuck) or the patient's head touches the examiner's hand, the test is terminated. Normal people should be able to hold for 39 ± 26 seconds while those with neck pain average 24 seconds.[94]

Tests for Neurological Symptoms

These tests are designed to provoke neurological symptoms in most cases (distraction test is the exception) to determine the effect of applying pressure or stretching to the nervous tissue. They are specific to neurological tissue (i.e., they produce neurological symptoms), but they do not necessarily tell where the pathology is originating. The pathology may be the result of trauma, degeneration, or anatomical anomalies that may occur anywhere along the path of the affected nerve or nerve root.[95,96]

Tests for neurological symptoms that involve movement of the nerve are called **neurodynamic tests,** because they assess the sensitivity of nerve roots and peripheral nerves to movement and tension caused by the movement. This sensitivity has also been called *neurologic mechanosensitivity.*[97]

Neck Disability Index (NDI)

This questionnaire has been designed to give the doctor information as to how your neck pain has affected your ability to manage in every-day life. Please answer every section and mark in each section only the ONE box which applies to you. We realize you may consider that two of the statements in any one section relate to you, but please just mark the box which most closely describes your problem.

Section 1 — Pain Intensity

☐ I have no pain at the moment. (0)
☐ The pain is very mild at the moment. (1)
☐ The pain is moderate at the moment. (2)
☐ The pain is fairly severe at the moment. (3)
☐ The pain is very severe at the moment. (4)
☐ The pain is the worst imaginable at the moment. (5)

Section 2 — Personal Care (Washing, Dressing, etc.)

☐ I can look after myself normally without causing extra pain. (0)
☐ I can look after myself normally but it causes extra pain. (1)
☐ It is painful to look after myself and I am slow and careful. (2)
☐ I need some help but manage most of my personal care. (3)
☐ I need help every day in most aspects of self care. (4)
☐ I do not get dressed. I wash with difficulty and stay in bed. (5)

Section 3 — Lifting

☐ I can lift heavy weights without extra pain. (0)
☐ I can lift heavy weights but it gives extra pain. (1)
☐ Pain prevents me from lifting heavy weights off the floor, but I can manage if they are conveniently positioned, for example on a table. (2)
☐ Pain prevents me from lifting heavy weights, but I can manage light to medium weights if they are conveniently positioned. (3)
☐ I can lift very light weights. (4)
☐ I cannot lift or carry anything at all. (5)

Section 4 — Reading

☐ I can read as much as I want to with no pain in my neck. (0)
☐ I can read as much as I want to with slight pain in my neck. (1)
☐ I can read as much as I want with moderate pain in my neck. (2)
☐ I cannot read as much as I want because of moderate pain in my neck. (3)
☐ I can hardly read at all because of severe pain in my neck. (4)
☐ I cannot read at all. (5)

Section 5 — Headaches

☐ I have no headaches at all. (0)
☐ I have slight headaches that come infrequently. (1)
☐ I have moderate headaches which come infrequently. (2)
☐ I have moderate headaches which come frequently. (3)
☐ I have severe headaches which come frequently. (4)
☐ I have headaches almost all the time. (5)

Section 6 — Concentration

☐ I can concentrate fully when I want to with no difficulty. (0)
☐ I can concentrate fully when I want to with slight difficulty. (1)
☐ I have a fair degree of difficulty in concentrating when I want to. (2)
☐ I have a lot of difficulty in concentrating when I want to. (3)
☐ I have a great deal of difficulty in concentrating when I want to. (4)
☐ I cannot concentrate at all. (5)

Section 7 — Work

☐ I can do as much work as I want to. (0)
☐ I can do my usual work, but no more. (1)
☐ I can do most of my usual work, but no more. (2)
☐ I cannot do my usual work. (3)
☐ I can hardly do any work at all. (4)
☐ I cannot do any work at all. (5)

Section 8 — Driving

☐ I can drive my car without any neck pain. (0)
☐ I can drive my car as long as I want with slight pain in my neck. (1)
☐ I can drive my car as long as I want with moderate pain in my neck. (2)
☐ I cannot drive my car as long as I want because of moderate pain in my neck. (3)
☐ I can hardly drive at all because of severe pain in my neck. (4)
☐ I cannot drive my car at all. (5)

Section 9 — Sleeping

☐ I have no trouble sleeping. (0)
☐ My sleep is slightly disturbed (less than 1 hr. sleepless). (1)
☐ My sleep is mildly disturbed (1–2 hrs. sleepless). (2)
☐ My sleep is moderately disturbed (2–3 hrs. sleepless). (3)
☐ My sleep is greatly disturbed (3–5 hrs. sleepless). (4)
☐ My sleep is completely disturbed (5–7 hrs. sleepless). (5)

Section 10 — Recreation

☐ I am able to engage in all my recreation activities with no neck pain at all. (0)
☐ I am able to engage in all my recreation activities, with some pain in my neck. (1)
☐ I am able to engage in most, but not all, of my usual recreation activities because of pain in my neck. (2)
☐ I am able to engage in a few of my usual recreation activities because of pain in my neck. (3)
☐ I can hardly do any recreation activities because of pain in my neck. (4)
☐ I cannot do any recreation activities at all. (5)

To use the NDI for patient decisions, a clinically important change has been calculated as 5 points, with a sensitivity of 0.78 and a specificity of 0.80.[81]

Scores (out of 50):   0–4 No disability
5–14 Mild disability
15–24 Moderate disability
25–34 Severe disability
>35 Complete disability

Figure 3-31 Neck Disability Index (NDI). (Modified from Vernon H, Mior S: The neck disability index: a study of reliability and validity. J Manip Physiol Ther 14:411, 1991.)

The following scales have been designed to find out about your neck pain and how it is affecting you. Please answer ALL the scales by circling ONE number on EACH scale that best describes how you feel:

1. Over the past week, on average how would you rate your neck pain?

No pain   Worst pain possible

0   1   2   3   4   5   6   7   8   9   10

2. Over the past week, how much has your neck pain interfered with your daily activities (housework, washing, dressing, lifting, reading, driving)?

No interference   Unable to carry out activities

0   1   2   3   4   5   6   7   8   9   10

3. Over the past week, how much has your neck pain interfered with your ability to take part in recreational, social, and family activities?

No interference   Unable to carry out activities

0   1   2   3   4   5   6   7   8   9   10

4. Over the past week, how anxious (tense, uptight, irritable, difficulty in cocentrating/relaxing) have you been feeling?

Not at all anxious   Extremely anxious

0   1   2   3   4   5   6   7   8   9   10

5. Over the past week, how depressed (down-in-the-dumps, sad, in low spirits, pessimistic, unhappy) have you been feeling?

Not at all depressed   Extremely depressed

0   1   2   3   4   5   6   7   8   9   10

6. Over the past week, how have you felt your work (both inside and outside the home) has affected (or would affect) your neck pain?

Have made it no worse   Have made it much worse

0   1   2   3   4   5   6   7   8   9   10

7. Over the past week, how much have you been able to control (reduce/help) your neck pain on your own?

Completely control it   No control whatsoever

0   1   2   3   4   5   6   7   8   9   10

Figure 3-32 **Global dimensions of the Neck Bournemouth Questionnaire.** (From Bolton JE, Humphreys BK: The Bournemouth Questionnaire: a short-form comprehensive outcome measure. II Psychometric properties in neck pain patients. J Manip Physiol Ther 25:148, 2002.)

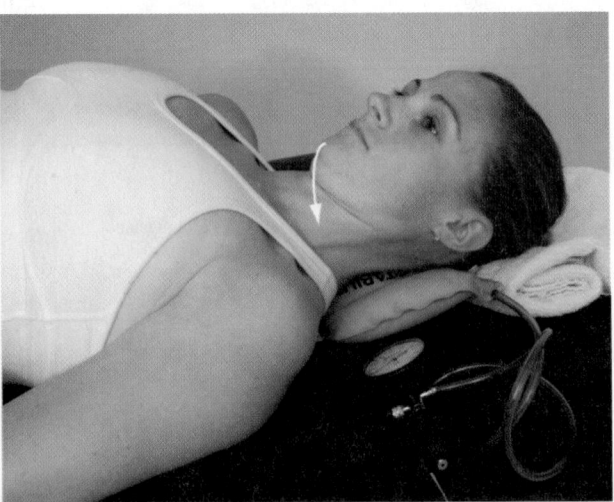

 Figure 3-33 Craniocervical flexion test.

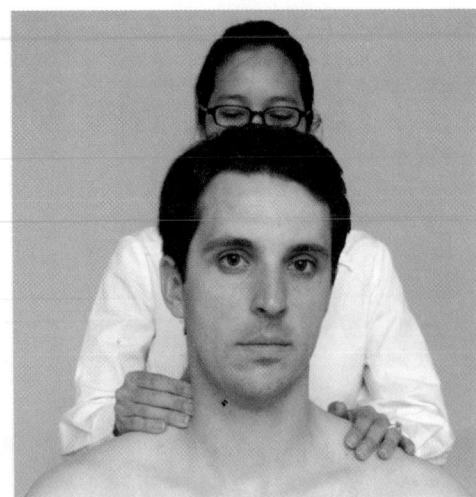

Figure 3-34 Maneuver to compress and squeeze the brachial plexus.

▼ Neurodynamic Tests[97]

During neurodynamic testing, a positive test is considered present only when one or more of the following occur:
- There is a reproduction of the patient's symptoms.
- There is asymmetric sensation between right and left limbs.
- There is significant deviation from normal sensation.
- Symptoms change with sensitizing movements.

❓ *Brachial Plexus Compression Test.*[98] The examiner applies firm compression to the brachial plexus by squeezing the plexus under the thumb or fingers (Figure 3-34). Pain at the site is not diagnostic; the test is positive only if pain radiates into the shoulder or upper extremity. It is positive for mechanical cervical lesions having a mechanical component.

✓ *Distraction Test.* The distraction test is used for patients who have complained of radicular symptoms in the history and show radicular signs during the examination. It is used to alleviate symptoms. To perform the distraction test, the examiner places one hand under the patient's chin and the other hand around the occiput, then slowly lifts the patient's head (Figure 3-35)—in effect, applying traction to the cervical spine. The test is classified as positive if the pain is relieved or decreased when the head is lifted or distracted, indicating pressure on nerve roots that has been relieved. This test may also be used to check radicular signs referred to the shoulder complex anteriorly or posteriorly. If the patient abducts the arms while traction is applied, the symptoms are often further relieved or lessened in the shoulder, especially if C4 or C5 nerve roots are involved. In this case, the test would still be indicative of nerve root pressure in the cervical spine, not shoulder pathology. Increased pain on distraction may be the result of muscle spasm,

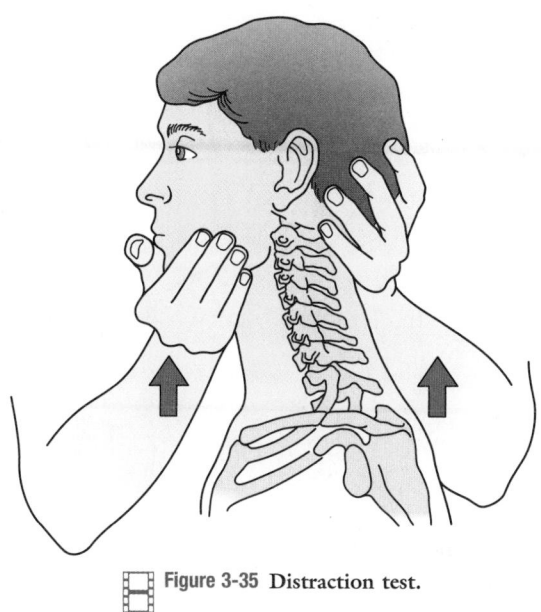

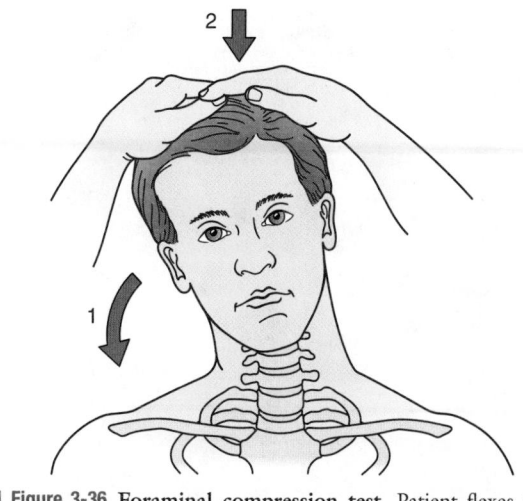

Figure 3-36 **Foraminal compression test.** Patient flexes head to one side *(1)*, and examiner presses straight down on head *(2)*.

Figure 3-35 **Distraction test.**

ligament sprain, muscle strain, dural irritability, or disc herniation.[13]

✓ *Foraminal Compression (Spurling's) Test.*[99] This test is performed if, in the history, the patient has complained of nerve root symptoms, which at the time of examination are diminished or absent. This test is designed to provoke symptoms. The patient bends or side flexes the head to the unaffected side first, followed by the affected side (Figure 3-36). The examiner carefully presses straight down on the head. Bradley and colleagues[55] advocate doing this test in three stages, each of which is increasingly provocative; if symptoms are produced, one does not proceed to the next stage. The first stage involves compression with the head in neutral. The second stage involves compression with the head in extension, and the final stage is with the head in extension and rotation to the unaffected side, then to the side of complaint with compression. The third part of the test more closely follows the test as described by Spurling.[99] A test result is classified as positive if pain radiates into the arm toward which the head is side flexed during compression; this indicates pressure on a nerve root (cervical radiculitis). **Radiculitis** implies pain in the dermatomal distribution of the nerve root affected.[55] Neck pain with no radiation into the shoulder or arm does not constitute a positive test. The dermatome distribution of the pain and altered sensation can give some indication as to which nerve root is involved. The test positions narrow the intervertebral foramen so that the following conditions may lead to symptoms: stenosis; cervical spondylosis; osteophytes; trophic, arthritic, or inflamed facet joints; herniated disc, which also narrow the foramen; or even vertebral fractures. If the pain is felt in the opposite side to which the head is taken, it is called a **reverse Spurling's sign** and is indicative of muscle spasm in conditions, such as tension myalgia and WADs.[100]

A very similar test is called the **maximum cervical compression test.** With this test, the patient side flexes the head and then rotates it to the same side. The test is repeated to the other side. A positive test is indicated if pain radiates into the arm.[29] If the head is taken into extension (as well as side flexion and rotation) and compression is applied, the intervertebral foramina close maximally to the side of movement and symptoms are accentuated. Pain on the concave side indicates nerve root or facet joint pathology, whereas pain on the convex side indicates muscle strain (Figure 3-37).[101] This second position may also compress the vertebral artery. If one is testing the vertebral artery, the position should be held for 20 to 30 seconds to elicit symptoms (e.g., dizziness, nystagmus, feeling faint, nausea) that would indicate compression of the vertebral artery.

✓ *Jackson's Compression Test.* This test is also a modification of the foraminal compression test. The patient rotates the head to one side. The examiner then carefully presses straight down on the head (Figure 3-38). The test is repeated with the head rotated to the other side. The test is positive if pain radiates into the arm, indicating pressure on a nerve root. The pain distribution (dermatome) can give some indication of which nerve root is affected.[53]

❓ *Scalene Cramp Test.*[45] The patient sits and rotates the head to the affected side and pulls the chin down into the hollow above the clavicle by flexing the cervical spine. If pain increases, it is usually in the trigger points of the scalenes toward which the head rotates. Radicular signs may indicate plexopathy or thoracic outlet symptoms.

⚠ *Shoulder Abduction (Relief) Test.* This test is used to test for radicular symptoms, especially those involving the C4 or C5 nerve roots. The patient is sitting or lying down, and the examiner passively or the patient actively

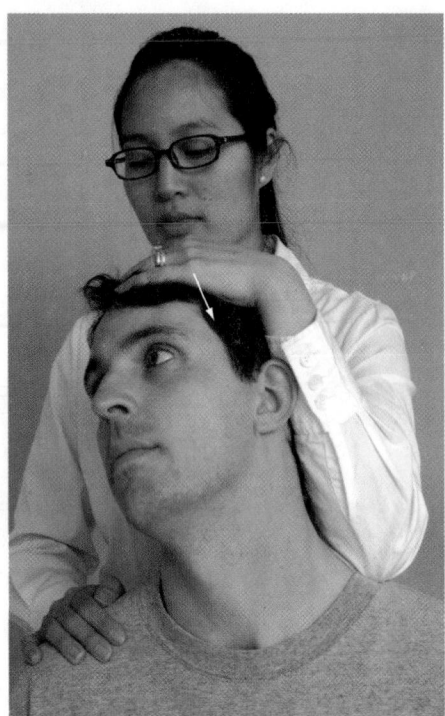

Figure 3-37 Maximum cervical compression test.

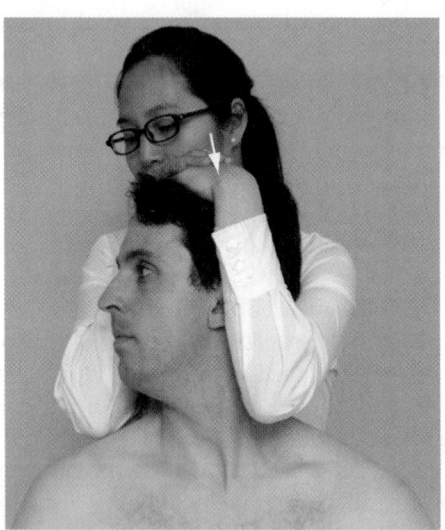

Figure 3-38 Jackson's compression test.

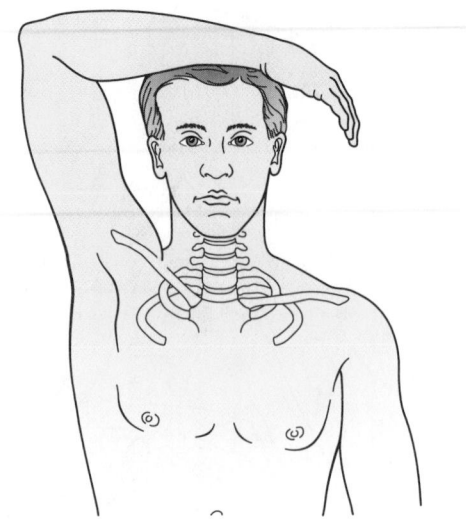

Figure 3-39 Shoulder abduction (Bakody's) test.

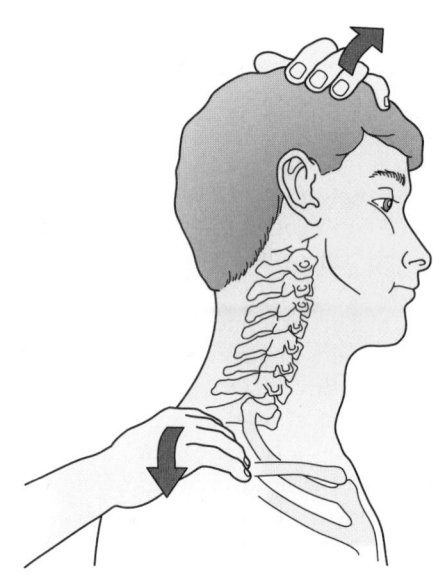

Figure 3-40 Shoulder depression test.

elevates the arm through abduction so that the hand or forearm rests on top of the head (Figure 3-39).[53,102] A decrease in or relief of symptoms indicates a cervical extra-dural compression problem, such as a herniated disc, epidural vein compression, or nerve root compression, usually in the C4–C5 or C5–C6 area. Differentiation is by the dermatome (and possible myotome) distribution of the symptoms. This finding is also called *Bakody's sign*.[54] Abduction of the arm decreases the length of the neurological pathway and decreases the pressure on the

lower nerve roots.[102,103] If the pain increases with the positioning of the arm, it implies that pressure is increasing in the interscalene triangle.[54]

? *Shoulder Depression Test.* This test may be used to evaluate for brachial plexus lesions (see Table 3-11), since the test position is the mechanism of injury for these lesions, plexopathies, and radiculopathies. With brachial plexus lesions, more than one nerve root is commonly affected. The examiner side flexes the patient's head to one side (e.g., the left) while applying a downward pressure on the opposite shoulder (e.g., the right) (Figure 3-40). If the pain is increased, it indicates irritation or compression of the nerve roots or foraminal encroachments, such as osteophytes in the area on the side being compressed, or adhesions around the dural sleeves of the nerve and adjacent joint capsule or a hypomobile joint capsule on the side being stretched. Differentiation is by the dermatome (and possibly myotome) distribution of symptoms.

❓ *Tinel Sign for Brachial Plexus Lesions.*[104] The patient sits with the neck slightly side flexed. The examiner taps the area of the brachial plexus (Figure 3-41) with a finger along the nerve trunks in such a way that the different nerve roots are tested. Pure local pain implies that there is an underlying cervical plexus lesion. A positive Tinel sign (tingling sensation in the distribution of a nerve) means the lesion is anatomically intact and some recovery is occurring. If pain is elicited in the distribution of a peripheral nerve, the sign is positive for a neuroma and indicates a disruption of the continuity of the nerve.

☑ *Upper Limb Neurodynamic (Tension) Tests (Brachial Plexus Tension or Elvey Test).* The upper limb neurodynamic tests (ULNT) are equivalent to the straight leg raising (SLR) test in the lumbar spine. They are tension tests designed to put stress on the neurological structures of the upper limb by stretching them, although, in truth, stress is put on all the tissues of the upper limb. The neurological tissue is differentiated by what is defined as sensitizing tests (e.g., neck flexion with the SLR test). This test, first described by Elvey,[72] has since been divided into four tests (Table 3-18). Modification of the position of the shoulder, elbow, forearm, wrist, and fingers places greater stress on specific nerves (nerve bias).[105]

Each test begins by testing the good side first and positioning the shoulder, followed by the forearm, wrist, fingers, and last, because of its large ROM, the elbow. Davis et al.[106] felt the tests should be considered positive only if neurological symptoms were manifested before 60° of elbow extension when elbow extension was the last movement performed. Each phase is added until symptoms are produced. To further "sensitize" the test, side flexion of the cervical spine may be performed.[72,101] Symptoms are more easily aggravated into the upper limb than the lower limb when doing tension tests,[105,107] and if the neurological signs are worsening or in the acute phase, or if a cauda equina or spinal cord lesion is present, these stress tests are contraindicated.[105]

When positioning the shoulder, it is essential that a constant depression force be applied to the shoulder girdle so that, even with abduction, the shoulder girdle remains depressed. If the shoulder is not held depressed, the test is less likely to work. While the shoulder girdle is

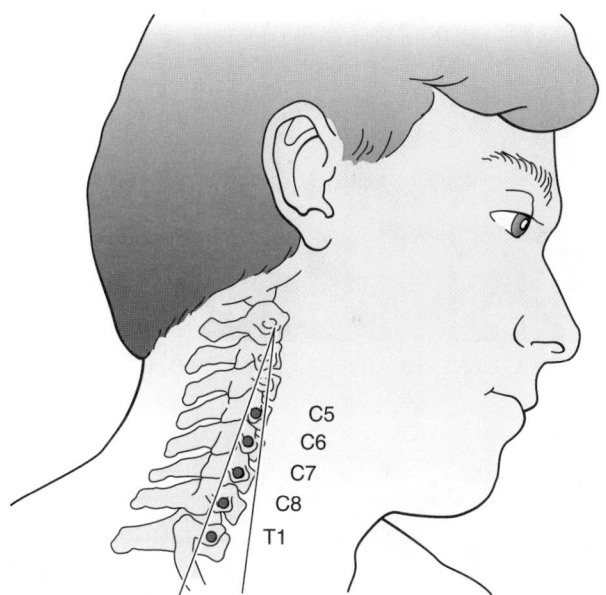

C5
C6
C7
C8
T1

Figure 3-41 Tinel sign for brachial plexus lesions. *Dots* indicate percussion points.

TABLE 3-18

Upper Limb Neurodynamic (Tension) Tests Showing Order of Joint Positioning and Nerve Bias

	ULNT1[96]	ULNT2	ULNT3	ULNT4
Shoulder	Depression and abduction (110°)	Depression and abduction (10°)	Depression and abduction (110°)	Depression and abduction (10° to 90°), hand to ear
Elbow	Extension	Extension	Extension	Flexion
Forearm	Supination	Supination	Pronation	Supination or pronation
Wrist	Extension	Extension	Flexion and ulnar deviation	Extension and radial deviation
Fingers and thumb	Extension	Extension	Flexion	Extension
Shoulder	—	Lateral rotation	Medial rotation	Lateral rotation
Cervical spine	Contralateral side flexion	Contralateral side flexion	Contralateral side flexion	Contralateral side flexion
Nerve bias	Median nerve, anterior interosseous nerve, C5, C6, C7	Median nerve, musculocutaneous nerve, axillary nerve	Radial nerve	Ulnar nerve, C8 and T1 nerve roots

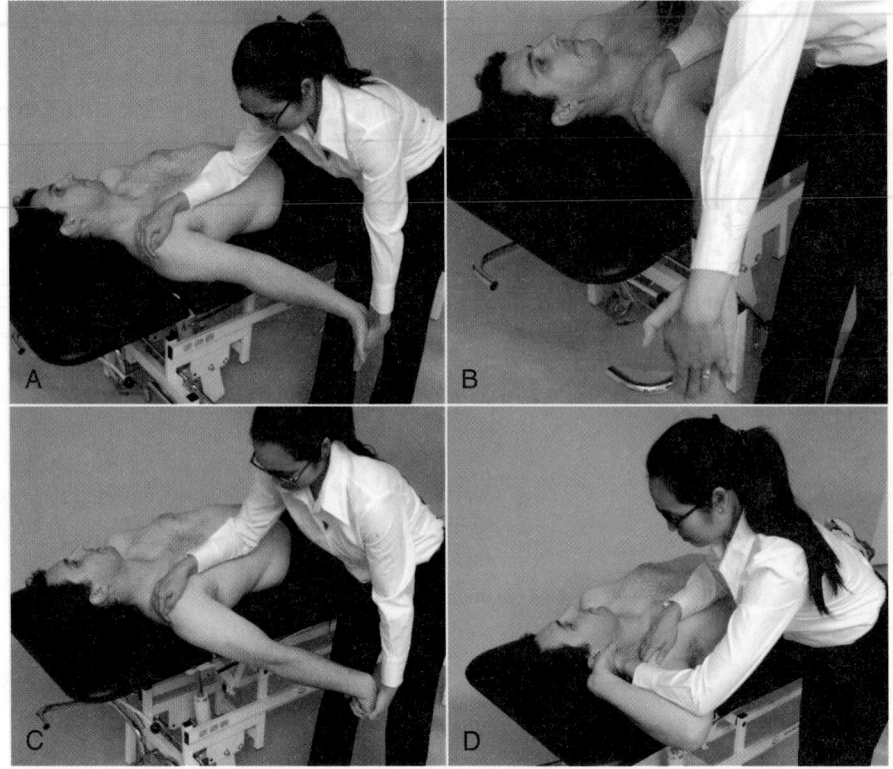

Figure 3-42 Upper limb neurodynamic (tension) tests (Elvey tests). **A,** ULNT1. **B,** ULNT2. **C,** ULNT3. **D,** ULNT4.

depressed, the glenohumeral joint is taken to the appropriate abduction position (110° or 10°, depending on the test), and the forearm, wrist, and fingers are taken to their appropriate end-of-range position; for example, in ULNT2 the wrist is in full extension (Figure 3-42). Elbow extension stresses the radial and median nerves, whereas flexion stresses the ulnar nerve. Wrist and finger extension stresses the median and ulnar nerve while releasing stress on the radial nerve.[105] If required (ULNT2, 3, and 4), the glenohumeral joint is appropriately rotated and held. The elbow position is often not performed until last because the large elbow ROM is easiest to measure when recording available range to show improvement over time. As the elbow is taken toward its extreme (end-of-range) position, symptoms are usually felt.[107] Some of these symptoms are normal (Table 3-19), and some are pathological. If symptoms are minimal or no symptoms appear, the head and cervical spine are taken into contralateral side flexion. This final movement is sometimes referred to as a **sensitizing test.** This sensitizing test may be within or near the test limb (e.g., neck side flexion in ULNT), or it may be in another quadrant (e.g., right ULNT and right SLR).

The tests are designed to stress tissues. Although they stress the neurological tissues, they also stress some contractile and inert tissues. Differentiation among the types of tissues depends on the signs and symptoms presented (Table 3-20).

TABLE **3-19**

Upper Limb Neurodynamic (Tension) Test: Normal and Pathological Signs and Symptoms

Normal (Negative)	Pathological (Positive)
• Deep ache or stretch in cubital fossa (99%) • Deep ache or stretch into anterior and radial aspect of forearm and radial aspect of hand (80%) • Tingling to the fingers supplied by appropriate nerve (nerve bias) • Stretch in anterior shoulder area • Above responses increased with contralateral cervical side flexion (90%) • Above responses decreased with ipsilateral cervical side flexion (70%)	• Production of patient's symptoms (most important feature) • A sensitizing test in the ipsilateral quadrant alters the symptoms • Different symptoms between right and left (contralateral quadrant)

Adapted from Butler DS: Mobilisation of the nervous system, Melbourne, 1991, Churchill Livingstone.

TABLE **3-20**

Differential Diagnosis of Contractile, Inert, and Nervous Tissue Based on Stretch or Tension

	Contractile Tissue	Inert Tissue (Ligament)	Neurogenic Tissue
Pain	Cramping, dull, ache	Dull→sharp	Burning, bright, lightning-like
Tingling	No	No	Yes
Constancy	Intermittent	Intermittent	Longer symptom duration
Dermatome pattern	No	No	Yes (if nerve root pathological)
Peripheral nerve sensory distribution	No	No	Yes (if peripheral nerve or nerve root is affected)
Resistance to stretch	Muscle spasm	Boggy, hard capsular	Soft tissue stretch

Finally, although specific ULNTs are described, if the patient describes neurological symptoms when doing functional movements (e.g., getting wallet out of back pocket) these movements should also be tested by positioning the limb and taking the joints toward their end range.

Evans[54] described a modification of the ULNT that he called the **brachial plexus tension test** ☑. The sitting patient abducts the arms with the elbows extended, stopping just short of the onset of symptoms. The patient laterally rotates the shoulder just short of symptoms, and the examiner then holds this position. Finally, the patient flexes the elbows so that the hands lie behind the head (Figure 3-43). Reproduction of radicular symptoms with elbow flexion is considered a positive test. This test is similar to ULNT4 and stresses primarily the ulnar nerve and the C8 and T1 nerve roots.

Evans[54] outlined a second similar test. The seated patient abducts the arm to 90° with the elbow fully flexed. The arm is extended at the shoulder and then the elbow is extended (Figure 3-44). If radicular pain results, the test is positive (**Bikele's sign**). This test in reality is a modification of the ULNT4 done actively.

☑ *Valsalva Test.* This test is used to determine the effect of increased pressure on the spinal cord. The examiner asks the patient to take a deep breath and hold it while bearing down, as if moving the bowels. A positive test is indicated by increased pain, which may be caused by increased intrathecal pressure. This increased pressure within the spinal cord usually results from a space-occupying lesion, such as a herniated disc, a tumor, stenosis, or osteophytes. Test results are very subjective. The test should be performed with care and caution because the patient may become dizzy and pass out during the test or shortly afterward if the procedure blocks the blood supply to the brain.

Tests for Upper Motor Neuron Lesions (Cervical Myelopathy)

In addition to the tests below, positive pathological reflexes (e.g., Babinski, Hoffman), hyperreflexia of the

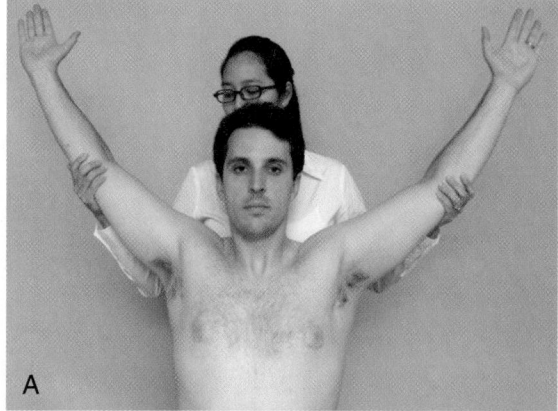

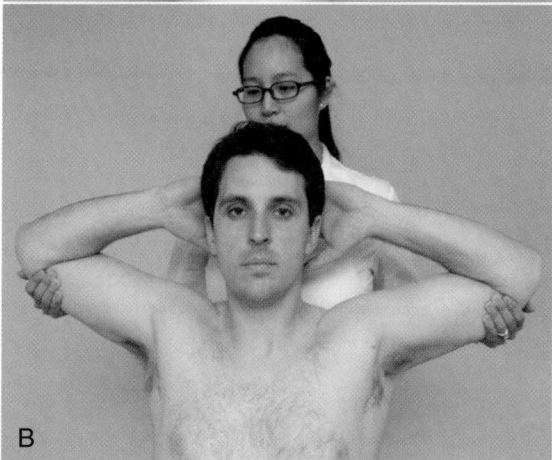

Figure 3-43 Brachial plexus tension test. A, The patient abducts and then laterally rotates the arms until symptoms are felt; the patient then lowers the arms until symptoms disappear, and the examiner holds the patient's arms in the position. **B,** While the shoulders are held in position, the patient flexes the elbows and places the hands behind the head. A positive test is indicated by return of symptoms.

deep tendon reflexes, and clonus may indicate a cervical myelopathy.[108]

❓ *Lhermitte Sign.* This is a test for the spinal cord itself and a possible upper motor neuron lesion. The patient is in the long leg sitting position on the examining table.

The examiner passively flexes the patient's head and one hip simultaneously with the leg kept straight (Figure 3-45). A positive test occurs if there is a sharp, electric shock-like pain down the spine and into the upper or lower limbs; it indicates dural or meningeal irritation in the spine or possible cervical myelopathy.[54] Coughing or sneezing may produce similar results. The test is similar to a combination of the Brudzinski test and the SLR test (see Chapter 9). If the patient actively flexes the head to the chest while in the supine lying position, the test is called the **Soto-Hall test.** If the hips are flexed to 135°, greater traction is placed on the spinal cord.[53]

✓ *Romberg Test.* For Romberg test, the patient is standing and is asked to close the eyes. The position is held for 20 to 30 seconds. If the body begins to sway excessively or the patient loses balance, the test is considered positive for an upper motor neuron lesion.

⚠ *Ten Second Step Test.*[109] The patient, while standing, is asked to step "in place" by lifting the thigh of one leg parallel to the floor (i.e., hip and knees at 90°) and then lifting the other leg in a similar manner as though walking at maximum speed while not holding on to any object. The number of steps in 10 seconds is counted (Table 3-21).

Tests for Vascular Signs (Vascular "Clearing" Tests)

Vertebral and internal carotid artery testing is an important component of the cervical spine assessment in cases where end range mobilization and manipulation treatment techniques are contemplated, especially if the techniques involve a rotary component (greater than 45°) and the upper cervical spine (C0 to C3).[110–112] The vertebral artery is especially vulnerable to injury as it transitions from its protective area in the foramen transversarium within the cervical spine transverse processes, then looping before it enters the cranial vault behind the first vertebra. Vertebrobasilar insufficiency leads to ischemic symptoms from the pons, medulla, and cerebellum (see Figure 3-1).[113] Several authors[110,113–117] have reported that the vertebral artery tests have not been conclusively proven to be effective in indicating stretching and occlusion of the vertebral artery or internal carotid artery but do say that the tests should be performed to decrease the risk of potentially catastrophic complications when doing

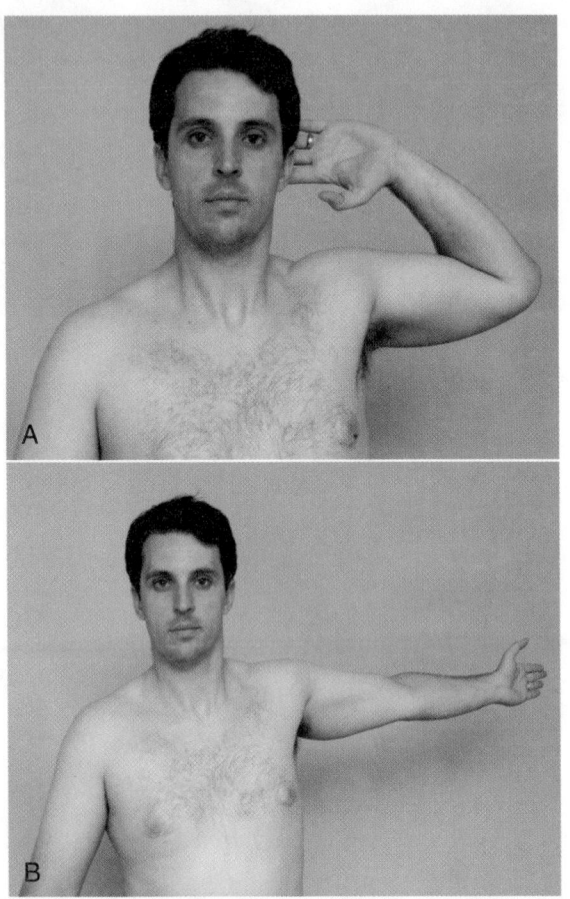

Figure 3-44 Bikele's sign. A, The arm is abducted to 90° with the elbow fully flexed. **B,** The arm and then the elbow are extended.

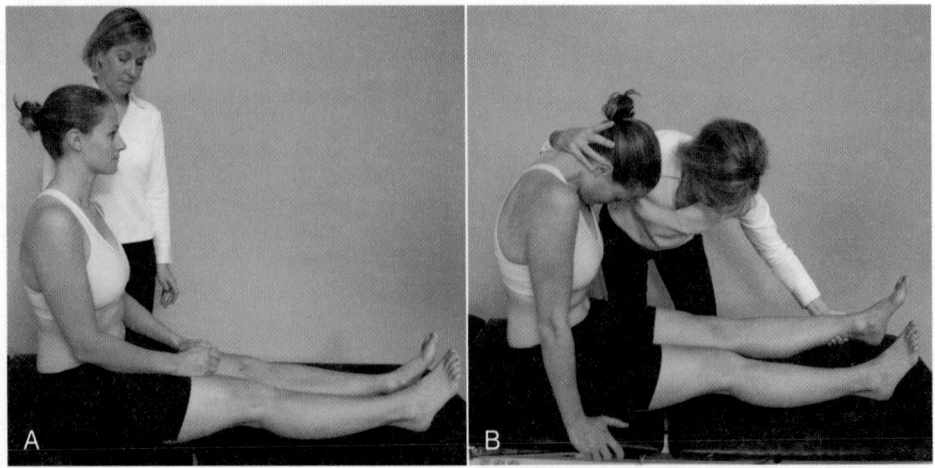

Figure 3-45 Lhermitte sign. A, Patient in long sitting position. **B,** Examiner flexes patient's head and hip simultaneously.

TABLE **3-21**

Normal Values of Ten Second Step Test in Each Gender and Age Group

Age	Male	Female
20 to 29	21.9 ± 2.6	20.6 ± 3.5
30 to 39	21.4 ± 3.7	20.9 ± 4.4
40 to 49	20.9 ± 3.5	19.9 ± 2.2
50 to 59	19.9 ± 3.1	19.0 ± 2.7
60 to 69	18.3 ± 2.8	18.2 ± 2.2
70 to 79	17.5 ± 3.1	16.9 ± 2.3
Average	20.0 ± 3.5	19.2 ± 3.3

Modified from Yukawa Y, Kato F, Ito K, et al: "Ten second step test" as a new quantifiable parameter of cervical myelopathy. Spine 34(1):82–86, 2009.

end-range mobilization or manipulation, especially of the upper cervical spine. Table 3-22 outlines vertebral and internal carotid artery signs and symptoms associated with pathology.[118] Although the following text discusses many vertebral artery tests, not all of them have to be performed. However, it is imperative that the patient be tested in the position in which the treatment will be given and held in that position for at least 10 to 30 seconds , especially if the technique is an end-range technique or involves the upper cervical spine.[6,119–121] Any of the signs and symptoms that indicate vertebral-basilar artery problems would indicate the treatment should not be given. When doing more than one test, 10 seconds should elapse between each test to ensure there are no latent symptoms from the previous test. It is recommended that if mobilization or manipulation of the cervical spine is contemplated, the clinician should follow the Australian Physiotherapy Association's protocol for premanipulative testing of the cervical spine.[122] If, when performing the vertebral artery tests, or if in the history, the patient complains of signs and symptoms that may be related to the vertebral artery, care should be taken when mobilizing the upper cervical spine.[111,123–125]

These tests are often more effective if performed with the patient sitting because the blood must flow against gravity and there is a restriction caused by the passive movement. However, the supine position allows greater passive range of movement.[126] Movements to the right tend to have more effect on the left vertebral artery, and movements to the left tend to have more effect on the right artery.[125]

? *Barre's Test.*[127] The patient stands with the shoulders forward flexed to 90°, elbows straight and forearms supinated, palms up and eyes closed, holding the position for 10 to 20 seconds. The test is considered positive if one arm slowly falls with simultaneous forearm pronation. The cause is thought to be diminished blood flow to the brainstem. This test is identical to the first part of Hautant's test.

Signs and Symptoms That May Indicate Possible Vertebral-Basilar Artery Problems[110,113]

- Dizziness/vertigo
- Dysphagia (difficulty swallowing)
- Drop attacks
- Malaise and nausea
- Vomiting
- Unsteadiness in walking, incoordination
- Visual disturbances
- Severe headaches
- Weakness in extremities
- Sensory changes in face or body
- Dysarthria (difficulty with speech)
- Unconsciousness, disorientation, lightheadedness
- Hearing difficulties
- Facial paralysis

NOTE: Similar symptoms may be seen with other conditions (e.g., benign paroxysmal positional vertigo, head injury, epilepsy, ear disease).

? *Hautant's Test.*[54,128] This test has two parts and is used to differentiate dizziness or vertigo caused by articular problems from that caused by vascular problems. The patient sits and forward flexes both arms to 90° (Figure 3-46). The eyes are then closed. The examiner watches for any loss of arm position. If the arms move, the cause is nonvascular. The patient is then asked to rotate, or extend and rotate, the neck; this position is held while the eyes are again closed. If wavering of the arms occurs, the dysfunction is caused by vascular impairment to the brain. Each position should be held for 10 to 30 seconds.

? *Naffziger Test.*[54,129] The patient is seated, and the examiner stands behind the patient with his or her fingers over the patient's jugular veins (Figure 3-47). The examiner compresses the veins for 30 seconds (Naffziger recommended 10 minutes!) and then asks the patient to cough. Pain may indicate a nerve root problem or space-occupying lesion (e.g., tumor). If lightheadedness or similar symptoms occur with compression of the jugular veins, the test should be terminated.

? *Static Vertebral Artery Tests.* The examiner may test the following passive movements with the patient supine or sitting, as advocated by Grant,[130] watching for eye nystagmus and complaints by the patient of dizziness, lightheadedness, or visual disturbances. Each of these tests is increasingly provocative; if symptoms occur with the first test, there is no need to progress to the next test.

In the sitting position:
1. Sustained full neck and head extension
2. Sustained full neck and head rotation, right and left (if this movement causes symptoms, it is sometimes called a positive **Barre-Lieou sign**)[54]
3. Sustained full neck and head rotation with extension right and left (**DeKleyn's test**)[54]

TABLE **3-22**

Vascular Pathology Signs and Symptoms Related to the Vertebral and Internal Carotid Arteries

Factors to Consider When Assessing Cervical Vascular Problems

- Risk factors
- Position testing (especially rotation and extension)
- Cranial nerve examination
- Eye examination
- Cognitive function
- Blood pressure examination
- "Headache like no other"

Vertebral Artery Non-Ischemic (Local) Signs and Symptoms

- Ipsilateral posterior neck pain
- Occipital headache
- C5–C6 cervical root impairment (rare)

Vertebral Artery Ischemic Signs and Symptoms

- "Headache like no other"
- Ipsilateral posterior upper cervical pain
- Occipital headache
- Hindbrain transient ischemia attack: dizziness, diplopia, dysarthria, dysphagia, drop attacks, nausea, nystagmus, facial numbness, ataxia, vomiting, hoarseness, loss of short-term memory, weakness, hypotonia/limb weakness (arm or leg), anhidrosis (lack of facial sweating), hearing disturbances, malaise, periodal dysthesia, photophobia, papillary changes, clumsiness, and agitation
- Hindbrain stroke: Wallenberg syndrome (a neurological condition caused by a stroke in the vertebral or posterior inferior cerebral artery of the brainstem), symptoms include difficulty in swallowing, hoarseness, dizziness, nausea and vomiting, rapid involuntary movements of the eyes (nystagmus), and problems with balance and gait coordination

Vascular Risk Factors

- Hypertension
- Hypercholesterolemia (high cholesterol)
- Hyperlipidemia (high fat)
- Hyperhomocysteinemia (hardening of the arteries)
- Diabetes mellitus
- General clotting disorders
- Infection
- Smoking
- Direct vessel trauma
- Iatrogenic causes (surgery, medical interventions)

Internal Carotid Non-Ischemic (Local) Signs and Symptoms

- Head/neck pain
- Horner's syndrome: a rare condition caused by injury to the sympathetic nerves of the face it involves a collection of symptoms including sinking of the eyeball into the face (enophthalmia), small (constricted) pupils (miosis), ptosis (drooping eyelid), anhidrosis (facial dryness)
- Pulsatile tinnitus
- Cranial nerve palsies (most commonly cranial nerve IX to XII)
- Ipsilateral carotid bruit (less common)
- Scalp tenderness (less common)
- Neck swelling (less common)
- Cranial nerve VI palsy (less common)
- Orbital pain (less common)

Internal Carotid Artery Ischemic Signs and Symptoms

- Ipsilateral frontal temporal headache (clusterlike, thunderclap, migraine without aura, or simply "different from previous headaches")
- Upper/middle and anterolateral cervical pain, facial pain and sensitivity (carotidynia)
- Transient ischemia attack (TIA)
- Ischemia stroke
- Retinal infarction
- Amaurosis fugax (transient episodic blindness caused by decreased blood flow to the retina)

Data from Kerry R, Taylor AJ: Cervical artery dysfunction assessment and manual therapy. Manual Therapy 11:243–253, 2006.

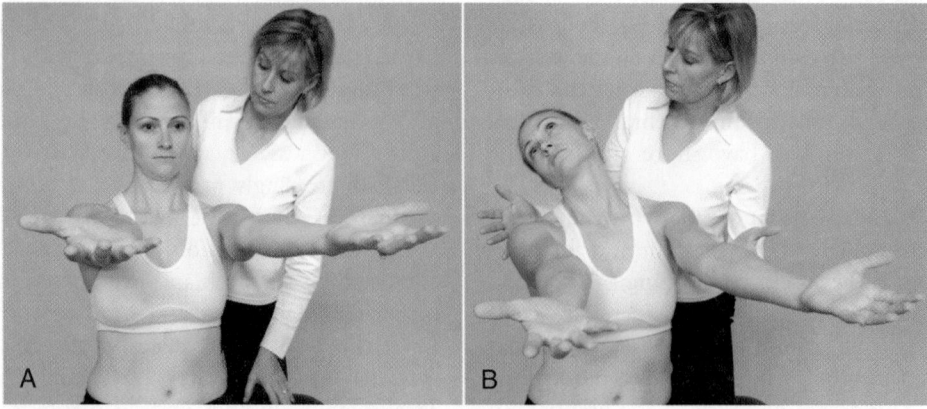

Figure 3-46 Positioning for Hautant's test. A, Forward flexion of both arms to 90°. **B,** Rotation and extension of neck with arms forward flexed to 90°.

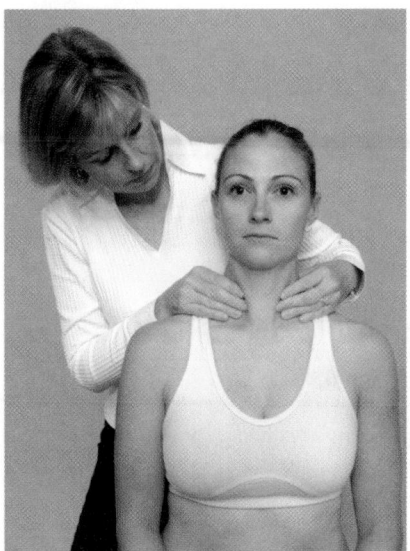

Figure 3-47 Naffziger test (compression of jugular veins).

TABLE 3-23

Relationship of Head Position to Blood Flow to Head and Neurological Function

Head Position	Blood Flow	Neurological Space
Neutral	Normal	Normal
Flexion	Normal	Normal
Extension	Usually normal	Decreased
Side flexion	Slight decrease in ipsilateral artery; normal in contralateral artery	Decrease on ipsilateral side; increase on contralateral side
Rotation	Slight decrease in ipsilateral artery; significant decrease in contralateral artery	Decrease on ipsilateral side; increase on contralateral side
Extension and rotation	Bilateral decrease, greater in contralateral artery	Bilateral decrease, greater on ipsilateral side
Flexion and rotation	Bilateral decrease	Decrease on ipsilateral side; increase on contralateral side

4. Provocative movement position*
5. Quick head movement into provocative position*
6. Quick repeated head movement into provocative position*
7. Head still, sustained trunk movement left and right (10 to 30 seconds)
8. Head still, repeated trunk movement left and right
   In supine position:
1. Sustained full neck and head extension
2. Sustained full neck and head rotation left and right
3. Sustained full neck and head rotation with extension left and right (if combined with side flexion, it is called the **Hallpike maneuver**[54]). Extension combined with rotation has been found to be the position most likely to occlude the vertebral artery.[110]
4. Unilateral posteroanterior oscillation (Maitland's grade IV) of C1 to C2 facet joints (prone lying) with head rotated left and right
5. Simulated mobilization and manipulation position

Each position should be held for at least 10 to 30 seconds unless symptoms are evoked. Extension in isolation is more likely to test the patency of the intervertebral foramen, whereas rotation and side flexion or, especially, rotation and extension are more likely to test the vertebral artery (Table 3-23).[10] If symptoms are evoked, care should be taken concerning any treatment to follow.

Aspinall[131] advocated the use of a progressive series of clinical tests to evaluate the vertebral artery. With these tests, the examiner progressively moves from the lower cervical spine and lower vertebral artery to the upper cervical spine and upper vertebral artery where it is more vulnerable to pathology. Table 3-24 demonstrates Aspinall's progressive clinical tests for the vertebral arteries.

❓ *Underburg's Test.*[54] The patient stands with the shoulders forward flexed to 90°, elbows straight and forearms supinated. The patient then closes the eyes and marches in place while holding the extended and rotated head to one side. The test is repeated with head movement to the opposite side. The test is considered positive if there is dropping of the arms, loss of balance, or pronation of the hands; a positive result indicates decreased blood supply to the brain.

❓ *Vertebral Artery (Cervical Quadrant) Test.* With the patient supine, the examiner passively takes the patient's head and neck into extension and side flexion (Figure 3-48).[132] After this movement is achieved, the examiner rotates the patient's neck to the same side and holds it for approximately 30 seconds. A positive test provokes referring symptoms if the opposite artery is affected. This test must be done with care. If dizziness or nystagmus occurs, it is an indication that the vertebral arteries are being compressed. The **DeKleyn-Nieuwenhuyse test**[55,127] ❓ performs a similar function but involves extension and rotation instead of extension and side flexion. Both tests may also be used to assess nerve root compression in the lower cervical spine. To test the upper cervical spine, the examiner "pokes" the patient's chin and follows with extension, side flexion, and rotation.

---

*Provocative position implies movement into the position that provokes symptoms.

TABLE **3-24**

Aspinall's Progressive Clinical Tests for Vertebral Artery Pathology

Vertebral Artery Area	POSITION		Test
	Sitting	Lying	
Area 1 (lower cervical spine)	X		Active cervical rotation
Area 2 (middle cervical spine)	X		Active cervical rotation
	X	X	Passive cervical rotation
	X		Active cervical extension
	X	X	Passive cervical extension
	X	X	Passive cervical extension with rotation
	X		Passive segmental extension with rotation
	X	X	Passive cervical flexion
	X	X	Cervical flexion with traction
		X	Accessory oscillatory anterior/posterior movement—transverse processes C2–C7 in combined extension and rotation
		X	Sustained manipulation position
Area 3 (upper cervical spine)	X		Active cervical rotation
	X	X	Passive cervical rotation
	X		Active cervical extension
	X	X	Passive cervical extension
	X	X	Passive cervical rotation with extension
	X	X	Cervical rotation with extension and traction
	X		Cervical rotation with flexion
		X	Accessory oscillatory anterior/posterior movement—transverse processes C1–C2 in combined rotation and extension
		X	Sustained manipulation position

From Aspinall W: Clinical testing for the craniovertebral hypermobility syndrome. J Orthop Sports Phys Ther 12:180–181, 1989.

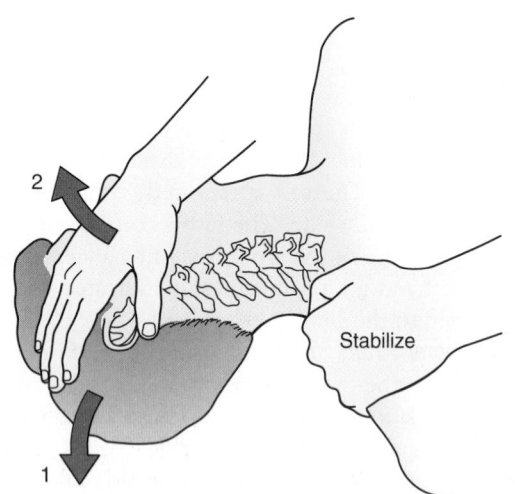

Figure 3-48 Vertebral artery (cervical quadrant) test. Examiner passively moves patient's head and neck into extension and side flexion *(1)*, then rotation *(2)*, holding for 30 seconds.

Tests for Vertigo and Dizziness

❓ *Dizziness Test.* The patient sits, and the examiner grasps the patient's head. The examiner actively rotates the patient's head as far as possible to the right and then to the left, holding the head at the extreme of motion for a short time (10 to 30 seconds) while the shoulders remain stationary. The patient's head is then returned to neutral. Next, the patient's shoulders are actively rotated as far to the right as possible, held for 10 to 30 seconds, and then to the left as far as possible, and held for 10 to 30 seconds while keeping the head facing straight ahead. If the patient experiences dizziness in both cases, the problem lies in the vertebral arteries, because in both cases the vertebral artery may be "kinked," decreasing the blood flow. If the patient experiences dizziness only when the head is rotated, the problem lies within the semicircular canals of the inner ear.

Fitz-Ritson[133] advocates a modification of this test. For the first part of the test, he advocates that the examiner hold the shoulders still while the patient rapidly rotates the head left and right with eyes closed. If vertigo results, the problem is in the vestibular nuclei or muscles and joints of the cervical spine. In addition, patients may lose their balance, veer to one side, or possibly vomit. The second stage is the same as previously mentioned, except that the eyes are closed. If vertigo is experienced this time, Fitz-Ritson believes that the problem is in the cervical spine because the vestibular apparatus is not being moved.

❓ *Hallpike-Dix Test.*[134,135] This test is used to identify benign paroxysmal positional vertigo (BPPV), a condition

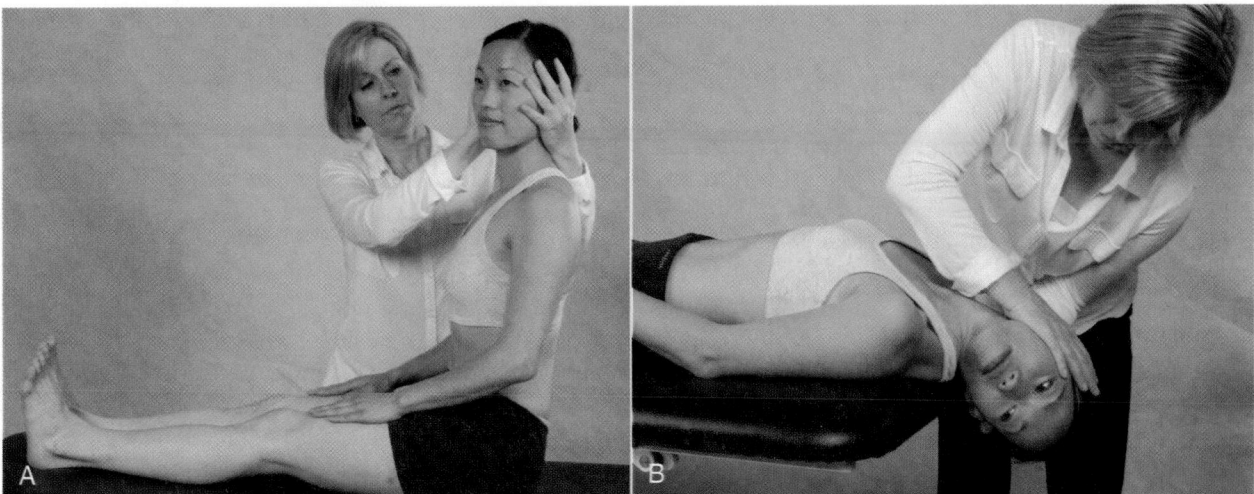

Figure 3-49 Hallpike-Dix Test. A, This test is performed by having the patient long-sit on a plinth with the head rotated approximately 30° to 45° to the unaffected side first. **B,** The patient is assisted into a supine position with the patient's head slightly below the horizontal plane while maintaining the rotation. The position is maintained for 30 to 60 seconds. Rotation both ways is tested.

in which patients experience episodes of dizziness, or vertigo, especially if the head and neck are moved to different positions. The test is performed by having the patient long-sit on a plinth with the head rotated approximately 30° to 45° (Figure 3-49, *A*). The examiner stands behind the patient with one hand supporting the head/neck and the other hand supporting the trunk. The patient is then assisted into a supine position with the patient's head slightly below the horizontal plane, and the position is maintained for 30 to 60 seconds (Figure 3-49, *B*). The test is performed with the head rotated to both sides starting with the unaffected side. Signs of dizziness and nystagmus (involuntary eye movement) are considered a positive test.

 Temperature (Caloric) Test. The examiner alternately applies hot and cold test tubes several times just behind the patient's ears on the side of the head; each side is done in turn. A positive test is associated with the inducement of vertigo, which indicates inner ear problems.

Tests for Cervical Instability (Instability "Clearing" Tests)

Instability in the cervical spine is most commonly the result of ligament damage (e.g., transverse ligament, alar ligaments), bone or joint damage (e.g., fracture or dislocation) or weak muscles (e.g., deep flexors or extensors). The instability may be the result of chronic arthritic conditions (e.g., rheumatoid arthritis), trauma, long-term corticosteroid use, congenital malformations, Down syndrome, and osteoporosis.[13] One commonly should have a high level of suspicion of instability if in the history the patient complains of instability, a lump in the throat, lip paresthesia, severe headache (especially with movement), muscle spasm, nausea, or vomiting.[13] If the examiner anticipates doing mobilization (especially end-range techniques) or manipulation techniques to the cervical spine,

especially the upper cervical spine, a selection of appropriate "clearing" tests should be performed to rule out instability. If instability is present, mobilization and/or manipulation should **not** be performed.

Signs and Symptoms of Cervical Instability

- Severe muscle spasm
- Patient does not want to move head (especially into flexion)
- Lump in throat
- Lip or facial paresthesia
- Severe headache
- Dizziness
- Nausea
- Vomiting
- Soft-end feel
- Nystagmus
- Pupil changes

 Anterior Shear or Sagittal Stress Test.[56,136,137] This test is designed to test the integrity of the supporting ligamentous and capsular tissues of the cervical spine. It is similar to the **posteroanterior central vertebral pressure (PACVP)** testing in the joint play section. The patient lies supine with the head in neutral resting on the bed. The examiner applies an anteriorly directed force through the posterior arch of C1 or the spinous processes of C2 to T1 or bilaterally through the lamina of each vertebral body. In each case, the normal end feel is tissue stretch with an abrupt stop (Figure 3-50). Positive signs, especially when the upper cervical spine is tested, include nystagmus, pupil changes, dizziness, soft end feel, nausea, facial or lip paresthesia, and a lump sensation in the throat.[55]

❓ *Lateral Flexion Alar Ligament Stress Test.*[88,128,136,138] The patient lies supine with the head in the physiological neutral position while the examiner stabilizes the axis with a wide pinch grip around the spinous process and lamina (Figure 3-51). The examiner then attempts to side flex the head and axis. Normally, if the ligament is intact, minimal side flexion occurs with a strong capsular end feel and a solid stop.

⚠ *Lateral (Transverse) Shear Test.*[128,136] This test is used to determine instability of the atlantoaxial articulation caused by odontoid dysplasia. The patient lies supine with the head supported. The examiner places the radial side of the second metacarpophalangeal (MCP) joint of one hand against the transverse process of the atlas and the MCP joint of the other hand against the opposite transverse process of the axis. The examiner's hands are then carefully pushed together, causing a shear of one bone on the other (Figure 3-52). Normally, minimal motion and no symptoms (cord or vascular) are produced. Because

this test is normally painful because of the compression of soft tissues against the bone, the patient should be warned beforehand that pain is a normal sensation to be expected. The test can also be used to test other levels of the cervical spine (i.e., C2 to C7).

❓ *Rotational Alar Ligament Stress Test.*[136,138] The patient is in sitting position. The examiner grips the lamina and spinous process of C2 between the finger and thumb. While stabilizing C2, the examiner passively rotates the patient's head left or right moving to the "no symptom" side first. If more than 20° to 30° rotation is possible without C2 moving, it is indicative of injury to the contralateral alar ligament especially if the lateral flexion alar stress test is positive in the same direction. If the excessive motion is in the opposite direction for both tests, the

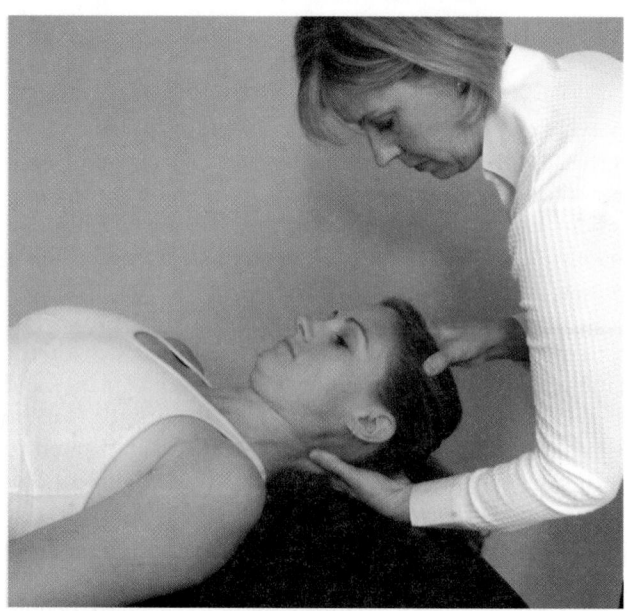

Figure 3-51 Lateral flexion alar ligament stress test. Examiner attempts to side flex the patient's head while stabilizing the axis.

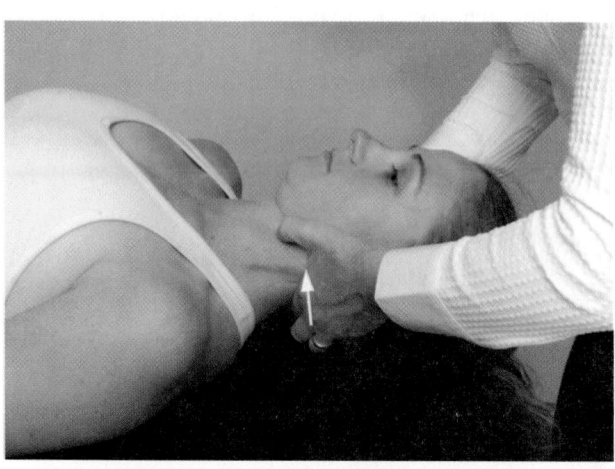

Figure 3-50 Anterior sagittal stress test.

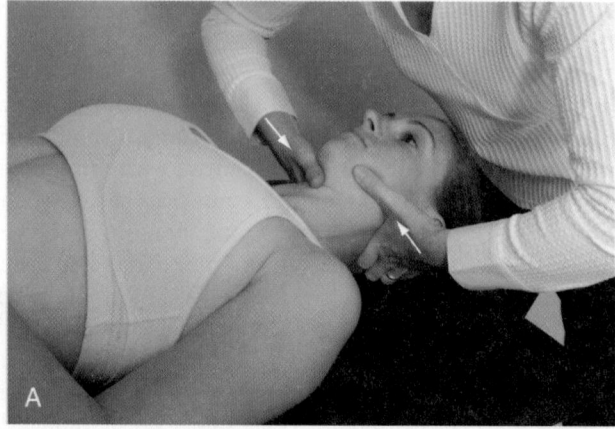

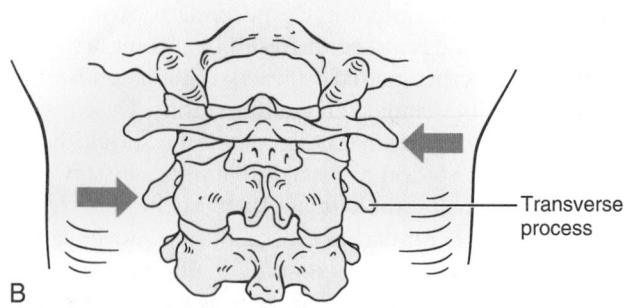

Transverse process

Figure 3-52 A, Atlantoaxial lateral shear test. **B,** Metacarpophalangeal joints against transverse processes.

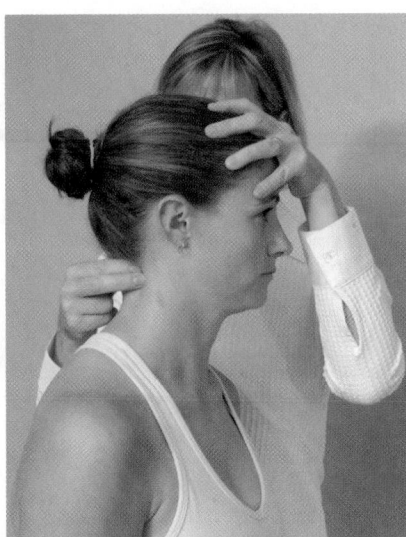

Figure 3-53 **Rotational alar ligament stress test.** While the examiner grips the lamina of C2, the patient's head is rotated left and right with the other hand.

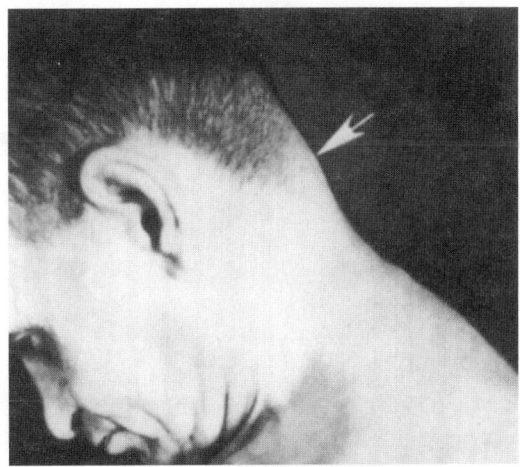

Figure 3-55 **Subluxation of the atlas on neck flexion.** Note the bulge in the posterior neck caused by the forward subluxation of the atlas, bringing the spinous process of the axis into prominence beneath the skin *(arrow)*. (Courtesy of Harold S. Robinson, MD, Vancouver, British Columbia.)

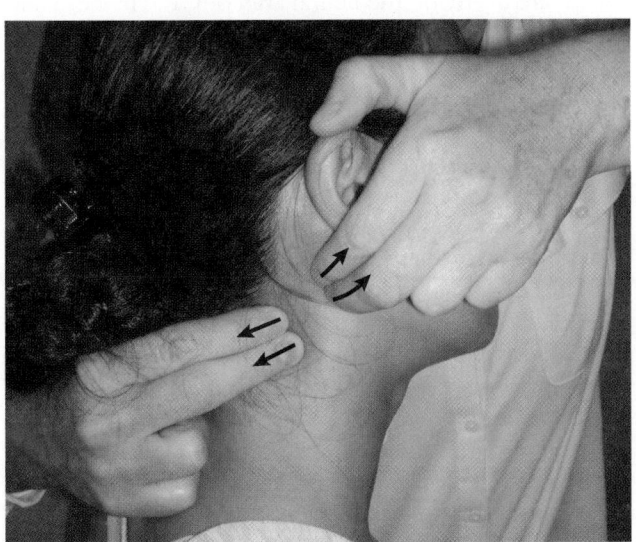

Figure 3-54 **Rotational alar ligament stress test.** Kaale's alternate method.

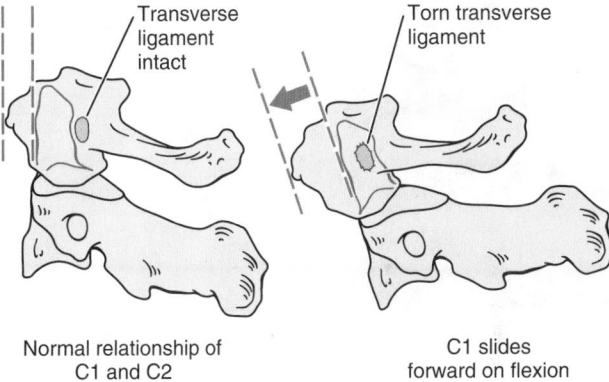

Figure 3-56 Forward translation of C1 on C2 on flexion as a result of torn transverse ligament.

instability is due to an increase in the neutral zone in the joint (Figure 3-53).

Kaale et al.[139] advocated doing the test ❓ in a different fashion. They advocate placing the patient in sitting position. The examiner supports the patient's head against his or her body and places both hands on the same side of the patient's occipitocervical junction. The lower hand (Figure 3-54) stabilizes C2 by pressing the second and third fingers against the lateral aspect of C2 pulling it backwards. The other hand is placed above with the third finger under the lateral mass of the atlas and the second finger under the mastoid process pulling upward into rotation (see Figure 3-54). The test is performed in

different angles of rotation to locate the position of maximum movement between C1 and C2.

⚠️ *Sharp-Purser Test.* This test should be performed *with extreme caution.* It is a test to determine subluxation of the atlas on the axis (Figure 3-55). If the transverse ligament that maintains the position of the odontoid process relative to C1 (Figure 3-56) is torn, C1 will translate forward (sublux) on C2 on flexion. Thus, the examiner may find the patient reticent to do forward flexion if the transverse ligament has been damaged. The examiner places one hand over the patient's forehead while the thumb of the other hand is placed over the spinous process of the axis to stabilize it (Figure 3-57). The patient is asked to slowly flex the head; while this is occurring, the examiner presses backward with the palm. A positive test is indicated if the examiner feels the head slide backward during the movement. The slide backward

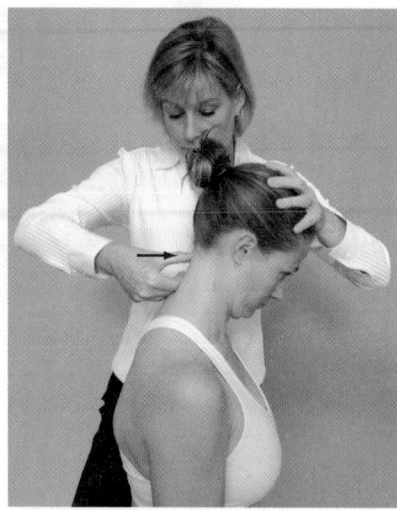

Figure 3-57 **The Sharp-Purser test** for subluxation of the atlas on the axis.

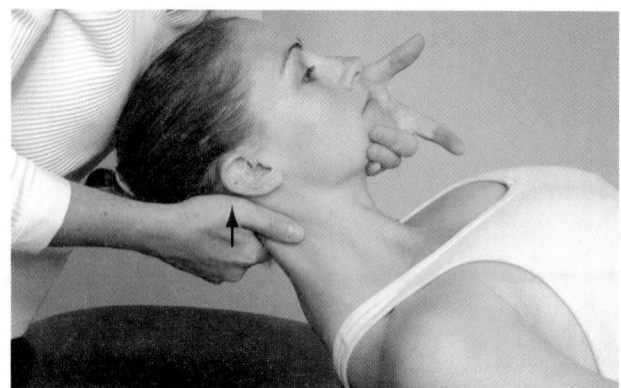

Figure 3-58 **Aspinall's transverse ligament test.**

indicates that the subluxation of the atlas has been reduced, and the slide may be accompanied by a "clunk."

Aspinall[140] advocates use of an additional test if the Sharp-Purser test is negative (**Aspinall's Transverse Ligament Test**). The patient is placed in supine. The examiner stabilizes the occiput on the atlas in flexion and holds the occiput in this flexed position. The examiner then applies an anteriorly directed force to the posterior aspect of the atlas (Figure 3-58). Normally, no movement or symptoms are perceived by the patient. For the test to be positive, the patient should feel a lump in the throat as the atlas moves toward the esophagus; this is indicative of hypermobility at the atlantoaxial articulation.

Rey-Einz et al.[141] advocated doing a similar test to test for hypomobility in the middle cervical spine (**posterior-anterior middle cervical spine gliding test**). The head and cervical spine are held in neutral and the examiner pushes anteriorly on the lamina of C3, C4, or C5. Hypomobility for the test was defined as abnormal resistance to movement, abnormal end feel and/or reproduction of local or referred pain.

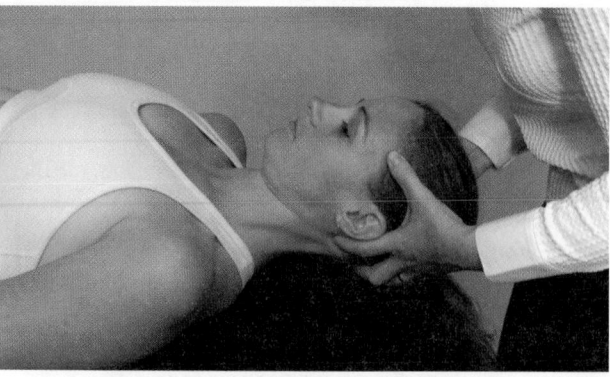

Figure 3-59 Testing the transverse ligament of C1. Examiner's hands support head and C1.

Transverse Ligament Stress Test.[128,136] The patient lies supine with the examiner supporting the occiput with the palms and the third, fourth, and fifth fingers. The examiner places the index fingers in the space between the patient's occiput and C2 spinous process so that the fingertips are overlying the neural arch of C1. The head and C1 are then carefully lifted anteriorly together, allowing no flexion or extension (Figure 3-59). This anterior shear is normally resisted by the transverse ligament (Figure 3-60). The position is held for 10 to 20 seconds to see whether symptoms occur, indicating a positive test. Positive symptoms include soft end feel; muscle spasm; dizziness; nausea; paresthesia of the lip, face, or limb; nystagmus; or a lump sensation in the throat. The test indicates hypermobility at the atlantoaxial articulation.

Kaale et al.[139] advocated doing the test by stabilizing C2 from the front of the neck with the fingers pressed against the anterior aspect of the side of the transverse process on one side and the thumb in the same position on the opposite side of C2 (Figure 3-61). *Do not choke the patient!* The examiner's other hand is similarly placed on the posterior aspect of the transverse processes of C1 and against the inferior part of the occiput. C1 is pressed forward while C2 is pressed backwards testing the translation of the dense of the atlas.

Tests for Upper Cervical Spine Mobility[69,142,143]

Cervical Flexion Rotation Test. The patient is in supine lying position. The examiner sits or stands at the head of the patient and flexes the cervical spine fully. While holding the flexed position, the examiner then rotates the head left and right. Normal rotation in the flexed position should be about 45° each way (Figure 3-62). Maintaining the flexed position is more likely to isolate the rotation to the C1–C2 area so that C1–C2 dysfunction may be evident if the rotation is less (hypomobility) or more (hypermobility) than normal.

Pettman's Distraction Test.[136,137] This test is used to test the tectorial membrane. The patient lies supine with the head in neutral position. The examiner applies gentle

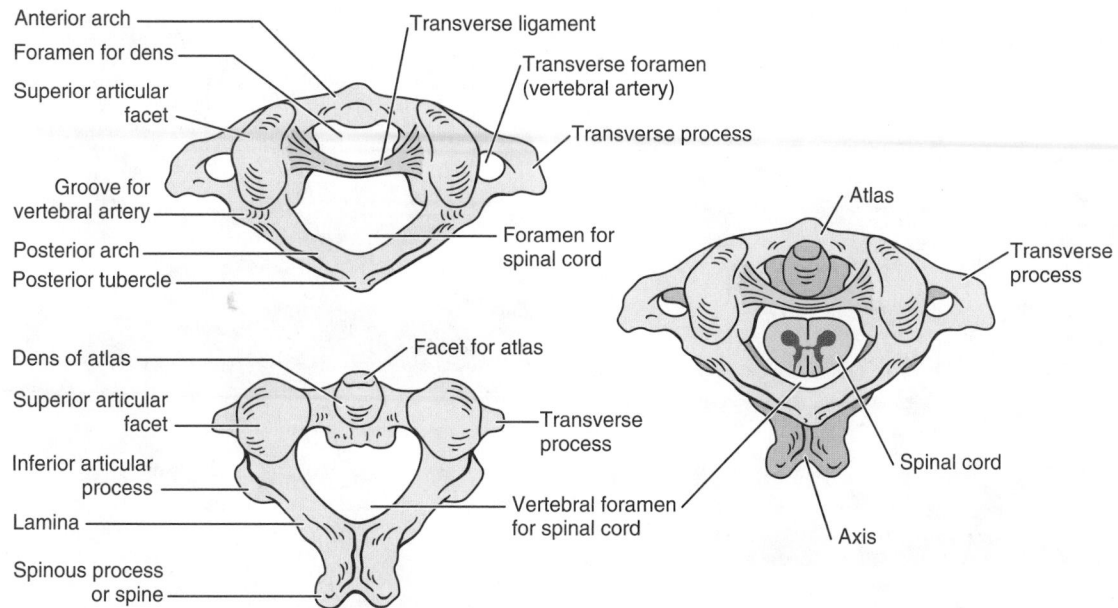

Figure 3-60 Relationship of C1 to C2 and the position of the transverse ligament.

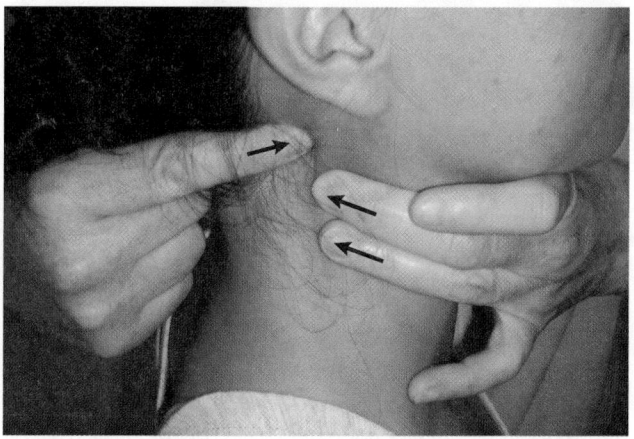

Figure 3-61 **Transverse ligament stress test.** Kaale's alternate method.

traction to the head. Provided no symptoms are produced, the patient's head is lifted forward, flexing the spine, and traction is reapplied. If the patient complains of symptoms, such as pain, or paresthesia in the second position, then the test is considered positive for a lax tectorial membrane (Figure 3-63).

Tests for First Rib Mobility
Although the first rib would normally be included with assessment of the thoracic spine, the examiner should always test for mobility of the first rib when examining the cervical spine, especially if side flexion is limited and there is pain or tenderness in the area of the first rib or T1.

✓ For the first test, the patient lies supine while fully supported. The examiner palpates the first rib bilaterally lateral to T1 and places his or her fingers along the path of the patient's ribs just posterior to the clavicles (Figure 3-64, *A*). While palpating the ribs, the examiner notes the movement of both first ribs as the patient takes a deep breath in and out, and any asymmetry is noted. The examiner then palpates one first rib and side flexes the head to the opposite side until the rib is felt to move up. The range of neck side flexion is noted. The side flexion is then repeated to the opposite side, and results from the two sides are compared. Asymmetry may be caused by hypomobility of the first rib or tightness of the scalene muscles on the same side.

For the second test, the patient lies prone, and the examiner again palpates the first rib (Figure 3-64, *B*). Using the thumb, reinforced by the other thumb, the examiner pushes the rib caudally, noting the amount of movement, end feel, and presence of pain. The other first rib is tested in a similar fashion, and the two sides are compared. Normally, a firm tissue stretch is felt with no pain, except possibly where the examiner's thumbs are compressing soft tissue against the rib.

Tests for Thoracic Outlet Syndrome
See Special Tests in Chapter 5.

Reflexes and Cutaneous Distribution
If the examiner suspects neurological involvement during the assessment, reflex testing and cutaneous sensation should be tested. For the cervical spine, the following reflexes should be checked for differences between the two sides, as shown in Figure 3-65: biceps (C5 to C6), the brachioradialis (C5 to C6), the triceps (C7 to C8),

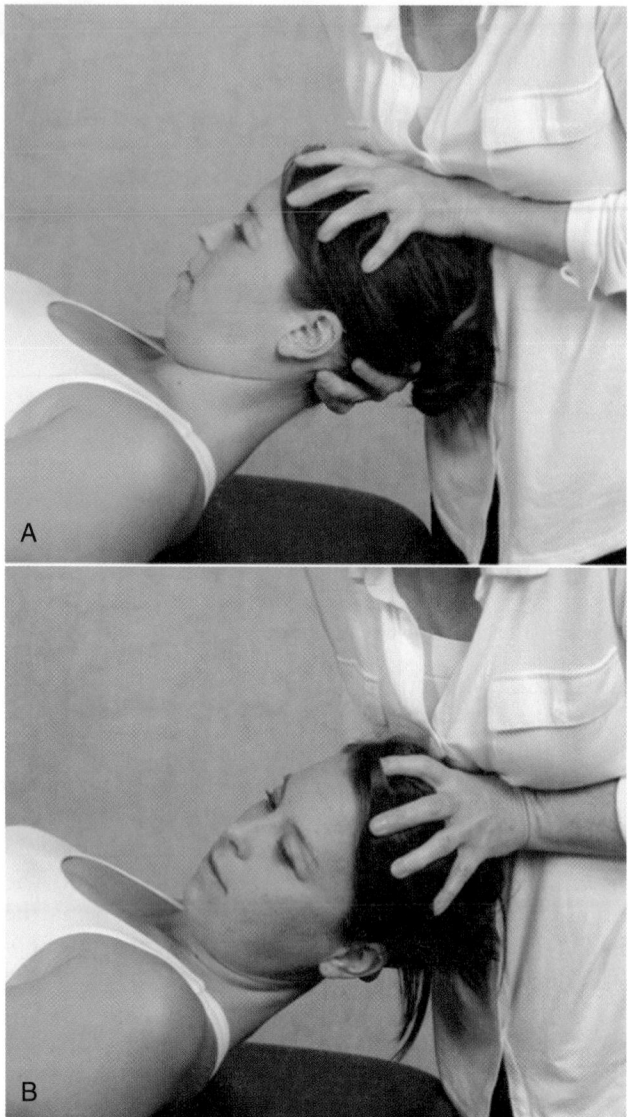

Figure 3-62 **Cervical flexion rotation test. A,** Flexion. **B,** Rotation in flexion.

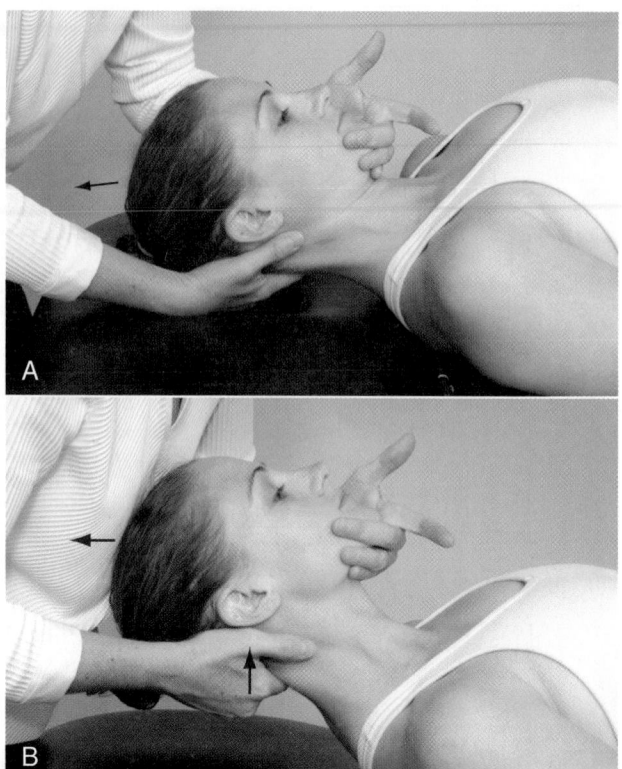

Figure 3-63 Pettman's distraction test. A, First position. **B,** Second (flexed) position.

and the jaw jerk (cranial nerve V). Bland[32] felt the jaw jerk was a useful diagnostic test. A normal (negative) jaw jerk combined with positive (exaggerated) tendon reflexes in the upper limb suggested the lesion was below the foramen magnum. If both reflexes were abnormal, then the lesion is above the pons.

Common Reflexes Checked in Cervical Spine Assessment

- Biceps (C5, C6)
- Triceps (C7, C8)
- Hoffmann sign (if upper motor neuron lesion suspected)

The reflexes are tested with a reflex hammer. The examiner tests the biceps and jaw jerk reflexes by placing his or her thumb over the patient's biceps tendon or at midpoint of the chin and then tapping the thumbnail with the reflex hammer to elicit the reflex. The jaw reflex may also be tested with a tongue depressor (see Figure 3-65, *B*). The examiner holds the tongue depressor firmly against the lower teeth while the patient relaxes the jaw and then strikes the tongue depressor with the reflex hammer. The brachioradialis and triceps reflexes are tested by directly tapping the tendon or muscle.

If an upper motor neuron lesion is suspected, the pathological reflexes (e.g., **Babinski reflex**) should be checked (see Table 1-33) and the deep tendon reflexes (see Table 1-31) may show hyperreflexia. **Hoffmann sign** is the upper limb equivalent of the Babinski test. To test for Hoffmann sign, the examiner holds the patient's middle finger and briskly flicks the distal phalanx. A positive sign is noted if the interphalangeal joint of the thumb of the same hand flexes/adducts. The fingers may also flex. Denno and Meadows[144] advocated a dynamic Hoffmann sign. The patient is asked to repeatedly flex and extend the head, and then the test is performed as described previously. Denno and Meadows believed that the dynamic test shows positive results earlier than the static or normal Hoffmann sign. Because an upper motor neuron lesion affects both the upper and lower limb, initially unilaterally and at later stages bilaterally, the Babinski test may be performed if desired. Clonus, most

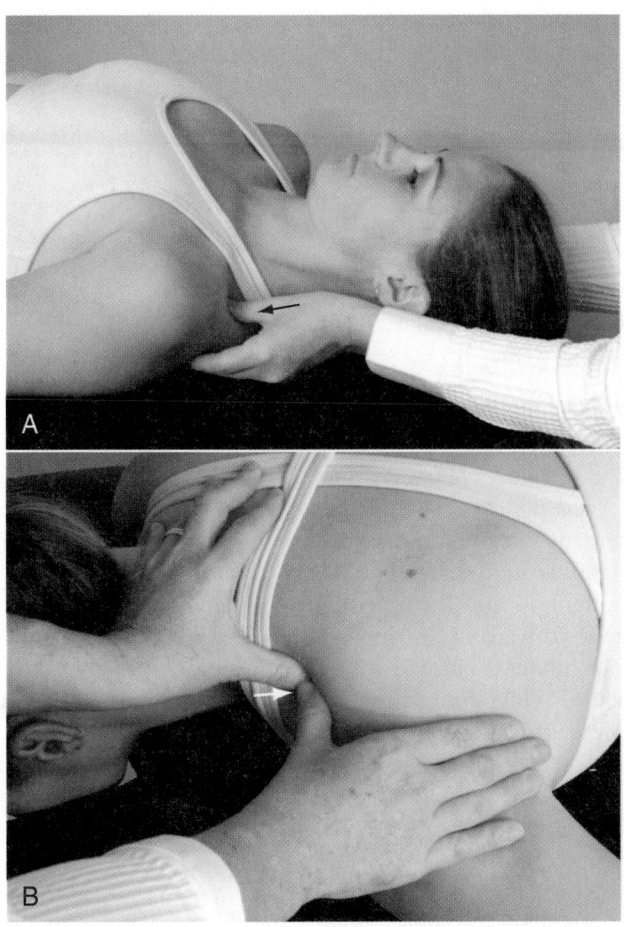

Figure 3-64 Testing mobility of the first rib. **A,** In supine. **B,** In prone.

easily seen by sudden dorsiflexion of the ankle resulting in three to five reflex twitches of the plantar flexors, is also a sign of an upper motor neuron lesion.[145,146]

The examiner then checks the dermatome pattern of the various nerve roots as well as the sensory distribution of the peripheral nerves (Figures 3-66 and 3-67) using a sensation scan (see previous discussion). Dermatomes vary from person to person and overlap a great deal, and the diagrams shown are estimations only. For example, C5 dermatome may stop distally on the radial side of the arm at the elbow, forearm, or wrist. Cervical radiculopathies may also show modified patterns. Levine et al.[47] point out that about 45% of patients have modified patterns and do not follow strict dermatome patterns. Classically, these patients also have referred pain into the trapezius and periscapular area posteriorly, and some will have pain into the breast area anteriorly.

Because of the spinal cord and associated nerve roots and their relation to the other bony and soft tissues in the cervical spine, referred pain is a relatively common experience in lesions of the cervical spine. Within the cervical spine, the intervertebral discs, facet joints, and other bony and soft tissues may refer pain to other segments of the neck (dermatomes) or to the head, the shoulder, the scapular area, and the whole of the upper limb (Figures 3-68 and 3-69).[45,61] Table 3-25 shows the muscles of the cervical spine and their referral of pain.

Brachial Plexus Injuries of the Cervical Spine[147,148]

Erb-Duchenne Paralysis. This paralysis is an upper brachial plexus injury involving injury to the upper nerve

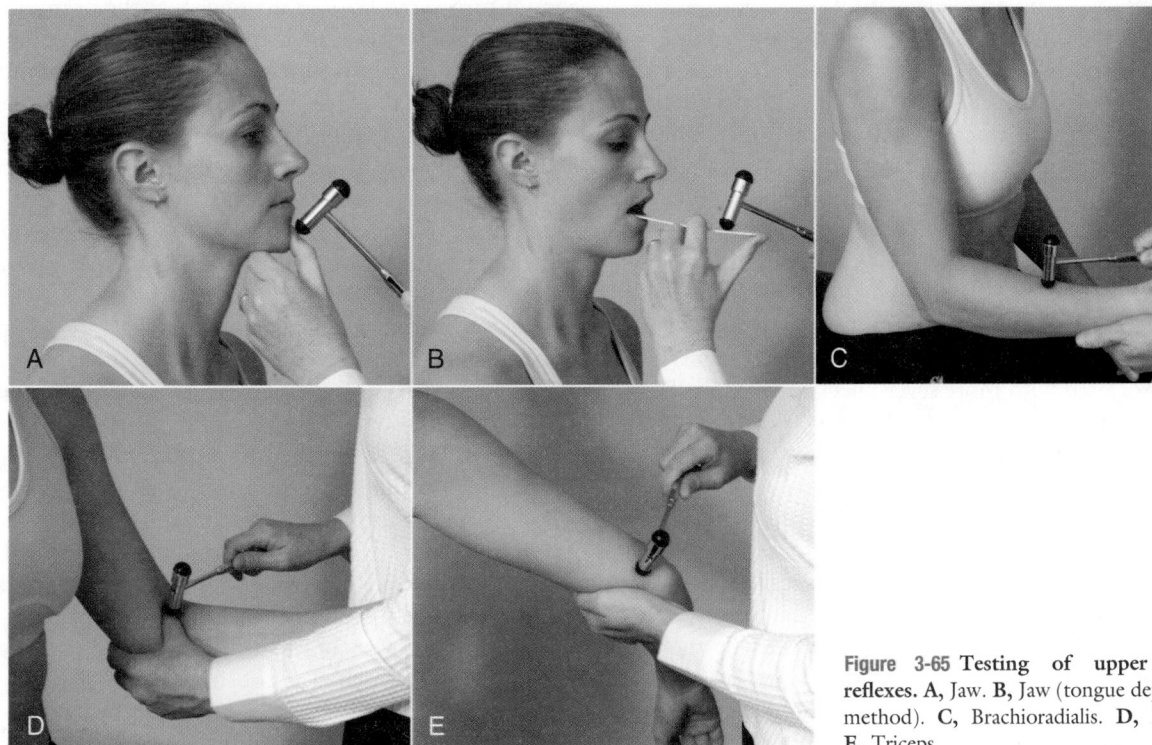

Figure 3-65 Testing of upper limb reflexes. A, Jaw. **B,** Jaw (tongue depressor method). **C,** Brachioradialis. **D,** Biceps. **E,** Triceps.

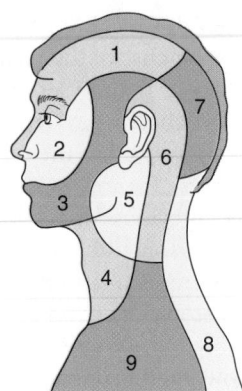

Figure 3-66 Sensory nerve distribution of the head, neck, and face. *1,* Ophthalmic nerve. *2,* Maxillary nerve. *3,* Mandibular nerve. *4,* Transverse cutaneous nerve of neck (C2–C3). *5,* Greater auricular nerve (C2–C3). *6,* Lesser auricular nerve (C2). *7,* Greater occipital nerve (C2–C3). *8,* Cervical dorsal rami (C3–C5). *9,* Suprascapular nerve (C5–C6).

roots (C5, C6) as a result of compression or stretching. The injury frequently occurs at Erb's point. With this injury, it is primarily the muscles of the shoulder region and elbow that are affected; the muscles of the hand (especially the intrinsic muscles) are not involved. However, sensation over the radial surfaces of the forearm and hand and the deltoid area are affected.

Klumpke (Dejerine-Klumpke) Paralysis. This injury involves the lower brachial plexus and results from compression or stretching of the lower nerve roots (C8, T1). Atrophy and weakness are evident in the muscles of the forearm and hand as well as in the triceps. The obvious changes are in the distal aspects of the upper limb. The resultant injury is a functionless hand. Sensory loss occurs primarily on the ulnar side of the forearm and hand.

Brachial Plexus Birth Palsy.[149] These injuries to the brachial plexus occur in 0.1% to 0.4% of births with the majority showing full recovery within 2 months. Those infants who have not recovered within 3 months are at considerable risk to decreased strength and range of motion in the upper limb.

Burners and Stingers.[150,151] These are transient injuries to the brachial plexus, which may be the result of trauma (see Figure 3-10) combined with factors, such as stenosis or a degenerative disc (spondylosis). Recurrent burners are not associated with more severe neck injury, but their effect on the nerve may be cumulative.[150]

Joint Play Movements

The joint play movements that are carried out in the cervical spine may be general movements (called **passive intervertebral movements [PIVMs]**) that involve the entire cervical spine (first four below) or specific movements isolated to one segment. As the joint play movements are performed, the examiner should note any decreased ROM, pain, or difference in end feel.

Joint Play Movements of the Cervical Spine

- Side glide of the cervical spine (general)
- Anterior glide of the cervical spine (general)
- Posterior glide of the cervical spine (general)
- Traction glide of the cervical spine (general)
- Rotation of the occiput on C1 (specific)
- Posteroanterior central vertebral pressure (specific)
- Posteroanterior unilateral vertebral pressure (specific)
- Transverse vertebral pressure (specific)

Side Glide. The examiner holds the patient's head and moves it from side-to-side, keeping the head parallel to the shoulders (Figure 3-70).[152]

Anterior and Posterior Glide. The examiner holds the patient's head with one hand around the occiput and one hand around the chin, taking care to ensure that the patient is not choked.[73] The examiner then draws the head forward in the same plane as the shoulders for anterior glide (Figure 3-71) and posteriorly for posterior glide. While doing these movements, the examiner must prevent flexion and extension of the head.

Traction Glide. The examiner places one hand around the patient's chin and the other hand on the occiput.[75] Traction is then applied in a straight longitudinal direction with the majority of the pull being through the occiput (Figure 3-72).

Vertebral Pressures. For the last three joint play movements (Figure 3-73), the patient lies prone with the forehead resting on the back of the hands.[132] These techniques are specific to each vertebra and are applied to each vertebra in turn, or at least to the ones that the examination has indicated may be affected by pathology. They are sometimes called **passive accessory intervertebral movements (PAIVMs)**.[71] The examiner palpates the spinous processes of the cervical spine, starting at the C2 spinous process and working downward to the T2 spinous process. The positions of the examiner's hands, fingers, and thumbs in performing PACVPs are shown in Figure 3-73, *A.* Pressure is then applied through the examiner's thumbs pushing carefully from the shoulders, and the vertebra is pushed forward. The examiner must take care to apply pressure slowly, with carefully controlled movements, in order to "feel" the movement, which in reality is minimal. This "springing test" may be repeated several times to determine the quality of the movement and the end feel. Hypomobility would be indicated by abnormal resistance to movement, abnormal end feel, or reproduction of local or referred pain.[141] End range can be determined by feeling the adjacent spinous process (above or below). When the adjacent spinous process begins to move, the end range of the vertebra to which the PACVP is being applied has been reached.

For **posteroanterior unilateral vertebral pressure (PAUVP)**, the examiner's fingers move laterally away

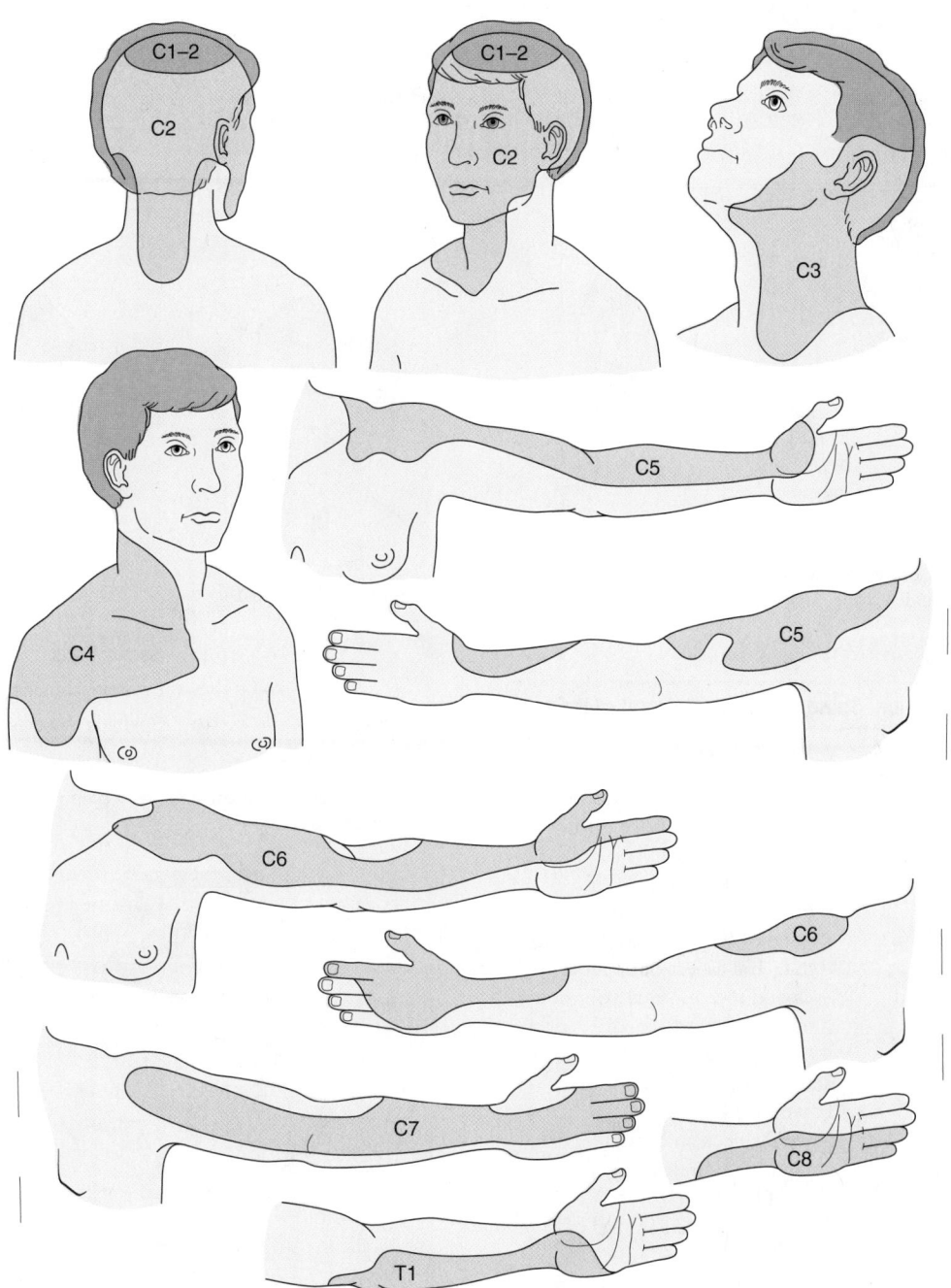

Figure 3-67 Dermatomes of the cervical spine.

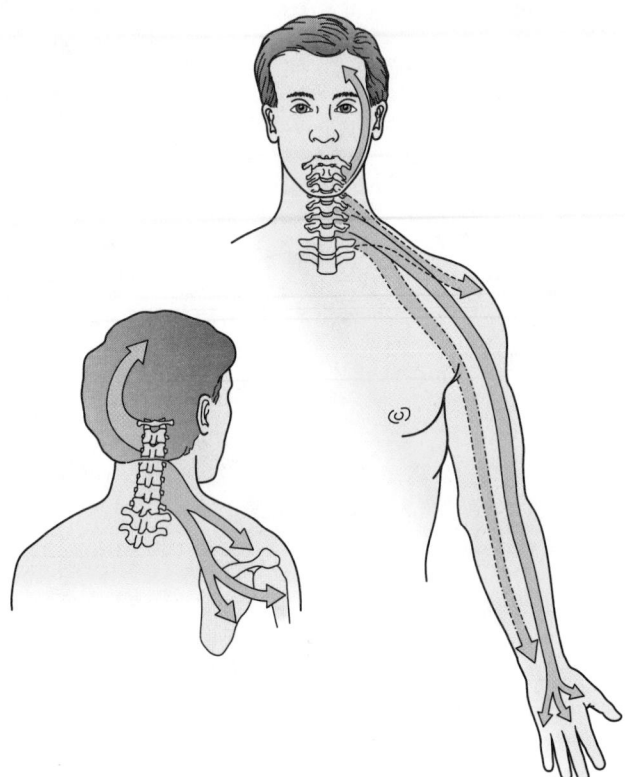

Figure 3-68 Referral of symptoms from the cervical spine to areas of the spine, head, shoulder girdle, and upper limb.

TABLE **3-25**

Muscles of the Cervical Spine and Their Referral of Pain

Muscle	Referral Pattern
Trapezius	Right and left occiput, lateral aspect of head above ear to behind eye, tip of jaw Spinous processes to medial border of scapula and along spine of scapula; may also refer to lateral aspect of upper arm
Sternocleidomastoid	Back and top of head, front of ear over forehead to medial aspect of eye; cheek Behind ear, ear to forehead
Splenius capitis	Top of head
Splenius cervicis	Posterior neck and shoulder angle, side of head to eye
Semispinalis cervicis	Back of head
Semispinalis capitis	Band around head at level of forehead
Multifidus	Occiput to posterior neck and shoulder angle to base of spine of scapula
Suboccipital	Lateral aspect of head to eye
Scalenes	Medial border of scapula and anterior chest down posterolateral aspect of arm to anterolateral and posterolateral aspect of hand

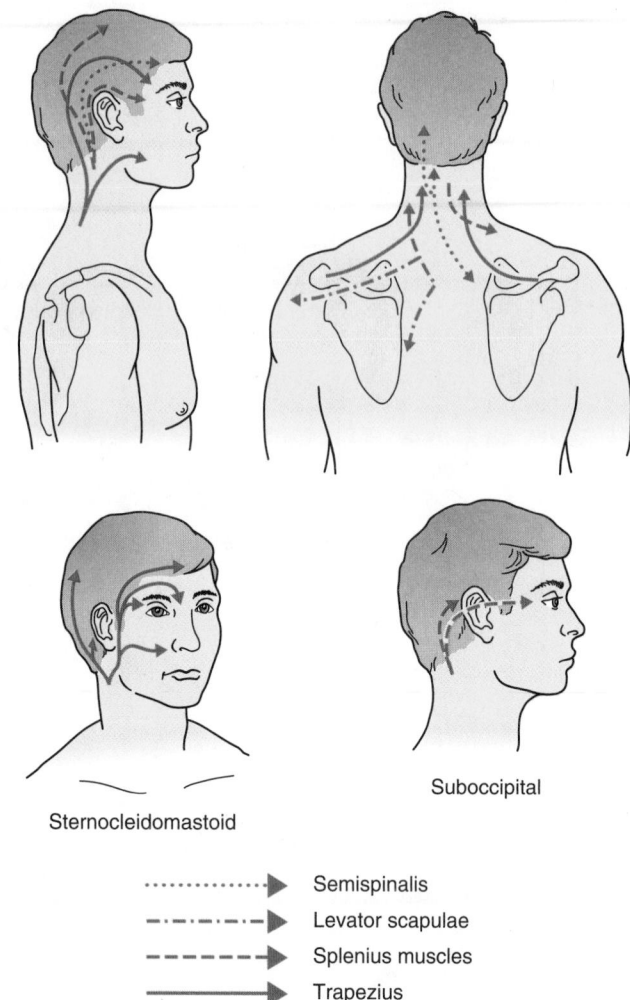

Suboccipital

Sternocleidomastoid

............▶ Semispinalis
—·—·—·—▶ Levator scapulae
— — — —▶ Splenius muscles
————————▶ Trapezius

Figure 3-69 Muscles and their referred pain patterns. Diagram shows primarily one side.

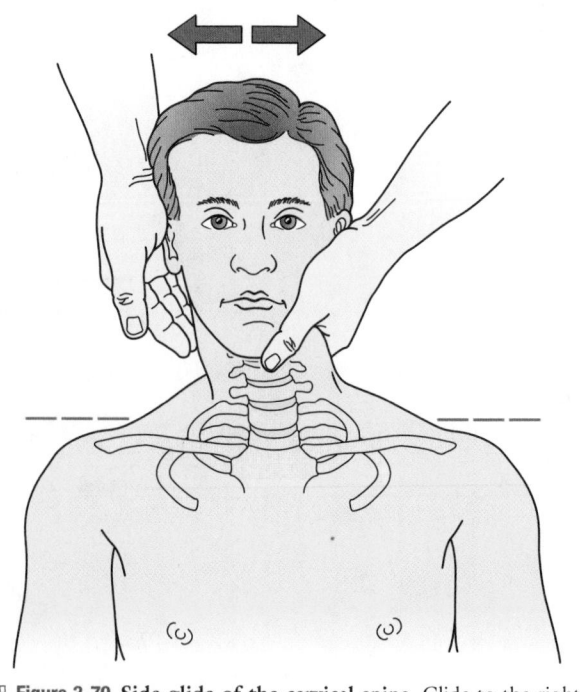

Figure 3-70 Side glide of the cervical spine. Glide to the right is illustrated.

from the tip of the spinous process so that the thumbs rest on the lamina or transverse process, about 2 to 3 cm (1 to 1.5 inches) lateral to the spinous process of the cervical or thoracic vertebra (see Figure 3-73, *B*). Anterior springing pressure is applied as in the central pressure technique. This pressure causes a minimal rotation of the vertebral body. If one was to palpate the spinous process while doing the technique, the spinous process would be felt to move to the side the pressure is applied. Similarly, end range can be determined by feeling the adjacent spinous process (above or below). When the adjacent spinous process begins to rotate, the end range of the

vertebra to which the PAUVP is being applied has been reached. Both sides should be done and compared.

For **transverse vertebral pressure,** the examiner's thumbs are placed along the side of the spinous process of the cervical or thoracic spine (see Figure 3-73, *C*). The examiner then applies a transverse springing pressure to the side of the spinous process, feeling for the quality of movement. This pressure also causes rotation of the vertebral body, and end range can be determined by feeling for rotation of the adjacent spinous process.

Palpation

If, after completing the examination of the cervical spine, the examiner decides the problem is in another joint, palpation should be delayed until that joint is completely examined. However, during palpation of the cervical spine, the examiner should note any tenderness, trigger points, muscle spasm, or other signs and symptoms that may indicate the source of the pathology. Pain provocation and landmark location has been found to have the greatest intrarater reliability with palpation.[153] As with any palpation, the examiner should note the texture of the skin and surrounding bony and soft tissues on the posterior, lateral, and anterior aspects of the neck. Usually, palpation is performed with the patient supine so that maximum relaxation of the neck muscles is possible. However, the examiner may palpate with the patient sitting (patient resting the head on forearms that are resting on something at shoulder height) or lying prone (on a table with a face hole) if it is more comfortable for the patient.

To palpate the posterior structures, the examiner stands at the patient's head behind the patient. With the patient lying supine, the patient's head is "cupped" in the examiner's hand while the examiner palpates with the fingers of both hands. For the lateral and anterior structures, the examiner stands at the patient's side. If the examiner suspects that the problem is in the cervical

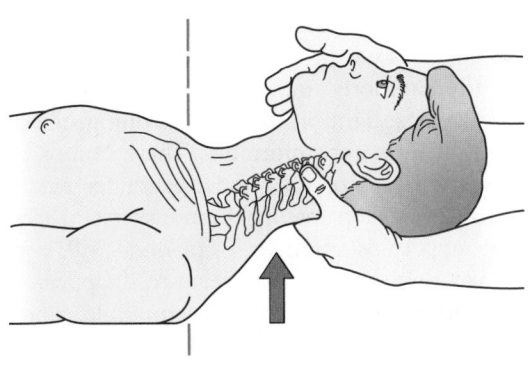

Figure 3-71 Anterior glide of the cervical spine.

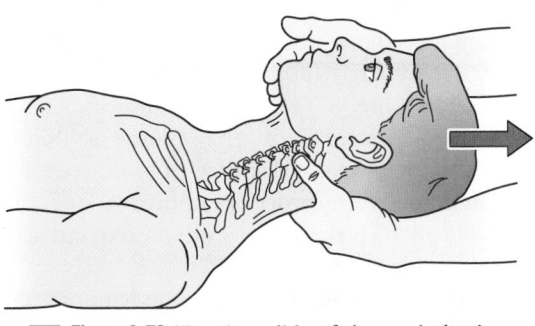

Figure 3-72 Traction glide of the cervical spine.

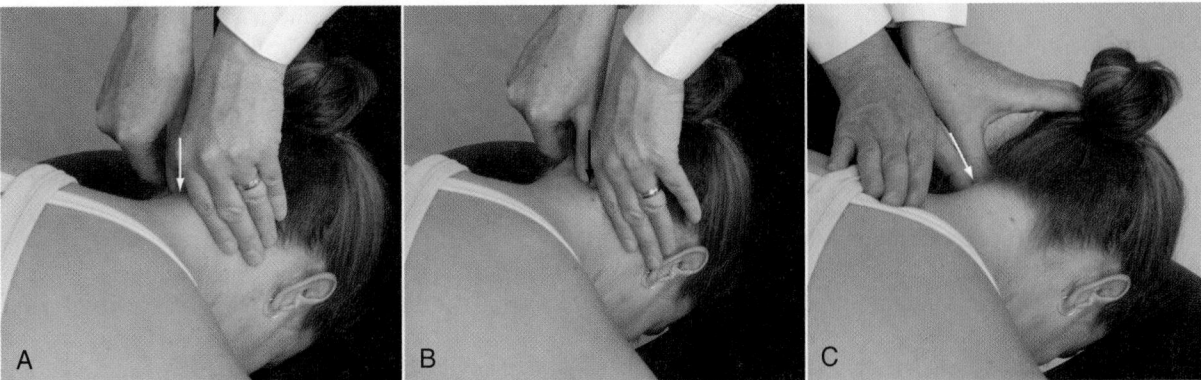

Figure 3-73 Vertebral pressures to the cervical spine. A, Posteroanterior central vertebral pressure on tip of spinous process. **B,** Posteroanterior unilateral vertebral pressure on posterior aspect of transverse process. **C,** Transverse vertebral pressure on side of spinous process.

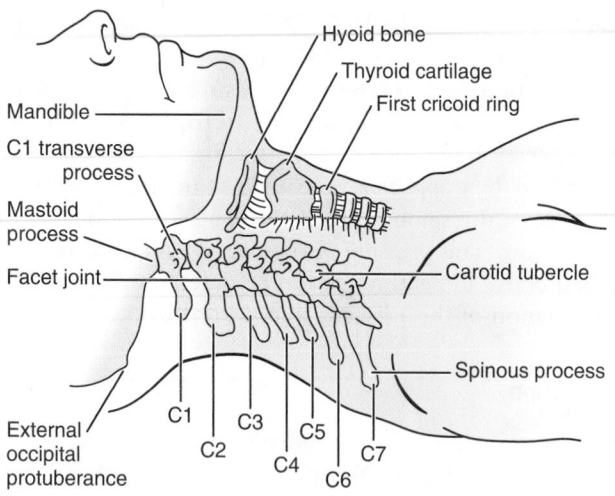

Figure 3-74 Palpation landmarks of the cervical spine.

spine, palpation is done on the following structures (Figure 3-74).

Posterior Aspect

External Occipital Protuberance. The protuberance may be found in the posterior midline. The examiner palpates the posterior skull in midline and moves caudally until coming to a point where the fingers "dip" inward. The part of the bone just before the dip is the external occipital protuberance. The inion, or "bump of knowledge," is the most obvious point on the external occipital protuberance and lies in the midline of the occiput.

Spinous Processes and Facet Joints of Cervical Vertebrae. The spinous processes of C2, C6, and C7 are the most obvious. If the examiner palpates the occiput of the skull and descends in the midline, the C2 spinous process will be palpated as the first bump. The next spinous processes that are most obvious are C6 and C7, although C3, C4, and C5 can be differentiated with careful palpation and by flexing the spine. The examiner can differentiate between C6 and C7 by passively flexing and extending the patient's neck. With this movement, the C6 spinous process moves in and out, and the C7 spinous process remains stationary. The movements between the spinous processes of C2 through C7 or T1 may be palpated by feeling between each set of spinous processes. While palpating between the spinous processes, the examiner can use the opposite hand or his/her chest to push the head into nodding flexion and releasing, causing the cervical spine to flex and extend; the palpating finger will feel the movement between the two spinous processes and tension (when flexing) in the interspinous and supraspinous ligaments. Relative movement between the cervical vertebrae can then be determined (i.e., hypomobility, normal movement, or hypermobility).[73] The facet joint may be palpated 1.3 to 2.5 cm (0.5 to 1 inch) lateral to the spinous process. Usually the facet joints are not felt as distinct structures but rather as a hard bony mass under the fingers. The muscles in the adjacent area may be palpated for tenderness, swelling, and other signs of pathology. Careful palpation should also include the suboccipital structures.

Mastoid Processes (Below and Behind Ear Lobe). If the examiner palpates the skull following the posterior aspect of the ear, there will be a point on the skull at which the finger again dips inward. The point just before the dip is the mastoid process.

Lateral Aspect

Transverse Processes of Cervical Vertebrae. The C1 transverse process is the easiest to palpate. The examiner first palpates the mastoid process and then moves inferiorly and slightly anteriorly until a hard bump is felt. If the examiner applies slight pressure to the bump, the patient should say it feels uncomfortable. These bumps are the transverse processes of C1. If the examiner rotates the patient's head while palpating the transverse processes of C1, the uppermost transverse process will protrude farther, and the lower one will seem to disappear. If this does not occur, the segment is hypomobile. The other transverse processes may be palpated if the musculature is sufficiently relaxed. After the C1 transverse process has been located, the examiner moves caudally, feeling for similar bumps. Normally, the bumps are not directly inferior but rather follow the lordotic path of the cervical vertebrae under the sternocleidomastoid muscle. These structures are situated more anteriorly than one might suspect (see Figure 3-74). During flexion, the space between the mastoid and the transverse processes increases. On extension, it decreases. On side flexion, the mastoid and transverse processes approach one another on the side to which the head is side flexed and separate on the other side.[73]

Lymph Nodes and Carotid Arteries. The lymph nodes are palpable only if they are swollen. The nodes lie along the line of the sternocleidomastoid muscle. The carotid pulse may be palpated in the midportion of the neck, between the sternocleidomastoid muscle and the trachea. The examiner should determine whether the pulse is normal and equal on both sides.

Temporomandibular Joints, Mandible, and Parotid Glands. The temporomandibular joints may be palpated anterior to the external ear. The examiner may either palpate directly over the joint or place the little or index finger (pulp forward) in the external ear to feel for movement in the joint. The examiner can then move the fingers along the length of the mandible, feeling for any abnormalities. The angle of the mandible is at the level of the C2 vertebra. Normally, the parotid gland is not palpable, because it lies over the angle of the mandible. If it is swollen, however, it is palpable as a soft, boggy structure.

Anterior Aspect

Hyoid Bone, Thyroid Cartilage, and First Cricoid Ring. The hyoid bone may be palpated as part of the superior part of the trachea above the thyroid cartilage anterior to the C2–C3 vertebrae. The thyroid cartilage lies anterior to the C4–C5 vertebrae. With the neck in a neutral position, the thyroid cartilage can be moved easily. In extension, it is tight and crepitations may be felt. Adjacent to the cartilage is the thyroid gland, which the examiner should palpate. If the gland is abnormal, it will be tender and enlarged. The cricoid ring is the first part of the trachea and lies above the site for an emergency tracheostomy. The ring moves when the patient swallows. Rough palpation of the ring may cause the patient to gag. While palpating the hyoid bone, the examiner should ask the patient to swallow; normally, the bone should move and cause no pain. The cricoid ring and thyroid cartilage also move when palpated as the patient swallows.

Paranasal Sinuses. Returning to the face, the examiner should palpate the paranasal sinuses (frontal and maxillary) for signs of tenderness and swelling (Figure 3-75).

First Three Ribs. The examiner palpates the manubrium sternum and, moving the fingers laterally, follows the path of the first three ribs posteriorly, feeling whether one rib is protruded more than the others. The examiner should palpate the ribs individually and with care, because it is difficult to palpate the ribs as they pass under the clavicle. The patient should be asked to breathe in and out deeply a few times so that the examiner can compare the movements of the ribs during breathing. Normally, there is equal mobility on both sides. The first rib is more prone to pathology than the second and third ribs and can refer pain to the neck and/or shoulder.

Supraclavicular Fossa. The examiner can palpate the supraclavicular fossa, which is superior to the clavicle. Normally, the fossa is a smooth indentation. The examiner should palpate for swelling after trauma (possible fractured clavicle), abnormal soft tissue (possible swollen glands), and abnormal bony tissue (possible cervical rib). In addition, the examiner should palpate the sternocleidomastoid muscle along its length for signs of pathology, especially in cases of torticollis.

Diagnostic Imaging

Imaging techniques should primarily be performed as an adjunct to the clinical examination. The appearance of many degenerative changes or anatomical or congenital variations is relatively high in the cervical spine, and many of the changes have no relationship with the patient's complaints.[154]

Plain Film Radiography

Normally, a standard set of x-rays for the cervical spine is made up of an anteroposterior (AP) view, a lateral view, and an open or odontoid ("through-the-mouth") view. Other views that may be included are the oblique view, flexion stress view (lateral view in flexion), and extension stress view (lateral view in extension). For osteoarthritis, the x-rays commonly taken are AP (C3 to C7), lateral, and oblique. In cases of trauma and an alert and stable

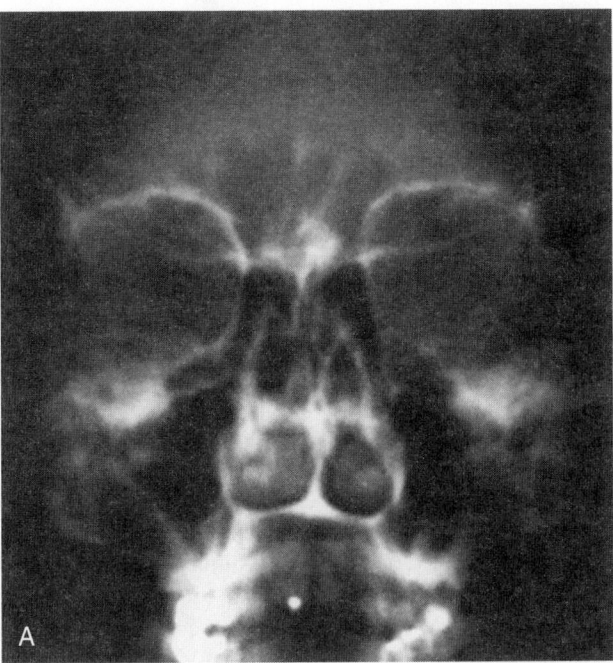
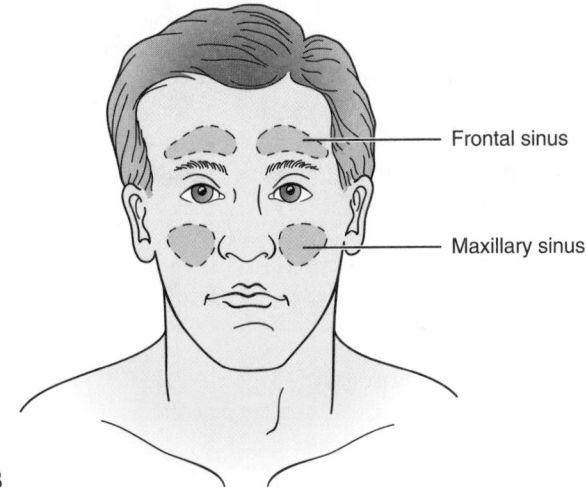

Figure 3-75 Paranasal sinuses. Radiograph (**A**) and illustration (**B**) of frontal and maxillary sinuses.

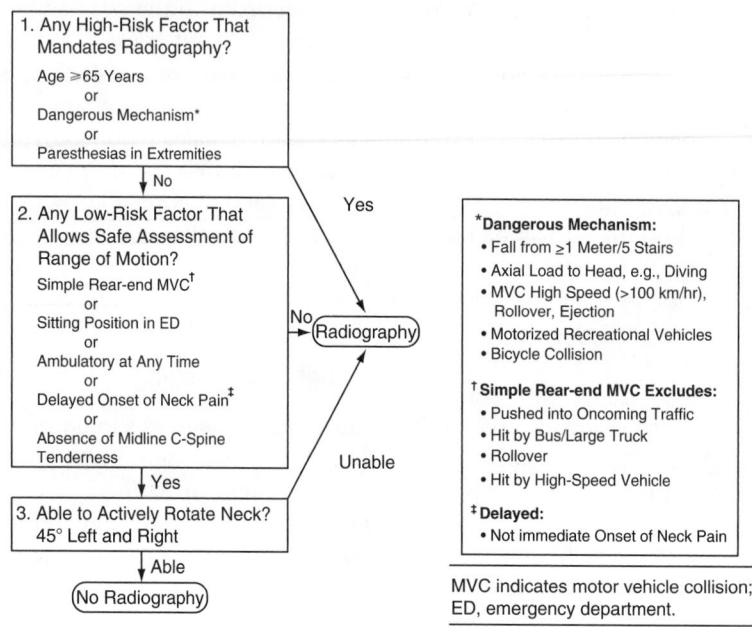

For Alert (Glasgow Coma Scale Score = 15)
and Stable Trauma Patients Where
Cervical Spine (C-Spine) Injury is a Concern

Figure 3-76 ✓ **The Canadian C-Spine Rule.** (From Stiell IG, Wells GA, Vandemheen KL, et al: The Canadian C-spine rule for radiography in alert and stable trauma patients. JAMA 286[15]:1846, 2001.)

patient, the Canadian C-Spine Rule[155,156] may be used to determine if diagnostic imaging is required (Figure 3-76). The National Emergency X-Radiography Utilization Study (NEXUS) low risk criteria is another clinical decision rule related to the use of x-rays.[157,158]

Common X-Ray Views of the Cervical Spine

- Anteroposterior view (see Figures 3-77 and 3-78)
- Lateral view (see Figure 3-79, A)
- Open mouth of odontoid view (following trauma) (see Figure 3-85)
- Oblique view (see Figure 3-87)
- Flexion stress view (lateral view in flexion) (see Figure 3-79, B)
- Extension stress view (lateral view in extension (see Figure 3-79, C)
- Swimmer's view (following trauma) (see Chapter 5, Figure 5-191, B)

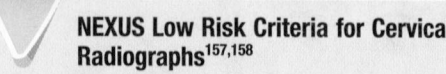

NEXUS Low Risk Criteria for Cervical Radiographs[157,158]

Cervical spine radiographs are indicated for patients with trauma unless they meet all of the following criteria:
- No posterior or midline cervical spine tenderness
- Normal levels of alertness
- No motor or sensory neurological deficit
- No clinically apparent painful injury that may distract patient from cervical injury
- No evidence of intoxication

NEXUS, National Emergency X-Radiography Utilization Study.

Anteroposterior View. The examiner should look for or note the following (Figures 3-77 and 3-78): the shape of the vertebrae, the presence of any lateral wedging or osteophytes, the disc space, and the presence of a cervical rib. Frontal alignment should also be ascertained.

Lateral View. Lateral views of the cervical spine give the greatest amount of radiological information. The examiner should look for or note the following (Figures 3-79 to 3-82):

1. *Normal or abnormal curvature.* The curvature may be highly variable, because 20% to 40% of normal spines have a straight or slightly kyphotic curve in neutral position.[159] McAviney et al.[160] reported the normal lordosis in the cervical spine as 30° to 40° (see Figure 3-7) when measuring the lines intersecting the posterior aspects of the vertebral bodies of C2 and C7. They felt patients with a lordosis of less than 20° were more likely to experience cervicogenic symptoms. Are the "lines" of the vertebrae normal? The line joining the anterior portion of the vertebral bodies (anterior vertebral line) should form a smooth, unbroken arc from C2 to C7 (see Figure 3-80). Similar lines should be seen for the posterior vertebral bodies (posterior vertebral line), which form the anterior aspect of the spinal canal, and the posterior aspect of the spinal canal (posterior canal line). Disruption of any of these lines would be an indication of instability possibly caused by ligamentous injury.

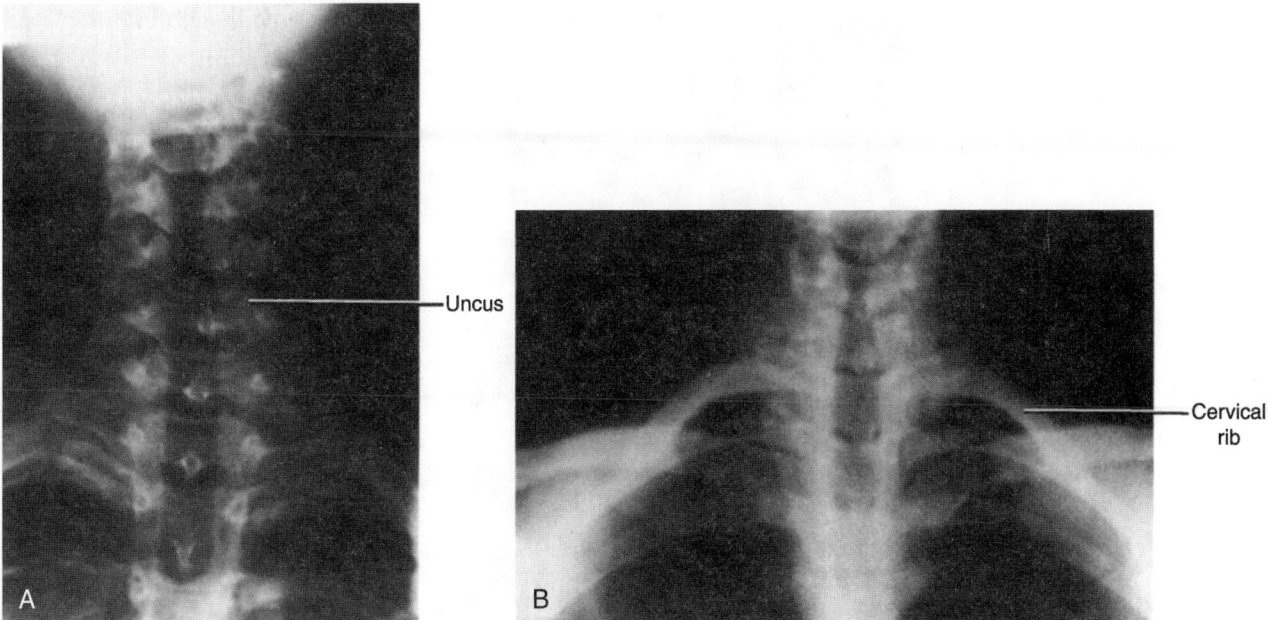

Figure 3-77 **Anteroposterior films of the cervical spine. A,** Normal spine. **B,** Cervical rib.

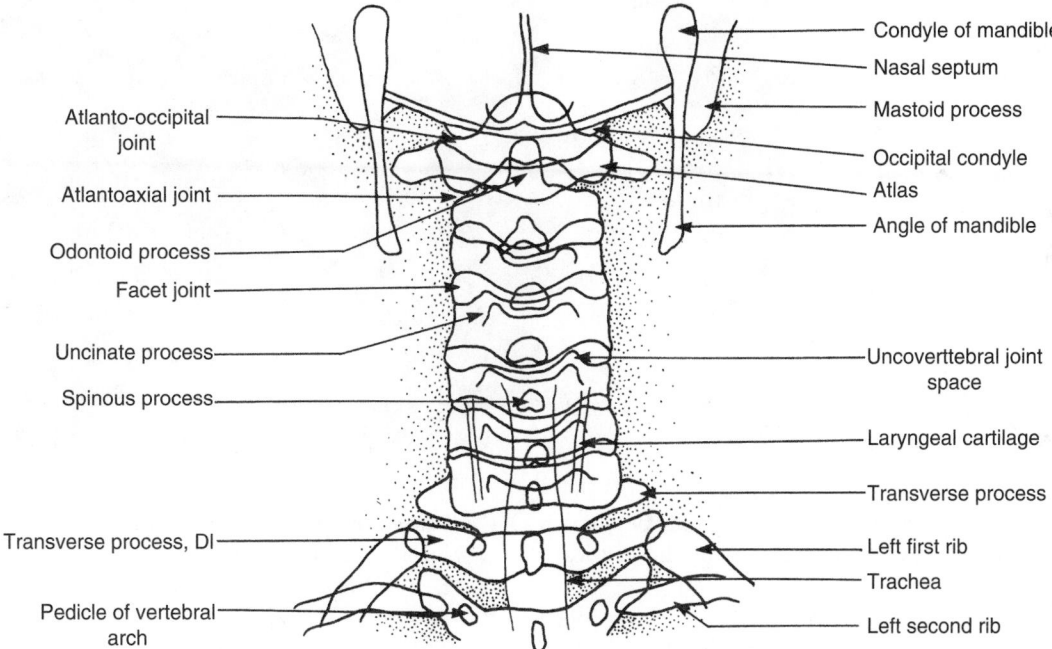

Figure 3-78 Diagram of structures seen on anteroposterior cervical spine film.

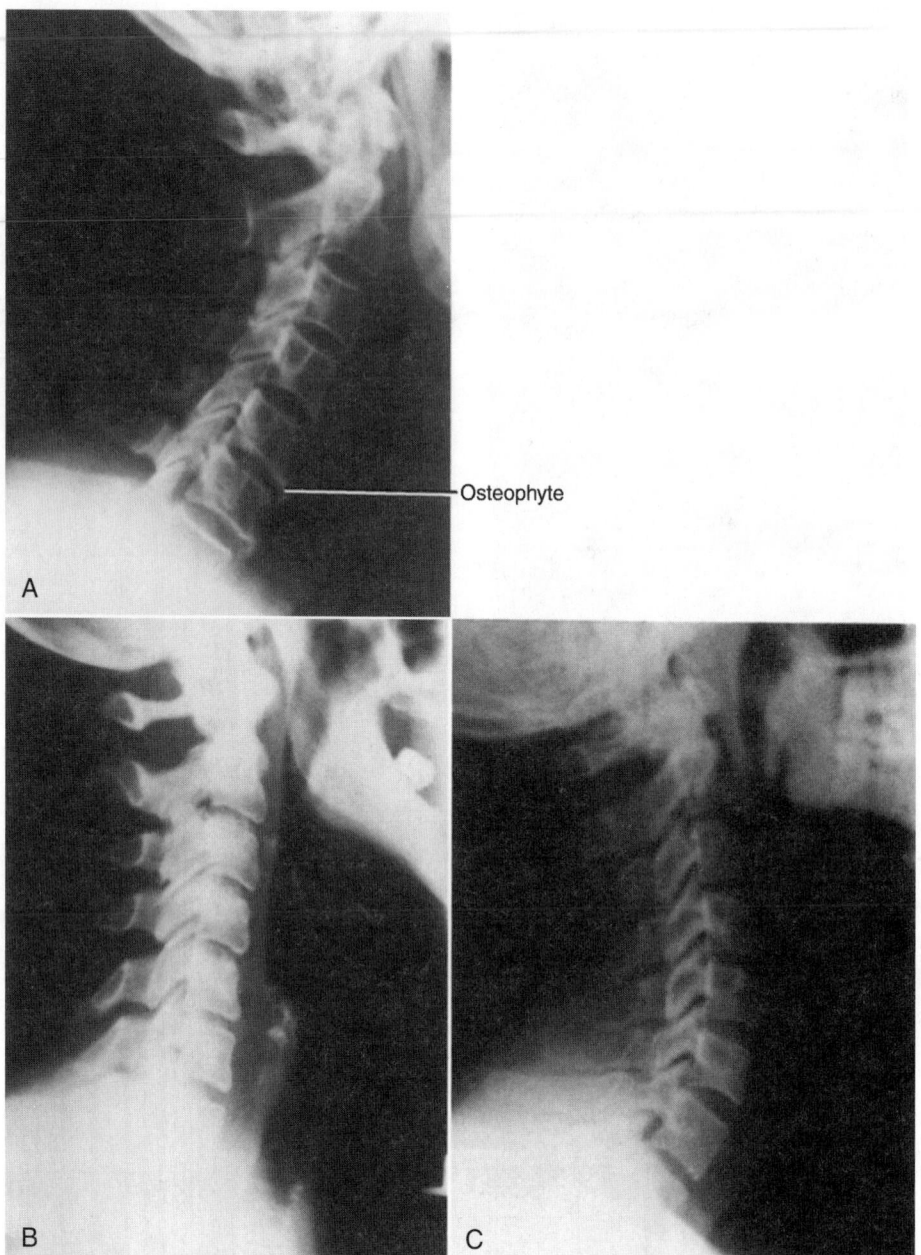

—Osteophyte

A

B

C

Figure 3-79 Lateral radiograph of the cervical spine. A, Normal curve showing osteophytic lipping. **B,** Cervical spine in flexion. **C,** Cervical spine in extension.

2. *"Kinking" of the cervical spine.* Kinking may be indicative of a subluxation or dislocation in the cervical spine.

3. *General shape of the vertebrae.* Is there any fusion, collapse, or wedging? The examiner should count the vertebrae, because x-ray films do not always show C7 or T1, and it is essential that they be visualized for a proper radiological examination.

4. *Displacement.* Do the vertebrae sit in normal alignment with one another (Figures 3-83 and 3-84)?

5. *Disc space.* Is it normal? Narrow? Narrowing may indicate cervical spondylosis (also called spondylosis deformans).

6. *Lipping at the vertebral edges.* Lipping indicates degeneration (see Figures 3-79, *A,* and 3-80).

7. *Osteophytes.* Osteophytes indicate degeneration or abnormal movement (instability) (see Figures 3-79, *A,* and 3-80).

8. *Ratio of the spinal canal diameter.* Normally, the ratio of the spinal canal diameter to the vertebral body diameter (Torg ratio) in the cervical spine is 1. If this ratio is less than 0.8, it is an indication of possible cervical stenosis.[50,161–164] This comparison is shown in Figure 3-81 (ratio AB:BC). Cantu[162] points out that this measurement is a static measurement and may not apply to stenosis that occurs during movement of the cervical spine.

9. *Prevertebral soft-tissue width.* Measured at the level of the anteroinferior border of the C3 vertebra, this width is normally 7 mm.[165] Edema or hemorrhage is

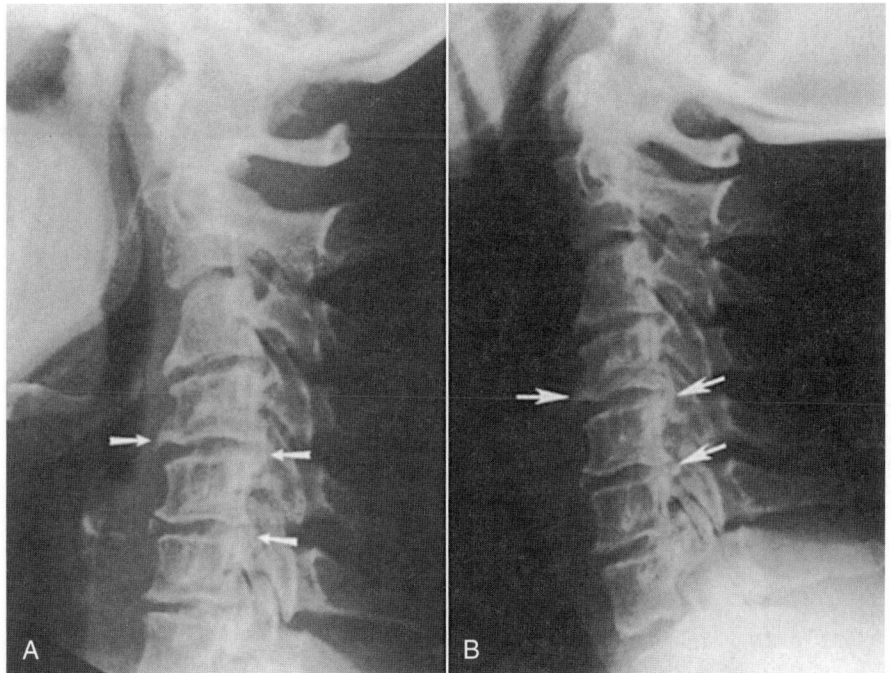

Figure 3-80 X-ray films of a 68-year-old man with multiple radiologic signs of cervical osteoarthritis *(arrows)*. **A,** The cervical spine in flexion, which is very limited. Note that the atlas tips up, as compared with that in **B.** All intervertebral disc spaces below C2–C3 are very narrow. Anterior and posterior osteophytes are apparent *(arrows)*. The spine extends very little in **B** and is quite straight in **A** (i.e., no significant flexion). (From Bland JH: Disorders of the cervical spine, Philadelphia, 1994, WB Saunders p. 213.)

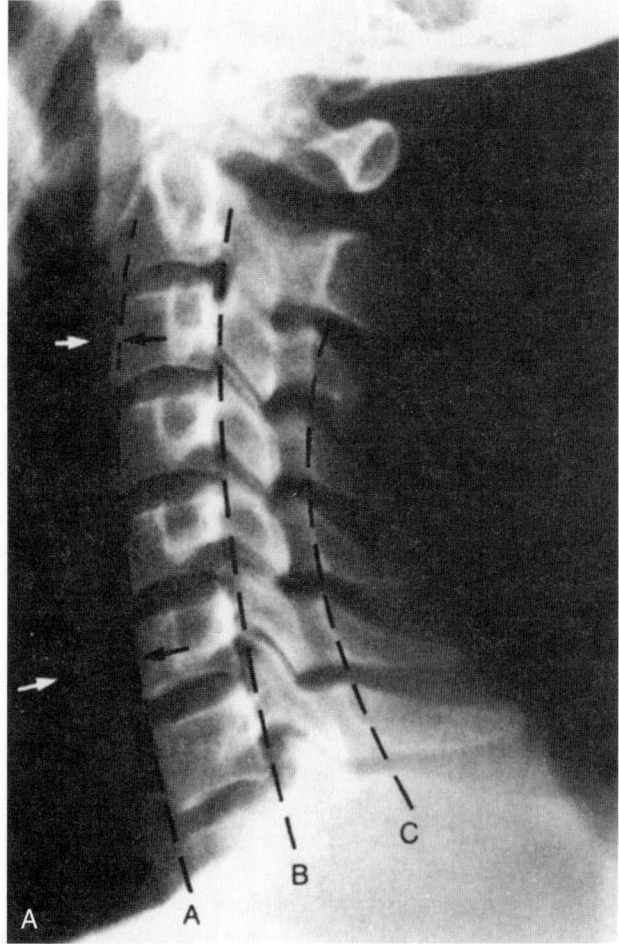

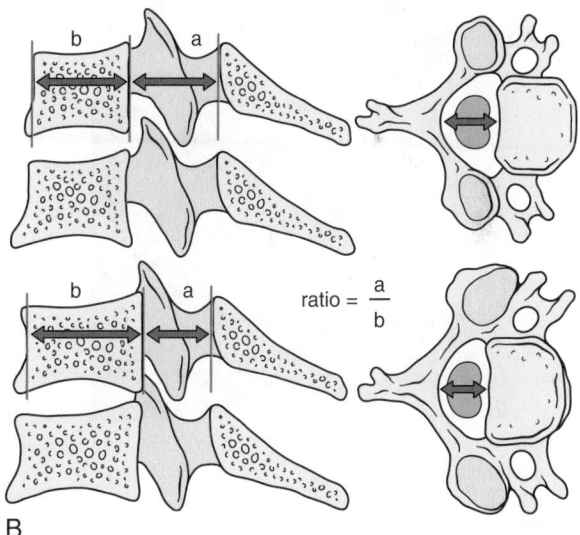

Figure 3-81 A, Normal cervical spine. Lateral projection. Note the alignment and appearance of the facet joints: *A,* anterior vertebral line; *B,* posterior vertebral line; *C,* posterior canal line. Retropharyngeal space *(between top arrows)* should not exceed 5 mm. Retrotracheal space *(between bottom arrows)* should not exceed 22 mm. **B,** The Torg ratio is calculated by dividing the shortest distance between the posterior vertebral body and the spinolaminar line *(a)* by the vertebral body width *(b)*. (**A,** Modified from Forrester DM, Brown JC: The radiology of joint disease, Philadelphia, 1987, W.B. Saunders, p. 408. **B,** Redrawn from McAlindon RJ: On field evaluation and management of head and neck injured athletes. Clin Sports Med 21:10, 2002. Adapted from Torg JS, Pavlov H: Cervical spinal stenosis with cord neuropraxia and transient quadriplegia. Clin Sports Med 6:115–133, 1987; with permission.)

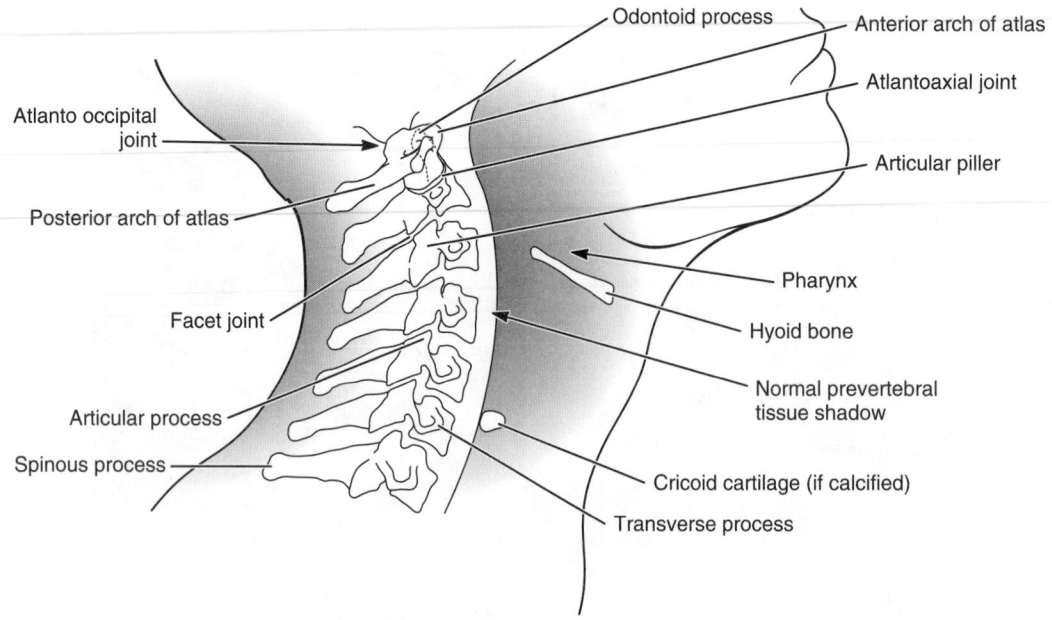

Figure 3-82 Diagram of structures seen on lateral film of the cervical spine.

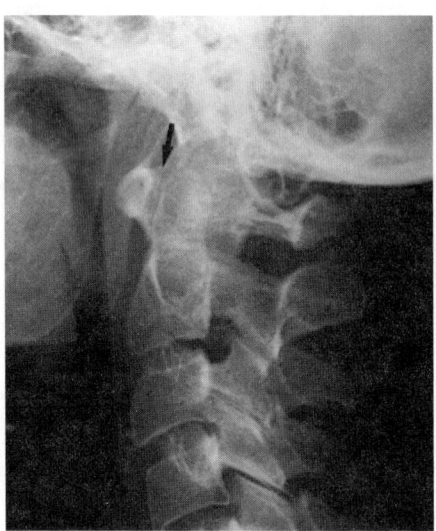

Figure 3-83 Atlantoaxial subluxation. Flexion view shows abnormal widening of the atlantoaxial space *(arrow)*, which measures 4 mm. (From Resnick D, Kransdorf MJ: Bone and joint imaging, Philadelphia, 2005, Saunders, p 883.)

suspected if the space is wider than 7 mm. The retropharyngeal space, lying between the anterior border of the vertebral body and the posterior border of the pharyngeal air shadow, should be 2 to 5 mm in width at C3. From C4 to C7, the space is called the **retrotracheal space** and should be 18 to 22 mm in width (see Figure 3-81).

10. *Subluxation of the facets.*
11. *Abnormal soft-tissue shadows.*
12. *Forward shifting of C1 on C2.* This finding indicates instability between C1 and C2. Normally, the joint

space between the odontoid process and the anterior arch of the atlas (sometimes called the **atlas-dens index** or **atlantodens interval [ADI]**) does not exceed 2.5 to 3 mm in the adult (4.5 to 5 mm in children). Instability is present when there is 3.5 mm ADI difference in flexion views. An ADI of more than 5 mm in adults commonly indicates a rupture of the transverse ligament. A 7 mm difference may imply disruption of alar ligaments. The **space available for cord (SAC)** is measured between the posterior dens and the anterior cortex of the posterior ring of the atlas. In adults and teenagers, the SAC should be greater than 13 mm.

13. *Instability.* Instability is present when more than 3.5 mm of horizontal displacement of one vertebra occurs in relation to the adjacent vertebra (see Figure 3-83).

Open or Odontoid ("Through-the-Mouth") View. This AP view enables the examiner to determine the state of the odontoid process of C2 and its relation with C1 (Figure 3-85; see Figure 3-84). It may also show the atlanto-occipital and atlantoaxial joints.

Oblique View. This view provides information on the neural foramen and posterior elements of the cervical spine. The examiner should look for or note the following (Figures 3-86 and 3-87):

1. Lipping of the joints of Luschka (osteophytes)
2. Overriding of the facet joints (subluxation, spondylosis)
3. Facet joints and intervertebral foramen (see Figure 3-87)

Pillar View. This special view is used to evaluate the lateral masses of the cervical spine and especially the facet

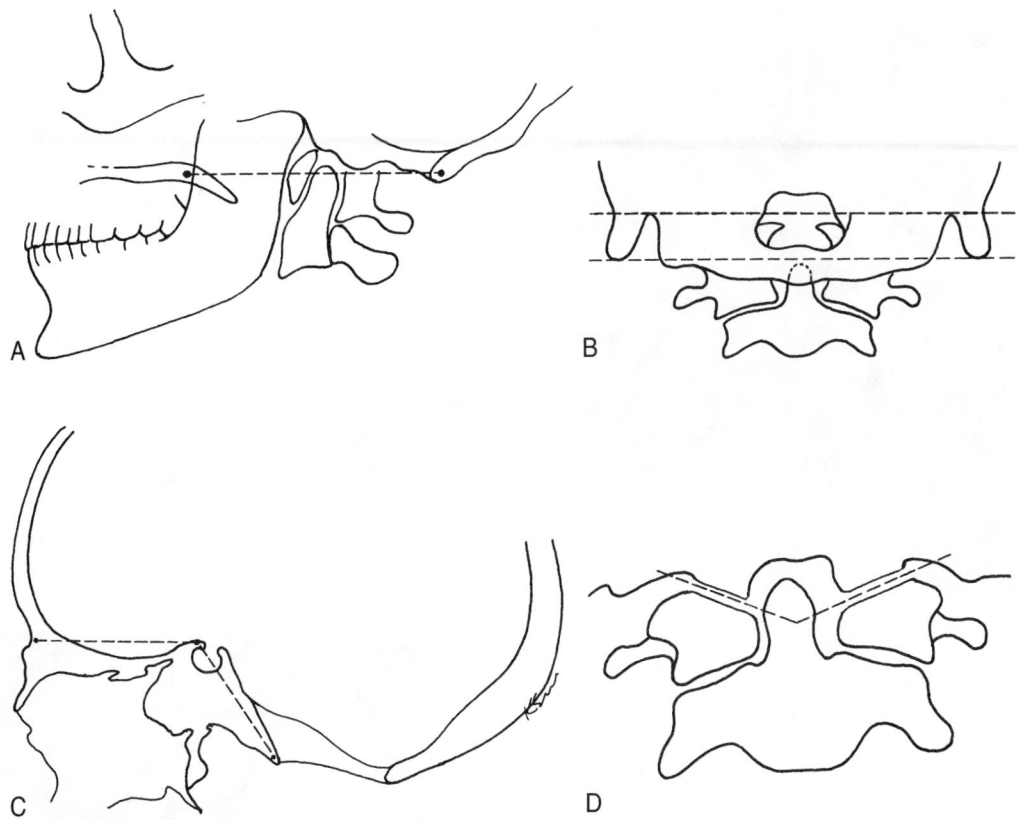

Figure 3-84 Cervicobasilar junction: Normal osseous relationships. A, Chamberlain's line is drawn from the posterior margin of the hard palate to the posterior border of the foramen magnum. The odontoid process normally does not extend more than 5 mm above this line. **B,** The bimastoid line *(lower line),* connecting the tips of the mastoids, is normally within 2 mm of the odontoid tip. The digastric line *(upper line),* connecting the digastric muscle fossae, is normally located above the odontoid process. **C,** The basilar angle, which normally exceeds 140°, is formed by the angle of intersection of two lines—one drawn from the nasion to the tuberculum sellae, and the second drawn from the tuberculum sellae to the anterior edge of the foramen magnum. **D,** The atlanto-occipital joint angle, constructed on frontal tomograms by the intersection of two lines drawn along the axes of these articulations, is normally not greater than 150°. (From Resnick D, Kransdorf MJ: Bone and joint imaging, Philadelphia, 2005, Saunders, p. 37.)

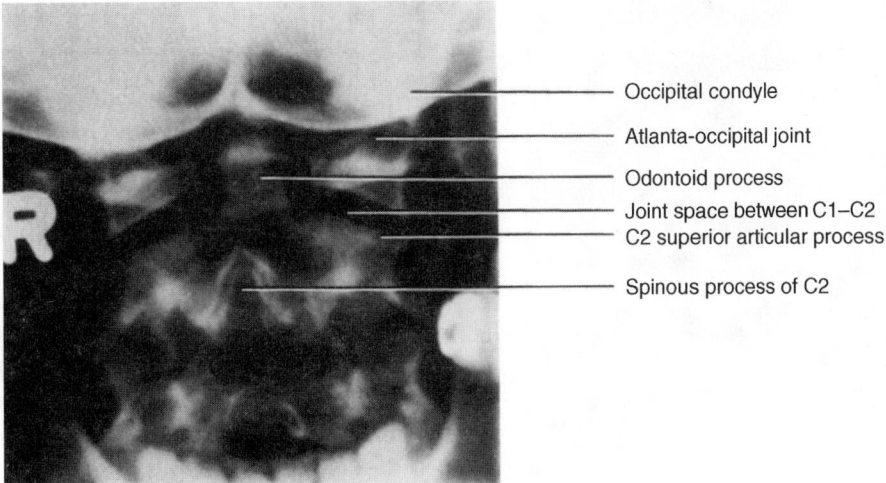

Figure 3-85 Through-the-mouth radiograph.

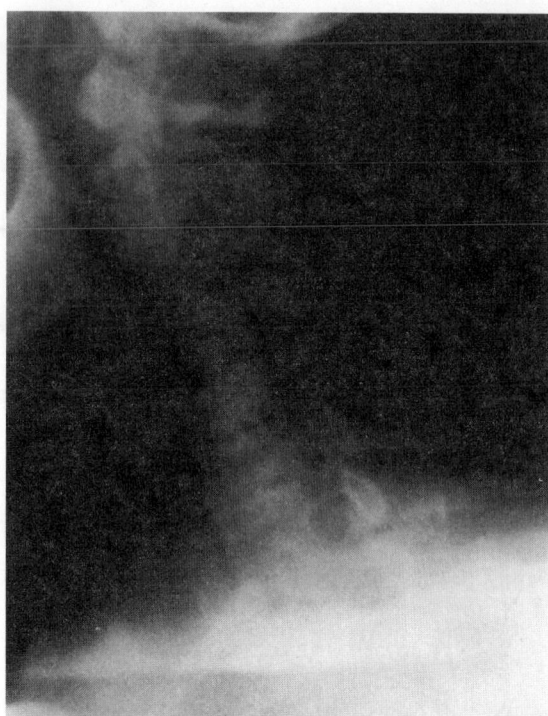

Figure 3-86 Abnormal x-ray findings on oblique view. Note loss of normal curve; narrowing at C4, C5, and C6; osteophytes and lipping of C4, C5, and C6; and encroachment on intervertebral foramen at C4–C5, C5–C6, and C6–C7.

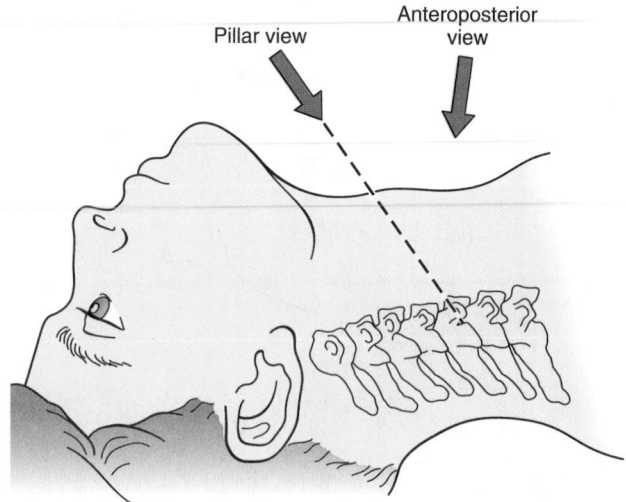

Figure 3-88 Diagram of pillar view showing orientation of facet joints.

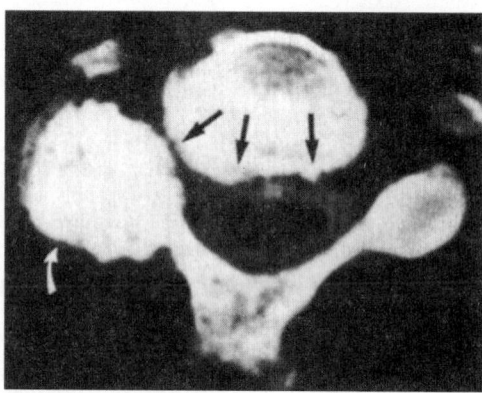

Figure 3-89 Foraminal stenosis caused by hypertrophic facet arthropathy and by spondylosis. Metrizamide-enhanced computed tomography scan through C5 foramina details the markedly overgrown facet *(white arrow)* and the bony "bar," or spondylotic spurring *(black arrows)*. The right foramen is almost occluded by abnormal bone. (From Dorwart RH, LaMasters DL: Application of computed tomographic scanning of the cervical spine. Orthop Clin North Am 16:386, 1985.)

joints (Figure 3-88). It is usually reserved for patients with suspected facet fractures.[166]

Computed Tomography

Computed tomography (CT) helps to delineate the bone and soft-tissue anatomy of the cervical spine in cross section and can show, for example, a disc prolapse. It also shows the true size and extent of osteophytes better than do plain x-rays (Figure 3-89). CT scans are especially useful for showing bone fragments in the spinal canal after a fracture and bony defects in the vertebral bodies and neural arches. CT scans may be combined with myelography to outline the spinal cord and nerve roots inside the thecal sac (Figure 3-90). CT scans are used only after conventional radiographs have been taken and a need for them is shown.

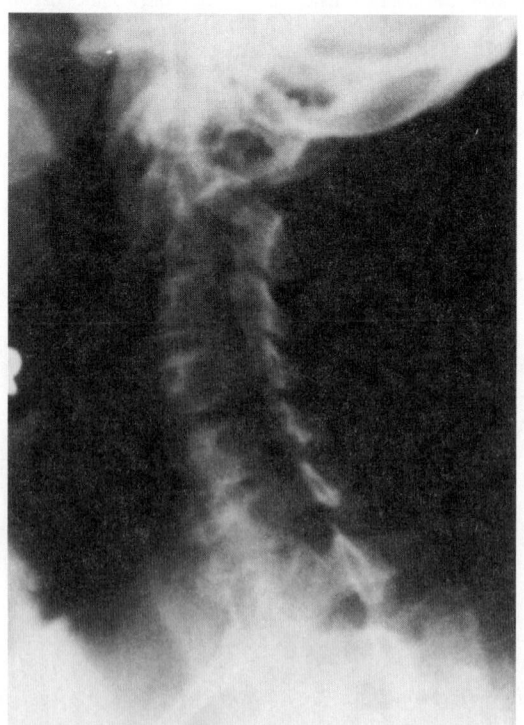

Figure 3-87 Oblique radiograph of the cervical spine showing intervertebral foramen and facet joints. Severe lipping in lower cervical spine and spondylosis are also evident.

Myelography

Myelograms are the modality of choice with brachial plexus avulsions, either Erb-Duchenne paralysis (C5 and C6) or Klumpke paralysis (C7, C8, and T1). They may also be used to demonstrate narrowing in the intervertebral foramen and cervical spinal stenosis. They may be used to outline the contour of the thecal sac, nerve roots, and spinal cord (Figure 3-91).

Magnetic Resonance Imaging

This noninvasive technique can differentiate between various soft tissues and bone (Figures 3-92 and 3-93). Because it shows differences based on water content, magnetic resonance imaging (MRI) can differentiate between the nucleus pulposus and the annulus fibrosus.

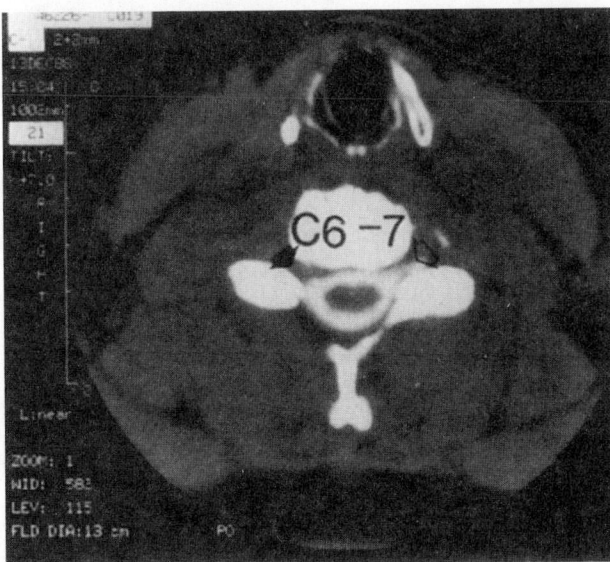

Figure 3-90 Postcontrast computed tomogram showing normally patent neural foramen at the C6–C7 level on the left side *(open arrow)*. The nerve root sleeve fills with contrast medium and enters the neural foramen. On the right side *(closed arrow)*, there is no evidence of filling of the nerve root sleeve within the neural foramen as a result of lateral C6 disc herniation. (From Bell GR, Ross JS: Diagnosis of nerve root compression: myelography, computed tomography, and MRI. Orthop Clin North Am 23:410, 1992.)

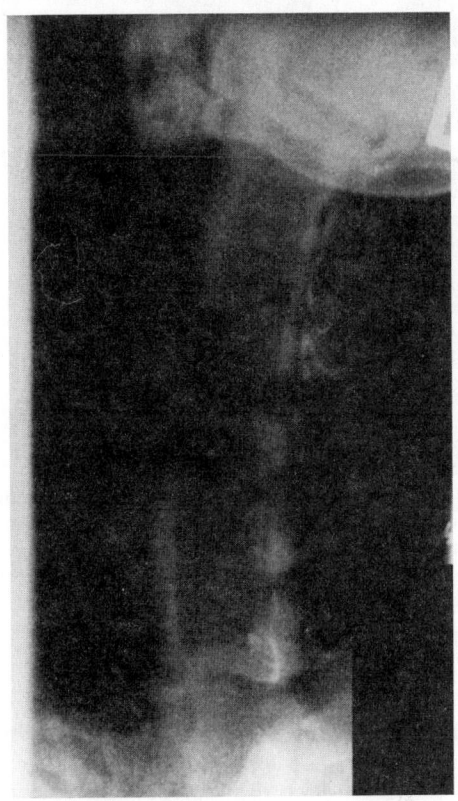

Figure 3-91 Myelogram of cervical spine.

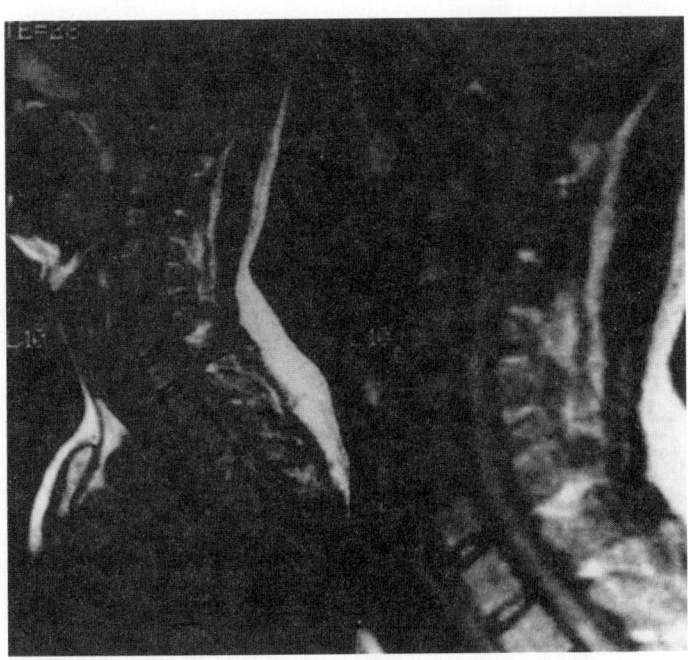

Figure 3-92 Magnetic resonance image of the cervical and upper thoracic spine. Sagittal view *(left)* with close-up of cervical spine *(right)*. (From Foreman SM, Croft AC: Whiplash injuries: the cervical acceleration/deceleration syndrome, Baltimore, 1988, Williams & Wilkins, p. 126.)

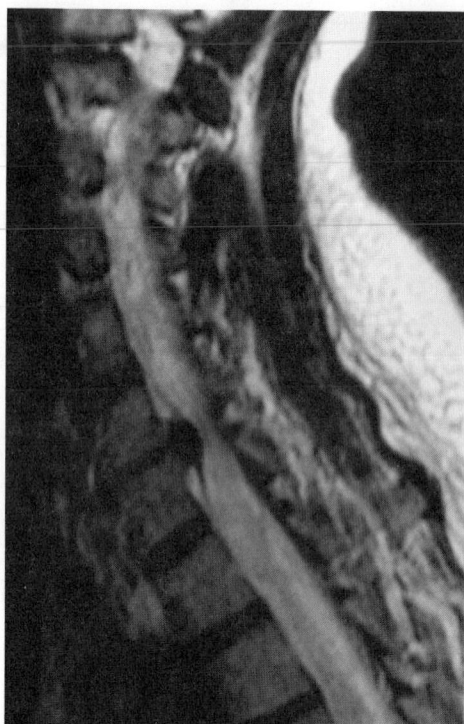

Figure 3-93 Posterior disc displacement: MR imaging findings. Sagittal T2-weighted (TR/TE, 2608/96) fast spin echo magnetic resonance image reveals an extruded paracentral disc of low signal intensity at the C6–C7 spinal level. (From Resnick D, Kransdorf MJ: Bone and joint imaging, Philadelphia, 2005, Saunders, p. 415. Courtesy of D. Goodwin, MD, Hanover, NH.)

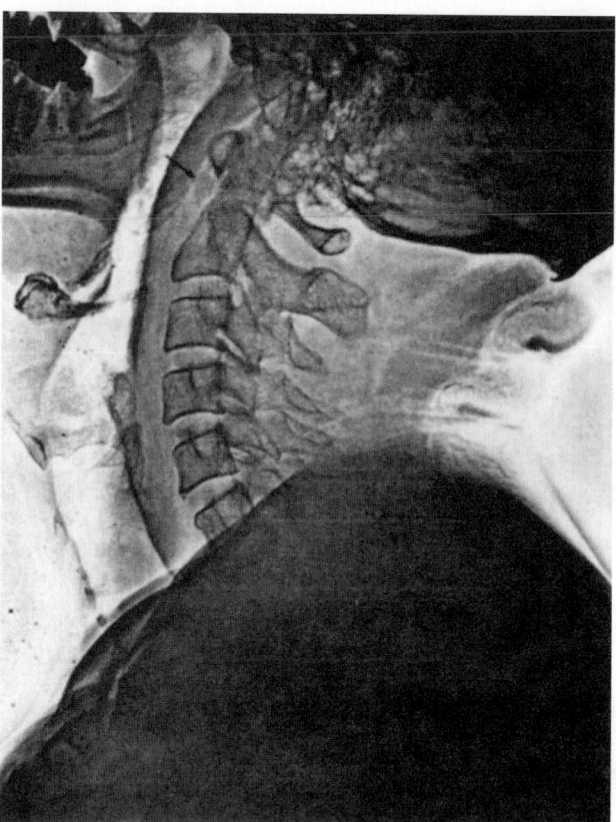

Figure 3-94 Xeroradiograph of cervical spine (lateral view). *Arrow* indicates calcified mass. (From Forrester DM, Brown JC: The radiology of joint disease, Philadelphia, 1987, WB Saunders, p. 420.)

MRI may be used to reveal disc protrusions, but it has been reported that patients showing these lesions are often asymptomatic, highlighting the fact that diagnostic imaging abnormalities should be considered only in relation to the history and clinical examination.[167] An MRI allows visualization of the nerve roots, spinal cord, and thecal sac as well as the bone and bone marrow. It is also used to identify postoperative scarring and disc herniation.[168] Magnetic resonance angiography is also useful for determining the patency and status of the vertebral artery.[169–171]

Xeroradiography

Xeroradiography helps to delineate bone and soft tissue by enhancing the interfaces between tissues (Figure 3-94).

PRÉCIS OF THE CERVICAL SPINE ASSESSMENT*

History
Observation (standing or sitting)
Examination (sitting)
  Active movements
    Flexion
    Extension
    Side flexion (right and left)
    Rotation (right and left)
    Combined movements (if necessary)
    Repetitive movements (if necessary)
    Sustained positions (if necessary)
  Resisted isometric movements (as in active movements)
  Scanning examination
    Peripheral joint
    Temporomandibular joints (open mouth and closed mouth)
    Shoulder girdle (elevation through abduction, elevation through forward flexion, elevation through plane of scapula, medial and lateral rotation with arm at side; medial and lateral rotation at 90° abduction)
    Elbow (flexion, extension, supination, pronation)
    Wrist (flexion, extension, radial, and ulnar deviation)
    Fingers and thumb (flexion, extension, abduction, adduction)
    Myotomes
    Neck flextion (C1, C2)
    Neck side flexion (C3)
    Shoulder elevation (C4)
    Shoulder abduction (C5)
    Elbow flexion (C6) and/or extension (C7)
    Wrist flexion (C7) and/or extension (C6)
    Thumb extension (C8) and/or ulnar deviation (C8)
    Hand intrinsics (abduction or adduction) (T1)
    Sensory scanning examination
  Functional assessment
  Special tests† (*sitting*)
    For neurological symptoms:
      Brachial plexus tension test
      Distraction test (if symptoms severe)
      Foraminal compression test (3 stages) (if symptoms absent or mild)
    For myelopathy:
      Romberg test
  Reflexes and cutaneous distribution
    Biceps (C5, C6)
    Triceps (C7, C8)

Hoffmann sign (or Babinski test)
Sensory scan
Examination, supine
  Passive movements
    Flexion
    Extension
    Side flexion
    Rotation
  Special tests† (*lying*)
    For cervical muscle (deep neck flexors) strength:
      Craniocervical flexion test (CCF)
      Deep neck flexor endurance test
    For neurological symptoms:
      Upper limb neurodynamic (tension) tests (specific to particular nerve/nerve root symptoms)
    For vascular signs:‡
      Hold planned mobilization/manipulation position for at least 30 seconds watching for vertebral-basilar artery signs
    For cervical instability:‡
      Anterior shear stress test
      Lateral shear test
      Lateral flexion alar ligament stress test
      Rotational alar ligament stress test
      Transverse ligament stress test
    For cervical spine mobility:
      Cervical flexion rotation test
    For first rib mobility:
      First rib mobility
  Joint play movements
    Side glide of cervical spine
    Anterior glide of cervical spine
    Posterior glide of cervical spine
    Traction glide of cervical spine
    Rotation of occiput on C1
  Palpation
Examination, prone
  Joint play movements
    Posteroanterior central vertebral pressure (PACVP)
    Posteroanterior unilateral vertebral pressure (PAUVP)
    Transverse vertebral pressure
  Palpation
  Diagnostic imaging
After any examination, the patient should be warned of the possibility of exacerbation of symptoms as a result of the assessment.

*The précis is shown in an order that limits the amount of moving that the patient has to do but ensures that all necessary structures are tested.

†The author recommends these key tests be learned by the clinician to facilitate a diagnosis.

‡These tests should be performed if the examiner anticipates doing end-range mobilization or manipulation techniques to the cervical spine, especially the upper cervical spine. If instability of vascular signs are present, mobilization and/or manipulation should *not* be performed.

CASE STUDIES

When doing these case studies, the examiner should list the appropriate questions to be asked and why they are being asked, what to look for and why, and what things should be tested and why. Depending on the answers of the patient (and the examiner should consider different responses), several possible causes of the patient's problems may become evident (examples are given in parentheses). A differential diagnosis chart should be made up (see Table 3-26 as an example). The examiner can then decide how different diagnoses may affect the treatment plan.

1. A 2-month-old baby is brought to you by a concerned parent. The child does not move the head properly, and the sternocleidomastoid muscle on the left side is prominent. Describe your assessment plan before beginning treatment (congenital torticollis versus Klippel-Feil syndrome).

2. A 54-year-old man comes to you complaining of neck stiffness, especially on rising; sometimes he has numbness into his left arm. Describe your assessment plan (cervical spondylosis versus subacromial bursitis).

3. An 18-year-old male football player comes to you complaining of a "dead arm" after a tackle he made 2 days ago. Although he can now move the left arm, it still does not feel right. Describe your assessment plan (brachial plexus lesion versus acromioclavicular sprain).

4. A 23-year-old woman comes to you after a motor vehicle accident. Her car was hit from behind while stopped for a red light. She could tell the accident was going to occur because she could see in the rearview mirror that the car behind her was not going to be able to stop. The car that hit her was going 50 kph (30 mph), and skid marks were visible for only 5 m from the location of her car. Describe your assessment plan (cervical sprain versus cervical facet syndrome).

5. A 35-year-old woman comes to you complaining of persistent headaches that last for days at a time. She has recently lost her job. She complains that she sometimes sees flashing lights and cannot stand having anyone around her when the pain is very bad. Describe your assessment plan for this patient (migraine versus tension headache).

6. A 26-year-old man comes to you complaining of pain in his neck. The pain was evident yesterday when he got up and has not decreased significantly since then. He thinks that he may have "slept wrong." There is no previous history of trauma. Describe your assessment plan for this patient (acquired torticollis versus cervical disc lesion).

7. A 75-year-old woman comes to you complaining primarily of neck pain but also of stiffness. She exhibits a dowager's hump. There is no history of trauma. Describe your assessment plan for this patient (osteoporosis versus cervical spondylosis).

8. A 47-year-old man comes to you complaining of elbow and neck pain. There is no recent history of trauma, but he remembers being in a motor vehicle accident 19 years ago. He now works at a desk all day. Describe your assessment for this patient (cervical spondylosis versus tennis elbow versus double crush injury).

9. A 16-year-old boy comes to you with a complaint of having hurt his neck. While "fooling" with some friends at the lake, he ran away from them and dove into the water to get away. The top of his head hit the bottom, and he felt a burning pain. The pain decreased as he came out of the water, but he still has a residual ache. Describe your plan for this patient (cervical fracture versus cervical sprain).

10. A 14-year-old girl comes to you complaining of neck pain. She has long hair. She states that when she "whipped" her hair out of her eyes, which she has done many times before, she felt a sudden pain in her neck. Although the pain intensity has decreased, it is still there, and she cannot fully move her neck. Describe your assessment plan for this patient (cervical sprain versus acquired torticollis).

TABLE **3-26**

Differential Diagnosis of Cervical Facet Syndrome, Cervical Nerve Root Lesion, and Thoracic Outlet Syndrome

Signs and Symptoms	Facet Syndrome	Cervical Nerve Root	Thoracic Outlet Syndrome
Pain referral	Possible	Yes	Possible
Pain on hyperextension and rotation	Yes (often without increased referral of symptoms)	Yes with increased symptoms	No
Spine stiffness	Yes	Possible	Possible
Paresthesia	No	Yes	Possible
Reflexes	Not affected	May be affected	May be affected
Muscle spasm	Yes	Yes	Yes
Tension tests	May or may not be positive	Positive	May be positive
Pallor and coolness	No	No	Possible
Muscle weakness	No	Possible	Not early (later small hand muscles)
Muscle fatigue and cramps	No	No	Possible

REFERENCES

1. Cyriax J: Textbook of orthopaedic medicine: diagnosis of soft tissue lesions, vol. 1, London, 1982, Bailliere Tindall.
2. Porterfield JA, DeRosa C: Mechanical neck pain—perspective in functional anatomy, Philadelphia, 1995, WB Saunders.
3. Radanov BP, Dvorak J, Valach L: Cognitive deficits in patients after soft tissue injury of the cervical spine. Spine 17:127–131, 1992.
4. Panjabi M, Dvorak J, Crisco J, et al: Flexion, extension, and lateral bending of the upper cervical spine in response to alar ligament transactions. J Spinal Disord 4(2):157–167, 1991.
5. Rieger P, Huber G: Fenestration and duplicate origin of the left vertebral artery in angiography: report of three cases. Neuroradiology 25(1):45–50, 1983.
6. Taylor AJ, Kerry R: Neck pain and headache as a result of internal carotid artery dissection: implications for manual therapists. Man Ther 10:73–77, 2005.
7. Castaigne P, Lhermitte F, Gautier JC, et al: Arterial occlusions in the vertebro-basilar system: a study of 44 patients with post-mortem data. Brain 96(1):133–154, 1973.
8. Toole J, Tucker SH: Influence of head position upon cerebral circulation. Arch Neurol 2:616–623, 1960.
9. Brown BS, Tissington-Tatlow WF: Radiographic studies of the vertebral arteries in cadavers. Radiology 81:80–88, 1963.
10. Haynes MJ: Doppler studies comparing the effects of cervical rotation and lateral flexion on vertebral artery blood flow. J Manip Physiol Ther 19:378–384, 1996.
11. Endo K, Ichimaru K, Shimura H, et al: Cervical vertigo after hair shampoo treatment at a hair dressing salon: a case report. Spine 25:632, 2000.
12. Nagler W: Vertebral artery obstruction by hyperextension of the neck: report of three cases. Arch Phys Med Rehabil 54:237–240, 1973.
13. Dutton M: Orthopedic examination, evaluation and intervention, New York, 2004, McGraw Hill.
14. Miyachi S, Okamura K, Watanabe M, et al: Cerebellar stroke due to vertebral artery occlusion after cervical spine trauma: two case reports. Spine 19:83–89, 1994.
15. Hart RG, Easton JD: Dissections. Stroke 16:925–927, 1985.
16. Hayes P, Gerlock AJ, Cobb CA: Cervical spine trauma: a cause of vertebral artery injury. J Trauma 20:904–905, 1980.
17. Schwarz N, Buchinger W, Gaudernak T, et al: Injuries of the cervical spine causing vertebral artery trauma: case reports. J Trauma 31:127–133, 1991.
18. Auer RN, Krcek J, Butt JC: Delayed symptoms and death after minor head trauma with occult vertebral artery injury. J Neurol Neurosurg Psychiatry 57:500–502, 1994.
19. Bose B, Northrup BE, Osteoholm JL: Delayed vertebrobasilar insufficiency following cervical spine injury. Spine 10:108–110, 1985.
20. Kapandji IA: The physiology of joints: the trunk and the vertebral column, vol. 3, New York, 1974, Churchill Livingstone.
21. Ishii T, Mukai Y, Hosono N, et al: Kinematics of the cervical spine in lateral bending in vivo three-dimensional analysis. Spine 31:155–160, 2006.
22. Ishii T, Mukai Y, Hosono N, et al: Kinematics of the subaxial cervical spine in rotation in vivo three-dimensional analysis. Spine 29:2826–2931, 2004.
23. Bogduk N: The innervation of the lumbar spine. Spine 8:286–293, 1983.
24. Boreadis AG, Gershon-Cohen J: Luschka joints of the cervical spine. Radiology 66:181–187, 1956.
25. Hall MC: Luschka's joint, Springfield, IL, 1965, Charles C Thomas.
26. Silberstein CE: The evolution of degenerative changes in the cervical spine and an investigation into the "joint of Luschka." Clin Orthop 40:184–204, 1965.
27. Willis TA: Luschka's joints. Clin Orthop 46:121–125, 1966.
28. Ferlic D: The nerve supply of the cervical intervertebral disc in man. Johns Hopkins Hosp Bull 113:347, 1963.
29. Mendel T, Wink CS, Zimny ML: Neural elements in human cervical intervertebral discs. Spine 17:132–135, 1992.
30. Rao RD, Currier BL, Albert TJ, et al: Degenerative cervical spondylosis: cervical syndromes, pathogenesis and management. J Bone Joint Surg Am 89:1360–1378, 2007.
31. Childs JD, Cleland JA, Elliott JM, et al: Neck pain: clinical guidelines linked to the international classification of functioning, disability and health. J Orthop Sports Phys Ther 38:A1–A34, 2008.
32. Bland JH: Disorders of the cervical spine, Philadelphia, 1994, WB Saunders.
33. Cleland J: Orthopedic clinical examination—an evidence based approach for physical therapists, Carlstadt, NJ, 2005, Icon Learning Systems.
34. Guzman J, Haldeman S, Carroll L, et al: Clinical practice implications of the Bone and Joint Decade 2000–2010 Task Force on Neck Pain and Its Associated Disorders: from concepts and findings to recommendations. J Manip Physiol Ther 32(2 Suppl): 227–243, 2009.
35. Watkins RG: Neck injuries in football. In Watkins RG, editor: The spine in sports, St Louis, 1996, Mosby-Year Book.
36. Buitenhuis J, de Jong PJ, Jaspers JP, et al: Catastrophizing and causal beliefs in whiplash. Spine 33:2427–2433, 2008.
37. Spitzer WO, Skovron ML, Salmi LR, et al: Scientific monograph of the Quebec Task Force on Whiplash-Associated Disorders: redefining "whiplash" and its management. Spine 20(8 Suppl):S1–S73, 1995.
38. Siegmund GP, Davis MB, Quinn KP, et al: Head-turned postures increase the risk of cervical facet capsule injury during whiplash. Spine 33:1643–1649, 2008.
39. Kitigawa T, Fujiwara A, Kobayashi N, et al: Morphologic changes in the cervical neural foramen due to flexion and extension–in vivo imaging study. Spine 29:2821–2825, 2004.
40. Benoist M: Natural evolution and resolution of the cervical whiplash syndrome. In Gunzburg R, Szpalski M, editors: Current concepts with prevention, diagnosis and treatment of cervical whiplash syndrome, Philadelphia, 1998, Lippincott-Raven.
41. Suissa S, Harder S, Veilleux M: The Quebec whiplash-associated disorders cohort study. Spine 20:S12–S20, 1995.
42. Evans RW: Some observations on whiplash injuries. Neurol Sci 10:975–997, 1992.
43. Deans GT, Magalliard JN, Kerr M, et al: Neck sprain—a major disability following car events. Injury 18:10–12, 1987.
44. Wiener SL: Differential diagnosis of acute pain by body region, New York, 1993, McGraw Hill.

45. Travell TG, Simons DG: Myofascial pain and dysfunction: the trigger point manual, vol. 1, Baltimore, 1983, Williams & Wilkins.

46. Malanga GA: The diagnosis and treatment of cervical radiculopathy. Med Sci Sports Exer 29:S236–S245, 1997.

47. Levine MJ, Albert TJ, Smith MD: Cervical radiculopathy diagnosis and nonoperative management. J Am Acad Orthop Surg 4:305–316, 1996.

48. Ellenberg MR, Honet JC, Treanor WJ: Cervical radiculopathy. Arch Phys Med Rehabil 75:342–352, 1994.

49. Carette S, Fehlings MG: Cervical radiculopathy. N Engl J Med 353:392–399, 2005.

50. Tsairis P, Jordan B: Neurological evaluation of cervical spinal disorders. In Camins MB, O'Leary PF, editors: Disorders of the cervical spine, Baltimore, 1992, Williams & Wilkins.

51. Dywer A, April C, Bogduk N: Cervical zygapophyseal joint pain patterns. Spine 15:453–457, 1990.

52. Petty NJ, Moore AP: Neuromusculoskeletal examination and assessment—a handbook for therapists, London, 1998, Churchill Livingstone.

53. Foreman SM, Croft AC: Whiplash injuries: the cervical acceleration/deceleration syndrome, Baltimore, 1988, Williams & Wilkins.

54. Evans RC: Illustrated essentials in orthopedic physical assessment, St Louis, 1994, Mosby-Year Books.

55. Bradley JP, Tibone JE, Watkins RG: History, physical examination, and diagnostic tests for neck and upper extremity problems. In Watkins RG, editor: The spine in sports, St Louis, 1996, Mosby-Year Book.

56. Meadows JT: Orthopedic differential diagnosis in physical therapy—a case study approach, New York, 1999, McGraw-Hill.

57. Levangie PK, Norkin CC: Joint structure and function: a comprehensive analysis, Philadelphia, 2005, FA Davis.

58. Watson D, Trott P: Cervical headache: an investigation of natural head posture and upper cervical flexor muscle performance. Cephalalgia 13:272–284, 1993.

59. Janda V: Muscles and motor control in cervicogenic disorders: assessment and management. In Grant R, editor: Physical therapy of the cervical and thoracic spine, New York, 1994, Churchill Livingstone.

60. Prushansky T, Dvir Z: Cervical motion testing: methodology and clinical implications. J Manip Physiol Ther 31:518–524, 2008.

61. Youdas JW, Garrett TR, Suman VJ, et al: Normal range of motion of the cervical spine: an initial goniometric study. Phys Ther 72:770–780, 1992.

62. Dvorak J, Antinnes JA, Panjabi M, et al: Age and gender related normal motion of the cervical spine. Spine 17:S393–S398, 1992.

63. Neumann DA: Kinesiology of the musculoskeletal system—foundations for physical rehabilitation, St Louis, 2002, CV Mosby.

64. Reese NB: Muscle and sensory testing, Philadelphia, 1999, WB Saunders.

65. Janda V: Muscles and cervicogenic pain syndrome. In Grant R, editor: Physical therapy of the cervical and thoracic spine, New York, 1988, Churchill Livingstone.

66. Smith K, Hall T, Robinson K: The influence of age, gender, lifestyle factors and sub-clinical neck pain on the cervical flexion rotation test and cervical range of motion. Man Ther 13:552–559, 2008.

67. Takasaki H, Hall T, Oshiro S, et al: Normal kinematics of the upper cervical spine during the flexion-rotation test—in vivo measurements using magnetic resonance imaging. Man Ther 16:167–171, 2011.

68. Hall T, Briffa K, Hopper D, et al: Long-term stability and minimal detectable change of the cervical flexion-rotation test. J Orthop Sports Phys Ther 40:225–229, 2010.

69. Hall T, Robinson K: The flexion-rotation test and active cervical mobility—a comparative measurement study in cervicogenic headache. Man Ther 9:147–202, 2004.

70. Yi-Kai L, Yun-Kun Z, Cai-Mo L, et al: Changes and implications of blood flow velocity of the vertebral artery during rotation and extension of the head. J Manip Physiol Ther 22:91–95, 1999.

71. Magarey ME: Examination of the cervical and thoracic spine. In Grant R, editor: Physical therapy of the cervical and thoracic spine, New York, 1988, Churchill Livingstone.

72. Elvey RL: The investigation of arm pain. In Boyling JD, Palastanga N, editors: Grieve's modern manual therapy: the vertebral column, ed 2, Edinburgh, 1994, Churchill Livingstone.

73. Magarey ME: Examination of the cervical spine. In Grieve GP, editor: Modern manual therapy of the vertebral column, Edinburgh, 1986, Churchill Livingstone.

74. Dvir Z, Pruchansky T: Cervical muscle strength testing: methods and clinical implications. J Manip Physiol Ther 31:518–524, 2008.

75. Schneider R, Gosch H, Norrell H, et al: Vascular insufficiency and differential distortion of brain and cord caused by cervicomedullary football injuries. J Neurosurg 33:363–375, 1970.

76. Pinfold M, Niere KR, O'Leary EF, et al: Validity and internal consistency of a whiplash-specific disability measure. Spine 29(3):263–268, 2004.

77. Willis C, Niere R, Hoving JL, et al: Reproducibility and responsiveness of the whiplash disability questionnaire. Pain 110(3):681–688, 2004.

78. Vernon H, Mior S: The neck disability index: a study of reliability and validity. J Manip Physiol Ther 14:409–415, 1991.

79. Vernon H: The neck disability index: state-of-the-art, 1991–2008. J Manip Physiol Ther 31:491–502, 2008.

80. Macdermid JC, Walton DM, Avery S, et al: Measurement properties of the neck disability index: a systemic review. J Orthop Sports Phys Ther 39:400–417, 2009.

81. Stratford PW, Riddle DL, Binkley JM, et al: Using the neck disability index to make decisions concerning individual patients. Physiother Can 51:107–112, 1999.

82. Manniche JA, Mosdal C, Hindsberger C: The Copenhagen Functional Disability Scale: a study of reliability and validity. J Manip Physiol Ther 21:520–527, 1998.

83. Leak AM, Cooper J, Dyer S, et al: The Norwick Park Neck Pain Questionnaire devised to measure neck pain and disability. Br J Rheumatol 33:469–474, 1994.

84. Hoving JL, O'Leary EF, Niere KR, et al: Validity of the neck disability index, Northwick Park neck pain questionnaire, and problem elicitation technique for measuring disability associated with whiplash associated disorders. Pain 102(3):273–281, 2003.

85. Bolton JE: Sensitivity and specificity of outcome measures in patients with neck pain: detecting clinically significant improvement. Spine 29:2410–2417, 2004.

86. Bolton JE, Humphreys BK: The Bournemouth Questionnaire: a short-form comprehensive outcome measure. II Psychometric properties in neck pain patients. J Manip Physiol Ther 25:141–148, 2002.

87. Cattrysse E, Swinkels RA, Oostendorp RA, et al: Upper cervical instability: are clinical tests reliable? Man Ther 2:91–97, 1997.

88. Olson KA, Paris SV, Spohr C, et al: Radiographic assessment and reliability study of the craniovertebral sidebending test. J Man Manip Ther 6:87–96, 1998.

89. Jull GA, O'Leary SP, Falla DL: Clinical assessment of the deep cervical flexor muscles: the craniocervical flexion test. J Manip Physiol Ther 31:525–533, 2008.

90. Falla DL, Jull GA, Hodges PW: Patients with neck pain demonstrate reduced electromyographic activity of the deep cervical flexor muscles during performance of the craniocervical flexion tests. Spine 29:2108–2114, 2004.

91. Jull GA: Physiotherapy management of neck pain of mechanical origin. In Giles LG, Singer KP, editors: Clinical anatomy and management of cervical spine pain, London, 1998, Butterworth-Heinemann.

92. Jull G, Barrett C, Magee R, et al: Further clinical clarification of the muscle dysfunction in cervical headache. Cephalalgia 19:179–185, 1999.

93. Uthaikhup S, Jull G: Performance in the craniocervical flexion test is altered in elderly subjects. Man Ther 14:475–479, 2009.

94. Harris KD, Heer DM, Roy TC, et al: Reliability of a measurement of neck flexor muscle endurance. Phys Ther 85:1349–1355, 2005.

95. Van Hoof T, Vangestel C, Forward M, et al: The impact of muscular variation on the neurodynamic test for the median nerve in a healthy population with Langer's axillary arch. J Manip Physiol Ther 31:414–483, 2008.

96. Vanti C, Conteddu L, Guccione A, et al: The upper limb neurodynamic test 1: intra- and inter-tester reliability and the effect of several repetitions on pain and resistance. J Manip Physiol Ther 33:292–299, 2010.

97. Boyd BS, Wanek L, Gray AT, et al: Mechanosensitivity of the lower extremity nervous system during straight leg raise neurodynamic testing in healthy individuals. J Orthop Sports Phys Ther 39:780–790, 2009.

98. Uchihara T, Furukawa T, Tsukagoshi H: Compression of brachial plexus as a diagnostic test of a cervical cord lesion. Spine 19:2170–2173, 1994.

99. Spurling RG, Scoville WB: Lateral rupture of the cervical intervertebral disc. Surg Gynec Obstet 78:350–358, 1944.

100. Kelly JJ: Neurological problems in the athlete's shoulder. In Pettrone FA, editor: Athletic injuries of the shoulder, New York, 1995, McGraw-Hill.

101. Wells P: Cervical dysfunction and shoulder problems. Physiotherapy 68:66–73, 1982.

102. Davidson RI, Dunn EJ, Metzmaker JN: The shoulder abduction test in the diagnosis of radicular pain in cervical extradural compressive monoradiculopathies. Spine 6:441–446, 1981.

103. Farmer JC, Wisneski RJ: Cervical spine nerve root compression: an analysis of neuroforaminal pressure with varying head and arm positions. Spine 19:1850–1855, 1994.

104. Landi A, Copeland S: Value of the Tinel sign in brachial plexus lesions. Ann R Coll Surg Engl 61:470–471, 1979.

105. Butler DS: Mobilisation of the nervous system, Melbourne, 1991, Churchill Livingstone.

106. Davis DS, Anderson IB, Carson MG, et al: Upper limb neural tension and seated slump tests: the false positive rate among healthy young adults without cervical or lumbar symptoms. J Man Manip Ther 16:136–141, 2008.

107. Slater H, Butler DS, Shacklock MO: The dynamic central nervous system: examination and assessment using tension tests. In Boyling JD, Palastanga N, editors: Grieve's modern manual therapy: the vertebral column, ed 2, Edinburgh, 1994, Churchill Livingstone.

108. Cook CE, Wilhelm M, Cook AE, et al: Clinical tests for screening and diagnosis of cervical spine myelopathy: a systemic review. J Manip Physiol Ther 34:539–546, 2011.

109. Yukawa Y, Kato F, Ito K, et al: "Ten second step test" as a new quantifiable parameter of cervical myelopathy. Spine 34:82–86, 2009.

110. Grant R: Vertebral artery testing—the Australian Physiotherapy Association Protocol after 6 years. Man Ther 1:149–153, 1996.

111. Kunnasmaa KT, Thiel HW: Vertebral artery syndrome: a review of the literature. J Orthop Med 16:17–20, 1994.

112. Bolton PS, Stick PE, Lord RS: Failure of clinical tests to predict cerebral ischemia before neck manipulation. J Manip Physiol Ther 12:304–307, 1989.

113. Magarey ME, Rebbeck T, Coughlan B, et al: Premanipulative testing of the cervical spine review, revision and new clinical guidelines. Man Ther 9:95–108, 2004.

114. Rivett DA, Sharples KJ, Milburn PD: Effects of premanipulative test on vertebral artery and internal carotid artery blood flow: a pilot study. J Manip Physiol Ther 22(6):368–375, 1999.

115. Thiel H, Rix G: Is it time to stop functional premanipulation testing of the cervical spine? Man Ther 10:154–158, 2005.

116. Kerry R, Taylor AJ, Mitchell J, et al: Cervical arterial dysfunction and manual therapy: a critical literature review to inform professional practice. Man Ther 13:278–288, 2008.

117. Bowler N, Shamley D, Davies R: The effect of a simulated manipulation position on internal carotid and vertebral artery blood flow in healthy individuals. Man Ther 16:87–93, 2011.

118. Willett GM, Wachholtz NA: A patient with internal carotid artery dissection. Phys Ther 91(8):1266–1274, 2011.

119. Arnold C, Bourassa R, Langer T, et al: Doppler studies evaluating the effect of a physical therapy screening protocol on vertebral artery blood flow. Man Ther 9:13–21, 2004.

120. Fast A, Zinicola DF, Marin EL: Vertebral artery damage complicating cervical manipulation. Spine 12:840–842, 1987.

121. Golueke P, Sclafani S, Phillips T, et al: Vertebral artery injury—diagnosis and management. J Trauma 27:856–865, 1987.

122. Australian Physiotherapy Association: Protocol for pre-manipulative testing of the cervical spine. Aust J Physiother 34:97–100, 1988.

123. Rivett DA: The premanipulative vertebral artery testing protocol. N Z J Physiother 23:9–12, 1995.

124. Barker S, Kesson M, Ashmore J, et al: Guidance for pre-manipulative testing of the cervical spine. Man Ther 5:37–40, 2000.

125. Mitchell J: Vertebral artery blood flow velocity changes associated with cervical spine rotation: a meta-analysis of the evidence with implications for professional practice. J Man Manip Ther 17:46–56, 2009.

126. Wadsworth CT: Manual examination and treatment of the spine and extremities, Baltimore, 1988, Williams & Wilkins.

127. Ombregt L, Bisschop P, ter Veer HJ, et al: A system of orthopedic medicine, London, 1995, WB Saunders.

128. Meadows JJ, Magee DJ: An overview of dizziness and vertigo for the orthopedic manual therapist. In Boyling JD, Palastanga N, editors: Grieve's modern manual therapy: the vertebral column, ed 2, Edinburgh, 1994, Churchill Livingstone.

129. Gird RB, Naffziger HC: Prolonged jugular compression: a new diagnostic test of neurological value. Trans Am Neurol Assoc 66:45–49, 1940.

130. Grant R: Vertebral artery insufficiency: a clinical protocol for pre-manipulative testing of the cervical spine. In Boyling JD, Palastanga N, editors: Grieve's modern manual therapy: the vertebral column, ed 2, Edinburgh, 1994, Churchill Livingstone.

131. Aspinall W: Clinical testing for cervical mechanical disorders which produce ischemic vertigo. J Orthop Sports Phys Ther 11:176–182, 1989.

132. Maitland GD: Vertebral manipulation, London, 1973, Butterworths.

133. Fitz-Ritson D: Assessment of cervicogenic vertigo. J Manip Physiol Ther 14:193–198, 1991.

134. Herdman SJ: Vestibular rehabilitation, ed 3, Philadelphia, 2007, FA Davis.

135. Johnson EG, Landel R, Kusunose RS, et al: Positive patient outcome after manual cervical spine management despite a positive vertebral artery test. Man Ther 13:367–371, 2008.

136. Pettman E: Stress tests of the craniovertebral joints. In Boyling JD, Palastanga N, editors: Grieve's Modern manual therapy: the vertebral column, ed 2, Edinburgh, 1994, Churchill Livingstone.

137. Osmotherly PG, Rivett DA, Rowe LJ: The anterior shear and distraction tests for craniocervical instability: an evaluation using magnetic resonance imaging. Man Ther 17:416–421, 2012.

138. Osmotherly PG, Rivett DA, Rowe LJ: Construct validity of clinical tests for alar ligament integrity: an evaluation using magnetic resonance imaging. Phys Ther 92:718–725, 2012.

139. Kaale BR, Krakenes J, Albrektsen G, et al: Clinical assessment techniques for detecting ligament and membrane injuries in the upper cervical spine region—a comparison with MRI results. Man Ther 13:397–403, 2008.

140. Aspinall W: Clinical testing for the craniovertebral hypermobility syndrome. J Orthop Sports Phys Ther 12:47–54, 1990.

141. Rey-Eiriz G, Alburque-Sendin F, Barrera-Mellado I, et al: Validity of the posterior-anterior middle cervical spine gliding test for the examination of the intervertebral joint hypomobility in mechanical neck pain. J Manip Phyiol Ther 33:279–285, 2010.

142. Hall TM, Robinson KW, Fujinawa O, et al: Intertester reliability and diagnostic validity of the cervical flexion-rotation test. J Manip Physiol Ther 31(4):293–300, 2008.

143. Ogince M, Hall T, Robinson K: The diagnostic validity of the cervical flexion-rotation test in C1/2 related cervicogenic headache. Man Ther 12:256–262, 2007.

144. Denno JJ, Meadows GR: Early diagnosis of cervical spondylotic myelopathy: a useful clinical sign. Spine 16:1353–1355, 1991.

145. Refshauge K, Gass E: The neurological examination. In Refshauge K, Gass E, editors: Musculoskeletal physiotherapy, Oxford, 1995, Butterworth-Heinemann.

146. Cook C, Roman M, Stewart KM, et al: Reliability and diagnostic accuracy of clinical special tests for myelopathy in patients seen for cervical dysfunction. J Orthop Sports Phys Ther 39:172–178, 2009.

147. Coene LN: Mechanisms of brachial plexus lesions. Clin Neuro Neurosurg 95S:S24–S29, 1993.

148. Benjamin K: Injuries to the brachial plexus: mechanisms of injury and identification of risk factors. Adv Neonatal Care 5:181–189, 2005.

149. Waters PM: Obstetric brachial plexus injuries: evaluation and management. J Am Acad Orthop Surg 5:205–214, 1997.

150. Cantu RC: Stingers, transient quadriplegia, and cervical spinal stenosis: return to play criteria. Med Sci Sports Exer 29:S233–S235, 1997.

151. Weinstein SM: Assessment and rehabilitation of the athlete with a "stinger." A model for the management of noncatastrophic athletic cervical spine injury. Clin Sports Med 17:127–135, 1998.

152. Mennell JM: Joint pain, Boston, 1964, Little, Brown.

153. Seffinger MA, Najm WI, Mishra SI, et al: Reliability of spinal palpation for diagnosis of back and neck pain. Spine 19:E413–E425, 2004.

154. Johnson MJ, Lucas GL: Value of cervical spine radiographs as a screening tool. Clin Orthop Relat Res 340:102–108, 1997.

155. Stiell IG, Wells GA, Vandemheen KL, et al: The Canadian C-spine rule for radiography in alert and stable trauma patients. JAMA 286(15):1841–1848, 2001.

156. Brehaut JC, Steill IG, Graham ID: Will a new clinical decision rule be widely used? The case of the Canadian C-spine rule. Acad Emerg Med 13:413–420, 2006.

157. Stiell IG, Clement CM, McKnight RD, et al: The Canadian C-spine rule versus the NEXUS low risk criteria in patients with trauma. New Eng J Med 349:2510–2518, 2003.

158. Cook CE, Hegedus EJ: Orthopedic physical examination tests—an evidence based approach, Upper Saddle River, NJ, 2008, Pearson/Prentice Hall.

159. Helliwell PS, Evans PF, Wright V: The straight cervical spine: does it indicate muscle spasm? J Bone Joint Surg Br 76:103–106, 1994.

160. McAviney J, Schulz D, Bock R, et al: Determining the relationship between cervical lordosis and neck complaints. J Manip Physiol Ther 28:187–193, 2005.

161. Pavlov H, Torg JS, Robie B, et al: Cervical spine stenosis: determination with vertebral body method. Radiology 164:771–775, 1987.

162. Cantu RC: Functional cervical spinal stenosis: a contraindication to participation in contact sports. Med Sci Sports Exerc 25:316–317, 1993.

163. Castro FP, Ricciardi J, Brunet ME, et al: Stingers, the Torg ratio, and the cervical spine. Am J Sports Med 25:603–608, 1997.

164. Torg JS, Pavlov H, Genuario SE, et al: Neurapraxia of the cervical spinal cord with transient quadriplegia. J Bone Joint Surg Am 68(9):1354–1370, 1986.

165. Templeton PA, Young JW, Mirvis SE, et al: The value of retropharyngeal soft tissue measurements in trauma of the adult cervical spine. Skeletal Radiol 18:98–104, 1987.

166. Harris JH: Radiographic evaluation of spinal trauma. Orthop Clin North Am 17:75–86, 1986.

167. Reid DC: Sports injury assessment and rehabilitation, New York, 1992, Churchill Livingstone.

168. Bigg-Wither G, Kelly P: Diagnostic imaging in musculoskeletal physiotherapy. In Refshauge K, Gass E, editors: Musculoskeletal physiotherapy, Oxford, 1995, Butterworth-Heinemann.

169. Vaccaro AR, Klein GR, Flanders AE, et al: Long-term evaluation of vertebral artery injuries following cervical spine trauma using magnetic resonance angiography. Spine 23:789–795, 1998.

170. Furumoto T, Nagase J, Takahashi K, et al: Cervical myelopathy caused by the anomalies vertebral artery—a case report. Spine 21:2280–2283, 1996.

171. Combs SB, Triano JJ: Symptoms of neck artery compromise: case presentations of risk estimate for treatment. J Manip Physiol Ther 20:274–278, 1997.

172. Wainner RS, Fritz JM, Irrgang JJ, et al: Reliability and diagnostic accuracy of the clinical examination and patient self-report measures for cervical radiculopathy. Spine 28(1):52–62, 2003.

173. Lauder TD, Dillingham TR, Andary M, et al: Predicting electrodiagnostic outcome in patients with upper limb symptoms: are the history and physical exam helpful? Arch Phys Med Rehabil 81:436–441, 2000.

174. Selvaratnam PJ, Matyas TA, Glasgow EF: Noninvasive discrimination of brachial plexus involvement in upper limb pain. Spine 19(1):26–33, 1994.

175. Viikari-Juntura E, Porras M, Laasonen EM: Validity of clinical tests in the diagnosis of root compression in cervical disc disease. Spine 14(3):253–257, 1989.

176. Nordin M, Carragee EJ, Hogg-Johnson S, et al: Assessment of neck pain and its associated disorders: results of the Bone and Joint Decade 2000–2010 Task Force on Neck Pain and Its Associated Disorders. J Manip Physiol Ther 32(2 Suppl):S117–S140, 2009.

177. Lindgren KA, Leino E, Manninen H: Cervical rotation lateral flexion test in brachialgia. Arch Phys Med Rehabil 73:735–737, 1992.

178. Cote P, Kreitz BG, Cassidy JD, et al: The validity of the extension-rotation test as a clinical screening procedure before neck manipulation: a secondary analysis. J Manip Physiol Ther 19(3):159–164, 1996.

179. Sandmark H, Nisell R: Validity of five common manual neck pain provoking tests. Scand J Rehab Med 27:131–136, 1995.

180. Tong HC, Haig AJ, Yamakawa K: The Spurling test and cervical radiculopathy. Spine 27:156–159, 2002.

181. Jull G, Bogduk N, Marsland A: The accuracy of manual diagnosis for cervical zygapophyseal joint pain syndromes. Med J Austr 148:233–236, 1988.

182. Viikari-Juntura E, Takala E-S, Riijimaki H, et al: Predictability of symptoms and signs in the neck and shoulders. J Clin Epidemiol 53:800–808, 2000.

183. Cleland JA, Fritz JM, Whitman JM, et al: The reliability and construct validity of the neck disability index and patient specific scale in patients with cervical radiculopathy. Spine 31(5):598–602, 2006.

184. Humphreys BK, Delahaye M, Pederson CK: An investigation into the validity of cervical spine motion palpation using subjects with congenital vertebrae as a "gold standard," BMC Musculoskelet Disord 5:19, 2004.

185. Singh A, Gnanalignham K, Casey A, et al: Quality of life assessment using the short form-12 (SF-12) questionnaire in patients with cervical spondylotic myelopathy: comparison with SF-36. Spine 31(6):639–643, 2006.

186. Uitvlugt G, Indenbaum S: Clinical assessment of atlantoaxial instability using the Sharp-Purser test. Arthr Rheum 31(7):918–922, 1988.

187. Bertilson BC, Grunnesjo M, Strender L-S: Reliability of clinical tests in the assessment of patients with neck/shoulder problems—impact of history. Spine 28:2222–2231, 2003.

188. Heide BVD, Zusman AM: Pain and muscular responses to a neural tissue provocation test in the upper limb. Man Ther 6(3):154–162, 2001.

189. Coppieters M, Stappaerts K, Janssens K, et al: Reliability of detecting "onset of pain" and "submaximal pain" during neural provocation testing of the upper quadrant. Physiother Res Int 7(3):146–156, 2002.

190. Kleinrensink GJ, Stoeckart R, Mulder PG, et al: Upper limb tension tests as tools in the diagnosis of nerve and plexus lesions: anatomical and biomechanical aspects. Clin Biomech 15(1):9–14, 2000.

191. Refshauge KM: Rotation: a valid premanipulative dizziness test? Does it predict safe manipulation. J Manip Physiol Ther 17(1):15–19, 1994.

SUGGESTED READINGS

Aprill C, Dwyer A, Bogduk N: Cervical zygapophyseal joint pain patterns: a clinical evaluation. Spine 15:458–461, 1990.

Bassett LW, Gold RH, Seeger LL: MRI atlas of the musculoskeletal system, London, 1989, Martin Dunitz.

Bateman JE: The shoulder and neck, Philadelphia, 1972, WB Saunders.

Beatty RM, Fowler FD, Hanson EJ: The abducted arm as a sign of ruptured cervical disc. Neurosurgery 21:731–732, 1987.

Bell GR, Ross JS: Diagnosis of nerve root compression: myelography, computed tomography, and MRI. Orthop Clin North Am 23:405–419, 1992.

Beggs I: Radiological assessment of degenerative diseases of the cervical spine. Semin Orthop 2:63–73, 1987.

Bogduk N, Marsland A: The cervical zygapophyseal joints as a source of neck pain. Spine 13:610–617, 1988.

Bonica JJ: The management of pain, Philadelphia, 1953, Lea & Febiger.

Breck LW, Van Norman RW: Medical legal aspects of cervical spine sprains. Clin Ortho Rel Res 74:124–128, 1971.

Butler D, Gifford L: The concept of adverse mechanical tension in the nervous system. Physiotherapy 75:622–636, 1989.

Cailliet R: Neck and arm pain, Philadelphia, 1964, FA Davis.

Campbell AM, Phillips DG: Cervical disc lesions with neurological disorder. Br Med J 2:480–485, 1960.

Carroll LJ, Holm LW, Hogg-Johnson S, et al: Course and prognostic factors for neck pain in whiplash-associated disorders (WAD): results of the Bone and Joint Decade 2000–2010 Task Force on Neck Pain and Its Associated Disorders. J Manip Physiol Ther 32(2 Suppl):S97–S107, 2009.

Cates JR, Soriano MM: Cervical spondylotic myelopathy. J Manip Physiol Ther 18:471–475, 1995.

Cervical Spine Research Society: The cervical spine, Philadelphia, 1989, JB Lippincott.

Cibulka MT: Evaluation and treatment of cervical spine injuries. Clin Sports Med 8:691–701, 1989.

Clark CR: Examination of the neck. In Clark CR, Bonfiglio M, editors: Orthopedics: essentials of diagnosis and treatment, New York, 1994, Churchill Livingstone.

Clark CR, Igram CM, El-Khoury GY, et al: Radiologic evaluation of cervical spine injuries. Spine 13:742–747, 1988.

Clark RN: Diagnosis and management of torticollis. Pediatr Ann 5:43–57, 1976.

Collins HR: An evaluation of cervical and lumbar discography. Clin Orthop 107:133–138, 1975.

Crouch JE: Functional human anatomy, Philadelphia, 1973, Lea & Febiger.

Darnell MW: A proposed chronology of events for forward head posture. J Craniomand Pract 1:50–54, 1983.

Dhimitri K, Brodeur S, Croteau M, et al: Reliability of the cervical range of motion device in measuring upper cervical motion. J Man Manip Ther 6:31–36, 1998.

Dorwart RH, LaMasters DL: Application of computed tomographic scanning of the cervical spine. Orthop Clin North Am 16:381–393, 1985.

Dvorak J: Soft tissue injuries of the cervical spine (whiplash injuries): classification and diagnosis. In Gunzburg R, Szpalski M, editors: Current concepts with prevention, diagnosis and treatment of cervical whiplash syndrome, Philadelphia, 1998, Lippincott-Raven.

Dvorak J, Dvorak V: Manual medicine: diagnostics, New York, 1984, Thieme-Stratton.

Edmeads J: Headaches and head pains associated with diseases of the cervical spine. Med Clin North Am 62:533–544, 1978.

Edwards BC: Combined movements in the cervical spine (C2–7): Their value in examination and technique choice. Aust J Physiother 26:165–171, 1980.

Edwards BC: Combined movements of the cervical spine in examination and treatment. In Grant R, editor: Physical therapy of the cervical and thoracic spine, New York, 1988, Churchill Livingstone.

Esposito CJ, Crim GA, Binkley TK: Headaches: a differential diagnosis. J Craniomand Pract 4:318–322, 1986.

Ferlic D: The range of motion of the "normal" cervical spine. Johns Hopkins Hosp Bull 110:59, 1962.

Fielding JW: Normal and selected abnormal motion of the cervical spine from the second cervical vertebra to the seventh cervical vertebra based on cineroentgenography. J Bone Joint Surg Am 46:1779–1781, 1964.

Fielding JW, Cochran GB, Lawsing JF, et al: Tears of the transverse ligament of the atlas: a clinical and biomechanical study. J Bone Joint Surg Am 56:1683–1691, 1974.

Forrester DM, Brown JC: The radiology of joint disease, Philadelphia, 1987, WB Saunders.

Franco JL, Herzog A: A comparative assessment of neck muscle strength and vertebral stability. J Orthop Sports Phys Ther 8:351–356, 1987.

Frykholm R: Lower cervical vertebrae and intervertebral discs: surgical anatomy and pathology. Acta Chir Scand 101(5):345–359, 1951.

Gould GA: The Spine. In Gould GA, editor: Orthopedic and sports physical therapy, St Louis, 1990, CV Mosby.

Grant R: Dizziness testing and manipulation of the cervical spine. In Grant R, editor: Physical therapy of the cervical and thoracic spine, New York, 1988, Churchill Livingstone.

Grieve GP: Common vertebral joint problems, New York, 1981, Churchill Livingstone.

Grieve GP: Mobilisation of the spine, ed 3, New York, 1979, Churchill Livingstone.

Gundry CR, Heithoff KB: Imaging evaluation of patients with spinal deformity. Orthop Clin North Am 25:247–264, 1994.

Harrelson GL: Evaluation of brachial plexus injuries. Sportsmed Update 4:3–9, 1989.

Hensinger RN: Congenital anomalies of the cervical spine. Clin Orthop 264:16–38, 1991.

Herrmann DB: Validity study of head and neck flexion-extension motion comparing measurements of a pendulum goniometer and roentgenograms. J Orthop Sports Phys Ther 11:414–418, 1990.

Hershman EB: Injuries to the brachial plexus. In Torg JS, editor: Athletic injuries to the head, neck and face, St Louis, 1991, Mosby-Year Book.

Hohl M: Normal motions in the upper portion of the cervical spine. J Bone Joint Surg Am 46:1777–1779, 1964.

Hohl M: Soft-tissue injuries of the neck. Clin Orthop 109:42–49, 1975.

Hohl M, Baker HR: The atlanto-axial joint: roentgenographic and anatomic study of normal and abnormal motion. J Bone Joint Surg Am 46:1739–1752, 1964.

Hollinshead WH, Jenkins DB: Functional anatomy of the limbs and back, Philadelphia, 1981, WB Saunders.

Hoppenfeld S: Physical examination of the spine and extremities, New York, 1976, Appleton-Century-Crofts.

Hu R, Burnham R, Reid DC, et al: Burners in contact sports. Clin J Sports Med 1:236–242, 1991.

Humphreys BK: Cervical outcome measures: testing for postural stability and balance. J Manip Physiol Ther 31:540–546, 2008.

Jackson R: The cervical syndrome, Springfield, IL, 1976, Charles C Thomas.

Jordon K: Assessment of published reliability studies for cervical spine range of motion measurement tools. J Manip Physiol Ther 23:180–195, 2000.

Judge RD, Zuidema GD, Fitzgerald FT: Clinical diagnosis: a physiological approach, Boston, 1982, Little, Brown.

Kaye JJ, Nance EP: Cervical spine trauma. Orthop Clin North Am 21:449–462, 1990.

Kaye S, Mason E: Clinical implications of the upper limb tension test. Physiotherapy 75:750–752, 1989.

Kenneally M, Rubenach H, Elvey R: The upper limb tension test: the SLR rest of the arm. In Grant R, editor: Physical therapy of the cervical and thoracic spine, New York, 1988, Churchill Livingstone.

Kettner NW: The radiology of cervical spine injury. J Manip Physiol Ther 14:518–526, 1991.

Law MD, Bernhardt M, White AA: Evaluation and management of cervical spondylotic myelopathy. J Bone Joint Surg Am 76:1420–1433, 1994.

Liebenson CS: Thoracic outlet syndrome: diagnosis and conservative management. J Manip Physiol Ther 11:493–499, 1988.

Liebgott B: The anatomical basis of dentistry, Philadelphia, 1982, WB Saunders.

Lysell E: Motion in the cervical spine. Acta Orthop Scand Supp 123:1–61, 1969.

Macnab I: Cervical spondylosis. Clin Orthop 109:69–77, 1975.

Maigne R: Diagnosis and treatment of pain of vertebral origin: a manual medicine approach, Baltimore, 1996, Williams & Wilkins.

Maigne R: Orthopaedic medicine: a new approach to vertebral manipulation, Springfield, IL, 1972, Charles C Thomas.

Mathews JA, Pemberton J: Radiologic anatomy of the neck. Physiotherapy 65:77–80, 1979.

Matsunaga S, Sakou T, Taketomi E, et al: The natural course of myelopathy caused by ossification of the posterior longitudinal ligament in the cervical spine. Clin Orthop 305:1668–1677, 1994.

McKinnis LN: Fundamentals of musculoskeletal imaging, Philadelphia, 2005, FA Davis.

McRae R: Clinical orthopaedic examination, New York, 1976, Churchill Livingstone.

Meyer SA, Schulte KR, Callaghan JJ, et al: Cervical spinal stenosis and stingers in collegiate football players. Am J Sports Med 22:158–166, 1994.

Miller JS, Polissar NL, Haas M: A radiographic comparison of neutral cervical posture with cervical flexion and extension ranges of motion. J Manip Physiol Ther 19:296–301, 1996.

Nilsson N, Christensen HW, Hartvigsen J: The interexaminer reliability of measuring passive cervical range of motion, revisited. J Manip Physiol Ther 19:302–305, 1996.

Nilsson N, Hartvigsen J, Christensen HW: Normal ranges of passive cervical motion for women and men 20–60 years old. J Manip Physiol Ther 19:306–309, 1996.

Palmer ML, Epler M: Clinical assessment procedures in physical therapy, Philadelphia, 1990, JB Lippincott.

Panjabi MM: Cervical spine mechanics as a function of transection of components. J Biomech 8:327–336, 1975.

Patterson RH: Cervical ribs and the scalenus muscle syndrome. Ann Surg 111:531–543, 1940.

Pavlov H: Radiographic evaluation of the cervical spine and related structures. In Torg JS, editor: Athletic injuries to the head, neck and face, St Louis, 1991, Mosby-Year Book.

Pavlov H, Torg JS, Robie B, et al: Cervical spinal stenosis: determination with vertebral body ratio method. Radiology 164:771–775, 1987.

Pedersen HE, Blunck CFJ, Gardner E: The anatomy of lumbosacral posterior rami and meningeal branches of spinal nerves (sinu-vertebral nerves). J Bone Joint Surg Am 38:377–391, 1956.

Penning L: Functional pathology of the cervical spine, New York, 1968, Excerpta Medica Foundation.

Penning L: Normal movements of the cervical spine. Am J Roentgenol 130:317–326, 1978.

Post M: Physical Examination of the musculoskeletal system, Chicago, 1987, Year Book Medical Publishers.

Rahim KA, Stambough JL: Radiographic evaluation of the degenerative cervical spine. Orthop Clin North Am 23:395–403, 1992.

Ratkovits BL: Radiographic assessment. In Bland JH, editor: Disorders of the lumbar spine, Philadelphia, 1994, WB Saunders.

Refshauge K: Testing adequacy of cerebral blood flow (vertebral artery testing). In Refshauge K, Gass E, editors: Musculoskeletal physiotherapy, Oxford, 1995, Butterworth-Heinemann.

Resnick D, Kransdorf MJ: Bone and joint imaging, Philadelphia, 2005, Saunders.

Rheault W, Albright B, Byers C, et al: Intertester reliability of the cervical range of motion device. J Orthop Sports Phys Ther 15:147–150, 1992.

Rockett FX: Observations on the "burner:" traumatic cervical radiculopathy. Clin Orthop 164:18–19, 1982.

Rorabech CH, Harris WR: Factors affecting the prognosis of brachial plexus injuries. J Bone Joint Surg Br 63:404–407, 1981.

Rothman RH: The acute cervical disc. Clin Orthop 109:59–68, 1975.

Rothman RH, Simeone FA: The spine, Philadelphia, 1982, WB Saunders.

Saunders HD, Saunders R: Evaluation, treatment and prevention of musculoskeletal disorders, Chaska, MN, 1995, Educational Opportunities.

Sherk HH, Watters WC, Zeiger L: Evaluation and treatment of neck pain. Orthop Clin North Am 13:439–452, 1982.

Southwick WO, Keggi K: The normal cervical spine. J Bone Joint Surg Am 46:1767–1777, 1964.

Speer KP, Bassett FH: The prolonged burner syndrome. Am J Sports Med 18:591–594, 1990.

Stanwood JE, Kraft GH: Diagnosis and assessment of brachial plexus injuries. Arch Phys Med Rehabil 52:52–60, 1971.

Stratton SA, Bryon JM: Dysfunction, evaluation and treatment of the cervical spine and thoracic inlet. In Donatelli R, Wooden MJ, editors: Orthopedic physical therapy, New York, 1989, Churchill Livingstone.

Sunderland S: Meningeal-neural relations in the intervertebral foramen. J Neurosurg 40:756–763, 1974.

Tardiff GS: Nerve injuries: testing and treatment tactics. Phys Sportsmed 23:61–72, 1995.

Tatlow WFT, Bammer HG: Syndrome of vertebral artery compression. Neurology 7:331–340, 1957.

Templeton PA, Young JW, Mirvis SE, et al: The value of retropharangeal soft tissue measurements in trauma of the adult cervical spine. Skeletal Radiol 16:98–104, 1987.

Torg JS, Pavlov H, Glasgow SG: Radiographic evaluation of athletic injuries to the cervical spine. In Camins MB, O'Leary PF, editors: Disorders of the cervical spine, Baltimore, 1992, Williams & Wilkins.

Torg JS, Ramsey-Emrhein JA: Cervical spine and brachial plexus injuries–return to play recommendations. Phys Sportsmed 25(7):61–88, 1997.

Troost BT: Dizziness and vertigo in vertebrobasilar disease. Stroke 11:413–415, 1980.

Vereschagin KS, Wiens JJ, Fanton GS, et al: Burners: don't overlook or underestimate them. Phys Sportsmed 19:96–106, 1991.

Waldron RL, Wood EH: Cervical myelography. Clin Orthop 97:74–89, 1973.

Wasenko JJ, Lanzieri CF: Plain radiographic examination in cervical spine trauma. In Camins MB, O'Leary PF, editors: Disorders of the cervical spine, Baltimore, 1992, Williams & Wilkins.

Weir DC: Roentgenographic signs of cervical injury. Clin Orthop 109:9–17, 1975.

White AA, Johnson RM, Panjabi MM, et al: Biomechanical analysis of clinical stability in the cervical spine. Clin Orthop 109:85–96, 1975.

White AA, Panjabi MM: The clinical biomechanics of the occipito-atlantoaxial complex. Orthop Clin North Am 9:867–878, 1978.

White AA, Panjabi MM: Clinical biomechanics of the spine, Philadelphia, 1978, JB Lippincott.

Williams P, Warwick R, editors: Gray's anatomy, ed 36, (British), Edinburgh, 1980, Churchill Livingstone.

Wong A, Nansel DD: Comparisons between active vs. passive end-range assessments in subjects exhibiting cervical range of motion asymmetries. J Manip Physiol Ther 15:159–163, 1992.

Worth DR: Movements of the head and neck. In Boyling JD, Palastanga N, editors: Grieve's modern manual therapy: the vertebral column, ed 2, Edinburgh, 1994, Churchill Livingstone.

Wyke B: Neurology of the cervical spine joints. Physiotherapy 65:72–76, 1979.

Yu YL, Woo E, Huang CY: Cervical spondylotic myelopathy and radiculopathy. Acta Neurol Scand 75:367–373, 1987.

Zatzkin HR, Kveton FW: Evaluation of the cervical spine in whiplash injuries. Radiology 75:577–583, 1960.

CHAPTER 4

Temporomandibular Joint

The temporomandibular joints are two of the most frequently used joints in the body, but they probably receive the least amount of attention. Without these joints, we would be severely hindered when talking, eating, yawning, kissing, or sucking. In any examination of the head and neck, the temporomandibular joints should be included. Temporomandibular disorders (TMDs) consist of several complex multifactorial ailments involving many interrelating factors including psychosocial issues.[1-3] Three cardinal features of TMD are orofacial pain, restricted jaw motion, and joint noise.[1] Much of the work in this chapter has been developed from the teachings of Rocabado.[4]

APPLIED ANATOMY

The temporomandibular joint is a synovial, condylar, modified ovoid, and hinge-type joint with fibrocartilaginous surfaces rather than hyaline cartilage[5] and an articular disc; this disc completely divides each joint into two cavities (Figure 4-1). Both joints, one on each side of the jaw, must be considered together in any examination. Along with the teeth, these joints are considered to be a "trijoint complex."

Gliding, translation, or **sliding movement** occurs in the upper cavity of the temporomandibular joint, whereas **rotation** or **hinge movement** occurs in the lower cavity (Figure 4-2). Rotation occurs from the beginning to the midrange of movement. The upper head of the lateral pterygoid muscle draws the disc, or **meniscus,** anteriorly and prepares for condylar rotation during movement. The rotation occurs through the two condylar heads between the articular disc and the condyle. In addition, the disc provides congruent contours and lubrication for the joint. Gliding, which occurs as a second movement, is a translatory movement of the condyle and disc along the slope of the articular eminence. Both gliding and rotation are essential for full opening and closing of the mouth (Figure 4-3). The capsule of the temporomandibular joints is thin and loose. In the resting position, the mouth is slightly open, the lips are together, and the teeth are not in contact but slightly apart. In the close-packed position, the teeth are tightly clenched, and the heads of the condyles are in the posterior aspect of the joint. **Centric occlusion** is the relation of the jaw and teeth when there is maximum contact of the teeth, and it is the position

assumed by the jaw in swallowing. The position in which the teeth are fully interdigitated is called the **median occlusal position.**[6]

Temporomandibular Joints	
Resting position:	Mouth slightly open, lips together, teeth not in contact
Close-packed position:	Teeth tightly clenched
Capsular pattern:	Limitation of mouth opening

The temporomandibular joints actively displace only anteriorly and slightly laterally. When the mouth is opening, the condyles of the joint rest on the disc in the articular eminences, and any sudden movement, such as a yawn, may displace one or both condyles forward. As the mandible moves forward on opening, the disc moves medially and posteriorly until the collateral ligaments and lateral pterygoid stop its movement. The disc is then "seated" on the head of the mandible, and both disc and mandible move forward to full opening. If this "seating" of the disc does not occur, full range of motion at the temporomandibular joint is limited. In the first phase, mainly rotation occurs, primarily in the inferior joint space. In the second phase, in which the mandible and disc move together, mainly translation occurs in the superior joint space.[7]

The hyoid bone, found in the anterior throat region, is sometimes referred to as the skeleton of the tongue.[6] It serves as an attachment for the extrinsic tongue muscles and infrahyoid muscles and, by so doing, provides reciprocal stabilization during swallowing and through its muscle attachments can affect cervical and even shoulder function. Figure 4-4 outlines the effect of a forward head posture and the relation to the hyoid bone and related muscles.

The temporomandibular joints are innervated by branches of the auriculotemporal and masseteric branches of the mandibular nerve. The disc is innervated along its periphery but is aneural and avascular in its intermediate (force-bearing) zone.

The **temporomandibular,** or **lateral, ligament** restrains movement of the lower jaw and prevents

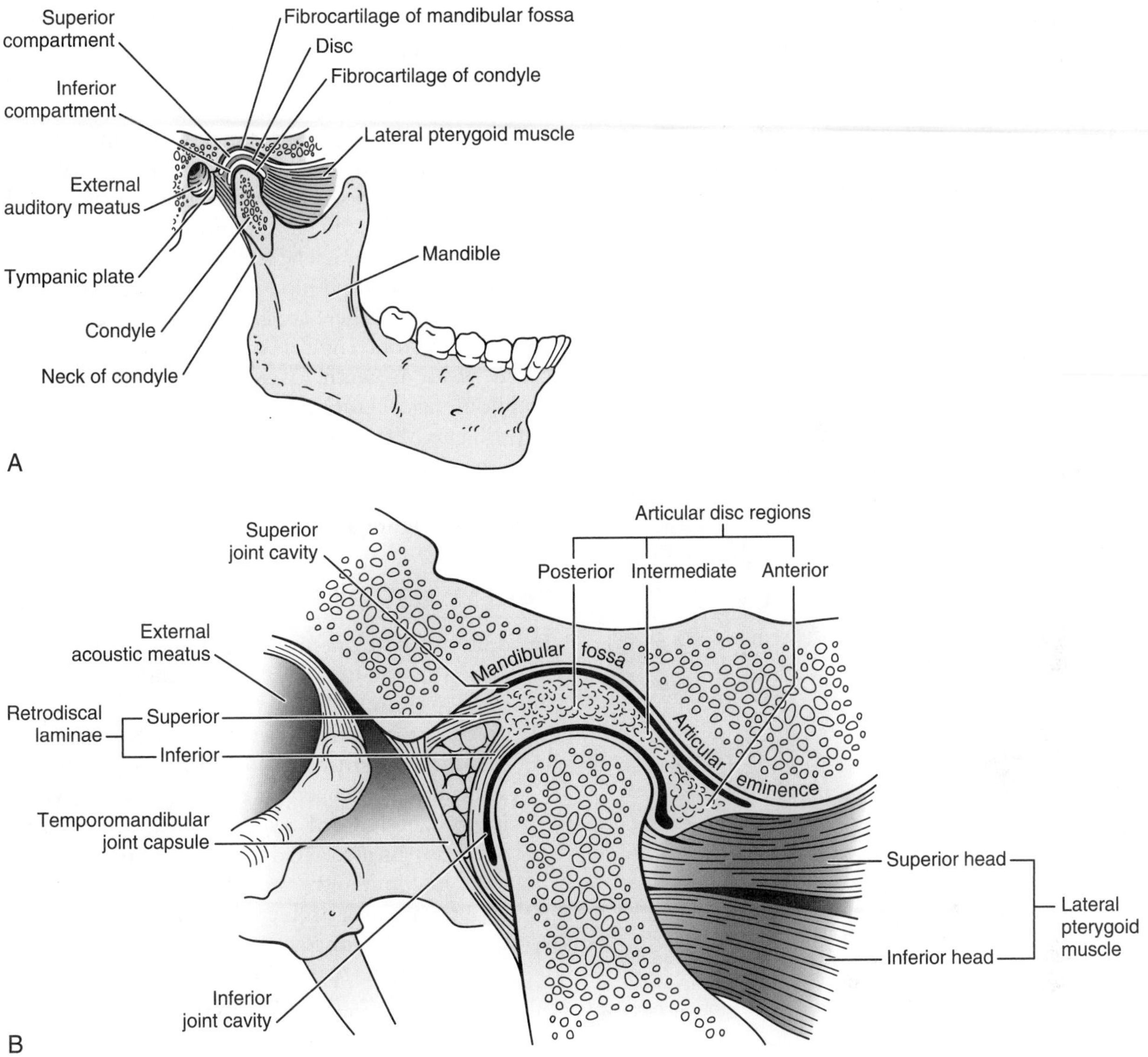

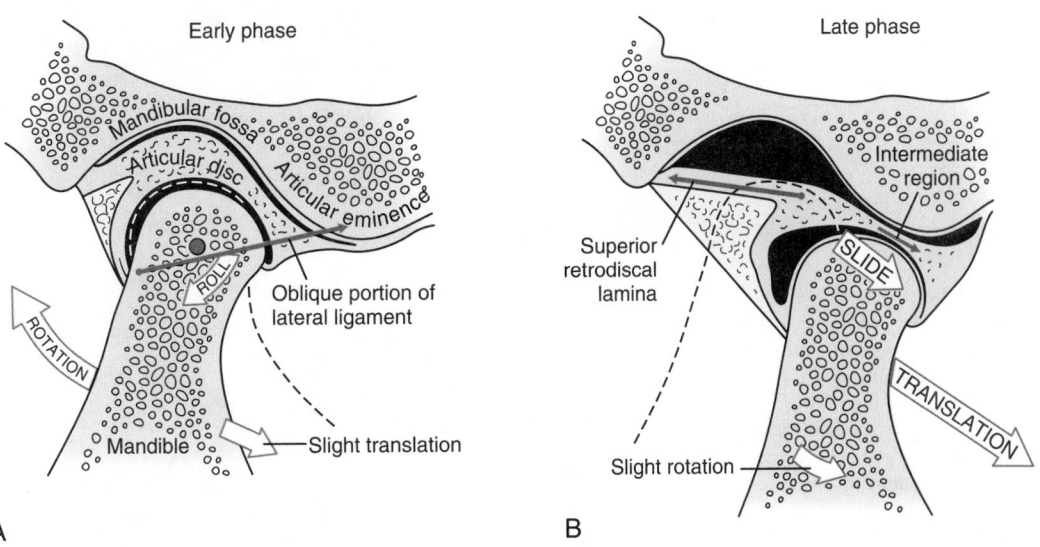

Superior compartment
Fibrocartilage of mandibular fossa
Disc
Inferior compartment
Fibrocartilage of condyle
Lateral pterygoid muscle
External auditory meatus
Tympanic plate
Mandible
Condyle
Neck of condyle

A

Superior joint cavity
Articular disc regions
Posterior   Intermediate   Anterior
External acoustic meatus
Mandibular fossa
Retrodiscal laminae — Superior
— Inferior
Articular eminence
Temporomandibular joint capsule
Superior head
Lateral pterygoid muscle
Inferior head
Inferior joint cavity

B

Figure 4-1 A, The temporomandibular joint. **B,** Close up of temporomandibular joint. (**B,** Redrawn from Neumann DA: Kinesiology of the musculoskeletal system—foundations for physical rehabilitation, St Louis, 2002, CV Mosby, p. 357.)

Early phase
Mandibular fossa
Articular disc
Articular eminence
ROLL
ROTATION
Oblique portion of lateral ligament
Mandible
Slight translation

A

Late phase
Intermediate region
Superior retrodiscal lamina
SLIDE
TRANSLATION
Slight rotation

B

Figure 4-2 Arthrokinematics of opening the mouth: A, Early phase. **B,** Late phase. (Modified from Neumann DA: Kinesiology of the musculoskeletal system—foundations for physical rehabilitation, St Louis, 2002, CV Mosby, p. 360.)

compression of the tissues behind the condyle. In reality, this collateral ligament is a thickening in the joint capsule. The **sphenomandibular** and **stylomandibular ligaments** act as "guiding" restraints to keep the condyle, disc, and temporal bone firmly opposed. The stylomandibular ligament is a specialized band of deep cerebral fascia with thickening of the parotid fascia.

In the human, there are 20 deciduous, or temporary ("baby"), teeth and 32 permanent teeth (Figure 4-5). The temporary teeth are shed between the ages of 6 and

13 years. In the adult, the incisors are the front teeth (four maxillary and four mandibular) with the maxillary incisors being larger than the mandibular incisors. The incisors are designed to cut food. The canine teeth (two maxillary and two mandibular) are the longest permanent teeth and are designed to cut and tear food. The premolars crush and break down the food for digestion; usually they have two cusps. There are eight premolars in all, two on each side, top and bottom. The final set of teeth is the molars, which crush and grind food for digestion. They have four or five cusps, and there are two or three on each side, top and bottom (total eight to twelve). The third molars are called **wisdom teeth.** Missing teeth, abnormal tooth eruption, malocclusion, or dental caries (decay) may lead to problems of the temporomandibular joint. By convention, the teeth are divided into four quadrants—the upper left, the upper right, the lower left, and the lower right quadrants (Figure 4-6).

PATIENT HISTORY

In addition to the questions listed under Patient History in Chapter 1, the examiner should obtain the following information from the patient:[8,9]

1. *Is there pain or restriction on opening or closing of the mouth?* Pain in the fully opened position (e.g., pain associated with opening to bite an apple, yawning) is probably caused by an extra-articular problem, whereas pain associated with biting firm objects (e.g., nuts, raw fruit and vegetables) is probably caused by an intra-articular problem.[10] Limited opening may be due to the disc displaced anteriorly, inert tissue tightness, or muscle spasm. Restriction can lead to anxiety in patients because of its effect on everyday activities (e.g., eating, talking).[3]

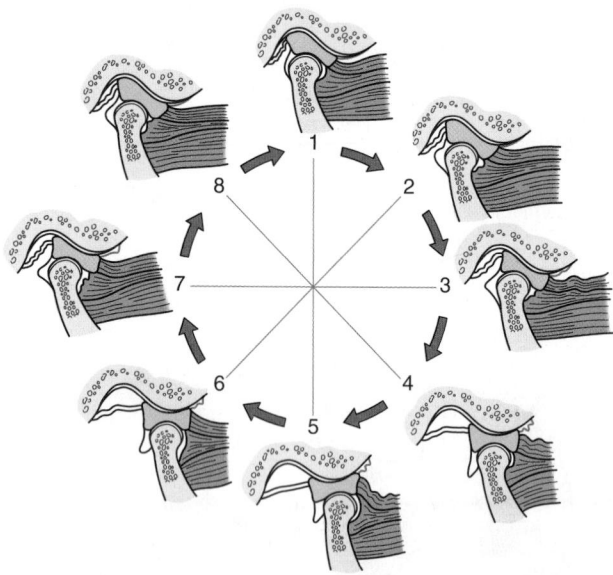

Figure 4-3 Normal functional movement of the condyle and disc during the full range of opening and closing. Note that the disc is rotated posteriorly on the condyle as the condyle is translated out of the fossa. The closing movement is the exact opposite of the opening movement.

Figure 4-4 A forward head posture shows one mechanism by which passive tension in selected suprahyoid and infrahyoid muscles alter the resting posture of the mandible. The mandible is pulled inferiorly and posteriorly, changing the position of the condyle within the temporomandibular joint. Note the interrelationship to the cervical spine and shoulder. (Modified from Neumann DA: Kinesiology of the musculoskeletal system—foundations for physical rehabilitation, St Louis, 2002, CV Mosby, p. 366.)

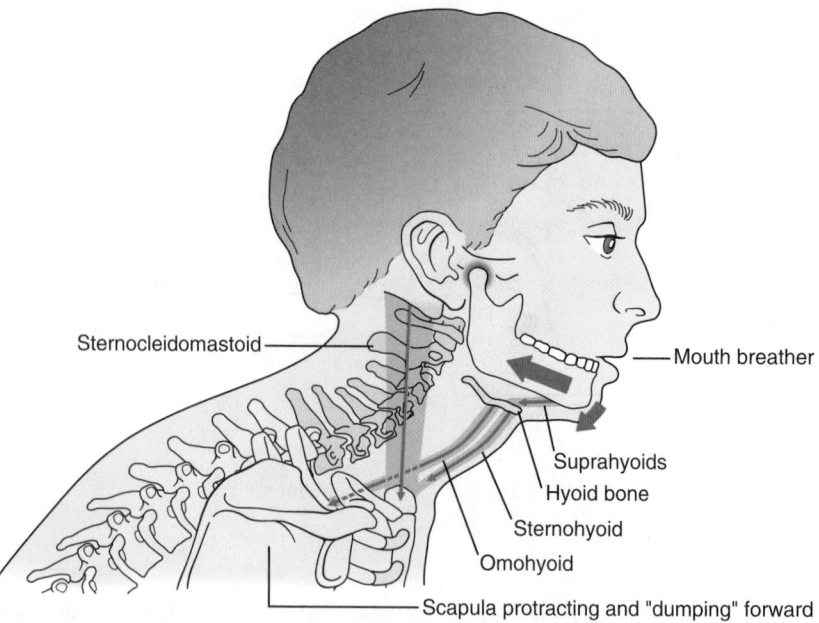

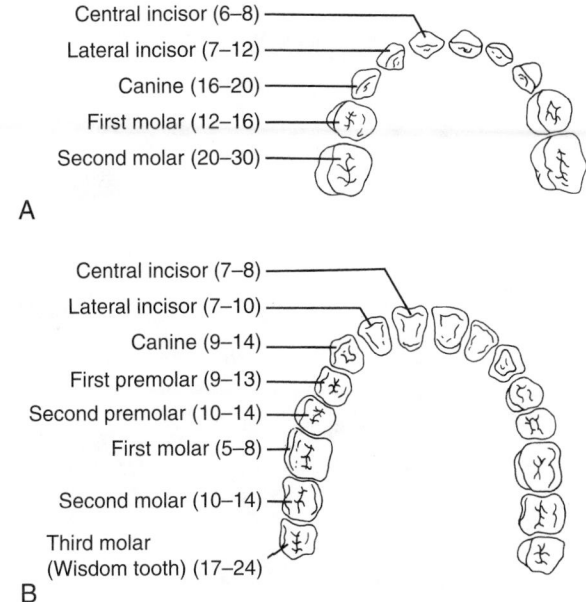

A

B

Figure 4-5 Teeth in a child (**A**) and in an adult (**B**). Numbers indicate age (in months for a child, in years for an adult) at which teeth erupt.

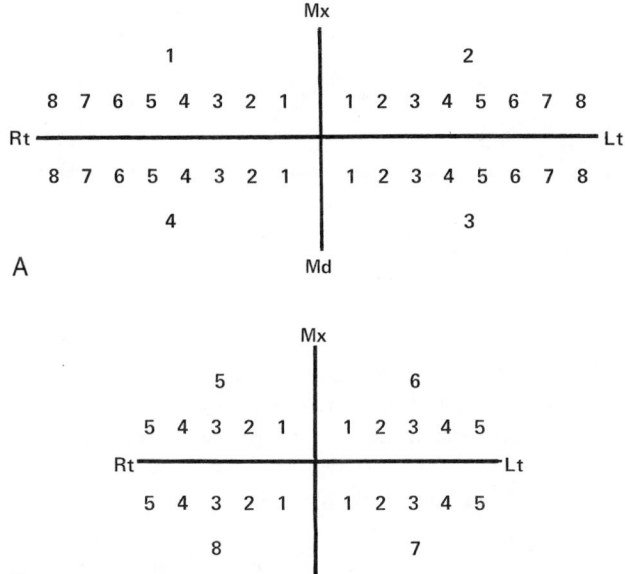

A

B

Figure 4-6 **Numeric symbols for dentition** in an adult (**A**) and in a child (**B**). (From Liebgott B: The anatomical basis of dentistry, St Louis, 1986, CV Mosby.)

2. *Is there pain on eating? Does the patient chew on the right? Left? Both sides equally?* Loss of molars or worn dentures can lead to loss of vertical dimension, which can make chewing painful. **Vertical dimension** is the distance between any two arbitrary points on the face, one of these points being above and the other below

the mouth, usually in midline. Often, chewing on one side is the result of malocclusion.[10]

3. *What movements of the jaw cause pain? Do the symptoms change over a 24-hour period?* The examiner should watch the patient's jaw movement while the patient is talking. A history of stiffness on waking with pain on function that disappears as the day goes on suggests osteoarthritis.[11]

4. *Do any of these actions cause pain or discomfort: yawning, biting, chewing, swallowing, speaking, or shouting? If so, where?* All of these actions cause movement, compression, and/or stretching of the soft tissues of the temporomandibular joints.

5. *Does the patient breathe through the nose or the mouth?* Normal breathing is through the nose with the lips closed and no "air gulping." If the patient is a "mouth breather," the tongue does not sit in the proper position against the palate. In the young, if the tongue does not push against the palate, developmental abnormalities may occur, because the tongue normally provides internal pressure to shape the mouth. The buccinator and orbicularis oris muscle complex provides external pressure to counterbalance the internal pressure of the tongue. Loss of normal neck balance often results in the individual's becoming a mouth breather and an upper respiratory breather, making greater use of the accessory muscles of respiration. Conditions (such as, adenoids, tonsils, and upper respiratory tract infections) may cause the same problem.

6. *Has the patient complained of any **crepitus** or **clicking**?* Normally, the condyles of the temporomandibular joint slide out of the concavity and onto the rim of the disc. Clicking is the result of abnormal motion of the disc and mandible. Early clicking implies a developing dysfunction, whereas late clicking is more likely to mean a chronic problem. Clicking may occur when the condyle slides back off the rim into the center (Figure 4-7).[12] If the disc sticks or is bunched slightly, opening causes the condyle to move abruptly over the disc and into its normal position, resulting in a single click (see Figure 4-7).[13] There may be a partial anterior displacement (subluxation) or dislocation of the disc, which the condyle must override to reach its normal position when the mouth is fully open (Figure 4-8). This override may also cause a click. Similarly, a click may occur if the disc is displaced anteriorly and/or medially, causing the condyle to override the posterior rim of the disc later than normal during mouth opening. This is referred to as **disc displacement with reduction.** If clicking occurs in both directions, it is called **reciprocal clicking** (Figure 4-9). The opening click occurs somewhere during the opening or protrusive path, and the click indicates the condyle is slipping over the thicker posterior border of the disc to its position

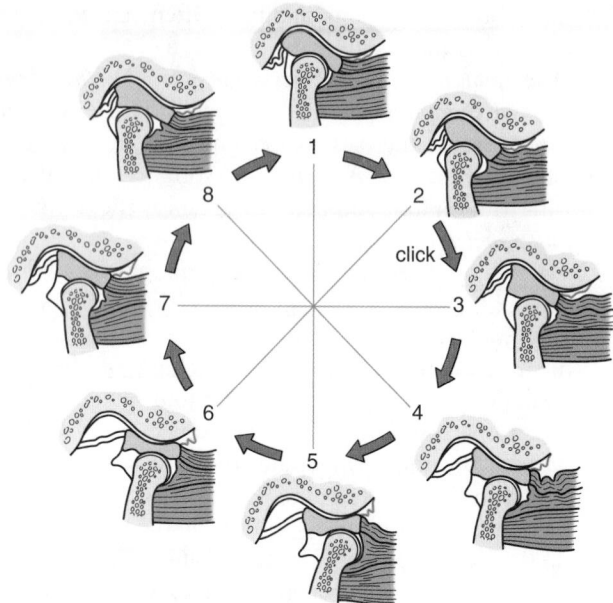

Figure 4-7 Single click. Between positions *2* and *3*, a click is felt as the condyle moves across the posterior border into the intermediate zone of the disc. Normal condyle-disc function occurs during the remaining opening and closing movement. In the closed joint position *(1)*, the disc is again displaced forward (and medially) by activity of the superior lateral pterygoid muscle.

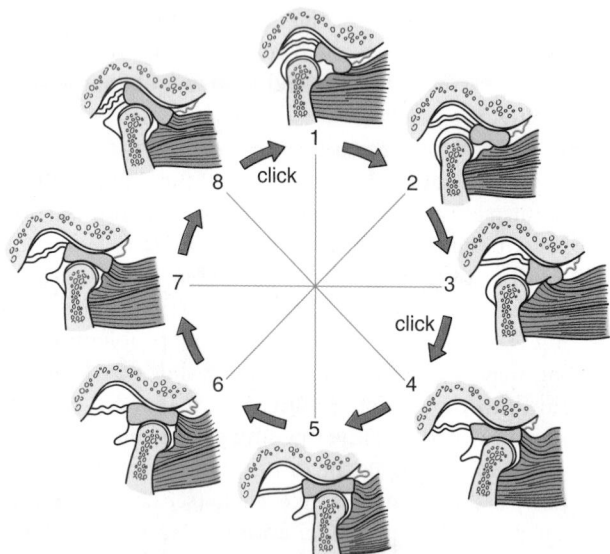

Figure 4-8 Functional dislocation of the disc with reduction. During opening, the condyle passes over the posterior border of the disc into the intermediate area of the disc, thus reducing the dislocated disc.

in the thinner middle or intermediate zone. The closing (reciprocal) click occurs near the end of the closing or retrusive path as the pull of the superior lateral pterygoid muscle causes the disc to slip more anteriorly and the condyle to move over its posterior border.

Clicks may also be caused by adhesions (Figure 4-10), especially in people who clench their teeth

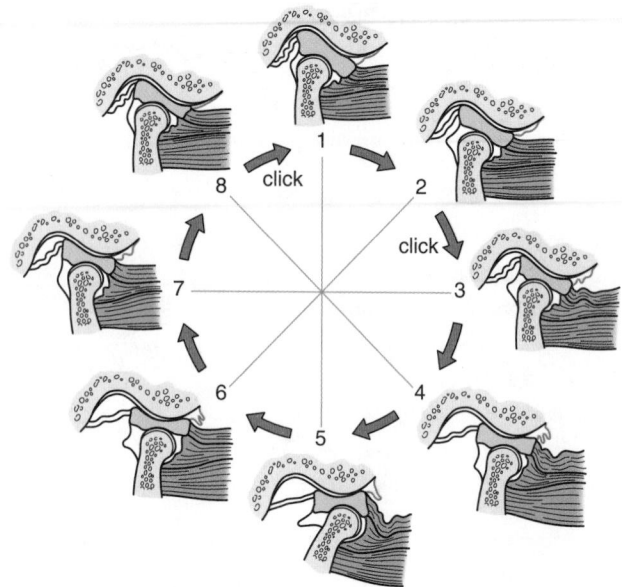

Figure 4-9 Reciprocal click. Between positions *2* and *3*, a click is felt as the condyle moves across the posterior border of the disc. Normal condyle-disc function occurs during the remaining opening and closing movement until the closed joint position is approached. A second click is heard as the condyle once again moves from the intermediate zone to the posterior border of the disc between positions *8* and *1*.

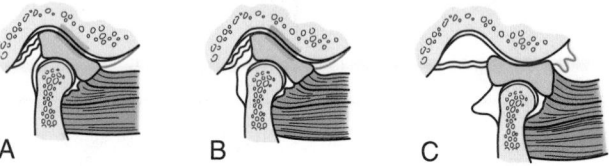

Figure 4-10 A, Adhesion in the superior joint space. **B,** The presence of the adhesion limits the joint to rotation only. **C,** If the adhesion is freed, normal translation can occur.

(bruxism). These "adhesive" clicks occur in isolation, after the period of clenching.[14] If adhesions occur in the superior or inferior joint space, translation or rotation will be limited. This presents as a temporary closed lock, which then opens with a click.

If the articular eminence is abnormally developed (i.e., short, steep posterior slope or long, flat anterior slope), the maximum anterior movement of the disc may be reached before maximum translation of the condyle has occurred. As the condyle overrides the disc, a loud crack is heard, and the condyle-disc leaps or jogs (subluxes) forward.[14]

"Soft" or "popping" clicks that are sometimes heard in normal joints are caused by ligament movement, articular surface separation, or sucking of loose tissue behind the condyle as it moves forward. These clicks usually result from muscle incoordination. "Hard" or "cracking" clicks are more likely to indicate joint pathology or joint surface defects. Soft crepitus (like rubbing knuckles together) is a sound

TABLE **4-1**

Temporomandibular Disc Dysfunction

Stage	Characteristics
Stage 1	Disc slightly anterior and medial on mandibular condyle
	Inconsistent click (may or may not be present)
	Mild or no pain
Stage 2	Disc anterior and medial
	Reciprocal click present (early on opening, late on closing)
	Severe consistent pain
Stage 3	Reciprocal consistent click present (later on opening, earlier on closing)
	Most painful stage
Stage 4	Click rare (disc no longer relocates)
	No pain

Data from Iglarsh ZA, Snyder-Mackler L: Tempormandibular joint and the cervical spine. In Richardson JK, Iglarsh ZA (editors): Clinical orthopedic physical therapy, Philadelphia, 1994, WB Saunders.

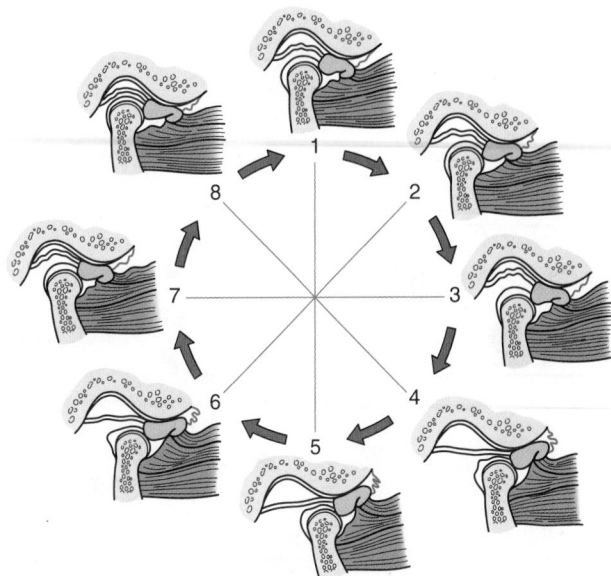

Figure 4-11 Closed lock. The condyle never assumes a normal relation to the disc but instead causes the disc to move forward ahead of it. This condition limits the distance the condyle can translate forward.

that sometimes occurs in symptomless joints and is not necessarily an indication of pathology.[15] Hard crepitus (like a footstep on gravel) is indicative of arthritic changes in the joints. The clicking may be caused by uncoordinated muscle action of the lateral pterygoid muscles, a tear or perforation in the disc, osteoarthrosis, or occlusal imbalance. Normally, the upper head of the lateral pterygoid muscle pulls the disc forward. If the disc does not move first, the condyle clicks over the disc as it is pulled forward by the lower head of the lateral pterygoid muscle. Iglarsh and Snyder-Mackler[7] have divided disc displacement into four stages (Table 4-1).

7. *Has the mouth or jaw ever locked?* Locking may imply that the mouth does not fully open or it does not fully close and is often related to problems of the disc or joint degeneration. Locking is usually preceded by reciprocal clicking. If the jaw has locked in the closed position, the locking is probably caused by a disc with the condyle being posterior or anteromedial to the disc. Even if translation is blocked (e.g., "locked" disc), the mandible can still open 30 mm by rotation. If there is functional dislocation of the disc with reduction (see Figure 4-8), the disc is usually positioned anteromedially, and opening is limited. The patient complains that the jaw "catches" sometimes, so the locking occurs only occasionally and, at those times, opening is limited. If there is functional anterior dislocation of the disc without reduction, a **closed lock** occurs. Closed lock implies there has been anterior and/or medial displacement of the disc so that the disc does not return to its normal position during the entire movement of the condyle.

In this case, opening is limited to about 25 mm, the mandible deviates to the affected side (Figure 4-11), and lateral movement to the uninvolved side is reduced.[14] If locking occurs in the open position, it is probably caused by subluxation of the joint or possibly by posterior disc displacement (see Figure 4-11). With an **open lock,** there are two clicks on opening, when the condyle moves over the posterior rim of the disc and then when it moves over the anterior rim of the disc, and two clicks on closing. If, after the second click occurs on opening, the disc lies posterior to the condyle, it may not allow the condyle to slide back (Figure 4-12).[16] If the condyle dislocates outside the fossa, it is a true dislocation with open lock; the patient cannot close the mouth, and the dislocation must be reduced.[16]

8. *Does the patient have any habits, such as smoking pipes, using a cigarette holder, leaning on the chin, chewing gum, biting the nails, chewing hair, pursing and chewing lips, continually moving the mouth, or any other nervous habits?* All these activities place additional stress on the temporomandibular joints.

9. *Does the patient grind the teeth or hold them tightly?* **Bruxism** is the forced clenching and grinding of the teeth, especially during sleep. This may lead to facial, jaw, or tooth pain, or headaches in the morning along with muscle hypertrophy. If the front teeth are in contact and the back ones are not, facial and temporomandibular pain may develop as a result of malocclusion. Normally, the upper teeth cover the upper one third of the bottom teeth (Figure 4-13).

10. *Does there appear to be any related psychosocial problems?* Temporomandibular dysfunction is often

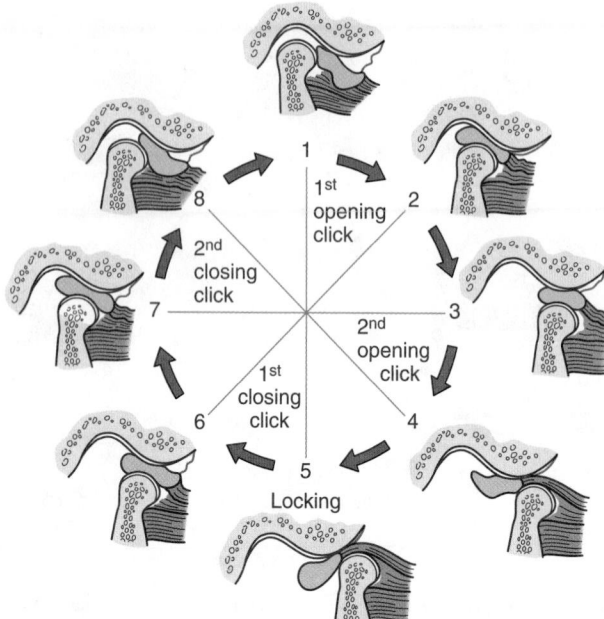

Figure 4-12 Open lock (disc incoordination). *1,* The disc always stays in anterior position with the jaw closed. *1-4,* Disc is displaced posterior to the condyle with one or two opening clicks. *5-6,* The disc disturbs jaw closing after maximum opening. *6-1,* The disc is again displaced to anterior position from the posterior with one or two clicks.

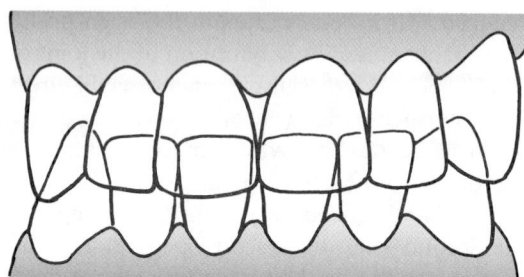

Figure 4-13 Normally the maxillary anterior teeth overlap the mandibular anterior teeth almost half the length of the mandibular crowns. (From Okeson JP: Management of temporomandibular disorders and occlusion, St Louis, 1998, CV Mosby, p. 84.)

accompanied by related psychosocial issues.[1,17] Table 4-2 outlines psychosocial factors that may affect the temporomandibular joint.

11. *Are any teeth missing? If so, which ones, and how many?* The presence or absence of teeth and their relation to one another must be noted on a table similar to the one shown in Figure 4-6. Their presence or absence can have an effect on the temporomandibular joints and their muscles. If some teeth are missing, others may deviate to fill in the space, altering the occlusion.

12. *Are any teeth painful or sensitive?* This finding may be indicative of dental caries or abscess. Tooth pain may lead to incorrect biting when chewing, which puts abnormal stresses on the temporomandibular joints.

TABLE 4-2

Checklist of Psychological and Behavioral Factors*

1. Clinically significant anxiety or depression
2. Evidence of drug abuse
3. Repeated failures with conventional therapies
4. Evidence of secondary gain
5. Major life events; for example, new job, marriage or divorce, death
6. Pain duration greater than 6 months
7. History of possible stress-related disorders
8. Inconsistency in response to drugs
9. Inconsistent, inappropriate, and vague reports of pain, or both
10. Overdramatization of symptoms
11. Symptoms that vary with life events

From McNeill C, Mohl ND, Rugh JD, et al: Temporomandibular disorders: diagnosis, management, education and research. J Am Dent Assoc 120:259, 1990.
*Note: The first two factors are the most significant and warrant further evaluation by a mental health professional; factors 3 to 6 need at least one more factor for consideration of referral; and factors 7 to 11 require three or more factors for consideration of referral to a mental health professional.

13. *Does the patient have any difficulty swallowing? Does the patient swallow normally or gulp? What happens to the tongue when the patient swallows? Does it move normally, anteriorly, or laterally? Is there any evidence of tongue thrust or thumb sucking?* For example, the facial nerve (cranial nerve VII) and the trigeminal nerve (cranial nerve V), which control facial expression and mastication and contribute to speech, also control anterior lip seal. If lip seal is weakened, the teeth may move anteriorly, an action that would be accentuated in "tongue thrusters." The normal resting position of the tongue is against the anterior palate (Figure 4-14). It is the position in which one would place the tongue to make a "clicking" sound.

14. *Are there any ear problems such as hearing loss, ringing in the ears, blocking of the ears, earache, or dizziness?* Symptoms such as these may be caused by inner ear, cervical spine, or temporomandibular joint problems.

15. *Does the patient have any habitual head postures?* For example, holding the telephone between the ear and the shoulder compacts the temporomandibular joint on that side. Reading or listening to someone while leaning one hand against the jaw has the same effect.

16. *Has the patient noticed any voice changes?* Changes may be caused by muscle spasm.

17. *Does the patient have headaches? If so, where?* Temporomandibular joint problems can refer pain to the head. Is there any history of infection or swollen glands?

18. *Does the patient ever feel dizzy or faint?*

19. *Has the patient ever worn a dental splint? If so, when? For how long?*
20. *Has the patient ever been seen by a dentist, such as a periodontist (a dentist who specializes in the study of tissues around the teeth and diseases of these tissues), an orthodontist (a dentist who specializes in correction and prevention of irregularities of the teeth), or an endodontist (a dentist who specializes in the treatment of diseases of the tooth pulp, root canal, and periapical areas)? If so, why did the patient see the specialist, and what was done?*

OBSERVATION

When assessing the temporomandibular joints, the examiner must also assess the posture of the cervical spine and head. For example, it is necessary that the head be "balanced" on the cervical spine and be in proper postural alignment.

1. Is the face symmetrical horizontally and vertically, and are facial proportions normal (Figure 4-15)? The examiner should check the eyebrows, eyes, nose, ears, and corners of the mouth for symmetry on both horizontal and vertical planes. Horizontally, the face of an adult is divided into thirds (Figure 4-16); this demonstrates normal vertical dimension. Usually the upper and lower teeth are used to measure vertical dimension. The horizontal bipupital, otic, and occlusive lines should be parallel to each other (Figure 4-17). Loss of teeth on one side can lead to convergence in which at least two of the lines may converge because the jaw line is short on one side relative to the other. A quick way to measure the vertical dimension is to measure from the lateral edge of the eye to the corner of the mouth and from the nose to the chin (Figure 4-18). Normally, the two measurements are equal. If the second measurement is smaller than the first by 1 mm

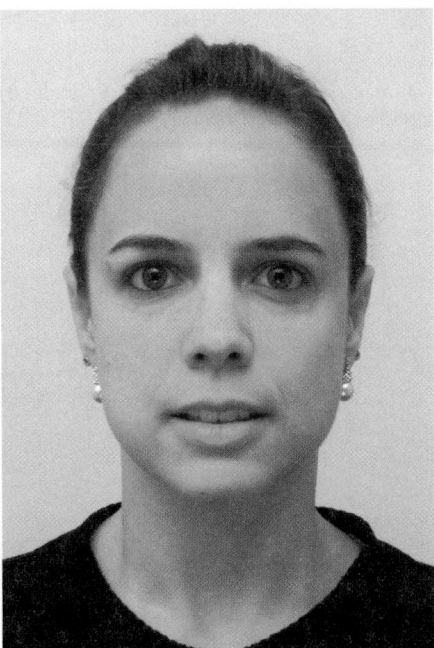

Figure 4-14 Normal resting position of the tongue. Tongue position cannot be seen because of teeth but upper and lower teeth are not in contact.

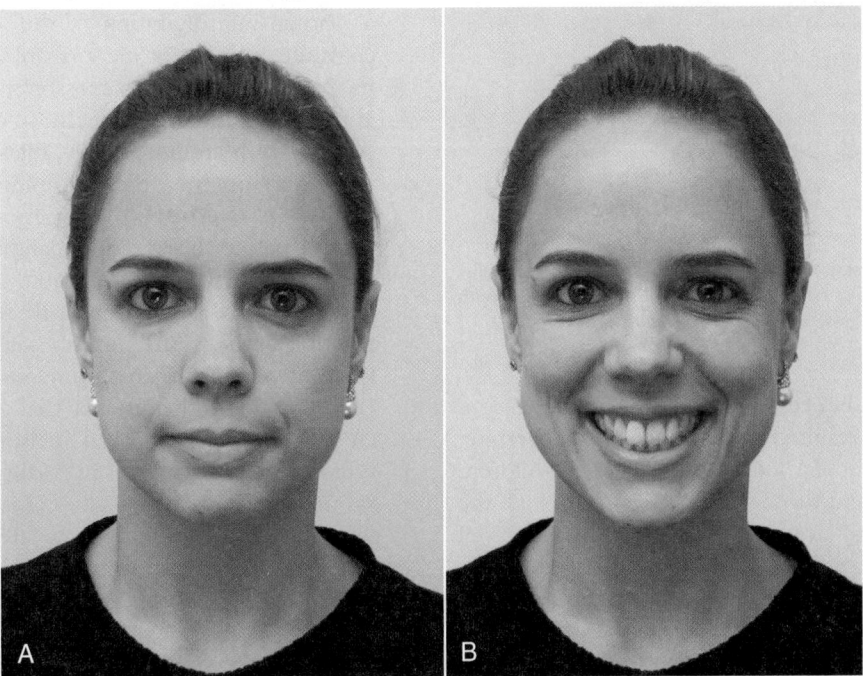

Figure 4-15 Facial symmetry. Look for asymmetry both vertically and horizontally. Asymmetrical changes may be seen with no smile (**A**) or with smile (**B**). These asymmetrical differences may or may not be related to pathology.

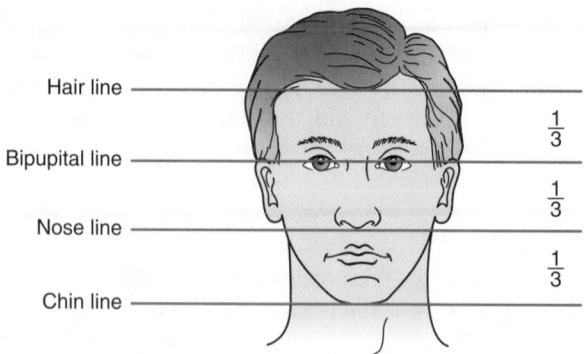

Figure 4-16 Divisions of the face (vertical dimension).

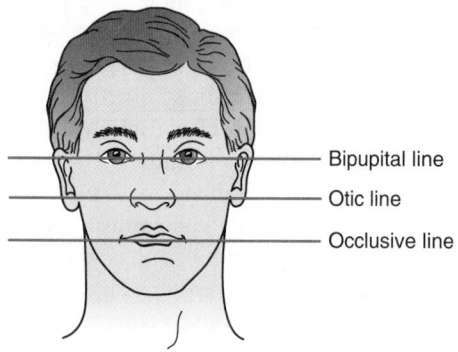

Figure 4-17 Normally, bipupital, otic, and occlusive lines are parallel.

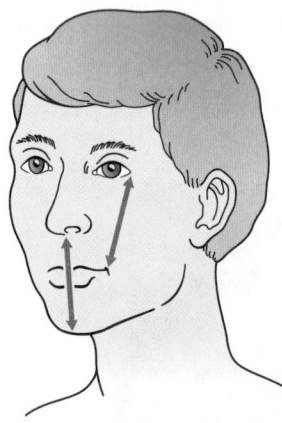

Figure 4-18 A quick measurement of vertical dimension. Normally, the distance from the lateral edge of the eye to the corner of the mouth equals the distance from nose to point of chin.

or more, there has been a loss of vertical dimension, which may have resulted from loss of teeth, overbite, or temporomandibular joint dysfunction. In children, elderly persons, and those with massive tooth loss, the lower third of the face is not well developed (lack of teeth) or has recessed (Figure 4-19). As the teeth grow, the lower third develops into its normal proportion. The examiner should notice whether there is any paralysis, which could be indicated by ptosis (drooping of an eyelid) or by drooping of the mouth on one side (Bell palsy).

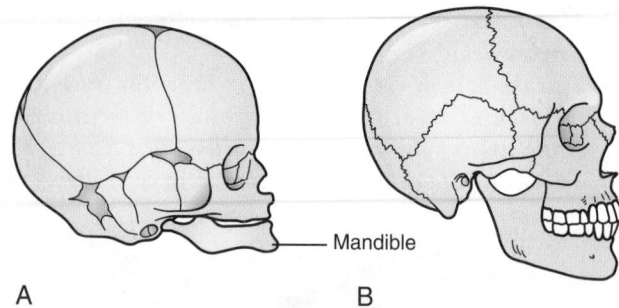

Figure 4-19 Human skull at birth (A) and in the adult (B). Note the difference brought about by development of the teeth and lower jaw in the adult.

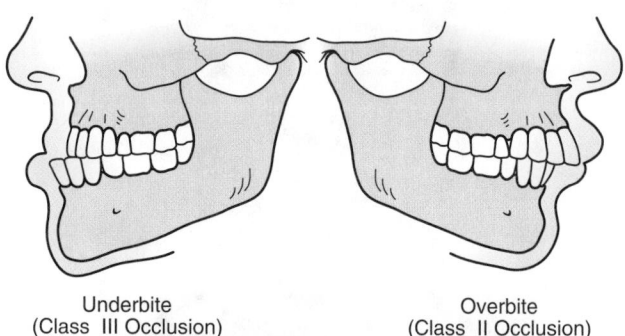

Figure 4-20 Underbite and overbite.

2. The examiner should note whether the teeth are normally aligned or there is any crossbite, underbite, or overbite (Figure 4-20). With **crossbite,** the teeth of the mandible are lateral to the upper (maxillary) teeth on one side and medial on the opposite side. There is abnormal interdigitation of the teeth. With anterior crossbite, the lower incisors are ahead of the upper incisors. With posterior crossbite, there is a transverse abnormal relation of the teeth. In **underbite,** the mandibular teeth are unilaterally, bilaterally, or in pairs in **buccoversion** (i.e., they lie anterior to the maxillary teeth). In **overbite,** the anterior maxillary incisors extend below the anterior mandibular incisors when the jaw is in centric occlusion. A small amount of overbite (2 to 3 mm) anteriorly is the most common position of the teeth. This is because the maxillary arch is slightly longer than the mandibular arch. **Overjet** (Figure 4-21) is the distance that the maxillary incisors close over the mandibular incisors when the mouth is closed. This distance is normally 2 to 3 mm. **Occlusal interference** refers to premature teeth contact, which tends to deflect the jaw laterally and/or anteriorly.[18] Any orthodontic appliances or false teeth present should also be evaluated for fit and possible sore spots.

3. The examiner should note whether there is any **malocclusion** that may result in a faulty bite. Malocclusion may be a major factor in the development of disc

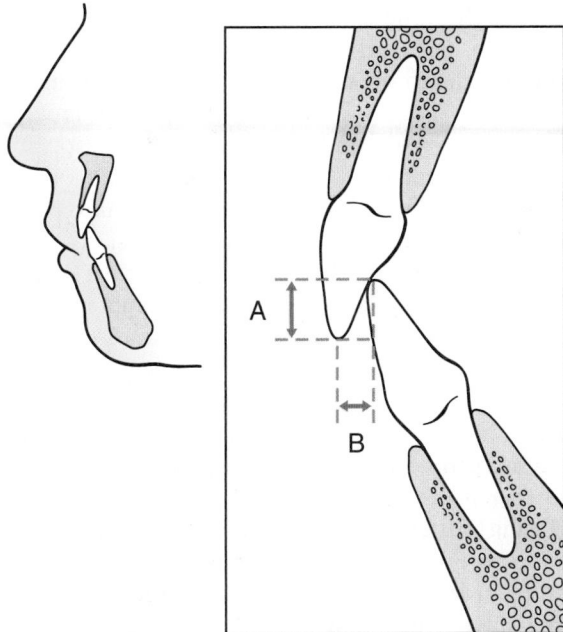

Figure 4-21 Overlap of maxillary anterior teeth. A, Vertical overlap (overbite). **B,** Horizontal overlap (overjet). (Redrawn from Friedman MH, Weisberg J: The temporomandibular joint. In Gould JA, editor: Orthopedics and sports physical therapy, St Louis, 1990, CV Mosby, p. 578.)

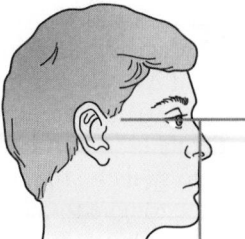

Orthognathic

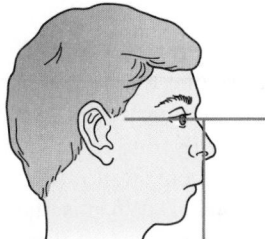

Retrognathic

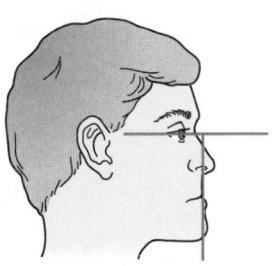

Prognathic

Figure 4-22 Facial profiles.

problems of the temporomandibular joints. Occlusion occurs when the teeth are in contact and the mouth is closed. Malocclusion is defined as any deviation from normal occlusion. Class I occlusion refers to the normal anteroposterior relation of the maxillary teeth to mandibular teeth. A slight modification with only the incisors affected and overjet slightly larger is sometimes classified as a Class I malocclusion. Class II malocclusion (overbite) occurs when the mandibular teeth are positioned posterior to their normal position relative to the maxillary teeth. This malocclusion deformity involves all the teeth, including the molars. The designation Class II Division 1 malocclusion (also called *large overjet* or **horizontal overlap**) indicates that the maxillary incisors demonstrate significant overjet. Class II Division 2 malocclusion (also called *deep overbite* or **vertical overlap**) implies that overjet is not significant but that there is overbite and lateral flaring of the lateral maxillary incisors.[19] Class III malocclusion (i.e., underbite) occurs when the mandibular teeth are positioned anterior to their normal position relative to the maxillary teeth. If maxillary and mandibular teeth are on the same vertical plane, a Class III malocclusion would be present.

4. What is the facial profile? The orthognathic profile is the normal, "straight-jawed" form. With this facial profile, a vertical line dropped perpendicular to the bipupital line would touch the upper and lower lips and the tip of the chin. In a person with a retrognathic profile, the chin would lie behind the vertical line and the person would be said to have a "receding chin." With the prognathic profile, the chin would be in front of the vertical line and the person would have a protruded or "strong" chin (Figure 4-22).[19]

5. The examiner should note whether the patient demonstrates normal bony and soft-tissue contours. When the patient bites down, do the masseter muscles bulge as they normally should? Hypertrophy caused by overuse may lead to abnormal wear of the teeth. When looking at the soft tissues, it is important to note symmetry. The upper lip should normally cover two thirds of the maxillary teeth at rest. If it does not, the lip is said to be short.[7] If the lip can be drawn over the upper teeth, however, the upper lip is said to be functional, and no treatment is necessary. The lower lip normally covers the mandibular teeth and, when the mouth is closed, part of the maxillary teeth.

6. Is the patient able to move the tongue properly? Can the patient move the tongue up to and against the palate? Can the tongue be protruded or rolled? Is the patient able to "click" the tongue? **Tongue thrusting** refers to forward movement of the tongue, usually to push against the lower teeth; it also occurs when the

tongue is pushed against the upper teeth and the lower teeth are closed firmly against it, creating an oral seal.[20] Tongue thrusters find it easier to thrust the tongue if the head is protruded. Therefore, to test for tongue thrusting, the patient's head posture is corrected and the patient is asked to swallow. In the tongue thruster, swallowing causes the tongue to move forward resulting in protrusion of the head. Tongue thrusting may be due to hyperactivity of the masticatory muscles. When one swallows, the hyoid bone should move up and down quickly. If it moves only upward and slowly, and the suboccipital muscles posteriorly contract, it is suggestive of a tongue thrust.[21]

7. Where does the tongue rest? Is the tongue bitten frequently? Does the tongue have any scalloping or ridges? Does the patient swallow normally? Do the lips part when swallowing? What is the tongue position when swallowing? Do the facial muscles tighten on swallowing? All of these factors give the examiner some idea of the mobility of the structures of the mouth and jaw and their neurological mechanisms.

EXAMINATION

The examiner must remember that many problems of the temporomandibular joints may be the result of or related to problems in the cervical spine or teeth. Therefore, the cervical spine is at least partially included in any temporomandibular assessment.

Active Movements

With the patient in the sitting position, the examiner watches the active movements, noting whether they deviate from what would be considered normal range of motion and whether the patient is willing to do the movement. The patient is first asked to carry out active movements of the cervical spine. The most painful movements, if any, should be done last.

Active Movements of the Cervical Spine

- Flexion
- Extension
- Side flexion left and right
- Rotation left and right
- Combined movements (if necessary)
- Repetitive movements (if necessary)
- Sustained positions (if necessary)

During flexion of the neck, the mandible moves up and forward, and the posterior structures of the neck become tight. During extension, the mandible moves down and back, and the anterior structures of the neck become tight. The examiner should note whether the patient can flex and extend the neck while keeping the mouth closed or whether the patient must open the mouth to do these movements. The patient should be asked to place a fist under the chin and then open the mouth while keeping the fist in place and the lower jaw against it. If the mouth opens in this way, movement of the neck into extension is occurring because the head is rotating backwards on the temporomandibular condyles. This test movement would be especially important if the patient subjectively feels that there is a loss of neck extension. With side flexion of the neck to the right, maximum occlusion occurs on the right. Side flexion and rotation of the neck occur to the same side, and so if these movements are carried out to the right, maximum occlusion also occurs to the right.

Having observed the neck movements, the examiner goes on to note the active movements of the temporomandibular joints. The movements of the mandible can be measured with a millimeter ruler, depth gauge, or vernier calipers. When using the ruler, the examiner should pick a midline point from which to measure opening and lateral deviation.[22] This same ruler can be used to measure protrusion and retrusion.

Active Movements of the Temporomandibular Joints

- Opening of the mouth
- Closing of the mouth
- Protrusion of the mandible
- Lateral deviation of the mandible right and left

Opening and Closing of the Mouth

With opening and closing of the mouth, the normal arc of movement of the jaw is smooth and unbroken; that is, both temporomandibular joints are working in unison with no asymmetry or sideways movement, and both joints are bilaterally rotating and translating equally. Any alteration may cause or indicate potential problems in the temporomandibular joints. To observe any asymmetries, opening and closing of the mouth must be done slowly. The first phase of opening is rotation, which can be tested by having the patient open the mouth as widely as possible while maintaining the tongue against the roof (hard palate) of the mouth. Usually this movement causes minimal pain and occurs even in the presence of acute temporomandibular dysfunction. The second phase of opening is translation and rotation as the condyles move along the slope of the eminence. This phase begins when the tongue loses contact with the roof of the mouth.[2] Most of the clicking sensations occur during this phase.

Normally, the mandible should open and close in a straight line (Figures 4-23 and 4-24), provided the

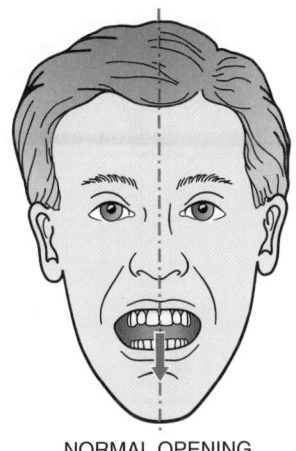 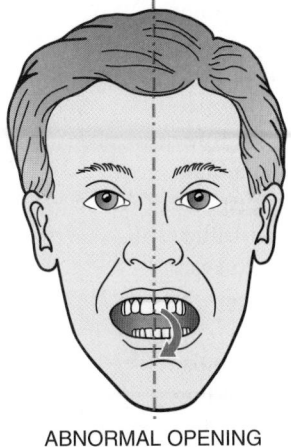 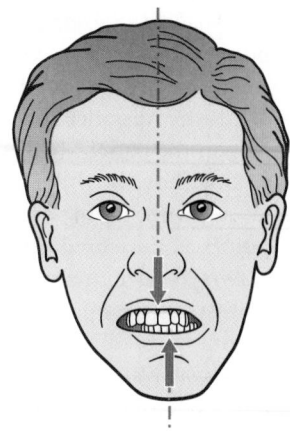

NORMAL OPENING   ABNORMAL OPENING   ABNORMAL CLOSED

Figure 4-23 Mandibular motion.

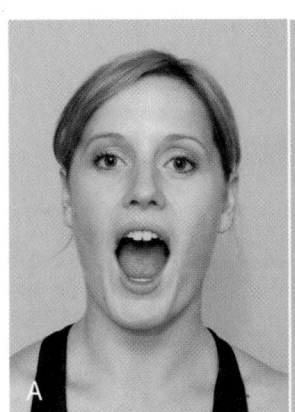 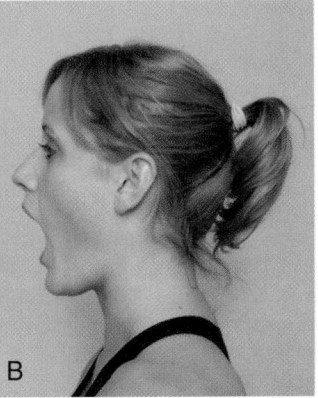

Figure 4-24 Active opening of mouth. A, Anteroposterior view. **B,** Side view.

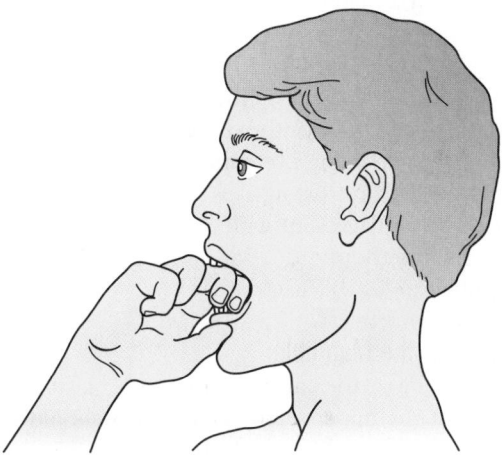

Figure 4-25 Functional opening "knuckle" test.

bilateral action of the muscles is equal and the inert tissues have normal pliability. If deviation occurs to the left on opening (see Figure 4-23) (a C-type curve) or to the right (a reverse C-type curve), hypomobility is evident toward the side of the deviation caused either by a displaced disc without reduction or unilateral muscle hypomobility;[9] if the deviation is an S-type or reverse S-type curve, the problem is probably muscular imbalance or medial displacement as the condyle "walks around" the disc on the affected side.[9] The chin deviates toward the affected side, usually because of spasm of the pterygoid or masseter muscles or an obstruction in the joint. Early deviation on opening is usually caused by muscle spasm, whereas late deviation on opening is usually a result of capsulitis or a tight capsule. Pain or tenderness, especially on closing, indicates posterior capsulitis.

The examiner should then determine whether the patient's mouth can functionally be opened. The **functional** or **full active opening** is determined by having the patient try to place two or three flexed proximal interphalangeal joints within the mouth opening (Figure 4-25).[23]

This opening should be approximately 35 to 55 mm.[3] Normally, only about 25 to 35 mm of opening is needed for everyday activity. If the patient has pain on opening, the examiner should also measure the amount of opening to the point of pain and compare this distance with functional opening.[8] If the space is less than this, the temporomandibular joints are said to be hypomobile. Kropmans et al.[24] have pointed out that for treatment, at least 6 mm of change has to be seen to be a detectable difference when doing more than one measurement or to determine the effect of treatment.

As the mouth opens, the examiner should palpate the external auditory meatus with the index or little finger (fleshy part anterior). The patient is then asked to close the mouth. When the examiner first feels the condyle touch the finger, the temporomandibular joints are in the resting position. This resting position of the temporomandibular joints is called the **freeway space,** or **interocclusal space.** The freeway space is the potential space or vertical distance that is found between the teeth when the mandible is in the resting position. To determine the freeway space, the examiner marks a point on the chin and a point vertically above on the upper lip below the nose. The patient closes the mouth into centric occlusion, and the distance between the two points is measured. Then the patient is asked to say three simple words (e.g., "boy, boy, boy") and then maintain this position of the jaw without moving. The distance between the two points is measured again. The difference between the two measurements is the freeway space.[18] Normally, the space between the front teeth at this point is 2 to 4 mm.

If rotation does not occur at the temporomandibular joint, the mouth cannot open fully. There may be gliding at the temporomandibular joint, but rotation has not occurred. If translation (gliding) does not occur, the mandible may still open up to 30 mm as a result of rotation. Normally, when the mouth opens, the disc moves forward approximately 7 mm, and the condyle moves forward approximately 14 mm.[25]

If clicking (see question 6 under the earlier History section) occurs on opening, the examiner should ask the patient to open the mouth with the jaw protruded and retruded. If the clicking is eliminated with protrusion and accentuated with retrusion, it is likely the problem is an anterior disc displacement with reduction.[26] Anterior disc displacement without reduction cannot be determined as confidently.[27]

Protrusion of the Mandible

The examiner asks the patient to protrude or jut the lower jaw out past the upper teeth. The patient should be able to do this without difficulty. The normal movement is more than 7 mm, measured from the resting position to the protruded position.[3] The normal values vary depending on the degree of overbite (greater movement) or underbite (less movement).

Retrusion of the Mandible

The examiner asks the patient to retrude or pull the lower jaw in or back as far as possible. In full retention or centric relation, the temporomandibular joint is in a close-packed position. The normal movement is 3 to 4 mm.[10]

Lateral Deviation or Excursion of the Mandible

For lateral deviation, the teeth are slightly disoccluded, and the patient moves the mandible laterally, first to one side and then to the other. With the joints in the resting position, two points are picked on the upper and lower teeth that are at the same level. When the mandible is laterally deviated, the two points, which have moved apart, are measured, giving the amount of lateral deviation. The normal lateral deviation is 10 to 15 mm.[3] During lateral deviation, the opposite condyle moves forward, down, and toward the motion side. The condyle on the motion side (e.g., left condyle on left lateral

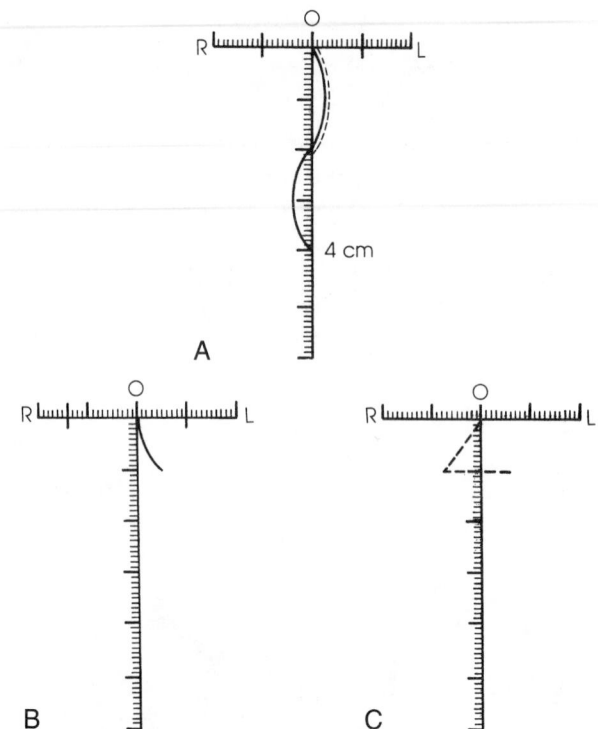

Figure 4-26 Charting temporomandibular motion. A, Deviation to both right *(R)* and left *(L)* on opening; maximum opening, 4 cm; lateral deviation equal (1 cm each direction); protrusion on functional opening *(dashed lines)*. **B,** Capsule-ligamentous pattern; opening limited to 1 cm; lateral deviation greater to right than left; deviation to left on opening. **C,** Protrusion is 1 cm; lateral deviation to right on protrusion (indicates weak lateral pterygoid on opposite side).

deviation) remains relatively stationary and becomes more prominent.[10] Any lateral deviation from the normal opening position or abnormal protrusion to one side indicates that the lateral pterygoid, masseter, or temporalis muscle, the disc, or the lateral ligament on the opposite side is affected.

When charting any changes, the examiner should note the type of opening deviation as well as the functional opening and any lateral deviation (Figure 4-26).

Mandibular Measurement

Next, the examiner should measure the mandible from the posterior aspect of the temporomandibular joint to the notch of the chin (Figure 4-27). Both sides are measured and compared for equality (the normal distance is 10 to 12 cm). Any difference indicates a developmental problem or structural change leading to left or right convergence; the patient may not be able to obtain balancing in the midline.

Swallowing and Tongue Position

The patient is asked to relax and then swallow. The patient is asked to leave the tongue in the position it assumed when swallowing occurred. The examiner,

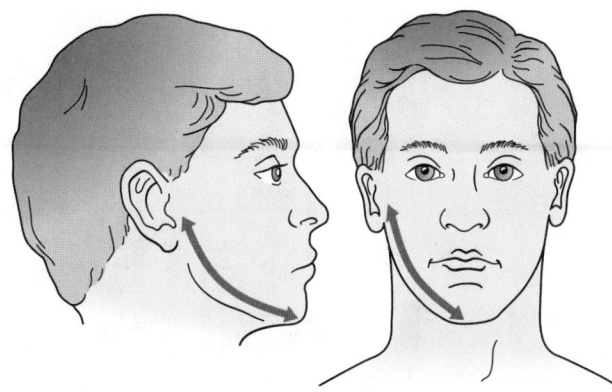

Figure 4-27 Measurement of the mandible.

wearing rubber gloves, then separates the lips and notes the position of the tongue (e.g., between teeth? at upper anterior palate?).[18]

Cranial Nerve Testing

If injury to the cranial nerves is suspected, the cranial nerves should be tested.

Cranial Nerve Testing	
CN I:	Smell coffee or some similar substance with eyes closed
CN II (optic nerve):	Read something with one eye closed
CN III, IV, VI:	Eye movements; note any ptosis
CN V (trigeminal nerve):	Contract muscles of mastication (masseter and temporalis)
CN VII (facial nerve):	Move eyebrows up and down, purse lips, show teeth. This cranial nerve is the most commonly injured one. If the patient is unable to whistle or wink or close an eye on one side, the symptoms may be indicative of Bell palsy (paralysis of the facial nerve).
CN VIII (auditory nerve):	Eyes closed; talk to patient and have him or her repeat what was said
CN IX:	Have patient swallow
CN X (vagus nerve):	Have patient swallow
CN XI (spinal accessory):	Have patient contract sternomastoid
CN XII:	Have patient stick out tongue, move it to right and left

Passive Movements

Very seldom are passive movements carried out for the temporomandibular joints except when the examiner is attempting to determine the end feel of the joints. The amount of passive opening (full passive stretch) may also be measured and compared with functional opening amount.[8] The normal end feel of these joints is tissue stretch on opening and teeth contact ("bone-to-bone") on closing. When the teeth are in maximum contact, the horizontal overjet is sometimes measured. The overjet is the horizontal distance from the edge of the upper central incisors to the lower central incisors (see Figure 4-21). If the lower teeth extend over the upper teeth, this malocclusion condition is called an *underbite*. Overbite is the vertical overlap of the teeth.

Normal End Feel at the Temporomandibular Joints

- Opening: Tissue stretch
- Closing: Bone to bone

Resisted Isometric Movements

Resisted isometric movements of the temporomandibular joints are relatively difficult to test. The jaw should be in the resting position. The examiner applies firm but gentle resistance to the joints and asks the patient to hold the position, saying "Don't let me move you."

Resisted Isometric Movements of the Temporomandibular Joints

- Depression (opening)
- Occlusion (closing)
- Lateral deviation left and right

Opening of the Mouth (Depression). This movement may be tested by applying resistance at the chin or, using a rubber glove, over the teeth with one hand while the other hand rests behind the head or neck or over the forehead to stabilize the head (Figure 4-28, *A*; Table 4-3).

Closing of the Mouth (Elevation or Occlusion). One hand is placed over the back of the head or neck to stabilize the head while the other hand is placed under the chin of the patient's slightly open mouth to resist the movement (Figure 4-28, *B*). In a second method, the examiner uses a rubber glove and places two fingers over the patient's lower teeth (mandible) to resist the movement (Figure 4-28, *C*).

Lateral Deviation of the Jaw. One of the examiner's hands is placed over the side of the head above the temporomandibular joint to stabilize the head. The other hand is placed along the jaw of the patient's slightly open mouth, and the patient pushes out against it (Figure 4-28, *D*). Both sides are tested individually.

Functional Assessment

After the basic movements of the temporomandibular joints have been tested, the examiner should test

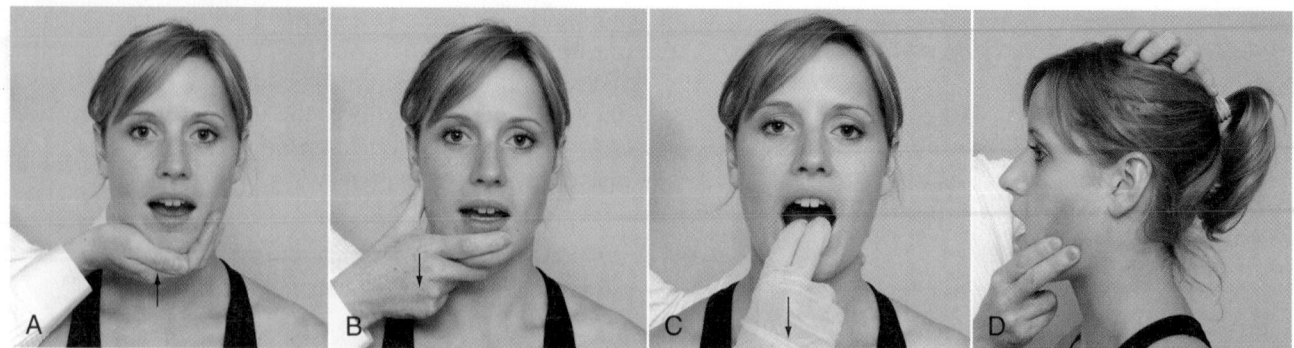

Figure 4-28 Resisted isometric movements for the muscles controlling the temporomandibular joint. **A,** Opening of the mouth (depression). **B,** Closing of the mouth (elevation or occlusion). **C,** Closing of the mouth (alternative method). **D,** Lateral deviation of the jaw.

TABLE 4-3

Muscles of the Temporomandibular Joint: Their Actions and Nerve Supply

Action	Muscles Acting	Nerve Supply
Opening of mouth (depression of mandible)	1. Lateral (external) pterygoid 2. Mylohyoid* 3. Geniohyoid* 4. Digastric*	Mandibular (CN V) Inferior alveolar (CN V) Hypoglossal (CN XII) Inferior alveolar (CN V) Facial (CN VII)
Closing of mouth (elevation of mandible or occlusion)	1. Masseter 2. Temporalis 3. Medial (internal) pterygoid	Mandibular (CN V) Mandibular (CN V) Mandibular (CN V)
Protrusion of mandible	1. Lateral (external) pterygoid 2. Medial (internal) pterygoid 3. Masseter* 4. Mylohyoid* 5. Geniohyoid* 6. Digastric* 7. Stylohyoid* 8. Temporalis (anterior fibers)*	Mandibular (CN V) Mandibular (CN V) Mandibular (CN V) Inferior alveolar (CN V) Hypoglossal (CN XII) Inferior alveolar (CN V) Facial (CN VII) Facial (CN VII) Mandibular (CN V)
Retraction of mandible	1. Temporalis (posterior fibers) 2. Masseter* 3. Digastric* 4. Stylohyoid* 5. Mylohyoid* 6. Geniohyoid*	Mandibular (CN V) Mandibular (CN V) Inferior alveolar (CN V) Facial (CN VII) Inferior alveolar (CN VII) Inferior alveolar (CN V) Hypoglossal (CN XII)
Lateral deviation of mandible	1. Lateral (external) pterygoid (ipsilateral muscle) 2. Medial (internal) pterygoid (contralateral muscle) 3. Temporalis* 4. Masseter*	Mandibular (CN V) Mandibular (CN V) Mandibular (CN V) Mandibular (CN V)

CN, Cranial nerve.
*Act only when assistance is required.

functional activities or activities of daily living involving the use of the temporomandibular joints. These activities include chewing, swallowing, coughing, talking, and blowing. If the patient complains of pain while eating, the examiner can ask the patient to bite down on a tongue depressor held between the teeth in different positions to see if the compressive movement is painful in the teeth or temporomandibular joint. Biting down on one side stresses the temporomandibular joint on the opposite side.[6]

In addition, there are a number of function questionnaires that may be used as part of the functional assessment: the Research Diagnostic Criteria for Temporomandibular Disorders (RDC/TMD),[28–33] the Limitations of Daily

Limitation of Daily Function Questionnaire for Patients with TMD
(LDF-TMD-Jaw Function Scale)

This questionnaire has been designed to give the doctor information as to how **"your jaw"** has affected your ability to manage in even daily life. Please answer every section and mark in each section only the ONE box, which applies to you. We realize you may consider that two of the statements in any one section relate to you, but please just mark the box that most closely describes your problem (**mark with a "X" in the option that applies to you**).

Name: *Date:*

ITEMS	No problem	Slightly difficult	Moderately difficult	Very difficult	Extremely difficult
• How much does your present jaw problem prevent or limit you for talking for a long period of time including telephone conversations?	○	○	○	○	○
• How much does your present jaw problem prevent or limit you from grinding thin foods?	○	○	○	○	○
• How much does your present jaw problem prevent or limit you from prolonged chewing during meals?	○	○	○	○	○
• How much does your present jaw problem prevent or limit you from activity at home, school, and/or work?	○	○	○	○	○
• How much does your present jaw problem prevent or limit you from clenching teeth when participating in sports (contact teeth together during sports)?	○	○	○	○	○
• How much does your present jaw problem prevent or limit you from opening your mouth widely?	○	○	○	○	○
• How much does your present jaw problem prevent or limit you from yawning?	○	○	○	○	○
• How much does your present jaw problem prevent or limit you from brushing your back teeth?	○	○	○	○	○
• How much does your present jaw problem prevent or limit you from falling asleep?	○	○	○	○	○
• How much does your present jaw problem prevent or limit you from sleeping through the night?	○	○	○	○	○

Figure 4-29 **Limitation of Daily Function Questionnaire for Patients with Temporomandibular Disorder (LDF-TMD-Jaw Function Scale).** (From Sugisaki M, Kino K, Yoshida N, et al: Development of a new questionnaire to assess pain-related limitations of daily functions in Japanese patients with temporomandibular disorders. Community Dent Oral Epidemiol 33[5]:384–395, 2005.)

Function Questionnaire (TMJ)[34] (Figure 4-29), the Jaw Functional Limitation Scale,[35] the Mandibular Function Impairment Questionnaire (MFIQ),[36,37] the History Questionnaire for Jaw Pain, and the TMJ Scale.

Special Tests

There are no routine special tests for the temporomandibular joints. The **Chvostek test** ❓ may be used to determine whether there is pathology involving the seventh cranial (facial) nerve (Figure 4-30). The examiner taps the parotid gland overlying the masseter muscle. If the facial muscles twitch, the test is considered positive.

If the patient is suffering from a facial nerve injury (Bell palsy), the examiner may use the facial nerve grading system (see Table 2-24) developed by the American Academy of Otolaryngology.[8]

The examiner can listen to (auscultate) the temporomandibular joints during movement (Figure 4-31). The movements "listened to" include opening and closing

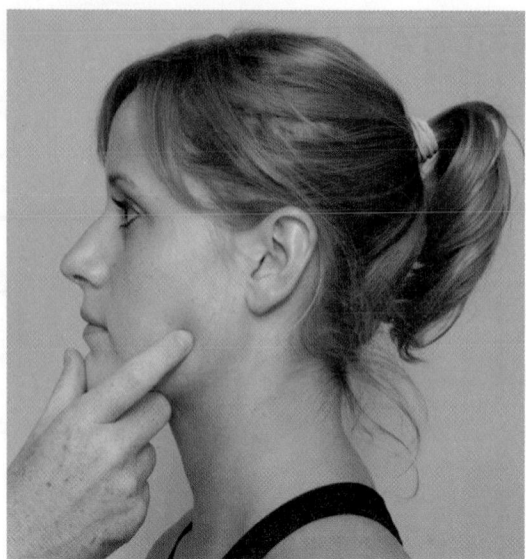

Figure 4-30 Chvostek test.

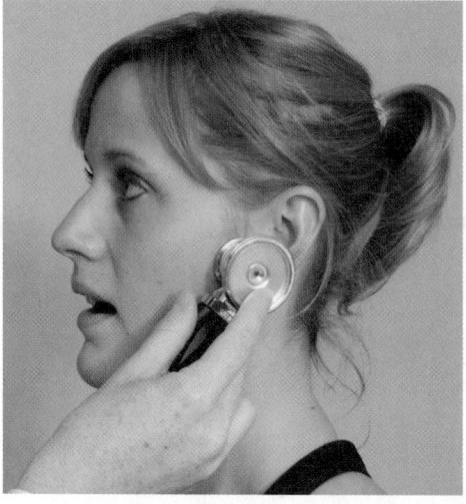

Figure 4-31 Auscultation of the left temporomandibular joint.

of the mouth, lateral deviation of the mandible to the right and left, and mandibular protrusion. Normally, a sound would be heard only on occlusion. This is a single, solid sound, not a "slipping" sound. A slipping sound could occur if the teeth are not "hitting" simultaneously. The most common joint noise is reciprocal clicking (see Figure 4-9), which occurs when the mouth opens and when it closes. The clicking ✓ is clinical evidence that the condyle is slipping over the disc and then self-reducing. The opening click results when the condyle slips under the posterior aspect of the disc (reduces) or slips anterior to the disc (subluxes) on opening. The second click, which is quieter, occurs when the condyle slips posterior to the disc (subluxes) or into its proper position and reduces. A single click may occur if the condyle gets caught behind the disc on opening (see

Figure 4-7) or if the condyle slips behind the disc on closing. On opening, the later the click occurs, the more anterior lies the disc. The later the opening click, the more the disc is displaced anteriorly, and the more likely it is to lock. A closing click is usually caused by loosening of the structures attaching the disc to the condyle. Clicking is more likely to occur in hypermobile joints.[38,39]

Grating noise (crepitus) is usually indicative of degenerative joint disease or a perforation in the disc. Painful crepitus usually means that the disc has eroded, the condyle bone and temporal bone are rubbing together, and much of the fibrocartilage has been lost. While the examiner is listening, each movement should be done four or five times to ensure a correct diagnosis.

For the reader who would like to review them, the reliability, validity, specificity, sensitivity, and odds ratios of some of the special tests used in the temporomandibular joint are available in on the Evolve website.

Reflexes and Cutaneous Distribution

The reflex of the temporomandibular joints is called the *jaw reflex*. The examiner's thumb is placed on the chin of the patient with the patient's mouth relaxed and open in the resting position. The patient is asked to close the eyes. If this is not done, the patient commonly tenses as he or she sees the reflex hammer being swung toward the examiner's thumb or the tongue depressor, and the test does not work. The examiner then taps the thumbnail with a neurological hammer (Figure 4-32, *A*). The jaw reflex may also be tested by using a tongue depressor (Figure 4-32, *B*). The examiner holds the tongue depressor firmly against the bottom teeth; while the patient relaxes the jaw muscles, the examiner taps the tongue depressor with the reflex hammer. The reflex closes the mouth and is a test of cranial nerve V.

The examiner must be aware of the dermatome patterns for the head and neck (Figure 4-33) as well as the sensory nerve distribution of the peripheral nerves (see Figure 3-66). Pain may be referred from the temporomandibular joint to the teeth, neck, or head, and vice versa (Figure 4-34). Table 4-4 shows the muscles of the temporomandibular joint and their referral of pain.

Joint Play Movements

The joint play movements of the temporomandibular joints are then tested. Pain on performing these tests may indicate articular problems or pathology to the retrodiscal tissues.[40]

Longitudinal Cephalad and Anterior Glide. Wearing rubber gloves, the examiner places the thumb on the patient's lower teeth inside the mouth with the index finger on the mandible outside the mouth. The mandible is then distracted by pushing down with the thumb and pulling down and forward with the index finger while the other

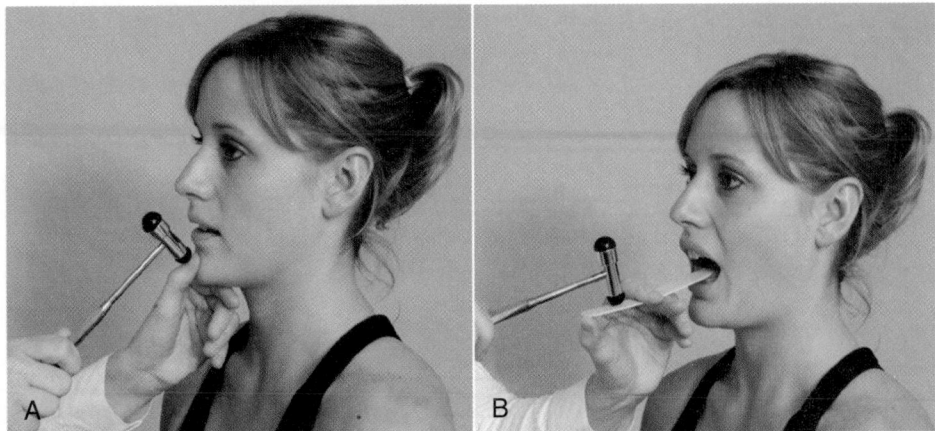

Figure 4-32 **Testing of the jaw reflex. A,** Hitting examiner's thumb. **B,** Hitting tongue depressor.

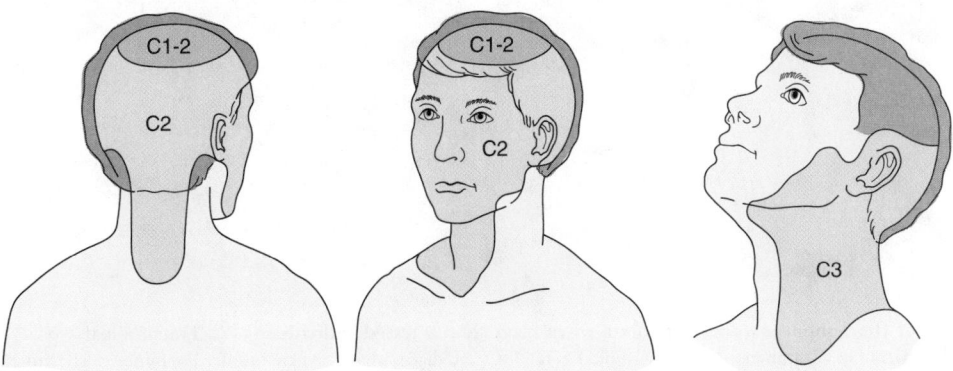

Figure 4-33 Dermatomes of the head.

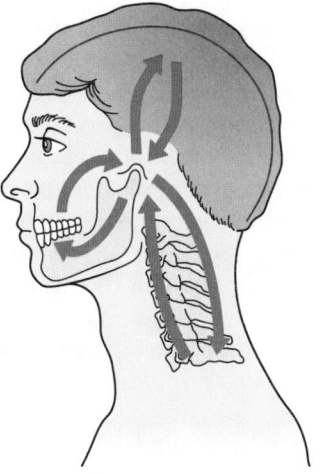

Figure 4-34 Referred pain patterns to and from the temporomandibular joint in the teeth, head, and neck.

TABLE 4-4

Temporomandibular Muscles and Referral of Pain

Muscle	Referral Pattern
Masseter	Cheek, mandible to forehead or ear
Temporalis	Maxilla to forehead and side of head above ear
Medial pterygoid	Posterior mandible to temporomandibular joint
Lateral pterygoid	Cheek to temporomandibular joint
Digastric	Lateral cervical spine to posterolateral skull
Occipitofrontal	Above eye, over eyelid, and up over lateral aspect of skull

fingers push against the chin, acting as a pivot point. The examiner should feel the tissue stretch of the joint. Each joint is done individually while the other hand and arm stabilize the head (Figure 4-35, *A*).

Lateral Glide of the Mandible. The patient lies supine with the mouth slightly open and the mandible relaxed. The examiner places the thumb inside the mouth along the medial side of the mandible and teeth. By pushing the thumb laterally, the mandible glides laterally.[21] Each joint is done individually (Figure 4-35, *B*).

Medial Glide of the Mandible. The patient is in side lying with the mandible relaxed. The examiner places the thumb (or overlapping thumbs) over the lateral aspect of the mandibular condyle outside the mouth and applies a

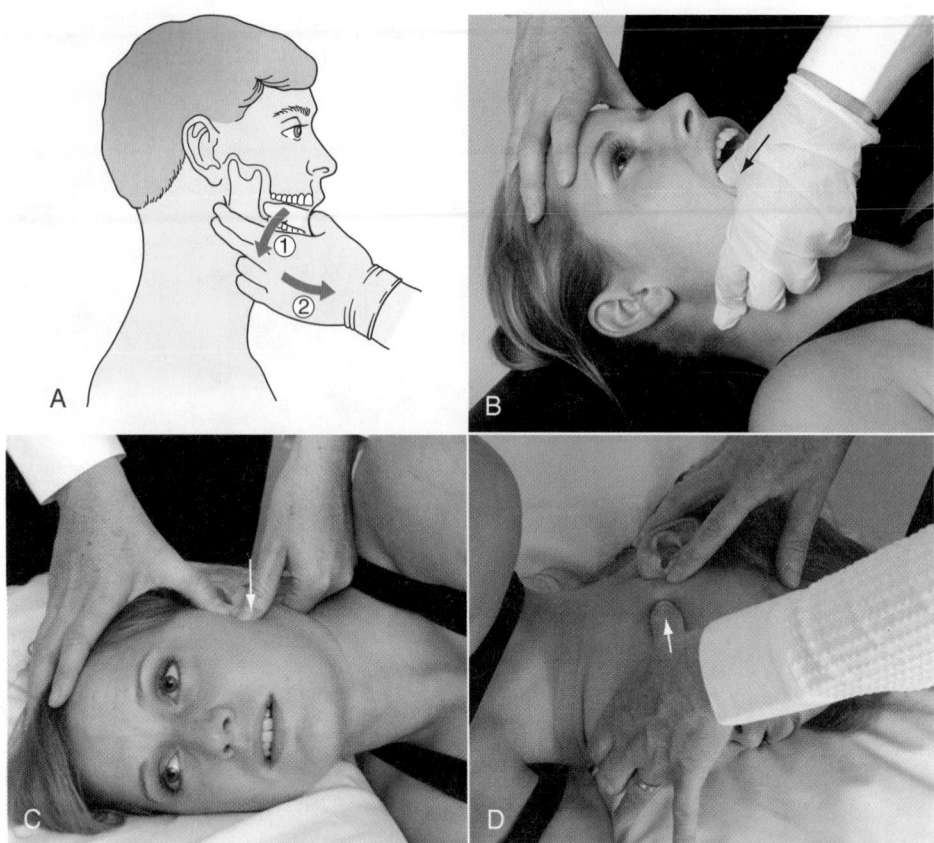

Figure 4-35 Joint play of the temporomandibular joints when each side is tested individually. A, Longitudinal cephalad and anterior glide. **B,** Lateral glide of the mandible. Examiner pushes mandible laterally. **C,** Medial glide of the mandible. Examiner pushes mandible medially while palpating temporomandibular joint with other thumb. **D,** Posterior glide of the mandible. Examiner pushes mandible posteriorly while palpating temporomandibular joint with other thumb.

medial pressure to the condyle, gliding the condyle medially.[21] Each joint is done individually (Figure 4-35, *C*).

Posterior Glide of the Mandible. The patient is in side lying with the mandible relaxed. The examiner places the thumb (or overlapping thumbs) over the anterior aspect of the mandibular condyle outside the mouth and applies a posterior pressure to the condyle, gliding the condyle posteriorly.[21] Each joint is done individually (Figure 4-35, *D*).

Palpation

To palpate the temporomandibular joints, the examiner places the fingers (padded part anteriorly) in the patient's external auditory canals and asks the patient to actively open and close the mouth. As this is being done, the examiner determines whether both sides are moving simultaneously and whether the movement is smooth. If the patient feels pain on closing, the posterior capsule is usually involved.

The examiner then places the index fingers over the mandibular condyles and feels for elicited pain or tenderness on opening and closing of the mouth. The examiner may also palpate the medial pterygoid, the medial and

lower border of the inferior head of the lateral pterygoid, the temporalis and its tendon, and the masseter muscles and any other soft tissues for tenderness or indications of pathology (Figure 4-36). This procedure is followed by palpation of the following structures.

Mandible. The examiner palpates the mandible along its entire length, feeling for any differences between the left and right sides. As the examiner moves along the superior aspect of the angle of the mandible, the fingers pass over the parotid gland. Normally, the gland is not palpable, but with pathology (e.g., mumps), the site feels "boggy" rather than having the normal hard and bony feel.

Teeth. The examiner should note the position, absence, or tenderness of the teeth. The examiner wears a rubber glove and palpates inside the patient's mouth. At the same time, the interior cheek region and gums may be palpated for pathology.

Hyoid Bone (Anterior to C2, C3 Vertebrae). While palpating the hyoid bone (Figure 4-37), the examiner asks the patient to swallow. Normally, the bone moves and causes no pain. The hyoid bone is part of the superior trachea.

Thyroid Cartilage (Anterior to C4, C5 Vertebrae). While the neck is in the neutral position, the thyroid cartilage

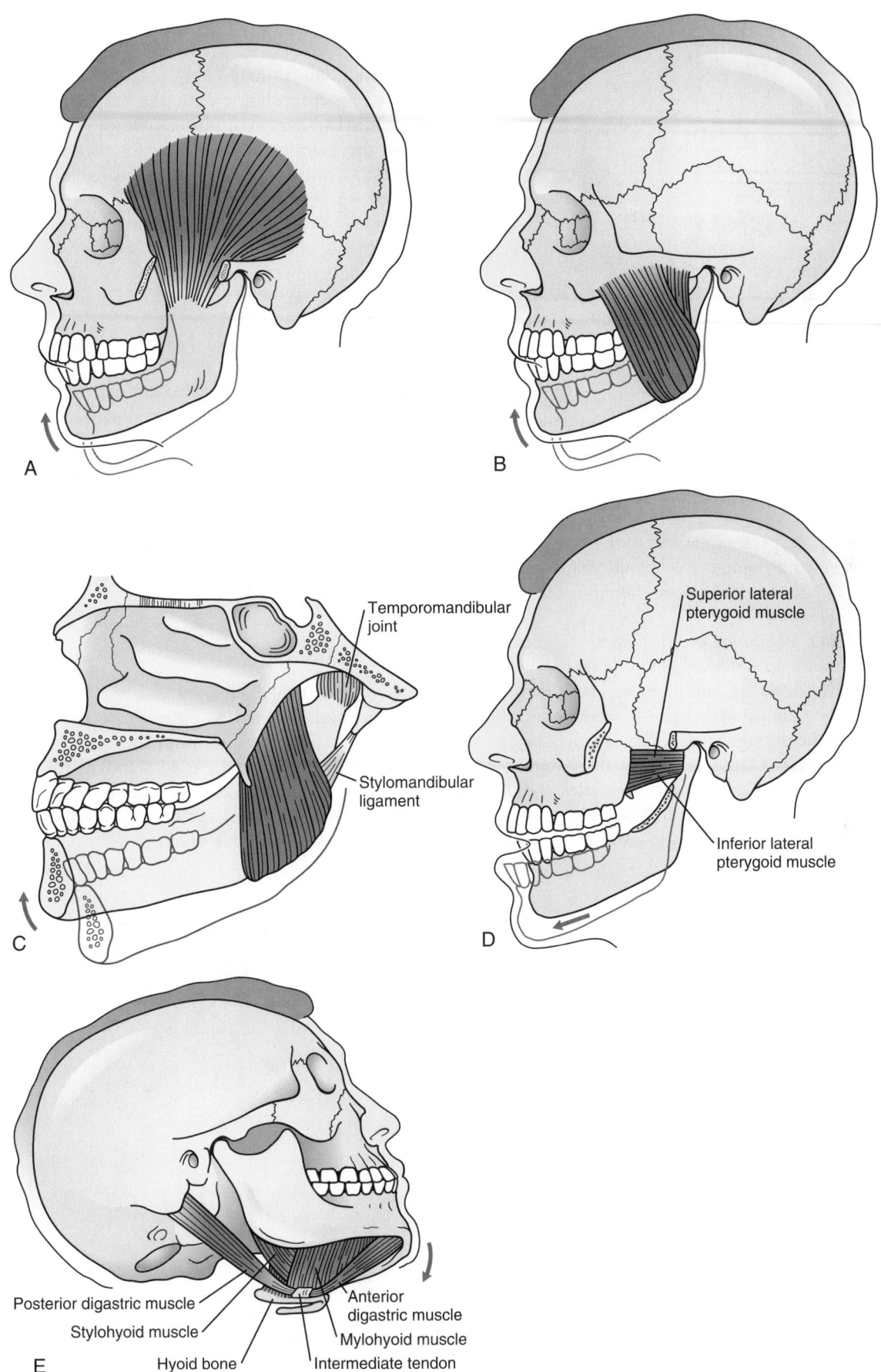

Figure 4-36 Muscles of the temporomandibular joint. A, Temporalis muscle. **B,** Masseter muscle. **C,** Medial pterygoid muscle. **D,** Inferior and superior lateral pterygoid muscles. **E,** Digastric muscle. (Modified from Okeson JP: Management of temporomandibular disorders and occlusion, St Louis, 1998, CV Mosby, pp. 18–20, 22.)

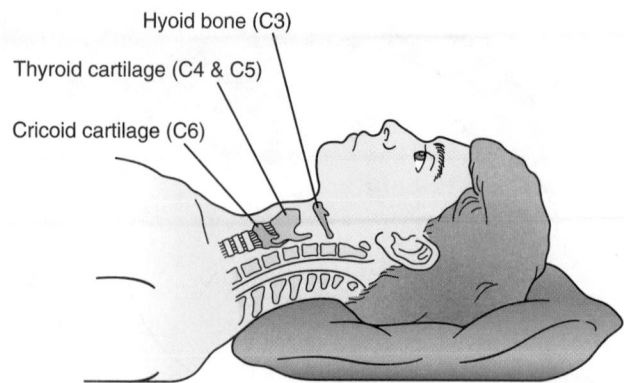

Figure 4-37 Position of hyoid bone, thyroid cartilage, and cricoid cartilage.

can be easily moved; while in extension, it is tight, and the examiner may feel crepitations. The thyroid gland, which is adjacent to the cartilage, may be palpated at the same time. If abnormal or inflamed, it will be tender and enlarged.

Mastoid Processes. The examiner should palpate the skull, following the posterior aspect of the ear. The examiner will come to a point on the skull where the finger dips inward. The point just before the dip is the mastoid process (see Figure 3-74).

Cervical Spine. Beginning on the posterior aspect at the occiput, the examiner systematically palpates the posterior structures of the neck (spinous processes, facet joints, and muscles of the suboccipital region), working from the head toward the shoulders. On the lateral aspect, the transverse processes of the vertebrae, the lymph nodes (palpable only if swollen), and the muscles should be palpated for tenderness. A more detailed description of the palpation of these structures is given in Chapter 3.

Diagnostic Imaging

Plain Film Radiography

On the anteroposterior view, the examiner should look for condylar shape and normal contours. On the lateral view, the examiner should look for condylar shape and contours, position of condylar heads in the opened and closed positions (Figure 4-38), amount of condylar movement (closed versus open), and relation of temporomandibular joint to other bony structures of the skull and cervical spine (Figure 4-39). X-ray views commonly taken for the temporomandibular joint are shown in the following box.

Common X-Ray Views of the Temporomandibular Joints

- Anteroposterior view (mouth closed) (Figure 4-40)
- Lateral view (open and closed mouth) of temporomandibular joint (Figure 4-41)
- Lateral view (closed mouth) (Figure 4-42)
- Lateral view (TMJ and cervical spine) (see Figure 4-39)
- Transcranial (lateral oblique) view (Figure 4-43)
- Submentovertex view (Figure 4-44)

Magnetic Resonance Imaging

This technique is used to differentiate the soft tissue of the joint, mainly the disc, from the bony structures and therefore has become the gold standard for testing the reliability of clinical findings in the temporomandibular joint.[41] It has the advantage of using nonionizing radiation (Figures 4-45 and 4-46).

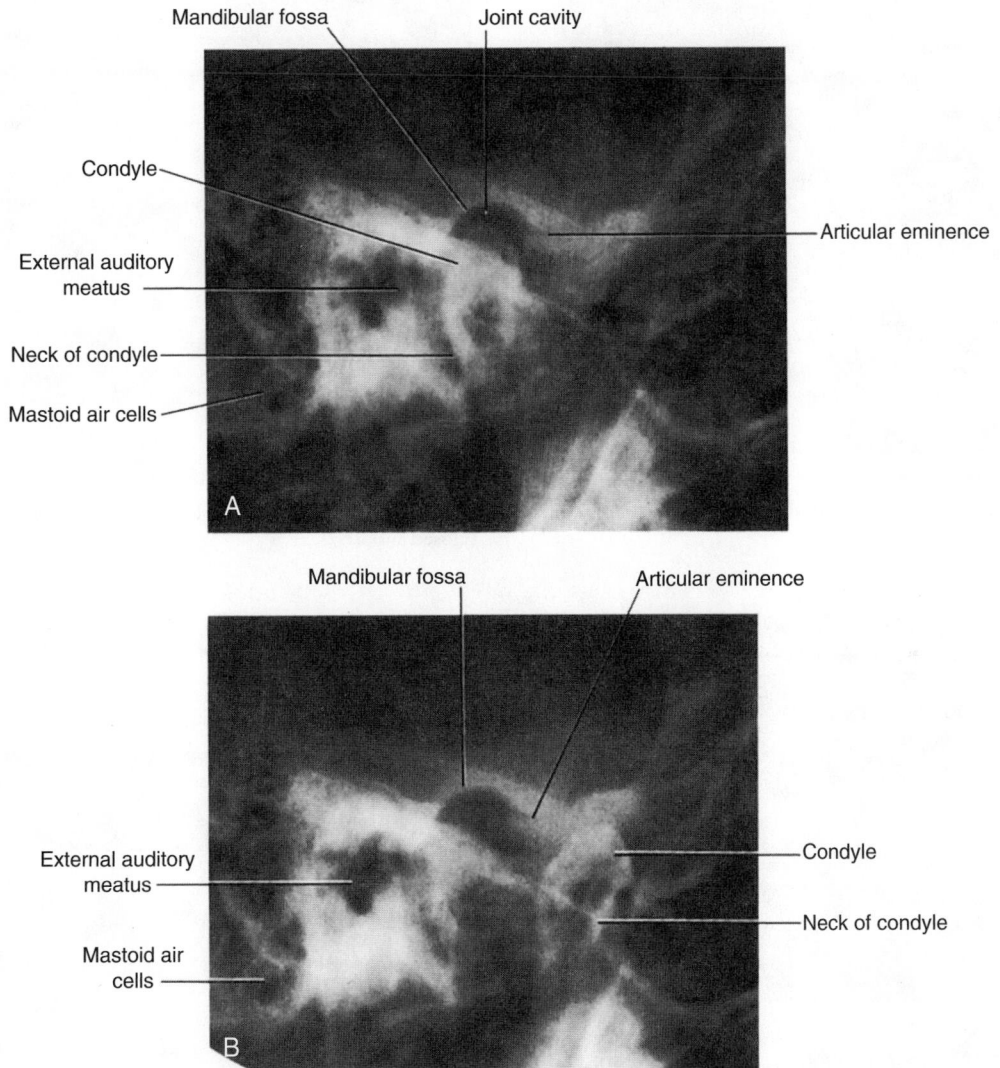

Figure 4-38 Radiographs of the right temporomandibular joint. A, Mouth closed. **B,** Mouth open. (From Liebgott B: The anatomical basis of dentistry, St Louis, 1986, CV Mosby, p. 295; courtesy of Dr. Friedman.)

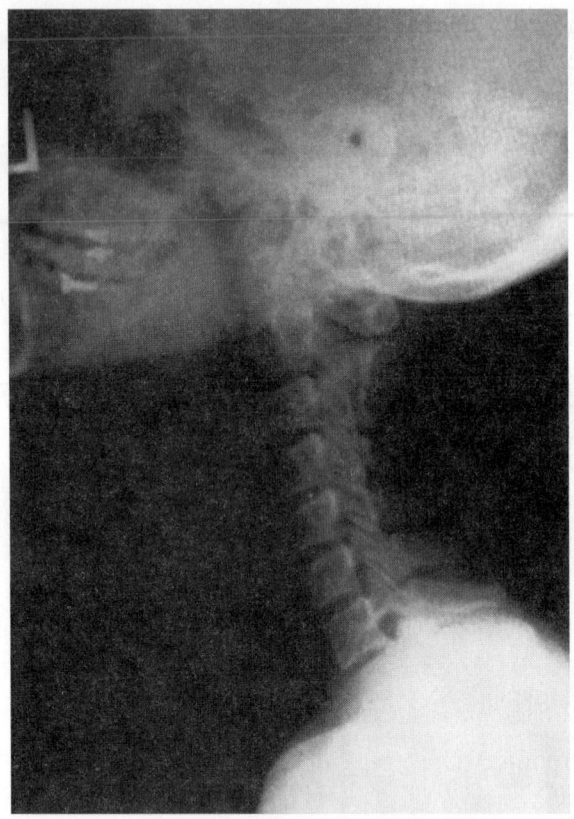

Figure 4-39 Lateral radiograph of the skull, left temporomandibular joint, and cervical spine.

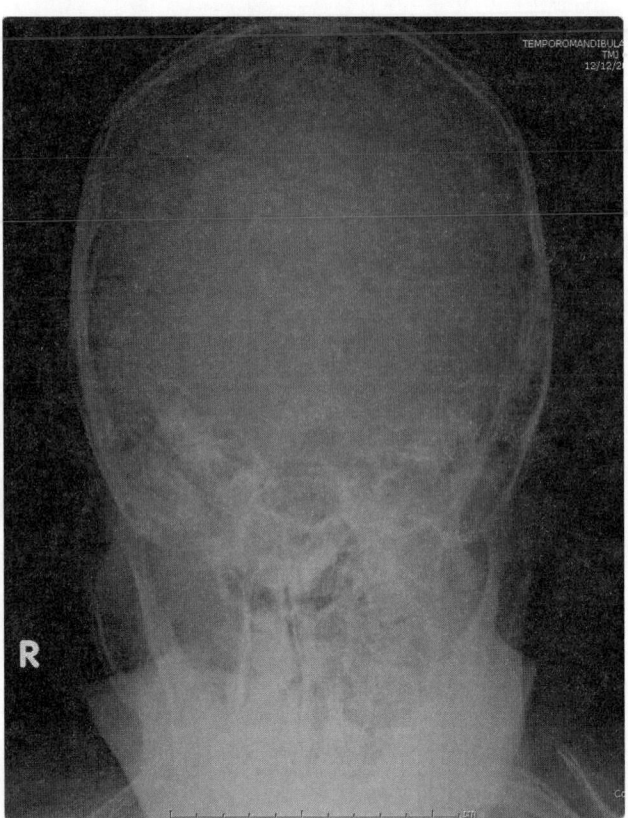

Figure 4-40 Anteroposterior view of the temporomandibular joints (closed mouth).

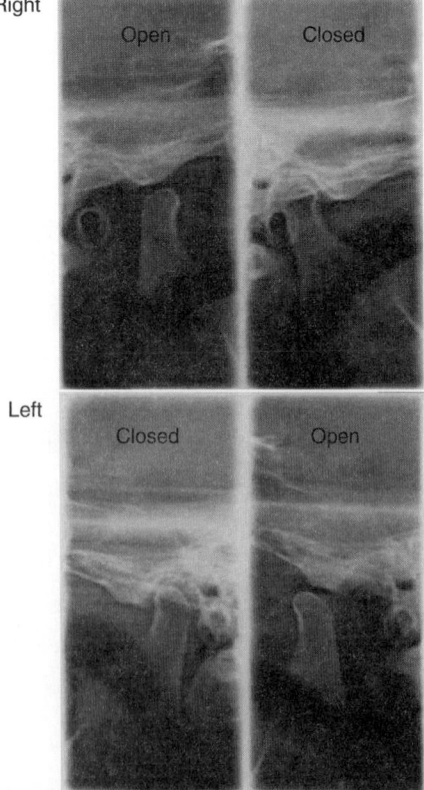

Figure 4-41 Lateral view of the temporomandibular joints (open and closed mouth).

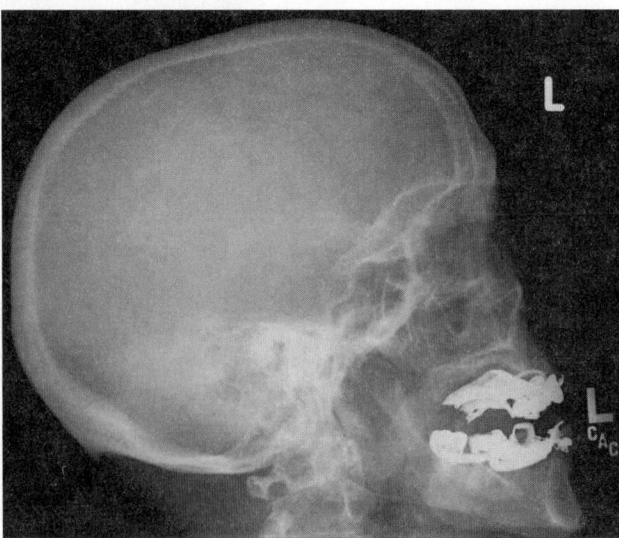

Figure 4-42 Lateral view of the skull (closed mouth).

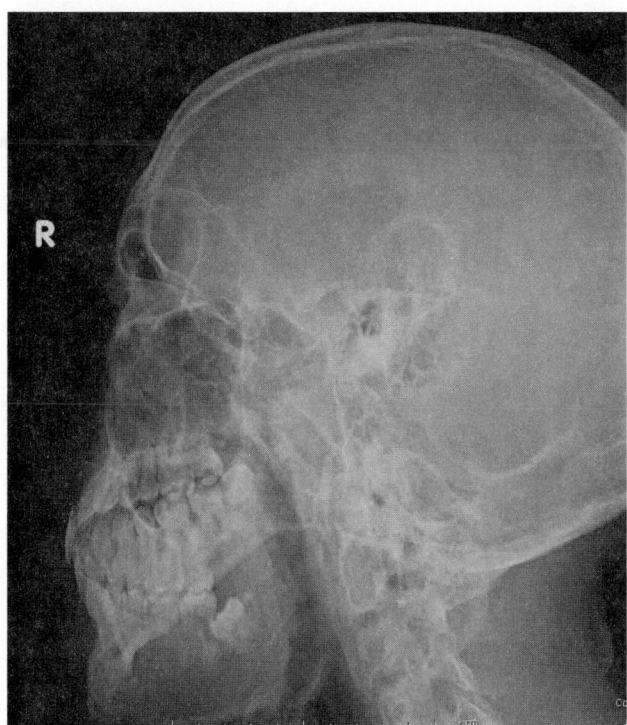

Figure 4-43 Transcranial (lateral oblique) view (closed mouth).

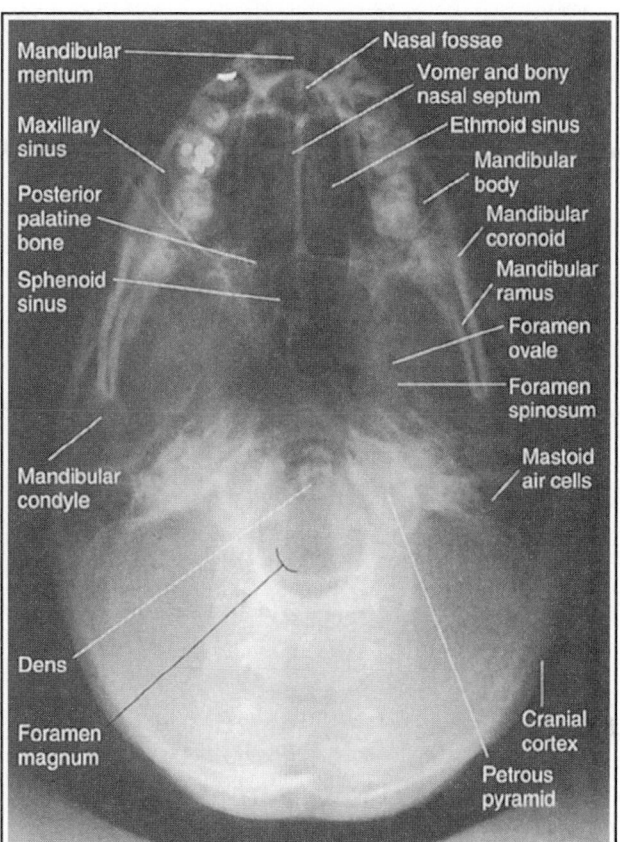

Mandibular mentum

Maxillary sinus

Posterior palatine bone

Sphenoid sinus

Mandibular condyle

Dens

Foramen magnum

Nasal fossae

Vomer and bony nasal septum

Ethmoid sinus

Mandibular body

Mandibular coronoid

Mandibular ramus

Foramen ovale

Foramen spinosum

Mastoid air cells

Cranial cortex

Petrous pyramid

Figure 4-44 Submentovertex (Schueller) cranial image with accurate positioning. (From McQuillen Martensen K: Radiographic image analysis, ed 3, St Louis, 2011, WB Saunders Company, p. 525.)

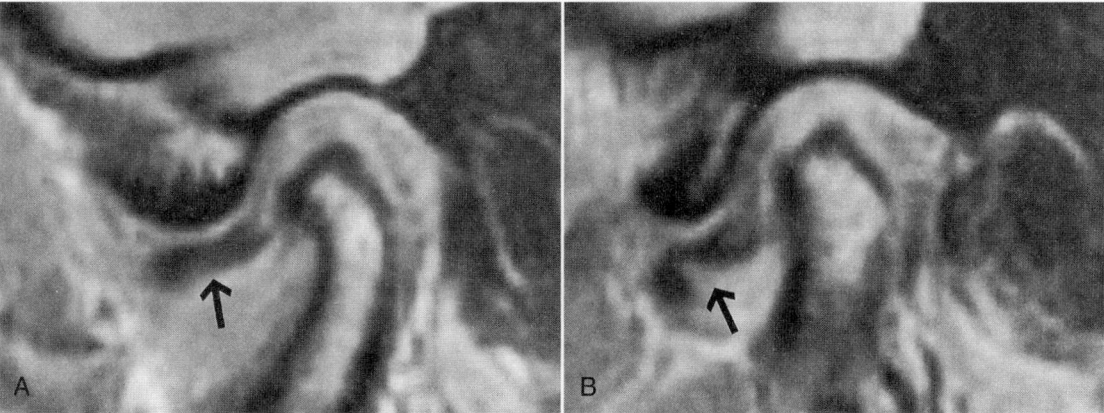

Figure 4-45 Acute temporomandibular joint lock from a nonreducing displaced disc. A, T1-weighted sagittal spin echo magnetic resonance image with the mouth closed shows the dislocated disc *(arrow)* anterior to the condyle. **B,** With attempted mouth opening, no appreciable anterior translation of the condyle occurs, but the disc folds on itself in the thin intermediate zone because of increased pressure from the condyle. The normal biconcave configuration of the disc and the normal intradiscal signal intensity are maintained *(arrow)*. (From Resnick D, Kransdorf MJ: Bone and joint imaging, Philadelphia, 2005, WB Saunders, p. 516.)

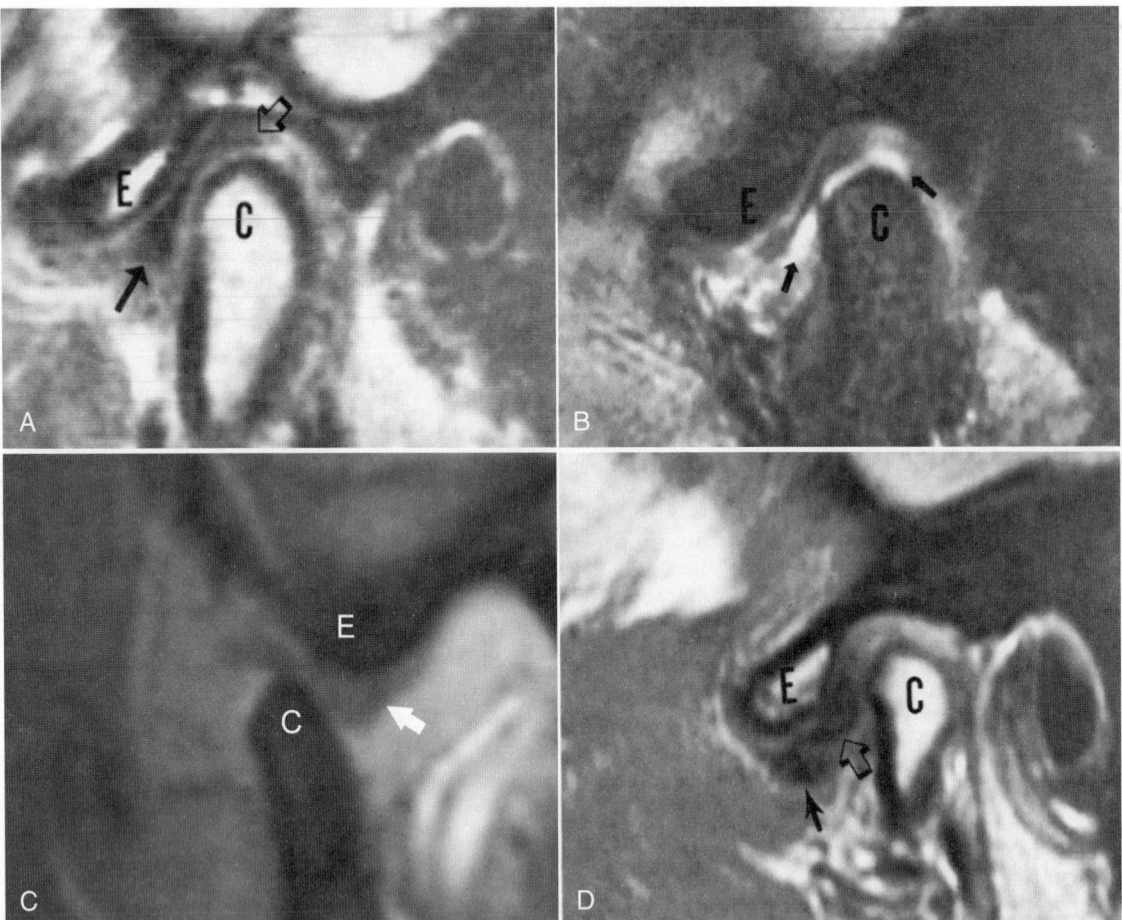

Figure 4-46 Magnetic resonance (MR) imaging of the temporomandibular joint (TMJ). A, T1-weighted sagittal spin echo MR image of a normal TMJ. View with the mouth closed shows high signal intensity from the condylar marrow *(C)* and articular eminence *(E).* Surrounding cortical bone is devoid of signal. The disc, of low signal intensity, is interposed between the condyle and the fossa; the intermediate zone articulates with the condyle and eminence where they are most closely apposed. The *solid arrow* points to the anterior band and the *open arrow* to the posterior band of the disc. **B,** Sagittal gradient echo MR image used for fast (pseudodynamic) scanning shows a normal position of the disc with the mouth closed. Marrow becomes low in signal intensity with this sequence, and fluid in the inferior joint space becomes bright *(arrows);* the disc remains low in signal intensity. **C,** Sagittal gradient image of a normal TMJ with the mouth open. The intermediate zone of the disc maintains its position between the condyle *(C)* and the eminence *(E),* whereas the posterior band slides posterior to the condyle *(arrow).* **D,** T1-weighted sagittal spin echo MR image in a patient with clicking and pain demonstrates internal derangement with both the anterior *(solid arrow)* and posterior *(open arrow)* bands of the disc displaced anteriorly relative to the condyle *(C). C,* Condyle; *E,* eminence. (From Resnick D, Kransdorf MJ: Bone and joint imaging, Philadelphia, 2005, WB Saunders, p. 509.)

PRÉCIS OF THE TEMPOROMANDIBULAR JOINT ASSESSMENT*

History
Observation
Examination
  Active movements
    Neck flexion
    Neck extension
    Neck side flexion (left and right)
    Neck rotation (left and right)
    Extend neck by opening mouth
    Assess functional opening
    Assess freeway space
    Open mouth
    Closed mouth (occlusion)
    Measure protrusion of mandible
    Measure retrusion of mandible

    Measure lateral deviation of mandible (left and right)
    Measure mandibular length
    Swallowing and tongue position
    Cranial nerve testing (if necessary)
  Passive movements (as in active movements, if necessary)
  Resisted isometric movements
    Open mouth
    Closed mouth (occlusion)
    Lateral deviation of jaw
  Functional assessment
  Special tests
  Reflexes and cutaneous distribution
  Joint play movements
  Palpation
  Diagnostic imaging

*Usually the entire assessment is done with the patient sitting. After any examination, the patient should be warned of the possibility of exacerbation of symptoms as a result of the assessment.

CASE STUDIES

When doing these case studies, the examiner should list the appropriate questions to be asked and why they are being asked, what to look for and why, and what things should be tested and why. Depending on the answers of the patient (and the examiner should consider different responses), several possible causes of the patient's problem may become evident (examples are given in parentheses). A differential diagnosis chart should be made up (see Table 4-5 as an example). The examiner can then decide how different diagnoses may affect the treatment plan.

1. A 49-year-old woman comes to you complaining of neck and left temporomandibular joint pain. The pain is worse when she eats, especially if she chews on the left. Describe your assessment plan for this patient (cervical spondylosis versus temporomandibular dysfunction; see Table 4-5).

2. A 33-year-old woman comes to you complaining of pain and clicking when opening her mouth, especially when the mouth is open wide. She states that there is a small click on closing but minimal pain. Describe your assessment plan for this patient (temporomandibular joint arthritis versus temporomandibular disc dysfunction).

3. An 18-year-old male hockey player comes to you stating that he was hit in the jaw while playing. He is in severe pain and has difficulty speaking. Describe your assessment plan for this patient (cervical sprain versus temporomandibular joint dysfunction).

4. A 35-year-old man comes to you with his jaw locked open. Describe your assessment plan for this patient (temporomandibular disc dysfunction versus temporomandibular arthritis).

5. A 42-year-old woman comes to you complaining of jaw pain and headaches. She slipped on some wet stairs 3 days ago and fell, hitting her chin on the stairs. Describe your assessment plan for this patient (temporomandibular joint dysfunction versus head injury).

6. A 27-year-old nervous woman with long hair comes to you complaining of jaw pain. She has recently had a new dental plate installed. Describe your assessment plan for this patient (cervical sprain versus temporomandibular joint dysfunction).

TABLE **4-5**

Differential Diagnosis of Cervical Spondylosis and Temporomandibular Joint Dysfunction

	Cervical Spondylosis	TMJ Dysfunction
History	Insidious onset	Insidious onset
	May complain of referred pain into shoulder, arm, or head	May be related to biting something hard
	Stiff neck	Pain may be referred to neck or head
Observation	Muscle guarding of neck muscles	Minimal or no muscle guarding
Active movements	Cervical spine movements limited	Cervical movements may be limited if they compress or stress TMJ
	TMJ movements normal	TMJ movements may or may not be painful but range of motion is altered
Passive movements	Restricted	Restricted
	May have altered end feel: muscle spasm or bone-to-bone	
Resisted isometric movements	Relatively normal	Normal
	Myotomes may be affected	
Special tests	Spurling's test may be positive	None
	Distraction test may be positive	
Reflexes and cutaneous distribution	Deep tendon reflexes may be hyporeflexic	No effect
	See history for referred pain	See history for referred pain

TMJ, Temporomandibular joint.

REFERENCES

1. Dimitroulis G: Temporomandibular disorders: a clinical update. BMJ 317:190–194, 1998.
2. Clark GT, Seligman DA, Solberg WK, et al: Guidelines for the examination and diagnosis of temporomandibular disorders. J Craniomand Disord 3:7–14, 1989.
3. Dimitroulis G, Dolwick MF, Gremillion HA: Temporomandibular disorders: clinical evaluation. Aust Dent J 40:301–305, 1995.
4. Rocabado M: Course notes: course on temporomandibular joints, Edmonton, Canada, 1979.
5. Rees LA: The structure and function of the mandibular joint. Br Dent J 96:125–133, 1954.
6. Dutton M: Orthopedic examination, evaluation and intervention, New York, 2004, McGraw Hill.
7. Iglarsh ZA, Snyder-Mackler L: Temporomandibular joint and the cervical spine. In Richardson JK, Iglarsh ZA, editors: Clinical orthopedic physical therapy, Philadelphia, 1994, W.B. Saunders.
8. House JW, Brackmann DE: Facial nerve grading system. Otolaryngol Head Neck Surg 93:146–147, 1985.
9. Okeson JP: Management of temporomandibular disorders and occlusion, St Louis, 1998, CV Mosby.
10. Trott PH: Examination of the temporomandibular joint. In Grieve G, editor: Modern manual therapy of the vertebral column, Edinburgh, 1986, Churchill Livingstone.
11. Day LD: History taking. In Morgan DH, House LR, Hall WP, et al, editors: Diseases of the temporomandibular apparatus, St Louis, 1982, C.V. Mosby.
12. Isberg-Holm AM, Westesson PL: Movement of the disc and condyle in temporomandibular joints with clicking. Acta Odontol Scand 40:151–164, 1982.
13. Bush FM, Butler JH, Abbott DM: The relationship of TMJ clicking to palpable facial pain. J Craniomand Pract 1:44–48, 1983.
14. Bourbon B: Craniomandibular examination and treatment. In Myers R, editor: Saunders manual of physical therapy practice, Philadelphia, 1995, W.B. Saunders.
15. Kaplan AS: Examination and diagnosis. In Kaplan AS, Assael LA, editors: Temporomandibular disorders—diagnosis and treatment, Philadelphia, 1991, W.B. Saunders.
16. Hondo T, Shimoda T, Moses JJ, et al: Traumatically induced posterior disc displacement without reduction of the TMJ. J Craniomand Pract 12:128–132, 1994.
17. McNeill C, Mohl ND, Rugh JD, et al: Temporomandibular disorders: diagnosis, management, education and research. J Am Dent Assoc 120:253–260, 1990.
18. Curnette DC: The role of occlusion in diagnoses and treatment planning. In Morgan DH, House LR, Hall WP, et al, editors: Diseases of the temporomandibular apparatus, St Louis, 1982, C.V. Mosby.
19. Enlow DH: Handbook of facial growth, Philadelphia, 1975, W.B. Saunders.
20. Mew J: Tongue posture. Br J Orthod 8:203–211, 1981.
21. Petty NJ, Moore AP: Neuromusculoskeletal examination and assessment—a handbook for therapists, London, 1998, Churchill Livingstone.
22. Walker N, Bohanen RW, Cameron D: Discriminant validity of temporomandibular joint range of motion measurements obtained with a ruler. J Orthop Sports Phys Ther 30:484–492, 2000.
23. Friedman M, Weisberg J: Screening procedures for temporomandibular joint dysfunction. Am Fam Physician 25:157–160, 1982.
24. Kropmans T, Dijkstra P, Stegenga B, et al: Smallest detectable difference of maximal mouth opening in patients with painful restricted temporomandibular joint function. Eur J Oral Sci 108:9–13, 2000.
25. Friedman MH, Weisberg J: The temporomandibular joint. In Gould JA, editor: Orthopedic and sports physical therapy, St Louis, 1990, C.V. Mosby.
26. Yatani H, Sonoyama W, Kuboki T, et al: The validity of clinical examination for diagnosing anterior disc displacement with reduction. Oral Surg Oral Med Oral Pathol Oral Radiol Endod 85:647–653, 1998.
27. Yatani H, Suzuki K, Kuboki T, et al: The validity of clinical examination for diagnosing anterior disc displacement without reduction. Oral Surg Oral Med Oral Pathol Oral Radiol Endod 85:654–660, 1998.
28. List T, Greene CS: Moving forward with the RDC/TMD. J Oral Rehab 37:731–733, 2010.
29. Schiffman EL, Truelove EL, Ohrbach R, et al: The research diagnostic criteria for temporomandibular disorders I: overview and methodology for assessment of validity. J Orofacial Pain 24:7–24, 2010.
30. Look JO, John MT, Tai F, et al: The research diagnostic criteria for temporomandibular disorders II: reliability of axis I diagnoses and selected clinical measures. J Orofacial Pain 24:25–34, 2010.
31. Ohrbach R, Turner JA, Sherman JJ, et al: The research diagnostic criteria for temporomandibular disorders IV: evaluation of psychometric properties of the axis II measures. J Orofacial Pain 24:48–62, 2010.
32. Schiffman EL, Ohrbach R, Truelove EL, et al: The research diagnostic criteria for temporomandibular disorders V: methods used to establish and validate revised axis I diagnostic algorithms. J Orofacial Pain 24:63–78, 2010.
33. Anderson GC, Gonzalez YM, Ohrbach R, et al: The research diagnostic criteria for temporomandibular disorders VI: future directions. J Orofacial Pain 24:79–88, 2010.
34. Sugisaki M, Kino K, Yoshida N, et al: Development of a new questionnaire to assess pain-related limitations of daily functions in Japanese patients with temporomandibular disorders. Community Dent Oral Epidemiol 33:384–395, 2005.
35. Ohrbach R, Larsson P, List T: The jaw functional limitation scale: development, reliability and validity of 8-item and 20-item versions. J Orofacial Pain 22:219–230, 2008.
36. Stegenga B, de Bont LG, de Lecuw R, et al: Assessment of mandibular function impairment associated with temporomandibular joint osteoarthrosis and internal derangement. J Orofacial Pain 7:183–195, 1993.
37. Kropmans TJ, Dijkstra PU, van Veen A, et al: The smallest detectable difference of mandibular function impairment in patients with a painfully restricted temporomandibular joint. J Dent Res 78:1445–1449, 1999.
38. Friedman MH, Weisberg J: Application of orthopedic principles in evaluation of the temporomandibular joint. Phys Ther 62:597–603, 1982.
39. Rocabado M: Arthrokinematics of the temporomandibular joint. Dent Clin North Am 27:573–594, 1983.
40. Langendoen J, Muller J, Jull GA: Retrodiscal tissue of the temporomandibular joint: clinical anatomy and its role in diagnosis and treatment of arthropathies. Man Ther 2:191–198, 1997.
41. Emshoff R, Brandlmaier I, Bosch R, et al: Validation of the clinical diagnostic criteria for temporomandibular disorders for the diagnostic subgroup—disc derangement with reduction. J Oral Rehab 29:1139–1145, 2002.

SUGGESTED READINGS

Anthony CP, Kotthoff NJ: Textbook of anatomy and physiology, St Louis, 1971, C.V. Mosby.
Atkinson TA, Vossler S, Hart DL: The evaluation of facial, head, neck and temporomandibular joint pain patients. J Orthop Sports Phys Ther 3:193–199, 1982.
Bassett LW, Gold RH, Seeger LL: MRI atlas of the musculoskeletal system, London, 1989, Martin Dunitz Ltd.
Bell WE: Understanding temporomandibular biomechanics. J Craniomand Pract 1:28–33, 1983.
Clarke GT: Examining temporomandibular disorder patients for cranio-cervical dysfunction. J Craniomand Pract 2:56–63, 1984.
Crawford WA: Centric relation reappraised. J Craniomand Pract 2:40–45, 1984.
Crouch JE: Functional human anatomy, Philadelphia, 1973, Lea & Febiger.
Curl DD: The visual range of motion scale: analysis of mandibular gait in a chiropractic setting. J Manipulative Physiol Ther 15:115–122, 1992.

Dawson PE: Evaluation, diagnosis, and treatment of occlusal problems, St Louis, 1984, C.V. Mosby.
de Leuw R, Boering G, Stegenga B, et al: Symptoms of temporomandibular joint osteoarthrosis and internal derangement 30 years after nonsurgical treatment. J Craniomand Pract 13:81–88, 1995.
Dworkin SF, Huggins KH, LeResche L, et al: Epidemiology of signs and symptoms in temporomandibular disorders: clinical signs in cases and controls. J Am Dent Assoc 120:273–281, 1990.
Eriksson L, Westesson PL, Sjoberg H: Observer performance in describing temporomandibular joint sounds. J Craniomand Pract 5:33–35, 1987.
Eversaul GA: Dental kinesiology, Las Vegas, 1977, G.A. Eversaul.
Fain WD, McKinney JM: The TMJ examination form. J Craniomand Pract 3:138–144, 1985.
Farrar WB, McCarty WL: Inferior joint space arthrography and characteristics of condylar paths in internal derangements of the TMJ. J Prosthet Dent 41:548–555, 1979.
Farrar WB, McCarty WL: The TMJ dilemma. J Alabama Dent Assoc 63:19–26, 1979.
Friedman MH, Weisberg J: Joint play movements of the temporomandibular joint: Clinical considerations. Arch Phys Med Rehabil 65:413–417, 1984.
Frumker SC: Determining masticatory muscle spasm and TMJ capsulitis. J Craniomand Pract 1:52–58, 1983.
Gelb H: Clinical management of head, neck and TMJ pain and dysfunction, Philadelphia, 1977, W.B. Saunders.
Gelb H: An orthopaedic approach to occlusal imbalance and temporomandibular joint dysfunction. Dent Clin North Am 23:181–197, 1979.
Gelb H, Tarte J: A two-year clinical dental evaluation of 200 cases of chronic headache: The craniocervical-mandibular syndrome. J Am Dent Assoc 91:1230–1236, 1975.

Graber TM: Overbite: The dentist's challenge. J Am Dent Assoc 79:1135–1145, 1969.

Helland MM: Anatomy and function of the temporomandibular joint. J Orthop Sports Phys Ther 1:145–152, 1980.

Helland MM: Anatomy and function of the temporomandibular joint. In Grieve G, editor: Modern manual therapy of the vertebral column, Edinburgh, 1986, Churchill Livingstone.

Hollinshead WH, Jenkins DB: Functional anatomy of the limbs and back, Philadelphia, 1981, W.B. Saunders.

Hoover D, Ritzlane P: The temporomandibular joint. In Levangie PK, Norkin CC, editors: Joint structure and function—a comprehensive analysis, Philadelphia, 2005, F.A. Davis.

Hoppenfeld S: Physical examination of the spine and extremities, New York, 1976, Appleton-Century-Crofts.

Humberger HC, Humberger NW: Physical therapy evaluation of the craniomandibular pain and dysfunction patient. J Craniomand Pract 10:138–143, 1992.

Iglarsh ZA: Temporomandibular joint pain. Orthop Phys Ther Clin North Am 4:471–484, 1995.

Klineberg I: Structure and function of temporomandibular joint innervation. Ann R Coll Surg Engl 49:268–288, 1971.

Liebgott B: The anatomical basis of dentistry, ed 2, St Louis, 1986, C.V. Mosby.

Maitland GD: The peripheral joints: examination and recording guide, Adelaide, Australia, 1973, Virgo Press.

McKinnism LN: Fundamentals of musculoskeletal imaging, Philadelphia, 2005, F.A. Davis.

Neumann DA: Kinesiology of the musculoskeletal system—foundations for physical rehabilitation, St Louis, 2002, C.V. Mosby.

Ombregt L, Bisschop P, ter Veer HJ, et al: A system of orthopedic medicine, London, 1995, W.B. Saunders.

Paesani D, Westesson PL, Hatala M, et al: Prevalence of temporomandibular joint internal derangement in patients with craniomandibular disorders. Am J Orthod Dentofac Orthop 101:41–47, 1992.

Palmer ML, Epler M: Clinical assessment procedures in physical therapy, Philadelphia, 1990, J.B. Lippincott.

Pollmann L: Sounds produced by the mandibular joint in young men. J Max Fac Surg 8:155–157, 1980.

Ranalli DW: Dental injuries in sports. Curr Sports Med Rep 4:12–17, 2005.

Raustia AM, Tervonen O, Pyhtinen J: Temporomandibular joint findings obtained by brain MRI. J Craniomand Pract 12:28–32, 1994.

Resnick D, Kransdorf MJ: Bone and joint imaging, Philadelphia, 2005, W.B. Saunders.

Sherriff J: Tongue posture. Br J Orthod 8:203–211, 1981.

Silver CM, Simon SD, Savastano AA: Meniscus injuries of the temporomandibular joint. J Bone Joint Surg Am 38:541–552, 1956.

Snow DF: Initial examination. In Morgan DH, House LR, Hall WP, et al, editors: Diseases of the temporomandibular apparatus, St Louis, 1982, C.V. Mosby.

Stein JL: The temporomandibular joint. In Little H, editor: Rheumatological physical examination, Orlando, 1986, Grune & Stratton.

Talley RL, Murphy GJ, Smith SD, et al: Standards for the history, examination, diagnosis and treatment of temporomandibular disorders: a position paper. J Craniomand Pract 8:60–77, 1990.

Thilander B: Innervation of the temporo-mandibular disc in man. Acta Odontol Scand 22:151–156, 1964.

Travell J: Temporomandibular joint pain referred muscles of the head and neck. J Prosthet Dent 10:745–763, 1960.

Travell JG, Simons DG: Myofacial pain and dysfunction: the trigger point manual, Baltimore, 1983, Williams & Wilkins.

Watt DM: Temporomandibular joint sounds. J Dent 8:119–127, 1980.

Weinberg LA: Temporomandibular joint injuries. In Foreman SM, Croft AC, editors: Whiplash injuries, Baltimore, 1988, Williams & Wilkins.

Williams P, Warwick R, editors: Gray's anatomy, ed 36, (British), Edinburgh, 1980, Churchill Livingstone.

Wright EF: A simple questionnaire and clinical examination to help identify possible non-craniomandibular disorders that may influence a patient's CMD symptoms. J Craniomand Pract 10:228–234, 1992.

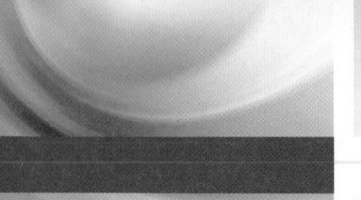

CHAPTER **5**

Shoulder

The prerequisite to any treatment of a patient with pain in the shoulder region is a precise and comprehensive picture of the signs and symptoms as they present during the assessment and as they existed until that time. This knowledge ensures that the techniques used will suit the condition and that the degree of success will be estimated against this background. Shoulder pain can be caused by intrinsic disease of the shoulder joints or pathology in the periarticular structures, or it may originate from the cervical spine, chest, or visceral structures. Pathology is commonly related to the level of activity, and age can play a significant role. The shoulder complex is difficult to assess because of its many structures (most of which are located in a small area), its many movements, and the many lesions that can occur either inside or outside the joints. Influences such as referred pain from the cervical spine and the possibility of more than one lesion being present at one time, as well as the difficulty in deciding what weight to give to each response, make the examination even more difficult to understand. Assessment of the shoulder region often necessitates an evaluation of the cervical spine (see Chapter 3) and thoracic spine (see Chapter 8), especially the ribs to rule out referred symptoms, and the examiner must be prepared to include the cervical spine and its scanning examination in any shoulder assessment.

APPLIED ANATOMY

The **glenohumeral joint** is a multiaxial, ball-and-socket, synovial joint that depends primarily on the muscles and ligaments rather than bones for its support, stability, and integrity.[1] Thus, the assessment of the muscles and ligaments/capsule can play a major role in the assessment of the shoulder. The **labrum,** which is the ring of fibrocartilage, surrounds and deepens the glenoid cavity of the scapula about 50% (Figure 5-1).[2] Only part of the humeral head is in contact with the glenoid at any one time. This joint has three axes and three degrees of freedom. The resting position of the glenohumeral joint is 55° of abduction and 30° of horizontal adduction. The close packed position of the joint is full abduction and lateral rotation. When relaxed, the humerus sits centered in the glenoid cavity; with contraction of the rotator cuff muscles, it is pushed or translated anteriorly, posteriorly, inferiorly,

superiorly, or in any combination of these movements. This movement is small, but if it does not occur, full movement is impossible. The glenoid in the resting position has a 5° superior tilt or inclination and a 7° retroversion (slight medial rotation). The angle between the humeral neck and shaft is about 130°, and the humeral head is retroverted 30° to 40° relative to the line joining the epicondyle (Figure 5-2).[3]

The rotator cuff muscles play an integral role in shoulder movement. Their positioning on the humerus may be visualized by "cupping" the shoulder with the thumb anteriorly, as shown in Figure 5-3. The biceps tendon (Figure 5-4) runs between the thumb and index finger just anterior to the index finger. The rotator cuff controls osteokinematic and arthrokinematic motion of the humeral head in the glenoid and along with the biceps depresses the humeral head during movements into elevation.

The primary ligaments of the glenohumeral joint—the superior, middle, and inferior glenohumeral ligaments—play an important role in stabilizing the shoulder (Figure 5-5).[3,4] The superior glenohumeral ligament's primary role is limiting inferior translation in adduction. It also restrains anterior translation and lateral rotation up to 45° abduction. The middle glenohumeral ligament, which is absent in 30% of the population, limits lateral rotation between 45° and 90° abduction. The inferior glenohumeral ligament is the most important of the three ligaments. It has an anterior and posterior band with a thin "axillary pouch" in between, so it acts much like a hammock or sling. It supports the humeral head above 90° abduction, limiting inferior translation while the anterior band tightens on lateral rotation and the posterior band tightens on medial rotation.[5] Excessive lateral rotation, as seen in throwing, may lead to stretching of the anterior portion of the ligament (and capsule), thereby increasing glenohumeral laxity.[6] The coracohumeral ligament primarily limits inferior translation and helps limit lateral rotation below 60° abduction. This ligament is found in the rotator interval between the anterior border of the supraspinatus tendon and the superior border of the subscapularis tendon, thus the ligament unites the two tendons anteriorly (Figure 5-6).[7-9] The **rotator interval** consists of fibers of the coracohumeral ligament, superior glenohumeral ligament, glenohumeral

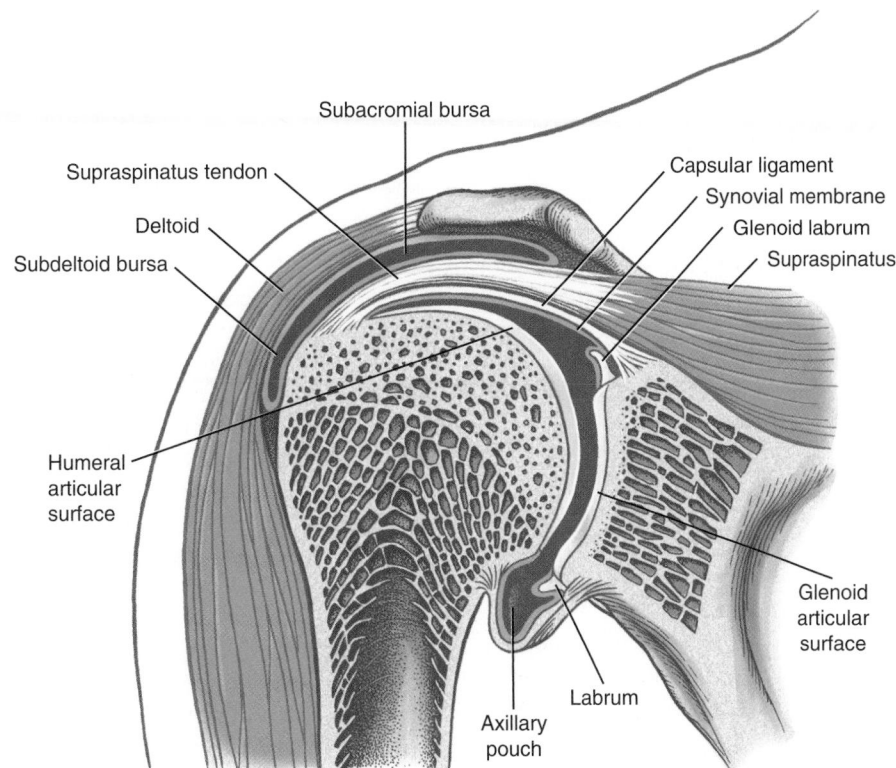

Figure 5-1 Anterior view of a frontal plane cross-section of the right glenohumeral joint. Note the subacromial and subdeltoid bursa within the subacromial space. Bursa and synovial lining are depicted in *blue*. The deltoid and supraspinatus muscles are also shown. (From Neuman DA: Kinesiology of the musculoskeletal system: foundations for rehabilitation, ed 2, St Louis, 2010, Mosby/Elsevier, p. 143.)

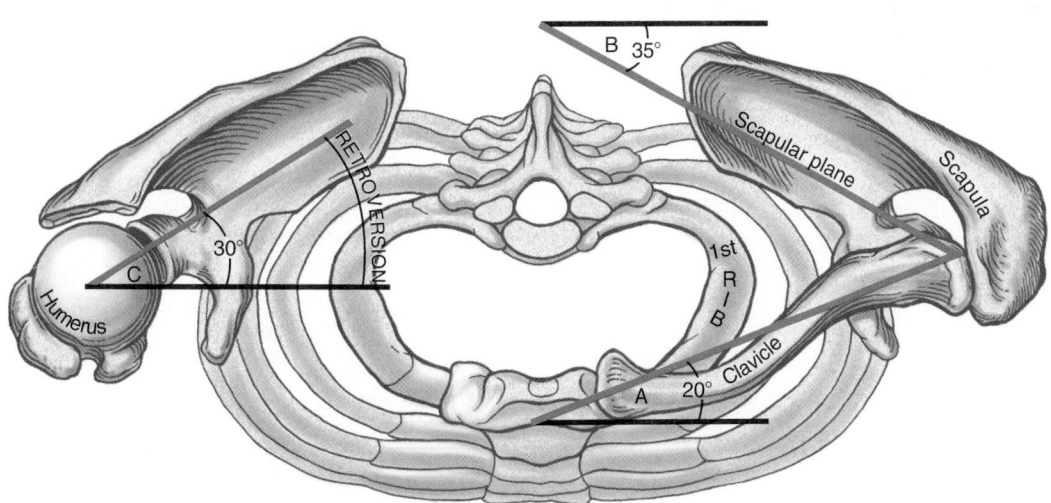

Figure 5-2 Superior view of both shoulders in the anatomic position. *Angle A:* The clavicle is deviated about 20° posterior to the frontal plane. *Angle B:* The scapula (scapular plane or "scaption") is deviated about 35° anterior to the front plane. *Angle C:* Retroversion of the humeral head about 30° posterior to the medial-lateral axis at the elbow. The right clavicle and acromion have been removed to expose the top of the right glenohumeral joint. (From Neuman DA: Kinesiology of the musculoskeletal system: foundations for rehabilitation, ed 2, St Louis, 2010, Mosby/Elsevier, p. 123.)

joint capsule, and part of the tendons of supraspinatus and subscapularis.[9] Injury to these structures can lead to contractures, biceps tendon instability, and anterior glenohumeral instability.[9] See Table 5-1 for structures limiting movement in different degrees of abduction.[5,10] The coracoacromial ligament forms an arch over the humeral head, acting as a block to superior translation.[11] The transverse humeral ligament forms a roof over the bicipital groove to hold the long head of biceps tendon within the groove. The capsular pattern of the glenohumeral joint is lateral rotation most limited, followed by abduction and medial rotation. Branches of the posterior cord of the brachial plexus and the suprascapular, axillary, and lateral pectoral nerves innervate the joint.

Glenohumeral Joint	
Resting position:	40° to 55° abduction, 30° horizontal adduction (scapular plane)
Close packed position:	Full abduction, lateral rotation
Capsular pattern:	Lateral rotation, abduction, medial rotation

The **acromioclavicular joint** is a plane synovial joint that augments the range of motion (ROM) of the humerus in the glenoid (Figure 5-7). The bones making up this joint are the acromion process of the scapula and the lateral end of the clavicle. The acromion may have different undersurface shapes or types: type I—flat (17%), type II—curved (43%), type III—hooked (39%), and type IV—convex (upturned) (1%) (Figure 5-8).[12] About 70% of rotator cuff tears are associated with a hooked acromion.[12] Some believe the hooked acromion is not an anatomical variant but is the result of ossification of the coracoacromial ligament at its attachment to the acromion.[13] The joint has three degrees of freedom. The capsule, which is fibrous, surrounds the joint. An articular disc may be found within the joint. Rarely does the disc separate the acromion and clavicular articular surfaces. This joint depends on ligaments for its strength. The acromioclavicular ligaments surround the joint and control horizontal motion of the clavicle.[14] These are commonly the first ligaments injured when the joint is stressed. The coracoclavicular ligament is the primary support of the acromioclavicular joint. It has two portions: the conoid (medial) and trapezoid (lateral) parts, and they control the vertical motion of the clavicle.[14,15] If a step deformity occurs, this ligament has been torn. In the resting position of the joint, the arm rests by the side in the normal, standing position. In the close packed position of the acromioclavicular joint, the arm is abducted to 90°. The indication of a capsular pattern in the joint

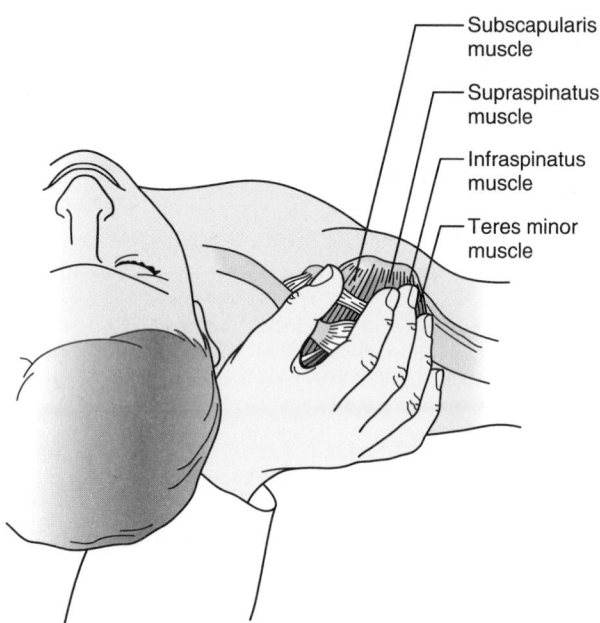

Figure 5-3 Positioning of the rotator cuff with thumb over subscapularis, index finger over supraspinatus, middle finger over infraspinatus, and ring finger over teres minor.

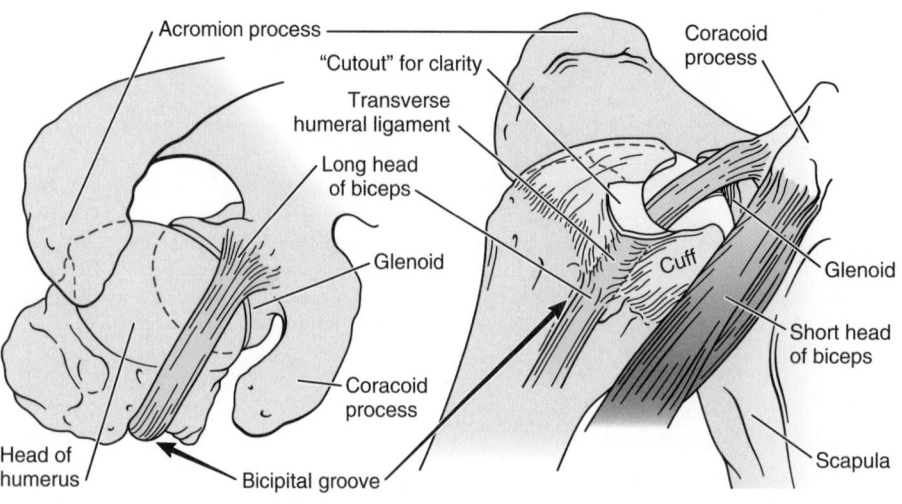

Figure 5-4 The biceps apparatus.

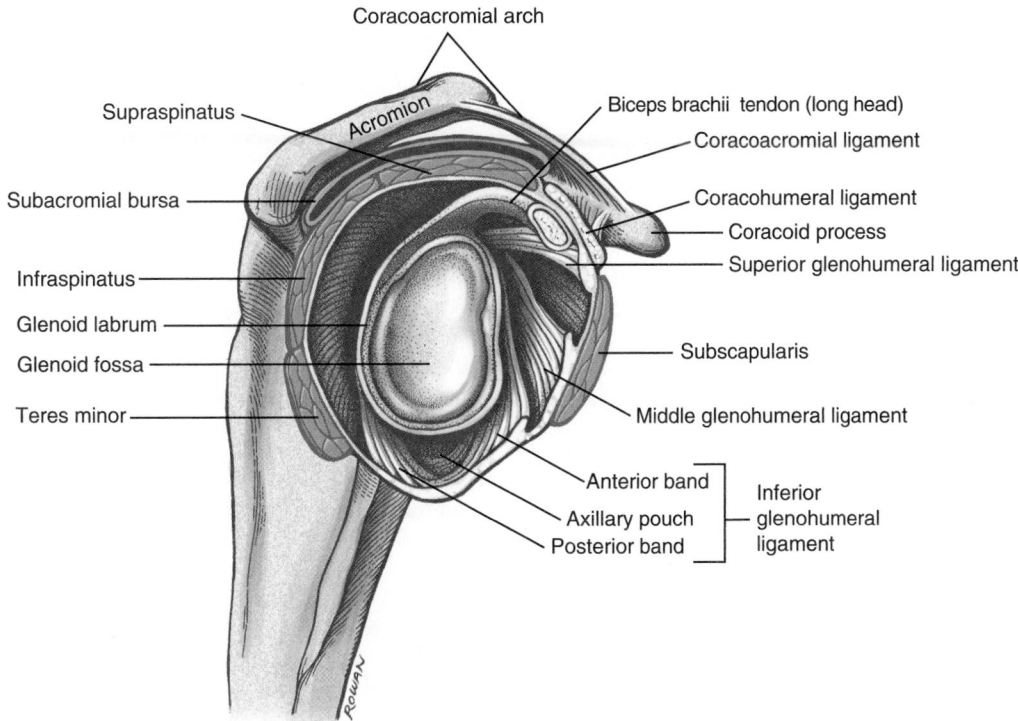

Figure 5-5 Lateral aspect of the internal surface of the right glenohumeral joint. The humerus has been removed to expose the capsular ligaments and the glenoid fossa. Note the prominent coracoacromial arch and underlying subacromial bursa *(blue)*. The four rotator cuff muscles are shown in *red*. (From Neuman DA: Kinesiology of the musculoskeletal system: foundations for rehabilitation, ed 2, St Louis, 2010, Mosby/Elsevier, p. 139.)

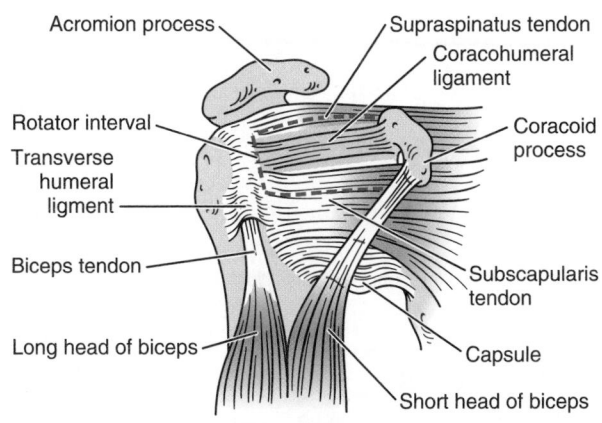

Figure 5-6 Rotator interval *(dashed lines)* showing the relationship between the supraspinatus tendon, subscapularis tendon, and the coracohumeral ligament.

is pain at the extreme ROM, especially in horizontal adduction (cross-flexion) and full elevation. This joint is innervated by branches of the suprascapular and lateral pectoral nerve.

The **sternoclavicular joint,** along with the acromioclavicular joint, enables the humerus in the glenoid to move through a full 180° of abduction (Figure 5-9). It is a saddle-shaped synovial joint with 3° of freedom and is made up of the medial end of the clavicle, the

Acromioclavicular Joint	
Resting position:	Arm resting by side in normal physiological position
Close packed position:	90° abduction
Capsular pattern:	Pain at extremes of ROM, especially horizontal adduction and full elevation

manubrium sternum, and the cartilage of the first rib. It is the joint that joins the appendicular skeleton to the axial skeleton.[16] A substantial disc is between the two bony joint surfaces, and the capsule is thicker anteriorly than posteriorly. The disc separates the articular surfaces of the clavicle and sternum and adds significant strength to the joint because of attachments, thereby preventing medial displacement of the clavicle. Like the acromioclavicular joint, the joint depends on ligaments for its strength. The ligaments of the sternoclavicular joint include the anterior and posterior sternoclavicular ligaments, which support the joint anteriorly and posteriorly, the interclavicular ligament, and the costoclavicular ligament running from the clavicle to the first rib and its costal cartilage. This is the main ligament maintaining the integrity of the sternoclavicular joint. The movements possible at this joint and at the acromioclavicular joint are

TABLE **5-1**

Structures Limiting Movement in Different Degrees of Abduction

Angle of Abduction	Lateral Rotation	Neutral	Medial Rotation
0°	Superior GH ligament Anterior capsule	Coracohumeral ligament Superior GH ligament Capsule (anterior and posterior) Supraspinatus	Posterior capsule
0° to 45° (note: 30° to 45° abduction in scapular plane [resting position]—maximum looseness of shoulder)	Coracohumeral ligament Superior GH ligament Anterior capsule	Middle GH ligament Posterior capsule Subscapularis Infraspinatus Teres minor	Posterior capsule
45° to 60°	Middle GH ligament Coracohumeral ligament Inferior GH ligament (anterior band) Anterior capsule	Middle GH ligament Inferior GH ligament (especially anterior portion) Subscapularis Infraspinatus Teres minor	Inferior GH ligament (posterior band) Posterior capsule
60° to 90°	Inferior GH ligament (anterior band) Anterior capsule	Inferior GH ligament (especially posterior portion) Middle GH ligament	Inferior GH ligament (posterior band) Posterior capsule
90° to 120°	Inferior GH ligament (anterior band) Anterior capsule	Inferior GH ligament	Inferior GH ligament (posterior band) Posterior capsule
120° to 180°	Inferior GH ligament (anterior band) Anterior capsule	Inferior GH ligament	Inferior -H ligament (posterior band) Posterior capsule

Data from Curl LA, Warren RF: Glenohumeral joint stability—selective cutting studies on the static capsular restraints. Clin Orthop Relat Res 330:54–65, 1996; and Peat M, Culham E: Functional anatomy of the shoulder complex. In Andrews JR, Wilks KE, editors: The athlete's shoulder, New York, 1994, Churchill Livingstone.
GH, Glenohumeral.

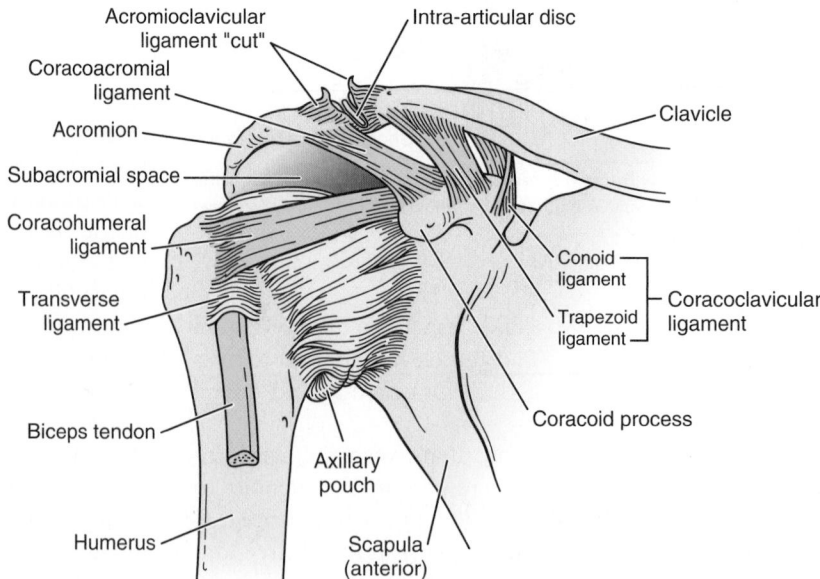

Figure 5-7 Anterior view of the right glenohumeral and acromioclavicular joints. Note the subacromial space or supraspinatus outlet located between the top of the humeral head and the underside of the acromion. (Modified from Neumann DA: Kinesiology of the musculoskeletal system: foundations for rehabilitation, St Louis, 2002, Mosby, p. 107.)

elevation, depression, protrusion, retraction, and rotation. The close packed position of the sternoclavicular joint is full or maximum rotation of the clavicle, which occurs when the upper arm is in full elevation. The resting position and capsular pattern are the same as with the acromioclavicular joint. The joint is innervated by branches of the anterior supraclavicular nerve and the nerve to the subclavius muscle. Major vessels and the trachea lie close behind the sternum and the sternoclavicular joint (see Figure 5-9, *B*).[16]

Sternoclavicular Joint

Resting position:	Arm resting by side in normal physiological position
Close packed position:	Full elevation and protraction
Capsular pattern:	Pain at extremes of ROM, especially horizontal adduction and full elevation

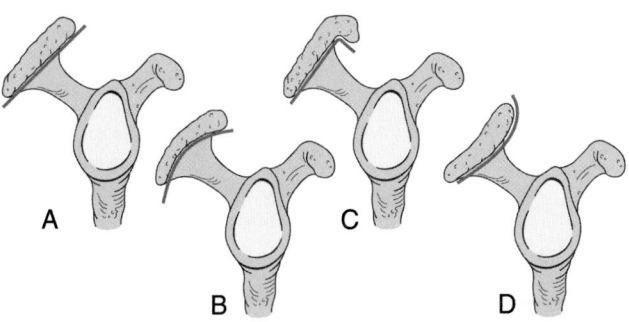

Figure 5-8 Acromion morphology. A, Flat. **B,** Curved. **C,** Hooked. **D,** Convex (upturn).

Although the **scapulothoracic joint** is not a true joint, it functions as an integral part of the shoulder complex and must be considered in any assessment because a stable scapula enables the rest of the shoulder to function correctly. Some texts call this structure the scapulocostal joint. This "joint" consists of the body of the scapula and the muscles covering the posterior chest wall. The muscles acting on the scapula help to control its movements. The medial border of the scapula is not parallel with the spinous processes but is angled about 3° away (top to bottom), and the scapula lies 20° to 30° forward relative to the sagittal plane.[3] Because it is not a true joint, it does not have a capsular pattern nor a close packed position. The resting position of this joint is the same as for the acromioclavicular joint. The scapula extends from the level of T2 spinous process to T7 or T9 spinous process, depending on the size of the scapula. Because the scapula acts as a stable base for the rotator cuff muscles, the muscles controlling its movements must be strong and balanced because the joint funnels the forces of the trunk and legs into the arm.[17]

PATIENT HISTORY

In addition to the questions listed under "Patient History" in Chapter 1, the examiner should obtain the following information from the patient.[18] Most commonly, the patient complains of pain, especially on movement, restricted motion, or shoulder instability.

1. *What is the patient's age?* Many problems of the shoulder can be age-related. For example, rotator cuff degeneration usually occurs in patients who are between 40 and 60 years of age. Rotator cuff tears,

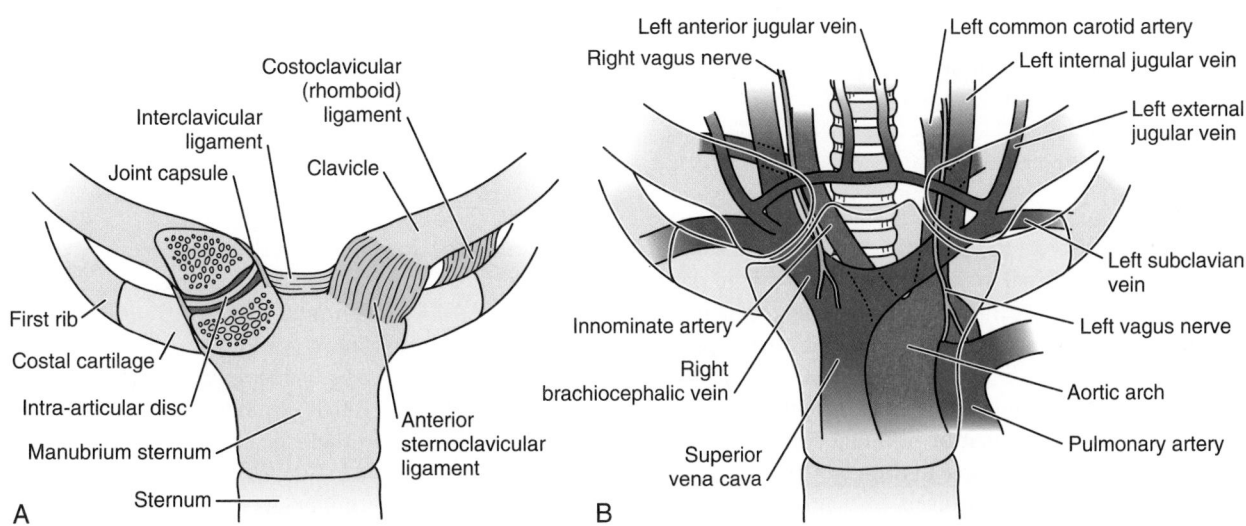

Figure 5-9 A, Bony and ligamentous anatomy of the sternoclavicular joint. The major supporting structures include the anterior capsule, the posterior capsule, the interclavicular ligament, the costoclavicular (rhomboid) ligament, and the intra-articular disc and ligament. **B,** Retrosternal anatomy. Note the proximity of the sternoclavicular joint to the trachea, aortic arch, and brachiocephalic vein. (Redrawn from Higginbotham TO, Kuhn JE: Atraumatic disorders of the sternoclavicular joint. J Am Acad Ortho Surg 13:139, 2005.)

TABLE **5-2**

Differential Diagnosis of Rotator Cuff Degeneration, Frozen Shoulder, Atraumatic Instability, and Cervical Spondylosis

	Rotator Cuff Lesions	Frozen Shoulder	Atraumatic Instability	Cervical Spondylosis
History	Age 30 to 50 years Pain and weakness after eccentric load	Age 45+ (insidious type) Insidious onset or after trauma or surgery Functional restriction of lateral rotation, abduction, and medial rotation	Age 10 to 35 years Pain and instability with activity No history of trauma	Age 50+ years Acute or chronic
Observation	Normal bone and soft tissue outlines Protective shoulder hike may be seen	Normal bone and soft-tissue outlines	Normal bone and soft-tissue outlines	Minimal or no cervical spine movement Torticollis may be present
Active movement	Weakness of abduction or rotation, or both Crepitus may be present	Restricted ROM Shoulder hiking	Full or excessive ROM	Limited ROM with pain
Passive movement	Pain if impingement occurs	Limited ROM, especially in lateral, rotation, abduction, and medial rotation (capsular pattern)	Normal or excessive ROM	Limited ROM (symptoms may be exacerbated)
Resisted isometric movement	Pain and weakness on abduction and lateral rotation	Normal, when arm by side	Normal	Normal, except if nerve root compressed Myotome may be affected
Special tests	Drop-arm test positive Empty can test positive	None	Load and shift test positive Apprehension test positive Relocation test positive Augmentation tests positive	Spurling's test positive Distraction test positive ULNT positive Shoulder abduction test positive
Sensory function and reflexes	Not affected	Not affected		Dermatomes affected Reflexes affected
Palpation	Tender over rotator cuff	Not painful unless capsule is stretched	Anterior or posterior pain	Tender over appropriate vertebra or facet
Diagnostic imaging	Radiography: Upward displacement of humeral head; acromial spurring MRI diagnostic	Radiography: Negative Arthrography: Decreased capsular size	Negative	Radiography: Narrowing osteophytes

MRI, Magnetic resonance imaging; *ROM,* range of motion; *ULNT,* upper limb neurodynamic (tension) test.

though, can occur at any age.[19] Litaker, et al.[20] suggested that external rotation weakness, night pain, and age over 65 are indicative of rotator cuff tears. Primary impingement due to degeneration and weakness is usually seen in patients older than 35, whereas secondary impingement due to instability caused by weakness in the scapular or humeral control muscles is more common in people in their late teens or twenties, especially those involved in vigorous overhead activities, such as swimmers or pitchers in baseball.[21] Calcium deposits may occur between the ages of 20 and 40.[22] Chondrosarcomas may be seen in those older than 30 years of age, whereas frozen shoulder is seen in persons between the ages of 45 and 60 years if it results from causes other than trauma (Tables 5-2 and 5-3). Frozen shoulder due to trauma can occur at any age but is more common with increased age.

2. *Does the patient support the upper limb in a protected position* (Figure 5-10) *or hesitate to move it?* This action could mean that one of the joints of the shoulder complex is unstable or that there is an acute problem in the shoulder. In some cases, patients with lax shoulders ask, "What happens when I do this?" In effect, the patient is subluxing the shoulder (Figure 5-11). This may or may not be pathological, but it is a sign of voluntary instability in which the patient

TABLE **5-3**

Differential Diagnosis of Shoulder Pathology

Pathology	Symptoms
External primary impingement (stage I)	Intermittent mild pain with overhead activities Over age 35
External primary impingement (stage II)	Mild to moderate pain with overhead activities or strenuous activities
External primary impingement (stage III)	Pain at rest or with activities Night pain may occur Scapular or rotator cuff weakness is noted
Rotator cuff tears (full thickness)	Classic night pain Weakness noted predominantly in abduction and lateral rotators Loss of motion
Adhesive capsulitis (idiopathic frozen shoulder)	Inability to perform ADLs owing to loss of motion Loss of motion may be perceived as weakness
Anterior instability (with or without external secondary impingement)	Apprehension to mechanical shifting limits activities Slipping, popping, or sliding may present as suitable instability Apprehension usually associated with horizontal abduction and lateral rotation Anterior or posterior pain may be present Weak scapular stabilizers
Posterior instability	Slipping or popping of the humerus out the back This may be associated with forward flexion and medial rotation while the shoulder is under a compressive load
Multidirectional instability	Looseness of shoulder in all directions This may be most pronounced while carrying luggage or turning over while asleep Pain may or may not be present

Modified from Maughon TS, Andrews JR: The subjective evaluation of the shoulder in the athlete. In Andrews JR, Wilk KE, editors: The athlete's shoulder, New York, 1994, Churchill-Livingstone, p. 36.
ADL, Activity of daily living.

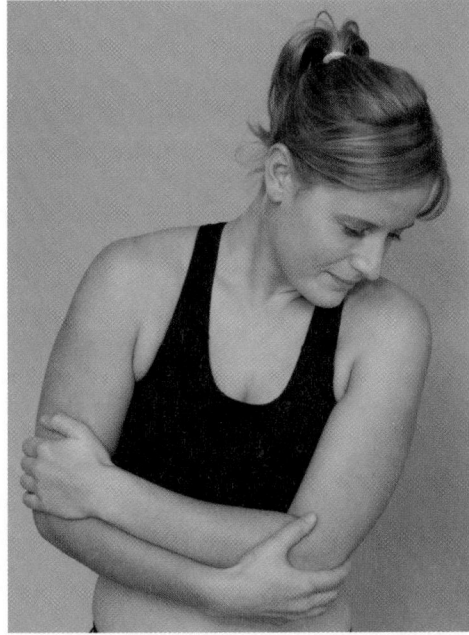

Figure 5-10 Patient supports the upper limb in protected position.

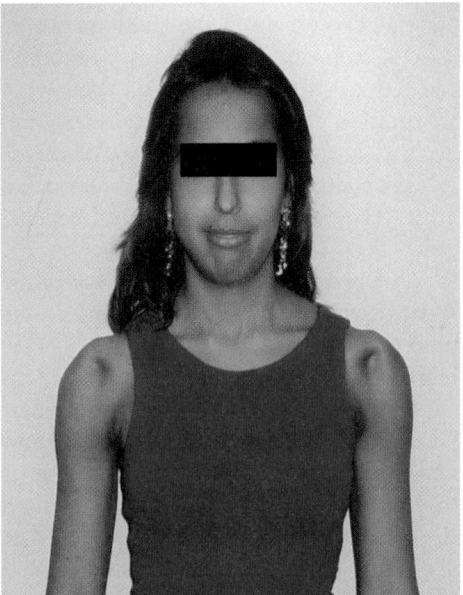

Figure 5-11 Voluntary instability. Note how the patient uses her muscles to sublux the humerus in the glenoid, resulting in an anterior sulcus in each shoulder.

uses his or her muscles to sublux the humerus in the glenoid, stressing the labrum and inert tissues.

3. *If there was an injury, what exactly was the mechanism of injury?* Did the patient injure themself with a fall on out-stretched hand (FOOSH), which could indicate a fracture or dislocation of the glenohumeral joint? Did the patient fall on or receive a blow to the tip of the shoulder, or did the patient land on the elbow, driving the humerus up against the acromion? This finding may indicate an acromioclavicular dislocation or subluxation.[23,24] Does the shoulder feel unstable or feel like it is "coming out" during movement? Does the arm "go dead" when doing activity? "Going dead" implies the patient cannot use the arm functionally because of pain and a subjective feeling of unease when using the arm.[25] Patients with instability may appear normal on clinical examination, especially if shoulder muscles are not fatigued. Many overuse injuries are more evident immediately after the patient does repeated activity.[26] This may indicate gross or anatomical instability, such as in recurrent shoulder dislocation, subluxation, or subtle translational instability. The spectrum of instability varies from gross or anatomical instability—the TUBS type (**T**raumatic onset, **U**nidirectional anterior with a **B**ankart lesion responding to **S**urgery) to a more subtle translational instability—the AMBRI type (**A**traumatic cause, **M**ultidirectional with **B**ilateral shoulder findings with **R**ehabilitation as appropriate treatment and, rarely, **I**nferior capsular shift surgery).

4. *Are there any movements or positions that cause the patient pain or symptoms?* If so, which ones? The examiner must keep in mind that cervical spine movements may cause pain in the shoulder. Persons who have had recurrent dislocations/instability of the shoulder may find that any movement involving lateral rotation bothers them, because this movement is involved in anterior dislocations of the shoulder. Questions related to instability should include[27]:
   a. How many episodes have there been in the last year?
   b. Was there an injury that precipitated this?
   c. What direction does the shoulder "go out" most times?
   d. Have you ever needed help getting the shoulder back into proper position within the joint?

   Recurrent dislocators may sometimes show pain at extreme of medial rotation when the humeral head is "tightened" against the anterior glenoid. Long head of biceps pathology causes pain that moves medially and laterally with medial and lateral rotation of the shoulder.[28] Excessive abduction and lateral rotation may lead to dead-arm syndrome in which the patient feels a sudden paralyzing pain and weakness in the shoulder.[25] This finding often indicates altered shoulder mechanics commonly involving a tight posterior capsule, altered arthrokinematics of the glenohumeral joint, and **scapular dyskinesia**.[25,29,30] In throwers, the condition may be referred to as a "SICK" scapula (malposition of **S**capula, prominence of **I**nferior medial border of scapula, **C**oracoid pain and malposition, and scapular dys**K**inesia).[31] If the patient complains of pain during specific phases of pitching (for example, during the late cocking and acceleration phases), anterior instability should be considered even in the presence of minimal clinical signs.[32] Commonly, instability and secondary impingement occur together. Secondary impingement implies that although impingement signs are present, they result from a primary problem somewhere else, commonly in the scapular or humeral control or stabilizer muscles. Primary impingement implies that impingement or pinching is the primary cause of the pain.

Causes of Shoulder Primary and Secondary Impingement Syndrome

- Abnormal glenohumeral arthrokinematics (secondary)
- Abnormal scapulothoracic arthrokinematics (secondary)
- "Slouched" (chin poking) posture (secondary)
- Muscle weakness or fatigue (secondary)
- Muscle hypomobility (secondary)
- Capsule tightness especially posterior (secondary)
- Inflammation in subacromial space (primary)
- Rotator cuff tendon degeneration (primary)
- Adhesions especially inferiorly (secondary)
- Osteophytes under acromioclavicular joint (primary)
- Hooked acromion (primary)
- Glenohumeral joint hypermobility (primary)

Stability of the shoulder depends on both dynamic stabilizers (the muscles) and static stabilizers (e.g., the capsule, labrum).[5] Night pain and resting pain are often related to rotator cuff tears and, on occasion, to tumors; activity-related pain usually signifies paratenonitis. Arthritis pain commonly shows, at least initially, at the extremes of motion. Acromioclavicular pain is especially evident at greater than 90° of abduction and tends to be localized to the joint. Similarly, sternoclavicular pain is localized to the joint and increases on horizontal adduction.

5. *What is the extent and behavior of the patient's pain?* For example, deep, boring, toothache-like pain in the neck, shoulder region, or both may indicate **thoracic outlet syndrome**[33] (Figure 5-12) or acute brachial plexus neuropathy. Strains of the rotator cuff usually cause dull, toothache-like pain that is worse at night, whereas acute calcific tendinitis usually causes a hot, burning type of pain. Sprain of the first or second rib from direct trauma or sudden contraction of the

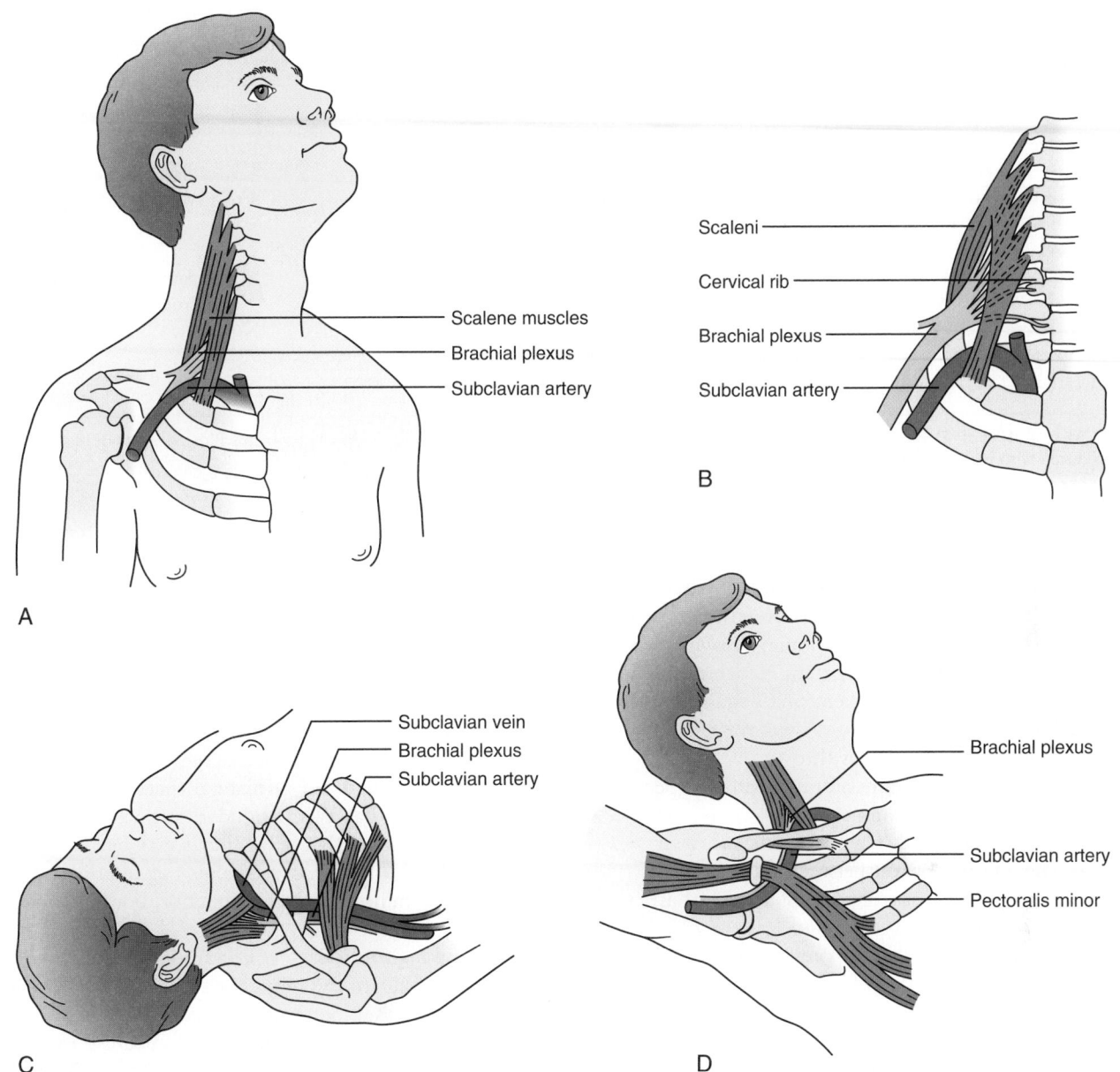

Figure 5-12 **Location and causes of thoracic outlet syndrome. A,** Scalenus anterior syndrome. **B,** Cervical rib syndrome. **C,** Costoclavicular space syndrome. **D,** Hyperabduction syndrome (abduction, extension, and lateral rotation).

scaleni may mimic an acute impingement or rotator cuff injury.[34]

6. *Are there any activities that cause or increase the pain?* For example, bicipital paratenonitis or tendinosis[35] are often seen in skiers and may result from holding on to a ski tow; in cross-country skiing, it may result from poling (using the pole for propulsion). Paratenonitis is inflammation of the paratenon of the tendon. The paratenon is the outer covering of the tendon whether or not it is lined with synovium. Tendinosis is actual degeneration of the tendon itself. With chronic overuse, tendinosis is more likely than paratenonitis[35,36] (Table 5-4; see Table 1-20). Elite swimmers may train for more than 15,000 m daily,

which can lead to stress overload (repetitive microtrauma) of the structures of the shoulder. Does throwing or reaching alter the pain? If so, what positions cause pain or discomfort? These questions may indicate which structures are injured.

7. *Do any positions relieve the pain?* Patients with nerve root pain may find that elevating the arm over the head relieves symptoms. For a patient with instability or inflammatory conditions, lifting the arm over the head usually exacerbates shoulder problems.

8. *What is the patient unable to do functionally?* Is the patient able to talk or swallow? Is the patient hoarse? These signs could indicate an injury to the sternoclavicular joint (if there is swelling) or a posterior

TABLE **5-4**

Implications of the Diagnosis of Tendinosis Compared with Tendinitis

Trait	Overuse Tendinosis	Overuse Tendinitis
Prevalence	Common	Rare
Time for recovery, early presentation	6 to 10 weeks	Several days to 2 weeks
Time for full recovery, chronic presentation	3 to 6 months	4 to 6 weeks
Likelihood of full recovery to sport from chronic symptoms	Approximately 80%	99%
Focus of conservative therapy	Encouragement of collagen-synthesis maturation and strength	Anti-inflammatory modalities and drugs
Role of surgery	Excise abnormal tissue	Not known
Prognosis for surgery	70% to 85%	95%
Time for recovery from surgery	4 to 6 months	3 to 4 weeks

From Khan KM, et al: Overuse tendinosis, not tendonitis. Part 1: a new paradigm for a difficult clinical problem. Phys Sportsmed 28:43, 2000. Reproduced with permission of McGraw-Hill.

dislocation of the joint because pressure is being applied to the trachea. In addition, determining whether the shoulder has been overstressed or overused is important.[37] For example, in swimmers and baseball pitchers, it is important to determine[38]:

a. The age when the patient first began the activity
b. The total years throwing/swimming
c. The number of pitches thrown per outing
d. The number of games/innings pitched per year
e. The distances swam per week
f. The strokes used/types of pitches thrown
g. The amount of rest between outings
h. Whether there was any complete rest from activity during year
i. Whether there was any previous injury related to the activity
j. The phase of activity that produces the symptoms

9. *How long has the problem bothered the patient?* For example, an idiopathic frozen shoulder goes through three stages: the condition becomes progressively worse, plateaus, and then progressively improves, with each stage lasting 3 to 5 months.[39,40]

10. *Is there any indication of muscle spasm, deformity, bruising, wasting, paresthesia, or numbness?*[41] These findings can help the examiner determine the acuteness of the condition and, potentially, the structures injured.

11. *Does the patient complain of weakness and heaviness in the limb after activity?* Does the limb tire easily? These findings may indicate vascular involvement. Are there any venous symptoms, such as swelling or stiffness, that may extend all the way to the fingers? Are there any arterial symptoms, such as coolness or pallor in the upper limb? These complaints may result from pressure on an artery, a vein, or both. An example is thoracic outlet syndrome (see Figure 5-12), in which pressure may be applied to the vascular or neurological structures as they enter the upper limb in three locations: at the scalene triangle, at the costoclavicular space, and under the pectoralis minor and the coracoid process.[42,43] Excessive repetitive demands placed on the shoulder (such as, those seen in pitching) may lead to thoracic outlet syndrome, axillary artery occlusion, effort thrombosis, or pressure in the quadrilateral space. (The quadrilateral space has as its boundaries the medial border of the humerus laterally, the lateral border of the long head of triceps medially, the inferior border of teres minor, and the superior border of teres major.)[44]

12. *Is there any indication of nerve injury?* The examiner should evaluate the nerves and the muscles supplied by the nerves to determine possible nerve injury. Any history of weakness, numbness, or paresthesia may indicate nerve injury (Table 5-5). For example, the suprascapular nerve may be injured as it passes through the suprascapular notch under the transverse scapular ligament, leading to atrophy and paralysis of the supraspinatus and infraspinatus muscles. The examiner should listen to the patient history carefully, because this condition could mimic a third-degree (rupture) strain of the supraspinatus tendon. Another potential nerve injury is one to the axillary (circumflex) nerve (Figure 5-13) or musculocutaneous nerve (Figure 5-14) after dislocation of the glenohumeral joint. With an axillary nerve injury, the deltoid muscle and the teres minor muscle are atrophied and weak or paralyzed. The radial nerve (see Figure 5-13) is sometimes injured as it winds around the posterior aspect of the shaft of the humerus. The injury frequently occurs when the humeral shaft is fractured. If the nerve is damaged in this location, the extensors of the elbow, wrist, and fingers are affected, and an

TABLE **5-5**

Peripheral Nerve Injuries (Neuropathy) About the Shoulder

Affected Nerve (Root)	Muscle Weakness	Sensory Alteration	Reflexes Affected	Mechanism of Injury
Suprascapular nerve (C5, C6)	Supraspinatus, infraspinatus (arm lateral rotation)	Top of shoulder from clavicle to spine of scapula Pain in posterior shoulder radiating into arm	None	Compression in suprascapular notch Stretch into scapular protraction plus horizontal adduction Compression in spinoglenoid notch Direct blow Space occupying lesion (e.g., ganglion)
Axillary (circumflex) nerve (posterior cord; C5, C6)	Deltoid, teres minor (arm abduction)	Deltoid area Anterior shoulder pain	None	Anterior glenohumeral dislocation or fracture of surgical neck of humerus Forced abduction Surgery for instability
Radial nerve (C5–C8, T1)	Triceps, wrist extensors, finger extensors (shoulder, wrist, and hand extension)	Dorsum of hand	Triceps	Fracture humeral shaft Pressure (e.g., crutch palsy)
Long thoracic nerve (C5, C6, [C7])	Serratus anterior (scapular control)			Direct blow Traction Compression against internal chest wall (backpack injury) Heavy effort above shoulder height Repetitive strain
Musculocutaneous nerve (C5–C7)	Coracobrachialis, biceps, brachialis (elbow flexion)	Lateral aspect of forearm	Biceps	Compression Muscle hypertrophy Direct blow Fracture (clavicle and humerus) Dislocation (anterior) Surgery (Putti-Platt, Bankart)
Spinal accessory nerve (cranial nerve XI; C3, C4)	Trapezius (shoulder elevation)	Brachial plexus symptoms possible because of drooping of shoulder Shoulder aching	None	Direct blow Traction (shoulder depression and neck rotation to opposite side) Biopsy
Subscapular nerve (posterior cord; C5, C6)	Subscapularis, teres major (medial rotation)	None	None	Direct blow Traction
Dorsal scapular nerve (C5)	Levator scapulae, rhomboid major, rhomboid minor (scapular retraction and elevation)	None	None	Direct blow Compression
Lateral pectoral nerve (C5, C6)	Pectoralis major, pectoralis minor	None	None	Direct blow
Thoracodorsal nerve (C6, C7, [C8])	Latissimus dorsi	None	None	Direct blow Compression
Supraclavicular nerve	—	Mild clavicular pain Sensory loss over anterior shoulder	None	Compression

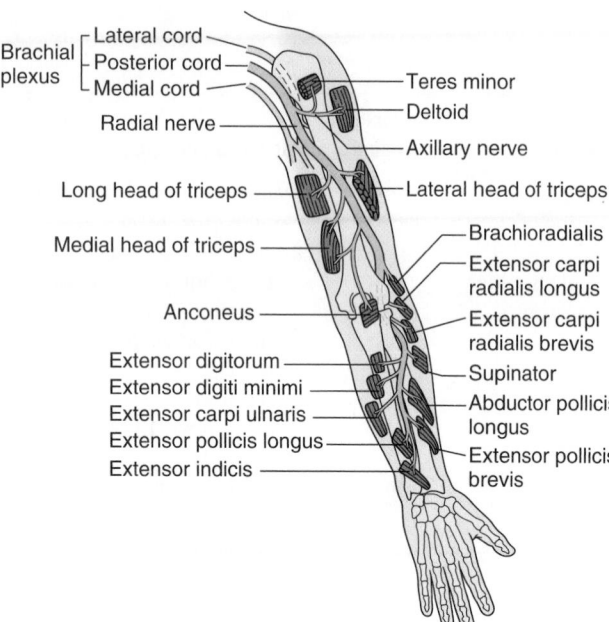

Figure 5-13 Motor distribution of the radial and axillary nerves.

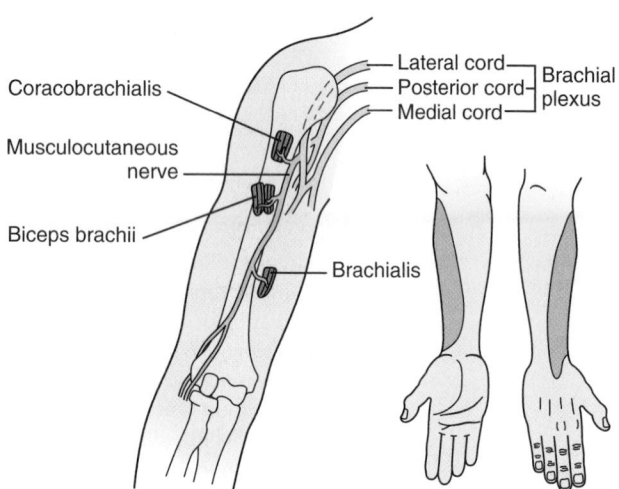

Figure 5-14 Motor and sensory distribution of musculocutaneous nerve.

altered sensation occurs in the radial nerve sensory distribution.

13. *Which hand is dominant?* Often the dominant shoulder is lower than the nondominant shoulder and the ROM may not be the same for both. Usually, the dominant shoulder shows greater muscularity and can show different ROM from the nondominant shoulder.[45]

OBSERVATION

The patient must be suitably undressed so that the examiner can observe the bony and soft-tissue contours of both shoulders and determine whether they are normal and symmetric. When observing the shoulder, the examiner looks at the head, the cervical spine, the thorax (especially the posterior aspect), and the entire upper limb. The hand, for example, may show vasomotor changes that result from problems in the shoulder, including shiny skin, hair loss, swelling, and muscle atrophy.

It is important to observe the patient as he or she removes clothes from the upper body and later replaces them. For example, does the patient undress the affected arm last or dress it first? This pattern indicates that the patient is limiting the movement of the arm as much as possible, signifying possible pathology. The patient's actions give some indication of functional restriction, pain, or weakness in the upper limb.

As part of the observation, noting whether the patient can assume a "neutral pelvis" position is important, because an abnormal pelvic position can lead to an abnormal scapulothoracic, glenohumeral, and cervical spine position and abnormal kinematics in these joints. In addition, kinematics plays a role in how much force can be generated by the lower quadrant that contributes to an activity. For example, about 50% of the force of throwing is normally generated by the lower quadrant. Three questions must be asked by the examiner related to the "neutral pelvic" position:

1. Can the patient get into the "neutral pelvis" position?
2. Can the patient hold the static "neutral pelvis" position while doing distal dynamic movement (e.g., shoulder movements)?
3. Can the patient control a dynamic "neutral pelvis" while doing dynamic shoulder movements?

If the answer to any of the questions is negative, the examiner has to consider including the pelvis in the treatment plan for the shoulder.

Anterior View

When looking at the patient from the anterior view (Figure 5-15, *A*), the examiner should begin by ensuring that the head and neck are in the midline of the body and observing their relation to the shoulders. A forward head posture is often associated with rounded shoulders, a medially rotated humerus and a protracted scapula resulting in the humeral head translating anteriorly, a tight posterior capsule, tightness of the pectoral, upper trapezius, and levator scapulae muscles, and weakness of the lower scapular stabilizers and deep neck flexors.[46] While observing the shoulder, the examiner should look for the possibility of a **step deformity** (Figure 5-16, *A*). Such a deformity may be caused by an acromioclavicular dislocation with the distal end of the clavicle lying superior to the acromion process. Seen at rest, a step deformity indicates both the acromioclavicular and coracoclavicular ligaments have been torn. The deformity may be accentuated by asking the patient to horizontally adduct the arm or to medially rotate the shoulder and bring the hand up the back as high as possible. Occasionally, swelling is

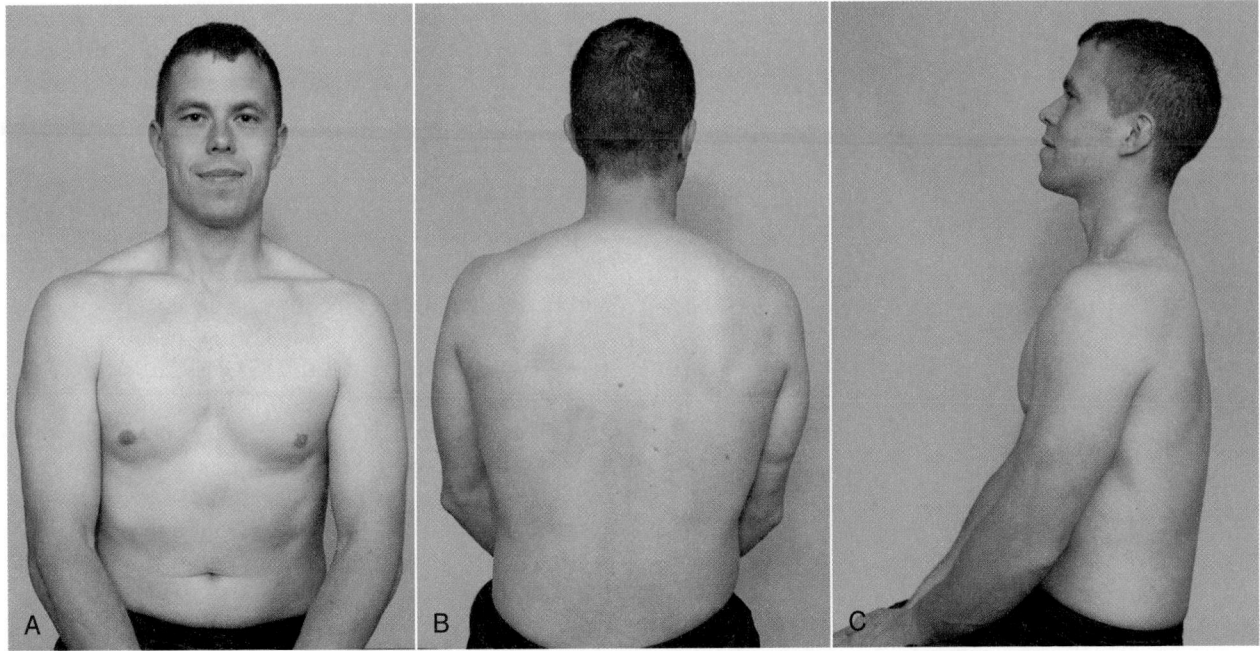

Figure 5-15 Views of the shoulder. A, Anterior. **B,** Posterior. **C,** Side.

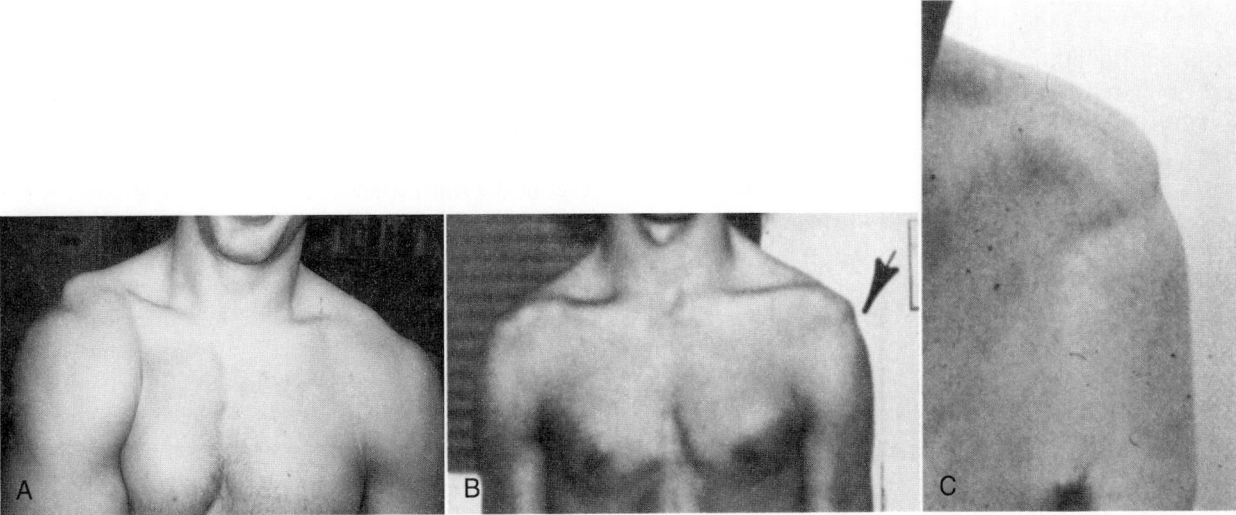

Figure 5-16 A, Step deformity resulting from acromioclavicular dislocation. **B,** Sulcus sign for shoulder instability. **C,** Subluxation of glenohumeral joint following a stroke (paralysis of deltoid muscle). (**B,** From Warren RF: Subluxation of the shoulder in athletes. Clin Sports Med 2:339, 1983.)

evident anterior to the acromioclavicular joint. This is called the **Fountain sign** and indicates that degeneration has caused communication between the acromioclavicular joint and swollen subacromial bursa underneath.[47] If a **sulcus deformity** appears when traction is applied to the arm, it may be caused by multidirectional instability or loss of muscle control due to nerve injury or a stroke, leading to inferior subluxation of the glenohumeral joint (Figure 5-16, *C*). This deformity is lateral to the acromion and should not be confused with a step deformity. This is also referred to as a *sulcus sign* because of the appearance of a sulcus or groove below the acromion

process (Figure 5-16, *B*). Flattening of the normally round deltoid muscle area may indicate an anterior dislocation of the glenohumeral joint or paralysis of the deltoid muscle (Figure 5-17). With an anterior dislocation, note also how the arm is held abducted because of the location of the humeral head below the glenoid. If the examiner palpated in the axilla, he or she would feel the head of the humerus. The examiner should note any abnormal bumps or malalignment in the bones that may indicate past injury, such as a healed fracture of the clavicle.

In most people, the dominant side is lower than the nondominant side. This difference may be caused by the

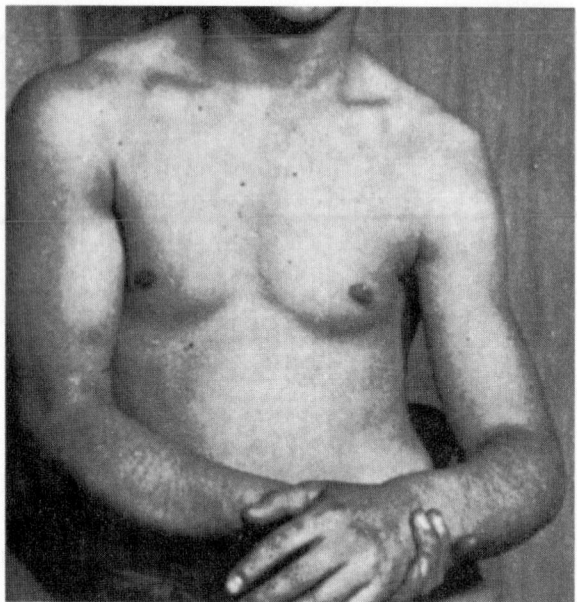

Figure 5-17 Subcoracoid dislocation of the shoulder. Note the prominent acromion, the arm held away from the side, and the flat deltoid. (From McLaughlin HL: Trauma, Philadelphia, 1959, WB Saunders, p. 246.)

tend to allow the tendon too much lateral movement, leading to inflammation of the paratenon (paratenonitis);[35] the deep grooves tend to be too narrow, compressing the tendon, especially if it becomes inflammed.[52]

Posterior View

When viewing the patient from behind (Figure 5-15, *B*), the examiner again notes bony and soft-tissue contours and body alignment especially scapular malpositioning.[53] The scapula plays a major role in the shoulder.[54] First, it provides an origin for the rotator cuff muscles as well as the biceps and triceps muscles and, therefore, provides a stable dynamic base from which these muscles act. Second, it maintains the glenohumeral alignment within physiological limits that facilitates congruency and concavity compression capability at the glenohumeral joint through the full ROM. Third, the attachment of the acromion to the clavicle leads to scapular upward rotation and posterior tilt to allow maximum arm elevation. Finally, the scapula facilitates force transfer from the shoulder to the core (and vice versa) acting like a funnel for efficient energy transfer. This transfer of forces can involve the whole kinetic chain, and by using this "chain" correctly, the patient can decrease the stresses to the shoulder itself.

Atrophy of the upper trapezius may indicate spinal accessory nerve palsy, whereas atrophy of supraspinatus or infraspinatus may indicate supraspinous nerve palsy.[55] The spines of the scapulae, which begin medially at the level of the third thoracic (T3) vertebra, should be at the same angle. The scapula itself should extend from the T2 or T3 spinous process to the T7 or T9 spinous process of the thoracic vertebrae. Sobush and associates developed a method for measuring the scapular position called the **Lennie test.**[56] In this test, they measured from the spinous processes horizontally to three scapular positions: the medial aspect of the most superior point (superior angle), the root of the spine of the scapula, and the inferior angle (Figure 5-22).[56] If the scapula is sitting lower than normal against the chest wall, the superior medial border of the scapula may "washboard" over the ribs, causing a snapping or clunking sound (snapping scapula) during abduction and adduction.[57-61] Other causes of snapping may be spinal kyphosis, rounded shoulders, forward tipped scapula, and a chin poking posture.[62] The inferior angles of the scapulae should be equidistant from the spine.

Scapular dyskinesia, or **scapular dysfunction,** although not an injury itself, can lead to altered glenohumeral joint angulation, abnormal stress on shoulder ligaments, altered subacromial space, overload of the acromioclavicular joint, increased strain on the scapular stabilizing muscles, altered muscle activation, and modified arm position and motion.[54] These alterations are commonly the result of an excessively protracted scapula during arm motion. Kibler, et al.[63] divided scapular

extra use of the dominant side, which stretches the ligaments, joint capsules, and muscles, allowing the arm to sag slightly. Tennis players[48] and others who stretch their upper limbs in a reaching action show even greater differences, along with gross hypertrophy of the muscles on the dominant side (Figure 5-18). If the patient is protective of the shoulder, however, it may appear that the injured shoulder, whether dominant or nondominant, is higher than the normal side (see Figure 5-10).

The examiner notes whether the patient is able to assume the normal functional position for the shoulder, which is in the scapular plane with 60° of abduction and the arm in neutral or no rotation. In this position, or with the arm abducted to 90°, rupture or congenital absence of the pectoralis major may be evident (Figures 5-19 and 5-20).[49-51] Rupture of the pectoralis major is often accompanied by a tearing sensation and pop along with weakness, painful limitation of movement, and ecchymosis.[49] If the patient's arm is medially rotated from this position to bring the hand into midline, the biceps tendon is forced against the lesser tuberosity of the medial wall of the bicipital (intertubercular) groove. If this position is maintained for long periods, there may be increased wear of the biceps tendon, which can lead to bicipital tendinitis or paratenonitis. If the arm is horizontally adducted while it is medially rotated, anterior pain indicates impingement symptoms (Hawkins-Kennedy test—see the "Special Tests" section). The width and depth of the bicipital groove may vary (Figure 5-21), possibly leading to problems if the shoulder is overused. Especially wide or deep grooves lead to the greatest problems. The wide grooves

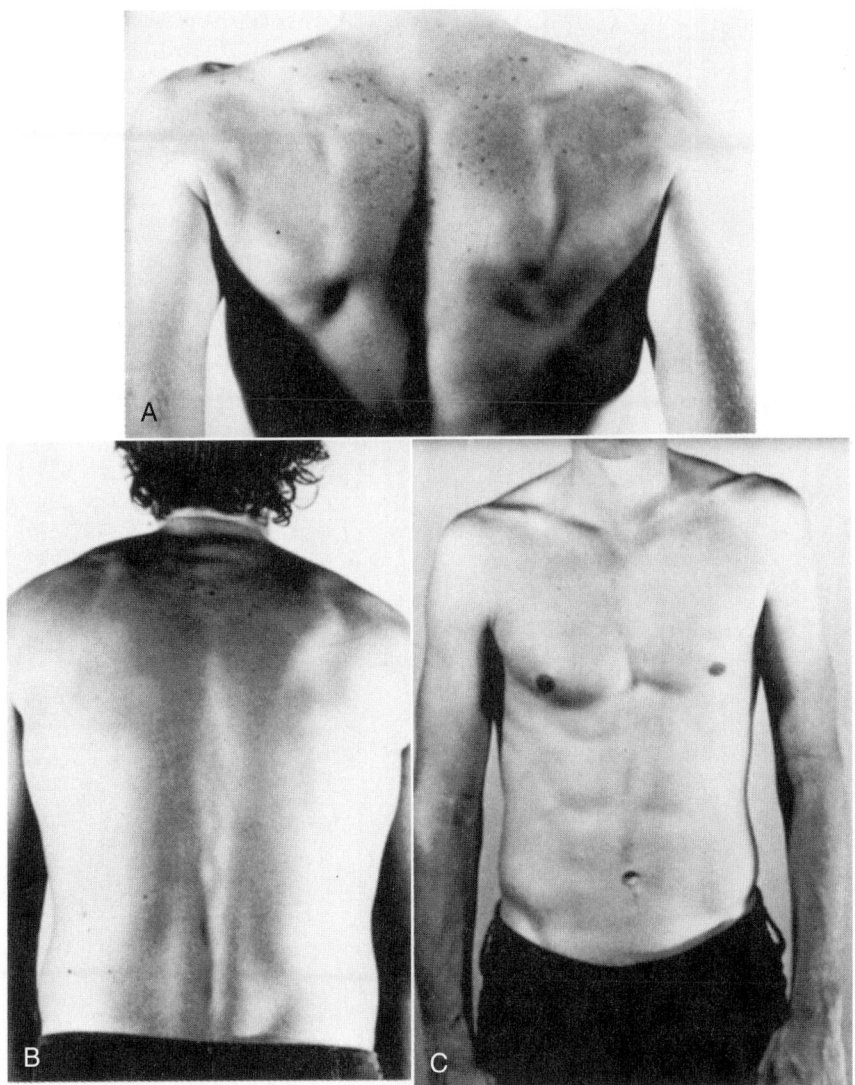

Figure 5-18 Depressed right shoulder in a right-dominant individual—in this case, a tennis player. **A,** Hypertrophy of playing shoulder muscles. **B,** With muscles relaxed, the distance between spinous processes and medial border of scapula is widened on the right. **C,** Depressed shoulder. (From Priest JD, Nagel DA: Tennis shoulder. Am J Sports Med 4:33, 1976.)

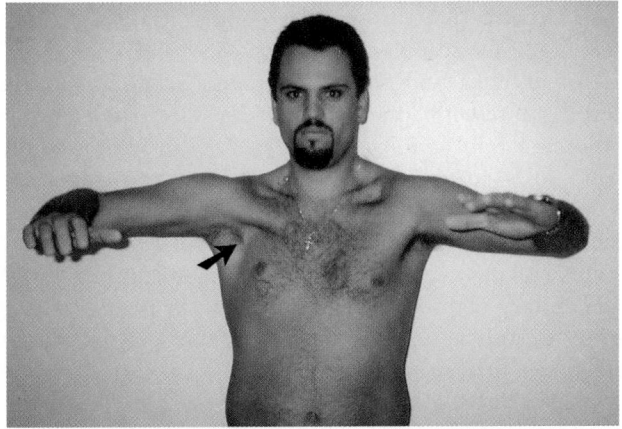

Figure 5-19 Congenital absence of sternal head of pectoralis major. Note fascial cord *(arrow).*

dysfunction or dyskinesia into four movement patterns. Type I shows the inferior medial border being prominent at rest and the inferior angle tilts dorsally with movement (scapular tilt), while the acromion tilts anteriorly over the top of the thorax. It may be seen at rest or during concentric or eccentric movement. If the inferior border tilts away from the chest wall, it may indicate the presence of weak muscles (e.g., lower trapezius, latissimus dorsi, serratus anterior) or a tight pectoralis minor or major pulling, or tilting, the scapula forward from above.[31] Type II is the classic winging of the scapula with the whole medial border of the scapula being prominent and lifting away from the posterior chest wall both statically and dynamically (Figure 5-23). It too may be seen at rest or during eccentric or concentric movements. This deformity may indicate the presence of a superior labrum anterior to posterior (SLAP) to the biceps lesion; weakness of the

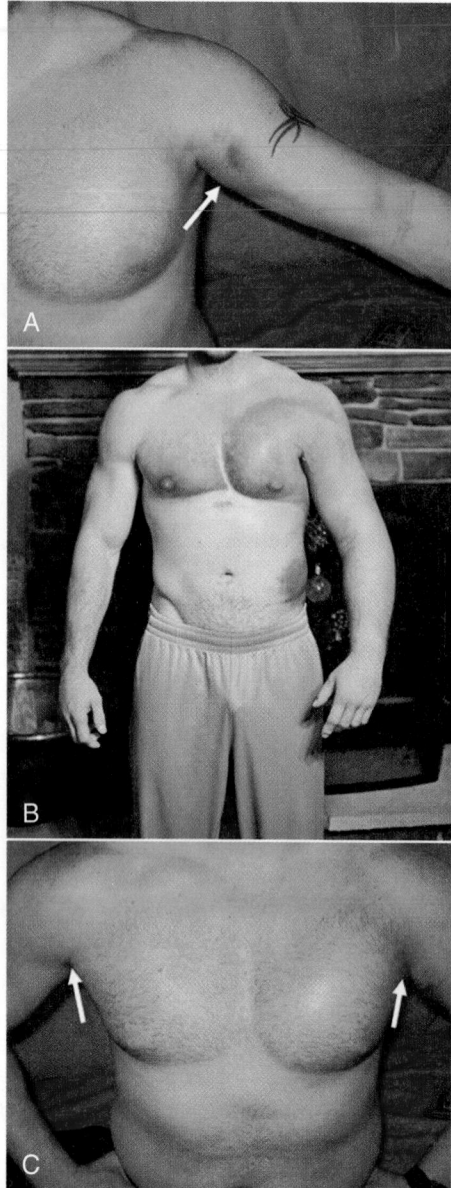

Figure 5-20 Pectoralis major rupture. A, Ecchymosis and swelling with *arrow* illustrating the sternal head rupture of pectoralis major. **B,** Massive swelling and bruising after pectoralis major rupture. **C,** Loss of axillary fold on the left side due to a pectoralis major tear creates an asymmetry compared with the normal right side. (From Provencher MT, et al: Injuries to the pectoralis major muscle—diagnosis and management. Am J Sports Med 38:1693–1705, 2010.)

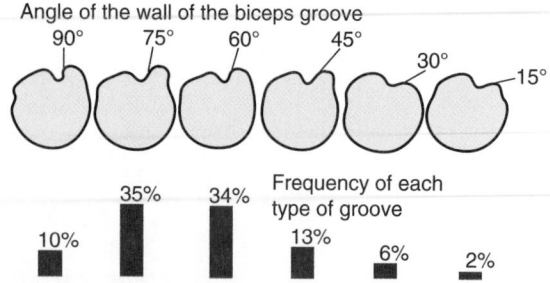

Figure 5-21 Different shapes of the bicipital groove. (Adapted from Hitchcock HH, Bechtol CO: Painful shoulder: observation on the role of the tendon of the long head of the biceps brachii in its causation. J Bone Joint Surg Am 30:267, 1948.)

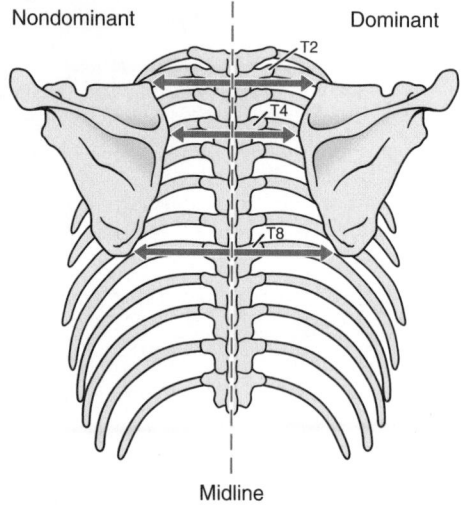

Figure 5-22 Lennie test. Measurements are taken at three positions on the scapula, and the dominant and nondominant sides are compared.

serratus anterior; rhomboids; lower, middle, and upper trapezius; a long thoracic nerve problem; or tight humeral rotators.[31] Type III is illustrated by the superior border of the scapula being elevated at rest and during movement; a shoulder shrug initiates the movement, and there is minimal winging. This deformity is seen with active movement and may result from overactivity of the levator scapula and upper trapezius along with imbalance of the upper and lower trapezius force couple (Figure 5-24). It is associated with impingement and rotator cuff lesions.[31] In the type IV pattern, both scapulae are symmetrical at rest and during motion; they rotate symmetrically upward with the inferior angles rotating laterally away from midline (rotary winging). It is seen during movement and may indicate that the scapular control muscles are not stabilizing the scapula.

Kibler, et al.[54] advocated a **dynamic scapular motion test** ☑ to test for scapular dyskinesia. The patient, while holding a 3 lb to 5 lb (1.4 kg to 2.3 kg) weight in the hand, is asked to fully elevate and lower the arms three to five times into forward flexion or scaption. The examiner watches for prominence of the medial border of the scapula (classic winging), which indicates a positive test.[64]

Primary scapular winging implies the winging is the result of muscle weakness of one of the scapular muscle stabilizers that, in turn, disrupts the normal muscle force couple balance of the scapulothoracic complex.[65] **Secondary scapular winging** implies that the normal movement of the scapula is altered because of pathology in the glenohumeral joint.[65] **Dynamic scapular winging** (i.e., winging with movement) may be caused by a lesion of

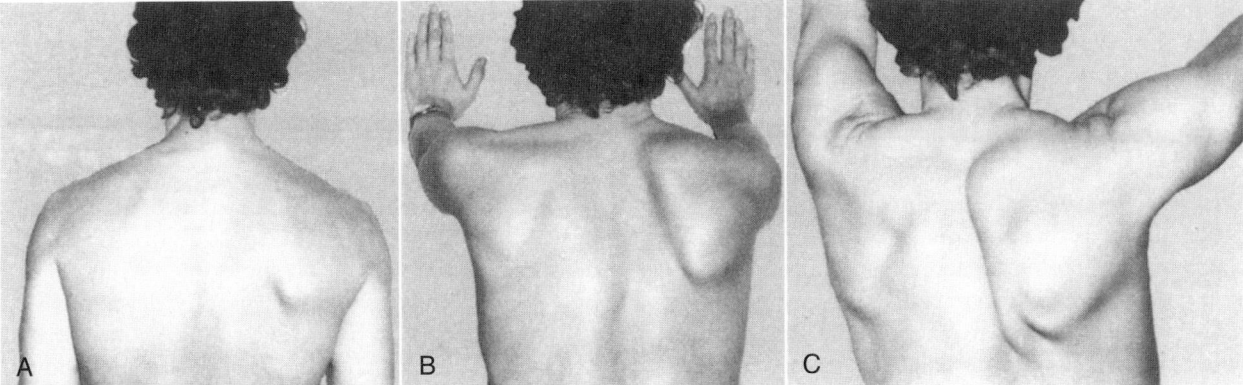

Figure 5-23 Winging of the scapula. A, The shoulders are at rest. **B,** Winging is apparent when the patient is pushing forward. **C,** Winging when attempting full abduction. (From Foo CL, Swann M: Isolated paralysis of the serratus anterior: a report of 20 cases. J Bone Joint Surg Br 65:554, 1983.)

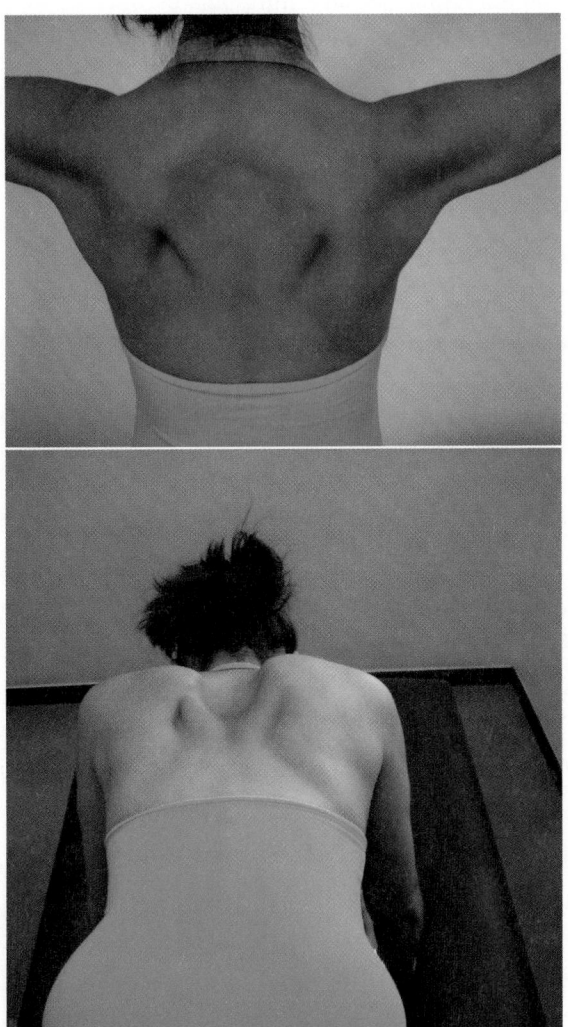

Figure 5-24 Imbalance pattern of the upper and lower trapezius. Note overdevelopment of upper trapezius and lower trapezius working to prevent rotary winging.

Causes of Scapular Dyskinesia[54]

BONY
- Thoracic kyphosis
- Clavicular fracture nonunion
- Clavicular fracture malunion

JOINT
- Acromioclavicular instability
- Acromioclavicular arthrosis
- Glenohumeral internal derangement

NEUROLOGICAL
- Cervical radiculopathy
- Long thoracic nerve palsy
- Spinal accessory nerve palsy

SOFT TISSUE
- Intrinsic muscle pathology (1°, 2°, or 3° strain)
- Hypomobility (e.g., short head of biceps, pectoralis minor)
- Glenohumeral internal rotation deficit (GIRD)
- Altered muscle activation patterns
- Altered muscle force-couple action

the long thoracic nerve affecting serratus anterior, trapezius palsy (spinal accessory nerve), rhomboid weakness, multidirectional instability, voluntary action, or a painful shoulder resulting in splinting of the glenohumeral joint, which in turn causes reverse scapulohumeral rhythm.[66] This splinting of the glenohumeral joint leads to reverse origin-insertion of the rotator cuff muscles so that instead of moving the humerus as they normally would, they work in reverse fashion and move the scapula. Commonly, with pathology, the scapular control muscles are weak and cannot counteract this action, resulting in protraction of the scapula and dynamic winging. The two other common causes of dynamic winging—long thoracic nerve palsy and spinal accessory nerve palsy—cause different scapula positioning and different winging patterns. Spinal accessory nerve palsy causes the scapula to depress and move laterally with the inferior angle rotated laterally. If the trapezius is weak or paralyzed, the winging of the scapula occurs before 90° abduction, and there is little winging on forward flexion.[67] Long thoracic nerve palsy causes the scapula to elevate and move medially with the inferior angle rotating medially (Figure 5-25).[68,69] If the serratus anterior is weak or paralyzed, the winging of the scapula occurs on abduction and forward flexion (especially with a "punch out" forward against resistance) (see Figure 5-23).[67,70] Radiculopathies at C3, C4 (trape-

zius), C5 (rhomboids), and C7 (serratus anterior, rhomboids) can also cause winging.[71,72]

Static winging (i.e., winging occurring at rest) is usually caused by a structural deformity of the scapula, clavicle, spine, or ribs.[73]

Sprengel's deformity, which is a developmental condition leading to a high or undescended scapula (Figure 5-26), is rare, but it is the most common congenital deformity of the shoulder complex.[74-77] With this deformity, the scapular muscles are poorly developed or are replaced by a fibrous band. The condition may be unilateral or bilateral, and the range of the shoulder abduction decreases, leading to decreased shoulder function. Usually, the scapula is smaller than normal and is medially rotated. It may be associated with other anomalies (e.g., scoliosis, Klippel-Feil syndrome, rib anomalies).[77]

The shoulder muscles may be accentuated by having the patient place the hands on the hips and contract the muscles. The examiner should check closely for wasting in the supraspinatus and infraspinatus muscles (suprascapular nerve palsy), the serratus anterior muscle (long thoracic nerve palsy), and the trapezius muscle (spinal accessory nerve palsy), all of which can lead to winging of the scapula.

EXAMINATION

Because assessment of the shoulder may include an assessment of the cervical spine, the examination can be an extensive one. If the examiner has any doubt as to the location of the lesion, a cervical spine assessment (see Chapter 3) should be performed. In addition, the examiner must remember that the arm, of which the

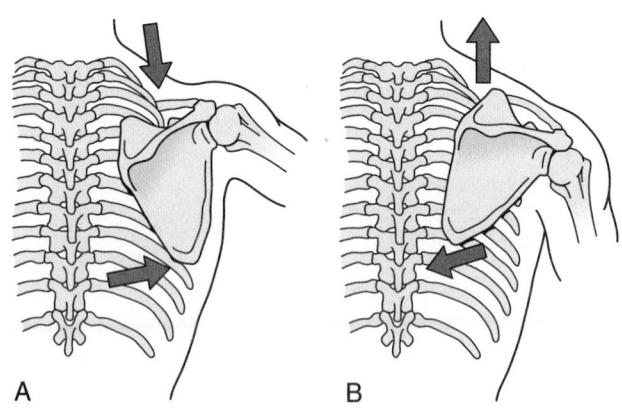

Figure 5-25 Scapular movement resulting in scapular winging caused by trapezius palsy **(A)** and serratus anterior palsy **(B).**

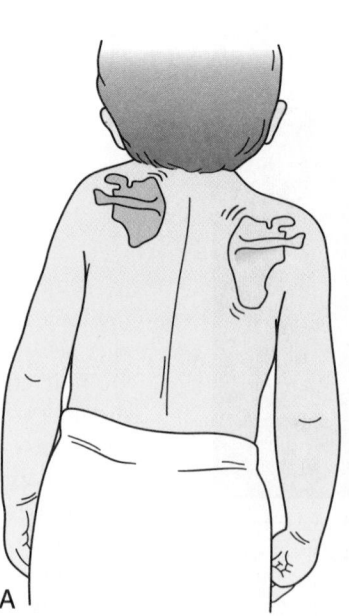
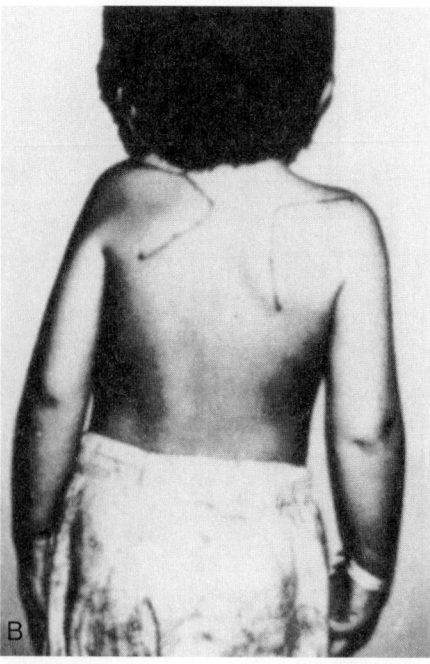

Figure 5-26 Sprengel's deformity. Diagram **(A)** and photograph **(B)** of child with Sprengel's deformity. Note elevated shoulder and poorly developed scapula on the left. (**A,** Modified from Gartland JJ: Fundamentals of orthopaedics, Philadelphia, 1979, WB Saunders, p. 73. **B,** Courtesy of Dr. Roshen Irani.)

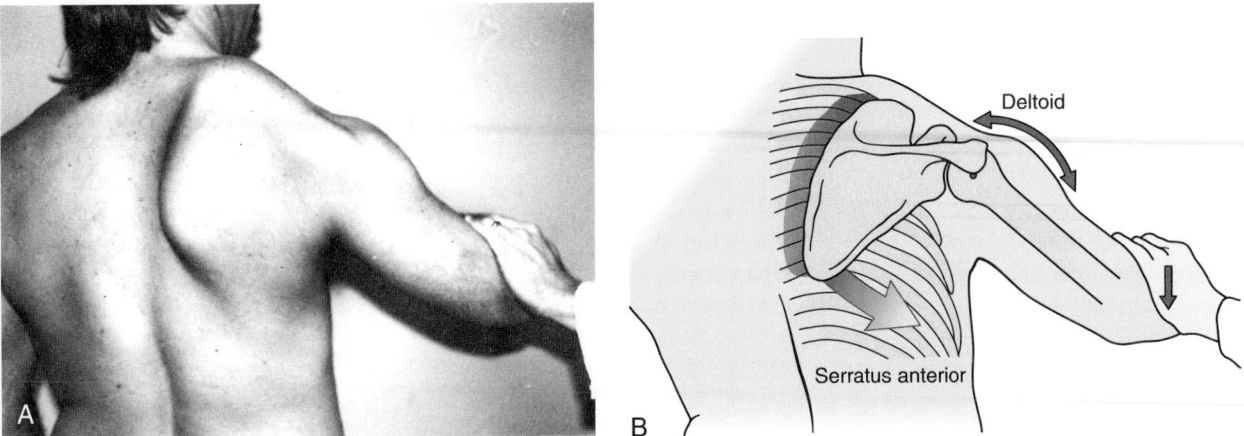

Figure 5-27 The pathomechanics of "classic winging" of the scapula. A, Winging of the right scapula caused by marked weakness of the right serratus anterior. The winging is exaggerated when resistance is applied against a shoulder abduction effort. Note how the stabilization occurs where the examiner's hand is offering resistance. Instead of the arm moving, the scapula moves because its stabilizing muscles are weak. **B,** Kinesiologic analysis of the winging scapula. Without an adequate upward rotation force from the serratus anterior *(fading arrow)*, the scapula becomes unstable and cannot resist the pull of the deltoid. Subsequently, the force of the deltoid *(bidirectional arrow)* causes the scapula to downwardly rotate and the glenohumeral joint to partially abduct (reverse origin-insertion). (From Neumann DA: Kinesiology of the musculoskeletal system: foundations for physical rehabilitation, St Louis, 2002, Mosby, p. 107.)

shoulder is an integral part, may act as an open kinetic chain when the hand is free to move, or as a closed kinetic chain when the hand is fixed to some relatively immovable object. For example, scapular instability may be evident in closed kinetic chain when the arm is fixed and the rotator cuff muscles work in reverse order (reverse origin-insertion; for example, the insertion of the muscles into the humerus becomes the stable part because the arm is fixed, whereas the scapula becomes the mobile part and is more likely to move) (Figure 5-27). It may also be evident in open kinetic chain, especially during high-speed movements when the scapula needs to be stabilized (e.g., when hitting a ball) or when the scapular muscles should be working eccentrically to slow or stop a movement (i.e., they are unable to do so because of weakness). In open kinetic chain, the scapula acts as the base or origin of the muscles, whereas the insertion into the humerus is more mobile. Knowledge of muscle balance and muscle force couples becomes imperative in determining a diagnosis. For example, the legs, pelvis, and trunk act as force generators, whereas the shoulder acts as a funnel and force regulator with the arm acting as the force delivery system.[31] These **kinetic chains** and the intricate and complex interplay of the components of the kinetic chain have different effects on the shoulder. Eating, reaching, and dressing are considered open kinetic chain activities, whereas crutch walking and pushing up from a chair are considered closed kinetic chain movements.

As with any assessment, the examiner is comparing one side of the body with the other. This comparison is necessary because of individual differences among normal people.

Active Movements

The first movements to be examined are the active movements. These movements are usually done in such a way that the painful movements are performed last so that pain does not carry over to the next movement. It is important to remember that shoulder movements are a combination of not only glenohumeral, scapulothoracic, acromioclavicular and sternoclavicular movements, but maximum end range movement may also involve the thoracic spine and ribs.[78] Thus, being able to differentiate between scapular movement and glenohumeral movements as well as these other movements when watching active movements is essential, because scapular movement often compensates for restricted glenohumeral movement leading to weak and often lengthened scapular control muscles.

Active Movements of the Shoulder Complex

- Elevation through abduction (170° to 180°)
- Elevation through forward flexion (160° to 180°)
- Elevation through the plane of the scapula (170° to 180°)
- Lateral (external) rotation (80° to 90°)
- Medial (internal) rotation (60° to 100°)
- Extension (50° to 60°)
- Adduction (50° to 75°)
- Horizontal adduction/abduction (cross-flexion/cross-extension; 130°)
- Circumduction (200°)
- Scapular protraction
- Scapular retraction
- Combined movements (if necessary)
- Repetitive movements (if necessary)
- Sustained positions (if necessary)

TABLE **5-6**

Force Couples About the Shoulder

Movement	Agonist/Stabilizer	Antagonist/Stabilizer
Protraction (scapula)	Serratus anterior* Pectoralis major[†] and minor[†]	Trapezius Rhomboids
Retraction (scapula)	Trapezius Rhomboids	Serratus anterior* Pectoralis major[†] and minor[†]
Elevation (scapula)	Upper trapezius[†] Levator scapulae[†]	Serratus anterior* Lower trapezius*
Depression (scapula)	Serratus anterior* Lower trapezius*	Upper trapezius[†] Levator scapulae[†]
Lateral rotation (upward rotation of inferior angle of scapula)	Trapezius (upper[†] and lower* fibers) Serratus anterior*	Levator scapulae[†] Rhomboids Pectoralis minor[†]
Medial rotation (downward rotation of inferior angle of scapula)	Levator scapulae[†] Rhomboids Pectoralis minor[†]	Trapezius (upper[†] and lower* fibers) Serratus anterior*
Scapular stabilization	Upper trapezius[†] Lower trapezius* Rhomboids	Serratus anterior*
Abduction (humerus)	Deltoid	Supraspinatus
Medial rotation (humerus)	Subscapularis[†] Pectoralis major[†] Latissimus doris Anterior deltoid	Infraspinatus* Teres minor Posterior deltoid
Lateral rotation (humerus)	Infraspinatus Teres minor Posterior deltoid	Subscapularis[†] Pectoralis major[†] Latissimus dorsi Anterior deltoid

*Muscles prone to weakness.
[†]Muscles prone to tightness.

An understanding of the **force couples** acting on the shoulder complex and the necessity of balancing the muscle strength and endurance of these muscles is especially important when assessing the shoulder.[79] Force couples are groups of counteracting muscles that show obvious action when a movement is loaded or done quickly.[80] With a particular movement, one group of muscles (the agonists) acts concentrically, whereas the other group (the antagonists) acts eccentrically in a controlled, harmonized fashion to produce smooth movement. In addition, these muscles may work by co-contraction or co-activation to provide a stabilizing effect and joint control. Table 5-6 gives examples of some of the force couples acting about the shoulder.

Active elevation through abduction is normally 170° to 180°. The extreme of the ROM occurs when the arm is abducted and lies against the ear on the same side of the head (Figure 5-28). As the patient elevates the upper extremity by abducting the shoulder, the examiner should note whether a **painful arc** ⚠ is present (Figure 5-29).[81] A painful arc may be caused by subacromial bursitis, calcium deposits, a peritenonitis or tendinosis[35,36] of the rotator cuff muscles, or most commonly by an unstable scapula. The pain results from pinching of inflamed or tender structures under the acromion process and the coracoacromial ligament. Initially, the structures are not pinched under the acromion process, so the patient is able to abduct the arm 45° to 60° with little difficulty. As the patient abducts further (60° to 120°), the structures (e.g., subacromial bursa, rotator cuff tendon insertions, especially supraspinatus) become pinched, and the patient is often unable to abduct fully because of pain. If full abduction is possible, however, the pain diminishes after approximately 120° because the pinched soft tissues have passed under the acromion process and are no longer being pinched. Often, the pain is greater going up (against gravity) than coming down, and there is more pain on active abduction than on passive abduction. If the movement is very painful, the patient often elevates the arm through forward flexion or hikes the shoulder using upper trapezius and levator scapulae in an attempt to decrease the pain. In some cases, retracting the scapula and holding it retracted slightly enlarges the space under the coracoacromial space, which may decrease pain. A second painful arc in the shoulder may be seen during the same abduction movement. This painful arc (see Figure 5-29) occurs

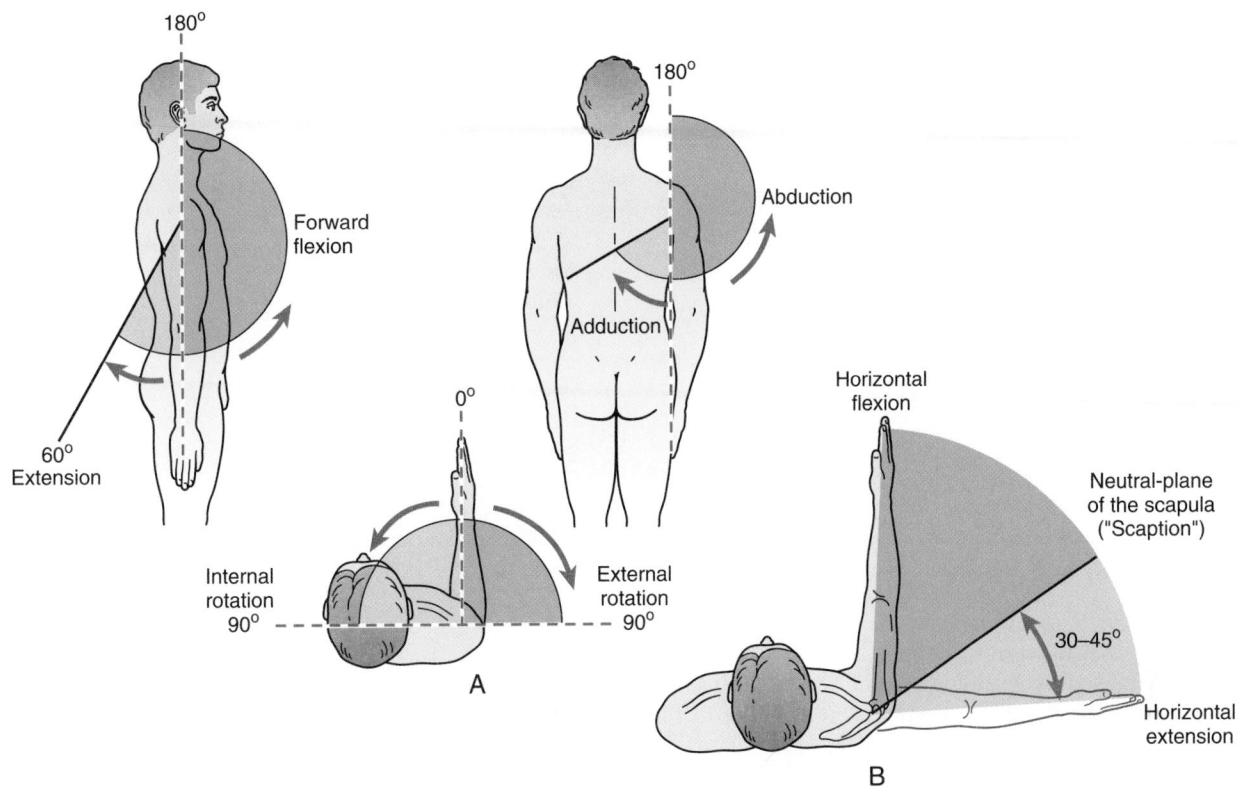

Figure 5-28 **Movement in the shoulder complex. A,** Range of motion (ROM) of the shoulder. **B,** Axes of arm elevation. (Adapted from Perry J: Anatomy and biomechanics of the shoulder in throwing, swimming, gymnastics, and tennis. Clin Sports Med 2:255, 1983.)

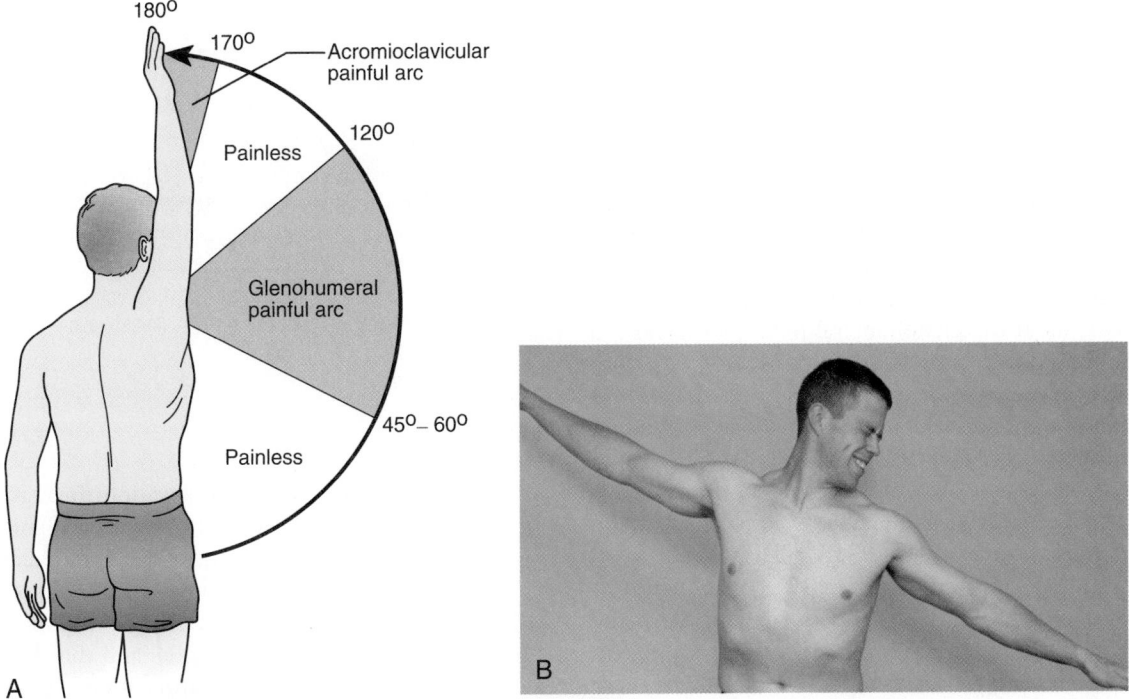

Figure 5-29 **Painful arc in the shoulder. A,** Painful arc of the glenohumeral joint. In the case of acromioclavicular joint problems only, the range of 170° to 180° would elicit pain. **B,** Note the impingement causing pain on the right at approximately 85°. (**A,** Modified from Hawkins RJ, Hobeika PE: Impingement syndrome in the athletic shoulder. Clin Sports Med 2:391, 1983.)

TABLE **5-7**

Classification of Glenohumeral Painful Arcs

	Anterior	Posterior	Superior
Night pain	Yes	Yes	Maybe
Age	50+	50+	40+
Sex ratio	F > M	F > M	M > F
Aggravated by	Lateral rotation and abduction	Medial rotation and abduction	Abduction
Tenderness	Lesser tuberosity	Posterior aspect of greater tuberosity	Greater tuberosity
Acromioclavicular joint involvement	No	No	Often
Calcification (if present)	Supraspinatus, infraspinatus, and/or subscapularis	Supraspinatus and/or infraspinatus	Supraspinatus and/or subscapularis
Third-degree strain biceps brachii (long head)	No	No	Occasional
Prognosis	Good	Very good	Poor (without surgery)

From Kessel L, Watson M: The painful arc syndrome. J Bone Joint Surg Br 59:166, 1977.

toward the end of abduction, in the last 10° to 20° of elevation, and is caused by pathology in the acromioclavicular joint or by a positive impingement test. In the case of the acromioclavicular joint lesion, the pain tends to be localized to the joint. With the impingement syndrome, the pain is usually found in the anterior shoulder region. Table 5-7 presents the signs and symptoms of three types of painful arc in the shoulder with the superior type being the most common. The arc of pain may be present also during elevation through forward flexion and scaption, although the pain is usually less severe on these movements. The interconnection of the subacromial, subcoracoid, and subscapularis bursae with each other and with the glenohumeral joint capsule often produces a broad area of signs and symptoms, which may result in a painful arc.

When examining the movement of elevation through abduction, the examiner must take time to observe **scapulohumeral rhythm** of the shoulder complex (Figure 5-30), both anteriorly and posteriorly.[82–84] That is, during 180° of abduction, there is roughly a 2:1 ratio of movement of the humerus to the scapula with 120° of movement occurring at the glenohumeral joint and 60° at the scapulothoracic joint; one should be aware, however, that there is a great deal of variability among individuals and may depend on the speed of movement,[85] and authors do not totally agree on the exact amounts of each movement.[83,84,86] Although all authors concede that there is more movement in the glenohumeral joint than in the scapulothoracic joint, Davies and Dickoff-Hoffman believe the ratio is greater, at least to 120° of abduction,[87] whereas Poppen and Walker[88] and others[7,89] believe the ratio is less (5:4 or 3:2) after 30° of abduction. During this total simultaneous movement at the four joints, there are three phases; the reader should understand that others will give values of the amount of each movement that vary from those noted here.

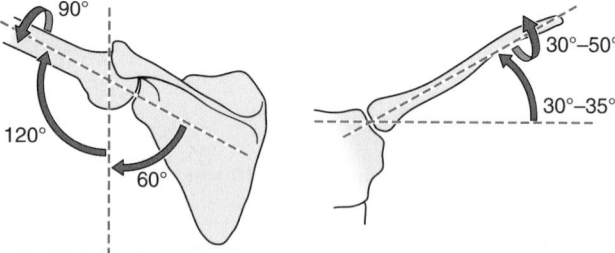

Figure 5-30 Movement of the scapula, humerus, and clavicle during scapulohumeral rhythm.

Scapulohumeral Rhythm

Phase 1:	Humerus	30° abduction
	Scapula	Minimal movement (setting phase)
	Clavicle	0° to 5° elevation
Phase 2:	Humerus	40° abduction
	Scapula	20° rotation, minimal protraction or elevation
	Clavicle	15° elevation
Phase 3:	Humerus	60° abduction, 90° lateral rotation
	Scapula	30° rotation
	Clavicle	30° to 50° posterior rotation, up to 15° elevation

1. In the first phase of 30° of elevation through abduction, the scapula is said to be "setting." This setting phase means that the scapula may rotate slightly in, rotate slightly out, or not move at all.[70] Thus, there is no 2:1 ratio of movement during this phase. The angle between the scapular spine and the clavicle may also increase up to 5° by elevating at the sternoclavicular and acromioclavicular joints,[82] but this depends on whether the scapula moves during this phase. The clavicle rotates minimally during this stage.

TABLE **5-8**

Summary of Scapular Kinematics During Arm Elevation in Healthy and Pathologic States

Group	Healthy (Normal)	Impingement or Rotator Cuff Disease	Glenohumeral Joint Instability	Adhesive Capsulitis
Primary scapular motion	Upward rotation	Lesser upward rotation	Lesser upward rotation	Greater upward rotation
Secondary scapular motion	Posterior tilting	Lesser posterior tilting	No consistent evidence for alteration	No consistent evidence for alteration
Accessory scapular motion	Variable medial/lateral rotation	Greater medial rotation	Greater medial rotation	No consistent evidence for alteration
Presumed implications	Maximize shoulder ROM and available sub-acromial space	Presumed contributory to subacromial or internal impingement	Presumed contributory to lesser inferior and anterior joint stability	Presumed compensatory to minimize functional shoulder ROM loss

Modified from Ludewig PM, Reynolds JF: The association of scapular kinematics and glenohumeral joint pathologies. J Orthop Sports Phys Ther 39:95, 2009.
ROM, Range of motion.

2. During the next 60° of elevation (second phase), the scapula rotates upward (inferior angle moves out) about 20°, and the humerus elevates 40° with minimal protraction or elevation of the scapula.[82] Thus, there is a 2:1 ratio of scapulohumeral movement. During phase 2, the clavicle elevates because of the scapular rotation[7,82] and begins to posteriorly rotate. During the second and third phase, the rotation of the scapula (total: 60°) is possible because there is 20° of motion at the acromioclavicular joint and 40° at the sternoclavicular joint.

3. During the final 90° of motion (third phase), the 2:1 ratio of scapulohumeral movement continues, and the angle between the scapular spine and the clavicle increases an additional 10°. Thus, the scapula continues to rotate and now begins to elevate. The amount of protraction continues to be minimal when the abduction movement is performed. It is in this stage that the clavicle rotates posteriorly 30° to 50° on a long axis and elevates up to a further 15°.[7] In reality, the clavicle only rotates 5° to 8° relative to the acromion because of scapular rotation.[90,91] Also, during this final stage, the humerus finishes its lateral rotation to 90° so that the greater tuberosity of the humerus avoids the acromion process. Tables 5-8 and 5-9 outline the shoulder kinematics in healthy and pathological states.[92]

In the unstable shoulder, scapulohumeral rhythm is commonly altered because of incorrect dynamic functioning of the scapular or humeral stabilizers or both.[93] This may be related to incorrect arthrokinematics at the glenohumeral joint, and so the examiner must be sure to check for normal joint play and the presence of hypomobile structures that could lead to these abnormal motions.[93]

Kibler pointed out that it is important to watch the movement, especially of the scapula, in both the ascending and descending phases of abduction.[94] Commonly,

TABLE **5-9**

Mechanisms of Scapular Dyskinesia

Mechanism	Associated Effects
Inadequate serratus anterior activation	Lesser scapular upward rotation and posterior tilt
Excess upper trapezius activation	Greater clavicular elevation
Pectoralis minor tightness	Greater scapular medial rotation and anterior tilt
Posterior glenohumeral joint soft tissue tightness	Greater scapular anterior tilt
Thoracic kyphosis or flexed posture	Greater scapular medial rotation and anterior tilt, lesser scapular upward rotation

Modified from Ludewig PM, Reynolds JF: The association of scapular kinematics and glenohumeral joint pathologies. J Orthop Sports Phys Ther 39:97, 2009.

weakness of the scapular control muscles is more evident during descent, and an instability jog, hitch, or jump may occur when the patient loses control of the scapula.

The speed of abduction may also have an effect on the ratio.[95] Therefore, it is more important to look for asymmetry between the injured and the good sides than to be concerned with the actual degrees of movement occurring at each joint. That being said, if the clavicle does not rotate and elevate, elevation through abduction at the glenohumeral joint is limited to 120°.[82] If the glenohumeral joint does not move, elevation through abduction is limited to 60°, which occurs totally in the scapulothoracic joint. If there is no lateral rotation of the humerus during abduction, the total movement available is 120°, 60° of which occurs at the glenohumeral joint and 60° of which occurs at the scapulothoracic articulation.[7] The

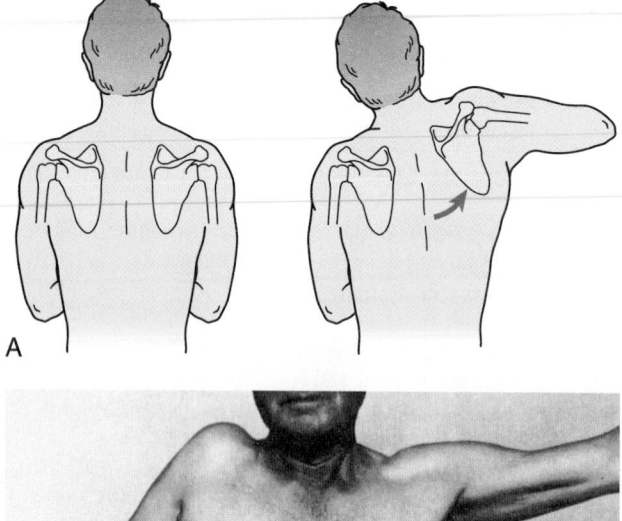

A

B

Figure 5-31 Reverse scapulohumeral rhythm (notice shoulder hiking) and excessive scapular movement. Examples include frozen shoulder (**A**) or tear of rotator cuff (**B**). (**B,** From Beetham WP, Polley HF, Slocum CH, et al: Physical examination of the joints. Philadelphia, 1965, WB Saunders, p. 41.)

normal end of ROM is reached when there is contact of a surgical neck of humerus with the acromion process. **Reverse scapulohumeral rhythm** (Figure 5-31) means that the scapula moves more than the humerus. This occurs in conditions like the frozen shoulder. The patient appears to "hike" the entire shoulder complex rather than produce a smooth coordinated abduction movement.

Active elevation through forward flexion is normally 160° to 180°, and at the extreme of the ROM, the arm is in the same position as for active elevation through abduction. Active elevation (170° to 180°) through the plane of the scapula (30° to 45° of forward flexion), termed **scaption,** is the most natural and functional motion of elevation (see Figure 5-28). Elevation in this position is sometimes called *neutral elevation*. The exact angle is determined by the contour of the chest wall on which the scapula rests. Often, movement into elevation is less painful in this position than elevation through abduction in which the glenohumeral joint is actually in extension, or elevation in forward flexion. Movement in the plane of the scapula puts less stress on the capsule and surrounding musculature and is the position in which most of the functions of daily activity are commonly performed. Strength testing in this plane also gives higher values. Patients with weakness spontaneously choose this plane when elevating the arm.[96,97] During scaption elevation, scapulohumeral rhythm is similar to

that of abduction although there is greater individual variability. The three phases are similar, but there are differences. For example, in scaption elevation, there is little or no lateral rotation of the head of the humerus in the third phase.[89] Also, the total elevation in scaption is about 170° with scapular rotation being about 65° and humeral abduction about 105°; although there is slightly more scapular rotation in scaption, this difference again may result from individual variation.[89] More scapular protraction is likely to occur in scaption elevation, especially in elevation through forward flexion.

Active lateral rotation is normally 80° to 90° but may be greater in some athletes, such as gymnasts and baseball pitchers. Care must be taken when applying overpressure with this movement, because it could lead to anterior dislocation of the glenohumeral joint, especially in those with recurrent dislocation problems. If glenohumeral lateral rotation is limited, the patient will compensate by retracting the scapula. To minimize scapular movement, lateral rotation may be measured in supine or side lying with the arm abducted 90° (Figure 5-32). Wilk, et al.[98] have recommended that rotation be tested in supine lying with the arm abducted to 90° and the scapula stabilized to increase reliability.

Active medial rotation is normally 60° to 100°. This is usually assessed by measuring the height of the "hitch-hiking" thumb (thumb in extension) reaching up the patient's back (Figure 5-33, *A* and *B*). Common reference points include the greater trochanter, buttock, waist, and spinous processes with T5 to T10 representing the normal degree of medial rotation.[99] When doing the test in this fashion, the examiner must be aware that, in reality, the range measured is not that of the glenohumeral joint alone. In fact, much of the range is gained by winging the scapula. In the presence of tight medial glenohumeral motion, greater winging and protraction of the scapula occurs.

Doing the rotation testing in 90° abduction (if the patient can achieve this position) will give a clearer indication of true glenohumeral joint medial and lateral rotation, which are measured when the scapula starts to move (Figure 5-33, *C*). If rotation is tested in 90° abduction and crepitus is present on rotation, it indicates abrasion of torn tendon margins against the coracoacromial arch and is called the **"abrasion sign."**[57]

It is important to compare medial and lateral rotation, especially in active people who use their dominant arm at extremes of motion and under high load situations. Normally, any gain in lateral rotation is commonly accompanied by a comparable loss in medial rotation. Thus, it is important to note any **glenohumeral internal (medial) rotation deficit (GIRD)** (Figure 5-34),[25] which is the difference in medial rotation between the patient's two shoulders. Small changes in GIRD can lead to biomechanical changes in passive glenohumeral motion.[100] For example, the loss of medial rotation may be due to

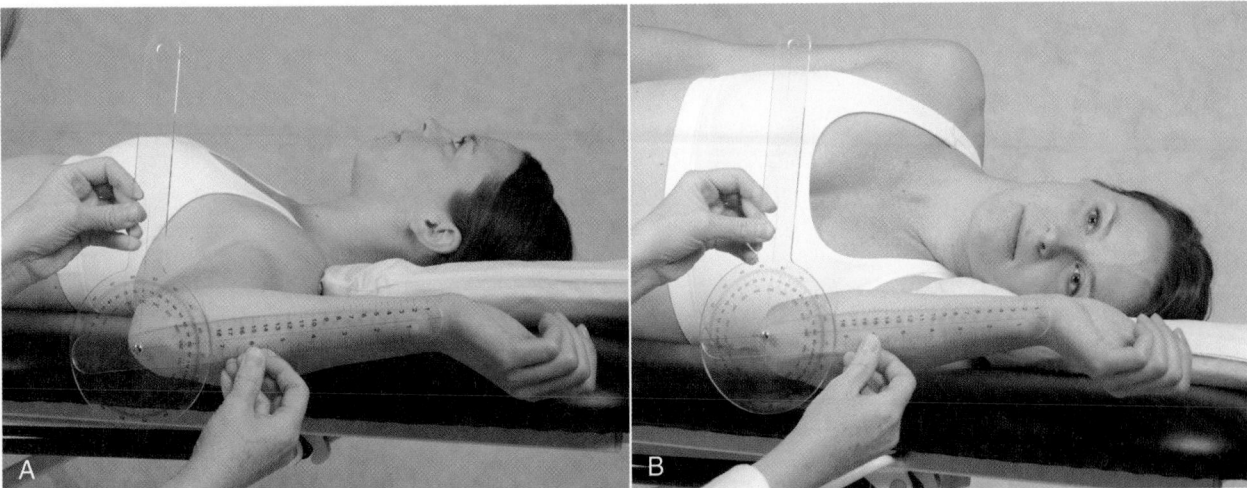

Figure 5-32 Measuring lateral rotation. A, Supine. The patient's arm is rotated until the scapula is felt to move and until an endpoint is reached. A handheld goniometer is used to measure medial and lateral rotation. **B,** Side lying. The examiner rotates the arm until the scapula is seen to move and resistance is felt. The amount of lateral and medial rotation can be examined in this manner with a handheld goniometer.

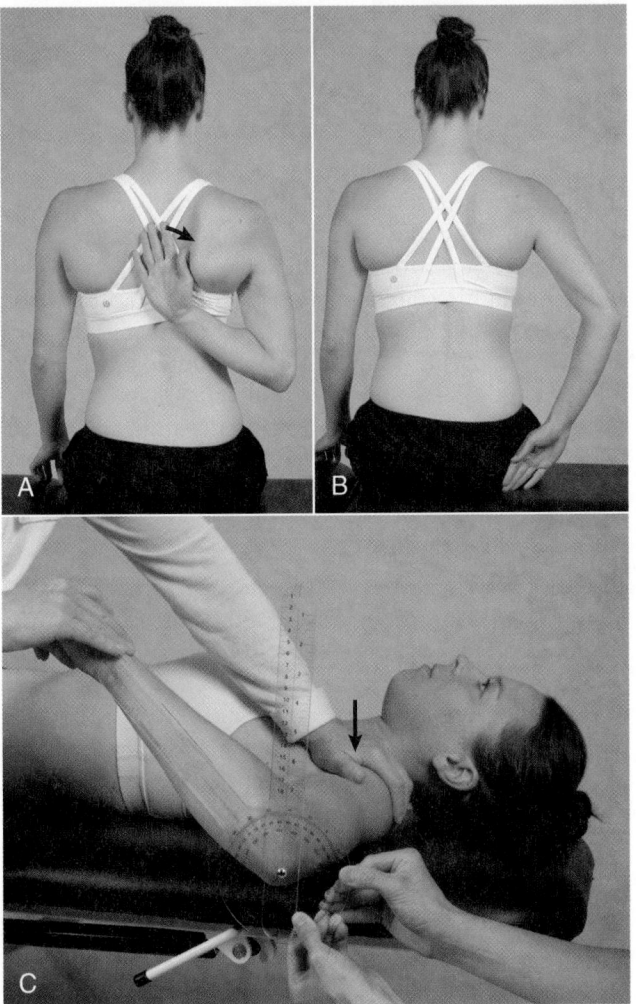

Figure 5-33 Measuring medial rotation. A, Reaching up the patient's back. Note winging of scapula (*arrow*). **B,** Position of hand when scapula begins to wing indicates end of true medial rotation at the glenohumeral joint. **C,** Supine. Glenohumeral medial rotation passive range of motion measurement using stabilization of the scapula by holding the coracoid process and the scapula down.

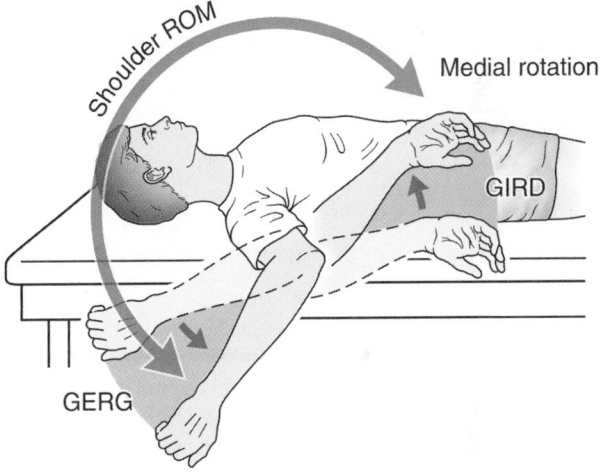

Figure 5-34 Range of shoulder motion showing glenohumeral internal (medial) rotation deficit (GIRD) and glenohumeral external (lateral) rotation gain (GERG).

contracture of the posteroinferior capsule, which in turn can lead to a SLAP lesion.[37] Normally, the difference should be within 20° or 10% of total rotation of the opposite arm.[25,101,102] This may also be compared with the **glenohumeral external (lateral) rotation gain (GERG)** (see Figure 5-34). If the GIRD/GERG ratio is greater than 1, the patient will probably develop shoulder problems.[31,103]

In the unstable shoulder, it has been advocated that the examiner do the **dynamic rotary stability test (DRST),** ⚠ which assesses the rotator cuff's ability to maintain the humeral head in the glenoid through the arc of rotation (i.e., the ability of the rotator cuff to maintain arthrokinematic control).[104–106] The patient is positioned in sitting or lying with the arm abducted to about 90° and the elbow flexed to about 90°. The examiner controls

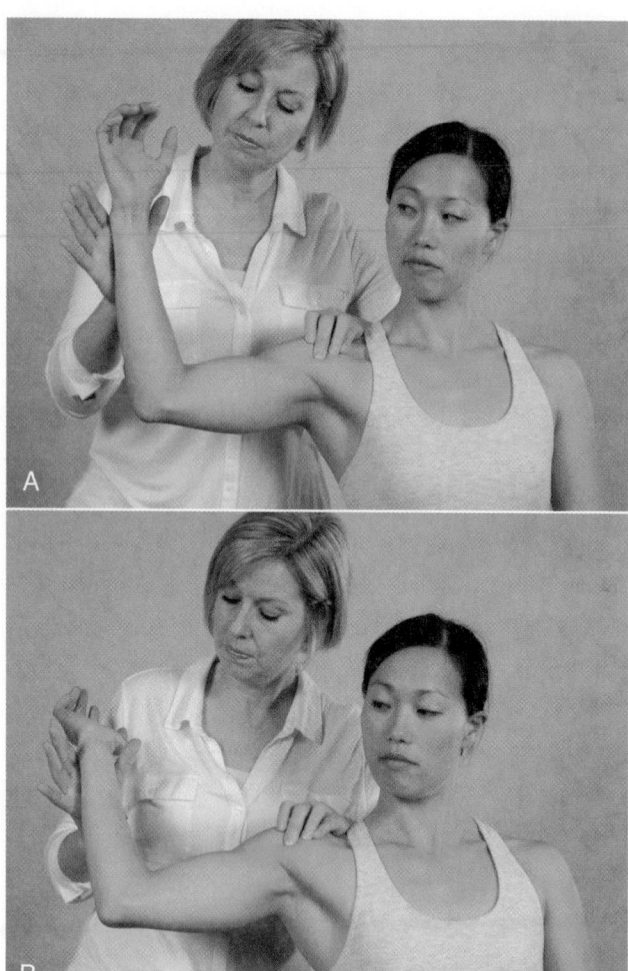

Figure 5-35 **Dynamic rotary instability test** demonstrating two different positions in which humeral head control can be evaluated. The examiner's left hand is placed over the humeral head in order to detect any translation that occurs during contraction of the rotators. Isometric lateral rotation is resisted in mid-range (**A**) and end-range (**B**) in a position functionally relevant for a thrower.

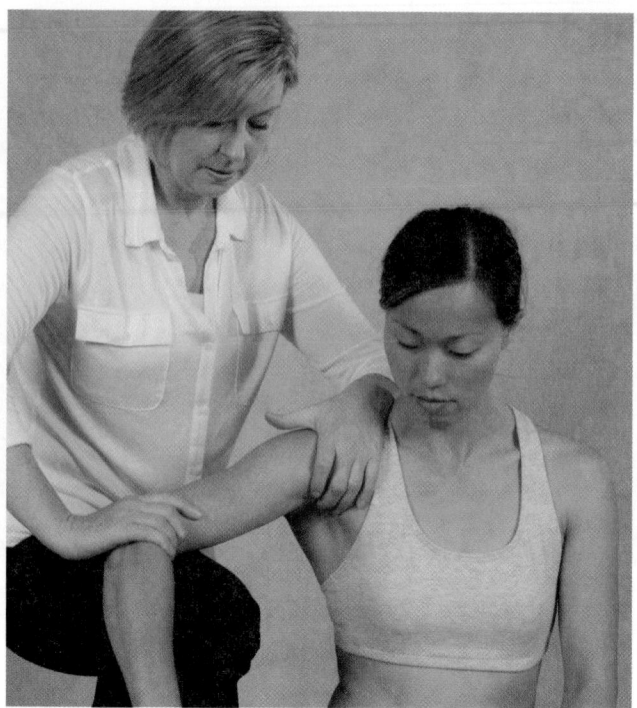

Figure 5-36 **Dynamic relocation test.**

the patient's arm position with one hand while the other hand palpates the position of the humerus in the glenoid (it is best to palpate the joint line). (Figure 5-35). The examiner places the patient's glenohumeral joint in different positions of flexion and abduction close to the position where the patient has symptoms. The patient is asked to do an isometric contraction against light to moderate resistance then isotonically (concentrically or eccentrically [eccentric break] depending on what movements caused the patient's symptoms). While the patient does the contraction, the examiner palpates the joint line to see if and when arthrokinematic control is lost (i.e., does the humeral head slip or translate?).[105] During the test, the scapula should be stable and not translate. If the scapula protracts during the test, it indicates lack of scapular control.

Magarey and Jones[105] also advocated doing the **Dynamic Relocation Test (DRT),** ⚠ which tests the

ability of the rotator cuff to stabilize the humeral head through co-contraction of the rotator cuff muscles. The patient is seated with the arm supported in 60° to 80° abduction in the scapular plane (scaption) (Figure 5-36). With the middle finger of one hand palpating the subscapularis and the thumb along the outer edge of the acromion, the examiner uses the other hand to apply traction (longitudinal distraction) to the arm while asking the patient to pull the arm up into the socket. As the patient pulls the arm in and up, the examiner should feel for contraction of the rotator cuff, especially the subscapularis. If the pectoral muscles are overactive, the examiner may palpate the rotator cuff posteriorly.[104] During the test, the scapula should not move. If the scapula protracts, it indicates an unstable scapula.

Active extension is normally 50° to 60°. The examiner must ensure that the movement is in the shoulder and not in the spine because some patients may flex the spine or bend forward, giving the appearance of increased shoulder extension. Similarly, retraction of the scapula increases the appearance of glenohumeral extension. Weakness of full extension commonly implies weakness of the posterior deltoid in one arm and is sometimes called the **swallow tail sign,** because both arms do not extend the same amount either due to injury to the muscle itself or to the axillary nerve.[107]

Adduction is normally 50° to 75° if the arm is brought in front of the body. Horizontal adduction, or cross-flexion, is normally 130°. To accomplish this movement, the patient first abducts the arm to 90° and then moves the arm across the front of the body. Horizontal

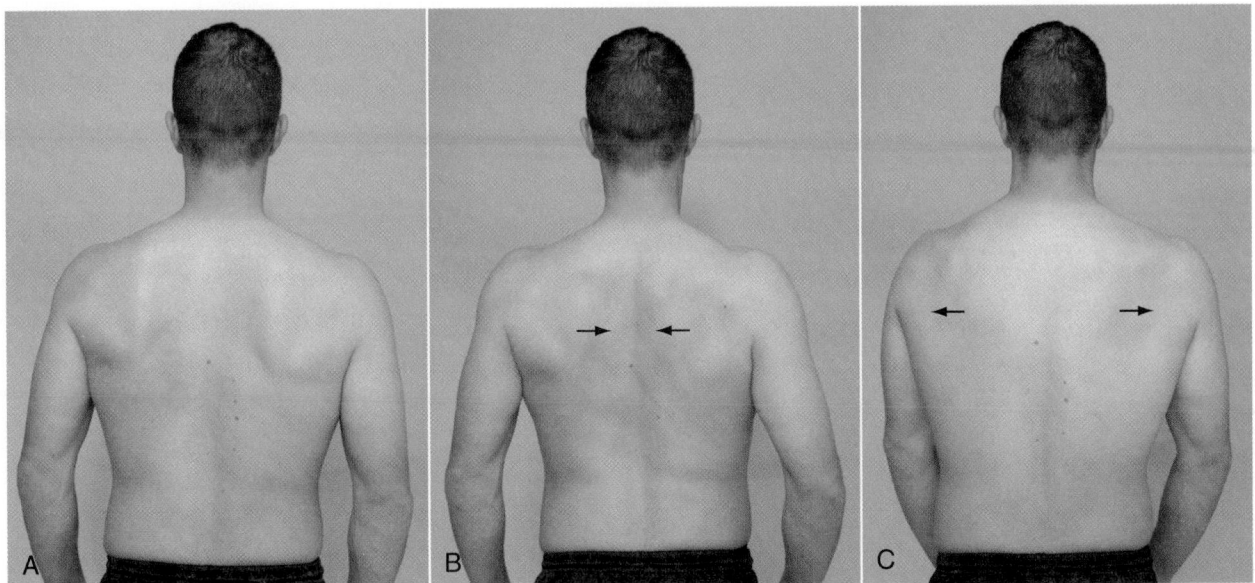

Figure 5-37 **A,** Resting position. **B,** Scapular retraction. **C,** Scapular protraction.

abduction, or cross-extension, is approximately 45°. After abducting the arm to 90°, the patient moves the straight arm in a backward direction. In both cases, the examiner should watch the relative amount of scapular movement between the normal and pathological sides. If movement is limited in the glenohumeral joint, greater scapular movement occurs. Circumduction is normally approximately 200° and involves taking the arm in a circle in the vertical plane.

In addition to the aforementioned movements, several of which involve movement of the humerus and scapula, the patient should actively perform two distinct movements of the scapulae: scapular retraction and scapular protraction (Figure 5-37). For scapular retraction, the examiner asks the patient to squeeze the shoulder blades (scapula) together. Normally, the medial borders of the scapula remain parallel to the spine but move toward the spine with the soft tissue bunching up between the scapula (see Figure 5-37, B). Ideally, the patient should be able to do this movement without excessive contraction of the upper trapezius muscles. For scapular protraction, the patient tries to bring the shoulders together anteriorly so that the scapula move away from midline with the inferior angle of the scapula commonly moving laterally more than the superior angle so that some lateral rotation of the inferior angle occurs (see Figure 5-37, C). This protraction/retraction cycle may cause a clicking or snapping near the inferior angle or supramedial corner, which is sometimes called a **snapping scapula,** caused by the scapula rubbing over the underlying ribs.[60]

Injury to the individual muscles can affect several movements. For example, if the serratus anterior muscle is weak or paralyzed, the scapula "wings" away from the thorax on its medial border. It also assists upper rotation of the scapula during abduction. Injury to the muscle or its nerve may therefore limit abduction. In fact, loss or weakness of serratus anterior affects all shoulder movements because scapular stabilization is lost.[80] Similarly, weakness of the lower trapezius muscle can alter scapular mechanics resulting in anterior secondary impingement. Many of the tests for these muscles are described in the "Special Tests" section.

When observing these movements, the examiner may ask the patient to perform them in combination, especially if the patient history has indicated that combined movements are bothersome. For example, **Apley's scratch test** combines medial rotation with adduction and lateral rotation with abduction (Figure 5-38). This method may decrease the time required to do the assessment. In addition, by having the patient do the combined movements, the examiner gains some idea of the functional capacity of the patient. For example, abduction combined with flexion and lateral rotation or adduction combined with extension and medial rotation is needed to comb the hair, to zip a back zipper, or to reach for a wallet in a back pocket. However, the examiner must take care to notice which movements are restricted and which ones are not, because several movements are performed at the same time. Some examiners prefer doing the same motion in both arms at the same time: neck reach (abduction, flexion, and lateral rotation at the glenohumeral joint) and back reach (adduction, extension, and medial rotation at the glenohumeral joint). Some believe this method makes comparison easier (Figure 5-39).[47] Often, the dominant shoulder shows greater restriction than the nondominant shoulder, even in normal people. An exception would be patients who continually use their arms at the extremes of motion (e.g., baseball pitchers). Because

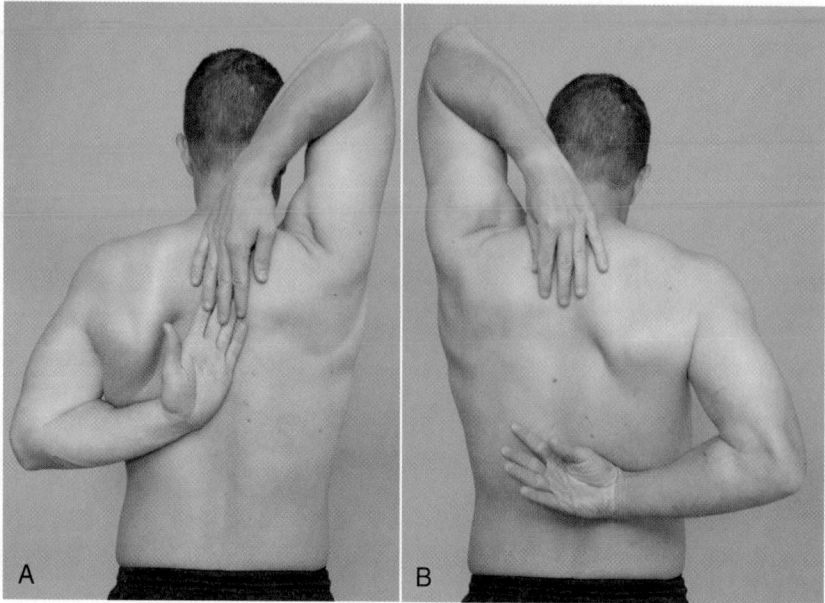

Figure 5-38 **Apley's scratch test. A,** The right arm is in lateral rotation, flexion, and abduction; and the left arm is in medial rotation, extension, and adduction. **B,** The left arm is in lateral rotation, flexion, and abduction; and the right arm is in medial rotation, extension, and adduction. Note the difference in medial rotation and scapular winging in the right arm compared to the left arm in **A.**

of the extra ROM developed over time doing the activity, the dominant arm may show greater ROM. However, the examiner must always be aware that shoulder movements include movements of the scapula and clavicle as well as the glenohumeral joint and that many of the perceived glenohumeral joint problems are, in reality, scapular muscle control problems, which may secondarily lead to glenohumeral joint problems, especially in people under 40 years of age. If, in the history, the patient has complained that shoulder movements in certain postures are painful or that sustained or repetitive movements increase symptoms, the examiner should consider having the patient hold a sustained arm position (10 to 60 seconds) or do the movements repetitively (ten to twenty repetitions). Ideally, these repeated movements should be performed at the speed and with the load that the patient was using when the symptoms were elicited. Thus, the volleyball player should do the spiking motion in which he or she jumps up to hit the imaginary ball.

Capsular tightness, although commonly tested during passive movement, can affect active movement by limiting some or all movements in the glenohumeral joint with compensating excessive movement of the scapula. Just as a frozen shoulder can affect all movements, selected tightness due to particular pathologies may affect only part of the capsule. For example, with anterior shoulder instability, posterior capsular tightness is a common finding combined with weak lower trapezius and serratus anterior muscles. Table 5-10 shows common selected capsular tightness and states their effect on movement.

Likewise, muscle tightness can affect both active and passive movement. For example, with anterior shoulder

instability, the following muscles may be found to be tight: subscapularis, pectoralis minor and major, latissimus dorsi, upper trapezius, levator scapulae, sternocleidomastoid, scalenes, and rectus capitus. Weak muscles include serratus anterior, middle and lower trapezius, infraspinatus, teres minor, posterior deltoid, rhomboids, longus colli, and longus capitus.[60]

The biceps tendon does not move in the bicipital groove during movement; rather, the humerus moves over the fixed tendon. From adduction to full elevation of abduction, a given point in the groove moves along the tendon at least 4 cm. If the examiner wants to keep excursion of the bicipital groove along the biceps tendon to a minimum, the arm should be elevated with the humerus in medial rotation; elevating the arm with the humerus laterally rotated causes maximum excursion of the bicipital groove along the biceps tendon. Patients who have deltoid or supraspinatus pathology sometimes use this laterally rotated position because lateral rotation allows the biceps tendon to be used as a shoulder abductor in a "cheating" movement.

As the patient does the various movements, the examiner watches to see whether the components of the shoulder complex move in normal, coordinated sequence and whether the patient exhibits any apprehension when doing a movement. With **anterior instability** of the shoulder, the shoulder girdle often droops, and excessive scapulothoracic movement may occur on abduction. With **posterior instability,** horizontal adduction (crossflexion) may cause excessive scapulothoracic movement. Any apprehension on movement suggests the possibility of instability. The examiner should also watch for **winging** of the scapula on active movements. Winging of the medial border of the scapula indicates injury to the serratus anterior muscle or the long thoracic nerve; rotary winging of the scapula or scapular tilt indicates upper trapezius pathology or injury to the spinal accessory nerve (cranial nerve XI; Table 5-11).[55,99,108] Scapular tilt (inferior angle of scapula moves away from rib cage) may also be caused by weak lower trapezius or a tight pectoralis minor. In some cases, it may be necessary to load the appropriate muscle isometrically (hold the contraction for 10 to 15 seconds) to demonstrate abnormal scapular stability. It has been reported that application of a resistance to adduction at 30° and at 60° of shoulder abduction is the best way to show scapular winging.[99] Eccentric loading of the shoulder in different positions, especially into horizontal adduction, may also demonstrate winging or loss of scapular control. Weakness of the scapular control muscles often leads to overactivity of the rotator cuff and biceps muscle leading to overuse pathology in those structures.

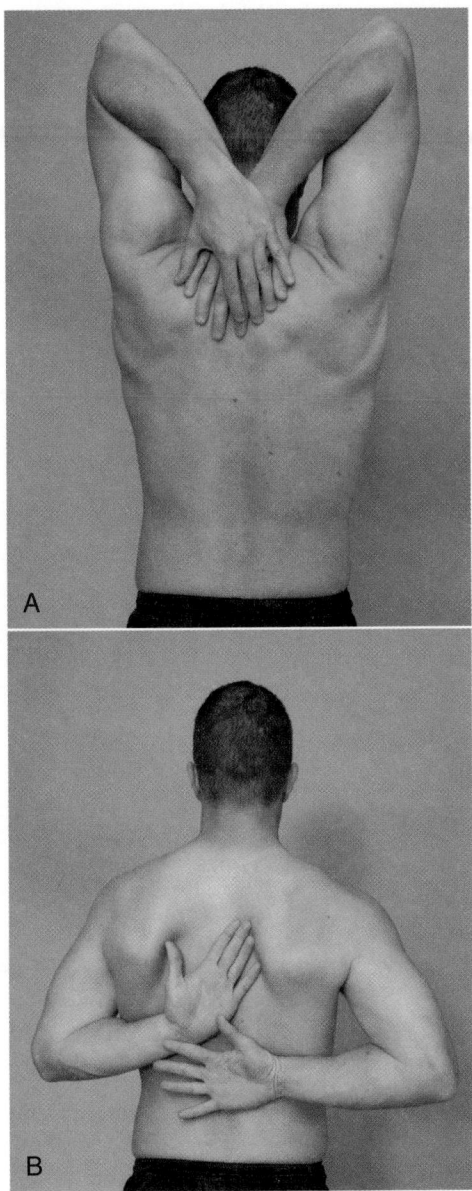

Figure 5-39 A, Neck reach. **B,** Back reach. Note the difference in medial rotation on both sides and greater winging of left scapula.

Causes of Scapular Imbalance Patterns

Increased protraction:	Tight pectoralis minor
	Weak/lengthened lower trapezius
	Weak/lengthened serratus anterior
Increased depression:	Weak upper trapezius
Loss of scapular stabilization:	Early/excessive protraction
	Early/excessive lateral rotation of scapula
	Early/excessive elevation of scapula
	Tight lateral rotators
	Secondary impingement

Indications of Loss of Scapular Control

- Scapula protracting along chest wall, especially under load
- Early contraction of upper trapezius on abduction, especially under load
- Increased work of rotator cuff and biceps, especially with closed chain activity (reverse origin-insertion)
- Altered scapulohumeral rhythm

Humeral Movement Faults

Superior humeral translation:	Scapular downward rotators are predominating
Anterior humeral translation:	Weak subscapularis and teres major; tight infraspinatus, teres minor
Inferior humeral translation:	Weak upward scapular rotators; poor glenohumeral rotation timing
Decreased lateral rotation:	Short pectoralis major and/or latissimus dorsi
Excessive scapular retraction during lateral rotation:	Tight anterior capsule; tight medial rotators; poor scapulothoracic muscle control

Scapular Winging Faults

On concentric elevation:	Long/weak serratus anterior
On eccentric forward flexion:	Overactive rotator cuff; underactive scapular control muscles
Tilting of inferior angle:	Tight pectoralis minor; weak lower trapezius

TABLE **5-10**

Capsular Tightness: Its Effect and Resulting Humeral Head Translation

Where	Effect (Signs and Symptoms)	Resulting Translation
Posterior	Cross flexion decreased Medial rotation decreased Flexion (end range) decreased Decreased posterior glide Impingement signs in medial rotation Weak external rotators Weak scapular stabilizers	Anterior (with medial rotation)
Posteroinferior	Elevation anteriorly Medial rotation of elevated arm decreased Horizontal adduction decreased	Superior Anterosuperior Anterosuperior
Posterosuperior	Medial rotation limited	Anterosuperior
Anterosuperior	Flexion (end range) decreased Extension (end range) decreased Lateral rotation decreased Horizontal extension decreased Abduction (end range) decreased Decreased posteroinferior glide Impingement in medial rotation and cross flexion Increased night pain Weak rotator cuff May have positive ULNT Biceps tests may be positive	Posterior (with lateral rotation)
Anteroinferior	Abduction decreased Extension decreased Lateral rotation decreased Horizontal extension decreased Increased posterior glide	Posterior (with lateral rotation of elevated arm)

Data from Matsen FA, et al: Practice evaluation and management of the shoulder, Philadelphia, 1994, WB Saunders.
ULNT, Upper limb neurodynamic test.

TABLE **5-11**

Winging of the Scapula: Dynamic Causes and Effects

Cause	Effect (Signs and Symptoms)
Trapezius or spinal accessory nerve lesion	Inability to shrug shoulder
Serratus anterior or long thoracic nerve lesion	Difficulty elevating arm above 120°
Strain of rhomboids	Difficulty pushing elbow back against resistance (with hand on hip)
Muscle imbalance or contractures	Winging of upper margin of scapula on adduction and lateral rotation

If the scapula appears to wing, the examiner asks the patient to forward flex the shoulder to 90°. The examiner then pushes the straight arm toward the patient's body while the patient resists. If there is weakness of the upper or lower trapezius muscle, the serratus anterior muscle, or the nerves supplying these muscles, their inability to contract will cause the scapula to wing. Another way to test winging of the scapula is to have the patient stand and lean against the wall. The examiner then asks the patient to do a pushup away from the wall while the examiner watches for winging (see Figure 5-23; Figure 5-40, *A*). Similarly, asking the patient to do a floor pushup may demonstrate this winging (Figure 5-40, *B*). The patient should be tested in a relaxed starting position and be asked to do the pushup. Sometimes the winging is visible at rest only (static winging), sometimes during rest and activity, and sometimes only with the activity (dynamic winging).

Injury to other nerves in the shoulder region must not be overlooked (Table 5-12). As previously mentioned, damage to the suprascapular nerve may affect both the supraspinatus and infraspinatus muscles, or it may affect only the infraspinatus, depending on where the pathology lies (see Figure 5-161), whereas injury to the musculocutaneous nerve can lead to paralysis of the coracobrachialis, biceps, and brachialis muscles. These changes affect elbow flexion and supination and forward flexion of the shoulder. There is also a loss of the biceps reflex. Injury to the axillary (circumflex) nerve leads to paralysis of the deltoid and teres minor muscles, affecting abduction and lateral

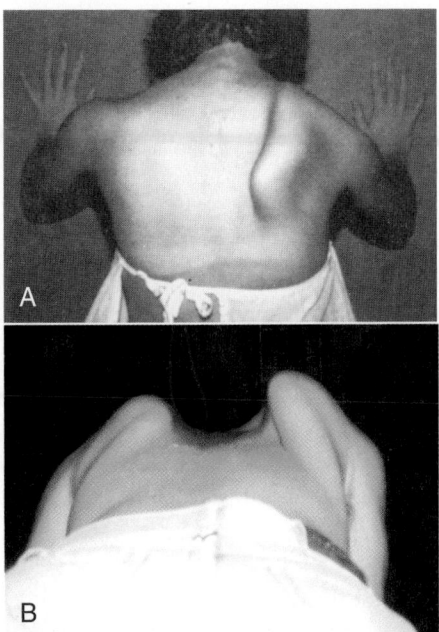

Figure 5-40 Scapular winging is demonstrated by having the patient push against a wall (unilateral weakness) (**A**) or the floor (bilateral weakness) (**B**) with both arms forward flexed to 90°. (**A**, From McClusky CM: Classification and diagnosis of glenohumeral instability in athletes. Sports Med Arthro Rev 8:163, 2000.)

TABLE **5-12**

Signs and Symptoms of Possible Peripheral Nerve Involvement

Spinal accessory nerve	Inability to abduct arm beyond 90°
	Pain in shoulder on abduction
Long thoracic nerve	Pain on flexing fully extended arm
	Inability to flex fully extended arm
	Winging starts at 90° forward flexion
Suprascapular nerve	Increased pain on forward shoulder flexion
	Shoulder weakness (partial loss of humeral control)
	Pain increases with scapular abduction
	Pain increases with cervical rotation to opposite side
Axillary (circumflex) nerve	Inability to abduct arm with neutral rotation
Musculocutaneous nerve	Weak elbow flexion with forearm supinated

rotation of the shoulder. A sensory loss over the deltoid insertion area also occurs. Damage to the radial nerve affects all of the extensor muscles of the upper limb, including the triceps. Triceps paralysis may be overlooked when examining the shoulder unless arm extension is attempted along with elbow extension against gravity. Both of these movements are affected in high radial nerve

palsy, although some triceps function may remain (e.g., in radial nerve palsy after a humeral shaft fracture).

Passive Movements

If the ROM is not full during the active movements and the examiner is unable to test the end feel, the examiner should perform all passive movements of the shoulder to determine the end feel, and any restriction should be noted. This passive examination should include not only the mobility of the four shoulder joints but also the ribs and spine as limitations in rib and spinal movement can restrict shoulder movement.

Passive Movements of the Shoulder Complex and Normal End Feel

- Elevation through forward flexion of the arm (tissue stretch)
- Elevation through abduction of the arm (bone-to-bone or tissue stretch)
- Elevation through abduction of the glenohumeral joint only (bone-to-bone or tissue stretch)
- Lateral rotation of the arm (tissue stretch)
- Medial rotation of the arm (tissue stretch)
- Extension of the arm (tissue stretch)
- Adduction of the arm (tissue approximation)
- Horizontal adduction (tissue stretch or approximation) and abduction of the arm (tissue stretch)
- Quadrant test

The end feel of capsular tightness is different from the tissue stretch end feel of muscle tightness.[109] Capsular tightness has a more hard elastic feel to it, and it usually occurs earlier in the ROM. If one is unsure of the end feel, the examiner can ask the patient to contract the muscles acting in the opposite direction 10% to 20% of maximum voluntary contraction (MVC) and then relax. The examiner then attempts to move the limb further into range. If the range increases, the problem was muscular not capsular.

If the problem is capsular, capsular tightness should be measured. For example, a tight posterior capsule can cause increased scapular protraction and depression leading to ante-tilting and insufficient scapular elevation, which in turn can lead to impingement.[37] In addition, it can limit horizontal adduction, and posteroinferior tightness can increase the risk of injury to the rotator cuff.[110] To measure posterior capsular tightness, the patient, suitably undressed (no shirt for males; bra for females), is placed in supine lying with the arm forward flexed to 90° and the elbow flexed to 90°. The examiner stands beside the patient and, while palpating the lateral edge of the scapula, horizontally adducts the patient's arm. As soon as the examiner feels the scapula begin to move, the horizontal adduction is stopped, and the angle relative to the

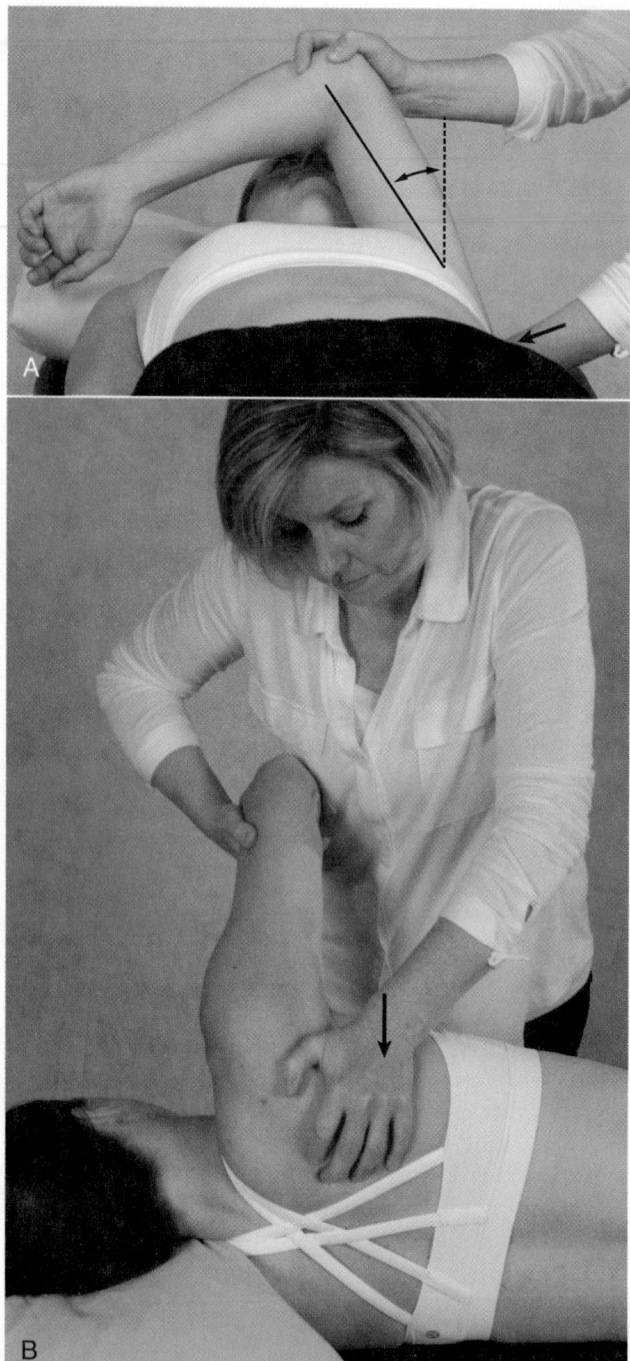

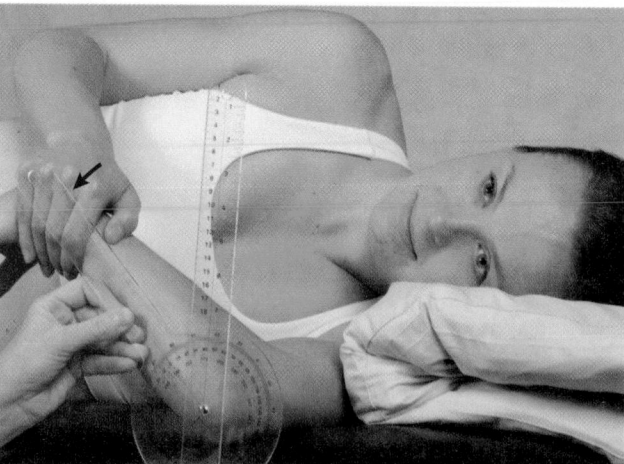

Figure 5-42 Measuring medial rotation in the sleeper stretch position.

Figure 5-41 **Testing for posterior capsular tightness. A,** Supine lying. Angle created by the end position of the humerus with respect to the starting position to determine glenohumeral horizontal adduction range of motion. Note stabilization of scapula (*arrow*). **B,** Starting position for the posterior shoulder flexibility measurement with the patient positioned in side lying. Note the scapular stabilization (*arrow*) with the torso perpendicular to the examining table. As soon as the scapula begins to move, the examiner stops.

vertical position is measured. Both sides, starting with the normal side, are measured (Figure 5-41, *A*).[111] The test may also be done in side lying but it is harder to stabilize the scapula (Figure 5-41, *B*).[112,113] The angle from the vertical to the arm indicates the passive ROM available.

If the pathological side has less ROM and the end feel is capsular, capsular tightness is present. This capsular tightness should correlate well with decreased medial rotation provided the scapula is not allowed to move in compensation.[112,113]

Particular attention must be paid to passive medial and lateral rotation if the examiner suspects a problem with the glenohumeral joint capsule (see previous discussion of GIRD). Lunden, et al.[114] have recommended that rotation, especially medial rotation, should be measured in side lying for greater reliability (Figure 5-42). Excessive scapular movement may be seen as compensation for a tight glenohumeral joint. **Subcoracoid bursitis** may limit full lateral rotation, and **subacromial bursitis** may limit full abduction because of compression or pinching of these structures. If lateral rotation of the shoulder is limited, the examiner should check forearm supination with the arm forward flexed to 90°. Patients who have a posterior dislocation at the glenohumeral joint exhibit restricted lateral rotation of the shoulder and limited supination in forward flexion (**Rowe sign** ❓).[115] Even if overpressure has been applied on active movement, it is still necessary for the examiner to perform elevation through abduction of the glenohumeral joint only (Figure 5-43) and the quadrant test.

The examiner performs passive elevation through abduction or scaption of the glenohumeral joint with the clavicle and scapula fixed to determine the amount of abduction in the glenohumeral joint alone. This can give an indication of capsular tightness or subacromial space pathology.[47] Normally, this movement should be up to 120°, although Gagey and Gagey[116] have stated that anything greater than 105° indicates laxity in the inferior glenohumeral ligament (**Gagey hyperabduction test** ❓).[117]

The rotation of the humerus in the quadrant position demonstrates Codman's "pivotal paradox"[97,118] and Mac-Conaill's[119] conjunct rotation (rotation that automatically

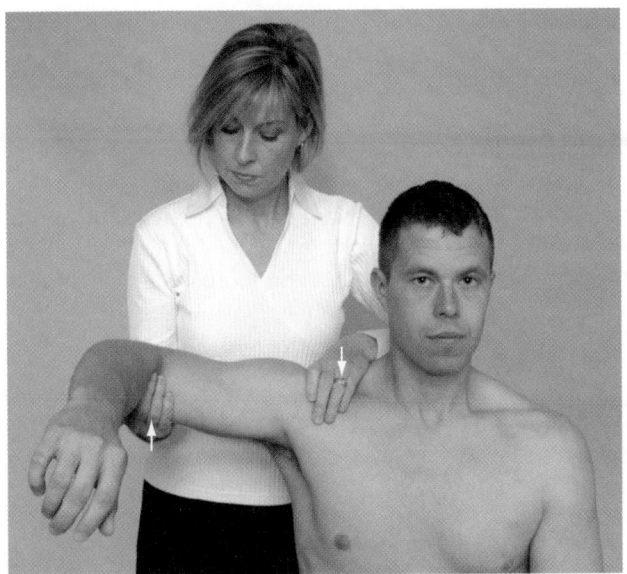

Figure 5-43 Passive abduction of the glenohumeral joint.

or subconsciously occurs with movement) in diadochal movement (a succession of two or more distinct movements). For example, if the arm, with the elbow flexed, is laterally rotated when the arm is at the side and then abducted in the coronal plane to 180°, the shoulder will be in 90° of medial rotation even though no apparent rotation has occurred. The path traced by the humerus during the quadrant test, in which the humerus moves forward at approximately 120° of abduction, is the unconscious rotation occurring at the glenohumeral joint. Thus, the quadrant test is designed to demonstrate whether the automatic or subconscious rotation is occurring during movement. The examiner should not only feel the movement but also determine the quality of the movement and the amount of anterior humeral movement. This test and the following locked quadrant test assess one area or quadrant of the 200° of circumduction. The humerus must rotate in the quadrant of the circumduction movement to allow full pain-free movement. Although both of these tests should normally be pain-free, the examiner should be aware that they place a high level of stress on the soft tissues of the glenohumeral joint, and discomfort should not be misinterpreted as pathological pain. If movement is painful and restricted, the tests indicate early stages of shoulder pathology.[120]

To test the **quadrant position**,[121,122] the examiner stabilizes the scapula and clavicle by placing the forearm under the patient's scapula on the side to be tested and extending the hand over the shoulder to hold the trapezius muscle and prevent shoulder shrugging (Figure 5-44). To test the position, the upper limb is elevated to rest alongside the patient's head with the shoulder laterally rotated. The patient's shoulder is then adducted. Because adduction occurs on the coronal plane, a point (the quadrant position) is reached at which the arm moves

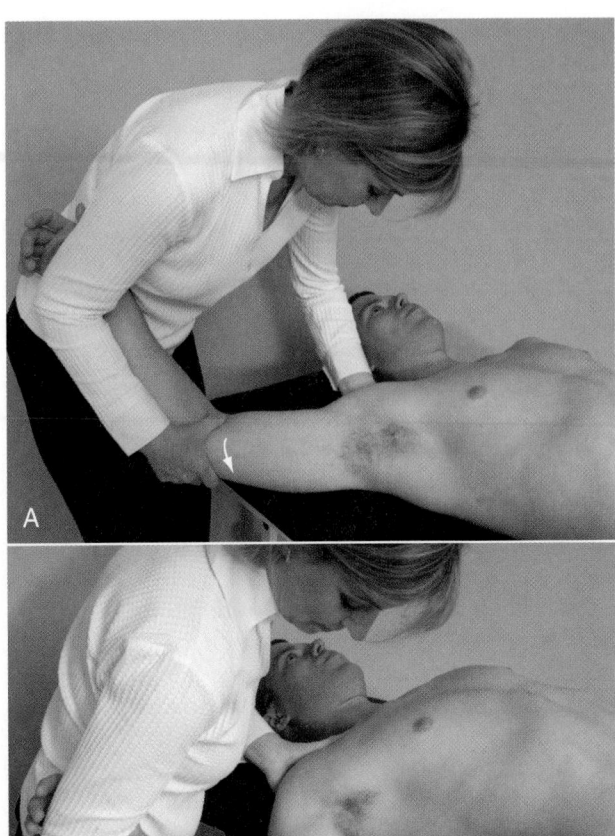

Figure 5-44 Quadrant position. **A,** Adduction test. **B,** Abduction test (locked quadrant).

forward slightly from the coronal plane. At approximately 60° of adduction (from the arm beside the head), this position of maximum forward movement occurs (i.e., at about 120° of abduction) even if a backward pressure is applied. As the shoulder is further adducted, the arm falls back to the previous coronal plane. The quadrant position indicates the position at which the arm has medially rotated during its descent to the patient's side.

The quadrant position also may be found by abducting the medially rotated shoulder while maintaining extension. In this case, the quadrant position is reached (at approximately 120° of abduction) when the shoulder no longer abducts, because it is prevented from laterally rotating by the catching of the greater tuberosity in the subacromial space. This position is referred to as the **locked quadrant position.**[122] If the arm is allowed to move forward, lateral rotation occurs and full abduction can be achieved. Both the quadrant and locked quadrant simply indicate where the rotation normally occurs during shoulder abduction/adduction.

The capsular pattern of the shoulder is lateral rotation showing the greatest restriction, followed by abduction and medial rotation. Each of these movements normally has a tissue-stretch end feel. Other movements may be limited, but not in the same order and not with as much restriction. Early capsular patterns may exhibit only limitations of lateral rotation or possibly lateral rotation and abduction. Finding of limitation, but not in the order described, indicates a noncapsular pattern.

Resisted Isometric Movements

Having completed the active and passive movements, which are done while the patient is standing, sitting, or lying supine (in the case of quadrant test), the patient lies supine to do the resisted isometric movements (Figure 5-45). The disadvantage of this position is that the examiner cannot observe the stabilization of the scapula during the testing. Normally, the scapula should not move during isometric testing. Scapular protraction, winging, or tilting during isometric testing indicates weakness of the scapular control muscles. Although all the muscles around the shoulder can be tested in supine lying, it has been advocated that the muscles should be tested in more than one position (for example, different amounts of abduction or forward flexion) to determine the mechanical effect of the contraction in different situations. If, in the history, the patient complained of pain in one or more positions, these positions should be tested as well. If the initial position causes pain, other positions (e.g., position of injury, position of mechanical advantage) may be tried to further differentiate the specific contractile tissue that has been injured. During the active movements, the examiner should have noted which movements caused discomfort or pain so that this information can be correlated with that obtained from resisted isometric movements. By carefully noting which movements cause pain on isometric testing, the examiner should be able to

determine which muscle or muscles are at fault (Table 5-13). For example, if the patient experiences pain primarily on medial rotation but also on abduction and adduction, the examiner would suspect a problem in the subscapularis muscle, because the other muscles involved in these actions were found to be pain-free in other movements. To do the initial resisted isometric tests, the examiner positions the patient's arm at the side with the elbow flexed to 90°. The muscles of the shoulder are then tested isometrically with the examiner positioning the patient and saying, "Don't let me move you."

Resisted Isometric Movements of the Shoulder Complex

- Forward flexion of the shoulder
- Extension of the shoulder
- Adduction of the shoulder
- Abduction of the shoulder
- Medial rotation of the shoulder
- Lateral rotation of the shoulder
- Flexion of the elbow
- Extension of the elbow

Resisted isometric elbow flexion and extension must be performed, because some of the muscles (e.g., biceps, triceps) act over the elbow as well as the shoulder. The examiner should watch for the possibility of a third-degree strain (rupture) of the long head of biceps tendon ("Popeye muscle" or **Popeye sign**) when testing isometric elbow flexion (Figure 5-46).

During testing, the examiner will find differences in the relative strengths of the various muscle groups around the shoulder. The relative percentages for isometric testing will be altered for tests at faster speeds and tests in different planes. If, in the history, the patient complained that concentric, eccentric, or econcentric (biceps and triceps) movements were painful or caused symptoms, these movements should also be tested, with loading or no loading, as required.

Relative Isometric Muscle Strengths

- Abduction should be 50% to 70% of adduction
- Forward flexion should be 50% to 60% of adduction
- Medial rotation should be 45% to 50% of adduction
- Lateral rotation should be 65% to 70% of medial rotation
- Forward flexion should be 50% to 60% of extension
- Horizontal adduction should be 70% to 80% of horizontal abduction

---

Functional Assessment

The shoulder complex plays an integral role in the ADLs, sometimes acting as part of an open kinetic chain and

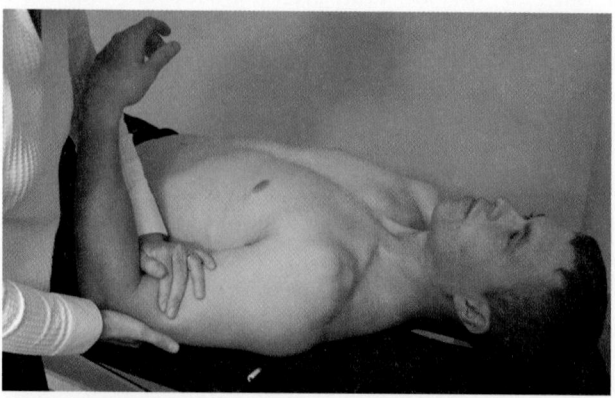

Figure 5-45 Positioning of the patient for resisted isometric movements.

TABLE **5-13**

Muscles About the Shoulder: Their Actions, Nerve Supply, and Nerve Root Derivation

Action	Muscles Acting	Nerve Supply	Nerve Root Derivation Retraction
Forward flexion	1. Deltoid (anterior fibers)	Axillary (circumflex)	C5, C6 (posterior cord)
	2. Pectoralis major (clavicular fibers)	Lateral pectoral	C5, C6 (lateral cord)
	3. Coracobrachialis	Musculocutaneous	C5–C7 (lateral cord)
	4. Biceps (when strong contraction required)	Musculocutaneous	C5–C7 (lateral cord)
Extension	1. Deltoid (posterior fibers)	Axillary (circumflex)	C5, C6 (posterior cord)
	2. Teres major	Subscapular	C5, C6 (posterior cord)
	3. Teres minor	Axillary (circumflex)	C5, C6 (posterior cord)
	4. Latissimus dorsi	Thoracodorsal	C6–C8 (posterior cord)
	5. Pectoralis major (sternocostal fibers)	Lateral pectoral / Medial pectoral	C5, C6 (lateral cord) / C8, T1 (medial cord)
	6. Triceps (long head)	Radial	C5–C8, T1 (posterior cord)
Horizontal adduction	1. Pectoralis major	Lateral pectoral	C5, C6 (lateral cord)
	2. Deltoid (anterior fibers)	Axillary (circumflex)	C5, C6 (posterior cord)
Horizontal abduction	1. Deltoid (posterior fibers)	Axillary (circumflex)	C5, C6 (posterior cord)
	2. Teres major	Subscapular	C5, C6 (posterior cord)
	3. Teres minor	Axillary (circumflex)	C5, C6 (brachial plexus trunk)
	4. Infraspinatus	Suprascapular	C5, C6 (brachial plexus trunk)
Abduction	1. Deltoid	Axillary (circumflex)	C5, C6 (posterior cord)
	2. Supraspinatus	Suprascapular	C5, C6 (brachial plexus trunk)
	3. Infraspinatus	Suprascapular	C5, C6 (brachial plexus trunk)
	4. Subscapularis	Subscapular	C5, C6 (posterior cord)
	5. Teres minor	Axillary (circumflex)	C5, C6 (posterior cord)
	6. Long head of biceps (if arm laterally rotated first, trick movement)	Musculocutaneous	C5–C7 (lateral cord)
Adduction	1. Pectoralis major	Lateral pectoral	C5, C6 (lateral cord)
	2. Latissimus dorsi	Thoracodorsal	C6–C8 (posterior cord)
	3. Teres major	Subscapular	C5, C6 (posterior cord)
	4. Subscapularis	Subscapular	C5, C6 (posterior cord)
Medial rotation	1. Pectoralis major	Lateral pectoral	C5, C6 (lateral cord)
	2. Deltoid (anterior fibers)	Axillary (circumflex)	C5, C6 (posterior cord)
	3. Latissimus dorsi	Thoracodorsal	C6–C8 (posterior cord)
	4. Teres major	Subscapular	C5, C6 (posterior cord)
	5. Subscapularis (when arm is by side)	Subscapular	C5, C6 (posterior cord)
Lateral rotation	1. Infraspinatus	Suprascapular	C5, C6 (brachial plexus trunk)
	2. Deltoid (posterior fibers)	Axillary (circumflex)	C5, C6 (posterior cord)
	3. Teres minor	Axillary (circumflex)	C5, C6 (posterior cord)
Elevation of scapula	1. Trapezius (upper fibers)	Accessory / C3, C4 nerve roots	Cranial nerve XI / C3, C4
	2. Levator scapulae	C3, C4 nerve roots / Dorsal scapular	C3, C4 / C5
	3. Rhomboid major	Dorsal scapular	(C4), C5
	4. Rhomboid minor	Dorsal scapular	(C4), C5
Depression of scapula	1. Serratus anterior	Long thoracic	C5, C6, (C7)
	2. Pectoralis major	Lateral pectoral	C5, C6 (lateral cord)
	3. Pectoralis minor	Medial pectoral	C8, T1 (medial cord)
	4. Latissimus dorsi	Thoracodorsal	C6–C8 (posterior cord)
	5. Trapezius (lower fibers)	Accessory / C3, C4 nerve roots	Cranial nerve XI / C3, C4

Continued

TABLE **5-13**

Muscles About the Shoulder: Their Actions, Nerve Supply, and Nerve Root Derivation—cont'd

Action	Muscles Acting	Nerve Supply	Nerve Root Derivation Retraction
Protraction (forward movement) of scapula	1. Serratus anterior 2. Pectoralis major 3. Pectoralis minor 4. Latissimus dorsi	Long thoracic Lateral pectoral Medial pectoral Thoracodorsal	C5, C6, (C7) C5, C6 (lateral cord) C8, T1 (medial cord) C6–C8 (posterior cord)
Retraction (backward movement) of scapula	1. Trapezius 2. Rhomboid major 3. Rhomboid minor	Accessory Dorsal scapular Dorsal scapular	Cranial nerve XI (C4), C5 (C4), C5
Lateral (upward) rotation of inferior angle of scapula	1. Trapezius (upper and lower fibers) 2. Serratus anterior	Accessory C3, C4 nerve roots Long thoracic	Cranial nerve XI C3, C4 C5, C6, (C7)
Medial (downward) rotation of inferior angle of scapula	1. Levator scapulae 2. Rhomboid major 3. Rhomboid minor 4. Pectoralis minor	C3, C4 nerve roots Dorsal scapular Dorsal scapular Dorsal scapular Medial pectoral	C3, C4 C5 (C4), C5 (C4), C5 C8, T1 (medial cord)
Flexion of elbow	1. Brachialis 2. Biceps brachii 3. Brachioradialis 4. Pronator teres 5. Flexor carpi ulnaris	Musculocutaneous Musculocutaneous Radial Median Ulnar	C5, C6, (C7) C5, C6 C5, C6, (C7) C6, C7 C7, C8
Extension of elbow	1. Triceps 2. Anconeus	Radial Radial	C6–C8 C7, C8, (T1)

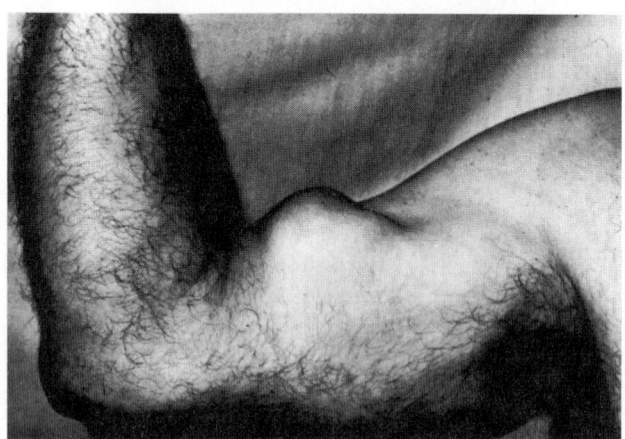

Figure 5-46 **Popeye sign.** Rupture of the long head of the biceps brachii caused by the patient's awkward catch of partner in gymnastics. Bunching of muscle is attended by complete loss of function of the long head of biceps. (From O'Donoghue DH: Treatment of injuries to athletes, ed 4, Philadelphia, 1984, WB Saunders, p. 53.)

sometimes acting as part of a closed kinetic chain. Assessment of function plays an important part of the shoulder evaluation.[123] Limitation of function can greatly affect the patient. For example, placing the hand behind the head (e.g., to comb the hair) requires almost full lateral rotation, whereas placing the hand in the small of the back (e.g., to get a wallet out of a back pocket or undo a bra) requires almost full medial rotation. Matsen, et al.[57] have listed the functional ROM necessary to do some of the functional ADLs (Table 5-14) and Mannerkorpi, et al.[124] and Dutton[125] have outlined functional movements of the arm (Table 5-15). The tables point out that although full ROM is desirable, most functional tasks can be performed with less than full ROM.[126] Test 1 in Table 5-15 measures the ability to do activities such as arm reach, pulling or hanging an object overhead, combing hair, or drinking from a cup. Test 2 measures the ability to do activities such as getting something out of a back pocket, scratching the back, or hooking a bra. Test 3 measures the ability to do such tasks as fastening a car seatbelt or turning a steering wheel.[124,125]

The functional assessment may be based on ADLs, work, or recreation and outcomes measures,[127] because these activities are of most concern to the patient (Figure 5-47),[128–130] or it may be based on numerical scoring charts (Figures 5-48 to 5-51 are examples), which are derived from clinical measures as well as functional measures. Some numerical evaluation scales are designed for specific populations, such as athletes (see Figure 5-48), level of disability[131–134] (see Figure 5-49), or specific

TABLE **5-14**

Range of Motion Necessary at the Shoulder to Do Certain Activities of Daily Living

Activity	Range of Motion	Activity	Range of Motion
Eating	70° to 100° horizontal adduction* 45° to 60° abduction	Hand behind head	10° to 15° horizontal adduction* 110° to 125° forward flexion 90° lateral rotation
Combing hair	30° to 70° horizontal adduction* 105° to 120° abduction 90° lateral rotation	Put something on shelf	70° to 80° horizontal adduction* 70° to 80° forward flexion 45° lateral rotation
Reach perineum	75° to 90° horizontal abduction 30° to 45° abduction 90°+ medial rotation	Wash opposite shoulder	60° to 90° forward flexion 60° to 120° horizontal adduction*
Tuck in shirt	50° to 60° horizontal abduction 55° to 65° abduction 90° medial rotation		

Adapted from Matsen FA, et al: Practical evaluation and management of the shoulder, Philadelphia, 1994, WB Saunders, pp. 20, 24.
*Horizontal adduction is from 0° to 90° of abduction.

TABLE **5-15**

Scoring for Functional Shoulder Movements of the Arm

Hand-To-Back of Neck (Test 1)

0   The fingers reach the posterior median line of the neck with the shoulder in full abduction and lateral rotation. The wrist is not dorsally extended.

1   The fingers reach the median line of the neck but do not have full abduction and/or lateral rotation.

2   The fingers reach the median line of the neck, but with compensation by adduction (over 20° in the horizontal plane) or by shoulder elevation.

3   The fingers touch the neck.

4   The fingers do not reach the neck.

Hand-To-Scapula (From Behind) (Test 2)

0   The hand reaches behind the trunk to the opposite scapula or 5 cm beneath it in full medial rotation. The wrist is not laterally deviated.

1   The hand reaches the opposite scapula 6 cm to 15 cm beneath it.

2   The hand reaches the opposite iliac crest.

3   The hand reaches the buttock.

4   Cannot move the hand behind the trunk.

Hand-To-Opposite Scapula (From in Front) (Test 3)

0   The hand reaches the spine of the opposite scapula in full adduction without wrist flexion.

1   The hand reaches the spine of the opposite scapula in full adduction.

2   The hand passes the midline of the trunk.

3   The hand cannot pass the midline of the trunk.

Modified from Mannerkorpi K, et al: Tests of functional limitations in fibromyalgia syndrome: a reliability study. Arthr Care Res 12(3):195, 1999; and Dutton M: Dutton's orthopedic examination, evaluation and intervention, ed 3, New York, 2012, McGraw-Hill, p. 511.

injuries, such as instability (see Figure 5-51). Other shoulder rating scales are also available.[135-146] When using numerical scoring charts, the examiner should not place total reliance on the scores, because most of these charts are based primarily on the examiner's clinical measures and not the patient's subjective functional, hoped-for outcome, which is the patient's primary concern.[147,148] Probably the most functional numerical shoulder tests from a patient's perspective are the **simple shoulder test** (Figure 5-52) developed by Lippitt, Matsen, and associates,[57,130,149,150] the **Disabilities of the Arm, Shoulder, and Hand (DASH) test** by Hudak, et al.[130,151] (Figure 5-53) and its modification—the **Quick DASH,**[152] the **Shoulder Pain and Disability Index (SPADI)** (see Figure 5-49),[133] and the **Penn Shoulder Score** by Leggin, et al.[153,154] Table 5-16 provides the examiner with a method of determining the patient's functional shoulder strength and endurance. This table is based on the general population and would not indicate a true functional reading of athletes or persons who do heavy work involving the shoulders. For athletes or those applying significant load to their shoulders while forward flexed, the **one-arm hop test** has been developed (Figure 5-54). To do this test, the patient assumes the pushup position, balancing on one arm. The patient then hops up onto a 10-cm (4-inch) step and then back to the floor. The hop is repeated five times and the time noted. The patient starts with the good arm and then uses the injured arm, and the two times are compared. Provided that the patient is trained, completing this action in less than 10 seconds is considered normal.[155]

Burkhart, et al. felt it was important to test core stability (i.e., testing kinetic chain function) and flexibility when assessing the shoulder to ensure the proper transfer

Please indicate with an "X" how often you performed each activity in your healthiest and most active state, in the past year.

	Never or less than once a month	Once a month	Once a week	More than once a week	Daily
Carrying objects 8 pounds or heavier by hand (such as a bag of groceries)					
Handling objects overhead					
Weight lifting or weight training with arms					
Swinging motion (as in hitting a tennis ball, golf ball, baseball, or similar object)					
Lifting objects 25 pounds or heavier (such as 3 gallons of water) NOT INCLUDING WEIGHT LIFTING					

For each of the following questions, please circle the letter that best describes your participation in that particular activity.

1) Do you participate in contact sports (such as, but not limited to, American football, rugby, soccer, basketball, wrestling, boxing, lacrosse, martial arts)?

   A No

   B Yes, without organized officiating

   C Yes, with organized officiating

   D Yes, at a professional level (i.e., paid to play)

2) Do you participate in sports that involve hard overhand throwing (such as baseball, cricket, or quarterback in American football), overhead serving (such as tennis or volleyball), or lap/distance swimming?

   A No

   B Yes, without organized officiating

   C Yes, with organized officiating

   D Yes, at a professional level (i.e., paid to play)

Figure 5-47 Shoulder activity scale. It includes five numerically-scored items and two alpha-scored items. (From Brophy RH, Beauvais RL, Jones EC, et al: Measurement of shoulder activity level. Clin Orthop Relat Res 439:105, 2005.)

of forces from the legs to the trunk and the shoulder as part of the kinetic chain.[31] They advocated testing one-legged stance (no Trendelenburg), one-legged squat (stable pelvis), one-legged step up and step down (stable pelvis), normal hip medial rotation bilaterally, and strength of hip abductors, trunk flexors, and abdominal muscles.

Special Tests

Special tests are often used in shoulder examinations to confirm findings or a tentative diagnosis. Many of the tests, especially those involving the labrum, have not shown high sensitivity or specificity; so, often a combination of tests (i.e., test clusters, clinical prediction rules) may be more helpful[156,157] although even in these cases, the tests are not necessarily definitive. The examiner must be proficient in those tests that he or she decides to use. Proficiency increases the reliability of the findings, although the reliability of some of the tests has been questioned.[158] Depending on the patient history, some tests are compulsory, and others may be used as confirming or excluding tests. As with all passive tests, results are more likely to be positive in the presence of pathology when the muscles are relaxed, the patient is supported, and there is minimal or no muscle spasm.

For the reader who would like to review them, the reliability, validity, specificity, sensitivity, and odds ratios of some of the special tests used in the shoulder are available on the Evolve website.

Instability and Pseudolaxity Impingement

Anterior shoulder pain is commonly seen in patients young and old complaining of shoulder pain and dysfunction. Instability at the shoulder manifests itself as symptomatic abnormal motion within the shoulder complex, including the scapula. This abnormal motion may be the result of abnormal scapular or glenohumeral muscle patterning, hypo- or hypermobility of the capsule (most commonly a tight posterior capsule) or ribs, a labral tear (a Bankart or SLAP lesion), a rotator cuff or biceps injury, altered surface area of contact between the glenoid and humeral head, and/or a problem with the central or peripheral nervous system.[104]

In the older patient (40-years-old or older), mechanical impingement occurs because of degenerative changes to the rotator cuff, the acromion process, the coracoid process, and the anterior tissues from stress overload resulting in impingement. In this case, impingement is the primary problem (thus, the term **primary impingement**). It may be intrinsic because of rotator cuff degeneration or extrinsic because of the shape of the acromion and degeneration of the coracoacromial ligament.[166]

In the young patient (15 to 35-years-old), anterior shoulder pain is primarily caused by problems with muscle dynamics with an upset in the normal force couple action leading to muscle imbalance and abnormal movement patterns at both the glenohumeral joint and the scapulothoracic articulation. These altered muscle dynamics lead to symptoms of anterior impingement (thus, the term **secondary impingement**). The impingement signs are a secondary result of altered muscle dynamics in the scapula or glenohumeral joint.[166]

Text continued on p. 299

Athletic Shoulder Outcome Rating Scale

Name _____ Age _____ Sex _____

Dominant Hand (R) _____ (L) _____ (Ambidextrous) _____

Date of Examination _____ Position Played _____

Surgeon _____ Years Played _____

Type of Sport _____ Prior Injury _____

Activity Level

1) Professional (major league)
2) Professional (minor league)
3) College
4) High school
5) Recreational (full time)
6) Recreational (occasionally)

Diagnosis

1) Anterior instability
2) Posterior instability
3) Multidirectional instability
4) Recurrent dislocations
5) Impingement syndrome
6) Acromioclavicular separation
7) Acromioclavicular arthrosis
8) Rotator cuff repair (partial)
9) Rotator cuff tear (complete)
10) Biceps tendon rupture
11) Calcific tendinitis
12) Fracture

Subjective (90 Points)

I. Pain	Points
No pain with competition	10
Pain after competing only	8
Pain while competing	6
Pain preventing competing	4
Pain with ADLs	2
Pain at rest	0

II. Strength/Endurance	Points
No weakness, normal competition fatigue	10
Weakness after competition, early competition fatigue	8
Weakness during competition, abnormal competition fatigue	6
Weakness or fatigue preventing competition	4
Weakness or fatigue with ADLs	2
Weakness or fatigue preventing ADLs	0

III. Stability	Points
No looseness during competition	10
Recurrent subluxations while competing	8
Dead-arm syndrome while competing	6
Recurrent subluxations prevent competition	4
Recurrent subluxations during ADLs	2
Dislocation	0

IV. Intensity	Points
Preinjury versus postinjury hours of competition (100%)	10
Preinjury versus postinjury hours of competition (less than 75%)	8
Preinjury versus postinjury hours of competition (less than 50%)	6
Preinjury versus postinjury hours of competition (less than 25%)	4
Preinjury and postinjury hours of ADLs (100%)	2
Preinjury and postinjury hours of ADLs (less than 50%)	0

V. Performance	Points
At the same level, same proficiency	50
At the same level, decreased proficiency	40
At the same level, decreased proficiency, not acceptable to athlete	30
Decreased level with acceptable proficiency at that level	20
Decreased level, unacceptable proficiency	10
Cannot compete, had to switch sport	0

Objective (10 Points)

Range of Motion	Points
Normal external rotation at 90°–90° position; normal elevation	10
Less than 5° loss of external rotation; normal elevation	8
Less than 10° loss of external rotation; normal elevation	6
Less than 15° loss of external rotation; normal elevation	4
Less than 20° loss of external rotation; normal elevation	2
Greater than 20° loss of external rotation, or any loss of elevation	0

Overall Results

Excellent:	90–100 points
Good:	70–89 points
Fair:	50–69 points
Poor:	Less than 50 points

Figure 5-48 Athletic shoulder outcome rating scale. (From Tibone JE, Bradley JP: Evaluation of treatment outcomes for the athlete's shoulder. In Matsen FA, Fu FH, Hawkins RJ, editors: The shoulder: a balance of mobility and stability, Rosemont, IL, 1993, American Academy of Orthopedic Surgeons, pp. 526–527.)

Shoulder Pain and Disability Index (SPADI)

Please place a mark on the line that best represents your experience during the last week attributable to your shoulder problem.

Pain scale

How severe is your pain?

Circle the number that best describes your pain where: 0 = no pain and 10 = the worst pain imaginable.

At its worst?	0	1	2	3	4	5	6	7	8	9	10
When lying on the involved side?	0	1	2	3	4	5	6	7	8	9	10
Reaching for something on a high shelf?	0	1	2	3	4	5	6	7	8	9	10
Touching the back of your neck?	0	1	2	3	4	5	6	7	8	9	10
Pushing with the involved arm?	0	1	2	3	4	5	6	7	8	9	10

Total pain score _____ /50 × 100 = _____ %

(Note: If a person does not answer all questions divide by the total possible score, e.g., if 1 question missed divide by 40.)

Disability scale

How much difficulty do you have?

Circle the number that best describes your experience where: 0 = no difficulty and 10 = so difficult it requires help.

Washing your hair?	0	1	2	3	4	5	6	7	8	9	10
Washing your back?	0	1	2	3	4	5	6	7	8	9	10
Putting on an undershirt or jumper?	0	1	2	3	4	5	6	7	8	9	10
Putting on a shirt that buttons down the front?	0	1	2	3	4	5	6	7	8	9	10
Putting on your pants?	0	1	2	3	4	5	6	7	8	9	10
Placing an object on a high shelf?	0	1	2	3	4	5	6	7	8	9	10
Carrying a heavy object of 10 pounds (4.5 kilograms)	0	1	2	3	4	5	6	7	8	9	10
Removing something from your back pocket?	0	1	2	3	4	5	6	7	8	9	10

Total disability score: _____ /80 × 100 = _____ %

(Note: If a person does not answer all questions divide by the total possible score, e.g., if 1 question missed divide by 70.)

Total Spadi score: _____ 130 × 100 = _____ %

(Note: If a person does not answer all questions divide by the total possible score, e.g., if 1 question missed divide by 120.)

Minimum Detectable Change (90% confidence) = 13 points
(Change less than this may be attributable to measurement error)

Figure 5-49 Shoulder Pain and Disability Index (SPADI). (From Roach KE, Budiman-Mak E, Songsiridej N, et al: Development of a shoulder pain and disability index. Arthritis Care Res 4[4]:143–149, 1991.)

American Shoulder and Elbow Surgeons' Shoulder Evaluation Form

Name _____ Hosp # _____ Date _____ Shoulder: R / L

I. Pain: (5 = none, 4 = slight, 3 = after unusual activity, 2 = moderate, 1 = marked, 0 = complete disability, NA = not available) _____

II. Motion:

A. Patient Sitting
1. Active total elevation of arm: _____ degrees*
2. Passive internal rotation:
(Circle segment of posterior anatomy reached by thumb)
(Note if reach restricted by limited elbow flexion)

1 = Less than trochanter	5 = L5	9 = L1	13 = T9	17 = T5
2 = Trochanter	6 = L4	10 = T12	14 = T8	18 = T4
3 = Gluteal	7 = L3	11 = T11	15 = T7	19 = T3
4 = Sacrum	8 = L2	12 = T10	16 = T6	20 = T2
				21 = T1

3. Active external rotation with arm at side: _____ degrees

4. Active external rotation at 90° abduction: _____ degrees
(Enter "NA" if cannot achieve 90° of abduction)

B. Patient Supine

1. Passive total elevation of arm: _____ degrees*

2. Passive external rotation with arm at side: _____ degrees

* Total elevation of arm measured by viewing patient from side and using goniometer to determine angle between *arm* and *thorax.*

III. Strength: (5 = normal, 4 = good, 3 = fair, 2 = poor, 1 = trace, 0 = paralysis)

A. Anterior deltoid _____   C. External rotation _____

B. Middle deltoid _____   D. Internal rotation _____

IV. Stability: (5 = normal, 4 = apprehension, 3 = rare subluxation, 2 = recurrent subluxation, 1 = recurrent dislocation, 0 = fixed dislocation, NA = not available)

A. Anterior _____   B. Posterior _____   C. Inferior _____

V. Function: (4 = normal, 3 = mild compromise, 2 = difficulty, 1 = with aid, 0 = unable, NA = not available)

A. Use back pocket   _____   I. Sleep on affected side   _____

B. Perineal care   _____   J. Pulling   _____

C. Wash opposite axilla   _____   K. Use hand overhead   _____

D. Eat with utensil   _____   L. Throwing   _____

E. Comb hair   _____   M. Lifting   _____

F. Use hand with arm at shoulder level   _____   N. Do usual work (specify _____)   _____

G. Carry 10–15 lb with arm at side   _____   O. Do usual sport (specify _____)   _____

H. Dress   _____

VI. Patient Response: (3 = much better, 2 = better, 1 = same, 0 = worse, NA = not available/applicable) _____

Figure 5-50 American Shoulder and Elbow Surgeons' shoulder evaluation form. (Courtesy the American Shoulder and Elbow Surgeons.)

12-Item Shoulder Instability Questionnaire

Item	Scoring Categories
1. During the last six months, how many times has your shoulder slipped out of joint (or dislocated?)	1 Not at all in 6 months 2 1 or 2 times in 6 months 3 1 or 2 times per month 4 1 or 2 times per week 5 More often than 1 or 2 times/week
2. During the last three months, have you had any trouble (or worry) dressing because of your shoulder?	1 No trouble at all 2 Slight trouble or worry 3 Moderate trouble or worry 4 Extreme difficulty 5 Impossible to do
3. During the last three months, how would you describe the worst pain you have had from your shoulder?	1 None 2 Mild ache 3 Moderate 4 Severe 5 Unbearable
4. During the last three months, how much has the problem with your shoulder interfered with your usual work (including school or college work, or housework)?	1 Not at all 2 A little bit 3 Moderately 4 Greatly 5 Totally
5. During the last three months, have you avoided any activities due to worry about your shoulder – feared that it might slip out of joint?	1 Not at all 2 Very occasionally 3 Some days 4 Most days or more than one activity 5 Every day or many activities
6. During the last three months, has the problem with your shoulder prevented you from doing things that are important to you?	1 No, not at all 2 Very occasionally 3 Some days 4 Most days or more than one activity 5 Every day or many activities
7. During the last three months, how much has the problem with your shoulder interfered with your social life (including sexual activity – if applicable)?	1 Not at all 2 Occasionally 3 Some days 4 Most days 5 Every day
8. During the last four weeks, how much has the problem with your shoulder interfered with your sporting activities or hobbies?	1 Not at all 2 A little/occasionally 3 Some of the time 4 Most of the time 5 All of the time
9. During the last four weeks, how often has your shoulder been "on your mind" – how often have you thought about it?	1 Never, or only if someone asks 2 Occasionally 3 Some days 4 Most days 5 Every day
10. During the last four weeks, how much has the problem with your shoulder interfered with your ability or willingness to lift heavy objects?	1 Not at all 2 Occasionally 3 Some days 4 Most days 5 Every day
11. During the last four weeks, how would you describe the pain which you usually had from your shoulder?	1 None 2 Very mild 3 Mild 4 Moderate 5 Severe
12. During the last four weeks, have you avoided lying in certain positions in bed at night, because of your shoulder?	1 No nights 2 Only 1 or 2 nights 3 Some nights 4 Most nights 5 Every night

TOTAL SCORE: _____   Maximum score: 60   Minimum score: 12

Figure 5-51 The twelve-item shoulder instability questionnaire. (Modified from Dawson J, Fitzpatrick R, Carr A: The assessment of shoulder instability: the development and validation of a questionnaire. J Bone Joint Surg Br 81:422, 1999.)

Last   First   M.I.

Name: _____ Date: __/__/__ Age: _____

Street/Apt #   City State Zip Code

Address: _____ Occupation: _____

Home   Business   Relative

Phone: ( ) - ( ) - ( ) -

Circle one   Circle one

Dominant Hand: Right / Left / Ambidextrous Shoulder Evaluated: Right / Left

Answer Each Question Below by Checking "Yes" or "No" **Response**

                 Yes No

1. Is your shoulder comfortable with your arm at rest by your side? ☐ ☐ 1
2. Does your shoulder allow you to sleep comfortably? ☐ ☐ 2
3. Can you reach the small of your back to tuck in your shirt with your hand? ☐ ☐ 3
4. Can you place your hand behind your head with the elbow straight out to the side? ☐ ☐ 4
5. Can you place a coin on a shelf at the level of your shoulder without bending your elbow? ☐ ☐ 5
6. Can you lift one pound (a full pint container) to the level of your shoulder without bending your elbow? ☐ ☐ 6
7. Can you lift eight pounds (a full gallon container) to the level of your shoulder without bending your elbow? ☐ ☐ 7
8. Can you carry twenty pounds at your side with the affected extremity? ☐ ☐ 8
9. Do you think you can toss a softball underhand ten yards with the affected extremity? ☐ ☐ 9
10. Do you think you can toss a softball overhand twenty yards with the affected extremity? ☐ ☐ 10
11. Can you wash the back of your opposite shoulder with the affected extremity? ☐ ☐ 11
12. Would your shoulder allow you to work full-time at your regular job? ☐ ☐ 12

Office Use Only

Diagnosis: DJD RA AVN IMP RCT FS TUBS AMBRII Other: _____

Dx Confirmed? _____ Pt# _____ Physician _____

SST: Initial / Pre-op / Follow-up: 6 mon 1 yr 18 mon 2 yr 3 yr 4 yr 5 yr Other: _____

Initial SST Date: __/__/__ Rx: _____ Surgery Date: __/__/__

Figure 5-52 Simple shoulder test questionnaire form. (From Lippitt SB, et al: A practical tool for evaluating function: the simple shoulder test. In Matsen FA, Fu FH, Hawkins RJ, et al, editors: The shoulder: a balance of mobility and stability, Rosemont, IL, 1993, American Academy of Orthopedic Surgeons, p. 514.)

Please rate your ability to do the following activities in the last week by circling the number below the appropriate response.

	No Difficulty	Mild Difficulty	Moderate Difficulty	Severe Difficulty	Unable
1. Open a tight or new jar.	1	2	3	4	5
2. Write.	1	2	3	4	5
3. Turn a key.	1	2	3	4	5
4. Prepare a meal.	1	2	3	4	5
5. Push open a heavy door.	1	2	3	4	5
6. Place an object on a shelf above your head.	1	2	3	4	5
7. Do heavy household chores (e.g., wash walls, wash floors).	1	2	3	4	5
8. Garden or do yard work.	1	2	3	4	5
9. Make a bed.	1	2	3	4	5
10. Carry a shopping bag or briefcase.	1	2	3	4	5
11. Carry a heavy object (over 10 lbs).	1	2	3	4	5
12. Change a light bulb overhead.	1	2	3	4	5
13. Wash or blow dry your hair.	1	2	3	4	5
14. Wash your back.	1	2	3	4	5
15. Put on a pullover sweater.	1	2	3	4	5
16. Use a knife to cut food.	1	2	3	4	5
17. Recreational activities which require little effort (e.g., cardplaying, knitting, etc.).	1	2	3	4	5
18. Recreational activities in which you take some force or impact through your arm, shoulder or hand (e.g., golf, hammering, tennis, etc.).	1	2	3	4	5
19. Recreational activities in which you move your arm freely (e.g., playing frisbee, badminton, etc.).	1	2	3	4	5
20. Manage transportation needs (getting from one place to another).	1	2	3	4	5
21. Sexual activities.	1	2	3	4	5

DISABILITIES OF THE ARM, SHOULDER, AND HAND

	Not at All	Slightly	Moderately	Quite a Bit	Extremely
22. During the past week, *to what extent* has your arm, shoulder, or hand problem interfered with your normal social activities with family, friends, neighbors or groups? (*circle number*)	1	2	3	4	5

	Not Limited At All	Slightly Limited	Moderately Limited	Very Limited	Unable
23. During the past week, were you limited in your work or other regular daily activities as a result of your arm, shoulder or hand problem? (*circle number*)	1	2	3	4	5

Please rate the severity of the following symptoms in the last week. (*circle number*)

	None	Mild	Moderate	Severe	Extreme
24. Arm, shoulder, or hand pain.	1	2	3	4	5
25. Arm, shoulder, or hand pain when you performed any specific activity.	1	2	3	4	5
26. Tingling (pins and needles) in your arm, shoulder, or hand.	1	2	3	4	5
27. Weakness in your arm, shoulder, or hand.	1	2	3	4	5
28. Stiffness in your arm, shoulder, or hand.	1	2	3	4	5

Figure 5-53 The DASH Questionnaire. (From Dutton M: Orthopedic examination, evaluation and intervention, New York, 2004, McGraw-Hill, pp. 449–450.)

DISABILITIES OF THE ARM, SHOULDER, AND HAND

	No Difficulty	Mild Difficulty	Moderate Difficulty	Severe Difficulty	So Much Difficulty That I Can't Sleep
29. During the past week, how much difficulty have you had sleeping because of the pain in your arm, shoulder or hand? (*circle number*)	1	2	3	4	5

	Strongly Disagree	Disagree	Neither Agree nor Disagree	Agree	Strongly Agree
30. I feel less capable, less confident or less useful because of my arm, shoulder, or hand problem. (*circle number*)	1	2	3	4	5

Scoring DASH function/symptoms: Add up circled responses (item 1–30); subtract 30; divide by 1.20 = DASH score.
SPORTS/PERFORMING ARTS MODULE (Optional)

The following questions relate to the impact of your arm, shoulder, or hand problem on playing *your musical instrument or sport*. If you play more than one sport or instrument (or play both), please answer with respect to that activity which is most important.

Please indicate the sport or instrument which is most important to you: _____

    I do not play a sport or an instrument. (You may skip this section.)

Please circle the number that best describes your physical ability in the past week. Did you have any difficulty:

	No Difficulty	Mild Difficulty	Moderate Difficulty	Severe Difficulty	Unable
1. Using your usual technique for playing your instrument or sport?	1	2	3	4	5
2. Playing your musical instrument or sport because of arm, shoulder, or hand pain?	1	2	3	4	5
3. Playing your musical instrument or sport as well as you would like?	1	2	3	4	5
4. Spending your usual amount of time practicing or playing your instrument or sport?	1	2	3	4	5

WORK MODULE (Optional)

The following questions ask about the impact of your arm, shoulder, or hand problem on your ability to work (including homemakers if that is your main work role).

    I do not work. (You may skip this section.)

Please circle the number that best describes your physical ability in the past week. Did you have any difficulty:

	No Difficulty	Mild Difficulty	Moderate Difficulty	Severe Difficulty	Unable
1. Using your usual technique for your work?	1	2	3	4	5
2. Doing your usual work because of arm, shoulder, or hand pain?	1	2	3	4	5
3. Doing your work as well as you would like?	1	2	3	4	5
4. Spending your usual amount of time doing your work?	1	2	3	4	5

Figure 5-53, cont'd

TABLE **5-16**

Functional Testing of the Shoulder

Starting Position	Action	Function Test*
Sitting	Forward flex arm to 90°	Lift 4 lb to 5 lb weight: Functional Lift 1 lb to 3 lb weight: Functionally fair Lift arm weight: Functionally poor Cannot lift arm: Nonfunctional
Sitting	Shoulder extension	Lift 4 lb to 5 lb weight: Functional Lift 1 lb to 3 lb weight: Functionally fair Lift arm weight: Functionally poor Cannot lift arm: Nonfunctional
Side lying (may be done in sitting with pulley)	Shoulder medial rotation	Lift 4 lb to 5 lb weight: Functional Lift 1 lb to 3 lb weight: Functionally fair Lift arm weight: Functionally poor Cannot lift arm: Nonfunctional
Side lying (may be done in sitting with pulley)	Shoulder lateral rotation	Lift 4 lb to 5 lb weight: Functional Lift 1 lb to 3 lb weight: Functionally fair Lift arm weight: Functionally poor Cannot lift arm: Nonfunctional
Sitting	Shoulder abduction	Lift 4 lb to 5 lb weight: Functional Lift 1 lb to 3 lb weight: Functionally fair Lift arm weight: Functionally poor Cannot lift arm: Nonfunctional
Sitting	Shoulder adduction (using wall pulley)	Lift 4 lb to 5 lb weight: Functional Lift 1 lb to 3 lb weight: Functionally fair Lift arm weight: Functionally poor Cannot lift arm: Nonfunctional
Sitting	Shoulder elevation (shoulder shrug)	5 to 6 Repetitions: Functional 3 to 4 Repetitions: Functionally fair 1 to 2 Repetitions: Functionally poor 0 Repetitions: Nonfunctional
Sitting	Sitting pushup (shoulder dysfunction)	5 to 6 Repetitions: Functional 3 to 4 Repetitions: Functionally fair 1 to 2 Repetitions: Functionally poor 0 Repetitions: Nonfunctional

Data from Palmer ML, Epler M: Clinical assessment procedures in physical therapy, Philadelphia, 1990, JB Lippincott, pp. 68–73.
*Younger, more fit patients should easily be able to do more than the values given for these tests. A comparison between the good side and the injured side gives the examiner some idea about the patient's functional strength capacity.

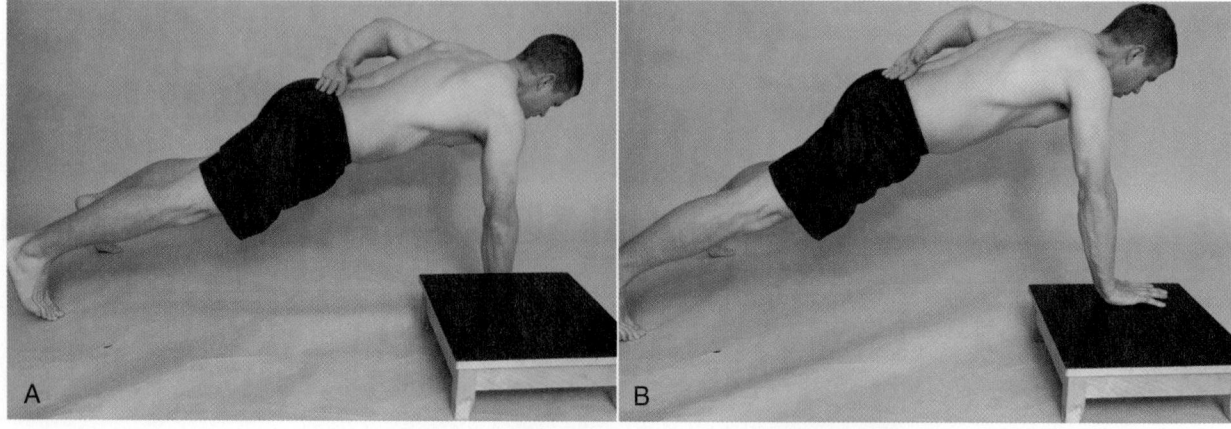

Figure 5-54 One-arm hop test. A, Start position. **B,** End position.

Key Tests Performed at the Shoulder Depending on Suspected Pathology*

- *For anterior shoulder (glenohumeral) instability:*
  - ✓ Anterior/apprehension release ("surprise") test
  - ⚠ Anterior drawer test
  - ✓ Crank (apprehension) and relocation test
  - ? Fulcrum test
  - ⚠ Load and shift test
- *For posterior shoulder (glenohumeral) instability:*
  - ✓ Jerk test
  - ⚠ Load and shift test
  - ? Norwood test
  - ? Posterior apprehension test
  - ? Posterior drawer test
- *For inferior and multidirectional shoulder (glenohumeral) instability:*
  - ? Feagin test
  - ✓ Sulcus sign
- *For anterior impingement:*
  - ✓ Coracoid impingement sign
  - ✓ Hawkins-Kennedy test
  - ✓ Neer test
  - ✓ Supine impingement test
  - ✓ Yokum test
  - ✓ Zaslav test (internal rotation resistance strength test [IRRST])
- *For posterior impingement:*
  - ? Posterior internal impingement test
- *For labral lesions:†*
  - ✓ Active compression test of O'Brien
  - ⚠ Anterior slide test
  - ⚠ Biceps tension test
  - ⚠ Biceps load test (Kim test II)
  - ⚠ Clunk test
  - ⚠ Compression rotation test
  - ? Dynamic labral shear test
  - ⚠ Forced shoulder abduction and elbow flexion test
  - ✓ Kim test I (biceps load test II)
  - ⚠ Mayo shear test
  - ⚠ Pain provocation test
  - ⚠ Resisted supination external rotation test (RSERT)
- *For scapular dyskinesia:*
  - ⚠ Lateral scapular slide test
  - ✓ Scapular load test
  - ⚠ Scapular retraction test (SRT)
  - ? Wall/floor pushup

- *For acromioclavicular joint pathology:*
  - ✓ Horizontal adduction test
  - ✓ Paxinos sign
- *For ligament pathology:*
  - ? Coracoclavicular ligament test
  - ✓ Crank test
- *For muscle pathology:†*
  Biceps
  - ✓ Speed's test
  - ✓ Yergason's test
  Supraspinatus
  - ⚠ Drop arm test
  - ✓ "Empty can" test
  Subscapularis
  - ? Bear-hug test
  - ? Belly press test (abdominal compression or Napolean test)
  - ✓ External rotation lag sign (ERLS)
  - ✓ Lift-off sign (Gerber's test)
  - ✓ Medial rotation lag or "spring back" test
  Infraspinatus
  - ⚠ Dropping sign
  - ✓ Infraspinatus test
  - ✓ Lateral rotation lag sign
  Teres Minor
  - ⚠ Hornblower's sign
  Rotator Cuff (general)
  - ✓ Rent test
  - ✓ Whipple test
  Trapezius
  - ✓ Trapezius test (three positions)
  Serratus Anterior
  - ✓ Punch out test
- *For neurological function:*
  - ✓ Upper limb neurodynamic (tension) test (ULNT)
    Median nerve (ULNTI)
    Median nerve (ULNTII)
    Radial nerve (ULNTIII)
    Ulnar nerve (ULNTIV)
- *For thoracic outlet syndrome:*
  - ⚠ Roos test

*See Chapter 1, p. 55, Key for Classifying Special Tests.
†Research has shown that no single test or even a group of tests can accurately diagnose a SLAP or rotator cuff lesion.[53,159–165]

As secondary impingement is primarily a problem with muscle dynamics, it commonly presents in conjunction with instability, either of the scapula or at the glenohumeral joint. A hypermobile or lax joint does not imply instability.[167] Laxity implies that there is a certain amount of nonpathological "looseness" in a joint so that ROM is greater in one or more directions and the shoulder complex functions normally. It is usually found bilaterally. Instability implies that the patient is unable to control or stabilize a joint during motion or in a static position either because static restraints have been injured (as would be noted in an anterior dislocation with tearing of the capsule and labrum, also called *gross* or *anatomical instability*), or because the muscles controlling the joint are weak or the force couples are unbalanced (also called *translational instability*).[168]

Both primary and second impingements occur anteriorly (thus, the terms **anterior primary impingement** or

TABLE **5-17**

Differential Diagnosis of Shoulder Instability (AMBRI) versus Traumatic Anterior Dislocation (TUBS)

	Shoulder Instability	Traumatic Anterior Dislocation
History	Feeling of shoulder slippage with pain Feeling of insecurity when doing specific activities No history of injury	Arm elevated and laterally rotated relative to body Feeling of insecurity when in specific position (of dislocation) Recurrent episodes of apprehension
Observation	Normal	Normal (if reduced) (if not, loss of rounding of deltoid caused by anterior dislocation)
Active movement	Normal ROM May be abnormal or painful at activity speed	Apprehension and decreased ROM in abduction and lateral rotation
Passive movement	Normal ROM Pain at extreme of ROM possible	Muscle guarding and decreased ROM in apprehension position
Resisted isometric movement	Normal in test position May be weak in provocative position	Pain into abduction and lateral rotation
Special tests	Load and shift test is positive	Apprehension positive Augmentation positive Relocation positive
Reflexes and cutaneous distribution	Normal reflexes and sensation	Reflexes normal Sensation normal, unless axillary or musculocutaneous nerve is injured
Palpation	Normal	Anterior shoulder is tender
Diagnostic imaging	Normal	Normal, unless still dislocated; defect possible

ROM, Range of motion.

anterior secondary impingement). Because the areas of impingement are in the supraspinatus outlet area, they are also called **outlet impingement syndromes.**[46]

Jobe and colleagues believed that impingement and instability often occur together in throwing athletes and, based on that assumption, developed the following classification[32,169]:
- Grade I: Pure impingement with no instability (often seen in older patients)
- Grade II: Secondary impingement and instability caused by chronic capsular and labral microtrauma
- Grade III: Secondary impingement and instability caused by generalized hypermobility or laxity
- Grade IV: Primary instability with no impingement

In this classification, secondary impingement implies the impingement occurs secondarily and that the main problem is instability.

A third type of impingement is termed **internal impingement** or nonoutlet impingement. This type of impingement is found posteriorly rather than anteriorly, mostly in overhead athletes. It involves contact of the undersurface of the rotator cuff (primarily supraspinatus and infraspinatus) with the posterosuperior glenoid labrum when the arm is abducted to 90° and laterally rotated fully.[155,170–175]

If the patient history indicates instability, then at least one test each for anterior, posterior, and multidirectional instability should be performed. Because of the interrelation of impingement and instability, tests for both should be applied if the patient history indicates that either condition may be present.[175] Traumatic, first-time subluxations and dislocations may result in a torn labrum (Bankart or SLAP), Hill-Sach lesion, osteochondral lesion, and/or capsular damage, and so the examiner should consider the possibility of these problems existing during the assessment.[176]

When looking at shoulder instability, it is important to realize that instability includes a spectrum of conditions from gross or anatomical instability (as seen with the TUBS lesion) to translational instability (muscle weakness) (as seen with AMBRI lesions)[57] (Table 5-17). Burkhart, et al.[25] also included **pseudolaxity,** which includes altered glenohumeral arthrokinematics because of the presence of a SLAP lesion, a tight posteroinferior capsule, and often scapular dyskinesia. They felt the apparent increased anterior laxity resulted from the decreased cam effect in the glenohumeral joint combined with functional lengthening of the anteroinferior capsule and glenohumeral ligament.[25] A posterosuperior SLAP lesion allows laxity on the opposite side (circle concept of instability).[25] With the instability tests, the examiner is trying to duplicate the patient's symptoms as well as feel for abnormal movement. Therefore, a response of "that's what my shoulder feels like when it bothers me" is much

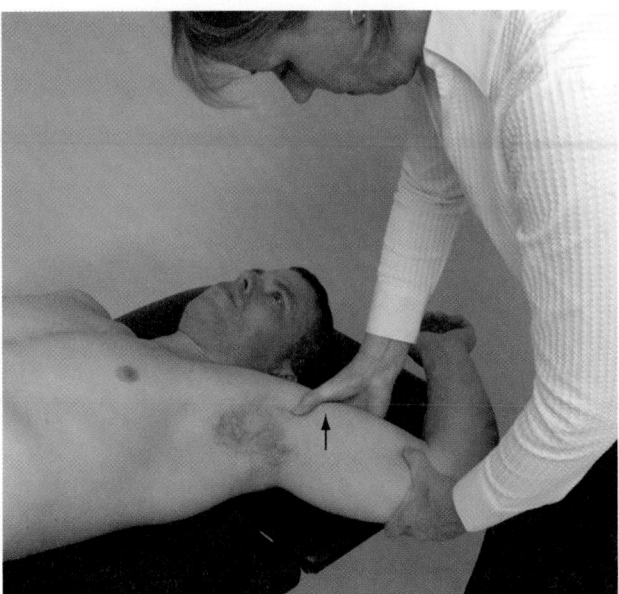

Figure 5-55 Andrews' anterior instability test.

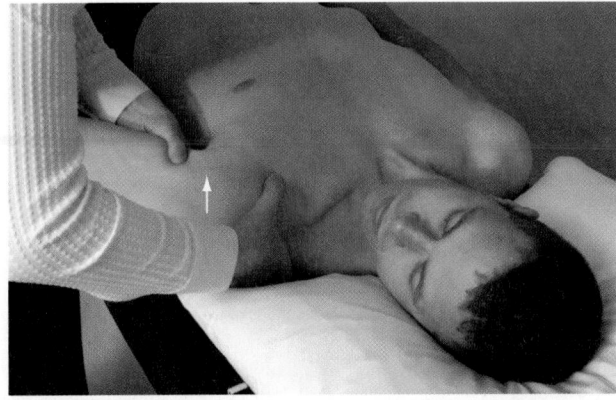

Figure 5-56 Anterior drawer test of the shoulder.

more significant than the degree of laxity or translation found.[57]

Tests for Anterior Shoulder Instability

Andrews' Anterior Instability Test.[177] The patient lies supine with the shoulder abducted 130° and laterally rotated 90°. The examiner stabilizes the elbow and distal humerus with one hand and uses the other hand to grasp the humeral head and lift it forward (Figure 5-55). A reproduction of the patient's symptoms gives a positive test for anterior instability. If the examiner hears a clunk, an anterior labral tear may be present. This test is a modification of the load and shift test.

Anterior Drawer Test of the Shoulder.[178] The patient lies supine. The examiner places the hand of the affected shoulder in the examiner's axilla, holding the patient's hand with the arm so that the patient remains relaxed. The shoulder to be tested is abducted between 80° and 120°, forward flexed up to 20°, and laterally rotated up to 30°. The examiner then stabilizes the patient's scapula with the opposite hand, pushing the spine of the scapula forward with the index and middle fingers. The examiner's thumb exerts counterpressure on the patient's coracoid process. Using the arm that is holding the patient's hand, the examiner places his or her hand around the patient's relaxed upper arm and draws the humerus forward. The movement may be accompanied by a click, by patient apprehension, or both. The amount of movement available is compared with that of the normal side. A positive test indicates anterior instability (Figure 5-56), depending on the amount of anterior translation. The click may indicate a labral tear or slippage of the humeral head over the glenoid rim. This test is a modification of the load and shift test.

Anterior Instability Test (Leffert's Test).[179] The examiner stands behind the shoulder being examined while the patient sits. The examiner places his or her near hand over the shoulder so that the index finger is over the head of the humerus anteriorly and the middle finger is over the coracoid process. The thumb is placed over the posterior humeral head. The examiner's other hand grasps the patient's wrist and carefully abducts and laterally rotates the arm (Figure 5-57). If, on movement of the arm, the finger palpating the anterior humeral head moves forward, the test is said to be positive for anterior instability. Normally, the two fingers remain in the same plane. With a positive test, when the arm is returned to the starting position, the index finger returns to the starting position as the humeral head glides backward.

Apprehension (Crank) Test for Anterior Shoulder Dislocation.[157] This test is primarily designed to check for traumatic instability problems causing gross or anatomical instability of the shoulder, although the relocation portion of the test is sometimes used to differentiate between instability and impingement. The examiner abducts the arm to 90° and laterally rotates the patient's shoulder slowly (Figure 5-58). By placing a hand under the glenohumeral joint to act as a fulcrum (Figure 5-59), the apprehension test becomes the **fulcrum test.**[180] Kvitne and Jobe[32] recommended applying a mild anteriorly-directed force to the posterior humeral head when in the test position to see if apprehension or pain increases (Figure 5-60). If posterior pain increases, this indicates posterior internal impingement.[174] Hamner, et al.[181] suggested that if posterior superior internal impingement is suspected, the relocation test should be done in 110° and 120° of abduction. Translation of the humeral head in the glenoid is less than with other tests, provided the joint is normal, because the test is taking the joint into the close packed position.[182] A positive test is indicated when the patient looks or feels apprehensive or alarmed and resists further motion. Thus, the patient's apprehension is greater than the complaint of pain (i.e., apprehension predominates). The patient may also state that the feeling resembles what it felt like when the shoulder was dislocated. This test *must* be done slowly.

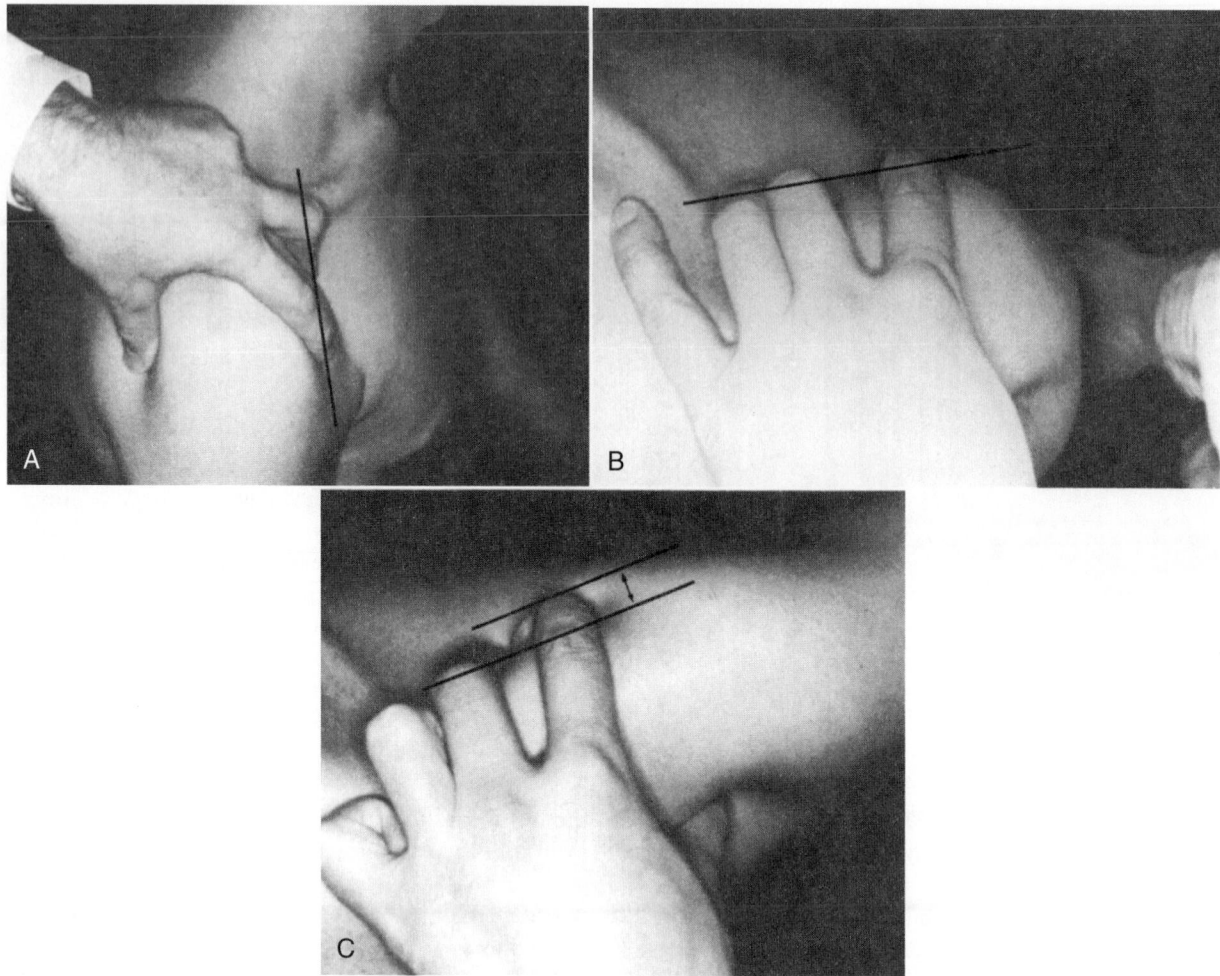

Figure 5-57 Anterior instability test. A, Side view. **B,** Superior view. With the patient's arm by the side, the examiner's fingers are in the same plane. **C,** With a positive test, on abduction and lateral rotation, the index and middle fingers are no longer in the same plane. (Adapted from Leffert RD, Gumbery G: The relationship between dead arm syndrome and thoracic outlet syndrome. Clin Orthop Relat Res 223: 22–23, 1987.)

If the test is done too quickly, the humerus may dislocate. Hawkins and Bokor noted that the examiner should observe the amount of lateral rotation that exists when the patient becomes apprehensive and compare the range with the uninjured side.[183]

If the examiner then applies a posterior translation stress to the head of the humerus or the arm **(relocation test),** the patient commonly loses the apprehension, any pain that is present commonly decreases, and further lateral rotation is possible before the apprehension or pain returns (see Figures 5-60, *A*, and 5-60, *C*). This relocation is sometimes referred to as the **Fowler sign or test** ☑ or the **Jobe relocation test** ☑. The test is considered positive if pain decreases during the maneuver, even if there was no apprehension.[184,185] If the patient's symptoms decrease or are eliminated when doing the relocation test, the diagnosis is glenohumeral instability, subluxation, dislocation, or impingement. If apprehension predominated when doing the crank test and disappears with the relocation test, the diagnosis is glenohumeral instability, subluxation, or dislocation. If pain predominated when doing the crank test and disappears with the relocation test, the diagnosis is pseudolaxity or anterior instability either at the glenohumeral joint or scapulothoracic joint with secondary impingement or a posterior SLAP lesion.[186] The relocation test does not alter the pain for patients with primary impingement.[32,169,187] If, when doing the relocation test posteriorly, posterior pain decreases, it is a positive test for posterior internal impingement.[174,188] If the arm is released **(anterior release** or **"surprise" test** ☑ [see Figure 5-60, *D*]) in the newly acquired range, pain and forward translation of the head are noted in positive tests.[175,185,189] The resulting pain from this release procedure may be caused by anterior shoulder instability, labral lesion (Bankart lesion or SLAP lesion—superior labrum, anterior posterior), or bicipital peritenonitis or tendinosus. Most commonly, it is related to anterior instability because the pain is temporarily produced by the anterior translation.[189] It has also been reported to cause pain in older patients with rotator cuff

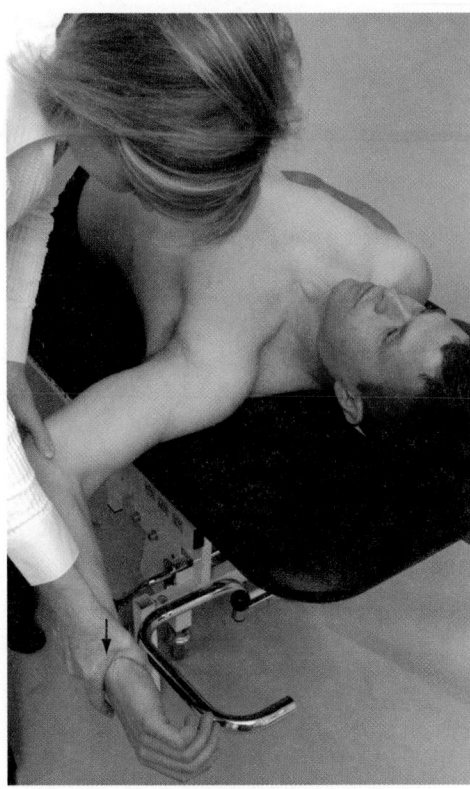

Figure 5-58 Anterior apprehension (crank) test.

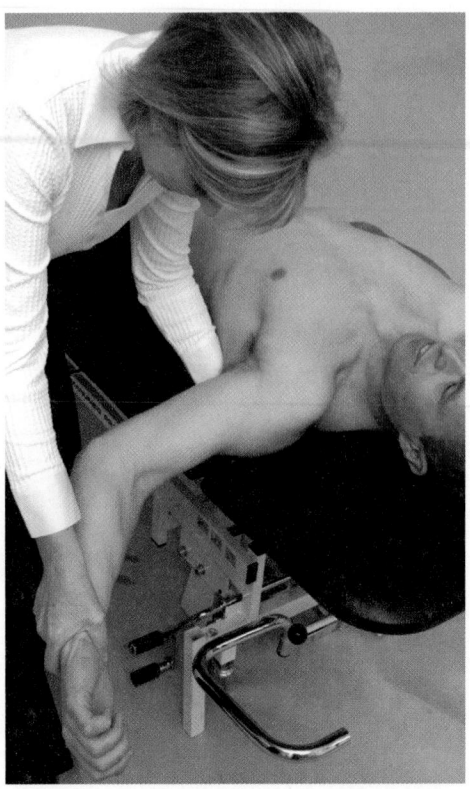

Figure 5-59 Fulcrum test with left fist pushing head of humerus anteriorly.

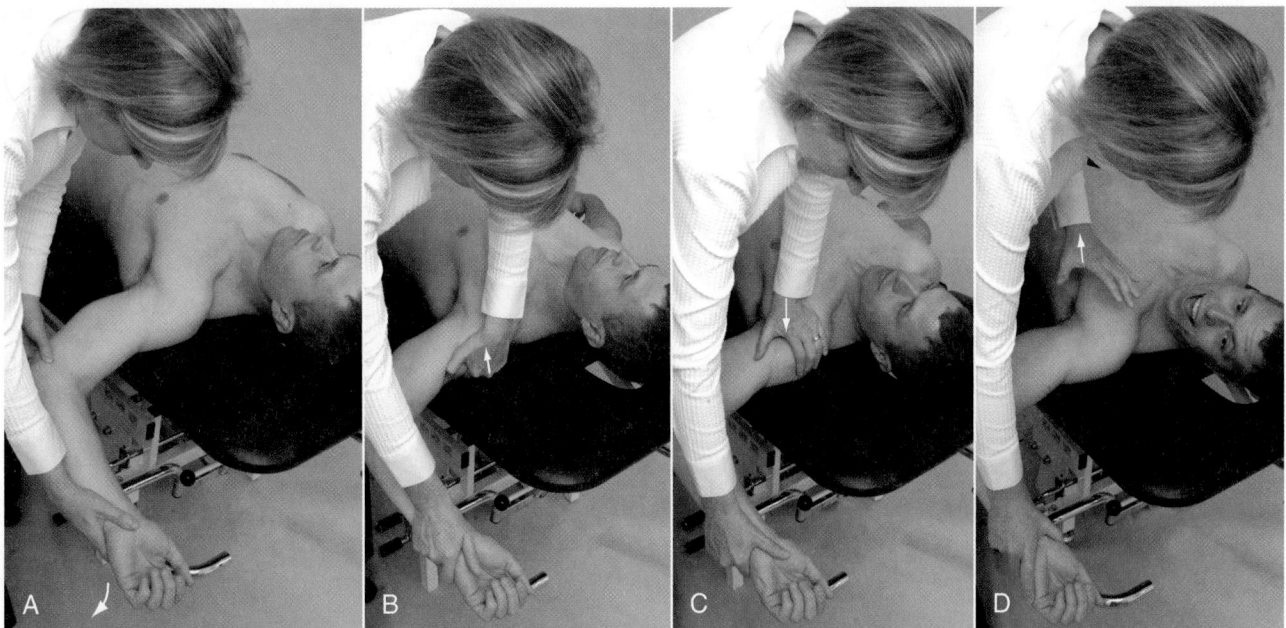

Figure 5-60 Crank and relocation test. A, Abduction and lateral rotation (crank test). **B,** Abduction and lateral rotation combined with anterior translation of humerus, which may cause anterior subluxation or posterior joint pain. **C,** Abduction and lateral rotation combined with posterior translation of the humerus (relocation test). **D,** "Surprise" test.

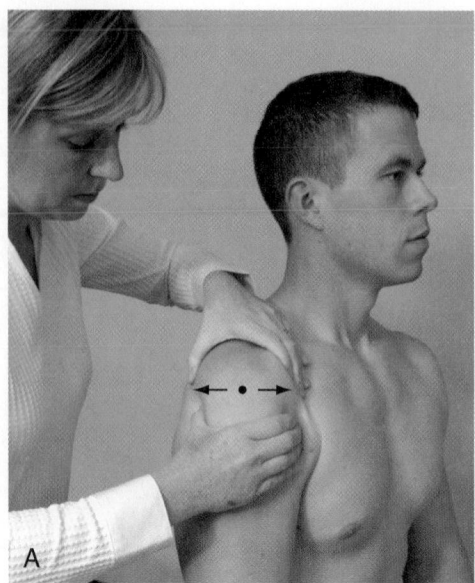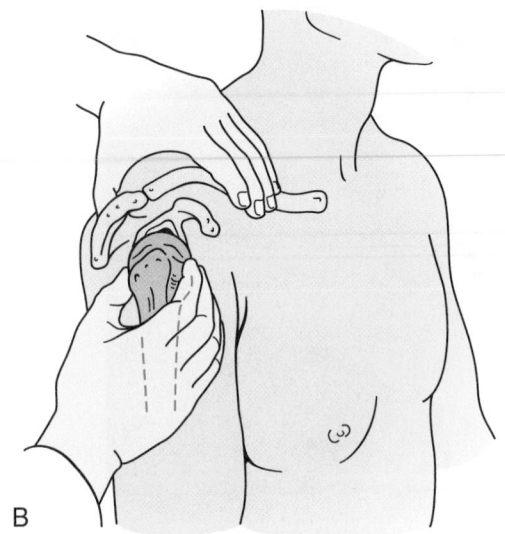

Figure 5-61 **A, Load and shift test** in sitting starting position. Note that the humerus is loaded or "centered" in the glenoid to begin. Examiner then shifts humerus anteriorly or posteriorly. **B,** Line drawing showing position of examiner's hands in relation to bones of patient's shoulder. Notice that examiner's left thumb holds the spine of the scapula for stability.

pathology and no instability.[190] This release maneuver should be done with care, because it often causes apprehension and distrust on the part of the patient, and it could cause a dislocation, especially in patients who have had recurrent dislocations. For most patients, therefore, when doing the relocation test, lateral rotation should be released before the posterior stress is released.

The crank test may be modified to test lateral rotation at different degrees of abduction, depending on the patient history and mechanism of injury.[191] The Rockwood test described later is simply a modification of the crank test.

? Dugas' Test.[192] This test is used if an unreduced anterior shoulder dislocation is suspected. The patient is asked to place the hand on the opposite shoulder and then attempt to lower the elbow to the chest. With an anterior dislocation, this is not possible, and pain in the shoulder results. If the pain is only over the acromioclavicular joint, problems in that joint should be suspected.

⚠ Load and Shift Test.[99,184] This test is designed to check primarily atraumatic instability problems of the glenohumeral joint. The patient sits with no back support and with the hand of the test arm resting on the thigh. Ideally, the patient should be sitting in a properly aligned posture (i.e., ear lobe, tip of acromion, and high point of iliac crest in a straight line). If the patient slouches forward, the scapula protracts, causing the humeral head to translate anteriorly in the glenoid and narrows the subacromial space.[193] For best results, the muscles about the shoulder should be as relaxed as possible. The examiner stands or sits slightly behind the patient and stabilizes

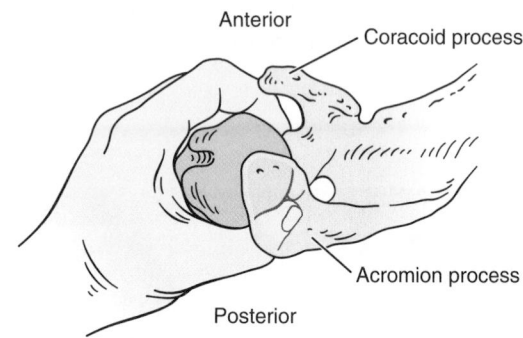

Figure 5-62 Superior view of the shoulder showing palpation of the anterior and posterior glenohumeral joint to ensure the humeral head is centered in the glenoid.

the shoulder with one hand over the clavicle and scapula (Figure 5-61, *A*). With the other hand, the examiner grasps the head of the humerus with the thumb over the posterior humeral head and the fingers over the anterior humeral head (Figure 5-61, *B*). The examiner runs the fingers along the anterior humerus and the thumb along the posterior humerus to feel where the humerus is seated relative to the glenoid (Figure 5-62). If the fingers "dip in" anteriorly as they move medially but the thumb does not, it indicates the humeral head is sitting anteriorly. Normally, the humeral head feels a bit more anterior (i.e., the "dip" is slightly greater anteriorly) when it is properly "seated" in the glenoid. Protraction of the scapula causes the glenoid head to shift anteriorly in the glenoid. The examiner must be careful with the finger and thumb placement. In the presence of anterior or posterior pathology, finger and thumb placement may cause pain. The humerus is then gently pushed anteriorly or posteriorly (most common) in the glenoid if necessary to seat it properly in the glenoid fossa.[175] The seating places the head of the humerus in its normal position relative to the glenoid.[47] This is the "load" portion of the test. If the load is not applied (as in the anterior drawer test), there is no "normal" or standard starting position for the test. The examiner then pushes the humeral head anteriorly (anterior instability) or posteriorly (posterior instability), noting the amount of translation and end feel. This is the "shift" portion of the test.

With anterior translation, if the head is not centered, posterior translation will be greater than anterior translation, giving a false negative test. If the head is properly centered first, however, with anterior instability present, anterior translation is possible, but posterior translation is virtually absent because of the tight posterior capsule that accompanies a positive anterior instability. Differences between affected and normal sides should be compared in terms of the amount of translation and the ease with which it occurs. This comparison, along with reproduction of the patient's symptoms, is often considered more important than the amount of movement obtained. If the patient has multidirectional instability, both anterior and posterior translation may be excessive on the affected side compared with the normal side. The test may also be done with the patient in supine lying position.

Translation of 25% or less, of the humeral head diameter anteriorly, is considered normal although results vary among patients.[183,194] Generally, anterior translation is less than posterior translation, although some authors disagree with this and say that anterior and posterior translation are virtually equal.[195,196] Sauers, et al.[196] and Ellenbecker, et al.[197] stated that hand dominance does not affect the amount of translation, but Lintner, et al.[198] disagreed saying that the nondominant shoulder shows more translation. Hawkins and Mohtadi,[184] Silliman and Hawkins,[175] and Altchek, et al.[199] advocated a three-grade system for anterior translation (Figure 5-63). These authors feel that the head normally translates 0% to 25% of the diameter of the humeral head. Up to 50% of humeral head translation, with the head riding up to the glenoid rim and spontaneous reduction, is considered grade I. For grade II, the humeral head has more than 50% translation; the head feels as though it is riding over the glenoid rim but spontaneously reduces. Normal hypermobile shoulders may show grade II translation in any direction.[198] Grade III implies that the humeral head rides over the glenoid rim and does not spontaneously reduce. For posterior translation, translation of 50% of the diameter of the humeral head is considered normal, although results vary among patients.[182] Thus, normally, one would expect greater posterior translation than anterior translation when doing the test. However, all authors do not support this view.

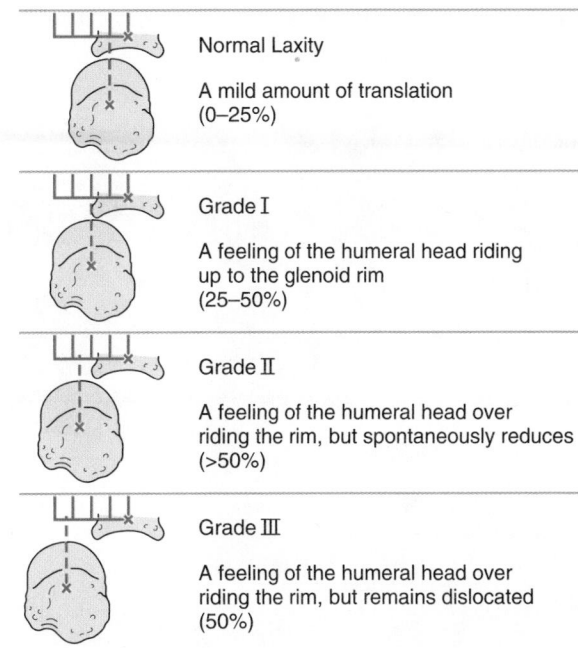

Figure 5-63 Grades of anterior glenohumeral translation.

Normal Laxity

A mild amount of translation (0–25%)

Grade I

A feeling of the humeral head riding up to the glenoid rim (25–50%)

Grade II

A feeling of the humeral head over riding the rim, but spontaneously reduces (>50%)

Grade III

A feeling of the humeral head over riding the rim, but remains dislocated (50%)

The load and shift test may also be done in supine lying position.[191] To test anterior translation, the patient's arm is taken to 45° to 60° scaption (abduction in the plane of the scapula) and in neutral rotation by the examiner holding the forearm near the wrist (Figure 5-64). The examiner then places the other hand around the patient's upper arm near the deltoid insertion with the thumb anterior and the fingers posterior feeling the movement of the humeral head in the glenoid while applying an anterior or anteroinferior translation force (with the fingers) or a posterior translation force (with the thumb). Ideally, the humerus should be "loaded" in the glenoid before starting the test. With the hand holding the forearm, the examiner controls the arm position and applies an axial load to the humerus. During the translation movements with the thumb or fingers, the scapula should not move. As the anterior or anteroinferior translation force is applied, the examiner, using the other hand (the one holding the forearm) incrementally, laterally rotates the humerus (Figure 5-64, *B*). This causes greater involvement of the anterior band of the inferior glenohumeral ligament, which, if intact, will limit movement so the amount of anterior translation decreases as lateral rotation increases. To test posterior translation (posterior instability), the arm is placed in scaption with 45° to 60° of lateral rotation (Figure 5-65). In this case, the thumb pushes the humerus posteriorly.[191,200] Incrementally, while applying the posterior translation, the examiner medially rotates the arm. Medial rotation causes the posterior band of the inferior glenohumeral ligament and the posteroinferior capsule to become increasingly tight so that posterior translation decreases as medial rotation increases.

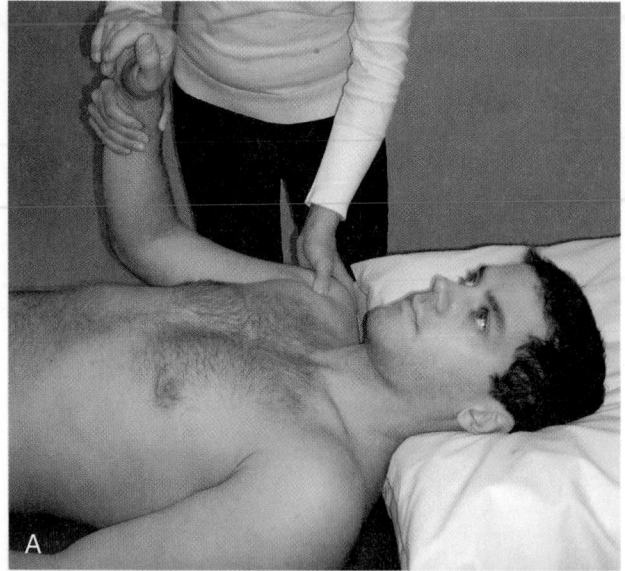

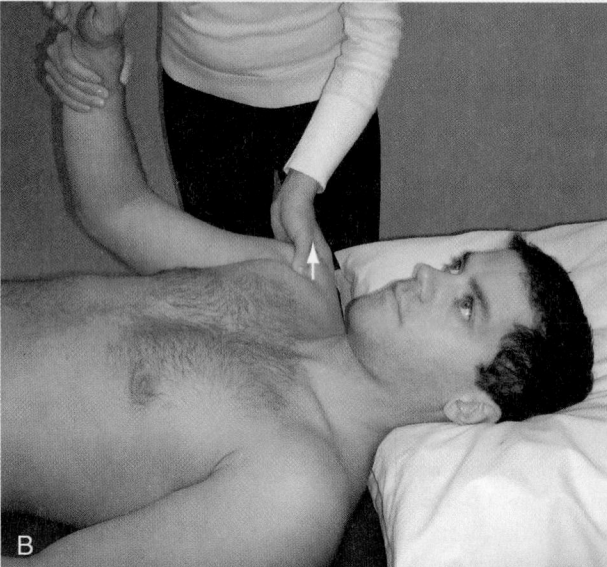

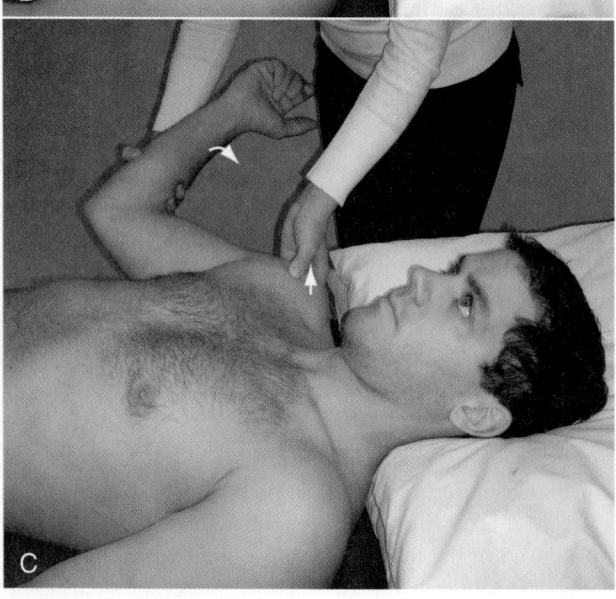

Figure 5-64 **A,** Initial position for load and shift test for anterior instability testing of the shoulder in supine lying position. The examiner's hand grasps the patient's upper arm with the fingers posterior. The examiner's arm positions the patient's arm and controls its rotation. The arm is placed in the plane of the scapula, abducted 45° to 60°, and maintained in 0° of rotation. The examiner's arm places an axial load to the patient's arm through the humerus. The examiner's fingers then shift the humeral head anteriorly, and anteroinferiorly over the glenoid rim. **B,** The second position for the load and shift test for anterior stability is as described in **A** for the initial position, except that the arm is progressively laterally rotated in 10° to 20° increments while the anterior dislocation force is alternatively applied and released. **C,** The examiner quantifies the degree of lateral rotation required to reduce the translation from grade 3 or 2 to grade 1. The examiner compares the normal and abnormal shoulders for this difference in translation with the humeral rotation. The degree of rotation required to reduce the translation is an indicator of the functional laxity of the anterior inferior capsular ligaments.

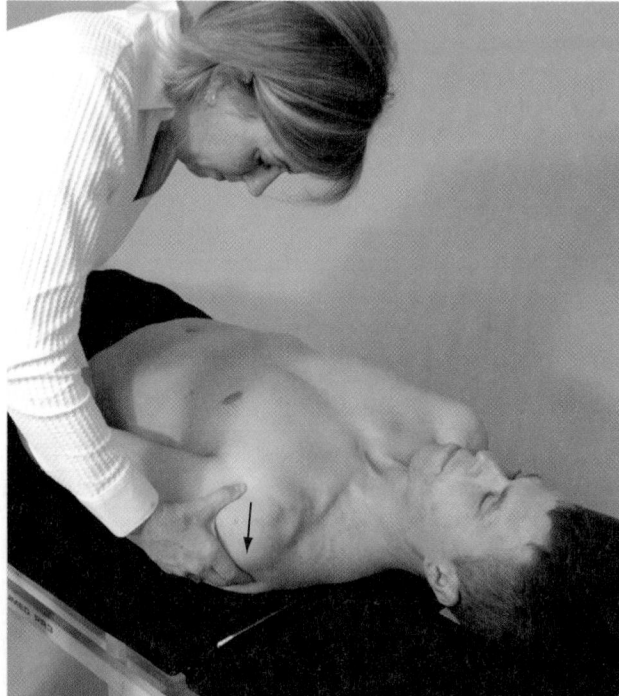

Figure 5-65 **Load and shift test for posterior instability testing of the shoulder in supine lying position.** The patient is supine on the examining table. The arm is brought into approximately 90° of forward elevation in the plane of the scapula. A posteriorly directed force is applied to the humerus with the arm in varying degrees of lateral rotation.

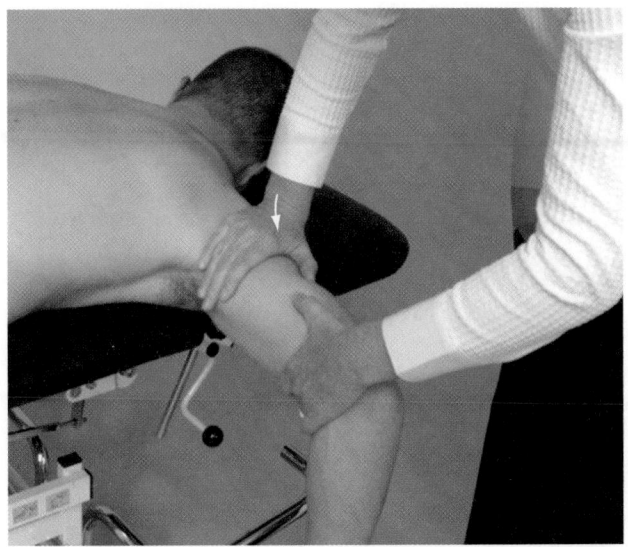

Figure 5-66 **Prone anterior instability test.** Examiner stabilizes the arm in 90° abduction and lateral rotation and then pushes anteriorly on the humerus.

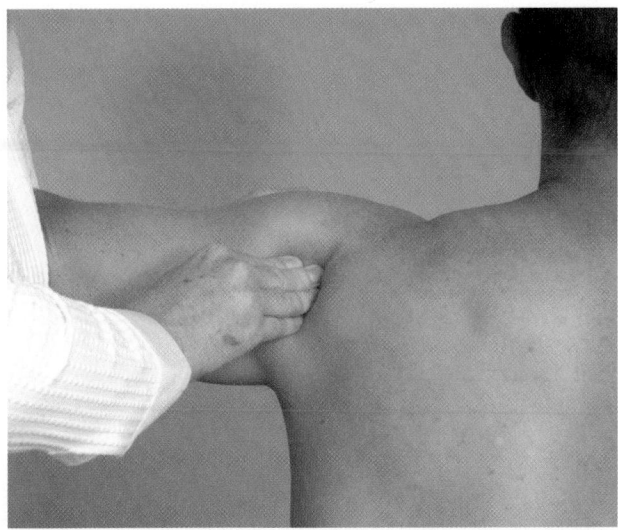

Figure 5-67 Protzman test for anterior instability (posterior view).

⍰ *Prone Anterior Instability Test.*[177] The patient lies prone. The examiner abducts the patient's arm to 90° and laterally rotates it 90°. While holding this position with one hand at the elbow, the examiner places the other hand over the humeral head and pushes it forward (Figure 5-66). A reproduction of the patient's symptoms indicates a positive test for anterior instability. This test is a modification of the load and shift test.

⍰ *Protzman Test for Anterior Instability.*[201] The patient is sitting. The examiner abducts the patient's arm to 90° and supports the arm against the examiner's hip so that the patient's shoulder muscles are relaxed. The examiner palpates the anterior aspect of the head of the humerus with the fingers of one hand deep in the patient's axilla while the fingers of the other hand are placed over the posterior aspect of the humeral head. The examiner then pushes the humeral head anteriorly and inferiorly (Figure 5-67). If this movement causes pain and if palpation indicates abnormal anteroinferior movement, the test is positive for anterior instability. Normally, anterior translation should be no more than 25% of the diameter of the humeral head.[202] A click may sometimes be palpated as the humeral head slides over the glenoid rim. The test may also be done with the patient in the supine lying position with the elbow supported on a pillow.

⍰ *Rockwood Test for Anterior Instability.*[203] The examiner stands behind the seated patient. With the arm at the patient's side, the examiner laterally rotates the shoulder. The arm is abducted to 45°, and passive lateral rotation is repeated. The same procedure is repeated at 90° and 120° (Figure 5-68). These different positions are performed because the stabilizers of the shoulder vary as the angle of abduction changes (see Table 5-1). For the test to be positive, the patient must show marked

apprehension with posterior pain when the arm is tested at 90°. At 45° and 120°, the patient shows some uneasiness and some pain; at 0°, there is rarely apprehension.

Similarly, the Rowe and fulcrum tests stress the anterior shoulder structures. They are more likely to bring on apprehension sooner, because they stress the anterior structures sooner (i.e., the examiner pushes the head of the humerus forward). In effect, they are the opposite of the relocation test; they are therefore called **augmentation tests.**

⍰ *Rowe Test for Anterior Instability.*[204] The patient lies supine and places the hand behind the head. The examiner places one hand (clenched fist) against the posterior humeral head and pushes up while extending the arm slightly (Figure 5-69). This part is similar to the fulcrum test. A look of apprehension or pain indicates a positive test for anterior instability. If a clunk or grinding sound may indicate a torn anterior labrum (see clunk test under "Tests for Labral Tears").

Tests for Posterior Shoulder Instability[205]

⍰ *Circumduction Test.*[206] The patient is in the standing position. The examiner stands behind the patient grasping the patient's forearm with the hand. The examiner begins circumduction by extending the patient's arm while maintaining slight abduction. As the circumduction continues into elevation, the arm is brought over the top and into the flexed and adducted position. As the arm moves into forward flexion and adduction from above, it is vulnerable to posterior subluxation if the patient is unstable posteriorly. If the examiner palpates the posterior aspect of the patient's shoulder as the arm moves downward in forward flexion and adduction, the humeral head will be felt to sublux posteriorly in a positive test, and the patient will say, "That's what it feels like when it bothers me" (Figure 5-70).

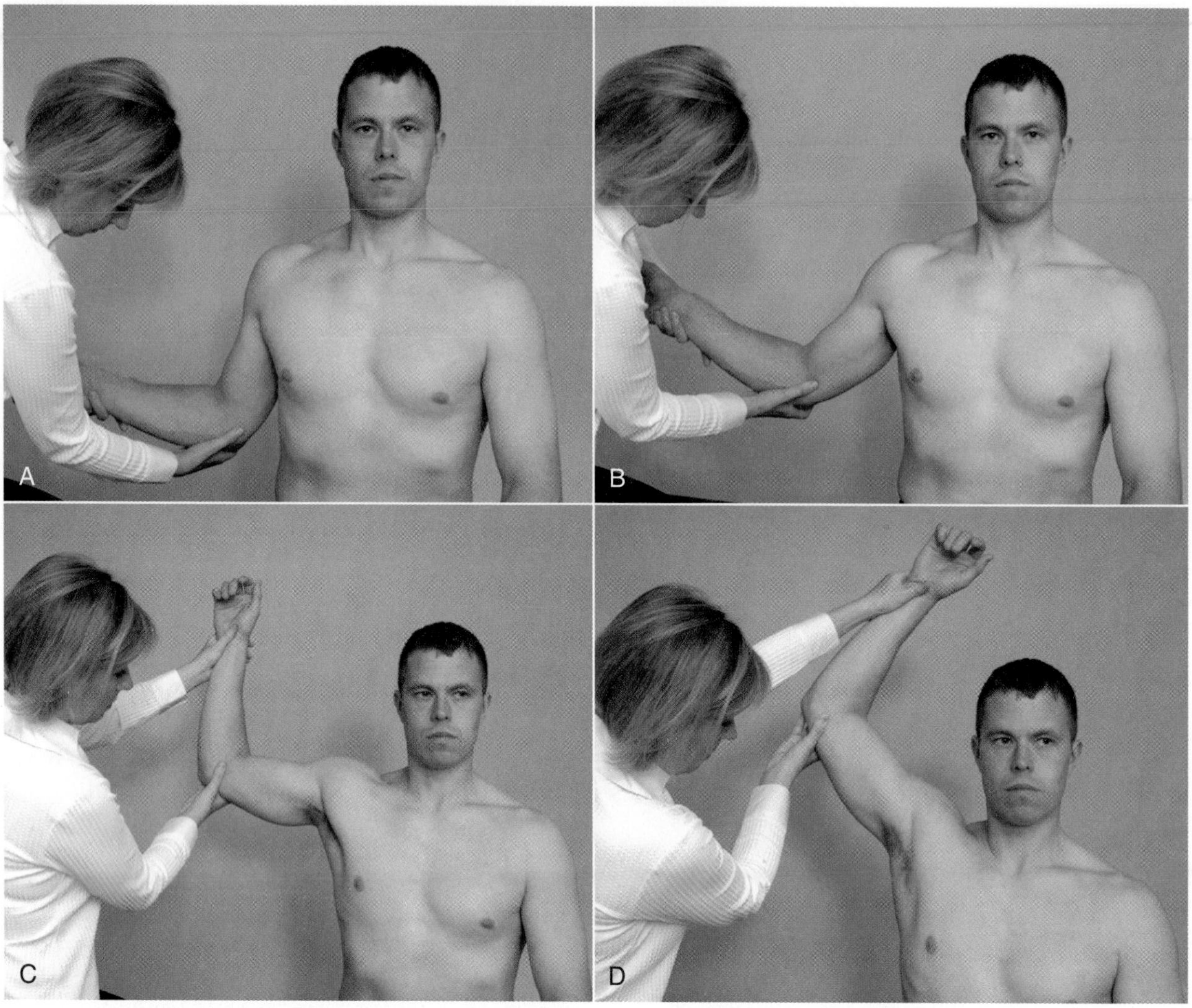

Figure 5-68 **Rockwood test for anterior instability. A,** Arm at side. **B,** Arm at 45°. **C,** Arm at 90°. **D,** Arm at 120°.

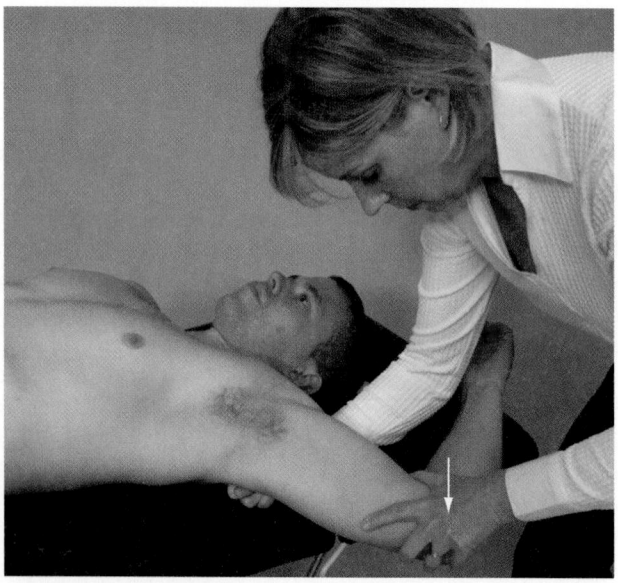

Figure 5-69 **Rowe test for anterior instability.**

✓ *Jerk Test.*[180,207,208] The patient sits with the arm medially rotated and forward flexed to 90°. The examiner grasps the patient's elbow and axially loads the humerus in a proximal direction. While maintaining the axial loading, the examiner moves the arm horizontally (cross-flexion/horizontal adduction) across the body (Figure 5-71). A positive test for recurrent posterior instability is the production of a sudden jerk or clunk as the humeral head slides off (subluxes) the back of the glenoid (Figure 5-72). When the arm is returned to the original 90° abduction position, a second jerk may be felt as the head reduces. Kim, et al.[208] reported that the positive signs also indicate a positive test for a posteroinferior labral tear.

⚠ *Load and Shift Test.* This test is described under anterior shoulder instability.

❓ *Miniaci Test for Posterior Subluxation.*[209] The patient lies supine with the shoulder off the edge of the examining table. The examiner uses one hand to flex (70° to 90°), adduct, and medially rotate the arm while pushing

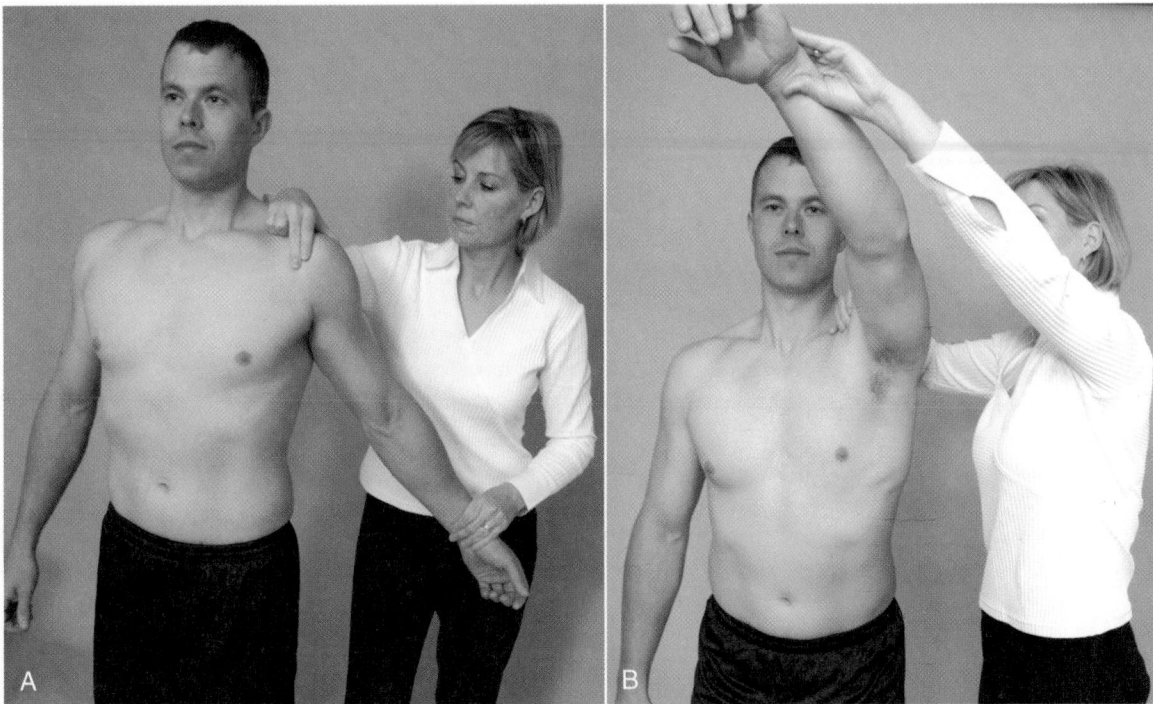

Figure 5-70 Circumduction test. **A,** Starting position. **B,** The flexed adducted position where the shoulder is vulnerable to posterior subluxation.

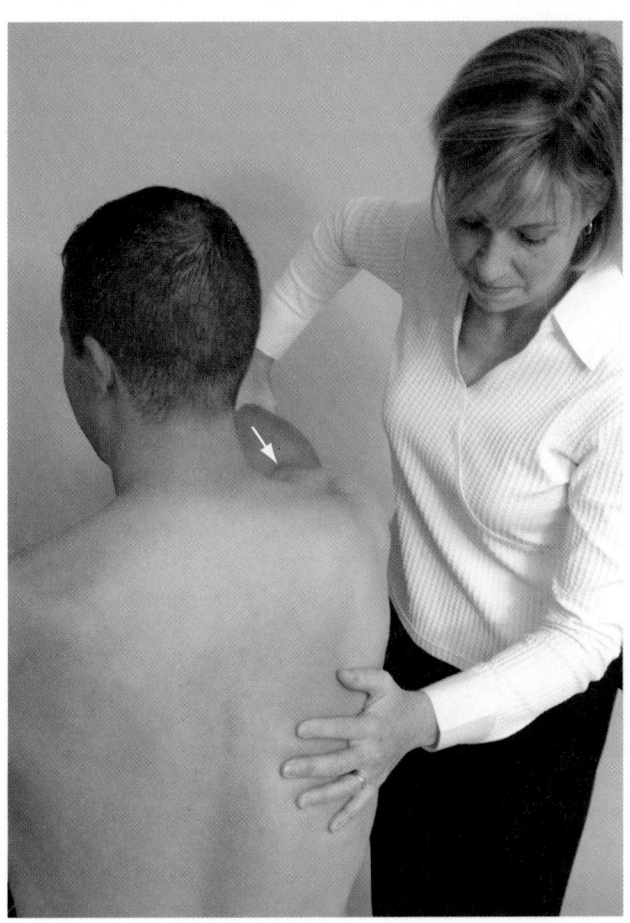

Figure 5-71 Jerk test.

the humerus posteriorly. The patient may become apprehensive during this maneuver, because these motions cause the humerus to sublux posteriorly. With the other hand, the examiner palpates the anterior and posterior shoulder. The examiner then abducts and laterally rotates the arm, a clunk is heard, and the humerus reduces (relocates), indicating a positive test (Figure 5-73).

Norwood Stress Test for Posterior Instability.[210] The patient lies supine with the shoulder abducted 60° to 100° and laterally rotated 90° and with the elbow flexed to 90° so that the arm is horizontal. The examiner stabilizes the scapula with one hand, palpating the posterior humeral head with the fingers, and stabilizes the upper limb by holding the forearm and elbow at the elbow or wrist. The examiner then brings the arm into horizontal adduction to the forward flexed position. At the same time, the examiner feels the humeral head slide posteriorly with the fingers (Figure 5-74). Cofield and Irving recommend medially rotating the forearm approximately 20° after the forward flexion then pushing the elbow posteriorly to enhance the effect of the test.[211] Similarly, the thumb may push the humeral head posteriorly as horizontal adduction in forward flexion is carried out to enhance the effect making the test similar to the posterior apprehension test. A positive test is indicated if the humeral head slips posteriorly relative to the glenoid. Care must be taken because the test does not always cause apprehension before subluxation or dislocation. The patient confirms that the sensation felt is the same as that

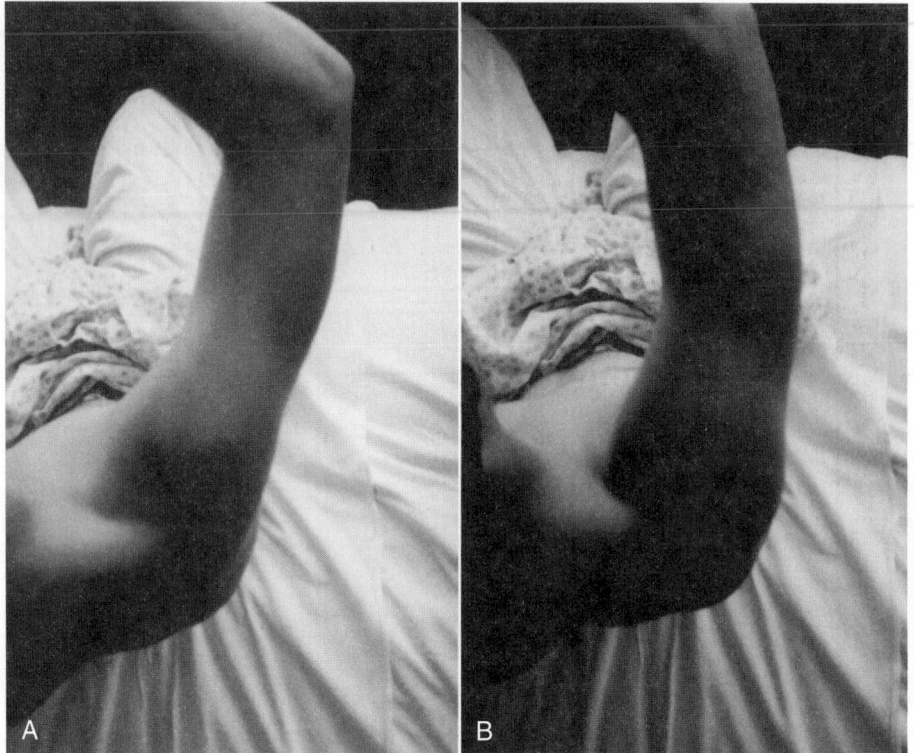

Figure 5-72 Positive jerk test. A, Normal appearance of the shoulder before the patient performs a jerk test. **B,** With axial loading and movement of the arm horizontally across the body, the humeral head slides off the back of the glenoid, as demonstrated by the prominence in the anterior aspect of the patient's shoulder. This maneuver resulted in a sudden jerk and some discomfort. (From Matsen FA, et al: Glenohumeral instability. In Rockwood CA, Matsen FA, editors: The shoulder, Philadelphia, 1990, WB Saunders, p. 551.)

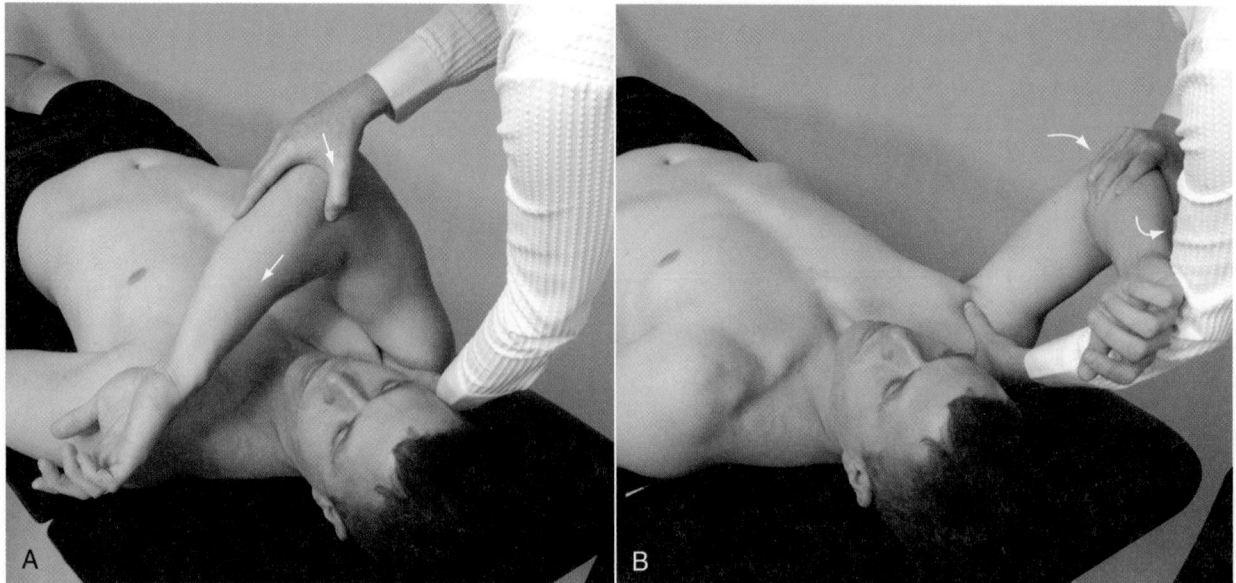

Figure 5-73 Miniaci test for posterior subluxation. A, To start, the examiner uses one hand to flex, adduct, and medially rotate the arm while pushing the humerus posteriorly. **B,** The arm is then abducted and laterally rotated while the examiner palpates for a clunk.

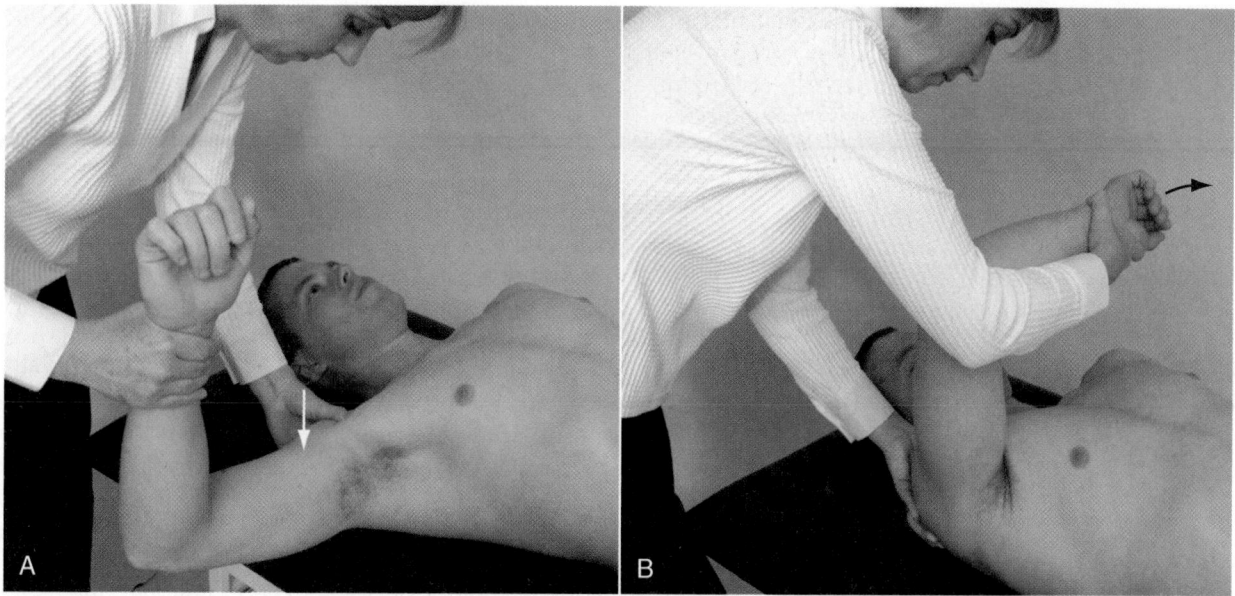

Figure 5-74 **Norwood stress test for posterior shoulder instability. A,** Arm is abducted 90°. **B,** Arm is horizontally adducted to the forward flexed position.

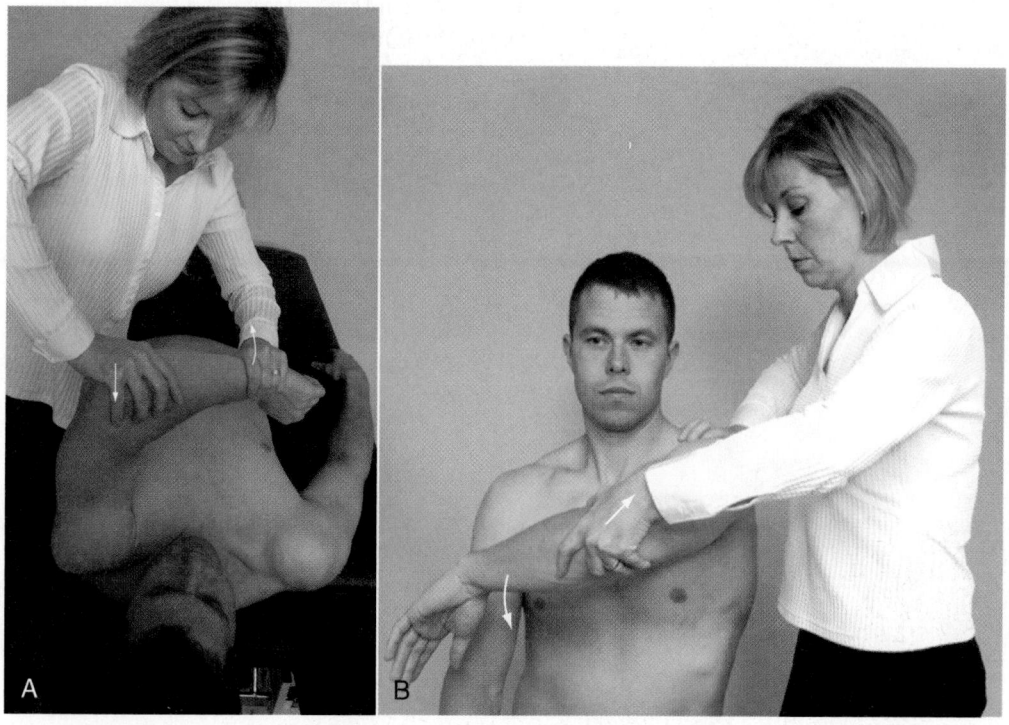

Figure 5-75 **Posterior apprehension test. A,** Supine. **B,** Sitting medially rotated and adducted.

felt during activities. The arm is returned to the starting position, and the humeral head is felt to reduce. A clicking caused by the passage of the head over the glenoid rim may accompany either subluxation or reduction.

Ⓠ *Posterior Apprehension or Stress Test.*[200,212] The patient is in a supine lying or sitting position. The examiner elevates the patient's shoulder in the plane of the scapula to 90° while stabilizing the scapula with the other

hand (Figure 5-75). The examiner then applies a posterior force on the patient's elbow. While applying the axial load, the examiner horizontally adducts and medially rotates the arm. A positive result is indicated by a look of apprehension or alarm on the patient's face and the patient's resistance to further motion or the reproduction of the patient's symptoms. Pagnani and Warren reported that pain production is more likely than apprehension in a positive test.[213] They reported that with atraumatic multidirectional (inferior) instability, the test is negative. If the test is done with the patient in the sitting position, the scapula must be stabilized. A positive test indicates a posterior instability or dislocation of the humerus. The

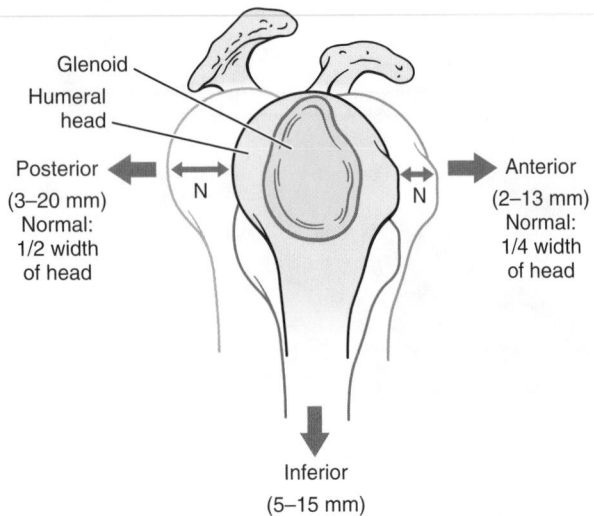

Figure 5-76 **Normal translation movement of humeral head in glenoid.** (Redrawn from Harryman DT 2nd, Slides JA, Harris SL, et al: Laxity of the normal glenohumeral joint: A quantitative in vivo assessment. J Shoulder Elbow Surg 1:73, 1992.)

test should also be performed with the arm in 90° of abduction. The examiner palpates the head of the humerus with one hand while the other hand pushes the head of the humerus posteriorly. Translation of 50% of the humeral head diameter or less is considered normal, although results vary among patients.[182] If the humeral head moves posteriorly more than 50% of its diameter (Figure 5-76), posterior instability is evident.[202] The movement may be accompanied by a clunk as the humeral head passes over the glenoid rim.

Posterior Drawer Test of the Shoulder.[178,214] The patient lies supine. The examiner stands at the level of the shoulder and grasps the patient's proximal forearm with one hand, flexing the patient's elbow to 120° and the shoulder to between 80° and 120° of abduction and between 20° and 30° of forward flexion. With the other hand, the examiner stabilizes the scapula by placing the index and middle fingers on the spine of the scapula and the thumb on the coracoid process. (The examining table partially stabilizes the scapula as well.) The examiner then rotates the upper arm medially and forward flexes the shoulder to between 60° and 80° while taking the thumb of the other hand off the coracoid process and pushing the head of the humerus posteriorly. The head of the humerus can be felt by the index finger of the same hand (Figure 5-77). The test is usually pain-free, but the patient may exhibit

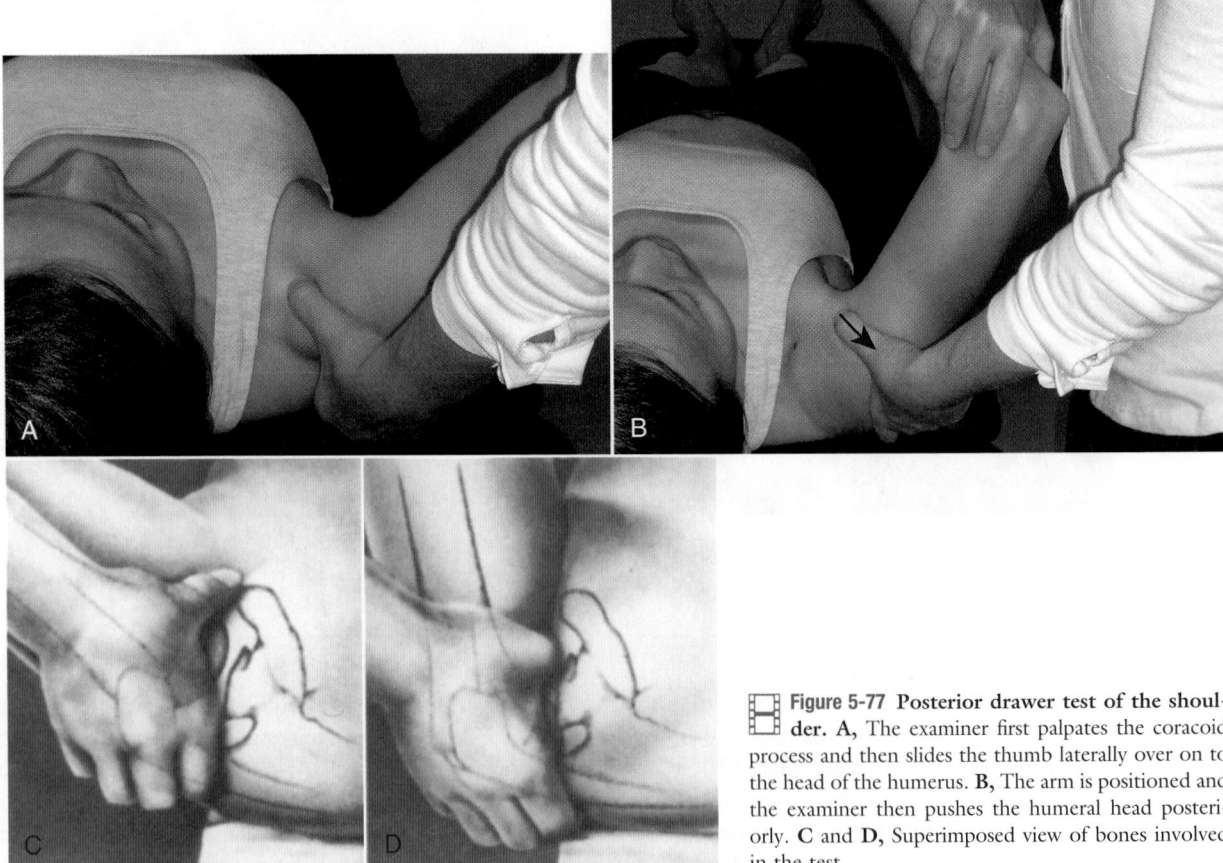

Figure 5-77 **Posterior drawer test of the shoulder. A,** The examiner first palpates the coracoid process and then slides the thumb laterally over on to the head of the humerus. **B,** The arm is positioned and the examiner then pushes the humeral head posteriorly. **C** and **D,** Superimposed view of bones involved in the test.

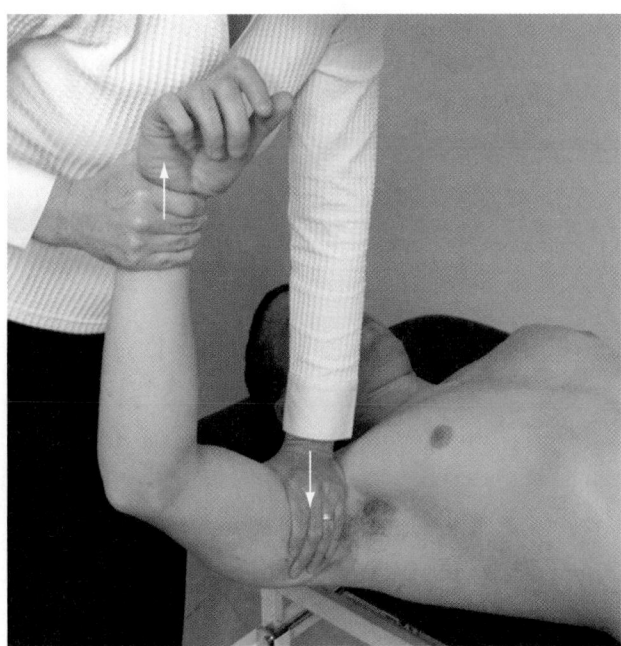

Figure 5-78 Push-pull test.

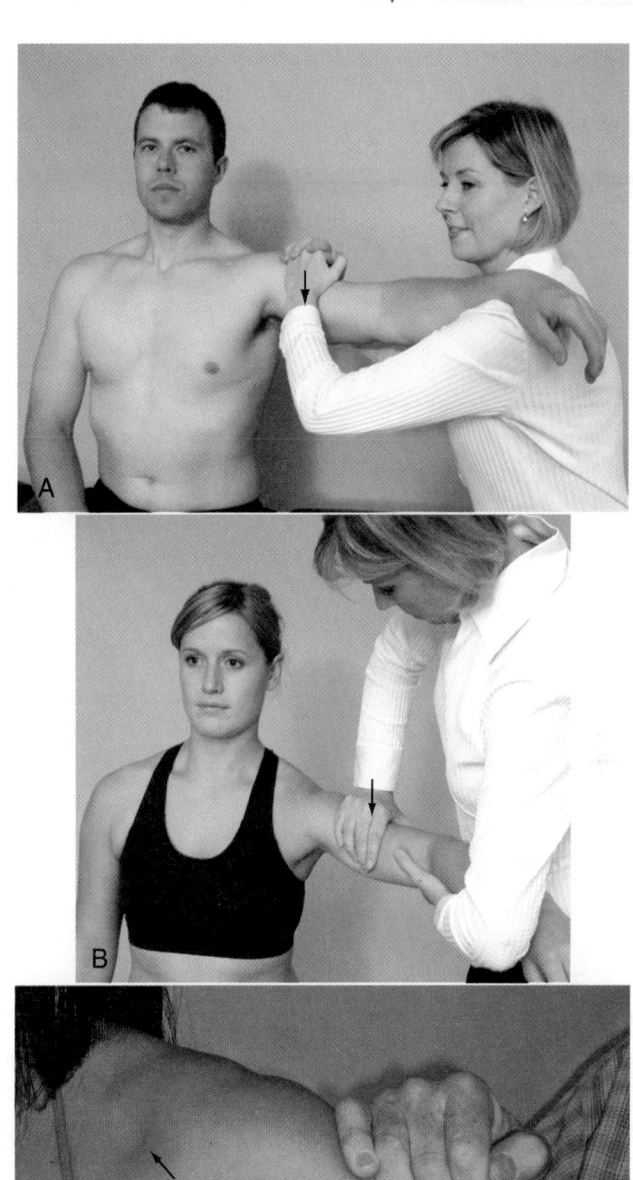

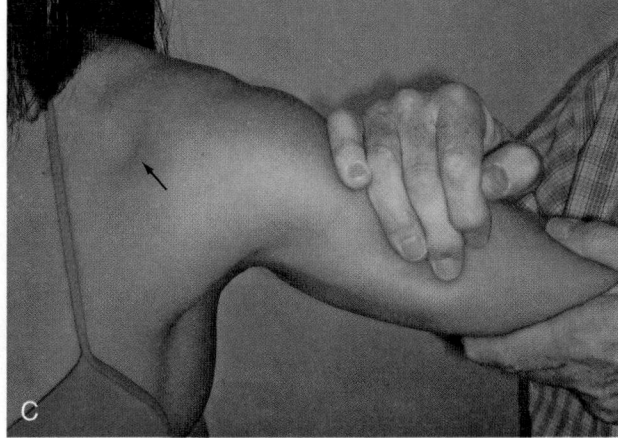

Figure 5-79 Feagin test. **A,** In standing. **B,** In sitting. **C,** Positive Feagin—note sulcus (*arrow*).

apprehension. A positive test indicates posterior instability and demonstrates significant posterior translation (more than 50% humeral head diameter). This test is similar to the Norwood test without the horizontal adduction.

? *Push-Pull Test.*[180] The patient lies supine. The examiner holds the patient's arm at the wrist, abducts the arm 90°, and forward flexes it 30°. The examiner places the other hand over the humerus close to the humeral head. The examiner then pulls up on the arm at the wrist while pushing down on the humerus with the other hand (Figure 5-78). Normally, 50% posterior translation can be accomplished. If more than 50% posterior translation occurs or if the patient becomes apprehensive or pain results, the examiner should suspect posterior instability.[203]

Tests for Inferior and Multidirectional Shoulder Instability

It is believed that if a patient demonstrates inferior instability, multidirectional instability is also present. Therefore, the patient with inferior instability also demonstrates anterior or posterior instability. The primary complaint of these patients is pain rather than instability with symptoms most commonly in midrange. Transient neurological symptoms may also be present.[215]

? *Feagin Test.*[203] The Feagin test is a modification of the sulcus sign test with the arm abducted to 90° instead of being at the side (Figure 5-79). Some authors consider it to be the second part of the sulcus test.[216] The patient stands with the arm abducted to 90° and the elbow extended and resting on the top of the examiner's shoulder. The examiner's hands are clasped together over the patient's humerus, between the upper and middle thirds.

The examiner pushes the humerus down and forward (see Figure 5-79, *A*). The test may also be done with the patient in a sitting position. In this case, the examiner holds the patient's arm at the elbow (elbow straight) abducted to 90° with one hand and arm holding the arm against the examiner's body. The other hand is placed just lateral to the acromion over the humeral head. Ensuring the shoulder musculature is relaxed, the examiner pushes the head of the humerus down and forward (see Figure 5-79, *B*). Doing the test this way often gives the examiner greater control when doing the test. A sulcus may also be seen above the coracoid process (Figure 5-80). A look of apprehension on the patient's face indicates a positive test

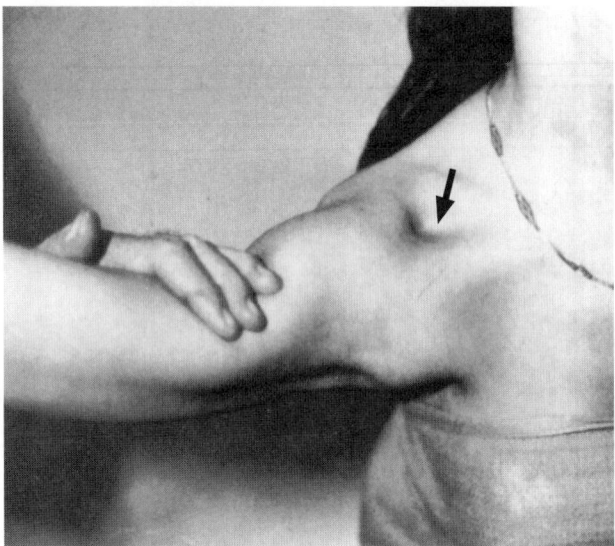

Figure 5-80 A 21-year-old woman whose shoulder could be dislocated inferiorly and anteriorly and subluxated posteriorly. Note sulcus *(arrow)* anteriorly. She was unable to carry books, reach overhead, or use the arm for activities, such as tennis or swimming. Associated episodes of numbness and weakness of the entire upper extremity lasted for 1 or 2 days at times. (From Neer CS, Foster CR: Inferior capsular shift for involuntary inferior and multidirectional instability of the shoulder. J Bone Joint Surg Am 62:900, 1980.)

and the presence of inferior capsular laxity.[217] If both the sulcus sign and Feagin test are positive, it is a greater indication of multidirectional instability rather than just laxity, but it should only be considered positive if the patient is symptomatic (e.g., pain/ache on activity, shoulder does not "feel right" with activity).[217] This test position also places more stress on the inferior glenohumeral ligament.

? *Rowe Test for Multidirectional Instability.*[204] The patient stands forward flexed 45° at the waist with the arms relaxed and pointing at the floor. The examiner places one hand over the shoulder so that the index and middle fingers sit over the anterior aspect of the humeral head and the thumb sits over the posterior aspect of the humeral head. The examiner then pulls the arm down slightly (Figure 5-81). To test for anterior instability, the humeral head is pushed anteriorly with the thumb while the arm is extended 20° to 30° from the vertical position. To test for posterior instability, the humeral head is pushed posteriorly with the index and middle fingers while the arm is flexed 20° to 30° from the vertical position. For inferior instability, more traction is applied to the arm, and the sulcus sign is evident.

✓ *Test for Inferior Shoulder Instability (Sulcus Sign).*[178,180] The patient stands with the arm by the side and shoulder muscles relaxed. The examiner grasps the patient's forearm below the elbow and pulls the arm distally (Figure 5-82). The presence of a **sulcus sign** (see Figure 5-82, *B*) may indicate inferior instability or glenohumeral laxity[218] but should only be considered positive for instability if the patient is symptomatic (e.g., pain/ache on activity,

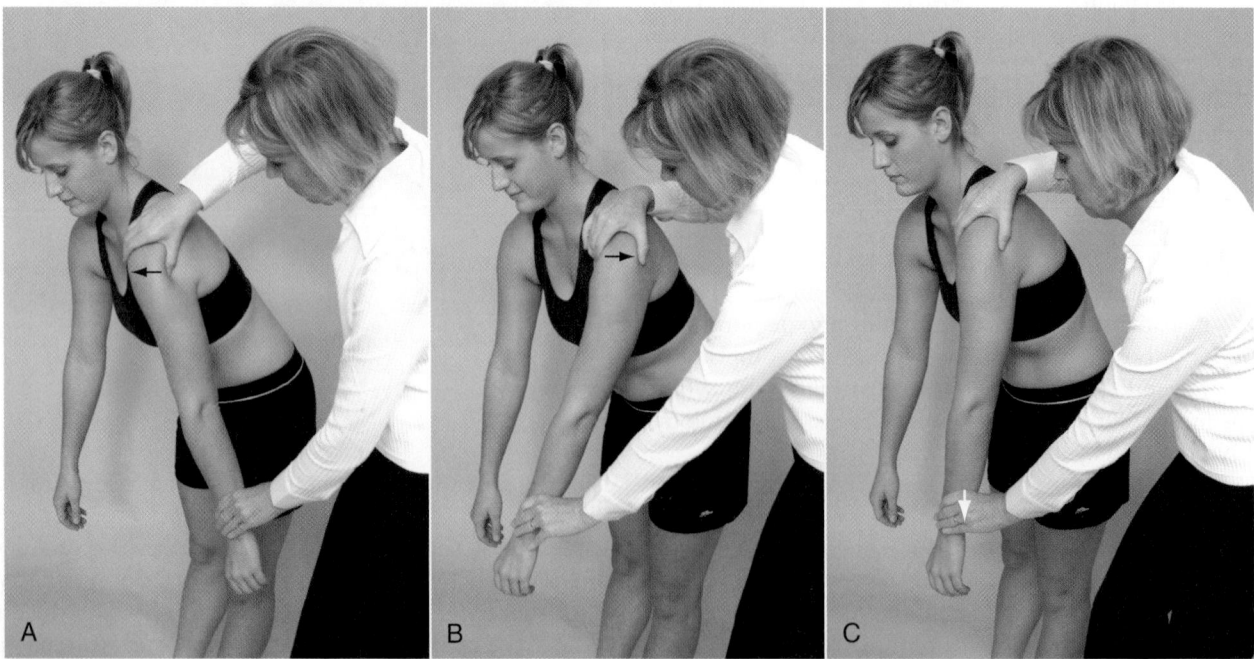

Figure 5-81 **Rowe test for multidirectional instability. A,** Testing for anterior instability. **B,** Testing for posterior instability. **C,** Testing for inferior instability.

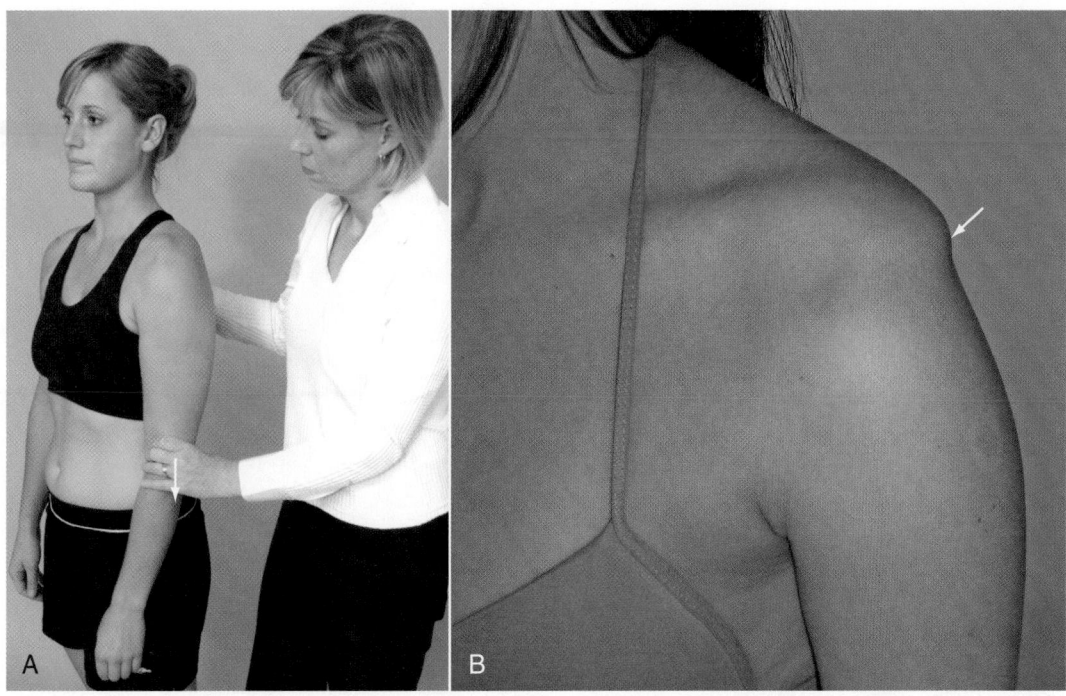

Figure 5-82 **A,** Test for inferior shoulder instability (**sulcus test**). **B,** Positive sulcus sign *(arrow).*

shoulder does not "feel right" with activity).[217] A bilateral sulcus sign is not as clinically significant as unilateral laxity on the affected side.[216] The sulcus sign with a feeling of subluxation is also clinically significant.[216] The sulcus sign may be graded by measuring from the inferior margin of the acromion to the humeral head. A +1 sulcus implies a distance of less than 1 cm; +2 sulcus, 1 to 2 cm; and +3 sulcus, more than 2 cm. Humeral head displacement of more than 2 cm from the acromion has been reported to be indicative of a high degree of glenohumeral laxity.[217]

The best position to test for inferior instability is at 20° to 50° of abduction with neutral rotation. Also, rotation causes the capsule to tighten anteriorly (lateral rotation) or posteriorly (medial rotation), and the sulcus distance decreases.[191] Thus, more than one position should be tested.[68,213,219] Depending on the patient history, the examiner should test the patient in the position in which the sensation of instability is reported.

Tests for Impingement

Anterior shoulder impingement, regardless of its cause (i.e., rotator cuff pathology, bicipital paratenonitis/tendinosis, scapular or humeral instability, labral pathology), results from structures being compressed in the anterior aspect of the humerus between the head of the humerus and the coracoid process under the acromion process (Figure 5-83).[220–225] Park, et al.[226] found that combining tests gave better results. They found that the Hawkins-Kennedy test, the painful arc sign, and a positive infraspinatus test gave the best probability of impingement, whereas the painful arc sign, drop arm test, and the infraspinatus test were best for full thickness rotator cuff tears.

✓ **Hawkins-Kennedy Impingement Test.**[38,157,227] The patient stands while the examiner forward flexes the arm to 90° and then forcibly medially rotates the shoulder (see Figure 5-87, *B*). This movement pushes the supraspinatus tendon against the anterior surface[228] of the coracoacromial ligament and coracoid process.[229–231] The test may also be performed in different degrees of forward flexion (vertically "circling the shoulder") or horizontal adduction (horizontally "circling the shoulder"). Pain indicates a positive test for supraspinatus paratenonitis/tendinosis or secondary impingement.[35] McFarland, et al.[232] described the **coracoid impingment sign** ✓, which is the same as the Hawkins-Kennedy test but involves horizontally adducting the arm across the body 10° to 20° before doing the medial rotation (Figure 5-84). This is more likely to approximate the lesser tuberosity of the humerus and the coracoid process. The **Yocum test** ✓ is a modification of this test in which the patient's hand is placed on the opposite shoulder and the examiner elevates the elbow.[48,233] Pain indicates a positive test.

❓ **Impingement Test.**[234] The patient is seated. The examiner takes the arm to 90° abduction and full lateral rotation. This is the same position as for the apprehension test. However, if there is no history of possible traumatic subluxation or dislocation, the movement also can cause anterior translation of the humerus, resulting in

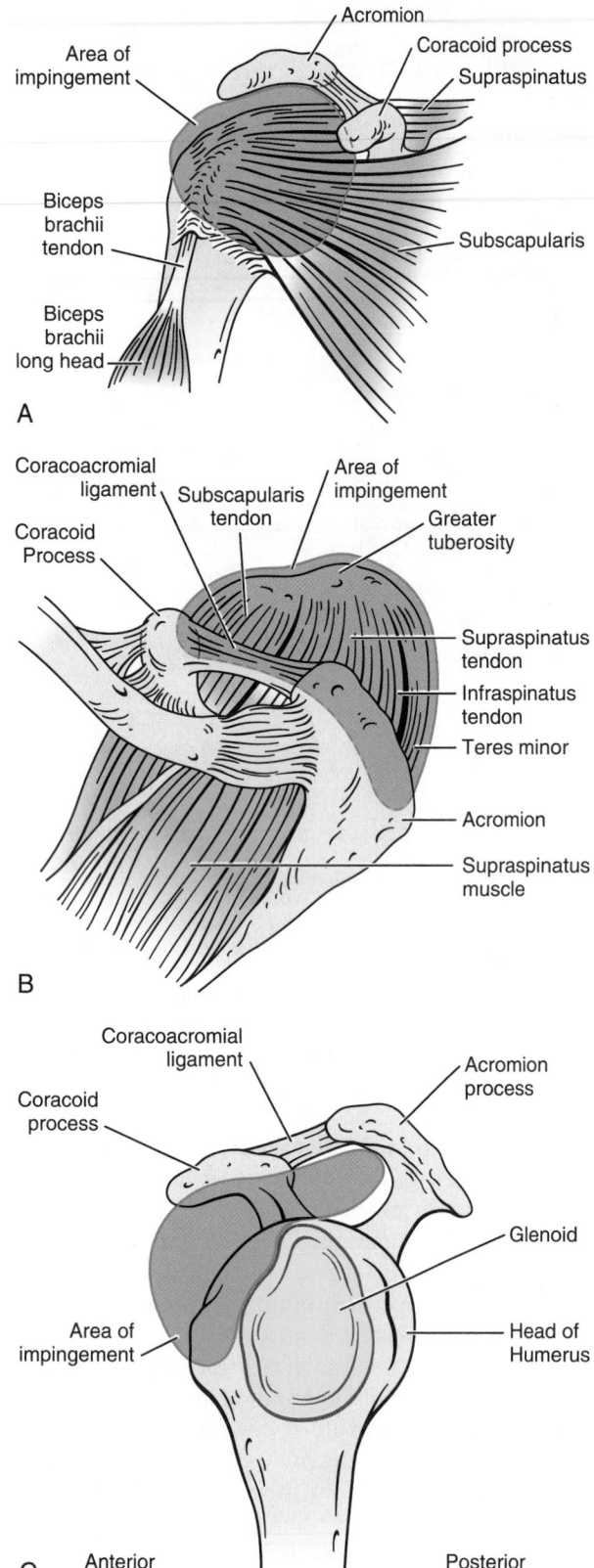

A

B

C Anterior   Posterior

Figure 5-83 **Impingement zone. A,** Anterior view. **B,** Superior view. **C,** Lateral view.

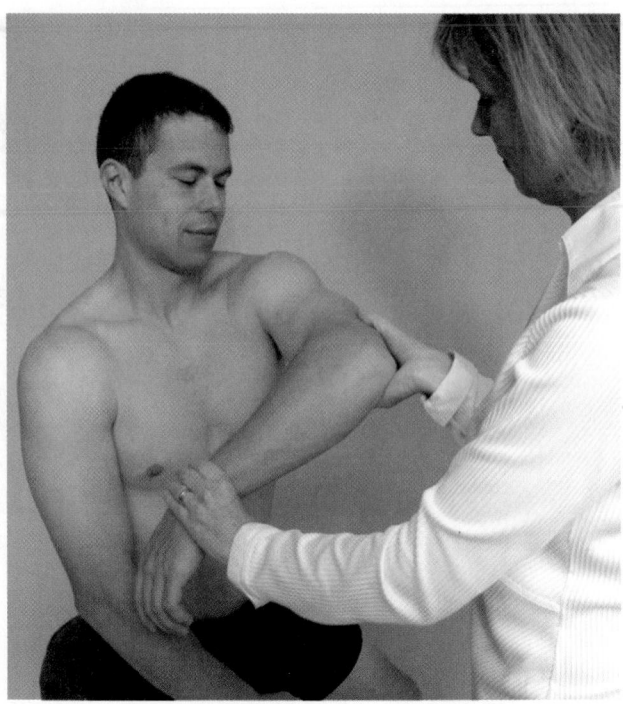

Figure 5-84 **The coracoid impingement sign** with the test performed with the arm flexed 90°, adducted 10°, and internally rotated. The test is positive if it produces pain in the area of the coracoid.

secondary impingement of the rotator cuff. Therefore, a positive test indicates a grade II or III shoulder lesion based on Jobe's classification (see the previous discussion).[169] A positive test depends on production of the patient's symptoms, anterior or posterior shoulder pain, or both.

Branch, et al.[235] advocated testing the anterior capsule in a position of 30° to 40° abduction and 0° to 10° flexion. Lateral rotation is then passively applied to stress the anterior capsule. To test the posterior capsule, they advocated placing the humerus in 60° to 70° abduction and 20° to 30° flexion, followed by passive medial rotation to stress the posterior capsule. By testing below 70° abduction, they felt impingement signs would be less.

☑ *Internal (Medial) Rotation Resistance Strength Test (IRRST) (Zaslav Test).*[236] This test is a follow-up to a Neer test. The patient stands with the arm abducted to 90° and laterally rotated 80° to 85°. The examiner then applies an isometric resistance into lateral rotation followed by isometric resistance into medial rotation (Figure 5-85). The test is considered positive in a patient who has a positive impingement test if the patient has good strength in lateral rotation but not medial rotation and indicates an internal impingement. If the patient exhibits more weakness on lateral rotation, it indicates a classic external anterior impingement. This test may be used to differentiate between an outlet (subacromial) impingement and an intra-articular (nonoutlet) problem when the examiner has found the Neer test to be positive.

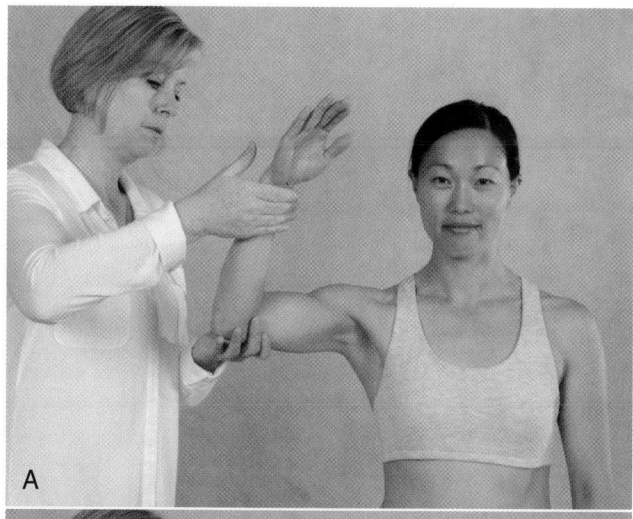

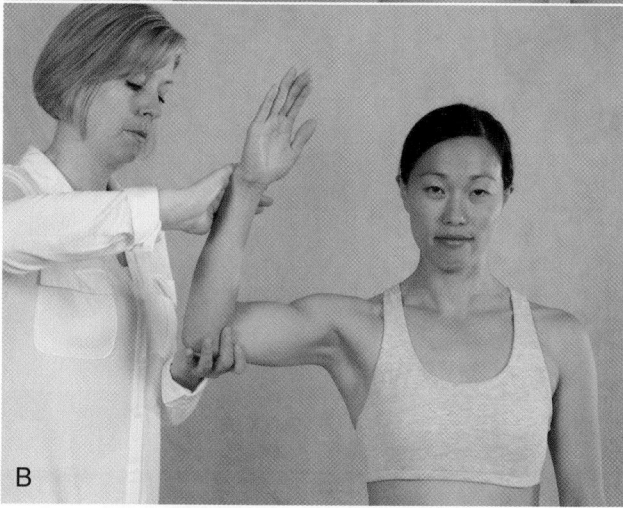

Figure 5-85 **Medial rotation resistance strength test.** The patient is asked to maximally resist lateral rotation (**A**) followed by medial rotation (**B**).

✓ *Neer Impingement Test.*[38,157,237] The patient's arm is passively and forcibly fully elevated in the scapular plane with the arm medially rotated by the examiner. This passive stress causes the greater tuberosity to jam against the anteroinferior border of the acromion (Figure 5-86).[229] The patient's face shows pain, reflecting a positive test result (Figure 5-87, *A*). The test indicates an overuse injury to the supraspinatus muscle and sometimes to the biceps tendon. If the test is positive when done with the arm laterally rotated, the examiner should check the acromioclavicular joint (**acromioclavicular differentiation test**).[238]

❓ *Posterior Internal Impingement Test.*[58,188,239–241] This type of impingement is found primarily in overhead athletes although it may be found in others who hold their arm in the vulnerable position. The impingement occurs when the rotator cuff impinges against the posterosuperior edge of the glenoid when the arm is abducted, extended beyond the coronal plane, and laterally rotated (Figure 5-88).[242–244] The result is of a "kissing" labral

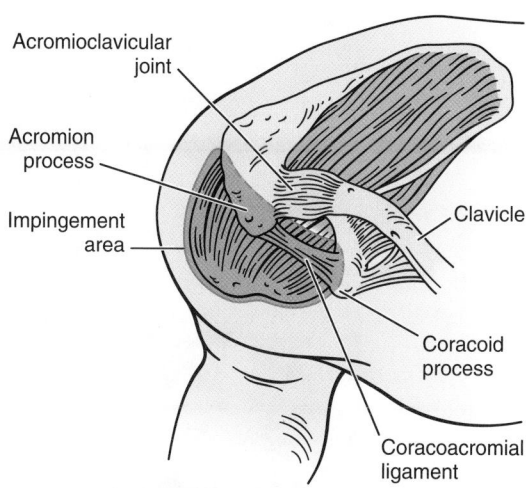

Figure 5-86 The functional arc of elevation of the proximal humerus is forward, as proposed by Neer. The greater tuberosity impinges against the anterior one-third of the acromial surface. This critical area comprises the supraspinatus and bicipital tendons and the subacromial bursa.

lesion posteriorly. The resulting impingement is between the rotator cuff and greater tuberosity on the one hand, and the posterior glenoid and labrum on the other. It often accompanies anterior instability or pseudolaxity, and the deltoid activity increases to compensate for weakened rotator cuff muscles. The patient complains of pain posteriorly in late cocking and early acceleration phase of throwing. To perform the test, the patient is placed in the supine lying position. The examiner passively abducts the shoulder to 90° to 110°, with 15° to 20° extension and maximum lateral rotation (Figure 5-89). The test is considered positive if it elicits localized pain in the posterior shoulder.[58]

❓ *Reverse Impingement Sign (Impingement Relief Test).*[190] This test is used if the patient has a positive painful arc or pain on lateral rotation. The patient lies supine. The examiner pushes the head of the humerus inferiorly as the arm is abducted or laterally rotated. Corso advocated doing the test in the standing position.[245] He also advocated an inferior glide of the humerus during abduction but suggested using a posteroinferior glide of the humeral head during forward flexion. He advocated applying the glide just before the ROM where pain occurred on active movement. If the pain decreases or disappears when repeating the movements with the humeral head depressed, it is considered a positive test for mechanical impingement under the acromion (Figure 5-90).

✓ *Supine Impingement Test.*[20,246] The patient is supine with the examiner at the side by the shoulder to be tested (Figure 5-91). The examiner holds the patient's wrist and humerus (near the elbow) and elevates the patient's arm to end range (approximately 170° to 180°). The examiner then laterally rotates the arm and adducts it into further elevation with the supinated arm against the patient's ear. The examiner then medially rotates the patient's arm. If

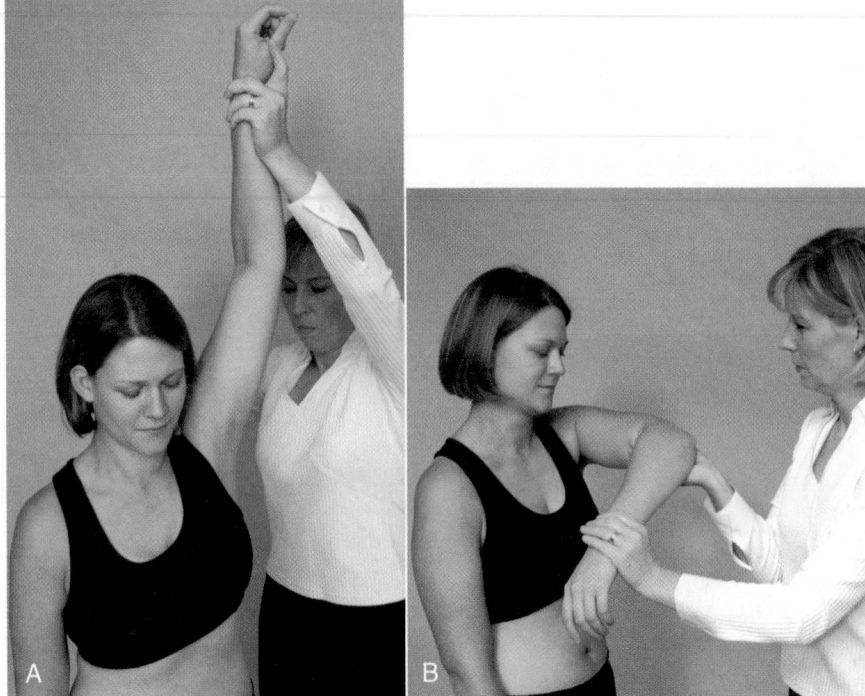

Figure 5-87 **Impingement sign. A,** A positive Neer impingement sign is present if pain and its resulting facial expression are produced when the examiner forcibly flexes the arm forward, jamming the greater tuberosity against the anteroinferior surface of the acromion. **B,** An alternative method (Hawkins-Kennedy impingement test) demonstrates the impingement sign by forcibly medially rotating the proximal humerus when the arm is forward flexed to 90°.

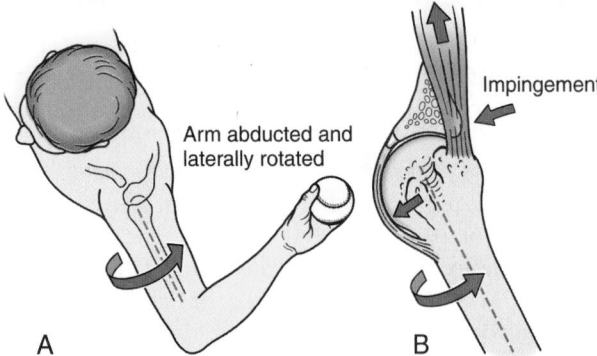

Figure 5-88 **Internal impingement** of the undersurface of the rotator cuff against the posterior aspect of the labrum in maximum lateral rotation and abduction.

the medial rotation causes a significant increase in pain, the test is considered positive for an impingement and rotator cuff pathology (nonspecific) because narrowing and compression in the subacromial space.

Tests for Labral Tears

Injuries to the labrum are relatively common, especially in throwing athletes where the labrum plays a key role in glenohumeral stability.[31] In the young, the tensile strength of the labrum is less than the capsule, so it is more prone to injury when anterior stress (e.g., anterior dislocation) is applied to the glenohumeral joint.[247] The

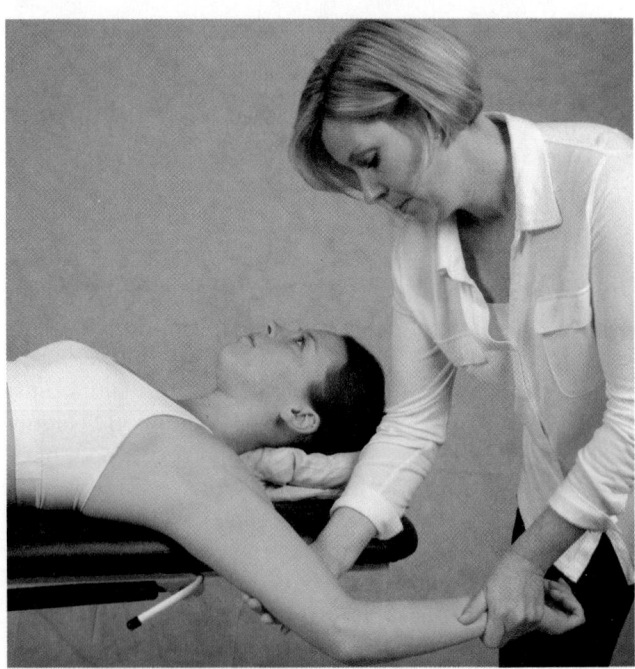

Figure 5-89 **Posterior internal impingement test.**

tear may be a **Bankart lesion,** in which the anteroinferior labrum is torn, or the superior labrum may have been injured, causing a **SLAP lesion** (to the biceps) (Figure 5-92).[248–250] These injuries are classic examples of the **circle concept of instability.** This concept suggests that

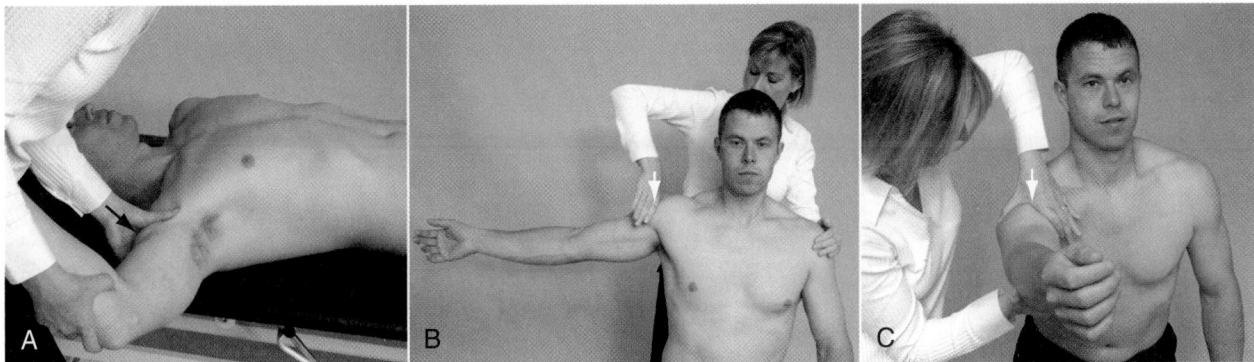

Figure 5-90 Reverse impingement sign (impingement relief test). A, In supine. **B,** In standing, doing test in abduction. **C,** In standing, doing test in forward flexion.

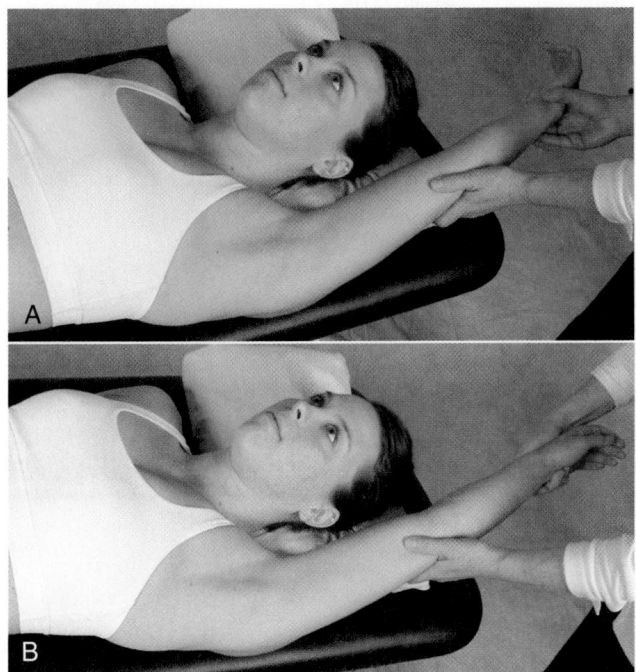

Figure 5-91 Supine impingement test. A, Arm in lateral rotation. **B,** Arm in medial rotation.

injury in one direction of the joint results in injury to structures on the other side of the joint. A Bankart lesion occurs most commonly with a traumatic anterior dislocation leading to anterior instability. In the right shoulder, for example, this injury results in the labrum being detached anywhere from the 3 o'clock to the 7 o'clock position resulting in both anterior and posterior structural injury (see Figure 5-92, *A*). Not only is the labrum torn, but the stability of the inferior glenohumeral ligament is lost.[251] The SLAP lesion has the labrum detaching (pulled or peeled depending on the mechanism) from the 10 o'clock to the 2 o'clock position (see Figure 5-92, *B*). The injury often results from a FOOSH injury, occurs during deceleration when throwing, or arises when sudden traction is applied to the biceps.[252,253] If the biceps tendon also detaches, the shoulder becomes unstable and

the support of the superior glenohumeral ligament is lost. Snyder and colleagues[254] have divided these SLAP lesions into four types:

- Type I: Superior labrum markedly frayed but attachments intact
- Type II: Superior labrum has small tear; instability of the labral-biceps complex (most common)
- Type III: Bucket-handle tear of labrum that may displace into joint; labral biceps attachment intact
- Type IV: Bucket-handle tear of labrum that extends to biceps tendon, allowing tendon to sublux into joint

Burkart, et al.[25,255] described a "peel back" mechanism that resulted in a posterior Type II SLAP lesion in overhead athletes who demonstrate increased lateral rotation, decreased medial rotation, and a tight posterior capsule that results in posterosuperior migration of the head during maximum lateral rotation, causing a tear of the posterosuperior labrum.[256-258] Figure 5-93 shows three possible mechanisms of SLAP injuries.

Research has shown that no single test can accurately diagnose a SLAP lesion.[53,159-162] There are several tests for labral lesions shown later. Labral lesion tests, especially those for SLAP lesions, show sensitivity but lack specificity. At present, there is no convincing evidence for accurate tests to detect a SLAP lesion.[163-165]

☑ ***Active Compression Test of O'Brien.***[38,58,161,186,259-262] This test is designed to detect SLAP (Type II) or superior labral lesions. The patient is placed in the standing position with the arm forward flexed to 90° and the elbow fully extended. The arm is then horizontally adducted 10° to 15° (starting position) and medially rotated so the thumb faces downward. The examiner stands behind the patient and applies a downward eccentric force to the arm (Figure 5-94). The arm is returned to the starting position and the palm is supinated so the shoulder is laterally rotated, and the downward eccentric load is repeated. If pain on the joint line or painful clicking is produced inside the shoulder (not over the acromioclavicular joint) in the first part of the test and eliminated or decreased in the second part, the test is considered positive for labral abnormalities. The test also "locks and loads" the

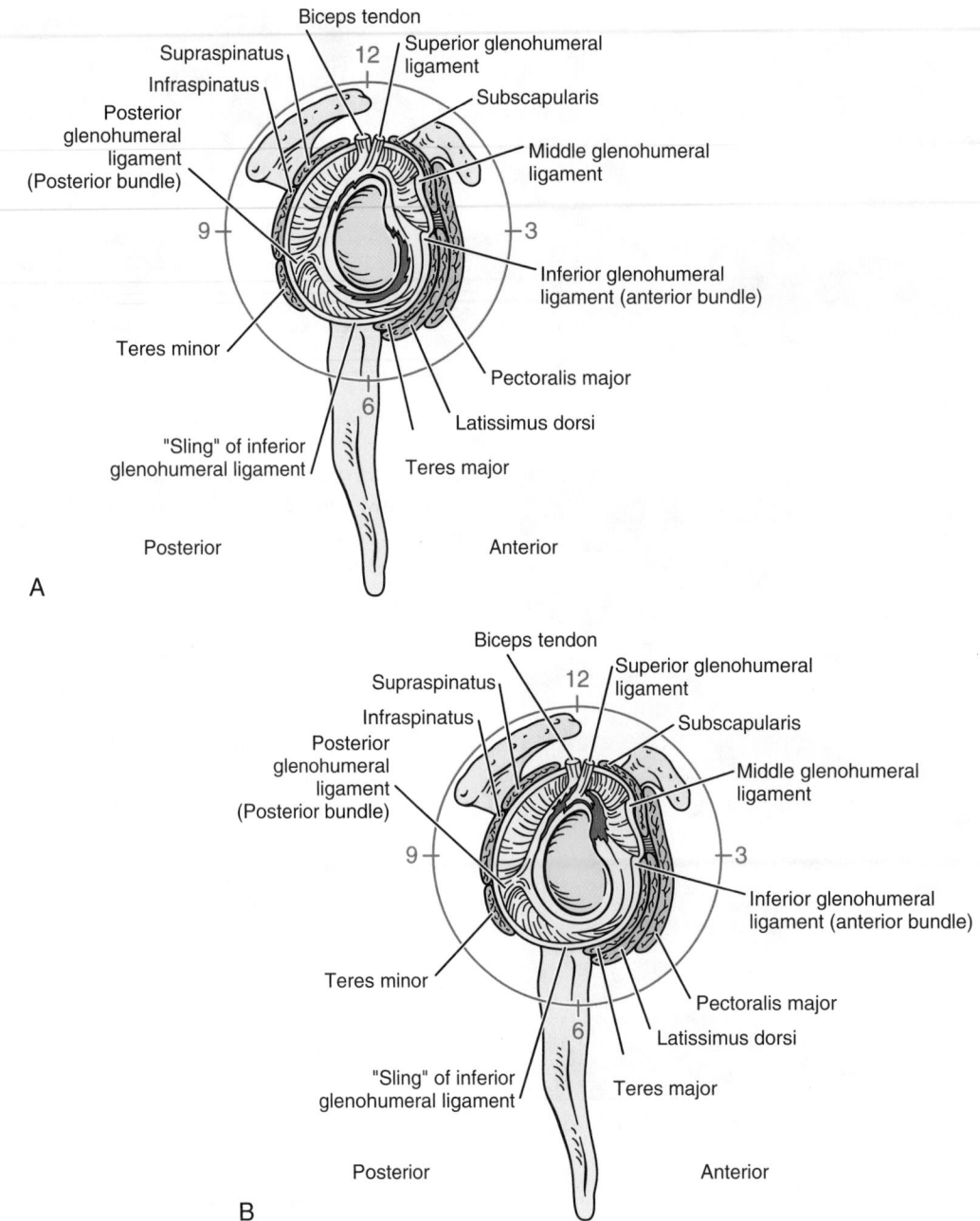

Figure 5-92 **Labral lesions to the right shoulder. A,** Bankart lesion. **B,** SLAP lesion.

acromioclavicular joint in medial rotation so that the examiner must take care to differentiate between labral and acromioclavicular (pain over acromioclavicular joint) pathology.[24]

▲ *Anterior Slide Test.*[38,260,263,264] The patient is sitting with the hands on the waist, thumbs posterior. The examiner stands behind the patient and stabilizes the scapula and clavicle with one hand. With the other hand, the examiner applies an anterosuperior force at the elbow (Figure 5-95, *A*). If the labrum is torn (SLAP lesion), the humeral head slides over the labrum with a pop or crack with pain on the joint line, and the patient complains of anterosuperior pain. McFarland, et al.[38] have described

the test as the examiner applying an axial upward load to the glenohumeral joint that the patient resists (Figure 5-95, *B*). The test is positive if a pain or click is produced deep in the shoulder.

▲ *Biceps Load Test (Kim Test II).*[160,265] This test is designed to check the integrity of the superior labrum. The patient is in the supine or seated position with the shoulder abducted to 120° and laterally rotated with the elbow flexed to 90° and the forearm supinated, as it is for the apprehension or crank test. The examiner performs an apprehension test on the patient by taking the arm into full lateral rotation. If apprehension appears, the examiner stops lateral rotation and holds the position. The patient is then asked to flex the elbow against the examiner's resistance at the wrist. If apprehension decreases or the patient feels more comfortable, the test is negative for a SLAP lesion. If the apprehension remains the same or the shoulder becomes more painful, the test is considered positive for SLAP lesions in the presence of recurrent dislocations (Figure 5-96). Wilk, et al.[266] also advocate doing the test with the forearm pronated (**pronated biceps load**

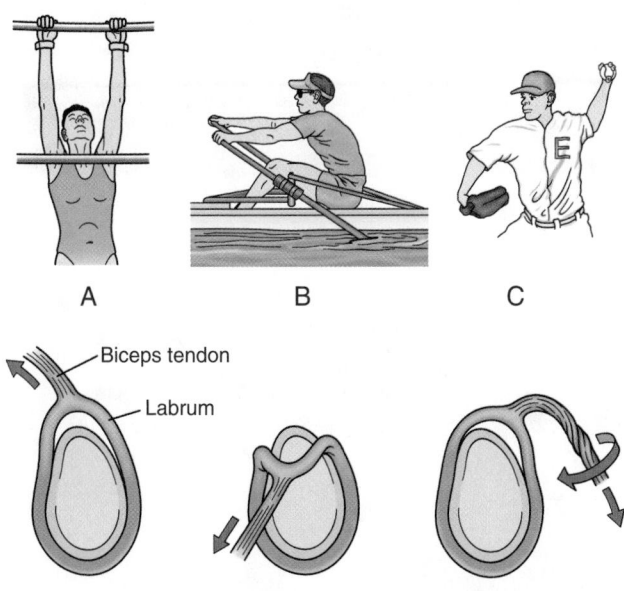

Figure 5-93 **Mechanisms of injury for SLAP lesions.**

test ❓). If the pain is located deep in the superior glenohumeral joint, the test is considered positive.

⚠ *Biceps Tension Test.*[157] This test determines whether a SLAP lesion is present. The patient, in standing, abducts and laterally rotates the arm to 90° with the elbow extended and forearm supinated. The examiner then applies an eccentric adduction force to the arm. A reproduction of the patient's symptoms is a positive test (Figure 5-97). The examiner should also do a Speed's test (discussed later) to rule out biceps pathology.

⚠ *Clunk Test.* The patient lies supine. The examiner places one hand on the posterior aspect of the shoulder over the humeral head. The examiner's other hand holds the humerus above the elbow. The examiner fully abducts the arm over the patient's head. The examiner then pushes anteriorly with the hand over the humeral head (a fist may be used to apply more anterior pressure) while the other hand rotates the humerus into lateral rotation (Figure 5-98). A clunk or grinding sound indicates both a positive test and a tear of the labrum.[267] The test may also cause apprehension if anterior instability is present. Walsh indicated that if the examiner follows these maneuvers with horizontal adduction that relocates the humerus, he or she may also hear a clunk or a click, indicating a tear of the labrum.[268]

The examiner may also position the arm in different amounts of abduction (vertically "circling the shoulder") and perform the test. This will stress different parts of the labrum.

⚠ *Compression Rotation Test.*[165,269,270] The patient is supine with the examiner standing beside the test

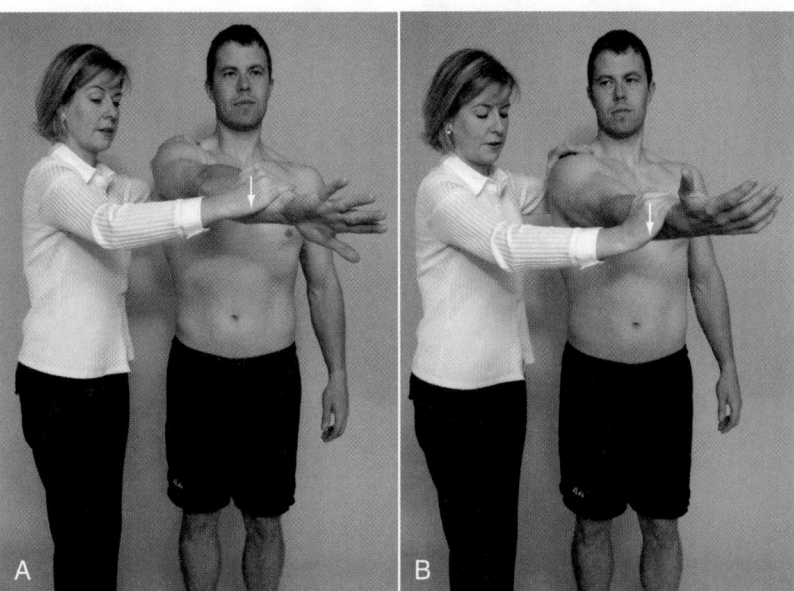

Figure 5-94 **Active compression test of O'Brien. A,** Position 1: The patient forward flexes the arm to 90° with the elbow extended and adducted 15° medial to the midline of the body and with the thumb pointed down. The examiner applies a downward force to the arm that the patient resists. **B,** Position 2: The test is performed with the arm in the same position, but the patient fully supinates the arm with the palm facing the ceiling. The same maneuver is repeated. The test is positive for a superior labral injury if pain is elicited in the first step and reduced or eliminated in the second step of this maneuver.

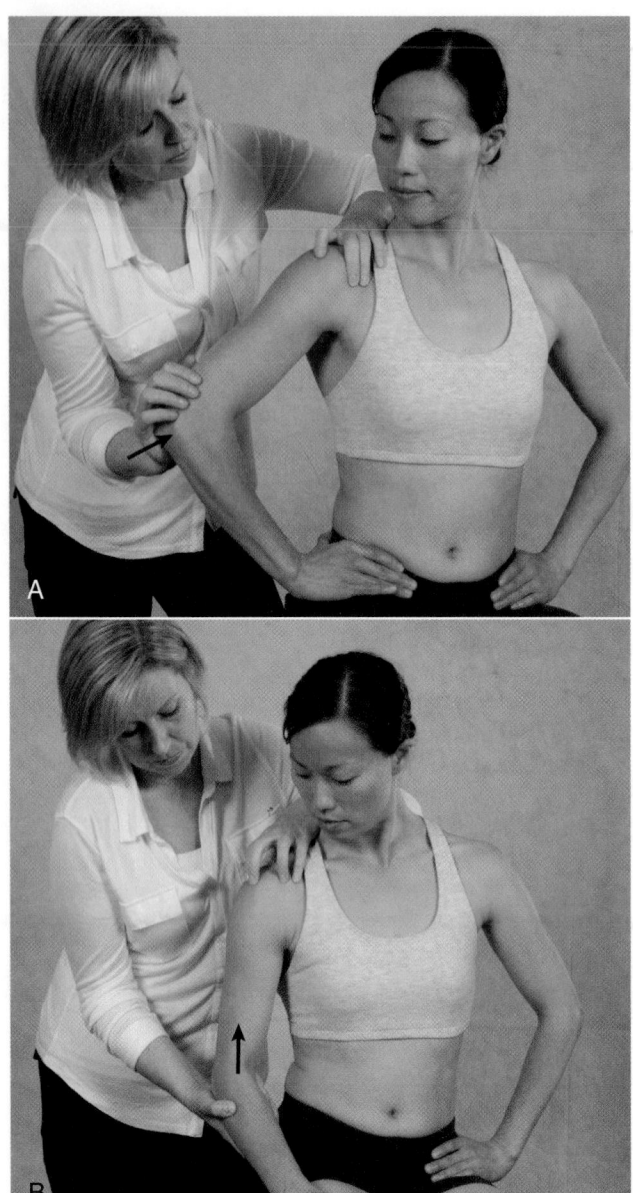

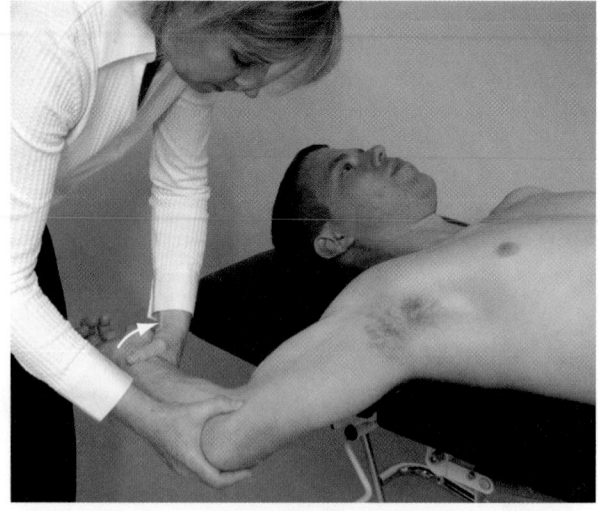

Figure 5-96 Biceps load test (Kim test II).

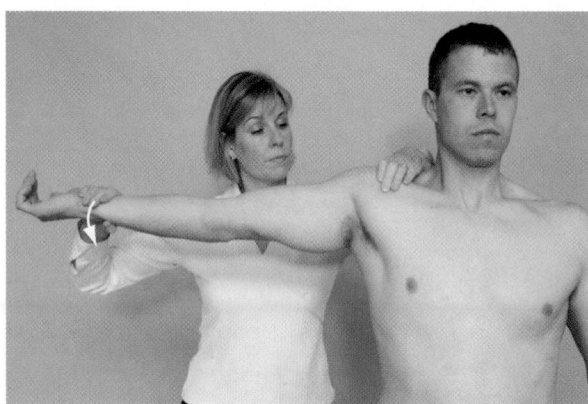

Figure 5-97 Biceps tension test. The patient's arm is abducted to 90° and laterally rotated. The examiner then applies an eccentric adduction force.

Figure 5-95 A, Anterior slide testing. Note the position of the examiner's hands and the patient's arms. **B,** McFarland's anterior slide test.

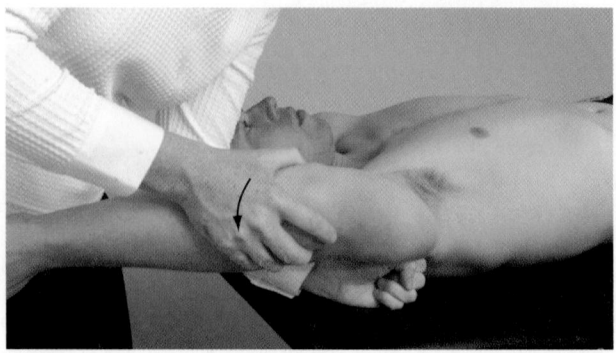

Figure 5-98 Clunk test.

shoulder. The examiner passively abducts the shoulder to between 20° and 90° with the patient's elbow at 90°. The examiner applies an axial compression force through the long axis of the humerus (pushing up through the elbow) while passively rotating the humerus back and forth (small and large circles) to try to trap the labrum within the joint (Figure 5-99). If pain, clicking, or a catching sensation is elicited, the test is considered positive for a torn labrum.

Dynamic Labral Shear Test (O'Driscoll's SLAP Test).[271] The patient is in supine or sitting with the arm at the side and the elbow flexed to 90°. If the patient is supine, the arm should not rest on the table. The examiner then laterally rotates the arm to tightness and takes the arm into 90° abduction in the scapular plane (Figure 5-100, *A*). Maintaining the flexed elbow, the examiner then abducts the arm to 120° and takes the arm into maximum horizontal abduction (Figure 5-100, *B*). While maintaining this position, the examiner applies a shear load to the joint by maintaining the horizontal abduction. A positive test

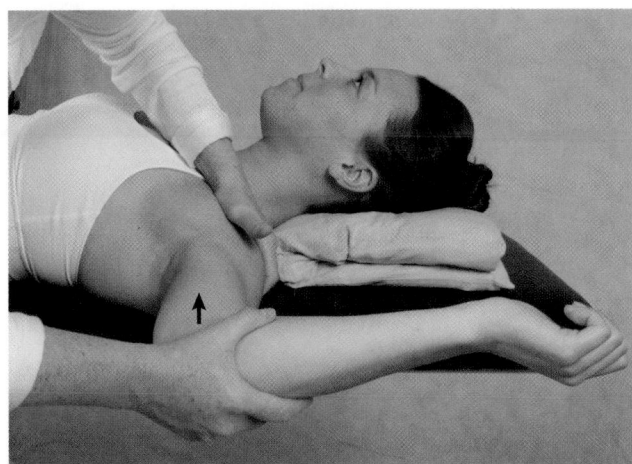

Figure 5-99 Compression rotation test.

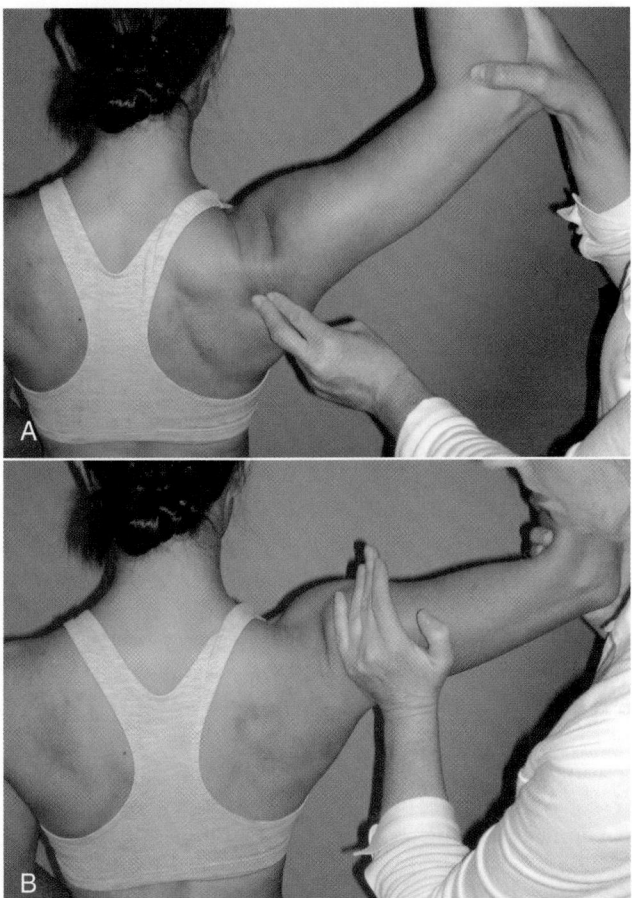

Figure 5-100 Dynamic labral shear test (O'Driscoll's test). **A,** Arm laterally rotated at 120° abduction with anterior shear force using fingers. **B,** Arm laterally rotated at 100° with anterior shear load using hypother eminence.

is indicated by pain and possibly a click between 90° and 120° of abduction. Kibler, et al.[260] modified the test by taking the arm above 120° before placing the arm in maximum horizontal abduction. The examiner then lowers the arm to 60° abduction.[272]

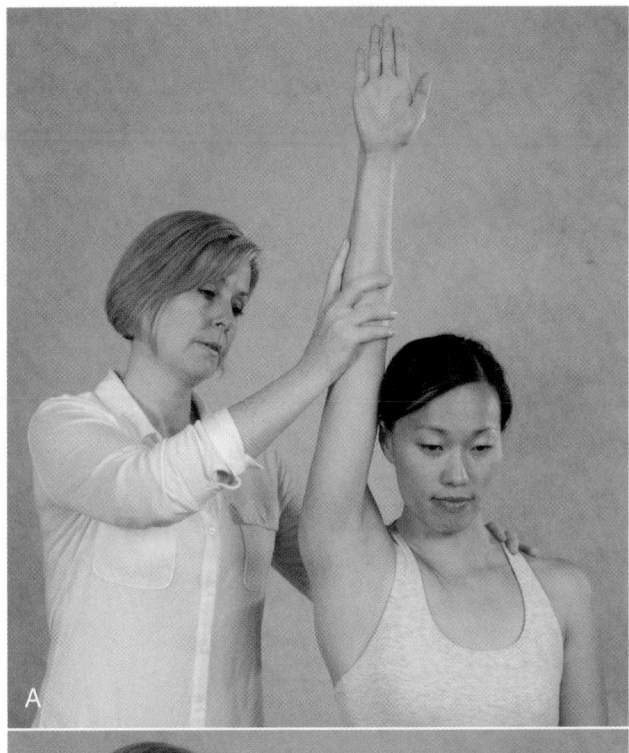

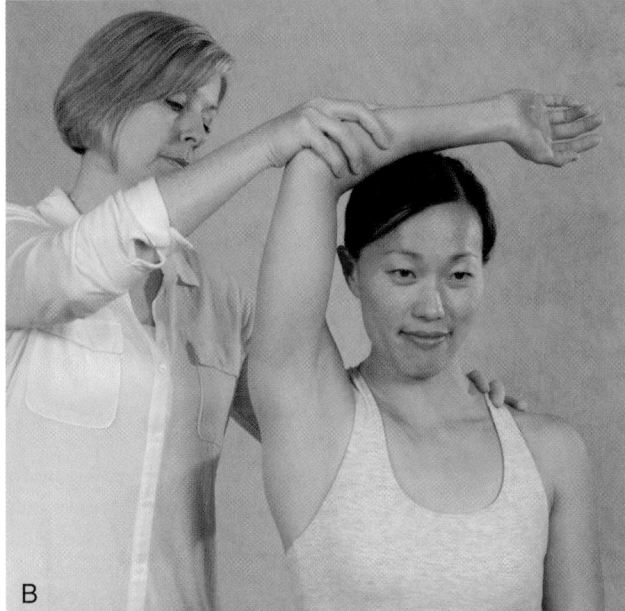

Figure 5-101 Forced shoulder abduction (**A**) and elbow flexion (**B**) test.

⚠ *Forced Shoulder Abduction and Elbow Flexion Test.*[273] The patient is seated with the examiner standing behind on the test side (Figure 5-101). The examiner passively abducts the patient's shoulder fully with the patient's elbow in full extension noting whether there is any pain in the posterosuperior aspect of the shoulder. The examiner then passively flexes the patient's elbow and notes whether the pain is decreased. If the pain is greater when the elbow is extended than when it is flexed, the test is considered positive for a superior labral tear.

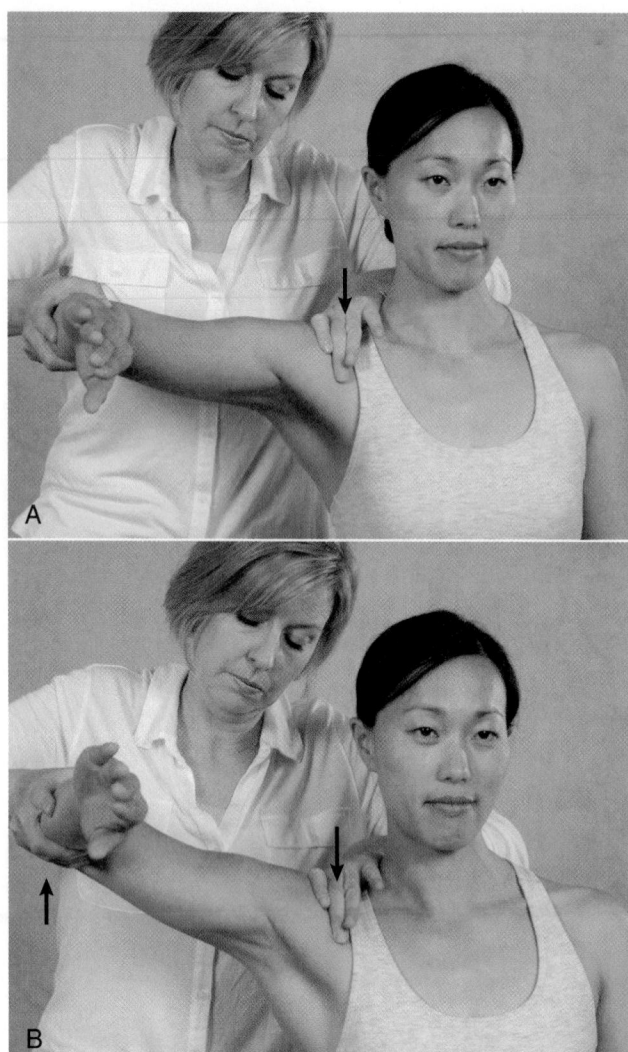

Figure 5-102 Hyperabduction test. **A,** Start position. **B,** End position.

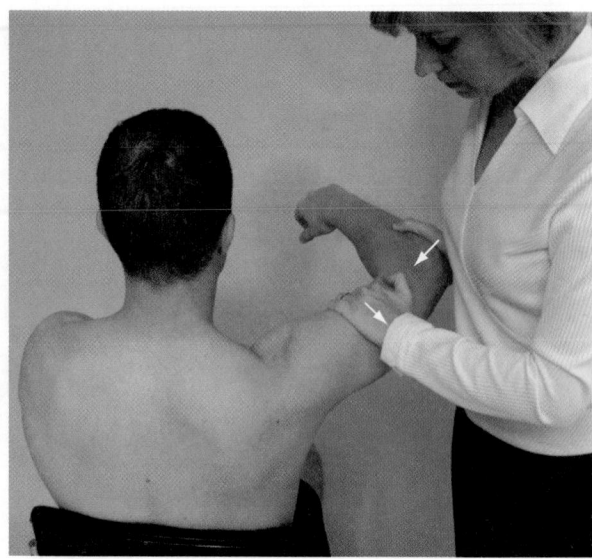

Figure 5-103 Kim test (Biceps load test I).

the other hand applies a downward and backward force to the proximal arm (Figure 5-103). A sudden onset of posterior shoulder pain and click indicates a positive test for a posteroinferior labral lesion.

? *Labral Crank Test.*[274] The patient is in the supine lying or sitting position. The examiner elevates the arm to 160° in the scapular plane. In this position, an axial load is applied to the humerus with one hand of the examiner while the other hand rotates the humerus medially and laterally. A positive test is indicated by pain on rotation, especially lateral rotation with or without a click or reproduction of the patient's symptoms (Figure 5-104).

? *Labral Tension Test.*[164] The patient lies supine. The examiner first places the patient's arm in 120° of abduction with the forearm in neutral and then into full lateral rotation (Figure 5-105). In this position, the examiner holds the patient's hand and asks the patient to supinate the forearm against resistance from the neutral forearm position. If the patient has increased pain on supination of the forearm, it is considered a positive test for a SLAP lesion.

⚠ *Mayo Shear Test.*[261] The patient stands with the examiner standing behind. The examiner elevates the patient's arm to about 70° and then laterally rotates the arm. Once laterally rotated, the patient's arm is taken into full elevation. The examiner then brings the arm down while maintaining lateral rotation and applying an anterior directed force with the hand on the posterior shoulder (Figure 5-106). The test is considered positive if the patient reports pain or a click in the posterior or posterosuperior shoulder and indicates a superior labral (SLAP) tear.

⚠ *Pain Provocation (Mimori) Test.*[275] The patient is seated and the arm is abducted to between 90° and 100°, and the examiner laterally rotates the arm by holding the

? *Hyperabduction Test.*[116] The patient is seated with the examiner standing behind. The examiner stabilizes the scapula with a downward force over the suprascapular region (Figure 5-102) and passively places the patient's elbow in 90° flexion with the forearm pronated. The examiner then passively abducts the arm maximally while restricting scapular movement with the downward pressure. If passive abduction is more than 105°, the test is considered positive for a torn labrum. It should be noted, however, that this is subjective as normal scapulohumeral rhythm shows that up to 120° of abduction normally occurs at the glenohumeral joint.

✓ *Kim Test (Biceps Load Test I).*[160,207,262] The patient sits with the back supported. The arm is abducted to 90° with the elbow supported in 90° flexion. The examiner's hand, while supporting the elbow and forearm, applies an axial compression force to the glenoid through the humerus. While maintaining the axial compression force, the arm is elevated diagonally upward using the same hand while

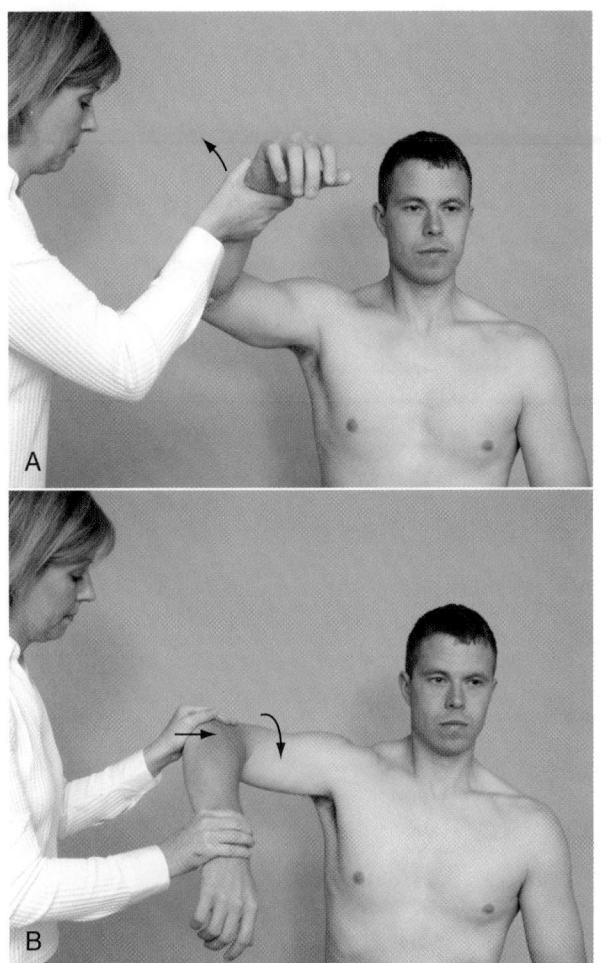

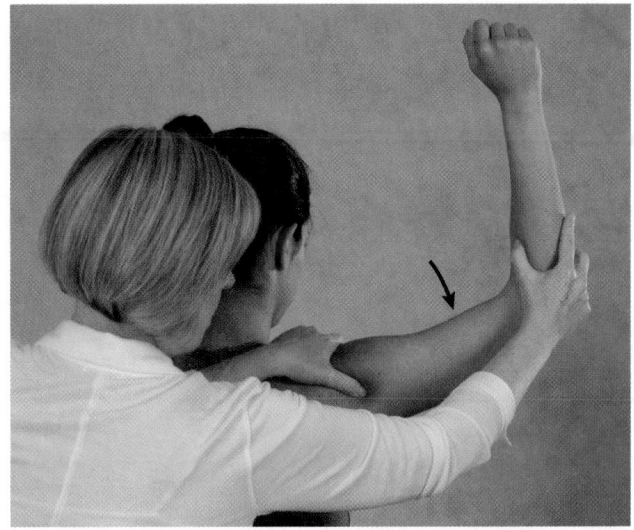

Figure 5-106 The Mayo shear test.

Figure 5-104 Labral crank test. A, Crank test in sitting with lateral humeral rotation. **B,** Crank test in sitting with medial humeral rotation.

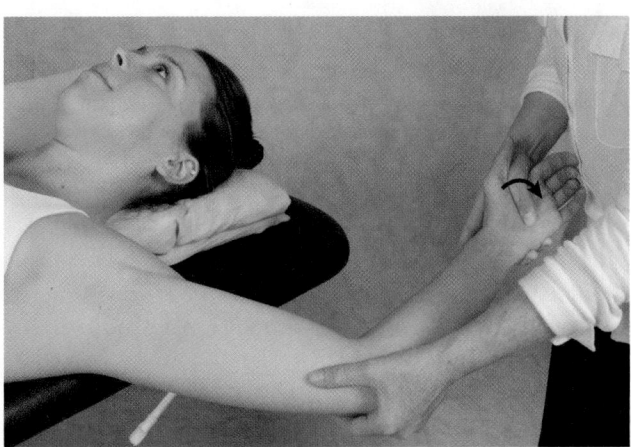

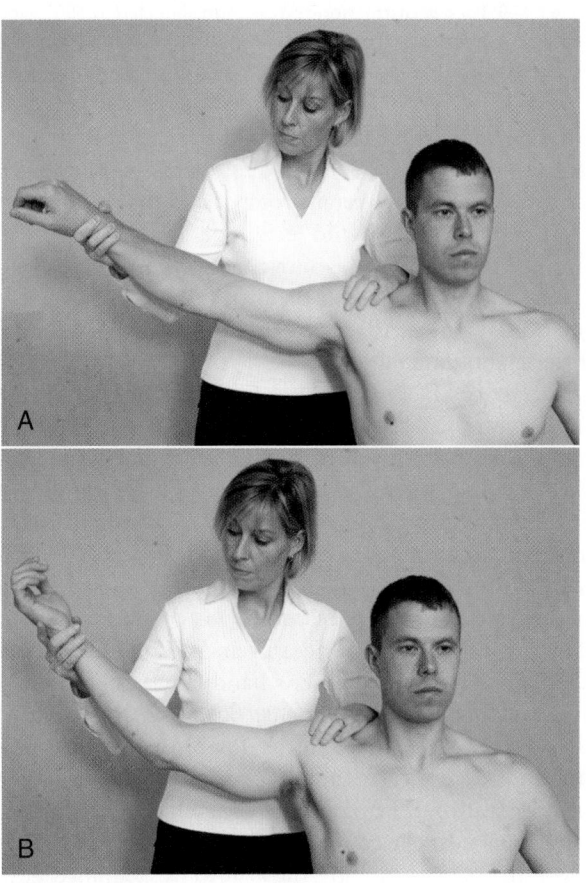

Figure 5-107 Pain provocation test. A, Test with forearm pronated. **B,** Test with forearm supinated.

Figure 5-105 Labral tension test.

wrist (Figure 5-107). The forearm is taken into maximum supination and then maximum pronation. If pain is provoked only in the pronated position or if the pain is more severe in the pronated position, the test is considered positive for a superior (SLAP) tear. As with other superior labral tests, the biceps must be tested (Speed's test) to rule out biceps pathology causing the pain.

***Passive Compression Test.*[276]** The patient is in side lying with the test arm uppermost and the examiner behind the patient. The examiner stabilizes the shoulder

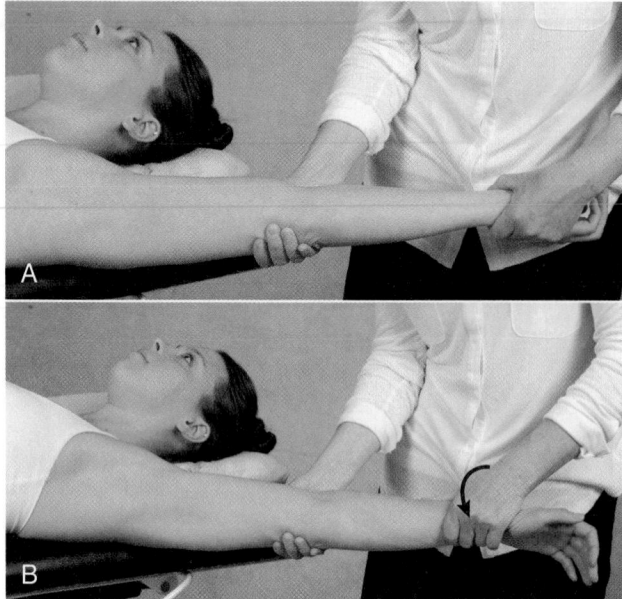

Figure 5-108 Passive distraction test. A, Arm abducted to 150°, elbow extended and forearm supinated. **B,** Forearm is pronated.

with one hand over the scapula and clavicle, and the other hand holds the arm in 30° abduction at the elbow. The patient's shoulder is laterally rotated and the patient's arm is pushed proximally and extended by the examiner's hand on the elbow. This movement causes compression of the superior labrum on the glenoid. A positive test for superior labral (SLAP) tears is indicated by a click or pain in the glenohumeral joint.

? *Passive Distraction Test (PDT).*[277] The patient lies supine with the test arm abducted to 150° with the elbow extended and the forearm supinated (Figure 5-108, *A*). The examiner stabilizes the upper arm (humerus) to prevent rotation. While maintaining the humerus in the same position, the forearm is pronated (Figure 5-108, *B*). Pain felt deep in the shoulder (anteriorly or posteriorly) is considered a positive test for a SLAP lesion. This test mimics the position of the arm and glenohumeral joint when a backstroke swimmer's hand enters the water.

⚠ *Resisted Supination External Rotation Test (RSERT).*[160,252] This test is designed to check for SLAP lesions and is thought to re-create the peel-back mechanism of the superior labrum. The patient is placed in supine lying with the scapula near the edge of the bed. The examiner stands beside the patient holding the arm to be examined at the elbow and hand. The patient's arm is placed with the shoulder abducted to 90°, the elbow flexed to 65° to 70°, and the forearm is neutral or slight pronation. The patient is then asked to maximally supinate the hand while the examiner resists. While the patient continues to supinate against the examiner's resistance, the examiner laterally rotates the shoulder to end range (Figure 5-109). The test is considered positive if the patient has anterior or deep shoulder pain, clicking or catching in the

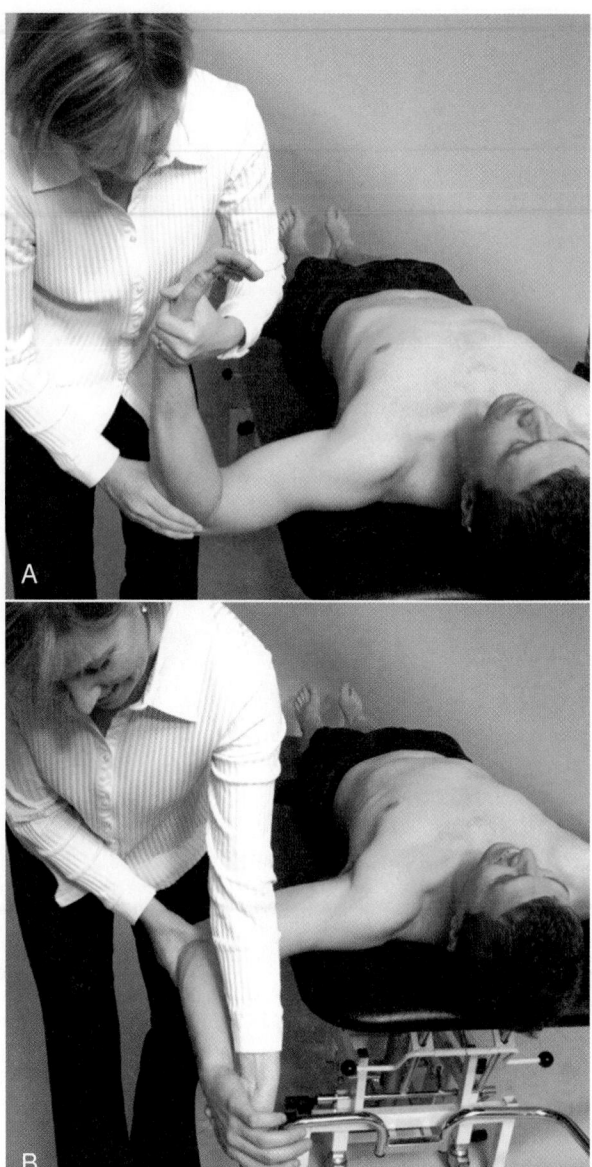

Figure 5-109 Resisted supination external rotation test (RSERT). A, The examiner supports the limb in the starting position. The patient attempts to supinate his hand as the examiner resists. **B,** The shoulder is then gently externally rotated to the maximal point.

shoulder, or reproduction of symptoms. It is considered negative if there is posterior shoulder pain, no pain, or apprehension.

? *SLAP Prehension Test.*[278] The patient is in the sitting or standing position. The arm is abducted to 90° with the elbow extended and the forearm pronated (thumb down and shoulder medially rotated). The patient is then asked to horizontally adduct the arm. The movement is repeated with the forearm supinated (thumb up and shoulder laterally rotated). If the patient feels pain in the bicipital groove in the first case (pronation) but the pain lessens or absent in the second case (supination), the test is considered positive for a SLAP lesion (Figure 5-110).

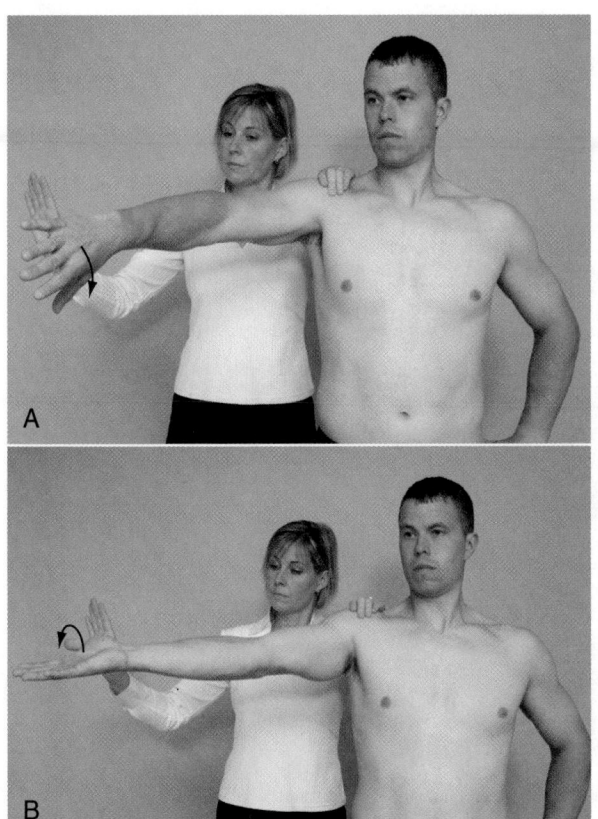

A

B

Figure 5-110 SLAP prehension test. A, Start position 1: Arm abducted to 90° with elbow extended and forearm pronated. The patient then horizontally adducts the arm. **B,** Start position 2: Same as position 1, but the forearm is supinated. The patient again horizontally adducts the arm. If position 1 is painful and position 2 is not, the test is considered positive.

Tests for Scapular Stability

For the muscles of the glenohumeral joint to work in a normal coordinated fashion, the scapula must be stabilized by its muscles to act as a firm base for the glenohumeral muscles. Thus, when doing these tests, the examiner is watching for movement patterns of the scapula as well as scapular dyskinesia.

"SICK" Scapula Signs and Symptoms[31]

- Insidious onset
- Prominence of inferior medial border of scapula
- Protraction of scapula
- Acromion less prominent
- Coracoid very tender to palpation
- Tight pectoralis minor
- Lack full forward flexion
- Tight short head of biceps

⚠ *Lateral Scapular Slide Test.*[61,87,279] This test determines the stability of the scapula during glenohumeral movements. The patient sits or stands with the arm resting

at the side. The examiner measures the distance from the base of the spine of the scapula to the spinous process of T2 or T3 (most common), from the inferior angle of the scapula to the spinous process of T7 to T9, or from T2 to the superior angle of the scapula. The patient is then tested holding two[279] (Figure 5-111) or four[87] other positions: 45° abduction (hands on waist, thumbs posteriorly),[87,279] 90° abduction with medial rotation,[87,279] 120° abduction,[87] and 150° abduction.[87] Davies and Dickoff-Hoffman[87] and Kibler[279] stated that in each position, the distance measured should not vary more than 1 cm to 1.5 cm (0.5 inch to 0.75 inch) from the original measure. However, there may be increased distances above 90° as the scapula rotates during scapulohumeral rhythm. Minimal protraction of the scapula should occur, however, during full elevation through abduction. Looking for asymmetry of movement between left and right sides is important, as well as noticing the amount of movement when determining scapular stability.

The test may also be performed by loading the arm (providing resistance) at 45° and greater abduction (**scapular load test** ✓) to see how the scapula stabilizes under dynamic load. This load may be applied anteriorly, posteriorly, inferiorly, or superiorly to the arm (Figure 5-112). Again, the scapula should not move more than 1.5 cm (0.75 inch). Odom and associates[280] have stated that the test has poor reliability for differentiating normal and pathological shoulders. However, loading the scapula, either by the weight of the arm or by applying a load to the arm, indicates the stabilizing ability of the scapular control muscles and whether abnormal winging or abnormal movement patterns occur.

In the different positions, the examiner may test for scapular and humeral stability by performing an eccentric movement at the shoulder by pushing the arm forward (**eccentric hold test**). One arm is tested at a time. As the arm is pushed forward eccentrically, the examiner should watch the relative movement at the scapulothoracic joint (protraction) and the glenohumeral joint (horizontal adduction). Normally, slightly more movement (relatively) occurs at the glenohumeral joint. If instability due to muscle weakness exists at either joint, excessive movement is evident at that joint relative to the other joint. In addition, the examiner should watch for winging of the scapula, which indicates scapular instability.

❓ *Scapular Assistance Test (SAT).*[54,61,94,281,282] This test evaluates scapular and acromial involvement in patients with impingement symptoms. The patient is in a standing position, and the examiner stands behind the patient. The examiner places the fingers of one hand over the clavicle with the heel of the hand over the spine of the scapula. This stabilizes the clavicle and scapula and holds the scapula retracted. The examiner's other hand holds the inferior angle of the scapula. As the patient actively abducts or forward flexes the arm, the examiner stabilizes and pushes the inferior medial border of the scapula up

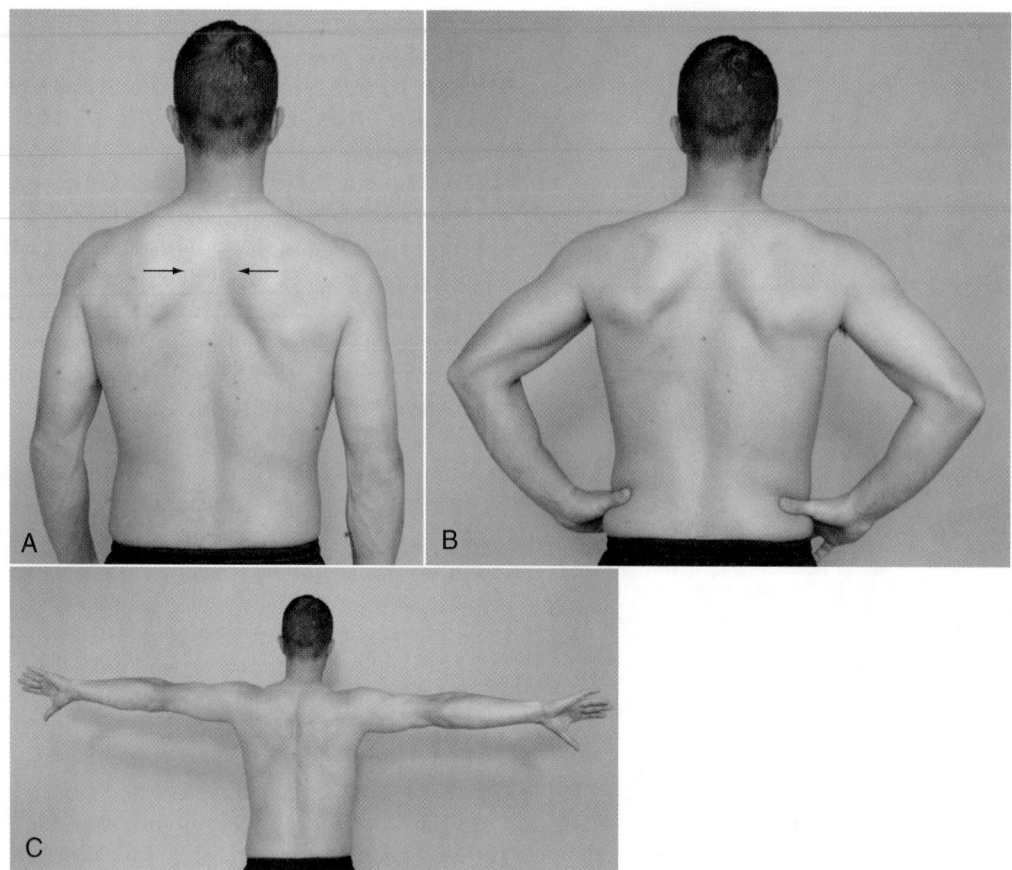

Figure 5-111 Lateral scapular slide test. The examiner measures from spinous process to scapula at level of base of spine of scapula (see *arrows* in **A**). **A,** Arms at side. **B,** Arms abducted, hands on waist, thumbs back. **C,** Arms abducted to 90°, thumbs down.

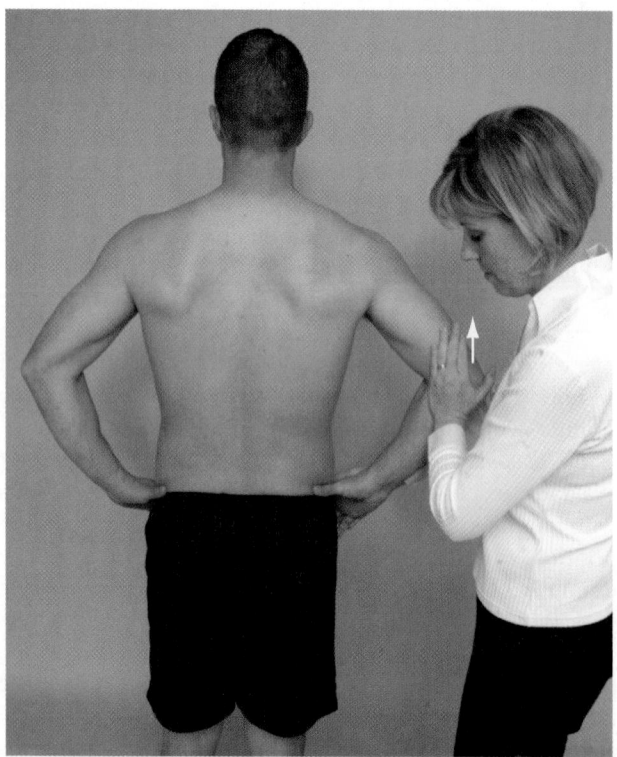

Figure 5-112 Scapular load test in 45° abduction.

and laterally while keeping the scapula retracted. Decreased pain would be a positive test and would indicate that the scapular control muscles are weak as the assistance by the examiner simulates the activity of serratus anterior and lower trapezius during elevation (Figure 5-113). During treatment, the test may be used as a method to increase the subacromial space.[283]

❓ *Scapular Isometric Pinch or Squeeze Test.*[94] The patient is in a standing position and is asked to actively "pinch" or retract the scapulae together as hard as possible and to hold the position for as long as possible (Figure 5-114). Normally, an individual can hold the contractions for 15 to 20 seconds with no burning pain or obvious muscle weakness. If burning pain occurs in less than 15 seconds, the scapular retractors are weak. When doing the test, the examiner must watch the patient carefully. Subconsciously, many patients will relax the contraction a slight amount, which is barely noticeable but allows the patient to hold the contraction in a comfort zone for longer periods with no burning.

⚠ *Scapular Retraction Test (SRT).*[54,61,94,281,282] The patient is in the standing position. The examiner, standing behind the patient, places the fingers of one hand over the clavicle with the heel of the hand over the spine of the scapula to stabilize the clavicle and scapula and to hold the scapula retracted. The examiner's other hand compresses the scapula against the chest wall (Figure 5-115). Holding the scapula in this position provides a firm stable base for the rotator cuff muscles, and often rotator cuff strength (if tested by a second examiner) improves. The test may also be positive in patients with a positive relocation test. If scapular retraction decreases the pain, when the relocation test is performed, it indicates that the weak scapular stabilizers must be addressed in the treatment.[282] This test

may also be done in supine. In patients with a SICK scapula, if the scapula is repositioned, forward flexion improves.[31]

Wall Pushup Test.[94,281] The patient stands arms length from a wall. The patient is then asked to do a "wall pushup" 15 to 20 times (Figure 5-116). Any weakness of the scapular muscles or winging usually shows up with 5 to 10 pushups. For stronger or younger people, a normal pushup on the floor shows similar scapular changes, usually with fewer repetitions. Goldbeck and Davies have taken this test further in what they describe as a **closed**

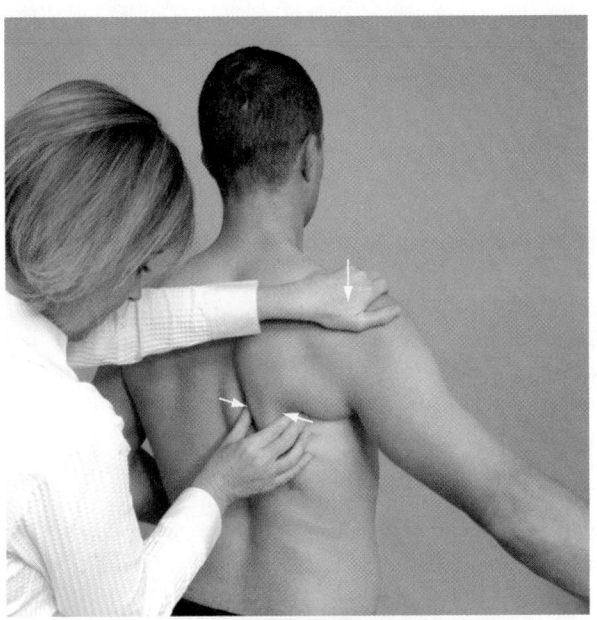

Figure 5-113 **Scapular assistance test (SAT).**

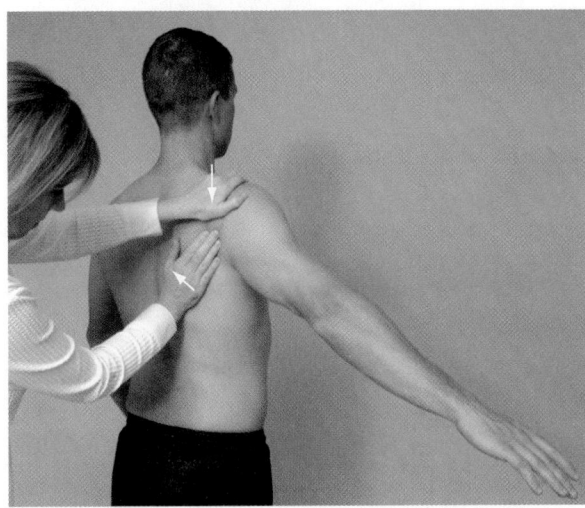

Figure 5-115 **Scapular retraction test.** Examiner uses hands to stabilize clavicle and scapula.

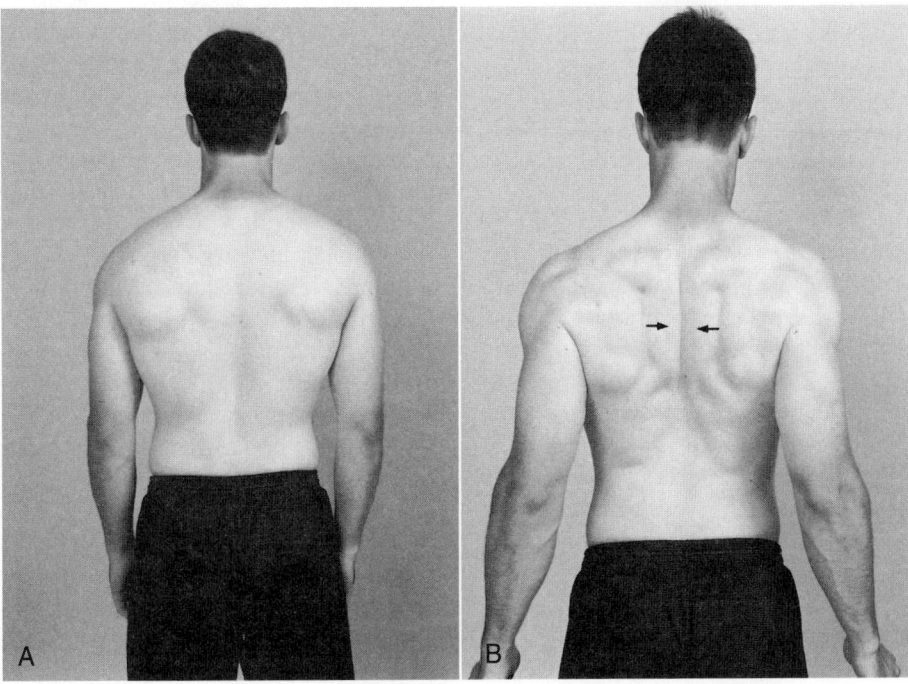

Figure 5-114 **Scapular isometric pinch test. A,** Start position. **B,** Pinch position.

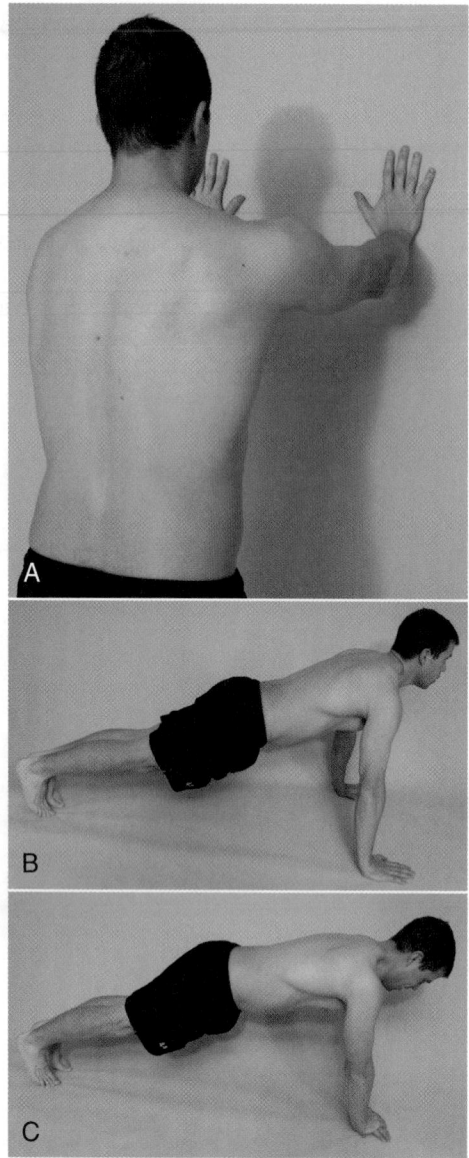

Figure 5-116 Wall (**A**) and floor (**B**) pushup tests. **C,** Closed kinetic chain upper extremity stability test touching opposite hand.

kinetic chain upper extremity stability test.[284] In this test, two markers (e.g., tape) are placed 91 cm (36 inches) apart. Patients assume the pushup position with one hand on each marker. When the examiner says "go," the subject moves one hand to touch the other, returns it to the original position, and then does the same with the other hand, repeating the motions for 15 seconds. The examiner counts the number of touches or crossovers made in the allotted time. The test is repeated three times, and the average is the test score. This test is designed primarily for young, active patients.

Other Shoulder Joint Tests

Scheibel, et al.[285] have developed an acromioclavicular joint instability (ACJI) scoring system to determine

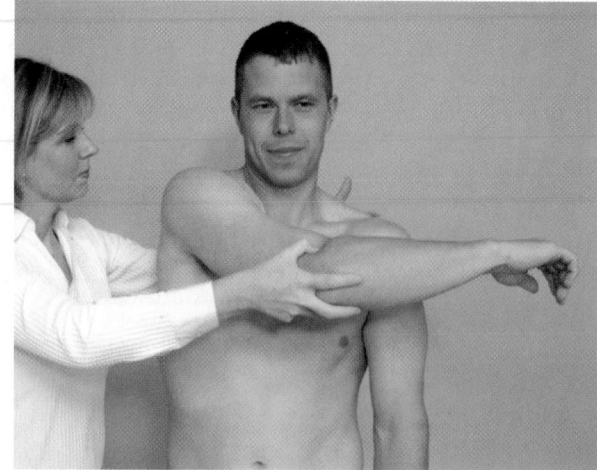

Figure 5-117 Acromioclavicular crossover, crossbody, or horizontal adduction test.

disability associated with injury to the acromioclavicular joint.

✓ *Acromioclavicular Crossover, Crossbody, or Horizontal Adduction Test.* The patient stands and reaches the hand across to the opposite shoulder. The examiner may also passively perform the test. With the patient in a sitting position, the examiner passively forward flexes the arm to 90° and then horizontally adducts the arm as far as possible (Figure 5-117).[47,266] If the patient feels localized pain over the acromioclavicular joint, the test is positive.[286–288] Localized pain in the sternoclavicular joint indicates that joint is at fault.

❓ *Acromioclavicular Shear Test.*[202] With the patient in the sitting position, the examiner cups his or her hands over the deltoid muscle with one hand on the clavicle and one hand on the spine of the scapula. The examiner then squeezes the heels of the hands together (Figure 5-118). Abnormal movement at the acromioclavicular joint indicates a positive test as well as acromioclavicular joint pathology.

❓ *Ellman's Compression Rotation Test.*[289,290] The patient lies on the unaffected side. The examiner compresses the humeral head into the glenoid while the patient rotates the shoulder medially and laterally. If the patient's symptoms are reproduced, glenohumeral arthritis is suspected (Figure 5-119).

✓ *Paxinos Sign.*[291] The patient is seated with the test arm relaxed at the side. The examiner stands beside the test arm and places one hand over the shoulder so that the thumb is under the posterolateral aspect of the acromion and the index and long fingers of the same hand (the fingers of the opposite hand may also be used instead) over the middle part of the clavicle on the same side (Figure 5-120). The examiner then applies pressure to the acromion with the thumb anterosuperiorly while applying an inferior directed counterforce to the clavicle with the fingers. The test is considered positive if pain in the area of acromioclavicular joint is increased.

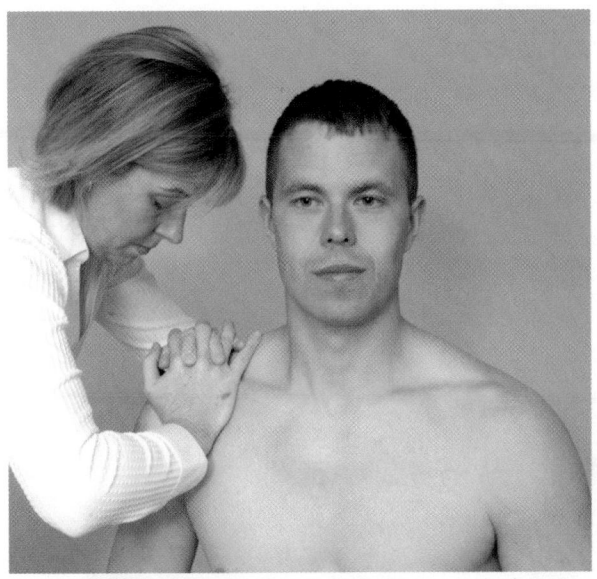

Figure 5-118 Acromioclavicular shear test.

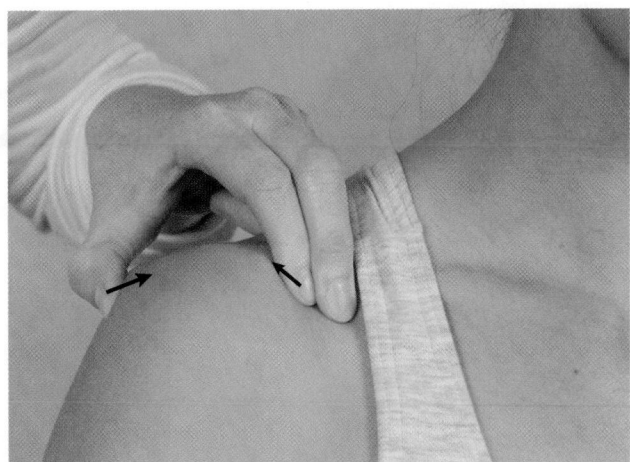

Figure 5-120 Paxinos sign.

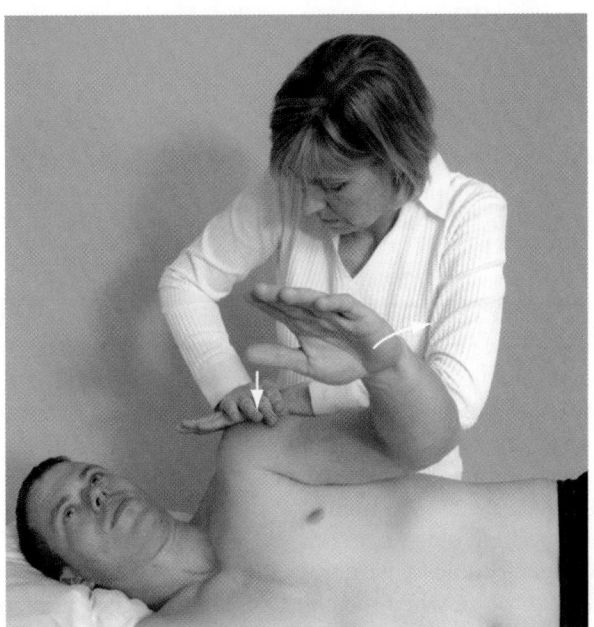

Figure 5-119 Ellman's compression-rotation test for glenohumeral arthritis.

Tests for Ligament Pathology

❓ *Coracoclavicular Ligament Test.* The integrity of the conoid portion of the coracoclavicular ligament may be tested by placing the patient in a side lying position on the unaffected side with the hand resting against the lower back. The examiner stabilizes the clavicle while pulling the inferior angle of the scapula away from the chest wall. The trapezoid portion of the ligament may be tested from the same position. The examiner stabilizes the clavicle and pulls the medial border of the scapula away from the chest wall (Figure 5-121). Pain in either case in

the area of the ligament (anteriorly under the clavicle between the outer one-third and inner two-thirds) constitutes a positive test.

✓ *Crank Test.* The crank test (see also under "Tests for Anterior Shoulder Instability") may also be used to evaluate the different glenohumeral ligaments (Figure 5-122). For example, when the crank test is done with the arm by the side, primarily the superior glenohumeral ligament and capsule are being tested. At 45° to 60° abduction, the middle glenohumeral ligament, the coracohumeral ligament, the inferior glenohumeral ligament (anterior band), and anterior capsule are being tested. Over 90° abduction, the inferior glenohumeral ligament and anterior capsule are being tested (see Table 5-1).[292,293]

❓ *Posterior Inferior Glenohumeral Ligament Test.*[263] Just as the crank test may be used to test the superior glenohumeral ligament, middle glenohumeral ligament, and the anterior portion of the inferior glenohumeral ligament; the posterior inferior glenohumeral test may be used to test the posterior portion of the inferior glenohumeral ligament. The patient sits while the examiner forward flexes the arm to between 80° and 90° and then horizontally adducts the arm 40° with medial rotation (Figure 5-123). While doing the movement, the examiner palpates the posteroinferior region of the glenoid. If the humerus protrudes or pain is felt in the area, the test is considered positive and indicates a lesion of the posterior portion of the inferior glenohumeral ligament. If movement (i.e., horizontal adduction) is restricted, it may also indicate a tight posterior capsule.

Tests for Muscle or Tendon Pathology

❓ *Abdominal Compression Test (Belly-Press or Napoleon Test).*[157,260,262,294–298] This test checks the subscapularis muscle, especially if the patient cannot medially rotate the shoulder enough to take it behind the back. The patient is in a standing position. The examiner places a hand on the abdomen below the xiphoid process so that

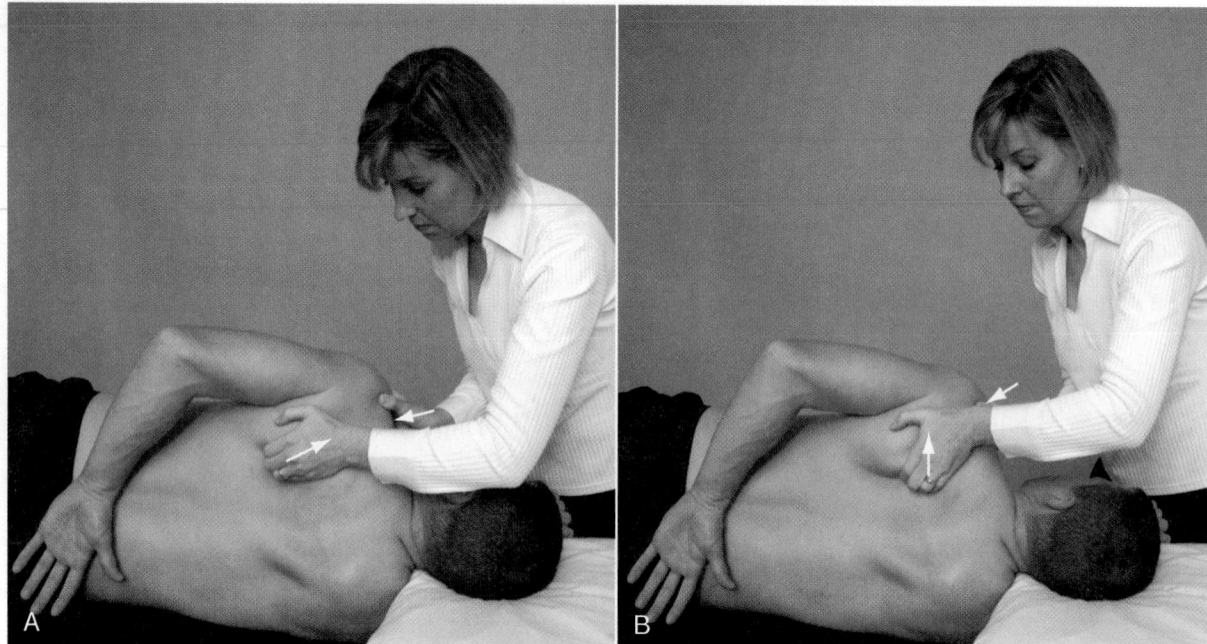

Figure 5-121 **Coracoclavicular ligament test. A,** Conoid portion. **B,** Trapezoid portion.

the examiner can feel how much pressure the patient is applying to the abdomen. The patient places his or her hand of the shoulder being tested on the examiner's hand and pushes the hand as hard as he or she can into the stomach (medial shoulder rotation). While pushing the hand into the abdomen, the patient attempts to bring the elbow forward to the scapular plane, causing greater medial shoulder rotation. If the patient is unable to maintain the pressure on the examiner's hand while moving the elbow forward, or posteriorly flexes the wrist or extends the shoulder, the test is positive for a tear of the subscapularis muscle (Figure 5-124).

? *Abrasion Sign.*[57] The patient sits and abducts the arm to 90° with the elbow flexed to 90°. The patient then medially and laterally rotates the arm at the shoulder. Normally, there are no signs and symptoms. If crepitus occurs, it is a sign that the rotator cuff tendons are frayed and are abrading against the under surfaces of the acromion process and the coracoacromial ligament.

? *Bear-Hug Test.*[157,260,298,299] The patient stands with the hand of the test shoulder on top of the other shoulder (Figure 5-125) with the fingers extended and the elbow in front of the body. The examiner stands in front of the patient and tries to lift the hand away from the shoulder applying a perpendicular lateral rotation force while the patient resists the movement. The examiner's other hand stabilizes the patient's elbow. If the patient cannot hold the hand on top of the shoulder because of weakness, it is considered a positive test for subscapularis strain.

⚠ *Biceps Tightness.* The patient lies supine with the shoulder in extension over the edge of the examining table with the elbow flexed and the forearm supinated.

The examiner then extends the elbow, which would normally have a bone-to-bone end feel if the biceps is normal. If the biceps is tight, full elbow flexion does not occur, and the end feel is a muscular tissue stretch (Figure 5-126).[300]

⚠ *Drop-Arm (Codman's) Test.* The examiner abducts the patient's shoulder to 90° and then asks the patient to slowly lower the arm to the side in the same arc of movement (Figure 5-127). A positive test is indicated if the patient is unable to return the arm to the side slowly or has severe pain when attempting to do so. A positive result indicates a tear in the rotator cuff complex.[301] A complete tear (3° strain) of the rotator cuff is more common in older patients (50-years-old or older). In younger people, a partial tear (1° or 2° strain) is more likely to occur when the patient is abducting the arm and a strong downward, eccentric load is applied to the arm.

⚠ *Dropping Sign.*[302] The patient stands with the test arm by the side. The examiner stands by the test side and passively places the patient's elbow in 90° flexion (Figure 5-128, *A*) with the arm in 45° lateral rotation. The patient is then asked to isometrically laterally rotate the arm against resistance and then relax. If the patient is not able to maintain the laterally rotated position and the arm drops back to the neutral position (Figure 5-128, *B*), the test is considered positive for an infraspinatus tear.

? *Gilchrest's Sign.*[202,303] While standing, the patient lifts a 2 kg to 3 kg (5 lb to 7 lb) weight over the head. The arm is laterally rotated fully and lowered to the side in the coronal plane. A positive test is indicated by discomfort or pain in the bicipital groove. A positive test indicates bicipital paratenonitis or tendinosis.[35] In some

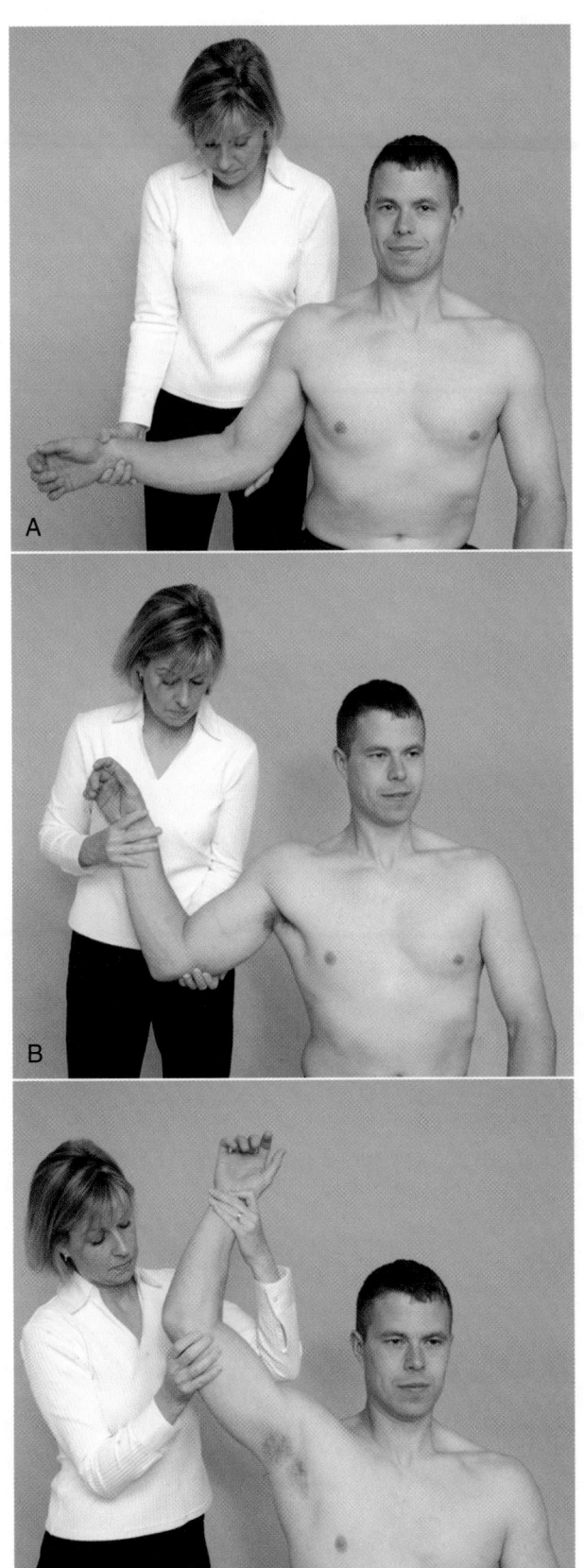

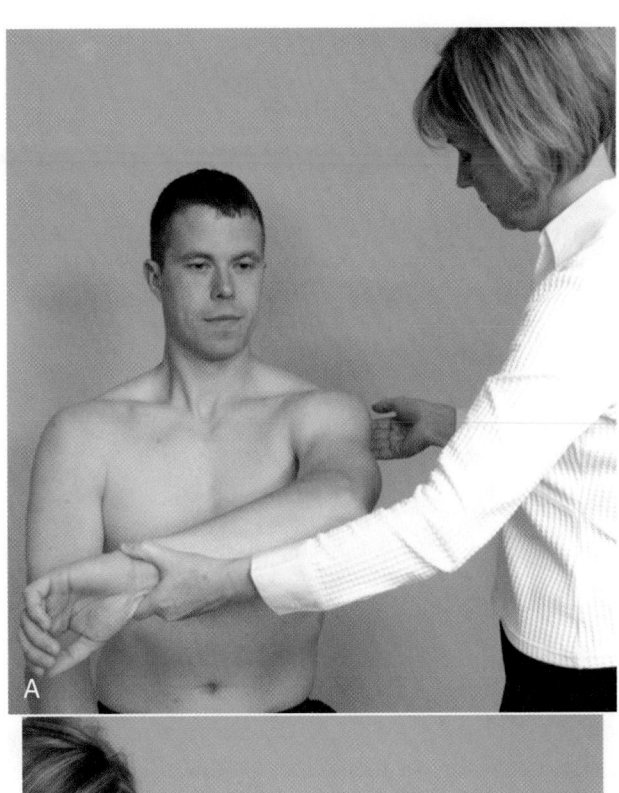

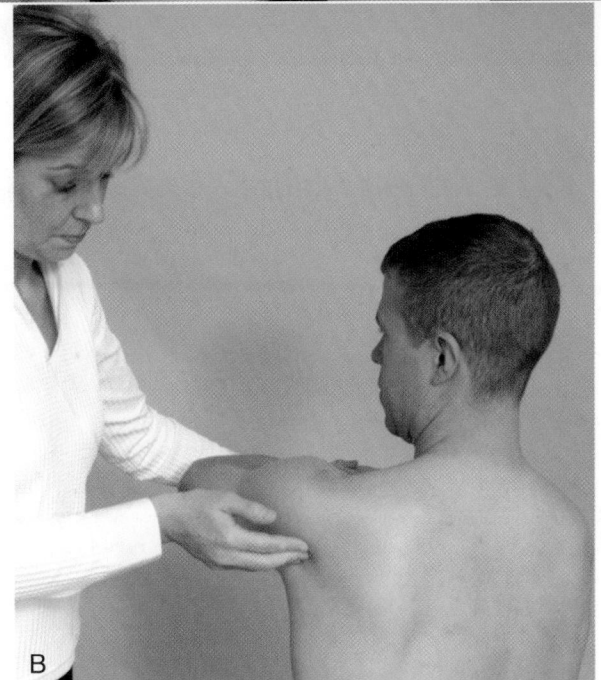

Figure 5-123 Posterior inferior ligament test. A, Anterior view. **B,** Posterior view.

Figure 5-122 Crank test used to test glenohumeral ligaments. A, Arm by the side—superior glenohumeral ligament tested. **B,** 45° to 60° abduction—middle glenohumeral ligament tested. **C,** Over 90° abduction—inferior glenohumeral ligament tested.

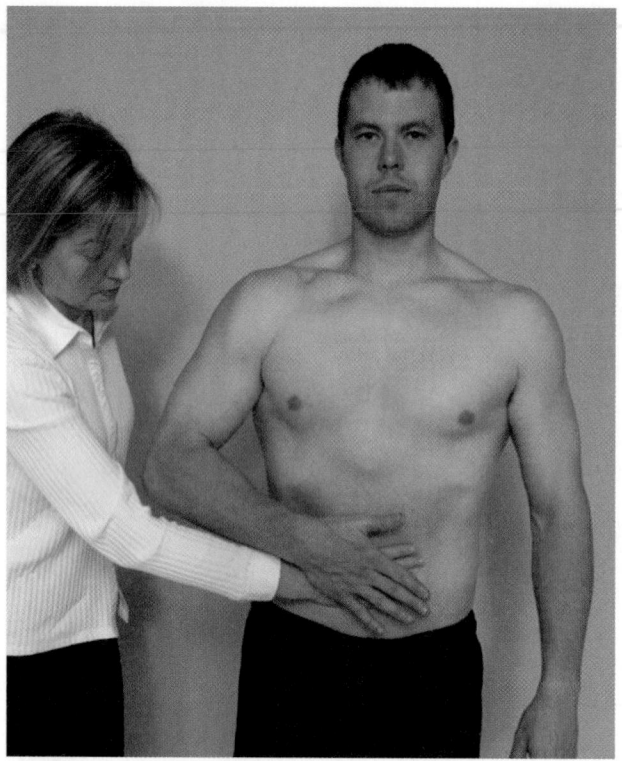

Figure 5-124 Abdominal compression test.

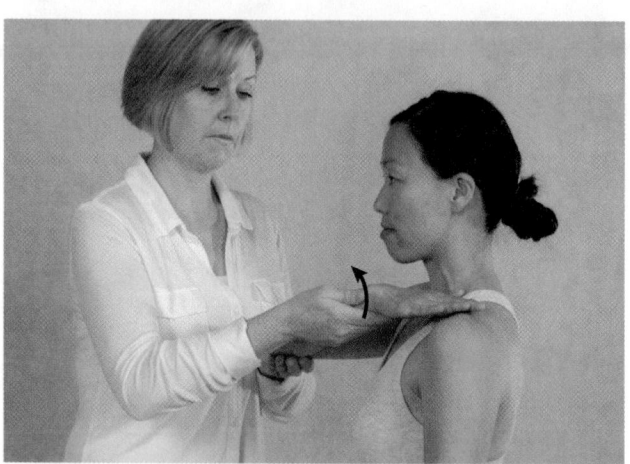

Figure 5-125 Bear-hug test.

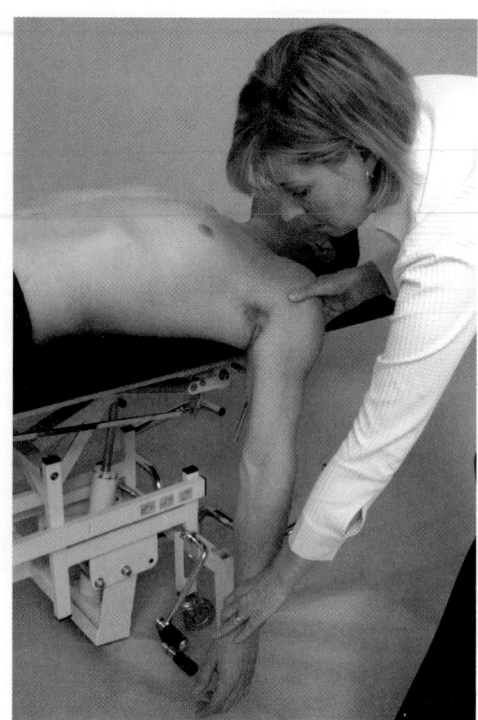

Figure 5-126 Testing for biceps tightness.

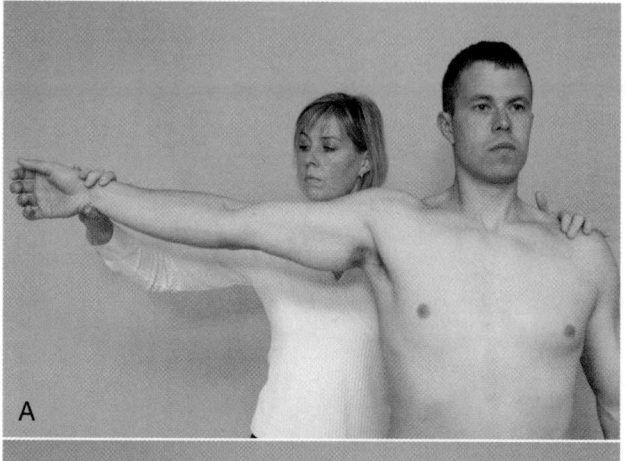

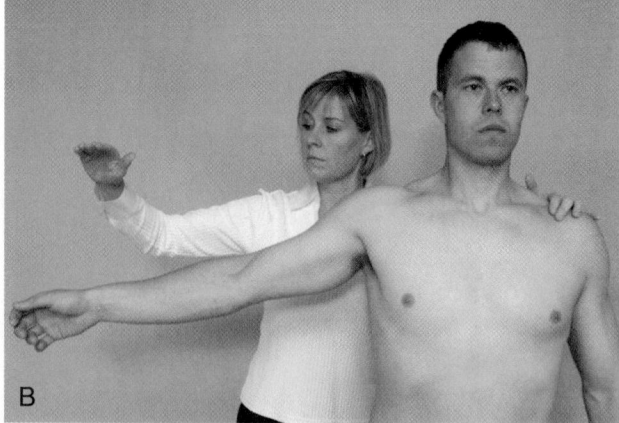

Figure 5-127 Drop-arm test. **A,** The patient abducts the arm to 90°. **B,** The patient tries to lower the arm slowly and is unable to do so; instead, the arm drops to his side. Examiner's hand illustrates the start position.

cases, an audible snap or pain may be felt at between 90° and 100° abduction.

Heuter's Sign.[303] Normally, if elbow flexion is resisted when the arm is pronated, some supination occurs as the biceps attempts to help the brachialis muscle flex the elbow. This supination movement is called *Heuter's sign*. If it is absent, the distal biceps tendon has been disrupted.

Hornblower's (Signe de Clairon) Sign.[168,302,304] This test, also called the *Patte test,* is designed to test the strength of teres minor. The patient is in a standing position

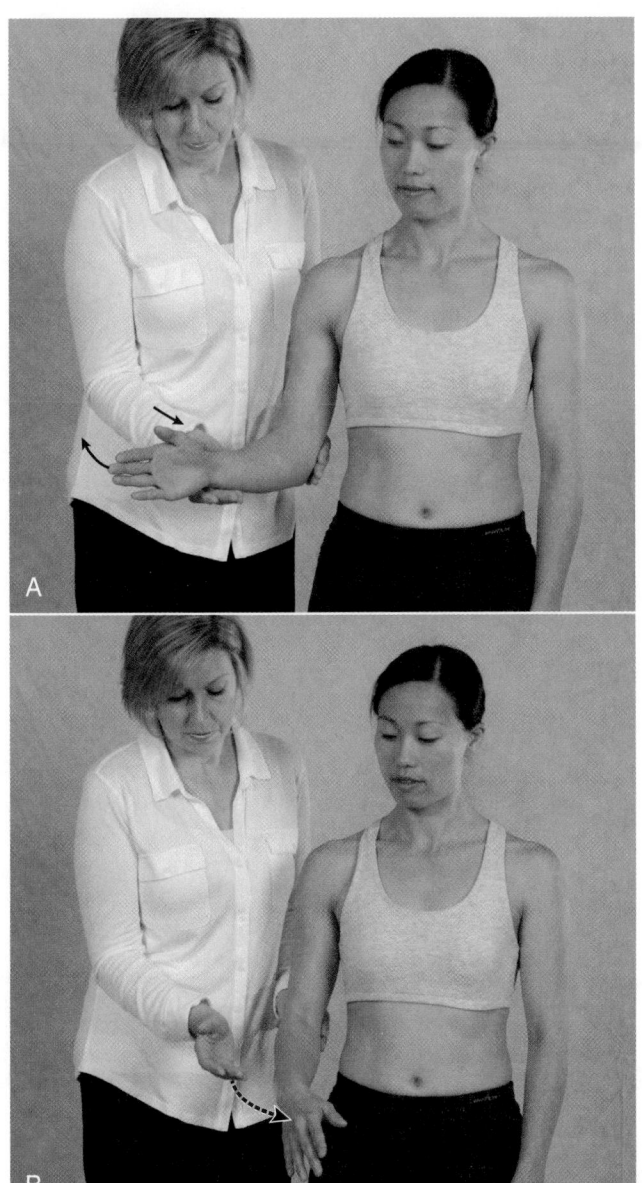

Figure 5-128 Dropping sign. A, Start position with examiner resisting patient's lateral rotation at 45° lateral rotation. **B,** Arm dropping back to neutral position *(arrow)* because of infraspinatus weakness.

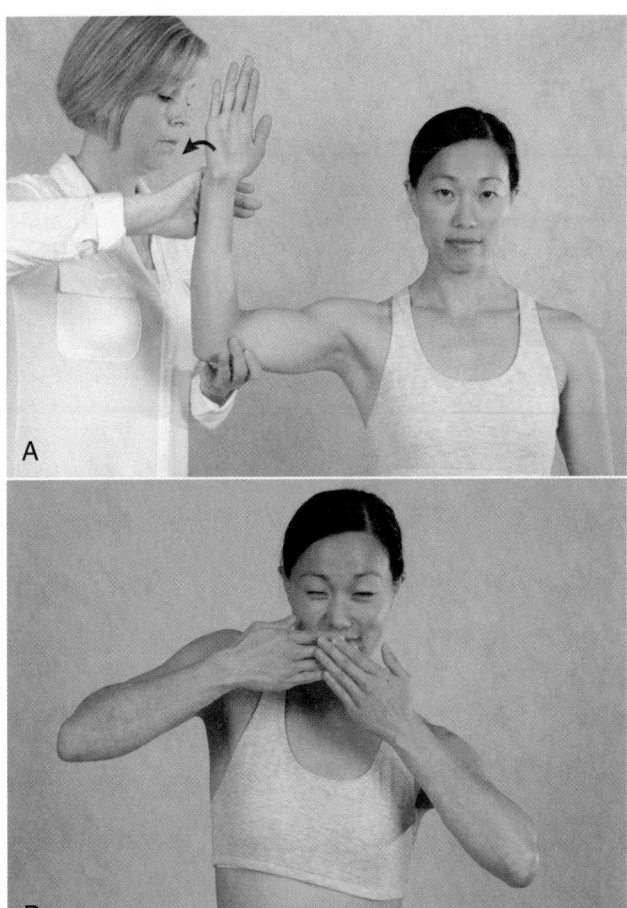

Figure 5-129 Hornblower's (Signe de Clairon) sign. A, The patient is in a standing position. The examiner elevates the patient's arm to 90° in the scapular plane (scaption). The examiner then flexes the elbow to 90°, and the patient is asked to laterally rotate the shoulder against resistance. **B,** McClusky modification: Patient is asked to abduct the arms to bring the hands to the mouth. A positive test is shown.

(Figure 5-129, *A*). The examiner elevates the patient's arm to 90° in the scapular plane (scaption). The examiner then flexes the elbow to 90°, and the patient is asked to laterally rotate the shoulder against resistance. A positive test is indicated when the patient is unable to laterally rotate the arm and indicates a tear of teres minor.[305]

McClusky offered a second way to do the test.[168] The patient is standing with the arms by the side and then is asked to bring the hands to the mouth. With a massive posterior rotator cuff tear, the patient is unable to do this without abducting the arm first (Figure 5-129, *B*). This abduction with hands to the mouth is called **hornblower's sign.**

✓ *Infraspinatus Test.* The patient stands with the arm at the side with the elbow at 90° and the humerus medially rotated to 45°. The examiner then applies a medial rotation force that the patient resists. Pain or the inability to resist medial rotation indicates a positive test for an infraspinatus strain (Figure 5-130).

✓ *Lateral Rotation Lag Sign (Infraspinatus "Spring Back" Test).*[168,306] The patient is seated or in standing position with the arm by the side and the elbow flexed to 90°. The examiner passively abducts the arm to 90° in the scapular plane, laterally rotates the shoulder to end range (some authors say 45°),[302] and asks the patient to hold it (Figure 5-131, *A*). For a positive test, the patient cannot hold the position and the hand springs back anteriorly toward midline, indicating infraspinatus and teres minor cannot hold the position due to weakness or pain (Figure 5-131, *B*).[307,308] The examiner will also find passive medial rotation will have increased on the affected side.

If the test is performed with the arm in 20° abduction or by the side in the scapular plane with the elbow at 90° and the shoulder laterally rotated, the examiner then takes the arm into maximum lateral rotation and asks the patient to hold the position (Figure 5-132, *A*). If the supraspinatus and infraspinatus are torn, the arm will medially rotate and spring back anteriorly indicating a positive test (Figure 5-132, *B*). This test has also been called the **external rotation lag sign (ERLS) test** ☑. Hertel, et al.[306] described a **drop sign** ☑ in which the patient is standing and abducts the arm to 90° with the elbow flexed to 90°. The examiner maximally laterally rotates the arm, and the patient is asked to hold the position. If the arm falls or drops into medial rotation, the test is considered positive for tears to infraspinatus and supraspinatus and perhaps subscapularis (Figure 5-133).[232,302,306] If the patient is able to hold the position, the strength of infraspinatus can be graded as three or greater, depending on the resistance to the examiner's medially rotated force.[302]

⚠ *Latissimus Dorsi Weakness.*[205] The patient is in a standing position with the arms elevated in the plane of the scapula to 160°. Against resistance of the examiner, the patient is asked to medially rotate and extend the arm downward as if climbing a ladder (Figure 5-134).

☑ *Lift-Off Sign.*[157,294,295,298,307,309,310] The patient stands and places the dorsum of the hand on the back pocket or against the midlumbar spine. Great subscapularis activity is shown with the second position (Figure 5-135).[311] The patient then lifts the hand away from the back. An inability to do so indicates a lesion of the subscapularis muscle. Abnormal motion in the scapula during the test may indicate scapular instability. If the patient is able to take the hand away from the back, the examiner should apply a load pushing the hand toward the back to test the strength of the subscapularis and to test how the scapula acts under dynamic loading. With a torn subscapularis tendon, passive (and active) lateral rotation increases.[310]

If the patient's hand is passively medially rotated as far as possible and the patient is asked to hold the position, it will be found that the hand moves toward the back (**subscapularis** or **medial rotation, "spring back,"** or

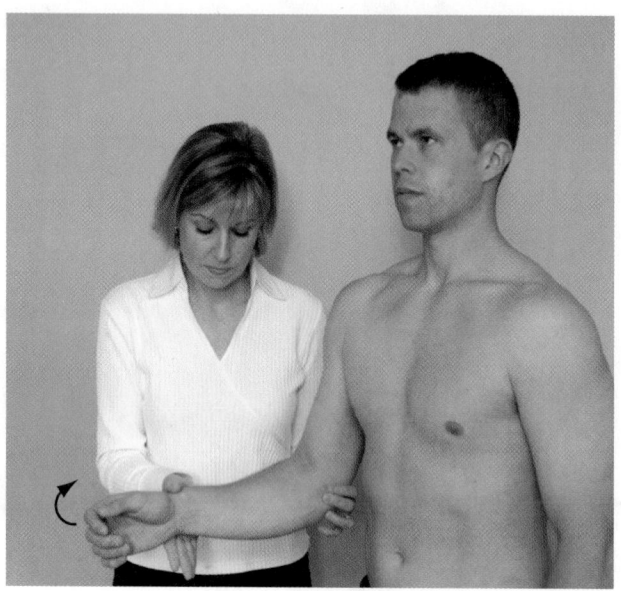

Figure 5-130 Infraspinatus test.

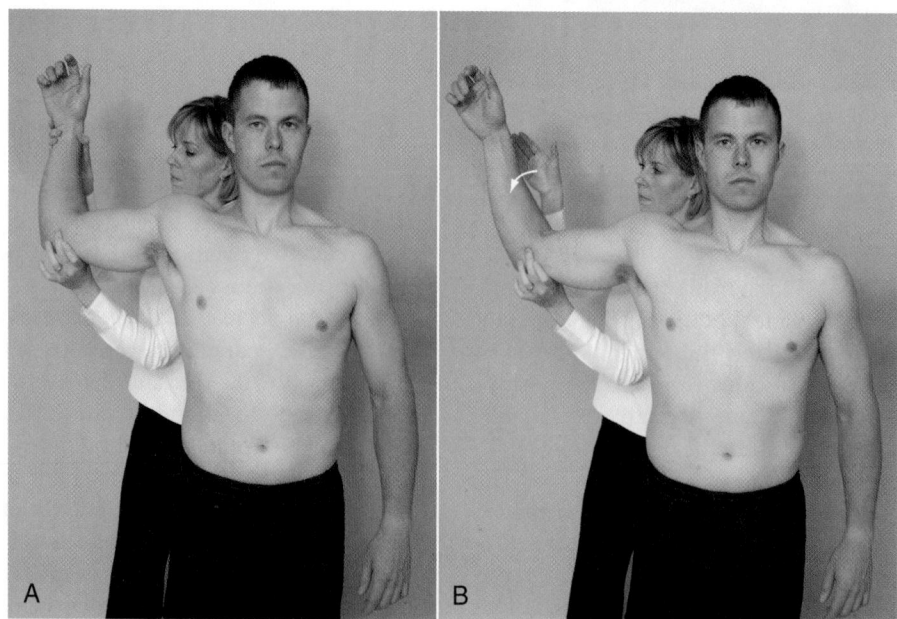

Figure 5-131 Lateral rotation lag test to test the teres minor and infraspinatus. **A,** Arm is abducted 90°. **B,** Note how hand springs forward when released by examiner.

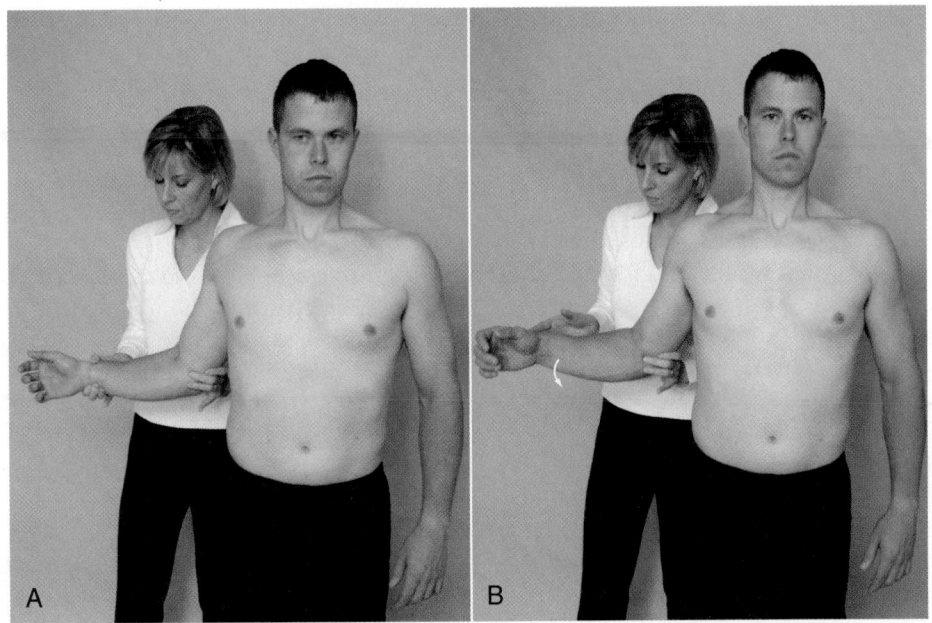

Figure 5-132 **External rotation lag sign (ERLS) or drop test. A,** Start position. **B,** Position in positive test.

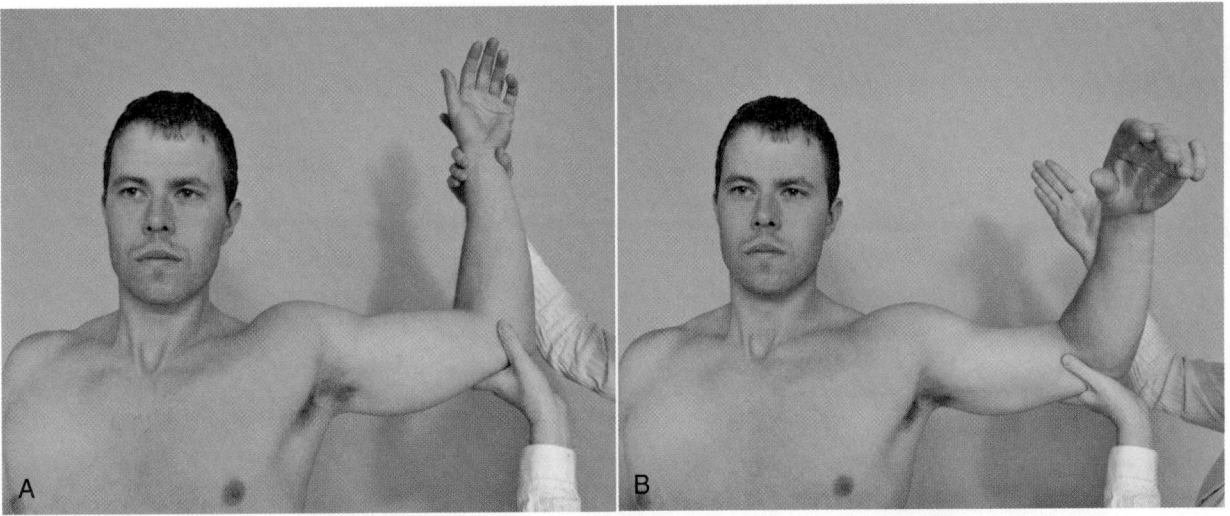

Figure 5-133 **The drop sign. A,** The test is performed by the examiner placing the arm in 90° of abduction and maximum external rotation and asking the patient to hold the position. **B,** If the patient cannot hold this position and the arm falls into internal rotation, the test is positive.

lag test ☑) because subscapularis cannot hold the position due to weakness or pain (Figure 5-136).[180,306] This test is also called the **modified lift-off test.**[304,310] A small lag between maximum passive medial rotation and active medial rotation implies a partial tear (1°, 2°) of subscapularis.[294] This modified test is reported to be more accurate in diagnosing rotator cuff tear.[306] The test may also be used to test the rhomboids. Medial border winging of the scapula during the test may indicate that the rhomboids are affected. Stefko, et al. reported that maximum isolation of the subscapularis was achieved by placing the hand against the posteroinferior border of the scapula (**maximum medial rotation test** ❓) and then attempting the lift off.[312] In the other positions for lift off, teres major, latissimus dorsi, posterior deltoid, or rhomboids may compensate for a weak subscapularis.

❓ *Lippman's Test.*[313] The patient sits or stands while the examiner holds the arm flexed to 90° with one hand. With the other hand, the examiner palpates the biceps tendon 7 cm to 8 cm (2.5 inches to 3 inches) below the glenohumeral joint and moves the biceps tendon from side-to-side in the bicipital groove. A sharp pain is a positive test and indicates bicipital paratenonitis or tendinosis.[35]

❓ *Ludington's Test.*[314] The patient clasps both hands on top of or behind the head, allowing the interlocking fingers to support the weight of the upper limbs (Figure 5-137). This action allows maximum relaxation of the biceps tendon in its resting position. The patient then alternately contracts and relaxes the biceps muscles. While the patient does the contractions and relaxations, the examiner palpates the biceps tendon, which will be felt on the uninvolved side but not on the affected side if the test result is positive. A positive result indicates that the long head of biceps tendon has ruptured.

⚠️ *Pectoralis Major Contracture Test.* The patient lies supine and clasps the hands together behind the head. The arms are then lowered until the elbows touch the examining table (Figure 5-138, *A*). A positive test occurs if the elbows do not reach the table and indicates a tight pectoralis major muscle.

⚠️ *Pectoralis Minor Tightness.* Pectoralis minor functions along with the rhomboids and levator scapulae to stabilize the scapula during arm extension. Tightness of the pectoralis minor can lead to increased scapular protraction and tilting of the inferior angle of the scapula posteriorly. Tightness of the pectoralis minor can be tested by having the patient in a supine lying position with arm forward flexed 30°.[315] The examiner places the heel of the hand over the coracoid process and pushes it toward the examining table retracting the scapula (Figure 5-138, *B*). Normally, the posterior movement occurs with no discomfort to the patient, and the scapula lies flat against the table. However, if there is tightness (muscle tissue stretch) over the pectoralis minor muscle during the posterior movement, the test is considered positive.

☑️ *Rent Test.*[316] The patient is seated with the arm by the side with the examiner standing behind (Figure 5-139). The examiner palpates the anterior margin of the patient's acromion with one hand while holding the patient's elbow at 90° with the other hand. The examiner then passively extends the patient's arm and slowly medially and laterally rotates the patient's humerus while palpating the greater tuberosity and rotator cuff tendons. The presence of a depression ("rent" or defect) of about

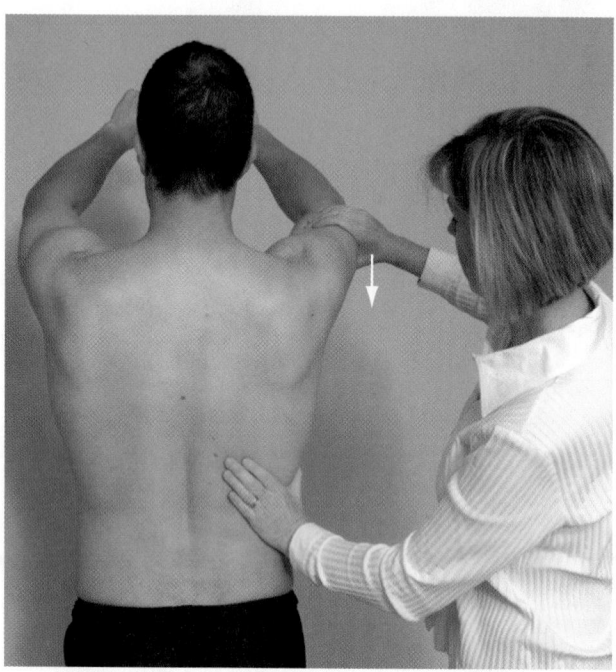

Figure 5-134 Testing for latissimus dorsi weakness.

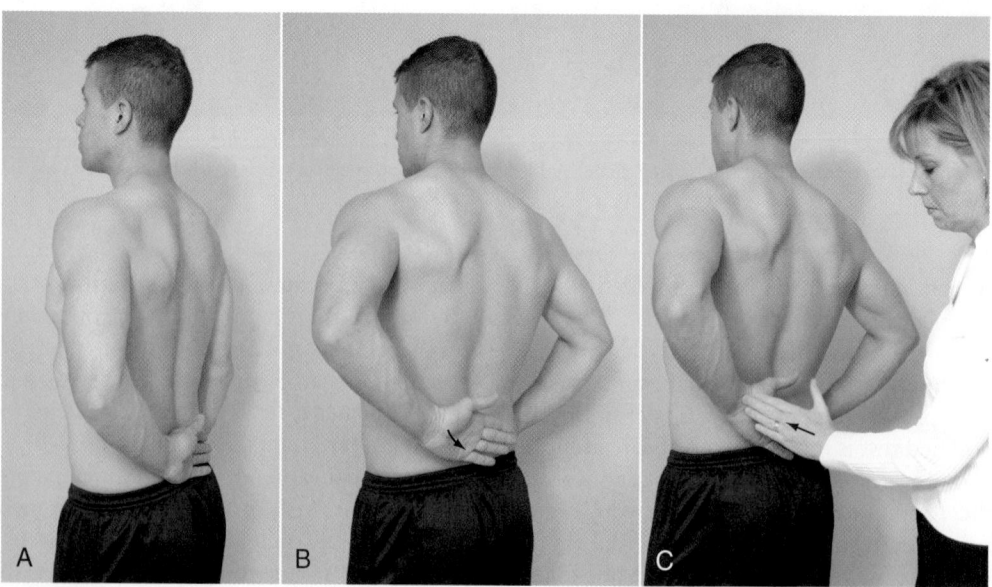

Figure 5-135 Lift-off sign. A, Start position. **B,** Lift-off position. **C,** Resistance to lift off provided by examiner. Examiner tests strength of subscapularis and watches positioning of scapula.

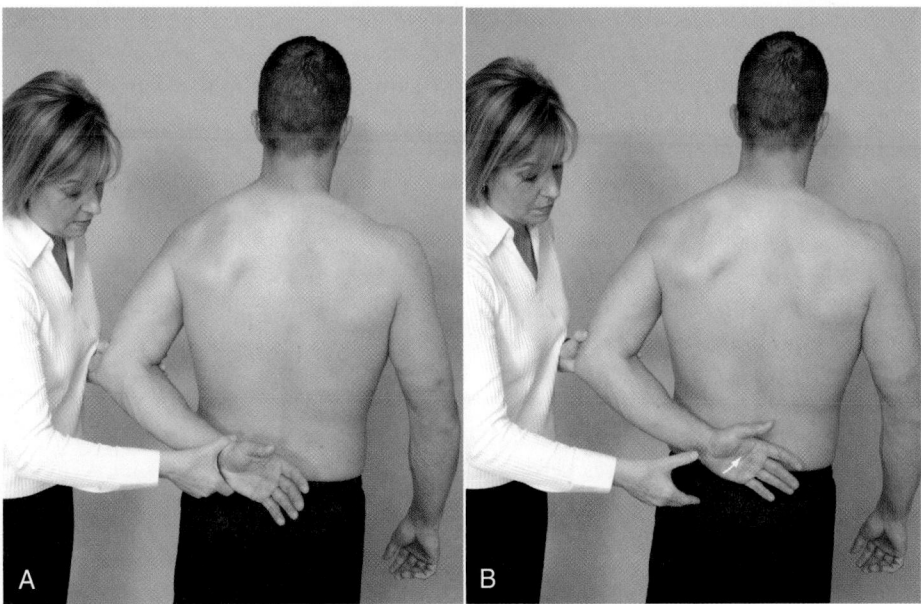

Figure 5-136 Subscapularis spring back or lag test. A, Start position. **B,** Patient is unable to hold the start position and hand springs back toward the lower back.

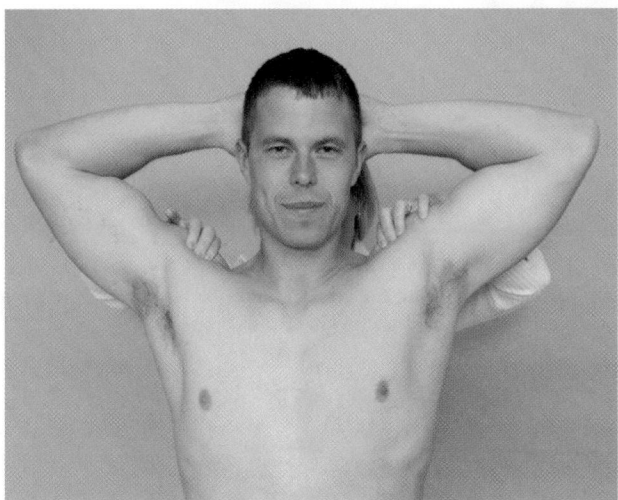

Figure 5-137 Ludington's test.

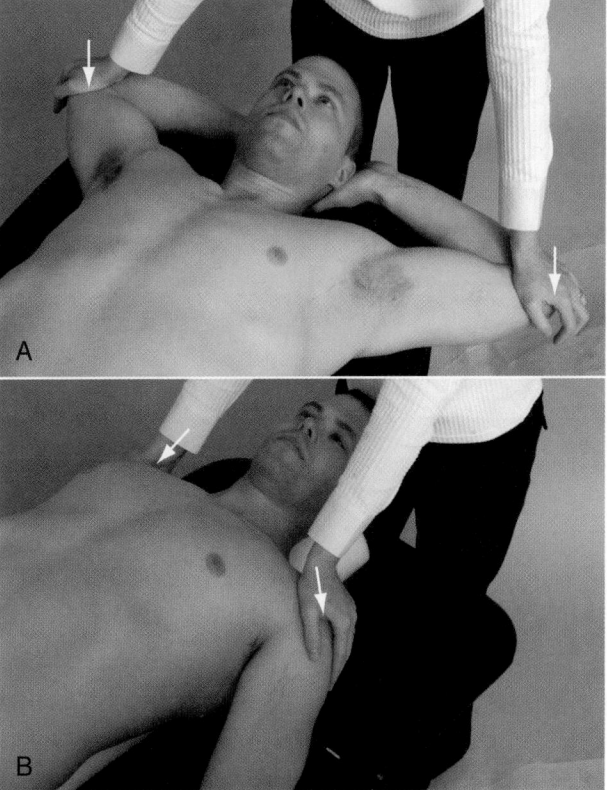

Figure 5-138 Testing for tightness of **(A)** pectoralis major and **(B)** pectoralis minor. Examiner is testing end feel. Note position of examiner's hand on **(A)** humerus and **(B)** coracoid process.

one finger width or a more prominent greater tuberosity (relative to the other side) indicates a positive test for a rotator cuff tear.

⚠ *Rhomboid Weakness.*[167,317] The patient is in a prone lying position or sitting with the test arm behind the body so that the hand is on the opposite side (opposite back pocket). The examiner places the index finger along and under the medial border of the scapula while asking the patient to push the shoulder forward slightly against resistance to relax the trapezius (Figure 5-140, *A*). The patient then is asked to raise the forearm and hand away from the body. If the rhomboids are normal, the fingers are pushed away from under the scapula (Figure 5-140, *B*).

Rhomboid and levator scapulae strength may also be tested by having the patient place the hands on the hips while the examiner pushes the elbows anteriorly.[65]

✓ *Serratus Anterior Weakness (Punch Out Test).*[317] The patient is in a standing position and forward flexes the arm to 90°. The examiner applies a backward force to the arm (Figure 5-141). If serratus anterior is weak or paralyzed, the medial border of the scapula wings (classic winging). The patient also has difficulty abducting or forward flexing the arm above 90° with a weak serratus anterior, but it still may be possible with lower trapezius compensation.[67] A similar finding may be accomplished by doing a wall or floor pushup.

To differentiate long thoracic nerve palsy (serratus anterior) from posterior instability that causes serratus anterior dysfunction, the examiner should ask the patient to laterally rotate the arm and then forward flex the arm. In this case, if scapular winging is eliminated, then the problem is posterior instability due to serratus anterior weakness.[65]

✓ *Speed's Test (Biceps or Straight-Arm Test).* The examiner resists shoulder forward flexion by the patient while

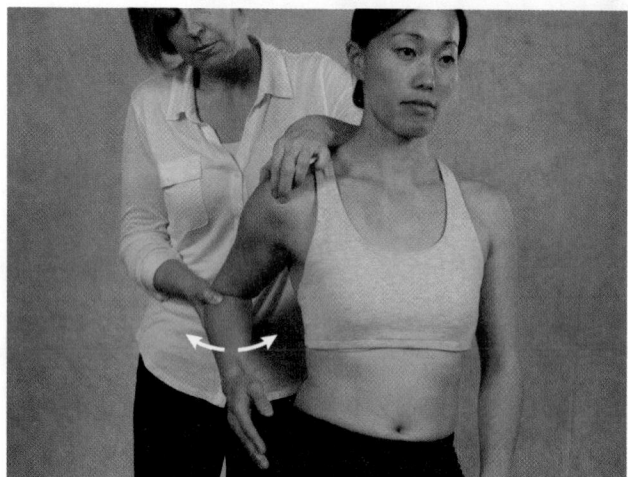

Figure 5-139 **Rent test for rotator cuff tear.**

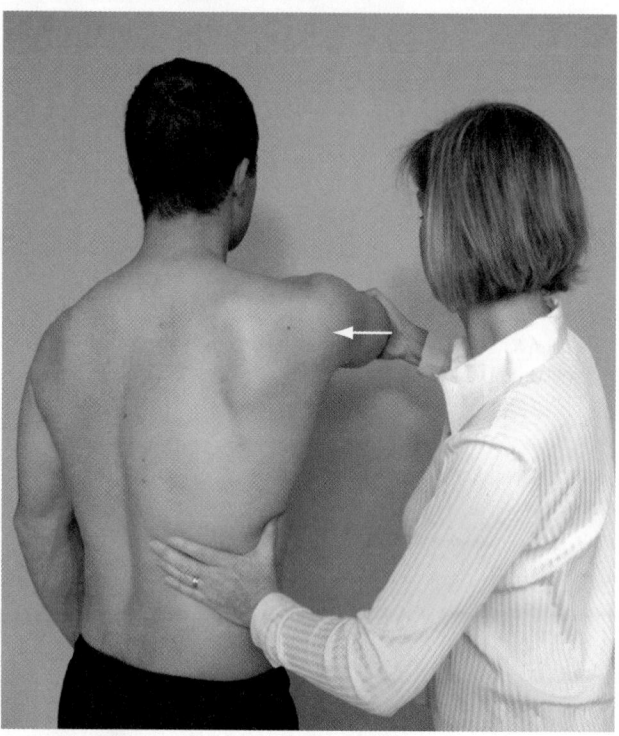

Figure 5-141 **Testing for serratus anterior weakness.** Punch out test: Examiner applies a backward force.

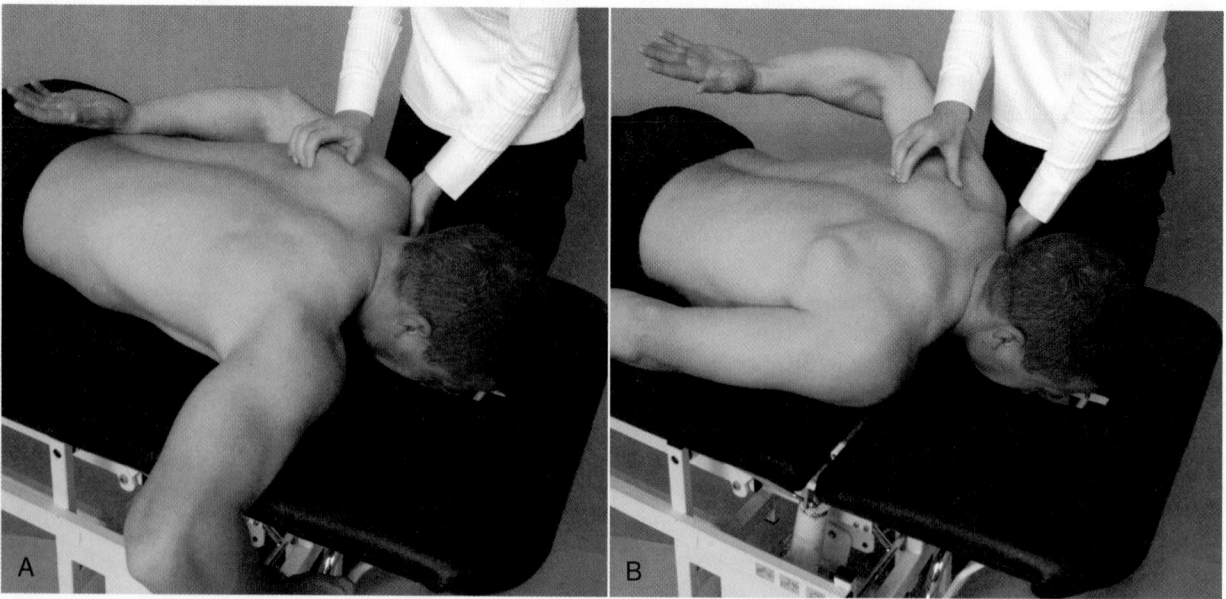

Figure 5-140 **Testing for rhomboid weakness. A,** Start position. **B,** Test position.

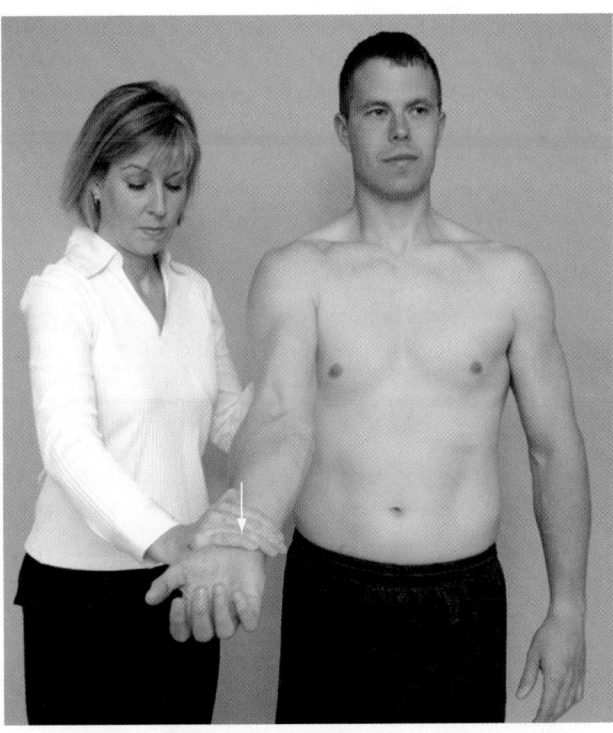

Figure 5-142 Speed's test (biceps or straight-arm test).

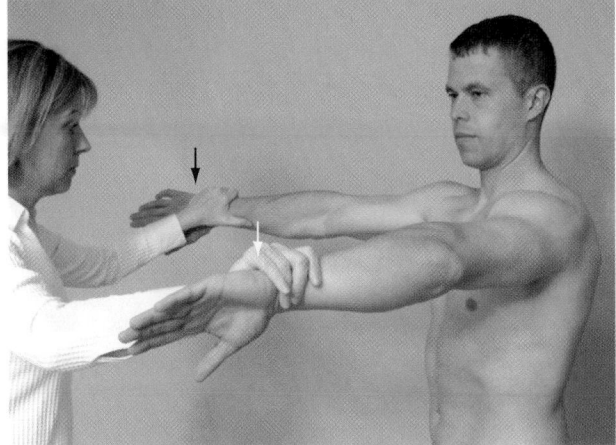

Figure 5-143 Supraspinatus "empty can" test.

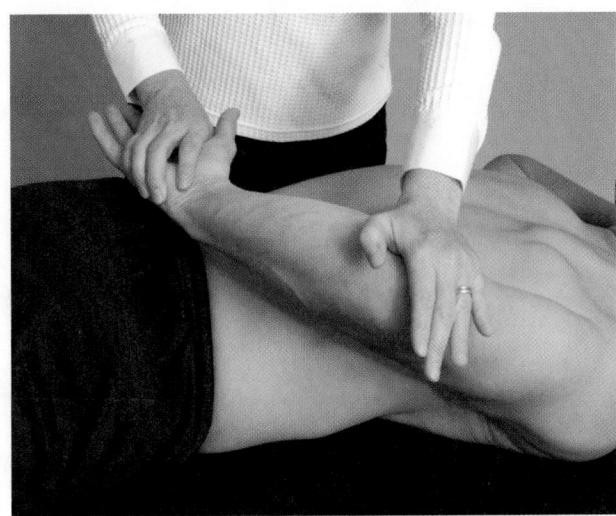

Figure 5-144 Teres minor test.

the patient's forearm is first supinated, then pronated, and the elbow is completely extended. The test may also be performed by forward flexing the patient's arm to 90° and then asking the patient to resist an eccentric movement into extension first with the arm supinated, then pronated[260,318] (Figure 5-142). A positive test elicits increased tenderness in the bicipital groove especially with the arm supinated and is indicative of bicipital paratenonitis or tendinosis.[35] Speed's test is more effective than Yergason's test because the bone moves over more of the tendon during the Speed's test. It has been reported that this test may cause pain and, therefore, is positive if a SLAP (type II) lesion is present.[218] If profound weakness is found on resisted supination, a severe second- or third-degree (rupture) strain of the distal biceps should be suspected.[319]

☑ *Supraspinatus ("Empty Can" or Jobe) Test.*[157,320] The patient's arm is abducted to 90° with neutral (no) rotation, and the examiner provides resistance to abduction. The shoulder is then medially rotated and angled forward 30° ("empty can" position) so that the patient's thumbs point toward the floor (Figure 5-143) in the plane of the scapula. Others have said that testing the arm with the thumb up ("full can") is best for maximum contraction of supraspinatus.[309] Resistance to abduction is again given while the examiner looks for weakness or pain, reflecting a positive test result. A positive test result indicates a tear of the supraspinatus tendon or muscle, or neuropathy of the suprascapular nerve.

❓ *Teres Minor Test.* The patient lies prone and places the hand on the opposite posterior iliac crest. The patient is then asked to extend and adduct the medially-rotated arm against resistance. Pain or weakness indicates a positive test for teres minor strain (Figure 5-144).

⚠ *Tightness of Latissimus Dorsi, Pectoralis Major, and Pectoralis Minor.* The patient is placed in a supine lying position and is asked to fully elevate the arms through forward flexion. If the three muscles have normal length, the arms will extend to rest against the examining table. If the scapula does not lie flat against the table, it indicates that the pectoralis minor, pectoralis major, or latissimus dorsi is tight (the scapula remains protracted) (Figure 5-145).[321]

☑ *Trapezius Weakness.*[317] The patient sits down and places the hands together over the head. The examiner stands behind the patient and pushes the elbows forward. Normally the three parts of the trapezius contract to

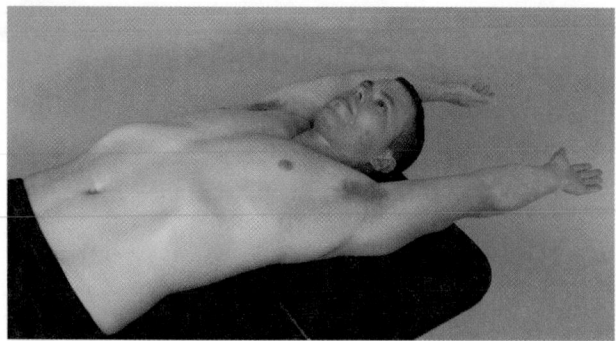

Figure 5-145 Testing for tightness of latissimus dorsi, pectoralis major, and pectoralis minor as a group.

stabilize the scapula (Figure 5-146, *A*). The upper trapezius can be tested separately by elevating the shoulder with the arm slightly abducted or to resisted shoulder abduction and head side flexion (Figure 5-146, *B*).[321,322] If the shoulder is elevated with the arm by the side, levator scapulae and rhomboids are more likely to be involved as well. The middle trapezius can be tested with the patient in a prone position with the arm abducted to 90° and laterally rotated. The test involves the examiner resisting horizontal extension of the arm watching for retraction of the scapula, which should normally occur (Figure 5-146, *C*).[321,322] If scapular protraction occurs,

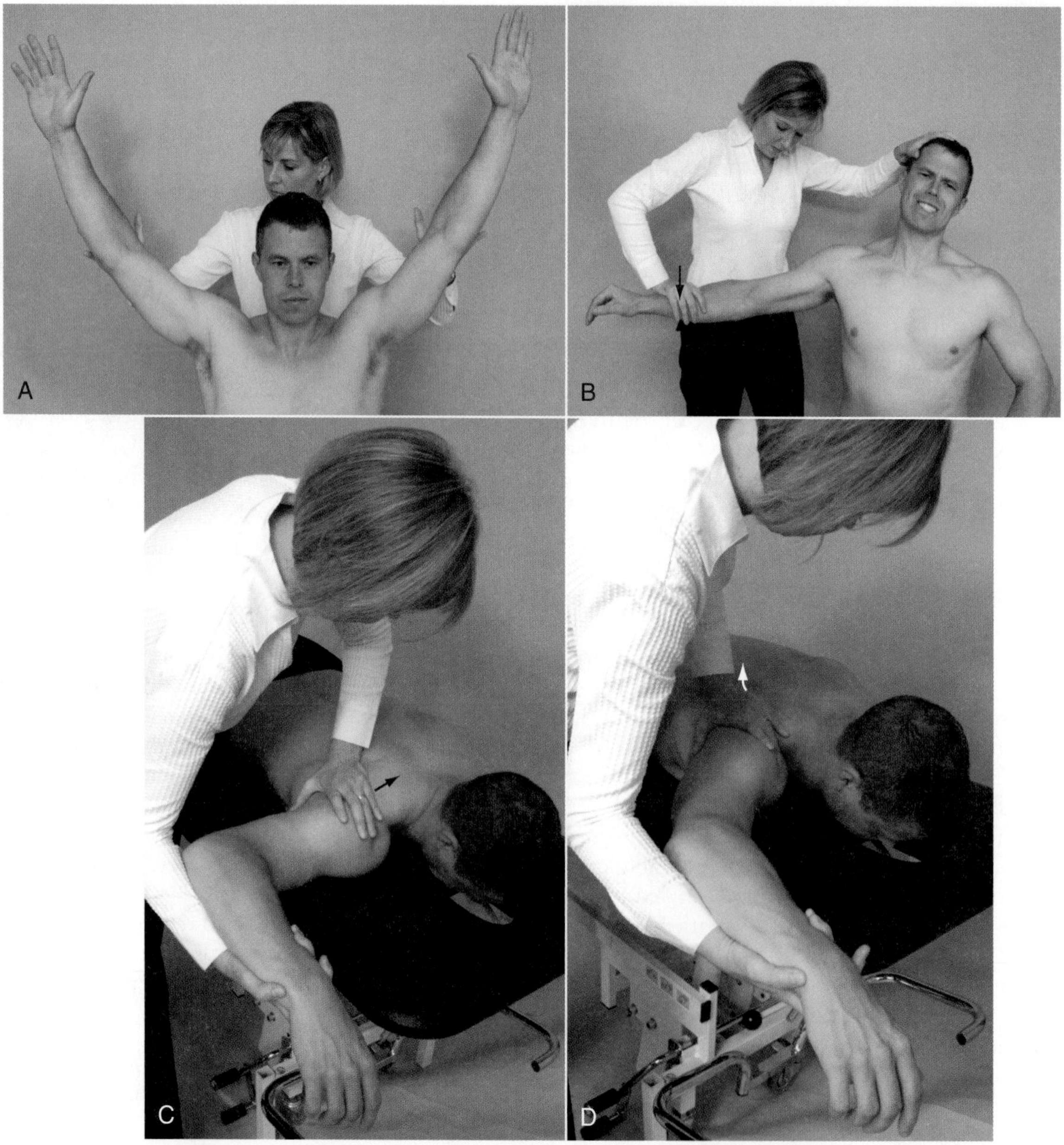

Figure 5-146 Testing for trapezius weakness. **A,** All portions of triceps. **B,** Upper trapezius. **C,** Middle trapezius. **D,** Lower trapezius.

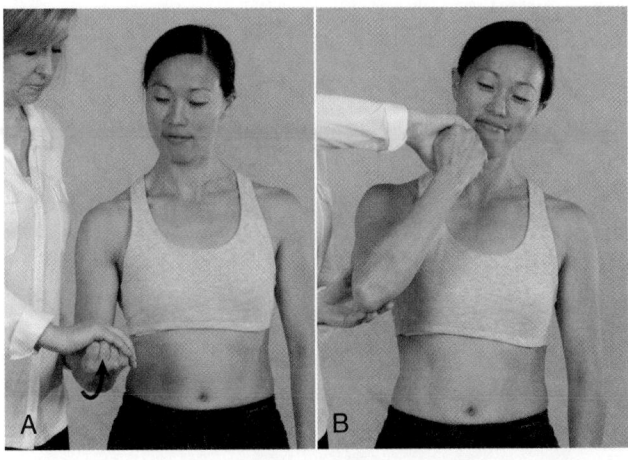

Figure 5-147 "Upper cut" test. A, Start position. B, End position.

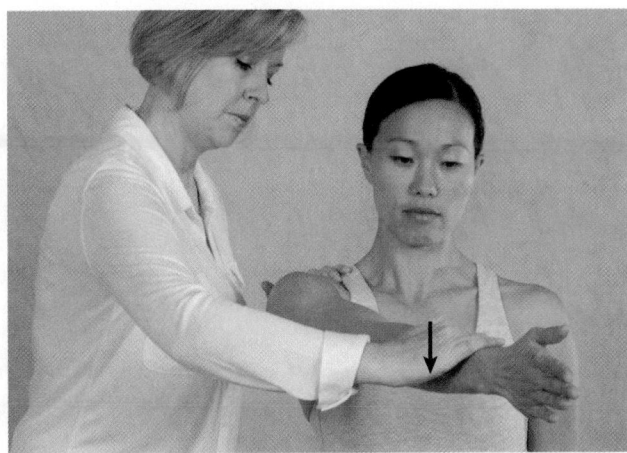

Figure 5-148 Whipple test for rotator cuff and superior labral tears.

the middle fibers of trapezius are weak. To test the lower trapezius, the patient is in prone lying with arm abducted to 120° and the shoulder laterally rotated. The examiner applies resistance to diagonal extension and watches for scapular retraction that should normally occur (Figure 5-146, D). If scapular protraction occurs, the lower trapezius is weak.[321] Paralysis of the trapezius muscle causes the scapula to translate inferiorly, and the inferior angle of the scapula is rotated laterally.[65] If the scapula is elevated more than normal, it may indicate a tight trapezius or the presence of cervical torticollis.

Triceps Tightness. The patient is in a sitting position. The arm is fully elevated through forward flexion and lateral rotation. While stabilizing the humerus, the examiner flexes the elbow (see Figure 6-16, B).[300] Normally, the end feel would be soft tissue approximation. If the triceps is tight, elbow flexion is limited and the end feel is muscular tissue stretch.

"Upper Cut" Test.[260] The patient stands with the shoulder in neutral by the side with the elbow flexed to 90°. The forearm is supinated and the hand is in a fist (Figure 5-147). The examiner puts a hand over the fist to resist the patient's movement. The patient then actively and quickly brings the hand up and toward the chin doing a "boxing upper cut punch." A positive test is indicated by pain or a painful pop over the anterior shoulder and is an indication of a biceps injury.

Whipple Test.[31] The patient stands with the arm forward flexed to 90° and adducted until the hand is opposite the other shoulder. The examiner pushes downward at the wrist while the patient resists (Figure 5-148). The test is considered positive for partial rotator cuff tears and/or superior labrum tears.

Yergason's Test. This test is primarily designed to check the ability of the transverse humeral ligament to hold the biceps tendon in the bicipital groove. With the patient's elbow flexed to 90° and stabilized against the thorax and with the forearm pronated, the examiner resists supination while the patient also laterally rotates

the arm against resistance (Figure 5-149).[323] If the examiner palpates the biceps tendon in the bicipital groove during the supination and lateral rotation movement, the tendon will be felt to "pop out" of the groove if the transverse humeral ligament is torn. Tenderness in the bicipital groove alone without the dislocation may indicate bicipital paratenonitis/tendinosis.[35] This test is not as effective as Speed's test when testing the biceps tendon, because the bicipital groove moves only slightly over the tendon affecting only a small part of the tendon during the test and because biceps tendon pain tends to occur with motion or palpation rather than with tension.

Tests for Neurological Function

Tinel Sign (at the Shoulder). The area of the brachial plexus above the clavicle in the area of the scalene triangle is tapped. A positive sign is indicated by a tingling sensation in one or more of the nerve roots.

Upper Limb Neurodynamic (Tension) Test (ULNT) (Brachial Plexus Tension Test).[324] This test is the upper limb equivalent of the straight leg raising test of the lower limb. It is used when the patient has presented with upper limb radicular signs or peripheral nerve symptoms. The patient is positioned to stress the neurological tissue entering the arm. The patient lies supine. The test may be performed by placing the joints of the upper limb in different positions to stress each of the neurological tissues differently.[325] There are, in effect, four upper limb tension tests (ULNT I to IV) (see Table 3-18 and Figure 3-42).[326] The key to performing the tests correctly is to ensure the shoulder is held in depression. If it is allowed to elevate, tension is taken off the neurological structures. Depending on the patient history, the examiner picks the ULNT that stresses the appropriate neurological tissue. Pain in the form of tingling or a stretch or ache in the cubital fossa indicates stretching of the dura mater in the cervical spine. The available range of passive movement at the elbow, when compared with the normal side, can indicate the restriction. Lateral or side flexion of the

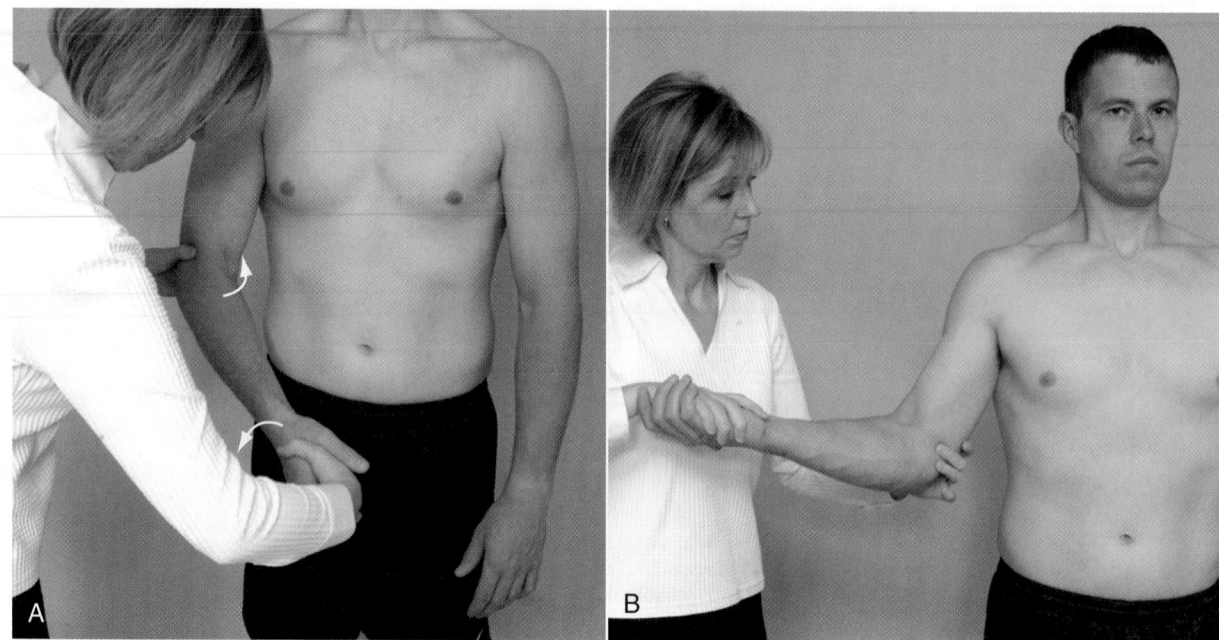

Figure 5-149 Yergason's test. A, Start position. **B,** End position.

cervical spine to the opposite side can enhance the effect. If full ROM is not available in the shoulder, the test can still be performed by taking the shoulder to the point just short of pain in abduction and lateral rotation and performing the other maneuvers of the arm or by passively side flexing the cervical spine. The upper limb tension tests put tension on the upper limb neurological tissues even in normal individuals. Therefore, reproduction of the patient's symptoms, rather than stretching, constitutes a positive sign. This finding indicates the neurological tissue is being stressed, but it does not tell the examiner where or why it is being stressed.

Tests for Thoracic Outlet Syndrome

Thoracic outlet syndromes may combine neurological and vascular signs, or the signs and symptoms of neurological deficit, restriction of arterial flow, or restriction of venous flow may be seen individually.[327] The patient may complain of fatigue in the shoulder, vague shoulder pain, achiness, and sense of heaviness in the shoulder, all of which can affect speed and control while doing activity (e.g., throwing, swimming) especially with the arm in abduction and lateral rotation (Table 5-18).[37] For this reason, a diagnosis of thoracic outlet syndrome is usually one of exclusion in which all other causes have been eliminated.[328-331] In fact, neurogenic signs are rare in thoracic outlet syndrome, and there is poor correlation between the vascular signs of the condition and neurological involvement. Thoracic outlet tests must not only decrease the pulse, they must also reproduce the patient's symptoms to be considered positive.[332] The tests do not show high reliability.

TABLE **5-18**

Thoracic Outlet Signs and Symptoms[330]

| | VASCULAR | |
Neurological	Arterial	Venous

• Numbness
• Tingling
• Weak grip
• Loss of manual
  dexterity (intrinsics)
	• Cool, pale
	  extremity
		• Swelling
		• Mottled
		  discoloration

With thoracic outlet tests that involve taking the pulse, the examiner must find the pulse before positioning the patient's arm or cervical spine. Because the pulse may be diminished even in a "normal" individual, looking for the reproduction of symptoms is more important than looking for diminution of the pulse. Unless stated, the duration of these provocative tests should be no more than 1 to 2 minutes.[329]

❓ *Adson Maneuver.*[33,333] This test is probably one of the most common methods of testing for thoracic outlet syndrome reported in the literature. The examiner locates the radial pulse. The patient's head is rotated to face the test shoulder (Figure 5-150). The patient then extends the head while the examiner laterally rotates and extends the patient's shoulder. The patient is instructed to take a deep breath and hold it. A disappearance of the pulse indicates a positive test.

❓ *Costoclavicular Syndrome (Military Brace) Test.*[33] The examiner palpates the radial pulse and then draws the

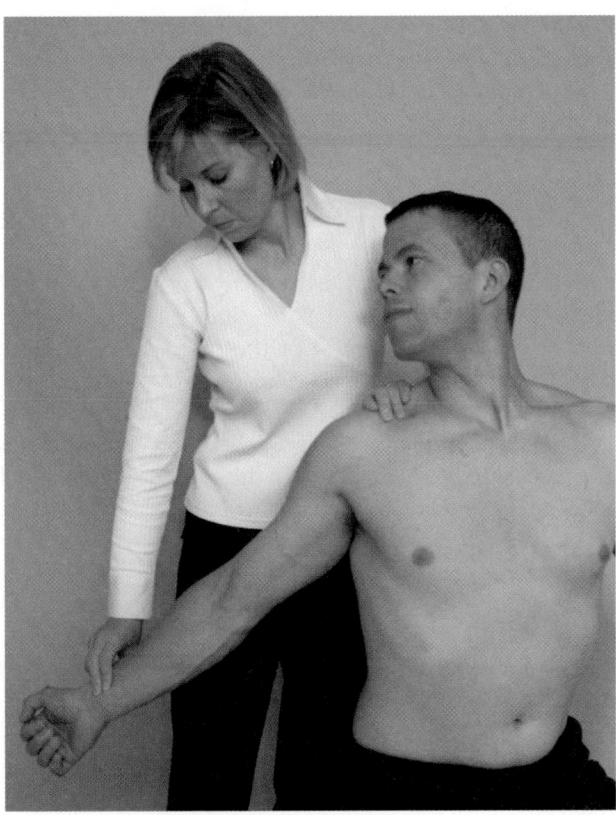

Figure 5-150 Adson maneuver.

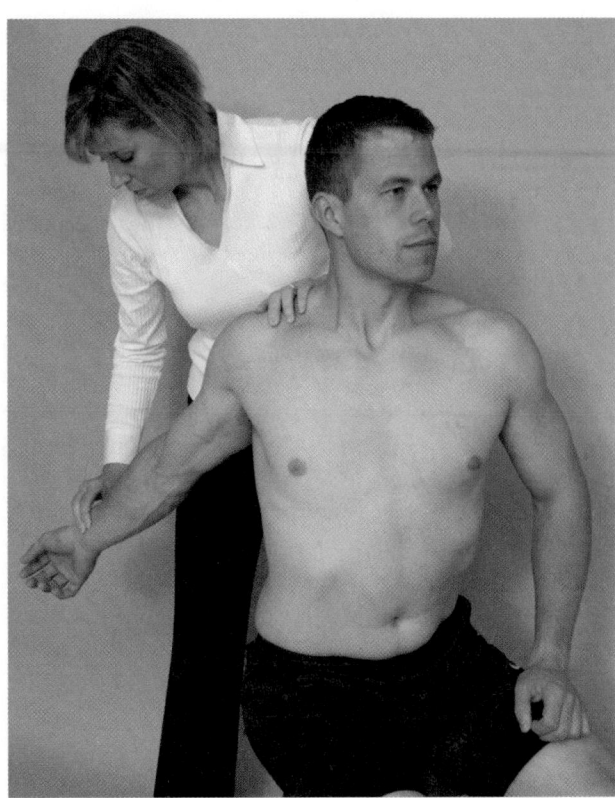

Figure 5-151 Costoclavicular syndrome test.

patient's shoulder down and back (Figure 5-151). A positive test is indicated by an absence of the pulse and implies possible thoracic outlet syndrome (costoclavicular syndrome). This test is particularly effective in patients who complain of symptoms while wearing a backpack or heavy coat.

❓ *Halstead Maneuver.* The examiner finds the radial pulse and applies a downward traction on the test extremity while the patient's neck is hyperextended and the head is rotated to the opposite side (Figure 5-152). Absence or disappearance of a pulse indicates a positive test for thoracic outlet syndrome.

❓ *Provocative Elevation Test.*[180] The patient elevates both arms above the horizontal and is asked to rapidly open and close the hands fifteen times. If fatigue, cramping, or tingling occurs during the test, the test is positive for vascular insufficiency and thoracic outlet syndrome. This test is a modification of the Roos test.

⚠ *Roos Test (Elevated Arm Stress Test [EAST]).*[33,334] The patient stands and abducts the arms to 90°, laterally rotates the shoulder, and flexes the elbows to 90° so that the elbows are slightly behind the frontal plane. The patient then opens and closes the hands slowly for 3 minutes (Figure 5-153). If the patient is unable to keep the arms in the starting position for 3 minutes or suffers ischemic pain, heaviness or profound weakness of the arm, or numbness and tingling of the hand during the 3

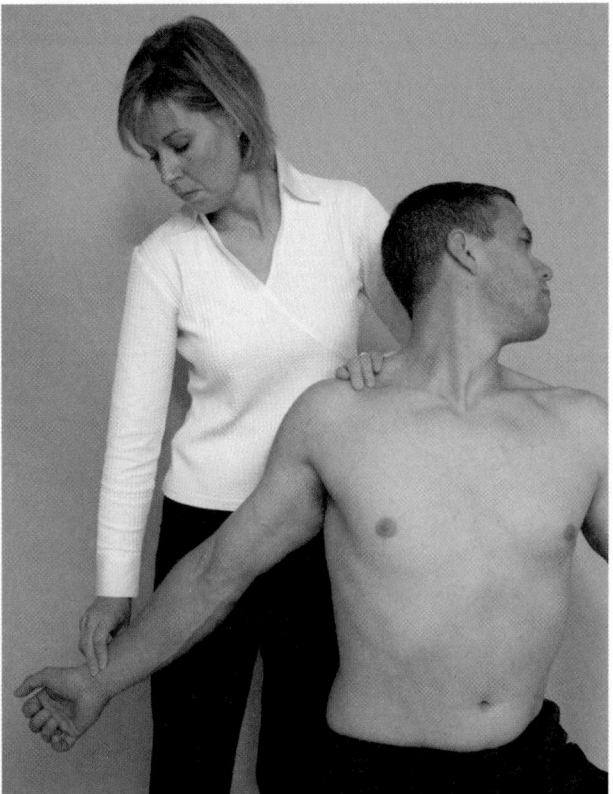

Figure 5-152 Halstead maneuver.

minutes, the test is considered positive for thoracic outlet syndrome on the affected side. Minor fatigue and distress are considered negative tests. The test is sometimes called the **positive abduction and external rotation (AER) position test,** the **"hands up" test,** or the **elevated arm stress test (EAST)** ▲.[334–337]

🔞 *Shoulder Girdle Passive Elevation.*[190] This test is used on patients who already present with symptoms. The patient sits, and the examiner grasps the patient's arms from behind and passively elevates the shoulder girdle up and forward into full elevation (a passive bilateral shoulder shrug); the position is held for 30 or more seconds (Figure 5-154). Arterial relief is evidenced by stronger pulse, skin color change (more pink), and increased hand temperature. Venous relief is shown by decreased cyanosis and venous engorgement. Neurological signs go from numbness to pins and needles or

tingling, as well as some pain, as the ischemia to the nerve is released. This is referred to as a *release phenomenon.*

🔞 *Wright Test or Maneuver.*[33] Wright advocated "hyperabducting" the arm so that the hand is brought over the head with the elbow and arm in the coronal plane with the shoulder laterally rotated (Figure 5-155, *A*).[338] He advocated doing the test in the sitting and then the supine positions. Having the patient take a breath or rotating or extending the head and neck may have an additional effect. The pulse is palpated for differences. This test is used to detect compression in the costoclavicular space and is similar to the costoclavicular syndrome test.

Examiners have modified this test over time so that it has come to be described as follows. The examiner flexes the patient's elbow to 90° while the shoulder is extended horizontally and rotated laterally (Figure 5-155, *B*). The patient then rotates the head away from the test side. The examiner palpates the radial pulse, which becomes absent (disappears) when the head is rotated away from the test side. The test done in this fashion has also been called the **Allen maneuver.** The pulse disappearance indicates a positive test result for thoracic outlet syndrome.

Reflexes and Cutaneous Distribution

The reflexes in the shoulder region that are often assessed include the pectoralis major, clavicular portion (C5 to C6), sternocostal portion (C7 to C8 and T1), the biceps (C5 to C6), and the triceps (C7 to C8) (Figure 5-156).

The examiner must be aware of the dermatome patterns of the nerve roots (Figure 5-157) as well as the cutaneous distribution of the peripheral nerves (Figure 5-158). Dermatomes vary from person to person, so the diagrams are estimations only. A scanning test for altered sensation is performed by running the relaxed

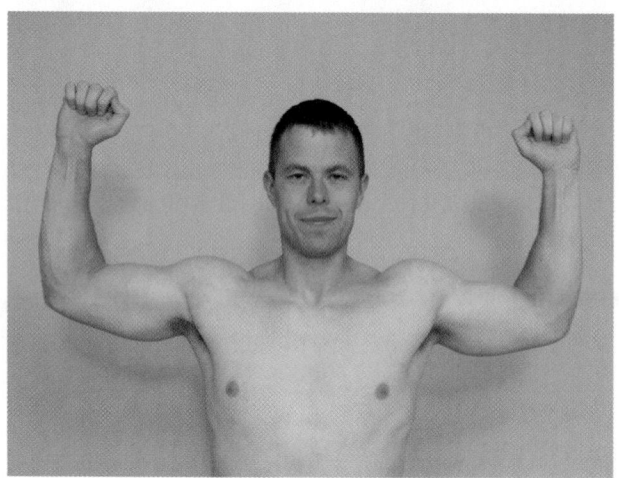

Figure 5-153 Roos test.

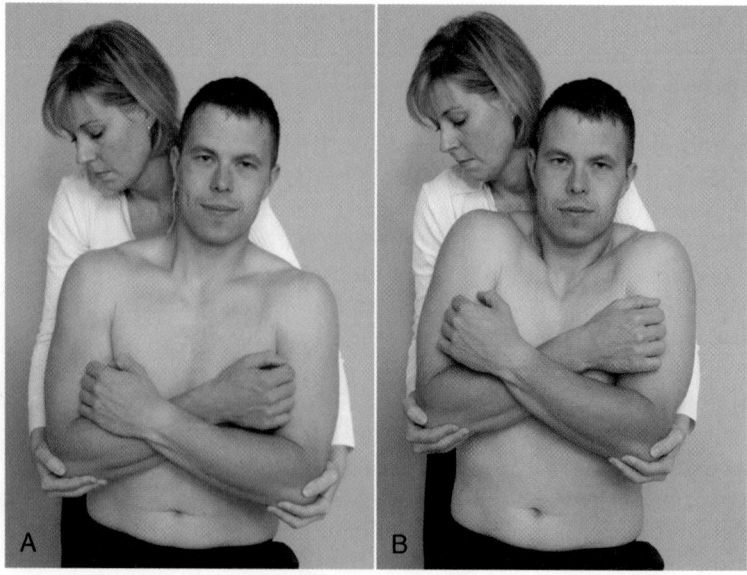

Figure 5-154 **Shoulder girdle passive elevation. A,** Start position. **B,** Relief position.

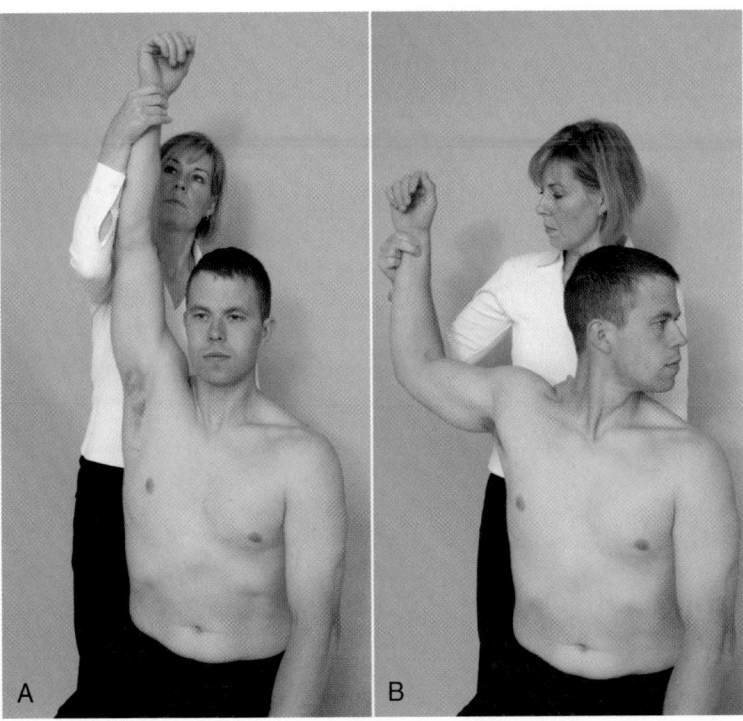

Figure 5-155 A, Wright test. **B,** Modified Wright test or maneuver (Allen maneuver).

hands and fingers over the neck, shoulders, and anterior and posterior chest area. Any difference in sensation between the two sides should be noted. These differences can be mapped more exactly using a pinwheel, a pin, a brush, or cotton batting. In this way, the examiner can use sensation to help differentiate between a peripheral nerve lesion and a nerve root lesion referred from the cervical spine.

True shoulder pain rarely extends below the elbow. Pain in the acromioclavicular or sternoclavicular joint tends to be localized to the affected joint and usually does not spread or radiate. Pain can be referred to the shoulder and surrounding tissues from many structures,[339] including the cervical spine, elbow, lungs, heart, diaphragm, gallbladder, and spleen (Figure 5-159; Table 5-19).

Peripheral Nerve Injuries About the Shoulder

Individual nerves can be injured about the shoulder as shown below. The examiner should not forget, however, that these nerves can be injured before they branch off the brachial plexus as individual nerves. Thus, thoracic outlet syndrome must be considered, especially in the throwing athlete, if symptoms arise with abduction and lateral rotation of the arm.[37]

Axillary (Circumflex) Nerve (C5 to C6). The axillary nerve is the most commonly injured nerve in the shoulder, and the most common cause of injury is anterior dislocation of the shoulder or fracture of the neck of the humerus.[340,341] The nerve injury may occur during the dislocation itself or during the reduction. Other traumatic events (e.g., fracture, bullet, or stab wounds) or brachial plexus

injuries, compression (e.g., crutches), quadrilateral space entrapment (Figure 5-160), or shoulder surgery also may affect the axillary nerve.[342]

Motor loss (see Tables 5-5 and 5-12) includes an inability to abduct the arm (deltoid), although the patient may attempt to laterally rotate the arm and use the long head of biceps to abduct the arm (trick movement). In some cases, a patient is asymptomatic, although he or she may demonstrate early fatigue with strenuous activities.[342] There is weakness of lateral rotation owing to the loss of teres minor.[342] The patient may attempt to use scapular movement (i.e., trapezius or serratus anterior) to compensate for the muscle loss (trick movement). Atrophy of the deltoid leads to loss of the lateral roundness (flattening) of the shoulder. Sensory loss is over the deltoid with the main loss being a small, 2 cm to 3 cm (1 inch) circular area at the deltoid insertion (see Figure 5-158).

Suprascapular Nerve (C5 to C6). The suprascapular nerve may be injured by a fall on the posterior shoulder, stretching, repeated microtrauma, or fracture of the scapula.[338,342,343] Commonly, the nerve is injured as it passes through the suprascapular notch under the transverse scapular (suprascapular) ligament or as it winds around the spine of the scapula under the spinoglenoid ligament (Figure 5-161).[66,342,344–349] Often, it is hard to distinguish from rotator cuff syndrome, and so the patient history and mechanism of injury become important for differential diagnosis. Most commonly, the condition is seen in people who work with their arms overhead or in activities involving cocking and following through (e.g., volleyball spiking, pitching).[58,345,350,351]

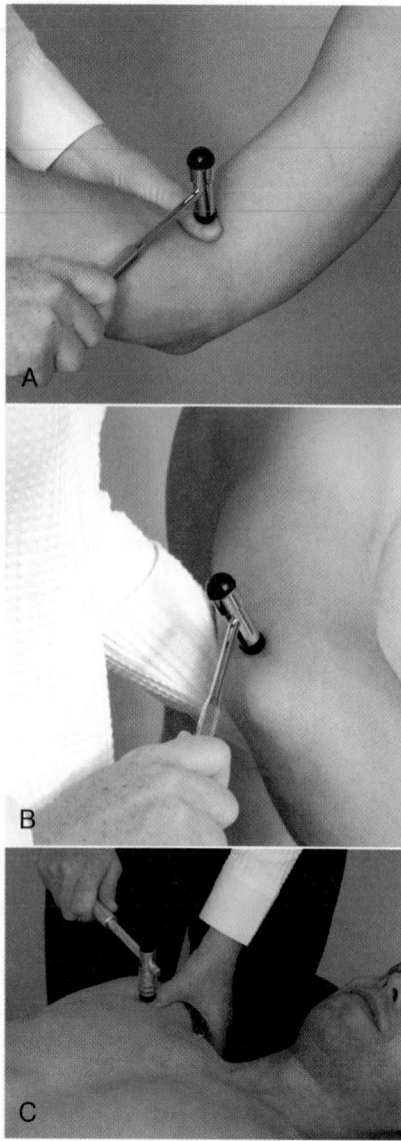

Figure 5-156 Positioning to test the reflexes around the shoulder. A, Biceps. **B,** Triceps. **C,** Pectoralis major.

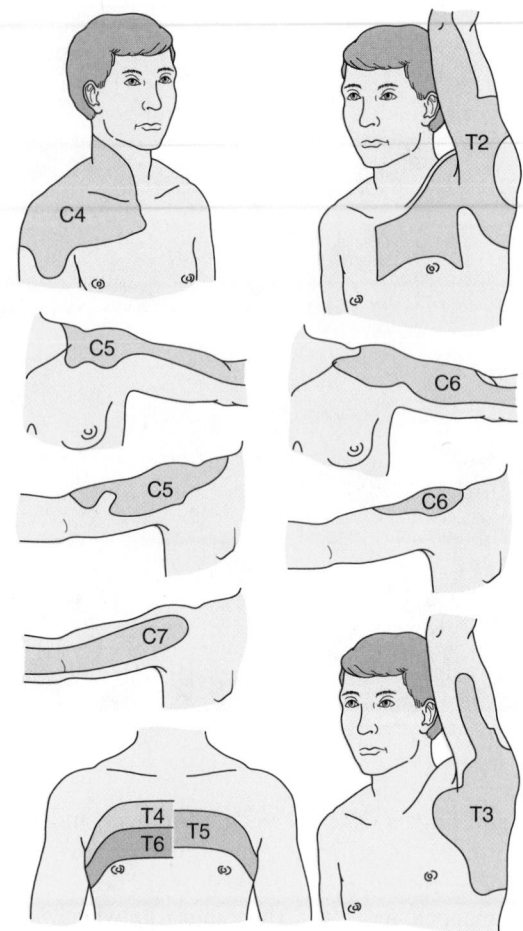

Figure 5-157 Dermatome pattern of the shoulder. Dermatomes on one side only are illustrated.

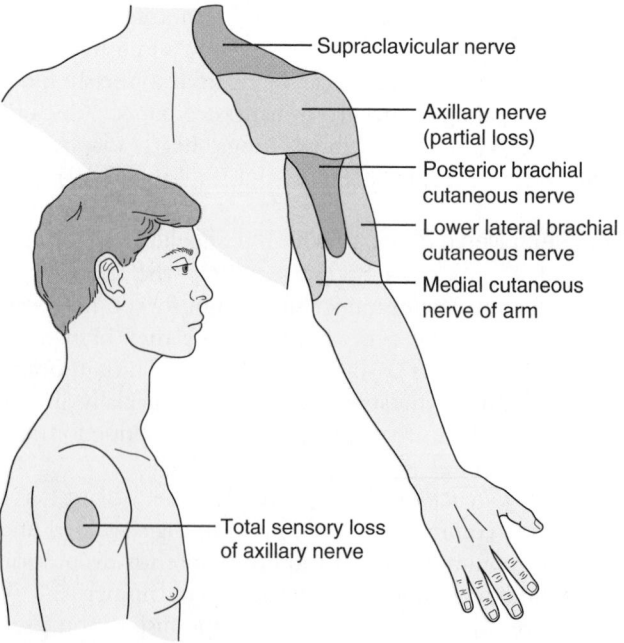

Figure 5-158 Cutaneous distribution of peripheral nerves around the shoulder.

Signs and symptoms include persistent rear shoulder pain and paralysis of the supraspinatus (suprascapular notch) and infraspinatus (suprascapular notch and spine of scapula), leading to decreased strength of abduction (supraspinatus) and lateral rotation (infraspinatus) of the shoulder. Wasting may also be evident in the muscles over the scapula.

Musculocutaneous Nerve (C5 to C6). This nerve is not commonly injured, although it may be injured by trauma (e.g., humeral dislocation or fracture) or in conjunction with injury to the brachial plexus or adjacent axillary artery. Injury to this nerve (see Tables 5-5 and 5-12) results primarily in loss of elbow flexion (biceps and brachialis), shoulder forward flexion (biceps and coracobrachialis), and decreased supination strength (biceps). In addition, injury to its sensory branch, the antebrachial

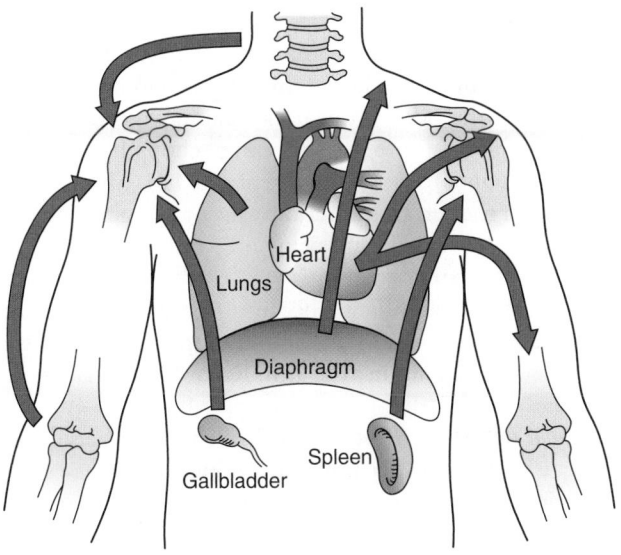

Figure 5-159 Structures referring pain to the shoulder.

TABLE **5-19**

Shoulder Muscles and Referral of Pain

Muscle	Referral Pattern
Levator scapulae	Over muscle to posterior shoulder and along medial border of scapula
Latissimus dorsi	Interior angle of scapula up to posterior and anterior shoulder into posterior arm; may refer to area above iliac crest
Rhomboids	Medial border of scapula
Supraspinatus	Over shoulder cap and above spine of scapula; sometimes down lateral aspect of arm to proximal forearm
Infraspinatus	Anterolateral shoulder and medial border of scapula; may refer down lateral aspect of arm
Teres minor	Near deltoid insertion, up to shoulder cap, and down lateral arm to elbow
Subscapularis	Posterior shoulder to scapula and down posteromedial and anteromedial aspects of arm to elbow
Teres major	Shoulder cap down lateral aspect of arm to elbow
Deltoid	Over muscle and posterior glenoid area of shoulder
Coracobrachialis	Anterior shoulder and down posterior arm

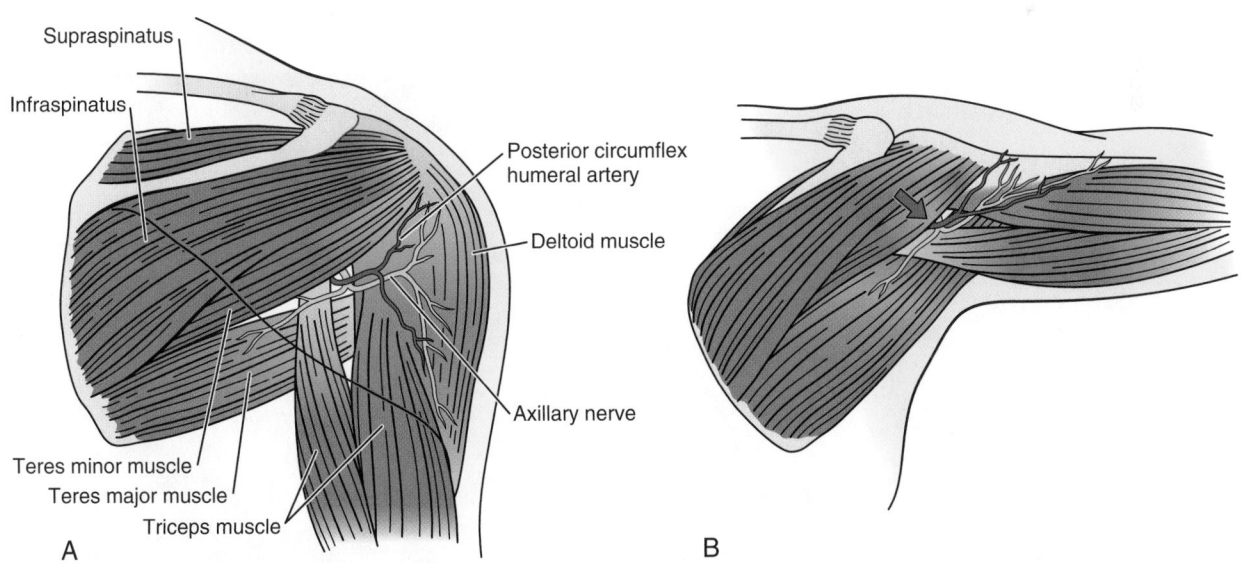

Figure 5-160 Quadrilateral space entrapment, posterior view of the shoulder. A, With the arm in adduction or at the side, there is no compression of the axillary nerve and posterior circumflex humeral artery. **B,** A mechanism of intermittent compression of the axillary nerve and posterior circumflex humeral artery as a result of shearing and closing down of the space by the teres major and teres minor. (Redrawn from Safran MR: Nerve injury about the shoulder in athletes. Part 1: suprascapular nerve and axillary nerve. Am J Sports Med 32:814, 2004.)

cutaneous nerve, leads to altered sensation in the antero-lateral aspect of the forearm (see Figure 5-14). This sensory branch is sometimes compressed as it passes under the distal biceps tendon, resulting in **musculocutaneous nerve tunnel syndrome.** The injury results in sensory loss in the forearm; it is usually the result of forced elbow hyperextension or repeated pronation (e.g., excessive screwdriving, backhand tennis strokes) and may be misdiagnosed as tennis elbow.

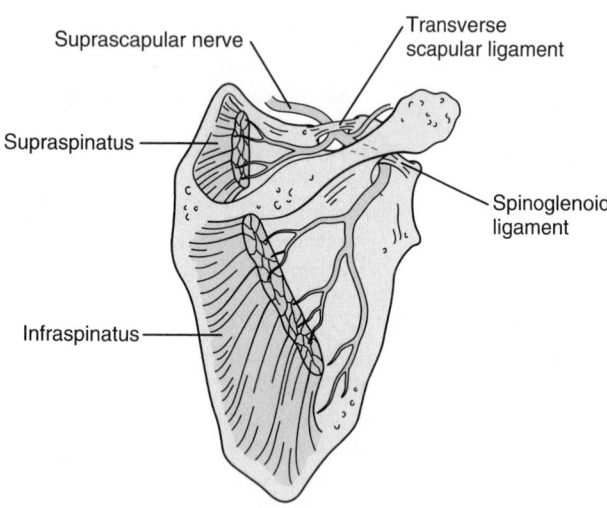

Figure 5-161 Suprascapular nerve.

Labels on figure:
- Suprascapular nerve
- Transverse scapular ligament
- Supraspinatus
- Spinoglenoid ligament
- Infraspinatus

Long Thoracic Nerve (C5 to C8). Injury to the long thoracic nerve, although not common, may occur from repetitive microtrauma with heavy effort above shoulder height, pressure on the nerve from backpacking, vigorous upper limb activities[331,352] (e.g., shoveling, chopping, stretching), or wounds (see Tables 5-5 and 5-12). The result is paralysis of the serratus anterior, causing winging (medial border) of the scapula and pain and weakness on forward flexion of the extended arm.[58,67,70,80,340,341,346,353,354] Abduction above 90° is difficult because of scapular winging. Stabilization of the scapula by the examiner enables the patient to further abduct the arm. Recovery time can be as long as 2 years.

Spinal Accessory Nerve (C3 to C4). The spinal accessory nerve is vulnerable to traumatic injury as it passes the posterior triangle of the neck; injury spares the sternocleidomastoid muscles but affects the trapezius muscle.[352] A common example would be abnormal pressure from a poorly fitting backpack (see Tables 5-5 and 5-12). Shoulder drooping (scapula is translated laterally and rotates downward) and scapular winging (medial superior portion) with medial rotation of the inferior angle, especially on abduction, may be evident, along with deepening of the supraclavicular fossa (asymmetric neck line) as a result of trapezius atrophy (Figure 5-162).[58,355,356] The patient has difficulty abducting the arm above 90°.[340] Interestingly, Safran reported that spinal accessory palsy results in scapular winging on abduction but not forward flexion.[331]

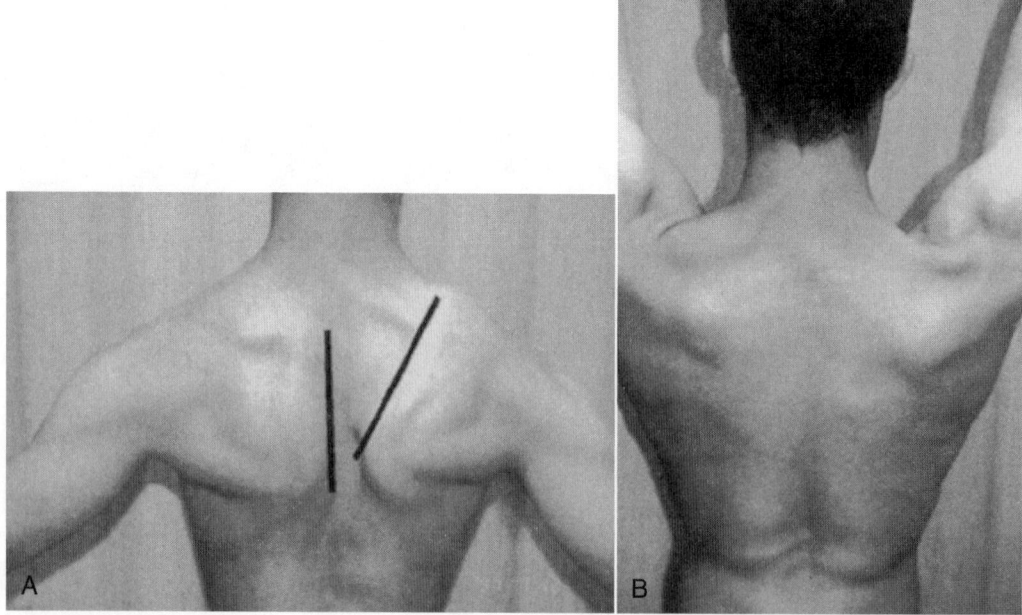

Figure 5-162 Spinal accessory nerve palsy. A 17-year-old male patient with a 1-year history of shoulder pain. **A,** Winging of the superior medial angle of the scapula with abduction. A line drawn along the medial border of the normal left shoulder is to be compared with the symptomatic right shoulder. **B,** Forward elevation does not result in winging in this patient, differentiating spinal accessory nerve palsy winging from long thoracic nerve palsy winging. (From Safran MR: Nerve injury about the shoulder in athletes. Part 2: long thoracic nerve, spinal accessory nerve, burners/stingers, thoracic outlet syndrome. Am J Sports Med 32:1065, 2004.)

Joint Play Movements

Joint play movements are usually performed with the patient lying supine.[70,357] The examiner compares the amount of available movement and end feel on the affected side with the movement on the unaffected side and notes whether the movements affect the patient's symptoms.

To perform the backward joint play movement of the humerus, the examiner grasps the patient's upper limb, placing one hand over the anterior humeral head. The other hand is placed around the humerus above and near the elbow while the patient's hand is held against the examiner's thorax by the examiner's arm (Figure 5-163, *A*). The examiner then applies a backward force (similar to a posterior shift), keeping the patient's arm parallel to the body so that no rotation or torsion occurs at the glenohumeral joint.

Forward joint play movement of the humerus is carried out in a similar fashion with the examiner's hands placed

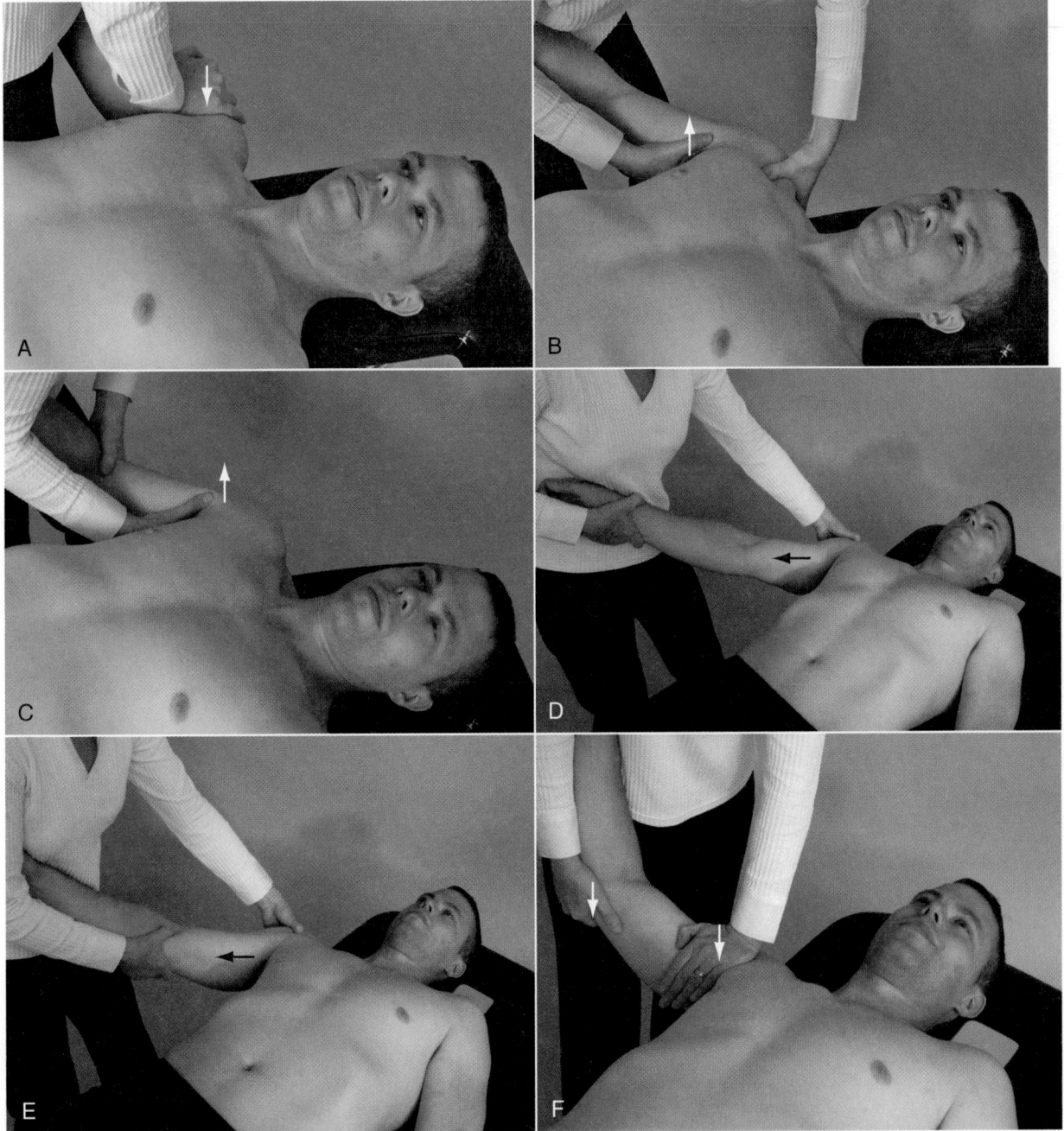

Figure 5-163 Joint play movements of the shoulder complex. A, Backward glide of the humerus. **B,** Forward glide of the humerus. **C,** Lateral distraction of the humerus. **D,** Long arm traction applied below elbow. **E,** Long arm traction applied above elbow. **F,** Backward glide of the humerus in abduction. Note that the examiner allows the elbow to drop the same amount as the movement at the shoulder to minimize torque at the shoulder. *Continued*

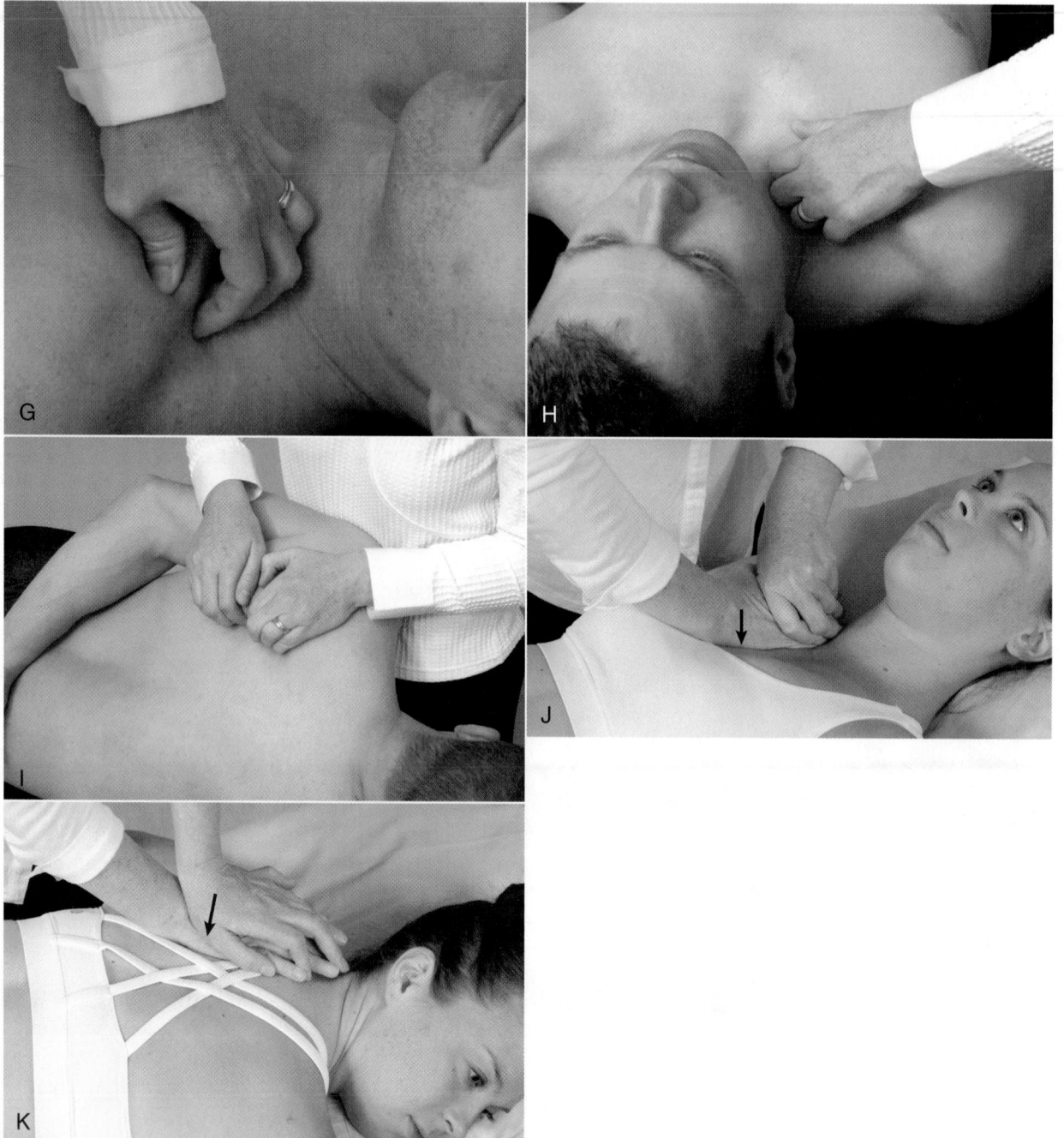

Figure 5-163, cont'd G, Joint play of the acromioclavicular joint. **H,** Joint play of the sternoclavicular joint. **I,** General movement of the scapula to determine mobility. **J,** Testing rib mobility—anteriorly. **K,** Testing rib mobility—posteriorly (be sure scapula is protracted).

as shown in Figure 5-163, *B.* The examiner applies an anterior force (anterior drawer), keeping the patient's arm parallel to the body so that no rotation or torsion occurs at the glenohumeral joint.

To apply a lateral distraction joint play movement to the humerus, the examiner's hands are placed as shown in Figure 5-163, *C.* A lateral distraction force is applied to the glenohumeral joint with the patient's arm kept parallel to the body so that no rotation or torsion occurs at the glenohumeral joint. The examiner must be careful

to apply the lateral distraction force with the flat of the hand, because one sometimes has a tendency, when applying a force, to turn the hand so the distraction is applied through the side of the index finger. This is uncomfortable for the patient.

Caudal glide (long arm traction) joint play movement is performed with the patient in the same supine position. The examiner grasps above the patient's wrist with one hand and palpates with the other hand, below the distal spine of the scapula posteriorly and below the distal

Joint Play Movements of the Shoulder Complex

- Backward glide of the humerus
- Forward glide of the humerus
- Lateral distraction of the humerus
- Caudal glide of the humerus (long arm traction)
- Backward glide of the humerus in abduction
- Lateral distraction of the humerus in abduction
- Anteroposterior and cephalocaudal movements of the clavicle at the acromioclavicular joint
- Anteroposterior and cephalocaudal movements of the clavicle at the sternoclavicular joint
- General movement of the scapula to determine mobility
- Ribs
- Thoracic spine

clavicle anteriorly over the glenohumeral joint line (Figure 5-163, D). The examiner then applies a traction force to the shoulder while palpating to see whether the head of the humerus drops down (moves distally) in the glenoid cavity as it normally should. If the patient complains of pain in the elbow, the test may be done with the hands positioned as in Figure 5-163, E.

The examiner then abducts the patient's arm to 90°, grasping above the patient's wrist with one hand while stabilizing the thorax with the other hand. The examiner applies a long arm traction force to determine joint play in this position.

With the patient's arm abducted to 90°, the examiner places one hand over the anterior humerus while stabilizing the patient's arm with the other hand and stabilizing the patient's hand against the thorax with the same arm. A backward force is then applied, keeping the patient's arm parallel to the body. This is a backward joint play movement of the humerus in abduction (Figure 5-163, F).

To assess the acromioclavicular and sternoclavicular joints (Figures 5-163, G, and 5-163, H, respectively), the examiner gently grasps the clavicle as close to the joint to be tested as possible and moves it in and out or up and down while palpating the joint with the other hand. Because the bone lies just under the skin, these techniques are uncomfortable for the patient where the examiner grasps the clavicle. The examiner should warn the patient before attempting this technique. A comparison of the amount of movement available is made between the two sides. Care should be taken not to squeeze the clavicle, because this too may cause pain.

For a determination of mobility of the scapula, the patient lies on one side to fixate the thorax with the arm relaxed and resting behind the low back (hand by opposite back pocket). The uppermost scapula is tested in this position. The examiner faces the patient, placing the lower hand along the medial border of the patient's scapula. The hand of the examiner's other arm holds the upper (cranial) dorsal surface of the patient's scapula. To relax the scapula further, the patient is asked to relax against the examiner and the examiner uses his or her body to push the patient's test shoulder posteriorly, retracting it to obtain a better hold on the scapula. By holding the scapula in this way, the examiner is able to move it medially, laterally, caudally, cranially, and away from the thorax (Figure 5-163, I).

With any shoulder examination, the ribs and spine should be checked for normal mobility as restrictions in these areas can restrict shoulder movement. To test the mobility of the ribs generally, the examiner can apply anterior rib springing using the side of the thenar eminance of the hand (Figure 5-163, J). By pressing down several times, the examiner can compare the bilateral mobility of the ribs. If done posteriorly (Figure 5-163, K), the examiner must ensure the scapula is protracted out of the way. Mobility of the thoracic spine is shown in Figure 8-38.

Palpation

When palpating the shoulder complex, the examiner should note any muscle spasm, tenderness, abnormal bumps, or other signs and symptoms that may indicate the source of pathology. The examiner should perform palpation in a systematic manner, beginning with the anterior structures and working around to the posterior structures. Findings on the injured side should be compared with those on the unaffected side. Any differences between the two sides should be noted, because they may indicate the cause of the patient's problems.

Anterior Structures

The anterior structures of the shoulder may be palpated with the patient in the supine lying or sitting position (Figure 5-164, A).

Clavicle. The clavicle should be palpated along its full length for tenderness or abnormal bumps, such as callus formation after a fracture, and to ensure that it is in its resting position relative to the uninjured side. That is, it may be rotated anteriorly or posteriorly more than the unaffected side, or one end may be higher than that of the uninjured side, indicating a possible subluxation or dislocation at the sternoclavicular or acromioclavicular joint.

Sternoclavicular Joint. The sternoclavicular joint should be palpated for normal positioning in relation to the sternum and first rib. Palpation should also include the supporting ligaments and sternocleidomastoid muscle. Adjacent to the joint, the suprasternal notch may be palpated. From the notch, the examiner moves the fingers laterally and posteriorly to palpate the first rib. The examiner should apply slight caudal pressure to the first rib on both sides and note any difference. Spasm of the scalene

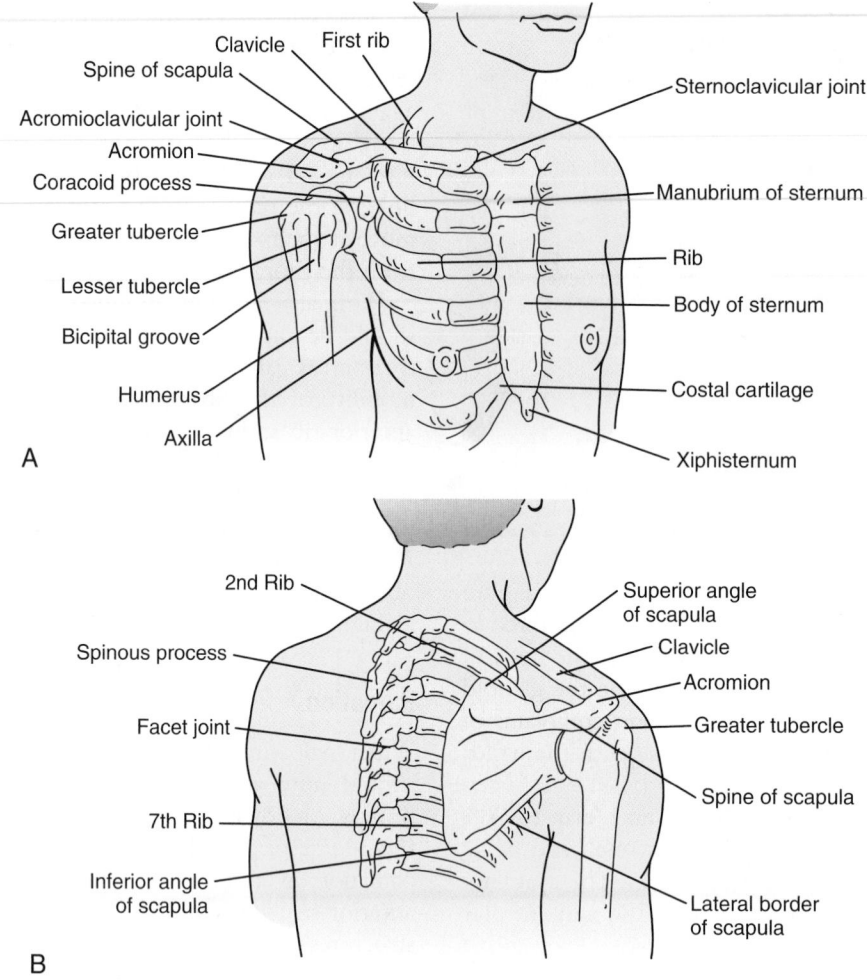

Figure 5-164 Bony landmarks of the shoulder region. **A,** Anterior view. **B,** Posterior view.

muscles or pathology in the area may elevate the first rib on the affected side.

Acromioclavicular Joint. Like the sternoclavicular joint, the acromioclavicular joint should be palpated for normal positioning and tenderness. Likewise, supporting ligaments (acromioclavicular and coracoclavicular) and the trapezius, subclavius, and deltoid (anterior, middle, and posterior fibers) muscles should be palpated for tenderness and spasm.

Coracoid Process. The coracoid process may be palpated approximately 2.5 cm (1 inch) below the junction of the lateral one-third and medial two-thirds of the clavicle. The short head of biceps and coracobrachialis muscles originate from, and the pectoralis minor inserts into, this process. With a SICK scapula syndrome, the coracoid is often very tender.[31]

Sternum. In the midline of the chest, the examiner should palpate the three portions of the sternum (manubrium, body, and xiphoid process), noting any abnormality or tenderness.

Ribs and Costal Cartilage. Adjacent to the sternum, the examiner should palpate the sternocostal and costochondral articulations, noting any swelling, tenderness, or other abnormality. These "articulations" are sometimes sprained or subluxed, or a costochondritis (Tietze syndrome) may be evident. The examiner should palpate the ribs as they extend around the chest wall, seeking any potential pathology and noting whether they are aligned with each other, or one protrudes more than the adjacent ones as sometimes occurs with anterior shoulder pathology.

Humerus and Rotator Cuff Muscles. Moving laterally from the chest and caudally from the acromion process, the examiner should palpate the humerus and its surrounding structures for potential pathology. The examiner first palpates the lateral tip of the acromion process and then moves inferiorly to the greater tuberosity of the humerus. The examiner should then laterally rotate the humerus. During palpation, the long head of the biceps in the bicipital groove will slip under the fingers, followed by the lesser tuberosity of the humerus (Figure 5-165). As with all palpation, the testing should be done gently and carefully to prevent causing the patient undue pain. By rotating the humerus alternately laterally and medially,

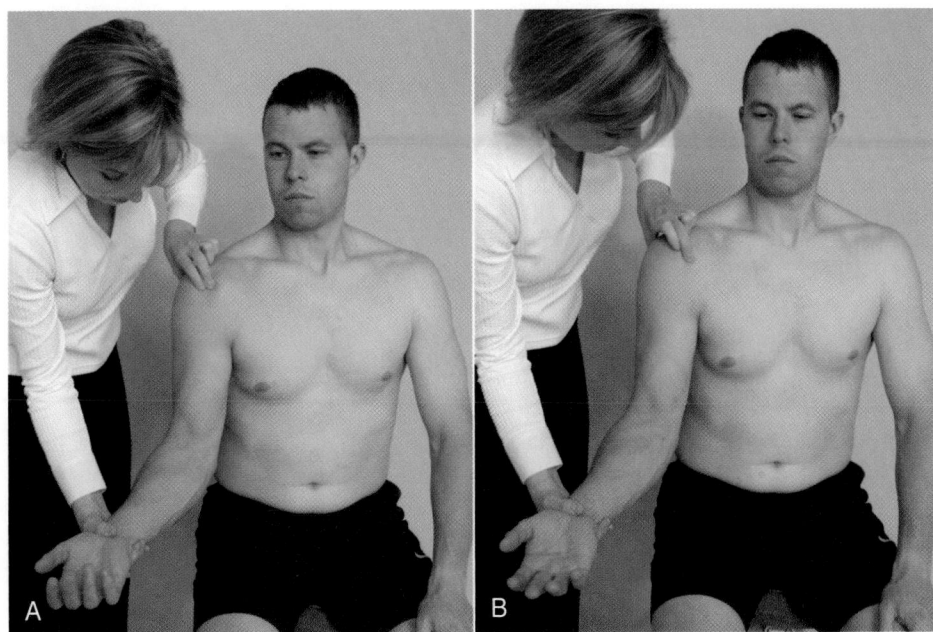

Figure 5-165 Palpation around the shoulder. A, Greater tuberosity. **B,** Lesser tuberosity. The bicipital groove lies between these two landmarks.

the smooth progression over the three structures is normally noted **(de Anquin test),** and the lesser tuberosity is felt at the level of the coracoid process. If the examiner then palpates along the lesser tuberosity and the lip of the bicipital groove, the fingers will rest on the tendon of the subscapularis muscle. The subscapularis may also be palpated in the triangle made up of the superior border of pectoralis major, the clavicle, and the medial border of the deltoid.[358] If the examiner places the thumb over the lesser tuberosity and "grips" the shoulder between the second, third, and fourth fingers (as shown in Figure 5-3), the fingers will be over the insertion of the other three rotator cuff muscles: supraspinatus, infraspinatus, and teres minor. Moving laterally over the bicipital groove to its other lip, the examiner may palpate the insertion of the pectoralis major muscle. The patient is then asked to further medially rotate the humerus so that the forearm rests behind the back, and the examiner palpates 2 cm inferior to the anterior aspect of the acromion process for the supraspinatus tendon. Any tenderness of the tendon should be noted. The examiner then passively abducts the patient's shoulder to between 80° and 90° and palpates the notch formed by the acromion and spine of the scapula with the clavicle. In the notch, the examiner is palpating the musculotendinous junction of the supraspinatus muscle. With the arm in the same position, the examiner can palpate the long head of biceps under the pectoralis major tendon by having the patient isometrically adducting and medially rotating the humerus to identify the pectoralis major tendon. The long head of biceps is then palpated under the tendon of pectoralis major in the axilla. Both sides should be compared.[50]

The examiner should then palpate the head of the humerus and its relationship to the glenoid cavity. By placing the fingers over the anterior humeral head and the thumb over the posterior humeral head, the examiner then slides the fingers and thumbs medially (see Figure 5-62). As the humeral head is larger than the glenoid with only about 25% to 30% of the head in contact with the glenoid at any one time, the examiner's fingers and thumb will "dip in" as they approach the glenohumeral joint. This "dipping in" should be slightly greater anteriorly. If there is no dipping anteriorly or posteriorly, it means the humeral head is sitting further posteriorly or anteriorly than it should. Once the examiner has found the glenohumeral joint (at the point of hardness after the "dip in"), he or she can palpate along the joint line superiorly and inferiorly on the anterior and posterior surface feeling for any pain or the presence of pathology (torn labrum, ligament, or capsule). The examiner can determine the joint line by medially and laterally rotating the humerus while palpating. The examiner should be able to differentiate the glenoid (does not move) from the humerus (rotates). As the technique is uncomfortable to the patient, the patient should be warned about possible discomfort, and the results should be compared with the normal side. With care, the examiner can palpate all of the glenoid edge except superiorly where the proximity of the acromion to the humerus does not allow it.

Axilla. With the shoulder slightly abducted (20° to 30°), the examiner palpates the structures of the axilla, latissimus dorsi muscle (posterior wall), pectoralis major muscle (anterior wall), serratus anterior muscle (medial wall), lymph nodes (palpable only if swollen), and brachial artery. The inferior glenohumeral joint and glenoid edge may also be palpated in the axilla. The patient is then asked to lie prone on the elbows (sphinx position) with the shoulders slightly laterally rotated and the elbow slightly adducted in relation to the shoulder. The examiner then palpates just inferior to the most lateral aspect of the scapula for the insertion of the infraspinatus muscle. Just distal to this insertion, the examiner may be able to palpate the insertion of the teres minor.

Posterior Structures

To complete the palpation, the patient may be either sitting or lying prone with the upper limb by the trunk (Figure 5-164, *B*).

Spine of Scapula. From the acromion process the examiner moves his or her hands along the spine of the scapula, noting any tenderness or abnormality.

Scapula. The examiner follows the spine of the scapula to the medial border of the scapula and then follows the outline of the scapula, which normally extends from the spinous process of T2 to the spinous process of T9, depending on the size of the scapula. The superior angle lies at the level of the T2 spinous process. The base or root of the spine of the scapula lies between T3 and T4, and the inferior angle lies between T7 and T9. Along the medial border and spine of the scapula, the examiner can palpate the trapezius muscle (upper, middle, and lower parts) and the rhomboids. At the inferior angle, the latissimus dorsi may be palpated. The examiner then moves around the inferior angle of the scapula and along its lateral border. Against the lateral border and along the ribs, the serratus anterior can be palpated. Near the glenoid, long head of triceps, and teres minor may be palpated. After the borders of the scapula have been palpated, the posterior surface (supraspinatus and infraspinatus muscles) may be palpated for tenderness, atrophy, or spasm. By positioning the arm in forward flexion (60°), adduction and lateral rotation, infraspinatus and teres minor may be palpated just under and slightly inferior to the posterior aspect of the acromion.[358]

Spinous Processes of Lower Cervical and Thoracic Spine. In the midline, the examiner may palpate the cervical and thoracic spinous processes for any abnormality or tenderness. This is followed by palpation of the trapezius muscle.

Diagnostic Imaging

Diagnostic imaging is used in conjunction with a physical examination to determine a diagnosis. It should never be used in isolation, but any findings should be related to clinical signs to rule out false positive indications or age-related changes.[359–361]

Plain Film Radiography[362–364]

Anteroposterior View. This may be a true anteriorposterior view or a tilt view (Figures 5-166 and 5-167).

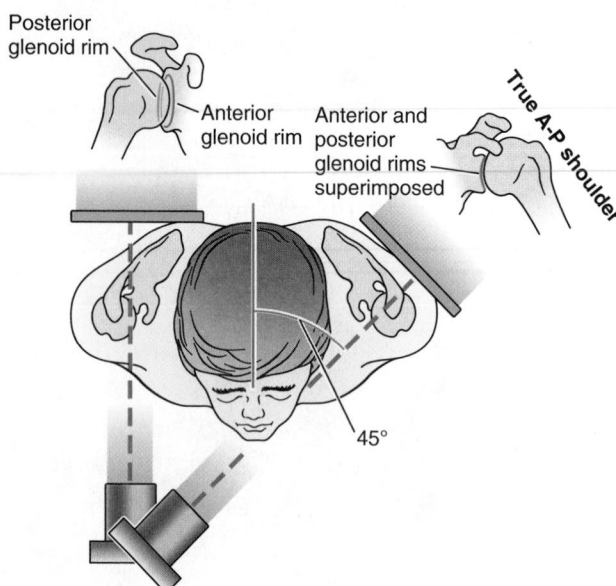

Routine A-P shoulder

Posterior glenoid rim

Anterior glenoid rim

Anterior and posterior glenoid rims superimposed

True A-P shoulder

45°

Figure 5-166 Positioning for the anteroposterior radiographic view.

Common X-Ray Views of the Shoulder

- Anteroposterior view (see Figures 5-166 and 5-167)
- Anteroposterior lateral rotation view (glenohumeral joint) (see Figure 5-169, *A*)
- Anteroposterior medial rotation view (glenohumeral joint) (see Figure 5-169, *B*)
- Transscapular (Y) lateral view (fracture or dislocation suspected) (see Figures 5-169, *D*, and 5-169, *E*)
- Stress x-ray of acromioclavicular joint (see Figure 5-175)
- Anteroposterior view (true) (glenohumeral joint) (also called Rockwood view) (Figures 5-176 and 5-177; see Figure 5-166)
- Anteroposterior view of sternoclavicular joint (Figure 5-178)
- Anteroposterior view of acromioclavicular joint (Figure 5-179)
- Lateral view of shoulder (Figure 5-180)
- Axillary lateral view (fracture or dislocation suspected) (see Figure 5-181)
- Stryker notch view (instability, Hill-Sach lesion) (see Figure 5-185)
- West point view (instability, anterior glenoid rim) (see Figure 5-187)
- Zanca view (10° to 15° cephalid anteroposterior) (see Figure 5-189)
- Swimmer's view (Figures 5-190 and 5-191)
- Serendipidy for sternoclavicular joint (beam 40° off vertical caudal, centered on sternum, patient supine)

This view may be used to assess the acromioclavicular joint width, spurring of the acromioclavicular undersurface, lateral tilt of the acromion and the distance between the humeral head and anterior acromion (Figure 5-168).[365] A great deal of information can be obtained from either view (Figure 5-169).

1. The relation of the humerus to the glenoid cavity should be examined. The "empty glenoid" sign may

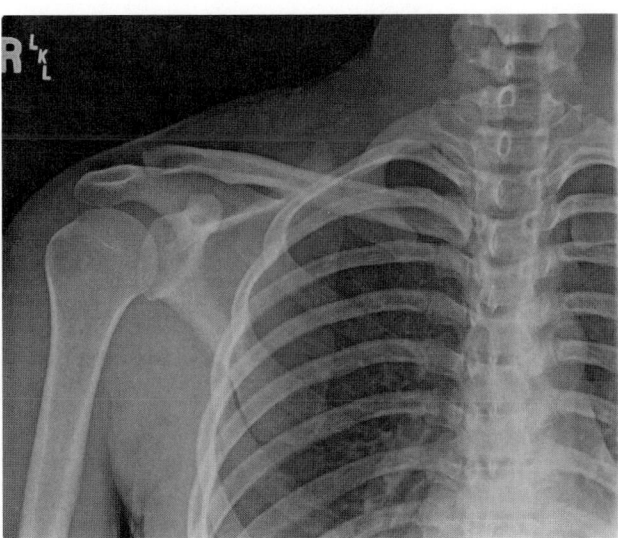

Figure 5-167 Anteroposterior view (routine) of the shoulder. Note glenoid sitting partially behind humerus.

recognize posterior dislocations. Normally, the radiograph shows overlapping shadows of the humerus and glenoid. With a posterior dislocation, this shadow is reduced or absent (Figure 5-170).[366]

2. The relation of the clavicle to the acromion process and the humerus to the glenoid should also be observed.

3. The examiner should determine whether the epiphyseal plate of the humeral head is present and, if so, whether it is normal.

4. The examiner should note whether there are any calcifications in any of the tendons (Figure 5-171), especially those of the supraspinatus or infraspinatus muscles, or fractures.[367,368]

5. The examiner should note the configuration of the undersurface of the acromion (see Figures 5-8 and 5-169, D)[369,370] and the presence of any subacromial spurs (Figure 5-172).

6. Medial rotation of the humerus with this view may show a defect on the lateral aspect of the humeral head

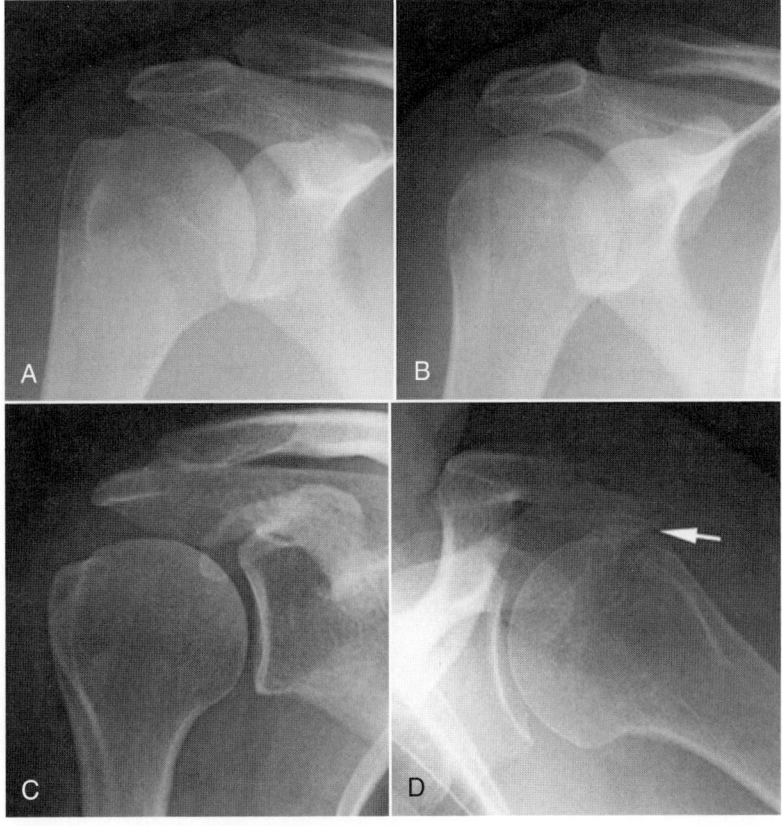

Figure 5-168 A, Anteroposterior lateral rotation. Note the greater tubercle in profile and the humeral-acromial distance and the coracoclavicular interspace. **B,** Anteroposterior medial rotation. Note the smooth rounded contour of the humeral head. **C,** Grashey projection. The glenohumeral joint appears more "open." **D,** Active abduction view. Note the narrowing of the acromiohumeral distance *(arrow)* in this patient with a rotator cuff tear (normal more than 2 mm). (From Anderson MW, Brennan C, Mittal A: Imaging evaluation of the rotator cuff. Clin Sports Med 31[4]:613, 2012.)

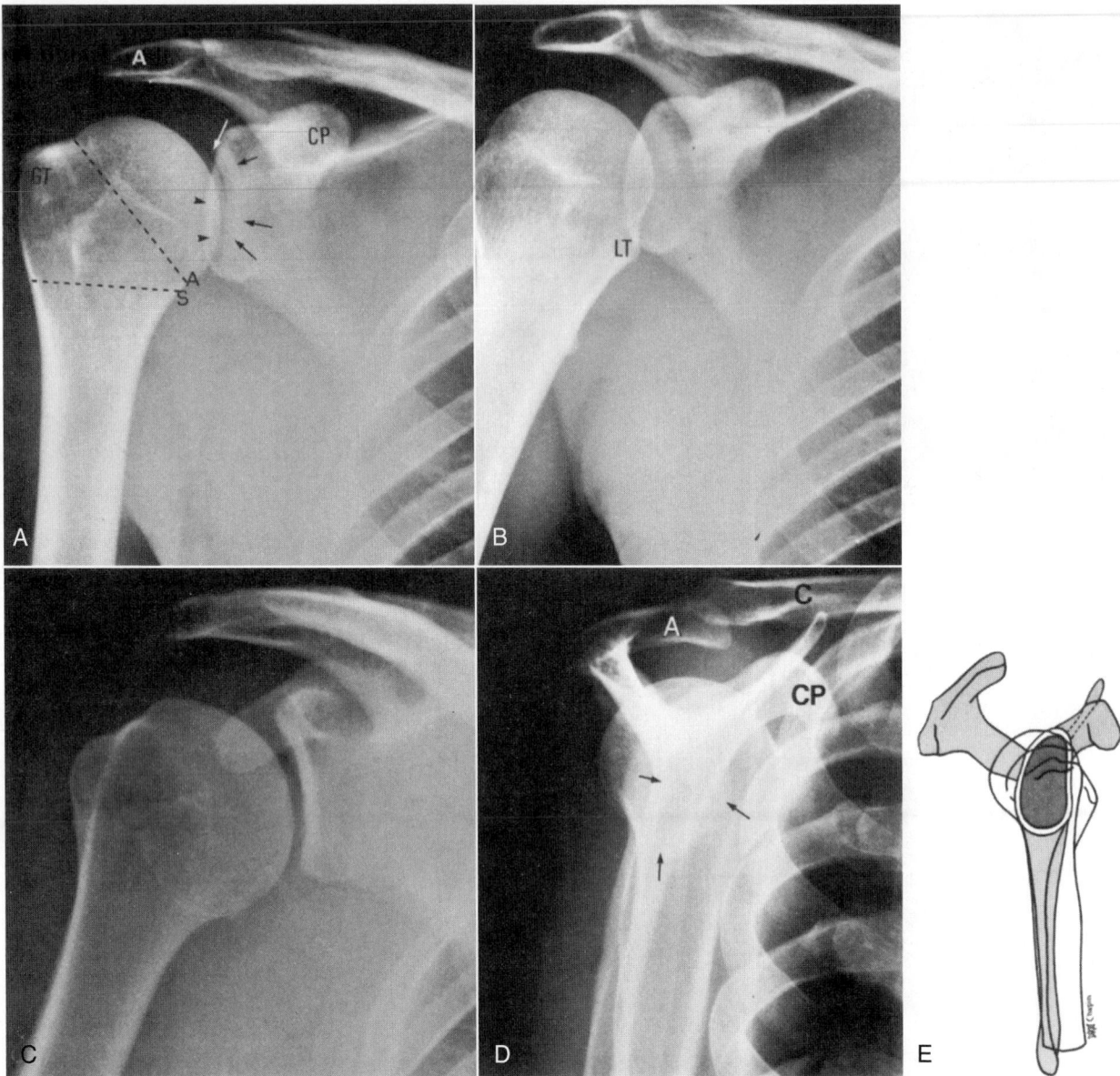

Figure 5-169 Normal radiographic examination. A, Lateral rotation. The greater tuberosity *(GT)* is shown in profile. The humeral head normally overlaps the glenoid on this view. The anterior *(black arrows)* and posterior *(arrowheads)* glenoid margins are well shown and do not overlap because of the anterior tilt of the glenoid. The anatomical *(black A)* and surgical *(S)* necks of the humerus are indicated. A vacuum phenomenon *(white arrow)* is present. **B,** Medial rotation. The overlap of the greater tuberosity and the humeral head produces a rounded appearance of the proximal humerus. A small exostosis is noted projecting from the humeral metaphysis. **C,** Posterior oblique. The glenohumeral cartilage space is shown in profile with no overlap of the humerus and glenoid. **D,** Normal scapular Y view. This true lateral view of the scapula (anterior oblique of the shoulder) shows the humeral head centered over the glenoid *(arrows)*. **E,** Diagram of normal scapular Y view.

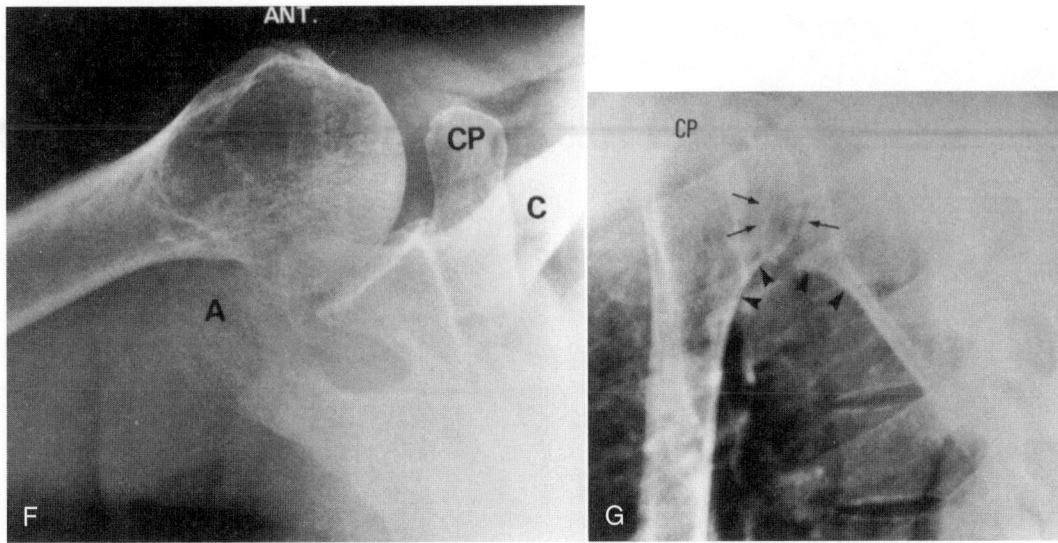

Figure 5-169, cont'd **F,** Axillary view. **G,** Normal transthoracic view. The smooth arch formed by the inferior border of the scapula and the posterior aspect of the humerus is indicated *(arrowheads)*. A faint view of the coracoid process *(CP)* is shown. The margins of the glenoid are indicated *(arrows)*. This view is slightly oblique, allowing the glenoid to be shown more en face than usual. *A,* Acromion; *A (white),* acromion process: *ANT,* anterior; *C,* clavicle; *CP,* coracoid process; *LT,* lesser tuberosity. (From Weissman BNW, Sledge CB: Orthopedic radiology. Philadelphia, 1986, WB Saunders, p. 219.)

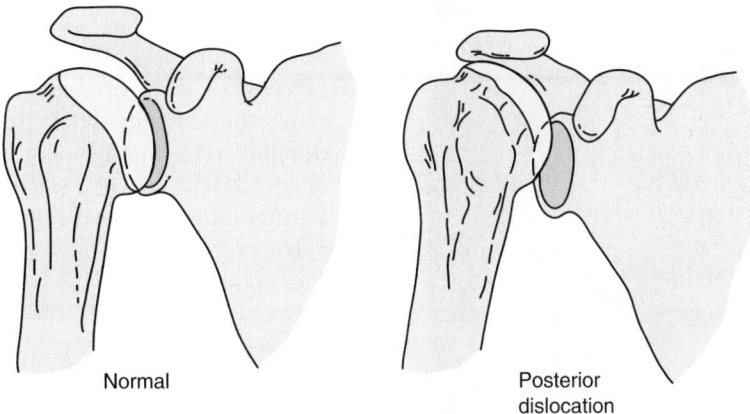

Normal

Posterior dislocation

Figure 5-170 **"Empty glenoid" sign of posterior dislocation on anteroposterior radiograph.** The head of the humerus fills the glenoid in the normal radiograph *(left)*. With a posterior dislocation, the glenoid is "empty," especially in its anterior portion *(right)*. (From Magee DJ, Reid DC: Shoulder injuries. In Zachazewski JE et al, editors: Athletic injuries and rehabilitation, Philadelphia, 1996, WB Saunders, p. 523.)

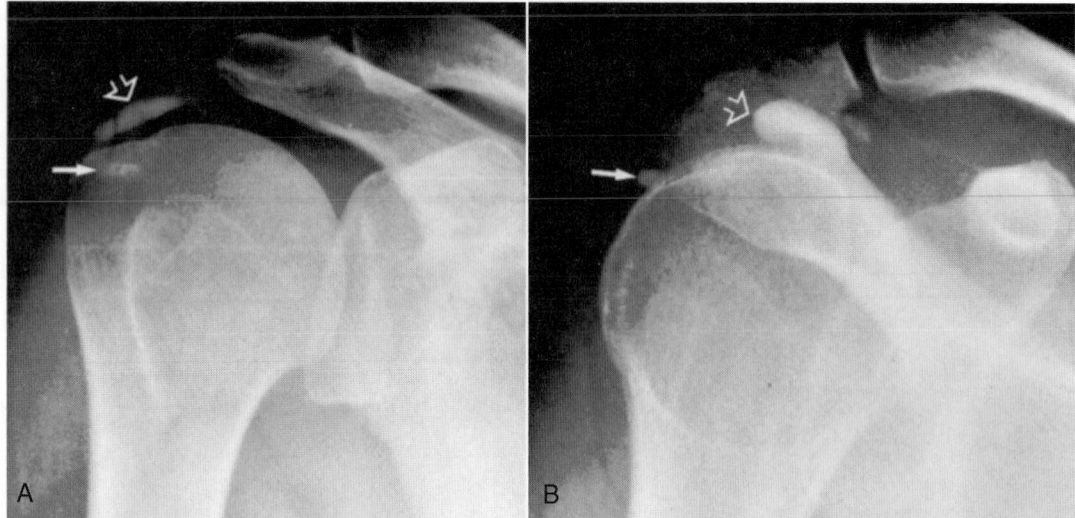

Figure 5-171 Calcific tendinitis—supraspinatus and infraspinatus. A, Lateral rotation view shows calcification projected over the base of the greater tuberosity *(white arrow)* and above the greater tuberosity *(open arrow).* **B,** Medial rotation view projects the infraspinatus calcification *(white arrow)* in profile and documents its posterior location. The supraspinatus calcification *(open arrow)* is rotated medially and maintains its superior location. (From Weissman BNW, Sledge CB: Orthopedic radiology, Philadelphia, 1986, WB Saunders, p. 227.)

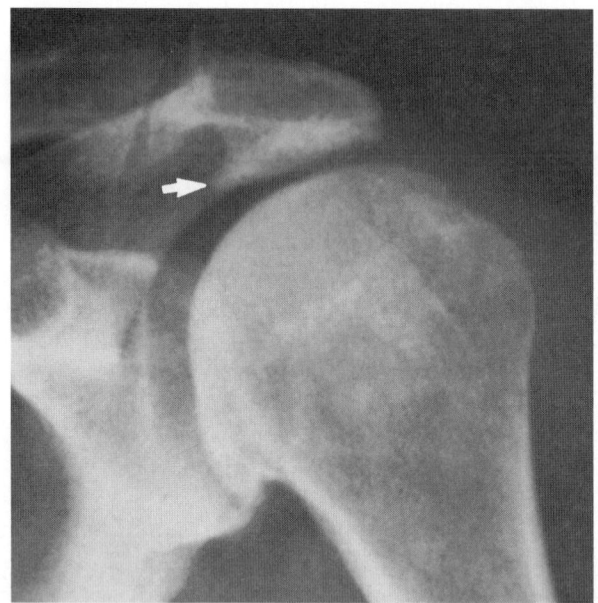

Figure 5-172 External subacromial impingement syndrome: Route radiographic abnormalities. Frontal radiograph of the shoulder shows a large enthesophyte *(arrow)* extending from the anteroinferior portion of the acromion and associated with osteophytes at the acromioclavicular joint and in the inferior portion of the humeral head. (From Resnick D, Kransdorf MJ: Bone and joint imaging, Philadelphia, 2005, WB Saunders, p. 922.)

from recurrent dislocations. This defect, in reality a compression fracture of the posterosuperolateral humeral head, is called a **Hill-Sachs lesion** (Figure 5-173) and may be classed as engaged or nonengaged.[371,372] Engaged implies the area of the lesion articulates with the glenoid when the arm is in

abduction and lateral rotation. The size of the defect may affect the stability of the joint.[373]

7. The examiner should look at the acromiohumeral interval (the space between the acromion and the humerus) and see whether it is normal.[374] The normal interval is 7 mm to 14 mm (Figure 5-174). If this distance decreases, it may indicate rotator cuff tears.[375] Likewise, if the arm is medially rotated and the view shows the coracohumeral distance of less than 11 mm, this indicates impingement and rotator cuff pathology.[376] If the arm is x-rayed in 90° abduction, the acromiohumeral distance is much less (see Figure 5-168, *D).*[365]

8. The normal coracoclavicular interspace (distance between the coracoid process and the clavicle) is 1.1 to 1.3 cm.[377]

9. A stress anteroposterior radiograph may be used to gap the injured acromioclavicular joint to see whether there has been a third-degree sprain or to show an inferior laxity at the glenohumeral joint (Figure 5-175). Equal weights of 9 kg (20 lbs) are tied to each of the patient's hands to apply traction to the arms. If a third-degree acromioclavicular sprain has occurred, the coracoclavicular distance will increase and a step deformity will be evident. These radiographs are not, however, routinely done.[24]

Axillary Lateral View. This view shows the relation of the humeral head to the glenoid and the coracohumeral distance[365] (Figure 5-181). It is used to diagnose anterior and posterior dislocations at the glenohumeral joint and to look for avulsion fractures of the glenoid or a Hill-Sachs lesion. It does, however, require the patient to be able to abduct the arm 70° to 90° (Figure 5-182).

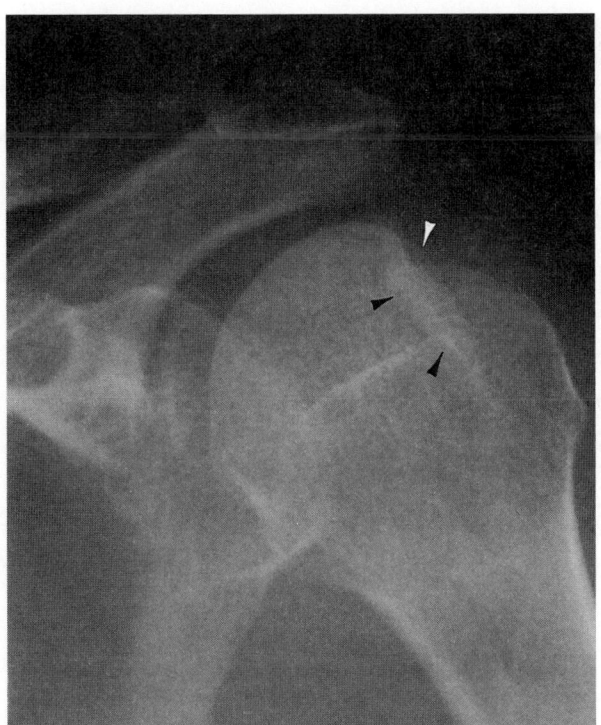

Figure 5-173 Glenohumeral joint: Hill-Sachs lesion. In a patient with a previous anterior dislocation, an internal rotation view reveals the extent of the Hill-Sachs lesion *(arrowheads)*. (From Resnick D, Kransdorf MJ: Bone and joint imaging, Philadelphia, 2005, WB Saunders, p. 833.)

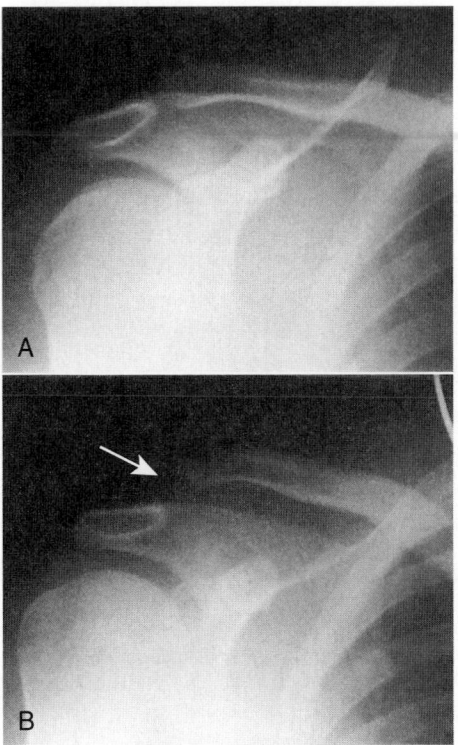

Figure 5-175 Stress radiograph for third-degree acromioclavicular sprain. A, No stress. **B,** Stress. Note the increase in the distance between the acromion process and the clavicle *(arrow)*.

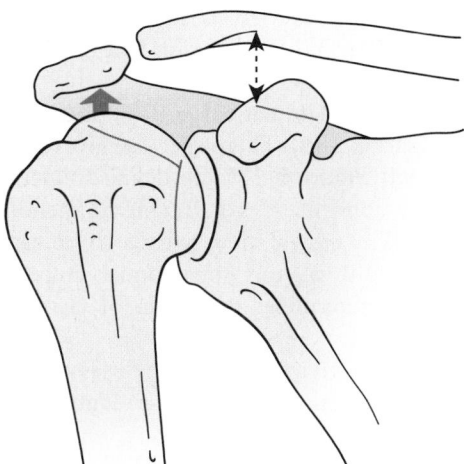

Figure 5-174 Acromiohumeral interval *(solid arrow)* and coracoclavicular interspace *(dashed arrows)*.

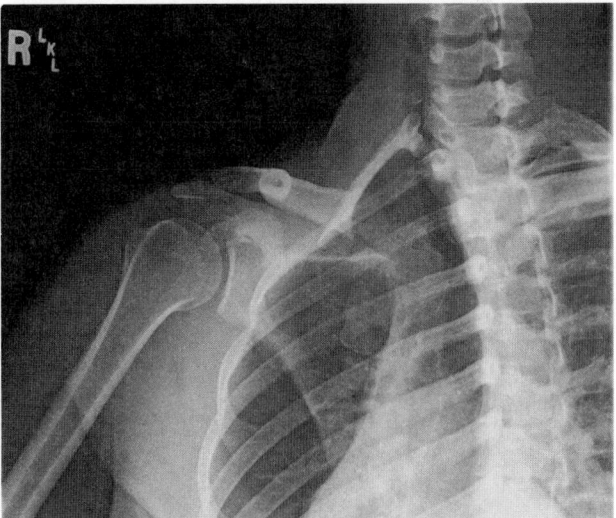

Figure 5-176 Anteroposterior view (true) of the glenohumeral joint (Rockwood view).

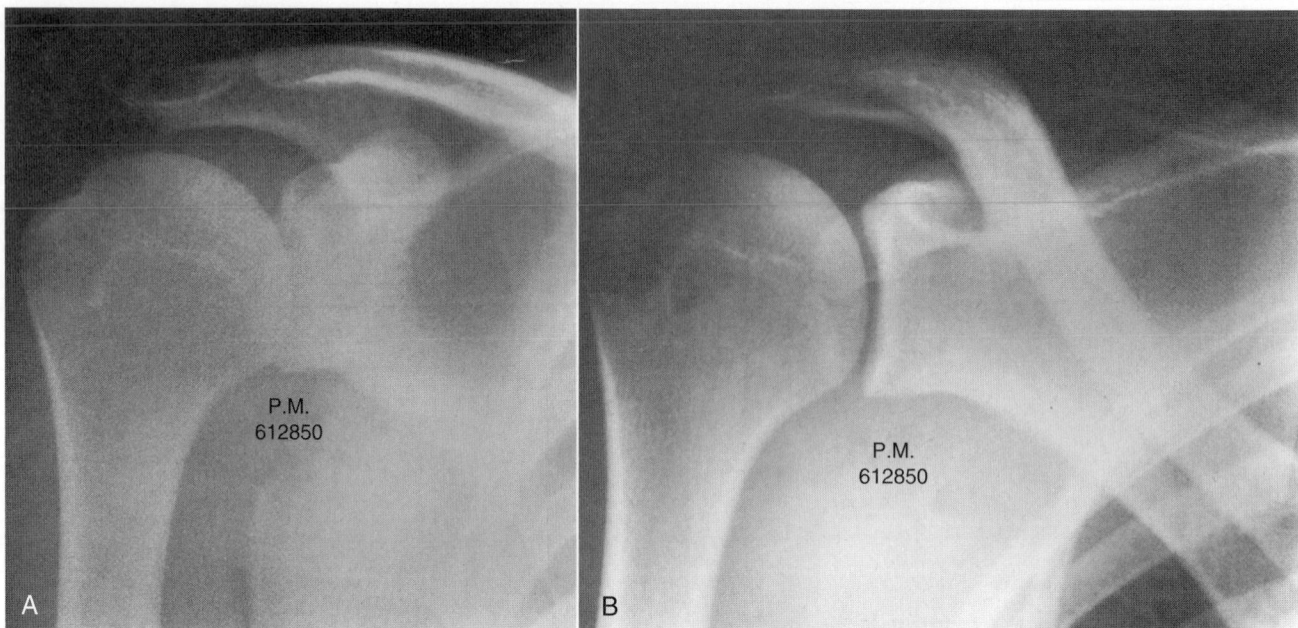

Figure 5-177 A, A radiograph of the shoulder in the plane of the thorax. **B,** A radiograph of the shoulder taken in the plane of the scapula. (Modified from Rockwood CA, Green DP [eds]: Fractures [3 vols], 2nd ed. Philadelphia: JB Lippincott, 1984.)

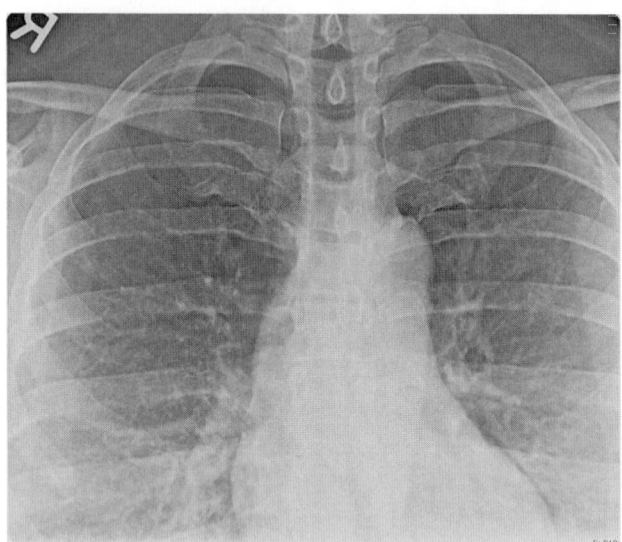

Figure 5-178 Anteroposterior view of the sternoclavicular joint.

This view is the best for observation of the acromioclavicular joint. In addition, the examiner should note the relations of the glenoid cavity, humerus, scapula, and clavicle and any calcifications in the subscapularis, infraspinatus, or teres minor muscles. A dynamic axillary view may be used to show horizontal instability of the acromioclavicular joint.[378]

Transscapular (Y) Lateral (Outlet) View. This view (Figure 5-183) shows the position of the humerus relative to the glenoid and the shape of the acromion and coracoid processes. This view is the true lateral view of the scapula (see Figure 5-169, *D*, and 5-169, *E*).

Stryker Notch View. For this view, the patient lies supine with the arm forward flexed and the hand on top of the head (Figure 5-184). The radiograph centers on the coracoid process. This view is used to assess fractures of the coracoid, a Hill-Sachs lesion (Figure 5-185) or a Bankart lesion.[24,365,379]

West Point View. The patient is positioned in a prone position (Figure 5-186). This projection gives a good view of the glenoid (Figure 5-187) to delineate glenoid fractures and bony abnormalities of the anterior glenoid rim.[380]

Arch View. This lateral view is used to determine the width and height of the subacromial arch. It helps the examiner determine the type of acromial arch (Figure 5-188).

Zanca View. This view is used to assess degenerative change in the acromioclavicular joint (Figure 5-189).

Arthrography

An arthrogram of the shoulder is useful for delineating many of the soft tissues and recesses around the glenohumeral joint (Figures 5-192 and 5-193).[209,381-383] The joint can normally hold approximately 16 mL to 20 mL of solution. With adhesive capsulitis (idiopathic frozen shoulder), the amount the joint can hold may decrease to 5 mL to 10 mL. The arthrogram shows a decrease in the capacity of the joint and obliteration of the axillary fold. Also, there is an almost complete lack of

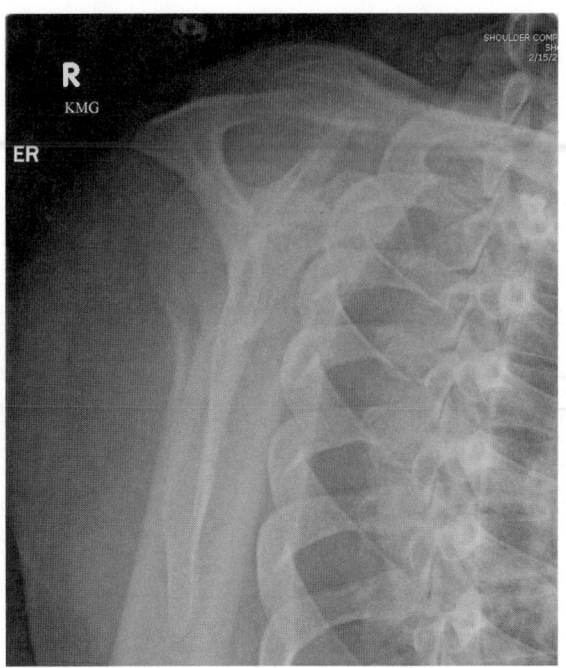

Figure 5-180 Lateral view of the shoulder.

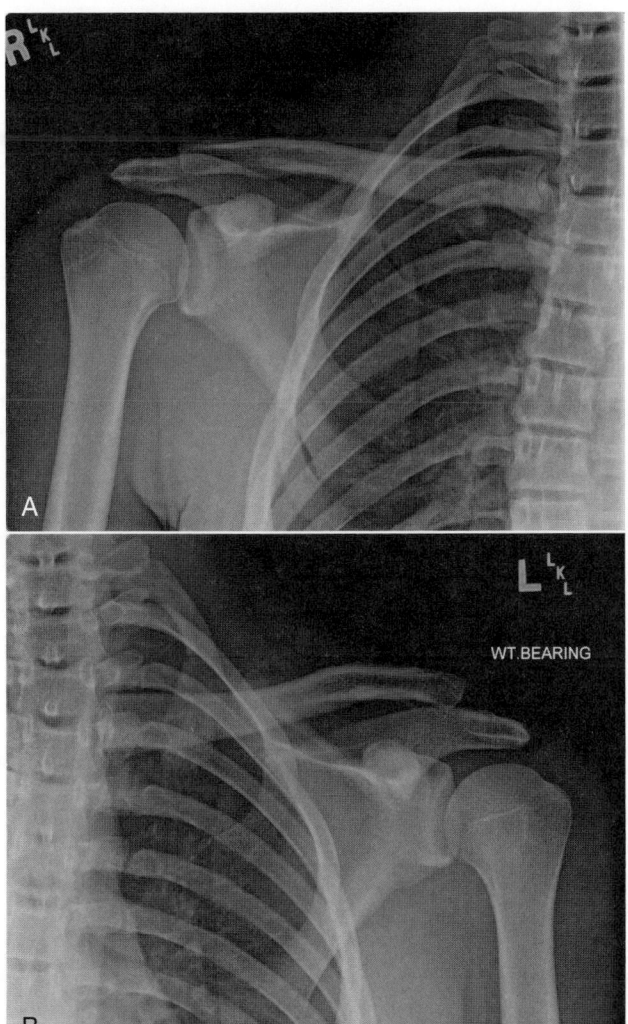

Figure 5-179 A, Anteroposterior view of the acromioclavicular joint. Note the clavicle is in line with the acromion. **B,** If there is a 3° sprain of the acromioclavicular joint and the arm is loaded, the clavicle will be seen to be above the acromion.

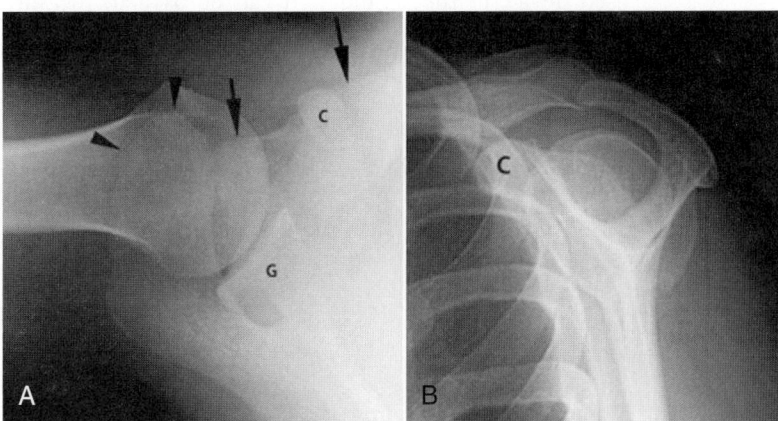

Figure 5-181 A, Axillary view reveals the relationship of the humeral head to the glenoid *(G)* as well as the coracoid *(C)*, acromion *(arrowheads)*, and distal clavicle *(arrows)*. **B,** Outlet view shows the humeral head centered on the glenoid, the coracoid process *(C)* anteriorly, and the acromioclavicular joint in profile. (From Anderson MW, Brennan C, Mittal A: Imaging evaluation of the rotator cuff. Clin Sports Med 31[4]:614, 2012.)

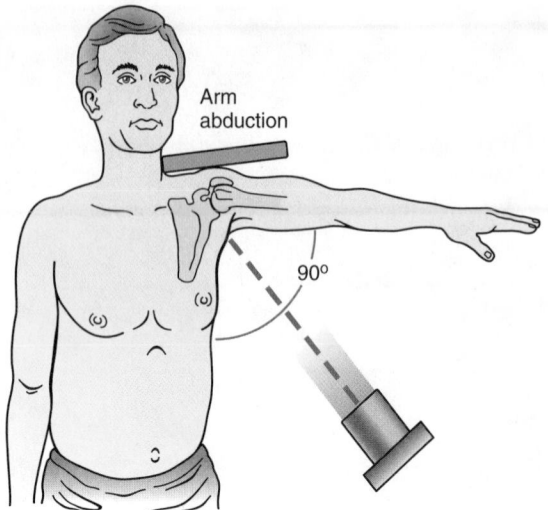

Figure 5-182 Axillary lateral view.

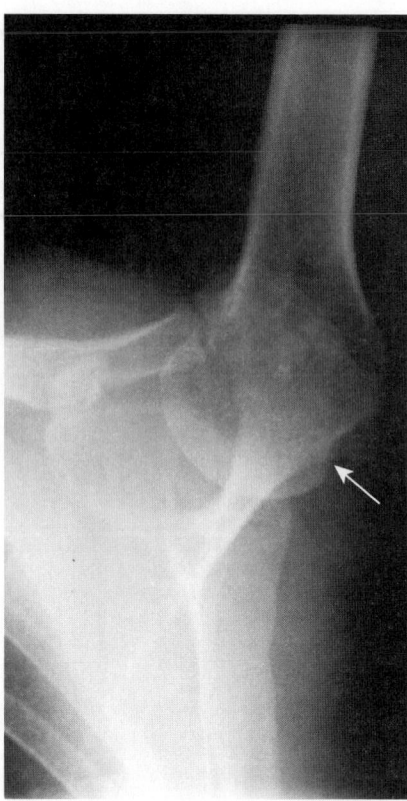

Figure 5-185 **Stryker notch view** demonstrates a notch in the postero-lateral aspect of the humeral head, representing a large Hill-Sachs lesion *(arrow)*.

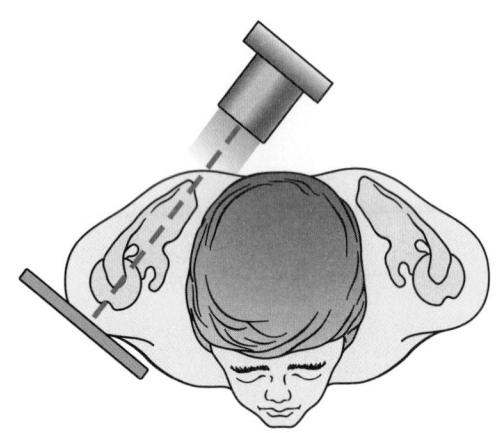

Figure 5-183 Positioning for transscapular (Y) lateral view.

filling of the subscapular bursa with adhesive capsulitis (Figure 5-194). Tearing of any structures, such as the supraspinatus tendon and rotator cuff, may result in extravasation of the radiopaque dye.[384]

Ultrasonography

Diagnostic ultrasound is becoming a more frequently used device in the shoulder. It can be used to measure the acromiohumeral distance,[385] amount of laxity,[386,387] and for rotator cuff tears.[388]

Computed Tomography

Computed tomography, especially when combined with radiopaque dye **(computed tomoarthrogram [CTA]),** is effective in diagnosing bone and soft-tissue anomalies and injuries around the shoulder, including tears of the labrum (Figures 5-195 through 5-197) and the rotator cuff.[375,389] This technique helps delineate capsular redundancy, glenoid rim abnormalities, and loose bodies.[368,390–392]

Magnetic Resonance Imaging

Magnetic resonance imaging (MRI) is proving to be useful in diagnosing soft-tissue injuries to the shoulder and

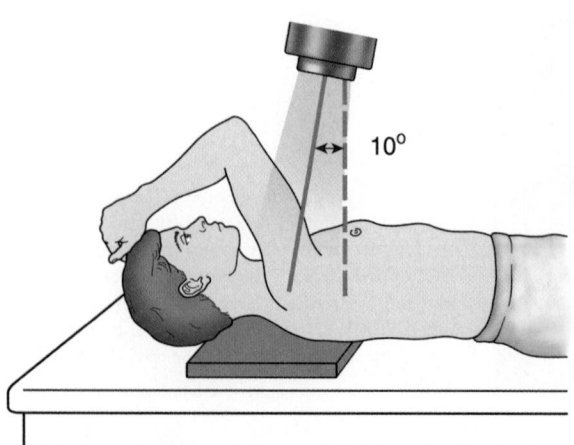

Figure 5-184 Positioning for Stryker notch view.

Text continued on p. 370

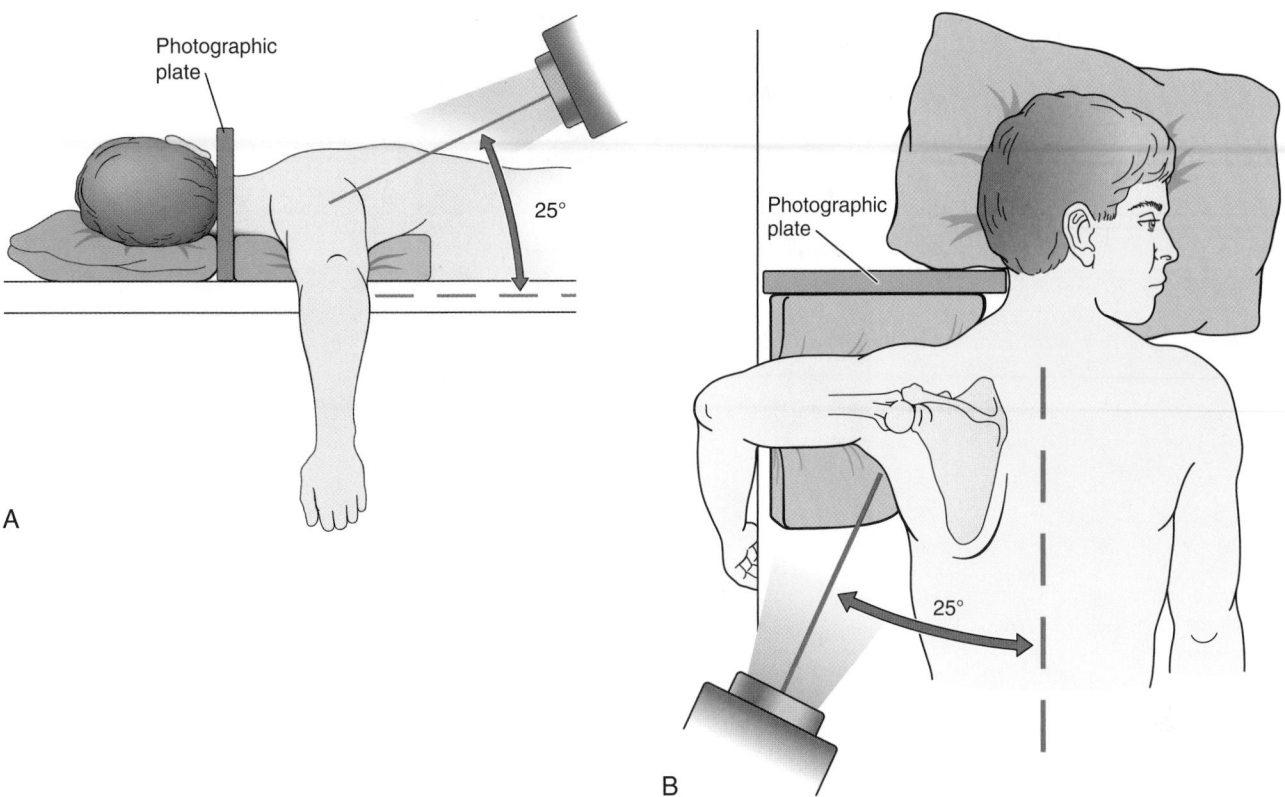

Photographic plate

25°

A

Photographic plate

25°

B

Figure 5-186 Positioning patient for West Point axillary view. A, Side view. **B,** The beam *(bottom left)* is angled downward to form an angle of 25° from the horizontal plane.

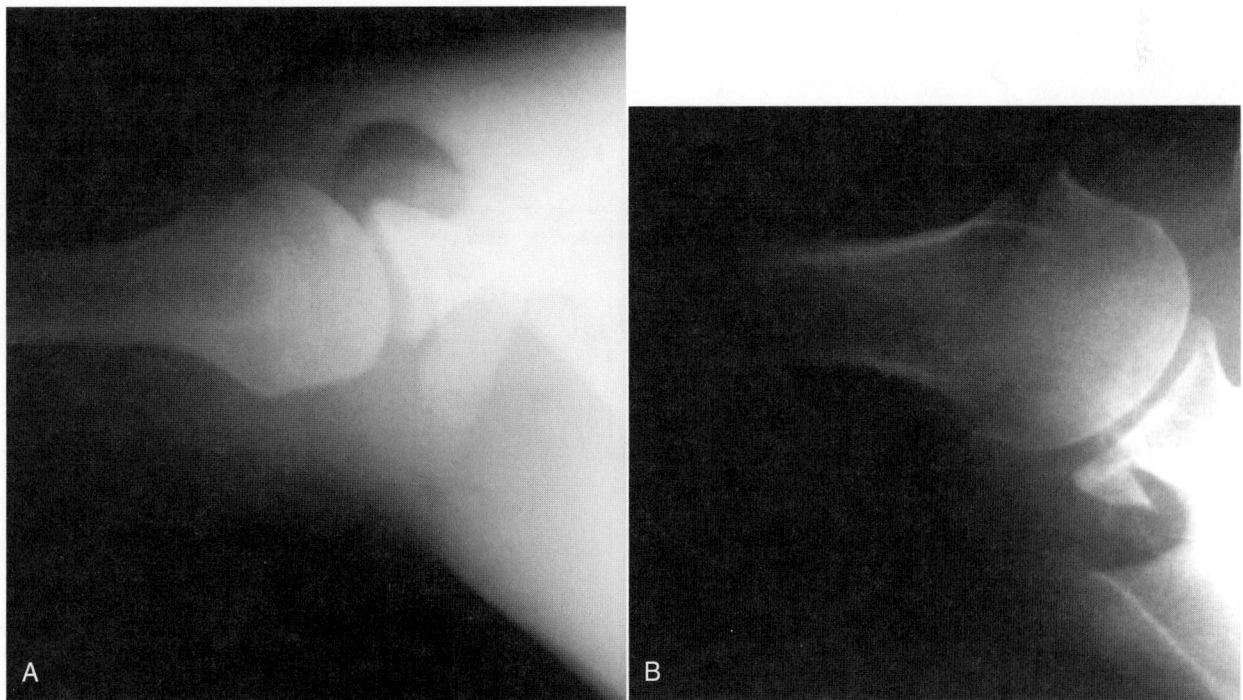

A

B

Figure 5-187 A, The result of a West Point view of the glenohumeral joint. Note the acromion superior to the glenoid and the coracoid process, which is inferior to the glenoid in this view. **B,** Plain film x-ray in an axillary or West Point view of a fracture of the glenoid, a Bankart fracture. (From Swain J, Bush KW: Diagnostic imaging for physical therapists, St Louis, 2009, Saunders/Elsevier, pp. 196, 208.)

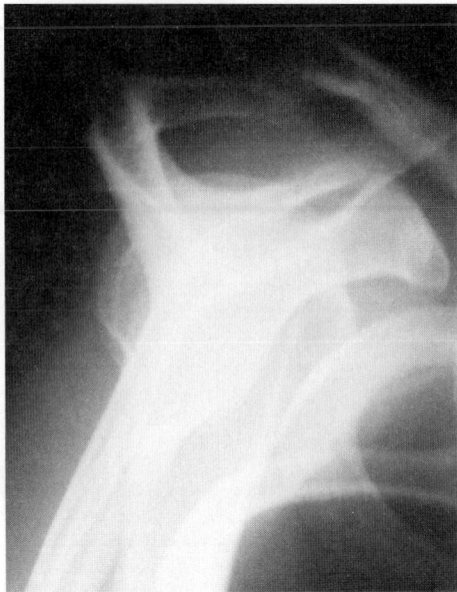

Figure 5-188 Arch view of acromioclavicular joint. Notice the separation of the clavicle and acromion. The view also shows the relation of the humerus to the glenoid (Y view).

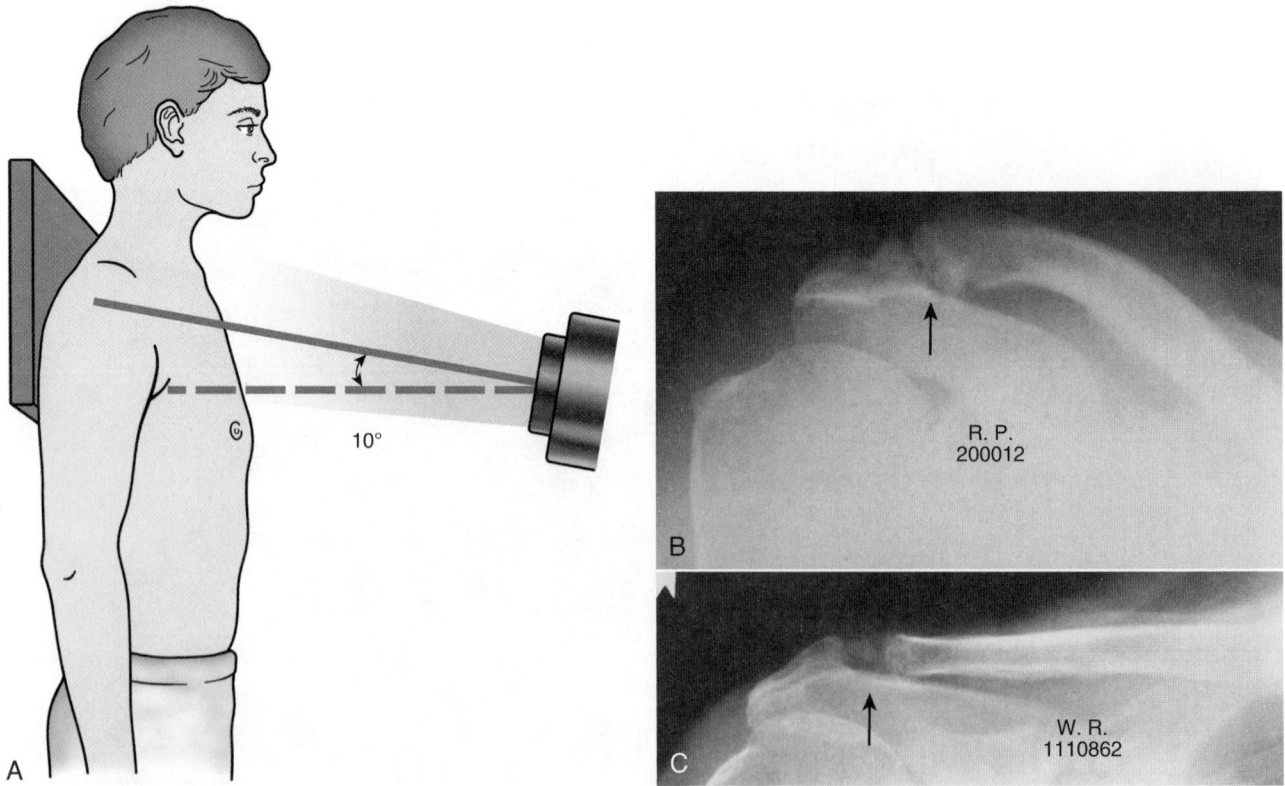

Figure 5-189 A, Positioning patient for a Zanca view of the acromioclavicular joint. **B,** A Zanca view of the joint reveals significant degenerative changes. **C,** With the Zanca view, a loose body is clearly noted within the joint. (**B** and **C,** From Rockwood CA: The shoulder, ed 4, Philadelphia, 2009, WB Saunders.)

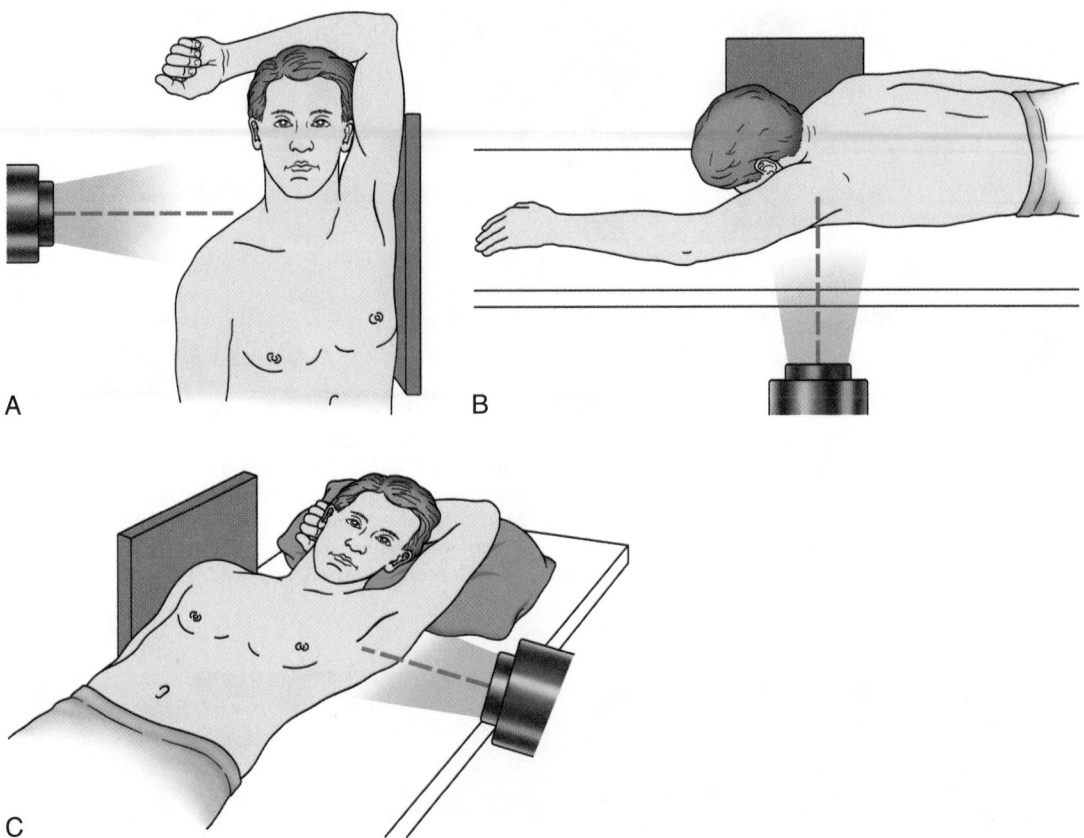

Figure 5-190 Patient positioning for swimmer's view. A, Lateral. **B,** Prone. **C,** Supine.

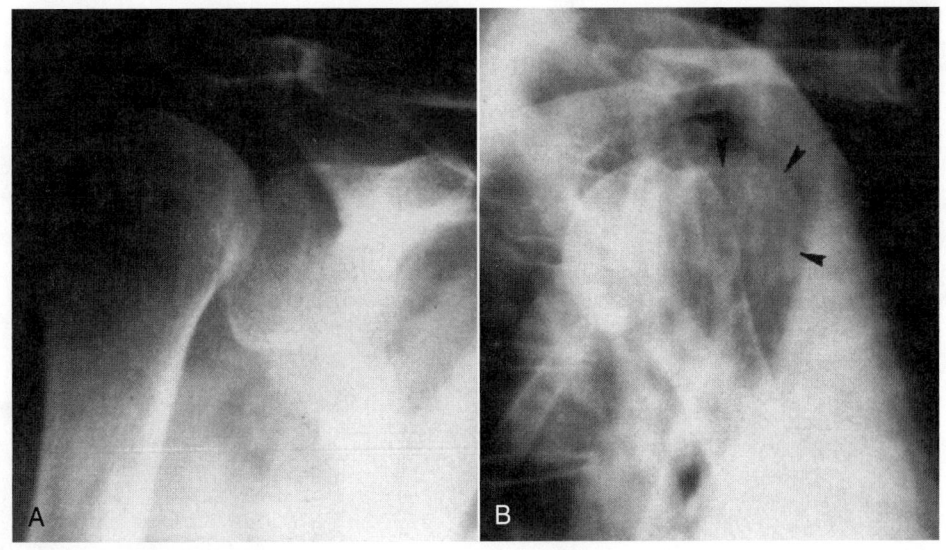

Figure 5-191 A, Posterior dislocation of the humerus. **B,** A swimmer's view (From Sutton D, Young JWR: A concise textbook of clinical imaging, ed 2, St Louis, 1995, Mosby).

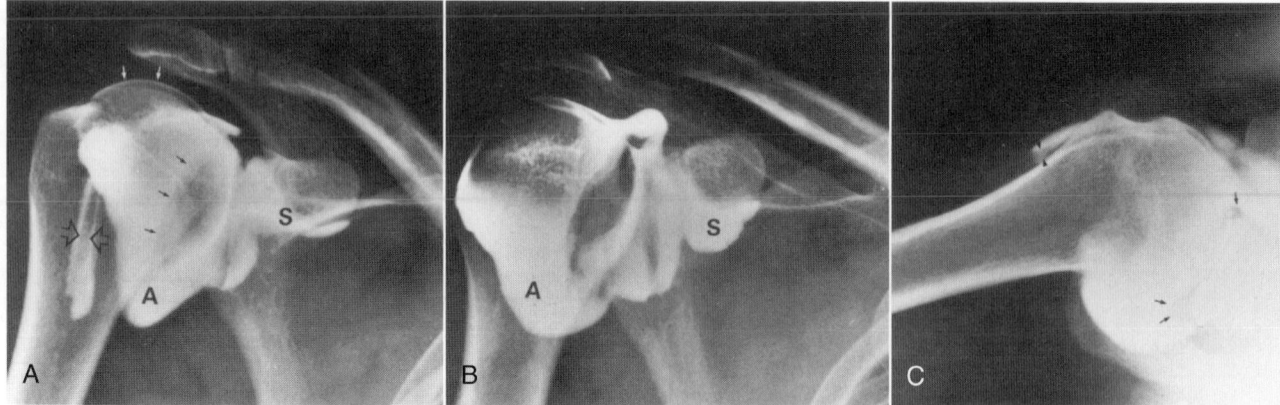

Figure 5-192 Normal single-contrast arthrogram. A, Lateral rotation. **B,** Medial rotation. The humeral articular cartilage is coated with contrast medium *(white arrows)*. There is no contrast agent in the subacromial-subdeltoid bursa. The defect created by the glenoid labrum *(black arrows)* is shown. Filling of the subscapularis recess is often poor on lateral rotation views because of bursal compression by the subscapularis muscle. **C,** In the axillary view, the anterior *(single arrow)* and posterior *(double arrows)* glenoid labral margins are shown. The biceps tendon *(arrowheads)* is surrounded by contrast medium in the biceps tendon sheath. No contrast agent overlies the surgical neck of the humerus. *A,* Axillary recess; *open arrows,* tendon of long head of biceps within biceps sheath; *S,* subscapularis recess. (From Weissman BNW, Sledge CB: Orthopedic radiology, Philadelphia, 1986, WB Saunders, p. 222.)

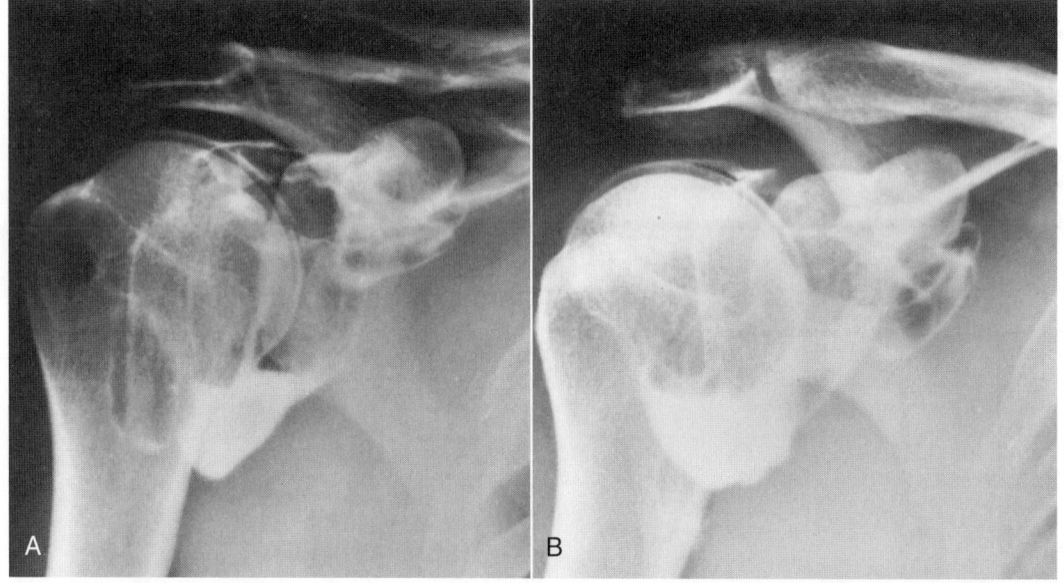

Figure 5-193 Normal double-contrast arthrogram. Upright views of the patient with a sandbag suspended from the wrist, and the humerus in lateral rotation **(A)** and medial rotation **(B)** show the structures noted on single-contrast examination and allow better appreciation of the articular cartilages. (From Weissman BNW, Sledge CB: Orthopedic radiology, Philadelphia, 1986, WB Saunders, p. 222.)

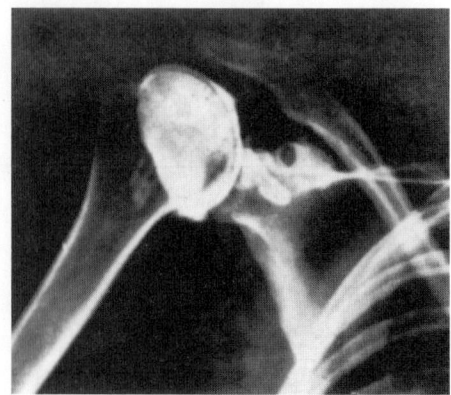

Figure 5-194 Typical arthrographic picture in adhesive capsulitis. Note the absence of a dependent axillary fold and poor filling of the biceps. (From Neviaser JS: Arthrography of the shoulder joint: study of the findings of adhesive capsulitis of the shoulder. J Bone Joint Surg Am 44:1328, 1962.)

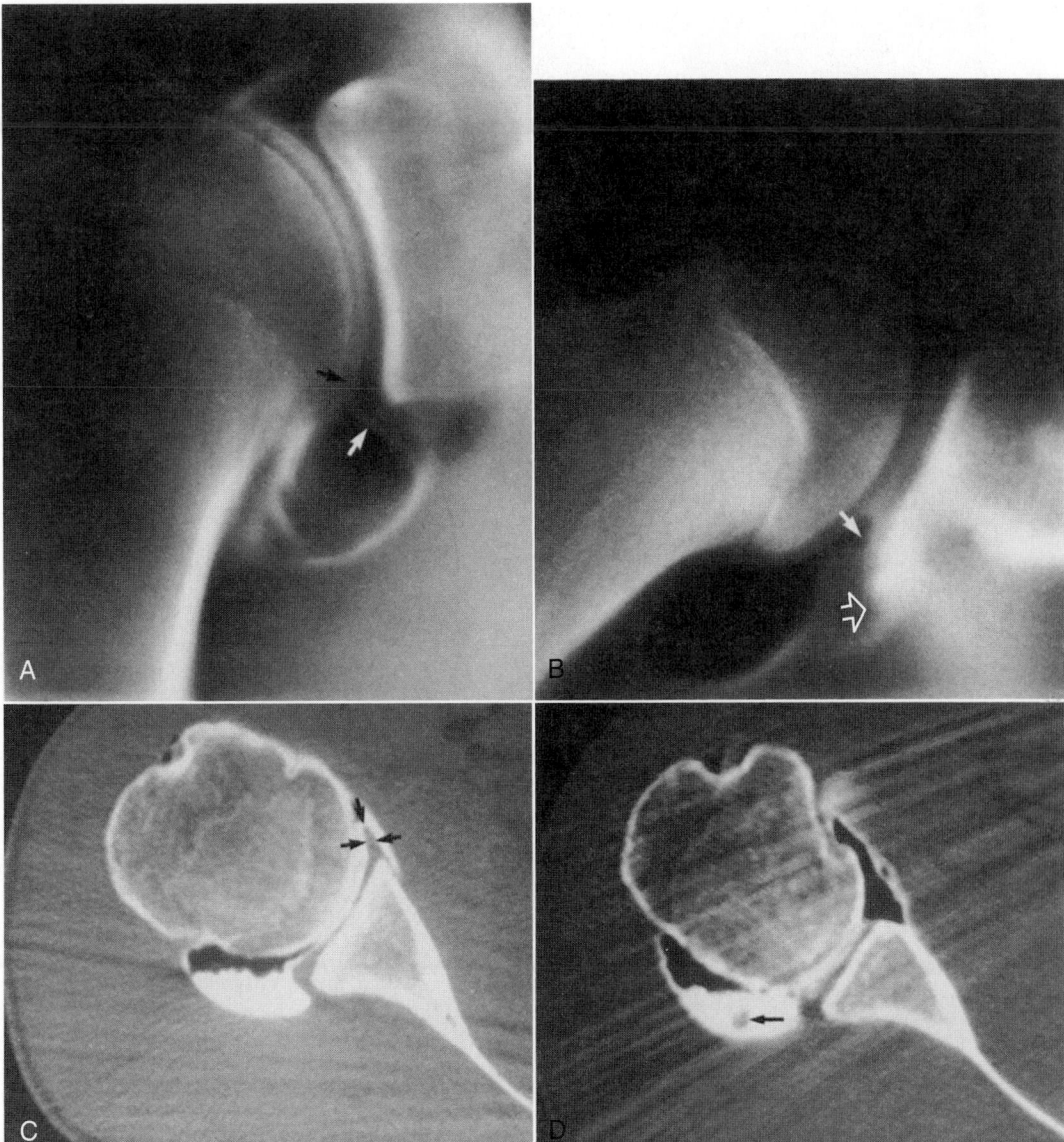

Figure 5-195 Tomogram and computed tomography scan of the glenoid labrum. A, Normal glenoid labrum on posterior oblique double-contrast arthrotomography. Tomographic section through the anterior margin of the glenoid in the posterior oblique position shows smooth articular cartilage on the humeral head *(black arrow)* and glenoid and a smooth contour to the glenoid labrum *(white arrow)*. **B,** Abnormal glenoid labrum. Tomographic section shows a triangular defect in the labrum *(white arrow)*. The bony margin of the glenoid is also irregular *(open arrow)*. The patient had suffered a single anterior dislocation. **C,** Normal glenoid labrum on computed tomography after double-contrast arthrography. The sharply pointed anterior *(arrows)* and slightly rounder posterior margins of the labrum are visible. **D,** Computed tomoarthrogram shows an absence of the anterior labrum and a loose body *(arrow)* posteriorly. (**B,** Courtesy Dr. Ethan Braunstein, Brigham and Women's Hospital, Boston, MA; **C** and **D,** Courtesy Dr. Arthur Newberg, Boston, MA. From Weissman BNW, Sledge CB: Orthopedic radiology, Philadelphia, 1986, WB Saunders, p. 257.)

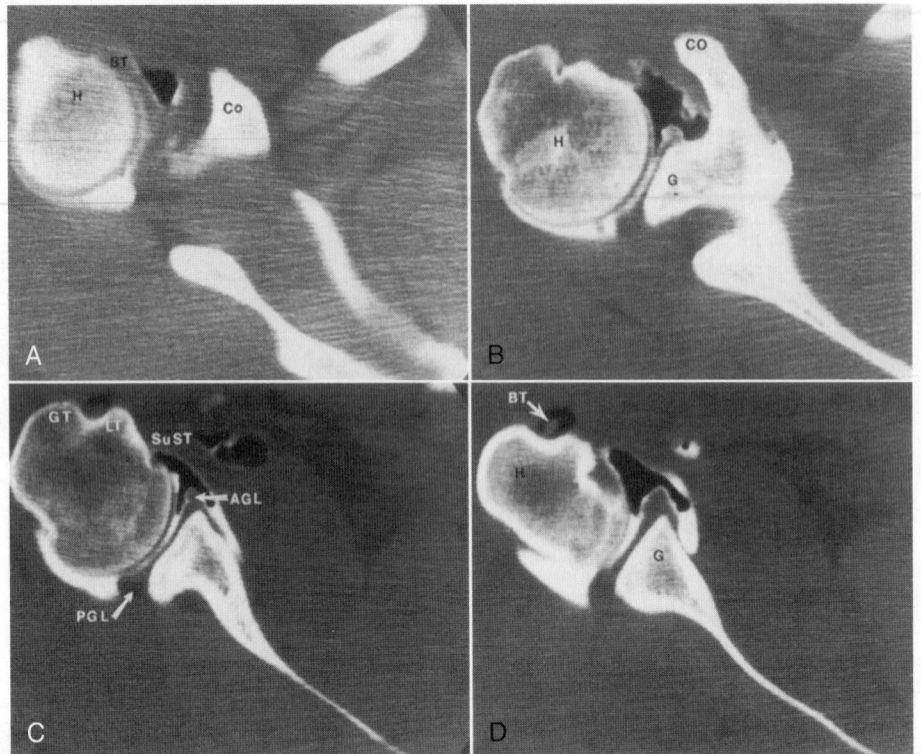

Figure 5-196 Normal shoulder, computed arthrotomography. Normal anatomy is demonstrated by computed arthrotomographic sections at the level of the bicipital tendon origin **(A)**, the coracoid process **(B)**, the subscapularis tendon, **(C)** and the inferior joint level **(D)**. *AGL,* Anterior glenoid labrum; *Bt,* bicipital tendon; *Co,* coracoid process; *G,* glenoid process; *GT,* greater tuberosity; *H,* humeral head; *LT,* lesser tuberosity; *PGL,* posterior glenoid labrum; *SuST,* subscapularis tendon. (From De Lee JC, Drez D, editors: Orthopedic sports medicine: principles and practice, Philadelphia, 1994, WB Saunders, p. 721.)

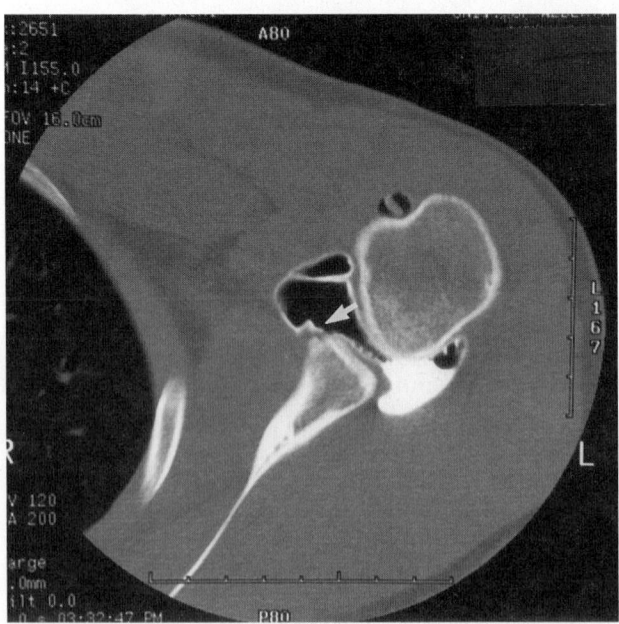

Figure 5-197 Computed tomography scan of labral tear *(arrow).*

has, in fact, become the method of choice for demonstrating soft-tissue abnormalities of the shoulder, such as labral and rotator cuff pathology.[364,393-398] However, it is important that these abnormalities be correlated with clinical findings.[394,398] It is possible to differentiate bursitis, peritenonitis/tendinosis, muscle strains, especially with injuries to the rotator cuff.[399] It is also useful for differentially diagnosing causes of impingement and instability syndromes. Labral tears, Hill-Sachs lesions, glenoid irregularities, and the state of bone marrow can also be diagnosed in the shoulder with the use of MRI (Figures 5-198 through 5-204).[208,364,368,400-405] Magnetic resonance arthrography has been found to increase the sensitivity to detecting partial thickness tears.[399,406]

Angiography

In the case of thoracic outlet syndromes and other syndromes involving arterial impingement, angiograms are sometimes used to demonstrate blockage of the subclavian artery during certain moves (Figure 5-205).

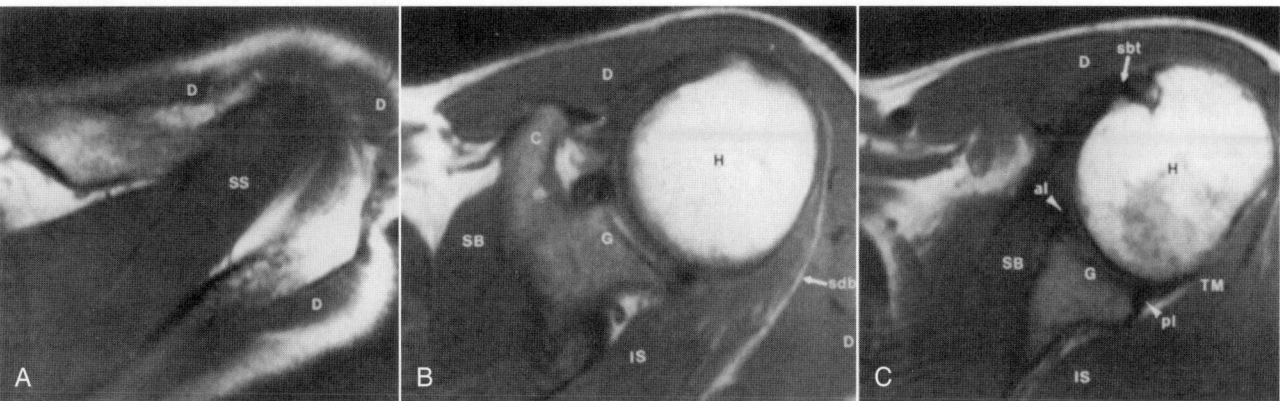

Figure 5-198 T1-weighted axial magnetic resonance images from cranial **(A)** to caudal **(C).** *al,* anterior labrum; *C,* coracoid; *D,* deltoid muscle; *G,* glenoid of scapula; *H,* humerus; *IS,* infraspinatus muscle; *pl,* posterior labrum; *SB,* subscapularis muscle; *sbt,* subscapularis tendon; *sdb,* subdeltoid-subacromial bursa; *SS,* supraspinatus muscle; *TM,* teres minor muscle. (From Meyer SJF, Dalinka MK: Magnetic resonance imaging of the shoulder. Orthop Clin North Am 21:499, 1990.)

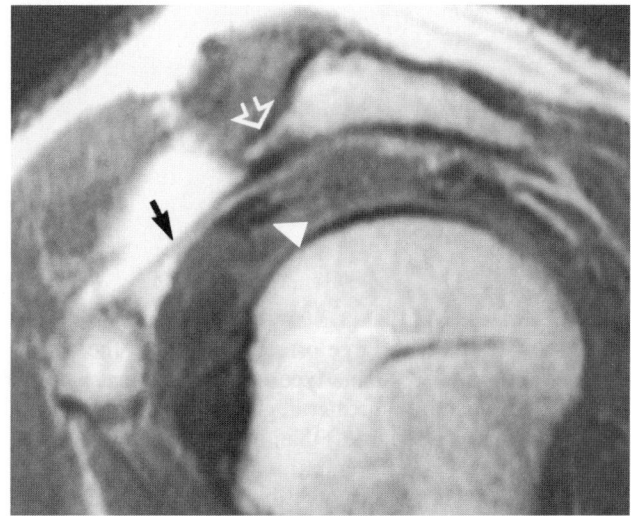

Figure 5-199 Shoulder impingement syndrome: Subacromial enthesophyte. Sagittal oblique T1-weighted (TR/TE, 800/20) spin echo magnetic resonance (MR) image shows the enthesophyte *(open arrow),* which is intimate with the coracoacromial ligament *(solid arrow)* and supraspinatus tendon *(arrowhead).* (From Resnick D, Kransdorf MJ: Bone and joint imaging, Philadelphia, 2005, WB Saunders, p. 375.)

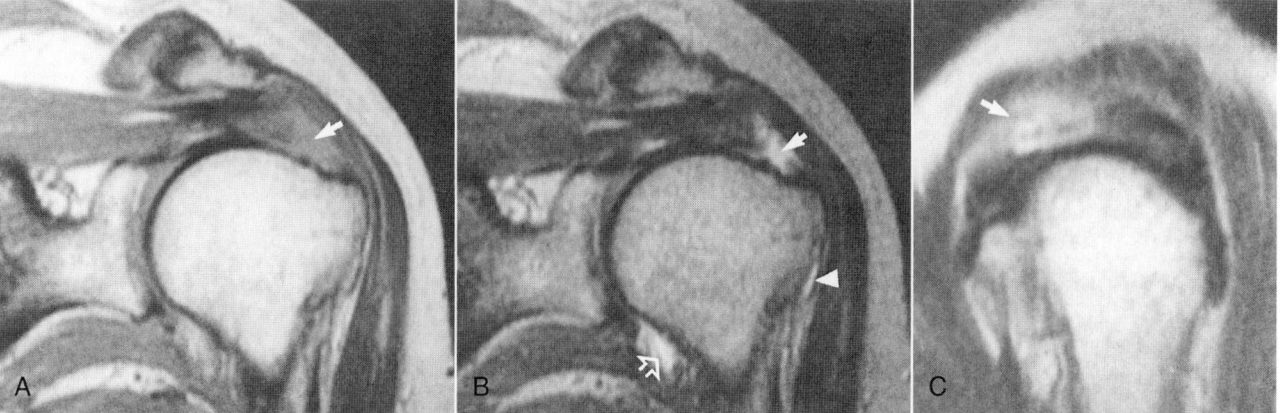

Figure 5-200 Full-thickness rotator cuff tear: Magnetic resonance (MR) imaging. In the coronal oblique plane, intermediate-weighted (TR/TE, 2000/20) **(A)** and T2-weighted (TR/TE, 2000/80) **(B)** spin echo MR images show fluid in a gap *(solid arrow)* in the supraspinatus tendon; the fluid is of increased signal intensity in **B.** Also in **B,** note the increased signal intensity related to fluid in the glenohumeral joint *(open arrow)* and subdeltoid bursa *(arrowhead).* Osteoarthritis of the acromioclavicular joint is evident. **C,** In the same patient, sagittal oblique T2-weighted (TR/TE, 2000/60) spin echo MR images show the site *(arrow)* of disruption of the supraspinatus tendon, which is of high signal intensity. (From Resnick D, Kransdorf MJ: Bone and joint imaging, Philadelphia, 2005, WB Saunders, p. 925.)

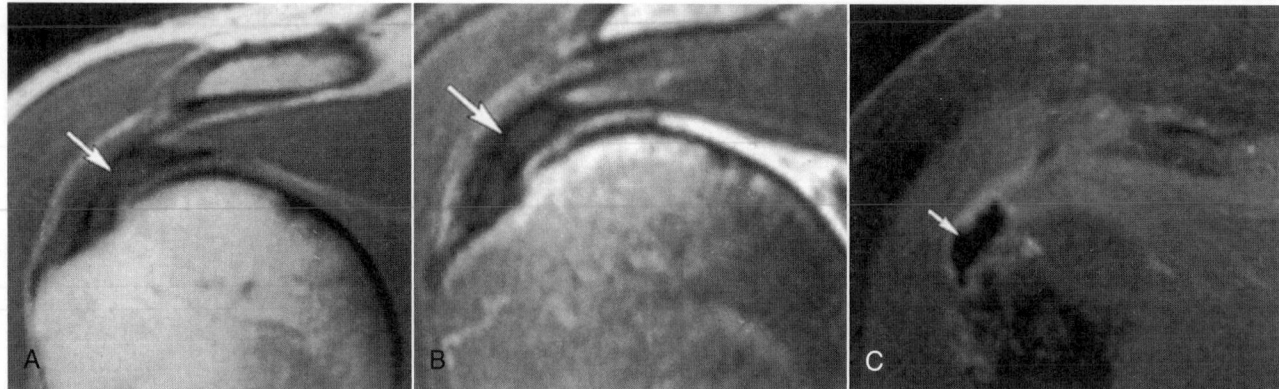

Figure 5-201 A, T1-weighted coronal image demonstrating mild thickening of the supraspinatus tendon with intermediate signal *(arrow)* present within the substance of the tendon. **B,** T2-weighted coronal image at the same level also demonstrating thickening of the tendon with intermediate signal *(arrow)* within the tendon. The presence of intermediate signal within the tendon is diagnostic of tendinopathy, whereas bright (fluid) signal within the tendon is diagnostic of a tear. **C,** A globular area of low signal abnormality *(arrow)* in the infraspinatus tendon and mild surrounding edema consistent with calcific bursitis. (From Sanders TG, Miller MD: A systematic approach to magnetic resonance imaging interpretation of sports medicine injuries of the shoulder. Am J Sports Med 33:1094, 2005.)

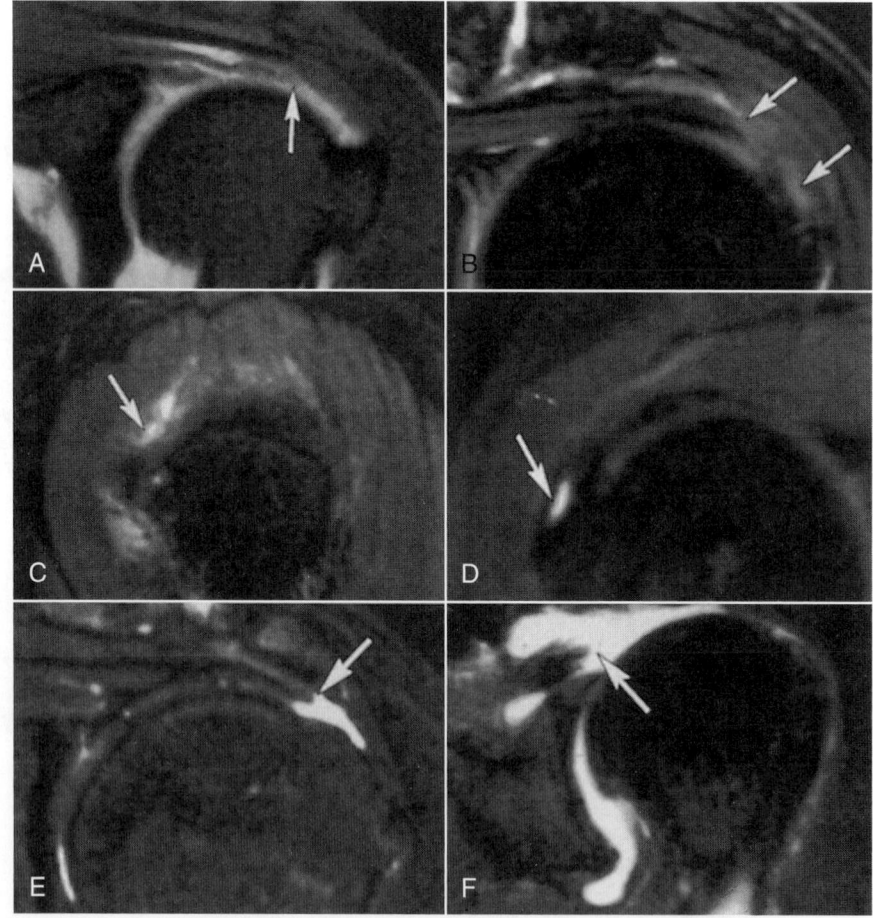

Figure 5-202 Rotator cuff tear. Criteria for diagnosing a rotator cuff tear on magnetic resonance (MR) imaging include the presence of fluid in the expected location of the tendon or retraction of the tendon. **A,** MR arthrogram of a partial-thickness articular surface tear of the supraspinatus tendon as contrast *(arrow)* extends into the substance of the tendon but not completely through the thickness of the tendon. **B,** Conventional T2-weighted coronal image. **C,** Sagittal image. Both **(B)** and **(C)** demonstrate fluid signal intensity *(arrows)* extending partially through the thickness of the tendon involving the bursal surface. **D,** An interstitial tear *(arrow)* of the supraspinatus tendon. Fluid signal intensity *(arrow)* is present within the substance of the tendon but does not extend to either the articular or bursal surface of the tendon. **E,** A full-thickness tear with bright fluid signal *(arrow)* extending all the way through the thickness of the tendon from top to bottom. **F,** A complete tear of the supraspinatus tendon extending from front to back, with approximately 3 cm of retraction of the musculotendinous junction *(arrow)*. (From Sanders TG, Miller MD: A systematic approach to magnetic resonance imaging interpretation of sports medicine injuries of the shoulder. Am J Sports Med 33:1094, 2005.)

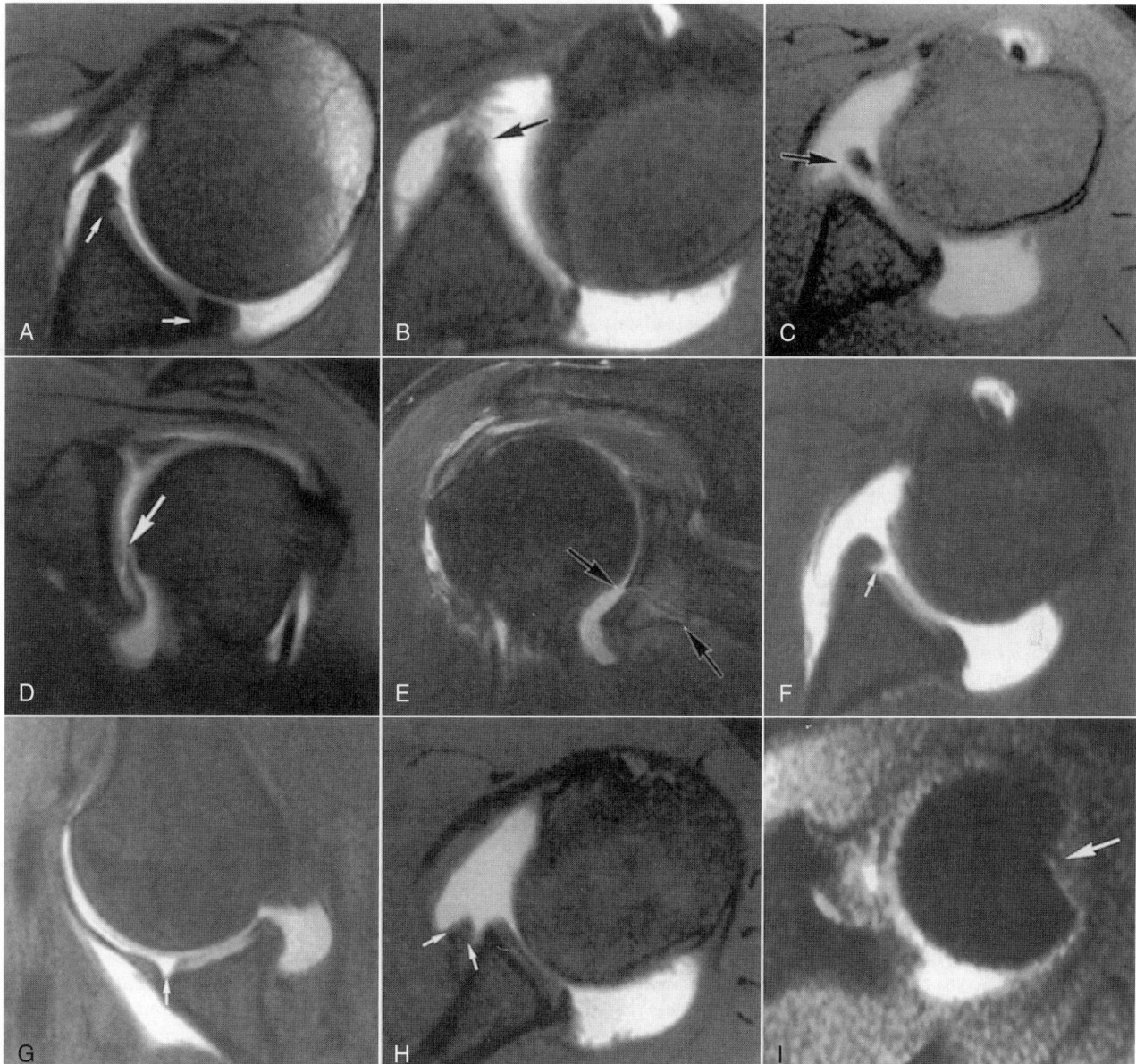

Figure 5-203 Bankart lesions. A, Cartilage undermining *(arrows)* the anterior and posterior labrum. The articular cartilage is intermediate in signal intensity and smooth and tapering, because it undermines the fibrocartilage of the glenoid labrum. This image should not be confused with a tear, which will be irregular in appearance and usually extends completely beneath the labrum. **B,** Marked irregularity and fraying *(arrow)* of the antero-inferior labrum. **C,** A displaced Bankart lesion *(arrow).* **D,** T2-weighted coronal image through the level of the anterior labrum demonstrating an irregular fluid collection *(arrow)* located within a tear of the anterior labrum, between the labrum and the glenoid. This irregularity is referred to as the "double axillary pouch" sign and is very for an anterior labral tear. **E,** A minimally displaced Bankart fracture *(arrows)* through the inferior glenoid. **F,** Axial image with intra-articular contrast. **G,** Abduction external rotation image with intra-articular contrast. Both **F** and **G** demonstrate a small collection of contrast *(arrows)* extending partially beneath the anterior labrum, representing a nondisplaced Bankart (Perthes) lesion. **H,** A medialized Bankart lesion *(arrows).* **I,** T2-weighted axial image through the superior aspect of the humeral head demonstrating a concavity *(arrow)* of the posterosuperior humeral head, representing a Hill-Sachs deformity. The humeral head should be round on the top three images with no flattening or concavity. (From Sanders TG, Miller MD: A systematic approach to magnetic resonance imaging interpretation of sports medicine injuries of the shoulder. Am J Sports Med 33:1097, 2005.)

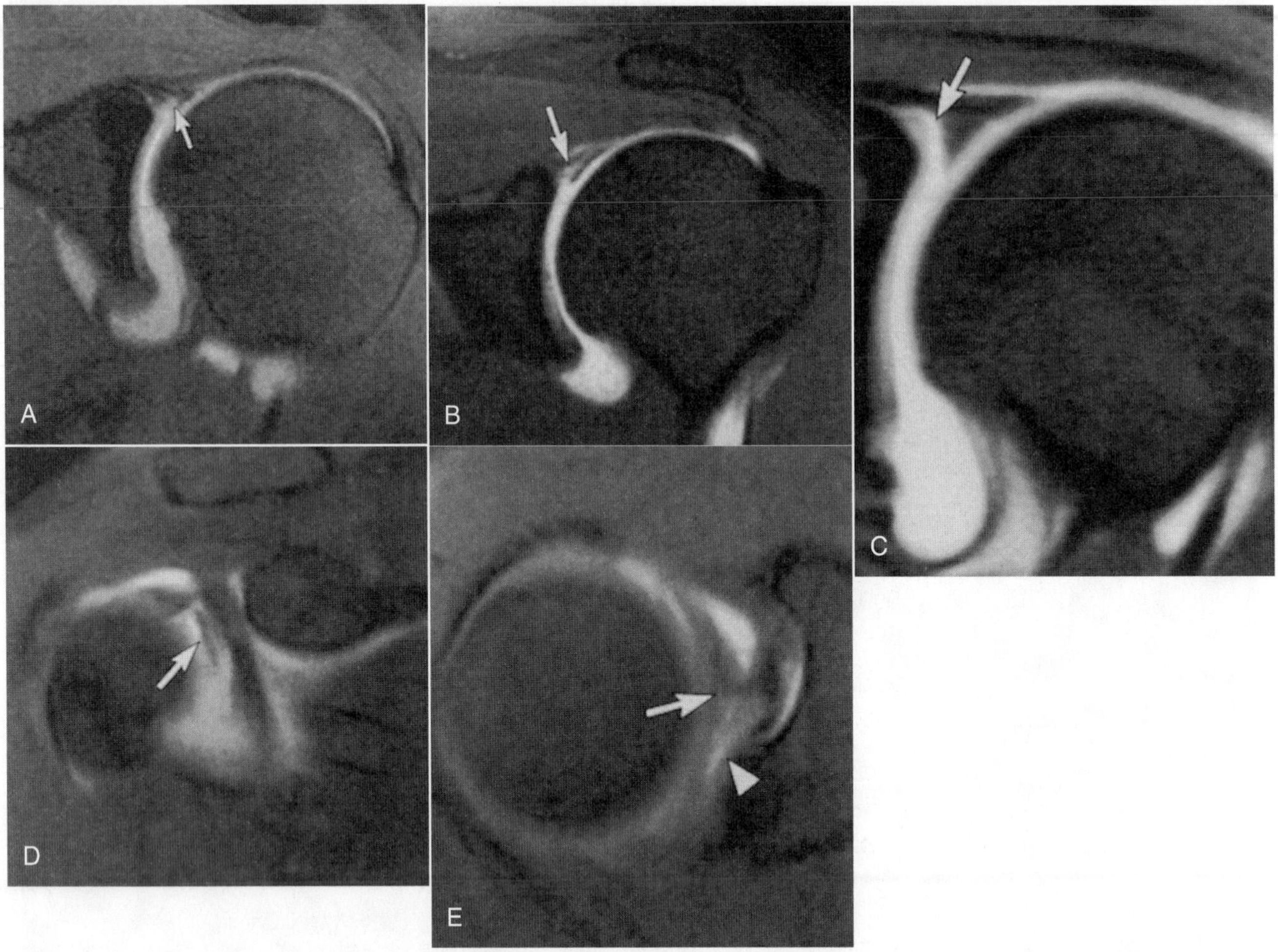

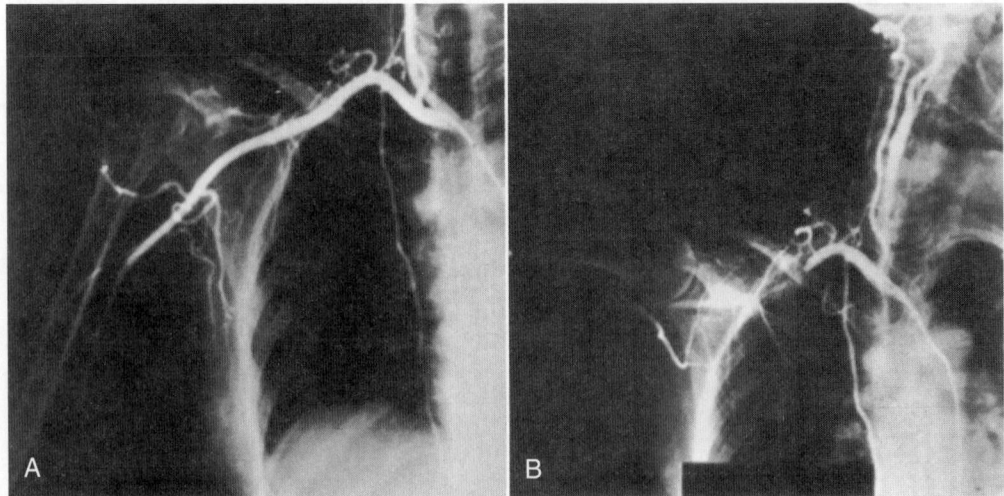

Figure 5-204 Superior labral anterior posterior (SLAP) tear. A, Fraying and irregularity *(arrow)* of the undersurface of the superior labrum, consistent with a SLAP tear. **B,** A linear area of high signal *(arrow)* extending into the substance of the superior labrum. The presence of any high signal within the substance of the superior labrum is diagnostic of a SLAP tear. **C,** Displacement *(arrow)* of the superior labrum away from the glenoid. This image represents a type II SLAP tear. **D,** A bucket-handle tear (type III SLAP tear) of the superior labrum with the bucket-handle fragment *(arrow)* dangling in the superior joint. **E,** Axial image demonstrating an irregular collection of contrast extending into the biceps anchor consistent with a type IV SLAP tear with involvement of the biceps anchor. (From Sanders TG, Miller MD: A systematic approach to magnetic resonance imaging interpretation of sports medicine injuries of the shoulder. Am J Sports Med 33:1096, 2005.)

Figure 5-205 Angiograms of the subclavian artery with the arm at rest **(A)** and abducted **(B).** Note complete obstruction of the subclavian artery in **B.** (From Brown C: Compressive, invasive referred pain to the shoulder. Clin Orthop 173:59, 1983.)

PRÉCIS OF THE SHOULDER ASSESSMENT*

Patient History (sitting)
Observation (sitting or standing)
Examination
    Active movements (sitting or standing)
        Elevation through forward flexion of the arm
        Elevation through abduction of the arm
        Elevation through the plane of the scapula (scaption)
        Medial rotation of the arm
        Lateral rotation of the arm
        Adduction of the arm
        Horizontal adduction and abduction of the arm
        Circumduction of the arm
    Passive movements (sitting)
        Elevation through abduction of the arm
        Elevation through forward flexion of the arm
        Elevation through abduction at the glenohumeral
          joint only
        Lateral rotation of the arm
        Medial rotation of the arm
        Extension of the arm
        Adduction of the arm
        Horizontal adduction and abduction of the arm
    Functional assessment
    Special tests† (sitting or standing)
        For anterior shoulder instability:
          Load and shift test
        For posterior shoulder instability:
          Jerk test
          Load and shift test
         For inferior and multidirectional shoulder instability:
          Feagin test
          Sulcus sign
        For anterior impingement:
          Coracoid impingement sign
          Hawkins-Kennedy test
          Neer test
          Yokum test
          Zaslav test (internal rotation resistance strength test
            [IRRST])
        For posterior impingement:
          Posterior internal impingement test
        For labral lesions‡:
          Active compression test of O'Brien
          Anterior slide test
          Biceps tension test
          Biceps load test (Kim test II)
          Dynamic labral shear test
          Forced shoulder abduction and elbow flexion test
          Jerk test
          Kim test I (biceps load test II)
          Mayo shear test
          Pain provocation test
        For scapular dyskinesia:
          Lateral scapular slide test
          Scapular load test
          Scapular retraction test (SRT)
          Wall/floor pushup
        For acromioclavicular joint pathology:
          Horizontal adduction test
          Paxinos sign
        For muscle pathology‡:
          Speed's test (biceps)
          Yergason's test (biceps)

          Drop arm test (supraspinatus)
          "Empty can" test (supraspinatus)
          Bear-hug test (subscapularis)
          Belly press test (abdominal compression or
            Napolean test) (subscapularis)
          External rotation lag sign (ERLS) (subscapularis)
          Lift-off sign (Gerber's test) (subscapularis)
          Medial rotation lag or "spring back" test
            (subscapularis)
          Dropping sign (infraspinatus)
          Infraspinatus test (infraspinatus)
          Lateral rotation lag sign (infraspinatus)
          Hornblower's sign (teres minor)
          Rent test (rotator cuff—general)
          Whipple test (rotator cuff—general)
          Trapezius test (three positions)
          Punch out test (serratus anterior)
        For thoracic outlet syndrome:
          Roos test
    Reflexes and cutaneous distribution (sitting)
        Reflexes
        Sensory scan
        Peripheral nerves
          Axillary nerve
          Suprascapular nerve
          Musculocutaneous nerve
          Long thoracic nerve
          Spinal accessory nerve
    Palpation (sitting)
    Resisted isometric movements (supine lying)
        Forward flexion of the shoulder
        Extension of the shoulder
        Abduction of the shoulder
        Adduction of the shoulder
        Medial rotation of the shoulder
        Lateral rotation of the shoulder
        Flexion of the elbow
        Extension of the elbow
    Special tests† (supine lying)
        For anterior shoulder instability:
          Anterior/apprehension release ("surprise") test
          Anterior drawer rest
          Crank (apprehension) and relocation test
          Fulcrum test
        For posterior shoulder instability:
          Norwood test
          Posterior apprehension test
          Posterior drawer test
        For anterior impingement:
          Supine impingement test
        For labral lesions‡:
          Clunk test
          Compression rotation test
          Resisted supination external rotation test (RSERT)
        For ligament pathology:
          Coracoclavicular ligament test
          Crank test
        For muscle pathology‡:
          Trapezius test (three positions) (prone lying)
        For neurological function:
          Upper limb neurodynamic (tension) test (ULNT)
            Median nerve (ULNT I)
            Median nerve (ULNT II)

Continued

PRÉCIS OF THE SHOULDER ASSESSMENT—cont'd

Radial nerve (ULNT III)
Ulnar nerve (ULNT IV)
Joint play movements (supine lying)
Backward glide of the humerus
Forward glide of the humerus
Lateral distraction of the humerus
Long arm traction
Backward glide of the humerus in abduction

Anteroposterior and cephalocaudal movements of the
clavicle at the acromioclavicular joint
Anteroposterior and cephalocaudal movements of the
clavicle at the sternoclavicular joint
General movement of the scapula to determine
mobility
Diagnostic imaging

*The précis is shown in an order that limits the amount of movement that the patient has to do but ensures that all necessary structures are tested. After any examination, the patient should be warned of the possibility that symptoms may exacerbate as a result of the assessment.

†The author recommends these key tests be learned by the clinician to facilitate a diagnosis.

‡Research has shown that no single test or even a group of tests can accurately diagnose a SLAP or rotator cuff lesion.[53,249–254]

CASE STUDIES

When doing these case studies, the examiner should list the appropriate questions to ask the patient and should specify why they are being asked, what to look for and why, what things should be tested, and why. Depending on the patient's answers (and the examiner should consider numerous responses), several possible causes of the patient's problem may become evident (examples are given in parentheses). The examiner should prepare a differential diagnosis chart. He or she can then decide how different diagnoses may affect the treatment plan. For example, a 23-year-old man comes to the clinic complaining of shoulder pain. He says that 2 days earlier he was playing touch football. When his friend threw the ball, he reached for it, lost his balance, and fell on the tip of his shoulder but managed to hang onto the ball. How would you differentiate between acromioclavicular sprain and supraspinatus tendinitis? Table 5-20 demonstrates a differential diagnosis chart for the two conditions.

1. A 47-year-old man comes to you complaining of pain in the left shoulder. There is no history of overuse activity. The pain that occurs when he elevates his shoulder is referred to his neck and sometimes down the arm to his wrist. Describe your assessment plan for this patient (cervical spondylosis versus subacromial bursitis).

2. An 18-year-old woman recently had a Putti-Platt procedure for a recurring dislocation of the left shoulder. When you see her, her arm is still in a sling, but the surgeon wants you to begin treatment. Describe your assessment for this patient.

3. A 68-year-old woman comes to you complaining of pain and restricted ROM in the right shoulder. She tells you that 3 months earlier she slipped on a rug on a tile floor and landed on her elbow. Both her elbow and shoulder hurt at that time. Describe your assessment plan for this patient (olecranon bursitis versus adhesive capsulitis).

4. Parents bring their 5-year-old son in to see you. They state that he was running around the recreation room chasing a friend when he tripped over a stool and landed on his shoulder. He refuses to move his arm and is crying, because the accident occurred only 2 hours earlier. Describe your assessment plan for this patient (clavicular fracture versus humeral epiphyseal injury).

5. A 35-year-old female master swimmer comes to you complaining of shoulder pain. She states that she has been swimming approximately 2000 m per day in two training sessions; she recently increased her swimming from 1500 m per day to get ready for a competition in 3 weeks. Describe your assessment plan for this patient (subacromial bursitis versus biceps tendinitis).

6. A 20-year-old male tennis player comes to you complaining that when he serves the ball, his arm "goes dead." He has had this problem for 3 weeks but never before. He has increased his training during the past month. Describe your assessment plan for this patient (thoracic outlet syndrome versus brachial plexus lesion).

7. A 15-year-old female competitive swimmer comes to you complaining of diffuse shoulder pain. She notices the problem most when she does the backstroke. She complains that her shoulder sometimes feels unstable when doing this stroke. Describe your assessment plan for this patient (anterior instability versus supraspinatus tendinitis).

8. A 48-year-old man comes to you complaining of neck and shoulder pain. He states that he has difficulty abducting his right arm. There is no history of trauma, but he remembers being in a car accident 10 years earlier. Describe your assessment plan for this patient (cervical spondylosis versus adhesive capsulitis).

TABLE **5-20**

Differential Diagnosis of Acromioclavicular Joint Sprain and Supraspinatus Paratenonitis

	Acromioclavicular Joint Sprain	Supraspinatus Paratenonitis
Observation	Step deformity (third-degree)	Normal
Active movement	Pain especially at extreme of motion (horizontal adduction and full elevation especially painful)	Pain on active movement, especially of abduction
Passive movement	Pain on horizontal adduction and elevation Muscle spasm end feel at end of ROM possible	No pain except if impingement occurs
Resisted isometric movement	May have some pain if test causes stress on joint (e.g., abduction)	Pain on abduction May have some pain on stabilizing for other movements
Functional tests	Pain on extremes of movement	Pain on any abduction movement
Special tests	Acromioclavicular shear test painful	"Empty can" test positive Impingement tests positive
Reflexes and cutaneous distribution	Negative	Negative
Joint play	Acromioclavicular joint play movements painful	Negative
Palpation	Acromioclavicular joint painful	Supraspinatus tendon and insertion tender or painful

ROM, Range of motion.

REFERENCES

1. Hess SA: Functional stability of the glenohumeral joint. Manual Therapy 5:63–71, 2000.
2. Tillman B, Petersen W: Clinical anatomy. In Wulker N, Mansat M, Fu F, editors: Shoulder surgery: an illustrated textbook, London, 2001, Martin Dunitz.
3. Warner JJ: The gross anatomy of the joint surfaces, ligaments, labrum and capsule. In Matsen FA, Fu FH, Hawkins RJ, editors: The shoulder: a balance of mobility and stability, Rosemont, IL, 1993, American Academy of Orthopedic Surgeons.
4. Bigliani LU, Kelkar R, Flatow EL, et al: Glenohumeral stability: biomechanical properties of passive and active stabilizers. Clin Orthop Relat Res 330:13–30, 1996.
5. Curl LA, Warren RF: Glenohumeral joint stability: selective cutting studies on the static capsular restraints. Clin Orthop Relat Res 330:54–65, 1996.
6. Mihata T, McGarry MH, Abe M, et al: Excessive humeral external rotation results in increased shoulder laxity. Am J Sports Med 32:1278–1285, 2004.
7. Lucas DB: Biomechanics of the shoulder joint. Arch Surg 107:425–432, 1973.
8. Peat M: Functional anatomy of the shoulder complex. Phys Ther 66:1855–1865, 1986.
9. Hunt SA, Kwon YW, Zuckerman JD: The rotator interval—anatomy, pathology and strategies for treatment. J Am Acad Orthop Surg 15:218–227, 2007.
10. Peat M, Culham E: Functional anatomy of the shoulder complex. In Andrews JR, Wilk KE, editors: The athlete's shoulder, New York, 1994, Churchill-Livingstone.
11. Soslowsky LJ, An CH, DeBano CM, et al: Coracoacromial ligament: in situ load and viscoelastic properties in rotator cuff disease. Clin Orthop Relat Res 330:40–44, 1996.
12. Bigliani LH, Morrison DS, April EW: The morphology of the acromion and its relation to rotator cuff tears. Orthop Trans 10:228, 1986.

13. Edelson JG: The "hooked" acromion revisited. J Bone Joint Surg Br 77:284–287, 1995.
14. Fukuda K, Craig EV, An KN, et al: Biomechanical study of the ligamentous system of the acromioclavicular joint. J Bone Joint Surg 68:434–440, 1986.
15. Izadpanah K, Weitzel E, Honal M, et al: In vivo analysis of coracoclavicular ligament kinematics during shoulder abduction. Am J Sports Med 40:185–192, 2012.
16. Higginbotham TO, Kuhn JE: Atraumatic disorders of the sternoclavicular joint. J Am Acad Ortho Surg 13:138–145, 2005.
17. Kibler WB: The role of the scapula in athletic shoulder function. Am J Sports Med 26:325–337, 1998.
18. Maughon TS, Andrews JR: The subjective evaluation of the shoulder in the athlete. In Andrews JR, Wilk KE, editors: The athlete's shoulder, New York, 1994, Churchill-Livingstone.
19. Tarkin IS, Morganti CM, Zillrner DA, et al: Rotator cuff tears in adolescent athletes. Am J Sports Med 33:596–601, 2005.
20. Litaker D, Pioro M, El Bilbeisi H, et al: Returning to the bedside: using the history and physical examination to identify rotator cuff tears. J Am Geriatr Soc 48(12):1633–1637, 2000.
21. Kauffman J, Jobe FW: Anterior capsulolabral reconstruction for recurrent anterior instability. Sports Med Arthro Rev 8:272–279, 2000.
22. Wolf WB: Calcific tendinitis of the shoulder: diagnosis and simple effective treatment. Phys Sportsmed 27:27–33, 1999.
23. Hutchinson MR, Ahuja CO: Diagnosing and treating clavicle injuries. Phys Sportsmed 24:26–36, 1996.
24. Simovitch R, Sanders B, Ozbzydar M, et al: Acromioclavicular joint injuries: diagnosis and management. J Am Acad Orthop Surg 17:207–219, 2009.
25. Burkhart SS, Morgan CD, Kibler WB: The disabled throwing shoulder: spectrum of pathology, part

one: pathoanatomy and biomechanics. Arthroscopy 19:404–420, 2003.
26. Su KA, Johnson MP, Gracely EJ, et al: Scapular rotation in swimmers with and without impingement syndrome: practice effects. Med Sci Sports Exerc 31:1117–1123, 2004.
27. Kuhn JE: A new classification system for shoulder instability. Br J Sports Med 44:341–346, 2010.
28. Krupp RJ, Kevern MA, Gaines MD, et al: Long head of biceps tendon pain: differential diagnosis and treatment. J Orthop Sports Phys Ther 39:55–70, 2009.
29. Kibler WB, Sciascia A: Current concepts: scapular dyskinesis. Br J Sports Med 44:300–305, 2010.
30. Borsa PA, Laudner KG, Sauers EL: Mobility and stability adaptations in the shoulder of the overhead athlete—a theoretical and evidence-based perspective. Sports Med 38:17–36, 2008.
31. Burkhart SS, Morgan CD, Kibler WB: The disabled throwing shoulder: spectrum of pathology, part three: the SICK scapula, scapular dyskinesia, the kinetic chain, and rehabilitation. Arthroscopy 19:641–661, 2003.
32. Kvitne RS, Jobe FW: The diagnosis and treatment of anterior instability in the throwing athlete. Clin Orthop 291:107–123, 1993.
33. Watson LA, Pizzari T, Balster S: Thoracic outlet syndrome. Part 1: clinical manifestations, differentiation and treatment pathways. Manual Therapy 14:586–595, 2009.
34. Boyle JJ: Is the pain and dysfunction of shoulder impingement lesion really second rib syndrome in disguise? Two case reports. Manual Therapy 4:44–48, 1999.
35. Khan KM, Cook JL, Taunton JE, et al: Overuse tendinosis, not tendinitis. Part 1: a new paradigm for a difficult clinical problem. Phys Sportsmed 28:38–48, 2000.

36. Khan KM, Cook JL, Bonar F, et al: Histopathology of common tendinopathies: update and implications for clinical management. Sports Med 27:393–408, 1999.

37. Seroyer ST, Nho SJ, Bach BR, et al: Shoulder pain in the overhead throwing athlete. Sports Health 1:108–120, 2009.

38. McFarland EG, Tanaka MJ, Papp DF: Examination of the shoulder in the overhead and throwing athlete. Clin Sports Med 27:553–578, 2008.

39. Cyriax J: Textbook of orthopaedic medicine, vol 1: diagnosis of soft tissue lesions, London, 1982, Bailliere Tindall.

40. Griggs SM, Ahn A, Green A: Idiopathic adhesive capsulitis: a prospective functional outcome study of non-operative treatment. J Bone Joint Surg Am 82:1398–1407, 2000.

41. Butcher JD, Siekanowicz A, Pettrone F: Pectoralis major rupture: ensuring accurate diagnosis and effective rehabilitation. Phys Sportsmed 24:37–44, 1996.

42. Nichols HM: Anatomic structures of the thoracic outlet syndrome. Clin Orthop 51:17–25, 1967.

43. Riddell DH: Thoracic outlet syndrome: thoracic and vascular aspects. Clin Orthop 51:53–64, 1967.

44. Baker CL, Liu SH: Neurovascular injuries to the shoulder. J Orthop Sports Phys Ther 18:360–364, 1993.

45. Conte AL, Marques AP, Cararotto RA, Amado-Joâo SM: Handedness influences passive shoulder range of motion in non athlete adult women. J Manip Physiol Ther 32:149–153, 2009.

46. Dutton M: Orthopedic examination, evaluation and intervention, New York, 2004, McGraw-Hill.

47. Rudert M, Wulker M: Clinical evaluation. In Wulker N, Mansat M, Fu F, editors: Shoulder surgery: an illustrated textbook, London, 2001, Martin Dunitz.

48. Priest JD, Nagel DA: Tennis shoulder. Am J Sports Med 4:28–42, 1976.

49. Petilon J, Carr DR, Sekiya JK, et al: Pectoralis major muscle injuries: evaluation and management. J Am Acad Ortho Surg 13:59–68, 2005.

50. Mazzocca AD, Cote MP, Arciero CL, et al: Clinical outcomes after subpectoral biceps tendonosis with an interference screw. Am J Sports Med 36:1922–1929, 2008.

51. Provencher MT, Handfield K, Boniquit NT, et al: Injuries to the pectoralis major muscle—diagnosis and management. Am J Sports Med 38:1693–1705, 2010.

52. Hitchcock HH, Bechtol CO: Painful shoulder: observation on the role of the tendon of the long head of the biceps brachii in its causation. J Bone Joint Surg Am 30:263–273, 1948.

53. McFarland EG, Garzon-Muvdi J, Jia X, et al: Clinical and diagnostic tests for shoulder disorders: a critical review. Br J Sports Med 44:328–332, 2010.

54. Kibler WB, Sciascia A, Wilkes T: Scapular dyskinesia and its relation to shoulder injury. J Am Acad Orthop Surg 20:364–372, 2012.

55. Silliman JF, Dean MT: Neurovascular injuries to the shoulder complex. J Orthop Sports Phys Ther 18:442–448, 1993.

56. Sobush DC, Simoneau GG, Dietz KE, et al: The Lennie test for measuring scapular position in healthy young adult females: a reliability and validity study. J Orthop Sports Phys Ther 23:39–50, 1996.

57. Matsen FA, Lippitt SB, Sidles JA, et al: Practical evaluation and management of the shoulder, Philadelphia, 1994, WB Saunders.

58. Meister K: Injuries to the shoulder in the throwing athlete. Part II: evaluation/treatment. Am J Sports Med 28:587–601, 2000.

59. Milch H: Snapping scapula. Clin Orthop Relat Res 20:139–150, 1961.

60. Manske RC, Reiman MP, Stovak ML: Nonoperative and operative management of snapping scapula. Am J Sports Med 32:1554–1565, 2004.

61. Kibler WB: Scapular dyskinesis and its relation to shoulder pain. J Am Acad Ortho Surg 11:142–151, 2003.

62. Lazar MA, Kwon YW, Rokuti AS: Snapping scapula syndrome. J Bone Joint Surg Am 91:2251–2262, 2009.

63. Kibler WB, Uhl TL, Maddux JW, et al: Qualitative clinical evaluation of scapular dysfunction: a reliability study. J Shoulder Elbow Surg 11:550–556, 2002.

64. Uhl TL, Kibler WB, Gecewich B, et al: Evaluation of clinical assessment methods for scapular dyskinesia. Arthroscopy 25:1240–1248, 2009.

65. Meininger AK, Figuerres BF, Goldberg BA: Scapular winging: an update. J Am Acad Orthop Surg 19:453–462, 2011.

66. Butters KP: Nerve lesions of the shoulder. In De Lee, JC, Drez D, editors: Orthopedic sports medicine: principles and practice, Philadelphia, 1994, WB Saunders.

67. Schultz JS, Leonard JA: Long thoracic neuropathy from athletic activity. Arch Phys Med Rehabil 73:87–90, 1992.

68. Bowen M, Warren R: Ligamentous control of shoulder stability based on selective cutting and static translation. Clin Sports Med 10:757–782, 1991.

69. Duralde X: Surgical management of neurologic and vascular lesions in the athlete's shoulder. Sports Med Arthro Rev 8:289–304, 2000.

70. Foo CL, Swann M: Isolated paralysis of the serratus anterior: a report of 20 cases. J Bone Joint Surg Br 65:552–556, 1983.

71. Makin GJ, Brown WF, Webers GC: C7 radiculopathy: importance of scapular winging in clinical diagnosis. J Neurol Neurosurg Psych 49:640–644, 1986.

72. Saeed MA, Gatens PF, Singh S: Winging of the scapula. Am Fam Physician 24:139–143, 1981.

73. Fiddian NJ, King RJ: The winged scapula. Clin Orthop 185:228–236, 1984.

74. Carson WC, Lovell WW, Whitesides TE: Congenital elevation of the scapula. J Bone Joint Surg Am 63:1199–1207, 1981.

75. Cavendish ME: Congenital elevation of the scapula. J Bone Joint Surg Br 54:395–408, 1972.

76. McMurtry I, Bennet GC, Bradish C: Osteotomy for congenital elevation of the scapula (Sprengel's deformity). J Bone Joint Surg Br 87:986–989, 2005.

77. Harvey EJ, Bernstein M, Desy NM, et al: Sprengel deformity: pathogenesis and management. J Am Acad Orthop Surg 20(3):177–186, 2012.

78. Miyashita K, Kobayashi H, Koshida S, et al: Glenohumeral, scapular and thoracic angles at maximum shoulder external rotation in throwing. Am J Sports Med 38:363–368, 2010.

79. Payne LZ, Deng XH, Craig EV, et al: The combined dynamic and static contributions to subacromial impingement: a biomechanical analysis. Am J Sports Med 25:801–808, 1997.

80. Watson CJ, Schenkman M: Physical therapy management of isolated serratus anterior muscle paralysis. Phys Ther 75:194–202, 1995.

81. Kessel L, Watson M: The painful arc syndrome. J Bone Joint Surg Br 59:166–172, 1977.

82. Inman VT, Saunders M, Abbott LC: Observations on the function of the shoulder joint. J Bone Joint Surg Br 26:1–30, 1944.

83. Reid DC: The shoulder girdle: its function as a unit in abduction. Physiotherapy 55:57–59, 1969.

84. Saha SK: Mechanism of shoulder movements and a plea for the recognition of "zero position" of glenohumeral joint. Clin Orthop 173:3–10, 1983.

85. Sugamoto K, Harada T, Machida A, et al: Scapulohumeral rhythm: relationship between motion velocity and rhythm. Clin Orthop Relat Res 401:119–124, 2002.

86. Boody SG, Freedman L, Waterland JC: Shoulder movements during abduction in the scapular plane. Arch Phys Med Rehabil 51:595–604, 1970.

87. Davies GJ, Dickoff-Hoffman S: Neuromuscular testing and rehabilitation of the shoulder complex. J Orthop Sports Phys Ther 18:449–458, 1993.

88. Poppen NK, Walker PS: Normal and abnormal motion of the shoulder. J Bone Joint Surg Am 58:195–201, 1976.

89. Freedman L, Munro RR: Abduction of the arm in the scapular plane: scapular and glenohumeral movements. J Bone Joint Surg Am 48:1503–1510, 1966.

90. Flatow EL: The biomechanics of the acromioclavicular, sternoclavicular and scapulothoracic joints. Instr Course Lect 42:237–245, 1993.

91. Stanley E, Rauh MJ, Michener LA, et al: Shoulder range of motion measures as risk factors for shoulder and elbow injuries in high school softball and baseball players. Am J Sports Med 39:1997–2006, 2011.

92. Ludewig PM, Reynolds JF: The association of scapular kinematics and glenohumeral joint pathologies. J Orthop Sports Phys Ther 39:90–104, 2009.

93. van Eisenhart-Rothe R, Matsen FA, Eckstein F, et al: Pathomechanics in atraumatic shoulder instability. Clin Orthop Relat Res 433:82–89, 2005.

94. Kibler WB: Evaluation and diagnosis of scapulothoracic problems in the athlete. Sports Med Arthro Rev 8:192–202, 2000.

95. Michiels I, Grevenstein J: Kinematics of shoulder abduction in the scapular plane: on the influence of abduction velocity and external load. Clin Biomech 10:137–143, 1995.

96. Perry J: Biomechanics of the shoulder. In Rowe CR, editor: The shoulder, Edinburgh, 1988, Churchill Livingstone.

97. Kapandji IA: The physiology of joints, vol 1: upper limb, New York, 1970, Churchill Livingstone.

98. Wilk KE, Reinold MM, Macrina LC, et al: Glenohumeral internal rotation measurements differ depending on stabilization techniques. Sports Health 1:131–136, 2009.

99. Boublik M, Silliman JF: History and physical examination. In Hawkins RJ, Misamore GW, editors: Shoulder injuries in the athlete, New York, 1996, Churchill Livingstone.

100. Gates JJ, Gupta A, McGarry MH, et al: The effect of glenohumeral internal rotation deficit due to posterior capsular contracture on passive glenohumeral joint motion. Am J Sports Med 40:2794–2800, 2012.

101. Lo IK, Nonweiler B, Woolfrey M, et al: An evaluation of the apprehension, relocation, and surprise tests for anterior shoulder instability. Am J Sports Med 32(2):301–307, 2004.

102. Naredo E, Aguado P, De Miguel E, et al: Painful shoulder: comparison physical examination and ultrasonographic findings. Ann Rheum Dis 61:132–136, 2002.

103. Wilk KE, Macrina LC, Fleisig GS, et al: Correlation of glenohumeral internal rotation deficit and total rotational motion to shoulder injuries in professional baseball players. Am J Sports Med 39:329–335, 2011.

104. Jaggi A, Lambert S: Rehabilitation of shoulder instability. Br J Sports Med 44:333–340, 2010.

105. Magarey ME, Jones MA: Dynamic evaluation and early management of altered motor control around the shoulder complex. Manual Therapy 8:195–206, 2003.

106. Howell SM, Galiant BJ, Renzi AJ, et al: Normal and abnormal mechanics of the glenohumeral joint in the horizontal plane. J Bone Joint Surg Am 70:227–232, 1988.

107. Nishijima N, Yamamuro T, Fujio K, et al: The swallow-tail sign: a test for deltoid function. J Bone Joint Surg Br 77:152–153, 1994.

108. Kuhn JE, Plancher KD, Hawkins RJ: Scapular winging. J Am Acad Orthop Surg 3:319–325, 1995.

109. Petersen CM, Hayes KW: Construct validity of Cyriax's selective tension examination: association of end feels with pain in the knee and shoulder. J Orthop Sports Phys Ther 30:512–521, 2000.

110. Muraki T, Yamamoto N, Zhao KD, et al: Effect of posteroinferior capsular tightness on contact pressure and area beneath the coracoacromial arch during pitching motion. Am J Sports Med 38:600–607, 2010.

111. Laudner KG, Meline MT, Meister K: The relationship between forward scapular posture and posterior shoulder tightness among baseball players. Am J Sports Med 38:2106–2112, 2010.

112. Tyler TF, Roy T, Nicholas SJ, et al: Reliability and validity of a new method of measuring posterior shoulder tightness. J Orthop Sports Phys Ther 29:262–274, 1999.

113. Tyler TF, Nicholas SJ, Roy T, et al: Quantification of posterior capsule tightness and motion loss in patients with shoulder impingement. Am J Sports Med 28:668–673, 2000.

114. Lunden JB, Muffenbier M, Giveans MR, et al: Reliability of shoulder internal rotation passive range of motion measurements in the supine vs sidelying position. J Orthop Sports Phys Ther 40:589–594, 2010.

115. Pagnani MJ, Galinat BJ, Warren RF: Glenohumeral instability. In De Lee JC, Drez D, editors: Orthopedic sports medicine: principles and practice, Philadelphia, 1994, WB Saunders.

116. Gagey OJ, Gagey N: The hyperabduction test: an assessment of the laxity of the inferior glenohumeral ligament. J Bone Joint Surg Br 83:69–73, 2001.

117. Cadet ER: Evaluation of glenohumeral instability. Orthop Clin North Am 41:287–295, 2010.

118. Rowe CR: Unusual shoulder conditions. In Rowe CR, editor: The shoulder, Edinburgh, 1988, Churchill Livingstone.

119. MacConaill MA, Basmajian JV: Muscles and movements: a basis for human kinesiology, Baltimore, 1969, Williams & Wilkins.

120. Corrigan B, Maitland GD: Practical orthopedic medicine, London, 1985, Butterworths.

121. Maitland GD: Peripheral manipulation, London, 1977, Butterworths.

122. Mullen F, Slade S, Briggs C: Bony and capsular determinants of glenohumeral "locking" and "quadrant" positions. Aust J Physio 35:202–206, 1989.

123. Richards RR: Outcomes analysis in the shoulder and elbow. In Norris TR, editor: Orthopedic knowledge update: shoulder and elbow, Rosemont, IL, 2002, American Academy of Orthopedic Surgeons.

124. Mannerkorpi K, Svantesson U, Carlsson J, et al: Tests of functional limitations in fibromyalgia syndrome: A reliability study. Arthr Care Res 12(3):193–199, 1999.

125. Dutton M: Dutton's orthopedic examination, evaluation and intervention, ed 3, New York, 2012, McGraw-Hill.

126. Namdari S, Yagnik G, Ebaugh DD, et al: Defining functional shoulder range of motion for activities of daily living. J Shoulder Elbow Surg 21:1177–1183, 2012.

127. Wright RW, Gaumgarten KM: Shoulder outcome measures. J Am Acad Orthop Surg 18:436–444, 2010.

128. Ellenbecker TS, Manske R, Davies GJ: Closed kinetic chain testing techniques of the upper extremities. Orthop Phys Ther Clin North Am 9:219–229, 2000.

129. Brophy RH, Beauvais RL, Jones EC, et al: Measurement of shoulder activity level. Clin Orthop Relat Res 439:101–108, 2005.

130. Roy JS, MacDermid JC, Woodhouse LJ: Measuring shoulder function: a systematic review of four questionnaires. Arthritis Rheum 61(5):623–632, 2009.

131. Roach KE, Budiman-Mak E, Songsiridej N, et al: Development of a shoulder pain and disability index. Arthritis Care Res 4(4):143–149, 1991.

132. Breckenridge JD, McAuley JH: Shoulder pain and disability index (SPADI). J Physiotherapy 57(3):197, 2011.

133. Williams JW, Holleman DR, Simel DL: Measuring shoulder function with the shoulder pain and disability index. J Rheumatol 22(4):727–732, 1995.

134. Heald SL, Riddle DL, Lamb RL: The shoulder pain and disability index: the construct validity and responsiveness of a region-specific disability measure. Phys Ther 77:1079–1089, 1997.

135. Ellman H, Hanker G, Bayer M: Repair of the rotator cuff: end result study of factors influencing reconstruction. J Bone Joint Surg Am 68:1136–1144, 1986.

136. Patte D: Directions for the use of the index of severity for painful and/or chronically disabled shoulder. In Abstracts from First Open Congress, European Society of Surgery of the Shoulder and Elbow, Paris, France, 1987, pp 36–41.

137. Rowe CR, Patel D, Southmayd WW: Bankart procedure: a long term end result study. J Bone Joint Surg Am 60:1–6, 1978.

138. Macdonald DA: The shoulder and elbow. In Pynsent PB, Fairbank JC, Carr A, editors: Outcome measures in orthopedics, appendices 8-1 through 8-7, Oxford, 1993, Butterworth-Heinemann.

139. Constant CR, Murley AHG: A clinical method of functional assessment of the shoulder. Clin Orthop 214:160–164, 1987.

140. Williams GH, Gangel TJ, Arciero RA, et al: Comparison of the single assessment numeric evaluation method and two shoulder rating scales: outcome measures after shoulder surgery. Am J Sports Med 27:214–221, 1999.

141. Richards RR, An KN, Bagliani LU, et al: A standardized method for the assessment of shoulder function. J Shoulder Elbow Surg 3:347–352, 1994.

142. L'Insalata JC, Warren RF, Cohen SB, et al: A self-administered questionnaire for assessment of symptoms and function of the shoulder. J Bone Joint Surg Am 79:738–748, 1997.

143. Leggin BG, Iannotti JP: Shoulder outcome measurement. In Iannotti JP, Williams CR, editors: Disorders of the shoulder, Philadelphia, 1999, Lippincott Williams & Wilkins.

144. Kirkley A, Alverez C, Griffin S: The development and evaluation of a disease-specific quality-of-life questionnaire for disorders of the rotator cuff: the Western Ontario Rotator Cuff Index. Clin J Sports Med 13:84–92, 2003.

145. Lopes AD, Ciconelli R, Carrera EF, et al: Validity and reliability of the Western Ontario Rotator Cuff Index (WORC) for use in Brazil. Clin J Sports Med 18:226–272, 2008.

146. Alberta FG, El Attrache NS, Bissell S, et al: The development and validcation of a functional assessment tool for the upper extremity in the overhead athlete. Am J Sports Med 38:903–911, 2010.

147. Romeo AA, Bach BR, O'Halloran KL: Scoring systems for shoulder conditions. Am J Sports Med 24:472–476, 1996.

148. Placzek JD, Lukens SC, Badalamenti S, et al: Shoulder outcome measures: a comparison of six functional tests. Am J Sports Med 32:1270–1277, 2004.

149. Lippitt SB, Harryman DT, Matsen FA: A practical tool for evaluating function: the simple shoulder test. In Matsen FA, Fu FH, Hawkins RJ, editors: The shoulder: a balance of mobility and stability, Rosemont, IL, 1993, American Academy of Orthopedic Surgeons.

150. Roy JS, Macdermid JC, Faber KJ, et al: The simple shoulder test is responsive in assessing change following shoulder arthroplasty. J Orthop Sports Phys Ther 40:143–421, 2010.

151. Hudak PL, Amadio PC, Bombardier C: Development of an upper extremity outcome measure: the DASH (disabilities of the arm, shoulder and hand) [corrected]: The Upper Extremity Collaborative Group (UECG). Am J Ind Med 29(6):602–608, 1996.

152. Beaton DE, Wright JG, Katz JN: Upper extremity collaborative group. Development of the Quick DASH: comparison of three item reduction approaches. J Bone Joint Surg Am 87:1038–1046, 2005.

153. Leggin BG, Iannotti JP: Shoulder outcome measurement. In Iannotti JP, Williams GR, editors: Disorders of the shoulder: diagnosis and management, Philadelphia, Lippincott, 1999, Williams & Wilkins.

154. Leggin BG, Michener LA, Shaffer MA, et al: The Penn shoulder score: reliability and validity. J Orthop Sports Phys Ther 36:138–151, 2006.

155. Falsone SA, Gross MT, Guskiewicz KM, et al: One-arm hop test: reliability and effects of arm dominance. J Orthop Sports Phys Ther 32:98–103, 2002.

156. Abrams GD, Safran MR: Diagnosis and management of superior labrum anterior osterior lesions in overhead athletes. Br J Sports Med 44:311–318, 2010.

157. Hegedus EJ, Goode A, Campbell S, et al: Physical examination tests of the shoulder: a systematic review with meta-analysis of individual tests. Br J Sports Med 42:80–92, 2008.

158. Levy AS, Lintner S, Kenter K, et al: Intra- and interobserver reproducibility of the shoulder laxity examination. Am J Sports Med 27:460–463, 1999.

159. Parentis MA, Glousman RE, Mohr KS, et al: An evaluation of the provocative tests for superior labral anterior posterior lesions. Am J Sports Med 34:265–268, 2006.

160. Dessaur WA, Magarey ME: Diagnostic accuracy of clinical tests for superior labral anterior posterior lesions: a systemic review. J Orthop Sports Phys Ther 38:341–352, 2008.

161. Meserve BB, Cleland JA, Boucher TR: A meta-analysis examining clinical test utility for assessing superior labral anterior posterior lesions. Am J Sports Med 37:2252–2258, 2009.

162. Munro W, Healy R: The validity and accuracy of clinical tests used to detect labral pathology of the shoulder—a systematic review. Manual Therapy 14:119–130, 2009.

163. Knesek M, Skendzel JG, Dines JS, et al: Diagnosis and management of superior labral anterior posterior tears in throwing athletes. Am J Sports Med 41:444–460, 2013.

164. Cook C, Beaty S, Kissenberth MJ, et al: Diagnostic accuracy of five orthopedic clinical tests for diagnosis of superior labrum anterior posterior (SLAP) lesions. J Shoulder Elbow Surg 21:13–22, 2012.

165. McFarland EG, Kim TK, Savino RM: Clinical assessment of three common tests for superior labral anterior-posterior lesions. Am J Sports Med 30(6): 810–815, 2002.

166. Cleeman E, Flatow EL: Classification and diagnosis of impingement and rotator cuff lesions in athletes. Sports Med Arthro Rev 8:141–157, 2000.

167. Brown GA, Tan JL, Kirkley A: The lax shoulders in females. Clin Orthop Relat Res 372:110–122, 2000.

168. McClusky CM: Classification and diagnosis of glenohumeral instability in athletes. Sports Med Arthro Rev 8:158–169, 2000.

169. Jobe FW, Kvitne RS: Shoulder pain in the overhand or throwing athlete: the relationship of anterior instability and rotator cuff impingement. Orthop Rev 18:963–975, 1989.

170. Walch G, Boileau P, Noel E, et al: Impingement of the deep surface of the supraspinatus tendon on the posterosuperior glenoid rim: an arthroscopic study. J Shoulder Elbow Surg 1:238–245, 1992.

171. Jobe CM: Posterior superior glenoid impingement: expanded spectrum. Arthroscopy J Arthro Relat Surg 11:530–536, 1995.

172. Davidson PA, Elattrache NS, Jobe CM, et al: Rotator cuff and posterosuperior glenoid labrum injury associated with increased glenohumeral motion: a new site of impingement. J Shoulder Elbow Surg 4:384–390, 1995.

173. Jobe CM: Evidence for a superior glenoid impingement upon the rotator cuff. J Shoulder Elbow Surg 2:319, 1993.

174. Jobe CM: Superior glenoid impingement. Orthop Clin North Am 28:137–143, 1997.

175. Silliman JF, Hawkins RJ: Classification and physical diagnosis of instability of the shoulder. Clin Orthop 291:7–19, 1993.

176. Owens BD, Nelson BJ, Duffey ML, et al: Pathoanatomy of first time, traumatic anterior glenohumeral subluxation events. J Bone Joint Surg 92:1605–1611, 2010.

177. Andrews JA, Timmerman LA, Wilk KE: Baseball. In Pettrone FA, editor: Athletic injuries of the shoulder, New York, 1995, McGraw-Hill.

178. Gerber C, Ganz R: Clinical assessment of instability of the shoulder. J Bone Joint Surg Br 66:551–556, 1984.

179. Leffert RD, Gumley G: The relationship between dead arm syndrome and thoracic outlet syndrome. Clin Orthop 223:20–31, 1987.

180. Matsen FA, Thomas SC, Rockwood CA: Glenohumeral instability. In Rockwood CA, Matsen FA, editors: The shoulder, Philadelphia, 1990, WB Saunders.

181. Hamner DL, Pink MM, Jobe FW: A modification of the relocation test: arthroscopic findings associated with a positive test. J Shoulder Elbow Surg 9:263–267, 2000.

182. Harryman DT, Sidles JA, Harris SL, et al: Laxity of the normal glenohumeral joint: a quantitative in vivo assessment. J Shoulder Elbow Surg 1:66–76, 1992.

183. Hawkins RJ, Bokor DJ: Clinical evaluation of shoulder problems. In Rockwood CA, Matsen FA, editors: The shoulder, Philadelphia, 1990, WB Saunders.

184. Hawkins RJ, Mohtadi NG: Clinical evaluation of shoulder instability. Clin J Sports Med 1:59–64, 1991.

185. Luime JJ, Verhagen AP, Miedema HS, et al: Does this patient have instability of the shoulder or a labrum lesion? JAMA 292:1989–1999, 2004.

186. Burkhart SS, Morgan CD, Kibler WB: The disabled throwing shoulder: spectrum of pathology, part two: evaluation and treatment of SLAP lesions in throwers. Arthroscopy 19:531–539, 2003.

187. Speer KP, Hannafin JA, Alteck DW, et al: An evaluation of the shoulder relocation test. Am J Sports Med 22:177–183, 1994.

188. Davidson PA, Elattrache NS, Jobe CM, et al: Rotator cuff and posterior-superior glenoid labrum injury associated with increased glenohumeral motion: a new site of impingement. J Shoulder Elbow Surg 4:384–390, 1995.

189. Gross ML, Distefano MC: Anterior release test: a new test for occult shoulder instability. Clin Orthop Relat Res 339:105–108, 1997.

190. Kelley MJ: Evaluation of the shoulder. In Kelley MJ, Clark WA, editors: Orthopedic therapy of the shoulder, Philadelphia, 1995, JB Lippincott.

191. Matthews LS, Pavlovich LJ: Anterior and anteroinferior instability: diagnosis and management. In Iannotti JP, Williams CR, editors: Disorders of the shoulder, Philadelphia, 1999, Lippincott Williams & Wilkins.

192. Evans RC: Illustrated essentials in orthopedic physical assessment, St Louis, 1994, Mosby Year Book.

193. Solem-Bertoft E, Thomas KA, Westerberg CE: The influence of scapular retraction and protraction on the width of the subacromial space. Clin Orthop Relat Res 296:99–103, 1993.

194. Borsa PA, Sauers EL, Herling DE: Patterns of glenohumeral joint laxity and stiffness in healthy men and women. Med Sci Sports Exerc 32:1685–1690, 2000.

195. Sauers EL, Borsa PA, Herling DE, et al: Instrumented measurement of glenohumeral joint laxity and its relationship to passive range of motion and generalized joint laxity. Am J Sports Med 29:143–150, 2001.

196. Sauers EL, Borsa PA, Herling DE, et al: Instrumental measurement of glenohumeral joint laxity: reliability and normative data. Knee Surg Sports Traumatol Arthros 9:34–41, 2001.

197. Ellenbecker TS, Maltalino AJ, Elam E, et al: Quantification of anterior translation of the humeral head in the throwing shoulder: manual assessment vs. stress radiography. Am J Sports Med 28:161–167, 2000.

198. Lintner SA, Levy A, Kenter K, et al: Glenohumeral translation in the asymptomatic athlete's shoulder and its relationship to other clinically measureable anthropometric variables. Am J Sports Med 24:716–720, 1996.

199. Altchek DA, Warren RF, Skyhar MJ, et al: T-plasty: a technique for treating multidirectional instability in the athlete. J Bone Joint Surg Am 73:105–112, 1991.

200. Ramsey ML, Klimkiewicz JJ: Posterior instability: diagnosis and management. In Iannotti JP, Williams CR, editors: Disorders of the shoulder, Philadelphia, 1999, Lippincott Williams & Wilkins.

201. Protzman RR: Anterior instability of the shoulder. J Bone Joint Surg Am 62:909–918, 1980.

202. Davies GJ, Gould JA, Larson RL: Functional examination of the shoulder girdle. Phys Sports Med 9:82–104, 1981.

203. Rockwood CA: Subluxations and dislocations about the shoulder. In Rockwood CA, Green DP, editors: Fractures in adults, Philadelphia, 1984, JB Lippincott.

204. Rowe CR: Dislocations of the shoulder. In Rowe CR, editor: The shoulder, Edinburgh, 1988, Churchill Livingstone.

205. Provencher MT, LeClere LE, King S, et al: Posterior instability of the shoulder—diagnosis and management. Am J Sports Med 39:874–886, 2011.

206. Arcand MA, Reider B: Shoulder and upper arm. In Reider B, editor: The orthopedic physical examination, Philadelphia, 1999, WB Saunders.

207. Kim SH, Park JS, Jeong WK, et al: The Kim test: a novel test for posteroinferior labral lesion of the shoulder—a comparison to the jerk test. Am J Sports Med 33:1188–1191, 2005.

208. Kim SH, Park JC, Park JS, et al: Painful jerk test: a predictor of success in nonoperative treatment of posteroinferior instability of the shoulder. Am J Sports Med 32:1849–1855, 2004.

209. Miniaci A, Salonen D: Rotator cuff evaluation: imaging and diagnosis. Orthop Clin North Am 28:43–58, 1997.

210. Norwood LA, Terry GC: Shoulder posterior and subluxation. Am J Sports Med 12:25–30, 1984.

211. Cofield RH, Irving JF: Evaluation and classification of shoulder instability. Clin Orthop 223:32–43, 1987.

212. Pollack RG, Bigliani LU: Recurrent posterior shoulder instability: diagnosis and treatment. Clin Orthop 291:85–96, 1993.

213. Pagnani MJ, Warren RF: Multidirectional instability in the athlete. In Pettrone FA, editor: Athletic injuries of the shoulder, New York, 1995, McGraw-Hill.

214. McFarland EG, Campbell C, McDowell J: Posterior shoulder laxity in asymptomatic athletes. Am J Sports Med 24:468–471, 1996.

215. Schenk TJ, Brems JJ: Multidirectional instability of the shoulder: pathophysiology, diagnosis and management. J Am Acad Orthop Surg 6:65–72, 1998.

216. McClusky GM: Classification and diagnosis of glenohumeral instability in athletes. Sports Med Artho Rev 8:158–169, 2000.

217. Gaskill TR, Taylor DC, Millett PJ: Management of multidirectional instability of the shoulder. J Am Acad Orthop Surg 19:758–767, 2011.

218. Bigliani LU, Codd TP, Conner PM, et al: Shoulder motion and laxity in the professional baseball player. Am J Sports Med 25:609–613, 1997.

219. Helmig P, Sojbjerg J, Kjaersgaard-Andersen P, et al: Distal humeral migration as a component of multidirectional shoulder instability. Clin Orthop 252:139–143, 1990.

220. Cleeman E, Flatow EL: Classification and diagnosis of impingement and rotator cuff lesions in athletes. Sports Med Arthro Rev 8:141–157, 2000.

221. Ferrick MR: Coracoid impingement: a case report and review of the literature. Am J Sports Med 28:117–119, 2000.

222. Lukasiewicz AC, McClure P, Michner L, et al: Comparison of 3-dimensional scapular position and orientation between subjects with and without shoulder impingement. J Orthop Sports Phys Ther 29:574–586, 1999.

223. Bigliani LU, Levine WN: Subacromial impingement syndrome. J Bone Joint Surg Am 79:1854–1868, 1997.

224. Harrison AK, Flatow EL: Subacromial impingement syndrome. J Am Acad Orthop Surg 19:701–708, 2011.

225. Ludewig PM, Braman JP: Shoulder impingement: biomechanical considerations in rehabilitation. Manual Therapy 16:33–39, 2011.

226. Park HB, Yokota A, Gill HS, et al: Diagnostic accuracy of clinical tests for the different degrees of subacromial impingement syndrome. J Bone Joint Surg Am 87:1446–1455, 2005.

227. Hawkins RJ, Kennedy JC: Impingement syndrome in athletics. Am J Sports Med 8:151–163, 1980.

228. Brossmann J, Preidler KW, Pedowitz KA, et al: Shoulder impingement syndrome: Influence of shoulder position on rotator cuff impingement: an anatomic study. Am J Roentgenol 167:1511–1515, 1996.

229. Valadic AL, Jobe CM, Pink MM, et al: Anatomy of provocative tests for impingement syndrome of the shoulder. J Shoulder Elbow Surg 9:36–46, 2000.

230. Gerber C, Terrier F, Ganz R: The role of the coracoid process in the chronic impingement syndrome. J Bone Joint Surg Br 67:703–708, 1985.

231. Tucker S, Taylor NF, Green RA: Anatomical validity of the Hawkins-Kennedy test—a pilot study. Manual Therapy 16:399–402, 2011.

232. McFarland EG, Selhi HS, Keyurapan E: Clinical evaluation of impingement: what to do and what works. J Bone Joint Surg Am 88:432–441, 2006.

233. Leroux JL, Thomas E, Bonnel F, et al: Diagnostic value of clinical tests for shoulder impingement. Rev Rheum 62:423–428, 1995.

234. Miniaci A, Dowdy PA: Rotator cuff disorders. In Hawkins RJ, Misamore GW, editors: Shoulder injuries in the athlete, New York, 1996, Churchill Livingstone.

235. Branch TP, Lawton RL, Jobst CA, et al: The role of glenohumeral capsular ligaments in internal and external rotation of the humerus. Am J Sports Med 23:632–637, 1995.

236. Zaslav KR: Internal rotation resistance strength tests: a new diagnostic test to differentiate intra-articular pathology from outlet (Neer) impingement syndrome in the shoulder. J Shoulder Elbow Surg 10:23–27, 2001.

237. Neer CS, Welsh RP: The shoulder in sports. Orthop Clin North Am 8:583–591, 1977.

238. Buchberger DJ: Introduction of a new physical examination procedure for the differentiation of acromioclavicular joint lesions and subacromial impingement. J Manip Physio Ther 22:316–321, 1999.

239. Jobe CM: Posterior superior glenoid impingement: expanded spectrum. Arthroscopy 11:530–536, 1995.

240. Jobe CM: Superior glenoid impingement. Clin Orthop Relat Res 330:98–107, 1996.

241. Giombini A, Rossi F, Pettrone FA, et al: Posterosuperior glenoid rim impingement as a cause of shoulder pain in top level waterpolo players. J Sports Med Phys Fit 37:273–278, 1997.

242. Mihata T, McGarry MH, Kinoshita M, et al: Excessive glenohumeral horizontal abduction as occurs during late cocking phase of the throwing motion can be critical for internal impingement. Am J Sports Med 38:369–374, 2010.

243. Heyworth BE, Williams RJ: Internal impingement of the shoulder. Am J Sports Med 37:1024–1037, 2009.

244. Castagna A, Garofalo R, Cesari E, et al: Posterior superior internal impingement: an evidence-based review. Br J Sports Med 44:382–388, 2009.

245. Corso G: Impingement relief test: an adjunctive procedure to traditional assessment of shoulder impingement syndrome. J Orthop Sports Phys Ther 22:183–192, 1995.

246. Moen MH, de Vos RJ, Ellenbecker TS, et al: Clinical tests in shoulder examination: how to perform them. Br J Sports Med 44:370–375, 2010.

247. Reeves B: Experiments on the tensile strength of the anterior capsular structures of the shoulder in man. J Bone Joint Surg Br 50:858–865, 1968.

248. Mileski RA, Snyder SJ: Superior labral lesions of the shoulder: pathoanatomy and surgical management. J Am Acad Orthop Surg 6:121–131, 1998.

249. Richards DB: Injuries to the glenoid labrum: a diagnostic and treatment challenge. Phys Sportsmed 22:73–85, 1999.

250. Huijbregts PA: SLAP lesions: structure, function and physical therapy diagnosis and treatment. J Man Manip Ther 9:71–83, 2001.

251. Pappas AM, Goss TP, Kleinman PK: Symptomatic shoulder instability due to lesions of the glenoid labrum. Am J Sports Med 11:279–288, 1983.

252. Myers TH, Zemanovic JR, Andrews JR: The resisted supination external rotation test: a new test for the diagnosis of superior labral anterior posterior lesions, Am J Sports Med 33:1315–1320, 2005.

253. Grossman MG, Tibone JE, McGarry MH, et al: A cadaveric model of the throwing shoulder: a possible etiology of superior labrum anterior-to-posterior lesions. J Bone Joint Surg Am 87:824–831, 2005.

254. Snyder SJ, Karzel RP, Del Pizzo W, et al: SLAP lesions of the shoulder. Arthroscopy 6:274–279, 1990.

255. Burkhart SS, Morgan CD: The peel-back mechanism—its role in producing and extending posterior type II SLAP lesions and its effect on SLAP repair rehabilitation. Arthroscopy 14:637–640, 1998.

256. Morgan CD, Burkhart SS, Palmari M, et al: Type II SLAP lesions: three subtypes and their relationships to superior instability and rotator cuff tears. Arthroscopy 14:553–565, 1998.

257. Braun S, Kokmeyer D, Millett PJ: Shoulder injuries in the throwing athlete. J Bone Joint Surg Am 91:966–978, 2009.

258. Keener JD, Brophy RH: Superior labral tears of the shoulder: pathogenesis, evaluation and treatment. J Am Acad Orthop Surg 17:627–637, 2009.

259. O'Brien SJ, Pagnoni MJ, Fealy S, et al: The active compression test: a new and effective test for diagnosing labral tears and acromioclavicular joint abnormality. Am J Sports Med 26:610–613, 1998.

260. Kibler WB, Sciascia AD, Hester P, et al: Clinical utility of traditional and new tests in the diagnosis of biceps tendon injuries and superior labrum anterior and posterior lesions in the shoulder. Am J Sports Med 37:1840–1847, 2009.

261. Pandya NK, Colton A, Webner D, et al: Physical examination and magnetic resonance imaging in the diagnosis of superior labrum anterior-posterior lesions of the shoulder: a sensitivity analysis. Arthroscopy 24:311–317, 2008.

262. Cadogan A, Laslett M, Hing W, et al: Interexaminer reliability of orthopedic special tests used in the assessment of shoulder pain. Manual Therapy 16:131–135, 2011.

263. Kibler WB: Clinical examination of the shoulder. In Pettrone FA, editor: Athletic injuries of the shoulder, New York, 1995, McGraw-Hill.

264. Kibler WB: Specificity and sensitivity of the anterior slide test in throwing athletes with superior glenoid labral tears. Arthroscopy 11:296–300, 1995.

265. Kim SH, Ha KI, Han KY: Biceps load test: a clinical test for superior labrum anterior and posterior lesions in shoulder with recurrent anterior dislocations. Am J Sports Med 27:300–303, 1999.

266. Wilk KE, Reinold MM, Dugas JR, et al: Current concepts in the recognition and treatment of superior labral (SLAP) lesions. J Orthop Sports Phys Ther 35:273–291, 2005.

267. Andrews JR, Gillogly S: Physical examination of the shoulder in throwing athletes. In Zarins B, Andrews JR, Carson WG, editors: Injuries to the throwing arm, Philadelphia, 1985, WB Saunders.

268. Walsh DA: Shoulder evaluation of the throwing athlete. Sports Med Update 4:24–27, 1989.

269. Guidi EJ, Suckerman JD: Glenoid labral lesions. In Andrews JR, Wilk KE, editors: The athlete's shoulder, New York, 1994, Churchill Livingstone.

270. Oh JH, Kim JY, Kim WS, et al: The evaluation of various physical examinations for the diagnosis of type II superior labrum anterior and posterior lesions. Am J Sports Med 36:353–359, 2008.

271. Cook C, Beaty S, Kissenberth MJ, et al: Diagnostic accuracy of five orthopedic clinical tests for diagnosis of superior labrum anterior posterior (SLAP) lesions. J Shoulder Elbow Surg 21:13–22, 2012.

272. Manske R, Prohaskab D: Superior labrum anterior and posterior (SLAP) rehabilitation in the overhead athlete. Physical Therapy in Sport 30:1–12, 2010.

273. Nakagawa S, Yoneda M, Hayashida K, et al: Forced shoulder abduction and elbow flexion test: a new simple clinical test to detect superior labral injury in the throwing shoulder. Arthroscopy 21:1290–1295, 2005.

274. Liu SH, Henry MH, Nuccion SL: A prospective evaluation of a new physical examination in predicting glenoid labral tears. Am J Sports Med 24:721–725, 1996.

275. Mimori K, Muneta T, Nakagawa T, et al: A new pain provocation test for superior labral tears of the shoulder. Am J Sports Med 27:137–142, 1999.

276. Kim YS, Kim JM, Ha KY, et al: The passive compression test—a new clinical test for superior labral tears of the shoulder. Am J Sports Med 35:1489–1494, 2007.

277. Schlechter JA, Summa S, Rubin BD: The passive distraction test: a new diagnostic aid for clinically significant superior labral pathology. Arthroscopy 25:1374–1379, 2009.

278. Berg EE, Ciullo JV: A clinical test for superior glenoid labral or "SLAP" lesions. Clin J Sports Med 8:121–123, 1998.

279. Kibler WB: Role of the scapula in the overhead throwing motion. Contemp Orthop 22:525–533, 1991.

280. Odom CJ, Taylor AB, Hurd CE, et al: Measurement of scapular asymmetry and assessment of shoulder dysfunction using the lateral scapular slide test: a reliability and validity study. Phys Ther 81:799–809, 2001.

281. Kibler WB: The role of the scapula in athletic shoulder function. Am J Sports Med 26:325–337, 1998.

282. Burkhart SS, Morgan CD, Kibler WB: Shoulder injuries in overhead athletes: the "dead arm" revisited. Clin Sports Med 19:125–158, 2000.

283. Seitz AL, McClure PW, Lynch SS, et al: Effects of scapular dyskinesis and scapular assistance test on subacromial space during static arm elevation. J Shoulder Elbow Surg 21:631–640, 2012.

284. Goldbeck TG, Davies GJ: Test-retest reliability of the closed kinetic chain–upper extremity stability test: a clinical field test. J Sports Rehab 9:35–43, 2000.

285. Scheibel M, Droschel S, Gerhardt C, et al: Arthroscopically assisted stabilization of acute high-grade acromioclavicular joint separations. Am J Sports Med 39:1507–1516, 2011.

286. Axe MJ: Acromioclavicular joint injuries in the athlete. Sports Med Arthro Rev 8:182–191, 2000.

287. Clark HD, McCann PD: Acromioclavicular joint injuries. Orthop Clin North Am 31:177–187, 2000.

288. Shaffer BS: Painful conditions of the acromioclavicular joint. J Am Acad Orthop Surg 7:176–188, 1999.

289. Petersen SA: Arthritis and arthroplasty. In Hawkins RJ, Misamore GW, editors: Shoulder injuries in the athlete, New York, 1996, Churchill Livingstone.

290. Ellman H, Harris E, Kay SP: Early degenerative joint disease simulating impingement syndrome: Arthroscopic findings. Arthroscopy 8:482–487, 1992.

291. Walton J, Mahajan S, Paxinos A, et al: Diagnostic values of tests for acromioclavicular joint pain. J Bone Joint Surg Am 86:807–812, 2004.

292. Blasier RB, Guldberg RE, Rothman ED: Anterior shoulder stability: contributions of rotator cuff forces and the capsular ligaments in a cadaver model. J Shoulder Elbow Surg 1:140–150, 1992.

293. Turkel SJ, Panio MW, Marshall JL, et al: Stabilizing mechanisms preventing anterior dislocation of the glenohumeral joint. J Bone Joint Surg Am 63: 1208–1217, 1981.

294. Gerber C, Krushell RJ: Isolated ruptures of the tendon of the subscapularis muscle. J Bone Joint Surg Br 73:389–394, 1991.

295. Lyons RP, Green A: Subscapularis tendon tears. J Am Acad Ortho Surg 13:353–363, 2005.

296. Williams GR: Complications of rotator cuff surgery. In Iannotti JP, Williams CR, editors: Disorders of the shoulder, Philadelphia, 1999, Lippincott Williams & Wilkins.

297. Tokish JM, Decker MJ, Ellis HB, et al: The belly-press test for the physical examination of the subscapularis muscle: electrodiagnostic validation and comparison to the lift-off test. J Shoulder Elbow Surg 12:427–430, 2003.

298. Pennock AT, Pennington WW, Torry MR, et al: The influence of arm and shoulder position on the bear-hug, belly-press and lift-off tests. Am J Sports Med 39:2338–2346, 2011.

299. Barth JR, Burkhart SS, DeBeer JF: The bear-hug test: a new and sensitive test for diagnosing a subscapularis tear. Arthroscopy 22:1076–1084, 2006.

300. Clarkson HM: Musculoskeletal assessment: joint range of motion and manual muscle strength, ed 3, Philadelphia, 2013, Lippincott Williams & Wilkins.

301. Moseley HF: Disorders of the shoulder. Clin Symp 12:1–30, 1960.

302. Walch G, Boulahia A, Calderone S, et al: The "dropping" and "hornblower's" signs in evaluating rotator cuff tears. J Bone Joint Surg Br 80:624–628, 1998.

303. Post M: Physical examination of the musculoskeletal system, Chicago, 1987, Year Book Medical.

304. Arroyo JS, Flatow EL: Management of rotator cuff disease: intact and repairable cuff. In Iannotti JP, Williams GR, editors: Disorders of the shoulder, Philadelphia, 1999, Lippincott Williams & Wilkins.

305. Pearl MD, Wong KA: Shoulder kinematics and kinesiology. In Norris TR, editor: Orthopedic knowledge update: shoulder and elbow, Rosemont, IL, 2002, American Academy of Orthopedic Surgeons.

306. Hertel R, Ballmer FT, Lambert SM, et al: Lag signs in the diagnosis of rotator cuff rupture. J Shoulder Elbow Surg 5:307–313, 1996.

307. Greis PE, Kuhn JE, Schultheis J, et al: Validation of the lift-off sign test and analysis of subscapularis activity during maximal internal rotation. Am J Sports Med 24:589–593, 1996.

308. Cordasco FA, Bigliani LU: Large and massive tears: technique of open repair. Orthop Clin North Am 28:179–193, 1997.

309. Kelly BT, Kadrmas WR, Speer KP: The manual muscle examination for rotator cuff strength: an electromyographic investigation. Am J Sports Med 24:581–588, 1996.

310. Ticker JB, Warner JJ: Single-tendon tears of the rotator cuff: evaluation and treatment of subscapularis tears. Orthop Clin North Am 28:99–116, 1997.

311. Greis PE, Kuhn JE, Schultheis J, et al: Validation of the lift-off test and analysis of subscapularis activity during maximal internal rotation. Am J Sports Med 24:589–593, 1996.

312. Stefko JM, Jobe FW, Vanderwilde RS, et al: Electromyographic and nerve block analysis of the subscapularis lift off test. J Shoulder Elbow Surg 6:347–355, 1997.

313. Lippman RK: Frozen shoulder: periarthritis, bicipital tendinitis. Arch Surg 7:283–296, 1943.

314. Ludington NA: Rupture of the long head of the biceps flexor cubiti muscle. Ann Surg 77:358–363, 1923.

315. Muraki T, Aoki M, Izumi T, et al: Lengthening of the pectoralis minor muscle during passive shoulder motions and stretching techniques—a cadaveric biomechanical study. Phys Ther 89:333–341, 2009.

316. Wolf EM, Agrawal V: Transdeltoid palpation (the rent test) in the diagnosis of rotator cuff tears. J Shoulder Elbow Surg 10:470–473, 2001.

317. Brunnstrom S: Muscle testing around the shoulder girdle: a study of the function of shoulder blade fixators in 17 cases of shoulder paralysis. J Bone Joint Surg Am 23:263–272, 1941.

318. Bennett WF: Specificity of the Speed's test: arthroscopic technique for evaluating the biceps tendon at the level of the bicipital groove. Arthroscopy 14:789–796, 1998.

319. Bell RH, Noble JB: Biceps disorders. In Hawkins RJ, Misamore GW, editors: Shoulder injuries in the athlete, New York, 1996, Churchill Livingstone.

320. Jobe FW, Moynes DR: Delineation of diagnostic criteria and a rehabilitation program for rotator cuff injuries. Am J Sports Med 10:336–339, 1982.

321. Kendall HO, Kendall FP: Muscles: testing and function, Baltimore, 1999, Williams & Wilkins.

322. Reese MB: Muscle and wensory testing, Philadelphia, 1999, WB Saunders.

323. Yergason RM: Supination sign. J Bone Joint Surg 13:160, 1931.

324. Elvey RL: The investigation of arm pain. In Grieve GP, editor: Modern manual therapy of the vertebral column, Edinburgh, 1986, Churchill Livingstone.

325. Coppieters MW, Stappaerts KH, Everaert DG, et al: Addition of test components during neurodynamic testing: effect of range of motion and sensory responses. J Orthop Sports Phys Ther 31:226–237, 2001.

326. Butler DS: Mobilisation of the nervous system, Melbourne, 1991, Churchill Livingstone.

327. Aval SM, Durand P, Shankwiler JA: Neurovascular injuries to the athlete's shoulder: part II. J Am Acad Orthop Surg 15:281–289, 2007.

328. Leffert RD, Perlmutter GS: Thoracic outlet syndrome: results of 282 transaxillary first rib resections. Clin Orthop Relat Res 368:66–79, 1999.

329. Atasoy E: Thoracic outlet compression syndrome. Orthop Clin North Am 27:265–303, 1996.

330. Ault J, Suutala K: Thoracic outlet syndrome. J Man Manip Ther 6:118–129, 1998.

331. Safran MR: Nerve injury about the shoulder in athletes. Part 2: long thoracic nerve, spinal accessory nerve, burners/stingers, thoracic outlet syndrome. Am J Sports Med 32:1063–1076, 2004.

332. Kozin SH: Injuries to the brachial plexus. In Iannotti JP, Williams CR, editors: Disorders of the shoulder, Philadelphia, 1999, Lippincott Williams & Wilkins.

333. Adson AW, Coffey JR: Cervical rib: a method of anterior approach for relief of symptoms by division of the scalenus anticus. Ann Surg 85:839–857, 1927.

334. Roos DB: Congenital anomalies associated with thoracic outlet syndrome. J Surg 132:771–778, 1976.

335. Liebenson CS: Thoracic outlet syndrome: diagnosis and conservative management. J Manip Physiol Ther 11:493–499, 1988.

336. Ribbe EB, Lindgren SH, Norgren NE: Clinical diagnosis of thoracic outlet syndrome: evaluation of patients with cervicobrachial symptoms. Manual Med 2:82–85, 1986.

337. Sallstrom J, Schmidt H: Cervicobrachial disorders in certain occupations with special reference to compression in the thoracic outlet. Am J Ind Med 6:45–52, 1984.

338. Wright IS: The neurovascular syndrome produced by hyperabduction of the arms. Am Heart J 29:1–19, 1945.

339. Brown C: Compressive, invasive referred pain to the shoulder. Clin Orthop 173:55–62, 1983.

340. Kelly JJ: Neurologic problems in the athlete's shoulder. In Pettrone FA, editor: Athletic injuries of the shoulder, New York, 1995, McGraw-Hill.

341. Perlmutter GS: Axillary nerve injury. Clin Orthop Relat Res 368:28–36, 1999.

342. Safran MR: Nerve injury about the shoulder in athletes. Part 1: suprascapular nerve and axillary nerve. Am J Sports Med 32:803–819, 2004.

343. Piasecki DP, Romeo AA, Bach BR, et al: Suprascapular neuropathy. J Am Acad Orthop Surg 17:665–676, 2009.

344. Plancher KD, Peterson RK, Johnston JC, et al: The spinoglenoid ligament: anatomy, morphology and histological findings. J Bone Joint Surg Am 87:361–365, 2005.

345. Ferretti A, De Carli A, Fontana M: Injury of the suprascapular nerve at the spinoglenoid notch: the natural history of infraspinatus atrophy in volleyball players. Am J Sports Med 26(6):759–763, 1998.

346. Kaminsky SB, Baker CL: Neurovascular injuries in the athlete's shoulder. Sports Med Arthro Rev 8:170–181, 2000.

347. Cummins CA, Messer TM, Nuber GW: Suprascapular nerve entrapment. J Bone Joint Surg Am 82:415–424, 2000.

348. Cummins CA, Bowen M, Anderson K, et al: Suprascapular nerve entrapment at the spinoglenoid notch in a professional baseball pitcher. Am J Sports Med 27:810–812, 1999.

349. Moen TC, Babatunde OM, Hsu SH, et al: Suprascapular neuropathy: what does the literature show? J Shoulder Elbow Surg 21:835–846, 2012.

350. Pecina MM, Krmpotic-Nemanic J, Markiewitz AD: Tunnel syndromes, Boca Raton, FL, 1991, CRC Press.

351. Fealy S, Altchek DW: Athletic injuries and the throwing athlete: shoulder. In Norris TR, editor: Orthopedic knowledge update: shoulder and elbow, Rosemont, IL, 2002, American Academy of Orthopedic Surgeons.

352. Aval SM, Durand P, Shankwiler JA: Neurovascular injuries to the athlete's shoulder: part I. J Am Acad Orthop Surg 15:249–256, 2007.

353. White SM, Witten CM: Long thoracic nerve palsy in a professional ballet dancer. Am J Sports Med 21:626–628, 1993.

354. Bertelli JA, Ghizoni MF: Long thoracic nerve: anatomy and functional assessment. J Bone Joint Surg Am 87:993–998, 2005.

355. Patten C, Hillel AD: The 11th nerve syndrome: accessory nerve palsy or adhesive capsulitis. Arch Otolaryngol Head Neck Surg 119:215–220, 1993.

356. Wiater JM, Biglian LU: Spinal accessory nerve injury. Clin Orthop Relat Res 368:5–16, 1999.

357. Kaltenborn EM: Mobilization of the extremity joints, Oslo, 1980, Olaf Norlis Bokhandle.

358. Mattingly GE, Mackarey PJ: Optimal methods of shoulder tendon palpation: a cadaver study. Phys Ther 76:166–174, 1996.

359. Bonsell S, Pearsall AW, Heitman RJ, et al: The relationship of age, gender and degenerative changes observed on radiographs of the shoulder in asymptomatic individuals. J Bone Joint Surg Br 82:1135–1139, 2000.

360. Liu SH, Henry MH, Nuccion S, et al: Diagnosis of glenoid labral tears: a comparison between magnetic resonance imaging and clinical examination. Am J Sports Med 24:149–154, 1996.

361. DiGiovine NM: Glenohumeral instability and imaging technique. Orthop Phys Ther Clin North Am 4:123–1995.

362. Schwartz ML: Diagnostic imaging of the shoulder complex. In Andrews JR, Wilk KE, editors: The

athlete's shoulder, New York, 1994, Churchill-Livingstone.

363. Terry GC, Patton WC: Radiographic views and imaging of the shoulder. Sports Med Arthro Rev 8:203–206, 2000.

364. Sanders TG, Morrison WB, Miller MD: Imaging techniques for the evaluation of glenohumeral instability. Am J Sports Med 28:414–434, 2000.

365. Anderson MW, Brennan C, Mittal A: Imaging evaluation of the rotator cuff. Clin Sports Med 31:605–631, 2012.

366. Magee DJ, Reid DC: Shoulder injuries. In Zachazewski JE, Magee DJ, Quillen WS, editors: Athletic injuries and rehabilitation, Philadelphia, 1996, WB Saunders.

367. Uhthoff HK, Loehr JW: Calcific tendinopathy of the rotator cuff: pathogenesis, diagnosis and management. J Am Acad Orthop Surg 5:183–191, 1997.

368. King LJ, Healy JC: Imaging of the painful shoulder. Manual Therapy 4:11–18, 1999.

369. Epstein RE, Schweitzer ME, Frieman BG, et al: Hooked acromion: prevalence on MR images of painful shoulders. Radiology 187:479–481, 1993.

370. Bigliani LU, Tucker JB, Flatow EL, et al: The relationship of acromial architecture to rotator cuff disease. Clin Sports Med 10:823–838, 1991.

371. Burkhart SS: Recurrent anterior shoulder instability. In Norris TR, editor: Orthopedic knowledge update: shoulder and elbow, Rosemont, IL, 2002, American Academy of Orthopedic Surgeons.

372. Provencher M, Frank RM, LeClere LE, et al: The Hill-Sach lesion: diagnosis, classification and management. J Am Acad Orthop Surg 20:242–252, 2012.

373. Kaar SG, Fening SD, Jones MH, et al: Effect of humeral head defect size on glenohumeral stability—a cadaveric study of simulated Hill-Sachs defects. Am J Sports Med 38:594–599, 2010.

374. Weiner DS, Macnab I: Superior migration of the humeral head. J Bone Joint Surg Br 52:524–527, 1970.

375. Nové-Josserand L, Edwards TB, O'Conner DP, et al: The acromioclavicular and coracohumeral intervals are abnormal in rotator cuff tears with muscular fatty degeneration. Clin Orthop Relat Res 433:90–96, 2005.

376. Bonutti PM, Norfray JF, Friedman RJ, et al: Kinematic MRI of the shoulder. J Comput Assist Tomogr 17:666–669, 1993.

377. Bearden JM, Hughston JC, Whatley GS: Acromioclavicular dislocation: method of treatment. J Sports Med 1:5–17, 1973.

378. Tauber M, Koller H, Hitzl W, et al: Dynamic radiographic evaluation of horizontal instability in acute acromioclavicular joint dislocations. Am J Sports Med 38:1188–1195, 2010.

379. Pavlov H, Warren RF, Weiss CB, et al: The roentgenographic evaluation of anterior shoulder instability. Clin Orthop 194:153–158, 1985.

380. Engebretsen L, Craig EV: Radiologic features of shoulder instability. Clin Orthop 291:29–44, 1993.

381. Kernwein GA, Rosenberg B, Sneed WR: Arthrographic studies of the shoulder joint. J Bone Joint Surg Am 39:1267–1279, 1957.

382. Neviaser JS: Arthrography of the shoulder joint: study of the findings of adhesive capsulitis of the shoulder. J Bone Joint Surg Am 44:1321–1330, 1962.

383. Reeves B: Arthrography of the shoulder. J Bone Joint Surg Br 48:424–435, 1966.

384. Nevasier TJ, Nevasier RJ, Nevasier JS: Incomplete rotator cuff tears: a technique of diagnosis and treatment. Clin Orthop 306:12–16, 1994.

385. Desmeules F, Minville L, Riederer B, et al: Acromiohumeral distance variation measured by ultrasonography and its association with the outcome of rehabilitation for shoulder impingement syndrome. Clin J Sport Med 14(4):197–205, 2004.

386. Borsa PA, Jacobson JA, Scibek JS, et al: Comparison of dynamic sonography to stress radiography for assessing glenohumeral laxity in asymptomatic shoulders. Am J Sports Med 33(5):734–741, 2005.

387. Borsa PA, Scibek JS, Jacobson JA, et al: Sonographic stress measurement of glenohumeral joint laxity in collegiate swimmers and age matched controls. Am J Sports Med 33:1077–1084, 2005.

388. Iannotti JP, Ciccone J, Buss DD, et al: Accuracy of office-based ultrasonography of the shoulder for the diagnosis of rotator cuff tears. J Bone Joint Surg Am 87:1305–1311, 2005.

389. Charousset C, Bellaiche L, Duranthon LD, et al: Accuracy of CT arthrography in the assessment of tears of the rotator cuff. J Bone Joint Surg Br 87:824–828, 2005.

390. Collaghan JJ, McNeish LM, Dehaven JP, et al: A prospective comparison study of double contrast computed tomography (CT) arthrography and arthroscopy of the shoulder. Am J Sports Med 16:13–20, 1988.

391. Bernageau J: Roentgenographic assessment of the rotator cuff. Clin Orthop 254:87–91, 1990.

392. Speer KP, Ghelman B, Warren RF: Computed tomography arthrography of the shoulder. In Andrews JR, Wilk KE, editors: The athlete's shoulder, New York, 1994, Churchill-Livingstone.

393. Sanders TG, Miller MD: A systematic approach to magnetic resonance imaging interpretation of sports medicine injuries of the shoulder. Am J Sports Med 33:1088–1105, 2005.

394. Jost B, Zumstein M, Pfirrmann CW, et al: MRI findings in throwing shoulders. Clin Orthop Relat Res 434:130–137, 2005.

395. Chiapat L, Palmer WE: Shoulder magnetic resonance imaging. Clin Sports Med 25:371–386, 2006.

396. Moosikasuwan JB, Miller TT, Hines DM: Imaging of the painful shoulder in throwing athletes. Clin Sports Med 25:433–444, 2006.

397. Bencardino JT, Rosenberg ZS: Entrapment neuropathies of the shoulder and elbow in the athlete. Clin Sports Med 25:465–488, 2006.

398. Murray PJ, Shaffer BS: MR imaging of the shoulder. Sports Med Arthrosc Rev 17:40–48, 2008.

399. Toyoda H, Ito Y, Tomo H, et al: Evaluation of rotator cuff tears with magnetic resonance arthrography. Clin Orthop Relat Res 439:109–115, 2005.

400. Oxner KG: Magnetic resonance imaging of the musculoskeletal system: part 6 the shoulder. Clin Orthop Relat Res 334:354–373, 1997.

401. Connell DA, Potter HG, Wickiewicz TL, et al: Non-contrast magnetic resonance imaging of superior labral lesions: 102 cases confirmed at arthroscopic surgery. Am J Sports Med 27:208–213, 1999.

402. Miniaci A, Burman ML, Mascia AT: Role of magnetic resonance imaging for evaluating shoulder injuries in the athlete. Sports Med Arthro Rev 8:207–218, 2000.

403. Wall MS, O'Brien SJ: Arthroscopic evaluation of the unstable shoulder. Clin Sports Med 14:817–839, 1995.

404. Herzog RJ: Magnetic resonance imaging of the shoulder. J Bone Joint Surg Am 79:934–953, 1997.

405. Kneeland JB: Magnetic resonance imaging: general principles and techniques. In Iannotti JP, Williams CR, editors: Disorders of the shoulder, Philadelphia, 1999, Lippincott Williams & Wilkins.

406. Stetson WB, Phillips T, Deutsch A: The use of magnetic resonance arthrography to detect partial-thickness rotator cuff tears. J Bone Joint Surg Am 87(52):81–88, 2005.

407. Chronopoulos E, Kim TK, Park HB, et al: Diagnostic value of physical tests for isolated chronic acromioclavicular lesions. Am J Sports Med 32(3):655–661, 2004.

408. Guanche CA, Jones DC: Clinical testing for tears of the glenoid labrum. Arthroscopy 19(5):517–523, 2003.

409. Stetson WB, Templin K: The crank test, the O'Brien test, and routine magnetic resonance imaging scans in the diagnosis of labral tears. Am J Sports Med 30(6):806–809, 2002.

410. Jia X, Petersen SA, Khosravi AH, et al: Examination of the shoulder: the past, the present and the future. J Bone Joint Surg Am 91(Suppl 6):10–18, 2009.

411. Michener LA, McClure PW, Sennet BJ: American shoulder and elbow surgeons standardized shoulder assessment form, patient self-reported selection: reliability, validity and responsiveness. J Shoulder Elbow Surg 11(6):587–594, 2002.

412. Beaton D, Richards RR: Assessing the reliability and responsiveness of 5 shoulder questionnaires. J Shoulder Elbow Surg 7(6):565–572, 1998.

413. Kocher MS, Horan MP, Briggs KK, et al: Reliability, validity, and responsiveness of the American Shoulder and Elbow Surgeons subjective shoulder scale in patients with shoulder instability, rotator cuff disease and glenohumeral arthritis. J Bone Joint Surg Am 87:2006–2011, 2005.

414. Tzannes A, Paxinos A, Callanan M, et al: An assessment of the interexaminer reliability of tests for shoulder instability. J Shoulder Elbow Surg 13(1):18–23, 2004.

415. Michael G, Michael D: Anterior release test: a new test for occult shoulder instability. Clin Orthop 339:105–108, 1997.

416. Farber AJ, Castillo R, Clough M, et al: Clinical assessment of three common tests for traumatic anterior shoulder instability. J Bone Joint Surg Am 88(7):1467–1474, 2006.

417. Kim SH, Ha KI, Ahn JH, et al: Biceps load test II: a clinical test for SLAP lesions of the shoulder. Arthroscopy 17(2):160–164, 2001.

418. Calis M, Akgun K, Birtane M, et al: Diagnostic values of clinical diagnostic tests in subacromial impingement syndrome. Ann Rheum Dis 59(1):44–47, 2000.

419. Beaton DE, Katz JN, Fossel AH, et al: Measuring the whole or the parts? Validity, reliability, and responsiveness of the disabilities of the arm, shoulder and hand outcome measure in different regions of the upper extremity. J Hand Ther 14:128–146, 2001.

420. Getahun TY, MacDermid JC, Patterson SD: Concurrent validity of patient rating scales in assessment of outcome after rotator cuff repair. J Musculoskelet Res 4:119–127, 2000.

421. Maier M, Maier-Bosse T, Schulz CU, et al: Inter and intraobserver variability in DePalma's classification of shoulder calcific tendinitis. J Rheumatol 30(5):1029–1031, 2003.

422. Itoi E, Kido T, Sano A, et al: Which is more useful, the "full can test" or the "empty can test" in detecting torn supraspinatus tendon? Am J Sports Med 27:65–68, 1999.

423. Hayes KW, Petersen CM: Reliability of assessing end-feel and pain and resistance sequence in subjects with painful shoulders and knees. J Orthop Sports Phys Ther 31(8):432–445, 2001.

424. Hicks GE, Fritz JM, Delitto A, et al: Interrater reliability of clinical examination measures for identification of lumbar segmental instability. Arch Phys Med Rehabil 84(12):1858–1864, 2003.

425. MacDonald PB, Clark P, Sutherland K: An analysis of the diagnostic accuracy of the Hawkins and Neer

subacromial impingement signs. J Shoulder Elbow Surg 9(4):299–301, 2000.

426. Dover G, Powers ME: Reliability of joint position sense and force reproduction measures during internal and external rotation of the shoulder. J Athl Train 38:304–310, 2003.

427. Koslow PA, Prosser LA, Strony GA, et al: Specificity of the lateral scapular slide test in asymptomatic competitive athletes. J Orthop Sports Phys Ther 33(6):331–336, 2003.

428. Jorgensen U, Bak K: Shoulder instability: assessment of anterior-posterior translation with a knee laxity tester. Acta Orthop Scand 66(5):398–400, 1995.

429. Pizzari T, Kolt GS, Remedios I: Measurement of anterior-to-posterior translation on the glenohumeral joint using the KT-1000. J Orthop Sports Phys Ther 29(10):602–608, 1999.

430. Jee WH, McCauley TR, Katz LD, et al: Superior labral anterior posterior (SLAP) lesions of the glenoid labrum: reliability and accuracy of MR arthrography for diagnosis. Radiology 218(1):127–132, 2001.

431. Teefey SA, Rubin DA, Middleton WD, et al: Detection and quantification of rotator cuff tears: comparison of ultrasonographic, magnetic resonance imaging, and arthroscopic findings in seventy-one consecutive cases. J Bone Joint Surg Am 86(4):708–716, 2004.

432. Walton J, Mahajan S, Paxinos A, et al: Diagnostic values of tests for acromioclavicular joint pain. J Bone Joint Surg Am 86:817–812, 2004.

433. Boyd EA, Torrance GM: Clinical measures of shoulder subluxation: their reliability. Can J Public Health 83(Suppl 2):S24–S28, 1992.

434. Meister K, Buckley B, Batts J: The posterior impingement sign: diagnosis of rotator cuff and posterior labral tears secondary to internal impingement in overhand athletes. Am J Orthop 33(8):412–415, 2004.

435. Wolf EM, Agrawal V: Trans-deltoid palpation (the rent test) in the diagnosis of rotator cuff tears. J Shoulder Elbow Surg 10:470–473, 2001.

436. Holtby R, Razmjou H: Accuracy of the Speed's and Yergason's tests in detecting biceps pathology and SLAP lesions: comparison with arthroscopic findings. Arthroscopy 20(3):231–236, 2004.

437. Bennett WF: Specificity of the speed's test: arthroscopic technique for evaluating the biceps tendon at the level of the bicipital groove. Arthroscopy 14:789–796, 1998.

438. Holtby R, Razmjou H: Validity of the supraspinatus test as a single clinical test in diagnosing patients with rotator cuff pathology. J Orthop Sports Phys Ther 34:194–200, 2004.

439. Reish R, Williams K: ULNT2—Median nerve bias: examiner reliability and sensory responses in asymptomatic subjects. J Man Manip Ther 13(1):44–55, 2005.

440. Patrik GE, Kuhn JE: Validation of the life-off test and analysis of subscapularis activity during maximal internal rotation. Am J Sports Med 24(5):589, 1996.

SUGGESTED READINGS

Adams JC: Outline of orthopaedics, London, 1968, E & S Livingstone.

Albert MS, Wooden MJ: Isokinetic evaluation and treatment of the shoulder. In Physical therapy of the shoulder, Edinburgh, 1991, Churchill Livingstone.

American Orthopaedic Association: Manual of orthopaedic surgery, Chicago, 1972, American Orthopaedic Association.

Anderson JE: Grant's atlas of anatomy, Baltimore, 1983, Williams & Wilkins.

Arrigo CA, Wilk KE, Andrews JR: Peak torque and maximum work repetition during isokinetic testing of the shoulder internal and external rotators. Isokin Exerc Sci 4:171–175, 1994.

Ault JL: Subacromial impingement syndrome. J Man Manip Ther 7:56–63, 1999.

Bassett LW, Gold RH, Seeger LL: MRI atlas of the musculoskeletal system, London, 1989, Martin Dunitz.

Bateman JE: Neurogenic painful conditions affecting the shoulder. Clin Orthop 173:44–54, 1983.

Bateman JE: The shoulder and neck, ed 2, Philadelphia, 1978, WB Saunders.

Beasley L, Faryniarz DA, Hannafin JA: Multidirectional instability of the shoulder in the female athlete. Clin Sports Med 19:331–349, 2000.

Beetham WP, Polley HF, Slocum CH, et al: Physical examination of the joints, Philadelphia, 1965, WB Saunders.

Bennett JB, Mehlhoff TL: Thoracic outlet syndrome. In De Lee JC, Drez D, editors: Orthopedic sports medicine: principles and practice, Philadelphia, 1994, WB Saunders.

Bigg-Wither G, Kelly P: Diagnostic imaging in musculoskeletal physiotherapy. In Refshauge K, Gass E, editors: Musculoskeletal physiotherapy, Oxford, 1995, Butterworth-Heinemann.

Bishop JY, Flatow EZ: Pediatric shoulder trauma. Clin Orthop Relat Res 432:41–48, 2005.

Black KP, Lombardo JA: Suprascapular nerve injuries with isolated paralysis of the infraspinatus. Am J Sports Med 18:225–228, 1990.

Boissonnault WG, Janos SC: Dysfunction, evaluation and treatment of the shoulder. In Donatelli RA, Wooden MJ, editors: Orthopedic physical therapy, Edinburgh, 1989, Churchill Livingstone.

Booth RE, Marvel JP: Differential diagnosis of shoulder pain. Orthop Clin North Am 6:353–379, 1975.

Borsa PA, Lephart SM, Kocher MS, et al: Functional assessment and rehabilitation of shoulder proprioception for glenohumeral instability. J Sports Rehab 3:84–104, 1994.

Borsa PA, Sauers EL, Herling DE: In vivo assessment of AP laxity in healthy shoulders using an instrumental arthrometer. J Sports Rehab 8:157–170, 1999.

Boublik M, Hawkins RJ: Clinical examination of the shoulder complex. J Orthop Sports Phys Ther 18:379–385, 1993.

Brown LP, Niehues SL, Harrah A, et al: Upper extremity range of motion and isokinetic strength of the internal and external shoulder rotators in major league baseball players. Am J Sports Med 16:577–585, 1988.

Cahill BR, Palmer RE: Quadrilateral space syndrome. J Hand Surg 8:65–69, 1983.

Cailliet R: Shoulder pain, Philadelphia, 1966, FA Davis.

Chen FS, Diaz VA, Loebenberg M, et al: Shoulder and elbow injuries in the skeletally immature athlete. J Am Acad Ortho Surg 13:172–185, 2005.

Chesworth BM, MacDermid JV, Roth JH, et al: Movement diagram and "end-feel" reliability when measuring passive lateral rotation of the shoulder in patients with shoulder pathology. Phys Ther 78:593–601, 1998.

Ciocca MF: Bilateral shoulder pain: psoriatic arthritis masquerading as overuse. Phys Sportsmed 26(9):50–55, 1998.

Cofield RH, Nessler JP, Weinstabl R: Diagnosis of shoulder instability by examination under anesthesia. Clin Orthop 291:45–53, 1993.

Collins K, Peterson K: Case report: diagnosing suprascapular neuropathy: pinpointing a shoulder injury site. Phys Sportsmed 22:59–69, 1994.

Cone RO: Imaging the glenohumeral joint. In De Lee JC, Drez D, editors: Orthopedic sports medicine: principles and practice, Philadelphia, 1994, WB Saunders.

Coppieters MW, Stappaerts KH, Staes FF, et al: Shoulder girdle elevation during neurodynamic testing: an assessible sign? Manual Therapy 6:88–96, 2000.

De Laat EA, Visser CP, Coene LN, et al: Nerve lesions in primary shoulder dislocations and humeral neck fractures. J Bone Joint Surg Br 76:381–383, 1994.

Dempster WT: Mechanisms of shoulder movement. Arch Phys Med Rehabil 46:49–70, 1965.

Deutsch AL, Resnick D, Mink JH: Computed tomography of the glenohumeral and sternoclavicular joints. Orthop Clin North Am 16:497–511, 1985.

Dickoff-Hoffman SA: Examination of the shoulder. Orthop Phys Ther Clin North Am 3:403–425, 1994.

DiVeta J, Walker ML, Skibinski B: Relationship between performance of selected scapular muscles and scapular abduction in standing subjects. Phys Ther 70:470–478, 1990.

Dodson CC, Altchek DW: SLAP lesions: an update on recognition and treatment. J Orthop Sports Phys Ther 39:71–80, 2009.

Drez D: Suprascapular neuropathy in the differential diagnosis of rotator cuff injuries. Am J Sports Med 4:43–45, 1976.

Drye C, Zachazewski JE: Peripheral nerve injuries. In Zachazewski JE, Magee DJ, Quillen WS, editors: Athletic injuries and rehabilitation, Philadelphia, 1996, WB Saunders.

Duralde XA, Bigliani LU: Neurologic disorders. In Hawkins RJ, Misamore GW, editors: Shoulder injuries in the athlete, New York, 1996, Churchill Livingstone.

Fallcel JE, Murphy TC, Malone TR: Shoulder injuries: sports injury management, Baltimore, 1988, Williams & Wilkins.

Ferreti A, Cerullo G, Russo G: Suprascapular neuropathy in volleyball players. J Bone Joint Surg Am 69:260–263, 1987.

Forrester DM, Brown JC: The radiology of joint disease, Philadelphia, 1987, WB Saunders.

Foster CR: Multidirectional instability of the shoulder in the athlete. Clin Sports Med 2:355–368, 1983.

Fowler PJ: Swimming. In Fu FH, Stone DA, editors: Sports injuries: mechanisms, prevention, treatment, Baltimore, 1994, Williams & Wilkins.

France MK: Anatomy and biomechanics of the shoulder. In Donatelli RA, editor: Physical therapy of the shoulder, Edinburgh, 1991, Churchill Livingstone.

Francis WR: Thoracic outlet syndrome. In Camins MB, O'Leary PF, editors: Disorders of the cervical spine, Baltimore, 1992, Williams & Wilkins.

Fritts HM, Cooper CR: Magnetic resonance and shoulder imaging. In Hawkins RJ, Misamore GW, editors: Shoulder injuries in the athlete, New York, 1996, Churchill Livingstone.

Garrick JG, Webb DR: Sports injuries: diagnosis and management, Philadelphia, 1990, WB Saunders.

Gartland JJ: Fundamentals of orthopaedics, Philadelphia, 1979, WB Saunders.

Gerber C: Integrated scoring systems for the functional assessment of the shoulder. In Matsen FA, Fu FH, Hawkins RJ, editors: The shoulder: a balance of mobility and stability, Rosemont, IL, 1993, American Academy of Orthopedic Surgeons.

Gibson MH, Goebel GV, Jordan TM, et al: A reliability study of measurement techniques to determine static scapular position. J Orthop Sports Phys Ther 21:100–106, 1995.

Gilliman JF, Hawkins RJ: Clinical examination of the shoulder complex. In Andrews JR, Wilk KE, editors: The athlete's shoulder, New York, 1994, Churchill Livingstone.

Graichen H, Stammberger T, Bonel H, et al: Magnetic resonance based motion analysis of the shoulder during elevation. Clin Orthop Relat Res 370:154–163, 2000.

Greenfield BH, Donatelli R, Wooden MJ, et al: Isokinetic evaluation of shoulder rotational strength between the plane of the scapula and the frontal plane. Am J Sports Med 18:124–128, 1990.

Gregg JR, Labosky D, Harty M, et al: Serratus anterior paralysis in the young athlete. J Bone Joint Surg Am 61:825–832, 1979.

Halback JW, Tank RT: The shoulder. In Gould JA, editor: Orthopedic and sports physical therapy, St Louis, 1990, Mosby.

Hallstrom E, Karrholm J: Shoulder kinematics in 25 patients with impingement and 12 controls. Clin Orthop Relat Res 48:22–27, 2006.

Hancock RE, Hawkins RJ: Applications of electromyography in the throwing shoulder. Clin Orthop Relat Res 330:84–97, 1996.

Harrison AL, Barry-Greb T, Wojtowicz G: Clinical measurement of hand and shoulder posture variables. J Orthop Sports Phys Ther 23:353–361, 1996.

Harryman DT, Sidles JA, Clark JM, et al: Translation of the humeral head on the glenoid with passive glenohumeral motion. J Bone Joint Surg Am 72:1334–1343, 1990.

Hawkins RJ: Musculoskeletal examination, St Louis, 1995, Mosby Year Book.

Hawkins RJ, Abrams JS: Impingement syndrome in the absence of rotator cuff tear (stage 1 and 2). Orthop Clin North Am 18:373–382, 1987.

Hawkins RJ, Hobeika PE: Impingement syndrome in the athletic shoulder. Clin Sports Med 2:391–405, 1983.

Hershman EB, Wilbourn AJ, Bergfeld JA: Acute brachial neuropathy in athletes. Am J Sports Med 17:655–659, 1989.

Hirayama T, Takemitsa Y: Compression of the suprascapular nerve by a ganglion at the suprascapular notch. Clin Orthop 155:95–96, 1981.

Hollinshead WH, Jenkins DB: Functional anatomy of the limb and back, Philadelphia, 1981, WB Saunders.

Hoppenfeld S: Physical examination of the spine and extremities, New York, 1976, Appleton-Century-Crofts.

Hughes RE, An KN: Force analysis of rotator cuff muscles. Clin Orthop Relat Res 330:75–83, 1996.

Hughes RE, Johnson ME, O'Driscoll PW, et al: Age-related changes in normal isometric shoulder strength. Am J Sports Med 27:651–657, 1999.

Iannotti JP: Lesions of the rotator cuff: pathology and pathogenesis. In Matsen FA, Fu FH, Hawkins RJ, editors: The shoulder: a balance of mobility and stability, Rosemont, IL, 1993, American Academy of Orthopedic Surgeons.

Iannotti JP, Zlatkin MB, Esterhai JL, et al: Magnetic resonance imaging of the shoulder. J Bone Joint Surg Am 73:17–29, 1991.

Itoi E, Minagawa H, Yamamoto N, et al: Are pain location and physical examinations useful in locating a tear site of the rotator cuff? Am J Sports Med 34:256–264, 2006.

Jobe CM: Superior glenoid impingement. Clin Orthop Relat Res 330:98–107, 1996.

Jobe FW, Bradley JP: Rotator cuff injuries in basketball. Sports Med 6:378–389, 1988.

Jobe FW, Jobe CM: Painful athletic injuries of the shoulder. Clin Orthop 173:117–124, 1983.

Johnson MP, McClure PW, Karduna AR: New method to assess scapular upward rotation in subjects with shoulder pathology. J Orthop Sports Phys Ther 31:81–89, 2001.

Johnson TR, Steinbach LS: Essentials of musculoskeletal imaging, Rosemont, IL, 2004, American Academy of Orthopaedic Surgeons.

Judge RD, Zuidema GD, Fitzgerald FT: Clinical diagnosis: a physiological approach, Boston, 1982, Little Brown.

Keskula DR, Perrin DH: Effect of test protocol on torque production of the rotators of the shoulder. Isokin Exerc Sci 4:176–181, 1994.

Kibler WB, Sciascia A: Rehabilitation of the athlete's shoulder. Clin Sports Med 27:821–831, 2008.

Kim TK, McFarland EG: Internal impingement of the shoulder in flexion. Clin Orthop Relat Res 421:112–119, 2004.

Kuhn JE, Bey MJ, Huston LJ, et al: Ligamentous restraints to external rotation of the humerus in the late cocking phase of throwing: a cadaveric biomechanical investigation. Am J Sports Med 28:200–205, 2000.

Kuijpers T, van derWindt DA, Boeke AJ, et al: Clinical prediction rules for the prognosis of shoulder pain in general practice. Pain 120:276–285, 2006.

Lear LJ, Gross MT: An electromyographical analysis of the scapular stabilizing synergists during a push-up progression. J Orthop Sports Phys Ther 28:146–157, 1998.

Lee KW, Debski RE, Chan CH, et al: Functional evaluation of the ligaments at the acromioclavicular joint during anteroposterior and superoinferior translation. Am J Sports Med 25:858–862, 1997.

Lee SB, Kim KJ, O'Driscoll SW, et al: Dynamic glenohumeral stability provided by the rotator cuff muscles in the mid range and end range of motion. J Bone Joint Surg Am 82:849–857, 2000.

Leffert RD: Clinical diagnoses, testing and electromyographic study in brachial plexus traction injuries. Clin Orthop 237:24–31, 1988.

Lemos MJ: The evaluation and treatment of the injured acromioclavicular joint in athletes. Am J Sports Med 26:137–144, 1998.

Levine WN, Flatow EL: The pathophysiology of shoulder instability. Am J Sports Med 28:910–917, 2000.

Lippman RK: Frozen shoulder; periarthritis; bicipital tenosynovitis. Arch Surg 47:283–296, 1943.

Ludewig PM, Cook TM: Alterations in shoulder kinematics and associated muscle activity in people with symptoms of shoulder impingement. Phys Ther 80:276–291, 2000.

Maday MG, Harner CD, Warner JJ: Shoulder injuries. In Fu FH, Stone DA, editors: Sports injuries: mechanisms, prevention, treatment, Baltimore, 1994, Williams & Wilkins.

Maki NJ: Cineradiographic studies with shoulder instabilities. Am J Sports Med 16:362–364, 1988.

Malerba JL, Adam ML, Harris BA, et al: Reliability of dynamic and isometric testing of shoulder external and internal rotators. J Orthop Sports Phys Ther 18:543–552, 1993.

Matava MJ, Purcell DB, Rudzki JR: Partial thickness rotator cuff tears. Am J Sports Med 33:1405–1417, 2005.

McConville OR, Iannotti JP: Partial thickness tears of the rotator cuff: evaluation and management. J Am Acad Orthop Surg 7:32–43, 1999.

McIlveen SJ, Duralde XA, D'Alessandro DF, et al: Isolated nerve injuries about the shoulder. Clin Orthop 306:54–63, 1994.

McKinnis LN: Fundamentals of musculoskeletal imaging, Philadelphia, 2005, FA Davis.

McMaster WC: Painful shoulder in swimmers: a diagnostic challenge. Phys Sportsmed 14:108–122, 1986.

Meister K: Injuries to the shoulder in the throwing athlete. Part one: biomechanics/pathophysiology/classification of injury. Am J Sports Med 28:265–275, 2000.

Meyer SJF, Dalinka MK: Magnetic resonance imaging of the shoulder. Orthop Clin North Am 21:497–513, 1990.

Michener LA, Boardman ND, Pidcoe PE, et al: Scapular muscle tests in subjects with shoulder pain and functional loss: reliability and construct validity. Phys Ther 85:1128–1138, 2005.

Moran CA, Saunders SR: Evaluation of the shoulder: a sequential approach. In Donatelli RA, editor: Physical therapy of the shoulder, Edinburgh, 1991, Churchill Livingstone.

Myers JB, Ju YY, Hwang JH, et al: Reflexive muscle activation alternations in shoulders with anterior glenohumeral instability. Am J Sports Med 32:1013–1021, 2004.

Myers JB, Landner KG, Pasquale MR, et al: Scapular position and orientation in throwing athletes. Am J Sports Med 33:263–271, 2005.

Naffziger HC, Grant WT: Neuritis of the brachial plexus mechanical in origin: the scalenus syndrome. Clin Orthop 51:7–15, 1967.

Neer CS: Anterior acromioplasty for the chronic impingement syndrome in the shoulder. J Bone Joint Surg Am 54:41–50, 1972.

Neer CS: Impingement lesions. Clin Orthop 173:70–77, 1983.

Neer CS, Foster CR: Inferior capsular shift for involuntary inferior and multidirectional instability of the shoulder. J Bone Joint Surg Am 62:897–908, 1980.

Neiers L, Worrell TW: Assessment of scapular position. J Sports Rehab 2:20–25, 1993.

Neumann DA: Kinesiology of the musculoskeletal system: foundations for physical rehabilitation, St Louis, 2002, Mosby.

Neviaser JS: Adhesive capsulitis and the stiff and painful shoulder. Orthop Clin North Am 11:327–331, 1980.

Neviaser RJ: Anatomic considerations and examination of the shoulder. Orthop Clin North Am 11:187–195, 1980.

Neviaser RJ: Lesions of the biceps and tendinitis of the shoulder. Orthop Clin North Am 11:343–348, 1980.

Neviaser RJ: Painful conditions affecting the shoulder. Clin Orthop 173:63–69, 1983.

Neviaser RJ: Tears of the rotator cuff. Orthop Clin North Am 11:295–306, 1980.

Neuman DA: Kinesiology of the musculoskeletal system—foundations for rehabilitation, ed 2, St Louis, 2010, Mosby/Elsevier.

Norris TR: History and physical examination of the shoulder. In Nicholas JA, Hershman EB, editors: The upper extremity in sports medicine, St Louis, 1990, Mosby.

Norris TR, Green A: Imaging modalities in the evaluation of shoulder disorders. In Matsen FA, Fu FH, Hawkin RJS, editors: The shoulder: a balance of mobility and stability, Rosemont, IL, 1993, American Academy of Orthopedic Surgeons.

O'Donoghue DH: Treatment of injuries to athletes, ed 4, Philadelphia, 1984, WB Saunders.

O'Driscoll SW: Atraumatic instability: pathology and pathogenesis. In Matsen FA, Fu FH, Hawkins RJ, editors: The shoulder: a balance of mobility and stability, Rosemont, IL, 1993, American Academy of Orthopedic Surgeons.

Oliashirazi A, Monsat P, Cofield RH, et al: Examination under anaesthesia for evaluation of anterior shoulder instability. Am J Sports Med 27:464–468, 1999.

Overton LM: The causes of pain in the upper extremities: a differential diagnosis study. Clin Orthop 51:27–44, 1967.

Palmer ML, Epler M: Clinical assessment procedures in physical therapy, Philadelphia, 1990, JB Lippincott.

Patla CE: Upper extremity. In Payton OD, Fabio RPD, Paris SV, editors: Manual of physical therapy, Edinburgh, 1989, Churchill Livingstone.

Pearl ML, Harris SL, Lippitt SB, et al: A system for describing positions of the humerus relative to the thorax and its use in the presentation of several functionally important arm positions. J Shoulder Elbow Surg 1:113–118, 1992.

Pellecchia GL, Paolino J, Connell J: Intertester reliability of the Cyriax evaluation assessing patients with shoulder pain. J Orthop Sports Phys Ther 23:34–38, 1996.

Perry J: Anatomy and biomechanics of the shoulder in throwing, swimming, gymnastics, and tennis. Clin Sports Med 2:247–270, 1983.

Peterson DE, Blankenship KR, Robb JB, et al: Investigation of the validity and reliability of four objective techniques for measuring forward shoulder posture. J Orthop Sports Phys Ther 25:34–42, 1997.

Piasecki DP, Nicholson GP: Tears of the subscapularis tendon in athletes—diagnosis and repair techniques. Clin Sports Med 27:731–745, 2008.

Pink M, Perry J, Browne A, et al: The normal shoulder during freestyle swimming: an electromyographic and cinemagraphic analysis of 12 muscles. Am J Sports Med 19:569–576, 1991.

Plafcan DM, Canavan PK, Sebastianelli WJ, et al: Relability of a new instrument to measure scapular position. J Man Manip Ther 8:183–192, 2000.

Plafcan DM, Turczany PJ, Guenin BA, et al: An objective measurement technique for posterior scapular displacement. J Orthop Sports Phys Ther 25:336–341, 1997.

Pollack RG, Bigliani LU: Glenohumeral instability: evaluation and treatment. J Am Acad Orthop Surg 1:24–32, 1993.

Pollard H, Lakay B, Tucker F, et al: Interexaminer reliability of the deltoid and psoas muscle test. J Manip Physiol Ther 28:52–56, 2005.

Post M, Mayer J: Suprascapular nerve entrapment: diagnosis and treatment. Clin Orthop 223:126–131, 1987.

Post M, Silver R, Singh M: Rotator cuff tear: diagnosis and treatment. Clin Orthop 173:78–91, 1983.

Rathbun JB, Macnab I: The microvascular pattern of the rotator cuff. J Bone Joint Surg Br 52:540–553, 1970.

Recht MP, Resnic D: Magnetic resonance imaging studies of the shoulder: diagnosis of lesions of the rotator cuff. J Bone Joint Surg Am 75:1244–1253, 1993.

Reid DC: Focusing the diagnosis of shoulder pain: pearls of practice. Phys Sportsmed 22:28–43, 1994.

Reid DC: Functional anatomy and joint mobilization, Edmonton, 1970, University of Alberta Press.

Reid DC: Sports injury assessment and rehabilitation, New York, 1992, Churchill Livingstone.

Resnick D, Kransdorf MJ: Bone and joint imaging, Philadelphia, 2005, WB Saunders.

Riddle DL, Rothstein JM, Lamb RL: Goniometric reliability in a clinical setting: shoulder measurements. Phys Ther 67:668–673, 1987.

Ringel SP, Treihaft M, Carry M, et al: Suprascapular neuropathy in pitchers. Am J Sports Med 18:80–86, 1990.

Robinson CM, Aderinto J: Posterior shoulder dislocations and fracture dislocations. J Bone Joint Surg Am 87:639–650, 2005.

Robinson CM, Aderinto J: Recurrent posterior shoulder instability. J Bone Joint Surg Am 87:883–892, 2005.

Rockwood CA, Szalay EA, Curtis RJ, et al: X-ray evaluation of shoulder problems. In Rockwood CA, Masten FA, editors: The shoulder, Philadelphia, 1990, WB Saunders.

Rowe C: Examination of the shoulder. In Rowe CR, editor: The shoulder, Edinburgh, 1988, Churchill Livingstone.

Rowe CR: Recurrent transient anterior subluxation of the shoulder: the dead arm syndrome. Clin Orthop 223:11–19, 1987.

St. John's Ambulance: First aid, Ottawa, 1963, The Runge Press.

Sarrafian SK: Gross and functional anatomy of the shoulder. Clin Orthop 173:11–19, 1983.

Schenkman M, de Cartaya VR: Kinesiology of the shoulder complex. J Orthop Sports Phys Ther 8:438–450, 1987.

Schenkman M, Lamb KC, Kuchibhatla M, et al: Measures of shoulder protraction and thoracolumbar rotation. J Orthop Sports Phys Ther 25:329–335, 1997.

Schmitt L, Snyder-Mackler L: Role of scapular stabilizers in etiology and treatment of impingement syndrome. J Orthop Sports Phys Ther 29:31–38, 1999.

Schob CJ: Suprascapular nerve entrapment. In Andrews JR, Wilk KE, editors: The athlete's shoulder, New York, 1994, Churchill Livingstone.

Schwartz E, Warren RF, O'Brien SJ, et al: Posterior shoulder instability. Orthop Clin North Am 18:409–419, 1987.

Schwartz ML: Diagnostic imaging of the shoulder complex. In Andrews JR, Wilk KE, editors: The athlete's shoulder, New York, 1994, Churchill Livingstone.

Scovazzo ML, Browne A, Pink M, et al: The painful shoulder during freestyle swimming: an electromyographic cinematographic analysis of 12 muscles. Am J Sports Med 19:577–582, 1991.

Seeger LL: Magnetic resonance imaging of the shoulder. Clin Orthop 244:48–59, 1989.

Sigman SA, Richmond JC: Office diagnosis of shoulder disorders. Phys Sportsmed 23(7):25–31, 1995.

Silliman JF, Hawkins RJ: Clinical examination of the shoulder complex. In Andrews JR, Wilk KE, editors: The athlete's shoulder, New York, 1994, Churchill-Livingstone.

Skurja M, Monlux JH: Case studies: the suprascapular nerve and shoulder dysfunction. J Orthop Sports Phys Ther 6:254–258, 1985.

Smith J, Padgett DJ, Kaufman KR, et al: Rhomboid muscle electromyography activity during three different manual muscle tests. Arch Phys Med Rehabil 85:987–992, 2004.

Souza TA: Sports injuries of the shoulder, 1994, New York, Churchill Livingstone.

Speer KP, Garrett WE: Muscular control of motion and stability about the pectoral girdle. In Matsen FA, Fu FH, Hawkins RJ, editors: The shoulder: a balance of mobility and stability, Rosemont, IL, 1993, American Academy of Orthopedic Surgeons.

Speer KP, Ghelman B, Warren RF: Computed tomography: arthrography of the shoulder. In Andrews JR, Wilk KE, editors: The athlete's shoulder, New York, 1994, Churchill Livingstone.

Starkey C, Ryan J: Evaluation of orthopedic and athletic injuries, Philadelphia, 1996, FA Davis.

Tank R, Halbach J: Physical therapy evaluation of the shoulder complex in athletes. J Orthop Sports Phys Ther 3:108–120, 1982.

Tardiff GS: Nerve injuries, testing and treatment tractics. Phys Sportsmed 23:61–72, 1995.

Tasto JP: Shoulder stability testing using the lateral decubitive position. Phys Sportsmed 24(12):75–76, 1998.

Tata GE, Ng L, Kramer JF: Shoulder antagonistic strength ratios during concentric and eccentric muscle actions in the scapular plane. J Orthop Sports Phys Ther 18:654–660, 1993.

Thompson RC, Schneider W, Kennedy T: Entrapment neuropathy of the inferior branch of the suprascapular nerve by ganglion. Clin Orthop 166:185–187, 1982.

Tibone JE, Bradley JP: Evaluation of treatment outcomes for the athlete's shoulder. In Matsen FA, Fu FH, Hawkins RJ, editors: The shoulder: a balance of mobility and stability, Rosemont, IL, 1993, American Academy of Orthopedic Surgeons.

Travell JG, Simons DG: Myofascial pain and dysfunction: the trigger point manual, Baltimore, 1983, Williams & Wilkins.

Tullos HS, Erwin WD, Woods GW, et al: Unusual lesions of the pitching arm. Clin Orthop Relat Res 88:169–182, 1972.

van Duijn AJ, Jensen RH: Reliability of inferior glide mobility testing of the glenohumeral joint. J Man Manip Ther 9:109–114, 2001.

Vastamaki M, Goransson H: Suprascapular nerve entrapment. Clin Orthop 297:135–143, 1993.

von Schroeder HP, Kuiper SD, Botte MJ: Osseous anatomy of the scapula. Clin Orthop Relat Res 383:131–139, 2001.

Wadsworth CT: Manual examination and treatment of the spine and extremities, Baltimore, 1988, Williams & Wilkins.

Warner JJ, Krushell RJ, Masquelet A, et al: Anatomy and relationships of the suprascapular nerve: anatomical constraints to mobilization of the supraspinatus and infraspinatus muscles in the management of massive rotator cuff tears. J Bone Joint Surg Am 74:36–45, 1992.

Wechsler LR, Busis NA: Sports neurology. In Fu FH, Stone DA, editors: Sports injuries: mechanisms, prevention, treatment, Baltimore, 1994, Williams & Wilkins.

Weiser WM, Lee TQ, McMaster WC, et al: Effects of simulated scapular protraction on anterior glenohumeral stability. Am J Sports Med 27:801–805, 1999.

Weissman BNW, Sledge CB: Orthopedic radiology, Philadelphia, 1986, WB Saunders.

Werner A, Mueller T, Boehm D, et al: The stabilizing sling for the long head of the biceps tendon in the rotator cuff interval: a histoanatomic study. Am J Sports Med 28:28–31, 2000.

Werner SL, Gill TJ, Murray TA, et al: Relationships between throwing mechanics and shoulder distraction in professional baseball players. Am J Sports Med 29:354–358, 2001.

White SM, Witten CM: Long thoracic nerve palsy in a professional ballet dancer. Am J Sports Med 21:626–628, 1993.

Wiles P, Sweetnam R: Essentials of orthopaedics, London, 1965, JA Churchill.

Wilk KE, Andrews JR, Arrigo CA: The physical examination of the glenohumeral joint: emphasis on the stabilizing structures. J Orthop Sports Phys Ther 25:380–389, 1997.

Wilk KE, Arrigo C: Current concepts in the rehabilitation of the athletic shoulder. J Orthop Sports Phys Ther 18:365–378, 1993.

Wilk KE, Arrigo CA, Andrews JR: Current concepts: the stabilizing structures of the glenohumeral joint. J Orthop Sports Phys Ther 25:364–379, 1997.

Wilk KE, Obma P, Simpson CD, et al: Shoulder injuries in the overhead athlete. J Orthop Sports Phys Ther 39:38–54, 2009.

Williams A, Evans R, Shirley PD: Imaging of sports injuries, London, 1989, Bailliere Tindall.

Williams GR, Iannotti JP: Diagnostic tests and surgical techniques. In Kelley MJ, Clark WA, editors: Orthopedic therapy of the shoulder, Philadelphia, 1995, JB Lippincott.

Williams GR, Shakil M, Klimkiewicz J, et al: Anatomy of the scapulothoracic articulation. Clin Orthop Relat Res 359:237–246, 1999.

Wilson RW: Entrapment neuropathy of the inferior supra-scapular nerve in a weight lifter. J Sports Rehab 2: 208–210, 1993.

Woo SL, McMahon PJ, Debski RE, et al: Factors limiting and defining shoulder motion: what keeps it from going farther? In Matsen FA, Fu FH, Hawkins RJ, editors: The shoulder: a balance of mobility and stability, Rosemont, IL, 1993, American Academy of Orthopedic Surgeons.

Wood VE, Brondi J: Double crush nerve compression in thoracic outlet syndrome. J Bone Joint Surg Am 72:85–87, 1990.

Wood VE, Twito R, Verska JM: Thoracic outlet syndrome. Orthop Clin North Am 19:131–146, 1988.

Yocum LA: Assessing the shoulder: history, physical examination, differential diagnosis, and special tests used. Clin Sports Med 2:281–289, 1983.

Yoon TN, Grabois M, Guillen M: Suprascapular nerve injury following trauma to the shoulder. J Trauma 21:652–655, 1981.

Zarins B: Anterior subluxation and dislocation of the shoulder. In AAOSS on Upper Extremity Injuries in Athletes, St Louis, 1986, CV Mosby.

Zarins B, McMahon MS, Rowe CR: Diagnosis and treatment of traumatic anterior instability of the shoulder. Clin Orthop 291:75–84, 1993.

Zemek MJ, Magee DJ: Comparison of glenohumeral joint laxity in elite and recreational swimmers. Clin J Sports Med 6:40–47, 1996.

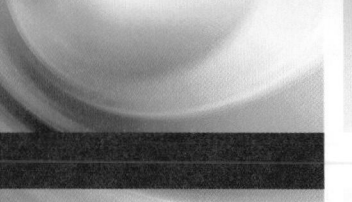

CHAPTER 6

Elbow

The elbow's primary role in the upper limb complex is to help an individual position his or her hand in the appropriate location to perform its function. Once the shoulder has positioned the hand in a gross fashion, the elbow allows for adjustments in height and length of the limb, allowing one to position the hand correctly. In addition, the forearm rotates, in part at the elbow, to place the hand in the most effective position to perform its function.

APPLIED ANATOMY

The elbow consists of a complex set of joints that require careful assessment for proper treatment. The treatment must be geared to the pathology of the condition, because the joint responds poorly to trauma, harsh treatment, or incorrect treatment.

Because they are closely related, the joints of the elbow complex make up a compound synovial joint with injury to any one part affecting the other components as well (Figure 6-1). In addition, the ulnar and humeral articulations "fit" together rather intimately, which does not allow much "give" as compensation when an injury occurs. Thus, this joint often does not respond well to trauma. The elbow articulations are made up of the ulnohumeral joint and the radiohumeral joint. In addition, the complexity and intricate relation of the elbow articulations are further increased by the superior radioulnar joint, which has continuity with the elbow articulations. These three joints make up the **cubital** articulations. The capsule and joint cavity are continuous for all three joints. The combination of these joints allows 2° of freedom at the elbow. The trochlear joint allows 1° of freedom (flexion-extension), and the radiohumeral and superior radioulnar joints allow the other degree of freedom (rotation).

The **ulnohumeral** or **trochlear joint** (see Figure 6-1) is found between the trochlea of the humerus and the trochlear notch of the ulna and is classified as a uniaxial hinge joint. The bones of this joint are shaped so that the axis of movement is not horizontal but instead passes downward and medially, going through an arc of movement. This position leads to the carrying angle at the elbow (Figure 6-2). The resting position of this joint is with the elbow flexed to 70° and the forearm supinated 10°. The neutral position (0°) is midway between supination and pronation in the thumb-up position (Figure 6-3). The capsular pattern is flexion more limited than extension, and the close packed position is extension with the forearm in supination. On full extension, the medial part of the olecranon process is not in contact with the trochlea; on full flexion, the lateral part of the olecranon process is not in contact with the trochlea. This change allows the side-to-side joint play movement necessary for supination and pronation. A small amount of rotation occurs at this joint. In early flexion, 5° of medial rotation occurs; in late flexion, 5° of lateral rotation occurs.

Ulnohumeral (Trochlear) Joint	
Resting position:	70° elbow flexion, 10° supination
Close packed position:	Extension with supination
Capsular pattern:	Flexion, extension

The **radiohumeral joint** is a uniaxial hinge joint between the capitulum of the humerus and the head of the radius (see Figure 6-1). The resting position is with the elbow fully extended and the forearm fully supinated. The close packed position of the joint is with the elbow flexed to 90° and the forearm supinated 5°. As with the trochlear joint, the capsular pattern is flexion more limited than extension.

Radiohumeral Joint	
Resting position:	Full extension and full supination
Close packed position:	Elbow flexed to 90°, forearm supinated to 5°
Capsular pattern:	Flexion, extension, supination, pronation

The ulnohumeral and radiohumeral joints are supported medially by the **ulnar collateral ligament,** a fan-shaped structure, and laterally by the **radial collateral ligament,** a cordlike structure (Figure 6-4).[1] These ligaments, along with the ulnohumeral articulation, are the primary restraints to instability in the elbow.[2] The lateral (radial) collateral ligament is the primary restraint to

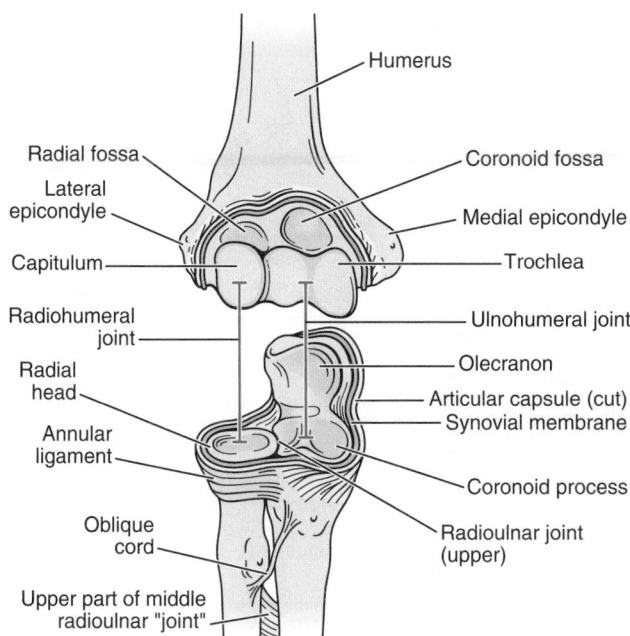

Figure 6-1 Anterior view of the right elbow disarticulated to expose the ulnohumeral and radiohumeral joints. The margin of the proximal radioulnar joint is shown within the elbow's capsule.

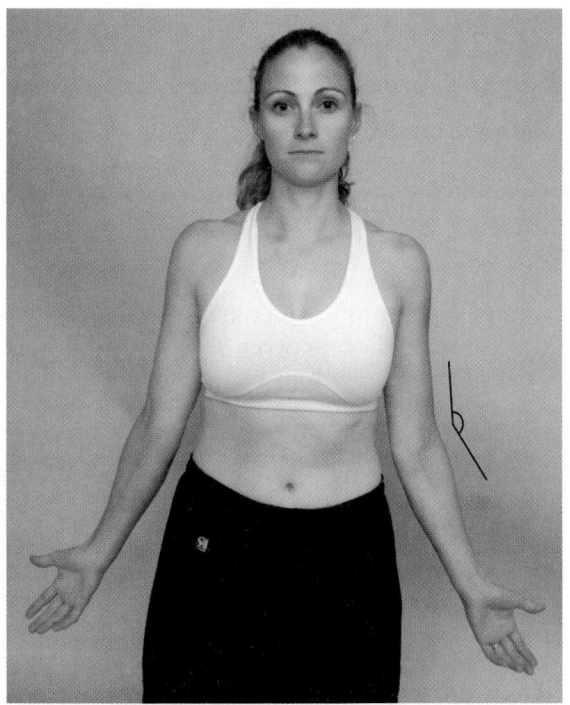

Figure 6-2 Carrying angle of the elbow.

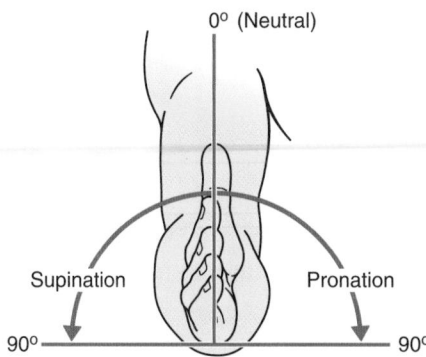

Figure 6-3 "Thumb-up" or neutral (zero) position between supination and pronation.

blow to the area or injury that increases the carrying angle puts an abnormal stress on the nerve as it passes through the tunnel. This can lead to problems such as **tardy ulnar palsy,** the symptoms of which can occur many years after the original injury and may be caused by the "double crush" phenomena of a cubital tunnel problem combined with a cervical spine problem.

The **superior radioulnar joint** is a uniaxial pivot joint. The head of the radius is held in proper relation to the ulna and humerus by the **annular ligament** (see Figures 6-1 and 6-4), which makes up four fifths of the joint.[3] The resting position of this joint is supination of 35° and elbow flexion of 70°. The close packed position is supination of 5°. The capsular pattern of this joint is equal limitation of supination and pronation.

Superior Radioulnar Joint	
Resting position:	35° supination, 70° elbow flexion
Close packed position:	5° supination
Capsular pattern:	Equal limitation of supination and pronation

The three elbow articulations are innervated by branches from the musculocutaneous, median, ulnar, and radial nerves. The **middle radioulnar articulation** is not a true joint but is made up of the radius and ulna and the interosseous membrane between the two bones. The **interosseous membrane** is tense only midway between supination and pronation (neutral position). Although this "joint" is not part of the elbow joint complex, it is affected by injury to the elbow joints; conversely, injury to this area can affect the mechanics of the elbow articulations. The interosseous membrane prevents proximal displacement of the radius on the ulna. The displacement is most likely to occur with pushing movements. The **oblique cord** connects the radius and ulna, running from the lateral side of the **ulnar tuberosity** to the radius slightly below the **radial tuberosity**. Its fibers run at

posterolateral instability (most common instability), whereas the medial (ulnar) collateral ligament is the primary restraint to valgus instability.[2] The ulnar collateral ligament has three parts, which along with the flexor carpi ulnaris muscle form the **cubital tunnel** through which passes the ulnar nerve (see Figure 6-4). Any injury or

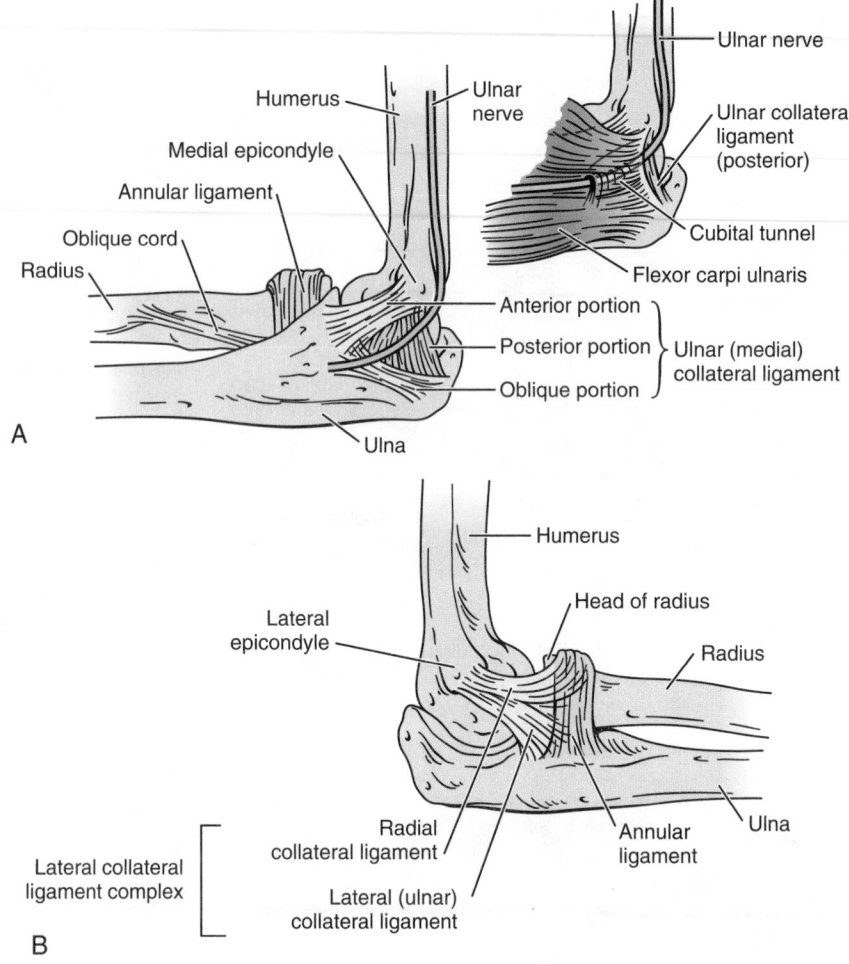

Figure 6-4 Ligaments of the elbow. A, Ligaments on medial side of elbow. Note the passage of the ulnar nerve through the cubital tunnel. **B,** Ligaments on the lateral side of elbow.

right angles to those of the interosseous membrane (see Figure 6-1). The cord assists in preventing displacement of the radius on the ulna, especially during movements involving pulling.

PATIENT HISTORY

In addition to the questions listed under the "Patient History" section in Chapter 1, the examiner should obtain the following information from the patient:

1. *How old is the patient? What is the patient's occupation?* Tennis elbow (lateral epicondylitis) problems usually occur in persons 35 years of age or older and in those who use a great deal of wrist flexion and extension in their occupations or activities, requiring wrist stabilization in slight extension (functional position). If the patient is a child who complains of pain in the elbow and lacks supination on examination, the examiner could suspect a dislocation of the head of the radius. This type of injury is often seen in young children. A parent may give the child a sharp "come-along" tug on the arm, or the child may trip

while the parent is holding the hand, dislocating the head of the radius. Between the ages of 15 and 20, osteochondritis dissecans may be found.[4]

2. *What was the mechanism of injury?* Did the patient experience a fall on out-stretched hand (FOOSH) injury or on the tip of the elbow? Catching oneself from falling (Figure 6-5) or repetitive stress in sports (e.g., throwing) can create a severe valgus force to the elbow causing a medial side traction injury (e.g., sprain of the medial collateral ligament) and a lateral side compression injury. This can lead to injury at the radiohumeral joint, abnormal stress at the medial epicondyle ("little leaguer's elbow"—if from repetitive stress from throwing), and osteochondral damage either on the olecranon process or olecranon fossa. Were any repetitive activities involved? Does the patient's job involve any repetitive activities? Did the patient perform any unusual activities in the previous week? Did the patient feel a "pop" when throwing or doing other activity? If the pop was followed by pain and swelling on the medial side of the elbow, it may indicate an ulnar collateral ligament sprain.[5] A

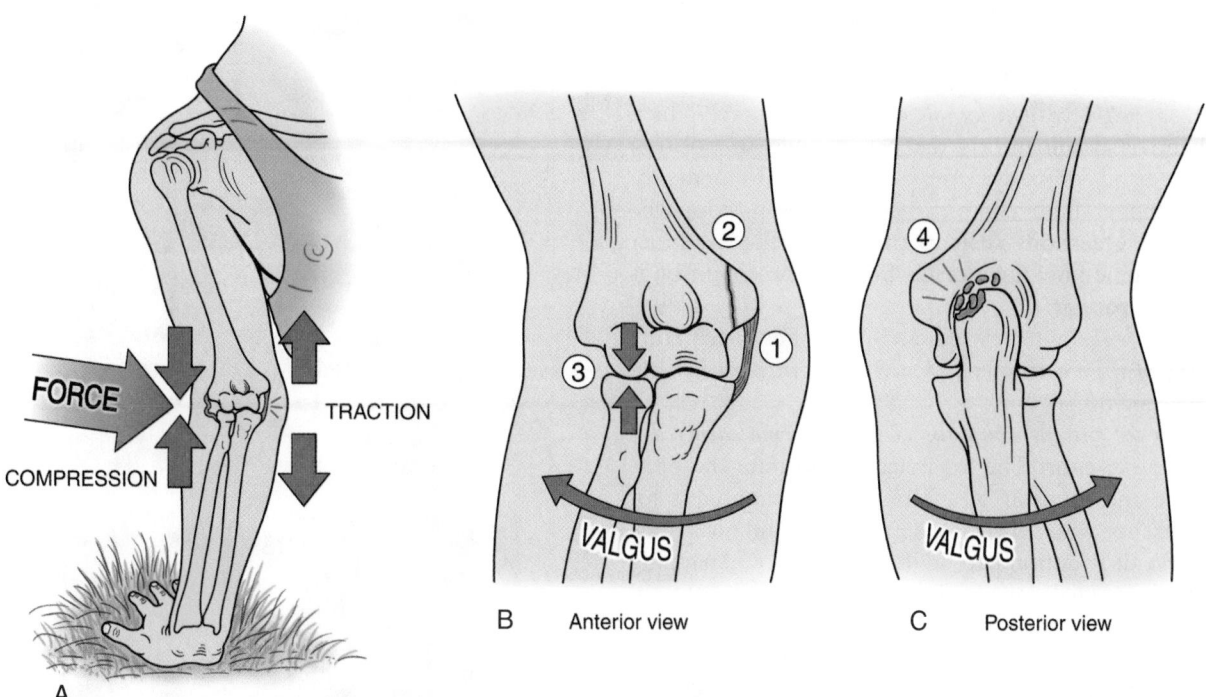

Figure 6-5 Valgus overload to the elbow. (A) Mechanism of injury. **(B)** Anterior view. **(C)** Posterior view. Injury may lead to 1) stretching of medial collateral ligament, 2) stress on epicondylar growth plate (pitcher's or little leaguer's elbow), 3) compression at radiohumeral joint, or 4) compression of the olecranon in the fossa, which may lead to osteophyte and loose body formation.

centralized "pop" and weakness of elbow flexion may be the result of a distal biceps rupture. Such questions help determine the structure injured and the degree of injury.

3. *How long has the patient had the problem? Does the condition come and go? What activities aggravate the problem?* Such questions indicate the seriousness of the condition and how much it bothers the patient.

4. *What are the details of the present pain and other symptoms?* What are the sites and boundaries of the pain? Is the pain radiating, does it ache, and is it worse at night? Aching pain over the lateral epicondyle that radiates may indicate a tennis elbow problem. Depending on the patient's age and past history, the examiner may want to consider referral of pain from the cervical spine or the possibility of a double crush neurological injury. Also, multiple joint diseases (e.g., rheumatoid arthritis, osteoarthritis) must be considered if the patient complains of pain in several joints.

5. *Are there any activities that increase or decrease the pain? Does pulling (traction), twisting (torque), or pushing (compression) alter the pain?* For example, writing, twisting motions of the arm (e.g., turning key, opening door), ironing, gripping, carrying, and leaning on forearm all stress the elbow.[6] Such questions may indicate the tissues being stressed or the tissues injured.

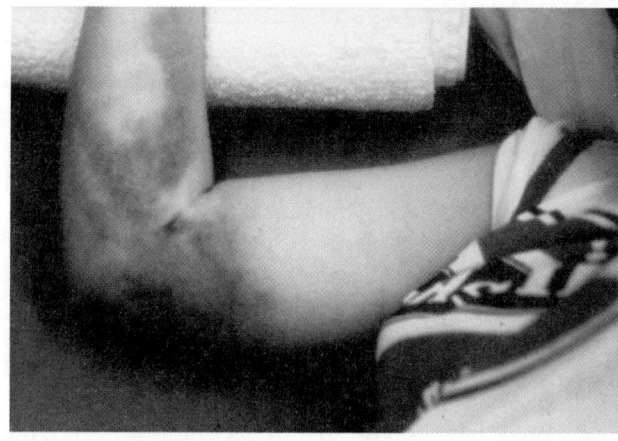

Figure 6-6 Bruising around elbow following dislocation *(now reduced).*

6. *Are there any positions that relieve the pain?* Patients often protectively hold the elbow to the side (in the resting position) and hold the wrist for support, especially in acute conditions.

7. *Is there any indication of deformity, bruising* (Figure 6-6), *wasting, or muscle spasm?*

8. *Are any movements impaired?* Which movements make the patient feel restricted? If flexion or extension is limited, two joints may be involved, the ulnohumeral or the radiohumeral. If supination or pronation is problematic, any one of five joints could

be involved: the radiohumeral, superior radioulnar at the elbow, middle radioulnar, inferior radioulnar, or ulnomeniscocarpal joints at the wrist.

9. *What is the patient unable to do functionally?* Which hand is dominant? Is the patient able to position the hand properly? Are abnormal movements of the upper limb complex necessary to position the hand? Questions such as these help the examiner determine how functionally limiting the condition is to the patient.

10. *What is the patient's usual activity or pastime? Have any of these activities been altered or increased in the past month?*

11. *Does the patient complain of any abnormal nerve distribution pain?* The examiner should note the presence and location of any tingling or numbness for reference when checking dermatomes and peripheral nerve distribution later in the examination. Snapping on the medial side may indicate recurrent dislocation of the ulnar nerve or the medial head of the triceps dislocating over the medial epicondyle.[4]

12. *Does the patient have a history of previous overuse injury or trauma?* This question is especially important in regard to the elbow because the ulnar nerve may be affected by tardy ulnar palsy.

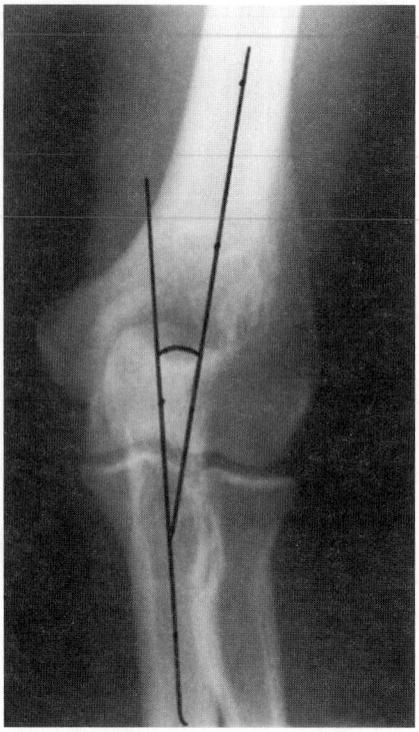

Figure 6-7 Carrying angle. The carrying angle may be determined by noting the angle of intersection between a line connecting midpoints in the distal humerus and a line connecting midpoints in the proximal ulna.

OBSERVATION

The patient must be suitably undressed so that both arms are exposed to allow the examiner to compare the two sides. If the history indicates an insidious onset of elbow problems, the examiner should take the time to observe full body posture, especially the neck and shoulder areas, for possible referral of symptoms.

The examiner first places the patient's arm in the anatomical position to determine whether there is a normal **carrying angle**[7] (see Figure 6-2). It is the angle formed by the long axis of the humerus and the long axis of the ulna and is most evident when the elbow is straight and the forearm is fully supinated (Figure 6-7). In the adult, this would be a slight valgus deviation between the humerus and the ulna when the forearm is supinated and the elbow is extended. In males, the normal carrying angle is 5° to 10°; in females, it is 10° to 15°. If the carrying angle is more than 15°, it is called **cubitus valgus;** if it is less than 5° to 10°, it is called **cubitus varus** (Figure 6-8). Because of the shape of the humeral condyles that articulate with the radius and ulna, the carrying angle changes linearly depending on the degree of extension or flexion. Cubitus valgus is greatest in extension. The angle decreases as the elbow flexes, reaching varus in full flexion.[8] If there has been a fracture or epiphyseal injury to the distal humerus and a cubitus varus results, a **gun stock deformity** may occur in full extension (Figure 6-9, see Figure 6-8).

If swelling exists, all three joints of the elbow complex are affected because they have a common capsule. Joint swelling is often most evident in the triangular space between the radial head, tip of olecranon, and lateral epicondyle (Figure 6-10). Swelling resulting from olecranon bursitis (student's elbow) is more discrete, being more sharply demarcated as a "goose egg" over the olecranon process (Figure 6-11). With swelling, the joint would be held in its resting position, with the elbow held in approximately 70° of flexion, because it is in the resting position that the joint has maximum volume.

The examiner should look for normal bony and soft-tissue contours anteriorly and posteriorly. Often, athletes (such as, pitchers, other throwers, and rodeo riders) have a much larger forearm because of muscle and bone hypertrophy on the dominant side.

The examiner should note whether the patient can assume the normal position of function of the elbow (Figure 6-12). A normal functional position is 90° of flexion with the forearm midway between supination and pronation.[9] The forearm may also be considered to be in a functional position when slightly pronated, as in writing. From this position, forward flexion of the shoulder along with slightly more elbow flexion (up to 120°) enables the person to bring food to the mouth; supination of the forearm decreases the amount of shoulder flexion necessary to accomplish this. At 90° of elbow flexion, the

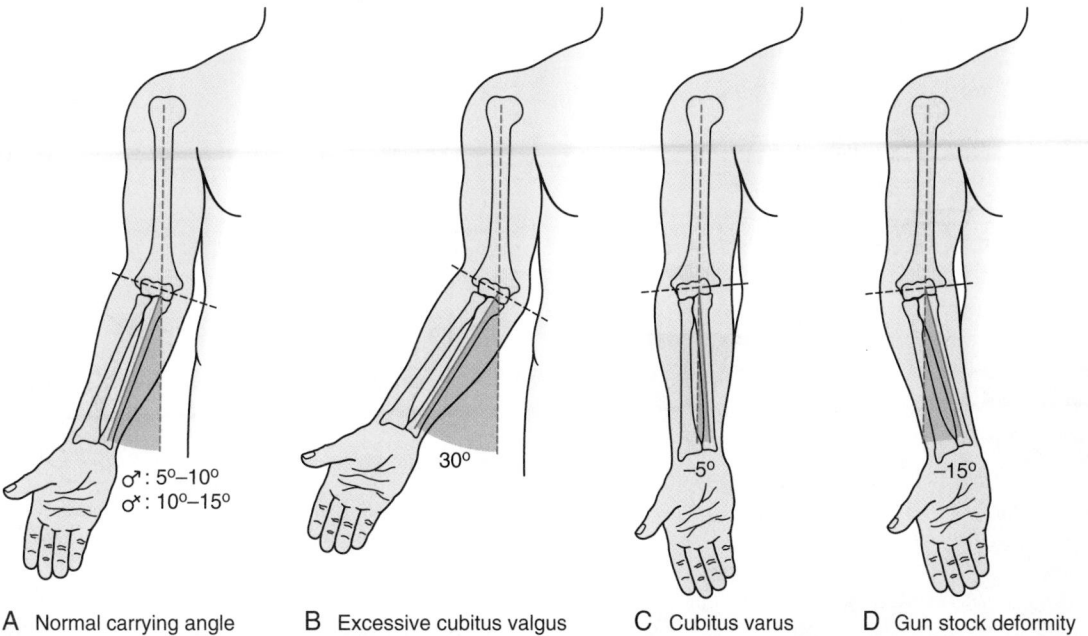

A Normal carrying angle	**B** Excessive cubitus valgus	**C** Cubitus varus	**D** Gun stock deformity

Figure 6-8 A, The elbow's axis of rotation extends slightly, obliquely in a medial-lateral direction through the capitulum and the trochlea. Normal carrying angle of the elbow is shown with the forearm deviated laterally from the longitudinal axis of the humerus axis between 5° and 15°. **B,** Excessive cubitus valgus deformity is shown with the forearm deviated laterally 30°. **C,** Cubitus varus deformity is depicted with the forearm deviated medially −5°. **D,** Gunstock deformity with −15° medial deviation. (**A** to **C,** Redrawn from Neumann DA: Kinesiology of the musculoskeletal system: foundations for physical rehabilitation, St Louis, 2002, Mosby, p. 138.)

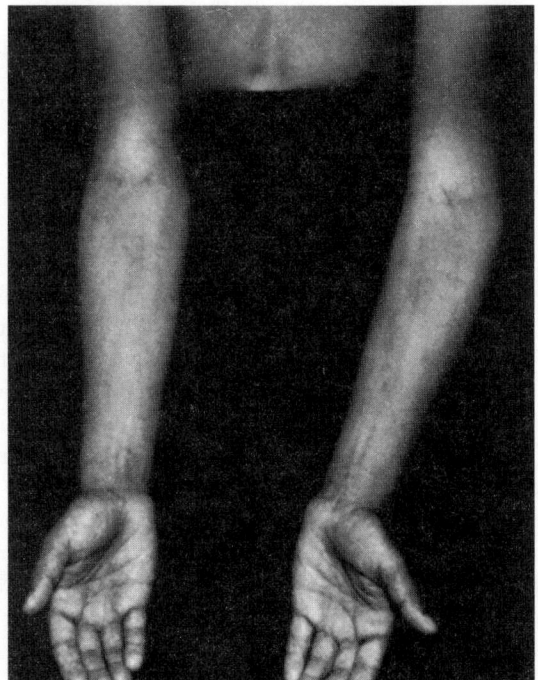

Figure 6-9 Cubitus varus with "gun stock" deformity on the left arm. (From Regan WD, Morrey BF: The physical examination of the elbow. In Morrey BF, editor: The elbow and its disorders, ed 2, Philadelphia, 1993, WB Saunders, p. 74.)

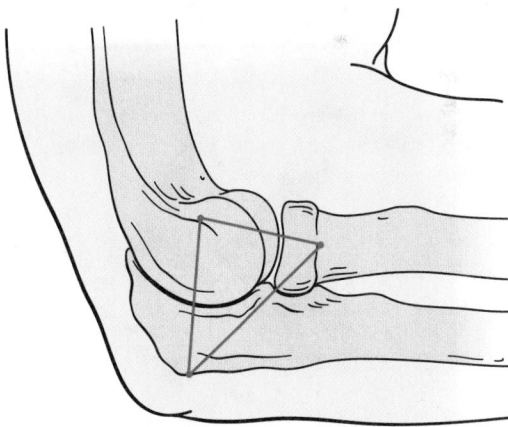

Figure 6-10 The triangular area in which intra-articular swelling is most evident in the elbow.

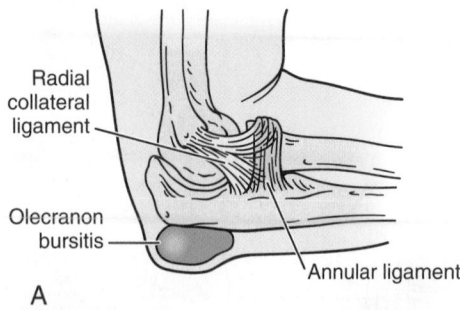

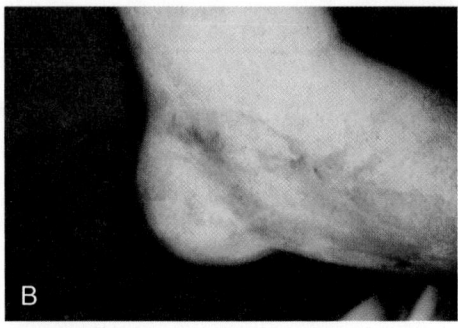

Figure 6-11 A, Olecranon bursitis. **B,** Actual inflamed bursa. The orange color is from disinfectant applied before aspiration.

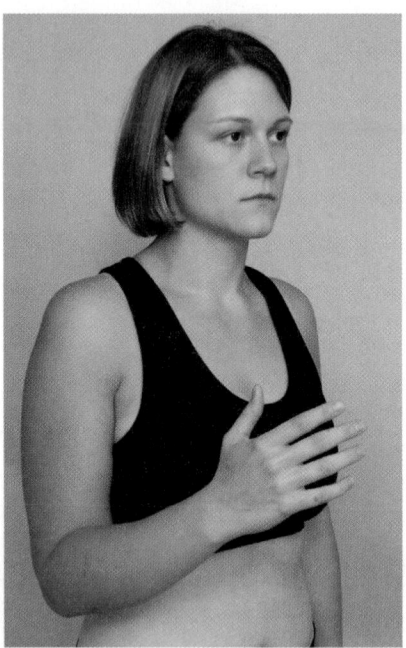

Figure 6-12 Position of most common function of the elbow—90° flexion, midway between supination and pronation.

olecranon process of the ulna and the medial and lateral epicondyles of the humerus normally form an isosceles triangle (Figure 6-13). When the arm is fully extended, the three points normally form a straight line.[10] The isosceles triangle is sometimes called the **triangle sign.** If there is a fracture, dislocation, or degeneration leading to loss of bone or cartilage, the distance between the apex

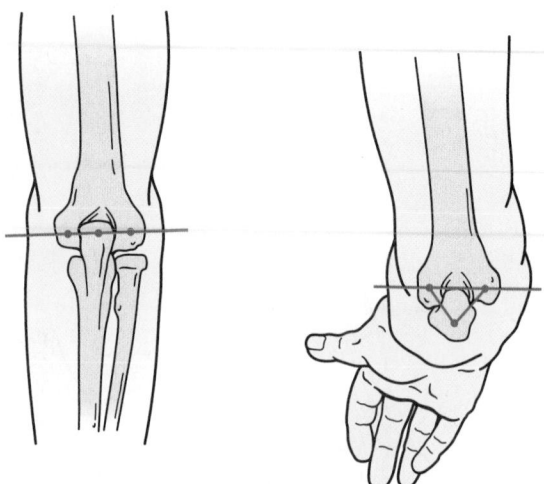

Figure 6-13 Relation of the medial and lateral epicondyles and the olecranon at the elbow in extension *(left)* and flexion *(right)*.

and the base decreases and the isosceles triangle no longer exists. The triangle can be measured on x-ray films.[8]

EXAMINATION

If the history indicates an insidious onset of elbow symptoms, and if the patient has complained of weakness and pain, the examiner may consider performing an examination of the cervical spine, which includes the upper limb peripheral joint scanning examination and myotome testing. Because of the potential referral of symptoms from the cervical spine and the necessity of differentiating nerve root symptoms from peripheral nerve lesions, the consideration of including cervical assessment is essential.

Active Movements

The examination is performed with the patient in the sitting position. As always, active movements are done first, and it is important to remember that the most painful movements are done last. In addition, structures outside the joint may affect range of motion (ROM). For example, with lateral epicondylitis, the long extensors of the forearm are often found to be tight or shortened, so the position of the wrist and fingers may affect movement.

Active Movements of the Elbow Complex

- Flexion of the elbow (140° to 150°)
- Extension of the elbow (0° to 10°)
- Supination of the forearm (90°)
- Pronation of the forearm (80° to 90°)
- Combined movements (if necessary)
- Repetitive movements (if necessary)
- Sustained positions (if necessary)

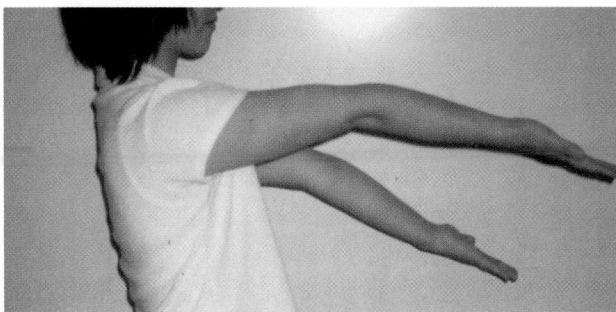

Figure 6-14 Normal elbow hyperextension.

Active elbow flexion is 140° to 150°. Movement is usually stopped by contact of the forearm with the muscles of the arm.

Active elbow extension is 0°, although up to a 10° hyperextension may be exhibited, especially in women. This hyperextension is considered normal if it is equal on both sides and there is no history of trauma. Normally, the movement is arrested by the locking of the olecranon process of the ulna into the olecranon fossa of the humerus. In some cases, under violent compressive loads (e.g., gymnastics, weight lifting), the olecranon process may act as a pivot, resulting in posterior dislocation of the elbow. This mechanism of injury is more likely to occur in someone with elbows that normally hyperextend (Figure 6-14). Loss of elbow extension is a sensitive indicator of intra-articular pathology. It is the first movement lost after injury to the elbow and the first regained with healing. However, terminal flexion loss is more disabling than the same degree of terminal extension loss because of the need of flexion for many activities of daily living (ADLs). Loss of either motion affects the area of reach of the hand, which in turn affects function.

Active supination should be 90° so that the palm faces up. The examiner should ensure that the shoulder is not adducted further in an attempt to give the appearance of increased supination or to compensate for a lack of sufficient supination (Figure 6-15).[11]

For active pronation, the ROM is approximately the same (80° to 90°) so that the palm faces down. The examiner should be sure that the patient does not abduct the shoulder in an attempt to increase the amount of pronation or to compensate for a lack of sufficient pronation.[11] However, for both supination and pronation, only about 75° of movement occurs in the forearm articulations. The remaining 15° is the result of wrist action.

If, in the history, the patient has complained that combined movements, repetitive movements, or sustained positions cause pain, these specific movements should be included in the active movement assessment. If the patient has difficulty or cannot complete a movement, but it is pain free, the examiner must consider a severe injury to the contractile tissue (rupture) or a neurological injury, and further testing is necessary.

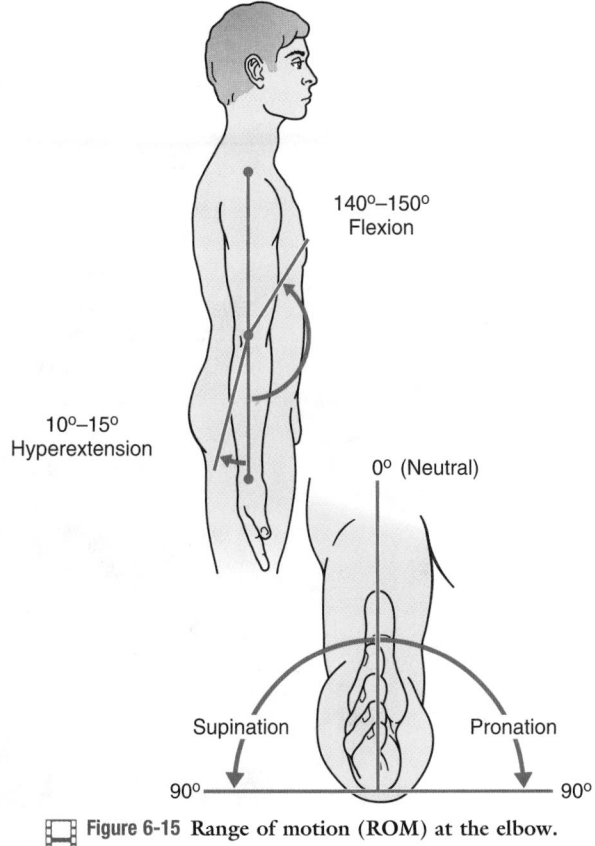

Figure 6-15 Range of motion (ROM) at the elbow.

Passive Movements

If the ROM is full on active movements, overpressure may be gently applied to test the end feel in each direction. If the movement is not full, passive movements should be carried out carefully to test the end feel and to test for a capsular pattern.

Passive Movements of the Elbow Complex and Normal End Feel

- Elbow flexion (tissue approximation)
- Elbow extension (bone-to-bone)
- Forearm supination (tissue stretch)
- Forearm pronation (tissue stretch)

It should be pointed out that although tissue approximation is the normal end feel of elbow flexion, in thin patients the end feel may be bone to bone as a result of the coronoid process hitting in the coronoid fossa. Likewise, in thin individuals, pronation may be bone to bone.

In addition to the end feel tests during passive movements, the examiner should note whether a capsular pattern is present. The capsular pattern for the elbow complex as a whole is more limitation of flexion than extension.

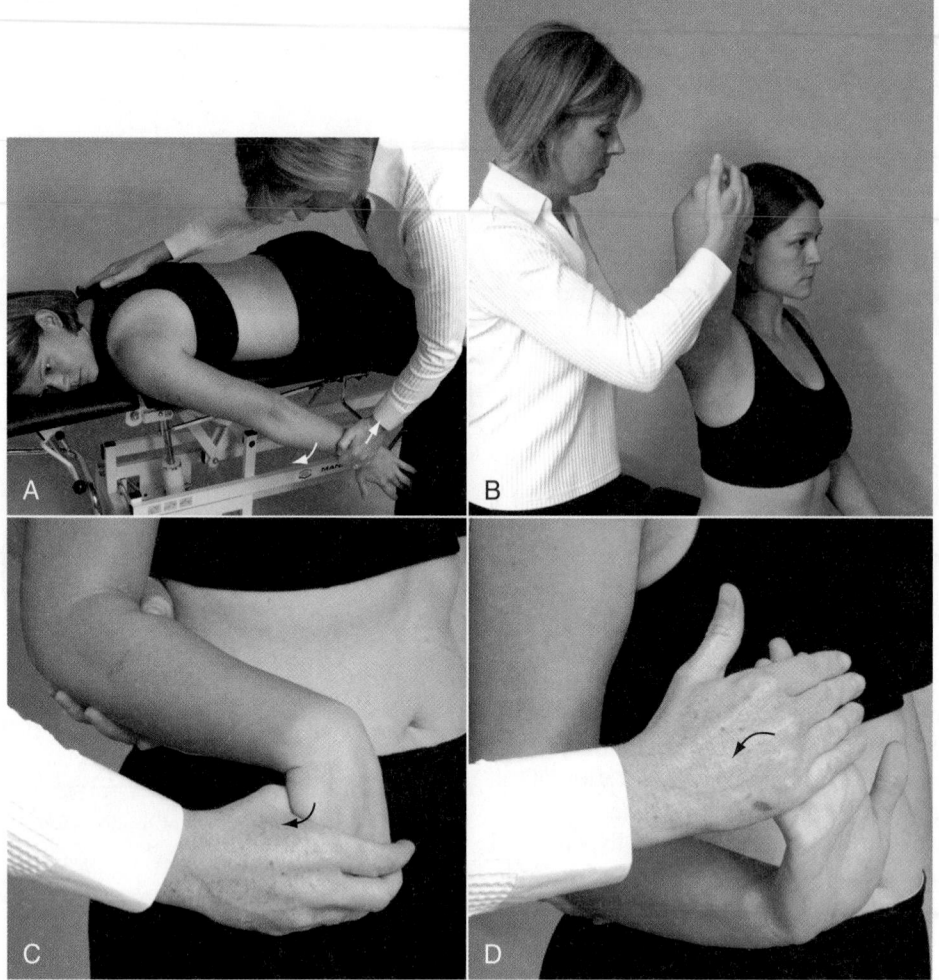

Figure 6-16 Testing length of tight muscles. A, Biceps. **B,** Triceps. **C,** Long wrist extensors. **D,** Long wrist flexors.

In some cases, the examiner may want to determine whether muscles crossing the elbow are tight. If the muscles are tight, the end feel will be a muscle stretch, and ROM at one of the joints that the muscle passes over will be restricted (usually the joint that is the last to be stretched). If the muscle is normal, the end feel will be the normal joint tissue stretch end feel and the ROM will be normal. To test biceps length (Figure 6-16, *A*), the patient is placed in supine with the shoulder to be tested off the edge of the bed. The shoulder is passively extended to end range and then the elbow is extended.[12] Normally, elbow extension should be the same as that seen with active movement.

To test triceps length (Figure 6-16, *B*), the patient is placed in sitting. The examiner passively forward flexes the arm to full elevation while the elbow is in extension. The elbow is then passively flexed.[9] Normally, elbow flexion should be similar to that seen with active movement.

To test the length of the long wrist extensors (as one would want to do with lateral epicondylitis), the patient is placed in supine lying with the elbow extended (Figure 6-16, *C*). The examiner passively flexes the fingers and then flexes the wrist.[12] Normally, wrist flexion and finger flexion should be the same as found with active movement.

To test the length of the long wrist flexors (Figure 6-16, *D*), the patient is placed in supine lying with the elbow extended. The examiner passively extends the fingers and then the wrist.[12] Normally, wrist extension and finger extension should be the same as that found with active movement.

Resisted Isometric Movements

For proper testing of the muscles of the elbow complex, the movement must be resisted and isometric. Muscle flexion power around the elbow is greatest in the range of 90° to 110° with the forearm supinated. At 45° and 135°, flexion power is only 75% of maximum.[9] Isometrically, research shows that men are two times stronger than women at the elbow; extension is 60% of flexion, and pronation is about 85% of supination.[13] To perform the resisted isometric tests, the patient is seated (Figure 6-17).

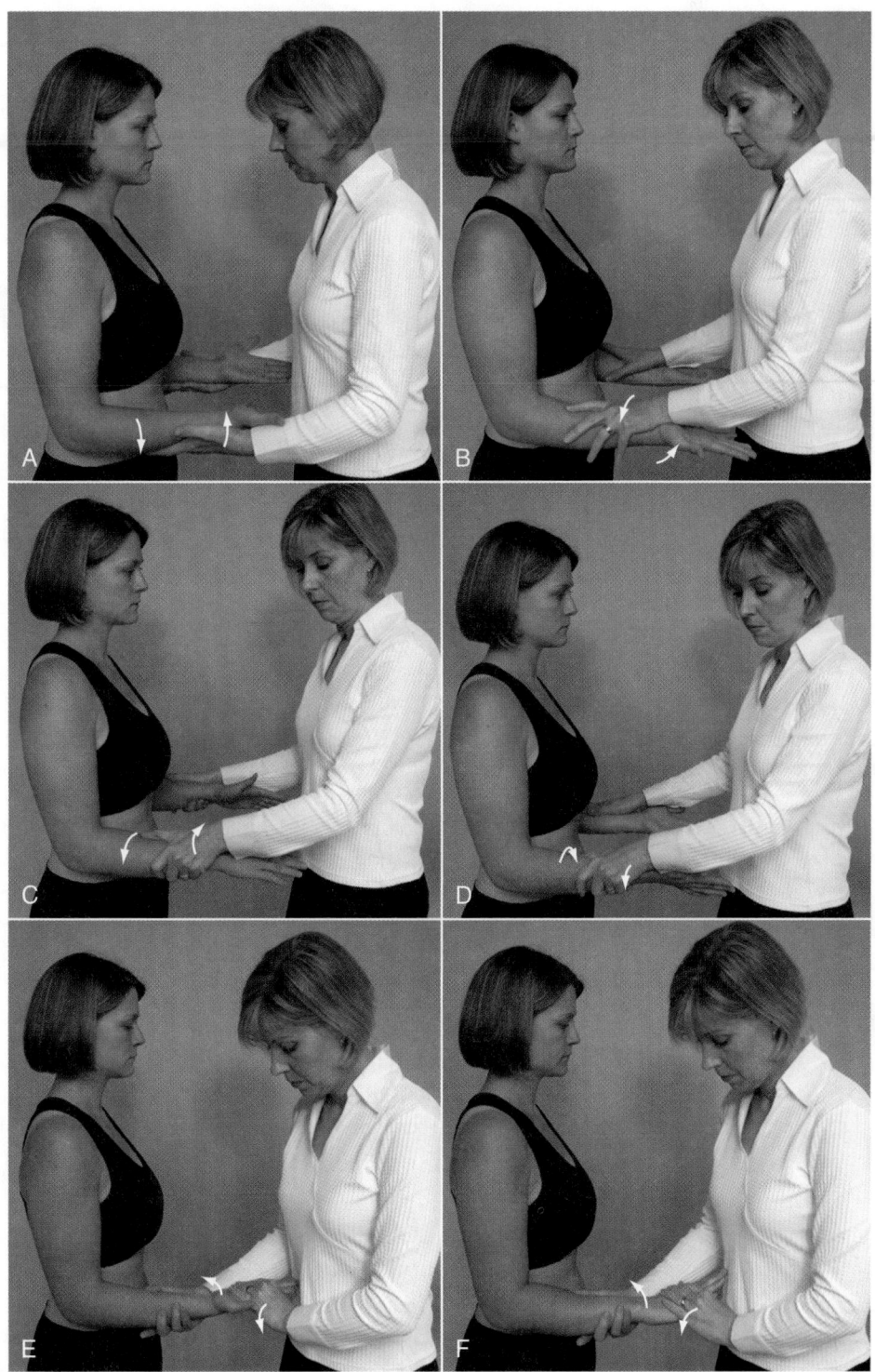

Figure 6-17 **Positioning for resisted isometric movements. A,** Elbow extension. **B,** Elbow flexion. **C,** Forearm supination. **D,** Forearm prona-tion. **E,** Wrist flexion. **F,** Wrist extension.

TABLE **6-1**

Muscles about the Elbow: Their Actions, Nerve Supply, and Nerve Root Derivation

Action	Muscles Acting	Nerve Supply	Nerve Root Derivation
Flexion of elbow	1. Brachialis	Musculocutaneous	C5, C6, (C7)
	2. Biceps brachii	Musculocutaneous	C5, C6
	3. Brachioradialis	Radial	C5, C6, (C7)
	4. Pronator teres	Median	C6, C7
	5. Flexor carpi ulnaris	Ulnar	C7, C8
Extension of elbow	1. Triceps	Radial	C6–C8
	2. Anconeus	Radial	C7, C8, (T1)
Supination of forearm	1. Supinator	Posterior interosseous (radial)	C5, C6
	2. Biceps brachii	Musculocutaneous	C5, C6
Pronation of forearm	1. Pronator quadratus	Anterior interosseous (median)	C8, T1
	2. Pronator teres	Median	C6, C7
	3. Flexor carpi radialis	Median	C6, C7
Flexion of wrist	1. Flexor carpi radialis	Median	C6, C7
	2. Flexor carpi ulnaris	Ulnar	C7, C8
Extension of wrist	1. Extensor carpi radialis longus	Radial	C6, C7
	2. Extensor carpi radialis brevis	Posterior interosseous (radial)	C7, C8
	3. Extensor carpi ulnaris	Posterior interosseous (radial)	C7, C8

If the examiner finds that a particular movement or movements cause pain, Table 6-1 can be used to help differentiate the cause. Carrying out wrist extension and flexion is also necessary, because a large number of muscles act over the wrist as well as the elbow.

Resisted Isometric Movements of the Elbow Complex

- Elbow flexion
- Elbow extension
- Supination
- Pronation
- Wrist flexion
- Wrist extension

If, in the history, the patient has complained that combined movements under load, repetitive movements under load, or sustained positions under load cause pain, the examiner should carefully examine these resisted isometric movements and positions as well, but only after the basic movements have been tested isometrically. For example, the biceps is a strong supinator and flexor of the elbow, but its ability to generate force depends on the position of the elbow. The biceps play a greater role in elbow flexion when the forearm is supinated than when it is pronated. At 90° of elbow flexion, biceps makes its greatest contribution to supination.[14] If the history indicates that concentric, eccentric, or econcentric movements have caused symptoms, these movements should also be tested with load or no load, as required.

If the resisted isometric contraction is weak and pain free, the examiner must consider a major injury to the contractile tissue (third-degree strain) or neurological injury. For example, weakness of elbow flexion and supination may occur with a rupture of the distal biceps tendon, especially if these findings follow a sudden sharp pain in the antecubital fossa when an extension force is applied to the flexing elbow.[14] If there is no history of trauma, the most likely cause is neurological, either a nerve root or peripheral nerve lesion. By selectively testing the muscles and sensory distribution (Table 6-2) and by having a knowledge of nerve compression sites (see the "Reflexes and Cutaneous Distribution" section), the examiner should be able to determine the neurological tissue injured and where the injury has occurred.

Functional Assessment

When assessing the elbow, it is important to remember that the elbow is the middle portion of an integral upper limb kinetic chain. It allows the hand to be positioned in space, helps stabilize the upper extremity for power and detailed work activities, and provides power to the arm for lifting activities.[15] Motion in the elbow allows the hand to be positioned so that daily functions can be performed easily. Thus, functionally, the elbow is often one part of a functional assessment that may also involve the shoulder and/or hand. This is especially true for athletes who put several joints in the kinetic chain under stress at the same time. For example, the Kerlan-Jobe Orthopaedic Clinic (KJOC) shoulder and elbow score (Figure 6-18) is a function score that is designed to look

TABLE **6-2**

Nerve Injuries About the Elbow

Nerve	Motor Loss	Sensory Loss	Functional Loss
Median nerve (C6 to C8,T1)	Pronator teres Flexor carpi radialis Palmaris longus Flexor digitorum superficialis Flexor pollicis longus Lateral half of flexor digitorum profundus Pronator quadratus Thenar eminence Lateral two lumbricals	Palmar aspect of hand with thumb, index, middle, and lateral half of ring finger Dorsal aspect of distal third of index, middle, and lateral half of ring finger	Pronation weak or lost Weak wrist flexion and abduction Radial deviation at wrist lost Inability to oppose or flex thumb Weak thumb abduction Weak grip Weak or no pinch (ape hand deformity)
Anterior interosseous nerve (branch of median nerve)	Flexor pollicis longus Lateral half of flexor digitorum profundus Pronator quadratus Thenar eminence Lateral two lumbricals	None	Pronation weak especially at 90° elbow flexion Weak opposition and flexion of thumb Weak finger flexion Weak pinch (no tip-to-tip)
Ulnar nerve (C7 to C8,T1)	Flexor carpi ulnaris Medial half of flexor digitorum profundus Palmaris brevis Hypothenar eminence Adductor pollicis Medial two lumbricals All interossei	Dorsal and palmar aspect of little and medial half of ring finger	Weak wrist flexion Loss of ulnar deviation at wrist Loss of distal flexion of little finger Loss of abduction and adduction of fingers Inability to extend second and third phalanges of little and ring fingers (benediction hand deformity) Loss of thumb adduction
Radial nerve (C5 to C8,T1)	Anconeus Brachioradialis Extensor carpi radialis longus and brevis Extensor digitorum Extensor pollicis longus and brevis Abductor pollicis longus Extensor carpi ulnaris Extensor indices Extensor digiti minimi	Dorsum of hand (lateral two-thirds) Dorsum and lateral aspect of thumb Proximal two-thirds of dorsum of index, middle, and half ring finger	Loss of supination Loss of wrist extension (wrist drop) Inability to grasp Inability to stabilize wrist Loss of finger extension Inability to abduct thumb
Posterior interosseous nerve (branch of radial nerve)	Extensor carpi radialis brevis Extensor digitorum Extensor pollicis longus and brevis Abductor pollicis longus Extensor carpi ulnaris Extensor indices Extensor digiti minimi	None	Weak wrist extension Weak finger extension Difficulty stabilizing wrist Difficulty with grasp Inability to abduct thumb

Kerlan-Jobe Orthopedic Clinic Shoulder & Elbow Score

Name _____ Age _____ Sex _____ Dominant Hand (R) _____ (L) _____ (Ambidextrous)

_____ Date of Examination _____ Sport _____ Position _____ Years Played _____

Please answer the following questions related to your history of injuries to **YOUR ARM ONLY:**

	YES	NO
1. Is your arm currently injured?	☐	☐
2. Are you currently active in your sport?	☐	☐
3. Have you missed game or practice time in the last year due to an injury to your shoulder or elbow?	☐	☐
4. Have you been diagnosed with an injury to your shoulder or elbow other than a strain or sprain? If yes, what was the diagnosis? _____	☐	☐
5. Have you received treatment for an injury to your shoulder or elbow? If yes, what was the treatment? (Check all that apply) ☐ Rest ☐ Therapy ☐ Surgery (please describe): _____	☐	☐

Please describe your level of competition in your current sport:

(Use Professional Major League, Professional Minor League, Intercollegiate, High School as the choices)

6. What is the highest level of competition you've participated at? _____

7. What is your current level of competition? _____

8. If your current level of competition is not the same as your highest level, do you feel it is due to an injury to your arm?	☐	☐

Please check the **ONE category only** that best describes your current status:

☐ Playing without any arm trouble ☐ Playing, but with arm trouble
☐ Not playing due to arm trouble

Instructions to athletes:

The following questions concern your physical functioning during game and practice conditions. Unless otherwise specified, all questions relate to your **shoulder or elbow.** Please answer with an X along the horizontal line that corresponds to your current level.

1. How difficult is it for you to get loose or warm prior to competition or practice?

●━━━━━━━━━━━━━━━━━━━━━━●

Naver feel loose during   Normal warm-up
games or practice   time

2. How much pain do you experience in your shoulder or elbow?

●━━━━━━━━━━━━━━━━━━━━━━●

Pain at rest   No pain with
competition

3. How much weakness and/or fatigue (i.e., loss of strength) do you experience in your shoulder or elbow?

●━━━━━━━━━━━━━━━━━━━━━━●

Weakness or   No weakness, normal
fatigue preventing   competition fatigue
any competition

4. How unstable does your shoulder or elbow feel during competition?

●━━━━━━━━━━━━━━━━━━━━━━●

"Popping out"   No instability
routinely

Figure 6-18 Kerlan-Jobe Orthopedic Clinic (KJOC) shoulder and elbow score. (From Alberta FG, et al: The development and validation of a functional assessment tool for the upper extremity in the overhead athlete. Am J Sports Med 38:906–907, 2010.)

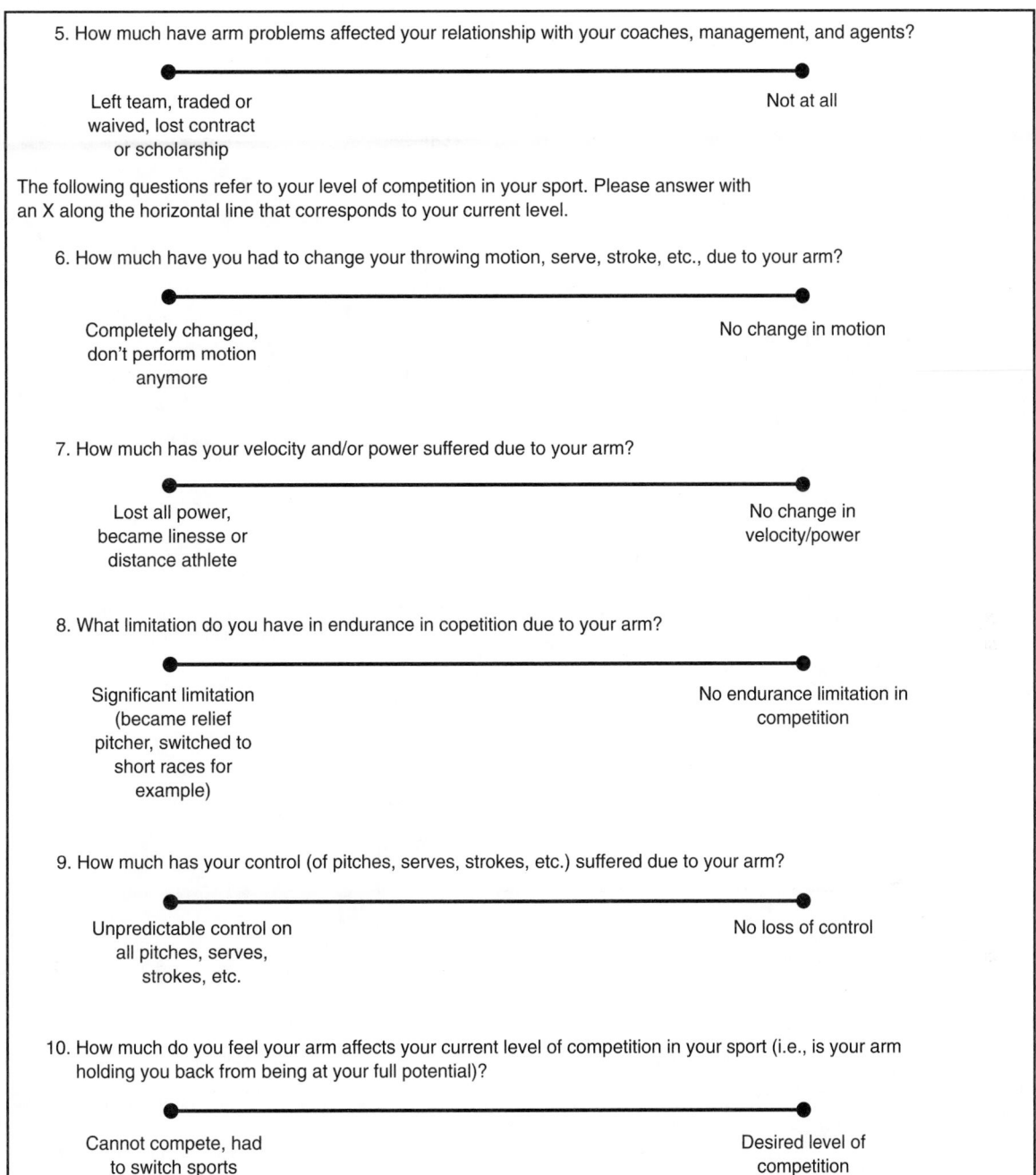

5. How much have arm problems affected your relationship with your coaches, management, and agents?

Left team, traded or
waived, lost contract
or scholarship

Not at all

The following questions refer to your level of competition in your sport. Please answer with an X along the horizontal line that corresponds to your current level.

6. How much have you had to change your throwing motion, serve, stroke, etc., due to your arm?

Completely changed,
don't perform motion
anymore

No change in motion

7. How much has your velocity and/or power suffered due to your arm?

Lost all power,
became linesse or
distance athlete

No change in
velocity/power

8. What limitation do you have in endurance in copetition due to your arm?

Significant limitation
(became relief
pitcher, switched to
short races for
example)

No endurance limitation in
competition

9. How much has your control (of pitches, serves, strokes, etc.) suffered due to your arm?

Unpredictable control on
all pitches, serves,
strokes, etc.

No loss of control

10. How much do you feel your arm affects your current level of competition in your sport (i.e., is your arm holding you back from being at your full potential)?

Cannot compete, had
to switch sports

Desired level of
competition

Figure 6-18, cont'd

at a functional outcome score involving the shoulder and elbow in overhead athletes.[16,17]

The full range of elbow movements is not necessary to perform these activities; most ADLs are performed at between 30° and 130° of flexion and between 50° of pronation and 50° of supination (Figures 6-19 and 6-20). To reach the head, approximately 140° of flexion is needed. The activities of combing or washing the hair, reaching a back zipper, and walking with crutches require a greater ROM. Activities, such as pouring fluid, drinking from a container, cutting with a knife, reading a newspaper, and using a screwdriver, require an adequate range of supination and pronation. Figures 6-21 and 6-22 show the ROM or arc of movement necessary to do certain activities or the ROM needed to touch parts of the body. Examiners must remember that elbow injuries may preclude lifting objects as light as a cup of coffee, owing to lifting mechanics. Because of the length of the lever arm of the forearm when the elbow is at 90°, loads at the hand are magnified tenfold at the elbow.[18] Figure 6-23 is a numerical scoring assessment form that can be used to assess the elbow and includes an important functional component. Table 6-3 demonstrates functional tests of strength for the elbow.

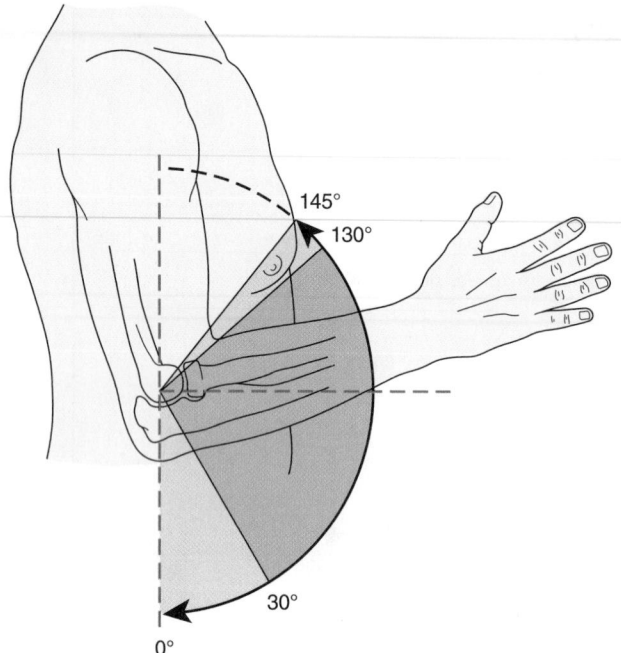

Figure 6-19 Normal range of elbow flexion is approximately 0° to 145°. However, the functional arc of motion is somewhat less, and most activities can be performed with flexion of 30° to 130°. (Redrawn from Regan WD, Morrey BF: The physical examination of the elbow. In Morrey BF, editor: The elbow and its disorders, ed 2, Philadelphia, 1993, WB Saunders, p. 81.)

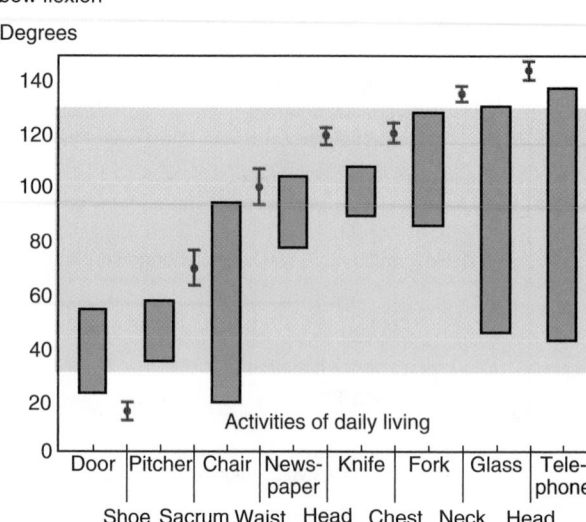

Figure 6-21 The arc and position of elbow flexion required to accomplish fifteen daily activities. Most of these activities are accomplished within a flexion range of 30° to 130°. (Modified from Morrey BF, Askew LJ, Chao EY: A biomechanical study of normal functional elbow motion. J Bone Joint Surg Am 63:873, 1981.)

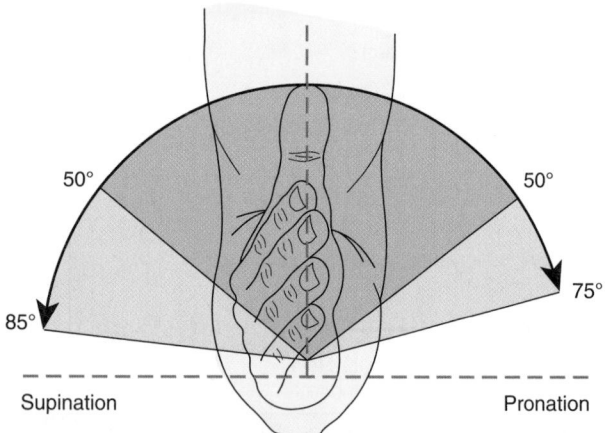

Figure 6-20 Pronation and supination motions average 75° and 85°, respectively. Most activities of daily living (ADLs), however, can be accomplished with 50° of each motion. (Redrawn from Regan WD, Morrey BF: The physical examination of the elbow. In Morrey BF, editor: The elbow and its disorders, ed 2, Philadelphia, 1993, WB Saunders, p. 81.)

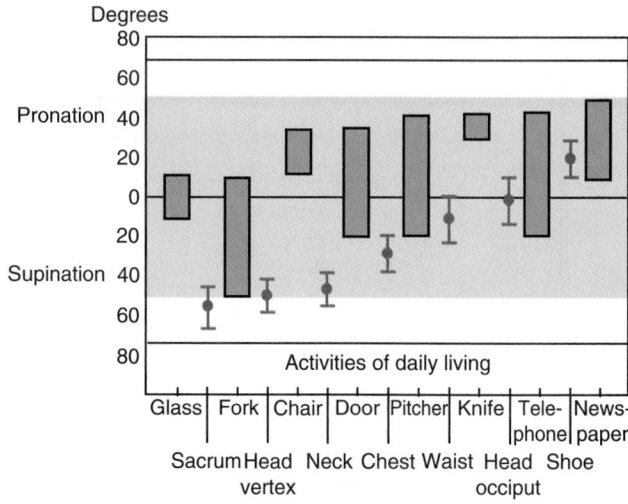

Figure 6-22 Fifteen activities of daily living (ADLs) accomplished with pronation and supination of up to 50° each. (Modified from Morrey BF, Askew LJ, Chao EY: A biomechanical study of normal functional elbow motion. J Bone Joint Surg Am 63:874, 1981.)

Special Tests

An examiner should perform only those special tests that have relevance or will help to confirm the diagnosis. If the history has not indicated any trauma or repetitive movement that could be associated with problems, the examiner, depending on the age of the patient, may want to include some of the nerve root compression tests (see Chapter 3) to rule out the possibility of referred symptoms from the cervical spine or the possibility of a "double crush" injury.

For the reader who would like to review them, the reliability, validity, specificity, sensitivity, and odds ratios of some of the special tests used in the elbow joint are available on the Evolve website.

Elbow Evaluation

Name: _____ UH#: _____ Elbow: R/L

Procedure: _____ Date: _____ Dominant: R/L

Date of Exam (month/day/year)	/ /	/ /	/ /	/ /	/ /
Pain (maximum points) 5 = none (30); 4 = slight—with continuous activity, no medication (25); 3 = moderate—with occasional activity, some medication (15); 2 = moderately severe—much pain, frequent medication (10); 1 = severe—constant pain, markedly limited activity (5); 0 = complete disability (0)	_____ ( )				
Motion degrees (37 points maximum) Extension (8 pts max) Flexion (17 pts max) Pronation/Supination (pt) = 0.1 per degree—6 maximum	Extension _____°( ) Flexion _____°( ) Pronation _____°( ) Supination _____°( )				
Strength (15 points maximum) 5 = normal; 4 = good; 3 = fair; 2 = poor; 1 = trace; 0 = paralysis; NA = not available Flex. Ext. Pro. Sup. Normal 5 (5) (4) (3) (3) Good 4 (4) (3) (2) (2) Fair 3 (3) (2) (1) (1) Poor 2 (2) (1) (0) (0) Trace 1 (1) (0) (0) (0) None 0 (0) (0) (0) (0)	Extension _____( ) Flexion _____( ) Pronation _____( ) Supination _____( )				
Instability (6 points maximum) Ant./Post. Med./Lat. None 3 3 Mild <5 mm, <5° 2 2 Moderate <10 mm, <10° 1 1 Severe >10 mm, >10° 0 0	Ant./Post. _____ Med./Lat. _____				
Function (12 points maximum) 4 = normal (1); 3 = mild compromise (0.75); 2 = difficulty (0.5); 1 = with aid (0.25); 0 = unable (0); NA = not applicable (Index—multiply × 0.25) 1. Use back pocket 2. Rise from chair 3. Perineal care 4. Wash opposite axilla 5. Eat with utensil 6. Comb hair 7. Carry 10–15 pounds with arm at side 8. Dress 9. Pulling 10. Throwing 11. Do usual work Specify work: 12. Do usual sport Specify sport:	_____( ) _____( ) _____( ) _____( ) _____( ) _____( ) _____( ) _____( ) _____( ) _____( ) _____( ) _____( )				
Patient Response 3 = much better; 2 = better; 1 = same; 0 = worse; NA = not available/not applicable	_____				
Completed By: Name of Examiner					
Index Key: 95–100 = excellent; 80–95 = good; 50–80 = fair; <50 = poor	( )	( )	( )	( )	( )

Figure 6-23 Clinical elbow evaluation form that provides objective data and grading as well as functional information. The use of such a rating index in the clinical setting provides an objective means of comparing different treatment options. (From Morrey BF, et al: Functional evaluation of the elbow. In Morrey BF, editor: The elbow and its disorders, Philadelphia, 1985, WB Saunders, pp. 88–89. Copyright Mayo Clinic Foundation, Rochester, MN.)

TABLE **6-3**

Functional Testing of the Elbow

Starting Position	Action	Functional Test*
Sitting	Bring hand to mouth lifting weight (elbow flexion)	Lift 2.3 kg to 2.7 kg: Functional Lift 1.4 kg to 1.8 kg: Functionally fair Lift 0.5 kg to 0.9 kg: Functionally poor Lift 0 kg: Nonfunctional
Standing 90 cm from wall, leaning against wall	Push arms straight (elbow extension)	5 to 6 Repetitions: Functional 3 to 4 Repetitions: Functionally fair 1 to 2 Repetitions: Functionally poor 0 Repetitions: Nonfunctional
Standing, facing closed door	Open door starting with palm down (supination of arm)	5 to 6 Repetitions: Functional 3 to 4 Repetitions: Functionally fair 1 to 2 Repetitions: Functionally poor 0 Repetitions: Nonfunctional
Standing, facing closed door	Open door starting with palm up (pronation of arm)	5 to 6 Repetitions: Functional 3 to 4 Repetitions: Functionally fair 1 to 2 Repetitions: Functionally poor 0 Repetitions: Nonfunctional

Data from Palmer ML, Epler M: Clinical assessment procedures in physical therapy, Philadelphia, 1990, JB Lippincott, pp. 109–111.
*Younger patients should be able to lift more (2.7 kg to 4.5 kg) more often (6 to 10 repetitions). With age, weight and repetitions decrease.

Key Tests Performed at the Elbow Depending on Suspected Pathology*[19,20]

- *For ligamentous instability:*
  - Lateral pivot shift test of the elbow
  - Ligamentous valgus instability test
  - Ligamentous varus instability test
  - Milking maneuver
  - Moving valgus stress test
- *For biceps rupture (third-degree strain):*
  - Hook (distal biceps) test
  - Popeye sign (proximal long head of biceps) (see Chapter 5)
- *For lateral epicondylitis (epicondylalgia):*
  - Cozen's test
  - Mill's test
- *For plica:*
  - Extension-supination plica test
  - Flexion-pronation plica test
- *For posterior impingement:*
  - Arm bar test
  - Extension impingement test
- *For neurological dysfunction:*
  - Elbow flexion test (ulnar nerve)
  - Pinch grip test (anterior interosseous branch of median nerve)
  - Tinel sign at elbow (ulnar nerve)

*The author recommends these key tests be learned by the clinician to facilitate a diagnosis. See Chapter 1, p. 55, Key for Classifying Special Tests.

Tests for Ligamentous Instability

These tests are designed to test for valgus and varus instability in the elbow.

Lateral Pivot Shift Test of the Elbow.[2,21] The patient lies supine with the arm to be tested overhead. The examiner grasps the patient's wrist and forearm with the elbow extended and the forearm fully supinated.[22] The patient's elbow is then flexed while a valgus stress and axial compression is applied to the elbow while maintaining supination. This causes the radius (and ulna) to sublux off the humerus leading to a prominent radial head posterolaterally and a dimple between the radial head and capitellum (Figure 6-24, *A*).[2,22] If the examiner continues flexing the elbow, at about 40° to 70°, there is a sudden reduction (clunk) of the joint, which can be palpated and seen (Figure 6-24, *B*).[23] If the patient is unconscious, subluxation and a clunk on reduction when the elbow is extended may occur, but these symptoms seldom present in the conscious patient.

Ligamentous Valgus Instability Test. To test for valgus instability, the patient's arm is stabilized with one of the examiner's hands at the elbow and the other hand placed above the patient's wrist. An abduction or valgus force at the distal forearm is applied to test the medial collateral ligament (valgus instability) while the ligament is palpated (Figure 6-25, *B*).[2] Regan and Morrey advocate doing the valgus stress test with the humerus in full lateral rotation.[18] The examiner should note any laxity, decreased mobility, or altered pain that may be present compared with the uninvolved elbow.

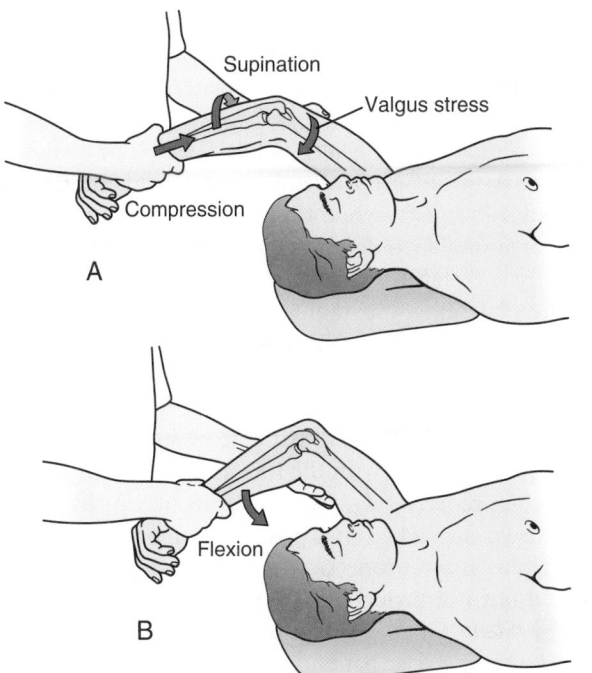

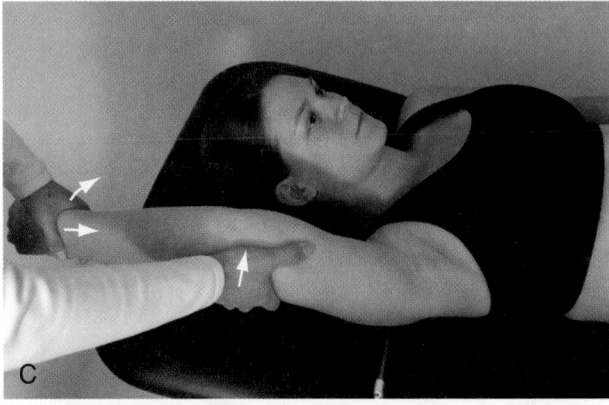

Figure 6-24 **Posterolateral pivot-shift apprehension test of the elbow. A,** The patient lies supine with the arm overhead. A mild supination force is applied to the forearm at the wrist. The patient's elbow is then flexed while a valgus stress and compression is applied to the elbow. **B,** If the examiner continues flexing the elbow at about 40° to 70°, subluxation and a clunk on reduction when the elbow is extended may occur, but usually only in the unconscious patient. **C,** Actual test with elbow positioned to resemble knee.

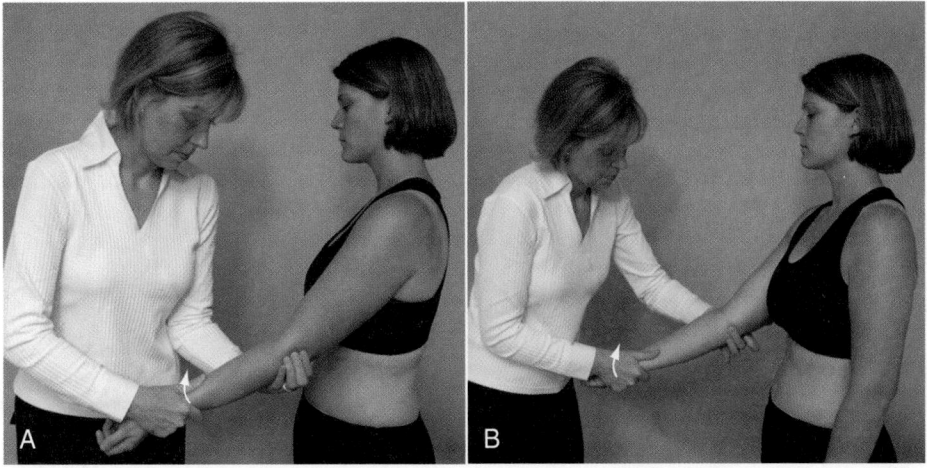

Figure 6-25 **Testing the collateral ligaments of the elbow. A,** Lateral collateral ligament. **B,** Medial collateral ligament.

✓ *Ligamentous Varus Instability Test.* With the patient's elbow slightly flexed (20° to 30°) and stabilized with the examiner's hand, an adduction or varus force is applied by the examiner to the distal forearm to test the lateral collateral ligament (varus instability) while the ligament is palpated (Figure 6-25, *A*). Normally, the examiner feels the ligament tense when stress is applied. Regan and Morrey advocated doing the varus stress test with the humerus in full medial rotation.[18] The examiner applies the force several times with increasing pressure while noting any alteration in pain or ROM. If excessive laxity

is found when doing the test or a soft end feel is felt, it indicates injury to the ligament (1°, 2°, or 3° sprain) and may, especially with a 3° sprain, indicate posterolateral joint instability. Posterolateral elbow instability is the most common pattern of elbow instability in which there is displacement of the ulna (accompanied by the radius) on the humerus, so the ulna supinates or laterally rotates away from or off the trochlea.[21]

⚠ *Milking Maneuver.*[2] The patient sits with the elbow flexed to 90° or more and the forearm supinated. The examiner grasps the patient's thumb under the forearm and pulls it imparting a valgus stress to the elbow (Figure 6-26). Reproduction of symptoms indicates a positive test and a partial tear of the medial collateral ligament.

☑ *Moving Valgus Stress Test.*[2,24] The patient lies supine or stands with the arm abducted and elbow flexed fully. While maintaining a valgus stress, the examiner quickly extends the patient's elbow. Reproduction of the patient's pain between 120° to 70° indicates a positive test and a partial tear of the medial collateral ligament (Figure 6-27).

❓ *Posterolateral Rotary Apprehension Test.*[2,21–23,25,26] The patient lies supine with the arm to be tested overhead. The elbow is supinated at the wrist, and a valgus stress is applied to the elbow while the examiner flexes the elbow. This movement (between 20° and 30° flexion) and stress cause the patient to be apprehensive that the

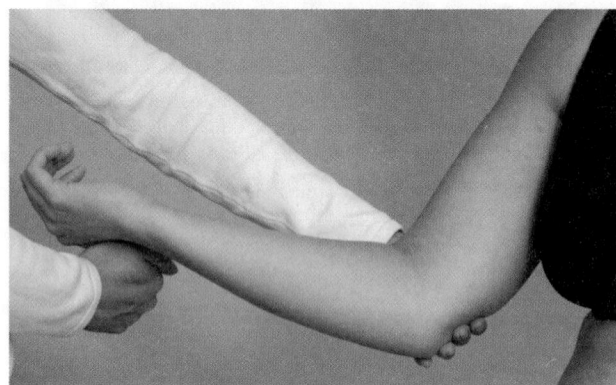

Figure 6-26 Milking maneuver to test medial collateral ligament.

elbow will dislocate while reproducing the patient's symptoms. In the conscious patient, actual subluxation is rare. A positive test indicates posterolateral rotary instability (Figure 6-28).

❓ *Posterolateral Rotary Drawer Test.*[2] The patient lies supine with the arm to be tested overhead and the elbow flexed 40° to 90° while the examiner holds the forearm and arm similar to doing a drawer test at the knee. As the humerus is stabilized and the radius and ulna are pushed posterolaterally, the radius and ulna rotate around an intact medial collateral ligament indicating a tear of the lateral collateral ligament and posterolateral instability at the elbow (Figure 6-29).

❓ *Pushup Test.*[27] The patient, in supine, attempts to do a pushup—first with the forearms maximally supinated and then repeated with the forearms maximally pronated (Figure 6-30). The test is positive for posterolateral rotary instability if symptoms occur when the forearms are supinated but not pronated.

❓ *Stand Up Test.*[2,4] The patient is seated in a chair without arms. The patient is asked to push up on the seat with his or her hands with the forearms fully supinated into standing. If the patient's symptoms are reproduced, the test is positive for injury to the posterior band of the medial collateral ligament (Figure 6-31).

Tests for Biceps Rupture (Third-Degree Strain)

❓ *Biceps Squeeze Test.*[27,28] The patient's elbow is flexed to between 60° and 80°. The examiner then squeezes the biceps muscle belly (Figure 6-32). If the biceps tendon is ruptured, the patient's forearm will not supinate.

⚠ *Hook Test.*[27,29] The patient abducts the shoulder to 90° with the elbow flexed to 90° and the arm supinated

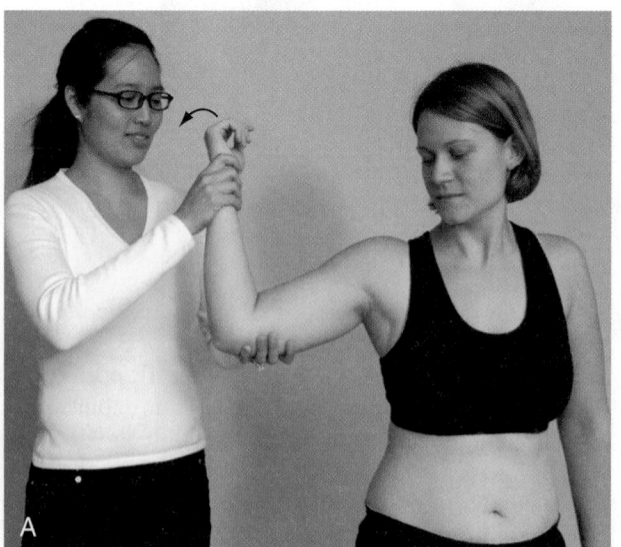

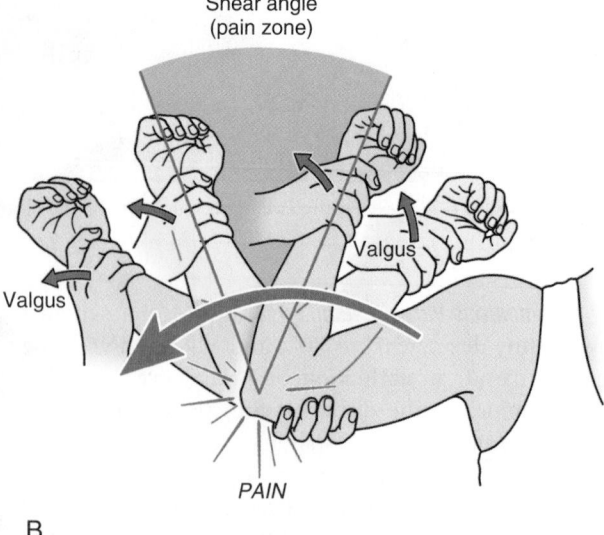

Shear angle (pain zone)

Valgus

Valgus

PAIN

B

Figure 6-27 A, The moving valgus stress test. **B,** Schematic representation of the moving valgus stress test. The shear range refers to the range of motion (ROM) that causes pain while the elbow is being extended with valgus stress. The shear angle is the point that causes maximum pain. (**B,** Redrawn with permission of the Mayo Foundation.)

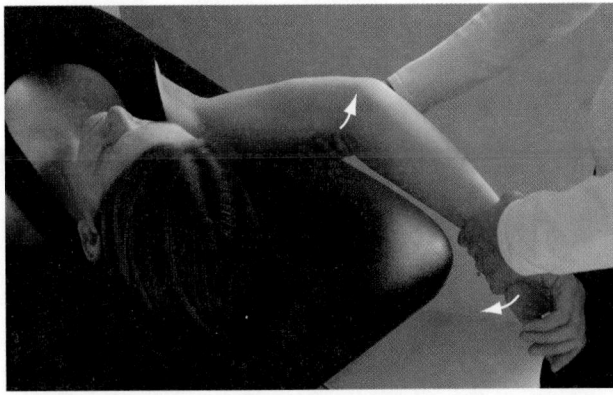

Figure 6-28 Posterolateral rotary apprehension test.

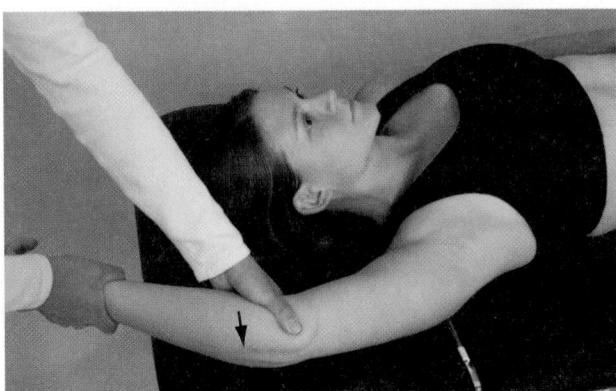

Figure 6-29 Posterolateral rotary drawer test.

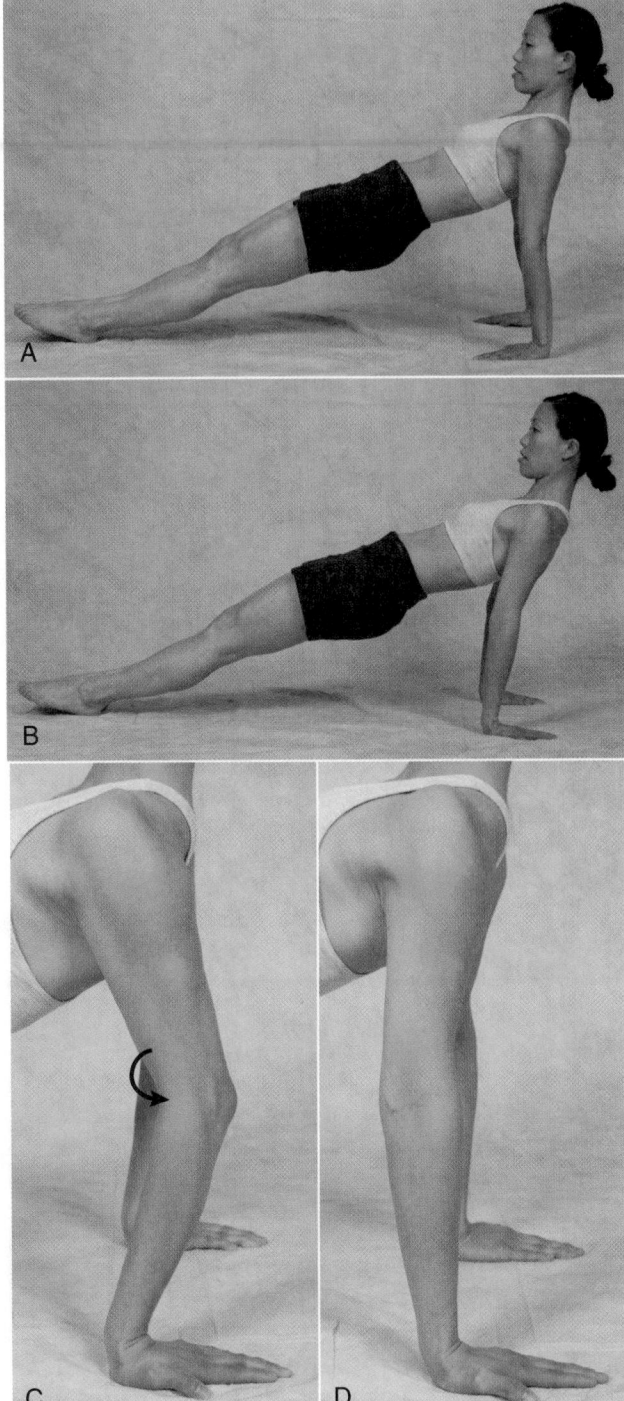

Figure 6-30 Pushup test. **A,** With forearms maximally supinated. **B,** With forearms maximally pronated. **C,** Elbow flexed. **D,** Elbow straight. Note how elbow has rotated which will show instability if present.

so that the thumb faces up (Figure 6-33). The patient is then asked to actively supinate the forearm against resistance of the examiner. With the index finger of the other hand, the examiner attempts to "hook" underneath the biceps tendon, "hooking" from lateral to medial at the same time. If no cord like structure can be hooked, the test is positive for a rupture of the distal biceps.

Tests for Epicondylitis

Chronic overuse injury to the extensor (tennis elbow, or lateral epicondylitis) or flexor (golfer's elbow, or medial epicondylitis) tendons at the elbow result from repeated microtrauma to the tendon leading to disruption and degeneration of the tendon's internal structure (tendinosus).[30] It appears to be a degenerative condition in which the tendon has failed to heal properly after repetitive microtrauma injury.[30,31]

When testing for epicondylitis, whether medial or lateral, the examiner must keep in mind that there may be referral of pain from the cervical spine or peripheral nerve involvement. If the epicondylitis does not respond to treatment, the examiner would be wise to check for neurological pathology.

⚠ **Lateral Epicondylitis (Tennis Elbow or Cozen's) Test (Method 1).** The patient's elbow is stabilized by the examiner's thumb, which rests on the patient's lateral epicondyle (Figure 6-34). The patient is then asked to actively make a fist, pronate the forearm, and radially deviate and extend the wrist while the examiner resists the motion. A

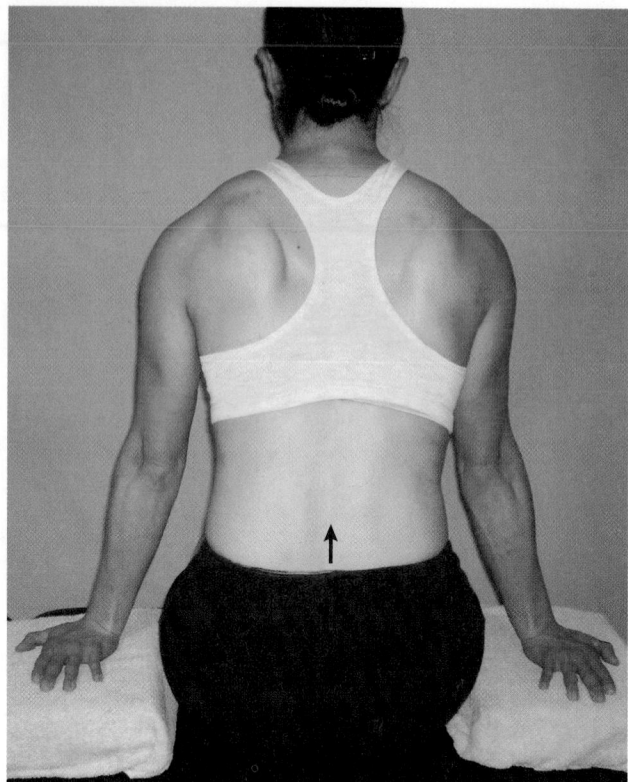

Figure 6-31 Stand up test for medial collateral ligament of the elbow. Note the scapular winging as well.

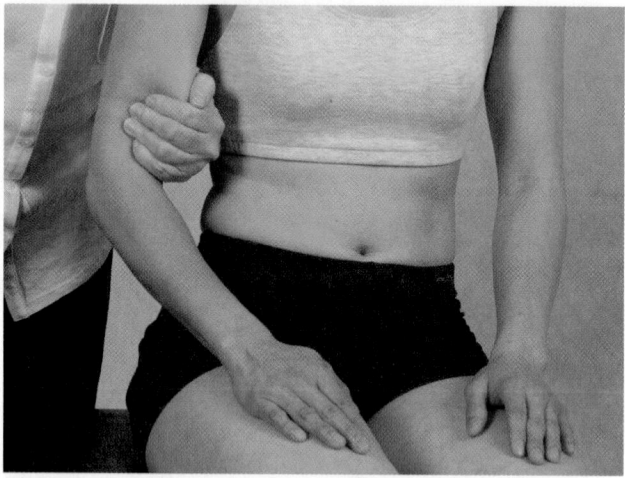

Figure 6-32 Biceps squeeze test. Muscle is squeezed near insertion at the elbow.

sudden severe pain in the area of the lateral epicondyle of the humerus is a positive sign. The epicondyle may be palpated to indicate the origin of the pain.

⚠ *Lateral Epicondylitis (Tennis Elbow or Mill's) Test (Method 2).* While palpating the lateral epicondyle, the examiner passively pronates the patient's forearm, flexes the wrist fully, and extends the elbow (see Figure 6-34). Pain over the lateral epicondyle of the humerus indicates a positive test. This maneuver also puts stress on the radial nerve

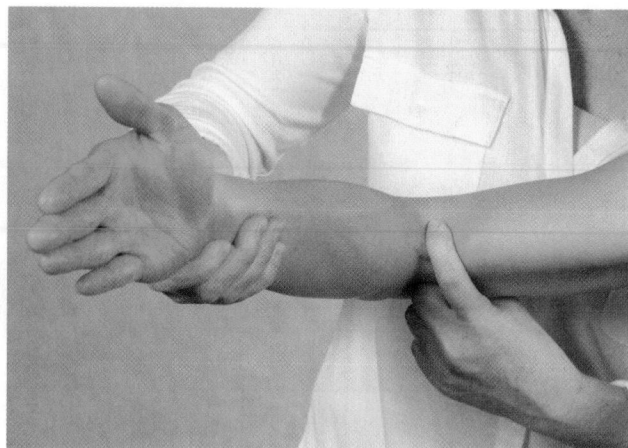

Figure 6-33 Hook test for biceps rupture at the elbow.

and, in the presence of compression of the radial nerve, causes symptoms similar to those of tennis elbow.[32] Electrodiagnostic studies help differentiate the two conditions.

❓ *Lateral Epicondylitis (Tennis Elbow or Maudsley's) Test (Method 3).* The examiner resists extension of the third digit of the hand distal to the proximal interphalangeal joint, stressing the extensor digitorum muscle and tendon (see Figure 6-34). A positive test is indicated by pain over the lateral epicondyle of the humerus.

❓ *Medial Epicondylitis (Golfer's Elbow) Test.* While the examiner palpates the patient's medial epicondyle, the patient's forearm is passively supinated and the examiner extends the elbow and wrist. A positive sign is indicated by pain over the medial epicondyle of the humerus.

Tests for Plica

❓ *Plica Impingement Test.*[27,33] The examiner applies a valgus load to the elbow while passively flexing the elbow with the forearm held in pronation (Figure 6-35, *A*). Pain or snapping between 90° and 110° of flexion indicates a positive test for the anterior radiocapitellar plica (**flexion-pronation plica test** ❓). To test the posterior radiocapitellar plica, the examiner applies a valgus load to the elbow while passively extending the elbow with the forearm held in supination (Figure 6-35, *B*) (**extension-supination plica test** ❓). Pain or a snap would indicate a positive test indicating a possible plica problem or radiocapitellar chondromalacia.

Tests for Posterior Impingement

❓ *Arm Bar Test.*[27] The patient rests the hand of the test arm on the examiner's shoulder with the elbow extended and shoulder medially rotated. The examiner pulls down on the olecranon to simulate forced extension (Figure 6-36). Reproduction of pain especially posteromedially along the olecranon is a positive test for posterior impingement. The patient may also lack full extension.

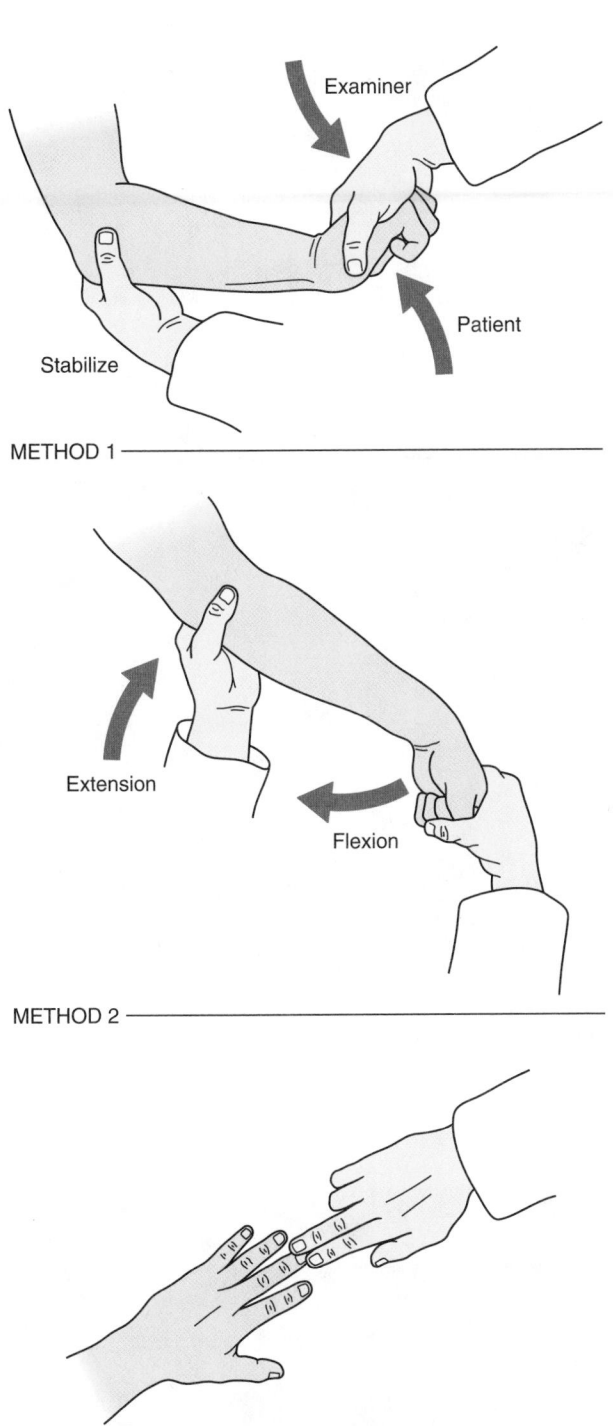

METHOD 1

METHOD 2

METHOD 3

Figure 6-34 Tests for tennis elbow.

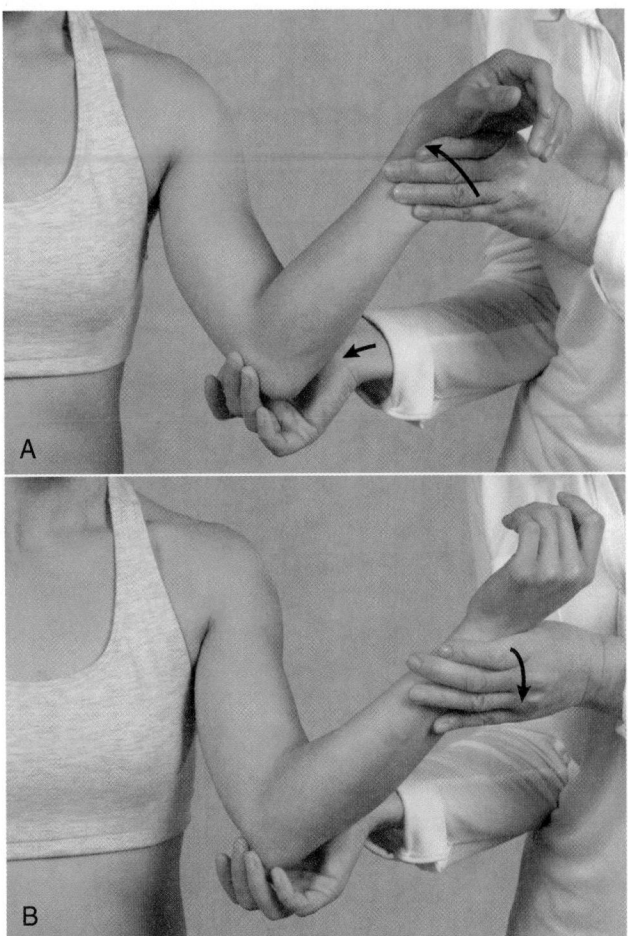

Figure 6-35 Plica impingement tests. A, Flexion-pronation plica test to test the anterior radiocapitellar plica. **B,** Extension-supination plica test to test the posterior radiocapitellar plica.

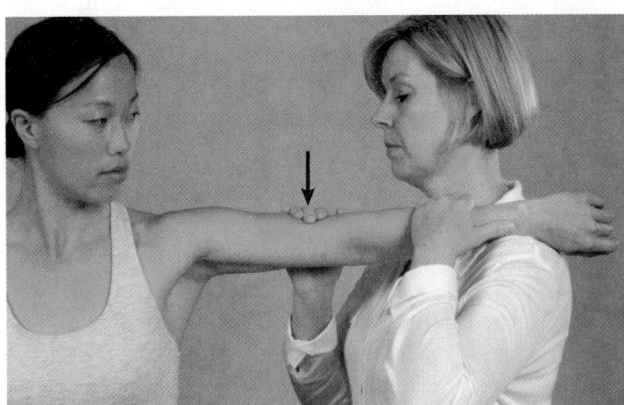

Figure 6-36 Arm bar test for posterior impingement.

❓ *Extension Impingement Test.*[27] The examiner applies a valgus stress to the elbow while quickly extending and flexing the elbow from 20° to 30° flexion to terminal flexion repeatedly (Figure 6-37). The test is then repeated without the valgus stress while the posteromedial olecranon is palpated for tenderness. This palpation differentiates tender impingement due to instability from pain over the medial olecranon without instability.

Tests for Joint Dysfunction

If the patient complains of pain in the elbow joint, especially on elbow movement, the examiner can perform two tests to differentiate between the radiohumeral and ulnohumeral joints. **To test the radiohumeral joint ❓,** the

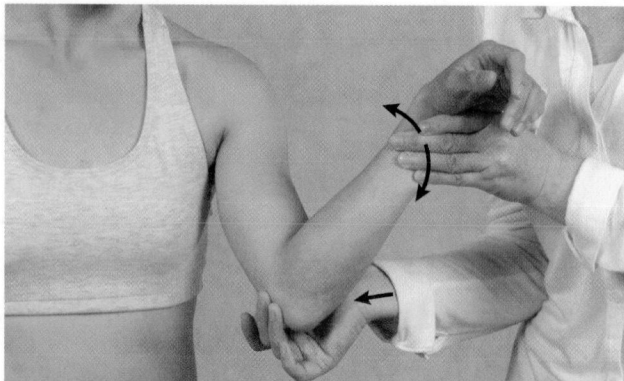

Figure 6-37 Extension impingement test. Valgus stress shown.

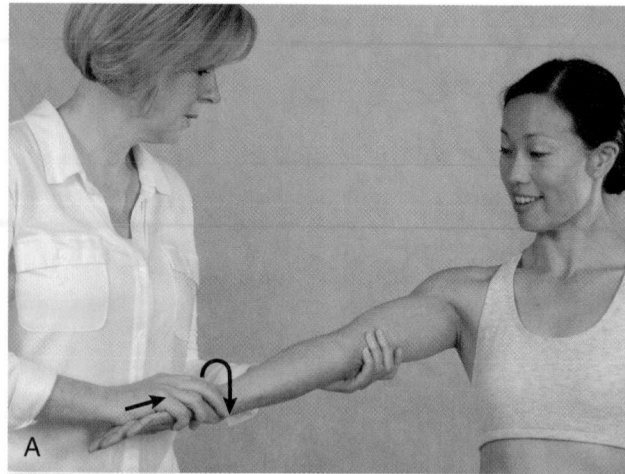

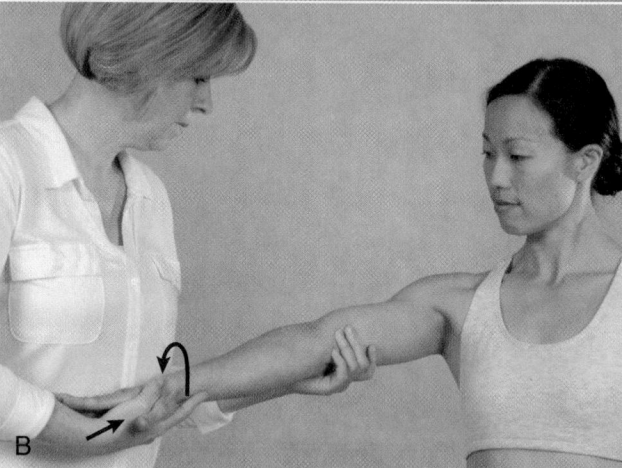

Figure 6-38 Active radiocapitellar compression test. A, Supination. **B,** Pronation.

examiner positions the elbow joint at the position of pain and then radially deviates the wrist to compress the radial head against the humerus. The production of pain would be considered a positive test. **To test the ulnohumeral joint ❓**, the examiner again positions the elbow joint at the position of discomfort and causes compression of the ulnohumeral joint by ulnar deviation at the wrist.[6] Again, pain indicates a positive test.

❓ *Active Radiocapitellar Compression Test.*[27] The examiner applies an axial (compression) load to the elbow in full extension. The patient is asked to actively supinate and pronate the forearm while the compression is maintained (Figure 6-38). Pain in the lateral compartment of the elbow is a positive test and may indicate an osteochondritis dissecans of the capitellum.

Tests for Neurological Dysfunction

✓ *Elbow Flexion Test.* The patient is asked to fully flex the elbow with extension of the wrist and shoulder girdle abduction (90°) and depression[34,35] and to hold this position for 3 to 5 minutes (Figure 6-39). Ochi, et al.[36] modified the test to include medial rotation of the shoulder calling it the **shoulder internal (medial) rotation elbow flexion test** ⚠ (Figure 6-40). They state that symptoms should develop in less than 5 seconds. Tingling or paresthesia in the ulnar nerve distribution of the forearm and hand indicates a positive test. The test helps to determine whether a cubital tunnel (ulnar nerve) syndrome is present. The test may be modified by the examiner applying direct pressure over the ulnar nerve with the index and middle finger between the posteromedial olecranon and the medial epicondyle (**elbow flexion compression test** or **cubital tunnel compression test** ❓) (Figure 6-41).

❓ *MacKinnon's Scratch Collapse Test.* The patient stands with the elbow flexed to 90° and by the side. The patient is asked to laterally rotate and abduct the forearms against resistance and then relaxes (Figure 6-42). The examiner then scratches along the course of the ulnar nerve at the elbow and then asks the patient to repeat the movement

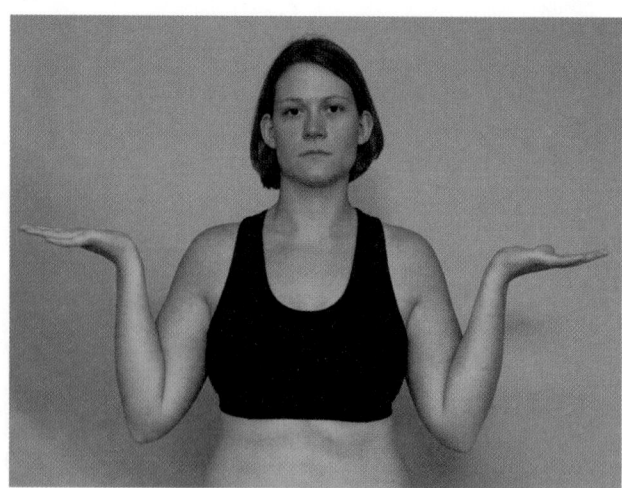

Figure 6-39 Elbow flexion test for ulnar nerve pathology.

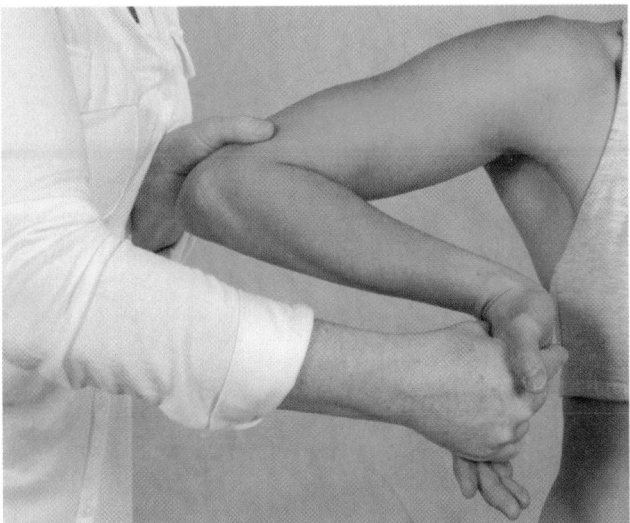

Figure 6-40 Shoulder medial rotation elbow flexion test. Medial rotation of the shoulder, maximum elbow flexion, maximum forearm supination, and maximum wrist extension.

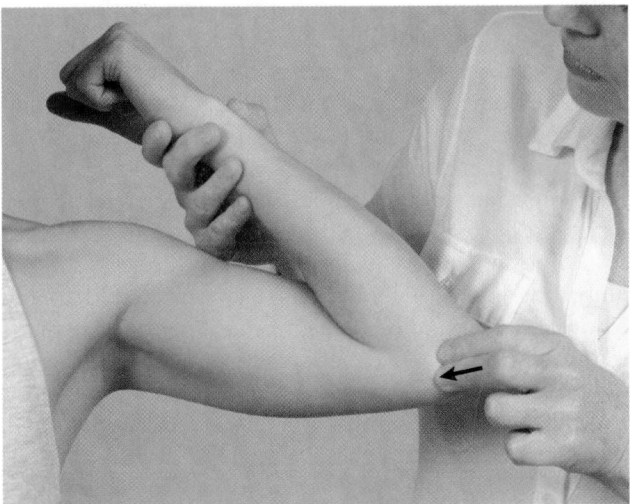

Figure 6-41 Elbow flexion compression test for ulnar nerve.

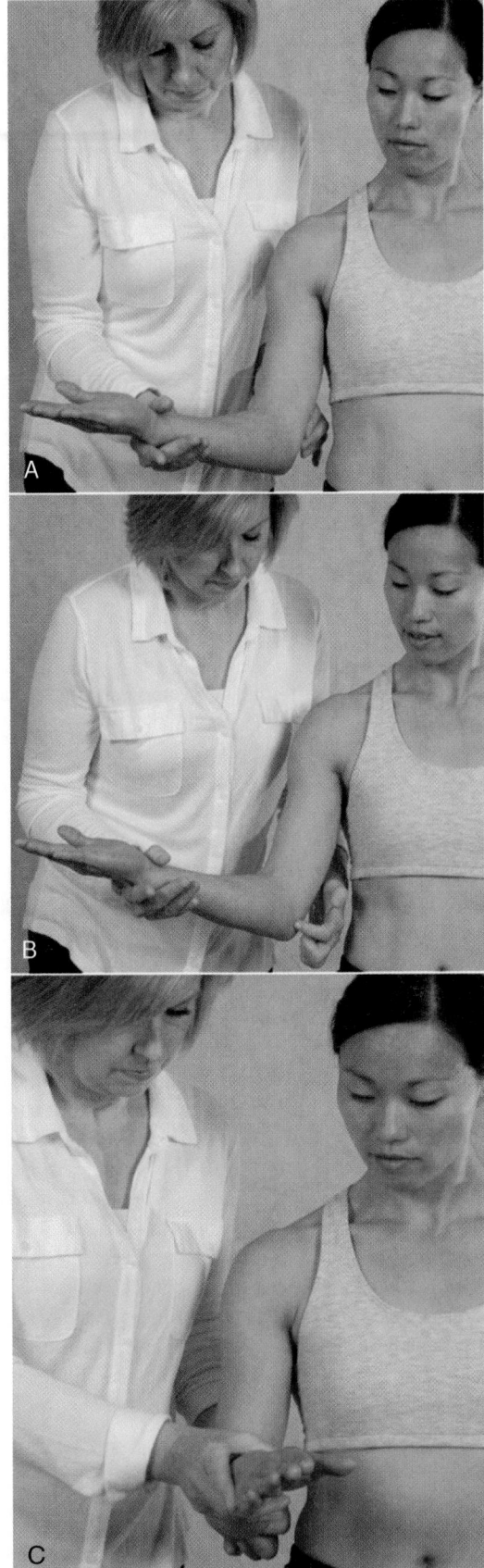

Figure 6-42 MacKinnon's scratch collapse test. A, The patient laterally rotates and abducts the forearm against resistance. **B,** The examiner scratches along the ulnar nerve pathway. **C,** The patient attempts to laterally rotate but cannot indicating a positive test.

against resistance. If the patient cannot momentarily laterally rotate against the examiner, it is considered a positive test.[37,38]

✓ *Pinch Grip Test.* The patient is asked to pinch the tips of the index finger and thumb together. Normally, there should be a tip-to-tip pinch. If the patient is unable to pinch tip-to-tip and instead has an abnormal pulp-to-pulp pinch of the index finger and thumb, this is a positive sign for pathology to the anterior interosseous nerve, which is a branch of the median nerve (Figure 6-43). This finding may indicate an entrapment of the anterior interosseous nerve as it passes between the two heads of the pronator teres muscle.[39]

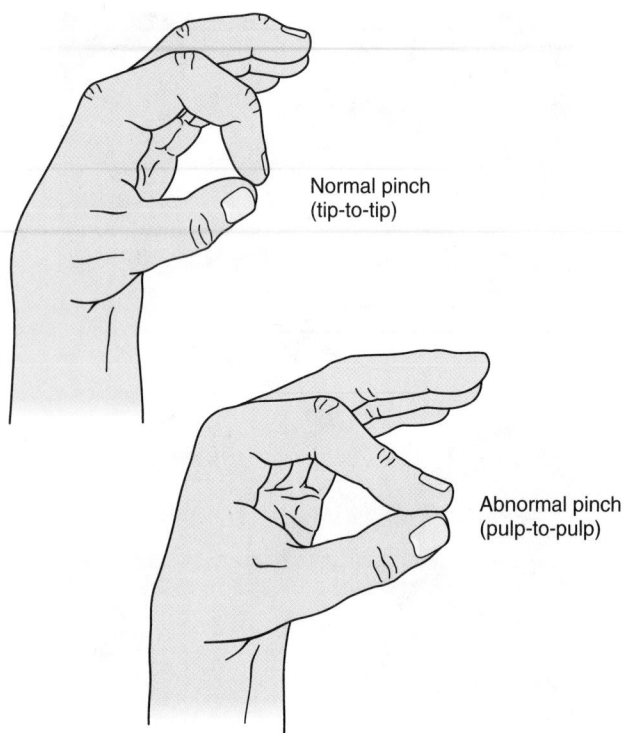

Figure 6-43 Normal tip-to-tip pinch compared with the abnormal pulp-to-pulp pinch seen in anterior interosseous nerve syndrome.

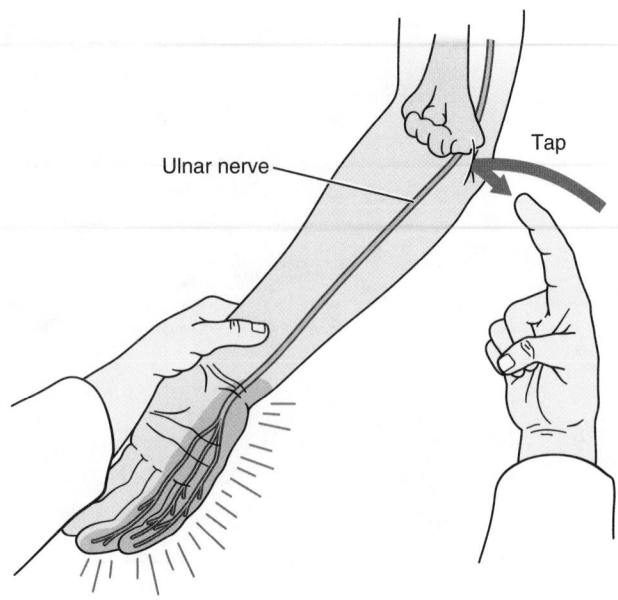

Figure 6-44 Tinel sign at the elbow for the ulnar nerve.

(?) Test for Pronator Teres Syndrome.[18] The patient sits with the elbow flexed to 90°. The examiner strongly resists pronation as the elbow is extended. Tingling or paresthesia in the median nerve distribution in the forearm and hand indicates a positive test.

⚠ Tinel Sign (at the Elbow). The area of the ulnar nerve in the groove (between the olecranon process and medial epicondyle) is tapped. A positive sign is indicated by a tingling sensation in the ulnar distribution of the forearm and hand distal to the point of compression of the nerve (Figure 6-44). The test indicates the point of regeneration of the sensory fibers of a nerve. The most distal point at which the patient feels the abnormal sensation represents the limit of nerve regeneration.

(?) Wartenberg Sign. The patient sits with his or her hands resting on the table. The examiner passively spreads the fingers apart and asks the patient to bring them together again. Inability to squeeze the little finger to the remainder of the hand indicates a positive test for ulnar neuropathy.[18,37]

Reflexes and Cutaneous Distribution

The reflexes around the elbow that are often checked (Figure 6-45) include the biceps (C5–C6), brachioradialis (C5–C6), and triceps (C7–C8). The examiner should also assess the dermatomes around the elbow and the cutaneous distribution of the various nerves, noting any difference (Figures 6-46 and 6-47). When looking at the dermatomes, the examiner should realize there is a great deal of variability in the distribution patterns. Except for T2 dermatome, which commonly ends at the elbow, all other dermatomes extend distally to the forearm, wrist, and hand; therefore, the elbow cannot be looked at in isolation when viewing dermatomes. Similarly, the peripheral nerves extend into the forearm, wrist, and hand, and so testing for sensory loss must involve the whole upper limb, not just the elbow. Pain may be referred to the elbow and surrounding tissues from the neck (often mimicking tennis elbow), the shoulder, or the wrist (Figure 6-48; Table 6-4).

In the extremities, the neurological tissues (nerve roots and peripheral nerves) play a significant role in function. Injury, pinching, or stress to these structures can have dire consequences functionally for the patient. The next section is a review of the peripheral nerves and how and where they may be traumatized about the elbow.

Peripheral Nerve Injuries About the Elbow

Median Nerve (C6–C8, T1). In the elbow region, the median nerve proper can be injured by trauma (e.g., lacerations, fractures, dislocations), by systemic disease, and especially by compression and/or traction.[40–42]

The median nerve may also be pinched or compressed above the elbow as it passes under the **ligament of Struthers,** an anomalous structure found in approximately 1% of the population (Figure 6-49).[43] The ligament runs from an abnormal spur on the shaft of the humerus to the medial epicondyle of the humerus. Because the brachial artery sometimes accompanies the nerve through this tunnel, it may also be compressed,

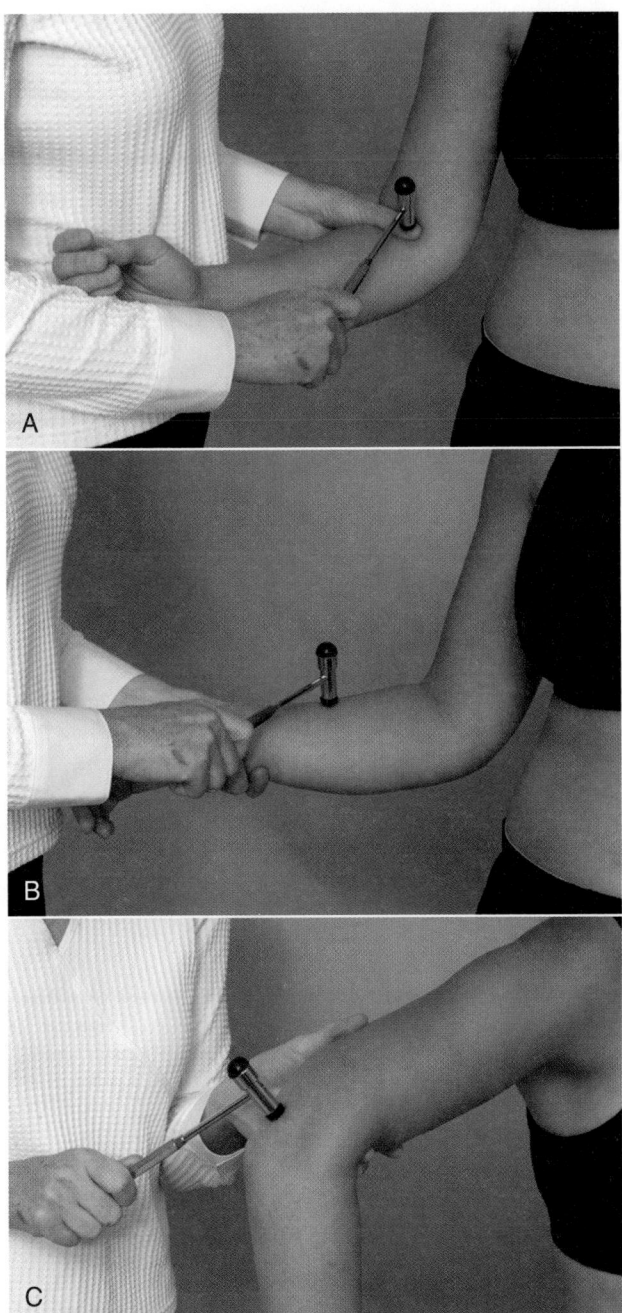

Figure 6-45 **Reflexes around the elbow. A,** Biceps. **B,** Brachioradialis. **C,** Triceps.

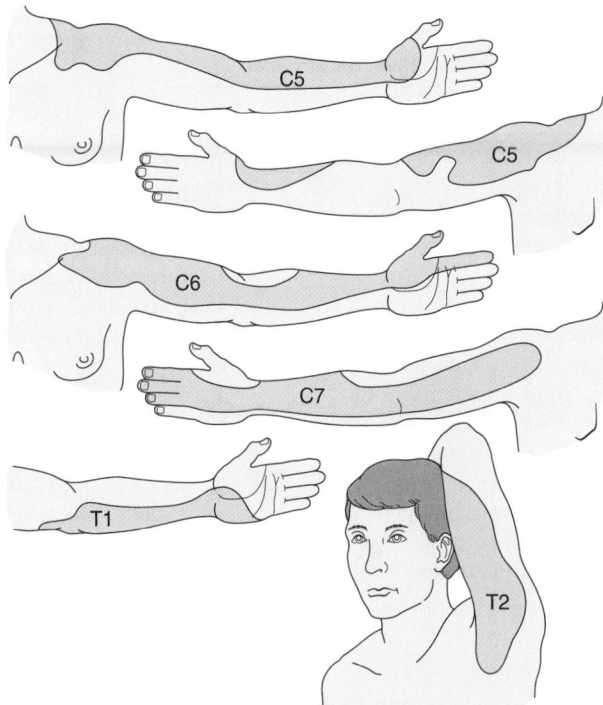

Figure 6-46 Dermatomes around the elbow.

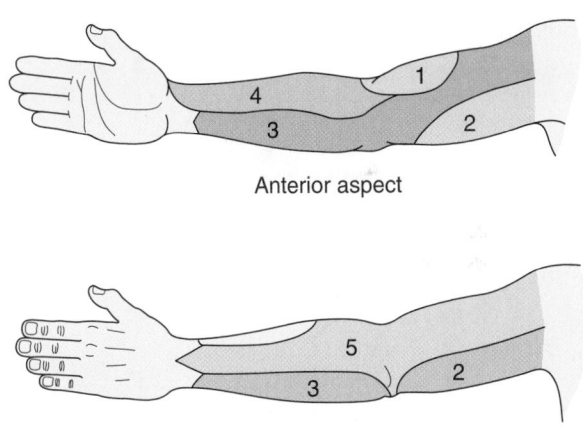

Anterior aspect

Posterior aspect

Figure 6-47 **Sensory nerve distribution around the elbow.** *1,* Lower lateral cutaneous nerve of arm (radial): *2,* medial cutaneous nerve of arm; *3,* medial cutaneous nerve of forearm; *4,* lateral cutaneous nerve of forearm (musculocutaneous nerve); *5,* posterior cutaneous nerve of forearm (radial nerve).

resulting in possible vascular as well as neurological symptoms. In this case, the neurological involvement would include weakness of the pronator teres muscle and of those muscles affected by the pronator syndrome (see later discussion). The condition may also be called the **humerus supracondylar process syndrome.** Pressure in the ligament of Struthers area leads to motor loss (see Table 6-2) and sensory loss (see Figure 7-81) of the median nerve. Initially, the patient complains of pain and paresthesia in the elbow and forearm; abnormality of

motor function is secondary. With time, however, motor function is also affected, with wrist and finger flexion as well as thumb movements being most affected.

A second area of compression of the median nerve as it passes through the elbow occurs where it passes through the two heads of pronator teres **(pronator syndrome).** In this case, the pronator teres remains normal, but the other muscles supplied by the median nerve (see Table 6-2) are affected, as is its sensory distribution. Pronation is possible, but weakness is evident as pronation is loaded.

TABLE **6-4**

Elbow Muscles and Referral of Pain

Muscles	Referral Pattern
Biceps	Upper shoulder (bicipital groove) to anterior elbow
Brachialis	Anterior arm, elbow to lateral thenar eminence
Triceps	Posterior shoulder, arm, elbow, and forearm to medial two fingers, medial epicondyle
Brachioradialis	Lateral epicondyle, lateral forearm to posterior web space between thumb and index finger
Anconeus	Lateral epicondyle area
Supinator	Lateral epicondyle and posterior web space between thumb and index finger
Pronator teres	Anterior forearm to wrist and part of anterior thumb
Extensor carpi ulnaris	Medial wrist
Extensor carpi radialis brevis	Posterior forearm to posterior wrist
Extensor carpi radialis longus	Lateral epicondyle to posterolateral wrist
Extensor indices	Posterior forearm to appropriate digit
Palmaris longus	Anterior forearm to palm
Flexor digitorum superficialis	Palm to appropriate digit
Flexor carpi ulnaris	Anteromedial wrist
Flexor carpi radialis	Anteromedial wrist

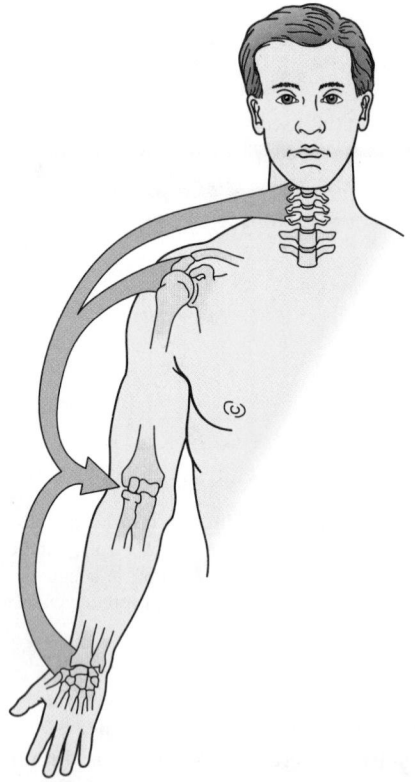

Figure 6-48 Pain referred to the elbow.

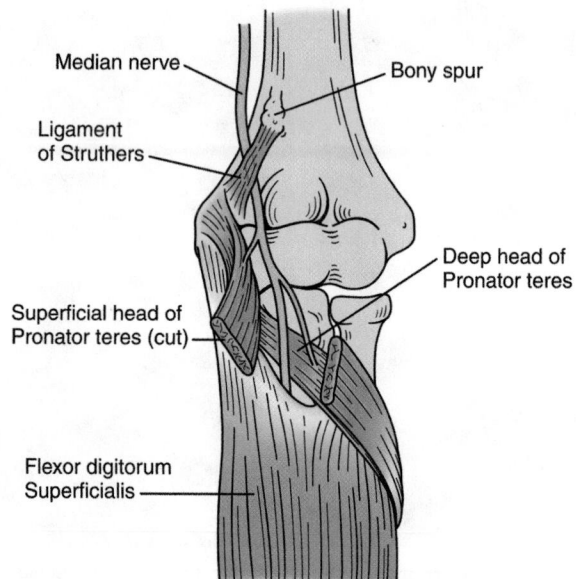

Figure 6-49 Compression of the median nerve under ligament of Struthers and in pronator syndrome. In the pronator syndrome, the median nerve may be kinked against the flexor digitorum superficialis muscle or compressed by the forceful action or structural hypertrophy of the deep head of the pronator teres. Compression of the nerve above the elbow (ligament of Struthers) leads to weakness of the pronator teres while this muscle is spared in the pronator syndrome, because the branches to the two heads of the pronator teres arise proximally to the muscle.

If the elbow is flexed to 90° and pronation is tested, noticeable weakness occurs, because in this position the action of pronator teres is minimized.

Butlers and Singer[44] reported four possible ways of eliciting median nerve symptoms if the nerve is suffering from pathology:
- Resisted pronation with elbow and wrist flexion for 30 to 60 seconds
- Resisted elbow flexion and supination
- Resisted long finger flexion at the proximal interphalangeal joint
- Direct pressure over the proximal aspect of pronator teres during pronation

It is interesting to note that one of the tests is similar to Mill's test for lateral epicondylitis. The results should be compared with the good side, and production of the patient's symptoms is considered a positive test.

Anterior Interosseous Nerve. The anterior interosseous nerve, which is a branch of the median nerve, is sometimes pinched or entrapped as it passes between the two heads of the pronator teres muscle, leading to pain and functional impairment of the flexor pollicis longus, the lateral half of the flexor digitorum profundus, and the pronator quadratus muscles. The condition is called **anterior interosseous nerve syndrome** or **Kiloh-Nevin syndrome** (Figure 6-50)[45,46] and is characterized by a pinch deformity (see Figure 6-43). The deformity results from the paralysis of the flexors of the index finger and thumb.

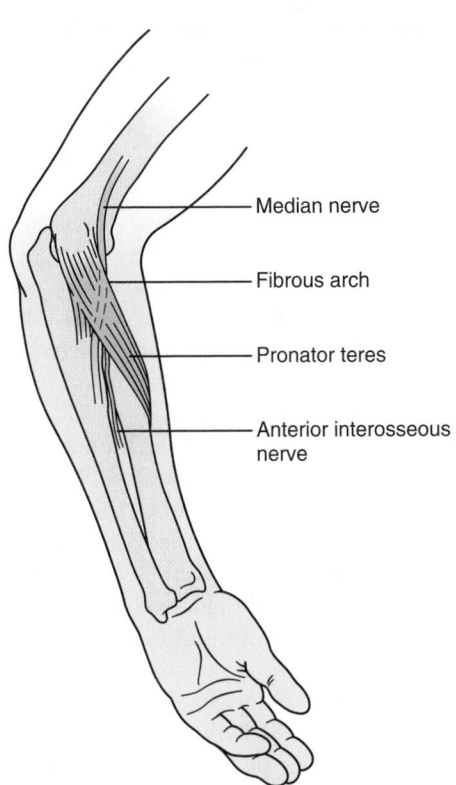

Median nerve

Fibrous arch

Pronator teres

Anterior interosseous nerve

Figure 6-50 Anterior interosseous syndrome.

This leads to extension of the distal interphalangeal joint of the index finger and the interphalangeal joint of the thumb. The resulting pinch is pulp to pulp rather than tip to tip. It has been reported that the nerve may also be injured with a forearm fracture (Monteggia fracture).[47] With anterior interosseous syndrome, there is no sensory loss, because the anterior interosseous nerve is a motor nerve; signs and symptoms of the condition are related to motor function.

Ulnar Nerve (C7–C8, T1). In the elbow region, the ulnar nerve is most likely to be injured, compressed, or stretched in the **cubital tunnel** (see Figure 6-4, *A*).[37,42,43,48-52] In fact, it is a common entrapment neuropathy, second only to carpal tunnel syndrome. The ulnar nerve may be injured or compressed as a result of swelling (e.g., trauma, pregnancy), osteophytes, arthritic diseases, trauma, or repeated microtrauma. This tunnel, which is relatively long, can compress the nerve as the nerve passes through the tunnel or between the two heads of the flexor carpi ulnaris muscle. Compression is altered as the elbow moves from extension (decreased) to flexion (increased), causing traction on the nerve, and is further enhanced if a significant cubitus valgus is present.[53,54] Symptoms therefore are more likely to occur when the elbow is flexed. It is usually in the cubital tunnel area that the ulnar nerve is affected, leading to tardy ulnar palsy. If the problem is the result of restriction in the cubital tunnel, direct pressure over the tunnel may reproduce or exacerbate the symptoms (see "Cubital Tunnel Compression Test").[42]

Tardy ulnar palsy implies that the symptoms of nerve injury come on long after the patient has been injured; this delayed reaction seems to be unique to the ulnar nerve. Although most common in adults, it has been reported in children, and in children the delay has been up to 29 months.[55] In adults, the possibility of a double crush injury (at cervical spine and elbow) should always be considered.

Injury to the ulnar nerve in the cubital tunnel affects the flexor carpi ulnaris and the ulnar half of the flexor digitorum profundus in the forearm, the hypothenar eminence in the hand (flexor digiti minimi, abductor digiti minimi, opponens digiti minimi, and adductor pollicis), the interossei, and the third and fourth lumbrical muscles (see Table 6-2). Commonly, patients cannot fully adduct the little finger and hold the finger abducted and extended, because the denervated palmar interosseous muscle cannot oppose the abductor digiti minimi (see "Wartenberg Sign").[37] Although these muscles show weakness and atrophy over time, the earliest and most obvious symptoms are sensory with pain and paresthesia in the medial elbow and forearm and paresthesia in the ulnar sensory distribution of the hand (see Figure 7-81).

Calfee, et al.[56] recommended testing for a hypermobile ulnar nerve which is reported to be found in over 30% of the population (**hypermobile ulnar nerve test** ❓). The patient maximally flexes the elbow with the forearm supinated. The examiner then places a finger on the proximal, posteromedial aspect of the medial epicondyle. While holding the finger in place, the patient is asked to extend the elbow. If the ulnar nerve stays anterior to the examiner's finger, it is said to dislocate. If the nerve is below the examiner's finger, it is perched on the medial humeral epicondyle. If the nerve cannot be palpated, it is stable in the groove.

Radial Nerve (C5–C8, T1). The radial nerve may be injured near the elbow if there is a fracture of the shaft of the humerus. The nerve may be damaged as it winds around behind the humerus in the radial groove. Injury may occur at the time of the fracture, or the nerve may get caught in the callus of fracture healing. Because the radial nerve supplies all of the extensor muscles of the arm, only the triceps is spared with this type of injury, and even it may show some weakness.

The major branch of the radial nerve in the forearm is the **posterior interosseous nerve,** which is given off in front of the lateral epicondyle of the humerus.[43,57] This branch may compress as it passes between the two heads of the supinator in the **arcade** or **canal of Frohse,** a fibrous arch in the supinator muscle occurring in 30% of the population (Figure 6-51). Compression can lead to functional involvement of the forearm extensor muscles (see Table 6-2) and functional wrist drop, and so the patient has difficulty or is unable to stabilize the wrist for proper hand function. Diagnosis of this condition is often delayed because there is no sensory deficit. Direct pressure over the supinator muscle while resisting supination may elicit weakness of supination or tenderness (**supinator compression test** ?).[42] This compression zone is one of five sites in the tunnel through which the radial nerve passes. The nerve may also be compressed at the entrance to the tunnel anterior to the head of the radius, near where the nerve supplies brachioradialis and extensor carpi radialis longus, between the ulnar half of the tendon

of extensor carpi radialis brevis and its fascia, and at the distal border of supinator.[58,59] This condition, sometimes called **radial tunnel syndrome,** may mimic tennis elbow.[32,58,60–63] If the patient has a persistent form of tennis elbow, a possible nerve lesion or cervical problem should be considered.

A third area of pathology is compression of the superficial branch of the radial nerve as it passes under the tendon of the brachioradialis. This branch is sensory only, and the patient complains primarily of nocturnal pain along the dorsum of the wrist, thumb, and web space. Trauma, a tight cast, any swelling in the area, or forearm pronation with wrist flexion and ulnar deviation may cause the compression and produce paresthesia.[42] Direct pressure at the junction of extensor carpi radialis longus and brachioradialis may also reproduce the paresthesia or numbness.[42] The condition is referred to as **cheiralgia paresthetica** or **Wartenberg disease/sign.**[51]

Joint Play Movements

When examining the joint play movements (Figure 6-52), the examiner must compare the injured side with the normal side.

Joint Play Movements of the Elbow Complex

- Radial deviation of the ulna and radius on the humerus
- Ulnar deviation of the ulna and radius on the humerus
- Distraction of the olecranon from the humerus in 90° of flexion
- Anteroposterior glide of the radius on the humerus

Radial and ulnar deviations of the ulna and radius on the humerus are performed in a fashion similar to those in the collateral ligament tests but with less elbow flexion. The examiner stabilizes the patient's elbow by holding the patient's humerus firmly and places the other hand above the patient's wrist, abducting and adducting the forearm (see Figure 6-52, *A*). The patient's elbow is almost straight (extended) during the movement, and the end feel should be bone-to-bone.

To distract the olecranon from the humerus, the examiner flexes the patient's elbow to 90°. Wrapping both hands around the patient's forearm close to the elbow, the examiner then applies a distractive force at the elbow, ensuring that no torque is applied (see Figure 6-52, *B*). If the patient has a sore shoulder, counter force should be applied with one hand around the humerus.

To test anteroposterior glide of the radius on the humerus, the examiner stabilizes the patient's forearm. The patient's arm is held between the examiner's body and arm. The examiner places the thumb of his or her hand over the anterior radial head while the flexed index finger is over the posterior radial head. The examiner then

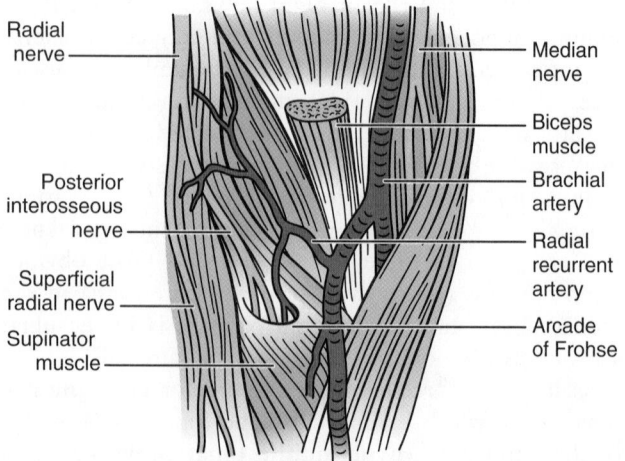

Radial nerve

Posterior interosseous nerve

Superficial radial nerve

Supinator muscle

Median nerve

Biceps muscle

Brachial artery

Radial recurrent artery

Arcade of Frohse

Figure 6-51 Canal, or arcade, of Frohse.

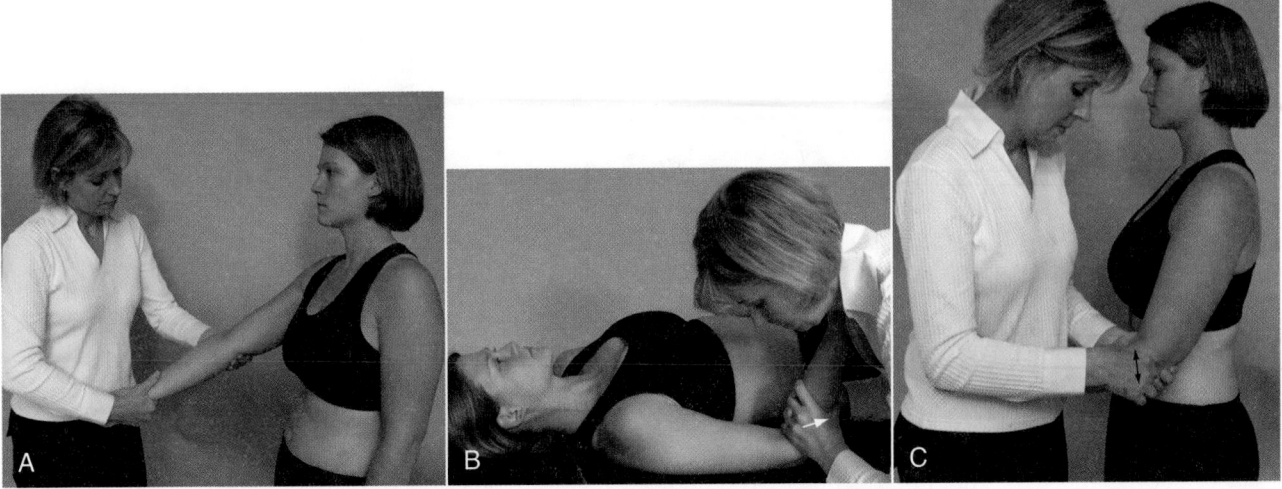

Figure 6-52 Joint play movements of the elbow complex. A, Radial and ulnar deviation of the ulna on the humerus. **B,** Distraction of the olecranon process from the humerus. **C,** Anteroposterior movement of the radius.

pushes the radial head posteriorly with the thumb and anteriorly with the index finger (see Figure 6-52, *C*). Commonly, posterior movement is easier to obtain with anterior movement in normal clients, being the result of the radial head returning to its normal position with a tissue stretch end feel. This movement must be performed with care, because it can be very painful as a result of pinching of the skin between the examiner's digits and the bone. In addition, pain may result from the force being applied even in the normal arm, so both sides must be compared.

The anterior and posterior glide of the radius may be tested in a slightly different way as well. To do anteroposterior glide of the head of the radius, the patient is placed in supine with the arm by the side. The examiner stands beside the patient, facing the patient's head, and holds the patient's arm slightly flexed by holding the hand between the examiner's thorax and elbow. The examiner places the thumbs over the head of the radius and carefully applies an anteroposterior pressure to the head of the radius feeling the amount of movement and end feel. To do posteroanterior glide, the patient is in supine lying with the arm at the side and the hand resting on the stomach. The examiner places the thumbs over the posterior aspect of the radial head and carefully applies a posteroanterior pressure (Figure 6-53).

Palpation

With the patient's arm relaxed, the examiner begins palpation on the anterior aspect of the elbow and moves to the medial aspect, the lateral aspect, and finally the posterior aspect (Figure 6-54). The patient may sit or lie supine, whichever is more comfortable. The joint line is located about 2 cm below an imaginary line joining the

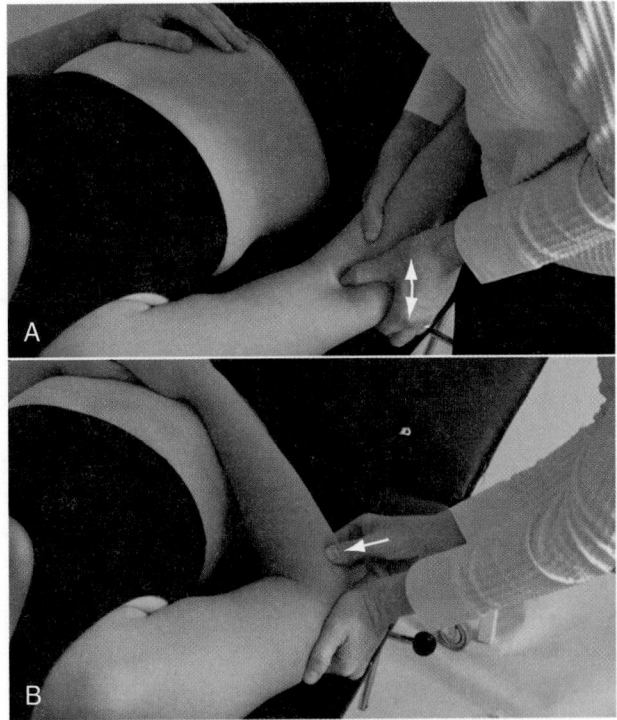

Figure 6-53 Joint play of the head of the radius (method 2). Anteroposterior **(A)** and posteroanterior **(B)** glide of the radius.

two epicondyles.[4] The examiner is looking for any tenderness, abnormality, change in temperature or in texture of the tissues, or abnormal bumps. As with all palpation, the injured side must be compared with the normal or uninjured side.

Anterior Aspect

Cubital Fossa. The fossa is bound by the pronator teres muscle medially, the brachioradialis muscle laterally, and

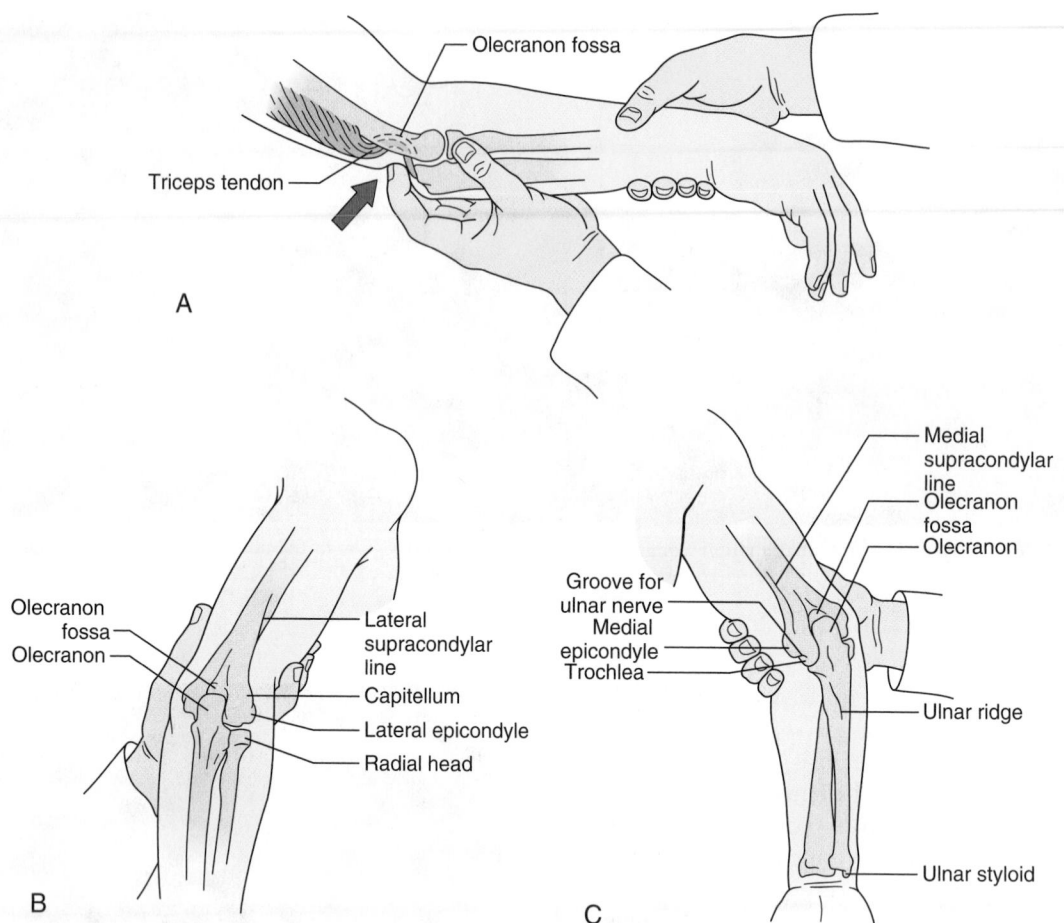

Figure 6-54 Palpation around the elbow. A, Olecranon fossa. **B,** Posterolateral aspect of the elbow. **C,** Posteromedial aspect of the elbow.

an imaginary line joining the two epicondyles superiorly. Within the fossa, the biceps tendon, brachialis, and brachial artery may be palpated. After crossing the elbow joint, the **brachial artery** divides into two branches, the radial artery and the ulnar artery. The examiner must be aware of the brachial artery, because it has the potential for being injured as a result of severe trauma at the elbow (e.g., fracture, dislocation). Trauma to this area may lead to compartment syndromes, such as **Volkmann ischemic contracture.** The median and musculocutaneous nerves are also found in the fossa, but they are not palpable. Pressure on the median nerve may cause symptoms in its cutaneous distribution.

Coronoid Process and Head of Radius. Within the cubital fossa, if the examiner palpates carefully so as not to hurt the patient, the coronoid process of the ulna and the head of the radius may be palpated. Palpation of the radial head is facilitated by supination and pronation of the forearm. The examiner may palpate the head of the radius from the posterior aspect at the same time by placing the fingers over the head on the posterior aspect and the thumb over it on the anterior aspect. In addition to the muscles previously mentioned, the biceps and brachialis

muscles may be palpated for potential abnormality. If the patient is complaining of pain and/or tenderness along the anteromedial humerus, radius, or ulna especially after repeated stress, the examiner should palpate the specific area. This tenderness or pain may be due to periostitis resulting in **humeral shin splints** or **"forearm splints,"** which may be precursors to stress fractures.

Medial Aspect

Medial Epicondyle. Originating from the medial epicondyle are the **wrist flexor-forearm pronator** groups of muscles. Both the muscle bellies and their insertions into bone should be palpated. Tenderness over the epicondyle where the muscles insert is sometimes called *golfer's elbow* or *tennis elbow of the medial epicondyle.*

Medial (Ulnar) Collateral Ligament. This fan-shaped ligament may be palpated, because it extends from the medial epicondyle to the medial margin of the coronoid process anteriorly and to the olecranon process posteriorly.

Ulnar Nerve. If the examiner moves posteriorly behind the medial epicondyle, the fingers will rest over the ulnar nerve in the cubital tunnel (proximal part). Usually, the nerve is not directly palpable, but pressure on the nerve often causes abnormal sensations in its cutaneous distribution. It is this nerve that is struck when someone hits his or her "funny bone."

Lateral Aspect

Lateral Epicondyle. The wrist extensor muscles originate from the lateral epicondyle, and their muscle bellies as well as their insertions into the epicondyle should be palpated. It is at this point of insertion of the common extensor tendon that lateral epicondylitis originates. When palpating, the examiner should remember that the extensor carpi radialis longus muscle inserts above the epicondyle along a short ridge extending from the epicondyle to the humeral shaft. The examiner palpates the brachioradialis and supinator muscles on the lateral aspect of the elbow at the same time. If the examiner palpates the lateral epicondyle, the posterior radial head and the olecranon tip, the anconeus "soft spot" will be found within this triangle (Figure 6-55).[27]

Lateral (Radial) Collateral Ligament. This cordlike ligament may be palpated as it extends from the lateral epicondyle of the humerus to the annular ligament and lateral surface of the ulna.

Annular Ligament. Distal to the lateral epicondyle, the annular ligament and head of the radius may be palpated if this has not previously been done. The palpation is facilitated by supination and pronation of the forearm.

Posterior Aspect

Palpation of posterior structures is shown in Figure 6-54.

Olecranon Process and Olecranon Bursa. The olecranon process is best palpated with the elbow flexed to 90°. If the examiner then grasps the skin overlying the process, the olecranon bursa can be palpated. Normally, it just feels like slippery tissue as the skin is moved. The examiner should note any synovial thickening, swelling, or presence of any rice bodies, which are small seeds of fragmented fibrous tissue that can act as further irritants to the bursa should it be affected.

Triceps Muscle. The triceps muscle, which inserts into the olecranon process, should be palpated both at its insertion and along its length for any signs of abnormality.

Diagnostic Imaging

Plain Film Radiography

Anteroposterior View. The examiner should note the relation of the epicondyles, trochlea, capitulum, radial head, radial tuberosity, coronoid process, and olecranon process (Figure 6-56). Any loose bodies, calcification, myositis ossificans, joint space narrowing, or osteophytes should be identified. If the patient is a young child, the examiner should check the epiphyseal plate to see if it is normal for each bone.

Lateral View. The examiner should note the relation of the epicondyles, trochlea, capitulum, radial head, radial tuberosity, coronoid process, and olecranon process. As

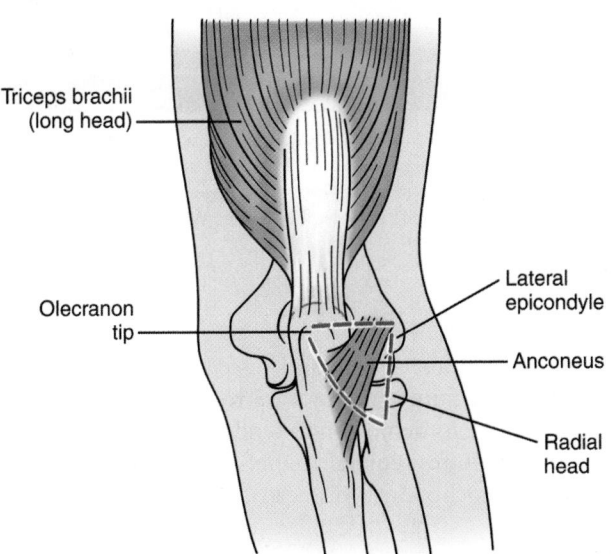

Figure 6-55 Palpation of anconeus in triangle of olecranon tip, lateral epicondyle, and radial head.

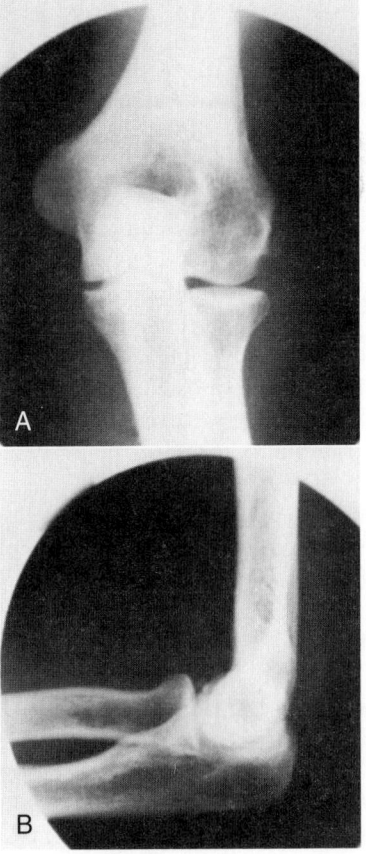

Figure 6-56 Anteroposterior (**A**) and lateral (**B**) radiographs of the elbow.

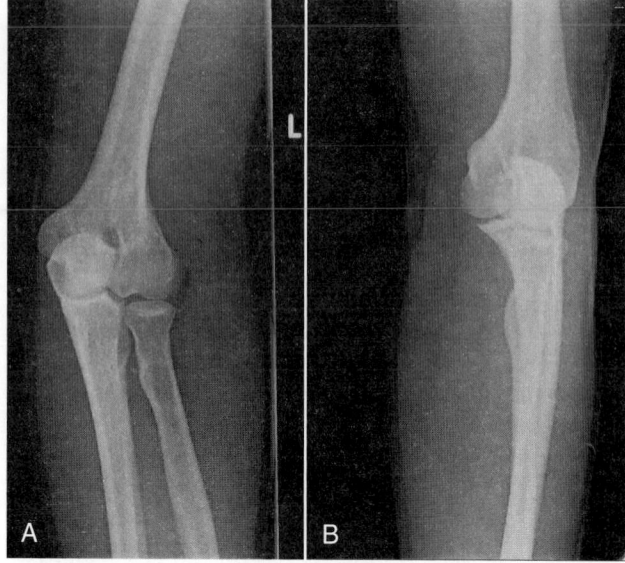

Figure 6-57 A, Anteroposterior external oblique view of the elbow. **B,** Anteroposterior internal oblique view of the elbow.

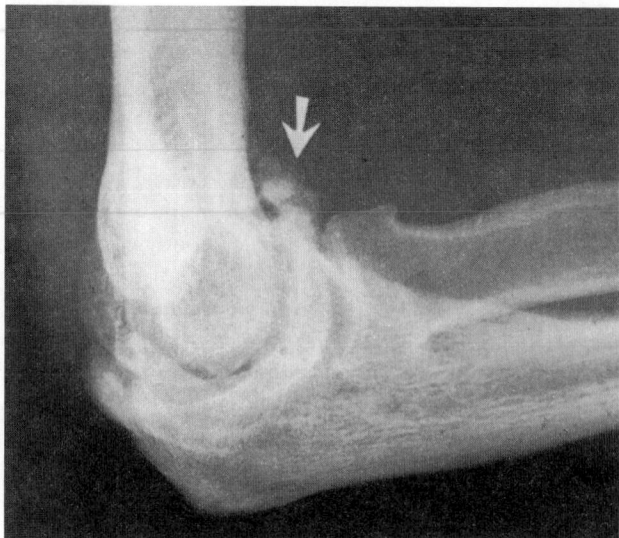

Figure 6-58 Excessive ossification *(arrow)* after dislocation of elbow treated by early active use. (From O'Donoghue DH: Treatment of injuries to athletes, ed 4, Philadelphia, 1984, WB Saunders, p. 232.)

Common X-Ray Views of the Elbow (Depending on Pathology)

- Anteroposterior view (see Figure 6-56, *A*)
- Lateral view at 90° flexion (see Figure 6-56, *B*)
- Cubital tunnel view (see Figure 6-61)
- Anteroposterior internal oblique view (trauma) (Figure 6-57, *B*)
- Anteroposterior external oblique view (trauma) (Figure 6-57, *A*)

---

with the anteroposterior view, any loose bodies, calcifications in or around the joint (Figure 6-58), myositis ossificans, dislocations (Figure 6-59), joint space narrowing, or osteophytes should be noted. The presence of the fat pad sign (Figure 6-60) occurs with elbow joint effusion and may indicate, for example, a fracture, acute rheumatoid arthritis, infection, or osteoid osteoma.[64] Plain radiographs may also be used to visualize the cubital tunnel (Figure 6-61) and to measure the carrying angle (see Figure 6-7).

Axial View. This view is taken with the elbow flexed to 45°. It shows the olecranon process and epicondyles. It is useful for showing osteophytes and loose bodies.[39]

Arthrography

Figure 6-62 illustrates the views seen in normal elbow arthrograms. With the advent of magnetic resonance imaging (MRI), this technique is seldom used today.

Magnetic Resonance Imaging

MRI is used to differentiate bone and soft tissues. Because of its high soft-tissue contrast, MRI, a noninvasive technique, is able to discriminate among bone marrow,

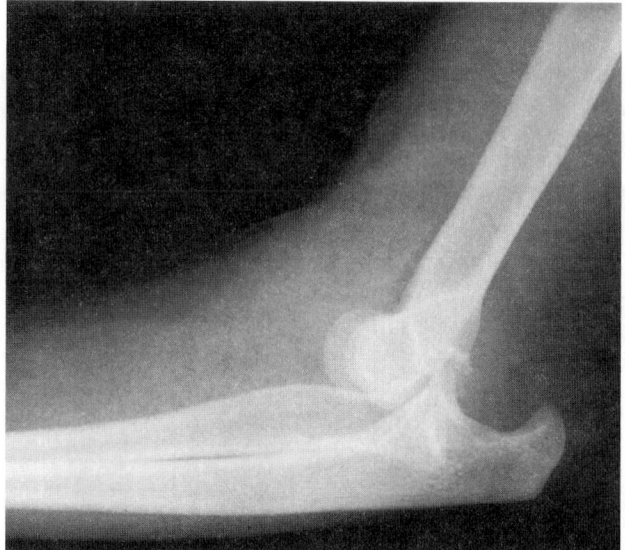

Figure 6-59 Lateral film of a dislocated elbow, showing the lower end of the humerus resting on the ulna in front of the coronoid. Note fragmentation of the coronoid. (From O'Donoghue DH: Treatment of injuries to athletes, ed 4, Philadelphia, 1984, WB Saunders, p. 227.)

cartilage, tendons, nerves, and vessels without the use of a contrast medium (Figures 6-63 to 6-65).[65,66] The technique is used to demonstrate tendon ruptures, collateral ligament ruptures, cubital tunnel pathology, epicondylitis, and osteochondritis dissecans.[67-69]

Xerography

Figure 6-66 illustrates the detailed borders of the various structures around the elbow.

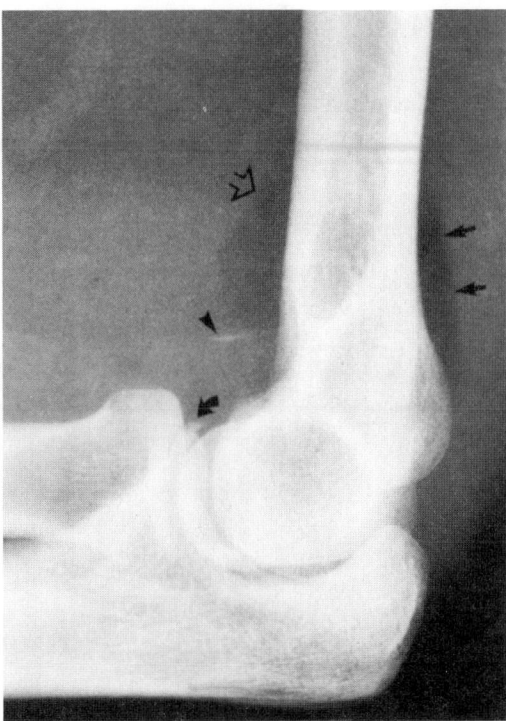

Figure 6-60 Coronoid process fracture with hemarthrosis. The posterior fat pad *(arrows)* is shown clearly on this lateral view with the arm flexed to 90°, indicating joint effusion. The anterior fat pad *(open arrow)* is clearly visible. There is a fracture of the coronoid process *(curved arrow)* and a loose body *(arrowhead)*. (From Weissman BNW, Sledge CB: Orthopedic radiology, Philadelphia, 1986, WB Saunders, p. 179.)

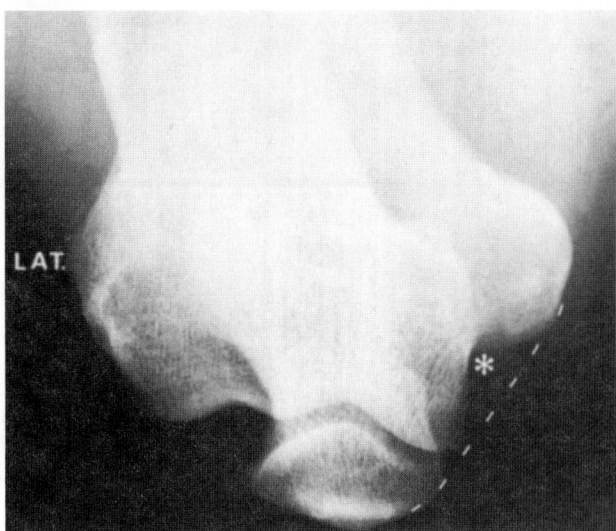

Figure 6-61 Cubital tunnel. The ulnar nerve *(asterisk)* lies in a tunnel bridged by the arcuate ligament *(dashed line)*, which extends from the medial epicondyle to the olecranon process. *LAT,* Lateral.

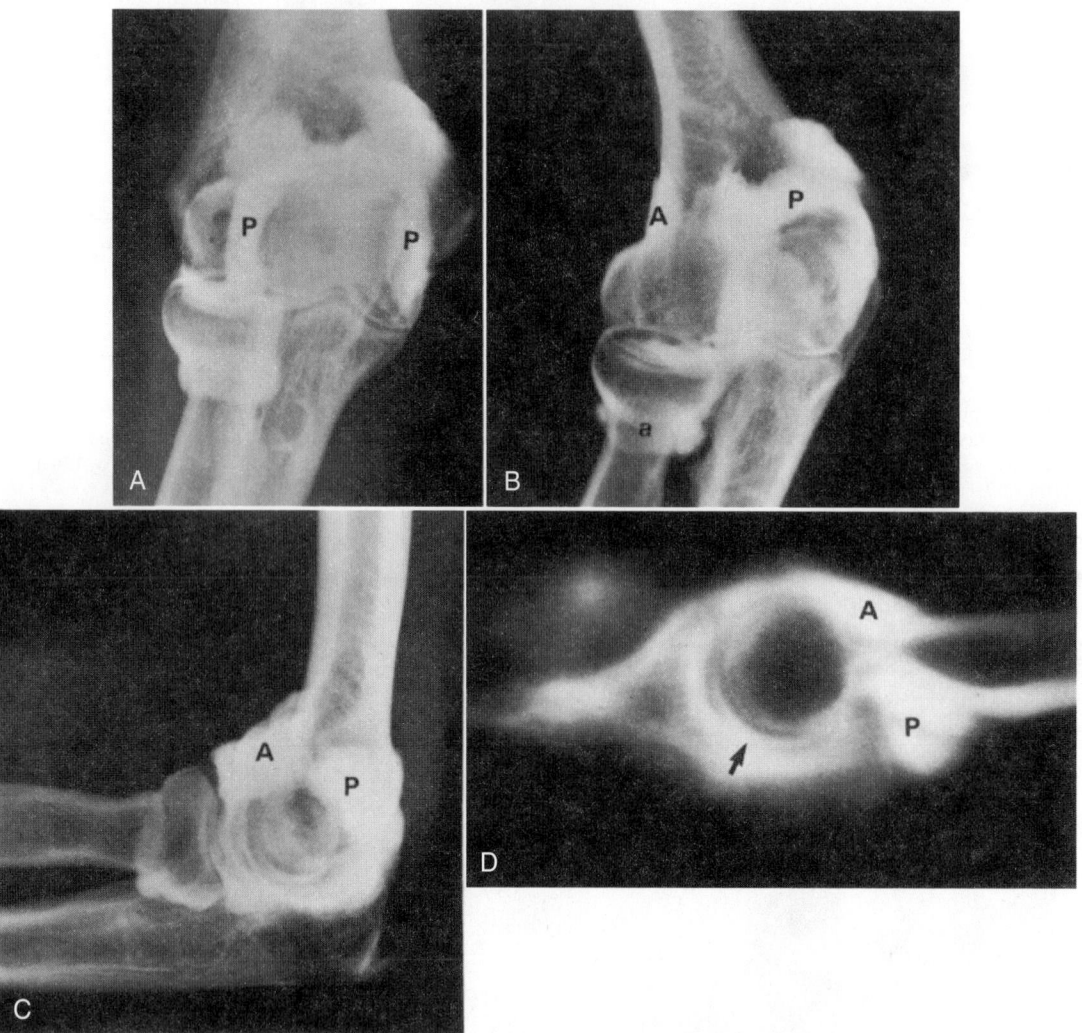

Figure 6-62 Normal elbow arthrogram. Anteroposterior **(A)**, external oblique **(B)**, and lateral **(C)** views in extension show the normal annular *(a)*, anterior *(A)*, and posterior *(P)* recesses. **D,** Lateral tomogram with the arm extended. The area of the trochlea that is devoid of cartilage *(arrow)* is shown. (From Weissman BNW, Sledge CB: Orthopedic radiology, Philadelphia, 1986, WB Saunders, p. 178.)

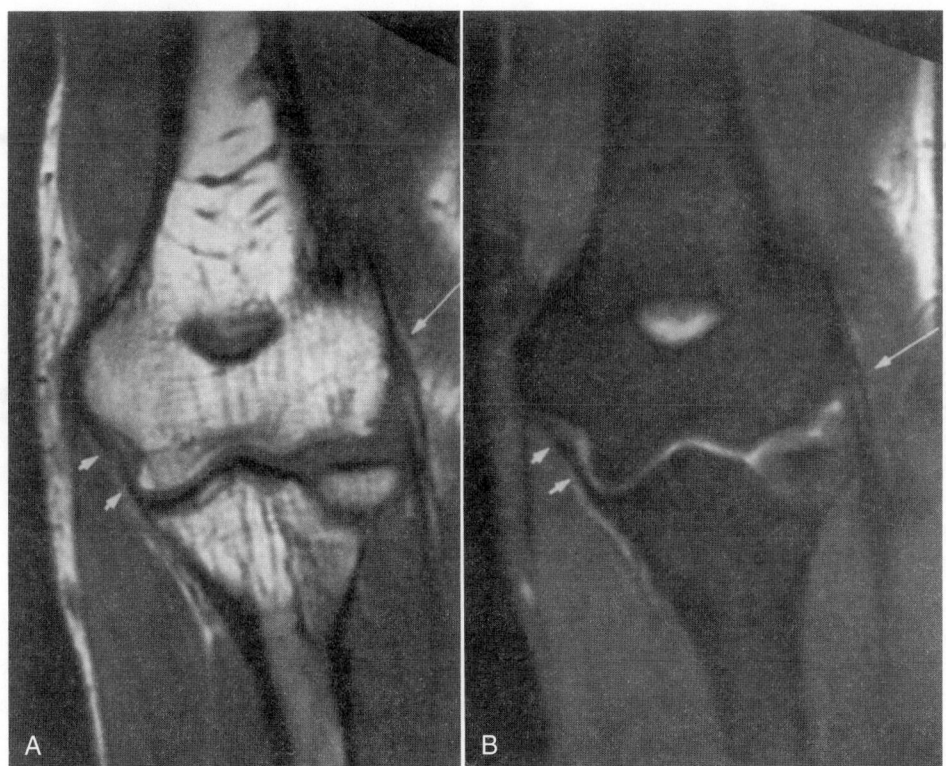

Figure 6-63 Normal common extensor tendon and the medial collateral ligament (MCL). A, Oblique coronal T1-weighted A spine echo and fat-saturated proton density. **B,** Fast spin echo image demonstrates the normal, smooth, thin contour and low signal of the common extensor tendon *(long arrow)* and anterior bundle of the MCL *(short arrows)*. (From Schenk M, Dalinka MK: Imaging of the elbow: an update. Orthop Clin North Am 28:519, 1997.)

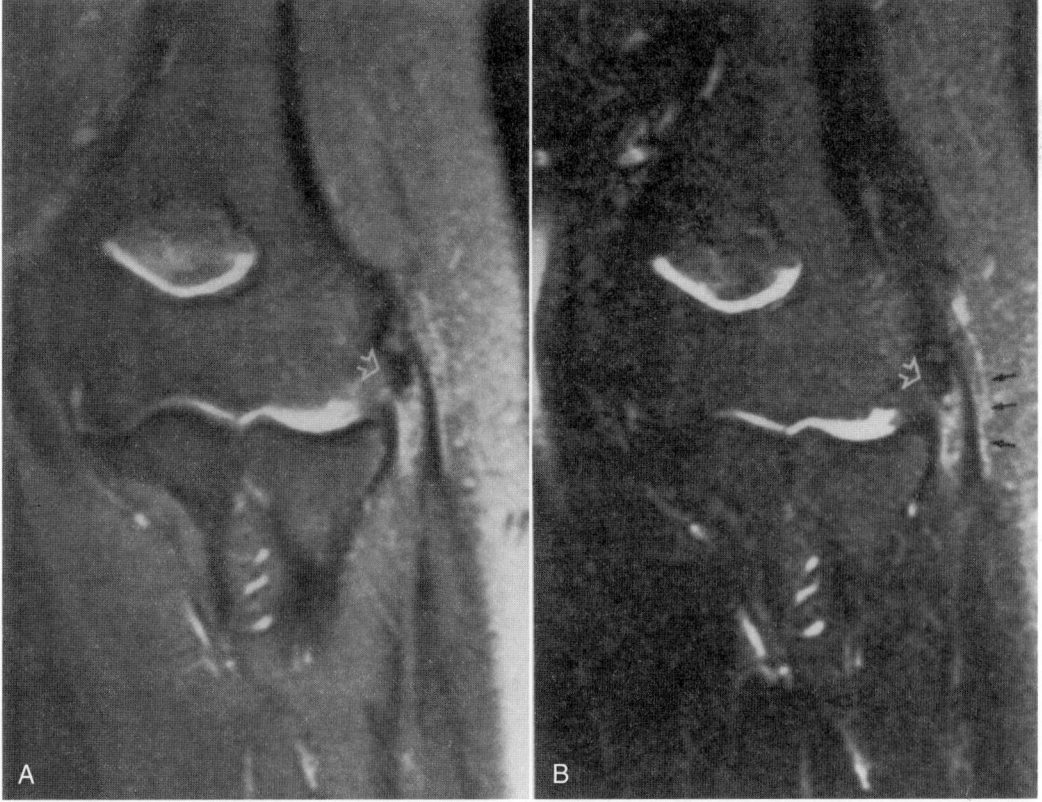

Figure 6-64 Lateral epicondylitis tendinitis. Oblique coronal fat-saturated proton density **(A)** and T2-weighted **(B)** fast spin echo images. Focal calcification within the common extensor tendon *(white arrow)*. There is a moderately increased signal within the tendon, without fiber disruption. Note the edema in the peritendinous tissues *(black arrows)*, suggesting active inflammation. (From Schenk M, Dalinka MK: Imaging of the elbow: an update. Orthop Clin North Am 28:524, 1997.)

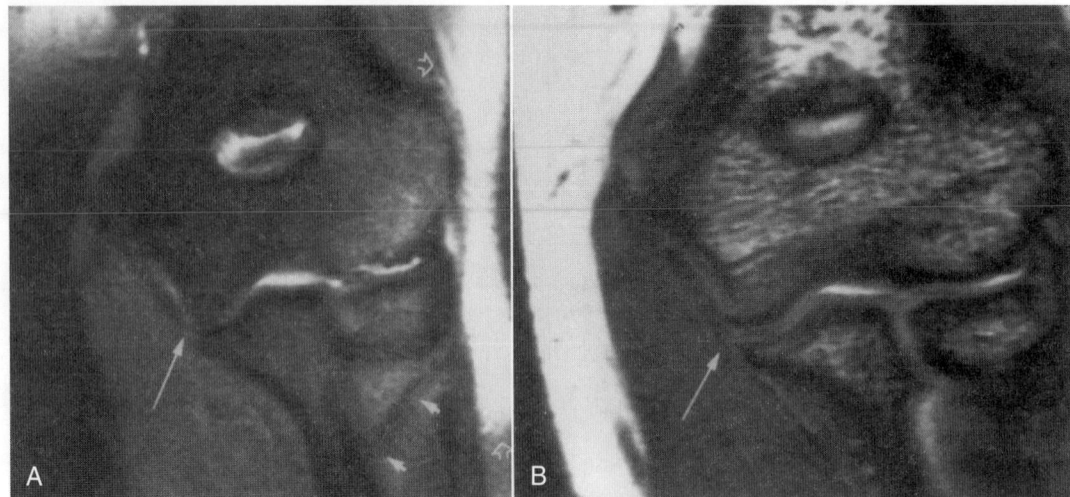

Figure 6-65 A and **B**, Medial collateral ligament (MCL) tear. Surgically proven tear in an athlete who was injured 3 months before imaging and complained of persistent pain with throwing. Oblique coronal fat-saturated proton density image shows a complete tear of the anterior bundle at its distal attachment to the ulna *(long arrow)*. Note the lateral ulna collateral ligament inserting into the ulna *(short arrows)*. Also note the bright signal within the subcutaneous fat laterally *(open arrows)*, which is secondary to incomplete fat suppression and should not be mistaken for edema. Three-dimensional gradient echo image reformatted along the plane of the MCL also demonstrates the distal tear *(arrow)*. (From Schenk M, Dalinka MK: Imaging of the elbow: an update. Orthop Clin North Am 28:528, 1997.)

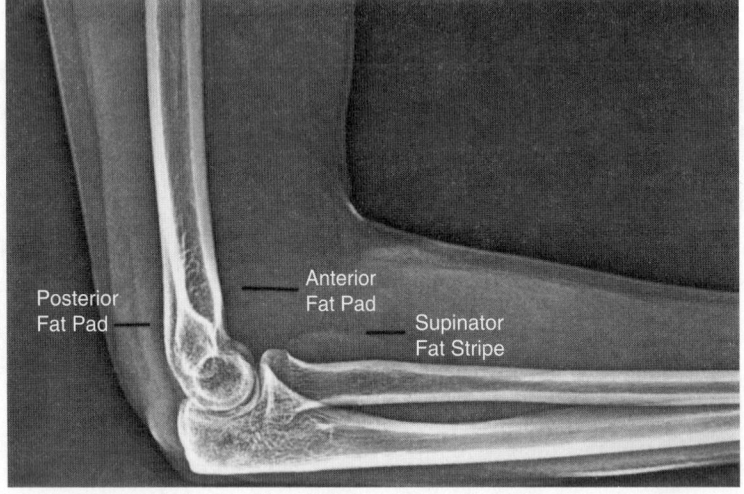

Figure 6-66 Xerogram of the elbow demonstrating the fat pads and supinator fat stripe resulting from subtle radial head fracture. (From Berquist TH: Diagnostic radiographic techniques of the elbow. In Morrey BF, editor: The elbow and its disorders, Philadelphia, 1993, WB Saunders, p. 106.)

PRÉCIS OF THE ELBOW ASSESSMENT*

History
Observation
Examination
  Active movements
    Elbow flexion
    Elbow extension
    Supination
    Pronation
    Combined movements (if necessary)
    Repetitive movements (if necessary)
    Sustained positions (if necessary)
  Passive movements (as in active movements, if necessary)
  Resisted isometric movements
    Elbow flexion
    Elbow extension
    Supination
    Pronation
    Wrist flexion
    Wrist extension
  Functional assessment
  Special tests
    For ligamentous instability:
      Lateral pivot shift test of the elbow
      Ligamentous valgus instability test
      Ligamentous varus instability test
      Milking maneuver
      Moving valgus stress test
    For biceps rupture (third-degree strain):
      Hook test
      Popeye sign (proximal longhead of biceps)

  For lateral epicondylitis (epicondylalgia):
    Cozen's test
    Mill's test
  For plica:
    Extension-supination plica test
    Flexion-pronation plica test
  For posterior impingement:
    Arm bar test
    Extension impingement test
  For neurological dysfunction:
    Elbow flexion test (ulnar nerve)
    Pinch grip test (anterior interosseous branch of
      median nerve)
    Tinel sign at elbow (ulnar nerve)
  Reflexes and cutaneous distribution
    Reflexes
    Sensory scan
    Peripheral nerves
      Median nerve and branches
      Ulnar nerve
      Radial nerve and branches
  Joint play movements
    Radial deviation of ulna and radius on humerus
    Ulnar deviation of ulna and radius on humerus
    Distraction of olecranon process on humerus in 90° of
      flexion
    Anteroposterior glide of radius on humerus
  Palpation
  Diagnostic imaging

*The entire assessment may be done with the patient in sitting position. After any examination, the patient should be warned of the possibility that symptoms may exacerbate as a result of the assessment.

CASE STUDIES

When doing these case studies, the examiner should list the appropriate questions to ask the patient and should specify why they are being asked, what to look for and why, and what things should be tested and why. Depending on the patient's answers (and the examiner should consider numerous different responses), several possible causes of the patient's problem may become evident (examples are given in parentheses). The examiner should prepare a differential diagnosis chart (Table 6-5 is an example for question 1). The examiner can then decide how different diagnoses may affect the treatment plan.

1. A 24-year-old woman comes to you complaining of pain in her right elbow on the medial side. The pain sometimes extends into the forearm and is often accompanied by tingling into the little finger and half of the ring finger. The pain and paresthesia are particularly bothersome when she plays recreational volleyball, which she enjoys very much. Describe your assessment plan for this patient (ulnar neuritis versus medial epicondylitis).

2. A 52-year-old man is referred to you with a history of right elbow pain. He complains of tenderness over the lateral epicondyle. He informs you that he has not done any repetitive forearm activity and does not play tennis. He has some restriction of neck movement. Describe your assessment plan for this patient (cervical spondylosis versus lateral epicondylitis).

3. A 26-year-old male football player is referred to you after surgery for a ruptured (third-degree strain) left biceps tendon at its insertion. His cast has been removed, and you have been asked to restore the patient to normal function. Describe your assessment plan for this patient.

4. Parents bring their 4-year-old daughter in to see you. They state that about 2 hours previously they were out shopping, and the mother was holding the little girl's arm. The little girl tripped, and the mother "yanked" her up as she fell. The little girl started to cry and would not move her elbow.

Continued

CASE STUDIES—cont'd

Describe your assessment plan for this patient (radial head dislocation versus ligamentous sprain).

5. A 46-year-old man comes to you complaining of diffuse left elbow pain. When he carries a briefcase for three or four blocks, his elbow becomes stiff and sore. When he picks up things with his left hand, the pain increases dramatically. Describe your assessment plan for this patient (lateral epicondylitis versus osteoarthritis).

6. A 31-year-old man comes to you complaining of posterior elbow pain. He says he banged his elbow on the table 10 days earlier, and he has had posterior swelling for 8 or 9 days. Describe your assessment plan for this patient (olecranon bursitis versus joint synovitis).

7. A 14-year-old female gymnast comes to you complaining of elbow pain. She explains she was doing a vault and bent her elbow backward, at which time she heard a snap. The injury occurred 1 hour earlier, and there is some swelling; she does not want to move the elbow. Describe your assessment plan for this patient (biceps tendon rupture versus epiphyseal fracture).

TABLE **6-5**

Differential Diagnosis of Ulnar Neuritis and Medial Epicondylitis

	Ulnar Neuritis	Medial Epicondylitis
History	May follow repetitive activity May follow bumped elbow May follow previously injured elbow Pain in forearm and into ulnar distribution of hand	Usually follows repetitive activity Pain in forearm, may radiate to wrist
Observation	Normal	Normal
Active movements	Weakness of ulnar deviation Weakness of little and ring finger flexion	Slight pain on wrist flexion
Passive movements	Normal, or pain may come on with elbow flexion and wrist flexion	Normal, but pain may occur with elbow extension and wrist extension
Resisted isometric movements	Weakness of ulnar deviation Weakness of little and ring finger flexion	Pain on wrist extension with elbow extension Pain on supination and wrist and finger flexion
Special tests	Tinel sign positive Wartenberg sign positive Elbow flexion test positive	Golfer's elbow test positive
Sensation	Paresthesia and pain in forearm, little finger, and half of ring finger	Pain in forearm, possibly to wrist

REFERENCES

1. Cohen MS, Bruno RJ: The collateral ligaments of the elbow: anatomy and clinical correlation. Clin Orthop Relat Res 383:123–130, 2001.
2. O'Driscoll SW: Acute, recurrent and chronic elbow instabilities. In Norris TR, editor: Orthopedic knowledge update 2: shoulder and elbow, Rosemont, IL, 2002, American Academy of Orthopedic Surgeons.
3. Bozkurt M, Acar HI, Apaydin N, et al: The annular ligament: an anatomical study. Am J Sports Med 33:114–118, 2005.
4. Dutton M: Orthopedic examination, evaluation and intervention, New York, 2004, McGraw-Hill.
5. Andrews JR, Wilk KE, Satterwhite YE, et al: Physical examination of the thrower's elbow. J Orthop Sports Phys Ther 17:296–304, 1993.
6. Petty NJ, Moore AP: Neuromusculoskeletal examination and assessment, London, 1998, Churchill Livingstone.
7. Beals RK: The normal carrying angle of the elbow. Clin Orthop 1190:194–196, 1976.

8. Charton A: The elbow: the rheumatological physical examination, Orlando, FL, 1986, Grune & Stratton.
9. Kapandji AI: The physiology of the joints, vol. 1: upper limb, New York, 1970, Churchill Livingstone.
10. American Orthopaedic Association: Manual of orthopaedic surgery, Chicago, 1972, American Orthopaedic Association.
11. Tarr RR, Garfinkel AI, Sarmiento A: The effects of angular and rotational deformities of both bones of the forearm. J Bone Joint Surg Am 66:65–70, 1984.
12. Clarkson HM: Musculoskeletal assessment: joint range of motion and manual muscle strength, Philadelphia, 2000, Lippincott Williams & Wilkins.
13. Askew LJ, An KN, Morrey BF, et al: Isometric elbow strength in normal individuals. Clin Orthop 222:261–266, 1987.
14. Ramsey ML: Distal biceps tendon injuries: diagnosis and management. J Am Acad Orthop Surg 7:199–207, 1999.

15. Morrey BF, An KN, Chao EYS: Functional evaluation of the elbow. In Morrey BF, editor: The elbow and its disorders, Philadelphia, 1993, WB Saunders.
16. Alberta FG, El Attrache NS, Bissell S, et al: The development and validation of a functional assessment tool for the upper extremity in the overhead athlete. Am J Sports Med 38:903–911, 2010.
17. Domb BG, David JT, Alberta FG, et al: Clinical follow up of professional baseball players undergoing ulnar collateral ligament reconstruction using the new Kerlan-Jobe Orthopedic Clinic overhead athlete shoulder and elbow score (KJOC score). Am J Sports Med 38:1558–1563, 2010.
18. Regan WD, Morrey BF: The physical examination of the elbow. In Morrey BF, editor: The elbow and its disorders, Philadelphia, 1993, WB Saunders.
19. Cook CE, Hegedus EJ: Orthopedic physical examination tests—an evidence based approach, Upper Saddle River, NJ, 2008, Pearson/Prentice Hall.

20. Cleland JA, Koppenhaver S: Netter's orthopedic clinical examination—an evidence-based approach, ed 2, Philadelphia, 2011, Saunders/Elsevier.

21. O'Driscoll SW: Classification and evaluation of recurrent instability of the elbow. Clin Orthop Relat Res 370:34–43, 2000.

22. Mehta JA, Bain GI: Posterolateral rotary instability of the elbow. J Am Acad Ortho Surg 12:405–415, 2004.

23. O'Driscoll SW, Bell DF, Morrey BF: Posterolateral rotary instability of the elbow. J Bone Joint Surg Am 73:440–446, 1991.

24. O'Driscoll SW, Lawton RM, Smith AM: The "moving valgus stress test" for medial collateral ligament tears of the elbow. Am J Sports Med 33:231–239, 2005.

25. Lee ML, Rosenwasser MP: Chronic elbow instability. Orthop Clin North Am 30:81–89, 1999.

26. Kalainov DM, Cohen MS: The posterolateral rotary instability of the elbow in association with lateral epicondylitis: a report to three cases. J Bone Joint Surg Am 87:1120–1125, 2005.

27. Hsu SH, Moen TC, Levine WN, et al: Physical examination of the athlete's elbow. Am J Sports Med 40:699–708, 2012.

28. Ruland RT, Dunbar RP, Bowen JD: The biceps squeeze test for diagnosis of distal biceps tendon ruptures. Clin Orthop Relat Res 437:128–131, 2005.

29. O'Driscoll SW, Goncalves LB, Dietz P: The hook test for distal biceps tendon avulsion. Am J Sports Med 35:1865–1869, 2007.

30. Kraushaar BS, Nirschl RP: Tendinosis of the elbow (tennis elbow). J Bone Joint Surg Am 81:259–278, 1999.

31. Johnstone AJ: Tennis elbow and upper limb tendinopathies. Sports Med Arthro Rev 8:69–79, 2000.

32. Roles NC, Maudsley RH: Radial tunnel syndrome: resistant tennis elbow as a nerve entrapment. J Bone Joint Surg Br 54:499–508, 1972.

33. Antuna SA, O'Driscoll SW: Snapping plica associated with radiocapitellar chondromalacia. Arthroscopy 17:491–495, 2001.

34. Buehler MJ, Thayer DT: The elbow flexion test: a clinical test for the cubital tunnel syndrome. Clin Orthop 233:213–216, 1988.

35. Butler DS: Mobilisation of the nervous system, Melbourne, 1991, Churchill Livingstone.

36. Ochi K, Horiuchi Y, Tanabe A, et al: Shoulder internal rotation elbow flexion test for diagnosing cubital tunnel syndrome. J Shoulder Elbow Surg 21:777–781, 2012.

37. Kroonen LT: Cubital tunnel syndrome. Orthop Clin North Am 43:475–486, 2012.

38. Cheng CJ, Mackinnon-Patterson B, Beck JL, et al: Scratch collapse test for evaluation of carpal and cubital tunnel syndrome. J Hand Surg Am 33:1518–1524, 2008.

39. Bigg-Wither G, Kelly P: Diagnostic imaging in musculoskeletal physiotherapy. In Refshauge K, Gass E, editors: Musculoskeletal physiotherapy: clinical science and practice, Oxford, 1995, Butterworth-Heinemann.

40. Limb D, Hodkinson SL, Brown RF: Median nerve palsy after posterolateral elbow dislocation. J Bone Joint Surg Br 76:987–988, 1994.

41. Conrad RW, Spinner RJ: Snapping brachialis tendon associated with median neuropathy. J Bone Joint Surg Am 77:1891–1893, 1995.

42. Popinchalk SP, Schaffer AA: Physical examination of upper extremity compression neuropathies. Orthop Clin North Am 43:417–430, 2012.

43. Spinner M, Spencer PS: Nerve compression lesions of the upper extremity: a clinical and experimental review. Clin Orthop 104:46–67, 1974.

44. Butlers KP, Singer KM: Nerve lesions of the arm and elbow. In De Lee JC, Drez D, editors: Orthopedic sports medicine: principles and practice, Philadelphia, 1994, WB Saunders.

45. Rask MR: Anterior interosseous nerve entrapment (Kiloh-Nevin Syndrome). Clin Orthop 142:176–181, 1979.

46. Wiens E, Lau SCK: The anterior interosseous nerve syndrome. Can J Surg 21:354–357, 1978.

47. Engher WD, Keene JS: Anterior interosseous nerve palsy associated with a Monteggia fracture. Clin Orthop 174:133–137, 1983.

48. O'Driscoll SW, Horii E, Carmichael SW, et al: The cubital tunnel and ulnar neuropathy. J Bone Joint Surg Br 73:613–617, 1991.

49. McPherson SA, Meals RA: Cubital tunnel syndrome. Orthop Clin North Am 23:111–123, 1992.

50. Wadsworth TG: The external compression syndrome of the ulnar nerve at the cubital tunnel. Clin Orthop 124:189–204, 1977.

51. Pecina MM, Krmpotic-Nemanic J, Markiewitz AD: Tunnel syndromes, Boca Raton, FL, 1991, CRC Press.

52. Khoo D, Carmichael SW, Spinner RJ: Ulnar nerve anatomy and compression. Orthop Clin North Am 27:317–338, 1996.

53. Gelberman RH, Eaton R, Urbaniak JR: Peripheral nerve compression. J Bone Joint Surg Am 75:1854–1878, 1993.

54. Apfelberg DB, Larsen SJ: Dynamic anatomy of the ulnar nerve by the deep flexor-pronator aponeurosis. Plast Reconstr Surg 51:79–81, 1973.

55. Holmes JC, Hall JE: Tardy ulnar nerve palsy in children. Clin Orthop 135:128–131, 1978.

56. Calfee RP, Manske PR, Gelberman RH, et al: Clinical assessment of the ulnar nerve at the elbow: reliability of instability testing and the association of hypermobility with clinical symptoms. J Bone Joint Surg Am 92:2801–2808, 2010.

57. Wadsworth TG: The elbow, New York, 1982, Churchill Livingstone.

58. Plancher KD, Peterson RK, Steichen JB: Compressive neuropathies and tendinopathies in the athletic elbow and wrist. Clin Sports Med 15:331–372, 1996.

59. Weinstein SM, Herring SA: Nerve problems and compartment syndromes in the hand, wrist and forearm. Clin Sports Med 11:161–188, 1992.

60. Lutz FR: Radial tunnel syndrome: an etiology of chronic lateral elbow pain. J Orthop Sports Phys Ther 14:14–17, 1991.

61. Ferlec DC, Morrey BF: Evaluation of the painful elbow: the problem elbow. In Morrey BF, editor: The elbow and its disorders, Philadelphia, 1993, WB Saunders.

62. Lister GD, Belsole RB, Kleinert HE: The radial tunnel syndrome. J Hand Surg 4:52–59, 1979.

63. Van Rossum J, Buruma OJ, Kamphuisen HA, et al: Tennis elbow: a radial tunnel syndrome? J Bone Joint Surg Br 60:197–198, 1978.

64. Quinton DN, Finlay D, Butterworth R: The elbow fat pad sign: brief report. J Bone Joint Surg Br 69:844–845, 1987.

65. Herzog RJ: Efficacy of magnetic resonance imaging of the elbow. Med Sci Sports Exerc 26:1193–1202, 1994.

66. Miller TT: Imaging of elbow disorders. Orthop Clin North Am 30:21–36, 1999.

67. Fritz RC, Brody GA: MR imaging of the wrist and elbow. Clin Sports Med 14:315–352, 1995.

68. Schenk M, Dalinka MK: Imaging of the elbow: an update. Orthop Clin North Am 28:517–535, 1997.

69. Tuite MJ, Kijowski R: Sports related injuries of the elbow: an approach to MRI interpretation. Clin Sports Med 25:387–408, 2006.

70. Novak CB, Lee GW, Mackinnon SE, et al: Provocative testing for cubital tunnel syndrome. J Hand Surg Am 19:817–820, 1994.

71. Hawksworth CR, Freeland P: Inability to fully extend the injured elbow: an indicator of significant injury. Arch Emerg Med 8(4):253–256, 1991.

72. Docherty MA, Schwab RA, Ma OJ: Can elbow extension be used as a test of clinically significant injury? Southern Med J 95:539–541, 2002.

73. Irshad F, Shaw NJ, Gregory RJ: Reliability of fat pad sign in radial head/neck fractures of the elbow. Injury 28:433–435, 1997.

74. Patla CE, Paris SV: Reliability of interpretation of the Paris classification of normal end-feel for elbow flexion and extension. J Man Manip Ther 1:60–66, 1993.

75. Smidt N, van der Windt DA, Assendelft WJ, et al: Intraobserver reproducibility of the assessment of severity of complaints, grip strength, and pressure pain threshold in patients with lateral epicondylitis. Arch Phys Med Rehabil 83:1145–1150, 2002.

76. Stratford PW, Norman GR, McIntosh JM: Generalizability of grip strength measurements in patients with tennis elbow. Phys Ther 69:276–281, 1989.

77. Overend TJ, Wupri-Fearn JL, Kramer JF, et al: Reliability of a patient-rated forearm evaluation questionnaire for patients with lateral epicondylitis. J Hand Ther 12:31–37, 1999.

SUGGESTED READINGS

Aeurbach DM, Collins ED, Kunkle KL, et al: The radial sensory nerve: an anatomic study. Clin Orthop 308:241–249, 1994.

Amir D, Frankel U, Pogrund H: Pulled elbow and hypermobility of joints. Clin Orthop 257:94–99, 1990.

An KN, Morrey BF: Biomechanics of the elbow. In Morrey BF, editor: The elbow and its disorders, Philadelphia, 1993, WB Saunders.

Anderson TE: Anatomy and physical examination of the elbow. In Nicholas JA, Hershman EB, editors: The upper extremity in sports medicine, St Louis, 1990, Mosby.

Andrews JR, Meister K: Overuse injuries of the athlete's elbow. In Griffin LY, editor: Orthopedic knowledge update: sports medicine, Rosemont, IL, 1994, American Academy of Orthopaedic Surgeons.

Bassett LW, Gold RH, Seeger LL: MRI atlas of the musculoskeletal system, London, 1989, Martin Dunitz.

Belhobek GH: Roentgenographic evaluation of the elbow. In Nicholas JA, EB Hershman, editors: The upper extremity in sports medicine, St Louis, 1990, Mosby.

Berg EE, DeHoll D: The lateral elbow ligaments: a correlative radiographic study. Am J Sports Med 27:796–800, 1999.

Berquist TH: Diagnostic radiographic techniques of the elbow. In Morrey BF, editor: The elbow and its disorders, Philadelphia, 1993, WB Saunders.

Bledsoe RC, Izenstark JL: Displacement of fat pads in disease and injury of the elbow. Radiology 73:717–724, 1959.

Booker JM, Thibodeau GA: Athletic injury assessment, St Louis, 1989, Times Mirror/Mosby.

Bowling RW, Rockar PA: The elbow complex. In Gould JA, editor: Orthopedic and sports physical therapy, St Louis, 1990, Mosby.

Bunnell DH, Fisher DA, Bassett LW, et al: Elbow joint: normal anatomy on MR images. Radiology 165:527–531, 1987.

Cabrera JM, McCue FC: Nonosseous athletic injuries of the elbow, forearm, and hand. Clin Sports Med 5:681–700, 1986.

Chusid JG, McDonald JJ: Correlative neuroanatomy and functional neurology, Los Altos, CA, 1961, Lange Medical.

Clark CB: Cubital tunnel syndrome. JAMA 241:801–802, 1979.

Colman WW, Strauch RJ: Physical examination of the elbow. Orthop Clin North Am 30:15–20, 1999.

Conwell HE: Injuries to the elbow. Clin Symp 22:35–54, 1970.

Coutu R: Evaluating adolescent elbow injuries. Sports Med Update 13:10–13, 1998.

Cyriax J: Textbook of orthopaedic medicine, vol. 1: diagnosis of soft tissue lesions, London, 1982, Bailliere Tindall.

Del Pizzo W, Jobe FW, Norwood L: Ulnar nerve entrapment in baseball players. Am J Sports Med 5:182–185, 1977.

Dellon AL, Mackinnon SE: Radial sensory nerve entrapment in the forearm. J Hand Surg 11:199–205, 1986.

Dilorenzo CE, Parker JC, Chmelar RD: The importance of shoulder and cervical dysfunction in the etiology and treatment of athletic elbow injuries. J Orthop Sports Phys Ther 11:402–409, 1990.

Evans RC: Illustrated essentials in orthopedic physical assessment, St Louis, 1994, Mosby.

Forrester DM, Brown JC: The radiology of joint disease, Philadelphia, 1987, WB Saunders.

Garrick JG, Webb DR: Sports injuries: diagnosis and management, Philadelphia, 1990, WB Saunders.

Gunn CC, Milbrandt WE: Tennis elbow and the cervical spine. Can Med Assoc J 114:803–809, 1976.

Hollinshead WH, Jenkins DB: Functional anatomy of the limbs and back, Philadelphia, 1981, WB Saunders.

Hoppenfeld S: Physical examination of the spine and extremities, New York, 1976, Appleton-Century-Crofts.

Ishizuki M: Functional anatomy of the elbow joint and three-dimensional quantitative motion analysis of the elbow joint. J Jpn Orthop Assoc 53:989, 1979.

Jameson GG, Fleisig GS: Ulnar collateral ligament demands: investigating the biomechanics of UCL injuries. Sports Med Update 12:4–7, 1997.

Jobe FW, Fanton GS, Elaltrache NS: Ulnar nerve injury. In Morrey BF, editor: The elbow and its disorders, Philadelphia, 1993, WB Saunders.

Johnson RK, Spinner M, Shrewsburg MM: Median nerve entrapment syndrome in the proximal forearm. J Hand Surg 4:48–51, 1979.

Judge RD, Zuidema GD, Fitzgerald FT: Clinical diagnosis: a physiological approach, Boston, 1982, Little, Brown.

Kaltenborn FM: Mobilization of the extremity joints, Oslo, 1980, Olaf Norlis Bokhandel.

Kaminski TW, Powers ME, Buckley B: Differential assessment of elbow injuries. Athl Ther Today 5:6–11, 2000.

Kiloh LG, Nevin S: Isolated neuritis of the anterior interosseous nerve. Br Med J 1:850–851, 1952.

Leach RE, Miller JK: Lateral and medial epicondylitis of the elbow. Clin Sports Med 6:259–272, 1987.

London JT: Kinematics of the elbow. J Bone Joint Surg Am 63:529–535, 1981.

Macdonald DA: The shoulder and elbow. In Pynsent P, Fairbank J, Carr A, editors: Outcome measures in orthopedics, Oxford, 1993, Butterworth-Heinemann.

Maitland GD: The peripheral joints: examination and recording guide, Adelaide, Australia, 1973, Virgo Press.

Maloney MD, Mohr KJ, El Ahrache NS: Elbow injuries in the throwing athlete: difficult diagnosis and surgical complications. Clin Sports Med 18:795–809, 1999.

McFarland EG, Mamanee P, Queale WS, et al: Olecranon and prepatellar bursitis: treating acute, chronic and inflamed. Phys. Sportsmed 28:40–52, 2000.

Morrey BF: Loose bodies. In Morrey BF, editor: The elbow and its disorders, Philadelphia, 1993, WB Saunders.

Morrey BF: Physical examination of the elbow. In Post M, editor: Physical examination of the musculoskeletal system, Chicago, 1987, Year Book Medical.

Moss SH, Switzer HE: Radial tunnel syndrome: a spectrum of clinical presentations. J Hand Surg 8:414–420, 1983.

Nelson AJ, Izzi JA, Green A, et al: Traumatic nerve injuries about the elbow. Orthop Clin North Am 30:91–94, 1999.

Neumann DA: Kinesiology of the musculoskeletal system: foundations for physical rehabilitation, St Louis, 2002, Mosby.

Newberg AH: The radiographic examination of shoulder and elbow pain in the athlete. Clin Sports Med 6:785–809, 1987.

Nolan R: Cubital tunnel syndrome. Sports Med Update 5:21–23, 1990.

O'Donoghue DH: Treatment of injuries to athletes, Philadelphia, 1984, WB Saunders.

Ombregt L, Bisschop P: Atlas of orthopedic examination of the peripheral joints, Philadelphia, 1999, WB Saunders.

Omer GE: Physical diagnosis of peripheral nerve injuries. Orthop Clin North Am 12:207–228, 1981.

Palmer ML, Epler M: Clinical assessment procedures in physical therapy, Philadelphia, 1990, JB Lippincott.

Plancher KD, Halbrecht J, Lourie GM: Medial and lateral epicondylitis in the athlete. Clin Sports Med 15:283–303, 1996.

Radwin RG, Sesto ME, Zachary SV: Functional tests to quantify recovery following carpal tunnel release. J Bone Joint Surg Am 86:2614–2620, 2004.

Regan WD: Lateral elbow pain in the athlete: a clinical review. Clin J Sports Med 1:53–58, 1991.

Reid DC: Sports injury assessment and rehabilitation, New York, 1992, Churchill Livingstone.

Reid DC, Kushner S: The elbow region. In Donatelli R, Wooden MJ, editors: Orthopedic physical therapy, Edinburgh, 1989, Churchill Livingstone.

Roles NC, Madusley RH: Radial tunnel syndrome: resistant tennis elbow as a nerve entrapment. J Bone Joint Surg Br 54:499–508, 1972.

Skaggs DL, Mirzayan R: The posterior fat pad sign in association with occult fracture of the elbow in children. J Bone Joint Surg Am 81:1429–1433, 1999.

Spinner M: The arcade of Frohse and its relationship to posterior interosseous nerve paralysis. J Bone Joint Surg Br 50:809–812, 1968.

Spinner M, Linscheid RL: Nerve entrapment syndromes. In Morrey BF, editor: The elbow and its disorders, Philadelphia, 1993, WB Saunders.

Sprofkin BE: Cheiralgia paresthetica: Wartenberg's disease. Neurology 4:857–862, 1954.

Steinberg BD, Plancher KD: Clinical anatomy of the wrist and elbow. Clin Sports Med 14:299–313, 1995.

Stroyan M, Wilk KE: The functional anatomy of the elbow complex. J Orthop Sports Phys Ther 17:279–288, 1993.

Terzis JK, Noah EM: Anatomy and morphology of upper extremity nerves and frequent sites of compression. In Gordon SL, Blair SJ, Fine LJ, editors: Repetitive motion disorders of the upper extremity, Rosemont, IL, 1995, American Academy of Orthopaedic Surgeons.

Tomberlin JP, Saunders HD: Evaluation, treatment and prevention of musculoskeletal disorders: the extremities, Chaska, MN, 1994, The Saunders Group.

Tullos HS, Bryan WJ: Examination of the throwing elbow. In Zarins B, Andrews JR, Carson WG, editors: Injuries to the throwing arm, Philadelphia, 1985, WB Saunders.

Wadsworth CT: Manual examination and treatment of the spine and extremities, Baltimore, 1988, Williams & Wilkins.

Weissman BNW, Sledge CB: Orthopedic radiology, Philadelphia, 1986, WB Saunders.

Williams PL, Warwick R, editors: Gray's anatomy, ed 36, British, Edinburgh, 1980, Churchill Livingstone.

Yocum LA: The diagnosis and nonoperative treatment of elbow problems in the athlete. Clin Sports Med 8:439–451, 1989.

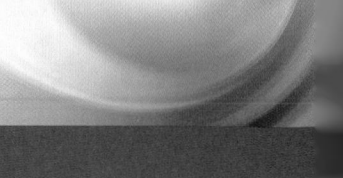

CHAPTER 7

Forearm, Wrist, and Hand

The hand and wrist are the most active and intricate parts of the upper extremity. Because of this, they are vulnerable to injury, which can lead to large functional difficulties, and they do not respond well to serious trauma. Their mobility is enhanced by a wide range of movement at the shoulder and complementary movement at the elbow. The 28 bones, numerous articulations, and 19 intrinsic and 20 extrinsic muscles of the wrist and hand provide a tremendous variability of movement. In addition to being an expressive organ of communication, the hand has a protective role and acts as both a motor and a sensory organ, providing information, such as temperature, thickness, texture, depth, and shape as well as the motion of an object. It is this sensual acuity that enables the examiner to accurately examine and palpate during an assessment.

The assessment of the hand and wrist should be performed with two objectives in mind. First, the injury or lesion should be assessed as accurately as possible to ensure proper treatment. Second, the examiner should evaluate the remaining function to determine whether the patient will have any incapacity in everyday life.

Although the joints of the forearm, wrist, and hand are discussed separately, they do not act in isolation but rather as functional groups. The position of one joint influences the position and action of the other joints. For example, if the wrist is flexed, the interphalangeal joints do not fully flex, primarily because of passive insufficiency of the finger extensors and their tendons. Each articulation depends on balanced forces for proper positioning and control. If this balance or equilibrium is not present because of trauma, nerve injury, or other factors, the loss of counterbalancing forces results in deformities. In addition, the entire upper limb should be considered a kinetic chain that enables the hand to be properly positioned. The actions of the shoulder, elbow, and wrist joints enable the hand to be placed on almost any area of the body.

APPLIED ANATOMY

The **distal radioulnar joint** is a uniaxial pivot joint that has one degree of freedom.[1] Although the radius moves over the ulna, the ulna does not remain stationary. It moves back and laterally during pronation and forward and medially during supination. The resting position of the joint is 10° of supination, and the close packed position is 5° of supination. The capsular pattern of the distal radioulnar joint is full range of motion (ROM) with pain at the extreme of rotation.

Distal Radioulnar Joint

Resting position:	10° of supination
Close packed position:	5° of supination
Capsular pattern:	Full ROM, pain at extremes of rotation

The **radiocarpal (wrist) joint** is a biaxial ellipsoid joint.[1,2] The radius articulates with the scaphoid and lunate. The distal radius is not straight but is angled toward the ulna (15° to 20°), and its posterior margin projects more distally to provide a "buttress effect."[3] The lunate and triquetrum also articulate with the triangular cartilaginous disc (triangular fibrocartilage complex [TFCC]) (Figures 7-1 and 7-2) and not the ulna. The disc extends from the ulnar side of the distal radius and attaches to the ulna at the base of the ulnar styloid process. The disc adds stability to the wrist. It creates a close relation between the ulna and carpal bones and binds together and stabilizes the distal ends of the radius and ulna.[4,5] With the disc in place, the radius bears 60% of the load and the ulna bears 40%. If the disc is removed, the radius transmits 95% of the axial load and the ulna transmits 5%.[6] Therefore, the cartilaginous disc acts as a cushion for the wrist joint and as a major stabilizer of the distal radioulnar joint.[3,7] The disc can be damaged by forced extension and pronation. The distal end of the radius is concave and the proximal row of carpals is convex, but the curvatures are not equal. The joint has 2° of freedom, and the resting position is neutral with slight ulnar deviation. The close packed position is extension, and the capsular pattern is equal limitation of flexion and extension.

Radiocarpal (Wrist) Joint

Resting position:	Neutral with slight ulnar deviation
Close packed position:	Extension with radial deviation
Capsular pattern:	Flexion and extension equally limited (works with midcarpal joints)

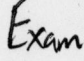

Exam

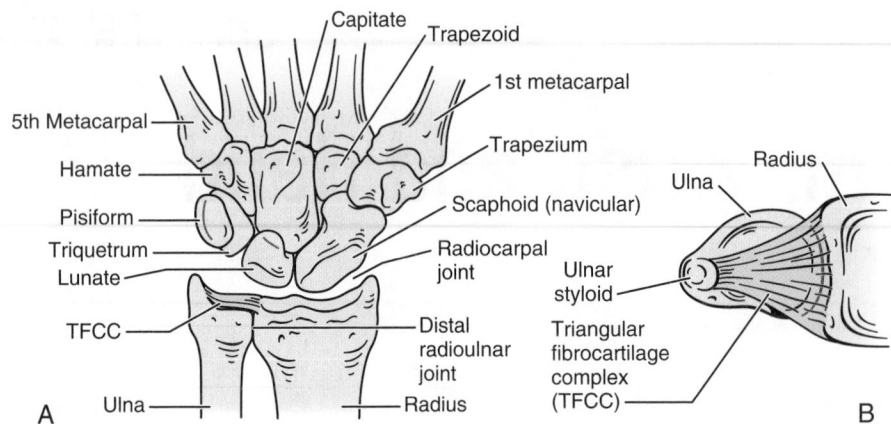

Figure 7-1 Bones and triangular fibrocartilage complex (TFCC). **A,** Palmar view. **B,** End view of TFCC and radius and ulna.

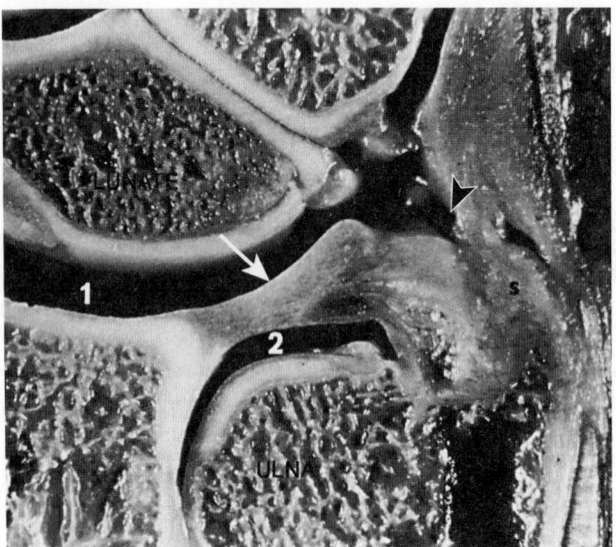

Figure 7-2 Articulations of the wrist: specific compartments. Ulnar limit of the radiocarpal compartment (coronal section). Note the extent of this compartment *(1),* its relationship to the inferior radioulnar compartment *(2),* the intervening triangular fibrocartilage *(arrow),* and the prestyloid recess *(arrowhead),* which is intimate with the ulnar styloid(s). (From Resnick D, Kransdorf MJ: Bone and joint imaging, Philadelphia, 2005, WB Saunders, p. 27.)

The stability of the carpals (wrist) is primarily maintained by a complex configuration of ligaments (Figure 7-3).[8] The ligaments stabilizing the scaphoid, lunate, and triquetrum are the most important.[9] Of these ligaments, the radioscapholunate ligament is one of the most important, because it is commonly injured and, when intact, maintains carpal stability.[10] This ligament is most likely to be injured with a pronated fall on out-stretched hand (FOOSH) injury (wrist extension, ulnar deviation, and intercarpal supination).[9,11] Lunotriquetral injuries are more likely to occur with wrist extension, radial deviation, and intercarpal supination.[9] The palmar ligaments are much stronger than the dorsal ligaments. The palmar extrinsic ligaments control the movement of the wrist and

scaphoid with the radioscapholunate ligament acting as a sling for the scaphoid.[10] This ligament along with the radiolunate ligament allows the scaphoid to rotate around them, and both stabilize the scaphoid at the extremes of motion.[10] On the ulnar side, the ligaments (palmar lunotriquetral, capitotriquetral, dorsal intercarpal, and the fibrocartilaginous disc) control the triquetrum.

The **intercarpal joints** include the joints between the individual bones of the proximal row of carpal bones (scaphoid, lunate, and triquetrum) and the joints between the individual bones of the distal row of carpal bones (trapezium, trapezoid, capitate, and hamate). Perilunate injuries involve the lunate and its relation with the other carpals as well as the radius and ulna.[12] They are bound together by small intercarpal ligaments (dorsal, palmar, and interosseous), which allow only a slight amount of gliding movement between the bones. The close packed position is extension, and the resting position is neutral or slight flexion. The **pisotriquetral joint** is considered separately, because the pisiform sits on the triquetrum and does not take a direct part in the other intercarpal movements.

Intercarpal Joints

Resting position:	Neutral or slight flexion
Close packed position:	Extension
Capsular pattern:	None

The **midcarpal joints** form a compound articulation between the proximal and distal rows of carpal bones with the exception of the pisiform bone. On the medial side, the scaphoid, lunate, and triquetrum articulate with the capitate and hamate, forming a compound sellar (saddle-shaped) joint. On the lateral aspect, the scaphoid articulates with the trapezoid and trapezium, forming another compound sellar joint. As with the intercarpal joints,

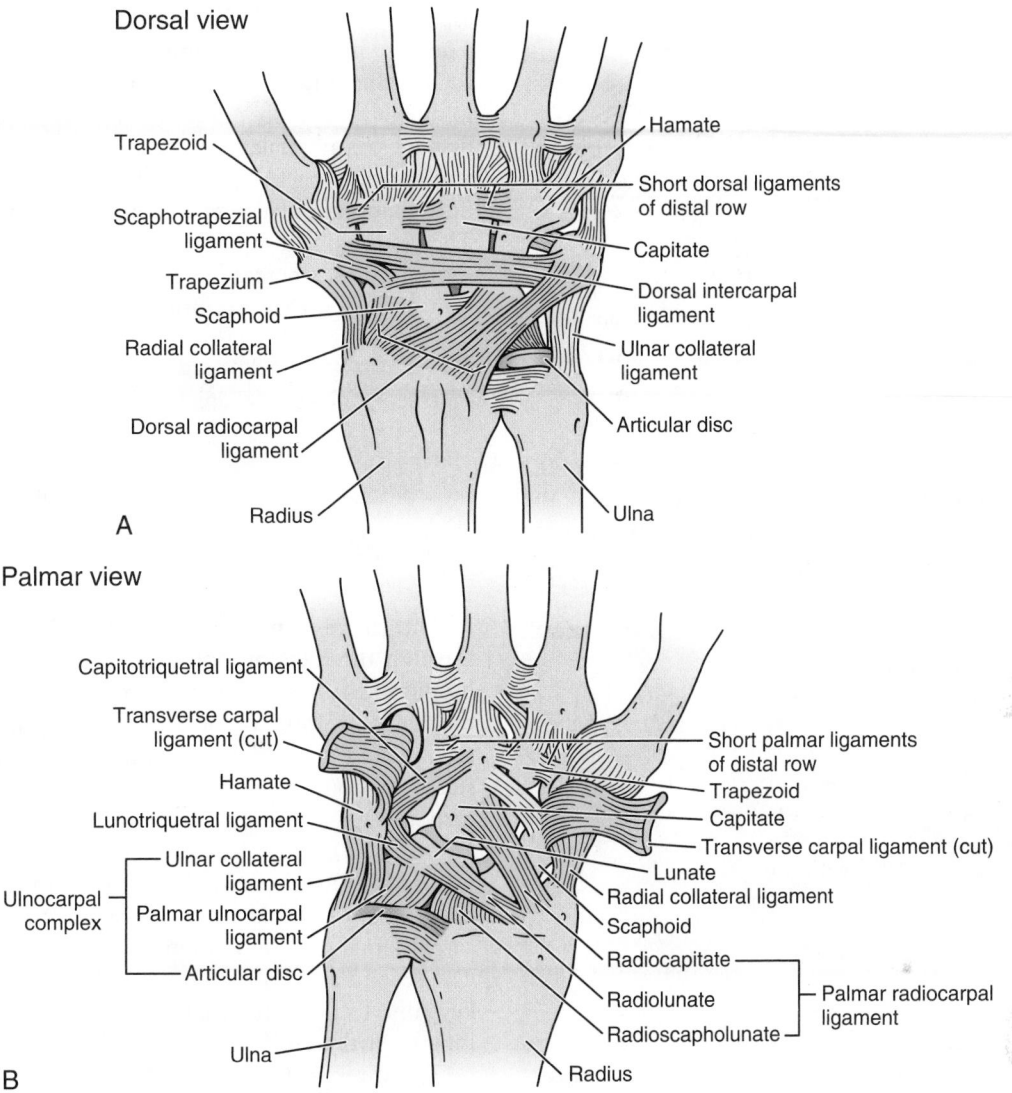

Figure 7-3 Ligaments of the wrist. A, Dorsal aspect of the right wrist. **B,** Palmar aspect of the right wrist. The transverse carpal ligament has been cut and reflected to show the underlying ligaments. (Redrawn from Neumann DA: Kinesiology of the musculoskeletal system—foundations for physical rehabilitation, St Louis, 2002, CV Mosby, pp. 178–179.)

these articulations are bound together by dorsal and palmar ligaments; however, there are no interosseous ligaments between the proximal and distal rows of bones. Therefore, greater movement exists at the midcarpal joints than between the individual bones of the two rows of the intercarpal joints. The close packed position of these joints is extension with ulnar deviation, and the resting position is neutral or slight flexion with ulnar deviation.

Midcarpal Joints

Resting position:	Neutral or slight flexion with ulnar deviation
Close packed position:	Extension with ulnar deviation
Capsular pattern:	Equal limitation of flexion and extension (works with radiocarpal joints)

The **proximal transverse arch** (Figure 7-4) that forms the carpal tunnel is formed by the distal row of carpal bones. In this relatively rigid arch, the capitate bone acts as a central keystone structure.[13]

At the thumb, the **carpometacarpal joint** is a sellar joint that has 3° of freedom, whereas the second to fifth carpometacarpal joints are plane joints.[14] The capsular pattern of the carpometacarpal joint of the thumb is abduction most limited, followed by extension. The resting position is midway between abduction and adduction and midway between flexion and extension. The close packed position of the carpometacarpal joint of the thumb is full opposition. For the second to fifth carpometacarpal joints, the capsular pattern of restriction is equal limitation in all directions. The bones of these joints are held together by dorsal and palmar ligaments. In addition, the thumb articulation has a strong lateral ligament

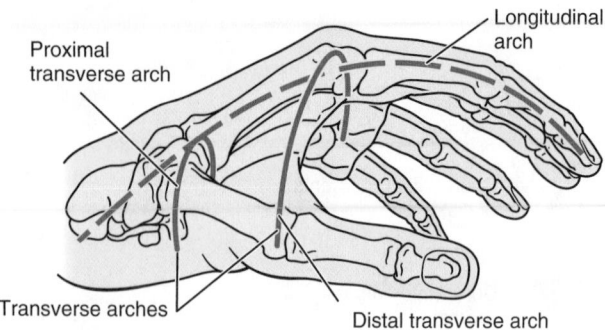

Figure 7-4 Longitudinal and transverse arches of the hand (lateral view).

extending from the lateral side of the trapezium to the radial side of the base of the first metacarpal, and the medial four articulations have an interosseous ligament similar to that found in the carpal articulation.

Carpometacarpal Joints

Resting position:	Thumb, midway between abduction and adduction, and midway between flexion and extension
	Fingers, midway between flexion and extension
Close packed position:	Thumb, full opposition
	Fingers, full flexion
Capsular pattern:	Thumb, abduction, extension
	Fingers, equal limitation in all directions

The carpometacarpal articulations of the fingers allow only gliding movement. The second and third carpometacarpal joints tend to be relatively immobile and are the primary "stabilizing" joints of the hand, whereas the fourth and fifth joints are more mobile to allow the hand to adapt to different shaped objects during grasping. The carpometacarpal articulation of the thumb is unique in that it allows flexion, extension, abduction, adduction, rotation, and circumduction. It is able to do this because the articulation is saddle shaped. Because of the many movements possible at this joint, the thumb is able to adopt any position relative to the palmar aspect of the hand.[14]

The plane **intermetacarpal joints** have only a small amount of gliding movement between them and do not include the thumb articulation. They are bound together by palmar, dorsal, and interosseous ligaments.

The **metacarpophalangeal joints** are condyloid joints. The collateral ligaments of these joints are tight on flexion and relaxed on extension. These articulations are also bound by palmar ligaments and deep transverse metacarpal ligaments. The **dorsal** or **extensor hood** (Figure 7-5) reinforces the dorsal aspect of the metacarpophalangeal joints while **volar** or **palmar plates** reinforce the palmar

aspect (see Figure 7-5).[3] Each joint has 2° of freedom. The first metacarpophalangeal joint has 3° of freedom, thus facilitating the movement of the carpometacarpal joint of the thumb.[14] The close packed position of the first metacarpophalangeal joint is maximum opposition, and the close packed position for the second through the fifth metacarpophalangeal joints is maximum flexion.[15] The resting position of the metacarpophalangeal joints is slight flexion, whereas the capsular pattern is more limitation of flexion than extension.

Metacarpophalangeal Joints

Resting position:	Slight flexion
Close packed position:	Thumb, full opposition
	Fingers, full flexion
Capsular pattern:	Flexion, extension

The **distal transverse arch** (see Figure 7-4) passes through the metacarpophalangeal joints and has greater mobility than the proximal transverse arch allowing the hand to form or fit around different objects. The second and third metacarpophalangeal joints form the stable portion of the arch while the fourth and fifth metacarpophalangeal joints form the mobile portion (see Figure 7-27).[13]

The **longituginal arch** follows the more rigid portion of the hand running from the carpals to the carpometacarpal joints providing longitudinal stability to the hand. The second and third metacarpophalangeal joints are the keystone to both the distal transverse arch and the distal longitudinal arch.[13]

The **interphalangeal joints** are uniaxial hinge joints, each having 1° of freedom. The close packed position of the proximal interphalangeal joints and distal interphalangeal joints is full extension; the resting position is slight flexion. The capsular pattern of these joints in flexion is more limited than extension. The bones of these joints are bound together by a fibrous capsule and by the palmar and collateral ligaments. During flexion, there is some rotation in these joints so that the pulp of the fingers faces more fully the pulp of the thumb. If the metacarpophalangeal joints and the proximal interphalangeal joints of the fingers are flexed, they converge toward the scaphoid tubercle (Figure 7-6). This is sometimes referred to as a **cascade sign.** If one or more fingers do not converge, it usually indicates trauma (e.g., fracture) to the digits that has altered their normal alignment.

Interphalangeal Joints

Resting position:	Slight flexion
Close packed position:	Full extension
Capsular pattern:	Flexion, extension

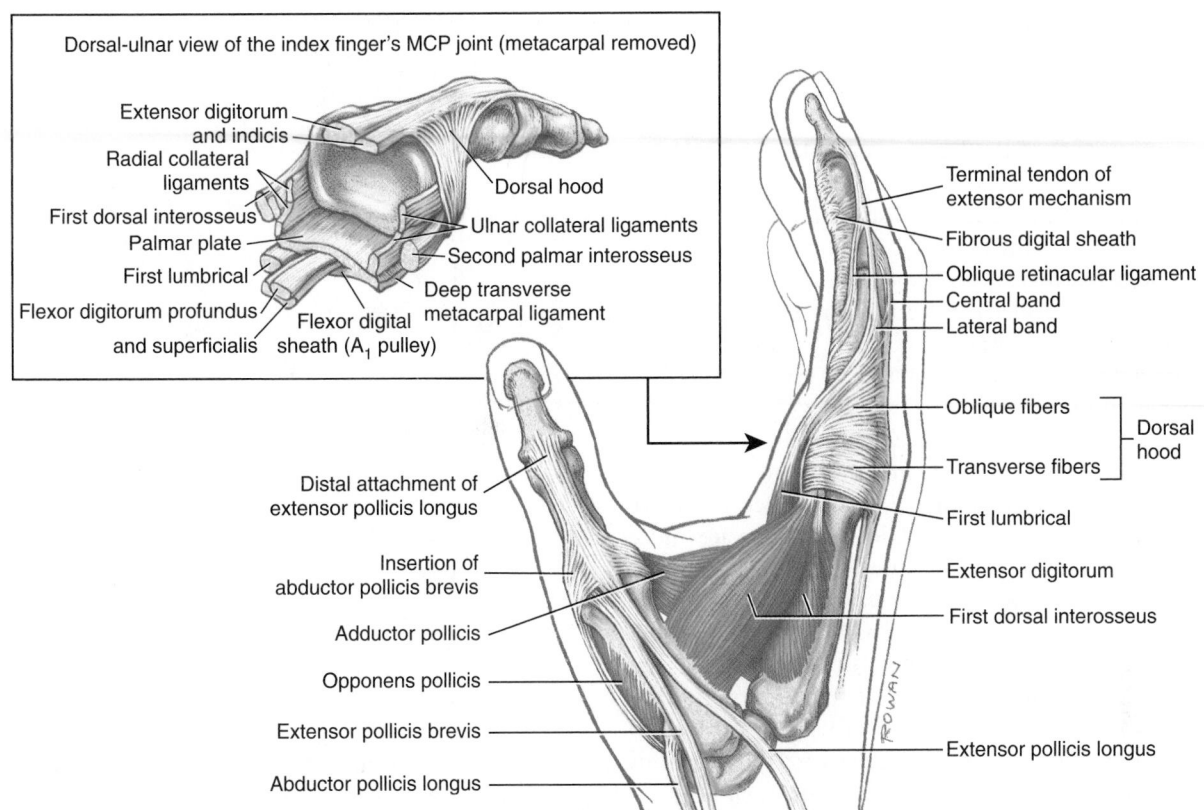

Dorsal-ulnar view of the index finger's MCP joint (metacarpal removed)

Extensor digitorum and indicis
Radial collateral ligaments
First dorsal interosseus
Palmar plate
First lumbrical
Flexor digitorum profundus and superficialis
Flexor digital sheath (A₁ pulley)
Dorsal hood
Ulnar collateral ligaments
Second palmar interosseus
Deep transverse metacarpal ligament

Terminal tendon of extensor mechanism
Fibrous digital sheath
Oblique retinacular ligament
Central band
Lateral band
Oblique fibers
Transverse fibers
Dorsal hood
First lumbrical
Extensor digitorum
First dorsal interosseus
Extensor pollicis longus

Distal attachment of extensor pollicis longus
Insertion of abductor pollicis brevis
Adductor pollicis
Opponens pollicis
Extensor pollicis brevis
Abductor pollicis longus

Figure 7-5 A lateral view of the muscles, tendons, and extensor mechanism of the right hand. The illustration in the box highlights the anatomy associated with the metacarpophalangeal joint of the index finger. (From Neumann DA: Kinesiology of the musculoskeletal system—foundations for physical rehabilitation, ed 2, St Louis, 2010, CV Mosby, p. 269.)

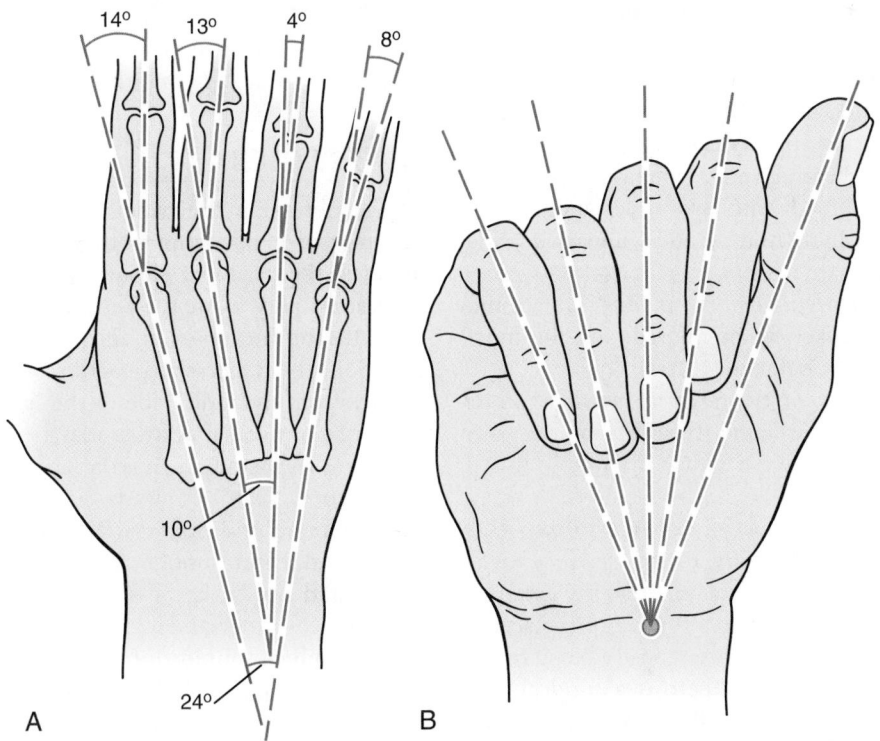

14° 13° 4° 8°
10°
24°
A
B

Figure 7-6 Alignment of the fingers. A, Normal physiological alignment. **B,** Oblique flexion of the last four digits. Only the index ray flexes toward the median axis. When the last four digits are flexed separately at the metacarpophalangeal and proximal interphalangeal joints, their axes converge toward the scaphoid tubercle. (Redrawn from Tubiana R: The hand, Philadelphia, 1981, WB Saunders, p. 22.)

PATIENT HISTORY

The assessment of the forearm, wrist, and hand often takes longer than that of other joints of the body because of the importance of the hand to everyday function and because of the many structures and joints involved.

In addition to the questions listed under the "Patient History" section in Chapter 1, the examiner should obtain the following information from the patient:

1. *What is the patient's age?* Certain conditions are more likely to occur at different ages. For example, arthritic changes are most commonly seen in patients who are older than 40 years of age.[16]

2. *What is the patient's occupation?* Certain occupations are more likely to affect the wrist and hand. For example, typists are more likely to suffer repetitive strain injuries, and automobile mechanics are more likely to suffer traumatic injuries.

3. *What was the mechanism of injury?*[16,17] For example, a FOOSH injury may lead to a lunate dislocation, Colles fracture, or scaphoid fracture, or extension of the fingers may cause dislocation of the fingers. A rotational force applied to the wrist or near it may lead to a Galeazzi fracture, which is a fracture of the radius and dislocation of the distal end of the ulna.

4. *What tasks is the patient able or unable to perform?* For example, is there any problem with buttoning, dressing, tying shoelaces, or any other everyday activity? This type of question gives an indication of the patient's functional limitations.

5. *When did the injury or onset occur, and how long has the patient been incapacitated?* These questions are not necessarily the same; for instance, a burn may occur at a certain time, but incapacity may not occur until hypertrophic scarring appears. The wrist is commonly injured by weight bearing (e.g., gymnastics), by rotational stress combined with ulnar deviation (e.g., hitting a racquet), by twisting, and by impact loading (FOOSH injury).[17,18]

6. *Which hand is the patient's dominant hand?* The dominant hand is more likely to be injured, and the functional loss, at least initially, is greater.

7. *Has the patient injured the forearm, wrist, or hand previously?* Was it the same type of injury? Was the mechanism of injury the same? If so, how was it treated?

8. *Which part of the forearm, wrist, or hand is injured?* If the flexor tendons (which are round, have synovial sheaths, and have a longer excursion than the extensor tendons) are injured, they respond much more slowly to treatment than do extensor tendons (which are flat or ovoid). Within the hand, there is a surgical "no man's land" (Figure 7-7), which is a region between the distal palmar crease and the midportion of the middle phalanx of the fingers. Damage to the flexor tendons in this area require surgical repair and usually

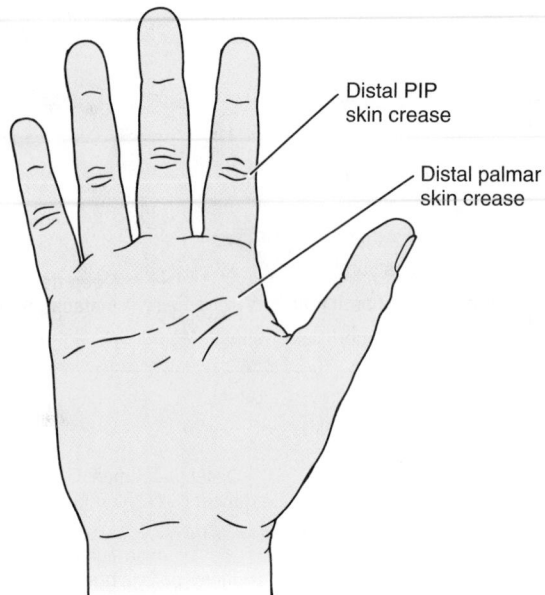

Distal PIP
skin crease

Distal palmar
skin crease

Figure 7-7 Surgical "no-man's land" (palmar view).

lead to the formation of adhesive bands that restrict gliding. In addition, the tendons may become ischemic, being replaced by scar tissue. Because of this, the prognosis after surgery in this area is poor.

9. *Does pain or abnormal sensation (e.g., tingling, pins and needles) predominate?* In the hand and fingers, the examiner must take the time to differentiate exactly where the symptoms are to differentiate peripheral nerve neuropathy, nerve root symptoms, and other painful localized conditions.[19,20]

OBSERVATION

While observing the patient and viewing the forearms, wrists, and hands from both the anterior and posterior aspects, the examiner should note the patient's willingness and ability to use the hand. Normally, when the hand is in the resting position and the wrist is in the normal position, the fingers are progressively more flexed as one moves from the radial side of the hand to the ulnar side. Loss of this normal attitude may be caused by pathology affecting the hand, such as a lacerated tendon, or by a contracture, such as Dupuytren contracture.

The bone and soft-tissue contours of the forearm, wrist, and hand should be compared for both upper limbs, and any deviation should be noted. The cosmetic appearance of the hand is very important to some patients. The examiner should note the patient's reaction to the appearance of the hand and be prepared to provide a cosmetic evaluation. This evaluation should always be included with the more important functional assessment. The posture of the hand at rest often demonstrates common deformities. Are the normal skin creases present?

Skin creases occur because of movement at the various joints. The examiner should note any muscle wasting on the thenar eminence (median nerve), first dorsal interosseous muscle (C7 nerve root), or hypothenar eminence (ulnar nerve) that may be indicative of peripheral nerve or nerve root injury.

Any localized swellings (e.g., ganglion) that are seen on the dorsum of the hand should be recorded (Figure 7-8).[21] In the wrist and hand, effusion and synovial thickening are most evident on the dorsal and radial aspects. Swelling of the metacarpophalangeal and interphalangeal joints is most obvious on the dorsal aspect.

The dominant hand tends to be larger than the nondominant hand. If the patient has an area on the fingers that lacks sensation, this area is avoided when the patient lifts or identifies objects, and the patient uses another finger instead with normal sensitivity. Therefore, the examiner should watch for abnormal or different patterns of movement, which may indicate adaptations or modifications necessitated by the presence of pathology.

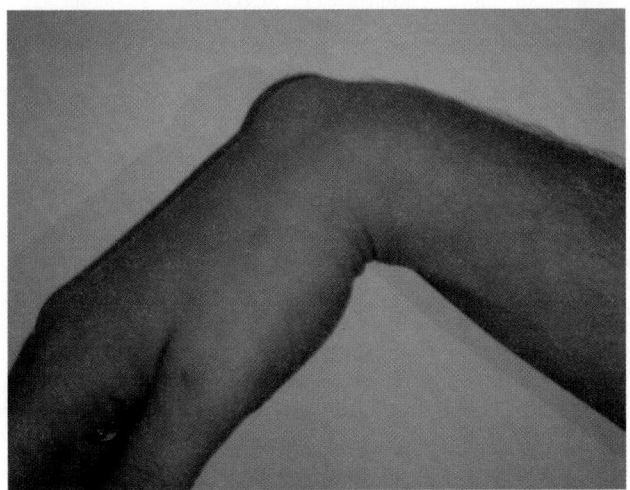

Figure 7-8 Ganglion or small cystic swelling on the dorsum of the right hand just distal to the wrist joint.

Any vasomotor, sudomotor, pilomotor, and trophic changes should be recorded. These changes may be indicative of a peripheral nerve injury, peripheral vascular disease, diabetes mellitus, Raynaud disease, or reflex neurovascular syndromes (also called *complex regional pain syndrome, reflex sympathetic dystrophy, shoulder-hand syndrome,* and *Sudeck atrophy*). The changes seen could include loss of hair on the hand, brittle fingernails, increase or decrease in sweating of the palm, shiny skin, radiographic evidence of osteoporosis, or any difference in temperature between the two limbs. Table 7-1 illustrates vasomotor, sudomotor, pilomotor, and trophic changes that occur in the hand when sympathetic nerve function has been affected.

The examiner should note any hypertrophy of the fingers. Hypertrophy of the bone may be seen in Paget disease, neurofibromatosis, or arteriovenous fistula.

The presence of Heberden or Bouchard nodes (Figure 7-9) should be recorded. Heberden nodes appear on the dorsal surface of the distal interphalangeal joints and are associated with osteoarthritis. Bouchard nodes are on the dorsal surface of the proximal interphalangeal joints. They are often associated with gastrectasis and osteoarthritis.

Any ulcerations may indicate neurological or circulatory problems. Any alteration in the color of the limb with changes in position may indicate a circulatory problem.

The examiner should note any rotational or angulated deformities of the fingers, which may be indicative of previous fracture. The nail beds are normally parallel to one another. The fingers, when extended, are slightly rotated toward the thumb to aid pinch. Ulnar drift (Figure 7-10) may be seen in rheumatoid arthritis, owing to the shape of the metacarpophalangeal joints and the pull of the long tendons.

The presence of any wounds or scars should be noted because they may indicate recent surgery or past trauma.

TABLE **7-1**

Sympathetic Changes after Nerve Injury

Sympathetic Function	Feature	Early Changes	Late Changes
Vasomotor	Skin color	Rosy	Mottled or cyanotic
	Skin temperature	Warm	Cool
Sudomotor	Sweating	Dry skin	Dry or overly moist
Pilomotor	Gooseflesh response	Absent	Absent
Trophic	Skin texture	Soft, smooth	Smooth, nonelastic
	Soft-tissue atrophy	Slight	More pronounced, especially in finger pulps
	Nail changes	Blemishes	Curved in longitudinal and horizontal planes, "talonlike"
	Hair growth	May fall out or become longer and finer	May fall out or become longer and finer
	Rate of healing	Slowed	Slowed

From Callahan AD: Sensibility assessment for nerve lesions-in-continuity and nerve lacerations. In Hunter J, Schneider LH, Mackin EJ, et al, editors: Rehabilitation of the hand and upper extremity, St Louis, 2002, Mosby, p. 225.

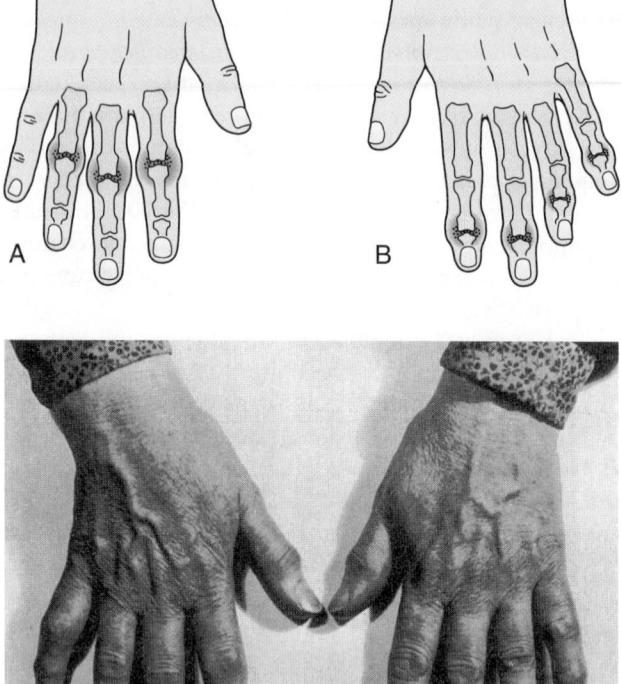

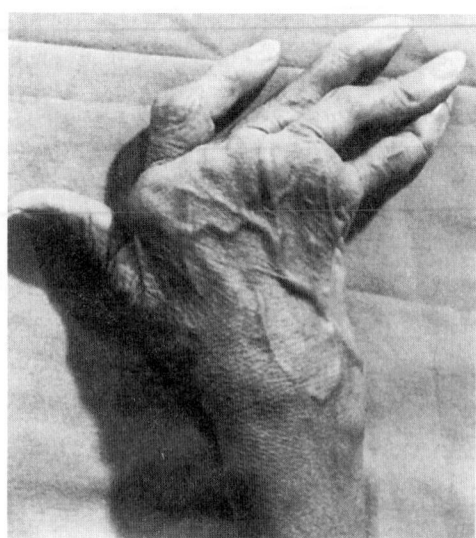

Figure 7-10 The most common deformities occurring in rheumatoid arthritis are ulnar drift and palmar subluxation at the metacarpophalangeal joints. Note swan neck and boutonnière deformities present in digits. (From Swanson AB: Pathomechanics of deformities in hand and wrist. In Hunter J, Schneider LH, Mackin EJ, et al, editors: Rehabilitation of the hand: surgery and therapy, St Louis, 1990, CV Mosby, p. 895.)

Figure 7-9 A, Bouchard nodes. **B,** Heberden nodes. **C,** Degenerative joint disease (osteoarthritis) of both hands. Osteoarthritic enlargement of the distal interphalangeal joints (Heberden nodes) and the proximal interphalangeal joints (Bouchard nodes) is present. The metacarpophalangeal joints are not affected. (**C,** From Polley HF, Hunder GG: Rheumatologic interviewing and physical examination of the joints, Philadelphia, 1978, WB Saunders, p. 120.)

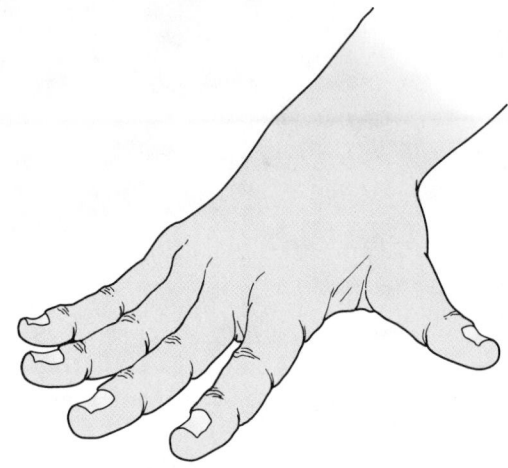

Figure 7-11 Spoon-shaped nails.

Common Hand and Finger Deformities

Ape Hand Deformity. Wasting of the thenar eminence of the hand occurs as a result of a median nerve palsy, and the thumb falls back in line with the fingers as a result of the pull of the extensor muscles. The patient is also unable to oppose or flex the thumb (Figure 7-13).

Bishop's Hand or Benediction Hand Deformity. Wasting of the hypothenar muscles of the hand, the interossei muscles, and the two medial lumbrical muscles occurs because of ulnar nerve palsy (Figure 7-14). Flexion of the fourth and fifth fingers is the most obvious resulting change.

Boutonnière Deformity. Extension of the metacarpophalangeal and distal interphalangeal joints and flexion of the

If wounds are present, are they new or old? Are they healing properly? Is the scar red (new) or white (old)? Is the scar mobile or adherent? Is it normal, hypertrophic, or keloid? Palmar scars may interfere with finger extension. Web space scars may interfere with finger separation and metacarpophalangeal joint flexion.

The examiner should take time to observe the fingernails. "Spoon-shaped" nails (Figure 7-11) are often the result of fungal infection, anemia, iron deficiency, long-term diabetes, local injury, developmental abnormality, chemical irritants, or psoriasis. They may also be a congenital or hereditary trait. "Clubbed" nails (Figure 7-12) may result from hypertrophy of the underlying soft tissue or respiratory or cardiac problems, such as chronic obstructive pulmonary disease, severe emphysema, congenital heart defects, or cor pulmonale. Table 7-2 shows other pathological processes that may affect the fingernails.

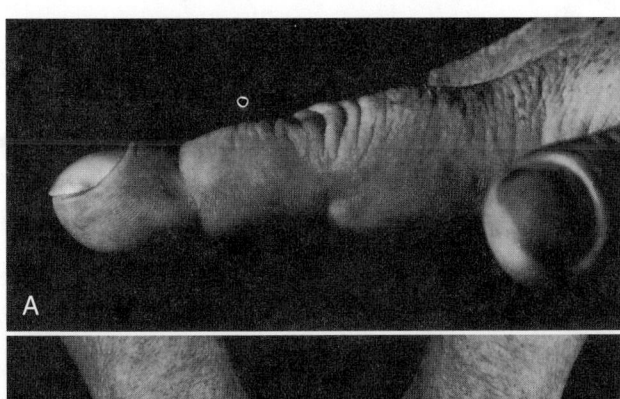

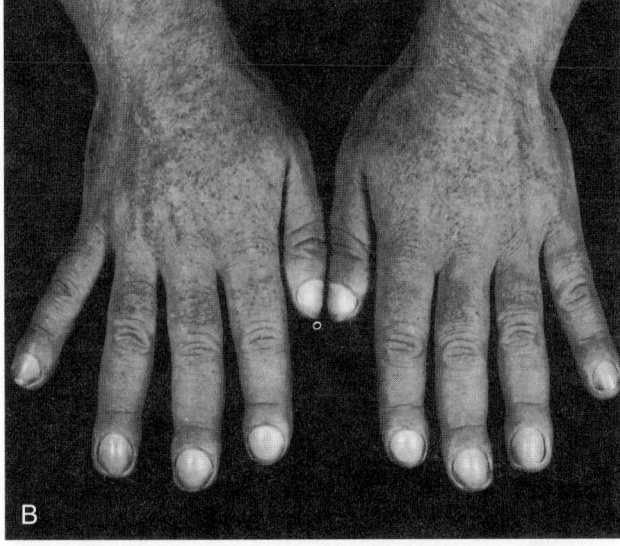

Figure 7-12 Clubbing of the distal interphalangeal joints and rounding of the nails in a patient with hypertrophic osteoarthropathy. **A,** Close-up side view of index finger. **B,** Dorsal aspect of both hands. (From Polley HF, Hunder GG: Rheumatologic interviewing and physical examination of the joints, Philadelphia, 1978, WB Saunders, p. 122.)

proximal interphalangeal joint (primary deformity) are seen with this deformity. The deformity is the result of a rupture of the central tendinous slip of the extensor hood and is most common after trauma or in rheumatoid arthritis (Figure 7-15).

Claw Fingers. This deformity results from the loss of intrinsic muscle action and the overaction of the extrinsic (long) extensor muscles on the proximal phalanx of the fingers. The metacarpophalangeal joints are hyperextended, and the proximal and distal interphalangeal joints are flexed (Figure 7-16). If intrinsic function is lost, the hand is called an **intrinsic minus hand.** The normal cupping of the hand is lost, both the longitudinal and the transverse arches of the hand (see Figure 7-4) disappear, and there is intrinsic muscle wasting. The deformity is most often caused by a combined median and ulnar nerve palsy.

Drop-Wrist Deformity. The extensor muscles of the wrist are paralyzed as a result of a radial nerve palsy, and the wrist and fingers cannot be actively extended by the patient (Figure 7-17).

Dupuytren Contracture. This progressive disease of genetic origin results in contracture of the palmar fascia.[22] There is a fixed flexion deformity of the metacarpophalangeal and proximal interphalangeal joints (Figure 7-18). Dupuytren contracture is usually seen in the ring or little finger, and the skin is often adherent to the fascia. It affects men more often than women and is usually seen in the 50- to 70-year-old age group.

Extensor Plus Deformity. This deformity is caused by adhesions or shortening of the extensor communis tendon proximal to the metacarpophalangeal joint. It results in the inability of the patient to simultaneously flex the metacarpophalangeal and proximal interphalangeal joints, although they may be flexed individually.

Mallet Finger.[23] A mallet finger deformity is the result of a rupture or avulsion of the extensor tendon where it inserts into the distal phalanx of the finger. The distal phalanx rests in a flexed position (Figure 7-19).

Myelopathy Hand. This deformity is a dysfunction of the hand caused by cervical spinal cord pathology in conjunction with cervical spondylosis. The patient shows an inability to extend and adduct the ring and little finger and sometimes the middle finger, especially rapidly, despite good function of the wrist, thumb, and index finger. In addition, the patient shows an exaggerated triceps reflex and positive pathological reflexes (e.g., Hoffman reflex).[24]

Polydactyly and Triphalangism. Polydactyly is a congenital anomaly characterized by the presence of more than the normal number of fingers or, in the case of the foot, toes. Triphalangism implies there are three phalanges instead of the normal two as would be seen in the thumb.[25]

Swan Neck Deformity. This deformity usually involves only the fingers. There is flexion of the metacarpophalangeal and distal interphalangeal joints, but the real deformity is extension of the proximal interphalangeal joint. The condition is a result of contracture of the intrinsic muscles or tearing of the volar plate and is often seen in patients with rheumatoid arthritis or following trauma (Figure 7-20).

Trigger Finger.[26] Also known as digital tenovaginitis stenosans, this deformity is the result of a thickening of the flexor tendon sheath (Notta's nodule), which causes sticking of the tendon when the patient attempts to flex the finger. A low-grade inflammation of the proximal fold of the flexor tendon leads to swelling and constriction (stenosis) in the digital flexor tendon. When the patient attempts to flex the finger, the tendon sticks, and the finger "lets go," often with a snap. As the condition worsens, eventually the finger will flex but not let go, and it will have to be passively extended until finally a fixed flexion deformity occurs. The condition is more likely to occur in middle-aged women, whereas **"trigger thumb"** with a flexion deformity of the interphalangeal joint is more common in young children.[27] The condition usually occurs in the third or fourth finger. In adults, it is most

TABLE **7-2**

Glossary of Nail Pathology

Condition	Description	Occurrence
Beau lines	Transverse lines or ridges marking repeated disturbances of nail growth	Systemic diseases, toxic or nutritional deficiency states of many types, trauma (from manicuring)
Defluvium unguium (onychomadesis)	Complete loss of nails	Certain systemic diseases, such as scarlet fever, syphilis, leprosy, alopecia areata, exfoliative dermatitis
Diffusion of lunula unguis	"Spreading" of lunula	Dystrophies of the extremities
Eggshell nails	Nail plate thin, semitransparent bluish-white with a tendency to curve upward at the distal edge	Syphilis
Fragilitas unguium	Friable or brittle nails	Dietary deficiency, local trauma
Hapalonychia	Nails very soft, split easily	Following contact with strong alkalis; endocrine disturbances, malnutrition, syphilis, chronic arthritis
Hippocratic nails	"Watch-glass nails" associated with "drumstick fingers"	Chronic respiratory and circulatory diseases, especially pulmonary tuberculosis; hepatic cirrhosis
Koilonychia	"Spoon nails;" nails are concave on the outer surface	Dysendocrinisms (acromegaly), trauma, dermatoses, syphilis, nutritional deficiencies, hypothyroidism
Leukonychia	White spots or striations or rarely the whole nail may turn white (congenital type)	Local trauma, hepatic cirrhosis, nutritional deficiencies, and many systemic diseases
Mees' lines	Transverse white bands	Hodgkin's granuloma, arsenic and thallium toxicity, high fevers, local nutritional derangement
Moniliasis of nails	Infections (usually paronychial) caused by yeast forms (*Candida albicans*)	Occupational (common in food-handlers, dentists, dishwashers, and gardeners)
Onychatrophia	Atrophy or failure of development of nails	Trauma, infection, dysendocrinism, gonadal aplasia, and many systemic disorders
Onychauxis	Nail plate is greatly thickened	Mild persistent trauma, systemic diseases, such as peripheral stasis, peripheral neuritis, syphilis, leprosy, hemiplegia; or at times may be congenital
Onychia	Inflammation of the nail matrix causing deformity of the nail plate	Trauma, infection, many systemic diseases
Onychodystrophy	Any deformity of the nail plate, nail bed, or nail matrix	Many diseases, trauma, or chemical agents (poisoning, allergy)
Onchogryposis	"Claw nails"—extreme degree of hypertrophy, sometimes with horny projections arising from the nail surface	May be congenital or related to many chronic systemic diseases (see onychauxis)
Onycholysis	Loosening of the nail plate beginning at the distal or free edge	Trauma, injury by chemical agents, many systemic diseases
Onychomadesis	Shedding of all the nails (defluvium unguium)	Dermatoses, such as exfoliative dermatitis, alopecia areata, psoriasis, eczema, nail infection, severe systemic diseases, arsenic poisoning
Onychophagia	Nail biting	Neurosis
Onychorrhexis	Longitudinal ridging and splitting of the nails	Dermatoses, nail infections, many systemic diseases, senility, injury by chemical agents, hyperthyroidism
Onychoschizia	Lamination and scaling away of nails in thin layers	Dermatoses, syphilis, injury by chemical agents
Onychotillomania	Alteration of the nail structures caused by persistent neurotic picking of the nails	Neurosis
Pachyonychia	Extreme thickening of all the nails; the nails are more solid and more regular than in onychogryposis	Usually congenital and associated with hyperkeratosis of the palms and soles
Pterygium unguis	Thinning of the nail fold and spreading of the cuticle over the nail plate	Associated with vasospastic conditions, such as Raynaud phenomenon and occasionally with hypothyroidism

From Berry TJ: The hand as mirror of systemic disease, Philadelphia, 1963, FA Davis.

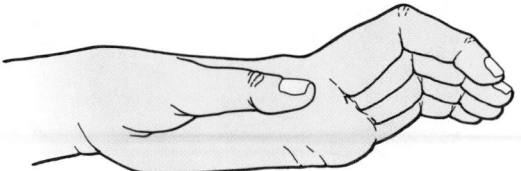

Figure 7-13 **Ape hand deformity.**

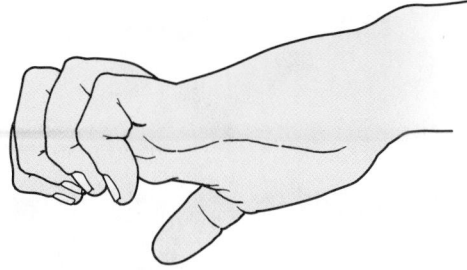

Figure 7-16 **Claw fingers (intrinsic minus hand).** Fingers are hyperextended at the metacarpophalangeal joints and flexed at the interphalangeal joints.

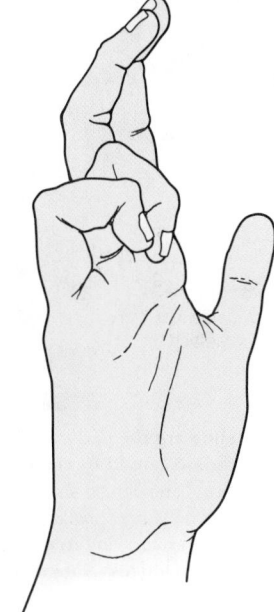

Figure 7-14 **Bishop's hand or benediction hand deformity.**

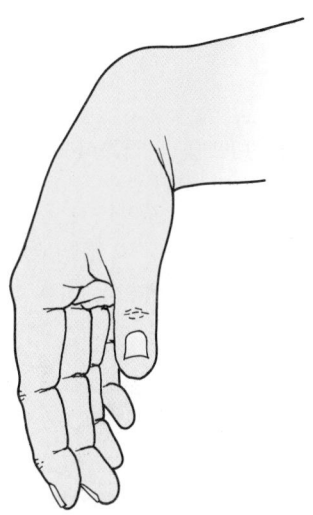

Figure 7-17 **Drop-wrist deformity.**

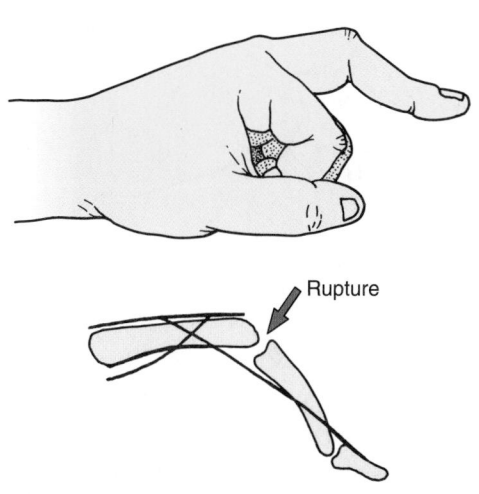

Figure 7-15 **Boutonnière deformity.** Note the flexion deformity at the proximal interphalangeal joint.

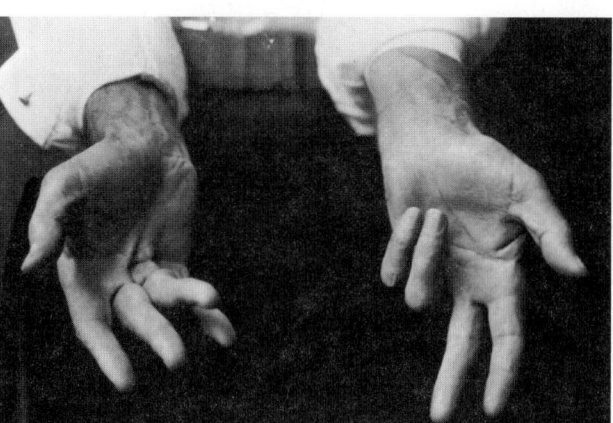

Figure 7-18 **Dupuytren contracture in both hands,** showing flexion contractures of the fourth and fifth digits of the left hand and less severe contractures in the third, fourth, and fifth digits of the right hand. Note the puckering of palmar skin and the presence of bands extending from the concavity of the palm to the proximal interphalangeal joints of the third and fourth digits of the right hand. (From Polley HF, Hunder GG: Rheumatologic interviewing and physical examination of the joints, Philadelphia, 1978, WB Saunders, p. 98.)

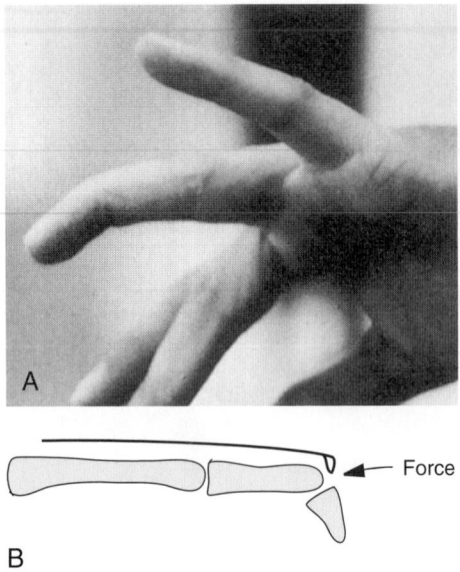

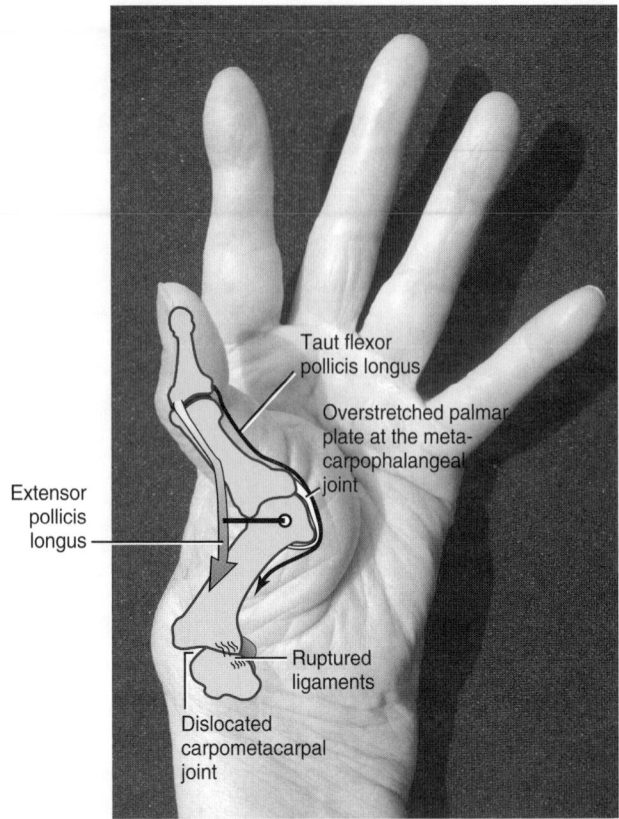

Figure 7-19 Mallet finger. A, Patient actively attempting to extend finger. **B,** Mechanism of injury. Tendon is ruptured or avulsed from bone.

Figure 7-21 Palmar view showing the pathomechanics of a common zigzag deformity of the thumb caused by rheumatoid arthritis. The thumb metacarpal dislocates laterally at the carpometacarpal joint, causing hyperextension at the metacarpophalangeal joint. The interphalangeal joint remains partially flexed owing to the passive tension in the stretched and taut flexor pollicis longus. Note that the "bowstringing" of the tendon of the extensor pollicis longus across the metacarpophalangeal joint creates a large extensor moment arm, thereby magnifying the mechanics of the deformity. (From Neumann DA: Kinesiology of the musculoskeletal system—foundations for physical rehabilitation, St Louis, 2002, CV Mosby, p. 237.)

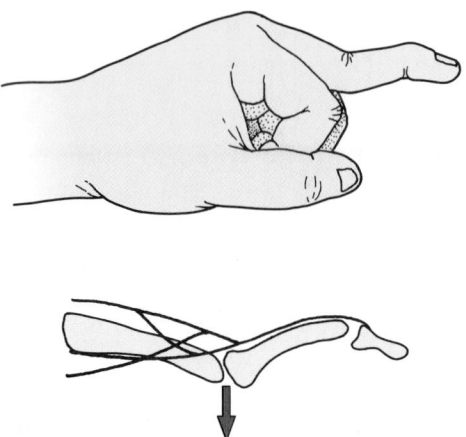

Figure 7-20 Swan neck deformity. Note the hyperextension at the proximal interphalangeal joint.

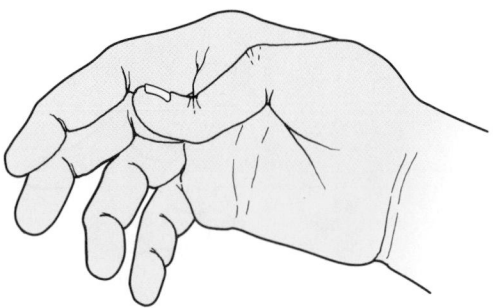

Figure 7-22 "Z" deformity of the thumb.

often associated with rheumatoid arthritis and tends to be worse in the morning.

Ulnar Drift. This deformity, which is commonly seen in patients with rheumatoid arthritis but can occur with other conditions, results in ulnar deviation of the digits because of weakening of the capsuloligamentous structures of the metacarpophalangeal joints and the accompanying "bowstring" effect of the extensor communis tendons (see Figure 7-10).

Zigzag Deformity of the Thumb. The thumb is flexed at the carpometacarpal joint and hyperextended at the metacarpophalangeal joint (Figure 7-21). The deformity is associated with rheumatoid arthritis. A "Z" deformity is due to hypermobility and may be familial (Figure 7-22).

Other Physical Findings

The hand is the terminal part of the upper limb. Many pathological conditions manifest themselves in this structure and may lead the examiner to suspect pathological conditions elsewhere in the body. It is important for the examiner to take the time to view the hands when

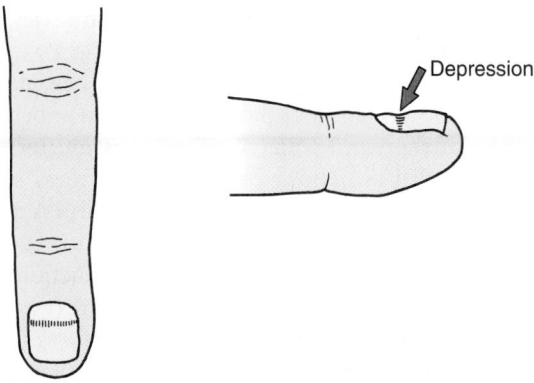

Figure 7-23 **Beau lines.**

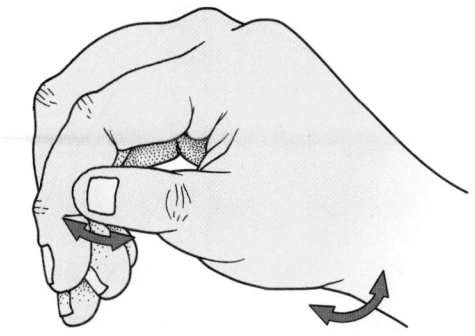

Figure 7-24 **"Pill rolling hand,"** seen in Parkinson disease.

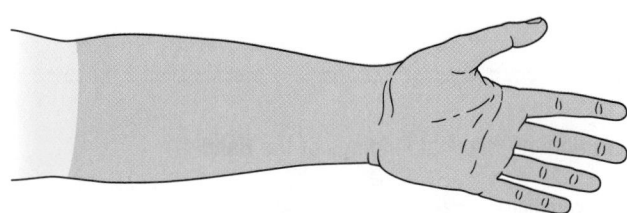

Figure 7-25 **"Opera glove anesthesia,"** showing area of abnormal sensation.

assessing any joint, especially if an abnormal pattern is presented or the history gives an indication that more than one joint may be involved. For example, if a patient presents with insidious neck pain and demonstrates nail changes that indicate psoriasis, the examiner should consider the possibility of psoriatic arthritis affecting the cervical spine as well as the hand. Some conditions involving the hand include the following:

1. Generalized or continued body exposure to radiation produces brittle nails, longitudinal nail ridges, skin keratosis (thickening), and ulceration.
2. The Plummer-Vinson syndrome produces spoon-shaped nails (see Figure 7-11). This condition is a dysphagia with atrophy in the mouth, pharynx, and upper esophagus.
3. Psoriasis may cause scaling, deformity, and fragmentation and detachment of the nails. Psoriasis may lead to psoriatic arthritis affecting spinal and peripheral joints.
4. Hyperthyroidism produces nail atrophy and ridging with warm, moist hands.
5. Vasospastic conditions produce a thin nail fold and pterygium (abnormal extension) of the cuticle.
6. Trauma to the nail bed, toxic radiation, acute illness, prolonged fever, avitaminosis, and chronic alcoholism produce transverse lines, or Beau lines, in the nails (Figure 7-23).
7. Many arterial diseases produce a lack of linear growth with thick, dark nails.
8. Lues (syphilis) produces a hypertrophic overgrowth of the nail plate. The nails break and crumple easily.
9. Chronic respiratory disorders produce clubbing of the nails (see Figure 7-12).
10. Subacute bacterial endocarditis may produce Osler nodes, which are small, tender nodes in the finger pads.
11. Congenital heart disease may produce cyanosis and nail clubbing.
12. Neurocirculatory aesthesia (loss of strength and energy) produces cold, damp hands.

13. Parkinson disease produces a typical hand tremor known as "pill rolling hand" (Figure 7-24).
14. Causalgic states produce a painful, swollen, hot hand.
15. "Opera glove" anesthesia is seen in hysteria, leprosy, and diabetes. It is a condition in which there is numbness from the elbow to the fingers (Figure 7-25).
16. Raynaud disease produces a cold, mottled, painful hand. It is an idiopathic vascular disorder characterized by intermittent attacks of pallor and cyanosis of the extremities brought on by cold or emotion.
17. Rheumatoid arthritis produces a warm, wet hand as well as joint swelling, dislocations or subluxations, and ulnar deviation or drift of the wrist (see Figure 7-10).
18. The deformed hand of Volkmann ischemic contracture is one that is very typical for a compartment syndrome after a fracture or dislocation of the elbow (Figure 7-26).[28]

Box 7-1 gives further examples of physical findings of the hand.

EXAMINATION

The examination of the forearm, wrist, and hand may be very extensive, or it may be limited to one or two joints, depending on the area and degree of injury. Regardless, because of its functional importance, the examiner must take extra care when examining this area. Not only must clinical limitations be determined, but functional limitations brought on by trauma, nerve injuries, or other factors must be carefully considered to have an appropriate outcome functionally, cosmetically, and clinically.

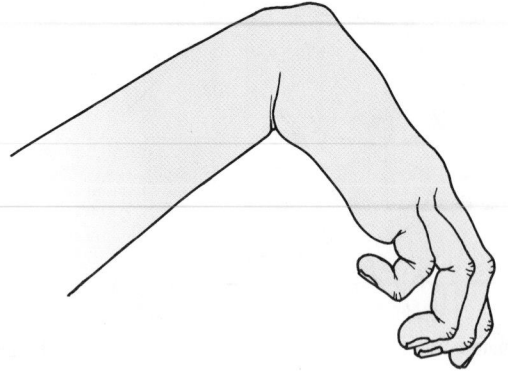

Figure 7-26 Deformity seen with Volkmann ischemic contracture. Note clawed fingers.

Because there are so many joints, bones, muscles, and ligaments involved, the examiner must develop a working knowledge of all of these tissues and how they interact with one another. The examiner should remember that adduction of the hand (ulnar deviation) is greater than abduction (radial deviation) because of shortness of the ulnar styloid process. Supination of the forearm is stronger than pronation, whereas abduction has a greater ROM in supination than pronation. Adduction and abduction ROM is minimal when the wrist is fully extended or flexed. Both flexion and extension at the fingers are maximal when the wrist is in a neutral position (not abducted or adducted); flexion and extension of the wrist are minimal when the wrist is in pronation.

BOX 7-1

Outline of Physical Findings of the Hand

I. **Variations in size and shape of hand**
 A. *Large, blunt fingers (spade hand)*
  1. Acromegaly
  2. Hurler's disease (gargoylism)
 B. *Gross irregularity of shape and size*
  1. Paget disease of bone
  2. Maffucci's syndrome
  3. Neurofibromatosis
 C. *Spider fingers, slender palm (arachnodactyly)*
  1. Hypopituitarism
  2. Eunuchism
  3. Ehlers-Danlos syndrome, pseudoxanthoma elasticum
  4. Tuberculosis
  5. Asthenic habitus
  6. Osteogenesis imperfecta
 D. *Sausage-shaped phalanges*
  1. Rickets (beading of joints)
  2. Granulomatous dactylitis (tuberculosis, syphilis)
 E. *Spindliform joints (fingers)*
  1. Early rheumatoid arthritis
  2. Systemic lupus erythematosus
  3. Psoriasis
  4. Rubella
  5. Boeck's sarcoidosis
  6. Osteoarthritis
 F. *Cone-shaped fingers*
  1. Pituitary obesity
  2. Fröhlich's dystrophy
 G. *Unilateral enlargement of hand*
  1. Arteriovenous aneurysm
  2. Maffucci's syndrome
 H. *Square, dry hands*
  1. Cretinism
  2. Myxedema
 I. *Single, widened, flattened distal phalanx*
  1. Sarcoidosis
 J. *Shortened fourth and fifth metacarpals (bradymetacarpalism)*
  1. Pseudohypoparathyroidism
  2. Pseudopseudohypoparathyroidism

 K. *Shortened, incurved fifth finger (symptom of Du Bois)*
  1. Mongolism
  2. "Behavioral problem"
  3. Gargoylism (broad, short, thick-skinned hand)
 L. *Malposition and abduction, fifth finger*
  1. Turner's syndrome (gonadal dysgenesis, webbed neck, etc.)
 M. *Syndactylism*
  1. Congenital malformations of the heart, great vessels
  2. Multiple congenital deformities
  3. Laurence-Moon-Biedl syndrome
  4. In normal individuals as an inherited trait
 N. *Clubbed fingers*
  1. Subacute bacterial endocarditis
  2. Pulmonary causes
   a. Tuberculosis
   b. Pulmonary arteriovenous fistula
   c. Pulmonic abscess
   d. Pulmonic cysts
   e. Bullous emphysema
   f. Pulmonary hypertrophic osteoarthropathy
   g. Bronchogenic carcinoma
  3. Alveolocapillary block
   a. Interstitial pulmonary fibrosis
   b. Sarcoidosis
   c. Beryllium poisoning
   d. Sclerodermatous lung
   e. Asbestosis
   f. Miliary tuberculosis
   g. Alveolar cell carcinoma
  4. Cardiovascular causes
   a. Patent ductus arteriosus
   b. Tetralogy of Fallot
   c. Taussig-Bing complex
   d. Pulmonic stenosis
   e. Ventricular septal defect

BOX **7-1**

Outline of Physical Findings of the Hand—cont'd

5. Diarrheal states
   a. Ulcerative colitis
   b. Tuberculous enteritis
   c. Sprue
   d. Amebic dysentery
   e. Bacillary dysentery
   f. Parasitic infestation (gastrointestinal tract)
6. Hepatic cirrhosis
7. Myxedema
8. Polycythemia
9. Chronic urinary tract infections (upper and lower)
   a. Chronic nephritis
10. Hyperparathyroidism (telescopy of distal phalanx)
11. Pachydermoperiostosis (syndrome of Touraine, Solente, and Golé)

O. Joint disturbances
   1. Arthritides
      a. Osteoarthritis
      b. Rheumatoid arthritis
      c. Systemic lupus erythematosus
      d. Gout
      e. Psoriasis
      f. Sarcoidosis
      g. Endocrinopathy (acromegaly)
      h. Rheumatic fever
      i. Reiter's syndrome
      j. Dermatomyositis
   2. Anaphylactic reaction-serum sickness
   3. Scleroderma

II. **Edema of the hand**
   A. Cardiac disease (congestive heart failure)
   B. Hepatic disease
   C. Renal disease
      1. Nephritis
      2. Nephrosis
   D. Hemiplegic hand
   E. Syringomyelia
   F. Superior vena caval syndrome
      1. Superior thoracic outlet tumor
      2. Mediastinal tumor or inflammation
      3. Pulmonary apex tumor
      4. Aneurysm
   G. Generalized anasarca, hypoproteinemia
   H. Postoperative lymphedema (radical breast amputation)
   I. Ischemic paralysis (cold, blue, swollen, numb)
   J. Lymphatic obstruction
      1. Lymphomatous masses in axilla
   K. Axillary mass
      1. Metastatic tumor, abscess, leukemia, Hodgkin's disease
   L. Aneurysm of ascending or transverse aorta, or of axillary artery
   M. Pressure on innominate or subclavian vessels
   N. Raynaud disease

O. Myositis
P. Cervical rib
Q. Trichiniasis
R. Scalenus anticus syndrome

III. **Neuromuscular effects**
   A. Atrophy
      1. Painless
         a. Amyotrophic lateral sclerosis
         b. Charcot-Marie-Tooth peroneal atrophy
         c. Syringomyelia (loss of heat, cold, and pain sensation)
         d. Neural leprosy
      2. Painful
         a. Peripheral nerve disease
            1. Radial nerve (wrist drop)
               a. lead poisoning, alcoholism, polyneuritis, trauma
               b. Diphtheria, polyarteritis, neurosyphilis, anterior poliomyelitis
            2. Ulnar nerve (benediction palsy)
               a. Polyneuritis, trauma
            3. Median nerve (claw hand)
               a. Carpal tunnel syndrome
                  1. Rheumatoid arthritis
                  2. Tenosynovitis at wrist
                  3. Amyloidosis
                  4. Gout
                  5. Plasmacytoma
                  6. Anaphylactic reaction
                  7. Menopause syndrome
                  8. Myxedema
   B. Extrinsic pressure on the nerve (cervical, axillary, supraclavicular, or brachial)
      1. Pancoast tumor (pulmonary apex)
      2. Aneurysms of subclavian arteries, axillary vessels, or thoracic aorta
      3. Costoclavicular syndrome
      4. Superior thoracic outlet syndrome
      5. Cervical rib
      6. Degenerative arthritis of cervical spine
      7. Herniation of cervical intervertebral disc
   C. Shoulder-hand syndrome
      1. Myocardial infarction
      2. Pancoast tumor
      3. Brain tumor
      4. Intrathoracic neoplasms
      5. Discogenetic disease
      6. Cervical spondylosis
      7. Febrile panniculitis
      8. Senility
      9. Vascular occlusion
      10. Hemiplegia
      11. Osteoarthritis
      12. Herpes zoster

Continued

BOX **7-1**

Outline of Physical Findings of the Hand—cont'd

D. *Ischemic contractures (sensory loss in fingers)*
   1. Tight plaster cast applications
E. *Polyarteritis nodosa*
F. *Polyneuritis*
   1. Carcinoma of lung
   2. Hodgkin's disease
   3. Pregnancy
   4. Gastric carcinoma
   5. Reticuloses
   6. Diabetes mellitus
   7. Chemical neuritis
      a. Antimony, benzene, bismuth, carbon tetrachloride, heavy metals, alcohol, arsenic, lead, gold, emetine
   8. Ischemic neuropathy
   9. Vitamin B deficiency
  10. Atheromata
  11. Arteriosclerosis
  12. Embolic
G. *Carpodigital (carpopedal spasm) tetany*
   1. Hypoparathyroidism
   2. Hyperventilation
   3. Uremia
   4. Nephritis
   5. Nephrosis
   6. Rickets
   7. Sprue
   8. Malabsorption syndrome
   9. Pregnancy
  10. Lactation
  11. Osteomalacia
  12. Protracted vomiting
  13. Pyloric obstruction
  14. Alkali poisoning
  15. Chemical toxicity
      a. Morphine, lead, alcohol
H. *Tremor*
   1. Parkinsonism
   2. Familial disorder
   3. Hypoglycemia
   4. Hyperthyroidism
   5. Wilson's disease (hepatolenticular degeneration)
   6. Anxiety
   7. Ataxia
   8. Athetosis
   9. Alcoholism, narcotic addiction
  10. Multiple sclerosis
  11. Chorea (Sydenham's, Huntington's)

Modified from Berry TJ: The hand as a mirror of systemic disease, Philadelphia, 1963, FA Davis.

The wrist and hand have both a fixed (stable) and a mobile segment. The fixed segment consists of the distal row of carpal bones (trapezium, trapezoid, capitate, and hamate) and the second and third metacarpals. This is the **stable segment** of the wrist and hand (Figure 7-27), and movement between these bones is less than that between the bones of the mobile segment. This arrangement allows stability without rigidity, enables the hand to move more discretely and with suppleness, and enhances the function of the thumb and fingers when they are used for power and/or precision grip. The **mobile segment** is made up of the five phalanges and the first, fourth, and fifth metacarpal bones.

The **functional position** of the wrist is extension to between 20° and 35° with ulnar deviation of 10° to 15°.[15] This position, sometimes called the **position of rest,** minimizes the restraining action of the long extensor tendons and allows complete flexion of the finger; thus, the greatest power of grip occurs when the wrist is in this position (Figure 7-28). In this position, the pulps of the index finger and thumb come into contact to facilitate thumb-finger action. The position of **wrist immobilization** (Figure 7-29) is further extension than is seen in the position of rest with the metacarpophalangeal joints more flexed and the interphalangeal joints extended. In this

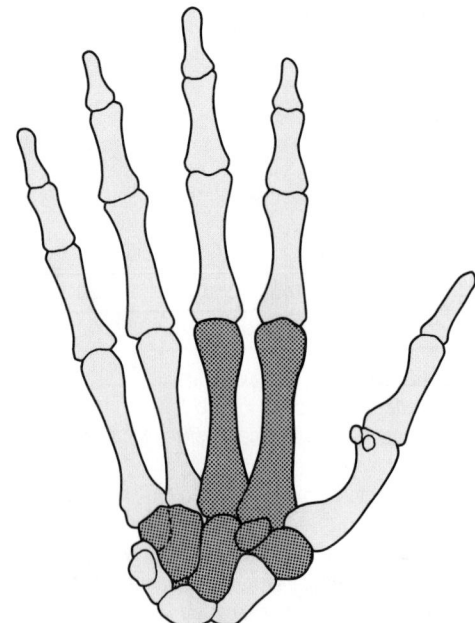

Figure 7-27 Palmar view of hand, showing stable segment *(stippled areas)*.

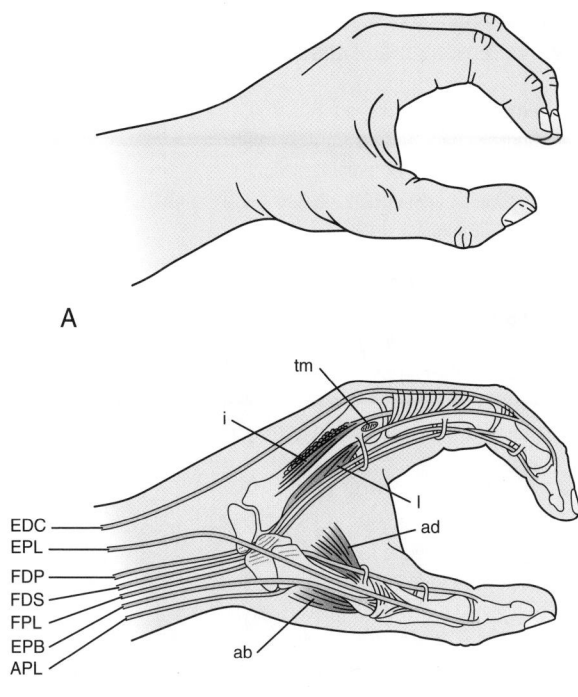

A

B

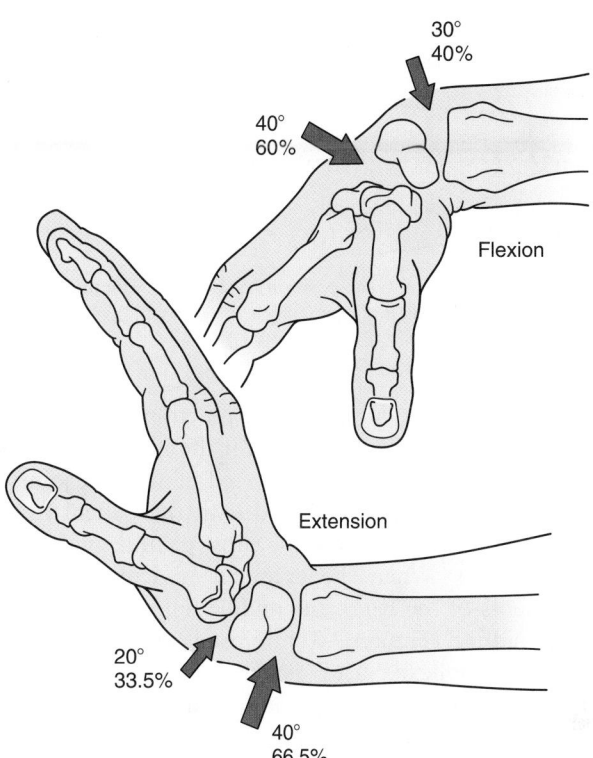

Figure 7-30 During flexion of the wrist, the motion is more mid-carpal and less radiocarpal. During extension of the wrist, the motion is more radiocarpal and less midcarpal. (Modified from Sarrafian SK, Melamed JL, Goshgarian GM: Study of wrist motion in flexion and extension. Clin Orthop 126:156, 1977.)

Figure 7-28 Position of function of the hand. A, Normal view. **B,** The hand is in the position of function. Notice in particular that a very small amount of motion in the thumb and fingers is useful motion in that it can be used in pinch and grasp. Notice the close relation of the tendons to bone. The flexor tendons are held close to bone by a pulley-like thickening of the flexor sheath as represented schematically. With the hand in this position, intrinsic and extrinsic musculature is in balance, and all muscles are acting within their physiological resting length. *ab,* Abductor pollicis brevis; *ad,* adductor pollicis brevis; *APL,* abductor pollicis longus; *EDC,* extensor digitorum communis; *EPB,* extensor pollicis brevis; *EPL,* extensor pollicis longus; *FDP,* flexor digitorum profundus; *FDS,* flexor digitorum sublimis; *FPL,* flexor pollicis longus; *i,* interossei; *l,* lumbrical; *tm,* transverse metacarpal ligament;. (**B,** Redrawn from O'Donoghue DH: Treatment of injuries to athletes, Philadelphia, 1984, WB Saunders, p. 287.)

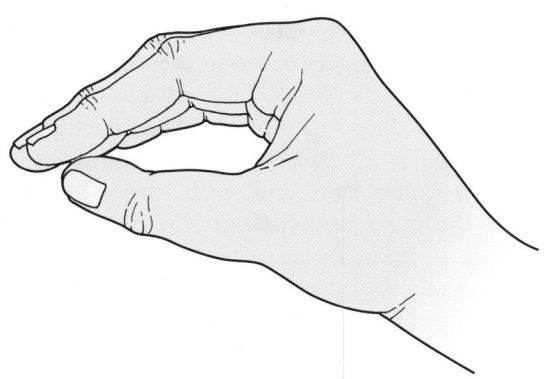

Figure 7-29 Position of immobilization.

way, when the joints are immobilized, the potential for contracture is kept to a minimum.

During extension at the wrist (Figure 7-30), most of the movement occurs in the radiocarpal joint (approximately 40°) and less occurs in the midcarpal joint

(approximately 20°).[14] The motion of extension is accompanied by slight radial deviation and pronation of the forearm. During wrist flexion (see Figure 7-30), most of the movement occurs in the midcarpal joint (approximately 40°) and less occurs in the radiocarpal joint (approximately 30°).[14] This movement is accompanied by slight ulnar deviation and supination of the forearm. Radial deviation occurs primarily between the proximal and distal rows of carpal bones (0° to 20°) with the proximal row moving toward the ulna and the distal row moving radially. Ulnar deviation occurs primarily at the radiocarpal joint (0° to 37°).[15]

Active Movements

Active movements are sometimes referred to as *physiological movements*. If there is pathology to only one area of the hand or wrist, only that area needs to be assessed, provided the examiner is satisfied that the pathology is not affecting or has not affected the function of the other areas of the forearm, wrist, and hand. For example, if the patient has suffered a FOOSH injury to the wrist, the examiner spends most of the examination looking at the wrist. However, because positioning of the wrist can affect the function of the rest of the hand and forearm,

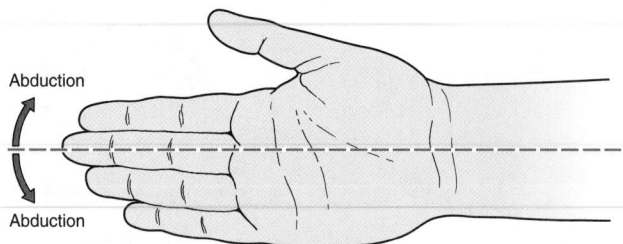

Figure 7-31 Axis or reference position of the hand. The middle finger provides a central reference from which the other fingers abduct and adduct.

the examiner must determine the functional effect of the injury to these other areas. Also, if the injury is chronic, adaptive changes may have occurred in adjacent joints.

Examination is accomplished with the patient in the sitting position. As always, the most painful movements are done last. When the examiner is determining the movements of the hand, the middle finger is considered to be midline (Figure 7-31). Wrist flexion decreases as the fingers are flexed just as finger flexion decreases as the wrist flexes, and movements of flexion and extension are limited, usually by the antagonistic muscles and ligaments. In addition, pathology to structures other than the joint may restrict ROM (e.g., muscle spasm, tight ligaments/capsules). If the examiner suspects these structures, passive movement end feels will help differentiate the problem. The patient should actively perform the various movements. Initially, the active movements of the forearm, wrist, and hand may be performed in a "scanning" fashion by having the patient make a fist and then open the hand wide. As the patient does these two movements, the examiner notes any restrictions, deviations, or pain. Depending on the results, the examiner can then do a detailed examination of the affected joints. This detailed examination is initiated by selection of the appropriate active movements to be performed, keeping in mind the effect one joint can have on others.

Active pronation and supination of the forearm and wrist are approximately 85° to 90°, although there is variability between individuals and it is more important to compare the movement with that of the normal side. Approximately 75° of supination or pronation occurs in the forearm articulations. The remaining 15° is the result of wrist action. If the patient complains of pain on supination, the examiner can differentiate between the distal radioulnar joint and the radiocarpal joints by passively supinating the ulna on the radius with no stress on the radiocarpal joint. If this passive movement is painful, the problem is in the distal radioulnar joint, not the radiocarpal joints. The normal end feel of both movements is tissue stretch, although in thin patients, the end feel of pronation may be bone-to-bone.

Radial and ulnar deviations of the wrist are 15° and 30° to 45°, respectively. The normal end feel of these movements is bone-to-bone.

Active Movements of the Forearm, Wrist, and Hand

- Pronation of the forearm (85° to 90°)
- Supination of the forearm (85° to 90°)
- Wrist abduction or radial deviation (15°)
- Wrist adduction or ulnar deviation (30° to 45°)
- Wrist flexion (80° to 90°)
- Wrist extension (70° to 90°)
- Finger flexion (MCP, 85° to 90°; PIP, 100° to 115°; DIP, 80° to 90°)
- Finger extension (MCP, 30° to 45°; PIP, 0°; DIP, 20°)
- Finger abduction (20° to 30°)
- Finger adduction (0°)
- Thumb flexion (CMC, 45° to 50°; MCP, 50° to 55°; IP, 85° to 90°)
- Thumb extension (MCP, 0°; IP, 0° to 5°)
- Thumb abduction (60° to 70°)
- Thumb adduction (30°)
- Opposition of little finger and thumb (tip-to-tip)
- Combined movements (if necessary)
- Repetitive movements (if necessary)
- Sustained positions (if necessary)

CMC, Carpometacarpal; *DIP*, distal interphalangeal; *IP*, interphalangeal; *MCP*, metacarpophalangeal; *PIP*, proximal interphalangeal.

Wrist flexion is 80° to 90°; **wrist extension** is 70° to 90°. The end feel of each movement is tissue stretch. Midcarpal instability may be evident on ulnar deviation. If there is midcarpal instability as the wrist is taken into ulnar deviation, the proximal row of carpals stays flexed longer and then audibly snaps or clunks into dorsiflexion (known as a "catch up clunk").[9,29,30] Instability at the radiocarpal and midcarpal joints involving groups of bones may be called **carpal instability nondissociative (CIND).** If there is instability of one bone relative to the other bones in the same row, it may be called **carpal instability dissociative (CID).**[31]

Flexion of the fingers occurs at the metacarpophalangeal joints (85° to 90°), followed by the proximal interphalangeal joints (100° to 115°) and the distal interphalangeal joints (80° to 90°). This sequence enables the hand to grasp large and small objects. **Extension** occurs at the metacarpophalangeal joints (30° to 45°), the proximal interphalangeal joints (0°), and the distal interphalangeal joints (20°). Hyperextension at the proximal interphalangeal joints can lead to a swan neck deformity. This hyperextension is usually prevented by the volar plates.[3] The end feel of finger flexion and extension is tissue stretch. **Finger abduction** occurs at the metacarpophalangeal joints (20° to 30°); the end feel is tissue stretch. **Finger adduction** (0°) occurs at the same joint.

The digits are medially deviated slightly in relation to the metacarpal bones (see Figure 7-6). When the fingers are flexed, they should point toward the scaphoid

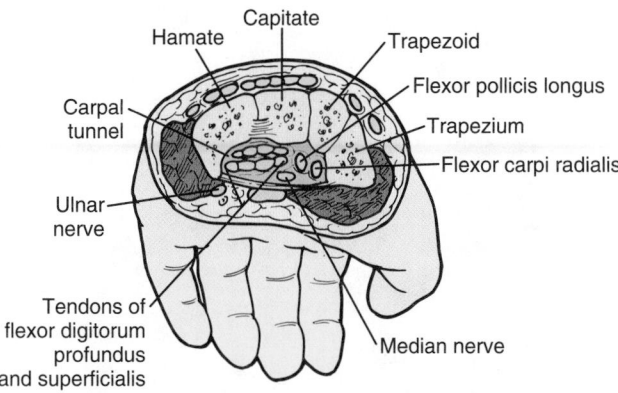

Figure 7-32 Cross section of the wrist showing the carpal tunnel.

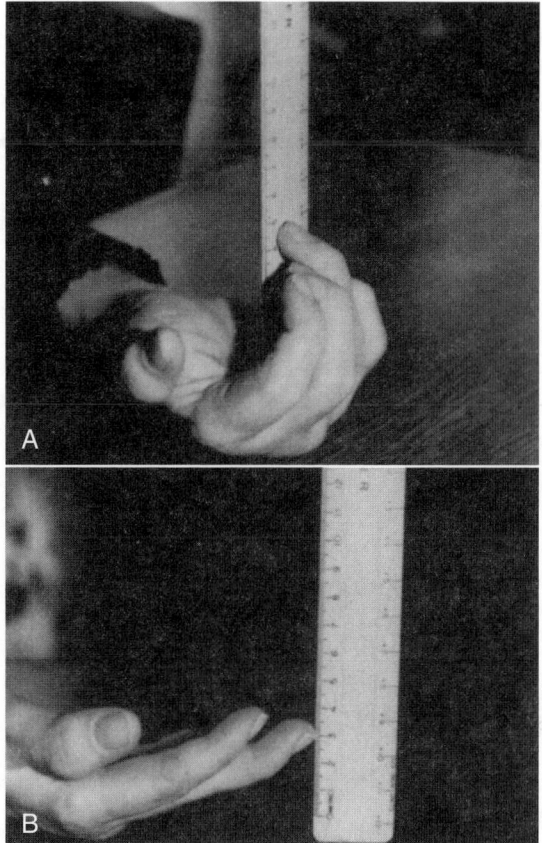

Figure 7-33 **A,** Gross flexion is measured as the distance between fingertips and proximal palmar crease. **B,** Gross extension is measured as the distance between fingertips and dorsal plane. (From Wadsworth CT: Wrist and hand examination and interpretation. J Orthop Sports Phys Ther 5:115, 1983.)

tubercle. In addition, the metacarpals are at an angle to each other. These positions increase the dexterity of the hand and oblique flexion of the medial four digits but contribute to deformities (e.g., ulnar drift) in conditions, such as rheumatoid arthritis.

Thumb flexion occurs at the carpometacarpal joint (45° to 50°), the metacarpophalangeal joint (50° to 55°), and the interphalangeal joint (80° to 90°). It is associated with medial rotation of the thumb as a result of the saddle shape of the carpometacarpal joint. **Extension of the thumb** occurs at the interphalangeal joint (0° to 5°); it is associated with lateral rotation. Flexion and extension take place in a plane parallel to the palm of the hand. **Thumb abduction** is 60° to 70°; **thumb adduction** is 30°. These movements occur in a plane at right angles to the flexion-extension plane.[15] The thumb is controlled by three nerves, a situation that is unique among the digits. The radial nerve controls extension and opening of the thumb as it does for the other digits. The ulnar nerve controls adduction, produces closure of pinch, and gives power to the grip; the median nerve controls flexion and opposition, producing precision with any grip.[3] The intrinsic muscles are stronger than the extrinsic muscles of the thumb; the opposite is true for the fingers.[3]

If the history has indicated that combined or repetitive movements and/or sustained postures have resulted in symptoms, these movements should also be tested.

The examiner must be aware that active movements may be affected because of neurological as well as contractile tissue problems. For example, the median nerve is sometimes compressed as it passes through the carpal tunnel (Figure 7-32), affecting its motor and sensory distribution in the hand and fingers. The condition is referred to as **carpal tunnel syndrome.**

If the patient does not have full active ROM and it is difficult to measure ROM because of swelling, pain, or contracture, the examiner can use a ruler or tape measure to record the distance from the fingertip to one of the palmar creases (Figure 7-33).[32] This measurement provides baseline data for any effect of treatment. It is important to note on the chart which crease was used in the measurement. The majority of functional activities of the hand require that the fingers and thumb to open at least 5 cm (2 inches), and the fingers should be able to flex within 1 to 2 cm (0.4 to 0.8 inch) of the distal palmar crease.[33]

Passive Movements

If, when watching the patient perform the active movements, the examiner believes the ROM is full, overpressure can be gently applied to test the end feel of the joint in each direction. If the movement is not full, passive movements must be carefully performed by the examiner to test the end feel. At the same time, the examiner must watch for the presence of a capsular pattern. The passive movements are the same as the active movements, and the examiner must remember to test each individual joint.

The capsular pattern of the distal radioulnar joint is full ROM with pain at the extremes of supination and pronation. At the wrist, the capsular pattern is equal limitation of flexion and extension. At the metacarpophalangeal and

Passive Movements of the Forearm, Wrist, and Hand and Normal End Feel

- Pronation (tissue stretch)
- Supination (tissue stretch)
- Radial deviation (bone-to-bone)
- Ulnar deviation (bone-to-bone)
- Wrist flexion (tissue stretch)
- Wrist extension (tissue stretch)
- Finger flexion (tissue stretch)
- Finger extension (tissue stretch)
- Finger abduction (tissue stretch)
- Thumb flexion (tissue stretch)
- Thumb extension (tissue stretch)
- Thumb abduction (tissue stretch)
- Thumb adduction (tissue approximation)
- Opposition (tissue stretch)

interphalangeal joints, the capsular pattern is flexion more limited than extension. At the trapeziometacarpal joint of the thumb, the capsular pattern is abduction more limited than extension.

In some cases, the examiner may want to test the length of the long extensor and flexor muscles of the wrist (Figure 7-34). If the length of the muscles is normal, the passive range on testing is full and the end feel is the normal joint tissue stretch end feel. If the muscles are tight, the end feel is muscle stretch, which is not as "stretchy" as tissue or capsular stretch, and the ROM is restricted.

To test the length of the long wrist extensors, the patient is placed in supine lying with the elbow extended. The examiner passively flexes the fingers and then flexes the wrist.[34] If the muscles are tight, wrist flexion is restricted.

To test the length of the long wrist flexors, the patient is placed in supine lying with the elbow extended. The examiner passively extends the fingers and then extends the wrist.[34] If the muscles are tight, wrist extension is limited.

Conjunct rotation can be tested by folding and fanning the hand (Figure 7-35). To do this, the examiner holds the scaphoid and trapezium with the index and middle finger of one hand and the pisiform and hamate of the other hand while the capitate is held with the thumbs on the dorsum of the hand. The examiner then folds and fans the hand feeling the movement.[35]

Resisted Isometric Movements

As with the active movements, the resisted isometric movements to the forearm, wrist, and hand are done with the patient in the sitting position. Not all resisted isometric movements need to be tested, but the examiner must keep in mind that the actions of the fingers and thumb

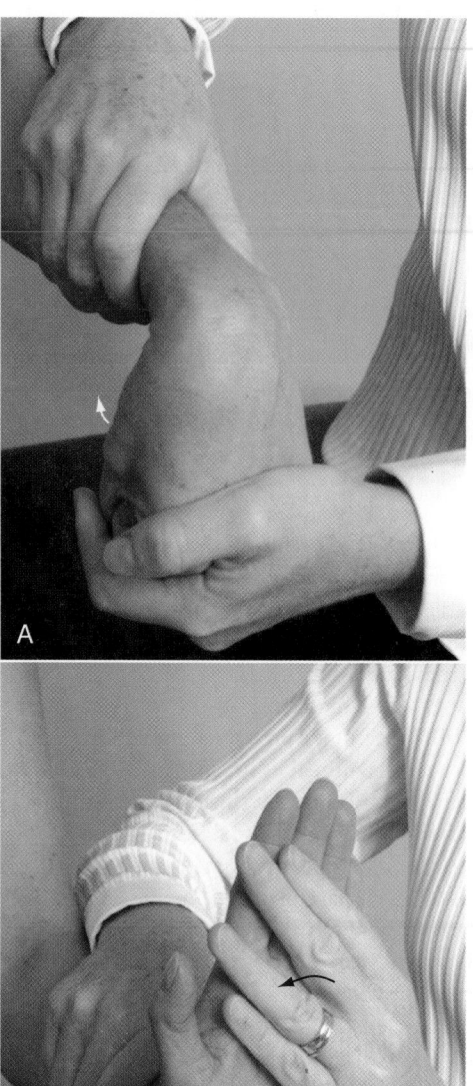

Figure 7-34 Testing the length of the long extensor (**A**) and flexor (**B**) muscles of the wrist.

and the wrist are controlled by extrinsic muscles (wrist, fingers, thumb) and intrinsic muscles (fingers, thumb), so injury affecting these structures requires testing of the appropriate muscles. The movements must be isometric and must be performed in the neutral position (Figures 7-36 and 7-37). If the history has indicated that concentric, eccentric, or econcentric movements have caused symptoms, these different types of resisted movement should be tested, but only after the movements have been tested isometrically.

Table 7-3 shows the muscles and their actions for differentiation during resisted isometric testing. If measured by test instruments, the strength ratio of wrist extensors to wrist flexors is approximately 50%, whereas the strength

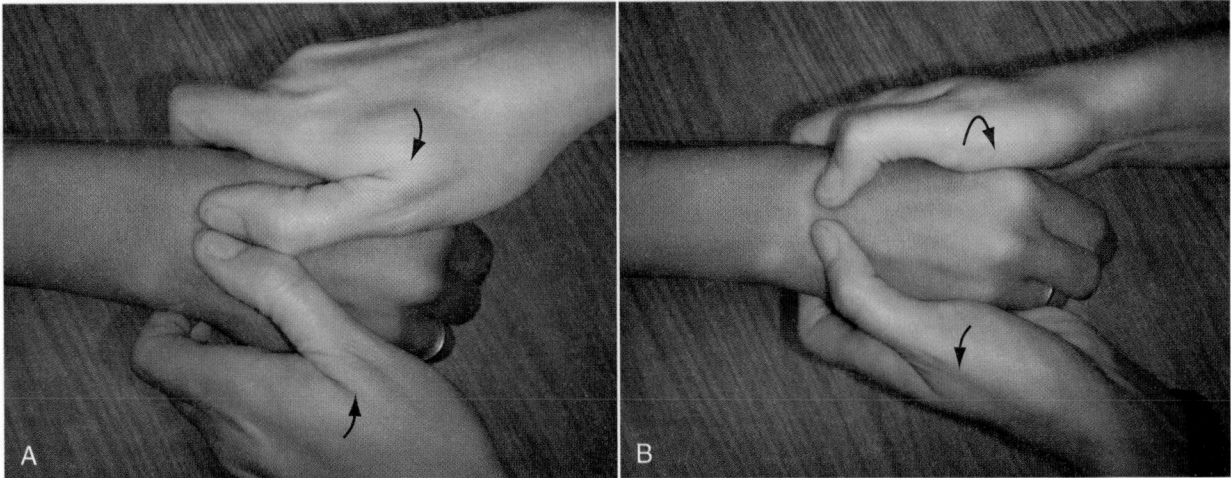

Figure 7-35 **A,** Fanning of the hand. **B,** Folding of the hand.

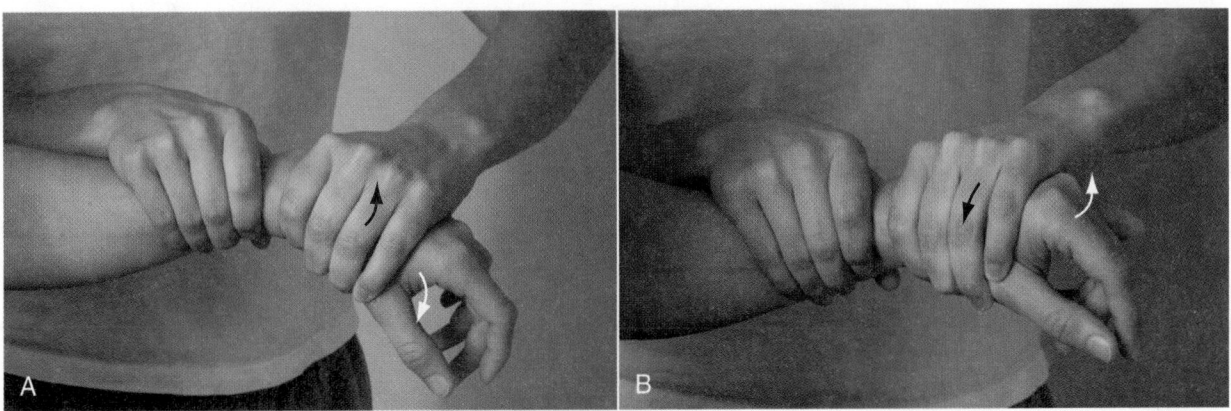

Figure 7-36 **Resisted isometric movements of the wrist. A,** Flexion. **B,** Extension.

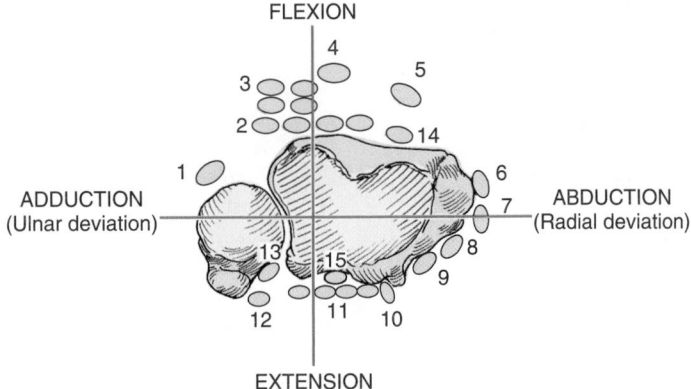

Figure 7-37 Muscles and their actions at the wrist. *1,* Flexor carpi ulnaris; *2,* flexor digitorum profundus; *3,* flexor digitorum superficialis; *4,* palmaris longus; *5,* flexor carpi radialis; *6,* abductor pollicis longus; *7,* extensor pollicis brevis; *8,* extensor carpi radialis longus; *9,* extensor carpi radialis brevis; *10,* extensor pollicis longus; *11,* extensor digitorum; *12,* extensor digiti minimi; *13,* extensor carpi ulnaris; *14,* flexor pollicis longus; *15,* extensor indices.

TABLE **7-3**

Muscles of the Forearm, Wrist, and Hand: Their Actions, Nerve Supply, and Nerve Root Derivation

Action	Muscles Acting	Nerve Supply	Nerve Root Deviation
Supination of forearm	1. Supinator	Posterior interosseous (radial)	C5, C6
	2. Biceps brachii	Musculocutaneous	C5, C6
Pronation of forearm	1. Pronator quadratus	Anterior interosseous (median)	C8, T1
	2. Pronator teres	Median	C6, C7
	3. Flexor carpi radialis	Median	C6, C7
Extension of wrist	1. Extensor carpi radialis longus	Radial	C6, C7
	2. Extensor carpi radialis brevis	Posterior interosseous (radial)	C7, C8
	3. Extensor carpi ulnaris	Posterior interosseous (radial)	C7, C8
Flexion of wrist	1. Flexor carpi radialis	Median	C6, C7
	2. Flexor carpi ulnaris	Ulnar	C7, C8
Ulnar deviation of wrist	1. Flexor carpi ulnaris	Ulnar	C7, C8
	2. Extensor carpi ulnaris	Posterior interosseous (radial)	C7, C8
Radial deviation of wrist	1. Flexor carpi radialis	Median	C6, C7
	2. Extensor carpi radialis longus	Radial	C6, C7
	3. Abductor pollicis longus	Posterior interosseous (radial)	C7, C8
	4. Extensor pollicis brevis	Posterior interosseous (radial)	C7, C8
Extension of fingers	1. Extensor digitorum communis	Posterior interosseous (radial)	C7, C8
	2. Extensor indices (second finger)	Posterior interosseous (radial)	C7, C8
	3. Extensor digiti minimi (little finger)	Posterior interosseous (radial)	C7, C8
Flexion of fingers	1. Flexor digitorum profundus	Anterior interosseous (median)	C8, T1
		Anterior interosseous (median): lateral two digits	C8, T1
		Ulnar: medial two digits	C8, T1
	2. Flexor digitorum superficialis	Median	C7, C8, T1 C8, T1
	3. Lumbricals	First and second: median; third and fourth: ulnar (deep terminal branch)	C8, T1
	4. Interossei	Ulnar (deep terminal branch)	C8, T1
	5. Flexor digiti minimi (little finger)	Ulnar (deep terminal branch)	C8, T1
Abduction of fingers (with fingers extended)	1. Dorsal interossei	Ulnar (deep terminal branch)	C8, T1
	2. Abductor digiti minimi (little finger)	Ulnar (deep terminal branch)	C8, T1
Adduction of fingers (with fingers extended)	1. Palmar interossei	Ulnar (deep terminal branch)	C8, T1
Extension of thumb	1. Extensor pollicis longus	Posterior interosseous (radial)	C7, C8
	2. Extensor pollicis brevis	Posterior interosseous (radial)	C7, C8
	3. Abductor pollicis longus	Posterior interosseous (radial)	C7, C8
Flexion of thumb	1. Flexor pollicis brevis	Superficial head: median (lateral terminal branch)	C8, T1
		Deep head: ulnar	C8, T1
	2. Flexor pollicis longus	Anterior interosseous (median)	C8, T1
	3. Opponens pollicis	Median (lateral terminal branch)	C8, T1
Abduction of thumb	1. Abductor pollicis longus	Posterior interosseous (radial)	C7, C8
	2. Abductor pollicis brevis	Median (lateral terminal branch)	C8, T1
Adduction of thumb	1. Adductor pollicis	Ulnar (deep terminal branch)	C8, T1
Opposition of thumb and little finger	1. Opponens pollicis	Median (lateral terminal branch	C8, T1
	2. Flexor pollicis brevis	Superficial head: median (lateral terminal branch)	C8, T1
	3. Abductor pollicis brevis	Median (lateral terminal branch)	C8, T1
	4. Opponens digiti minimi	Ulnar (deep terminal branch)	C8, T1

Resisted Isometric Movements of the Forearm, Wrist, and Hand

- Pronation of the forearm
- Supination of the forearm
- Wrist abduction (radial deviation)
- Wrist adduction (ulnar deviation)
- Wrist flexion
- Wrist extension
- Finger flexion
- Finger extension
- Finger abduction
- Finger adduction
- Thumb flexion
- Thumb extension
- Thumb abduction
- Thumb adduction
- Opposition of the little finger and thumb

ratio of ulnar deviators to radial deviators is approximately 80%. The greatest torque is produced by the wrist flexors, followed by the radial deviators, ulnar deviators, and finally the wrist extensors.[36]

Functional Assessment (Grip)

Having completed the basic movement testing of active, passive, and resisted isometric movements, the examiner then assesses the patient's functional active movements. Functionally, the thumb is the most important digit. Because of its relation with the other digits, its mobility, and the force it can bring to bear, its loss can affect hand function greatly. The index finger is the second most important digit because of its musculature, its strength, and its interaction with the thumb. Its loss greatly affects lateral and pulp-to-pulp pinch and power grip. In flexion, the middle finger is strongest, and it is important for both precision and power grips. The ring finger has the least functional role in the hand. The little finger, because of its peripheral position, greatly enhances power grip, affects the capacity of the hand, and holds objects against the hypothenar eminence.[3] In terms of **functional impairment,** the loss of thumb function affects about 40% to 50% of hand function. The loss of index finger function accounts for about 20% of hand function; the middle finger, about 20%; the ring finger, about 10%; and the little finger, about 10%. Loss of the hand accounts for about 90% loss of upper limb function.[37]

Hand function can be quickly assessed by performing a number of movements to test overall function of the wrist and hand (functional hand and wrist scan) (Figure 7-38).

Although the wrist, hand, and finger joints have the ability to move through a relatively large ROM, most functional daily tasks do not require full ROM. The

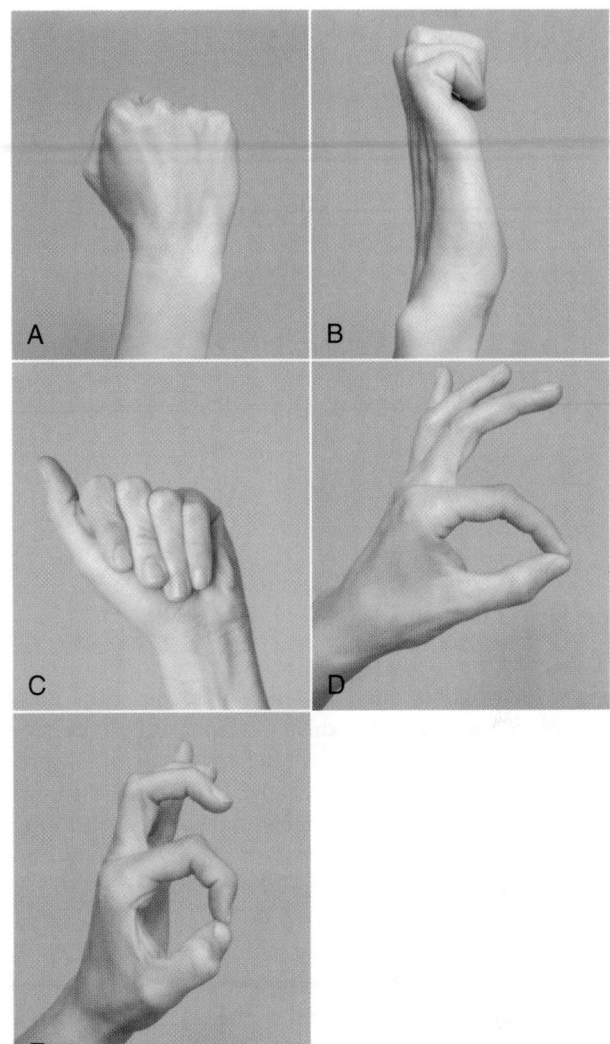

Figure 7-38 Parts of a functional wrist and hand scan. A, Standard fist. **B,** Hook grasp fist. **C,** Straight fist. **D,** Pulp-to-pulp pinch. **E,** Tip-to-tip pinch.

Functional Wrist and Hand Scan

- Wrist flexion and extension
- Wrist ulnar and radial deviation
- Making a standard fist
- Making a hook grasp
- Making a straight fist
- Pulp-to-pulp thumb to all fingers pinch
- Tip-to-tip thumb to all fingers pinch

optimum functional ROM at the wrist is approximately 10° flexion to 35° extension along with 10° of radial deviation and 15° of ulnar deviation.[38-41] Normally, the wrist is held in slight extension (10° to 15°) and slight ulnar deviation and is stabilized in this position to provide maximum function for the fingers and thumb. Excessive radial deviation, like ulnar drift of the fingers, can affect

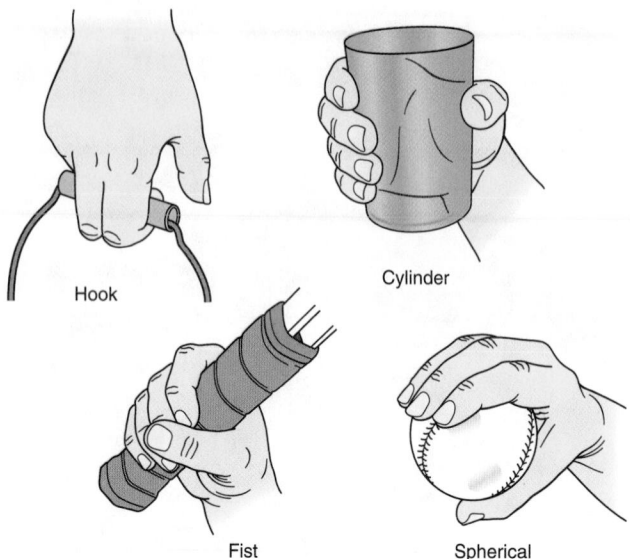

Figure 7-39 Types of power grips.

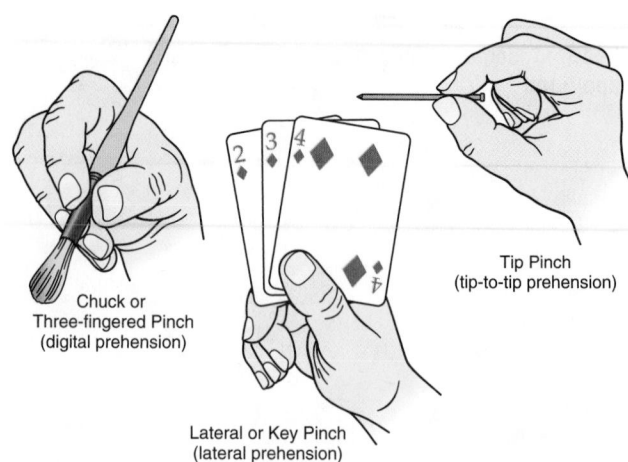

Figure 7-40 Types of precision grips or pinches.

grip strength adversely.[42] Functional flexion at the metacarpophalangeal and proximal interphalangeal joints is approximately 60°. Functional flexion at the distal interphalangeal joint is approximately 40°. For the thumb, functional flexion at the metacarpophalangeal and interphalangeal joints is approximately 20°.[33] Within these ROMs, the hand is able to perform most of its grip[15,43] and other functional activities.

The thumb, although not always used in gripping, adds another important dimension when it is used. It gives stability and helps control the direction in which the object moves. Both of these factors are necessary for precision movements. The thumb also increases the power of a grip by acting as a buttress, resisting the pressure of an object held between it and the fingers.

The nerve distribution and the functions of the digits also present interesting patterns. Flexion and sensation of the ulnar digits are controlled by the ulnar nerve and are more related to power grip. Flexion and sensation of the radial digits are controlled by the median nerve and are more related to precision grip. The muscles of the thumb, often used in both types of grip, are supplied by both nerves. In all cases of gripping, opening of the hand or release of grip depends on the radial nerve.

Power Grip. A power grip requires firm control and gives greater flexor asymmetry to the hand (Figure 7-39). During power grip, the ulnar side of the hand works with the radial side to give stronger stability. The ulnar digits tend to work together to provide support and static control.[3,15,43,44] This grip is used whenever strength or force is the primary consideration. With this grip, the digits maintain the object against the palm; the thumb may or may not be involved, and the extrinsic (forearm) muscles are more important. The combined effect of joint position brings the hand into line with the forearm. For

Stages of Grip

1. Opening of the hand, which requires the simultaneous action of the intrinsic muscles of the hand and the long extensor muscles
2. Positioning and closing of the fingers and thumb to grasp the object and adapt to the object's shape, which involves intrinsic and extrinsic flexor and opposition muscles
3. Exerted force, which varies depending on the weight, surface characteristics, fragility, and use of the object, again involving the extrinsic and intrinsic flexor and opposition muscles
4. Release, in which the hand opens to let go of the object, involving the same muscles as for opening of the hand

a power grip to be formed, the fingers are flexed and the wrist is in ulnar deviation and slightly extended. Examples of power grips include the **hook grasp,** in which all or the second and third fingers are used as a hook controlled by the forearm flexors and extensors. The hook grasp may involve the interphalangeal joints only or the interphalangeal and metacarpophalangeal joints (the thumb is not involved). In the **cylinder grasp,** a type of **palmar prehension,** the thumb is used, and the entire hand wraps around an object. With the **fist grasp,** or **digital palmar prehension,** the hand moves around a narrow object. Another type of power grip is the **spherical grasp,** another type of palmar prehension, in which there is more opposition and the hand moves around the sphere.

Precision or Prehension Grip. The precision grip is an activity limited mainly to the metacarpophalangeal joints and involves primarily the radial side of the hand (Figure 7-40).[15,43,44] This grip is used whenever accuracy and precision are required. The radial digits (index and long fingers) provide control by working in concert with the thumb to form a "dynamic tripod" for precision handling.[3] With precision grips, the thumb and fingers are used and the palm may or may not be involved; there is pulp-to-pulp contact between the thumb and fingers, and the thumb opposes the fingers. The intrinsic muscles are more important in precision than in power grips. The thumb is essential for precision grips, because it provides stability and control of direction and can act as a buttress, providing power to the grip.[3] There are three types of **pinch grip.** The first is called a **three-point chuck,** three-fingered, or **digital prehension,** in which palmar pinch, or subterminal opposition, is achieved. With this grip, there is pulp-to-pulp pinch, and opposition of the thumb and fingers is necessary (e.g., holding a pencil). This grip is sometimes called a **precision grip with power.** The second pinch grip is termed **lateral key, pulp-to-side pinch, lateral prehension,** or **subterminolateral opposition.** The thumb and lateral side of the index finger come into contact. No opposition is needed. An example of this movement is holding keys or a card. The third pinch grip is called the **tip pinch, tip-to-tip prehension,** or **terminal opposition.** With this positioning, the tip of the thumb is brought into opposition with the tip of another finger. This pinch is used for activities requiring fine coordination rather than power.

Estimated Use of Grips for Activities of Daily Living[43,45,46]

- 20% Pulp-to-pulp pinch: 20%
- Three lateral pinch: 20%
- Five-finger pinch: 15%
- Fist grip: 15%
- Cylinder grip: 14%
- Three-fingered (thumb, index finger, middle finger) pinch: 10%
- Spherical grip: 4%
- Hook grip: 2%

Testing Grip Strength

When testing grip strength using the grip dynamometer, the examiner should use the five adjustable hand spacings in consecutive order with the patient grasping the dynamometer with maximum force (Figure 7-41). Both hands are tested alternately, and each force is recorded.[47,48] Care must be taken to ensure that the patient does not fatigue. The results normally form a bell curve (Figure 7-42) with the greatest strength readings at the middle (second and third) spacings and the weakest at the beginning and at the end. There should be a 5% to 10% difference between the dominant and nondominant hands.[49] With injury, the bell curve should still be present, but the force exerted is less. If the patient does not exert maximum force for each test, the typical bell curve will not be produced, nor will the values obtained be consistent. Discrepancies of more than 20% in a test-retest situation indicate that the patient is not exerting maximal force.[48,50] Usually, the mean value

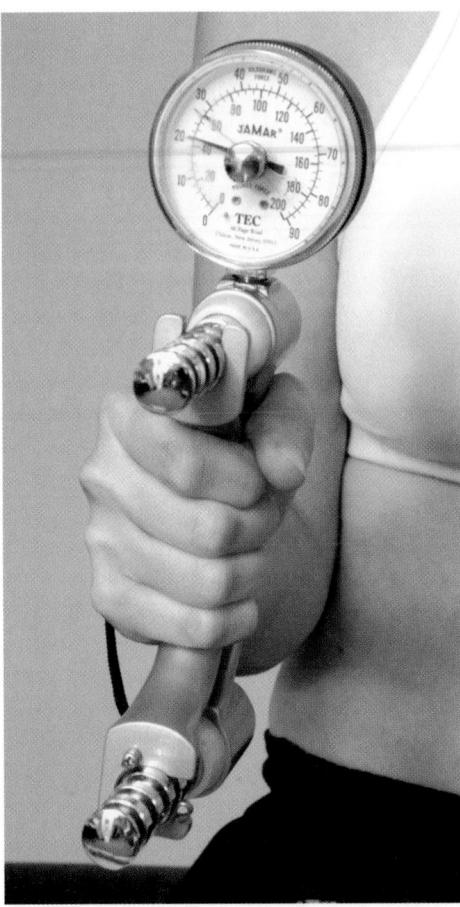

Figure 7-41 Jamar dynamometer. Arm should be held at the patient's side with elbow flexed at approximately 90° when grip is measured.

of three trials is recorded, and both hands are compared.[33] Table 7-4 gives normal values by age group and gender.

Testing Pinch Strength

The strength of the pinch may be tested with the use of a pinch meter (Figure 7-43). Average values are given for pulp-to-pulp pinch of each finger with the thumb (Table 7-5), lateral prehension (Table 7-6), and pulp-to-pulp pinch (Table 7-7) for different occupational levels. Normally, the mean value of three trials is recorded, and both hands are compared.

Other Functional Testing Methods

In addition to testing grip and pinch strength, the examiner may want to perform a full functional assessment of the patient. Figures 7-44 and 7-45 give examples of functional assessment forms for the hand. These forms are not numerical scoring charts, but they do include some functional aspects. Levine, et al.[51] have developed a severity questionnaire including a functional component to measure severity of symptoms and functional disability for a nerve—in this case, the median nerve in the carpal

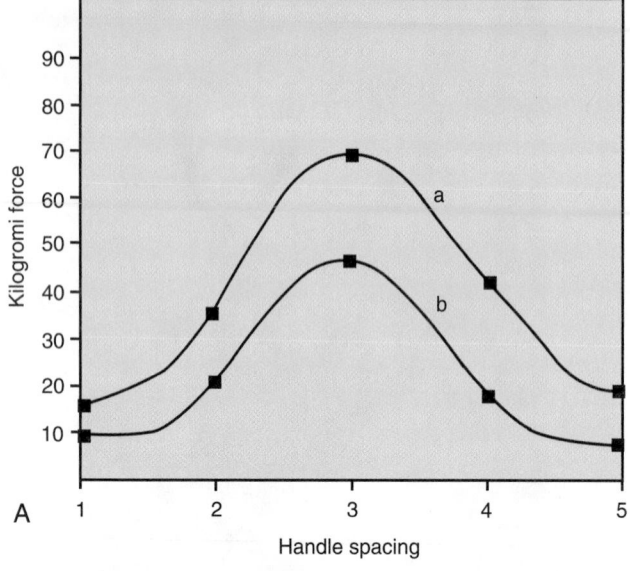

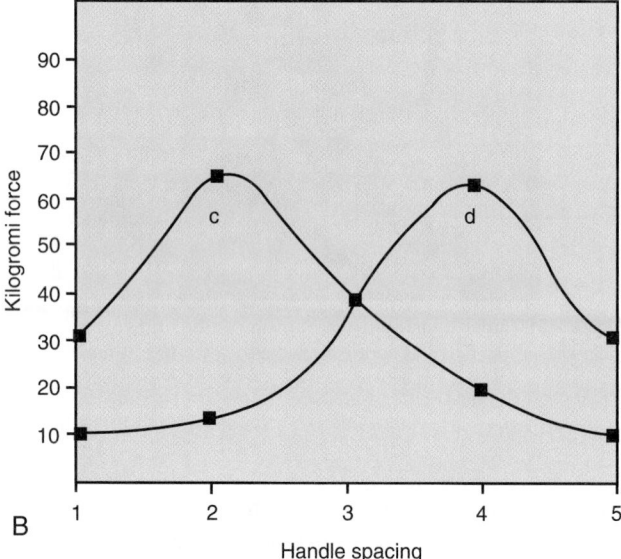

Figure 7-42 A, The grip strengths of a patient's uninjured hand (a) and injured hand (b) are plotted. Despite the patient's decrease in grip strength because of injury, *curve b* maintains a bell-shaped pattern and parallels that of the normal hand. These curves are reproducible in repeated examinations with minimal change in values. A great fluctuation in the size of the curve or absence of a bell-shaped pattern casts doubt on the patient's compliance with the examination and may indicate malingering. **B,** If the patient has an exceptionally large hand, the curve shifts to the right (d); with a very small hand, the curve shifts to the left (c). In both cases, the bell-shaped pattern is maintained. (Redrawn from Aulicino PL, DuPuy TE: Clinical examination of the hand. In Hunter J, Schneider LH, Mackin EJ, et al, editors: Rehabilitation of the hand: surgery and therapy, St Louis, 1990, CV Mosby, p. 45.)

tunnel (Figure 7-46). Chung, et al.[52] have developed a very comprehensive hand outcomes questionnaire—the Michigan Hand Outcomes Questionnaire, which gives the patient's evaluation of his or her outcome based on overall hand function, activities of daily living

(ADLs), pain, work performance, esthetics, and patient satisfaction (Figure 7-47). Likewise, Dias, et al.[53] have developed the Patient Evaluation Measure (PEM) Questionnaire (Figure 7-48). Table 7-8 provides a functional testing method. These strength values would be considered normal for an average population. They would be considered low for an athletic population or for persons in occupations subjecting the forearm, wrist, and hand to high repetitive loads.

Functional coordinated movements may be tested by asking the patient to perform simple activities, such as fastening a button, tying a shoelace, or tracing a diagram. Different prehension patterns are used regularly during daily activities.[46]

These tests may also be graded on a four-point scale.[47] This scale is particularly suitable if the patient has difficulty with one of the subtests, and the subtests can be scale-graded:

- Unable to perform task: 0
- Completes task partially: 1
- Completes task but is slow and clumsy: 2
- Performs task normally: 3

As part of the functional assessment, manual dexterity tests may be performed. Many standardized tests have been developed to assess manual dexterity and coordination. If comparison with other subjects is desired, the examiner must ensure that the patient is compared with a similar group of patients in terms of age, disability, and occupation. Each of these tests has its supporters and detractors. Some of the more common tests include the ones that follow.

Jebson-Taylor Hand Function Test. This easily administered test involves seven functional areas: 1) writing; 2) card turning; 3) picking up small objects; 4) simulated feeding; 5) stacking; 6) picking up large, light objects; and 7) picking up large, heavy objects. The subtests are timed for each limb. This test primarily measures gross coordination, assessing prehension and manipulative skills with functional tests. It does not test bilateral integration.[33,54-56] Anyone wishing to perform the test should consult the original article[57] for details of administration.

Minnesota Rate of Manipulation Test. This test involves five activities: 1) placing, 2) turning, 3) displacing, 4) one-hand turning and placing, and 5) two-hand turning and placing. The activities are timed for both limbs and compared with normal values. The test primarily measures gross coordination and dexterity.[33,54,55]

Purdue Pegboard Test. This test measures fine coordination with the use of small pins, washers, and collars. The assessment categories of the test are: 1) right hand, 2) left hand, 3) both hands, 4) right, left, and both, and 5) assembly. The subtests are timed and compared with normal values based on gender and occupation.[33,54,55]

Crawford Small Parts Dexterity Test. This test measures fine coordination, including the use of tools such as

Text continued on p. 465

TABLE **7-4**

Normal Values by Age Group (Years) and Gender for Combined Right and Left Hand Grip Strength (kg)

	AGES 15 TO 19		AGES 20 TO 29		AGES 30 TO 39		AGES 40 TO 49		AGES 50 TO 59		AGES 60 TO 69	
	Male	Female	Male	Female	Male	Female	Male	Female	Male	Female	Male	Female
Excellent	≥113	≥71	≥124	≥71	≥123	≥73	≥119	≥73	≥110	≥65	≥102	≥60
Above average	103–112	64–70	113–123	65–70	113–122	66–72	110–118	65–72	102–109	59–64	93–101	54–59
Average	95–102	59–63	106–112	61–64	105–112	61–65	102–109	59–64	96–101	55–58	86–92	51–53
Below average	84–94	54–58	97–105	55–60	97–104	56–60	94–101	55–58	87–95	51–54	79–85	48–50
Poor	≤83	≤53	≤96	≤54	≤96	≤55	≤93	≤54	≤86	≤50	≤78	≤47

Modified from Canadian Standardized Test of Fitness: Operations Manual, Ottawa, Fitness and Amateur Sport Canada, 1986, p. 36.

TABLE **7-5**

Average Strength of Chuck (Pulp-to-Pulp) Pinch with Separate Digits (100 Subjects)

	PULP-TO-PULP PINCH (kg)			
	MALE HAND		FEMALE HAND	
Digit	Major	Minor	Major	Minor
II	5.3	4.8	3.6	3.3
III	5.6	5.7	3.8	3.4
IV	3.8	3.6	2.5	2.4
V	2.3	2.2	1.7	1.6

From Hunter J, Schneider LH, Mackin EJ, et al, editors: Rehabilitation of the hand: surgery and therapy, St Louis, 1990, CV Mosby, p. 115.

TABLE **7-6**

Average Strength of Lateral Prehension Pinch by Occupation (100 Subjects)

	LATERAL PREHENSION PINCH (kg)			
	MALE HAND		FEMALE HAND	
Occupation	Major	Minor	Major	Minor
Skilled	6.6	6.4	4.4	4.3
Sedentary	6.3	6.1	4.1	3.9
Manual	8.5	7.7	6.0	5.5
Average	7.5	7.1	4.9	4.7

From Hunter J, Schneider LH, Mackin EJ, et al, editors: Rehabilitation of the hand: surgery and therapy, St Louis, 1990, CV Mosby, p. 114.

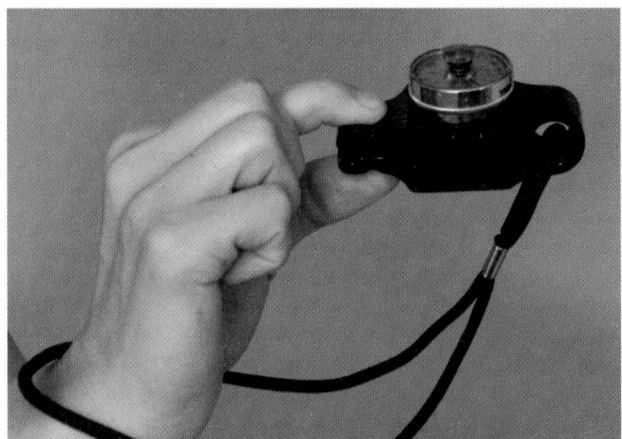

Figure 7-43 Commercial pinch meter to test pinch strength.

TABLE **7-7**

Average Strength of Chuck (Pulp-to-Pulp) Pinch by Occupation (100 Subjects)

	PULP-TO-PULP PINCH (kg)			
	MALE HAND		FEMALE HAND	
Occupation	Major	Minor	Major	Minor
Skilled	7.3	7.2	5.4	4.6
Sedentary	8.4	7.3	4.2	4.0
Manual	8.5	7.6	6.1	5.6
Average	7.9	7.5	5.2	4.9

From Hunter J, Schneider LH, Mackin EJ, et al, editors: Rehabilitation of the hand: surgery and therapy, St Louis, 1990, CV Mosby, p. 114.

Rheumatoid Arthritis Evaluation Record
Preoperative Silastic Implants

Name _____ Sex: [ ] Male [ ] Female Date _____ Birth date _____

Address _____

Occupation _____ Dominant hand: [ ] R [ ] L Hospital _____ Examiner _____

Diagnosis: [ ] Juvenile rheumatoid [ ] Adult rheumatoid [ ] Erosive arthritis [ ] Osteoarthritis [ ] Psoriatic arthritis
[ ] Ankylosing spondylitis [ ] Sjögren's syndrome [ ] Systemic lupus erythematosus [ ] Trauma

Onset date: _____ Sedimentation rate: [ ] Wintrobe [ ] Westergren [ ] Rourke

Rheumatoid test [ ] (+) [ ] (−)   Family Hx [ ] (+) [ ] (−)

Onset distribution: [ ] Peripheral [ ] Central [ ] Both: Remission [ ] Yes [ ] No: Anemia [ ] Yes [ ] No:

Check if the following has been completed: [ ] X-rays [ ] Photographs [ ] Movies [ ] Cineradiography

Range of motion (ROM): use neutral zero method of American Academy of Orthopedic Surgeons, 1965.
Codes 1–25 represent observed and measured abnormalities. Use as indicated in appropriate sections.
Severity indices mild, moderate, and severe are represented by a, b, and c and further categorize codes 1–25.
This evaluation record has been designed for computer analysis. Responses must be complete.

THUMB: Codes: 1, 2, 3, 9–14, 19, 22	Code		Joints		ROM	
	R	L	Abd (degrees) / Add (cm) / Opp (cm)		R	L
			MC	Abd		
				Add		
				Opp		
			MP			
			IP			

FINGER: Codes: 3–15, 19, 22–25

Index			MP		
			PIP		
			DIP		
Flex DIP crease to palmar crease (cm)					
Middle			MP		
			PIP		
			DIP		
Flex DIP crease to palmar crease (cm)					
Ring			MP		
			PIP		
			DIP		
Flex DIP crease to palmar crease (cm)					
Little			MP		
			PIP		
			DIP		
Flex DIP crease to palmar crease (cm)					
WRIST: Codes: 3, 7–14, 19, 20, 22, 23			Flex		
			Ext		
			U. Dev		
			R. Dev		

Prehensile patterns: Check if able to perform

		R	L
GRASP: Cylinders	2.5 cm		
	5 cm		
	7.5 cm		
	10 cm		
Spheres	5 cm		
	7.5 cm		
	10 cm		
	12.5 cm		

STRENGTH: [ ] Lb [ ] Kg [ ] mm Hg

		R	L
Pulp pinch	Index		
	Middle		
	Ring		
	Little		
Lateral or key pinch			
Grip			

ADL: I: Independent A: Assisted U: Unable

Dress	I	A	U	Hygiene	I	A	U
Upper ext				Teeth			
Trunk				Hair			
Lower ext				Shave			
Bathe				Pick up coin			
Shower				Turn key			
Eat				Doorknob			
Toilet				Car door			
Telephone				Screw-top jar			
Typewrite				Aerosol can			
Write				Fasteners			

Ambulatory status:
[ ] Independent [ ] Wheelchair with partial walking
[ ] Assisted walk [ ] Bedfast

Code for clinical abnormality:
1—Swan-neck, thumb
2—Thumb boutonnière
3—Subluxation–dislocation
4—Swan-neck, finger
5—Boutonnière, finger
6—Intrinsic tightness
7—Ulnar drift
8—Radial drift
9—Ankylosis
10—Instability
11—Tendon rupture
12—Constrictive tenosynovitis
13—Synovial hypertrophy
14—Crepitation with motion
15—Extensor tendon subluxation
16—Varus angle
17—Valgus angle
18—Rotational deformity
19—Erosions
20—Joint narrowing
21—Subchondral sclerosis
22—Painful joint with motion
23—Nerve compression—M, U, R
24—Vasculitis
25—Nodules

Severity index:
a—Mild
b—Moderate
c—Severe

Sketch implant into appropriate site

Palm R   Palm L

Figure 7-44 **Functional assessment form for the hand, designed for evaluation of rheumatoid and arthritic hands.** (Modified from Swanson AB: Flexible implant resection arthroplasty in the hand and extremities, St Louis, 1973, CV Mosby.)

HAND EVALUATION RECORD

Name _____ Age _____ Date _____ Major hand _____

Occupation _____ X-rays _____ Photographs _____

History:

Shoulder:	L	R	Wrist:			Circ:		
For	___	___		DF	___ ___	Biceps	___	___
Back	___	___		PF	___ ___	Forearm	___	___
Abd	___	___		RD	___ ___	Grip: L	___	___
Add	___	___		UD	___ ___	R	___	___
Rotation Int	___	___	Elbow:	Ext	___ ___	Forearm: Pro	___	___
Ext	___	___		Flex	___ ___	Sup	___	___

		MP	IP				% Impairment
Thumb	Ext			Abd			
	Flex			Add			
	Ankylosis			Opp			

		MP	PIP	DIP	Flex pulp to midpalmar crease	
Index	Ext					
	Flex					
	Ankylosis					
Middle	Ext					
	Flex					
	Ankylosis					
Ring	Ext					
	Flex					
	Ankylosis					
Little	Ext					
	Flex					
	Ankylosis					

Total % _____

Chart:
1. Amputations
2. Scars
3. Skin—subcutaneous loss
4. Nail bed injury
5. Major nerve loss: R, M, U
6. Digital bundle loss
7. Neuroma
8. Pain and tenderness
9. Bone damage
10. Joint damage
11. Flexor tendon loss
12. Extensor tendon loss
13. Ligament injury
14. Sensibility—pickup
         two-point
         Ninhydrin
15. Prehension:
    Grasp—small
        large
    Pinch—pulp
        tip
        lateral
    Hook—distal
        proximal
    Scoop
16. Maximum improvement
17. Rehabilitation needed
18. Further treatment
19. Classification

NOTE: Degrees of motion recorded as left/right

Dorsum R hand
or
Palmar L hand

Dorsum L hand
or
Palmar R hand

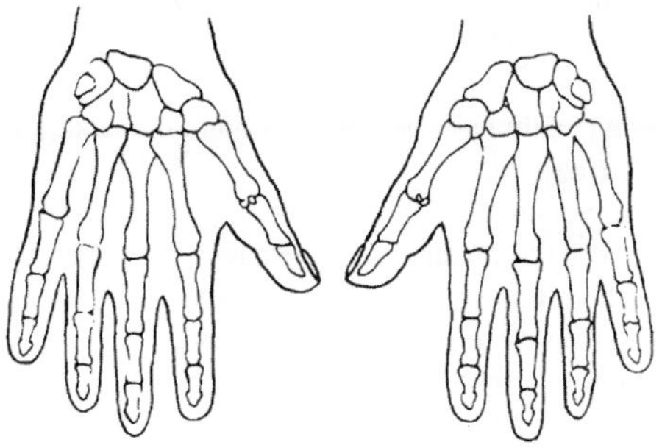

Figure 7-45 Hand Evaluation Record. This form is designed for posttraumatic conditions and other disorders of the hand. (Modified from Swanson AB: Flexible implant resection arthroplasty in the hand and extremities, St Louis, 1973, CV Mosby.)

Carpal Tunnel (Median Nerve) Function Disability Form

Symptom Severity Scale

The following questions refer to your symptoms for a typical twenty-four-hour period during the past two weeks (circle one answer to each question).

How severe is the hand or wrist pain that you have at night?
1   I do not have hand or wrist pain at night
2   Mild pain
3   Moderate pain
4   Severe pain
5   Very severe pain

How often did hand or wrist pain wake you up during a typical night in the past two weeks?
1   Never
2   Once
3   Two or three times
4   Four or five times
5   More than five times

Do you typically have pain in your hand or wrist during the daytime?
1   I never have pain during the day
2   I have mild pain during the day
3   I have moderate pain during the day
4   I have severe pain during the day
5   I have very severe pain during the day

How often do you have hand or wrist pain during the daytime?
1   Never
2   Once or twice a day
3   Three to five times a day
4   More than five times a day
5   The pain is constant

How long, on average, does an episode of pain last during the daytime?
1   I never get pain during the day
2   Less than 10 minutes
3   10 to 60 minutes
4   Greater than 60 minutes
5   The pain is constant throughout the day

Do you have numbness (loss of sensation) in your hand?
1   No
2   I have mild numbness
3   I have moderate numbness
4   I have severe numbness
5   I have very severe numbness

Do you have weakness in your hand or wrist?
1   No weakness
2   Mild weakness
3   Moderate weakness
4   Severe weakness
5   Very severe weakness

Do you have tingling sensations in your hand?
1   No tingling
2   Mild tingling
3   Moderate tingling
4   Severe tingling
5   Very severe tingling

Figure 7-46 Carpal tunnel (median nerve) function disability form. (Modified from Levine DW, Simmons BP, Koris MJ, et al: A self-administered questionnaire for the assessment of severity of symptoms and functional status in carpal tunnel syndrome. J Bone Joint Surg Am 75:1586–1587, 1993.)

Symptom Severity Scale *Continued*

How severe is numbness (loss of sensation) or tingling at night?
  1   I have no numbness or tingling at night
  2   Mild
  3   Moderate
  4   Severe
  5   Very severe

How often did hand numbness or tingling wake you up during a typical night during the past two weeks?
  1   Never
  2   Once
  3   Two or three times
  4   Four or five times
  5   More than five times

Do you have difficulty with the grasping and use of small objects such as keys or pens?
  1   No difficulty
  2   Mild difficulty
  3   Moderate difficulty
  4   Severe difficulty
  5   Very severe difficulty

Functional Status Scale

On a typical day during the past two weeks have hand and wrist symptoms caused you to have any difficulty doing the activities listed below? Please circle one number that best describes your ability to do the activity.

Activity	No Difficulty	Mild Difficulty	Moderate Difficulty	Severe Difficulty	Cannot Do at All Due to Hand or Wrist Symptoms
Writing	1	2	3	4	5
Buttoning of clothes	1	2	3	4	5
Holding a book while reading	1	2	3	4	5
Gripping of a telephone handle	1	2	3	4	5
Opening of jars	1	2	3	4	5
Household chores	1	2	3	4	5
Carrying of grocery bags	1	2	3	4	5
Bathing and dressing	1	2	3	4	5

Figure 7-46, cont'd

Michigan Hand Outcomes Questionnaire

Instructions: This survey asks for your views about your hands and your health. This information will help keep track of how you feel and how well you are able to do your usual activities. Answer *every* question by marking the answer as indicated. If you are unsure about how to answer a question, please give the best answer you can.

I. The following questions refer to the function of your hand(s)/wrist(s) *during the past week*. (Please circle one answer for each question.)

   A. The following questions refer to your *right* hand/wrist.

	Very Good	Good	Fair	Poor	Very Poor
1. Overall, how well did your *right* hand work?	1	2	3	4	5
2. How well did your *right* fingers move?	1	2	3	4	5
3. How well did your *right* wrist move?	1	2	3	4	5
4. How was the strength in your *right* hand?	1	2	3	4	5
5. How was the sensation (feeling) in your *right* hand?	1	2	3	4	5

   B. The following questions refer to your *left* hand/wrist.

	Very Good	Good	Fair	Poor	Very Poor
1. Overall, how well did your *left* hand work?	1	2	3	4	5
2. How well did your *left* fingers move?	1	2	3	4	5
3. How well did your *left* wrist move?	1	2	3	4	5
4. How was the strength in your *left* hand?	1	2	3	4	5
5. How was the sensation (feeling) in your *left* hand?	1	2	3	4	5

II. The following questions refer to the ability of your hand(s) to do certain tasks *during the past week*. (Please circle one answer for each question.)

   A. How difficult was it for you to perform the following activities using your *right* hand?

	Not at All Difficult	A Little Difficult	Somewhat Difficult	Moderately Difficult	Very Difficult
1. Turn a door knob	1	2	3	4	5
2. Pick up a coin	1	2	3	4	5
3. Hold a glass of water	1	2	3	4	5
4. Turn a key in a lock	1	2	3	4	5
5. Hold a frying pan	1	2	3	4	5

   B. How difficult was it for you to perform the following activities using your *left* hand?

	Not at All Difficult	A Little Difficult	Somewhat Difficult	Moderately Difficult	Very Difficult
1. Turn a door knob	1	2	3	4	5
2. Pick up a coin	1	2	3	4	5
3. Hold a glass of water	1	2	3	4	5
4. Turn a key in a lock	1	2	3	4	5
5. Hold a frying pan	1	2	3	4	5

   C. How difficult was it for you to perform the following activities using *both of your hands*?

	Not at All Difficult	A Little Difficult	Somewhat Difficult	Moderately Difficult	Very Difficult
1. Open a jar	1	2	3	4	5
2. Button a shirt/blouse	1	2	3	4	5
3. Eat with a knife/fork	1	2	3	4	5
4. Carry a grocery bag	1	2	3	4	5
5. Wash dishes	1	2	3	4	5
6. Wash your hair	1	2	3	4	5
7. Tie shoelaces/knots	1	2	3	4	5

Figure 7-47 Michigan Hand Outcomes Questionnaire. (From Chung KC, Pillsbury MS, Walter MR, et al: Reliability and validity testing of the Michigan hand outcomes questionnaire. J Hand Surg Am 23:584–587, 1998.)

III. The following questions refer to how you did in your *normal work* (including both housework and school work) during the *past 4 weeks*. (Please circle one answer for each question.)

	Always	Often	Sometimes	Rarely	Never
1. How often were you unable to do your work because of problems with your hand(s)/wrist(s)?	1	2	3	4	5
2. How often did you have to shorten your work day because of problems with your hand(s)/wrist(s)?	1	2	3	4	5
3. How often did you have to take it easy at your work because of problems with your hand(s)/wrist(s)?	1	2	3	4	5
4. How often did you accomplish less in your work because of problems with your hand(s)/wrist(s)?	1	2	3	4	5
5. How often did you take longer to do the tasks in your work because of problems with your hand(s)/wrist(s)?	1	2	3	4	5

IV. The following questions refer to how much *pain* you had in your hand(s)/wrist(s) *during the past week*. (Please circle one answer for each question.)

1. How often did you have pain in your hand(s)/wrist(s)?
   1. Always
   2. Often
   3. Sometimes
   4. Rarely
   5. Never

If you answered *never* to question IV-1 above, please skip the following questions and go to the next page.

2. Please describe the pain you have in your hand(s)/wrist(s)?
   1. Very mild
   2. Mild
   3. Moderate
   4. Severe
   5. Very severe

	Always	Often	Sometimes	Rarely	Never
3. How often did the pain in your hand(s)/wrist(s) interfere with your sleep?	1	2	3	4	5
4. How often did the pain in your hand(s)/wrist(s) interfere with your daily activities (such as eating or bathing)?	1	2	3	4	5
5. How often did the pain in your hand(s)/wrist(s) make you unhappy?	1	2	3	4	5

V. A. The following questions refer to the appearance (look) of your *right* hand *during the past week*. (Please circle one answer for each question.)

	Strongly Agree	Agree	Neither Agree Nor Disagree	Disagree	Strongly Disagree
1. I was satisfied with the appearance (look) of my *right* hand.	1	2	3	4	5
2. The appearance (look) of my *right* hand sometimes made me uncomfortable in public.	1	2	3	4	5
3. The appearance (look) of my *right* hand made me depressed.	1	2	3	4	5
4. The appearance (look) of my *right* hand interfered with my normal social activities.	1	2	3	4	5

Figure 7-47, cont'd *Continued*

B.   The following questions refer to the appearance (look) of your *left* hand *during the past week.*
     (Please circle one answer for each question.)

	Strongly Agree	Agree	Neither Agree Nor Disagree	Disagree	Strongly Disagree
1. I was satisfied with the appearance (look) of my *left* hand.	1	2	3	4	5
2. The appearance (look) of my *left* hand sometimes made me uncomfortable in public.	1	2	3	4	5
3. The appearance (look) of my *left* hand made me depressed.	1	2	3	4	5
4. The appearance (look) of my *left* hand interfered with my normal social activities.	1	2	3	4	5

VI. A.   The following questions refer to your satisfaction with your *right* hand/wrist *during the past week.*
          (Please circle one answer for each question.)

	Very Satisfied	Somewhat Satisfied	Neither Satisfied Nor Dissatisfied	Somewhat Dissatisfied	Very Dissatisfied
1. Overall function of your *right* hand	1	2	3	4	5
2. Motion of the fingers in your *right* hand	1	2	3	4	5
3. Motion of your *right* wrist	1	2	3	4	5
4. Strength of your *right* hand	1	2	3	4	5
5. Pain level of your *right* hand	1	2	3	4	5
6. Sensation (feeling) of your *right* hand	1	2	3	4	5

B.   The following questions refer to your satisfaction with your *left* hand/wrist *during the past week.*
     (Please circle one answer for each question.)

	Very Satisfied	Somewhat Satisfied	Neither Satisfied Nor Dissatisfied	Somewhat Dissatisfied	Very Dissatisfied
1. Overall function of your *left* hand	1	2	3	4	5
2. Motion of the fingers in your *left* hand	1	2	3	4	5
3. Motion of your *left* wrist	1	2	3	4	5
4. Strength of your *left* hand	1	2	3	4	5
5. Pain level of your *left* hand	1	2	3	4	5
6. Sensation (feeling) of your *left* hand	1	2	3	4	5

VII. Please provide the following information about yourself. (Please circle one answer for each question.)

1. Are you right-handed or left-handed?
    a.   Right-handed
    b.   Left-handed
    c.   Both

2. Which hand gives you the most problem?
    a.   Right hand
    b.   Left hand
    c.   Both

3. Have you changed your job since you had problems with your hand(s)?
    a.   Yes
    b.   No

    Please describe the type of job you did *before* you had problems with your hand(s) _____

    _____

    Please describe the type of job you are doing *now* _____

    _____

Figure 7-47, cont'd

Part one – treatment

Please put a circle around the number that is closest to the way you feel about how things have been for you. There are no right or wrong answers.

1. Throughout my treatment I have seen the same doctor:

    1   2   3   4   5   6   7
    Every time   Not at all

2. When the doctor saw me, he or she knew about my case:

    1   2   3   4   5   6   7
    Very well   Not at all

3. When I was with the doctor, he or she gave me the chance to talk:

    1   2   3   4   5   6   7
    As much as I wanted   Not at all

4. When I did talk to the doctor, he or she listened and understood me:

    1   2   3   4   5   6   7
    Very much   Not at all

5. I was given information about my treatment and progress:

    1   2   3   4   5   6   7
    All that I wanted   Not at all

Part two – how is your hand now

Hand health profile

1. The feeling in my hand is now:

    1   2   3   4   5   6   7
    Normal   Absent

2. When my hand is cold and/or damp, the pain is now:

    1   2   3   4   5   6   7
    Non-existent   Unbearable

3. Most of the time, the pain in my hand is now:

    1   2   3   4   5   6   7
    Non-existent   Unbearable

4. The duration my pain is present is:

    1   2   3   4   5   6   7
    Never   All the time

(Part two *cont'd*)

5. When I try to use my hand for fiddly things, it is now:

    1   2   3   4   5   6   7
    Skillful   Clumsy

6. Generally, when I move my hand it is:

    1   2   3   4   5   6   7
    Flexible   Stiff

7. The grip in my hand is now:

    1   2   3   4   5   6   7
    Strong   Weak

8. For everyday activities, my hand is now:

    1   2   3   4   5   6   7
    No problem   Useless

9. For my work, my hand is now:

    1   2   3   4   5   6   7
    No problem   Useless

10. When I look at the appearance of my hand now, I feel:

    1   2   3   4   5   6   7
    Unconcerned   Embarrassed & self-conscious

11. Generally, when I think about my hand I feel:

    1   2   3   4   5   6   7
    Unconcerned   Very upset

Part three – overall assessment

1. Generally, my treatment at the hospital has been:

    1   2   3   4   5   6   7
    Very satisfactory   Very unsatisfactory

2. Generally, my hand is now:

    1   2   3   4   5   6   7
    Very satisfactory   Very unsatisfactory

3. Bearing in mind my original injury or condition, I feel my hand is now:

    1   2   3   4   5   6   7
    Better than I expected   Worse than I expected

Figure 7-48 The Patient Evaluation Measure (PEM) Questionnaire. (From Dias JJ, Bhowal B, Wildin CJ, et al: Assessing the outcome of disorders of the hands—is the patient evaluation measure reliable, responsive, and without bias? J Bone Joint Surg Br 83:236, 2001.)

TABLE **7-8**

Functional Testing of the Wrist and Hand

Starting Position	Action	Functional Test
1. Forearm supinated, resting on table	Wrist flexion	Lift 0 lbs: Nonfunctional Lift 1 to 2 lbs: Functionally poor Life 3 to 4 lbs: Functionally fair Lift 5+ lbs: Functional
2. Forearm pronated, resting on table	Wrist extension lifting 1 to 2 lbs	0 Repetitions: Nonfunctional 1 to 2 Repetitions: Functionally poor 3 to 4 Repetitions: Functionally fair 5+ Repetitions: Functional
3. Forearm between supination and pronation, resting on table	Radial deviation lifting 1 to 2 lbs	0 Repetitions: Nonfunctional 1 to 2 Repetitions: Functionally poor 3 to 4 Repetitions: Functionally fair 5+ Repetitions: Functional
4. Forearm between supination and pronation, resting on table	Thumb flexion with resistance from rubber band* around thumb	0 Repetitions: Nonfunctional 1 to 2 Repetitions: Functionally poor 3 to 4 Repetitions: Functionally fair 5+ Repetitions: Functional
5. Forearm resting on table, rubber band around thumb and index finger	Thumb extension against resistance of rubber band*	0 Repetitions: Nonfunctional 1 to 2 Repetitions: Functionally poor 3 to 4 Repetitions: Functionally fair 5+ Repetitions: Functional
6. Forearm resting on table, rubber band around thumb and index finger	Thumb abduction against resistance of rubber band*	0 Repetitions: Nonfunctional 1 to 2 Repetitions: Functionally poor 3 to 4 Repetitions: Functionally fair 5+ Repetitions: Functional
7. Forearm resting on table	Thumb adduction, lateral pinch of piece of paper	Hold 0 s: Nonfunctional Hold 1 to 2 s: Functionally poor Hold 3 to 4 s: Functionally fair Hold 5+ s: Functional
8. Forearm resting on table	Thumb opposition, pulp-to-pulp pinch of piece of paper	Hold 0 s: Nonfunctional Hold 1 to 2 s: Functionally poor Hold 3 to 4 s: Functionally fair Hold 5+ s: Functional
9. Forearm resting on table	Finger flexion, patient grasps mug or glass using cylindrical grasp and lifts off table	0 Repetitions: Nonfunctional 1 to 2 Repetitions: Functionally poor 3 to 4 Repetitions: Functionally fair 5+ Repetitions: Functional
10. Forearm resting on table	Patient attempts to put on rubber glove keeping fingers straight	21+ s: Nonfunctional 10 to 20 s: Functionally poor 4 to 8 s: Functionally poor 2 to 4 s: Functional
11. Forearm resting on table	Patient attempts to pull fingers apart (finger abduction) against resistance of rubber band* and holds	Hold 0 s: Nonfunctional Hold 1 to 2 s: Functionally poor Hold 3 to 4 s: Functionally fair Hold 5+ s: Functional
12. Forearm resting on table	Patient holds piece of paper between fingers while examiner pulls on paper	Hold 0 s: Nonfunctional Hold 1 to 2 s: Functionally poor Hold 3 to 4 s: Functionally fair Hold 5+ s: Functional

Data from Palmer ML, Epler M: Clinical assessment procedures in physical therapy, Philadelphia, 1990, JB Lippincott, pp. 140–144.
lbs, Pounds; *s*, seconds.
*Rubber band should be at least 1 cm wide.

tweezers and screwdrivers to assemble things, to adjust equipment, and to do engraving.[33,54]

Simulated Activities of Daily Living Examination. This test consists of nineteen subtests, including standing, walking, putting on a shirt, buttoning, zipping, putting on gloves, dialing a telephone, tying a bow, manipulating safety pins, manipulating coins, threading a needle, unwrapping a Band-Aid, squeezing toothpaste, and using a knife and fork. Each subtask is timed.[46]

Moberg's Pickup Test. An assortment of nine or ten objects (e.g., bolts, nuts, screws, buttons, coins, pens, paper clips, keys) is used. The patient is timed for the following tests:

1. Putting objects in a box with the affected hand
2. Putting objects in a box with the unaffected hand
3. Putting objects in a box with the affected hand with eyes closed

The examiner notes which digits are used for prehension. Digits with altered sensation are less likely to be used. The test is used for median or combined median and ulnar nerve lesions.[58]

Box and Block Test. This is a test for gross manual dexterity in which 150 blocks, each measuring 2.5 cm (1 inch) on a side, are used. The patient has 1 minute in which to individually transfer the blocks from one side of a divided box to the other. The number of blocks transferred is given as the score. Patients are given a 15-second practice trial before the test.[56]

Nine-Hole Peg Test. This test is used to assess finger dexterity. The patient places nine 3.2-cm (1.3-inch) pegs in a 12.7 × 12.7 cm (5 × 5 inch) board and then removes them. The score is the time taken to do this task. Each hand is tested separately.[56]

Special Tests

For the forearm, wrist, and hand, no special tests exist that are commonly done with each assessment. Depending on the history, observation, and examination to this point, certain special tests may be performed. The examiner picks the appropriate test or tests to help confirm the diagnosis. As with all special tests, however, the examiner must keep in mind that they are confirming tests. When they are positive, they are highly suggestive that the problem exists, but if they are negative, they do not rule out the problem. This is especially true for the tests of neurological dysfunction.

For the reader who would like to review them, the reliability, validity, specificity, sensitivity, and odds ratios of some of the special tests used in the forearm, wrist and hand are available on the Evolve website.

Tests for Ligament, Capsule, and Joint Instability

❓ *Axial Load Test.* The patient sits while the examiner stabilizes the patient's wrist with one hand. With the other hand, the examiner carefully grasps the patient's

---

Key Tests Performed at the Forearm, Wrist, and Hand Depending on Suspected Pathology*[59,60]

- *For ligament, capsule and joint instability:*
  - ❓ Axial load test
  - ❓ Catch-up clunk test
  - ❓ Dorsal capitate displacement apprehension test
  - ⚠ Ligamentous instability test (fingers)
  - ⚠ Lunotriquetral ballottement (Reagan's) test
  - ⚠ Murphy's sign
  - ❓ Sitting hands test
  - ❓ Supination lift test
  - ⚠ Thumb ulnar collateral ligament laxity or instability test
  - ❓ Triangular fibrocartilage complex load test (Sharpey's test)
  - ⚠ Ulnar fovea sign test
  - ⚠ Ulnar styloid triquetral impaction (USTI) provocation test
  - ✓ Ulnomeniscotriquetral dorsal glide test
  - ✓ Watson (scaphoid shift) test
- *For tendons and muscles:*
  - ✓ Finkelstein test
  - ⚠ Sweater finger sign
- *For neurological dysfunction:*
  - ✓ Carpal compression test
  - ⚠ Froment's "paper" sign
  - ✓ Phalen's (wrist flexion) test
  - ⚠ Reverse Phalen's (prayer) test
  - ⚠ Tinel sign at wrist
  - ✓ Weber's (Moberg's) two-point discrimination test
- *For circulation and swelling:*
  - ✓ Allen test
  - ✓ Digital blood flow
  - ✓ Figure of eight measurement for swelling

*The author recommends these key tests be learned by the clinician to facilitate a diagnosis. See Chapter 1, p. 55, Key for Classifying Special Tests.

---

thumb and applies axial compression. Pain and/or crepitation indicate a positive test for a fracture of metacarpal or adjacent carpal bones or joint arthrosis. A similar test may be performed for the fingers.

❓ *Catch-Up Clunk Test.*[61] The patient has the forearm in pronation while radially and ulnarly deviating the wrist. Normally, during this movement, the proximal row of carpals rotates from flexion to extension while the distal row translates from anterior (palmar) to posterior when going from radial deviation to ulnar deviation. If there is midcarpal or radiocarpal instability during the movement from radial deviation to ulnar deviation, the proximal row remains flexed and the distal row remains anteriorly and takes longer to translate. As the soft tissue restraints become tighter, there is a sudden "catch-up" of the proximal row into extension and the distal row posteriorly often accompanied by a "clunk" indicating a positive test.

❓ *Dorsal Capitate Displacement Apprehension Test.* This test is used to determine the stability of the capitate bone.[62] The patient sits facing the examiner. The

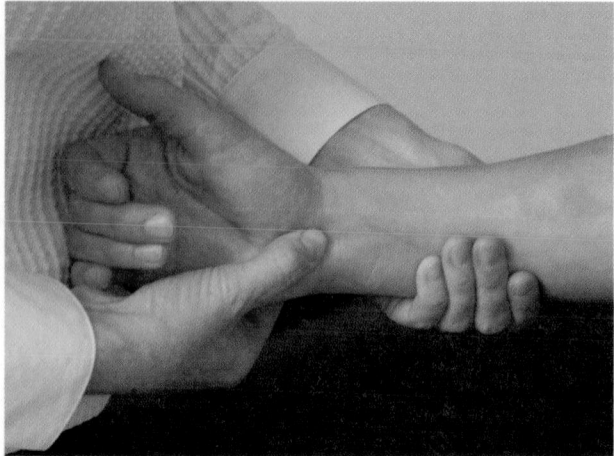

Figure 7-49 Dorsal capitate displacement apprehension test. Note the position of the examiner's thumb over the capitate to push it posteriorly.

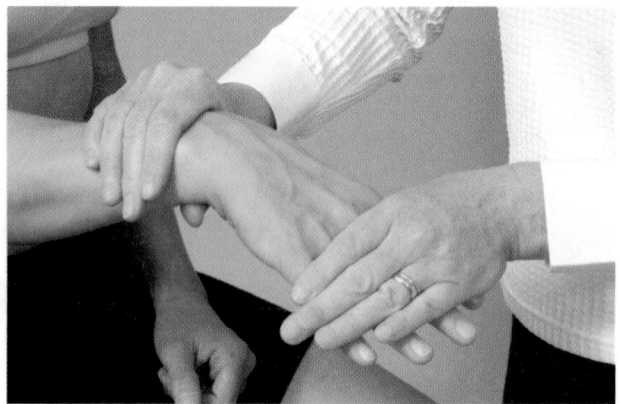

Figure 7-50 Finger extension or "shuck" test.

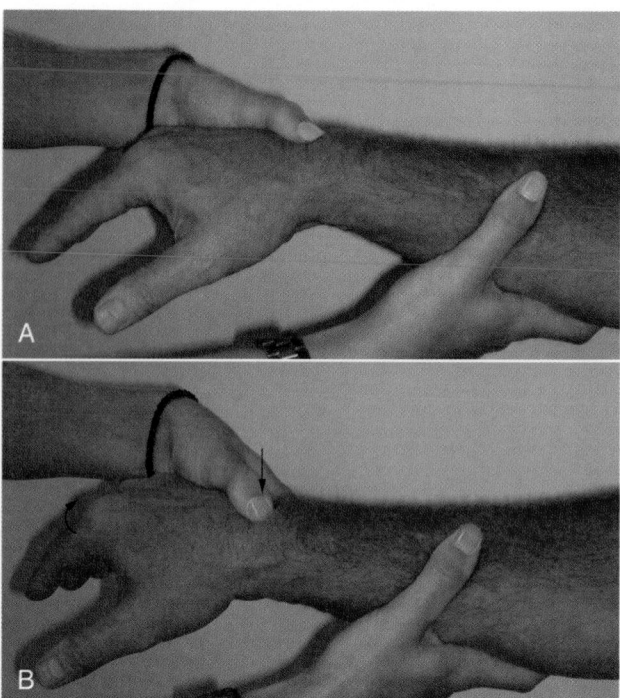

Figure 7-51 Lichtman (midcarpal shift) test. A, Start position. The forearm is pronated, wrist is in neutral. **B,** The examiner applies an anterior directed force to the capitate with axial compression while passively moving the wrist from radial deviation to ulnar deviation.

examiner holds the forearm (radius and ulna) with one hand. The thumb of the examiner's other hand is placed over the palmar aspect of the capitate while the fingers of that hand hold the patient's hand in neutral (no flexion or extension, no radial or ulnar deviation) and apply a counter pressure when the examiner pushes the capitate posteriorly with the thumb (Figure 7-49). Reproduction of the patient's symptoms, apprehension, or pain indicates a positive test. A click or snap may also be heard when pressure is applied.

Finger Extension or "Shuck" Test.[63] The patient is placed in sitting. The examiner holds the patient's wrist flexed and asks the patient to actively extend the fingers against resistance-loading the radiocarpal joints. Pain would indicate a positive test for radiocarpal or midcarpal instability, scaphoid instability, inflammation, or Kienböck disease (Figure 7-50).

Lichtman (Midcarpal Shift) Test.[30,35,61,64] The test is used to detect midcarpal instability. The patient's forearm is pronated with the hand held in support by the examiner. The examiner moves the patient's hand from radial to ulnar deviation while axially compressing the carpus into the radius while applying an anterior directed force to the capitate (Figure 7-51). If the distal carpal row jumps or snaps dorsally (from its subluxed position palmarly) and reproduces the patient's symptoms, the test is considered positive.

Ligamentous Instability Test for the Fingers. The examiner stabilizes the finger with one hand proximal to the joint to be tested. With the other hand, the examiner grasps the finger distal to the joint to be tested. The examiner's distal hand is then used to apply a varus or valgus stress to the joint (proximal or distal interphalangeal) to test the integrity of the collateral ligaments. The results are compared for laxity with those of the uninvolved hand, which is tested first.

Linscheid Test.[65,66] This test is used to detect ligamentous instability of the second and third carpometacarpal joints. The examiner supports the metacarpal shafts with one hand. With the other hand, the examiner pushes the metacarpal heads dorsally, then palmarly (Figure 7-52). Pain localized to the carpometacarpal joints is a positive test.

Lunotriquetral Ballottement (Reagan's) Test. This test is used to determine the integrity of the lunotriquetral ligament.[67] The examiner grasps the triquetrum between the thumb and second finger of one hand and the lunate with the thumb and second finger of the other hand (Figure 7-53). The examiner then moves the lunate up

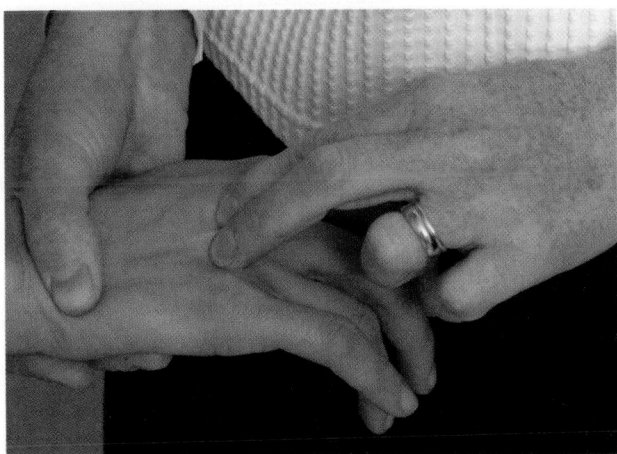

Figure 7-52 Linscheid test.

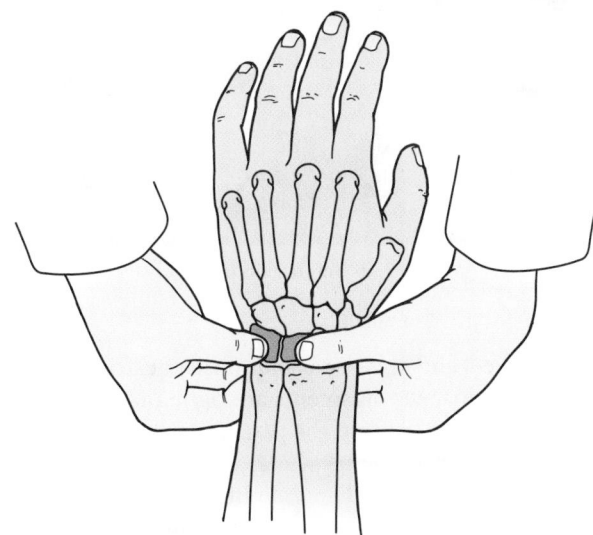

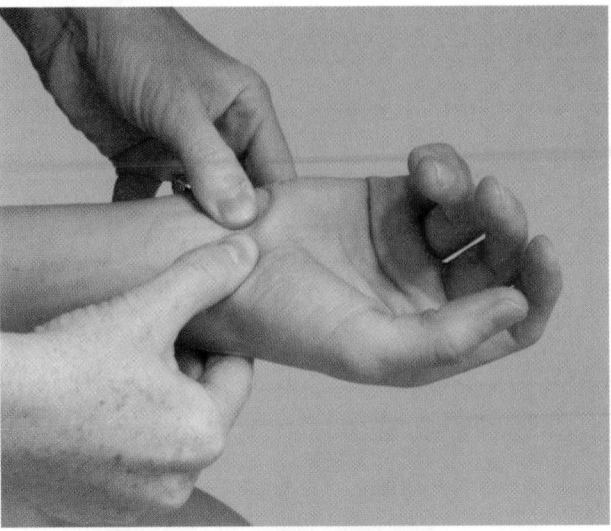

Figure 7-54 Lunotriquetral shear test.

Figure 7-53 Lunatotriquetral ballottement test for lunatotriquetral interosseous membrane dissociations.

and down (anteriorly and posteriorly), noting any laxity, crepitus, or pain, which indicates a positive test for lunotriquetral instability.[68,69]

❓ Lunotriquetral Shear Test.[67,70] This test also tests the integrity of the lunotriquetral ligament. The patient is seated with the elbow flexed in neutral rotation and resting on the examining table. With one hand, the examiner grasps the patient's wrist so that the thumb rests in the patient's palm and the fingers are placed over the dorsum of the proximal row of carpals to support the lunate. The thumb of the examiner's opposite hand loads the pisotriquetral joint on the palmar aspect, applying a shearing force to the lunotriquetral joint (Figure 7-54). Pain, crepitus, or abnormal movement are considered positive tests.

⚠ Murphy's Sign. The patient is asked to make a fist. If the head of the third metacarpal is level with the second and fourth metacarpals, the sign is positive and indicative

of a lunate dislocation.[71] Normally, the third metacarpal would project beyond (or further distally) the second and fourth metacarpals.

❓ "Piano Keys" Test. The patient sits with both arms in pronation. The examiner stabilizes the patient's arm with one hand so that the examiner's index finger can push down on the distal ulna. The examiner's other hand supports the patient's hand. The examiner pushes down on the distal ulna as one would push down on a piano key. The results are compared with the nonsymptomatic side. A positive test is indicated by a difference in mobility and the production of pain and/or tenderness. A positive test indicates instability of the distal radioulnar joint.[17]

❓ Pivot Shift Test of the Midcarpal Joint. The patient is seated with the elbow flexed to 90° and resting on a firm surface and the hand fully supinated. The examiner stabilizes the forearm with one hand and with the other hand takes the patient's hand into full radial deviation with the wrist in neutral. While the examiner maintains the patient's hand position, the patient's hand is taken into full ulnar deviation. A positive test results if the capitate "shifts" away from the lunate, indicating injury to the anterior capsule and interosseous ligaments.[3]

❓ Scaphoid Stress Test. This test is a modification of the Watson test, done actively by the patient. The patient sits and the examiner holds the patient's wrist with one hand so that the thumb applies pressure over the distal pole of the scaphoid. The patient then attempts to radially deviate the wrist. Normally, the patient is unable to deviate the wrist. If excessive laxity is present, the scaphoid is forced (shifted) posteriorly out of the scaphoid fossa of the radius with a resulting "clunk" and pain, indicating a positive test for scapholunate instability or a scaphoid fracture.[72,73] The test done passively by the examiner is called the **scaphoid shift test.**

❓ Sitting Hands (Press) Test.[65,74] The patient places both hands on the arms of a stable chair and pushes off,

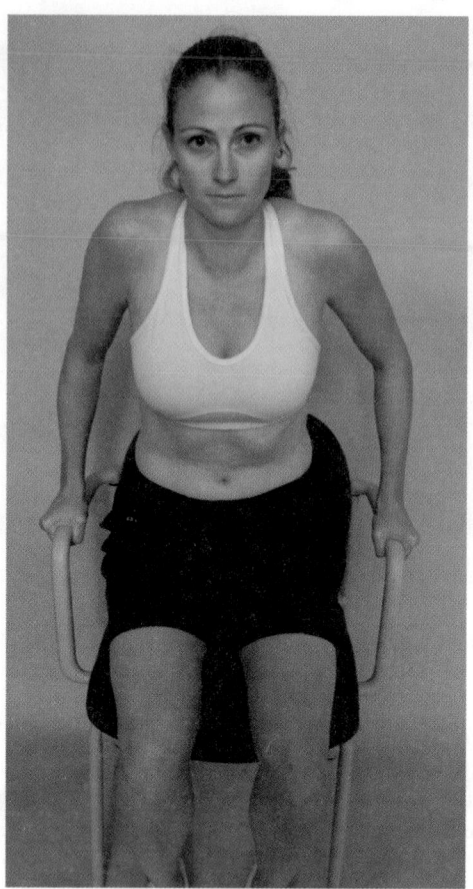

Figure 7-55 Sitting hands test.

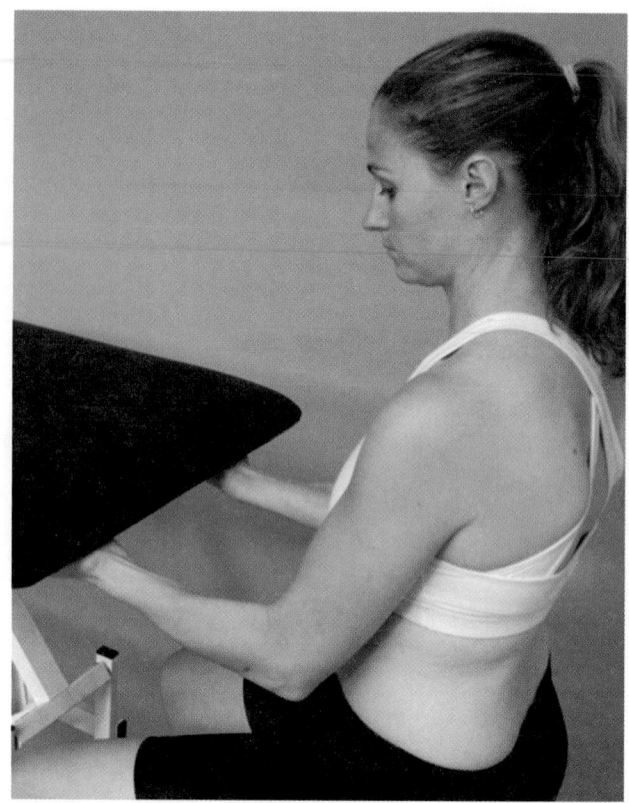

Figure 7-56 Supination lift test.

suspending the body while using only the hands for support (Figure 7-55). This test places a great deal of stress (axial ulnar load) at the wrist (and elbow; see elbow instability tests in Chapter 6) and is too difficult to do in the presence of significant wrist synovitis or wrist pathology.

❓ *Supination Lift Test.*[75] This test is used to determine pathology in the TFCC (also called the *triangular cartilaginous disc*). The patient is seated with elbows flexed to 90° and forearms supinated. The patient is asked to place the palms flat on the underside of a heavy table (or flat against the examiner's hands). The patient is then asked to lift the table (or push up against the resisting examiner's hands). Localized pain on the ulnar side of the wrist and difficulty applying the force are positive indications for a dorsal TFCC tear. Pain on forced ulnar deviation causing ulnar impaction is a symptom of TFCC tears (Figure 7-56).

❓ *Test for Tight Retinacular (Collateral) Ligaments (Haines-Zancolli Test).*[76] This test tests the structures around the proximal interphalangeal joint. The proximal interphalangeal joint is held in a neutral position while the distal interphalangeal joint is flexed by the examiner (Figure 7-57). If the distal interphalangeal joint does not flex, the retinacular (collateral) ligaments or proximal interphalangeal capsule are tight. If the proximal interphalangeal

joint is flexed and the distal interphalangeal joint flexes easily, the retinacular ligaments are tight and the capsule is normal. During the test, the patient remains passive and does no active movements.

❓ *Thumb Grind Test.* The examiner holds the patient's hand with one hand and grasps the patient's thumb below the metacarpophalangeal joint with the other hand. The examiner then applies axial compression and rotation to the metacarpophalangeal joint. If pain is elicited, the test is positive and indicative of degenerative joint disease in the metacarpophalangeal or metacarpotrapezial joint.[50,77] Axial compression with rotation to any of the wrist and hand joints may also indicate positive tests to those joints for the same condition.

⚠️ *Thumb Ulnar Collateral Ligament Laxity or Instability Test.* The patient sits while the examiner stabilizes the patient's hand with one hand and takes the patient's thumb into extension with the other hand. While holding the thumb in extension, the examiner applies a valgus stress to the metacarpophalangeal joint of the thumb, stressing the ulnar collateral ligament and accessory collateral ligament. If the valgus movement is greater than 30° to 35°, it indicates a complete tear of the ulnar collateral and accessory collateral ligaments.[78] If the ligament is only partially torn, the laxity would be less than 30° to 35°. In this case, laxity would still be greater than the unaffected side (normal laxity in extension is about 15°) but not as much as with a complete tear. To test the collateral ligament in isolation, the carpometacarpal joint is flexed to 30° and a valgus stress is applied.[79] This is a test for gamekeeper's or skier's thumb[80] (Figure 7-58).

❓ *Triangular Fibrocartilage Complex Load Test (Sharpey's Test).*[65] The examiner holds the patient's forearm with one hand and the patient's hand with the other hand. The examiner then axially loads and ulnarly deviates the wrist while moving it dorsally and palmarly or by rotating the forearm. A positive test is indicated by pain, clicking, or crepitus in the area of the TFCC.

⚠ *Ulnar Fovea Sign Test.* The patient stands or sits. The examiner presses a thumb or finger into the interval or depression (fovea) between the ulnar styloid process and the flexor carpi ulnaris tendon between the anterior surface of the ulnar head and the pisiform (Figure 7-59). The test is considered positive if the patient's pain is replicated or the area is very tender compared to the unaffected side.[81] The pain is believed to be due to distal radioulnar ligaments and ulnotriquetral ligament. Ulnotriquetral ligament tears are commonly associated with a stable distal radioulnar joint and fovea disruptions are associated with an unstable distal radioulnar joint.[81,82]

❓ *Ulnar Impaction Test.*[35] The patient is seated with the elbow flexed to 90° and the wrist in ulnar deviation. The examiner holds the patient's forearm with one hand and then applies an axial compression force through the fourth and fifth metacarpals (Figure 7-60). A positive test is indicated by pain and may be related to a TFCC injury or ulnar impaction syndrome.

⚠ *Ulnar Styloid Triquetral Impaction (USTI) Provocation Test.*[61] The patient is seated. The examiner holds the patient's elbow in one hand while the patient's wrist is extended and the forearm pronated. While maintaining the extension, the forearm is supinated (Figure 7-61). Pain at the ulnar styloid indicates a positive test for pathological impaction.

☑ *Ulnomeniscotriquetral Dorsal Glide Test.* The patient sits or stands with the arm pronated. The examiner places a thumb over the ulna dorsally and places the proximal interphalangeal joint of the index finger of the same hand over the pisotriquetral complex anteriorly. While stabilizing the ulna, the examiner applies a posteriorly directed force through the pisotriquetral complex stressing the TFCC (Figure 7-62). Excessive laxity or pain when the

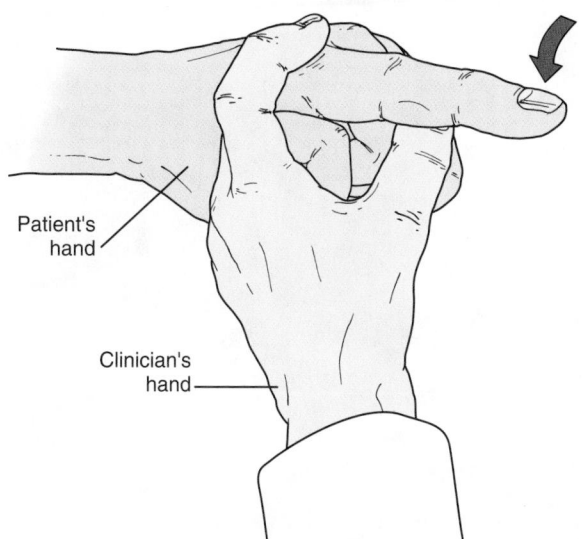

Patient's hand

Clinician's hand

Figure 7-57 Test for retinacular ligaments.

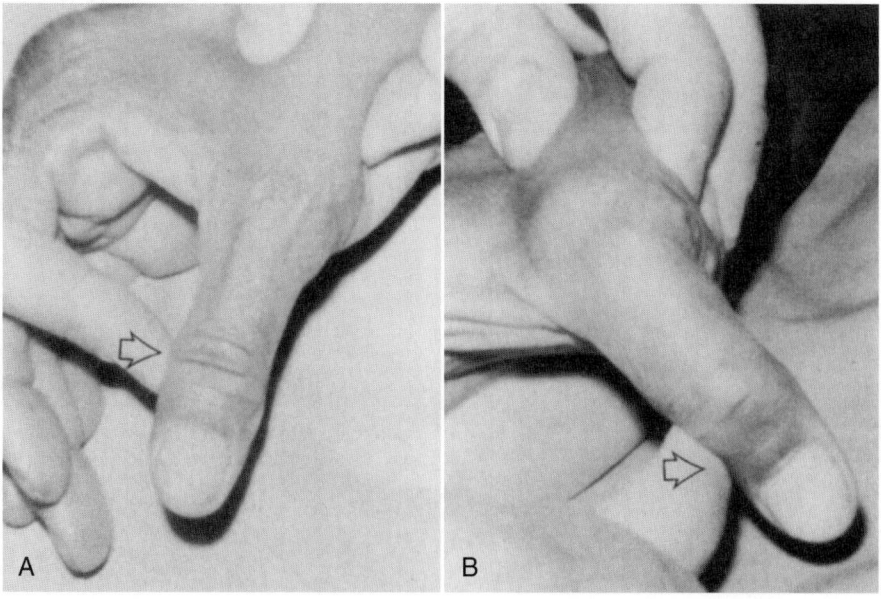

A   B

Figure 7-58 A and **B,** Testing stability of the ulnar collateral ligament in the thumb of a normal individual. In extension, the thumb was stable, but in flexion, it appeared to be unstable. This was caused by the laxity of the dorsal capsule at the metacarpophalangeal joint. (From Nicholas JA, Hershman EB, editors: Upper extremity in sports medicine, St Louis, 1989, CV Mosby, p. 580.)

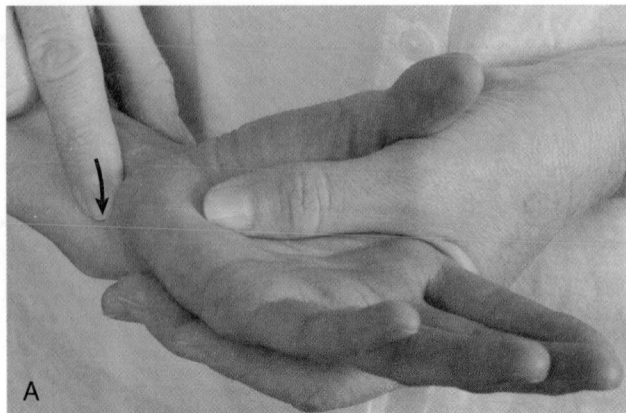

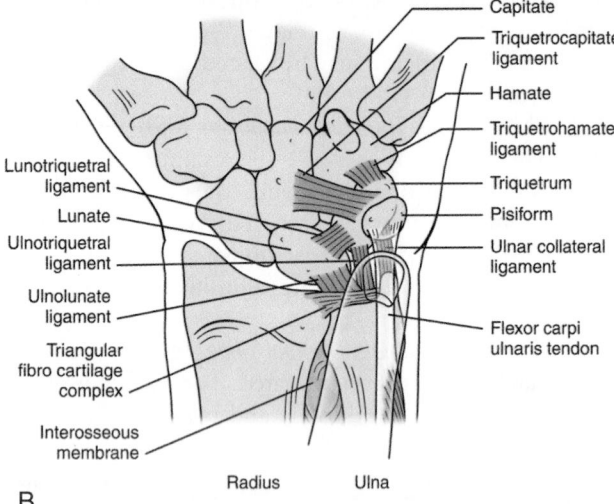

Capite
Triquetrocapitate ligament
Hamate
Triquetrohamate ligament
Triquetrum
Pisiform
Ulnar collateral ligament
Flexor carpi ulnaris tendon

Lunotriquetral ligament
Lunate
Ulnotriquetral ligament
Ulnolunate ligament
Triangular fibro cartilage complex
Interosseous membrane

Radius   Ulna

Figure 7-59 Ulnar fovea sign test. A, Area of palpation. **B,** Anatomical area of palpation (*line art*).

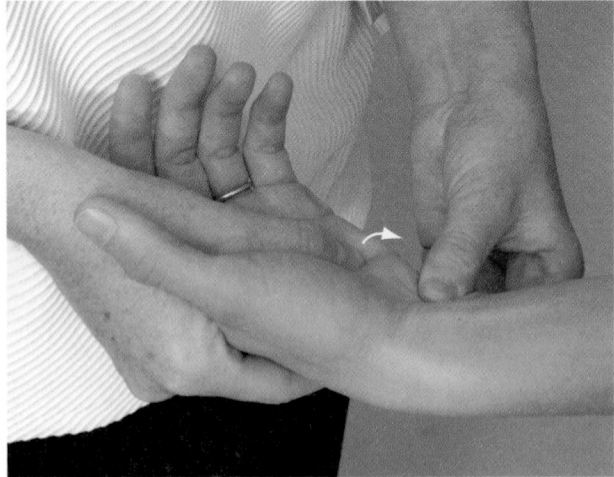

Figure 7-60 Ulnar impaction test.

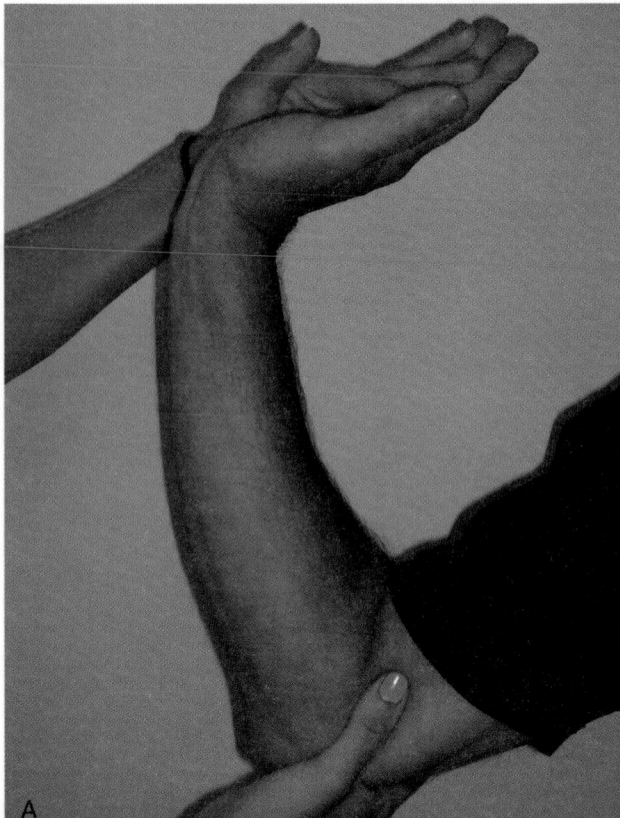

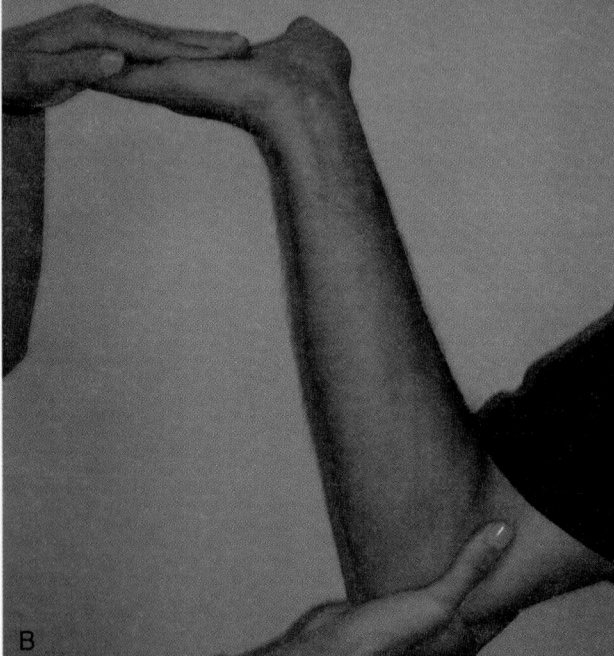

Figure 7-61 Ulnar styloid triquetral impaction (USTI) provocation test. A, Start position: wrist extension and forearm pronation. **B,** End position: wrist extension and forearm supination.

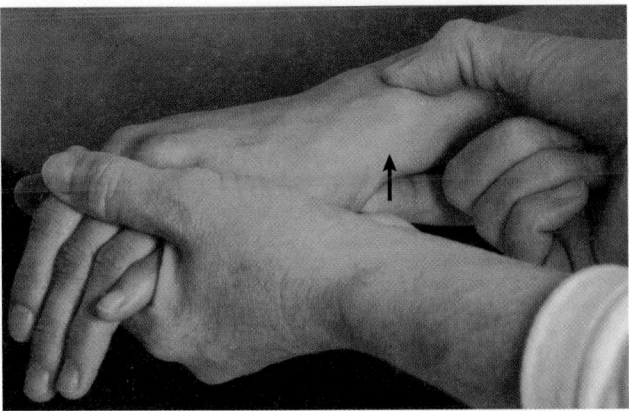

Figure 7-62 Ulnomeniscotriquetral dorsal glide test.

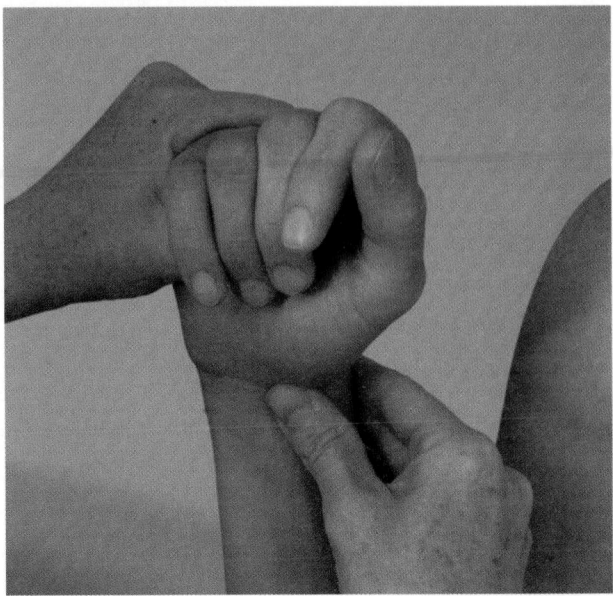

Figure 7-63 Watson (scaphoid shift) test.

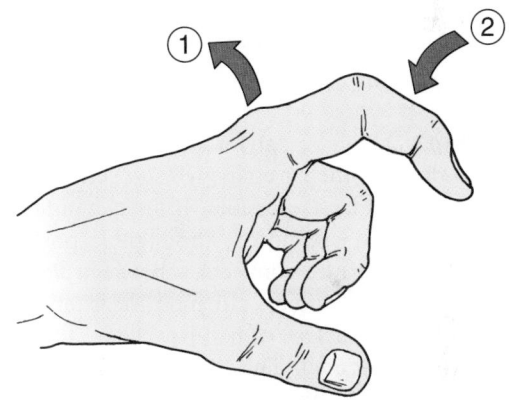

Figure 7-64 Positioning for the Bunnel-Littler test.

posteriorly directed force is applied indicates a positive test for TFCC pathology.[83]

✓ *Watson (Scaphoid Shift) Test.*[84] The patient sits with the elbow resting on the table and forearm pronated. The examiner faces the patient. With one hand, the examiner takes the patient's wrist into full ulnar deviation and slight extension while holding the metacarpals. The examiner presses the thumb of the other hand against the distal pole of the scaphoid on the palmar side to prevent it from moving toward the palm while the fingers provide a counter pressure on the dorsum of the forearm. With the first hand, the examiner radially deviates and slightly flexes the patient's hand while maintaining pressure on the scaphoid. This creates a subluxation stress if the scaphoid is unstable. If the scaphoid (and lunate) are unstable, the dorsal pole of the scaphoid subluxes or "shifts" over the dorsal rim of the radius and the patient complains of pain, indicating a positive test (Figure 7-63).[18,69,72,85] If the scaphoid subluxes with the thumb pressure when the thumb is removed, the scaphoid commonly returns to its normal position with a "thunk." If the ligamentous tissue is intact, the scaphoid normally moves forward, pushing the thumb forward with it. The test may also be used if a scaphoid fracture is suspected. In this case, pain occurs without the "thunk."

Tests for Tendons and Muscles

❓ *Boyes Test.*[86,87] This test also tests the central slip of the extensor hood. The examiner holds the finger to be examined in slight extension at the proximal interphalangeal joint. The patient is then asked to flex the distal interphalangeal joint. If the patient is unable or has difficulty flexing the distal interphalangeal joint, it is considered a positive test.

❓ *Bunnel-Littler (Finochietto-Bunnel) Test.* This test tests the structures around the metacarpophalangeal joint. The metacarpophalangeal joint is held slightly extended while the examiner moves the proximal interphalangeal joint into flexion, if possible (Figure 7-64).[88] If the test is positive (which is indicated by inability to flex the proximal interphalangeal joint), there is a tight intrinsic muscle or contracture of the joint capsule. If the metacarpophalangeal joints are slightly flexed, the proximal interphalangeal joint flexes fully if the intrinsic muscles are tight, but it does not flex fully if the capsule is tight. The patient remains passive during the test. This test is also called the *intrinsic-plus test.*[3]

✓ *Finkelstein Test.* The Finkelstein test[89] is used to determine the presence of de Quervain or Hoffmann disease, a paratenonitis in the thumb.[26] The patient makes a fist with the thumb inside the fingers (Figure 7-65). The examiner stabilizes the forearm and deviates the wrist toward the ulnar side. A positive test is indicated by pain over the abductor pollicis longus and extensor pollicis brevis tendons at the wrist and is indicative of a paratenonitis of these two tendons. Because the test can cause some discomfort in normal individuals, the examiner should compare the pain caused on the

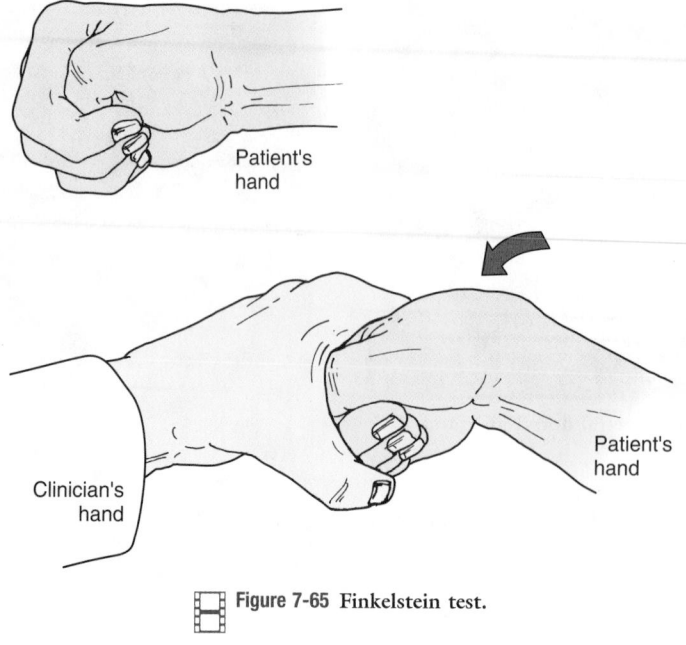

Figure 7-65 Finkelstein test.

affected side with that of the normal side. Only if the patient's symptoms are produced is the test considered positive.

Linburg's Sign. The patient flexes the thumb maximally onto the hypothenar eminence and actively extends the index finger as far as possible. If limited index finger extension and pain are noted, the sign is positive for paratenonitis at the interconnection between flexor pollicis longus and flexor indices (an anomalous tendon condition seen in 10% to 15% of hands).[68,90]

Sweater Finger Sign. The patient is asked to make a fist. If the distal phalanx of one of the fingers does not flex, the sign is positive for a ruptured flexor digitorum profundus tendon (Figure 7-66). It occurs most often to the ring finger.

Test for Extensor Hood Rupture.[86] The finger to be examined is flexed to 90° at the proximal interphalangeal joint over the edge of a table. The finger is held in position by the examiner. The patient is asked to carefully extend the proximal interphalangeal joint while the examiner palpates the middle phalanx. A positive test for a torn central extensor hood is the examiner's feeling little pressure from the middle phalanx while the distal interphalangeal joint is extending.

Tests for Neurological Dysfunction

Tests for neurological dysfunction are highly suggestive of a particular nerve lesion if they are positive, but they do not rule out the problem if they are negative. In fact, they may be negative 50% of the time, or more, when the condition actually exists with the symptoms varying during the day and daily.[20] Electrodiagnostic tests are more conclusive.[91,92] Keith et al.[20] noted that clinical tests

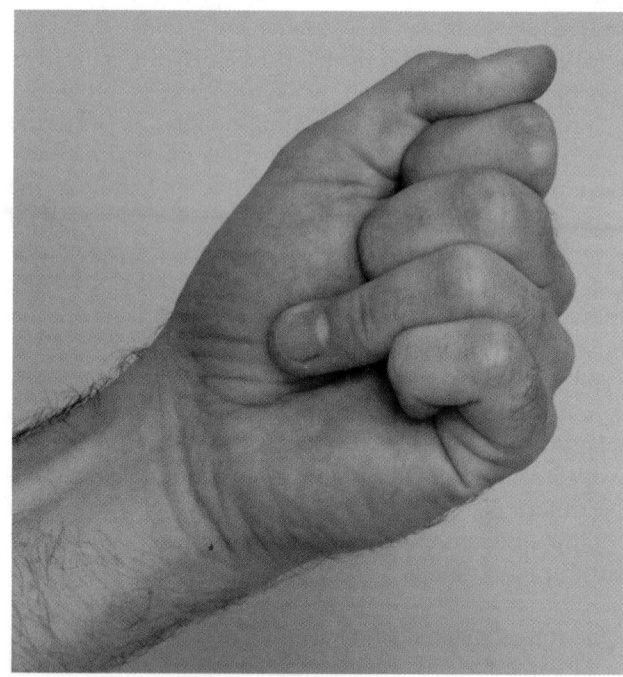

Figure 7-66 Sweater finger sign. Rupture of the flexor profundus tendon in the ring finger of a football player.

by themselves are not reliable, but when symptoms, clinical tests, and electrodiagnosis are combined, the diagnosis is more reliable.

Carpal Compression Test.[93] The examiner holds the supinated wrist in both hands and applies direct, even pressure over the median nerve in the carpal tunnel for up to 30 seconds (Figure 7-67). Production of the patient's symptoms is considered to be a positive test for

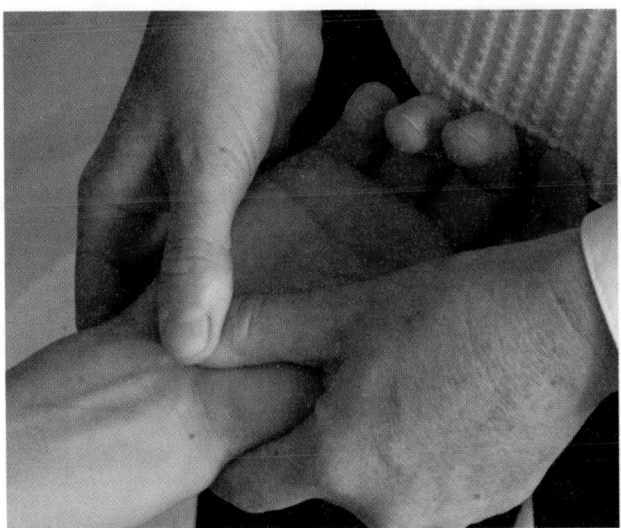

Figure 7-67 Carpal compression test.

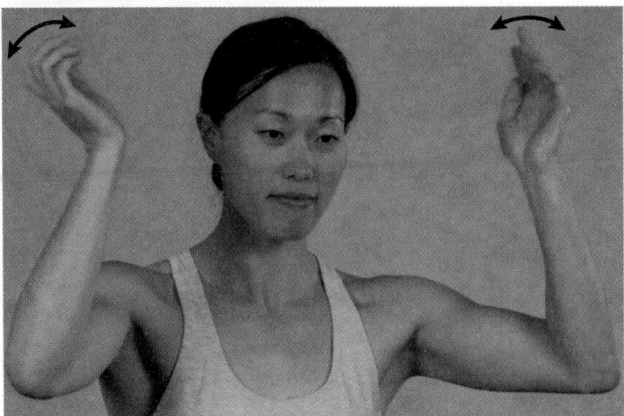

Figure 7-68 Flick maneuver.

carpal tunnel syndrome. This test is a modification of the reverse Phalen's test. The test may also involve flexing the wrist 60° before applying the pressure and whether symptoms are relieved when the examiner lets go (it may take a few minutes for the symptoms to be relieved).[94] The wrist flexion is felt to make the test more sensitive.

Dellon's Moving Two-Point Discrimination Test. This test is used to predict functional recovery; it measures the quickly adapting mechanoreceptor system.[43] The test is similar to Weber's two-point discrimination test except that the two points are moved during the test. This test is best for hand sensation related to activity and movement. The examiner moves two blunt points from proximal to distal along the long axis of the limb or digit, starting with a distance of 8 mm between the points. The distance between the points is increased or decreased, depending on the response of the patient, until the two points can no longer be distinguished. During the test, the patient's eyes are closed and the hand is cradled in the examiner's hand. The two smooth points, whether paper clip, two-point discriminator, or calipers, are gently placed longitudinally. There should be no blanching of the skin indicating too much pressure when the points are applied. The patient is asked whether one or two points are felt. If the patient is hesitant to respond or becomes inaccurate, the patient is required to respond accurately 7 or 8 of 10 times before the distance is narrowed and the test repeated.[33,58,95,96]

Normal discrimination distance recognition is 2 to 5 mm.[97] The values obtained for this test are slightly lower than those obtained for Weber's static two-point discrimination test.[95] Although the entire hand may be tested, it is more common to test only the anterior digital pulp.

Egawa's Sign. The patient flexes the middle digit and then alternately deviates the finger radially and ulnarly. If the patient is unable to do this, the interossei are affected. A positive sign is indicative of ulnar nerve palsy.

Flick Maneuver.[98] The patient is seated or standing and complains of paresthesia in the hand in the median nerve distribution. The patient is asked to vigorously shake the hands or flick the wrists (Figure 7-68). A resolution of the symptoms after flicking or shaking the hands is considered a positive test.

Froment's "Paper" Sign. The patient attempts to grasp a piece of paper between the thumb and index finger (Figure 7-69).[99] When the examiner attempts to pull away the paper, the terminal phalanx of the thumb flexes because of paralysis of the adductor pollicis muscle, indicating a positive test. If, at the same time, the metacarpophalangeal joint of the thumb hyperextends, the hyperextension is noted as a positive Jeanne's sign.[50] Both tests, if positive, are indicative of ulnar nerve paralysis.

Hand Elevation Test.[100,101] The patient raises both hands over the head and maintains the position for at least 3 minutes (Figure 7-70). A positive test is indicated if symptoms are reproduced in the median nerve distribution in less than 2 minutes.

Ninhydrin Sweat Test. The patient's hand is cleaned thoroughly and wiped with alcohol. The patient then waits 5 to 30 minutes with the fingertips not in contact with any surface. This allows time for the sweating process to ensue. After the waiting period, the fingertips are pressed with moderate pressure against good-quality bond paper that has not been touched. The fingertips are held in place for 15 seconds and traced with a pencil. The paper is then sprayed with triketohydrindene (Ninhydrin) spray reagent and allowed to dry (24 hours). The sweat areas stain purple. If the change in color (from white to purple) does not occur, it is considered a positive test for a nerve lesion.[58,102] The reagent must be fixed if a permanent record is required.

Phalen's (Wrist Flexion) Test.[103] The examiner flexes the patient's wrists maximally and holds this position for 1 minute by pushing the patient's wrists together

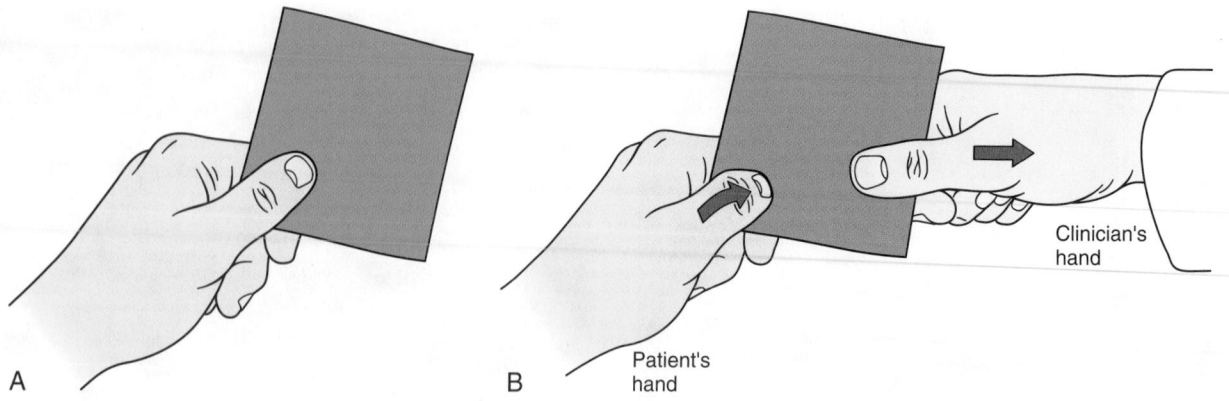

Figure 7-69 Froment's "paper" sign. **A,** Start position. **B,** Thumb flexes when paper is pulled away (positive test).

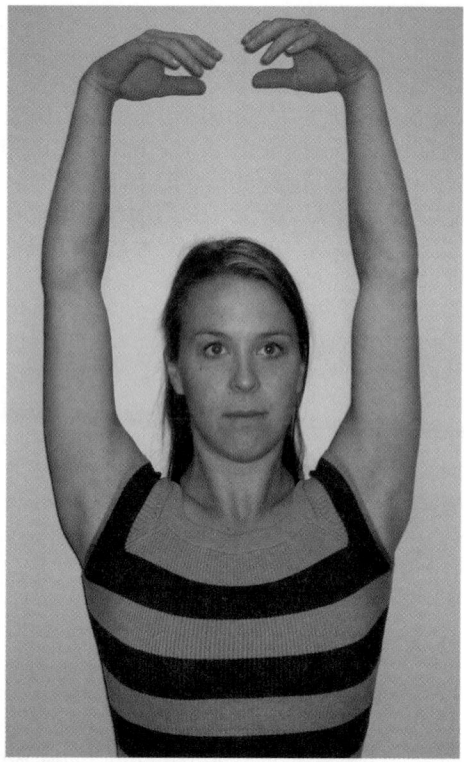

Figure 7-70 Hand elevation test for median nerve.

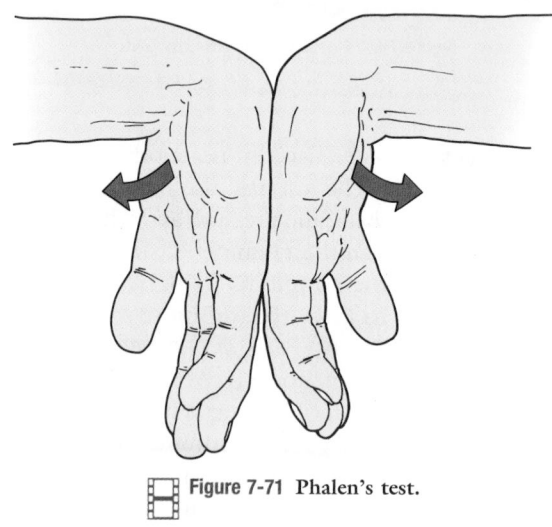

Figure 7-71 Phalen's test.

(Figure 7-71). A positive test is indicated by tingling in the thumb, index finger, and middle and lateral half of the ring finger and is indicative of carpal tunnel syndrome caused by pressure on the median nerve.[104]

⚠ **Reverse Phalen's (Prayer) Test.** The examiner extends the patient's wrist while asking the patient to grip the examiner's hand. The examiner then applies direct pressure over the carpal tunnel for 1 minute. The test is also described by having the patient put both hands together and bringing the hands down toward the waist while keeping the palms in full contact, causing extension of the wrist. Doing the test this way does not put as much pressure on the carpal tunnel. A positive test produces the same symptoms as those seen in Phalen's test and is indicative of pathology of the median nerve.[68]

⚠ **Tethered Median Nerve Stress Test.**[105] For the teathered median nerve stress test (TMNST), the patient stands or sits with the elbow flexed and forearm supinated with wrist in slight extension. The examiner then hyperextends the index finger at the distal interphalangeal joint (Figure 7-72). If anterior radiating forearm pain is felt, the test is considered positive for median nerve pathology.[105] Positive results are more likely in chronic conditions.[106,107]

⚠ **Tinel Sign (at the Wrist).**[89,108] The examiner taps over the carpal tunnel at the wrist (Figure 7-73). A positive test causes tingling or paresthesia into the thumb, index finger (forefinger), and middle and lateral half of the ring finger (median nerve distribution). Tinel sign at the wrist is indicative of a carpal tunnel syndrome. The tingling or paresthesia must be felt distal to the point of pressure for a positive test. The test gives an indication of the rate of regeneration of sensory fibers of the median nerve. The most distal point at which the abnormal sensation is felt represents the limit of nerve regeneration.

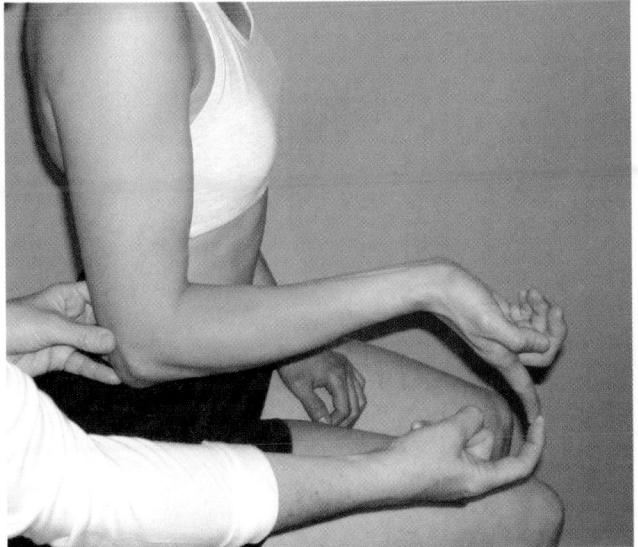

Figure 7-72 Tethered median nerve stress test (TMNST).

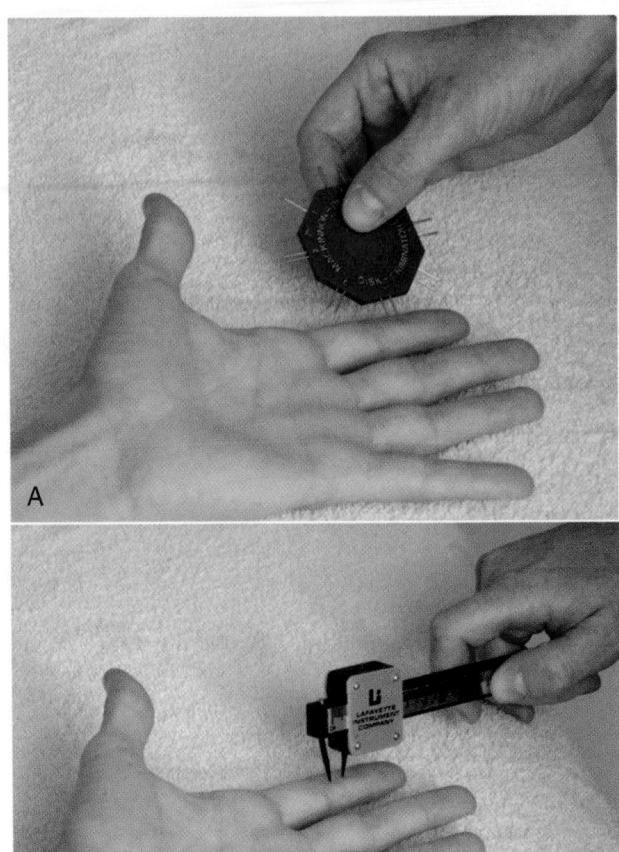

Figure 7-74 **Devices used to test two-point discrimination. A,** The Disk-Criminator is a set of two plastic discs, each containing a series of metal rods at varying intervals from 1 mm to 25 mm apart. This device evaluates both moving and static two-point discrimination. **B,** Two-point esthesiometer.

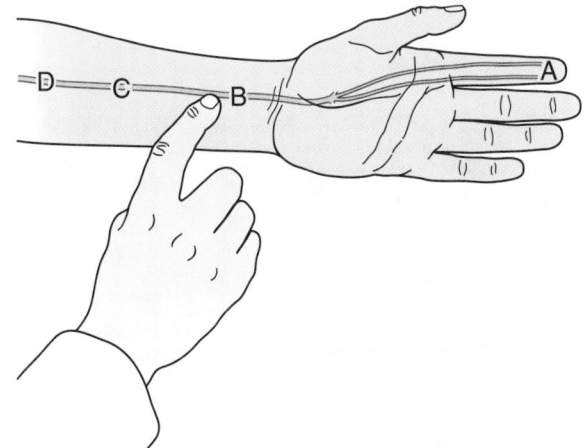

Figure 7-73 **Tinel sign at the wrist.** Light percussion is applied along nerve starting at "A" and progressing proximally. The point at which paresthesia is elicited is the level of axonal regrowth.

✓ *Weber's (Moberg's) Two-Point Discrimination Test.* The examiner uses a paper clip, two-point discriminator, or calipers (Figure 7-74) to simultaneously apply pressure on two adjacent points in a longitudinal direction or perpendicular to the long axis of the finger; the examiner moves proximal to distal in an attempt to find the minimal distance at which the patient can distinguish between the two stimuli.[43] This distance is called the *threshold for discrimination.* Coverage values are shown in Figure 7-75. The patient must concentrate on feeling the points and must not be able to see the area being tested. Only the fingertips need to be tested. The patient's hand should be immobile on a hard surface. For accurate results, the examiner must ensure that the two points touch the skin simultaneously. There should be no blanching of the skin indicating too much pressure when the points are applied. The distance between the points is decreased or increased depending on the response of the patient. The starting distance between the points is one that the patient can easily distinguish (e.g., 15 mm). If the patient is hesitant to respond or becomes inaccurate, the patient is required to respond accurately on 7 or 8 of 10 trials before the distance is narrowed and the test repeated.[33,58,95,97] Normal discrimination distance recognition is less than 6 mm, but this varies from person to person. This test is best for hand sensation involving static holding of an object between the fingers and thumb and requiring pinch strength. Table 7-9 demonstrates some two-point discrimination normal values and distances required for certain tasks.

❓ *Wrinkle (Shrivel) Test.* The patient's fingers are placed in warm water for approximately 5 to 20 minutes. The examiner then removes the patient's fingers from the water and observes whether the skin over the pulp is wrinkled (Figure 7-76). Normal fingers show wrinkling,

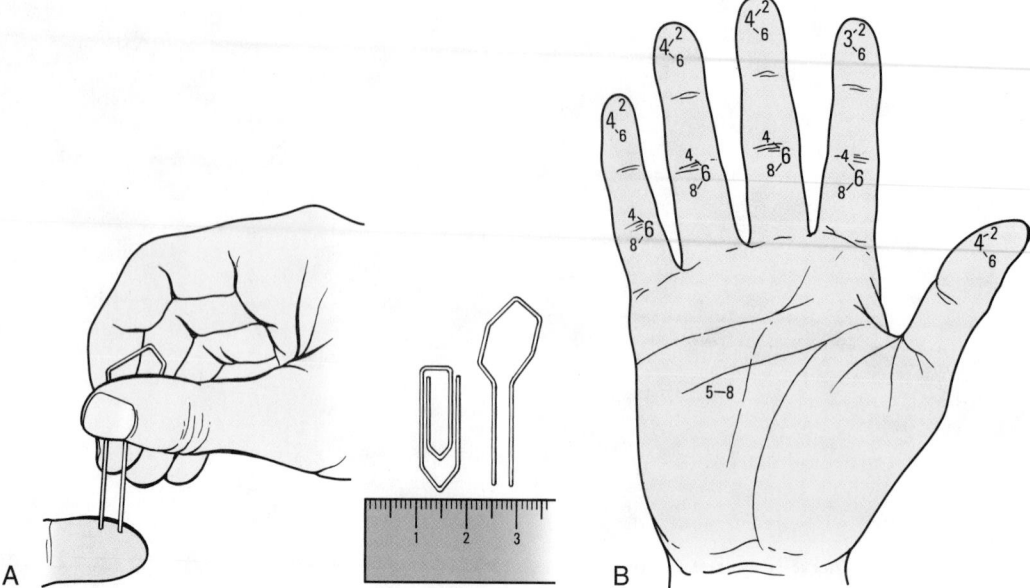

Figure 7-75 Two-point discrimination. A, Technique of performing the two-point discrimination test of Weber (after Moberg). **B,** Values of discrimination in the Weber test in millimeters in the different zones of the palm. The largest figure indicates the average values, the other two figures the minimum and maximum values (after Moberg). (From Tubiana R: The hand, Philadelphia, 1981, WB Saunders, pp. 645–646.)

TABLE **7-9**

Two-Point Discrimination Normal Values and Discrimination Distances Required for Certain Tasks

Normal	Less than 6 mm
Fair	6 to 10 mm
Poor	11 to 15 mm
Protective	1 point perceived
Anesthetic	0 points perceived
Winding a watch	6 mm
Sewing	6 to 8 mm
Handling precision tools	12 mm
Gross tool handling	Greater than 15 mm

Adapted from Callahan AD: Sensibility assessment for nerve lesions-in-continuity and nerve lacerations. In Hunter J, Schneider LH, Mackin EJ, et al, editors: Rehabilitation of the hand and upper extremity, St Louis, 2002, Mosby, p. 233.

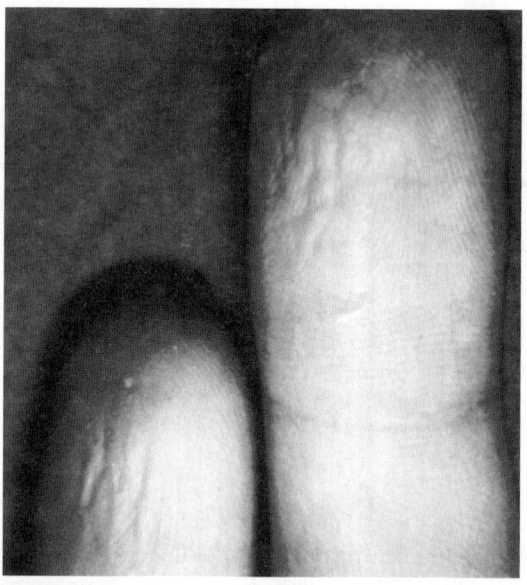

Figure 7-76 The wrinkle test may be reliable for digital nerve sympathetic function if the fingers (in this case, the radial digital nerve of the fourth and fifth digits) are completely denervated. (From Waylett-Rendall J: Sensibility evaluation and rehabilitation. Orthop Clin North Am 19:48, 1988.)

but denervated ones do not. The test is valid only within the first few months after injury.[109]

Tests for Circulation and Swelling

✓ ***Allen Test.*** The patient is asked to open and close the hand several times as quickly as possible and then squeeze the hand tightly (Figure 7-77).[104,110] The examiner's thumb and index finger are placed over the radial and ulnar arteries, compressing them. As an alternative technique, the examiner may use both hands, placing one thumb over each artery to compress the artery and placing the fingers on the posterior aspect of the arm for stability. The patient then opens the hand while pressure is maintained over the arteries. One artery is tested by releasing the pressure over that artery to see if the hand flushes. The other artery is then tested in a similar fashion. Both hands should be tested for comparison. This test determines the patency of the radial and ulnar arteries and determines which artery provides the major blood supply to the hand.

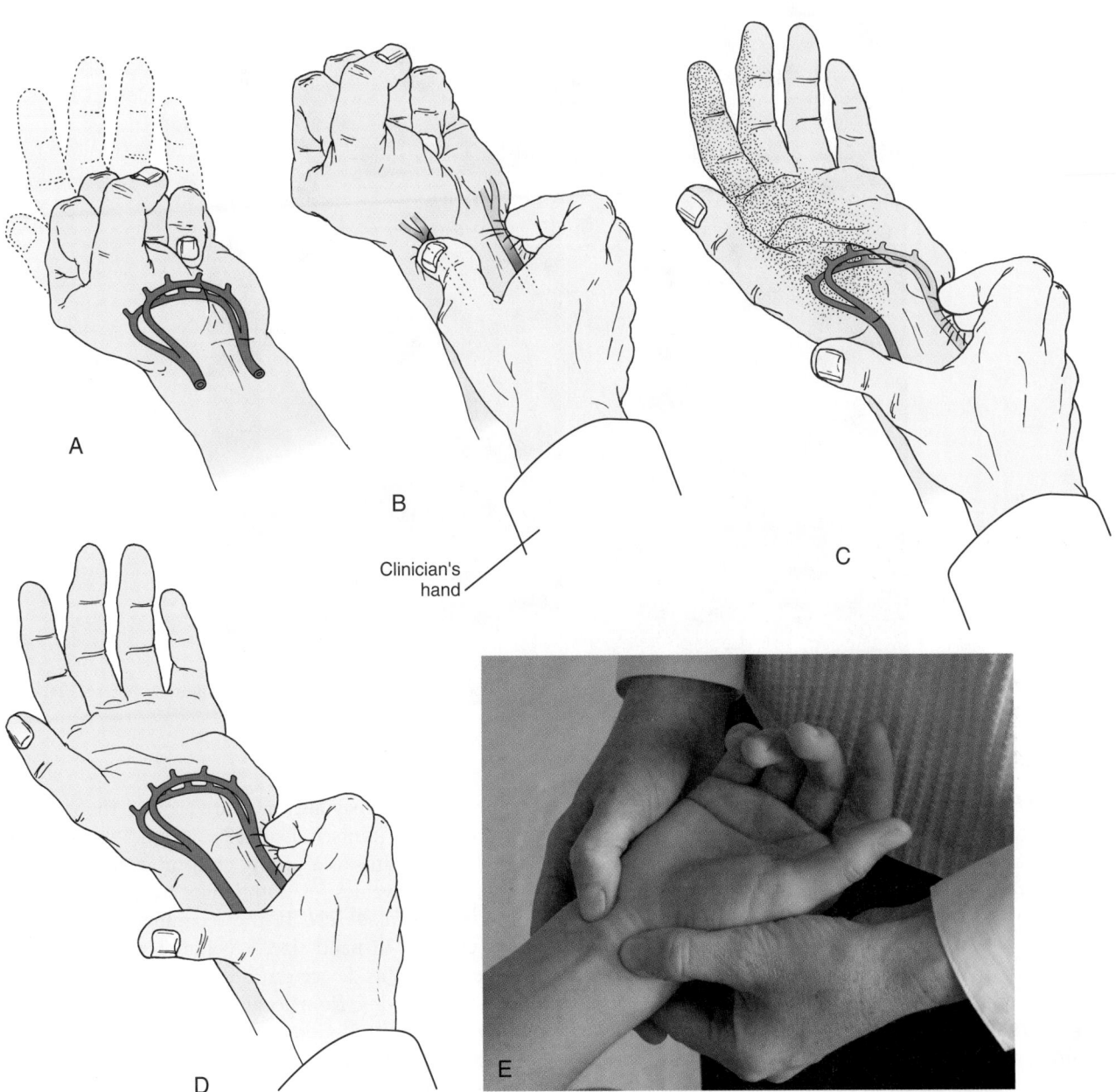

Clinician's
hand

Figure 7-77 Allen test. A, The patient opens and closes the hand. **B,** While the patient holds the hand closed, the examiner compresses the radial and ulnar arteries. **C,** One artery (in this case, the radial artery) is then released, and the examiner notes the filling pattern of the hand until the circulation is normal. **D,** The process is then repeated with the other artery. **E,** Alternative hand hold.

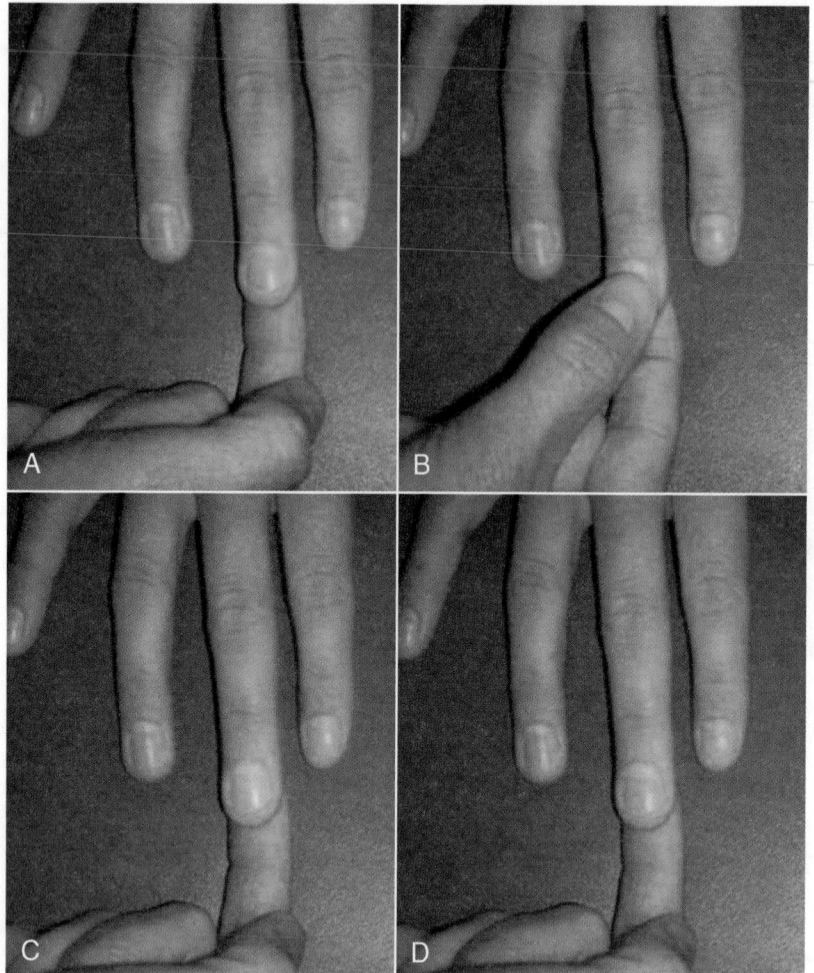

Figure 7-78 Checking digital blood flow. A, Starting position. **B,** Compression on finger. **C,** Immediately after pressure released. **D,** Three seconds after pressure released. Note darker color of nail as blood flow returns.

☑ *Digit Blood Flow.* To test distal blood flow, the examiner compresses the nail bed and notes the time taken for color to return to the nail (Figure 7-78). Normally, when the pressure is released, color should return to the nail bed within 3 seconds. If return takes longer, arterial insufficiency to the fingers should be suspected. Comparison with the normal side gives some indication of restricted flow.

☑ *Figure of Eight Measurement.* Swelling may also be measured with a tape measure. The examiner places a mark on the distal aspect of the ulnar styloid process as a starting point. The examiner then takes the tape measure across the anterior wrist to the most distal aspect of the radial styloid process (Figure 7-79, *A*). From there, the tape is brought diagonally across the back (dorsum) of the hand and over the fifth metacarophalangeal joint line (Figures 7-79, *B*, palmar view; and 7-79, *C*, dorsal view), across the anterior surface of the metacarpophalangeal joints (Figure 7-79, *D*) and then diagonally across the back of the hand to where the tape started (Figure 7-79, *E*).[111,112]

The examiner may also measure around the proximal interphalangeal joints individually, around the metacarpophalangeal joints as a group, and/or around the palm and wrist. The values for both hands are compared.

☑ *Hand Volume Test.* If the examiner is concerned about changes in hand size, a volumeter (Figure 7-80) may be used. This device can be used to assess change in hand size resulting from localized swelling, generalized edema, or atrophy.[54] Comparisons with the normal limb give the examiner an idea of changes occurring in the affected hand. Care must be taken when doing this test to ensure accurate readings. There is often a 10-mL difference between right and left hands and between dominant and nondominant hands. If swelling is the problem, differences of 30 to 50 mL can be noted.[33,113]

Reflexes and Cutaneous Distribution

Although it is possible to obtain reflexes from the tendons crossing the wrist, this is not commonly done. In fact, no deep tendon reflexes are routinely tested in the

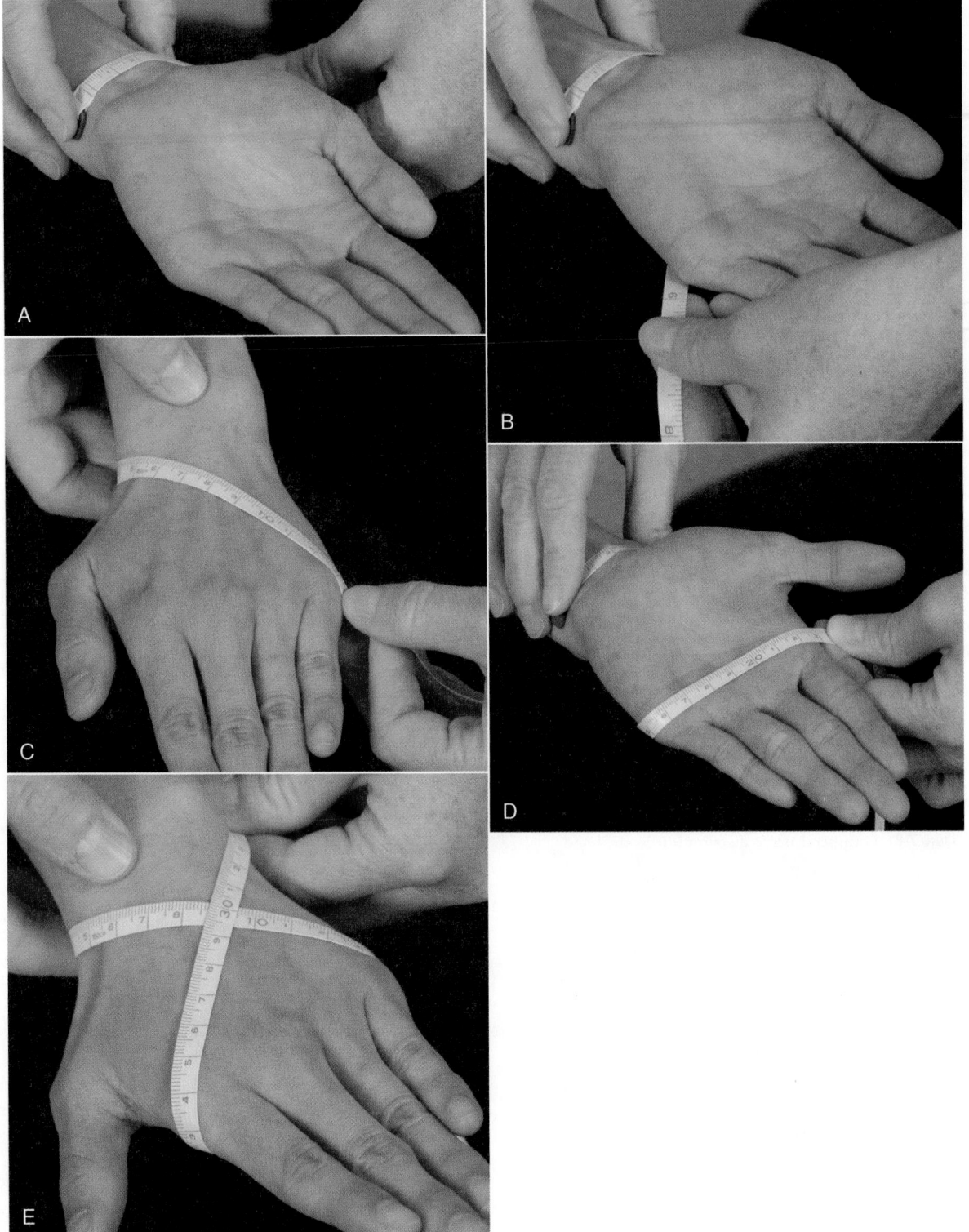

Figure 7-79 Figure of 8 measurement for hand swelling. A, Across wrist. **B,** Across back of hand (supinated view). **C,** Across back of hand (pronated view). **D,** Across anterior metacarpal head. **E,** Across back of hand to start point.

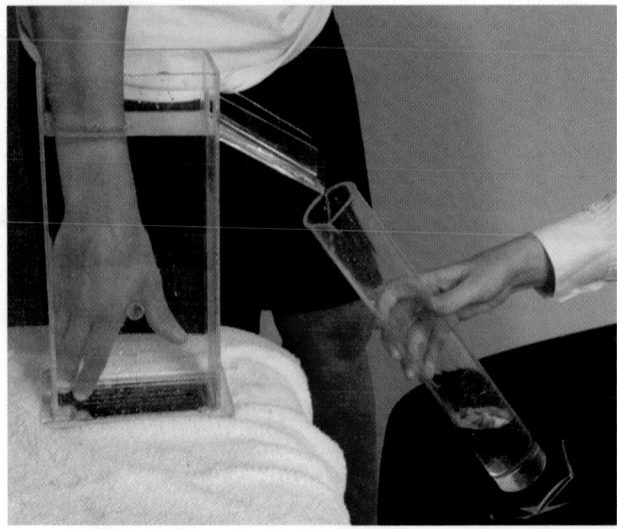

Figure 7-80 Volumeter used to measure hand volume.

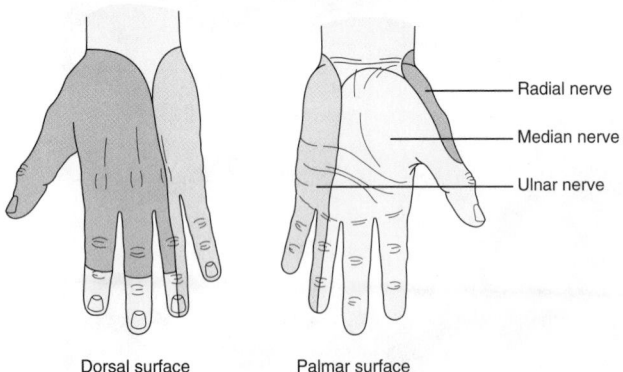

Dorsal surface   Palmar surface

Figure 7-81 Peripheral nerve distribution in the hand.

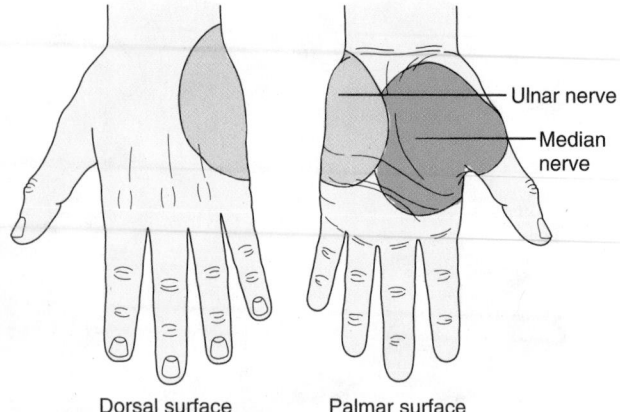

Dorsal surface   Palmar surface

Figure 7-82 Sensory distribution of branches of the ulnar and median nerves given off above the wrist.

TABLE **7-10**

Tests for Cutaneous Sensibility

Test	Sensation	Fiber/Receptor Type
Pin	Pain	Free nerve endings
Warm/cold	Temperature	Free nerve endings
Cotton wool	Moving touch	Quick adapting
Finger stroking	Moving touch	Quick adapting
Dellon's	Moving touch	Quick adapting
Tuning fork	Vibration	Quick adapting
Von Frey	Constant touch	Slow adapting
Weber's	Constant touch	Slow adapting
Pick-up	Constant touch	Slow adapting
Precision sensory grip	Constant touch	Slow adapting
Gross grip	Constant touch	Slow adapting

Modified from Dellon AL: The paper clip: light hardware to evaluate sensibility in the hand. Contemp Orthop 1:40, 1979.

forearm, wrist, and hand. The only reflex that may be tested in the hand is Hoffman reflex, which is a pathological reflex. This reflex may be tested if an upper motor neuron lesion is suspected. To test the reflex, the examiner "flicks" the terminal phalanx of the index, middle, or ring finger. A positive test is indicated by reflex flexion of the distal phalanx of the thumb or a finger that was not "flicked."

The examiner must be aware of the sensory distribution of the ulnar, median, and radial nerves in the hand (Figure 7-81) and must be prepared to compare peripheral nerve sensory distribution with nerve root sensory (dermatome) distributions. As previously mentioned, there is variability in both distributions. It has been reported, however, that each peripheral nerve of the upper limb has a "constant" area in the hand that is always affected if the nerve is injured. For the radial nerve, it is on the dorsum of the thumb near the apex of the anatomical snuff box; for the median nerve, it is the tip of the index finger; and for the ulnar nerve, it is the tip of the little finger.[114]

The median nerve gives off a sensory branch above the wrist before it passes through the carpal tunnel. This sensory branch supplies the skin of the palm (Figure 7-82). Thus, most commonly, carpal tunnel syndrome does not affect the median sensory distribution in the palm but results in altered sensation in the fingers.

Several sensation tests may be carried out in the hand. Table 7-10 illustrates the tests used and the sensation and nerve fibers tested. Pinprick is used to test for pain. Constant light touch, which is a component of fine discrimination, may be tested in the hand using a **Semmes-Weinstein** pressure esthesiometer (**Von Frey test** ✓). This kit has 20 probes, each with different thicknesses of nylon monofilament (Figure 7-83). The patient is blindfolded or otherwise unable to see the hand, and each filament is applied perpendicularly to the finger with the smallest filament being used first. The filament is pushed

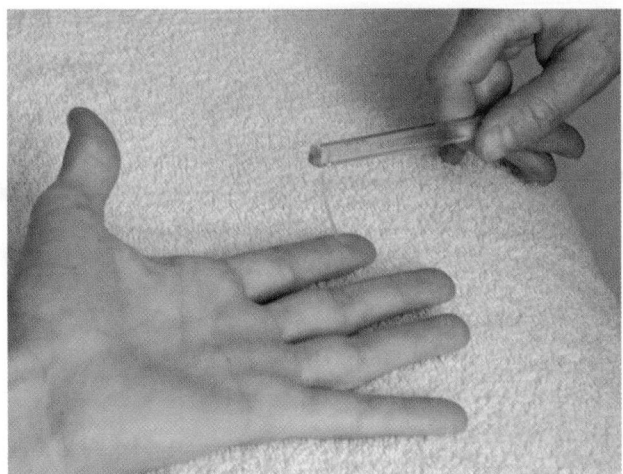

Figure 7-83 The Semmes-Weinstein monofilament is applied perpendicular to the skin for 1 to 1.5 seconds, held in place for 1 to 1.5 seconds, and lifted for 1 to 1.5 seconds.

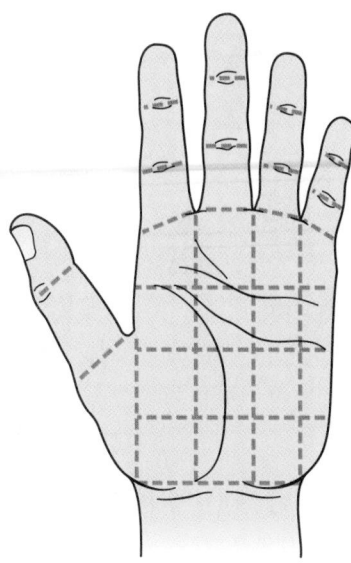

Palmar aspect

Figure 7-84 Grid pattern used for recording results of light touch sensation testing.

against the finger until the filament bends. The next filament is then used, and so on until the patient feels one before or just as it bends.[34,78] The test is repeated three times to ensure a positive result.[97] Normal values vary between probes 2.44 and 2.83 (Table 7-11). When doing the Semmes-Weinstein test, the hand and fingers are commonly divided into a grid (Figure 7-84), and only one point (usually in the center) is tested in each square. It is primarily the palmar aspect of the hand that is tested.

Stereognosis or tactile gnosis, which is the ability to identify common objects by touch, should also be tested. Objects are placed in the patient's hand while the patient is blindfolded or otherwise unable to see the object. The time taken to recognize the object is noted. Normal subjects can usually name the object within 3 seconds of contact.[95]

Vibratory sense is tested using a 256-cps (high frequency) or 30-cps (low-frequency) tuning fork. The patient, who cannot see the test site, indicates when vibration is felt as the examiner touches the skin with the vibrating tuning fork and whether the vibration feels the same. The score is the number of correct responses divided by the total number of presentations.[115]

To test moving touch, the examiner's fingers stroke the patient's finger. The patient notes whether the stroking was felt and what it felt like.

It must be remembered that pain may be referred to the wrist and hand from the cervical or upper thoracic spine, shoulder, and elbow. Seldom is wrist or hand pain referred up the limb (Figure 7-85). Table 7-12 shows the muscles acting on the forearm, wrist, and hand and their pain referral patterns when injured.

The examiner can attempt a differential diagnosis of paresthesia in the hand if altered sensation is present. A comparison with a normal dermatome chart should be made, and the examiner should remember that there is a

TABLE 7-11

Light Touch Testing Using Semmes-Weinstein Pressure Esthesiometer

Esthesiometer Probe Number	Calculated Pressure (g/mm²)	Interpretation
2.44–2.83	3.25–4.86	Normal light touch
3.22–4.56	11.1–47.3	Diminished light touch, point localization* intact
4.74–6.10	68.0–243.0	Minimal light touch, area localization† intact
6.10–6.65	243.0–439.0	Sensation but no localization sensibility

From Omer GE: Report of the committee for evaluation of the clinical result in peripheral nerve injury. J Hand Surg Am 8:755, 1983.
*Point localization: The dowel is in contact with the skin point stimulated.
†Area localization: The dowel is in contact with any point inside the zone of the area being tested (in the hand or foot).

fair amount of variability and overlap with dermatomes (Figure 7-86). In addition, there are areas of the hand where sensation is more important (Figure 7-87). Abnormal sensation may mean the following:

1. Numbness in the thumb only may be caused by pressure on the digital nerve on the outer aspect of the thumb.
2. A "pins and needles" feeling in the thumb may be caused by a contusion of the thenar branch of the median nerve.

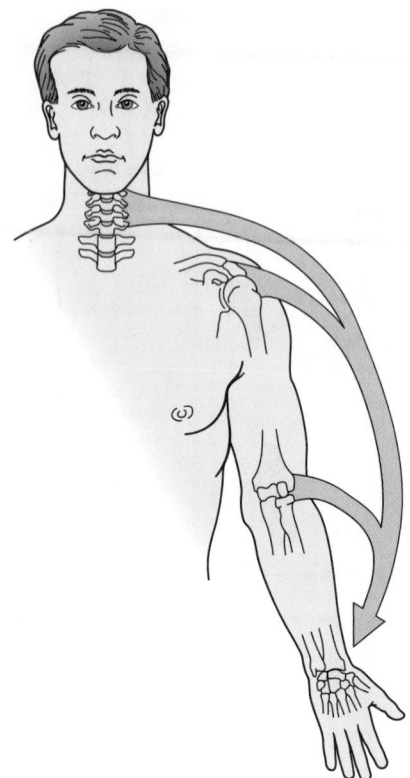

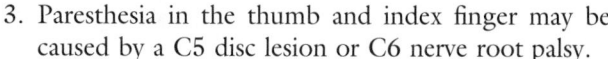

Figure 7-85 Symptoms can be referred to the wrist and hand from the elbow, shoulder, and cervical spine.

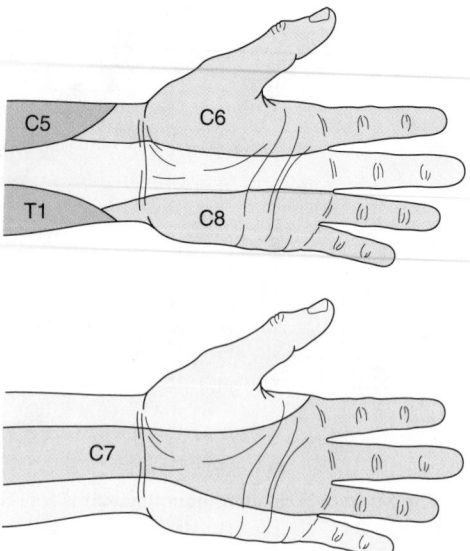

Figure 7-86 **Dermatomes of the hand.** Note overlap at dermatomes. Both views are palmar.

3. Paresthesia in the thumb and index finger may be caused by a C5 disc lesion or C6 nerve root palsy.
4. Paresthesia in the thumb, index finger, and middle finger may be caused by a C5 disc lesion, C6 nerve root palsy, or thoracic outlet syndrome.
5. Paresthesia of the thumb, index finger, middle finger, and half of the ring finger on the palmar aspect may be caused by an injury to the median nerve, possibly through the carpal tunnel; on the dorsal aspect, it could be caused by injury to the radial nerve.
6. Numbness of the thumb and middle finger may be caused by a tumor of the humerus.
7. Paresthesia on all five digits in one or both hands may be caused by a thoracic outlet syndrome. If it is in both hands, it may be caused by a central cervical disc protrusion. The level of protrusion would be indicated by the distribution of the paresthesia.
8. Paresthesia of the index and middle fingers may be caused by a trigger finger or "stick" palsy, if it is on the palmar aspect, or by a C6 disc lesion or C7 nerve root palsy. On the dorsal aspect of the hand, it may be caused by a carpal exostosis or subluxation. Stick palsy is the result of an inordinate amount of pressure from a cane or crutches on the ulnar nerve as it passes through the palm.

TABLE **7-12**

Forearm, Wrist, and Hand Muscles and Referral of Pain

Muscles	Referral Pattern
Brachioradialis	Lateral epicondyle, lateral forearm, and web space between thumb and index finger
Extensor carpi ulnaris	Medial side of dorsum of wrist
Extensor carpi radialis brevis	Middle of dorsum of wrist
Extensor carpi radialis longus	Lateral epicondyle, forearm, and lateral dorsum of hand
Extensor digitorum	Forearm, wrist to appropriate digit
Extensor indices	Dorsum of wrist to index finger
Palmaris longus	Anterior aspect of forearm to palm
Flexor carpi ulnaris	Anteromedial wrist into lateral palm
Flexor carpi radialis	Forearm to anterolateral wrist
Flexor digitorum superficialis	Palm into appropriate digit
Flexor pollicis longus	Thumb
Adductor pollicis	Anterolateral and posterolateral palm into thumb
Opponens pollicis	Anterolateral wrist into anterior thumb
Abductor digiti minimi	Dorsomedial surface of hand into little finger
Interossei	Into adjacent digit, and for first interossei, dorsum of hand

9. Paresthesia of the index, middle, and ring fingers may be caused by a C6 disc lesion, C7 nerve root injury, or carpal tunnel syndrome.
10. Paresthesia of all four fingers may be caused by a C6 disc lesion or injury to the C7 nerve root.
11. Paresthesia of the middle finger only may be caused by a C6 disc lesion or C7 nerve root lesion.
12. Paresthesia of the middle and ring fingers may be caused by a C6 disc lesion, C7 nerve root lesion, or stick palsy.
13. Paresthesia of the middle, ring, and little fingers may be caused by a C7 disc lesion or C8 nerve root palsy. The same would be true if there were paralysis of the ring and little fingers. This paresthesia may also be the result of a thoracic outlet syndrome.
14. Paresthesia on the ulnar side of the ring finger and the entire little finger may be caused by pressure of the ulnar nerve at the elbow or in the palm.

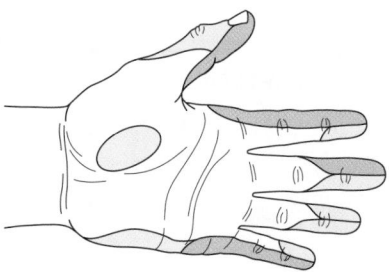

Figure 7-87 Importance of hand sensation. *Darker areas* indicate where sensation is most important; *lighter areas,* where sensation is a little less important; and *white areas,* where sensation is least important. (Redrawn from Tubiana R: The hand, Philadelphia, 1981, WB Saunders, p. 74.)

Peripheral Nerve Injuries of the Forearm, Wrist, and Hand

Carpal Tunnel Syndrome. The most common "tunnel" syndrome in the body is the carpal tunnel syndrome, in which the median nerve is compressed under the flexor retinaculum at the wrist (see Figure 7-32). This compression may follow trauma (for example, a Colles fracture or lunate dislocation), flexor tendon paratenonitis, a ganglion, arthritis (osteoarthritis or rheumatoid arthritis), or collagen disease. As many as 20% of pregnant women may experience median nerve symptoms because compression of the nerve as a result of fluid retention causes swelling in the carpal tunnel. With carpal tunnel syndrome, the symptoms, which are primarily distal to the wrist, are usually worse at night and include burning, tingling, pins and needles, and numbness into the median nerve sensory distribution (Table 7-13). In severe cases, pain may be referred to the forearm. Symptoms are often aggravated by wrist movements, and long-standing cases show atrophy and weakness of the thenar muscles (flexor and abductor pollicis brevis, opponens pollicis) and the lateral two lumbricals. The condition is most common in women between 40 and 60 years of age, and, although it may occur bilaterally, it is seen most commonly in the dominant hand. It is also commonly seen in younger patients who use their wrists a great deal in repetitive manual labor or are exposed to vibration.[116] Because of the apparent connection between carpal tunnel syndrome and cervical lesions resulting in double crush syndromes, the examiner should take care to include cervical assessment if the history appears to warrant such inclusion.[117-119]

Guyon (Pisohamate) Canal. The ulnar nerve is sometimes compressed as it passes through the pisohamate, or Guyon canal (Figure 7-88). The condition may also be called **ulnar tunnel syndrome,** because the nerve may

TABLE **7-13**

Nerve Injuries (Neuropathy) about the Wrist and Hand

Nerve	Motor Loss	Sensory Loss	Functional Loss
Median nerve (C6 to C8, T1; carpal tunnel)	Flexor pollicis brevis Abductor pollicis brevis Opponens pollicis Lateral two lumbricals	Palmar and dorsal thumb, index, middle and lateral half of ring finger If lesion above carpal tunnel, palmar sensation also affected	Thumb opposition Thumb flexion Weak or no pinch Weak grip
Ulnar nerve (C7, C8, T1; pisohamate canal)	Flexor digiti minimi Abductor digiti minimi Opponens digiti minimi Adductor pollicis Interossei Medial two lumbricals Palmaris brevis	Little finger, half of ring finger Palm often not affected	Thumb adduction Inability to extend PIP and DIP joints of fourth and fifth fingers Finger abduction Finger adduction Flexion of little finger

DIP, Distal interphalangeal; *PIP,* proximal interphalangeal.

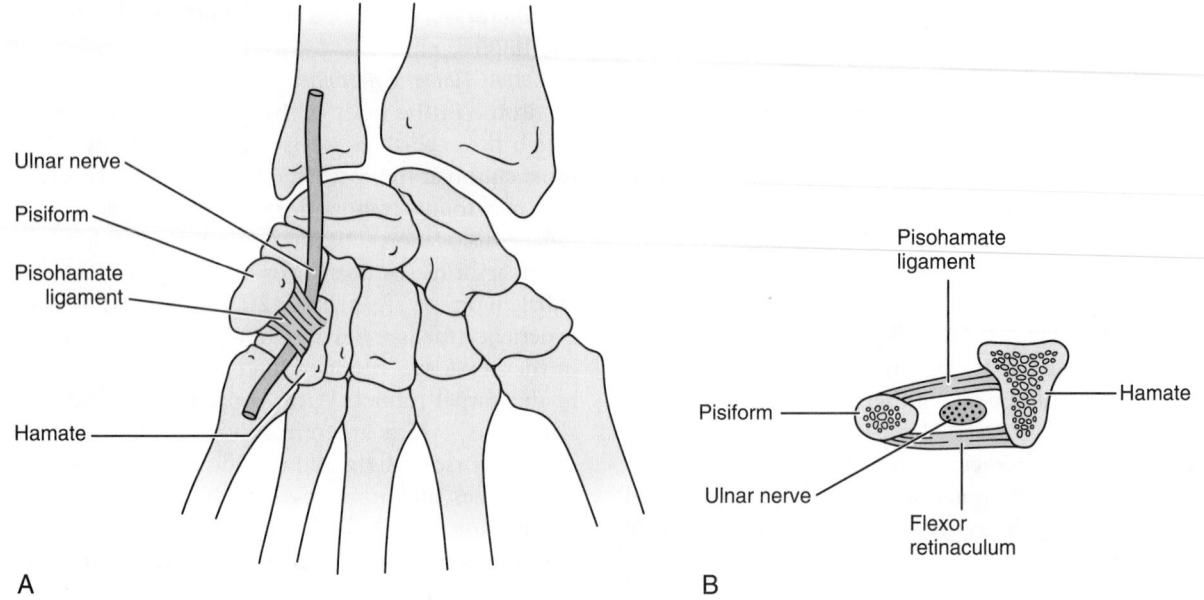

Figure 7-88 Guyon canal. **A,** Palmar view. **B,** Section view showing position of nerve relative to pisohamate ligament and flexor retinaculum.

be compressed in the wrist from trauma (acute or repetitive), a space occupying lesion, or vascular lesion.[120] The nerve may be compressed from trauma (e.g., fractured hook of hamate), use of crutches, or chronic pressure, as in people who cycle long distances while leaning on the handlebars or who use pneumatic jackhammers. If the problem is in the Guyon canal, direct pressure over the canal may reproduce or exacerbate the symptoms (**Guyon canal compression test** ❓).[121] The ulnar nerve gives off two sensory branches above the wrist. These branches supply the palmar and dorsal aspects of the hand, as illustrated in Figure 7-82, and do not pass through Guyon canal. Therefore, if the ulnar nerve is compressed in the canal, only the fingers show an altered sensation (see Table 7-13). Motor loss includes the muscles of the hypothenar eminence (flexor digiti minimi, abductor digiti minimi, and opponens digiti minimi), adductor pollicis, the interossei, medial two lumbricals, and palmaris brevis.

Joint Play Movements

When assessing joint play movements, the examiner should remember that if the patient complains of inability or pain on wrist flexion, the lesion is probably in the midcarpal joints. If the patient complains of inability or pain on wrist extension, the lesion is probably in the radiocarpal joints, because it is in these joints that most of the movement occurs during these actions. If the patient complains of pain or inability on supination and pronation, the lesion is probably in the ulnameniscocarpal joint or inferior radioulnar joint.

The amount of movement obtained by the joint play should be compared with that of the normal side and

> **Joint Play Movements of the Hand**
>
> **WRIST**
> - Long-axis extension (traction or distraction)
> - Anteroposterior glide
> - Side glide
> - Side tilt
>
> **INTERMETACARPAL JOINTS**
> - Anteroposterior glide
>
> **FINGERS**
> - Long-axis extension (traction or distraction)
> - Anteroposterior glide
> - Rotation
> - Side glide

considered significant only if there is a difference between the two sides. Reproduction of the patient's symptoms would also give an indication of the joints at fault.

Wrist

To perform **long-axis extension** at the wrist, the examiner stabilizes the radius and ulna with one hand (the patient's elbow may be flexed to 90°, and stabilization may be applied at the elbow if there is no pathology at the elbow) and places the other hand just distal to the wrist. The examiner then applies a longitudinal traction movement with the distal hand (Figure 7-89).

Anteroposterior glide is applied at the wrist in two positions. The examiner first places the stabilizing hand

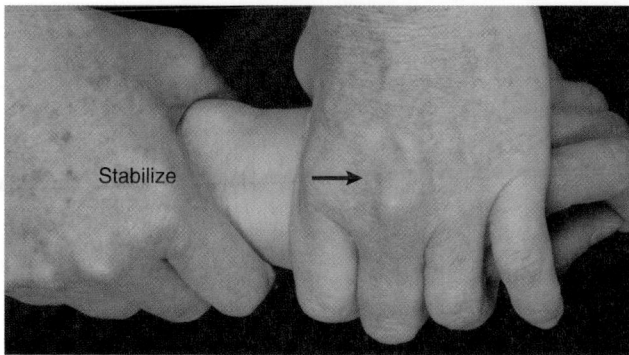

Figure 7-89 Long-axis extension (traction) of the wrist.

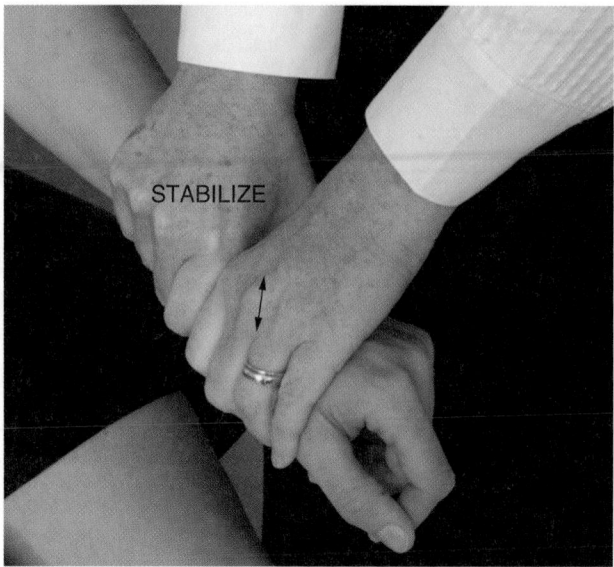

Figure 7-90 **Position for testing joint play movements of the wrist.** Note that there is no gap between the web spaces of the two hands.

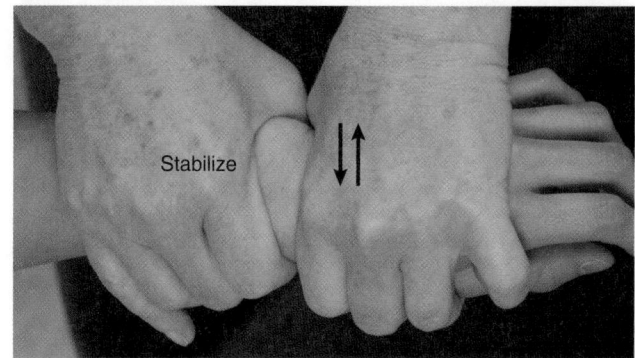

Figure 7-91 Wrist side glide.

around the distal end of the radius and ulna just proximal to the radiocarpal joint and then places the other hand around the proximal row of carpal bones. If the examiner's hands are positioned properly, they should touch each other (Figure 7-90). The examiner applies an anteroposterior gliding movement of the proximal row of carpal bones on the radius and ulna, testing the amount of movement and end feel. Then, the stabilizing hand is moved slightly distally (less than 1 cm) so that it is around the proximal row of carpal bones. The examiner places the mobilizing hand around the distal row of carpal bones. An anteroposterior gliding movement is applied to the distal row of carpal bones on the proximal row to test the amount of movement and end feel. These movements are sometimes called the **anteroposterior drawer tests** of the wrist.[3] If the examiner then moves the stabilizing hand slightly distally (less than 1 cm) again, the hand will be around the distal carpal bones. The mobilizing hand is then placed around the metacarpals, and an anteroposterior gliding movement is applied to the base of the metacarpals to test the amount of joint play and end feel.

Side glide is performed in a similar fashion, except that a side-to-side movement is performed instead of an anteroposterior movement. To perform **side tilting** of the carpals on the radius and ulna, the examiner stabilizes the radius and ulna by placing the stabilizing hand around the distal radius and ulna just proximal to the radiocarpal joint and the mobilizing hand around the patient's hand and then radially and ulnarly deviating the hand on the radius and ulna (Figure 7-91).

The joint play movements just described are general ones involving different "rows" of carpal bones. To check the joint play movements of the individual carpal bones, a technique such as **Kaltenborn's technique** should be used. Kaltenborn[122] suggested ten tests to determine the mobility of each of the carpal bones. The movement of each of the bones is determined in a sequential manner, and both sides are tested for comparison. These tests are sometimes referred to as **ballottement tests** or **shear**

tests (Figure 7-92).[3] The examiner may use Kaltenborn's order or any other order as long as each bone and its relationship to adjacent bones is tested individually for amount of accessory movement and end feel.[123] For example, some people start by testing the movement of the lunate relative to the radius, and then move to the capitate (relative to the lunate), followed by scaphoid-radius, scaphoid-trapezoid/trapezium, triquetrum-radius, and triquetrum-hamate. Pisiform may be tested individually. Pain on any of these joint play movements done in neutral, flexion, or extension could indicate pathology in the joint between the two bones.[35]

Intermetacarpal Joints

To accomplish **anteroposterior glide** at the intermetacarpal joints, the examiner stabilizes one metacarpal bone and moves the adjacent metacarpal anteriorly and

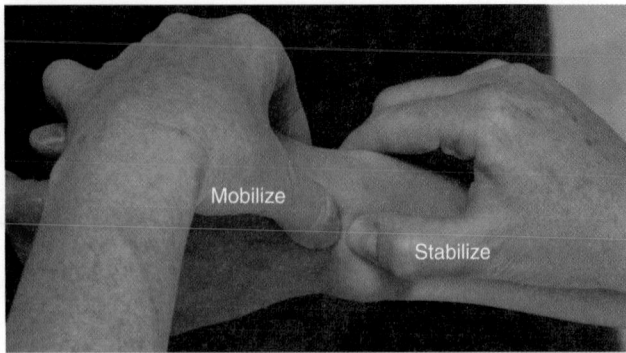

Figure 7-92 Individual carpal bone shear tests. Anteroposterior shear (glide) of lunate on radius demonstrated.

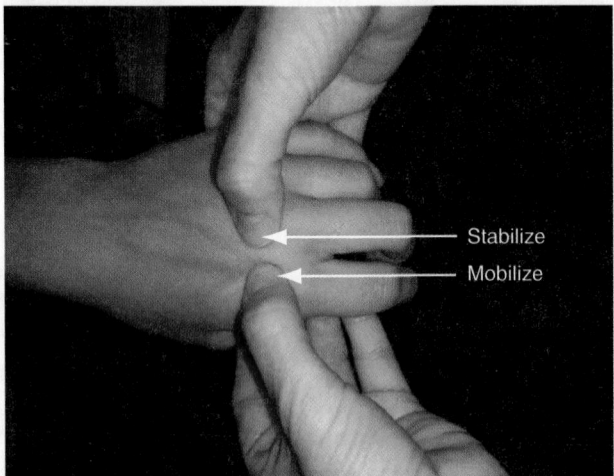

Figure 7-93 Anteroposterior glide of the intermetacarpal joints.

Kaltenborn's Carpal Mobilization

- Fixate the capitate, and move the trapezoid
- Fixate the capitate, and move the scaphoid
- Fixate the capitate, and move the lunate
- Fixate the capitate, and move the hamate
- Fixate the scaphoid, and move the trapezoid and trapezium
- Fixate the radius, and move the scaphoid
- Fixate the radius, and move the lunate
- Fixate the ulna, and move the triquetrum
- Fixate the triquetrum, and move the hamate
- Fixate the triquetrum, and move the pisiform

posteriorly in relation to the fixed bone to determine the amount of joint play and the end feel. The process is repeated for each joint (Figure 7-93).

Fingers

The joint play movements for the fingers are the same for the metacarpophalangeal, proximal interphalangeal, and distal interphalangeal joints; the hand position of the examiner simply moves farther distally.

To perform **long-axis extension,** the examiner stabilizes the proximal segment or bone using one hand while placing the second hand around the distal segment or bone of the particular joint to be tested. With the mobilizing hand, the examiner applies a longitudinal traction to the joint (Figure 7-94).

Anteroposterior glide is accomplished by stabilizing the proximal bone with one hand. The mobilizing hand is placed around the distal segment of the joint, and the examiner applies an anterior and/or posterior movement to the distal segment, being sure to maintain the joint surfaces parallel to one another while determining the amount of movement and end feel (Figure 7-95). A minimal amount of traction may be applied to bring about slight separation of the joint surfaces.

Rotation of the joints of the fingers is accomplished by stabilizing the proximal segment with one hand. With the other hand, the examiner applies slight traction to the joint to distract the joint surfaces and then rotates the distal segment on the proximal segment to determine the end feel and joint play (Figure 7-96).

To perform **side glide** joint play to the joints of the fingers, the proximal segment is stabilized with one hand. The examiner then applies slight traction to the joint with the mobilizing hand to distract the joint surfaces and then moves the distal segment sideways, keeping the joint surfaces parallel to one another to determine joint play and end feel (Figure 7-97).

Palpation

To palpate the forearm, wrist, and hand, the examiner starts proximally and works distally, first on the dorsal surface and then on the anterior surface (Figure 7-98). The muscles of the forearm are palpated first for any signs of tenderness or pathology.

Dorsal Surface

On the dorsal aspect, the examiner begins on the thumb side of the hand and palpates the "snuff box," the carpal bones, and the metacarpal bones and phalanges.

Anatomic Snuff Box. The snuff box is located between the tendons of extensor pollicis longus and extensor pollicis brevis and can best be seen by having the patient actively extend the thumb (Figure 7-99). The scaphoid bone may be palpated inside the snuff box. Tenderness of the scaphoid bone is often treated as a fracture until proven otherwise because of the possibility of avascular necrosis of the bone, especially the anterior fragment or pole.[124] With the wrist in anatomic position, proximal palpation is used to find the radial styloid on the lateral aspect. Moving medially over the radius, the examiner comes to the radial (Lister) tubercle. The extensor pollicis longus tendon moves around the tubercle to enter the

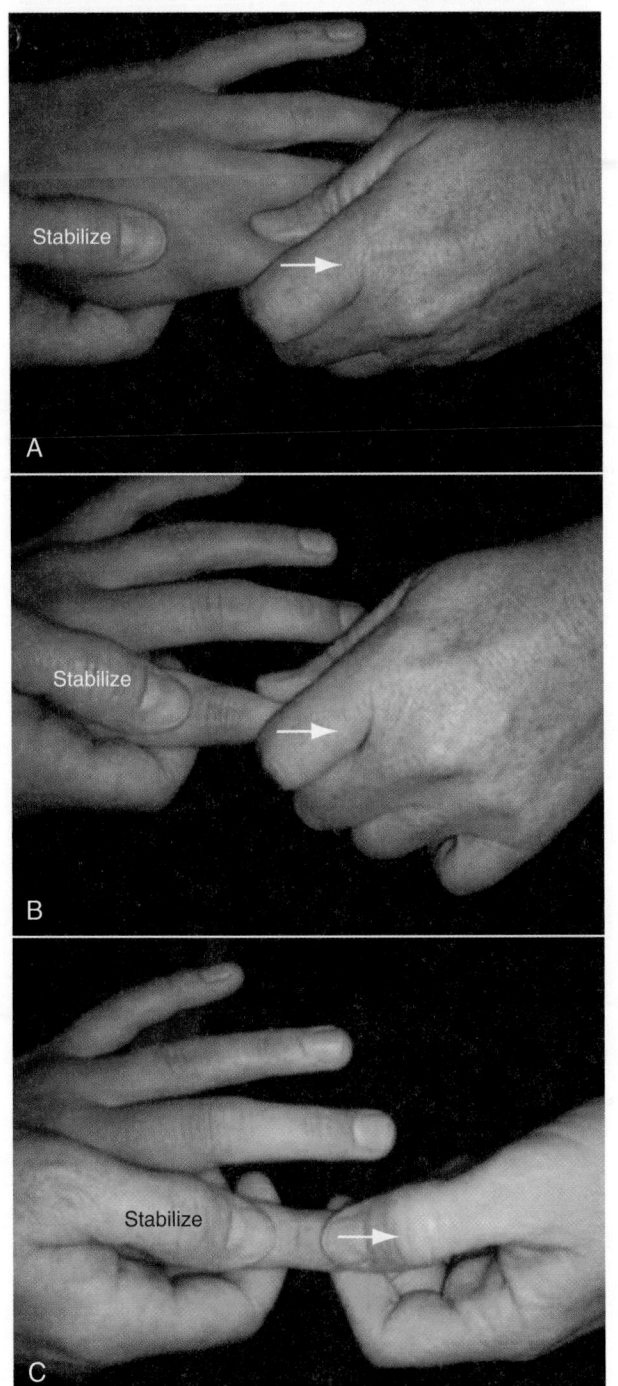

Figure 7-94 Long axis extension (traction) of the joints of the fingers. **A,** Metacarpophalangeal joint. **B,** Proximal interphalangeal joint. **C,** Distal interphalangeal joint.

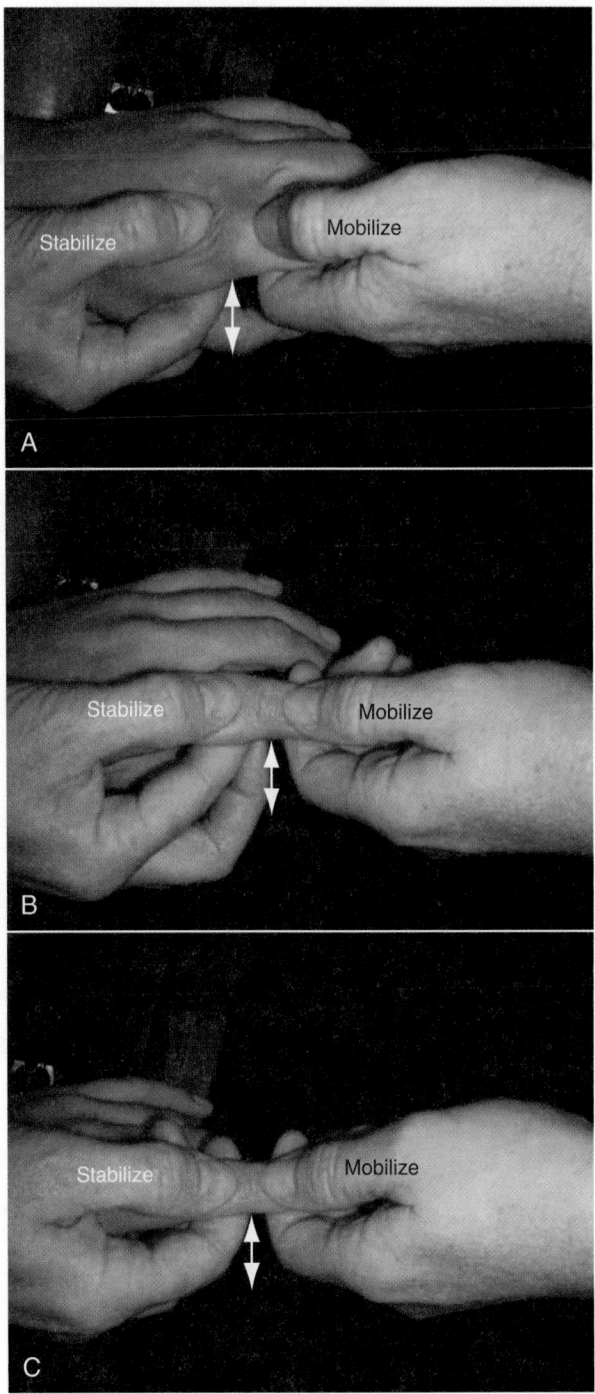

Figure 7-95 Anteroposterior glide of the joints of the fingers. **A,** Metacarpophalangeal joint. **B,** Proximal interphalangeal joint. **C,** Distal interphalangeal joint.

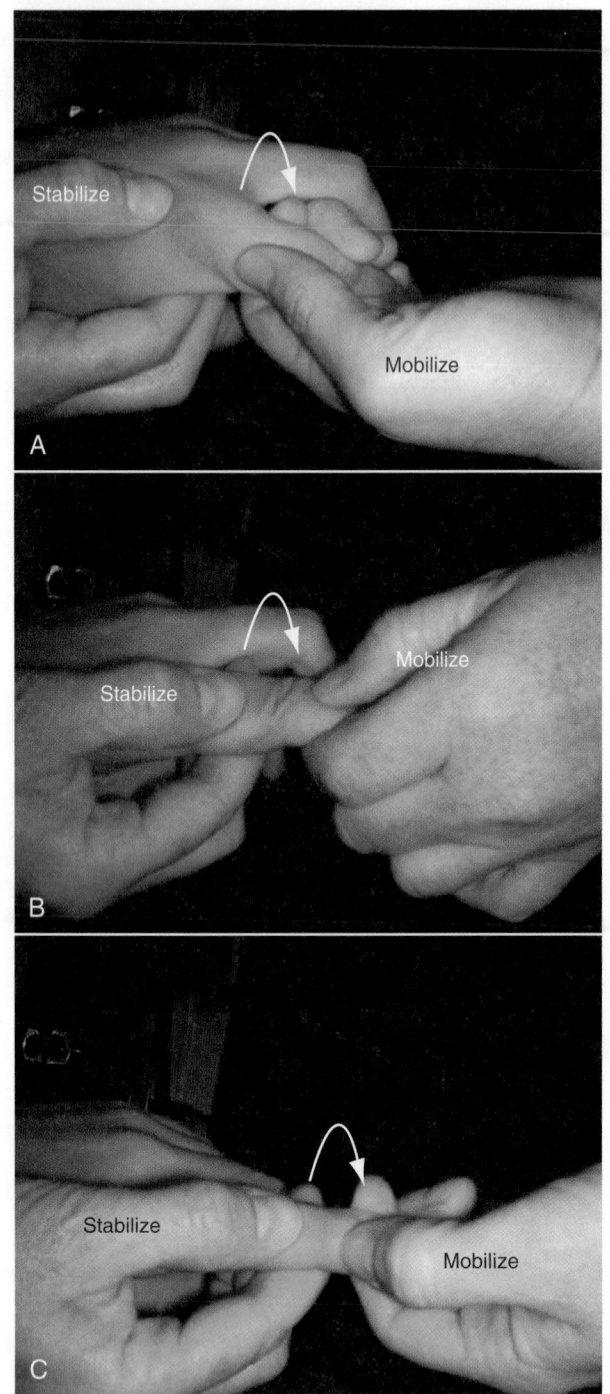

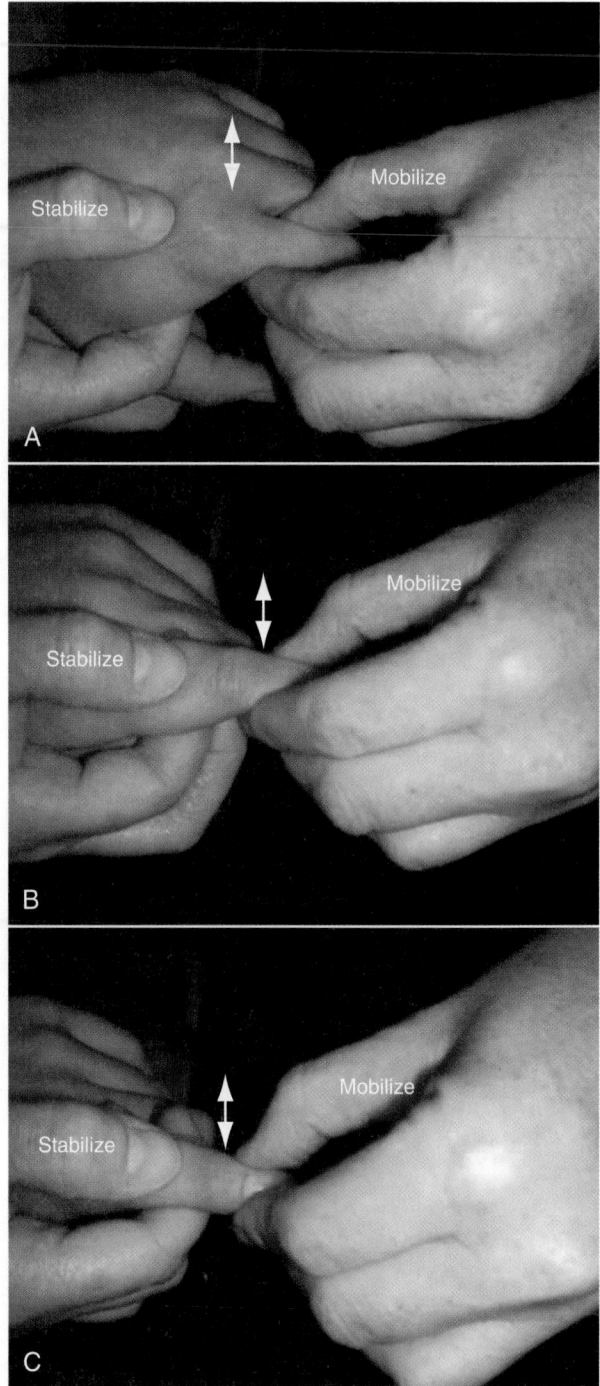

Figure 7-96 Rotation of the joints of the fingers. A, Metacarpophalangeal joint. **B,** Proximal interphalangeal joint. **C,** Distal interphalangeal joint.

Figure 7-97 Side glide of the joints of the fingers. A, Metacarpophalangeal joint. **B,** Proximal interphalangeal joint. **C,** Distal interphalangeal joint.

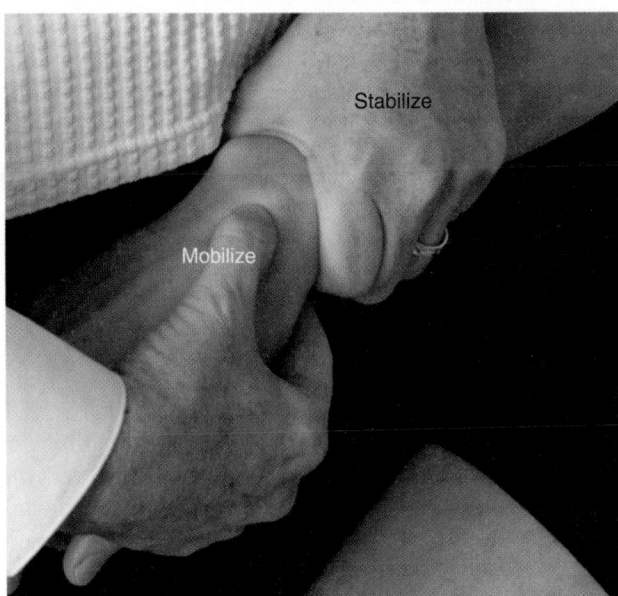

Figure 7-98 Palpation of the wrist.

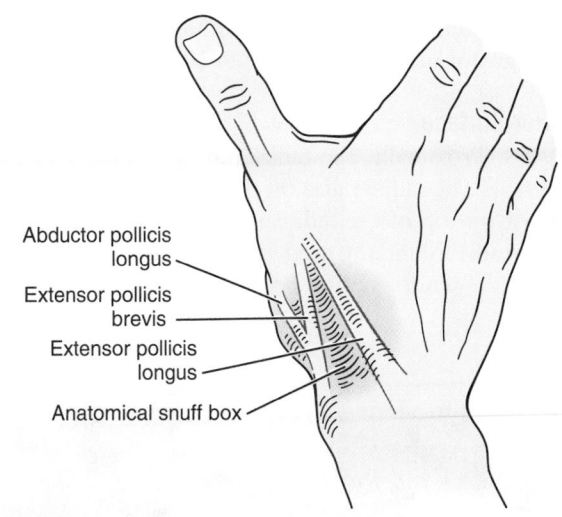

Figure 7-99 The anatomic snuff box. Note how the tendons of the abductor pollicis longus and extensor pollicis brevis diverge in proceeding distally. (Redrawn from Gardner E, et al: Anatomy: a regional study of human structure, London, 1975, WB Saunders, p. 135.)

thumb, which gives it a different angle of pull from that of the extensor pollicis brevis. With the wrist in anatomic position, the ulnar styloid is palpated on the medial aspect. The radial styloid extends farther distally than the ulnar styloid. By palpating over the dorsum of the wrist, crossing the radius and ulna, the examiner should attempt to palpate the six extensor tendon tunnels (noting any crepitus or restriction to movement), moving lateral to medial (see Figure 7-37):

- Tunnel 1: Abductor pollicis longus and extensor pollicis brevis
- Tunnel 2: Extensor carpi radialis longus and brevis
- Tunnel 3: Extensor pollicis longus
- Tunnel 4: Extensor digitorum and extensor indices
- Tunnel 5: Extensor digiti minimi
- Tunnel 6: Extensor carpi ulnaris

Carpal Bones. In the anatomic snuff box, the examiner can begin palpating the proximal row of carpal bones, starting with the scaphoid bone. When palpating the carpal bones, the examiner usually palpates them on the anterior and dorsal surfaces at the same time by applying anteroposterior joint play-like movements. The proximal row of carpal bones from lateral to medial (in the anatomic position) are the scaphoid, lunate, triquetrum (just below the ulnar styloid), and pisiform.

On the anterior aspect, the examiner should take care to ensure proper positioning of the lunate bone. If it dislocates or subluxes, it tends to move anteriorly into the carpal tunnel, which may lead to symptoms of carpal tunnel syndrome. The pisiform is often easier to palpate if the patient's wrist is flexed. The examiner may then palpate the pisiform where the flexor carpi ulnaris tendon inserts into it. Tenderness in the hollow between

the pisiform and ulnar styloid may indicate TFCC pathology.[11]

Returning to the anatomic snuff box and moving distally, the examiner palpates the trapezium bone. As this is done, the radial pulse is often palpated in the anatomic snuff box. The distal row of carpal bones from lateral to medial (in the anatomic position) is palpated individually: trapezium, trapezoid, capitate (distal to lunate and a slight indentation before the metacarpal), and hamate (distal to triquetrum; the hook of the hamate on the anterior surface is the easiest part to palpate). The hamate is most commonly injured by direct trauma.[76,125]

On the dorsal aspect, the examiner could begin palpation at the distal row of carpals. If the examiner places a finger over the middle metacarpal and slides along it until the finger drops into a "hole" or depression, this depression is the capitate bone. Moving medially (hamate) and laterally (trapezoid, trapezium), the other bones of the distal row may be palpated again by making anteroposterior joint play-like movements. If the examiner then moves proximally from the capitate, the finger rests on the lunate. Moving medially (triquetrum) and laterally (scaphoid), these carpals may be palpated.

Metacarpal Bones and Phalanges. The examiner returns to the trapezium bone and moves farther distally to palpate the first metacarpal joint and the first metacarpal bone. Moving medially, the examiner palpates each metacarpal bone on the anterior and dorsal surface in turn. A similar procedure is carried out for the metacarpophalangeal and interphalangeal joints and the phalanges. These structures are also palpated on their medial and lateral aspects for tenderness, swelling, altered temperature, or other signs of pathology (Figure 7-100).

Anterior Surface

Pulses. Proximally, the radial and ulnar pulses are palpated first. The radial pulse on the anterolateral aspect of the wrist on top of the radius is easiest to palpate and is the one most frequently used when taking a pulse. It runs between the tendons of flexor carpi radialis and abductor

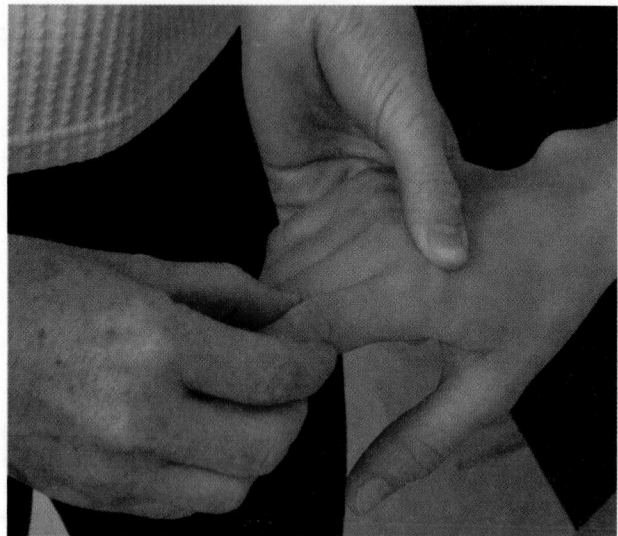

Figure 7-100 Palpation of the proximal interphalangeal joint of the second finger.

pollicis longus. The ulnar pulse may be palpated lateral to the tendon of flexor carpi ulnaris. It is more difficult to palpate because it runs deeper and lies under the pisiform and the palmar fascia.

Tendons. Moving across the anterior aspect, the examiner may be able to palpate the long flexor tendons (see Figure 7-37) in a lateral-to-medial direction: flexor carpi radialis, flexor pollicis longus, flexor digitorum superficialis, flexor digitorum profundus, palmaris longus, and flexor carpi ulnaris (inserts into pisiform). The examiner should also palpate the hollow between the flexor carpi ulnaris, the pisiform, and the ulnar styloid. In this hollow lies the triangular cartilaginous disc or TFCC.[75] The palmaris longus (if present) lies over the tendons of the flexor digitorum superficialis, which lie over the tendons of the flexor digitorum profundus. The palmaris longus tendon may sometimes be used for tendon repairs or transfers.

Palmar Fascia and Intrinsic Muscles. The examiner should then move distally to palpate the palmar fascia and intrinsic muscles of the thenar and hypothenar eminences for indications of pathology.

Skin Flexion Creases. From an anatomic point of view, the examiner should note the various skin flexion creases of the wrist, hand, and fingers (Figure 7-101). The flexion creases indicate lines of adherence between the skin and fascia with no intervening adipose tissue. The following creases should be noted:

1. The proximal skin crease of the wrist indicates the upper limit of the synovial sheaths of the flexor tendons.

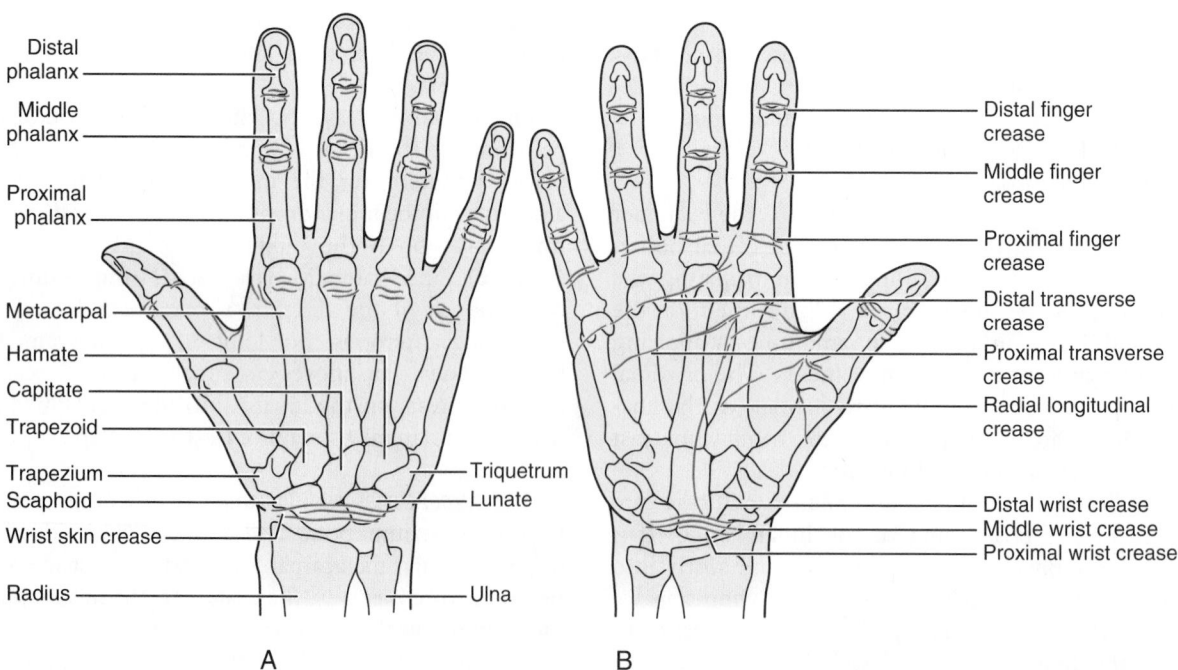

Figure 7-101 Bony landmarks and skin creases of the hand and wrist. **A,** Dorsal view. **B,** Palmar view. (Adapted from Tubiana R: The hand, Philadelphia, 1981, WB Saunders, p. 619.)

2. The middle skin crease of the wrist indicates the wrist (radiocarpal) joint.
3. The distal skin crease of the wrist indicates the upper margin of the flexor retinaculum.
4. The radial longitudinal skin crease of the palm encircles the thenar eminence. (Palm readers refer to this line as the "life line.")
5. The proximal transverse line of the palm runs across the shafts of the metacarpal bones, indicating the superficial palmar arterial arch. (Palm readers refer to this line as the "head line.")
6. The distal transverse line of the palm lies over the heads of the second to fourth metacarpals. (Palm readers refer to this line as the "love line.")
7. The proximal skin crease of the fingers is 2 cm (0.8 inch) distal to the metacarpophalangeal joints.
8. The middle skin crease of the fingers is made up of two lines and lies over the proximal interphalangeal joints.
9. The distal skin crease of the fingers lies over the distal interphalangeal joints.
10. On the flexor and extensor aspects, the skin creases over the proximal and distal interphalangeal joints lie proximal to the joint. On the extensor aspect, the metacarpophalangeal creases lie proximal to the joint; on the flexor aspect, they lie distal to the joint.

Arches. In addition, the examiner should ensure the viability of the arches of the hand (see Figure 7-4). The carpal transverse arch is the result of the shape of the carpal bones, which in part forms the carpal tunnel. The flexor retinaculum forms the roof for the tunnel. The metacarpal transverse arch is formed by the metacarpal bones, and its shape can have great variability because of the mobility of these bones. This arch is most evident when the palm is cupped. The longitudinal arch is made of the carpal bones, metacarpal bones, and phalanges. The keystone of this arch is the metacarpophalangeal joints, which provide stability and support for the arch. Weakness or atrophy of the intrinsic muscles of the hand leads to a loss of these arches. The deformity is most obvious with paralysis of the median and ulnar nerve, which results in an "ape hand" deformity.

Diagnostic Imaging

Plain Film Radiography

A routine wrist series of x-rays involves the following views; anteroposterior (AP), lateral, and scaphoid.[126] Motion views are sometimes taken, especially if instability is suspected. Common forearm, wrist, and hand x-ray views are shown in the following box.

Anteroposterior View.[127] The examiner should note the shape and position of the bones (Figure 7-102), watching for any evidence of fractures (Figure 7-107) or displacement, decrease in the joint spaces, or change in bone density, which may be caused by avascular necrosis.

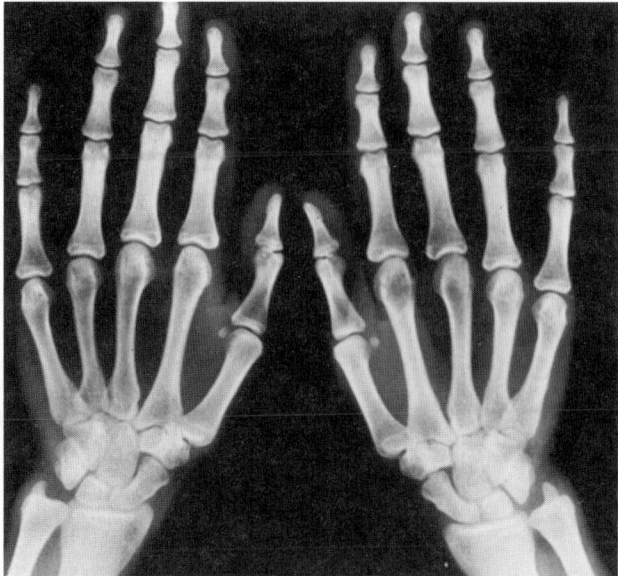

Figure 7-102 Radiograph showing the bones of both hands. The thumb metacarpal is the shortest, and the index metacarpal is by far the longest. The first and second phalanges of the middle and ring fingers are longer than those of the index finger. Note the interlocking design of the carpometacarpal articulations and the saddle shape in opposing planes of the articular surfaces of the trapezium and the base of the first metacarpal. (From Tubiana R: The hand, Philadelphia, 1981, WB Saunders, p. 21.)

Common X-Ray Views of the Forearm, Wrist, and Hand

- Anteroposterior/posteroanterior view
  - Forearm (Figure 7-103, *B*)
  - Wrist (in neutral) (Figure 7-104, *B*)
  - Hand (Figure 7-105)
  - Digits (Figure 7-106, *C*)
- Lateral view
  - Forearm (Figure 7-103, *A*)
  - Wrist (in neutral) (see Figure 7-107, *B*)
  - Hand (see Figure 7-110, *B*)
  - Digits (Figure 7-106, *A*)
- Scaphoid view (see Figure 7-109, *A*)
- Carpal tunnel (axial) view (see Figure 7-116)
- Clenched fist view (see Figure 7-117)
- Posteroanterior oblique view (Figure 7-104, *A*)
- Ulnar deviation of wrist (see Figure 7-110, *A*)
- Radial deviation of wrist (see Figure 7-110, *A*)
- Oblique view of digit (Figure 7-106, *B*)

The arcs of the wrist (Figure 7-108) show the normal relation of the carpal bones in the AP view. If avascular necrosis is present, there is rarefaction and increased density of the bone (increased whiteness) and possibly sclerosis (patchy appearance) of the bone. Avascular necrosis is often seen in the scaphoid bone (Figures 7-109 and 7-110, *A*) after a fracture or in the lunate in Kienböck disease (Figure 7-110, *B*).[56] In some cases, the TFCC may

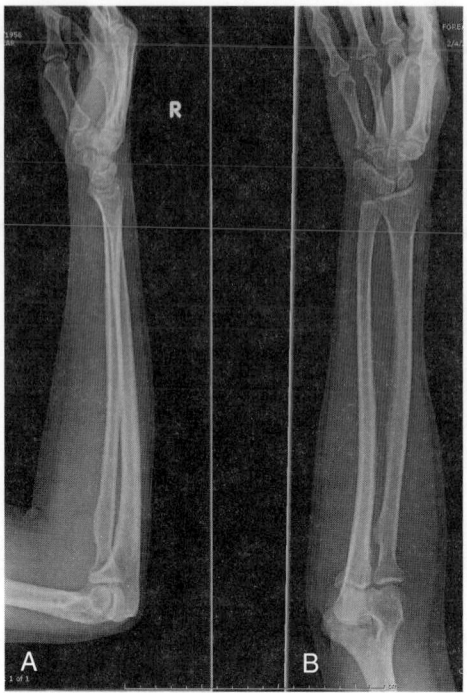

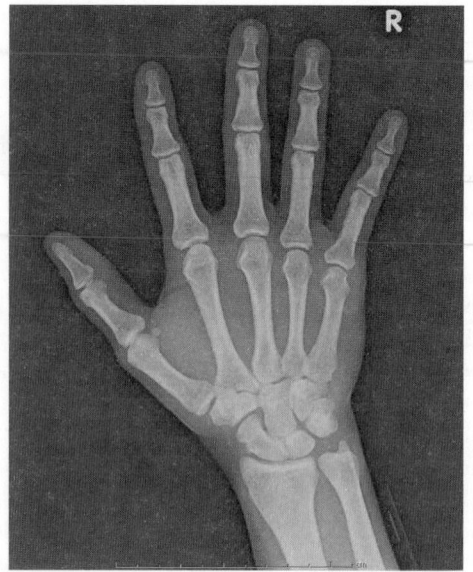

Figure 7-105 Posteroanterior view of the hand.

Figure 7-103 Radiographic views of the forearm. A, Lateral.
B, Posteroanterior.

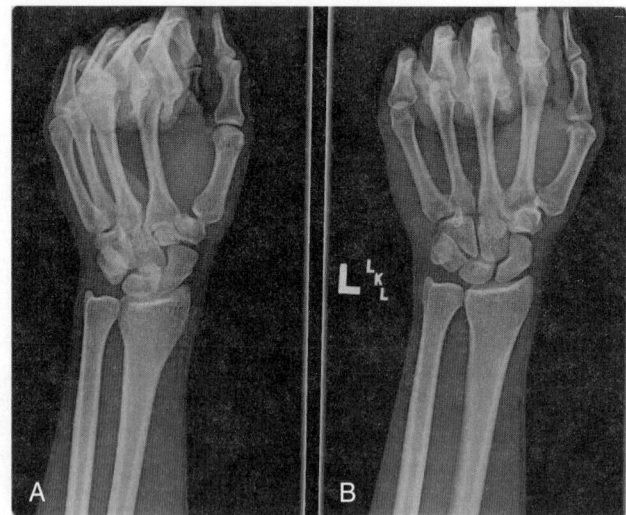

Figure 7-104 Radiographic views of the wrist (in neutral). A, Oblique. **B,** Posteroanterior.

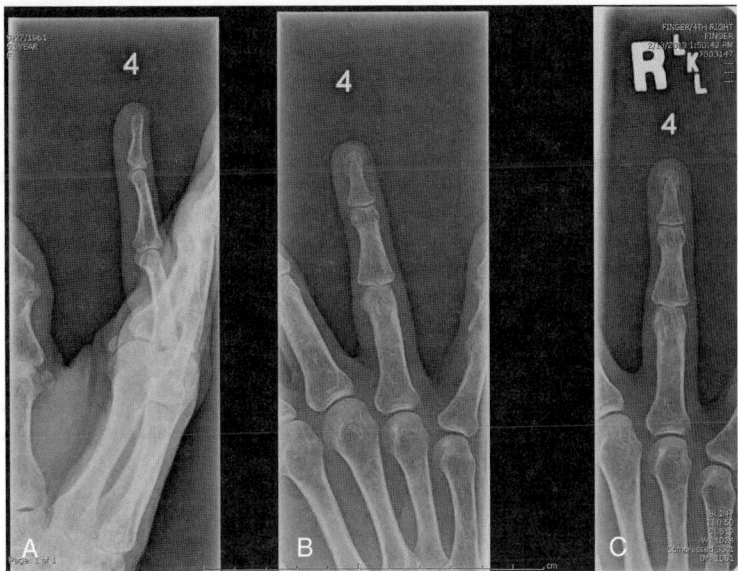

Figure 7-106 Radiographic views of the digits. A, Lateral. **B,** Oblique. **C,** Anteroposterior.

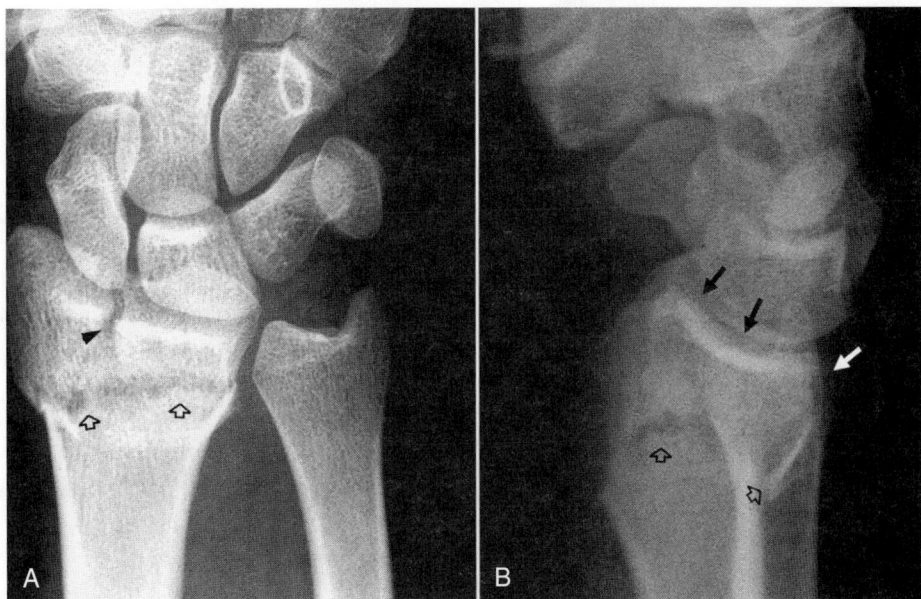

Figure 7-107 Wrist fracture: Colles' fracture. A, Observe the transverse fracture of the distal portion of the radius *(open arrows)* with extension into the radiocarpal joint *(arrowhead)*. **B,** In the lateral projection, dorsal angulation of the articular surface of the radius *(solid arrows)* is apparent and caused by compaction of bone dorsally. This injury is a three-part fracture. The ulnar styloid process is intact, and no evidence of subluxation of the distal portion of the ulna can be seen. (From Resnick D, Kransdorf MJ: Bone and joint imaging, Philadelphia, 2005, WB Saunders, p. 851.)

be visualized (Figure 7-111). The AP view may also be used to show dislocations of the lunate (Figure 7-112, *A*), the distal ulna (Figure 7-112, *B*), the lunatotriquetral relation (Figure 7-112, *C*), and ulnar variance (length of ulna in relation to radius).[128]

The AP view of the wrist and hand is also used to determine the skeletal age of a patient.[49] The left hand and wrist are used for study because they are thought to be less influenced by environmental factors. The method used in this technique is based on the fact that after an **ossification center** appears (Figure 7-113), it changes its

shape and size in a systematic manner as the ossification gradually spreads throughout the cartilaginous parts of the skeleton. The wrist and hand are studied because several bones are available for overall comparison, including the carpal bones, the metacarpal growth plates (seen at distal end of bone), and the phalangeal growth plates (seen at proximal end of bone). The patient's hand is compared with standard plates[76] until one plate is found that best approximates that of the patient. There is one standard for males and another for females. In two-thirds of the population, skeletal age is no more than 1 year above or below chronologic age. Acceleration or retardation of 3 years or more is considered abnormal. At birth, none of the carpal bones is visible (see Figure 1-27). This method may be used up to age 20 when the bones of the hand and wrist have fused.

Lateral View. The examiner should note the shape and position of bones for any evidence of fracture and/or displacement (Figure 7-114, *A*). The lateral view is also useful in detecting swelling around the carpal bones and for measuring the relation of the scaphoid and lunate to the radius and metacarpals (Figure 7-115).[128]

Scaphoid View. This view isolates the scaphoid to show a possible fracture (see Figure 7-109, *A*).

Carpal Tunnel (Axial) View. This view is used to show the margins of the carpal tunnel and is useful for determining fractures of the hook of hamate and trapezium (Figure 7-116).

Clenched-Fist (Anteroposterior) View. This view is sometimes useful to show increased gapping between the carpal bones, indicating instability (Figure 7-117).[129]

Arthrography

If the history and clinical assessment suggest a ligament or fibrocartilage problem of the wrist, arthrography can

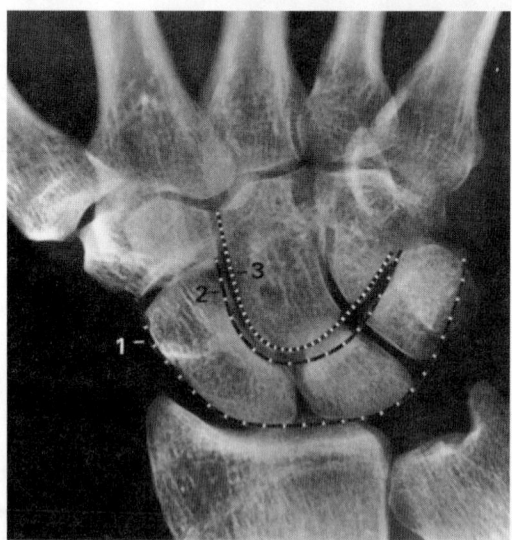

Figure 7-108 Wrist arcs. Three arcuate lines can normally be constructed along the carpal articular surfaces: *1,* Along the proximal margins of the scaphoid, lunate, and triquetrum; *2,* along the distal aspects of these bones; *3,* along the proximal margins of the capitate and hamate. (From Weissman BNW, Sledge CB: Orthopedic radiology, Philadelphia, 1986, WB Saunders, p. 117.)

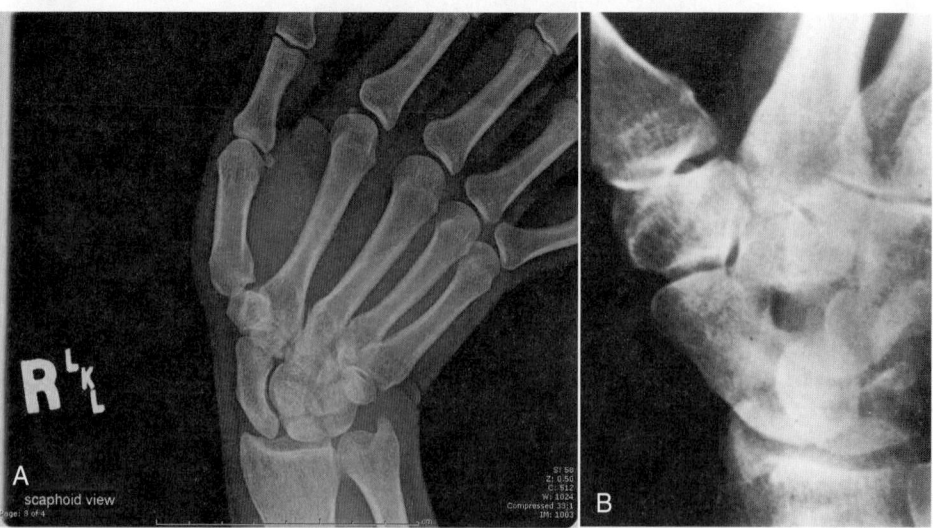

Figure 7-109 Radiographs of the normal scaphoid. A, Scaphoid view. **B,** Lateral view. (**B,** From Tubiana R: The hand, Philadelphia, 1981, WB Saunders, p. 659.)

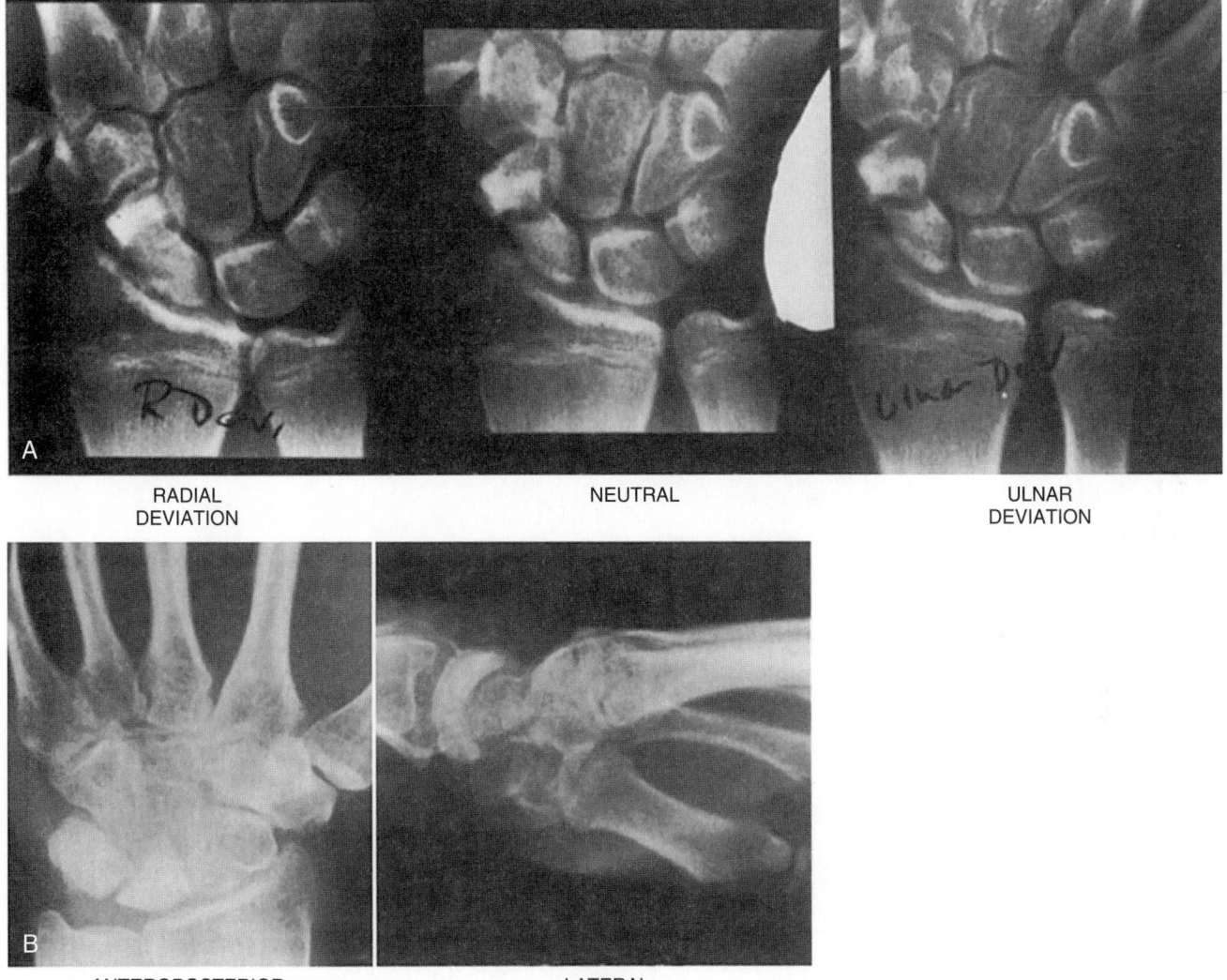

RADIAL
DEVIATION

NEUTRAL

ULNAR
DEVIATION

ANTEROPOSTERIOR
VIEW

LATERAL
VIEW

Figure 7-110 Avascular necrosis of the carpal bones. A, Scaphoid fracture shown in three positions. **B,** Lunate fracture and sclerosis in Kienböck disease. (**A,** From Cooney WP, Dobyns JH, Linscheid RL: Fractures of the scaphoid: a rational approach to management. Clin Orthop 149:92, 1980. **B,** From Beckenbaugh RD, Shives TC, Dobyns JH, et al: Kienböck's disease, the natural history of Kienböck's disease and consideration of lunate fractures. Clin Orthop 149:99, 1980.)

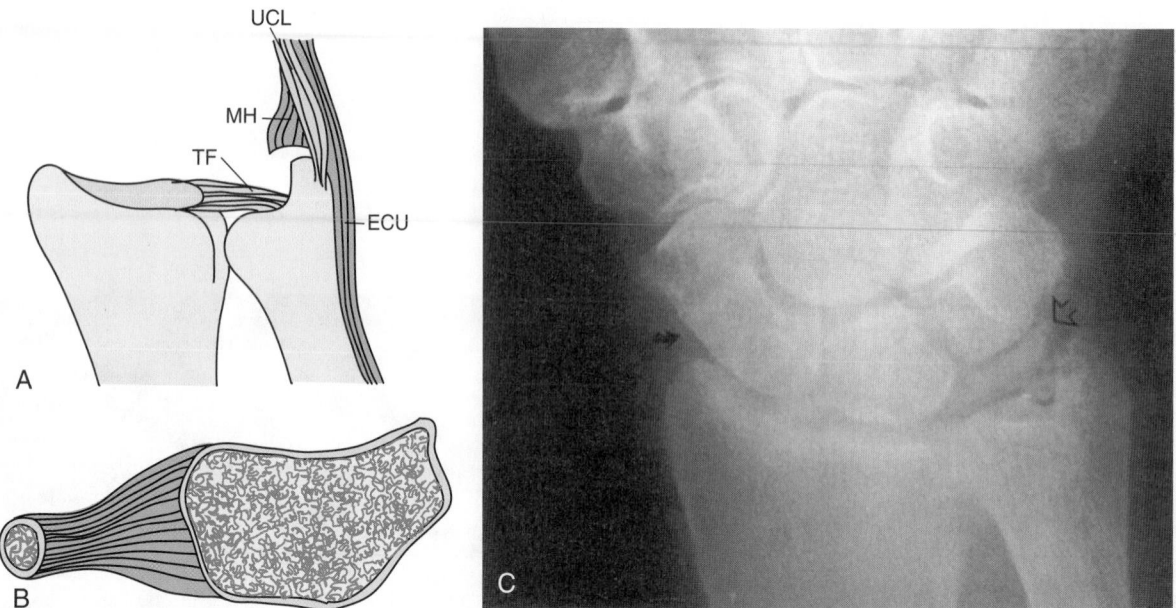

Figure 7-111 Triangular fibrocartilage complex (TFCC). A, This complex includes the triangular fibrocartilage *(articular disc, TF)*, the meniscus homolog *(MH)*, the ulnar collateral ligament *(UCL)*, and the dorsal and volar radioulnar ligaments (not shown). The extensor carpi ulnaris tendon *(ECU)* is shown. **B,** The triangular fibrocartilage *(dotted area)* attaches to the ulnar border of the radius and the distal ulna. The triangular shape is evident on this transverse section through the radius and ulnar styloid. The volar aspect of the wrist is at the top. **C,** Chondrocalcinosis. There is heavy calcification of the articular cartilage *(curved arrow)* and the area of the TFCC *(open arrow)*. (From Weissman BNW, Sledge CB: Orthopedic radiology, Philadelphia, 1986, WB Saunders, p. 115.)

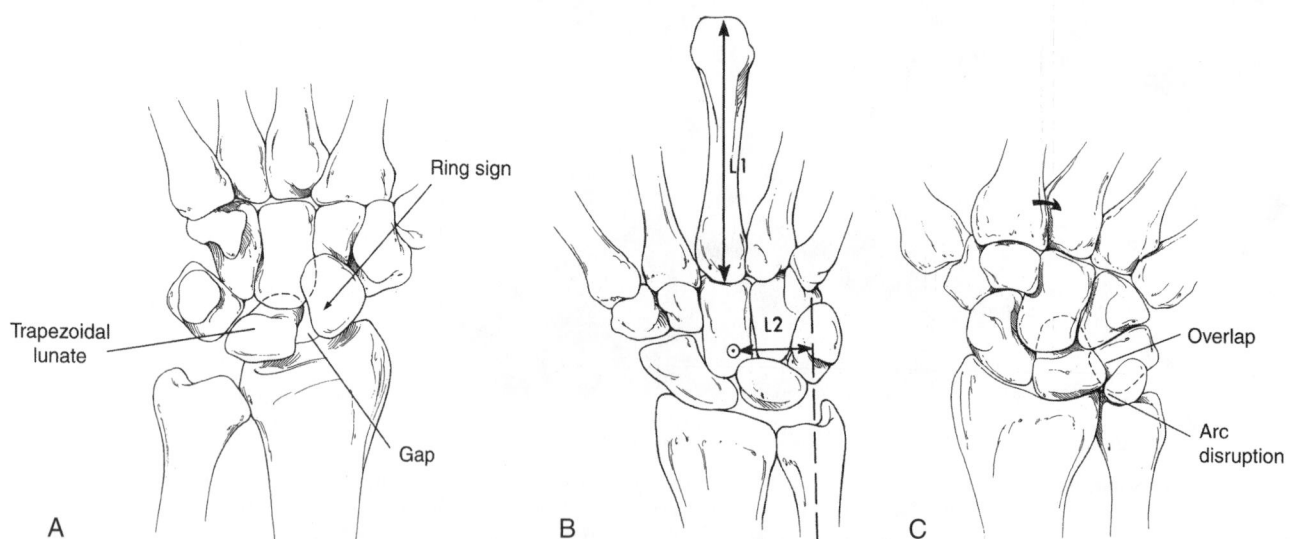

Figure 7-112 A, Scapholunate dissociation. The scaphoid is palmar flexed, producing a cortical ring sign. A gap is present between the scaphoid and the lunate. The lunate appears trapezoidal. **B,** Ulnar translocation can be identified radiographically from the ratio of the distance between the center of the capitate and a line along the longitudinal axis of the ulna *(L2)* divided by the length of the third metacarpal *(L1)*. In normal wrists, this ratio is 0.30 ± 0.03; it is decreased in wrists with ulnar translocation. **C,** Lunatotriquetral instability. Shortened scaphoid and cortical ring sign are present without scapholunate widening. Lunate appears triangular. Lunatotriquetral widening is not present. (© 1993 American Academy of Orthopaedic Surgeons. Reprinted from the Journal of the American Academy of Orthopaedic Surgeons: A Comprehensive Review, 1[1], pp. 14–15 with permission.)

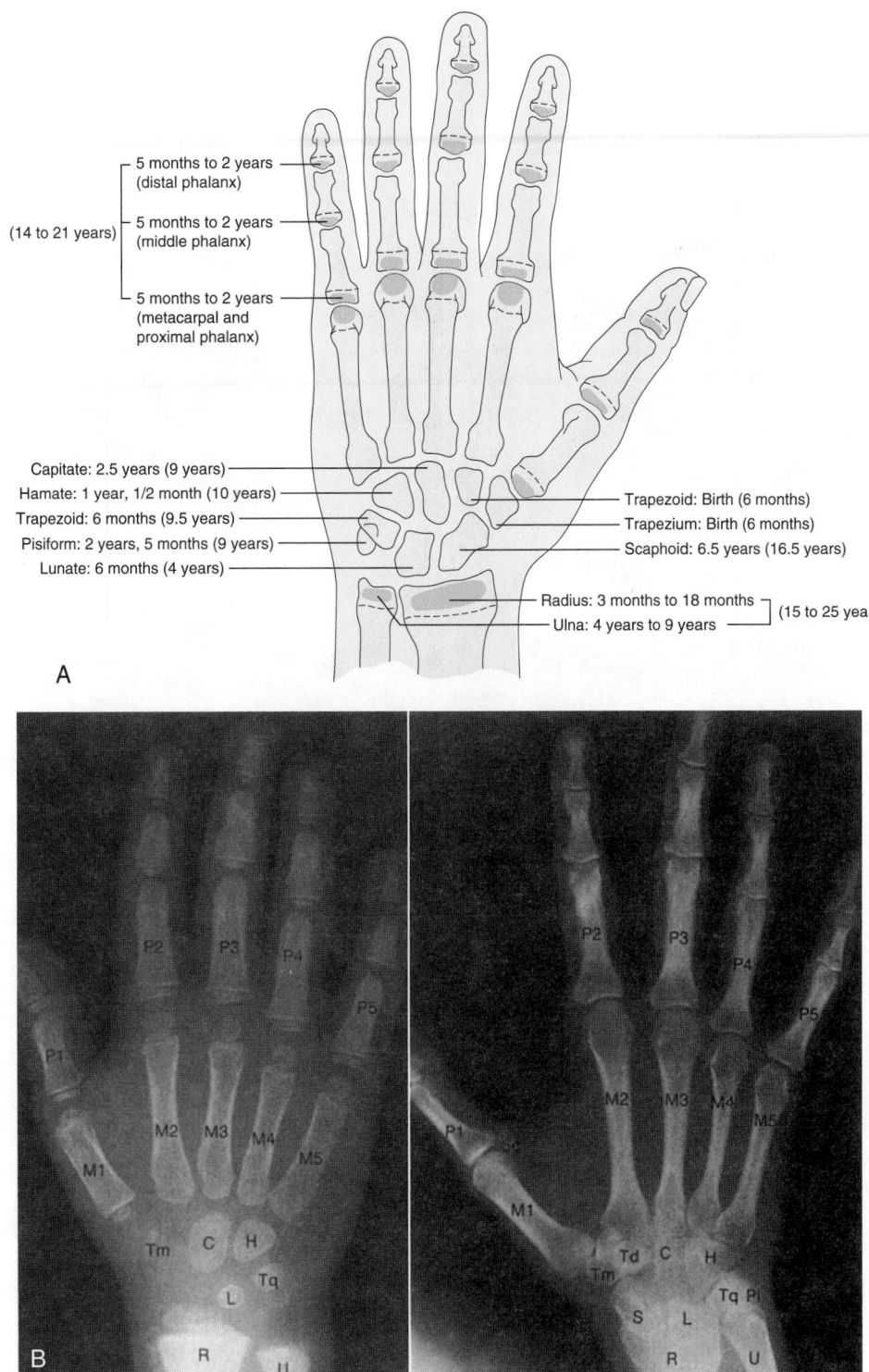

Figure 7-113 Ossification centers of the hand. A, Dates of appearance of ossification centers are shown with dates of fusion in parentheses. Note the different proximal and distal locations of growth plates. **B,** Radiographs of the hand and wrist of a 4- to 5-year-old boy or 3- to 4-year-old girl *(left)* and of an adult *(right)*. *C,* Capitate; *H,* hamate; *L,* lunate; *M,* metacarpal; *P,* phalanx; *Pi,* pisiform; *R,* radius; *S,* scaphoid; *Td,* trapezoid; *Tm,* trapezium; *Tq,* triquetrum; *U,* ulna. (**A,** Redrawn from Tubiana R: The hand, Philadelphia, 1981, WB Saunders, p. 11. **B,** From Liebgott B: The anatomical basis of dentistry, St Louis, 1986, CV Mosby.)

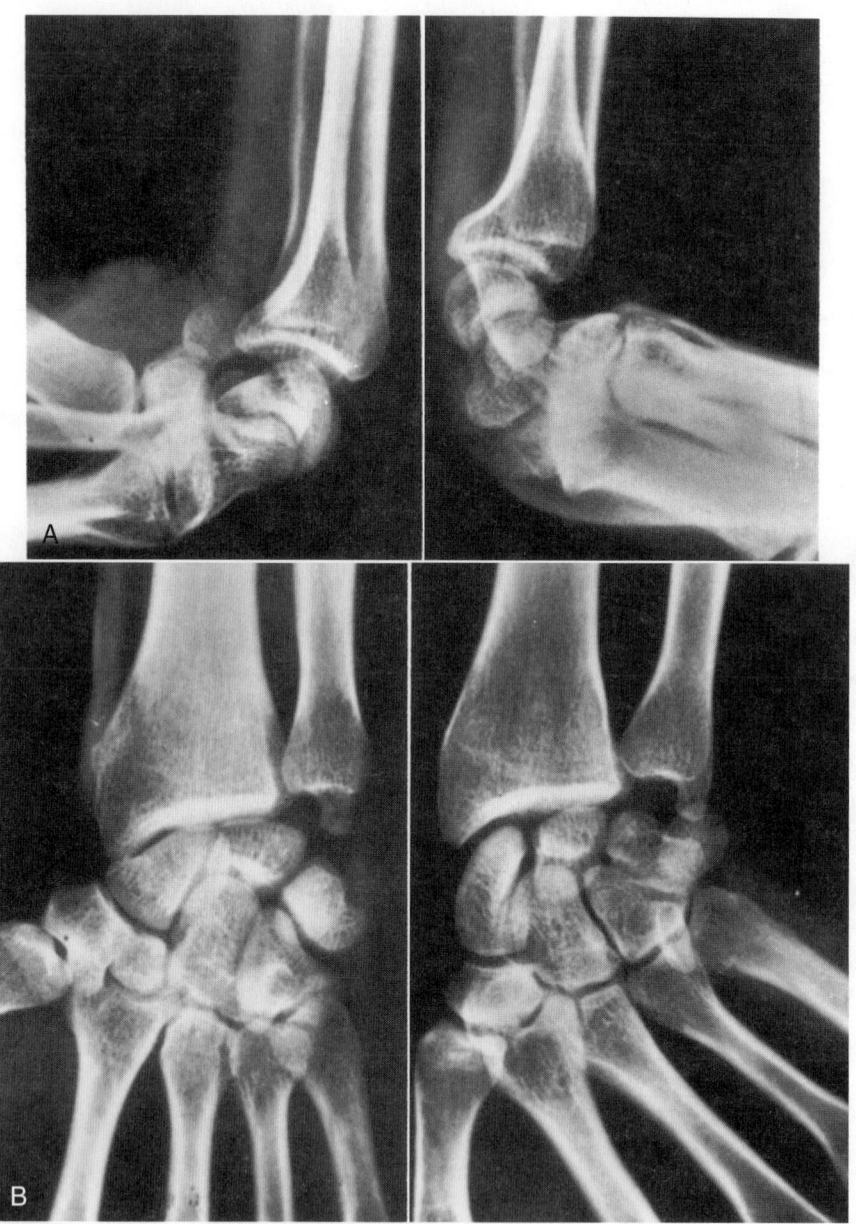

Figure 7-114 A, Lateral radiographs showing wrist flexion *(left)* and extension *(right)*. **B,** Posteroanterior views of wrist in radial *(left)* and ulnar *(right)* deviation. Note the change in the form of the lunate, indicating a slipping toward the front in the radial slant and toward the rear in the ulnar slant. (From Tubiana R: The hand, Philadelphia, 1981, WB Saunders, p. 655.)

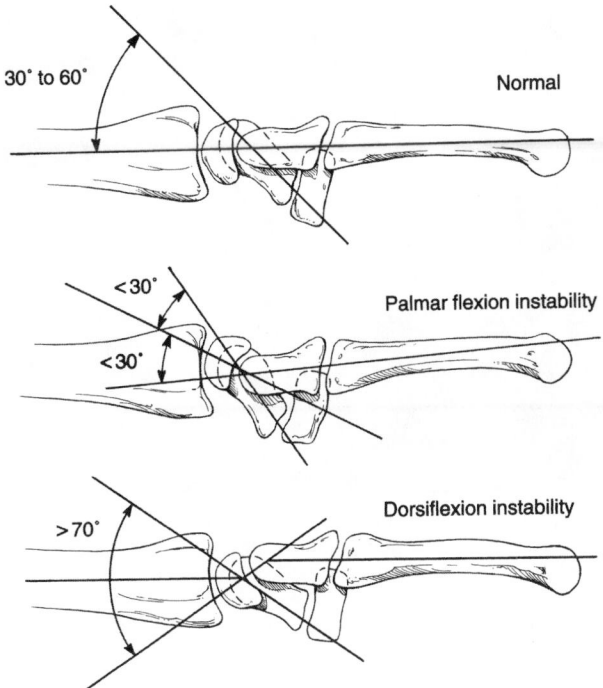

Figure 7-115 Scapholunate angle measurement in normal wrist and in carpal instability. (© 1993 American Academy of Orthopaedic Surgeons. Reprinted from the Journal of the American Academy of Orthopaedic Surgeons: A Comprehensive Review, 1[1], p. 14 with permission.)

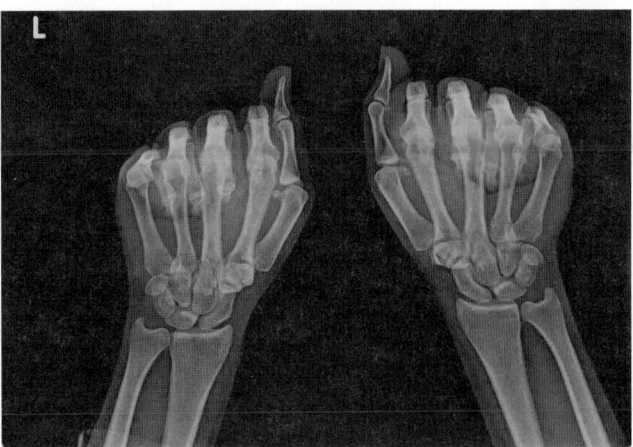

Figure 7-117 Clenched fist view.

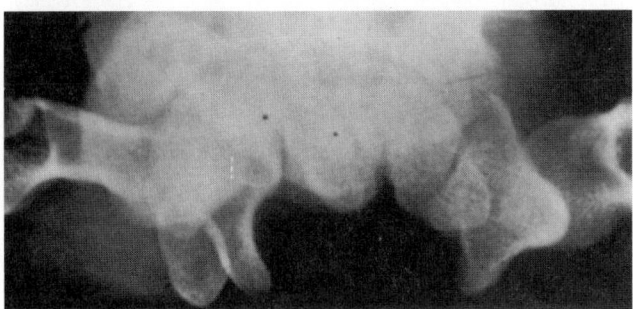

Figure 7-116 Carpal tunnel or axial radiographic view. (From Tubiana R: The hand, Philadelphia, 1981, WB Saunders, p. 662.)

help to confirm the diagnosis (Figure 7-118). Arthrograms, especially of the wrist, can demonstrate compartment communication, tendon sheaths, synovial irregularity, loose bodies, and cartilage abnormalities.

Computed Tomography

Computed tomography (CT) can be used to visualize bones and soft tissue; by making computer-assisted "slices," it allows tissues to be better visualized (Figure 7-119).

Magnetic Resonance Imaging

Magnetic resonance imaging (MRI) is a noninvasive technique that is useful for visualizing the soft tissues of the wrist and hand and provides the best means of delineating the soft tissues (primarily ligaments and the TFCC), as well as showing instability problems and bone.[130–132] For example, it can show swelling of the median nerve in carpal tunnel syndrome, tears in the triangular fibrocartilage (Figure 7-120), and thickening of tendon sheaths (Figure 7-121).

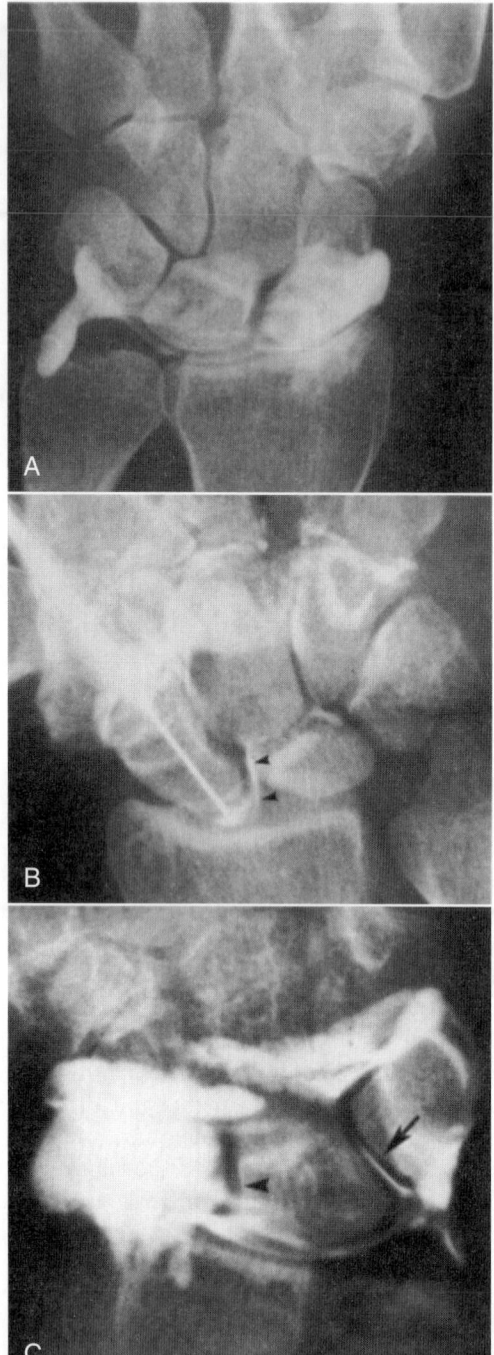

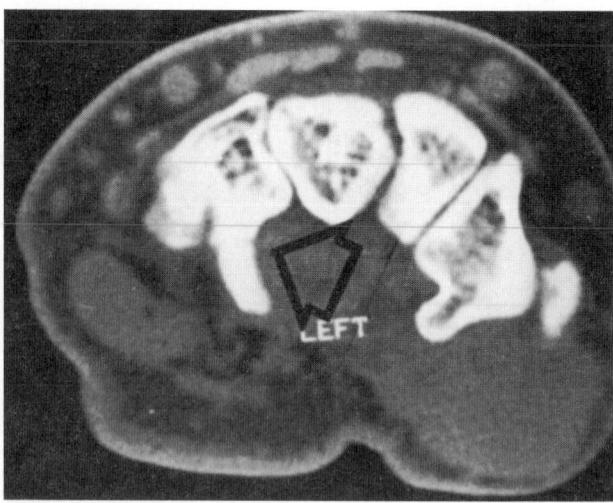

Figure 7-119 A fracture of the left hamate hook *(arrow)* as shown by a computed tomographic (CT) scan. In this instance, fracture was suspected on the carpal tunnel view but was not demonstrated as well as it was by CT scan. (From Zemel NP, Stark HH: Fractures and dislocations of the carpal bones. Clin Sports Med 5:720, 1986.)

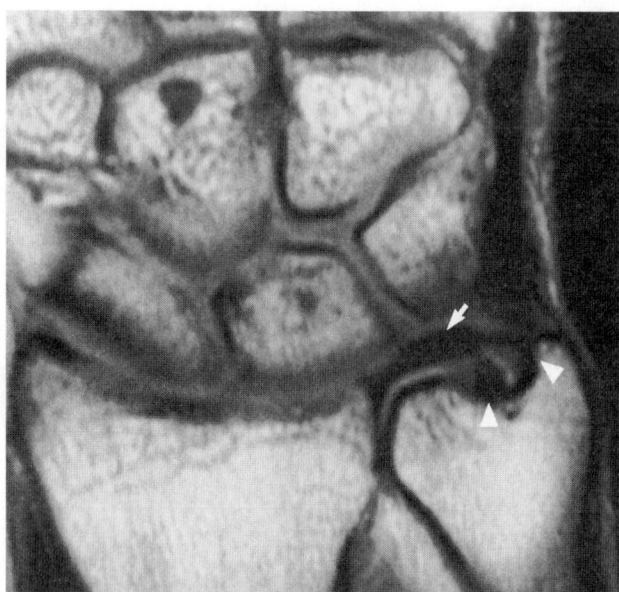

Figure 7-118 A, Posteroanterior view of the wrist after a normal radio-carpal joint arthrogram. Contrast remains confined to the radiocarpal space. **B,** After a radiocarpal joint space injection, contrast tracks *(arrowheads)* through a disrupted scapholunate ligament to fill the midcarpal and carpometacarpal joint spaces. **C,** After a radiocarpal joint space arthrogram, the scapholunate ligament is intact because contrast has not yet filled the scapholunate space *(arrowhead);* however, contrast tracks through the lunatotriquetral joint space *(arrow)* as a result of lunato-triquetral ligament disruption. (From Lightman DM: The wrist and its disorders, Philadelphia, 1988, WB Saunders, p. 89.)

Figure 7-120 Triangular fibrocartilage complex (TFCC): Normal appearance. On a coronal intermediate-weighted (TR/TE, 2000/20) spin echo magnetic resonance image, observe the low-signal intensity of the triangular fibrocartilage *(arrow)* with bifurcated bands of low-signal intensity *(arrowheads)* attaching to or near the styloid process of the ulna. The scapholunate and lunotriquetral interosseous ligaments are not well seen on this image. Note the two bone islands, which appear as foci of low-signal intensity, in the lunate and capitate. (From Resnick D, Kransdorf MJ: Bone and joint imaging, Philadelphia, 2005, WB Saunders, p. 907. Courtesy of AG Bergman, MD, Stanford, CA.)

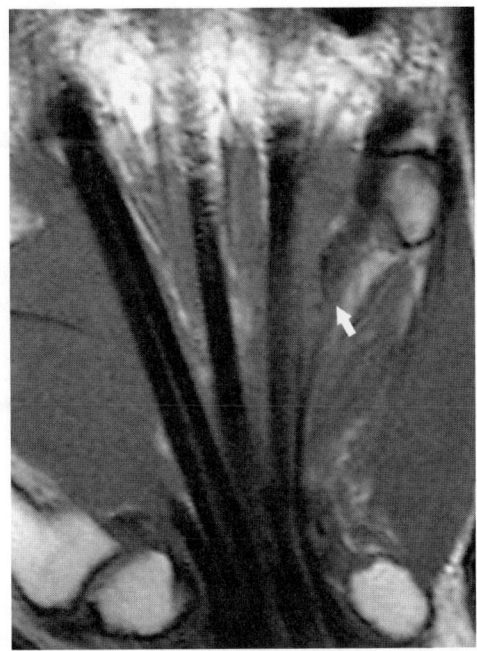

Figure 7-121 Tendon rupture. Coronal T1-weighted (TR/TE, 500/14) spin echo from magnetic resonance image of the hand shows rupture of the flexor tendon of the little finger. The free edge of the thickened, retracted, ruptured tendon *(arrow)* is well seen. (From Resnick D, Kransdor MJ: Bone and joint imaging, Philadelphia, 2005, WB Saunders, p. 913.)

PRÉCIS OF THE FOREARM, WRIST, AND HAND ASSESSMENT*

History (sitting)
Observation (sitting)
Examination (sitting)
  Active movements
    Pronation of the forearm
    Supination of the forearm
    Wrist flexion
    Wrist extension
    Radial deviation of wrist
    Ulnar deviation of wrist
    Finger flexion (at MCP, PIP, and DIP joints)
    Flexion extension (at MCP, PIP, and DIP joints)
    Finger abduction
    Finger adduction
    Thumb flexion
    Thumb extension
    Thumb abduction
    Thumb adduction
    Opposition of the thumb and little finger
  Passive movements (as in active movements)
  Resisted isometric movements (as in active movements, in
    the neutral position)
  Functional testing
    Functional grip tests
    Pinch tests
    Coordination tests
  Special tests (sitting)
    For ligament, capsule and joint instability:
      Axial load test
      Catch-up clunk test
      Dorsal capitate displacement apprehension test

      Ligamentous instability test (fingers)
      Lunotriquetral ballottement (Reagan's) test
      Murphy's sign
      Sitting hands test
      Supination lift test
      Thumb ulnar collateral ligament laxity or
        instability test
      Triangular fibrocartilage complex load test
        (Sharpey's test)
      Ulnar fovea sign test
      Ulnar styloid triquetral impaction (USTI)
        provocation test
      Ulnomeniscotriquetral dorsal glide test
      Watson (scaphoid shift) test
    For tendons and muscles:
      Finkelstein test
      Sweater finger sign
    For neurological dysfunction:
      Carpal compression test
      Froment paper sign
      Phalen's (wrist flexion) test
      Reverse phalen's (prayer) test
      Tinel sign at wrist
      Weber's (Moberg's) two-point discrimination test
    For circulation and swelling:
      Allen test
      Digital blood flow
      Figure of eight measurement for swelling
  Reflexes and cutaneous distribution (sitting)
    Reflexes
    Sensory scan

Continued

PRÉCIS OF THE FOREARM, WRIST, AND HAND ASSESSMENT—cont'd

Nerve injuries
Median nerve
Ulnar nerve
Radial nerve
Joint play movements (sitting)
   Long-axis extension at the wrist and fingers (MCP, PIP, and DIP joints)
   Anteroposterior glide at the wrist and fingers (MCP, PIP, and DIP joints)

Side glide at the wrist and fingers (MCP, PIP, and DIP joints)
Side tilt at the wrist
Anteroposterior glide at the intermetacarpal joints
Rotation at the MCP, PIP, and DIP joints
Individual carpal bone mobility
Palpation (sitting)
Diagnostic imaging

DIP, distal interphalangeal; *MCP*, metacarpophalangeal; *PIP*, proximal interphalangeal.

*After any examination, the patient should be warned of the possibility of exacerbation of symptoms as a result of the assessment.

CASE STUDIES

When doing these case studies, the examiner should list the appropriate questions to be asked and why they are being asked, what to look for and why, and what things should be tested and why. Depending on the answers of the patient (and the examiner should consider different responses), several possible causes of the patient's problem may become evident (examples are given in parentheses). A differential diagnosis chart should be made up. The examiner can then decide how different diagnoses may affect the treatment plan. For example, a 26-year-old man comes to you complaining of pain and clicking in his wrist. He is a carpenter, and it especially bothers him when he uses a screwdriver. See Table 7-14 for an example of a differential diagnosis chart for this patient.

1. A 31-year-old pregnant woman complains of pain in the right hand with a duration of 3 months. The pain awakens her at night and is relieved only by vigorous rubbing of her hand and motion of the fingers and wrist. There is some tingling in the index and middle fingers. Describe your assessment for this patient (carpal tunnel syndrome versus lunate subluxation).

2. An 18-year-old man comes to you after suffering a right scaphoid fracture. He has been in a cast for 12 weeks, and clinical union has been achieved. Describe your assessment for this patient.

3. A 16-year-old girl comes to you complaining of thumb pain. She was skiing during the weekend and fell, landing on her ski pole. She hurt her thumb when she fell. Describe your assessment for this patient (ulnar collateral ligament sprain versus Bennett fracture).

4. A 48-year-old man comes to you complaining of a painful hand. He happened to hit it against a metal door jam as he was going outside. During the next few days, the hand became swollen and painful, and he has become very protective of it.

Describe your assessment of this patient (Sudeck atrophy versus hand aneurysm).

5. A 52-year-old woman who has rheumatoid arthritis comes to you because her hands hurt and she has difficulty doing things functionally. Describe your assessment of this patient.

6. A 14-year-old boy comes to you complaining of wrist pain with swelling on the dorsum of the hand. He says he tripped and fell on the outstretched hand. He states the wrist hurt, the pain decreased, and then the swelling came on over 2 or 3 days. Describe your assessment of this patient (scaphoid fracture versus ganglion).

7. A 28-year-old man was in an industrial accident and lacerated the flexor tendons in the palm of his hand. Describe your assessment of this patient.

8. A 37-year-old woman comes to you complaining of pain and grating on the radial side of the wrist. Describe your assessment of this patient (cartilaginous disc versus scaphoid fracture).

9. A 72-year-old woman comes to you with a left Colles fracture. Describe your assessment of this patient.

TABLE **7-14**

Differential Diagnosis of Wrist Cartilaginous Disc and Degenerative Osteoarthritis

	Wrist Cartilaginous Disc	Degenerative Osteoarthritis
Mechanism of injury	Compression and pronation	Vibration, repetitive compression
Age affected	25 years and older	35 years and older
Active movement	Pain on compression and pronation Limited wrist extension more than flexion	Limited wrist flexion and extension
Passive movement	Pain on extension overpressure Pain on compression and pronation Tissue stretch end feel	Capsular pattern of wrist End feel is soft early, hard later
Resisted isometric movement	Pain on pronation	Possibly weak on wrist movements
Special tests	None	None
Reflexes and sensory distribution	Normal	Normal
Joint play	Pain on anteroposterior glide of radiocarpal joint	Pain on anteroposterior glide of radiocarpal and midcarpal joints
Palpation	Pain over lunate	Pain over affected carpal bones

REFERENCES

1. Chidgey JK: The distal radioulnar joint: problems and solutions. J Am Acad Orthop Surg 3:95–109, 1995.
2. Berger RA: The anatomy and basic biomechanics of the wrist joint. J Hand Surg 9:84–93, 1996.
3. Tubiana R, Thomiene JM, Mackin E: Examination of the hand and wrist, St Louis, 1996, CV Mosby.
4. Halikis MN, Taleisnik J: Soft-tissue injuries of the wrist. Clin Sports Med 15:235–259, 1996.
5. Gan BS, Richards RS, Roth JH: Arthroscopic treatment of triangular fibrocartilage tears. Orthop Clin North Am 26:721–729, 1995.
6. Palmer AD, Werner FW: The triangular fibrocartilage complex of the wrist: Anatomy and function. J Hand Surg Am 6:153–162, 1981.
7. Palmer AR, Werner FW: Biomechanics of the distal radioulnar joint. Clin Orthop 187:26–35, 1984.
8. Berger RA: The anatomy of the ligaments of the wrist and distal radioulnar joints. Clin Orthop Relat Res 383:32–40, 2001.
9. Rettig AC: Athletic injuries of the wrist and hand. Part I: traumatic injuries of the wrist. Am J Sports Med 31:1038–1048, 2003.
10. Steinberg BD, Plancher KD: Clinical anatomy of the wrist and elbow. Clin Sports Med 14:299–313, 1995.
11. Mayfield JK, Johnson RP, Kilcoyne RK: Carpal dislocations: pathomechanics and progressive perilunar instability. J Hand Surg Am 5:226–241, 1980.
12. Kozin SH: Perilunate injuries: Diagnosis and treatment. J Am Acad Orthop Surg 6:112–120, 1998.
13. Neumann DA: Kinesiology of the musculoskeletal system, ed 2, St Louis, 2010, CV Mosby.
14. Sarrafian SK, Melamed JL, Goshgarian GM: Study of wrist motion in flexion and extension. Clin Orthop 126:153–159, 1977.
15. Kapandji IA: The physiology of joints, vol. 1: upper limb, New York, 1970, Churchill Livingstone.
16. Nagle DJ: Evaluation of chronic wrist pain. J Am Acad Orthop Surg 8:45–55, 2000.
17. Rettig AC: Wrist injuries: avoiding diagnostic pitfalls. Phys Sportsmed 22:33–39, 1994.
18. Burton RI, Eaton RG: Common hand injuries in the athlete. Orthop Clin North Am 4:309–338, 1975.

19. Gonzalez-Iglesias J, Huijbregts P, Fernandez-de-las-Panas C, et al: Differential diagnosis and physical therapy management of a patient with radial wrist pain of 6 months duration: a case report. J Orthop Sports Phys Ther 40:361–368, 2010.
20. Keith MW, Masear V, Chung K, et al: Diagnosis of carpal tunnel syndrome. J Am Acad Orthop Surg 17:389–396, 2009.
21. Thornburg LE: Ganglions of the hand and wrist. J Am Acad Orthop Surg 7:231–238, 1999.
22. Black EM, Blazar PE: Dupuytren disease: an evolving understanding of an age-old disease. J Am Acad Orthop Surg 19:746–757, 2011.
23. Bendre AA, Hartigan BJ, Kalainov DM: Mallet finger. J Am Acad Ortho Surg 13:336–344, 2005.
24. Ono K, Ebara S, Fuji T, et al: Myelopathy hand-new clinical signs of cervical cord damage. J Bone Joint Surg Br 69:215–219, 1987.
25. Brown JA, Lichtman DM: Midcarpal instability. Hand Clin 3:135–140, 1987.
26. Johnstone AJ: Tennis elbow and upper limb tendinopathies. Sports Med Arthro Rev 8:69–79, 2000.
27. Shah AS, Bae DS: Management of pediatric trigger thumb and trigger finger. J Am Acad Orthop Surg 20:206–213, 2012.
28. Prasarn ML, Ouellette EA: Acute compartment syndrome of the upper extremity. J Am Acad Orthop Surg 19:49–58, 2011.
29. Cowell HR: Polydactyly, triphalangism of the thumb, and carpal abnormalities in the family. Clin Orthop Relat Res 434:16–25, 2005.
30. Lichtman DM, Schneider JR, Swafford AR, et al: Ulnar midcarpal instability—clinical and laboratory analysis. J Hand Surg Am 6:515–523, 1981.
31. Wolfe SW, Garcia-Elias M, Kitay A: Carpal instability nondissociative. J Am Acad Orthop Surg 20(9):575–585, 2012.
32. Wadsworth CT: Wrist and hand examination and interpretation. J Orthop Sports Phys Ther 5:108–120, 1983.
33. Blair SJ, McCormick E, Bear-Lehman J, et al: Evaluation of impairment of the upper extremity. Clin Orthop 221:42–58, 1987.

34. Clarkson HM: Musculoskeletal assessment—joint range of motion and manual muscle strength, Philadelphia, 2000, Lippincott Williams & Wilkins.
35. Dutton M: Orthopedic examination, evaluation and intervention, New York, 2004, McGraw Hill.
36. Vanswearingen JM: Measuring wrist muscle strength. J Orthop Sports Phys Ther 4:217–228, 1983.
37. Hume MC, Gellman H, McKellop H, et al: Functional range of motion of the joints of the hand. J Hand Surg Am 15:240–243, 1990.
38. Brumfield RH, Champoux JA: A biomechanical study of normal functional wrist motion. Clin Orthop 187:23–25, 1984.
39. Ryu JY, Cooney WP, Askew JL, et al: Functional range of motion of the wrist joint. J Hand Surg 16:409–419, 1991.
40. Palmer AK, Werner FW, Murphy D, et al: Functional wrist motion: a biomechanical study. J Hand Surg Am 10:39–46, 1985.
41. Nelson DL: Functional wrist motion. Hand Clin 13:83–92, 1997.
42. Lamereaux L, Hoffer MM: The effect of wrist deviation on grip and pinch strength. Clin Orthop 314:152–155, 1995.
43. Tubiana R: The hand, Philadelphia, 1981, WB Saunders.
44. Reid DC: Functional anatomy and joint mobilization, Edmonton, 1970, University of Alberta Press.
45. Sollerman C, Sperling L: Evaluation of activities of daily living function—especially hand function. Scand J Rehab Med 10:139–145, 1978.
46. McPhee SD: Functional hand evaluations: a review. Am J Occup Ther 41:158–163, 1987.
47. Bechtal CD: Grip test: the use of a dynamometer with adjustable handle spacing. J Bone Joint Surg Am 36:820–832, 1954.
48. Mathiowetz V, Weber K, Volland G, et al: Reliability and validity of grip and pinch strength evaluations. J Hand Surg Am 9:222–226, 1984.
49. Hansman CF, Mresh MM: Appearance and fusion of ossification centers in the human skeleton. Am J Roentgenol 88:476–482, 1962.

50. Aulicino PL, DuPuy TE: Clinical examination of the hand. In Hunter J, Schneider LH, Mackin EJ, et al, editors: Rehabilitation of the hand: surgery and therapy, St Louis, 1990, CV Mosby.

51. Levine DW, Simmons BP, Koris MJ, et al: A self-administered questionnaire for the assessment of severity of symptoms and functional status in carpal tunnel syndrome. J Bone Joint Surg Am 75:1585–1592, 1993.

52. Chung KC, Pillsbury MS, Walter MR, et al: Reliability and validity testing of the Michigan hand outcomes questionnaire. J Hand Surg Am 23:575–587, 1998.

53. Dias JJ, Bhowal B, Wildin CJ, et al: Assessing the outcome of disorders of the hands—is the patient evaluation measure reliable, responsive, and without bias? J Bone Joint Surg Br 83:235–240, 2001.

54. Fess EE: Documentation: essential elements of an upper extremity assessment battery. In Hunter J, Schneider LH, Mackin EJ, et al, editors: Rehabilitation of the hand: surgery and therapy, St Louis, 1990, CV Mosby.

55. Baxter-Petralia PL, Blackmore SM, McEntee PM: Physical capacity evaluation. In Hunter J, Schneider LH, Mackin EJ, et al, editors: Rehabilitation of the hand: surgery and therapy, St Louis, 1990, CV Mosby.

56. Beckenbaugh RD, Shives TC, Dobyns JH, et al: Kienböck's disease: the natural history of Kienböck's disease and consideration of lunate fractures. Clin Orthop 149:98–106, 1980.

57. Jebsen RH, Taylor N, Trieschmann RB, et al: An objective and standardized test of hand function. Arch Phys Med Rehabil 50:311–319, 1969.

58. Callahan AD: Sensibility testing. In Hunter J, Schneider LH, Mackin EJ, et al, editors: Rehabilitation of the hand: surgery and therapy, St Louis, 1990, CV Mosby.

59. Cleland JA, Koppenhaver S: Netter's orthopedic clinical examination—an evidence based approach, ed 2, Philadelphia, 2011, Saunders/Elsevier.

60. Cook CE, Hegedus EJ: Orthopedic physical examination tests—an evidence based approach, Upper Saddle River, NJ, 2008, Prentice Hall/Pearson.

61. Young D, Papp S, Giachimo A: Physical examination of the wrist. Orthop Clin North Am 38:149–165, 2007.

62. Johnson RP, Carrera GP: Chronic capitolunate instability. J Bone Joint Surg Am 68:1164–1176, 1986.

63. Nguyen DT, McCue FC, Urch SE: Evaluation of the injured wrist on the field and in the office. Clin Sports Med 17:421–432, 1998.

64. Lichtman DM, Bruckner JD, Culp RW, Alexander CE: Palmar midcarpal instability: results of surgical reconstruction. J Hand Surg Am 18:307–315, 1993.

65. Skirven T: Clinical examination of the wrist. J Hand Surg 9:96–107, 1996.

66. Beckenbaugh RD: Accurate evaluation and management of the painful wrist following injury. Orthop Clin North Am 15:289–306, 1984.

67. Shin AY, Battaglia MJ, Bishop AT: Lunotriquetral instability: diagnosis and treatment. J Am Acad Orthop Surg 8:170–179, 2000.

68. Post M: Physical examination of the musculoskeletal system, Chicago, 1987, Year Book Medical.

69. Taliesnik J: Soft tissue injuries of the wrist. In Strickland JW, Rettig AC, editors: Hand injuries in athletes, Philadelphia, 1992, WB Saunders.

70. Kleinman WB: The lunotriquetral shuck test. Am Soc Surg Hand Corr News 51, 1985.

71. Booher JM, Thibodeau GA: Athletic injury assessment, St Louis, 1989, CV Mosby.

72. Watson HK, Ashmead D, Makhlouf MV: Examination of the scaphoid. J Hand Surg Am 13:657–660, 1988.

73. Chidgey LK: Chronic wrist pain. Orthop Clin North Am 23:49–64, 1992.

74. Lester B, Halbrecht J, Levy IM, et al: "Press test" for office diagnosis of triangular fibrocartilage complex tears of the wrist. Ann Plast Surg 35:41–45, 1995.

75. Buterbaugh GA, Brown TR, Horn PC: Ulnar-sided wrist pain in athletes. Clin Sports Med 17:567–583, 1998.

76. Murray PM, Cooney WP: Golf-induced injuries of the wrist. Clin Sports Med 15:85–109, 1996.

77. Swanson A: Disabling arthritis at the base of the thumb: treatment by resection of the trapezium and flexible implant arthroplasty. J Bone Joint Surg Am 54:456–471, 1972.

78. Heyman P, Gelberman RH, Duncan K, et al: Injuries of the ulnar collateral ligament of the thumb metacarpophalangeal joint. Clin Orthop 292:165–171, 1993.

79. Heyman P: Injuries to the ulnar collateral ligament of the thumb metacarpophalangeal joint. J Am Acad Orthop Surg 5:224–229, 1997.

80. Tang P: Collateral ligament injuries of the thumb metacarpophalangeal joint. J Am Acad Orthop Surg 19:287–296, 2011.

81. Tay SC, Tomita K, Berger RA: The "ulnar fovea sign" for defining ulnar wrist pain: an analysis of sensitivity and specificity. J Hand Surg Am 32:438–444, 2007.

82. Sachar K: Ulnar sided wrist pain: evaluation and treatment of triangular fibrocartilage complex tears, ulnocarpal impaction syndrome and lunotriquetral ligament tears. J Hand Surg Am 37:1489–1500, 2012.

83. LaStayo P, Howell J: Clinical provocation tests used in evaluating wrist pain: a descriptive study. J Hand Ther 8:10–17, 1995.

84. Watson HK, Ballet FL: The SLAC wrist: scapulolunate advanced collapse pattern of degenerative arthritis. J Hand Surg Am 9:358–365, 1984.

85. Taleisnik J: Carpal instability. J Bone Joint Surg Am 70:1262–1268, 1988.

86. Elson RA: Rupture of the central slip of the extensor hood of the finger: a test for early diagnosis. J Bone Joint Surg Br 68:229–231, 1986.

87. Boyes J: Bunnell's surgery of the hand, Philadelphia, 1970, JB Lippincott.

88. Hoppenfeld S: Physical examination of the spine and extremities, New York, 1976, Appleton-Century-Crofts.

89. Finkelstein H: Stenosing tendovaginitis at the radial styloid process. J Bone Joint Surg 12:509, 1930.

90. Linburg RM, Comstock BE: Anomalous tendon slips from the flexor pollicis longus to the flexor digitorum profundus. J Hand Surg Am 4:79–83, 1979.

91. Golding DN, Rose DM, Selvarajah K: Clinical tests for carpal tunnel syndrome: an evaluation. Br J Rheum 25:388–390, 1986.

92. Gunnarsson LG, Amilon A, Hellstrand P, et al: The diagnosis of carpal tunnel syndrome-sensitivity and specificity of some clinical and electrophysiological tests. J Hand Surg Br 22:34–37, 1997.

93. Durkan JA: A new diagnostic test for carpal tunnel syndrome. J Bone Joint Surg Am 73:535–538, 1991.

94. Tetro AM, Evanoff BA, Hollstein SB, et al: A new provocative test for carpal tunnel syndrome: assessment of wrist flexion and nerve compression. J Bone Joint Surg Br 80:493–498, 1998.

95. Jones LA: The assessment of hand function: A critical review of techniques. J Hand Surg Am 14:221–228, 1989.

96. Dellon AL, Kallman CH: Evaluation of functional sensation in the hand. J Hand Surg Am 8:865–870, 1983.

97. Omer GE: Report of the Committee for Evaluation of the Clinical Result in Peripheral Nerve Injury. J Hand Surg Am 8:754–759, 1983.

98. Hansen PA, Micklesen P, Robinson LR: Clinical utility of the flick maneuver in diagnosing carpal tunnel syndrome. Am J Phys Med Rehabil 83:363–367, 2004.

99. Moldaver J: Tinel's sign: its characteristics and significance. J Bone Joint Surg Am 60:412–414, 1978.

100. Ahn DS: Hand elevation: a new test for carpal tunnel syndrome. Ann Plast Surg 46:120–124, 2001.

101. Ma H, Kim I: The diagnostic assessment of hand elevation test in carpal tunnel syndrome. J Korean Neurosurg Soc 52:472–475, 2012.

102. Stromberg WB, McFarlane RM, Bell JL, et al: Injury of the median and ulnar nerves: 150 cases with an evaluation of Moberg's ninhydrin test. J Bone Joint Surg Am 43:717–730, 1961.

103. MacDermid JC, Wessel J: Clinical diagnosis of carpal tunnel syndrome: a systematic review. J Hand Surg 17:309–319, 2004.

104. American Society for Surgery of the Hand: The hand: examination and diagnosis, Aurora, CO, 1978, American Society for Surgery of the Hand.

105. LaBan MM, Mackenzie JR, Zemenick GA: Anatomic observations in carpal tunnel syndrome as they relate to the tethered median nerve stress test. Arch Phys Med Rehabil 70:44–46, 1989.

106. LaBan MM, Friedman NA, Zemenick GA: "Tethered" median nerve stress test in chronic carpal tunnel syndrome. Arch Phys Med Rehabil 67:803–804, 1986.

107. Raudino F: Tethered median nerve stress test in the diagnosis of carpal tunnel syndrome. Electromyogr Clin Neurophysiol 40:57–60, 2000.

108. Kuschner SH, Ebramzadeh E, Johnson D, et al: Tinel's sign and Phalen's test in carpal tunnel syndrome. Orthopedics 15:1297–1302, 1992.

109. O'Riain S: Shrivel test: a new and simple test of nerve function in the hand. Br Med J 3:615–616, 1973.

110. Allen EV: Thromboangiitis obliterans: methods of diagnosis of chronic occlusive arterial lesions distal to the wrist with illustrative cases. Am J Med Sci 178:237–244, 1929.

111. Pellecchia GL: Figure of eight method of measuring hand size: reliability and concurrent validity. J Hand Ther 16:300–304, 2003.

112. Leard JS, Breglio L, Fraga L, et al: Reliability and concurrent validity of the figure-of-eight method of measuring hand size in patients with hand pathology. J Orthop Sports Phys Ther 34:335–340, 2004.

113. Bell-Krotoski JA, Breger DE, Beach RB: Application of biomechanics for evaluation of the hand. In Hunter J, Schneider LH, Mackin EJ, et al, editors: Rehabilitation of the hand: surgery and therapy, St Louis, 1990, CV Mosby.

114. Halpern JS: Upper extremity peripheral nerve assessment. J Emerg Nurs 15:261–265, 1989.

115. Trombly CA, Scott AD: Evaluation of motor control. In Trombly CA, editor: Occupational therapy for physical dysfunction, Baltimore, 1989, Williams & Wilkins.

116. Szabo RM, Madison M: Carpal tunnel syndrome. Orthop Clin North Am 23:103–109, 1992.

117. Murray-Leslie CF, Wright V: Carpal tunnel syndrome, humeral epicondylitis and the cervical spine: a study of clinical and dimensional relations. Br Med J 1:1439–1442, 1976.

118. Hurst LC, Weissberg D, Carroll RE: The relationship of the double crush to carpal tunnel syndrome. J Hand Surg Br 10:202–204, 1985.

119. Massey EW, Riley TL, Pleet AB: Co-existent carpal tunnel syndrome and cervical radiculopathy (double crush syndrome). South Med J 74:957–959, 1981.

120. Bachoura A, Jacoby SM: Ulnar tunnel syndrome. Orthop Clin North Am 43:467–474, 2012.

121. Popinchalk SP, Schaffer AA: Physical examination of upper extremity compressive neuropathies. Orthop Clin North Am 43:417–430, 2012.

122. Kaltenborn FM: Mobilization of the extremity joints, Oslo, 1980, Olaf Norlis Bokhandel.

123. Staes FF, Banks KJ, DeSmet L, et al: Reliability of accessory motion testing at the carpal joints. Man Ther 14:292–298, 2009.

124. Panagis JS, Gelberman RH, Taleisnik J, et al: The arterial anatomy of the human carpus. Part II: the interosseous vascularity. J Hand Surg Am 8:375–382, 1983.

125. Bishop AT, Beckenbaugh RD: Fracture of the hamate bone. J Hand Surg Am 13:135–139, 1988.

126. Peterson JJ, Bancroft LW: Injuries of the fingers and thumb in the athlete. Clin Sp Med 25:527–542, 2006.

127. Schuind FA, Linscheid RL, An KN, et al: A normal database of posteroanterior roentgenographic measurements of the wrist. J Bone Joint Surg Am 74:1418–1429, 1992.

128. Bednar JM, Osterman AL: Carpal instability: evaluation and treatment. J Am Acad Orthop Surg 1:10–17, 1993.

129. Weiss AP, Akelman E: Diagnostic imaging and arthroscopy for chronic wrist pain. Orthop Clin North Am 26:759–767, 1995.

130. Siegel S, White LM, Brahme S: Magnetic resonance imaging of the musculoskeletal system—the wrist. Clin Orthop Relat Res 332:281–300, 1996.

131. Bencardino JT, Rosenberg ZS: Sports related injuries of the wrist: an approach to MRI interpretation. Clin Sports Med 25:409–432, 2006.

132. Coggins CA: Imaging of the ulnar-sided wrist pain. Clin Sports Med 25:505–526, 2006.

133. Wainner RS, Fritz JM, Irrgang JJ, et al: Development of a clinical prediction rule for the diagnosis of carpal tunnel syndrome. Arch Phys Med Rehabil 86:609–618, 2005.

134. Kuhlman KA, Hennessey WJ: Sensitivity and specificity of carpal tunnel syndrome signs. Am J Phys Med Rehabil 76(6):451–457, 1997.

135. Grover R: Clinical assessment of scaphoid injuries and the detection of fractures. J Hand Surg Br 21:341–343, 1996.

136. Desrosiers J, Bravo G, Hebert R, et al: Validation of the box and block test as a measure of dexterity of elderly people: reliability, validity, and norms studies. Arch Phys Med Rehabil 75(7):751–755, 1994.

137. Priganc VW, Henry SM: The relationship among five common carpal tunnel syndrome tests and the severity of carpal tunnel syndrome. J Hand Ther 16:225–236, 2003.

138. Szabo RM, Slater RR, Farver TB, et al: The value of diagnostic testing in carpal tunnel syndrome. J Hand Surg Am 24(4):704–714, 1999.

139. Modelli M, Passero S, Giannini F: Provocative tests in different stages of carpal tunnel syndrome. Clin Neurol Neurosurg 103:170–183, 2001.

140. Del Pino JG, Delgado-Martinez AD, Gonzalez I, et al: Value of the carpal compression test in the diagnosis of carpal tunnel syndrome. J Hand Surg Br 20:38–41, 1997.

141. Fertl E, Wober C, Zeitlhofer J: The serial use of two provocative tests in the clinical diagnosis of carpal tunel syndrome. Acta Neurol Scand 98(5):328–332, 1998.

142. Farrell K, Johnson A, Duncan H, et al: The intertester and intratester reliability of hand volumetrics. J Hand Ther 16(4):292–299, 2003.

143. Doods RL, Nielsen KA, Shirley AG, et al: Test-retest reliability of the commercial volumeter. Work 22(2):107–110, 2004.

144. MacDermid JC, Kramer JF, Woodbury MG, et al: Interrater reliability of pinch and grip strength measurements in patients with cumulative trauma disorders. J Hand Surg 7:10–14, 1994.

145. Haward BM, Griffin MJ: Repeatability of grip strength and dexterity tests and the effects of age and gender. Int Arch Occup Environ Health 75(1–2):111–119, 2002.

146. Schreuders TA, Roebroeck ME, Goumans J, et al: Measurement error in grip and pinch force measurements in patients with hand injuries. Phys Ther 83:806–815, 2003.

147. Brown A, Cramer LD, Eckhaus D, et al: Validity and reliability of the Dexter hand evaluation and therapy system in hand-injured patients. J Hand Ther 25:37–45, 2000.

148. Agre JC, Magness JL, Hull SZ, et al: Strength testing with a portable dynamometer: reliability for upper and lower extremities. Arch Phys Med Rehabil 68:454–458, 1987.

149. Karl AI, Carney ML, Kaul MP: The lumbrical provocation test in subjects with median inclusive paresthesia. Arch Phys Med Rehabil 82(7):935–937, 2001.

150. Wiederien RC, Feldman TD, Heusel LD, et al: The effect of the median nerve compression test on median nerve conduction across the carpal tunnel. Electromyogr Clin Neurophysiol 42(7):413–421, 2002.

151. Chung KC, Pillsbury MS, Walters MR, et al: Reliability and validity testing of the Michigan Hand Outcomes Questionnaire. J Hand Surg Am 23(4):575–587, 1998.

152. Chung KC, Hamill JB, Walters MR, et al: The Michigan Hand Outcomes Questionnaire (MHQ): assessment of responsiveness to clinical change. Ann Plast Surg 42(6):619–622, 1999.

153. Feinstein WK, Lichtman DM, Noble PC, et al: Quantitative assessment of the midcarpal shift test. J Hand Surg Am 24(5):977–983, 1999.

154. Desrosiers J, Rochette A, Hebert R, et al: The Minnesota Manual Dexterity Test: reliability, validity and reference values studies with healthy elderly people. Can J Occup Ther 64(5):270–276, 1997.

155. Ruengsakulrach P, Brooks M, Hare DL, et al: Preoperative assessment of hand circulation by means of Doppler ultrasonography and the modified Allen test. J Thorac Cardiovasc Surg 121(3):526–531, 2001.

156. Bovend'Eerdt TJ, Dawes H, Johansen-Berg H, et al: Evaluation of the Modified Jebsen Test of Hand Function and the University of Maryland Arm Questionnaire for Stroke. Clin Rehabil 18(2):195–202, 2004.

157. MacDermid JC, Kramer JF, McFarlane RM, et al: Inter-rater agreement and accuracy of clinical tests used in diagnosis of carpal tunnel syndrome. Work 8:37–44, 1997.

158. Buch-Jaeger N, Foucher G: Correlation of clinical signs with nerve conduction tests in the diagnosis of carpal tunnel syndrome. J Hand Surg Br 19(6):720–724, 1994.

159. Smith YA, Hong E, Presson C: Normative and validation studies of the Nine-hole Peg Test with children. Percept Mot Skills 90:823–843, 2000.

160. Waeckerle JF: A prospective study identifying the sensitivity of radiographic findings and the efficacy of clinical findings in carpal navicular fractures. Ann Emerg Med 16(7):733–777, 1987.

161. MacDermid JC, Turgeon T, Richards RS, et al: Patient rating of wrist pain and disability: a reliable and valid measurement tool. J Orthop Trauma 12(8):577–586, 1998.

162. Marx RG, Hudak PL, Bombardier C, et al: The reliability of physical examination for carpal tunnel syndrome. J Hand Surg Br 23(4):499–502, 1998.

163. Katz JN, Larson MG, Sabra A, et al: The carpal tunnel syndrome: diagnostic utility of the history and physical examination findings. Channels Int Med 112:321–327, 1990.

164. Gellman H, Gellman RH, Tan AM, et al: Carpal tunnel syndrome—an evaluation of the provocative diagnostic tests. J Bone Jone Surg Am 68:735–737, 1980.

165. Heller L, Ring H, Costeff H, et al: Evaluation of Tinel's and Phalen's sign in diagnosis of the carpal tunnel syndrome. Eur Neurol 25:40–42, 1986.

166. Williams TM, Mackinnon SE, Novak CB: Verification of the pressure provocative test in carpal tunnel syndrome. Ann Plast Surg 29:8–11, 1992.

167. Fong PW, Ng GY: Effect of wrist positioning on the repeatability and strength of power grip. Am J Occup Ther 55(2):212–216, 2001.

168. Reddon JR, Gill DM, Gauk SE, et al: Purdue Pegboard: test-retest estimates. Percept Mot Skills 66(2):503–506, 1988.

169. Desrosiers J, Hebert R, Bravo G, et al: The Purdue Pegboard Test: normative data for people aged 60 and over. Disabil Rehabil 17(5):217–224, 1995.

170. Gallus J, Mathiowetz V: Test-retest reliability of the Purdue Pegboard for persons with multiple sclerosis. Am J Occup Ther 57(1):108–111, 2003.

171. Buddenberg LA, Davis C: Test-retest reliability of the Purdue Pegboard Test. Am J Occup Ther 54(5):555–558, 2000.

172. Sharar RB, Kizony R, Nota A: Validity of the Purdue Pegboard Test in assessing patients after traumatic hand injury. Work 11:315–320, 1998.

173. Powell JM, Lloyd GJ, Rintoul RF: New clinical test for fracture of the scaphoid. Can J Surg 31:237–238, 1988.

174. Novak CB, Lee GW, Mackinnon SE, et al: Provocative testing for cubital tunnel syndrome. J Hand Surg Am 19:817–820, 1994.

175. Kingery WS, Park KS, Wu PB, et al: Electromyographic motor Tinel's sign in ulnar mononeuropathies at the elbow. Am J Phys Med Rehabil 74(6):419–426, 1995.

176. Bohannon RW, Andrews AW: Interrater reliability of hand-held dynamometry. Phys Ther 67:931–933, 1987.

177. Wadsworth CT, Krishnan R, Sear M, et al: Intrarater reliability of manual muscle testing in hand-held dynametric muscle testing. Phys Ther 7:1342–1347, 1987.

178. Rheault W, Beal JL, Kubic KR, et al: Intertester reliability of the hand-held dynamometer for wrist flexion and extension. Arch Phys Med Rehabil 70:907–910, 1989.

SUGGESTED READINGS

American Orthopaedic Association: Manual of orthopaedic surgery, Chicago, 1972, AOA.

Anatomy and Biomechanics Committee: Definition of carpal instability. J Hand Surg Am 24:866–867, 1999.

Aulicino PL: Neurovascular injuries in the hands of athletes. Hand Clin 6:455–466, 1990.

Backhouse KM: Functional anatomy of the hand. Physiotherapy 4:114–117, 1968.

Balogun JA, Adenlola SA, Akinloye AA: Grip strength normative data for the Harpenden dynamometer. J Orthop Sports Phys Ther 14:155–160, 1991.

Beach RB: Measurement of extremity volume by water displacement. Phys Ther 57:286–287, 1977.

Beetham WP, Polley HF, Slocumb CH, et al: Physical examination of the joints, Philadelphia, 1965, WB Saunders.

Bell-Krotoski J, Tomancik E: The repeatability of testing with Semmes-Weinstein monofilaments. J Hand Surg Am 12:155–161, 1987.

Bohannon RW: Measurement of hand grip strength: manual muscle testing versus dynamometry. Physiother Can 51:268–272, 1999.

Bora FW, Osterman AL: Compression neuropathy. Clin Orthop 163:20–37, 1982.

Boscheinen-Morrin J, Davey V, Conolly WB: The hand: fundamentals of therapy, Oxford, 1992, Butterworth-Heinemann.

Brand PW: Clinical mechanisms of the hand, St Louis, 1985, CV Mosby.

Brown DE, Lightman DM: Physical examination of the wrist. In Lichtman D, editor: The wrist and its disorders, Philadelphia, 1988, WB Saunders.

Cailliet R: Hand pain and impairment, Philadelphia, 1971, FA Davis.

Canadian Standardized Test of Fitness: Operations manual, Ottawa, 1986, Fitness and Amateur Sport Canada.

Clawson DK, Souter WA, Carthum CJ, et al: Functional assessment of the rheumatoid hand. Clin Orthop 77:203–210, 1971.

Coleman HM: Injuries of the articular disc at the wrist. J Bone Joint Surg Br 42:522–529, 1960.

Cooney WP, Dobyns JH, Linschied RL: Fractures of the scaphoid: A rational approach to management. Clin Orthop 149:90–97, 1980.

Cooney WP, Lucca MJ, Chao EYS, et al: Kinesiology of the thumb trapeziometacarpal joint. J Bone Joint Surg Am 63:1371–1381, 1981.

Cyriax J: Textbook of orthopaedic medicine, vol. 1: diagnosis of soft tissue lesions, London, 1982, Bailliere Tindall.

Dellon AL: Clinical use of vibratory stimuli to evaluate peripheral nerve injury and compression neuropathy. Plast Reconstr Surg 65:466–475, 1980.

Dellon AL: The paper clip: light hardware to evaluate sensibility in the hand. Contemp Orthop 1:39–42, 1979.

Dellon AL: The moving two point discrimination test: clinical evaluation of the quickly adapting fiber/receptor system. J Hand Surg Am 3:474–481, 1978.

Destouet JM, Gilula LA, Reinus WR: Roentgenographic diagnosis of wrist pain and instability. In Lichtman D, editor: The wrist and its disorders, Philadelphia, 1988, WB Saunders.

Ellem D: Assessment of the wrist, hand and finger complex. J Manip Physiol Ther 3:9–14, 1995.

Ericson WB: Computerized evaluation of the hand. Semin Orthop 7:58–67, 1992.

Evans RC: Illustrated essentials in orthopedic physical assessment, St Louis, 1994, CV Mosby.

Ferris BD, Stanton J, Zamora J: Kinematics of the wrist: evidence of two types of movement. J Bone Joint Surg Br 82:242–245, 2000.

Forrester DM, Brown JC: The radiology of joint disease, Philadelphia, 1987, WB Saunders.

Garrick JG, Webb DR: Sports injuries: diagnosis and treatment, Philadelphia, 1990, WB Saunders.

Gelberman RH, Eaton R, Urbaniak JR: Peripheral nerve compression. J Bone Joint Surg Am 75:1854–1878, 1993.

Gelberman RH, Szabo RM, Williamson RV, et al: Sensibility testing in peripheral nerve compression syndromes. J Bone Joint Surg Am 65:632–637, 1983.

Gilula LA, Destouet JM, Weeks PM, et al: Roentgenographic diagnosis of the painful wrist. Clin Orthop 187:52–64, 1984.

Gilula LA, Weeks PM: Post-traumatic ligamentous instabilities of the wrist. Diagn Radiol 129:641, 1978.

Goodman CC, Snyder TE: Differential diagnosis in physical therapym, Philadelphia, 1995, WB Saunders.

Greulich WW, Pyle SU: Radiographic atlas of skeletal development of the wrist and hand, Stanford, CA, 1959, Stanford University Press.

Hackel ME, Wolfe GA, Bang SM, et al: Changes in hand function in the aging adult as determined by the Jebsen test of hand function. Phys Ther 72:373–377, 1992.

Hanson EC, Wood VE, Thiel AE, et al: Adhesive capsulitis of the wrist-diagnosis and treatment. Clin Orthop Relat Res 234:51–55, 1988.

Henderson WR: Clinical assessment of peripheral nerve injuries: Tinel's test. Lancet 2:801–805, 1948.

Holguin PH, Rico AA, Gomez LP, et al: The coordinate movements of the interphalangeal joints—a cinematic study. Clin Orthop Relat Res 362:117–124, 1999.

Hollinshead WH, Jenkins DB: Functional anatomy of the limbs and back, Philadelphia, 1981, WB Saunders.

Howard FM: Controversies in the nerve entrapment syndrome in the forearm and wrist. Orthop Clin North Am 17:375–381, 1986.

Jacobs JL: Hand and wrist. In Richardson JK, Iglarsh ZA, editors: Clinical orthopedic physical therapy, Philadelphia, 1994, WB Saunders.

Jacobs P: Atlas of hand radiographs, Baltimore, 1973, University Park Press.

Jacobsen C, Sperling L: Classification of the hand grip: a preliminary study. J Occup Med 18:395–398, 1976.

Johnson RP: The acutely injured wrist and its residuals. Clin Orthop 149:33–44, 1980.

Johnson TR, Steinbach LS: Essentials of musculoskeletal imaging, Rosemont, IL, 2004, American Academy of Orthopedic Surgeons.

Judge RD, Zuidema GD, Fitzgerald FT: Clinical diagnosis: a physiological approach, Boston, 1982, Little Brown.

Kauer JMG: Functional anatomy of the wrist. Clin Orthop 149:9–20, 1980.

Kendall EP, McCreary BK: Muscles: testing and function, Baltimore, 1983, Williams & Wilkins.

Khan KM, Cook JL, Taunton JE, et al: Overuse tendinosis, not tendinitis. Part 1: a new paradigm for a difficult clinical problem. Phys Sportsmed 28(9):38–48, 2000.

Koris K, Gelberman RH, Duncan K, et al: Carpal tunnel syndrome: evaluation of a quantitative provocational diagnostic test. Clin Orthop 251:157–161, 1990.

Kricum ME: Wrist arthrography. Clin Orthop 187:65–71, 1984.

La Stayo PC, Wheeler DL: Reliability of passive wrist flexion and extension goniometric measurements: a multicentre study. Phys Ther 74:162–176, 1994.

Levin S, Pearsall G, Ruderman RJ: Von Frey's method of measuring pressure sensibility in the hand: an emergency analysis of the Weinstein-Semmes pressure aesthesiometer. J Hand Surg Am 3:211–216, 1978.

Liebgott B: The anatomical basis of dentistry, Philadelphia, 1982, WB Saunders.

Linn MR, Mann FA, Gilula LA: Imaging the symptomatic wrist. Orthop Clin North Am 21:515–543, 1990.

Long C, Conrad PW, Hall EA, et al: Intrinsic-extrinsic muscle control of the hand in power grip and precision handling: an electromyographic study. J Bone Joint Surg Am 52:853–867, 1970.

Macey A, Kelly C: The hand. In Pynsent P, Fairbank J, Carr A, editors: Outcome measures in orthopedics, Oxford, 1994, Butterworth-Heinemann.

Macey AC, Burke FD: Outcomes of hand surgery. J Hand Surg Br 20:841–855, 1995.

Maitland GD: The peripheral joints: examination and recording guide, Adelaide, Australia, 1973, Virgo Press.

Mayer V: Evaluation and rehabilitation of athletic injuries of the hand and wrist: hand and wrist injuries and treatment. Sports Inj Manage 2:1–28, 1989.

Mayer V, Gieck JH: Rehabilitation of hand injuries in athletics. Clin Sports Med 5:783–794, 1986.

McCue FC, Bruce JF: The wrist. In De Lee JC, Drez D, editors: Orthopedic sports medicine: principles and practice, Philadelphia, 1994, WB Saunders.

McKinnis LN: Fundamentals of musculoskeletal imaging, Philadelphia, 2005, FA Davis.

McMurtry RY: The wrist. In Little H, editor: The rheumatological physical examination, Orlando, FL, 1986, Grune & Stratton.

McMurtry RY, Youm Y, Flatt AE, et al: Kinematics of the wrist, II: clinical applications. J Bone Joint Surg Am 60:955–961, 1978.

McRae R: Clinical orthopaedic examination, New York, 1976, Churchill Livingstone.

Mennell JM: Joint pain, Boston, 1964, Little Brown.

Mennell JM: Manipulation of the joints of the wrist. Physiotherapy 57:246–254, 1971.

Middleton WD, Kneeland JB, Kellman GM, et al: MRI imaging of the carpal tunnel: normal anatomy and preliminary findings in the carpal tunnel syndrome. Am J Radiol 148:307–316, 1987.

Mikic ZD: Detailed anatomy of the articular disc of the distal radioulnar joint. Clin Orthop 245:123–132, 1989.

Mirabello SC, Loeb PE, Andrews JR: The wrist: field evaluation and treatment. Clin Sports Med 11:1–25, 1992.

Moberg E: Criticism and study of methods for examining sensibility in the hand. Neurology 12:8–19, 1962.

Mooney JF, Siegel DB, Koman LA: Ligamentous injuries of the wrist in athletes. Clin Sports Med 11:129–139, 1992.

Moran CA, Callahan AD: Sensibility measurement and management. In Moran C, editor: Hand rehabilitation: clinics in physical therapy, Edinburgh, 1986, Churchill Livingstone.

Napier JR: The prehensile movements of the human hand. J Bone Joint Surg Br 38:902–913, 1956.

Newland CC: Gamekeeper's thumb. Orthop Clin North Am 23:41–48, 1992.

Newport ML: Extensor tendon injuries in the hand. J Am Acad Orthop Surg 5:59–66, 1997.

Nicholas JA, Hershman EB, editors: Upper extremity in sports medicine, St Louis, 1989, CV Mosby.

Nicholas JS: The swollen hand. Physiotherapy 63: 285–286, 1977.

Nuber GW, McCarthy WJ, Yao JS, et al: Arterial abnormalities of the hand in athletes. Am J Sports Med 18:520–523, 1990.

O'Donoghue DH: Treatment of injuries to athletes, ed 4, Philadelphia, 1984, WB Saunders.

Omer GE: Physical diagnosis of peripheral nerve injuries. Orthop Clin North Am 12:207–228, 1981.

Omer GE: Sensation and sensibility in the upper extremity. Clin Orthop 104:30–36, 1974.

Pagonis JF: Imaging for the wrist and hand. Orthop Phys Ther Clin North Am 4:95–121, 1995.

Palmer AK, Werner FW: Biomechanics of the distal radio-ulnar joint. Clin Orthop 187:26–35, 1984.

Palmer ML, Epler M: Clinical assessment procedures in physical therapy, Philadelphia, 1990, JB Lippincott.

Petly NJ, Moore AP: Neuromusculoskeletal examination and assessment—a handbook for therapists, Edinburgh, 1998, Churchill-Livingstone.

Phelps PE, Walker E: Comparison of the finger wrinkling test results to established sensory tests in peripheral nerve injury. Am J Occup Ther 31:565–572, 1977.

Porter RW: New test for finger-tip sensation. Br Med J 2:927–928, 1966.

Radwi RG, Sesto ME, Zachary SV: Functional tests to quantify recovery following carpal tunnel release. J Bone Joint Surg Am 86:2614–2620, 2004.

Reagan DS, Linscheid RL, Dobyn JHS: Lunotriquetral sprains. J Hand Surg Am 9:502–514, 1984.

Recht MP, Burk DL, Dalinka MK: Radiology of wrist and hand injuries in athletes. Clin Sports Med 6:811–828, 1987.

Reid DC: Sports injury assessment and rehabilitation, New York, 1992, Churchill Livingstone.

Renfrew S: Fingertip sensation: a routine neurological test. Lancet 1:396–397, 1969.

Resnick D, Kransdorf MJ: Bone and joint imaging, Philadelphia, 2005, WB Saunders.

Ruby LK: Carpal instability. J Bone Joint Surg Am 77:476–487, 1995.

Samman PD: The nails in disease, London, 1965, Wm. Heinemann Medical Books.

Schuett AM, Gieck J, McCue FC: Evaluation and treatment of injuries to the thumb and fingers. Orthop Phys Ther Clin North Am 3:367–383, 1994.

Schuind FG, Linscheid RL, An KN, et al: A normal data base of posteroanterior roentgenographic measurements of the wrist. J Bone Joint Surg Am 74:1418–1429, 1992.

Smith HB: Smith hand function evaluation. Am J Occup Ther 27:244–251, 1973.

Smith RJ: Balance and kinetics of the fingers under normal and pathological conditions. Clin Orthop 104:92–111, 1974.

Sperling L, Jacobson-Sollerman C: The grip pattern of the healthy hand during eating. Scand J Rehab Med 9:115–121, 1977.

Stahelin A, Pfeiffer K, Sennwald G, et al: Determining carpal collapse: an improved method. J Bone Joint Surg Am 71:1400–1405, 1989.

Stanley JK, Trail IA: Carpal instability. J Bone Joint Surg Br 76:691–700, 1994.

Sunderland S: The nerve lesion in the carpal tunnel syndrome. J Neurol Neurosurg Psych 39:615–626, 1976.

Swanson AB: Pathomechanics of deformities in hand and wrist. In Hunter J, Schneider LH, Mackin EJ, et al, editors: Rehabilitation of the hand: surgery and therapy, St Louis, 1990, CV Mosby.

Swanson AB, de Groof Swanson G, Goren-Hagert C: Evaluation of impairment of hand function. In Hunter J, Schneider LH, Mackin EJ, et al, editors: Rehabilitation of the hand: surgery and therapy, St Louis, 1990, CV Mosby.

Szabo RM, Madison M: Carpal tunnel syndrome as a work-related disorder. In Gordon SL, Blair SJ, Fine LJ: Repetitive motion disorders of the upper extremity, Rosemont, IL, 1995, American Academy of Orthopaedic Surgeons.

Szabo RM, Steinberg DR: Nerve entrapment syndromes at the wrist. J Am Acad Orthop Surg 2:115–123, 1994.

Tanzer RC: The carpal tunnel syndrome. J Bone Joint Surg Am 41:626–634, 1959.

Tardiff GS: Nerve injuries: testing and treatment tactics. Phys Sportsmed 23:61–72, 1995.

Terrono AL, Feldon PG, Hills W, et al: Evaluation and treatment of the rheumatoid wrist. J Bone Joint Surg Am 77:1116–1128, 1995.

Thiru-Pathi RG, Ferlic DC, Clayton MC, et al: Arterial anatomy of the triangular fibrocartilage of the wrist and its surgical significance. J Hand Surg Am 11:258–263, 1986.

Todd TW: Atlas of skeletal maturation, St Louis, 1937, CV Mosby.

Tucker WE: Manipulative techniques employed in the treatment of injury and osteoarthritis of the fingers and hands. Physiotherapy 57:255–258, 1971.

Volz RG, Lieb M, Benjamin J: Biomechanics of the wrist. Clin Orthop 149:112–117, 1980.

Wadsworth CT: Elbow, forearm, wrist, and hand. In Myers RS, editor: Saunders manual of physical therapy practice, Philadelphia, 1995, WB Saunders.

Wadsworth CT: The wrist and hand. In Gould JA, editors: Orthopedic and sports physical therapy, St Louis, 1990, CV Mosby.

Wadsworth CT: Manual examination and treatment of the spine and extremities, Baltimore, 1988, Williams & Wilkins.

Wadsworth CT: Wrist and hand examination and interpretation. J Orthop Sports Phys Ther 5:108–120, 1983.

Waylett-Rendall J: Sensibility evaluation and rehabilitation. Orthop Clin North Am 19:43–56, 1988.

Weiss KL, Beltran J, Lubbers LM: High-field MR surface-coil imaging of the hand and wrist: pathologic correlations and clinical relevance. Radiology 160:147–152, 1986.

Weissman BNW, Sledge CB: Orthopedic radiology, Philadelphia, 1986, WB Saunders.

Williams P, Warwick R: Gray's anatomy, ed 36, British, Edinburgh, 1980, Churchill Livingstone.

Wynn Parry CB: Rehabilitation of the hand, London, 1981, Butterworths.

Youm Y, McMurtry RY, Flatt AE, et al: Kinematics of the wrist: I. an experimental study of radioulnar deviation and flexion-extension. J Bone Joint Surg Am 60:423–431, 1978.

Zdavkovic V, Sennwald GR: A new radiographic method of measuring carpal collapse. J Bone Joint Surg Br 79:167–169, 1997.

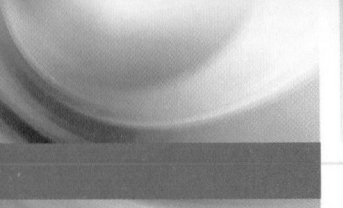

CHAPTER 8

Thoracic (Dorsal) Spine

Assessment of the thoracic spine involves examination of the part of the spine that is most rigid because of the associated rib cage. The rib cage in turn provides protection for the heart and lungs. Normally, the thoracic spine, being one of the primary curves, exhibits a mild **kyphosis** (posterior curvature); the cervical and lumbar sections, being secondary curves, exhibit a mild **lordosis** (anterior curvature). When the examiner assesses the thoracic spine, it is essential that the cervical and/or lumbar spines be evaluated at the same time (Figure 8-1; see Figure 3-7).

APPLIED ANATOMY

The **costovertebral joints** are synovial plane joints located between the ribs and the vertebral bodies (Figure 8-2). There are 24 of these joints, and they are divided into two parts. Ribs 1, 10, 11, and 12 articulate with a single vertebra. The other articulations have no intra-articular ligament that divides the joint into two parts, so each of ribs 2 through 9 articulates with two adjacent vertebrae and the intervening intervertebral disc. The main ligament of the costovertebral joint is the radiate ligament, which joins the anterior aspect of the head of the rib radiating to the sides of the vertebral bodies and disc in between. For ribs 10, 11, and 12, it attaches only to the adjacent vertebral body. The intra-articular ligament divides the joint and attaches to the disc.

The **costotransverse joints** are synovial joints found between the ribs and the transverse processes of the vertebra of the same level for ribs 1 through 10 (see Figure 8-2). Because ribs 11 and 12 do not articulate with the transverse processes, this joint does not exist for these two levels. The costotransverse joints are supported by three ligaments. The superior costotransverse ligament runs from the lower border of the transverse process above to the upper border of the rib and its neck. The costotransverse ligament runs between the neck of the rib and the transverse process at the same level. The lateral costotransverse ligament runs from the tip of the transverse process to the adjacent rib.

The **costochondral joints** lie between the ribs and the costal cartilage (Figure 8-3). The **sternocostal joints** are found between the costal cartilage and the sternum. Joints 2 through 6 are synovial, whereas the first costal cartilage is united with the sternum by a synchondrosis.

Where a rib articulates with an adjacent rib or costal cartilage (ribs 5 through 9), a synovial interchondral joint exists.

As in the cervical and lumbar spines, the two **apophyseal** or **facet joints** make up the main tri-joint complex along with the disc between the vertebrae. The superior facet of the T1 vertebra is similar to a facet of the cervical spine. Because of this, T1 is classified as a **transitional vertebra.** The superior facet faces up and back; the inferior facet faces down and forward. The T2 to T11 superior facets face up, back, and slightly laterally; the inferior facets face down, forward, and slightly medially (Figure 8-4). This shape enables slight rotation in the thoracic spine. Thoracic vertebrae T11 and T12 are classified as transitional, and the facets of these vertebrae become positioned in a way similar to those of the lumbar facets. The superior facets of these two vertebrae face up, back, and more medially; the inferior facets face forward and slightly laterally. The ligaments between the vertebral bodies include the ligamentum flavum, the anterior and posterior longitudinal ligaments, the interspinous and supraspinous ligaments, and the intertransverse ligament. These ligaments are found in the cervical, thoracic, and lumbar spine. The close packed position of the facet joints in the thoracic spine is extension.

Facet Joints of the Thoracic Spine

Resting position:	Midway between flexion and extension
Close packed position:	Full extension
Capsular pattern:	Side flexion and rotation equally limited, extension

Within the thoracic spine, there are 12 vertebrae, which diminish in size from T1 to T3 and then increase progressively in size to T12. These vertebrae are distinctive in having facets on the body and transverse processes for articulation with the ribs. The spinous processes of these vertebrae face obliquely downward (Figure 8-5). T7 has the greatest spinous process angulation, whereas the upper three thoracic vertebrae have spinous processes that project directly posteriorly. In other words, the spinous

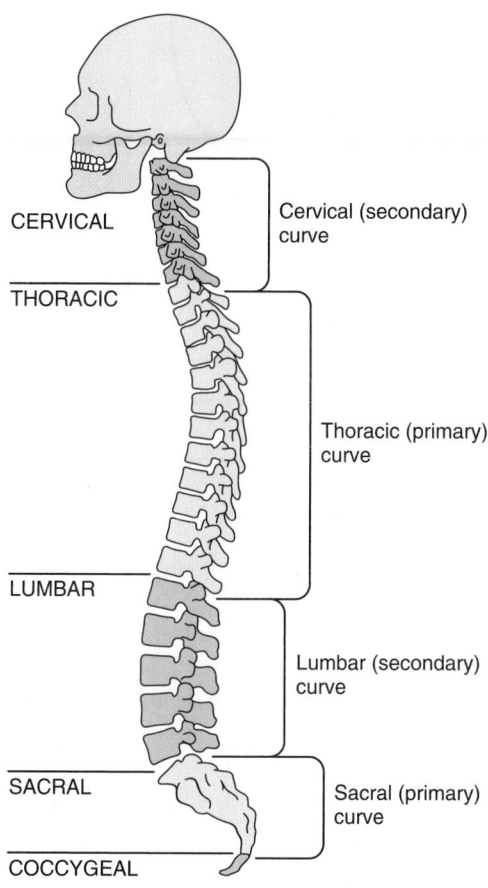

CERVICAL

Cervical (secondary) curve

THORACIC

Thoracic (primary) curve

LUMBAR

Lumbar (secondary) curve

SACRAL

Sacral (primary) curve

COCCYGEAL

Figure 8-1 The articulated spine.

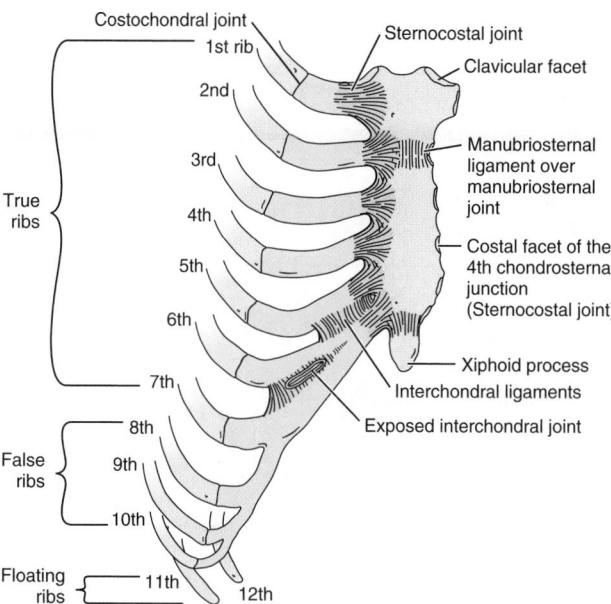

Costochondral joint

1st rib

2nd

3rd

4th

5th

6th

7th

True ribs

8th

9th

10th

False ribs

Floating ribs

11th

12th

Sternocostal joint

Clavicular facet

Manubriosternal ligament over manubriosternal joint

Costal facet of the 4th chondrosternal junction (Sternocostal joint)

Xiphoid process

Interchondral ligaments

Exposed interchondral joint

Figure 8-3 Anterior view of the part of the thoracic wall highlights the manubriosternal joint, sternocostal joints with costochondral and chondrosternal joints, and interchondral joints. The ribs are removed on the left side to expose the costal facets. (Modified from Neumann DA: Kinesiology of the musculoskeletal system—foundations for physical rehabilitation, St Louis, 2002, CV Mosby, p. 370.)

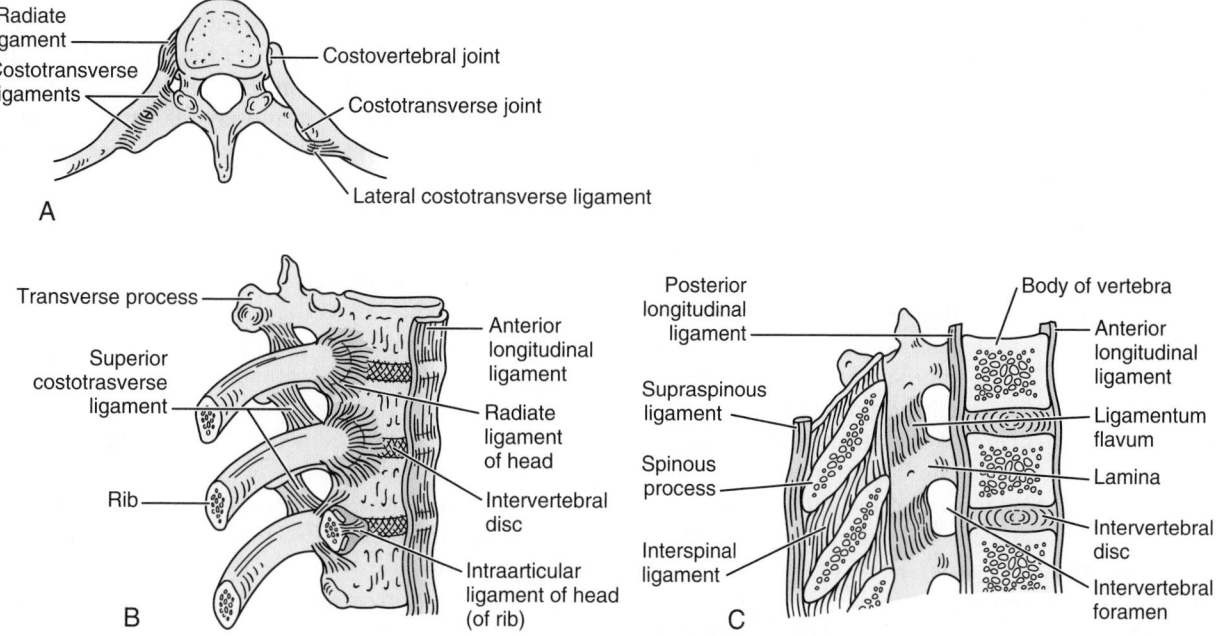

Radiate ligament

Costotransverse ligaments

Costovertebral joint

Costotransverse joint

Lateral costotransverse ligament

A

Transverse process

Superior costotrasverse ligament

Rib

Anterior longitudinal ligament

Radiate ligament of head

Intervertebral disc

Intraarticular ligament of head (of rib)

B

Posterior longitudinal ligament

Supraspinous ligament

Spinous process

Interspinal ligament

Body of vertebra

Anterior longitudinal ligament

Ligamentum flavum

Lamina

Intervertebral disc

Intervertebral foramen

C

Figure 8-2 Joints and ligaments of the thoracic vertebrae and ribs. A, Superior view. **B,** Anterolateral aspect. **C,** Median section through vertebra.

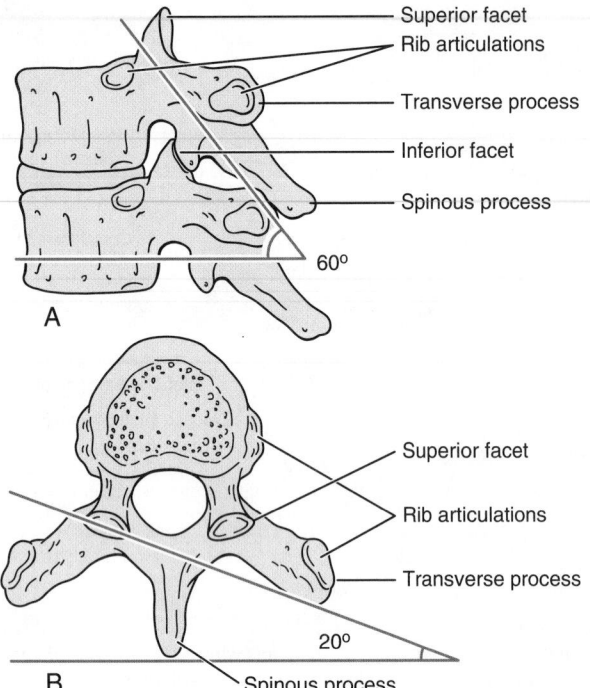

A

B

Figure 8-4 **Thoracic vertebra. A,** Side view. **B,** Superior view.

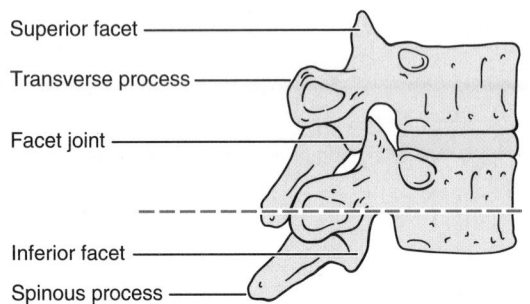

Figure 8-5 Spinous process of one thoracic vertebra at level of body of vertebra below (T7–T9).

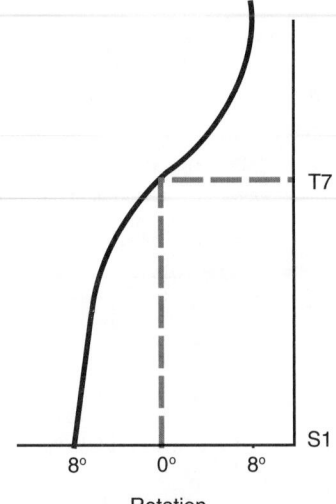

Figure 8-6 Axial rotation of the spine going from left to right on heel strike.

process of these vertebrae is on the same plane as the transverse processes of the same vertebrae.

T4 to T6 vertebrae have spinous processes that project downward slightly. In this case, the tips of the spinous processes are on a plane halfway between their own transverse processes and the transverse processes of the vertebrae below. For T7, T8, and T9 vertebrae, the spinous processes project downward, the tip of the spinous processes being on a plane of the transverse processes of the vertebrae below. For the T10 spinous process, the arrangement is similar to that of the T9 spinous process (i.e., the spinous process is level with the transverse process of the vertebra below). For T11, the arrangement is similar to that of T6 (i.e., the spinous process is halfway between the two transverse processes of the vertebra), and T12 is similar to T3 (i.e., the spinous process is level with the transverse process of the same vertebra). The location

of the spinous processes becomes important if the examiner wishes to perform posteroanterior central vertebral pressures (PACVPs). For example, if the examiner pushes on the spinous process of T8, the body of T9 also moves. In fact, the vertebral body of T8 probably arcs backwards slightly, whereas T9 will move in an anterior direction. T7 is sometimes classified as a transitional vertebra, because it is the point at which the lower limb axial rotation alternates with the upper limb axial rotation (Figure 8-6).

The ribs, which help to stiffen the thoracic spine, articulate with the demifacets on vertebrae T2 to T9. For T1 and T10, there is a whole facet for ribs 1 and 10, respectively. The first rib articulates with T1 only, the second rib articulates with T1 and T2, the third rib articulates with T2 and T3, and so on. Ribs 1 through 7 articulate with the sternum directly and are classified as **true ribs** (see Figure 8-3). Ribs 8 through 10 join directly with the costocartilage of the rib above and are classified as **false ribs.** Ribs 11 and 12 are classified as **floating ribs,** because they do not attach to either the sternum or the costal cartilage at their distal ends. Ribs 11 and 12 articulate only with the bodies of the T11 and T12 vertebrae, not with the transverse processes of the vertebrae, nor with the costocartilage of the rib above. The ribs are held by ligaments to the body of the vertebra and to the transverse processes of the same vertebrae. Some of these ligaments also bind the rib to the vertebra above.

At the top of the rib cage, the ribs are relatively horizontal. As the rib cage descends, they run more and more obliquely downward. By the 12th rib, the ribs are more vertical than horizontal. With inspiration, the ribs are pulled up and forward; this increases the anteroposterior diameter of the ribs. The first six ribs increase the anteroposterior dimension of the chest, mainly by rotating

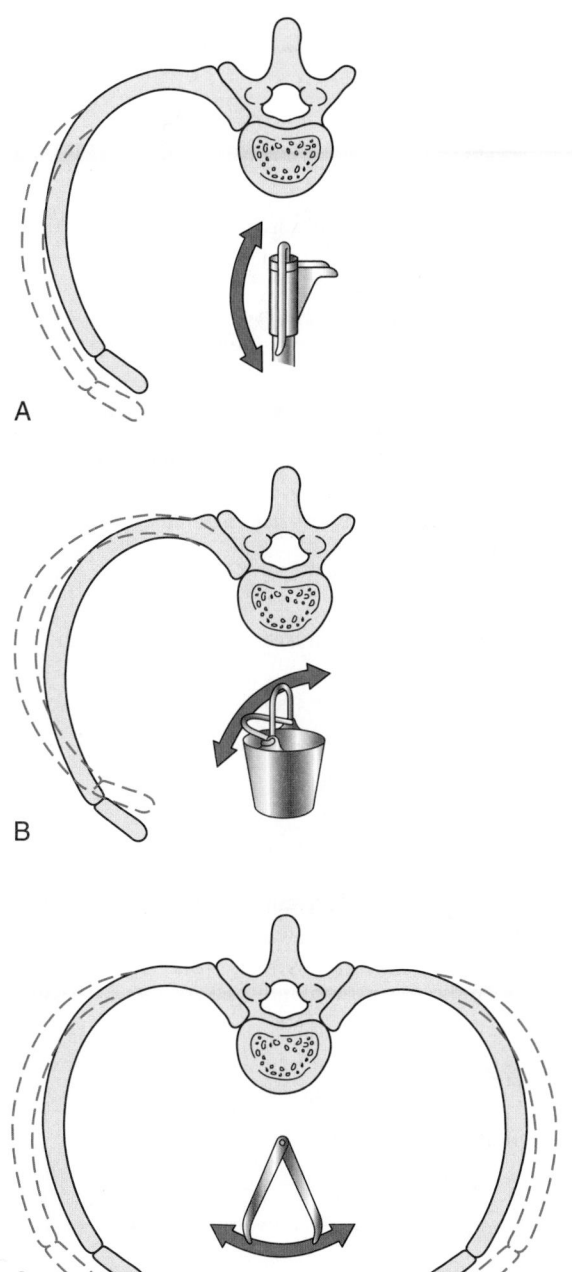

Figure 8-7 Actions of the ribs. A, Pump handle action (T1–T6). **B,** Bucket handle action (T7–T10). **C,** Caliper action (T11–T12). (**A** and **B,** Modified from Williams P, Warwick R, editors: *Gray's anatomy,* ed 37 British, Edinburgh, 1989, Churchill Livingstone, p. 498.)

around their long axes. Rotation downward of the rib neck is associated with depression, whereas rotation upward of the same portion is associated with elevation. These movements are known as a **pump handle action** and are accompanied by elevation of the manubrium sternum upward and forward (Figure 8-7, *A*).[1-3] Ribs 7 through 10 mainly increase in lateral, or transverse, dimension. To accomplish this, the ribs move upward, backward, and medially to increase the infrasternal angle, or they move downward, forward, and laterally to decrease

the angle. These movements are known as a **bucket handle action.** This action is also performed by ribs 2 through 6 but to a much lesser degree (Figure 8-7, *B*). The lower ribs (ribs 8 through 12) move laterally, in what is known as a **caliper action,** to increase lateral diameter (Figure 8-7, *C*).[2] The ribs are quite elastic in children, but they become increasingly brittle with age. In the anterior half of the chest, the ribs are subcutaneous; in the posterior half, they are covered by muscles.

PATIENT HISTORY

A thorough and complete history should include past and present problems. By listening carefully, the examiner is often able to identify the patient's problem, develop a working diagnosis, and then use the observation and examination to confirm or refute the impressions established from the history. All information concerning the present pain and its site, nature, and behavior is important. If any part of the history implicates the cervical or lumbar spine, the examiner must include these areas in the assessment as well.

In addition to the questions listed under the "Patient History" section in Chapter 1, the examiner should obtain the following information from the patient:

1. *What are the patient's age and occupation?* For example, conditions such as Scheuermann's disease typically occur in young people between 13 and 16 years of age. Idiopathic scoliosis is most commonly seen in adolescent females.

2. *What was the mechanism of injury?* Most commonly, rib injuries are caused by trauma. Thoracic spine problems may result from disease processes (e.g., scoliosis) and may have an insidious onset. Pain from true thoracic trauma tends to be localized to the area of injury. Facet syndromes present as stiffness and local pain, which can be referred.[4,5]

3. *What are the details of the present pain and other symptoms? What are the sites and boundaries of the pain?* Have the patient point to the location or locations. Is there any radiation of pain? The examiner should remember that many of the abdominal structures, such as the stomach, liver, and pancreas, may refer pain to the thoracic region (Tables 8-1 and 8-2 for thoracic spine and rib cage red flags and chest pain patterns). With thoracic disc lesions, because of the rigidity of the thoracic spine, active movements do not often show the characteristic pain pattern, and sensory and strength deficits are difficult if not impossible to detect.[6] Thoracic root involvement or spondylosis usually causes pain that follows the path of the ribs or a deep, "through-the-chest" pain.

4. *Does the pain occur on inspiration, expiration, or both?* Pain related to breathing may signal pulmonary problems or may be related to movement of the ribs.

TABLE **8-1**

Thoracic Spine and Rib Cage Red Flags

Condition	Red Flags
Myocardial infarction	Chest pain Pallor, sweating, dyspnea, nausea, or palpitations Presence of risk factors: previous history of coronary heart disease, hypertension, smoking, diabetes, and elevated blood serum cholesterol (>240 mg/dL) Men aged over 40 years and women aged over 50 years Symptoms lasting greater than 30 minutes and not relieved with sublingual nitroglycerin
Stable angina pectoris	Chest pain or pressure that occurs with predictable levels of exertion (if not, suspect unstable angina pectoris) Symptoms are also predictably alleviated with the rest or sublingual nitroglycerin (if not, suspect unstable angina pectoris)
Pericarditis	Sharp or stabbing chest pain that may be referred to the lateral neck or either shoulder Increased pan with left side lying Relieved with forward lean while sitting (supporting arms on knees or a table)
Pulmonary embolus	Chest, shoulder, or upper abdominal pain Dyspnea
Pleurisy	Severe, sharp knife-like pain with inspiration History of a recent or coexisting respiratory disorder (e.g., infection, pneumonia, tumor, or tuberculosis)
Pneumothorax	Chest pain that is intensified with inspiration, ventilation, or expanding rib cage Recent bout of coughing or strenuous exercise or trauma Hyperresonance upon percussion Decreased breath sounds
Pneumonia	Pleuritic pain that may be referred to shoulder Fever, chills, headache, malaise, or nausea Productive cough
Cholecystitis	Colicky pain in the right upper abdominal quadrant with accompanying right scapula pain Symptoms may worsen with ingestion of fatty foods Symptoms unaffected by activity of rest
Peptic ulcer	Dull, gnawing pain, or burning sensation in the epigastrium, mid-back, or suprasclavicular regions Symptoms relieved with food Localized tenderness at the right epigastrium Constipation, bleeding, vomiting, tarry colored stools, and coffee ground emeses
Pyelonephritis	Recent or coexisting urinary tract infection Enlarged prostate Kidney stone or past kidney stone
Nephrolithiasis (kidney stones)	Sudden, severe back, or flank pain Chills and fever Nausea or vomiting Renal colic Symptoms of urinary tract infection Reside in hot and humid environment Past episode(s) of kidney stone(s)

From Dutton M: Dutton's orthopedic examination, evaluation and intervention, ed 3, New York, 2012, McGraw Hill, p. 1247.

Pain referred around the chest wall tends to be costovertebral in origin. Does the patient have any difficulty in breathing? If a breathing problem exists, it may be caused by a structural deformity (e.g., scoliosis); thoracic trauma, such as disc lesions, fractures, or contusions; or thoracic pathology, such as pneumothorax, pleurisy, tumors, or pericarditis.

5. *Is the pain deep, superficial, shooting, burning, or aching?* Thoracic nerve root pain is often severe and is referred in a sloping band along an intercostal space. Pain between the scapulae may be the result of a cervical lesion. It has been reported that any symptoms above a line joining the inferior angles of the scapula should be considered of cervical origin

TABLE 8-2

Chest Pain Patterns

Origin of Pain	Site of Referred Pain	Type of Disorder
Substernal or retrosternal	Neck, jaw, back, left shoulder and arm, and abdomen	Angina
Substernal, anterior chest	Neck, jaw, back, and bilateral arms	Myocardial infarction
Substernal or above the sternum	Neck, upper back, upper trapezius, supraclavicular area, left arm, and costal margin	Pericarditis
Anterior chest (thoracic aneurysm); abdomen (abdominal aneurysm)	Posterior thoracic, chest, neck, shoulders, interscapular, or lumbar region	Dissecting aortic aneurysm
Variable	Variable, depending on structures involved	Musculoskeletal
Costochondritis (inflammation of the costal cartilage): sternum and rib margins	Abdominal oblique trigger points: pain referred up into the chest area	
Upper rectus abdominis trigger points (left side), pectoralis, serratus anterior, and sternalis muscles: precordial pain	Pectoralis trigger points: pain referred down medial bilateral arms along ulnar nerve distribution (fourth and fifth fingers)	
Precordium region (upper central abdomen and diaphragm)	Sternum, axillary lines, and either side of vertebrae; lateral and anterior chest wall; occasionally to one or both arms	Neurological
Substernal, epigastric, and upper abdominal quadrants	Around chest area, shoulders, and upper back region	Gastrointestinal
Within breast tissue; may be localized in pectoral and supraclavicular regions	Chest area, axilla, mid-back, and neck and posterior shoulder girdle	Breast pain
Commonly substernal and anterior chest region	No referred pain	Anxiety

From Dutton M: Dutton's orthopedic examination, evaluation and intervention, ed 3, New York, 2012, McGraw Hill, p. 1246.

until proven otherwise, especially if there is no history of trauma.[7]

6. *Is the pain affected by coughing, sneezing, or straining?* Dural pain is often accentuated by these maneuvers.

7. *Which activities aggravate the problem?* Active use of the arms sometimes irritates a thoracic lesion. Pulling and pushing activities can be especially bothersome to a patient with thoracic problems. Costal pain is often elicited by breathing and/or overhand arm motion.

8. *Which activities ease the problem?* For example, bracing the arms often makes breathing easier because this facilitates the action of the accessory muscles of respiration.

9. *Is the condition improving, becoming worse, or staying the same?*

10. *Does any particular posture bother the patient?*

11. *Is there any paresthesia or other abnormal sensation that may indicate a disc lesion or radiculopathy?*

12. *Are the patient's symptoms referred to the legs, arms, or head and neck?* If so, it is imperative that the examiner assess these areas as well. For example, shoulder movements may be restricted with thoracic spine problems.

13. *Does the patient have any problems with digestion?* Pain may be referred to the thoracic spine or ribs from pathological conditions within the thorax or abdomen. Visceral pain tends to be vague, dull, and indiscrete and may be accompanied by nausea and sweating. It tends to follow dermatome patterns in its referral. For example, cardiac pain is referred to the shoulder (C4) and posteriorly to T2. Stomach pain is referred to T6–T8 posteriorly. Ulcers may be referred to T4–T6 posteriorly.[4]

14. *Is the skin in the thorax area normal?* Conditions, such as herpes zoster, can cause unilateral, spontaneous pain. In the observation, the examiner should watch for erythema and grouped vesicles.[6]

OBSERVATION

The patient must be suitably undressed so that the body is exposed as much as possible. In the case of a female, the bra is often removed to provide a better view of the spine and rib cage. The patient is usually observed first standing and then sitting.

As with any observation, the examiner should note any alteration in the overall spinal posture (see Chapter 15), because it may lead to problems in the thoracic spine. It is important to observe the total body posture from the head to the toes and look for any deviation from normal (Figure 8-8). Posteriorly, the medial edge of the spine of

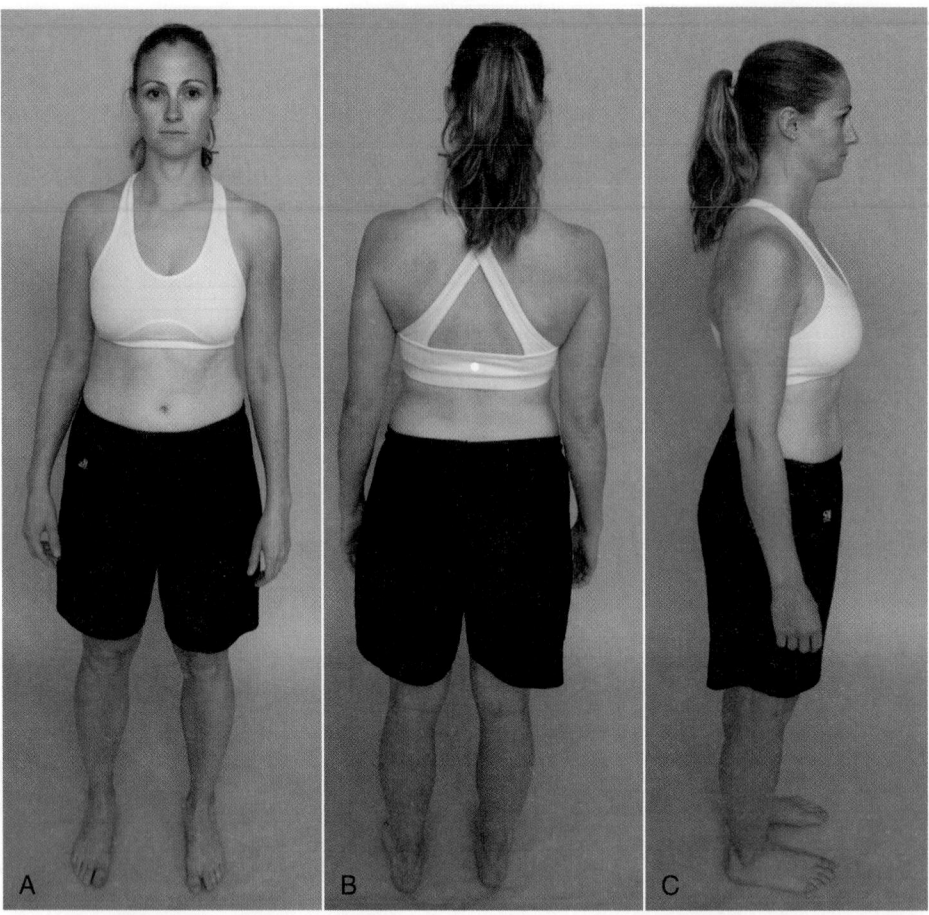

Figure 8-8 Normal posture. A, Front view. **B,** Posterior view. **C,** Side view.

the scapula should be level with the T3 spinous process, whereas the inferior angle of the scapula is level with the T7–T9 spinous process, depending on the size of the scapula. The medial border of the scapula is parallel to the spine and approximately 5 cm lateral to the spinous processes.

Kyphosis

Kyphosis is a condition that is most prevalent in the thoracic spine (Figure 8-9). The examiner must ensure that a kyphosis is actually present, remembering that a slight kyphosis, or posterior curvature, is normal and is found in every individual. Hyperkyphosis is a kyphotic angle of greater than 40° commonly measured by the Cobb method (see Figure 8-53) on a lateral x-ray measuring between T4 and T12.[8] After age 40, the thoracic kyphosis tends to increase.[8] In addition, some people have "flat" scapulae, which give the appearance of an excessive kyphosis, as does winging of the scapulae. The examiner must ensure that it is actually the spine that has the excessive curvature. Types of kyphotic deformities are shown in Figure 8-10 and listed below[9]:

1. **Round back** is decreased pelvic inclination (20°) with a thoracolumbar or thoracic kyphosis (Figure 8-11).

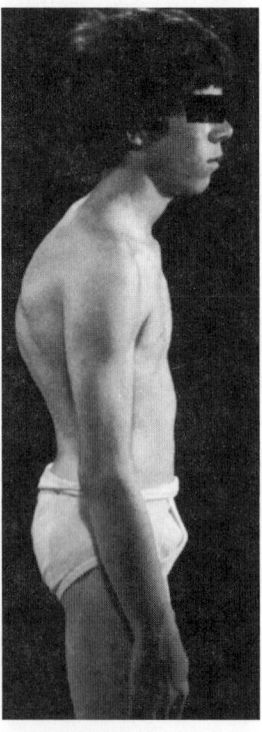

Figure 8-9 Congenital thoracic kyphosis. (From Bradford DS, Lonstein JE, Moe JH, et al: Moe's textbook of scoliosis and other spinal deformities, Philadelphia, 1987, WB Saunders, p. 263.)

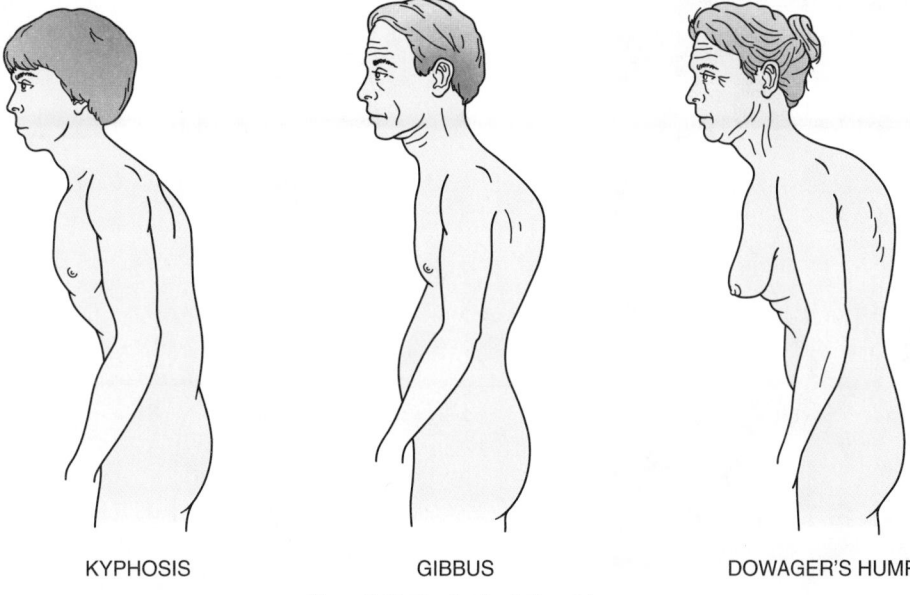

KYPHOSIS GIBBUS DOWAGER'S HUMP

Figure 8-10 **Kyphotic deformities.**

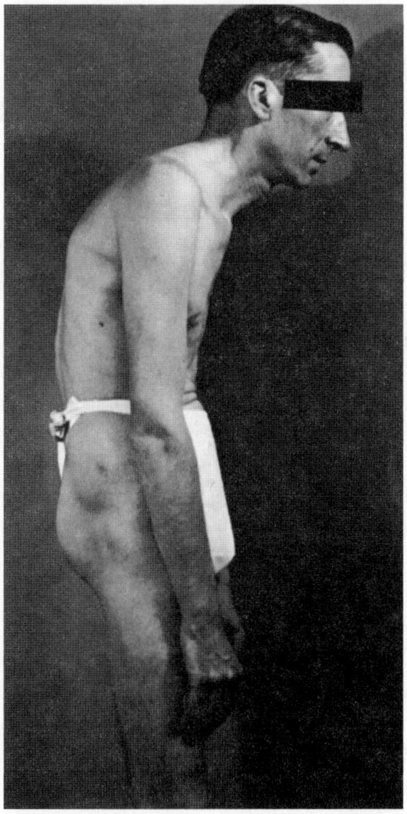

Figure 8-11 Lateral view of patient with ankylosing (rheumatoid) spondylitis showing forward protrusion of head, flattening of anterior chest wall, thoracic kyphosis, protrusion of abdomen, and flattening of lumbar lordosis. This patient also has slight flexion of the hips on the pelvis. (From Polley HF, Hunder GG: Rheumatologic interviewing and physical examination of the joints, Philadelphia, 1978, WB Saunders, p. 161.)

Most forms of kyphosis seen show a decreased pelvic inclination. To compensate and maintain the body's center of gravity, a structural kyphosis, usually caused by tight soft tissues from prolonged postural change or by a growth disturbance results, causing a round back deformity.

2. **Scheuermann's disease** is the most common structural kyphosis in adolescents but can occur in adults. Its etiology is unknown.[10]

3. **Hump back** is a localized, sharp, posterior angulation called a **gibbus**.[8] This kyphotic deformity is usually structural and often results from an anterior wedging of the body of one or two thoracic vertebrae. The wedging may be caused by a fracture, tumor, or bone disease. The pelvic inclination is usually normal (30°).

4. **Flat back** is decreased pelvic inclination (20°) with a mobile spine. This kyphotic deformity is similar to round back, except that the thoracic spine remains mobile and is able to compensate throughout its length for the altered center of gravity caused by the decreased pelvic inclination. Therefore, although a kyphosis is or should be present, it does not have the appearance of an excessive kyphotic curve.

5. **Dowager's hump**[8] results from postmenopausal osteoporosis. Because of the osteoporosis, anterior wedge fractures occur to several vertebrae, usually in the upper to middle thoracic spine, causing a structural scoliosis that also contributes to a decrease in height.

Scoliosis

Scoliosis is a deformity in which there are one or more lateral curvatures of the lumbar or thoracic spine; it is this spinal deformity that was suffered by the "Hunchback of

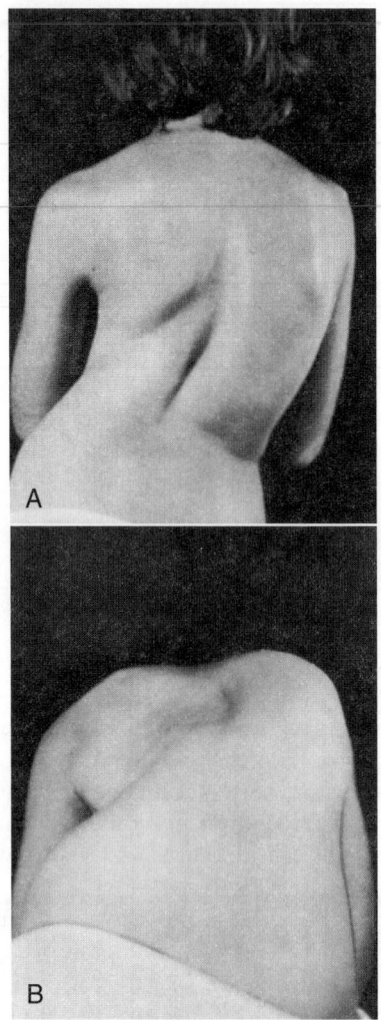

Figure 8-12 **Idiopathic scoliosis. A,** Postural deformity caused by idiopathic thoracolumbar scoliosis. **B,** Asymmetry of posterior thorax accentuated with patient flexed. Note "hump" on the right and "hollow" on the left. (From Gartland JJ: Fundamentals of orthopedics, Philadelphia, 1979, WB Saunders, p. 341.)

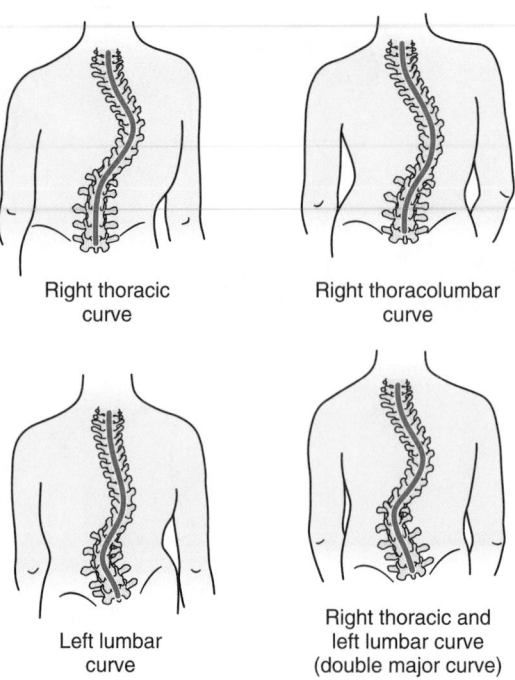

Right thoracic
curve

Right thoracolumbar
curve

Left lumbar
curve

Right thoracic and
left lumbar curve
(double major curve)

Figure 8-13 **Examples of scoliosis curve patterns.**

Notre Dame." (In the cervical spine, the condition is called **torticollis.**) The curvature may occur in the thoracic spine alone, in the thoracolumbar area, or in the lumbar spine alone (Figure 8-12). Scoliosis may be nonstructural (i.e., relatively easily correctable once the cause is determined) or structural. Poor posture, hysteria, nerve root irritation, inflammation in the spine area, leg length discrepancy, or hip contracture can cause nonstructural scoliosis. Structural changes may be genetic, idiopathic, or caused by some congenital problem, such as a wedge vertebra, hemivertebra, or failure of vertebral segmentation. In other words, there is a structural change in the bone, and normal flexibility of the spine is lost.[11]

A number of curve patterns may be present with scoliosis (Figure 8-13).[11] The curve patterns are designated according to the level of the apex of the curve (Table 8-3). A right thoracic curve has a convexity toward the

right, and the apex of the curve is in the thoracic spine. With a cervical scoliosis, or torticollis, the apex is between C1 and C6. For a cervicothoracic curve, the apex is at C7 or T1. For a thoracic curve, the apex is between T2 and T11. The thoracolumbar curve has its apex at T12 or L1. The lumbar curve has an apex between L2 and L4, and a lumbosacral scoliosis has an apex at L5 or S1. The involvement of the thoracic spine results in a very poor cosmetic appearance or greater visual defect as a result of deformation of the ribs along with the spine. The deformity can vary from a mild rib hump to a severe rotation of the vertebrae, causing a rib deformity called a **razorback spine.**

With a structural scoliosis, the vertebral bodies rotate to the convexity of the curve and become distorted.[12] If the thoracic spine is involved, this rotation causes the ribs on the convex side of the curve to push posteriorly, causing a rib "hump" and narrowing the thoracic cage on the convex side. As the vertebral body rotates to the convex side of the curve, the spinous process deviates toward the concave side. The ribs on the concave side move anteriorly, causing a "hollow" and a widening of the thoracic cage on the concave side (Figure 8-14). Lateral deviation may be more evident if the examiner uses a plumb bob (plumbline) from the C7 spinous process or external occipital protuberance (Figure 8-15).

The examiner should note whether the ribs are symmetric and whether the rib contours are normal and equal on the two sides. In idiopathic scoliosis, the rib contours are not normal, and there is asymmetry of the ribs. Muscle spasm resulting from injury may also be evident. The

TABLE **8-3**

Curve Patterns and Prognosis in Idiopathic Scoliosis

	CURVE PATTERN				
	Primary Lumbar	**Thoracolumbar**	**Combined Thoracic and Lumbar**	**Primary Thoracic**	**Cervicothoracic**
Incidence (%)	23.6	16	37	22.1	31.3
Average age curve noted (year)	13.25	14	12.3	11.1	15.3
Average age curve stabilized (year)	14.5	16	15.5	16.1	16.3
Extent of curve	T11–L3	T6 or T7–L1 or L1, L2	Thoracic, T6–T10 Lumbar, T11–L4	T6–T11	C7 or T1–T4 or T5
Apex of curve	L1 or L2	T11 or L2	Thoracic, T7 or T8 Lumbar, L2	T8 or T9 (rotation extreme, convexity usually to right)	T3
Average angular value at maturity (degrees)					
Standing	36.8	42.7	Thoracic, 51.9; Lumbar, 41.4	81.4	34.6
Supine	29.1	35	Thoracic, 41.4; Lumbar, 37.7	73.8	32.2
Prognosis	Most benign and least deforming of all idiopathic curves	Not severely deforming Intermediate between thoracic and lumbar curves	Good Body usually well aligned, curves even if severe tend to compensate each other High percentage of very severe scoliosis if onset before age of 10 years	Worst Progresses more rapidly, becomes more severe, and produces greater clinical deformity than any other pattern Five years of active growth during which curve could increase	Deformity unsightly Poorly disguised because of high shoulder, elevated scapula, and deformed thoracic cage

Adapted from Ponseti IV, Friedman B: Prognosis in idiopathic scoliosis. J Bone Joint Surg Am 32:382, 1950.

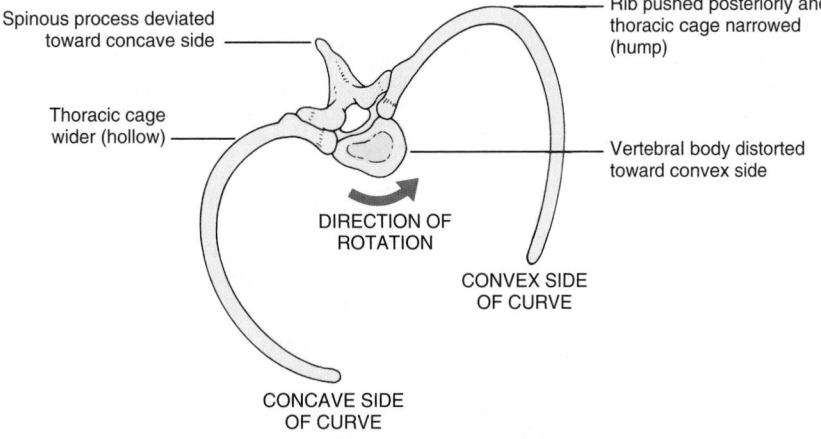

Figure 8-14 Pathological changes in the ribs and vertebra with idiopathic scoliosis in the thoracic spine.

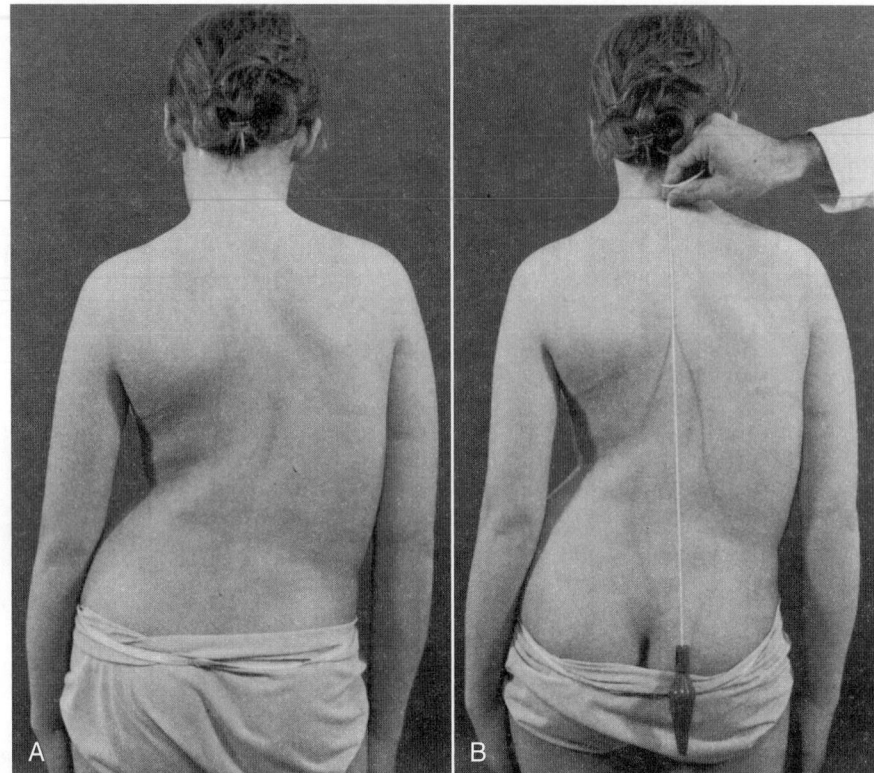

Figure 8-15 Right thoracic idiopathic scoliosis (posterior view). A, The left shoulder is lower, and the right scapula is more prominent. Note the decreased distance between the right arm and the thorax with the shift of the thorax to the right. The left iliac crest appears higher, but this results from the shift of the thorax with fullness on the right and elimination of the waistline; the "high" hip is only apparent, not real. **B,** Plumbline dropped from the prominent vertebra of C7 (vertebra prominens) measures the decompensation of the thorax over the pelvis. The distance from the vertical plumbline to the gluteal cleft is measured in centimeters and is recorded along with the direction of deviation. If there is a cervical or cervicothoracic curve, the plumb should fall from the occipital protuberance (inion). (From Moe JH, Winter RB, Bradford DS, et al: Scoliosis and other spinal deformities, Philadelphia, 1978, WB Saunders, p. 14.)

bony and soft-tissue contours should be observed for equality on both sides or for any noticeable difference.

The examiner should note whether the patient sits up properly with the normal spinal curves present (Figure 8-16, *A*); whether the tip of the ear, tip of the acromion process, and high point of the iliac crest are in a straight line as they should be; and whether the patient sits in a slumped position (i.e., sag sitting, as in Figure 8-16, *B*).

The skin should be observed for any abnormality or scars (Figure 8-17). If there are scars, are they a result of surgery or trauma? Are they new or old scars? If from surgery, what was the purpose of the surgery?

Breathing

As part of the observation, the examiner should note the patient's breathing pattern. Children tend to breathe abdominally, whereas women tend to do upper thoracic breathing. Men tend to be upper and lower thoracic breathers. In the aged, breathing tends to be in the lower thoracic and abdominal regions (Figure 8-18). The examiner should note the quality of the respiratory movements as well as the rate, rhythm, and effort required to inhale

and exhale. The examiner should also note whether the patient is using the primary muscles of respiration and/or the accessory muscles of respiration, because this will help indicate the ease of the patient's breathing (Table 8-4). In addition, the presence of any coughing or noisy or abnormal breathing patterns should be noted. Because the chest wall movement that occurs during breathing displaces the pleural surfaces, thoracic muscles, nerve, and ribs, pain is accentuated by breathing and coughing if any one of these structures is injured.

Chest Deformities

In addition to rib movements during breathing, the examiner should note the presence of any chest deformities. The more common deformities are shown in Figure 8-19 and are listed below:

1. With a **pigeon chest** (pectus carinatum) deformity, the sternum projects forward and downward like the heel of a boot, increasing the anteroposterior dimension of the chest. This congenital deformity impairs the effectiveness of breathing by restricting ventilation volume.

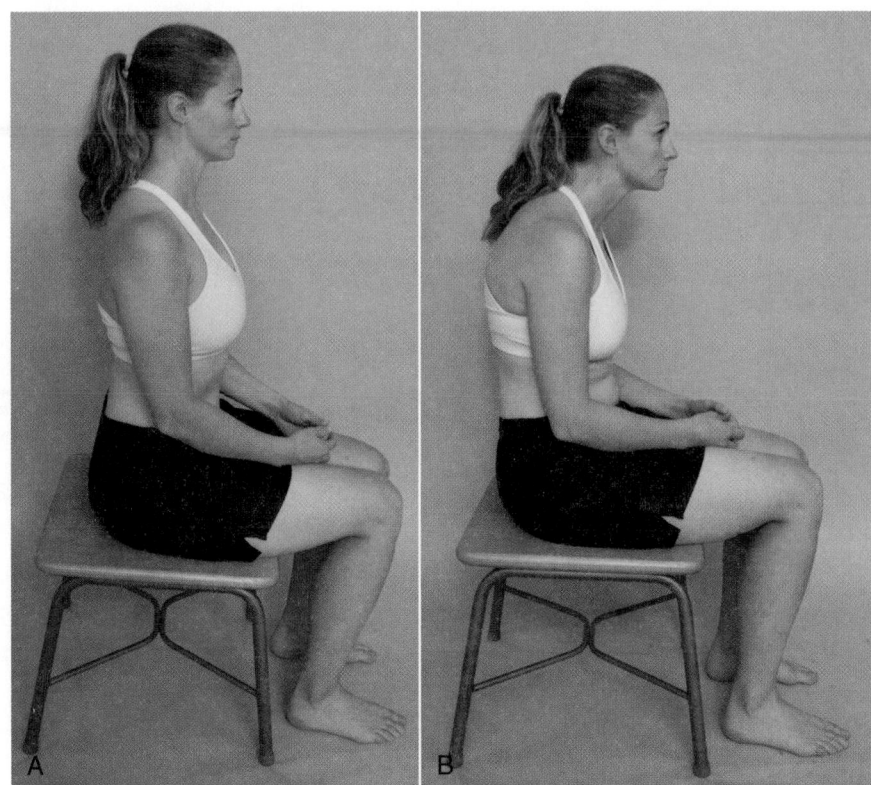

Figure 8-16 Sitting posture. A, Normal position. **B,** Sag sitting.

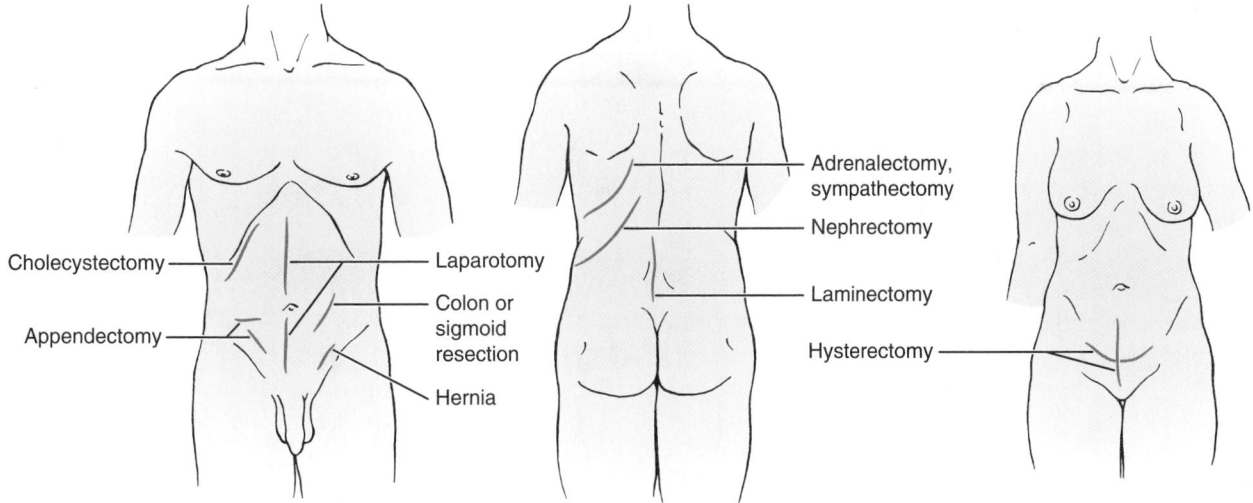

Cholecystectomy

Laparotomy

Appendectomy

Colon or
sigmoid
resection

Hernia

Adrenalectomy,
sympathectomy

Nephrectomy

Laminectomy

Hysterectomy

Figure 8-17 Common surgical scars of the abdomen and thorax. (Redrawn from Judge RD, Zuidema GD, Fitzgerald FT: Clinical diagnosis: a physiologic approach, Boston, 1982, Little Brown, p. 295.)

2. The **funnel chest** (pectus excavatum) is a congenital deformity that results from the sternum's being pushed posteriorly by an overgrowth of the ribs.[13] The anteroposterior dimension of the chest is decreased, and the heart may be displaced. On inspiration, this deformity causes a depression of the sternum that affects respiration and may result in kyphosis.

3. With the **barrel chest** deformity, the sternum projects forward and upward so that the anteroposterior

diameter is increased. It is seen in pathological conditions, such as emphysema.

EXAMINATION

Although the assessment is primarily of the thorax and thoracic spine, if the history, observation, or examination indicates symptoms into or from the neck, upper limb, or lumbar spine and lower limb, these structures must be

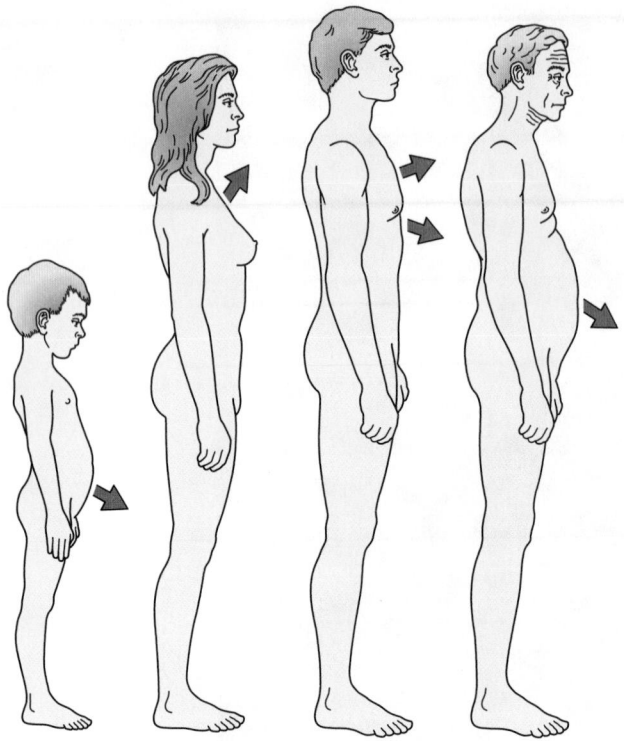

TABLE 8-4

Muscles of Respiration

	Primary	Secondary
Inspiration	Diaphragm	Scaleni
	Levator costorum	Sternocleidomastoid
	External intercostals	Trapezius
	Internal intercostals (anterior)	Serratus anterior and posterior
		Pectoralis major
		Pectoralis minor
		Subclavius
Both		Latissimus dorsi
Expiration	Internal obliques	Serratus posterior inferior
	External obliques	Quadratus lumborum
	Rectus abdominus	Iliocostalis lumborum
	Transverse abdominus	
	Transversus thoracis	
	Transverse intercostals	
	Internal intercostals (posterior)	

Figure 8-18 Normal breathing patterns for child, adult female, adult male, and elderly person. Occatemo lorenieniam quam, odit ima suscient

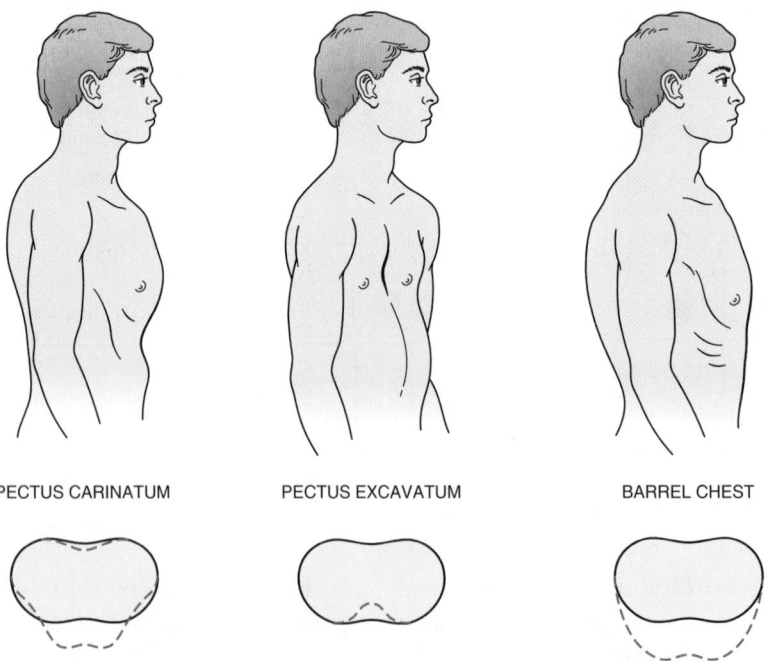

PECTUS CARINATUM   PECTUS EXCAVATUM   BARREL CHEST

Figure 8-19 Chest deformities. Lower vertical views show change in chest wall contours with deformity.

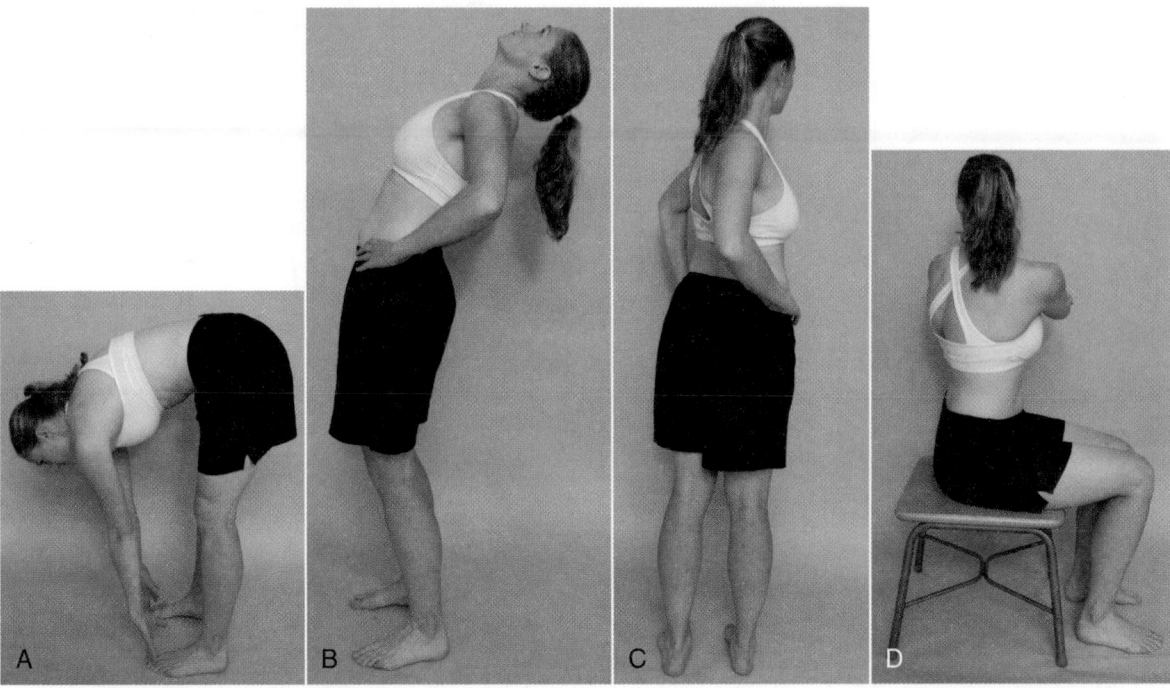

Figure 8-20 Active movements. A, Forward flexion. **B,** Extension. **C,** Rotation (standing). **D,** Rotation (sitting).

examined as well using an upper or lower scanning examination. If any signs or symptoms are elicited in the scanning exam, more detailed examination of the cervical or lumbar spine may be performed. Therefore, the examination of the thoracic spine may be an extensive one. Unless there is a history of specific trauma or injury to the thoracic spine or ribs, the examiner must be prepared to assess more than that area alone. If a problem is suspected above the thoracic spine, the scanning examination of the cervical spine and upper limb (as described in Chapter 3) should be performed. If a problem is suspected below the thoracic spine, the scanning examination of the lumbar spine and lower limb (as described in Chapter 9) should be performed. Only examination of the thoracic spine is described here.

Active Movements

The active movements of the thoracic spine are usually done with the patient standing. Movement in the thoracic spine is limited by the rib cage and the long spinous processes of the thoracic spine. When assessing the thoracic spine, the examiner should be sure to note whether the movement occurs in the spine or in the hips. A patient can touch the toes with a completely rigid spine if there is sufficient range of motion (ROM) in the hip joints. Likewise, tight hamstrings may alter the results. The movements may be done with the patient sitting, in which case the effect of hip movement is eliminated or decreased. Similarly, shoulder motion may be restricted if the upper thoracic segments or ribs are hypomobile.[14] As with any

examination, the most painful movements are done last. The active movements to be carried out in the thoracic spine are shown in Figure 8-20.

Active Movements of the Thoracic Spine

- Forward flexion (20° to 45°)
- Extension (25° to 45°)
- Side flexion, left and right (20° to 40°)
- Rotation, left and right (35° to 50°)
- Costovertebral expansion (3 cm to 7.5 cm)
- Rib motion (pump handle, bucket handle, and caliper)
- Combined movements (if necessary)
- Repetitive movements (if necessary)
- Sustained postures (if necessary)

Forward Flexion

The normal ROM of forward flexion (forward bending) in the thoracic spine is 20° to 45° (Figure 8-21). Because the ROM at each vertebra is difficult to measure, the examiner can use a tape measure to derive an indication of overall movement (Figure 8-22). The examiner first measures the length of the spine from the C7 spinous process to the T12 spinous process with the patient in the normal standing posture. The patient is then asked to bend forward and the spine is again measured. A 2.7-cm (1.1-inch) difference in tape measure length is considered normal.

If the examiner wishes, the spine may be measured from the C7 to S1 spinous process with the patient in the

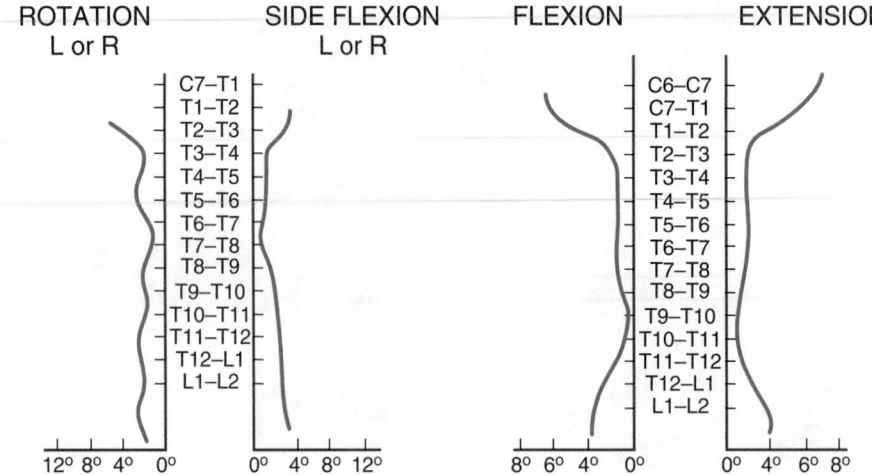

Figure 8-21 Average range of motion (ROM) in the thoracic spine. (Adapted from Grieve GP: Common vertebral joint problems, Edinburgh, 1981, Churchill Livingstone, pp. 41–42.)

normal standing position. The patient is then asked to bend forward, and the spine is again measured. A 10-cm (4-inch) difference in tape measure length is considered normal. In this case, the examiner is measuring movement in the lumbar spine as well as in the thoracic spine; most movement, approximately 7.5 cm (3 inches), occurs between T12 and S1.

A third method of measuring spinal flexion is to ask the patient to bend forward and try to touch the toes while keeping the knees straight. The examiner then measures from the fingertips to the floor and records the distance. The examiner must keep in mind that with this method, in addition to the thoracic spine movement, the movement may also occur in the lumbar spine and hips; in fact, movement could occur totally in the hips.

Each of these methods is indirect. To measure the ROM at each vertebral segment, a series of radiographs would be necessary. The examiner can decide which method to use. It is of primary importance, however, to note on the patient's chart how the measuring was done and which reference points were used.

While the patient is flexed forward, the examiner can observe the spine from the "skyline" view (Figure 8-23). With nonstructural scoliosis, the scoliotic curve disappears on forward flexion; with structural scoliosis, it remains. With the skyline view, the examiner is looking for a hump on one side (convex side of curve) and a hollow (concave side of curve) on the other. This "hump and hollow" sequence is caused by vertebral rotation in idiopathic scoliosis, which pushes the ribs and muscles out on one side and causes the paravertebral valley on the opposite side. The vertebral rotation is most evident in the flexed position.

When the patient flexes forward, the thoracic spine should curve forward in a smooth, even manner with no rotation or side flexion (Figure 8-24). The examiner should look for any apparent tightness or sharp

angulation, such as a gibbus, when the movement is performed. If the patient has an excessive kyphosis to begin with, very little forward flexion movement occurs in the thoracic spine. McKenzie[7] advocates doing flexion while sitting to decrease pelvic and hip movements. The patient then slouches forward flexing the thoracic spine. The patient can put the hands around the neck to apply overpressure at the end of flexion. If symptoms arise from forward flexion on the spine with the neck flexed by the hands, the examiner should repeat the movement with the neck slightly extended and the hands removed. This will help differentiate between cervical and thoracic pain.

Extension

Extension (backward bending) in the thoracic spine is normally 25° to 45°. Because this movement occurs over twelve vertebrae, the movement between the individual vertebrae is difficult to detect visually. As with flexion, the examiner can use a tape measure and obtain the distance between the same two points (the C7 and T12 spinous processes). Again, a 2.5-cm (1-inch) difference in tape measure length between standing and extension is considered normal. McKenzie[7] advocates having the patient place the hands in the small of the back to add stability while performing the backward movement or to do extension while sitting or prone lying (sphinx position).

As the patient extends, the thoracic curve should curve backward or at least straighten in a smooth, even manner with no rotation or side flexion. Lee[15] advocates asking the patient to fully forward flex the arms during extension to facilitate extension. The examiner should look for any apparent tightness or angulation when the movement is performed. If the patient shows excessive kyphosis (Figure 8-25), the kyphotic curvature remains on extension; that is, the thoracic spine remains flexed, whether the movement is tested while the patient is standing or lying prone (see Figure 8-25).

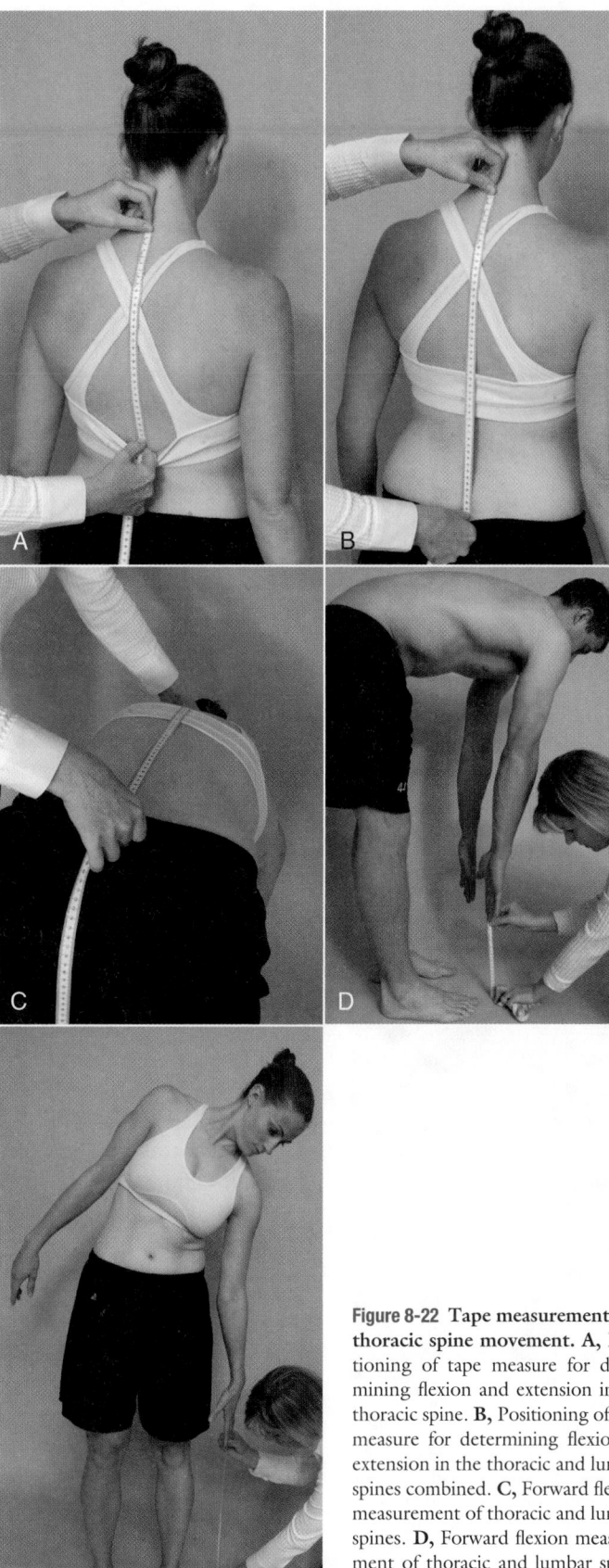

Figure 8-22 Tape measurements for thoracic spine movement. A, Positioning of tape measure for determining flexion and extension in the thoracic spine. **B,** Positioning of tape measure for determining flexion or extension in the thoracic and lumbar spines combined. **C,** Forward flexion measurement of thoracic and lumbar spines. **D,** Forward flexion measurement of thoracic and lumbar spines and hips (fingertips to floor). **E,** Side flexion measurement (fingertips to floor).

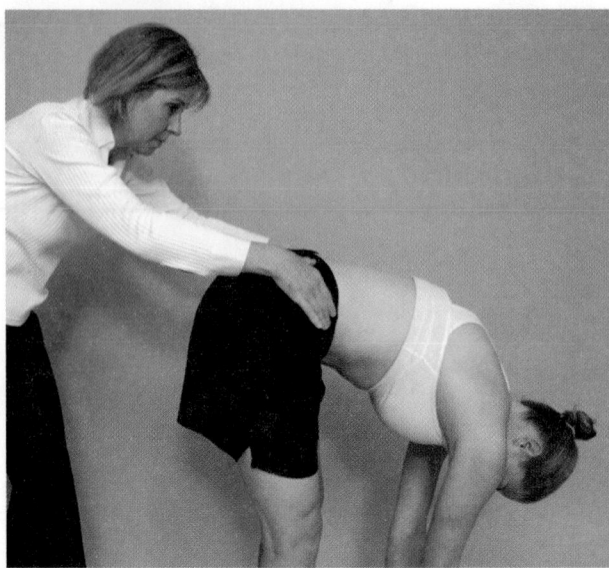

Figure 8-23 Examiner performing skyline view of spine for assessment of scoliosis.

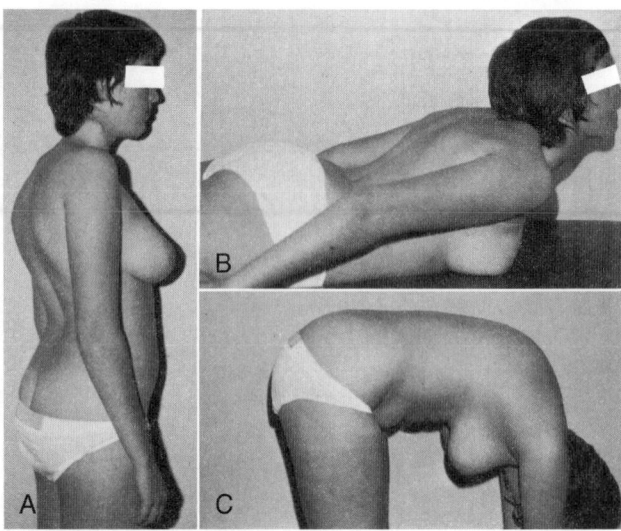

Figure 8-25 Kyphosis and lordosis. A, On physical examination, definite increases in thoracic kyphosis and lumbar lordosis are visualized. **B,** Thoracic kyphosis does not fully correct on thoracic extension. **C,** Lumbar lordosis, on the other hand, usually corrects on forward bending; in this case, some lordosis remains. (From Moe JH, Winter RB, Bradford DS, et al: Scoliosis and other spinal deformities, Philadelphia, 1978, WB Saunders, p. 339.)

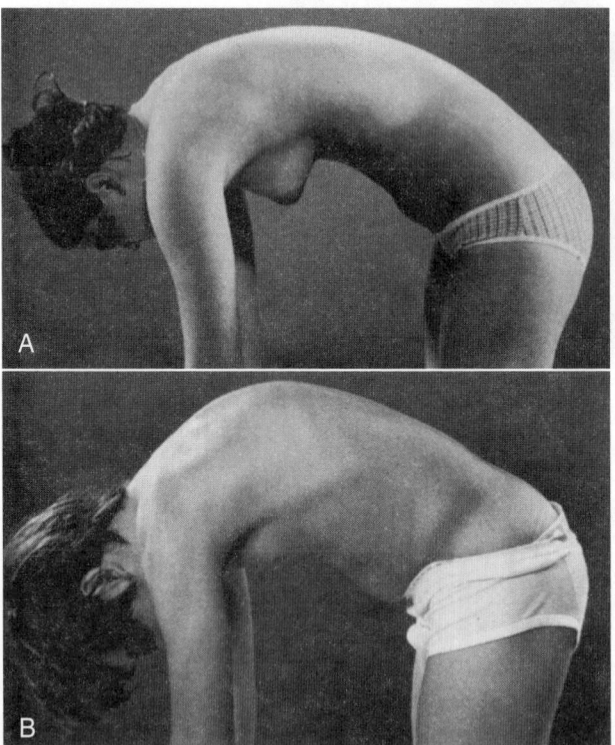

Figure 8-24 Side view in forward bending position for assessment of kyphosis. A, Normal thoracic roundness is demonstrated with a gentle curve to the whole spine. **B,** An area of increased bending is seen in the thoracic spine, indicating structural changes—Scheuermann disease, in this example. (From Moe JH, Winter RB, Bradford DS, et al: Scoliosis and other spinal deformities, Philadelphia, 1978, WB Saunders, p. 18.)

If extension is tested in prone lying, the normal thoracic kyphosis should, for the most part, disappear. If there is a structural kyphosis, the kyphotic curve will remain on extension. McKenzie[7] advocates doing prone extension by using a modified push up straightening the arms and allowing the spine to "sag down" toward the bed (Figure 8-26).

Side Flexion

Side (lateral) flexion is approximately 20° to 40° to the right and left in the thoracic spine. The patient is asked to run the hand down the side of the leg as far as possible without bending forward or backward. The examiner can then estimate the angle of side flexion or use a tape measure to determine the length from the fingertips to the floor and compare it with that of the other side (see Figure 8-22, *E*). Normally, the distances should be equal. In either case, the examiner must remember that movement in the lumbar spine as well as in the thoracic spine is being measured. As the patient bends sideways, the spine should curve sideways in a smooth, even, sequential manner. The examiner should look for any tightness or abnormal angulation, which may indicate hypomobility or hypermobility at a specific segment when the movement is performed. If, on side flexion, the ipsilateral paraspinal muscles tighten or their contracture is evident (Forestier's bowstring sign), ankylosing spondylitis or pathology causing muscle spasm should be considered.[16]

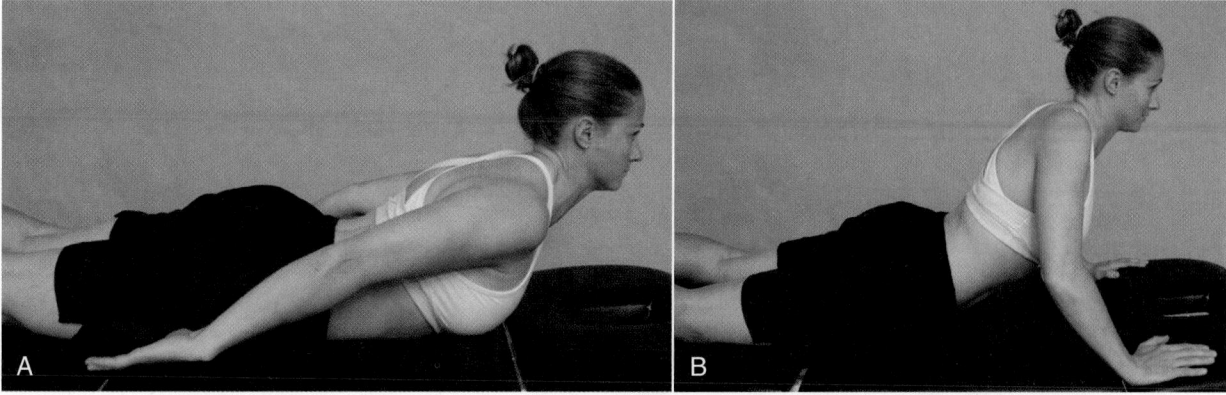

Figure 8-26 Thoracic extension in prone lying. A, Prone extension. **B,** McKenzie's prone extension.

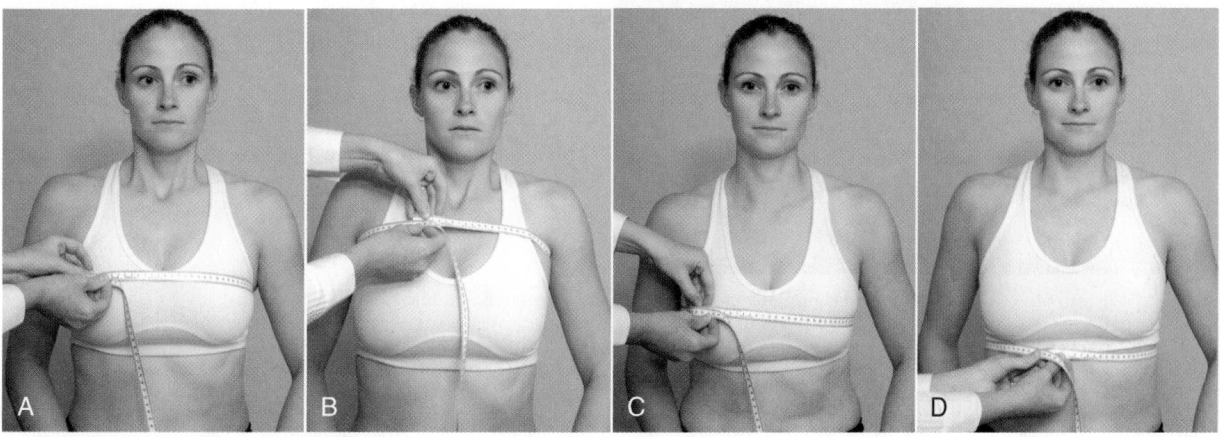

Figure 8-27 Measuring chest expansion. A, Fourth lateral intercostal space. **B,** Axilla. **C,** Nipple line. **D,** Tenth rib.

Rotation

Rotation in the thoracic spine is approximately 35° to 50°. The patient is asked to cross the arms in front or place the hands on opposite shoulders and then rotate to the right and left while the examiner looks at the amount of rotation, comparing both ways. Again, the examiner must remember that movement in the lumbar spine and hips as well as in the thoracic spine is occurring. To eliminate or decrease the amount of the hip movement, rotation may be done in sitting.

If the history indicated that repetitive motion, sustained postures, or combined movements caused aggravation of symptoms, then these movements should also be tested, but only after the original movements of flexion, extension, side flexion, and rotation have been completed. Combined movements that may be tested in the thoracic spine include forward flexion and side bending, backward bending and side flexion, and lateral bending with flexion and lateral bending with extension. Any restriction of motion, excessive movement (hypermobility) or curve abnormality should be noted. These movements would be similar to the H and I test described in the lumbar spine (see Chapter 9).

Costovertebral Expansion

Costovertebral joint movement is usually determined by measuring chest expansion (Figure 8-27). The examiner places the tape measure around the chest at the level of the fourth intercostal space. The patient is asked to exhale as much as possible, and the examiner takes a measurement. The patient is then asked to inhale as much as possible and hold the breath while the second measurement is taken. The normal difference between inspiration and expiration is 3 to 7.5 cm (1 to 3 inches).

A second method of measuring chest expansion is to measure at three different levels. If this method is used, the examiner must take care to ensure that the levels of measurement are noted for consistency. The levels are (1) under the axillae for apical expansion, (2) at the nipple line or xiphisternal junction for midthoracic expansion, and (3) at the T10 rib level for lower thoracic expansion. As before, the measurements are taken after expiration and inspiration.

After the measurement of chest expansion, it is worthwhile for the patient to take a deep breath and cough so that the examiner can determine whether this action causes or alters any pain. If it does, the examiner may

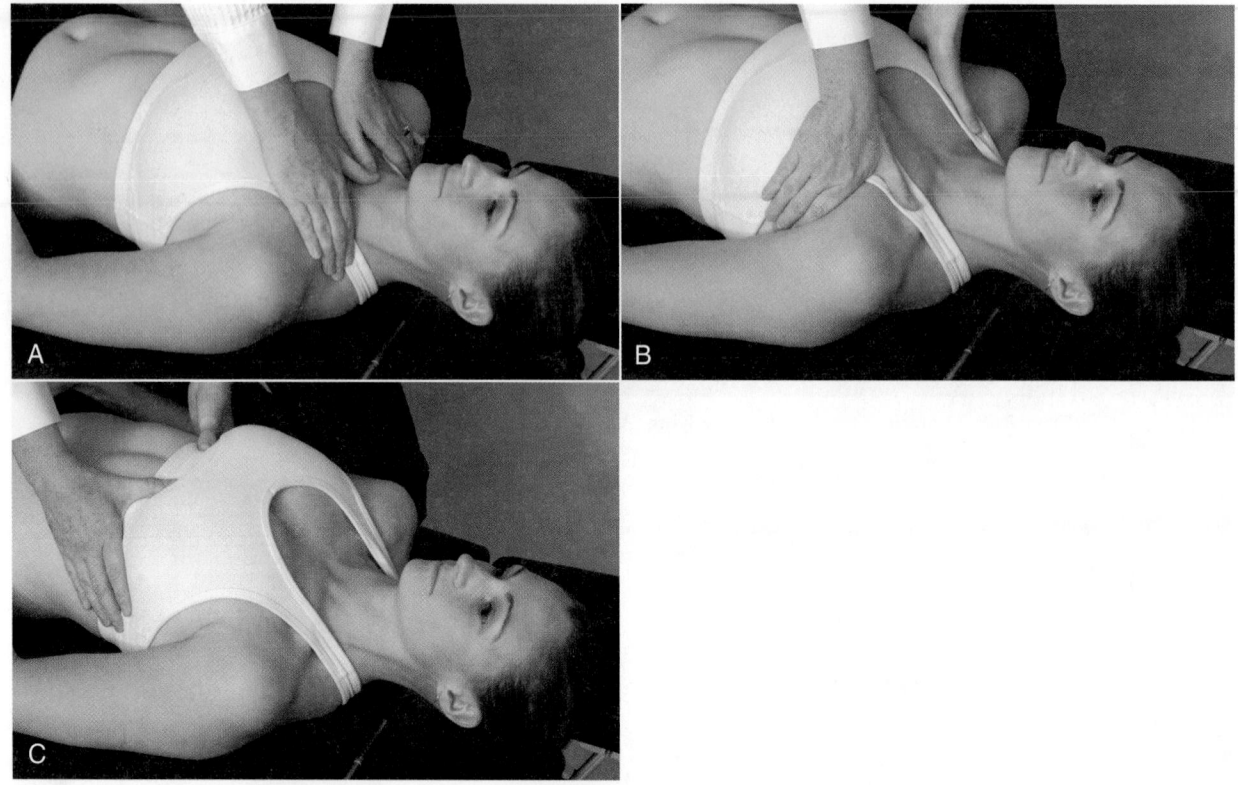

Figure 8-28 Feeling rib movement. A, Upper ribs. **B,** Middle ribs. **C,** Lower ribs.

suspect a respiratory-related problem or a problem increasing intrathecal pressure in the spine.

Evjenth and Gloeck[17] have noted a way to differentiate thoracic spine and rib pain during movement. If the patient has pain on flexion, the patient is returned to neutral and is asked to take a deep breath and hold it. While holding the breath, the patient flexes until pain is felt. At this point, the patient stops flexing and exhales. If further flexion can be accomplished after exhaling, the problem is more likely to be the ribs than the thoracic spine. Extension can be tested in a similar fashion.

Rib Motion

The patient is asked to lie supine. The examiner's hands are placed in a relaxed fashion over the upper chest. In this position, the examiner is feeling anteroposterior movement of the ribs (Figure 8-28). As the patient inhales and exhales, the examiner should compare both sides to see whether the movement is equal. Any restriction or difference in motion should be noted. If a rib stops moving relative to the other ribs on inhalation, it is classified as a **depressed rib.** If a rib stops moving relative to the other ribs on exhalation, it is classified as an **elevated rib.** It must be remembered that restriction of one rib affects the adjacent ribs. If a depressed rib is implicated, it is usually the highest restricted rib that causes the greatest problem. If an elevated rib is present, it is usually the lowest restricted rib that causes the greatest problem

although for both depressed and elevated rib the opposite may be true.[3,18] Rib springing or the presence of pain on stressing the rib joints will help to confirm the level that is hypomobile. The examiner then moves his or her hands down the patient's chest, testing the movement in the middle and lower ribs in a similar fashion.

To test lateral movement of the ribs, the examiner's hands are placed around the sides of the rib cage approximately 45° to the vertical axis of the patient's body. The examiner begins at the level of the axilla and works down the lateral aspect of the ribs, feeling the movement of the ribs during inspiration and expiration and noting any restriction.

Rib dysfunctions may be divided into structural, torsional, and respiratory (Table 8-5).[19] Structural rib dysfunctions are due to joint subluxation or dislocation. Torsional rib dysfunctions are due to thoracic vertebra dysfunction as a result of hypomobility or hypermobility. Respiratory rib dysfunctions are due to either hypomobility between the ribs (e.g., intercostal shortening) or hypomobility at the costotransverse or costovertebral joints.[19]

To test the movement of the ribs relative to the thoracic spine, the patient is placed in a sitting position. The examiner places one thumb or finger on the transverse process and the thumb of the other hand just lateral to the tubercle of the rib. The patient is asked to forward flex the head (for the upper thoracic spine) and thorax (for lower thoracic spine) while the examiner feels the

TABLE **8-5**

Rib Dysfunction

STRUCTURAL RIB DYSFUNCTION				
Dysfunction	**Rib Angle**	**Midaxillary Line**	**Intercostal Space**	**Anterior Rib**
Anterior subluxation	Less prominent	Symmetric	Tender, often with intercostal neuralgia	More prominent
Posterior subluxation	More prominent	Symmetric	Tender, often with intercostal neuralgia	Less prominent
Superior first rib subluxation	Superior aspect of first rib elevated (5 mm)	Hypertonicity of the scalene muscles on the same side	—	Marked tenderness of the superior aspect
Anterior-posterior rib compression	Less prominent	Prominent	Tender, often with intercostal neuralgia	Less prominent
Lateral compression	More prominent	Less prominent	Tender	More prominent
Laterally elevated	Tender	Prominent	Narrow above, wide below	Exquisitely tender at pectoral minor

TORSIONAL RIB DYSFUNCTION			
Dysfunction	**Rib Angle**	**Midaxillary Line**	**Intercostal Space**
External rib torsion	Superior border prominent and tender	Symmetric	Wide above, narrow below
Internal rib torsion	Inferior border prominent and tender	Symmetric	Narrow above, wide below

RESPIRATORY RIB FUNCTION		
Dysfunction	**Rib Angle**	**Key Rib**
Inhalation restriction	During inspiration the rib or group of ribs that cease rising	Top or superior rib
Exhalation restriction	During exhalation the rib or group of ribs that stop falling	Bottom or inferior rib

Modified from Bookhout MR: Evaluation of the thoracic spine and rib cage. In Flynn TW, editor: The thoracic spine and rib cage, Boston, 1996, Butterworth-Heinemann, pp. 163, 165, 166.

movement of the rib (Figure 8-29). Normally, the rib rotates anteriorly and the rib tubercle stays at the same level as the transverse process on the forward movement. If the rib is hypermobile, the rib elevates relative to the transverse process. If the rib is hypomobile, its motion stops before the thoracic spine.[15] Extension may also be tested in a similar fashion, but the rib rotates posteriorly.

Passive Movements

Because passive movements in the thoracic spine are difficult to perform in a gross fashion, the movement between each pair of vertebrae may be assessed. With the patient sitting, the examiner places one hand on the patient's forehead or on top of the head (Figure 8-30). With the other hand, the examiner palpates over and between the spinous processes of the lower cervical and upper thoracic spines (C5–T3) and feels for movement between the spinous processes while flexing (move apart) and extending (move together) the patient's head. Rotation (one side moves forward, the other moves back) and side flexion (one side moves apart, one side moves together) may be tested by rotating and side flexing the patient's head. To test the movement properly, the

examiner places the middle finger over the spinous process of the vertebra being tested and the index and ring fingers on each side of it, between the spinous processes of the two adjacent vertebrae. The examiner should feel the movement occurring, assess its quality, and note whether the movement is hypomobile or hypermobile relative to the adjacent vertebra. The hypomobility or hypermobility may be indicative of pathology.[18]

Passive Movements of the Thoracic Spine and Normal End Feel

- Forward flexion (tissue stretch)
- Extension (tissue stretch)
- Side flexion, left and right (tissue stretch)
- Rotation, left and right (tissue stretch)

If, when the spinous processes are palpated, one process appears to be out of alignment, the examiner can then palpate the transverse processes on each side and compare them with the levels above and below to determine whether the vertebrae is truly rotated or side flexed. For example, if the spinous process of T5 is shifted to the right and if rotation has occurred at that level, the left

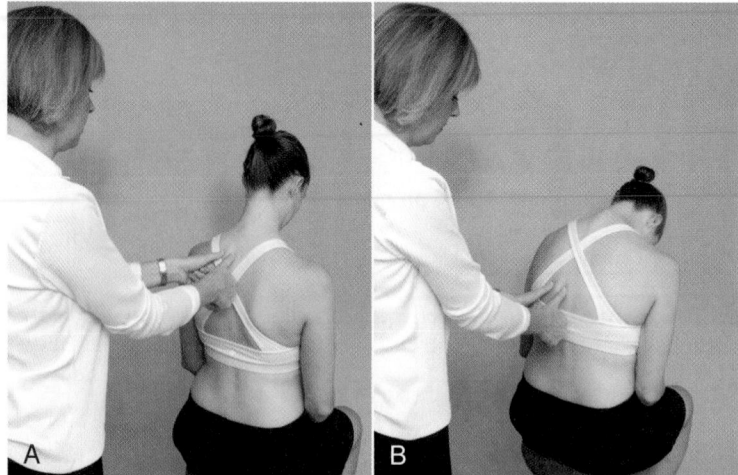

Figure 8-29 **Testing mobility of rib relative to thoracic vertebra.** Note one thumb is on the transverse process of the vertebra and one thumb is on the rib. **A,** Upper ribs. **B,** Lower ribs.

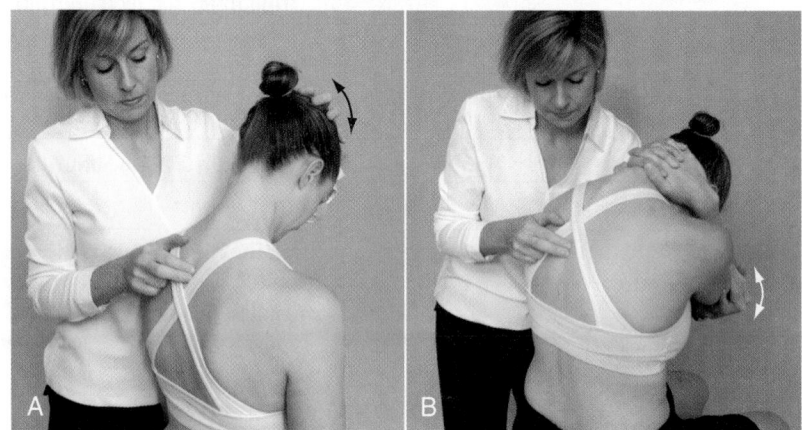

Figure 8-30 **Passive flexion/extension movement of the thoracic spine. A,** Upper thoracic spine. **B,** Middle and lower thoracic spine.

transverse process would be more superficial posteriorly, whereas the right one would appear deeper. If the spinous process rotation was an anomaly, the transverse processes would be equal as would the ribs. Passive or active movement of the spine while palpating the transverse processes also helps to indicate abnormal movement when comparing both sides or when comparing one level to another. If the alignment is normal to begin with and becomes abnormal with movement, or if it is abnormal to begin with and becomes normal with movement, it indicates a functional asymmetry rather than a structural one. Generally, a structural asymmetry would be evident if it remains through all movements.[19]

To test the movement of the vertebrae between T3 and T11, the patient sits with the fingers clasped behind the neck and the elbows together in front. The examiner places one hand and arm around the patient's elbows while palpating over and between the spinous processes, as previously described. The examiner then flexes and extends the spine by lifting and lowering the patient's elbows.

Side flexion and rotation of the trunk may be performed in a similar fashion to test these movements. The patient sits with the hands clasped behind the head. The examiner uses the thumb on one side of the spinous process and/or the index finger and/or the middle finger on the other side to palpate just lateral to the interspinous space. For side flexion, the examiner moves the patient into right side flexion and then left side flexion and by palpation compares the amount and quality of right and left movement including adjacent segments (Figure 8-31, *A*). For rotation, the examiner rotates the patient's shoulders to the right or left, comparing by palpation the amount and quality of movement of each segment as well as that of adjacent segments (Figure 8-31, *B*).[18]

Resisted Isometric Movements

Resisted isometric movements are performed with the patient in the sitting position. The examiner places one leg behind the patient's buttocks and the upper limbs around the patient's chest and back (Figure 8-32). The examiner then instructs the patient, "Don't let me move you," and isometrically tests the movements, noting any alteration in strength and occurrence of pain.

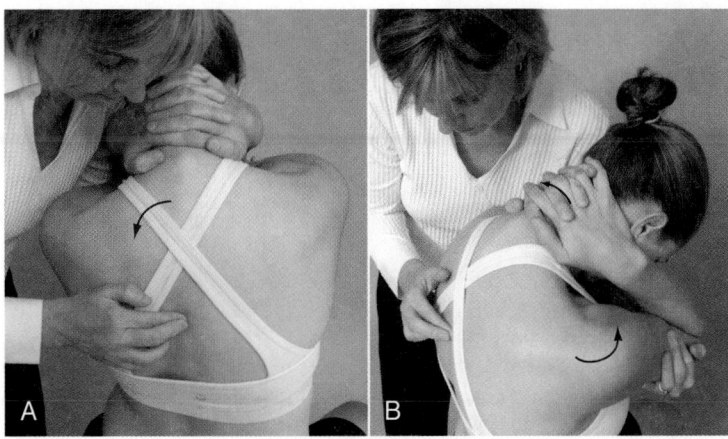

Figure 8-31 A, Passive side flexion of the thoracic spine. **B,** Passive rotation of the thoracic spine.

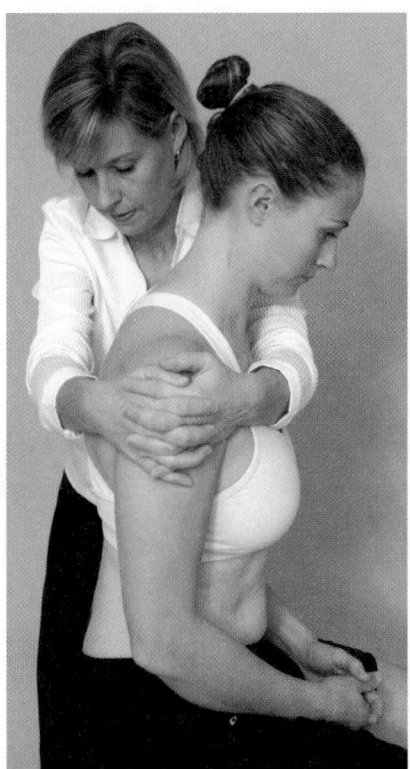

Figure 8-32 **Positioning for resisted isometric movements.**

Resisted Isometric Movements of the Thoracic Spine

- Forward flexion
- Extension
- Side flexion, left and right
- Rotation, left and right

The thoracic spine should be tested in a neutral position, and the most painful movements are done last. Table 8-6 lists the muscles of the thoracic spine, their actions, and their innervations. It must be remembered that the resisted isometric testing of the spine is in reality a very gross test, and subtle alterations in strength are almost impossible to detect. However, if the muscles being tested have been strained (1° or 2°), contraction of the muscle commonly produces pain. In some cases, however, the spine and thorax may have to be repositioned to isolate a particular muscle.

Functional Assessment

When doing specific activities, the thoracic spine primarily plays a stabilization role. Therefore, activities involving the cervical spine, lumbar spine, and shoulder may be impaired as a result of thoracic lesions. Functional activities involving these three areas should be reviewed or considered if functional impairment appears to be related to the thoracic spine or ribs. Activities such as lifting, rotating the thorax, doing heavy work, any activity requiring stabilization of the thorax, or any activity increasing cardiopulmonary output are most likely to provoke thoracic symptoms.

Functional disability scales, such as the Oswestry Disability Questionnaire[20] (see Chapter 9), although designed for the lumbar spine, could be used to test functional capacity in the thoracic spine as well.[20–22] The Oswestry Disability Questionnaire is better suited for persistent severe disability.[21] The Functional Rating Index (Figure 8-33) has been designed to show clinical change in conditions affecting the spine, whether cervical, thoracic, or lumbar.[23]

Special Tests

For the reader who would like to review them, the reliability, validity, specificity, sensitivity, and odds ratios of

TABLE **8-6**

Muscles of the Thorax and Abdomen: Their Actions and Nerve Root Derivation/Nerve Supply in the Thoracic Spine

Action	Muscles Acting	Nerve Root Derivation
Flexion of thoracic spine	1. Rectus abdominis	T6–T12
	2. External abdominal oblique (both sides acting together)	T7–T12
	3. Internal abdominal oblique (both sides acting together)	T7–T12, L1
Extension of thoracic spine	1. Spinalis thoracis	T1–T12
	2. Iliocostalis thoracis (both sides acting together)	T1–T12
	3. Longissimus thoracis (both sides acting together)	T1–T12
	4. Semispinalis thoracis (both sides acting together)	T1–T12
	5. Multifidus (both sides acting together)	T1–T12
	6. Rotatores (both sides acting together)	T1–T12
	7. Interspinalis	T1–T12
Rotation and side flexion of thoracic spine	1. Iliocostalis thoracis (to same side)	T1–T12
	2. Longissimus thoracis (to same side)	T1–T12
	3. Intertransverse (to same side)	T1–T12
	4. Internal abdominal oblique (to same side)	T7–T12, L1
	5. Semispinalis thoracis (to opposite side)	T1–T12
	6. Multifidus (to opposite side)	T1–T12
	7. Rotatores (to opposite side)	T1–T12
	8. External abdominal oblique (to opposite side)	T7–T12
	9. Transverse abdominis (to opposite side)	T7–T12, L1
Elevation of ribs	1. Scalenus anterior (first rib)	C4–C6
	2. Scalenus medius (first rib)	C3–C8
	3. Scalenus posterior (second rib)	C6–C8
	4. Serratus posterior superior (second to fifth ribs)	2 to 5 intercostal
	5. Iliocostalis cervicis (first to sixth rib)	C6–C8
	6. Levatores costarum (all ribs)	T1–T12
	7. Pectoralis major (if arm fixed)	Lateral pectoral (C6, C7)
		Medial pectoral (C7, C8, T1)
	8. Serratus anterior (lower ribs if scapula fixed)	Long thoracic (C5–C7)
	9. Pectoralis minor (second to fifth ribs if scapula fixed)	Lateral pectoral (C6, C7)
		Medial pectoral (C7, C8)
	10. Sternocleidomastoid (if head fixed)	Accessory C2, C3
Depression of ribs	1. Serratus posterior inferior (lower four ribs)	T9–T12
	2. Iliocostalis lumborum (lower six ribs)	L1–L3
	3. Longissimus thoracis	T1–T12
	4. Rectus abdominis	T6–T12
	5. External abdominal oblique (lower five to six ribs)	T7–T12
	6. Internal abdominal oblique (lower five to six ribs)	T7–T12, L1
	7. Transverse abdominal (all acting to depress lower ribs)	T7–T12, L1
	8. Quadratus lumborum (twelfth rib)	T12, L1–L4
	9. Transverse thoracis	T1–T12
Approximation of ribs	1. Iliocostalis thoracis	T1–T12
	2. Intercostals (internal and external)	1 to 11 intercostal
	3. Diaphragm	Phrenic
Inspiration	1. External intercostals	1 to 11 intercostal
	2. Transverse thoracis (sternocostalis)	1 to 11 intercostal
	3. Diaphragm	Phrenic
	4. Sternocleidomastoid	Accessory C2, C3
	5. Scalenus anterior	C4–C6
	6. Scalenus medius	C3–C8
	7. Scalenus posterior	C6–C8
	8. Pectoralis major	Lateral pectoral (C5, C6)
		Medial pectoral (C7, C8, T1)
	9. Pectoralis minor	Lateral pectoral (C6, C7)
		Medial pectoral (C7, C8)

TABLE **8-6**

Muscles of the Thorax and Abdomen: Their Actions and Nerve Root Derivation/Nerve Supply in the Thoracic Spine—cont'd

Action	Muscles Acting	Nerve Root Derivation
	10. Serratus anterior	Long thoracic (C5–C7)
	11. Latissimus dorsi	Thoracodorsal (C6–C8)
	12. Serratus posterior superior	2 to 5 intercostal
	13. Iliocostalis thoracis	T1–T12
Expiration	1. Internal intercostals	1 to 11 intercostal
	2. Rectus abdominis	T6–T12
	3. External abdominal oblique	T7–T12
	4. Internal abdominal oblique	T7–T12, L1
	5. Iliocostalis lumborum	L1–L3
	6. Longissimus	T1–L3
	7. Serratus posterior inferior	T9–T12
	8. Quadratus lumborum	T12, L1–L4

some of the special tests used in the thoracic spine are available in Appendix 8-1 on the Evolve website.

Key Tests Performed on the Thoracic Spine Depending on Suspected Pathology*[24,25]

- **For neurological involvement:**
  - ✓ Slump test
  - ✓ Upper limb neurodynamic (tension) tests (ULNT)
- **For thoracic outlet syndrome:**
  - ❓ Adson's test
  - ❓ Costoclavicular maneuver
  - ⚠ Hyperabduction (EAST) test
  - ⚠ Roos test
- **For rib mobility:**
  - ✓ First rib mobility
  - ✓ Rib springing
- **For failed load transfer (kinetic chain instability):**
  - ❓ Prone arm lift (PAL) test
  - ❓ Sitting arm lift (SAL) test

*The author recommends these key tests be learned by the clinician to facilitate a diagnosis. See Chapter 1, p. 55, Key for Classifying Special Tests.

Tests for Neurological Involvement

If the examiner suspects a problem with movement of the spinal cord, any of the neurodynamic tests that stretch the cord may be performed. These include the straight leg raising test and the Kernig sign (see Chapter 9). Either neck flexion from above or straight leg raising from below stretches the spinal cord within the thoracic spine. The following tests should be performed only if the examiner believes they are relevant.

❓ *First Thoracic Nerve Root Stretch.* The patient abducts the arm to 90° and flexes the pronated forearm to 90°.

No symptoms should appear in this position. The patient then fully flexes the elbow, putting the hand behind the neck. This action stretches the ulnar nerve and T1 nerve root. Pain into the scapular area or arm is indicative of a positive test for T1 nerve root.[26]

If the patient has upper limb symptoms that have become evident at the same time as thoracic symptoms, upper limb tension tests should also be considered to rule out referral of neurological symptoms from the thoracic spine.[27]

❓ *Passive Scapular Approximation.* The patient lies prone while the examiner passively approximates the scapulae by lifting the shoulders up and back. Pain in the scapular area may be indicative of a T1 or T2 nerve root problem on the side on which the pain is being experienced.[26]

✓ *Slump Test (Sitting Dural Stretch Test).* The patient sits on the examining table and is asked to "slump" so that the spine flexes and the shoulders sag forward while the examiner holds the chin and head erect. The patient is asked if any symptoms are produced. If no symptoms are produced, the examiner flexes the patient's neck and holds the head down and shoulders slumped to see if symptoms are produced. If no symptoms are produced, the examiner passively extends one of the patient's knees to see if symptoms are produced. If no symptoms are produced, the examiner then passively dorsiflexes the foot of the same leg to see if symptoms are produced (Figure 8-34). The process is repeated with the other leg. Symptoms of sciatic pain or reproduction of the patient's symptoms indicates a positive test, implicating impingement of the dura and spinal cord or nerve roots.[28] Butler[29] suggested that when testing the thoracic spine while the patient is in the slump position that trunk rotation left and right should be added. He felt this maneuver increased

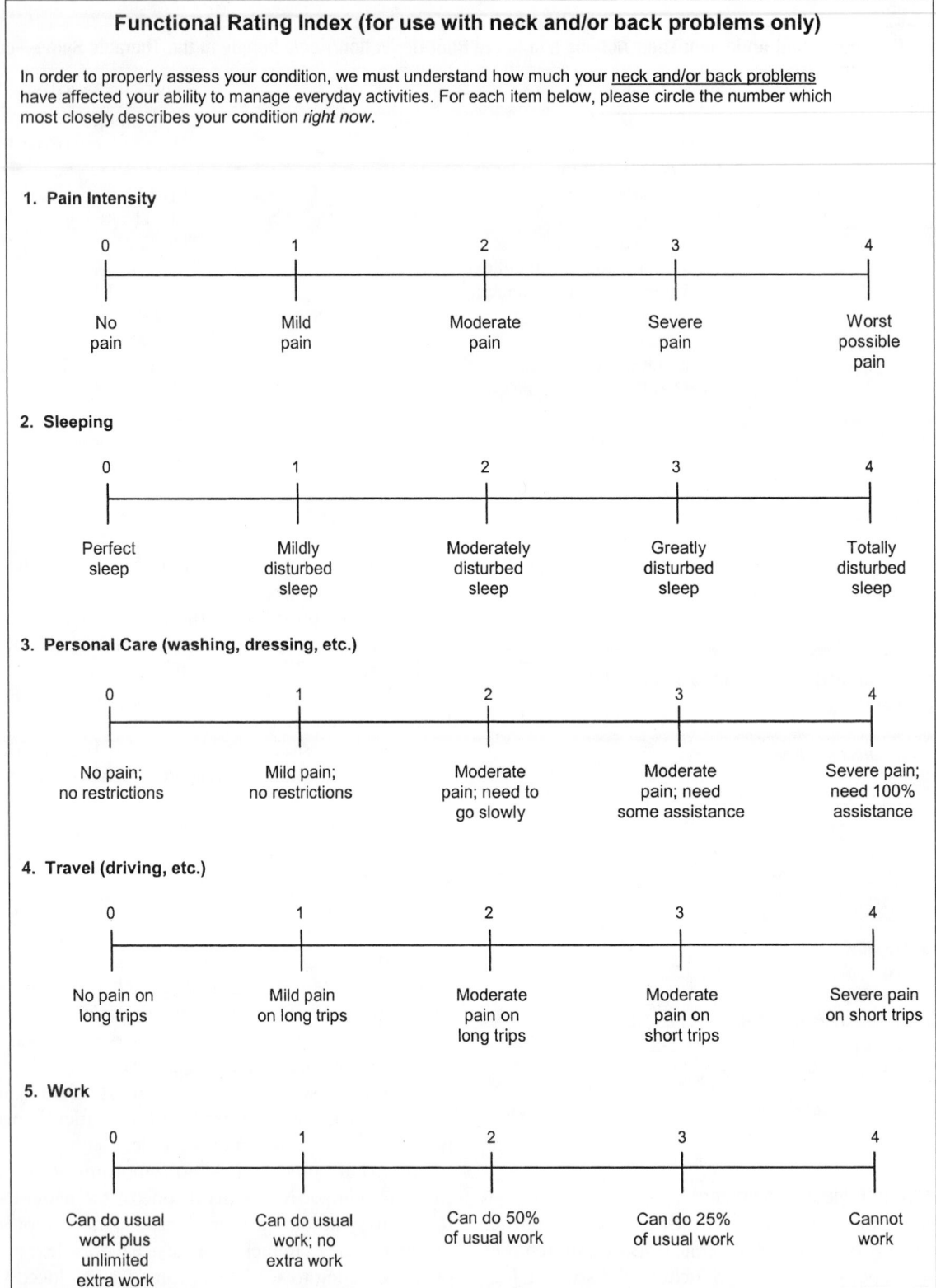

Functional Rating Index (for use with neck and/or back problems only)

In order to properly assess your condition, we must understand how much your <u>neck and/or back problems</u> have affected your ability to manage everyday activities. For each item below, please circle the number which most closely describes your condition *right now*.

1. Pain Intensity

0	1	2	3	4
No pain	Mild pain	Moderate pain	Severe pain	Worst possible pain

2. Sleeping

0	1	2	3	4
Perfect sleep	Mildly disturbed sleep	Moderately disturbed sleep	Greatly disturbed sleep	Totally disturbed sleep

3. Personal Care (washing, dressing, etc.)

0	1	2	3	4
No pain; no restrictions	Mild pain; no restrictions	Moderate pain; need to go slowly	Moderate pain; need some assistance	Severe pain; need 100% assistance

4. Travel (driving, etc.)

0	1	2	3	4
No pain on long trips	Mild pain on long trips	Moderate pain on long trips	Moderate pain on short trips	Severe pain on short trips

5. Work

0	1	2	3	4
Can do usual work plus unlimited extra work	Can do usual work; no extra work	Can do 50% of usual work	Can do 25% of usual work	Cannot work

Figure 8-33 Functional rating index. (Modified from Feise RJ, Menke JM: Functional rating index—a new valid and reliable instrument to measure the magnitude of clinical change in spinal conditions. Spine 26:85–86, 2001. © 1999 Institute of Evidence-Based Chiropractic; www.chiroevidence.com.)

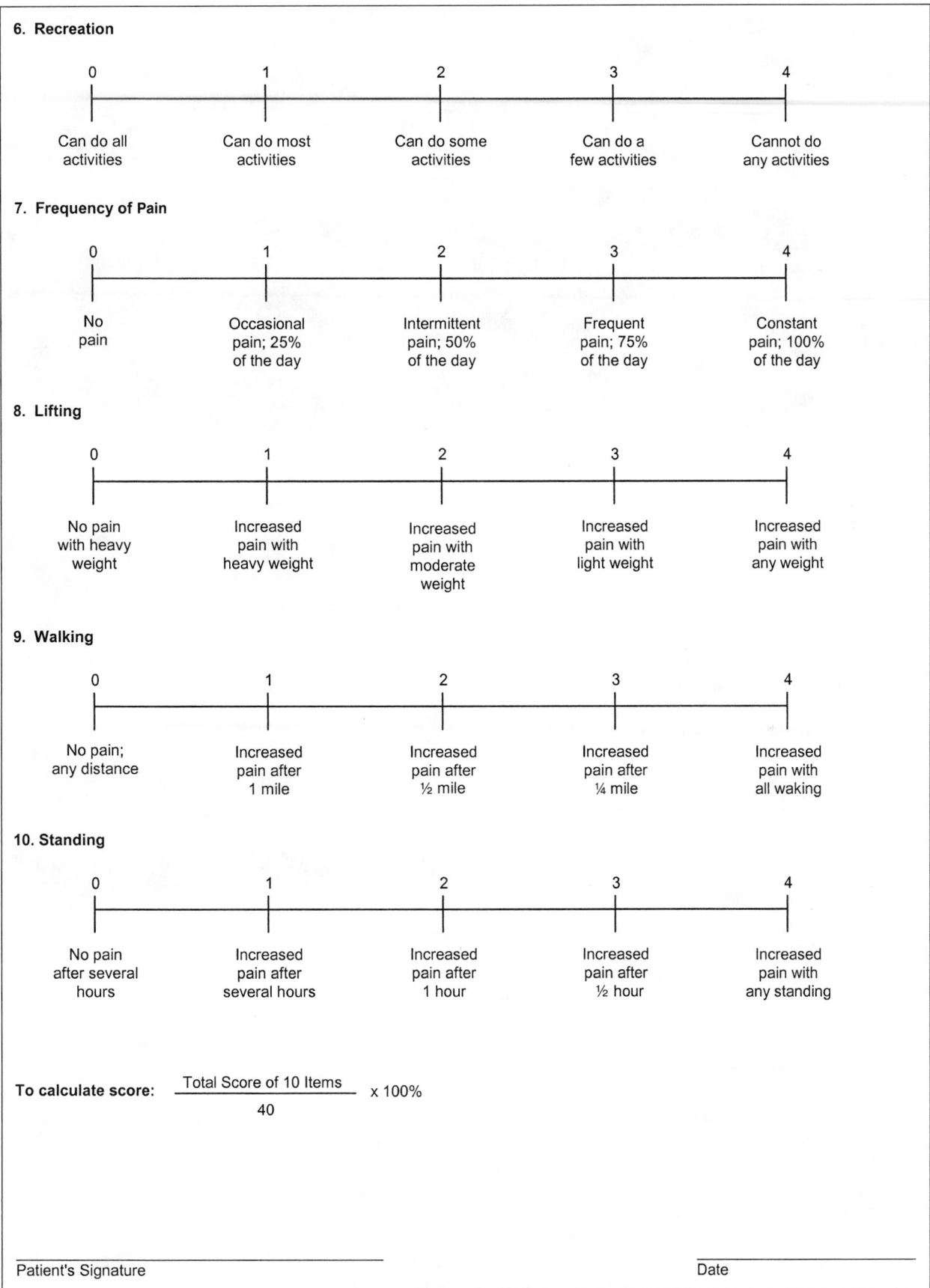

6. Recreation

0	1	2	3	4
Can do all activities	Can do most activities	Can do some activities	Can do a few activities	Cannot do any activities

7. Frequency of Pain

0	1	2	3	4
No pain	Occasional pain; 25% of the day	Intermittent pain; 50% of the day	Frequent pain; 75% of the day	Constant pain; 100% of the day

8. Lifting

0	1	2	3	4
No pain with heavy weight	Increased pain with heavy weight	Increased pain with moderate weight	Increased pain with light weight	Increased pain with any weight

9. Walking

0	1	2	3	4
No pain; any distance	Increased pain after 1 mile	Increased pain after ½ mile	Increased pain after ¼ mile	Increased pain with all waking

10. Standing

0	1	2	3	4
No pain after several hours	Increased pain after several hours	Increased pain after 1 hour	Increased pain after ½ hour	Increased pain with any standing

To calculate score: $\dfrac{\text{Total Score of 10 Items}}{40} \times 100\%$

Patient's Signature   Date

Figure 8-33, cont'd

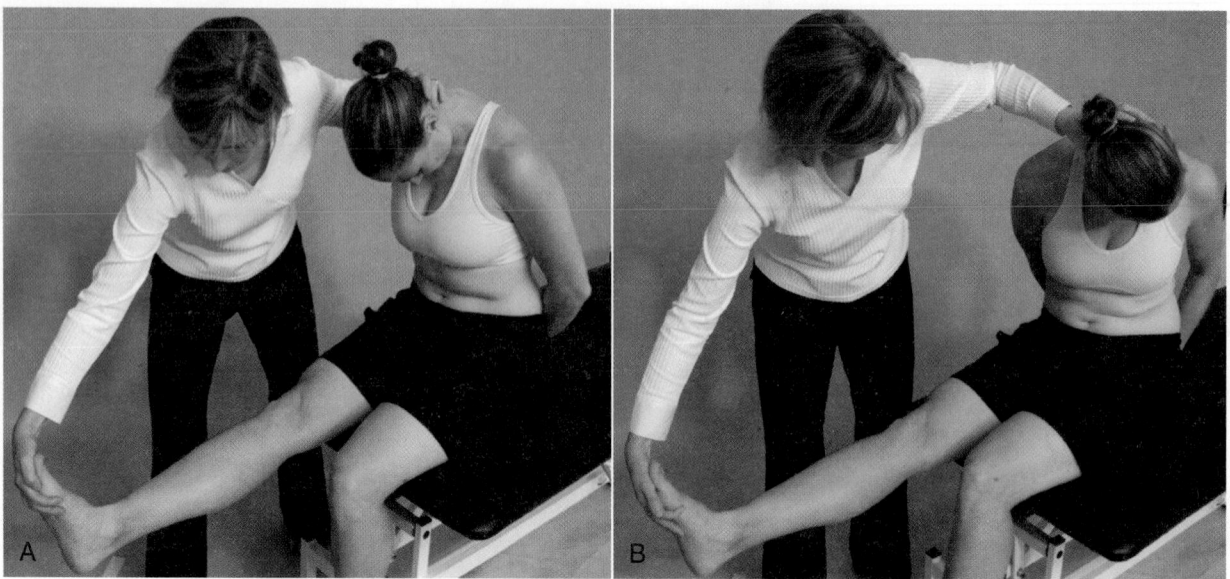

Figure 8-34 Slump test. A, Classic test. **B,** Trunk rotation added to classic test.

the stress on the intercostal nerves. The pain is usually produced at the site of the lesion in a positive test.

✓ *Upper Limb Neurodynamic (Tension) Test.* See Chapter 3 for a description of the upper limb neurodynamic (tension) test (ULNT4).

Tests for Thoracic Outlet Syndrome

There are several special tests that the examiner may consider if thoracic outlet syndrome is suspected. As all of the tests have questionable statistical value in terms of their reliability, the examiner should listen to the patient and use the test that best replicates the position or positions in which the patient has symptoms.

❓ *Adson Maneuver.* See Chapter 5 for a description of the test.

❓ *Costoclavicular Syndrome (Military Brace) Test.* See Chapter 5 for a description of the test.

⚠ *Cyriax Release Test.* The patient is sitting with elbows flexed. The examiner stands behind the patient and grasps under the patient's forearms while the patient's forearms, wrists, and hands are in neutral (Figure 8-35). The examiner then leans the patient's trunk backwards about 15° and lifts the patient's shoulder girdle to end range holding the position for 3 minutes. The production of symptoms or the disappearance of neurological signs **(release phenomenon)** indicates a positive test.

❓ *Halstead Maneuver.* See Chapter 5 for a description of the test.

⚠ *Roos Test (Elevated Arm Stress Test).* See Chapter 5 for a description of the test. The Roos test may also be used to test the arterial portion of thoracic outlet syndrome (testing the radial artery) by positioning the patient in the same position but while looking for neurological signs, the radial pulse is also taken. If the pulse

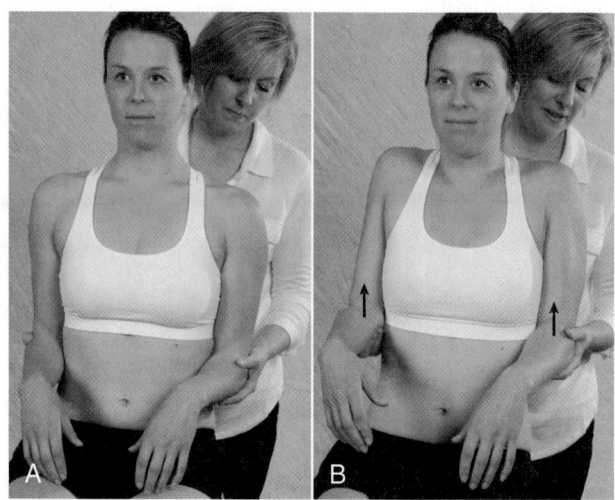

Figure 8-35 Cyriax release test. A, Start position. **B,** 3-minute hold position.

decreases when the patient is in the test position (called the **hyperabduction test** or **elevated arm stress test** **[EAST]** ⚠), it is considered a positive test for thoracic outlet syndrome.

❓ *Wright Test or Maneuver.* See Chapter 5 for a description of the test.

Tests for Rib Mobility

See Chapter 3.

Tests for Failed Load Transfer (Kinetic Chain Instability or Loss of Movement Control)

These tests have been designed to demonstrate the transfer of load through the thoracic spine as part of the kinetic chain. The tests identify the site within the thorax where there are load transfer problems and where in the thoracic area stabilization does not occur during movement.

❓ *Prone Arm Lift Test.*[30] The prone arm lift (PAL) test is a modification of the sitting arm lift (SAL) test. It assesses the ability of the arm to take a load in a higher angle of shoulder flexion. This test is especially useful in people who do overhead activities or who complain of problems when they try to lift heavy loads or try to move the arm too quickly. The patient lies prone with the arms overhead at approximately 140° of flexion and fully supported on the bed. The patient is then asked to lift one arm 2 cm and then lower it. This is repeated with the other side. If one arm is heavier than the other, it is considered the positive side. The examiner can then proceed to do an assessment like the second part of the SAL test, palpating the ribs for abnormal translation, watching the movement of the scapula for scapular dyskinesia, ensuring that the head of the humerus remains centralized in the glenoid, and palpating the cervical spine for abnormal translation.

❓ *Sitting Arm Lift Test.*[30] The patient sits on the bed with the hands resting on the thighs. The examiner asks the patient to lift one arm (the unaffected side first) into elevation through shoulder flexion with the arm straight and the thumb up. The patient then does the same movement with the opposite side. The examiner asks the patient whether one arm feels heavier to lift than the other. The examiner notes whether any symptoms are produced and which arm requires more effort to lift. If one arm is heavier and requires more effort to lift, the first part of the test is considered positive. The patient is then asked to repeat the movement several times while the examiner palpates the ribs individually by placing the thumb on the spinous process and index finger along the rib, noting whether there is any translation of the rib, especially in the first 90° of movement. Normally, when the patient lifts the arm, the muscles of the thorax are activated, stabilizing the thoracic spine so that there is no translation. A positive test for the second part of the test would be indicated by one or more of the thoracic rings (i.e., ribs or vertebrae) translating along any axis or rotating in any plane during the test. The examiner should note the level and direction of the loss of control. Normally what is seen is loss of rotational control with concurrent lateral translation either to the same side as the arm lift or to the contralateral side. This loss of control is usually seen between 0° and 90° of forward flexion.

The SAL test may also be used to demonstrate stability in the scapula, glenohumeral joint, and cervical spine. For the scapula, the examiner should watch the movement of the scapula to determine if there is any scapular dyskinesia indicating a loss of control. For the glenohumeral joint, the head of the humerus should remain centered in the glenoid fossa throughout the full forward flexion into elevation movement. To test the cervical spine, the examiner palpates the lateral aspect of the articular pillars of the cervical spine vertebra bilaterally while the patient does the movement. If there is translation of one vertebra relative to another when the patient does the SAL test, it indicates a lack of control of that individual segment.

Reflexes and Cutaneous Distribution

Within the thoracic spine, there is a great deal of overlap of the dermatomes (Figure 8-36). The dermatomes tend to follow the ribs, and the absence of only one dermatome may lead to no loss of sensation. Pain may be referred to the thoracic spine from various abdominal organs (Figure 8-37; Table 8-7). Although there are no reflexes to test in conjunction with the thoracic spine, the examiner would be wise to test the lumbar reflexes—the patellar reflex (L3–L4), the medial hamstrings reflex (L5–S1), and the Achilles reflex (S1–S2)—because pathology in the thoracic spine can affect these reflexes.

Thoracic nerve root symptoms tend to follow the course of the ribs and may be referred as follows[31]:
- T10 to T11: Pain in epigastric area
- T5: Pain around nipple
- T7 to T8: Pain in epigastric area
- T10 to T11: Pain in umbilical area
- T12: Pain in the groin

Muscles of the thoracic spine may also refer pain into adjacent areas (Table 8-8).

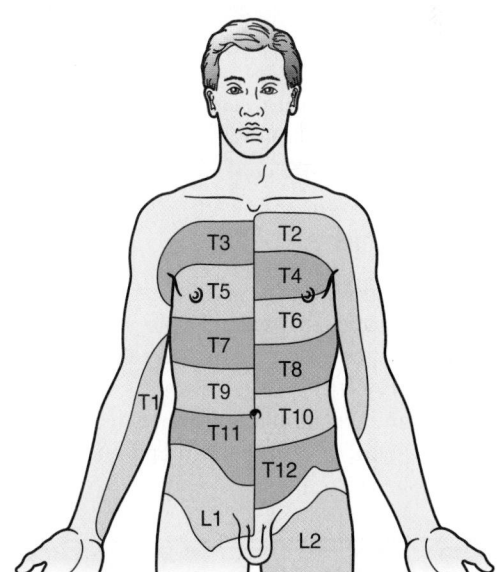

Figure 8-36 The cutaneous areas (dermatomes) supplied by the thoracic nerve roots (after Foerster). By comparing both sides, the degree of overlapping and the area of exclusive supply of any individual nerve root may be estimated. (Adapted from Williams P, Warwick R, editors: Gray's anatomy, ed 37 British, Edinburgh, 1989, Churchill Livingstone, p. 1150.)

TABLE **8-7**

Differences in Pain Perception

Structure	Effective Stimulus*	Conscious Pain Perception
Skin	Discrete touch, prick, heat, cold	Precisely localized, superficial, burning, sharp
Chest wall (muscles, ribs, ligaments, parietal pleura)	Movement, deep pressure	Intermediate in localization and depth; aching, sharp, or dull
Thoracic viscera	Ischemia, distension, muscle spasm	Vague, diffuse, deep, aching, usually dull

From Levene D.: Chest pain: an integrated diagnostic approach, Philadelphia, 1977, Lea & Febiger.
*The effectiveness of a stimuli is heightened by the presence of inflammation.

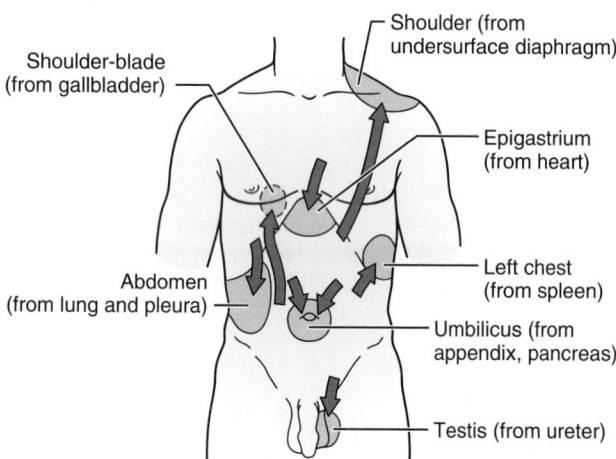

Figure 8-37 **Referred pain in the thorax and chest.** (Modified from Judge RD, Zuidema GD, Fitzgerald FT: Clinical diagnosis: a physiologic approach, Boston, 1982, Little Brown, p. 285.)

Joint Play Movements

The joint play movements performed on the thoracic spine are specific ones that were developed by Maitland.[31] They are sometimes called *passive accessory intervertebral movements (PAIVMs)*. When testing joint play movements, the examiner should note any decreased ROM, muscle spasm, pain, or difference in end feel. The normal end feel is tissue stretch.

Joint Play Movements of the Thoracic Spine

- Posteroanterior central vertebral pressure (PACVP)
- Posteroanterior unilateral vertebral pressure (PAUVP)
- Transverse vertebral pressure (TVP)
- Rib springing

TABLE **8-8**

Thoracic Muscles and Referral of Pain

Muscles	Referral Pattern
Levator scapulae	Neck shoulder angle to posterior shoulder and along medial edge of scapula
Latissimus dorsi	Inferior angle of scapula to posterior shoulder; iliac crest
Rhomboids	Medial border of scapula
Trapezius	Upper thoracic spine to medial border of scapula
Serratus anterior	Lateral chest wall to lower medial border of scapula
Serratus posterior	Medial border of arm to medial two fingers
Serratus superior	Scapular area to posterior and anterior arm down to little finger
Multifidus	Adjacent to spinal column
Iliocostalis	Spinal column to line along medial border of scapula

For the vertebral movements, the patient lies prone. The examiner palpates the thoracic spinous processes, starting at C6 and working down to L1 or L2. The occurrence of muscle spasm and/or pain on application of the vertebral pressure gives the examiner an indication of where the pathology may lie. The examiner must take care, however, because the pain and/or muscle spasm at one level may be the result of compensation for a lesion at another level. For example, if one level is hypomobile as a result of trauma, another level may become hypermobile to compensate for the decreased movement at the traumatized level. It is probable that both the hypomobile and the hypermobile segments will cause pain and/or muscle spasm. It is then important to determine which joint complex is hypomobile and which is hypermobile, because the treatment for each is different.

Posteroanterior Central Vertebral Pressure

The examiner's hands, fingers, and thumbs are positioned as in Figure 8-38, *A*. The examiner then applies pressure to the spinous process through the thumbs, pushing the vertebra forward. Care must be taken to apply pressure slowly and with careful control, so that the movement, which is minimal, can be felt. This springing test may be repeated several times to determine the quality of the movement. The load applied to the spinous process is primarily taken up by the thoracic spine, although part of it is taken up by the rib cage.[32] Each spinous process is done in turn, starting at C6 and working down to L1 or L2. When doing this test, the examiner must keep in mind that the thoracic spinous processes are not always at the level of the same vertebral body. For example, the spinous processes of T1, T2, T3, and T12 are at the same

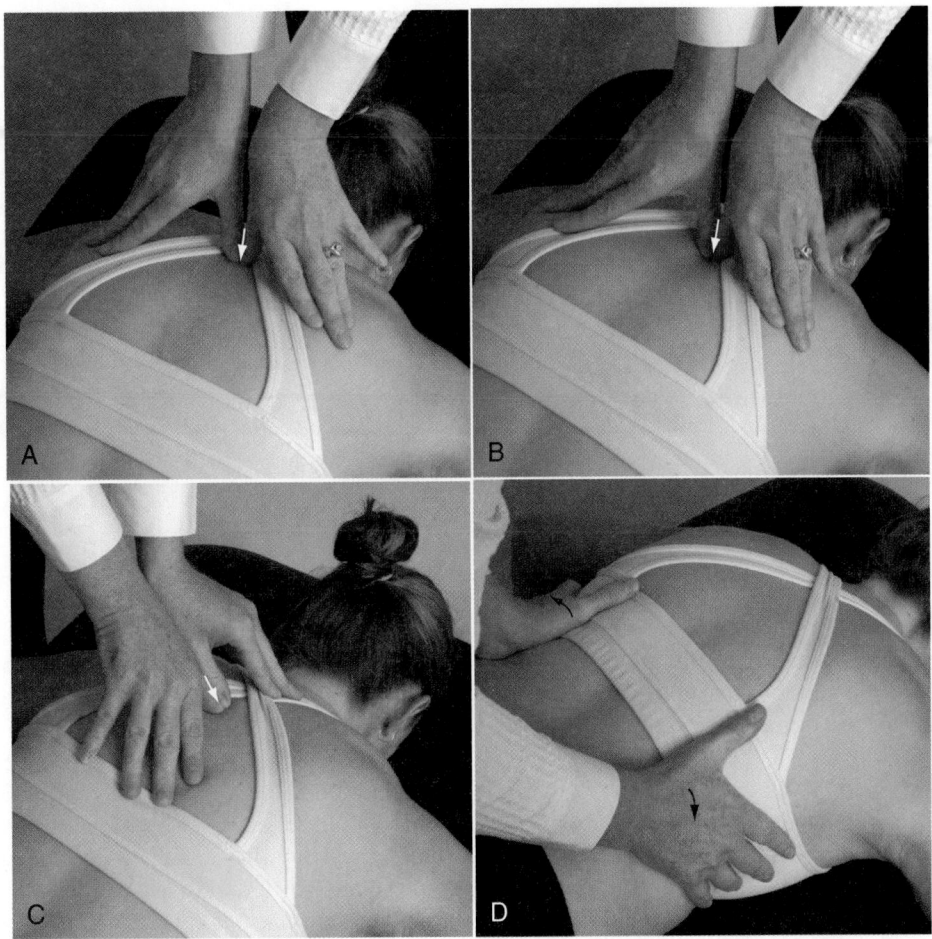

Figure 8-38 Hand, finger, and thumb positions for joint play movements. A, Posteroanterior central vertebral pressure (PACVP). **B,** Posteroanterior unilateral vertebral pressure (PAUVP). **C,** Transverse vertebral pressure. **D,** Rib springing (prone).

levels as the T1, T2, T3, and T12 vertebral bodies, but the spinous processes of T7, T8, T9, and T10 are at the same levels as the T8, T9, T10, and T11 vertebral bodies, respectively.

Posteroanterior Unilateral Vertebral Pressure

The examiner's fingers are moved laterally away from the tip of the spinous process so that the thumbs rest on the appropriate lamina or transverse process of the thoracic vertebra (see Figure 8-38, B; Figure 8-39). The same anterior springing pressure is applied as in the PACVP technique. Again, each vertebra is done in turn. The two sides should be examined and compared. It must be remembered that in the thoracic area, the spinous process is not necessarily at the same level as the transverse process on the same vertebra. For example, the T9 spinous process is at the level of the T10 transverse process. Therefore, it is necessary to move the fingers up and out from the tip of the T9 spinous process to the T9 transverse process, which is at the level of the T8 spinous process. This difference does not hold true for the entire thoracic spine. It is also important to realize that a posteroanterior

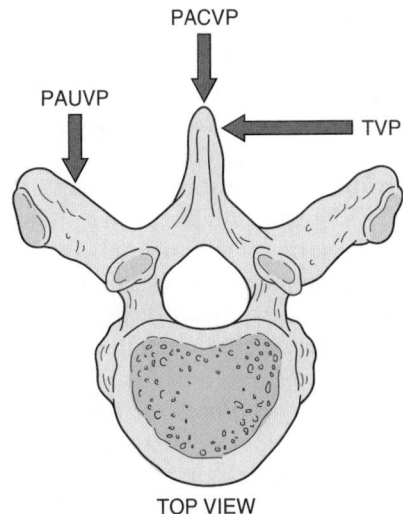

Figure 8-39 Direction of pressure during joint play movements. *PACVP,* Posteroanterior central vertebral pressure; *PAUVP,* posteroanterior unilateral vertebral pressure; *TVP,* transverse vertebral pressure.

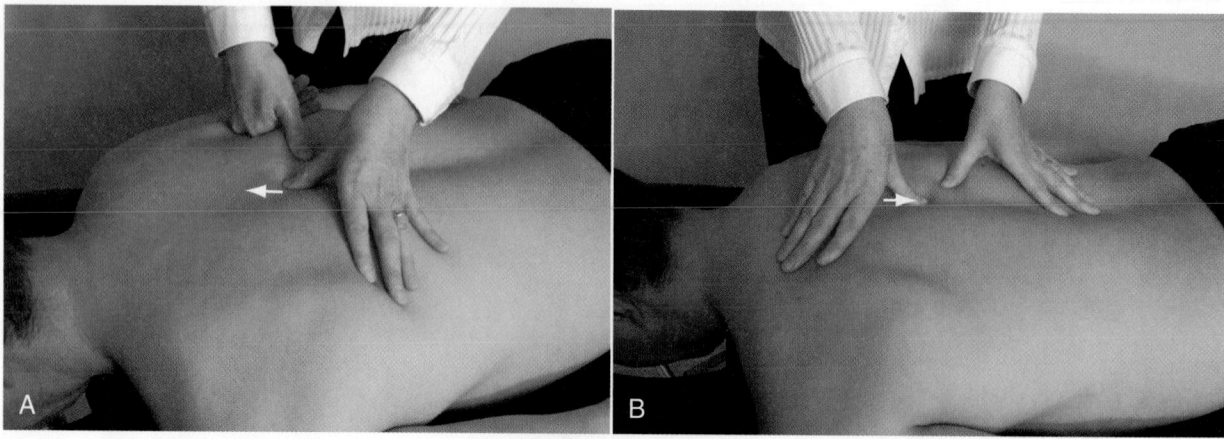

Figure 8-40 A, Superior glide of inferior facet of superior vertebra on inferior vertebra. **B,** Inferior glide of inferior facet of superior vertebra on inferior vertebra.

unilateral vertebral pressure (PAUVP) applies a rotary force to the vertebra; it therefore places a greater stress at the costotransverse joints, because the ribs are also stressed where they attach to the vertebrae. A PAUVP applied to the right transverse process causes the vertebral body to rotate to the left.

Transverse Vertebral Pressure

The examiner's fingers are placed along the side of the spinous process, as shown in Figures 8-38, *C* and 8-39. The examiner then applies a transverse springing pressure to the side of the spinous process, feeling for the quality of movement. As before, each vertebra is assessed in turn, starting at C6 and working down to L1 or L2. Pressure should be applied to both sides of the spinous process to compare the movement. This technique also applies a rotary force to the vertebra, but in the opposite direction to that caused by the PAUVP. A transverse vertebral pressure (TVP) applied to the right side of the spinous process causes the spinous process to rotate to the left and the vertebral body to rotate to the right.

The **individual apophyseal** joints may also be tested (Figure 8-40). The patient is placed in a prone lying position with the thoracic spine in neutral. To test the superior glide at the apophyseal joint (i.e., to test the ability of the inferior articular process of the superior vertebra [e.g., T6] to glide superiorly on the superior articular process of the inferior vertebra [e.g., T7]), the examiner stabilizes the transverse process of the inferior vertebra (e.g., T7) with one thumb while the other thumb glides the inferior articular process of the superior vertebra (e.g., T6) superoanteriorly, noting the end feel and quality of the motion (see Figure 8-40, *A*).[15]

To test the inferior glide at the apophyseal joint (i.e., to test the ability of the inferior articular process of the superior vertebra [e.g., T6] to glide inferiorly on the superior articular process of the inferior vertebra [e.g., T7]), the examiner stabilizes the transverse process of

the inferior vertebra (e.g., T7) with one thumb while the other thumb glides the inferior articular process of the superior vertebra (e.g., T6) inferiorly, noting the end feel and quality of the movement (see Figure 8-40, *B*).[15]

To test the costotransverse joints, the patient is placed in a prone lying position with the spine in neutral. The examiner stabilizes the thoracic vertebra by placing one thumb along or against the side of the transverse process. The other thumb is placed over the posterior and/or superior aspect of the rib just lateral to the tubercle. Some examiners may find it easier to cross thumbs. An anterior or inferior glide is applied to the rib, causing an anterior or inferior movement (Figure 8-41).

Rib Springing

The patient lies prone or on the side while the examiner's hands are placed around the posterolateral aspect of the rib cage (see Figure 8-38, *D*). The examiner's hands are approximately 45° to the vertical axis of the patient's body. The examination begins at the top of the rib cage and extends inferiorly, springing the ribs by pushing in with the hands on each side in turn and then quickly releasing. The amount and quality of movement occurring on both sides should be noted. If one rib appears hypomobile or hypermobile in relation to the others being tested, it or all the ribs can be tested individually by compressing them individually anteriorly and/or posteriorly.

See Chapter 3 for first rib mobility.

Palpation

As with any palpation technique, the examiner is looking for tenderness, muscle spasm, temperature alteration, swelling, or other signs that may indicate disease. Palpation should begin on the anterior chest wall, move around the lateral chest wall, and finish with the posterior structures (Figure 8-42). Palpation is usually done with the

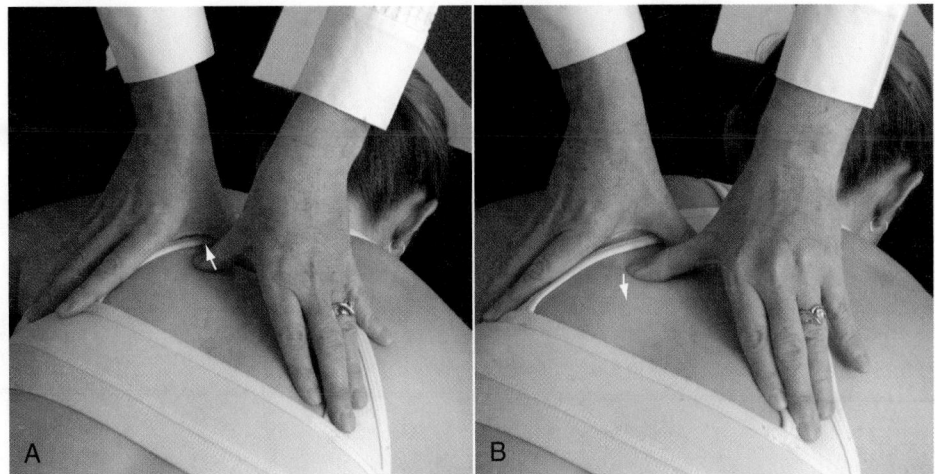

Figure 8-41 **Testing costotransverse joints. A,** Anterior glide with crossed thumbs. **B,** Inferior glide.

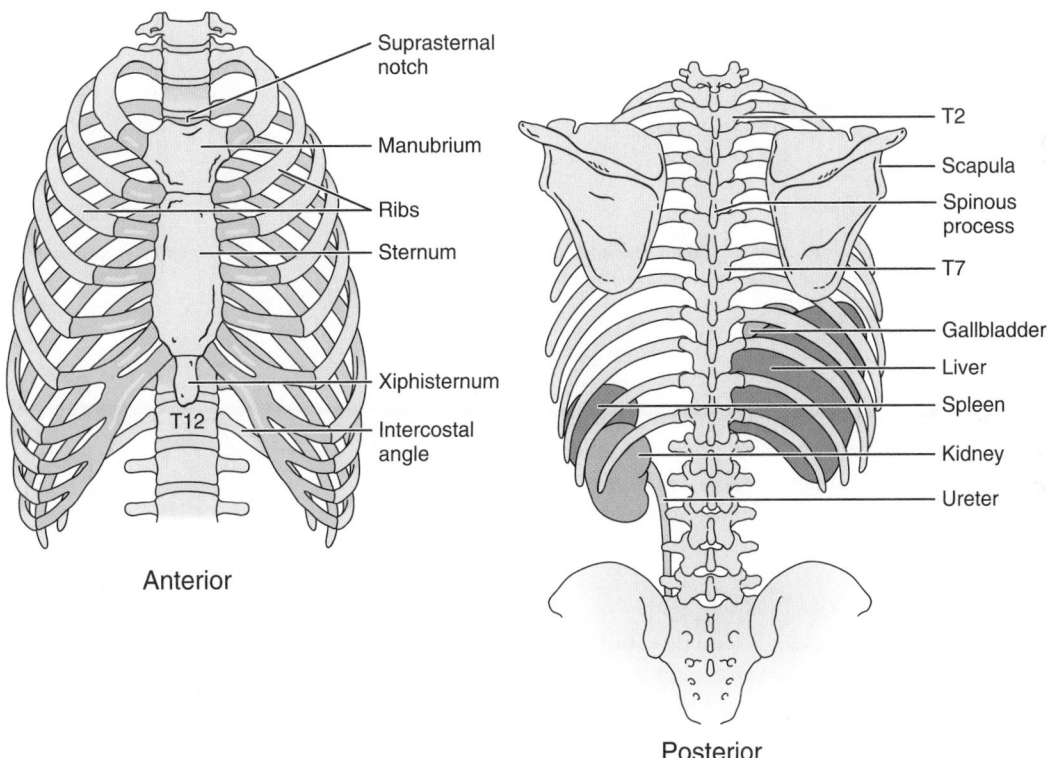

Figure 8-42 **Landmarks of the thoracic spine.**

patient sitting, although it may be done by combining the supine and prone lying positions. At the same time, the thorax may be divided into sections (Figure 8-43) to give some idea, in charting, where the pathology may lie.

Anterior Aspect

Sternum. In the midline of the chest, the manubrium sternum, body of the sternum, and xiphoid process should be palpated for any abnormality or tenderness.

Ribs and Costal Cartilage. Adjacent to the sternum, the examiner should palpate the sternocostal and costochondral articulations, noting any swelling, tenderness, or abnormality. These "articulations" are sometimes sprained or subluxed, or a costochondritis (e.g., Tietze syndrome) may be evident. The ribs should be palpated as they extend around the chest wall with any potential pathology or crepitations (e.g., subcutaneous emphysema) noted.

Clavicle. The clavicle should be palpated along its length for abnormal bumps (e.g., fracture, callus) or tenderness.

Abdomen. The abdomen should be palpated for tenderness or other signs indicating pathology. The palpation is done in a systematic fashion, using the fingers of one hand to feel the tissues while the other hand is used

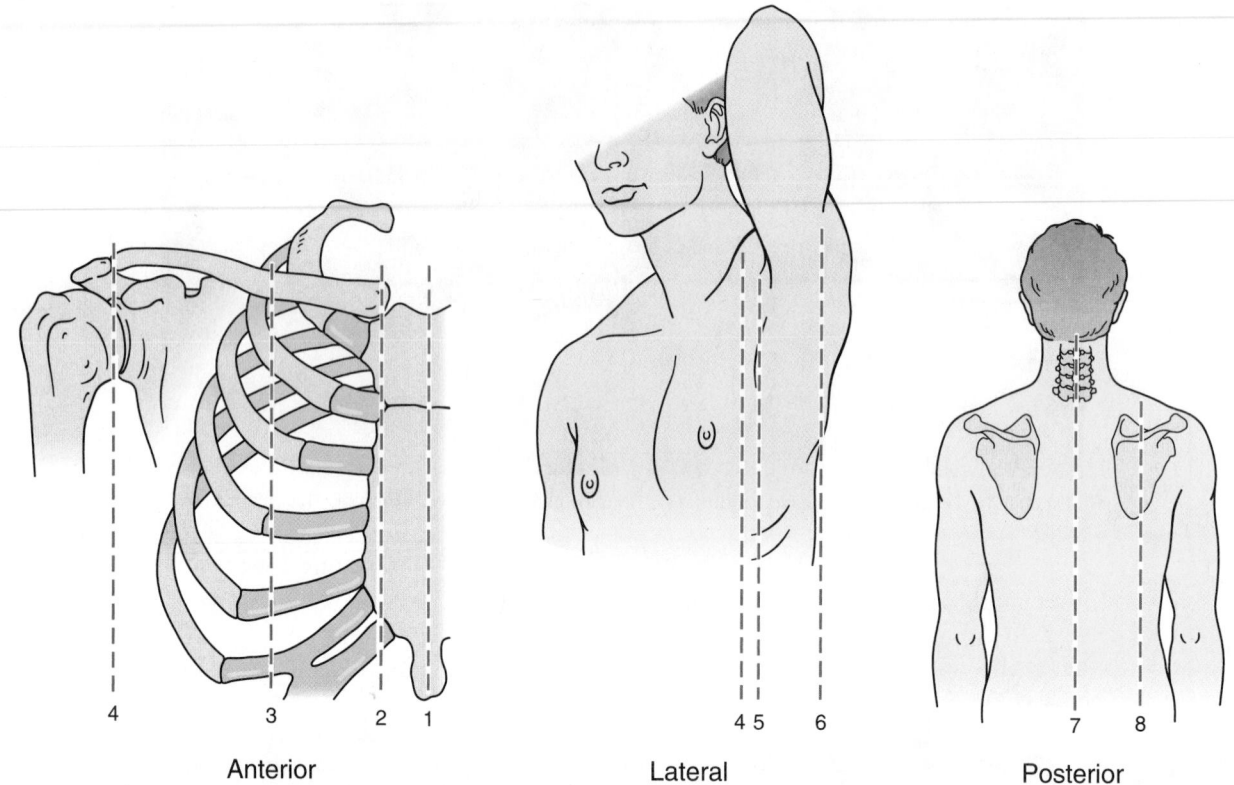

Figure 8-43 Lines of reference in the thoracic area: *1,* midtarsal line; *2,* parasternal line; *3,* midclavicular line; *4,* anterior axillary line; *5,* midaxillary line; *6,* posterior axillary line; *7,* midspinal (vertebral) line; *8,* midscapular line.

to apply pressure. Palpation is carried out to a depth of 1 to 3 cm (0.5 to 1.5 inches) to reveal areas of tenderness and abnormal masses. Palpation is usually carried out using the four quadrant or the nine-region system (Figure 8-44).

Posterior Aspect

Scapula. The medial, lateral, and superior borders of the scapula should be palpated for any swelling or tenderness. The scapula normally extends from the spinous process of T2 to that of T7–T9. After the borders of the scapula have been palpated, the examiner palpates the posterior surface of the scapula. Structures palpated are the supraspinatus and infraspinatus muscles and the spine of the scapula.

Spinous Processes of the Thoracic Spine. In the midline, the examiner may posteriorly palpate the thoracic spinous processes for abnormality. The examiner then moves laterally approximately 2 to 3 cm (0.8 to 1.2 inches) to palpate the thoracic facet joints. Because of the overlying muscles, it is usually very difficult to palpate these joints, although the examiner may be able to palpate for muscle spasm and tenderness. Muscle spasm may also be elicited if some internal structures are injured. For example, pathology affecting the following structures can cause muscle spasm in the surrounding area: gallbladder

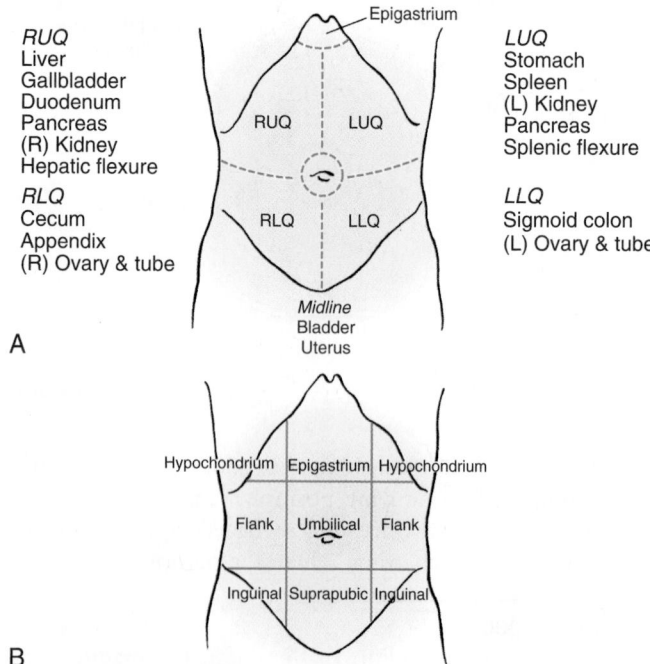

RUQ
Liver
Gallbladder
Duodenum
Pancreas
(R) Kidney
Hepatic flexure

RLQ
Cecum
Appendix
(R) Ovary & tube

LUQ
Stomach
Spleen
(L) Kidney
Pancreas
Splenic flexure

LLQ
Sigmoid colon
(L) Ovary & tube

Figure 8-44 Superficial topography of the abdomen. A, Four-quadrant system. *RUQ,* Right upper quadrant; *RLQ,* right lower quadrant; *LUQ,* left upper quadrant; *LLQ,* left lower quadrant. **B,** Nine-regions system. (From Judge RD, Zuidema GD, Fitzgerald FT: Clinical diagnosis: a physiologic approach, Boston, 1982, Little Brown, p. 284.)

(spasm on the right side in the area of the eighth and ninth costal cartilages), spleen (spasm at the level of ribs 9 through 11 on the left side), and kidneys (spasm at the level of ribs 11 and 12 on both sides at the level of the L3 vertebra). Evidence of positive findings with no comparable history of musculoskeletal origin could lead the examiner to believe the problem was not of a musculoskeletal origin.

Diagnostic Imaging

Plain Film Radiography

Common X-Ray Views of the Thoracic Spine

- Anteroposterior view (routine) (Figure 8-46)
- Lateral view (include ribs and sternum) (routine) (Figure 8-49)
- Lateral view (arm overhead)
- Oblique view (include ribs and sternum) (Figure 8-51)
- Swimmer's view (Figure 8-52)

Anteroposterior View. With this view (Figure 8-45), the examiner should note the following:

1. Any wedging of the vertebrae
2. Whether the disc spaces appear normal
3. Whether the ring epiphysis, if present, is normal
4. Whether there is a "bamboo" spine, indicative of ankylosing spondylitis (Figure 8-47)
5. Any scoliosis (Figure 8-48)
6. Malposition of heart and lungs
7. Normal symmetry of the ribs

Lateral View. The examiner should note the following:

1. A normal mild kyphosis
2. Any wedging of the vertebrae, which may be an indication of structural kyphosis resulting from conditions, such as Scheuermann's disease or wedge fracture from trauma or osteoporosis (Figure 8-50). Scheuermann's disease is radiologically defined as an anterior kyphosis in which there is a 5° or greater anterior wedging of at least three consecutive vertebral bodies.[10]
3. Whether the disc spaces appear normal
4. Whether the ring epiphysis, if present, is normal
5. Whether there are any **Schmorl nodules,** indicating herniation of the intervertebral disc into the vertebral body

6. Angle of the ribs
7. Any osteophytes

Diffuse Idiopathic Skeletal Hyperostosis (DISH). This condition of unknown etiology is indicated by ossification along the anterolateral aspect of at least four contiguous vertebrae leading to back pain and spinal stiffness. It is most common in the thoracic spine followed by cervical and lumbar spines. It does not involve the sacroiliac joints.

Measurement of Spinal Curvature for Scoliosis. With the Cobb method (Figure 8-53), an anteroposterior view is used.[11,33,34] A line is drawn parallel to the superior cortical plate of the proximal end vertebra and to the inferior cortical plate of the distal end vertebra. A perpendicular line is erected to each of these lines, and the angle of intersection of the perpendicular lines is the angle of spinal curvature resulting from scoliosis. Such techniques have led the Scoliosis Research Society to classify all forms of scoliosis according to the degree of curvature: group 1, 0° to 20°; group 2, 21° to 30°; group 3, 31° to 50°; group 4, 51° to 75°; group 5, 76° to 100°; group 6, 101° to 125°; and group 7, 126° or greater.[12] Other noninvasive methods of measuring the curve have been advocated. However, the examiner should use the same method each time for consistency and reliability.[35,36]

The rotation of the vertebrae may also be estimated from an anteroposterior view (Figure 8-54). This estimation is best done by the **pedicle method,** in which the examiner determines the relation of the pedicles to the lateral margins of the vertebral bodies. The vertebra is in neutral position when the pedicles appear to be at equal distance from the lateral margin of the peripheral bodies on the film. If rotation is evident, the pedicles appear to move laterally toward the concavity of the curve.

Computed Tomography

Computed tomography is of primary use in evaluating the bony spine, the spinal contents, and the surrounding soft tissues in cross-sectional views.

Magnetic Resonance Imaging

Magnetic resonance imaging (MRI) is a noninvasive technique that is useful for delineating soft tissue, including herniated discs and intrinsic spinal cord lesions, as well as bony tissue (Figure 8-55). However, MRI should be used only to confirm a clinical diagnosis, because conditions, such as disc herniation, have been demonstrated on MRI in the absence of clinical symptoms.[37,38]

Text continued on p. 546

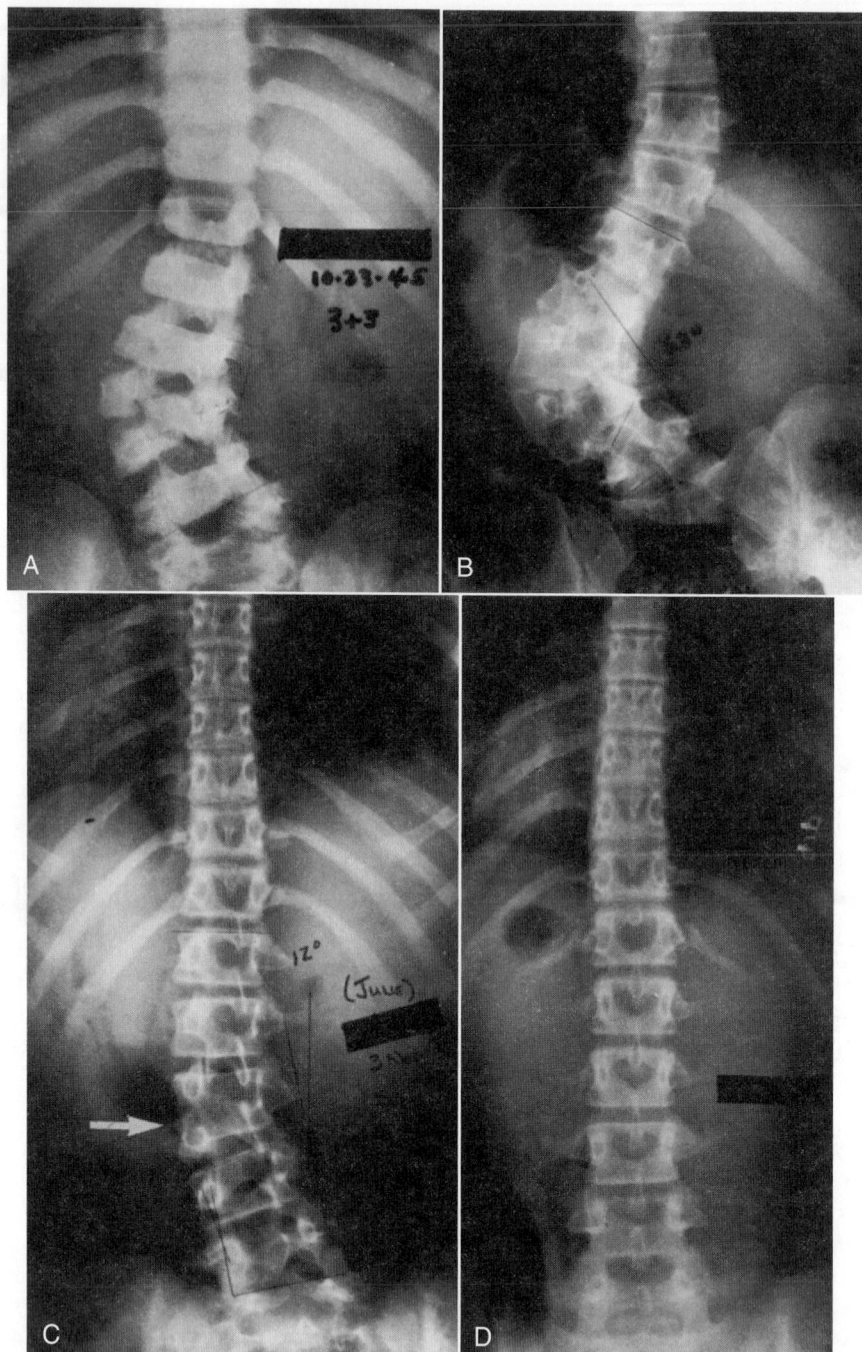

Figure 8-45 Structural scoliosis caused by congenital defect. A, Left midlumbar and right lumbosacral hemivertebrae in a 3-year-old child (example of hemimetameric shift). **B,** A first cousin also demonstrates a midlumbar hemivertebra as well as asymmetric development of the upper sacrum. **C,** This girl has a semisegmented hemivertebra *(arrow)* in the midlumbar spine with a mild 12° curve. **D,** Her identical twin sister showed no congenital anomalies of the spine. (From Moe JH, Winter RB, Bradford DS, et al: Scoliosis and other spinal deformities, Philadelphia, 1978, WB Saunders, p. 134.)

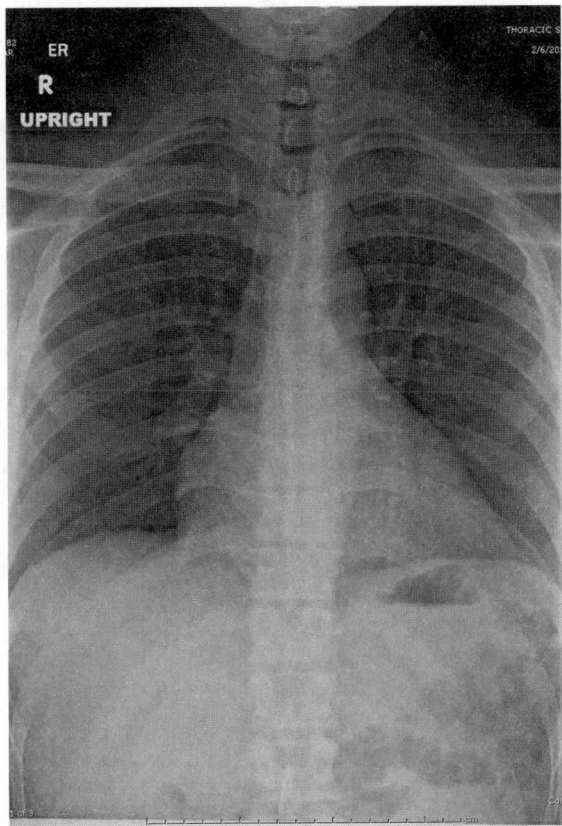

Figure 8-46 Anteroposterior view of the thoracic spine.

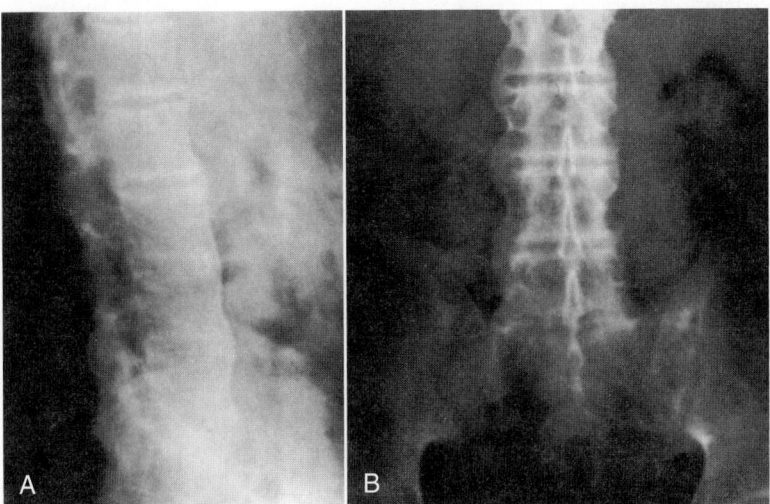

Figure 8-47 Ankylosing spondylitis of spine. Note the bony encasement of vertebral bodies on the lateral view **(A)** and the bamboo effect on the anteroposterior view **(B)**. (From Gartland JJ: Fundamentals of orthopedics, Philadelphia, 1979, WB Saunders, p. 147.)

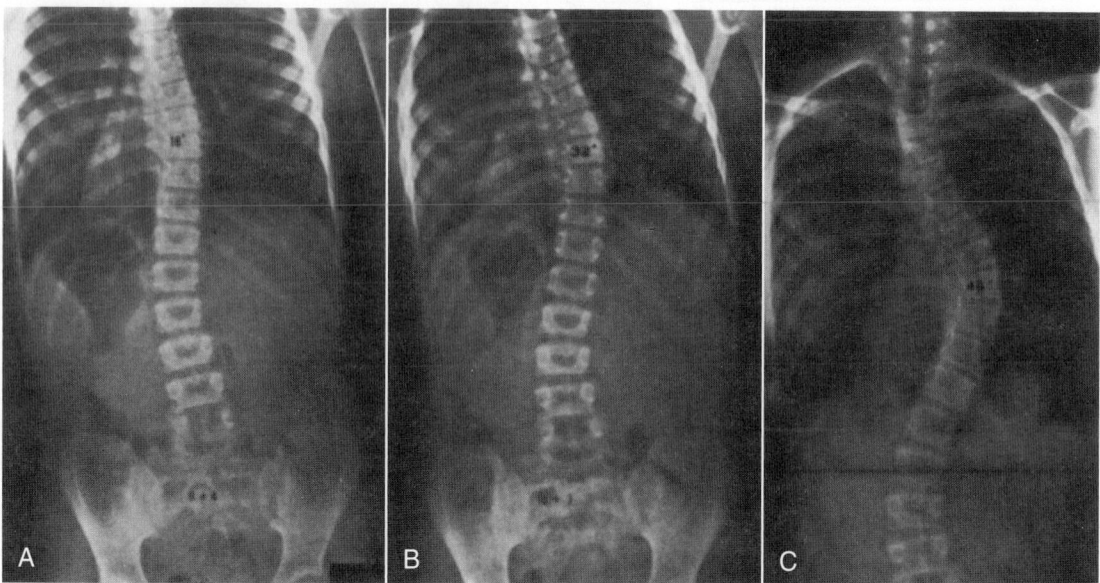

Figure 8-48 **The natural history of idiopathic scoliosis. A,** Note the mild degree of vertebral rotation and curvature and the imbalance of the upper torso. **B,** Note the rather dramatic increase in curvature and the increased rotation of the apical vertebrae 1 year later. **C,** Further progression of the curvature has occurred, and the opportunity for brace treatment has been missed. (From Bunnel WP: Treatment of idiopathic scoliosis. Orthop Clin North Am 10:817, 1979.)

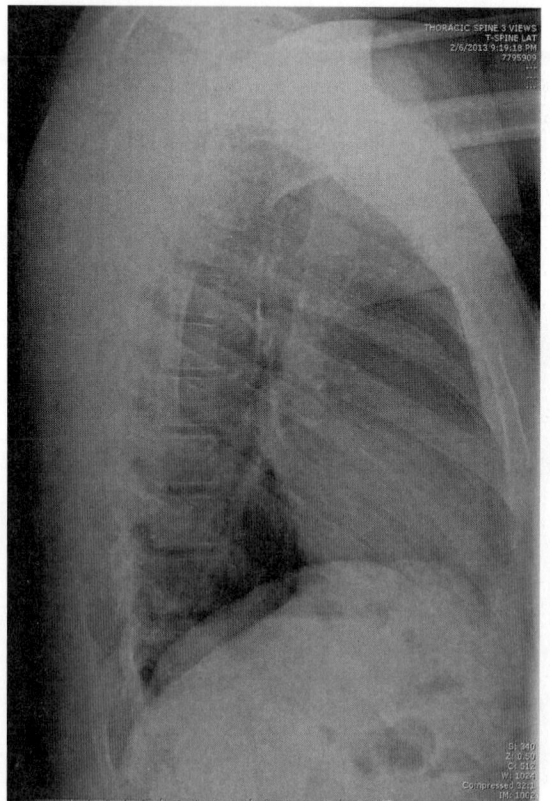

Figure 8-49 Lateral view of the thoracic spine (including ribs).

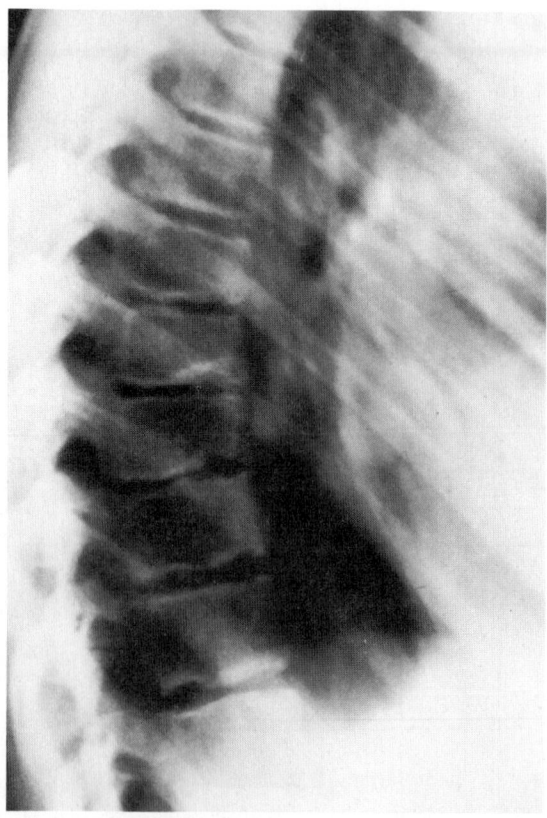

Figure 8-50 Classic radiographic appearance of the spine in a patient with Scheuermann disease. Note the wedged vertebra, Schmorl nodules, and marked irregularity of the vertebral end plates. (From Moe JH, Winter RB, Bradford DS, et al: Scoliosis and other spinal deformities, Philadelphia, 1978, WB Saunders, p. 32.)

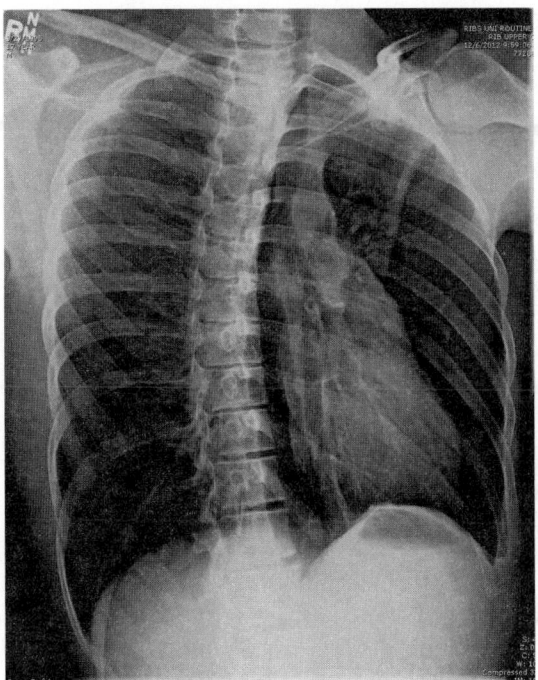

Figure 8-51 Oblique view of the thoracic spine (including ribs and sternum).

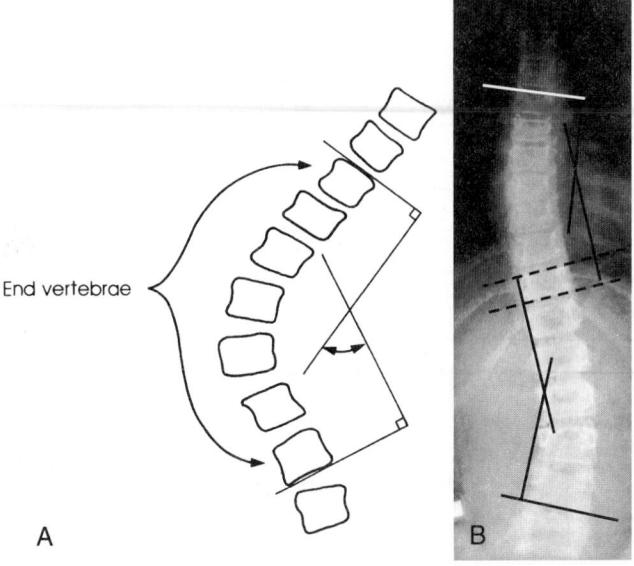

Figure 8-53 A, Cobb method of measuring scoliotic curve. **B,** Measurement of idiopathic scoliosis (Cobb's method). This 10-year-old girl has a T4–T11 right spinal curvature of 20° and a T11–L4 left spinal curvature of 27°. Note that T11 is included in both curve measurements. Minimal rotation occurs in the thoracic region, and essentially none in the lumbar segment. (**B,** From Ozonoff MB: Pediatric orthopedic radiology, ed 2, Philadelphia, 1992, WB Saunders.)

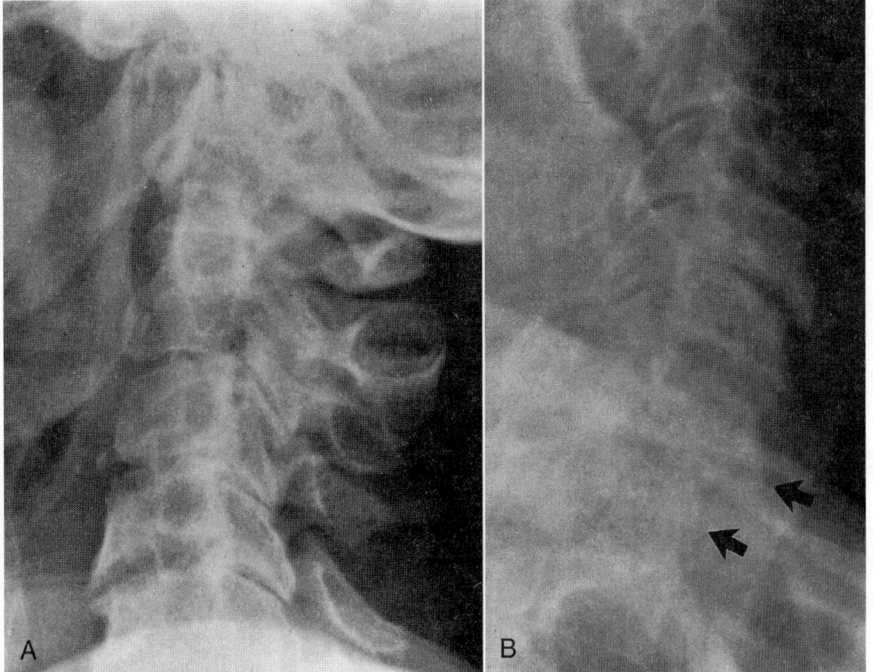

Figure 8-52 Swimmer's projection in demonstration of the cervicothoracic junction. A, Initial lateral radiograph includes only the first five cervical vertebrae. There is a small fracture from the anterior inferior margin of C3. **B,** A swimmer's projection clearly demonstrates dislocation at C7–T1 *(arrows).* (From Adam A, Dixon AK, editors: Grainger & Allison's diagnostic radiology: a textbook of medical imaging, ed 5, Edinburgh, 2008, Churchill Livingstone/Elsevier.)

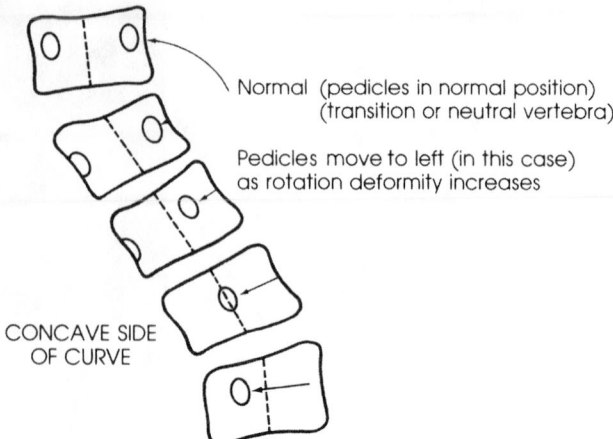

Figure 8-54 Rotation of vertebra in scoliosis. On radiography, the pedicles appear to be off center as the curve progresses.

Normal (pedicles in normal position) (transition or neutral vertebra)

Pedicles move to left (in this case) as rotation deformity increases

CONCAVE SIDE OF CURVE

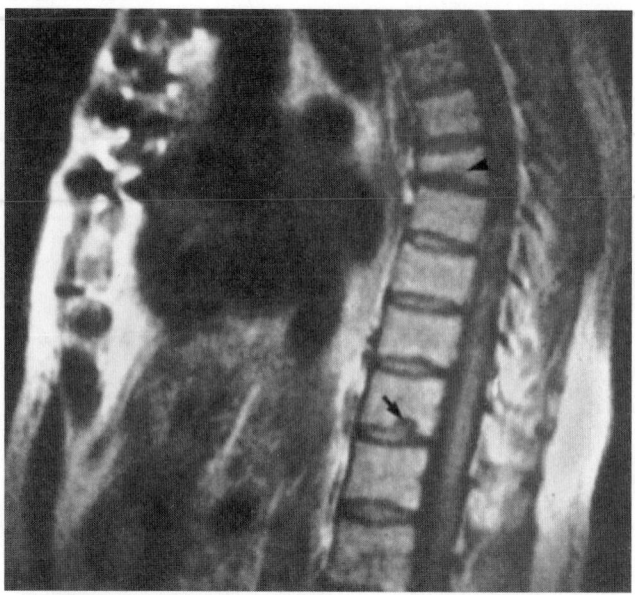

Figure 8-55 Osteoporotic compression fracture of thoracic spine. Midline sagittal T1-weighted magnetic resonance image (SE 500/30) shows compression fracture of upper thoracic vertebral body *(arrowhead)*, indicated by anterior wedging. Marrow signal intensity is maintained *(arrowhead)*. Schmorl nodule is incidentally noted at a lower level *(arrow)*. (From Bassett LW, Gold RH, Seeger LL: MRI atlas of the musculoskeletal system, London, 1989, Martin Dunitz, p. 49.)

PRÉCIS OF THE THORACIC SPINE ASSESSMENT*

History
Observation (standing)
Examination
  Active movements (standing or sitting)
    Forward flexion
    Extension
    Side flexion (left and right)
    Rotation (left and right)
    Combined movements (if necessary)
    Repetitive movements (if necessary)
    Sustained postures (if necessary)
  Passive movements (sitting)
    Forward flexion
    Extension
    Side flexion (left and right)
    Rotation (left and right)
  Resisted isometric movements (sitting)
    Forward flexion
    Extension
    Side flexion (left and right)
    Rotation (left and right)
  Functional assessment
  Special tests (sitting)
    Adson's test
    Costoclavicular maneuver

    Hyperabduction (EAST) test
    Roos test
    Slump test
  Reflexes and cutaneous distribution (sitting)
    Reflex testing
    Sensation scan
  Special tests (prone lying)
  Joint play movements (prone lying)
    Posteroanterior central vertebral pressure (PACVP)
    Posteroanterior unilateral vertebral pressure (PAUVP)
    Transverse vertebral pressure (TVP)
    Rib springing
  Palpation (prone lying)
  Special tests (supine lying)
    First rib mobility
    Rib springing
    Upper limb neurodynamic (tension) test 4 (ULNT4)
  Palpation (supine lying)
  Diagnostic imaging
After any assessment, the patient should be warned of the possibility of exacerbation of symptoms as a result of assessment.

*The précis is shown in an order that limits the amount of movement that the patient has to do but ensures that all necessary structures are tested.

CASE STUDIES

When doing these case studies, the examiner should list the appropriate questions to be asked and why they are being asked, what to look for and why, and what things should be tested and why. Depending on the answers of the patient (and the examiner should consider different responses), several possible causes of the patient's problems may be evident (examples are given in parentheses). If so, a differential diagnosis chart (see Table 8-9 as an example) should be made up. The examiner can then decide how different diagnoses may affect the treatment plan.

1. A 33-year-old patient comes to you complaining of stiffness in the lower spine that is extending into the thoracic spine. Describe your assessment plan for this patient (ankylosing spondylitis versus thoracic spinal stenosis).
2. A 14-year-old boy presents complaining of a severe aching pain in the middorsal spine of several weeks' duration. He is neurologically normal. X-rays reveal a narrowing and anterior wedging at T5 with a Schmorl nodule into T4. Describe your assessment plan for this patient (kyphosis versus Scheuermann disease).
3. A 23-year-old woman has a structural scoliosis with a single C curve having its apex at T7. Describe your assessment plan before beginning treatment. How would you measure the curve and the amount of rotation?
4. A 38-year-old woman comes to your clinic complaining of chest pain with tenderness at the costochondral junction of two ribs on the left side. Describe your assessment plan for this patient (Tietze syndrome versus rib hypomobility).
5. A 26-year-old male ice hockey player comes to you complaining of back pain that is referred around the chest. He explains that he was "boarded" (hit between another player and the boards). He did not notice the pain and stiffness until the next day. He has had the problem for 2 weeks. Describe your assessment plan for this patient (rib hypomobility versus ligament sprain).
6. A 21-year-old female synchronized swimmer comes to you complaining of pain in her side. She says she was kicked when she helped boost another athlete out of the water 5 days ago. Describe your assessment plan for this patient (rib fracture versus rib hypomobility).

TABLE **8-9**

Differential Diagnosis of Ankylosing Spondylitis and Thoracic Spinal Stenosis

	Ankylosing Spondylitis	Thoracic Spinal Stenosis
History	Morning stiffness Intermittent aching pain Male predominance Sharp pain → ache Bilateral sacroiliac pain may refer to posterior thigh	Intermittent aching pain Pain may refer to both legs with walking (neurogenic intermittent claudication)
Active movements	Restricted	May be normal
Passive movements	Restricted	May be normal
Resisted isometric movements	Normal	Normal
Special tests	None	Bicycle test of van Gelderen may be positive Stoop test may be positive
Reflexes	Normal	May be affected in long-standing cases
Sensory deficit	None	Usually temporary
Diagnostic imaging	Plain films are diagnostic	Computed tomography scans are diagnostic

REFERENCES

1. Williams P, Warwick R, editors: Gray's anatomy, ed 36, British, Edinburgh, 1980, Churchill Livingstone.
2. MacConaill MA, Basmajian JV: Muscles and movements: a basis for human kinesiology, Baltimore, 1969, Williams & Wilkins.
3. Mitchell FL, Moran PS, Pruzzo NA: An evaluation and treatment manual of osteopathic muscle energy procedures, Valley Park, MO, 1979, Mitchell, Moran & Pruzzo, Assoc.
4. Henderson JM: Ruling out danger: differential diagnosis of thoracic spine. Phys Sportsmed 20:124–132, 1992.
5. Dreyfuss P, Tibiletti C, Dreyer SJ: Thoracic zygapophyseal joint pain patterns: a study in normal volunteers. Spine 19:807–811, 1994.
6. Ombregt L, Bisschop P, ter Veer HJ, et al: A system of orthopedic medicine, London, 1995, WB Saunders.
7. McKenzie RA: The cervical and thoracic spine: mechanical diagnosis and therapy, Waikanae, New Zealand, 1981, Spinal Publications.
8. Katzman WB, Wanek L, Shepherd JA, et al: Age-related hyperkyphosis: its causes, consequences and management. J Orthop Sports Phys Ther 40:352–360, 2010.
9. Wiles P, Sweetnam R: Essentials of orthopaedics, London, 1965, JA Churchill.
10. Wood KB, Melikian R, Villamil F: Adult Scheuermann kyphosis: evaluation, management and new developments. J Am Acad Orthop Surg 20:113–121, 2012.
11. Keim HA: Scoliosis. Clin Symposia 25:1–25, 1973.
12. Keim HA: The adolescent spine, New York, 1982, Springer-Verlag.
13. Sutherland ID: Funnel chest. J Bone Joint Surg Br 40:244–251, 1958.
14. Dutton M: Orthopedic examination, evaluation and intervention, New York, 2004, McGraw-Hill.
15. Lee D: Manual therapy for the thorax—a biomechanical approach, Delta, BC, 1994, DOPC.
16. Evans RC: Illustrated essentials in orthopedic physical assessment, St Louis, 1994, CV Mosby.
17. Evjenth O, Gloeck C: Symptoms localization in the spine and the extremity joints, Minneapolis, 2000, OPTP.
18. Stoddard A: Manual of osteopathic technique, London, 1959, Hutchinson Medical Publications.
19. Bookhout MR: Evaluation of the thoracic spine and rib cage. In Flynn TW, editor: The thoracic spine and rib cage, Boston, 1996, Butterworth-Heinemann.
20. Fairbank JC, Pynsent PD: The Oswestry disability index. Spine 25:2940–2953, 2000.
21. Roland M, Fairbank J: The Roland-Morris disability questionnaire and the Oswestry disability questionnaire. Spine 25:3115–3124, 2000.
22. Fairbank JC, Couper J, Davies JB, et al: The Oswestry low back pain disability questionnaire. Physiotherapy 66:271–273, 1980.
23. Feise RJ, Menke JM: Functional rating index: A new valid and reliable instrument to measure the magnitude of clinical change in spinal conditions. Spine 26:78–87, 2001.
24. Cook CE, Hegedus EJ: Orthopedic physical examination tests—an evidence based approach, Upper Saddle River, NJ, 2008, Prentice Hall/Pearson.
25. Cleland JA, Koppenhaver S: Netter's orthopedic clinical examination—an evidence based approach, ed 2, Philadelphia, 2011, Saunders/Elsevier.
26. Cyriax J: Textbook of orthopaedic medicine, vol. 1: diagnosis of soft tissue lesions, London, 1982, Bailliere Tindall.
27. Wilke A, Wolf U, Lageard P, et al: Thoracic disc herniation: a diagnostic challenge. Man Ther 5:181–184, 2000.
28. Maitland GD: The slump test: examination and treatment. Aust J Physiother 31:215–219, 1985.
29. Butler DS: Mobilization of the nervous system, Melbourne, 1991, Churchill Livingstone.
30. Lee L-J, Lee D: The thoracic spine and ribs. In Magee DJ, Zachazewski J, Quillen W, editors: Musculoskeletal rehabilitation—pathology and intervention, St Louis, 2009, Elsevier.
31. Maitland GD: Vertebral manipulation, London, 1973, Butterworths.
32. Edmondston SJ, Allison GT, Althorpe BM, et al: Comparison of rib cage and posteroanterior thoracic spine stiffness: an investigation of the normal response. Man Ther 4:157–162, 1999.
33. Adam CJ, Izatt MT, Harvey JR, et al: Variability in Cobb angle measurements using reformatted computerized tomography scans. Spine 50:1664–1669, 2005.
34. Loder RT, Spiegel D, Gutknecht S, et al: The assessment of intraobserver and interobserver error in measurement of noncongenital scoliosis in children = 10 years of age. Spine 29:2548–2553, 2004.
35. Pearsall DJ, Reid JG, Hedden DM: Comparison of three noninvasive methods for measuring scoliosis. Phys Ther 72:648–657, 1992.
36. Pun WK, Luk KD, Lee W, et al: A simple method to estimate the rib hump in scoliosis. Spine 12:342–345, 1987.
37. Wood KB, Garvey TA, Gundry C, et al: Magnetic resonance imaging of the thoracic spine. J Bone Joint Surg Am 77:1631–1638, 1995.
38. Wood KB, Blair JM, Aepple DM, et al: The natural history of asymptomatic thoracic disc herniations. Spine 22:525–530, 1997.
39. Philip K, Lwe P, Matyas TA: The inter-therapist reliability of the slump test. Austr J Phys Ther 35(2):89–94, 1989.
40. Bridwell KH, Cats-Baril W, Harrast J, et al: The validity of the SRS-22 instrument in an adult spinal deformity population compared with the Oswestry and SF-12: a study of response distribution, concurrent validity, internal consistency and reliability. Spine 30(4):455–461, 2005.

SUGGESTED READINGS

Adams JC: Outline of orthopaedics, London, 1968, E & S Livingstone.

American Orthopaedic Association: Manual of orthopaedic surgery, Chicago, 1972, AOA.

Barrios C, Perez-Encinas C, Maruenda JI, et al: Significant ventilatory function restriction in adolescents with mild or moderate scoliosis during maximal exercise tolerance test. Spine 30:1610–1615, 2005.

Bassett LW, Gold RH, Seeger LL: MRI atlas of the musculoskeletal system, London, 1989, Martin Dunitz Ltd.

Beetham WP, Polley HF, Stocumb CH, et al: Physical examination of the joints, Philadelphia, 1965, WB Saunders.

Blair JM: Examination of the thoracic spine. In Grieve GP, editor: Modern manual therapy of the vertebral column, Edinburgh, 1986, Churchill Livingstone.

Bourdillon JR: Spinal manipulation, ed 4, New York, 1987, Appleton-Century-Crofts.

Bowling RW, Rockar P: Thoracic spine. In Richardson JK, Iglarsh ZA: Clinical orthopedic physical therapy, Philadelphia, 1994, WB Saunders.

Bradford DS: Juvenile kyphosis. Clin Orthop 128:45–55, 1977.

Bradford DS, Lonstein JE, Moe JH, et al: Moe's textbook of scoliosis and other spinal deformities, Philadelphia, 1987, WB Saunders.

Brashear HR, Raney RB: Shand's handbook of orthopaedic surgery, St Louis, 1978, CV Mosby.

Bunnel WP: Treatment of idopathic scoliosis. Orthop Clin North Am 10:813–827, 1979.

Burwell RG, James NJ, Johnson F, et al: Standardized trunk asymmetry scores: a study of back contour in healthy school children. J Bone Joint Surg Br 65:452–463, 1983.

Cacayorin ED, Hochhauser L, Petro GR: Lumbar and thoracic spine pain in the athlete: radiographic evaluation. Clin Sports Med 6:767–783, 1987.

Cailliet R: Scoliosis: diagnosis and management, Philadelphia, 1975, FA Davis.

Conroy JZ, Schneiders AG: The T4 syndrome—a case report. Man Ther 10:292–296, 2005.

Drummond DS, Rogala R, Gurr J: Spinal deformity: natural history and the role of school screening. Orthop Clin North Am 10:751–759, 1979.

Duval-Beaupre G: Rib hump and supine angle as prognostic factors for mild scoliosis. Spine 17:103–107, 1992.

Edgelow PE, Lescak AC, Jewell M: Trunk. In Myers RS, editor: Saunders manual of physical therapy practice, Philadelphia, 1995, WB Saunders.

Emans JB, Ciarlo M, Callahan M, et al: Prediction of thoracic dimensions and spinal length based on individual pelvic dimensions in children and adults. Spine 30:2824–2829, 2005.

Flynn TW: The thoracic spine and rib cage—musculoskeletal evaluation and treatment, Boston, 1996, Butterworth-Heinemann.

Flynn TW: Thoracic spine and rib cage disorders. Orthop Phys Ther Clin North Am 8:1–20, 1999.

Gartland JJ: Fundamentals of orthopaedics, London, 1968, E & S Livingstone.

Goldstein LA, Waugh TR: Classification and terminology of scoliosis. Clin Orthop 93:10–22, 1973.

Goodman CC, Snyder TE: Differential diagnosis in physical therapy, Philadelphia, 1995, WB Saunders.

Gould JA: The spine. In Gould JA, editor: Orthopedic and sports physical therapy, St Louis, 1990, CV Mosby.

Gregersen GG, Lucas DB: An in vivo study of the axial rotation of the human thoracolumbar spine. J Bone Joint Surg Am 49:247–262, 1967.

Grieve GP: Common vertebral joint problems, Edinburgh, 1981, Churchill Livingstone.

Grieve GP: Mobilisation of the spine, Edinburgh, 1979, Churchill Livingstone.

Grieve GP: Thoracic musculoskeletal problems. In Boyling JD, Palastanga N, editors: Grieve's modern manual therapy of the vertebral column, Edinburgh, 1994, Churchill Livingstone.

Hamzaoglu A, Talu U, Tezer M, et al: Assessment of curve flexibility in adolescent idiopathic scoliosis. Spine 30:1637–1642, 2005.

Hedequist D, Emans J: Congenital scoliosis. J Am Acad Orthop Surg 12:266–275, 2004.

Hollingshead WH, Jenkins DR: Functional anatomy of the limbs and back, Philadelphia, 1981, WB Saunders.

Hoppenfeld S: Physical examination of the spine and extremities, New York, 1976, Appleton-Century-Crofts.

Houpt JB: The shoulder girdle. In Little H, editor: The rheumatological physical examination, Orlando, FL, 1986, Grune & Stratton.

Howley P: The thoracic and abdominal region. In Zulauga M, Briggs C, Carlisle J, et al, editors: Sports physiotherapy: applied science and practice, Melbourne, 1995, Churchill Livingstone.

James JI: The etiology of scoliosis. J Bone Joint Surg Br 52:410–419, 1970.

Judge RD, Zuidema GD, Fitzgerald FT: Clinical diagnosis: a physiologic approach, Boston, 1982, Little Brown.

Kapandji IA: The physiology of the joints, vol. 3: the trunk and vertebral column, New York, 1974, Churchill Livingstone.

Kuklo TR, Potter BK, Polly Jr DW, et al: Reliability analysis for manual adolescent idiopathic scoliosis measurements. Spine 30(4):444–454, 2005.

Lane RE, Kroon P: Thoracic spine and ribs—anatomy and treatment. Orthop Phys Ther Clin North Am 7:525–539, 1998.

Lee DG: Rotational instability of the mid-thoracic spine: assessment and management. Man Ther 1:234–241, 1996.

Levange PK, Norkin CC: Joint structure and function—a comprehensive analysis, Philadelphia, 2005. FA Davis.

Levene DL: Chest pain: an integrated diagnostic approach, Philadelphia, 1977, Lea & Febiger.

Liebgott B: The anatomical basis of dentistry, Philadelphia, 1982, WB Saunders.

Loder RT, Urquhart A, Steen H, et al: Variability in Cobb angle measurements in children with congenital scoliosis. J Bone Joint Surg Br 77:768–773, 1995.

Love RM, Brodeur RR: Inter- and intra-examiner reliability of motion palpation for the thoracolumbar spine. J Manip Physiol Ther 10:1–4, 1987.

Lyu RK, Chang HS, Tang LM, et al: Thoracic disc herniation mimicking acute lumbar disc disease. Spine 24:416–418, 1999.

Magarey ME: Examination of the cervical and thoracic spine. In Grant R, editor: Physical therapy of the cervical and thoracic spine, clinics in physical therapy, Edinburgh, 1988, Churchill Livingstone.

Maigne R: Diagnosis and treatment of pain of vertebral origin: a manual medicine approach, Baltimore, 1996, Williams & Wilkins.

Maigne R: Orthopaedic medicine: a new approach to vertebral manipulation, Springfield, IL, 1972, Charles C. Thomas.

McKinnis LN: Fundamentals of musculoskeletal imaging, Philadelphia, 2005, FA Davis.

Meadows JT: Orthopedic differential diagnosis in physical therapy—a case study approach, New York, 1999, McGraw-Hill.

Moll JH, Wright V: Measurement of spinal movement. In Jayson M, editor: Lumbar spine and back pain, New York, 1976, Grune & Stratton.

Moll JMH, Wright V: An objective clinical study of chest expansion. Ann Rheum Dis 31:1, 1972.

Nash CL, Moe JH: A study of vertebral rotation. J Bone Joint Surg Am 51:223–229, 1969.

Neumann DA: Kinesiology of the musculoskeletal system—foundations for physical rehabilitation, St Louis, 2002, CV Mosby.

O'Donoghue DH: Treatment of injuries to athletes, ed 4, Philadelphia, 1984, WB Saunders.

O'Malley TP, Kamkar A: Manual examination and treatment of the cervicothoracic region. Orthop Phys Ther Clin North Am 7:499–523, 1998.

Papaioannu T, Stokes L, Kenwright J: Scoliosis associated with limb length inequality. J Bone Joint Surg Am 64:59–62, 1982.

Qiu G, Zhang J, Wang Y, et al: A new operative classification of idiopathic scoliosis: a peking union medical college method. Spine 30(12):1419–1426, 2005.

Raine S, Twomey LT: Validation of a non-invasive method of measuring the surface curvature of the erect spine. J Man Manip Ther 2:11–21, 1994.

Resnick D, Kransdorf MJ: Bone and joint imaging, Philadelphia, 2005, WB Saunders.

Rothman RH, Simeone FA: The spine, Philadelphia, 1982, WB Saunders.

Simmons EH: Kyphotic deformity of the spine in ankylosing spondylitis. Clin Orthop 128:65–77, 1977.

Spivak JM, Vaccaro AR, Cotler JM: Thoracolumbar spine trauma: evaluation and classification. J Am Acad Orthop Surg 3:345–352, 1995.

Stewart SG, Jull GA, Ng JKF, et al: An initial analysis of thoracic spine movement during unilateral arm elevation. J Man Manip Ther 3:15–20, 1995.

Sturrock RD, Wojtulewski JA, Hart FD: Spondylometry in a normal population and in ankylosing spondylitis. Rheumatol Rehabil 12:135–142, 1973.

Travell JG, Simons DG: Myofascial pain and dysfunction: the trigger point manual, Baltimore, 1983, Williams & Wilkins.

Tsou PM: Embryology of congenital kyphosis. Clin Orthop 128:18–25, 1977.

Tsou PM, Yau A, Hodgson AR: Embryogenesis and prenatal development of congenital vertebral anomalies and their classification. Clin Orthop 152:211–231, 1980.

Watkins RG: Thoracic pain syndromes. In Watkins RC, editor: The spine in sports, St Louis, 1996, CV Mosby.

White AA: Kinematics of the normal spine as related to scoliosis. J Biomech 4:405–411, 1971.

Whitesides TE: Traumatic kyphosis of the thoracolumbar spine. Clin Orthop 128:78–92, 1977.

Wyke B: Morphological and functional features of the innervation of the costovertebral joints. Folia Morphol (Warsz) 23:296, 1975.

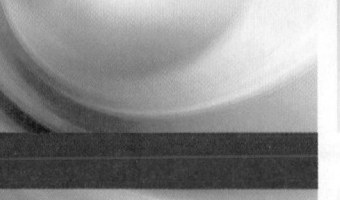

CHAPTER 9

Lumbar Spine

Back pain is one of the great human afflictions. Almost anyone born today in Europe or North America has a great chance of suffering a disabling back injury regardless of occupation.[1] The lumbar spine supports the upper body and transmits the weight of the upper body to the pelvis and lower limbs. Because of the strategic location of the lumbar spine, this structure should be included in any examination of the spine as a whole (i.e., posture) or in any examination of the hip or sacroiliac joints. Unless there is a definite history of trauma, determining whether an injury originates in the lumbar spine, sacroiliac joints, or hip joints is often difficult; therefore, all three should be examined in a sequential fashion.

APPLIED ANATOMY

There are ten (five pairs) facet joints (also called *apophyseal* or *zygoapophyseal joints*) in the lumbar spine (Figure 9-1).[2] These diarthrodial joints consist of superior and inferior facets and a capsule. The facets are located on the vertebral arches. With a normal intact disc, the facet joints carry about 20% to 25% of the axial load, but this may reach 70% with degeneration of the disc. The facet joints also provide 40% of the torsional and shear strength.[3] Injury, degeneration, or trauma to the **motion segment** (the facet joints and disc) may lead to **spondylosis**[4] (degeneration of the intervertebral disc), **spondylolysis**[5] (a defect in the pars interarticularis or the arch of the vertebra), **spondylolisthesis**[5] (a forward displacement of one vertebra over another), or **retrolisthesis** (backward displacement of one vertebra on another). The superior facets, or articular processes, face medially and backward and, in general, are concave; the inferior facets face laterally and forward and are convex (Figure 9-2). There are, however, abnormalities, or **tropisms,** that can occur in the shape of the facets, especially at the L5–S1 level (Figures 9-3 and 9-4).[6] In the lumbar spine, the transverse processes are virtually at the same level as the spinous processes.

These posterior facet joints direct the movement that occurs in the lumbar spine. Because of the shape of the facets, rotation in the lumbar spine is minimal and is accomplished only by a shearing force. Side flexion, extension, and flexion can occur in the lumbar spine, but the facet joints control the direction of movement. The close packed position of the facet joints in the lumbar spine is extension. Normally, the facet joints carry only a small amount of weight; however, with increased extension, they begin to have a greater weight-bearing function. The resting position is midway between flexion and extension. The capsular pattern is side flexion and rotation equally limited, followed by extension. However, if only one facet joint in the lumbar spine has a capsular restriction, the amount of observable restriction is minimal. The first sacral segment is usually included in discussions of the lumbar spine, and it is at this joint that the fixed segment of the sacrum joins with the mobile segments of the lumbar spine. In some cases, the S1 segment may be mobile. This occurrence is called **lumbarization** of S1, and it results in a sixth "lumbar" vertebra. At other times, the fifth lumbar segment may be fused to the sacrum or ilium, resulting in a **sacralization** of that vertebra. Sacralization results in four mobile lumbar vertebrae. These abnormalities are sometimes called transitional vertebra.[7]

Lumbar Spine

Resting position:	Midway between flexion and extension
Close packed position:	Full extension
Capsular pattern:	Side flexion and rotation equally limited extension

---

The main ligaments of the lumbar spine are the same as those in the lower cervical and thoracic spine (excluding the ribs). These ligaments include the anterior and posterior longitudinal ligaments, the ligamentum flavum, the supraspinous and interspinous ligaments, and the intertransverse ligaments (Figure 9-5). In addition, there is an important ligament unique to the lumbar spine and pelvis—the iliolumbar ligament (Figure 9-6), which connects the transverse process of L5 to the posterior ilium.[8] This ligament helps stabilize L5 with the ilium and helps prevent anterior displacement of L5.[9]

The intervertebral discs make up approximately 20% to 25% of the total length of the vertebral column. The function of the intervertebral disc is to act as a shock absorber distributing and absorbing some of the load

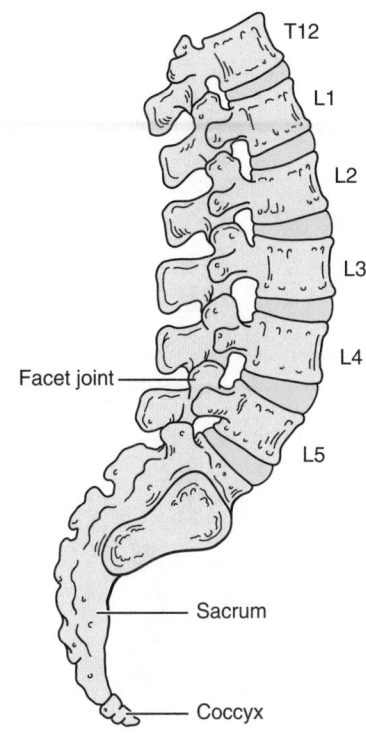

Figure 9-1 Lateral view of the lumbar spine.

applied to the spine, to hold the vertebrae together and allow movement between the bones, to separate the vertebra as part of a **functional segmental unit** acting in concert with the facet joints (Figure 9-7), and, by separating the vertebrae, to allow the free passage of the nerve roots out from the spinal cord through the intervertebral foramina. With age, the percentage of spinal length attributable to the discs decreases as a result of disc degeneration and loss of hydrophilic action in the disc.

The **annulus fibrosus,** the outer laminated portion of the disc, consists of three zones: 1) an outer zone made up of fibrocartilage (classified as **Sharpey fibers**) that attaches to the outer or peripheral aspect of the vertebral body and contains increasing numbers of cartilage cells in the fibrous strands with increasing depth, 2) an intermediate zone made up of another layer of fibrocartilage, and 3) an inner zone primarily made up of fibrocartilage and containing the largest number of cartilage cells.[10] The annulus fibrosus contains twenty concentric, collar-like rings of collagenous fibers that crisscross each other to increase their strength and accommodate torsion movements.[11]

The **nucleus pulposus** is well developed in both the cervical and the lumbar spines. At birth, it is made up of

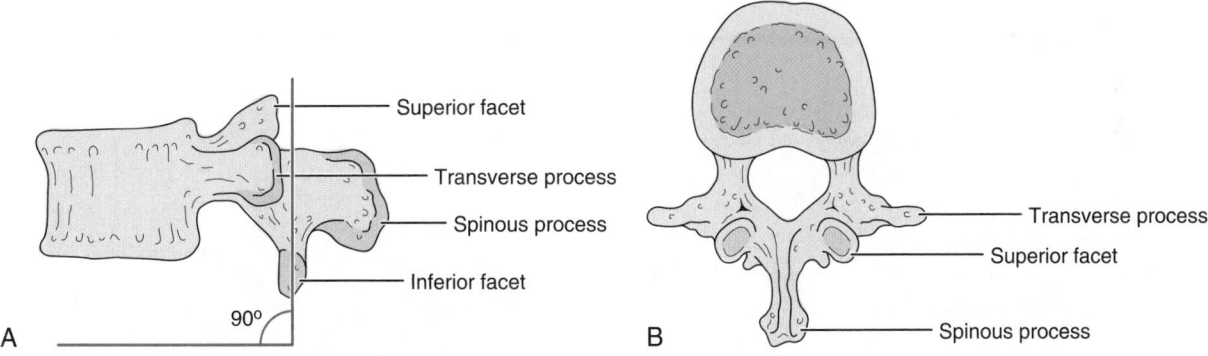

Figure 9-2 Lumbar vertebra. A, Side view. **B,** Superior view.

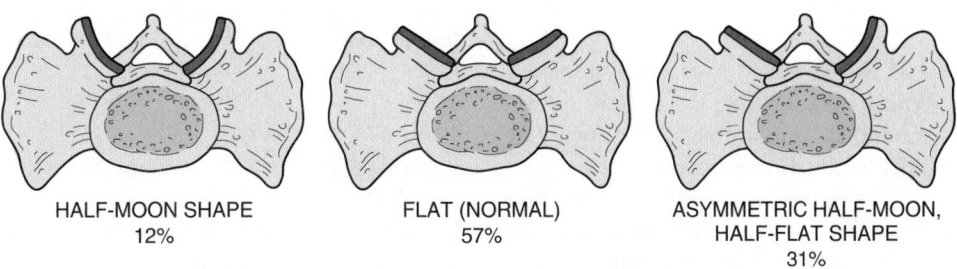

Figure 9-3 Facet anomalies (tropisms) at L5–S1.

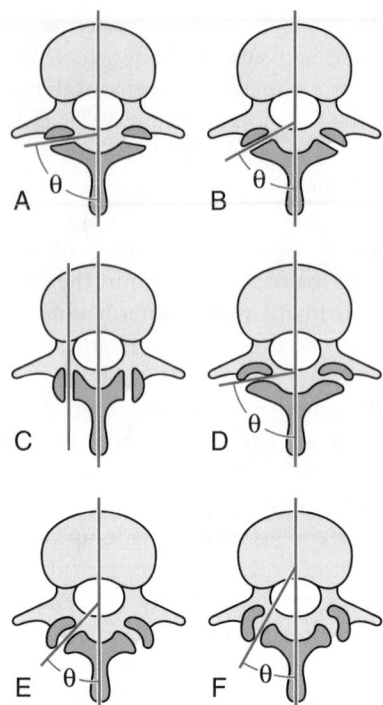

Figure 9-4 The varieties of orientation and curvature of the lumbar zygapophyseal joints. **A,** Flat joints oriented close to 90° to the sagittal plane. **B,** Flat joints orientated at 60° to the sagittal plane. **C,** Flat joints orientated parallel (0°) to the sagittal plane. **D,** Slightly curved joints with an average orientation close to 90° to the sagittal plane. **E,** "C"-shaped joints orientated at 45° to the sagittal plane. **F,** "J"-shaped joints orientated at 30° to the sagittal plane. (Redrawn from Bogduk N, Twomey LT: Clinical anatomy of the lumbar spine, New York, 1987, Churchill Livingstone, p. 26.)

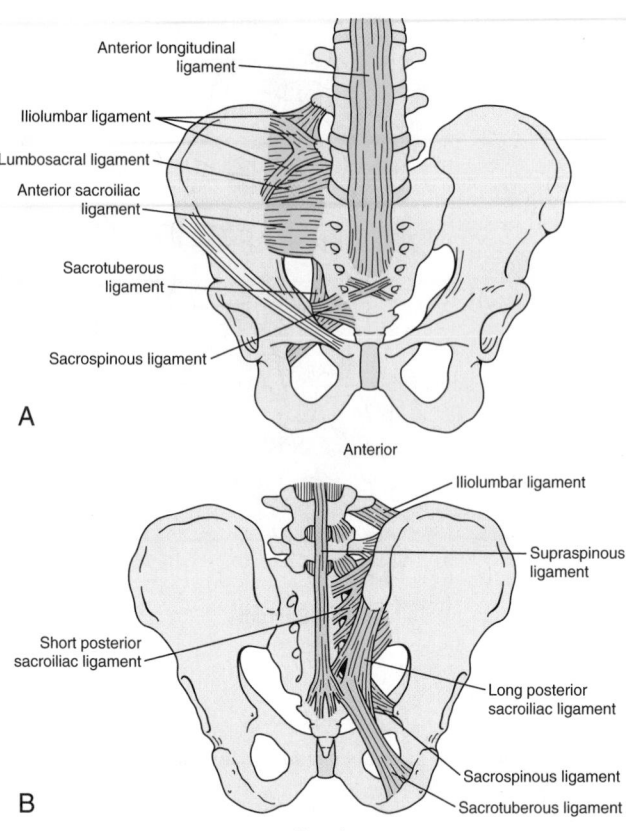

Figure 9-6 Ligaments of the sacrum, coccyx, and some in the lumbar spine.

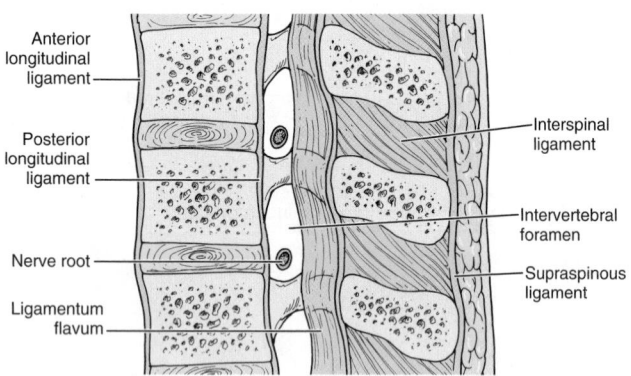

Figure 9-5 Ligaments of the lumbar spine.

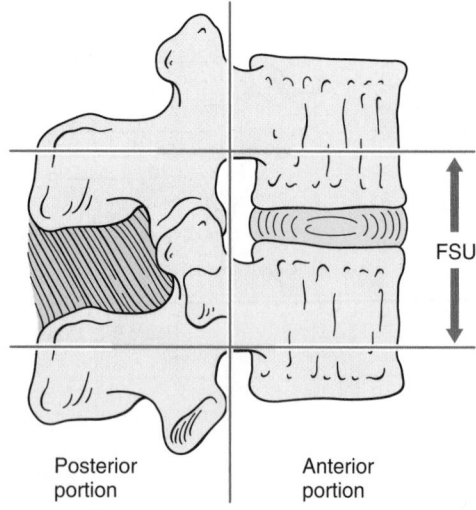

Figure 9-7 Functional segmental unit (three-joint complex) in the lumbar spine. Such a complex may also be seen in the cervical and thoracic spines.

a hydrophilic mucoid tissue, which is gradually replaced by fibrocartilage. With increasing age, the nucleus pulposus increasingly resembles the annulus fibrosus. The water-binding capacity of the disc decreases with age, and degenerative changes (spondylosis) begin to occur after the second decade of life. Initially, the disc contains approximately 85% to 90% water, but the amount decreases to 65% with age.[12] In addition, the disc contains

a high proportion of mucopolysaccharides, which cause the disc to act as an incompressible fluid. However, these mucopolysaccharides decrease with age and are replaced with collagen. The nucleus pulposus lies slightly posterior to the center of rotation of the disc in the lumbar spine.

The shape of the disc corresponds to that of the body to which it is attached. The disc adheres to the vertebral body by means of the cartilaginous end plate. The end plates consist of thin layers of cartilage covering the majority of the inferior and superior surfaces of the vertebral body. The cartilaginous end plates are approximately 1 mm thick and allow fluid to move between the disc and the vertebral body. The discs are primarily avascular with only the periphery receiving a blood supply. The remainder of the disc receives nutrition by diffusion, primarily through the cartilaginous end plate. Until the age of 8 years, the intervertebral discs have some vascularity; however, with age this vascularity decreases.

Usually, the intervertebral disc has no nerve supply, although the peripheral posterior aspect of the annulus fibrosus may be innervated by a few nerve fibers from the sinuvertebral nerve.[13,14] The lateral aspects of the disc are innervated peripherally by the branches of the anterior rami and gray rami communicants. The pain-sensitive structures around the intervertebral disc are the anterior longitudinal ligament, posterior longitudinal ligament, vertebral body, nerve root, and cartilage of the facet joint.

With the movement of fluid vertically through the cartilaginous end plate, the pressure on the disc decreases as the patient assumes the natural lordotic posture in the lumbar spine. Direct vertical pressure on the disc can cause the disc to push fluid into the vertebral body. If the pressure is great enough, defects may occur in the cartilaginous end plate, resulting in **Schmorl nodules,** which are herniations of the nucleus pulposus into the vertebral body. These are found in 20% to 30% of individuals.[15] Normally, an adult is 1 to 2 cm (0.4 to 0.8 inch) taller in the morning than in the evening (20% diurnal variation).[3,16] This change results from fluid movement in and out of the disc during the day through the cartilaginous end plate. This fluid shift acts as a pressure safety valve to protect the disc.

If there is an injury to the disc, four problems can result, all of which can cause symptoms.[17] There may be a **protrusion** of the disc, in which the disc bulges

Activity and Percentage Increase in Disc Pressure at L3	
• Coughing or straining:	5% to 35%
• Laughing:	40% to 50%
• Walking:	15%
• Side bending:	25%
• Small jumps:	40%
• Bending forward:	150%
• Rotation:	20%
• Lifting a 20-kg weight with the back straight and knees bent:	73%
• Lifting a 20-kg weight with the back bent and knees straight:	169%

posteriorly without rupture of the annulus fibrosus. In the case of a disc **prolapse,** only the outermost fibers of the annulus fibrosus contain the nucleus. With a disc **extrusion,** the annulus fibrosus is perforated, and discal material (part of the nucleus pulposus) moves into the epidural space. The fourth problem is a **sequestrated** disc, or a formation of discal fragments from the annulus fibrosus and nucleus pulposus outside the disc proper (Figure 9-8).[18] These injuries can result in pressure on the spinal cord itself (upper lumbar spine) leading to a myelopathy, pressure on the cauda equina leading to **cauda equina syndrome** (saddle anesthesia [Figure 9-9], bowel/bladder dysfunction),[19] or pressure on the nerve roots (most common). The amount of pressure on the neurological tissues determines the severity of the neurological deficit.[20] The pressure may be the result of the disc injury itself or in combination with the inflammatory response of the injury. Saal has outlined favorable, unfavorable, and neutral factors for positive-outcome prognostic factors for nonoperative lumbar disc herniation (Table 9-1).[17]

Within the lumbar spine, different postures can increase the pressure on the intervertebral disc (Figure 9-10). This information is based on the work of Nachemson and colleagues,[21,22] who performed studies of intradiscal pressure

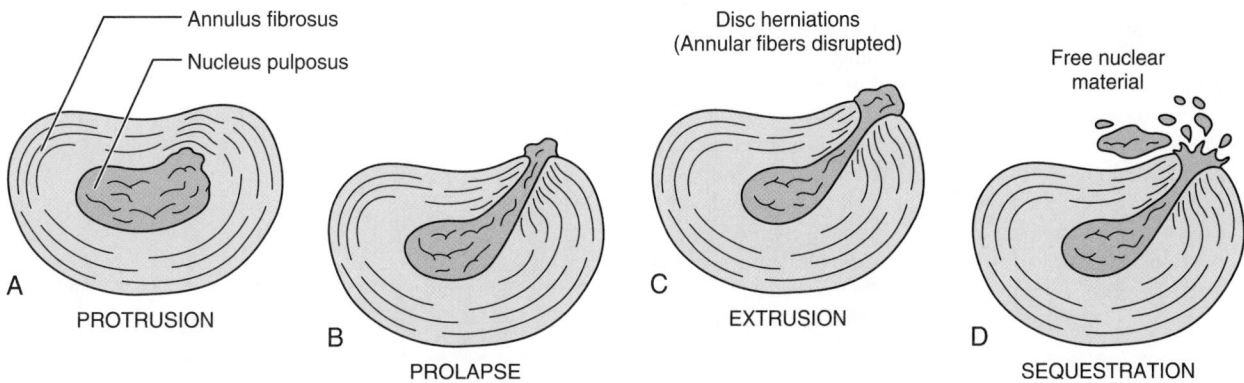

Figure 9-8 Types of disc herniations.

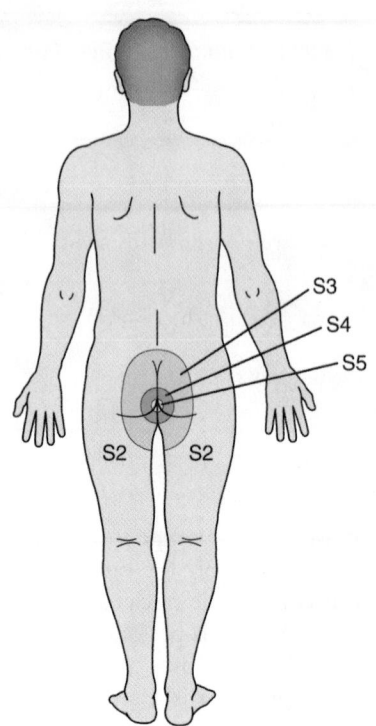

Figure 9-9 Saddle anesthesia. The S3, S4, and S5 nerves provide sensory innervation to the inner thigh, perineum, and rectum.

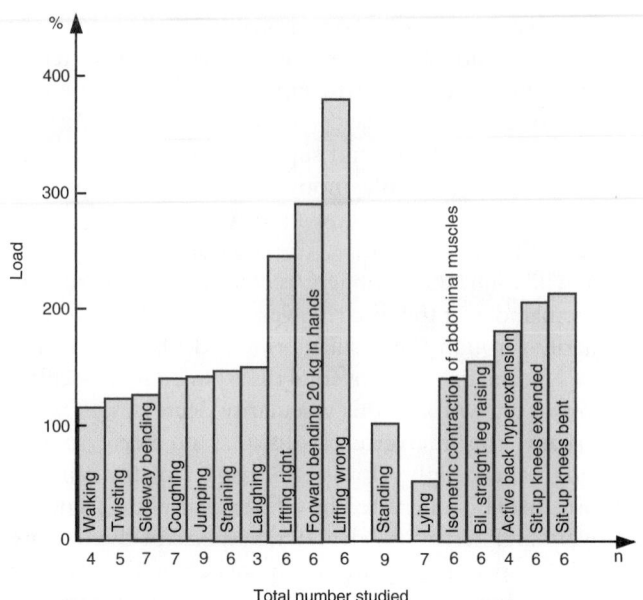

Figure 9-10 Mean change in load on L3 disc with various activities, compared with upright standing. (From Nachemson A, Elfstrom C: Intravital dynamic pressure measurements in lumbar discs. Scand J Rehabil Med [suppl. 1]:31, 1970.)

TABLE 9-1

Prognostic Factors for Positive Outcome with Nonoperative Care for Lumbar Disc Herniation

Favorable Factors	Unfavorable Factors	Neutral Factors	Questionable Factors
• Absence of crossed SLR • Spinal motion in extension that does not reproduce leg pain • Large extrusion or sequestration • Relief of >50% reduction in leg pain within the first 6 weeks of onset • Positive response to corticosteroid treatment • Limited psychosocial issues • Self-employed • Motivated to recover and return to function • Educational level >12 years • Good fitness level • Motivated to exercise and participate in recovery • Absence of spinal stenosis • Progressive return from neurologic deficit within the first 12 weeks	• Positive crossed SLR • Leg pain produced in spinal extension • Subligamentous contained LDH • Lack of >50% reduction in leg pain within the first 6 weeks of onset • Negative response to corticosteroid treatment • Overbearing psychosocial issues • Worker's compensation • Unmotivated to return to function • Educational level <12 years • Illiteracy • Unreasonable expectation of recovery time frames • Poorly motivated and passive in recovery process • Concomitant spinal stenosis • Progressive neurologic deficit • Cauda equina syndrome	• Degree of SLR • Response to bed rest • Response to passive care • Gender • Age • Degree of neurologic deficit (except progressive deficit and cauda equina syndrome)	• Actual size of LDH • Canal position of LDH • Spinal level of LDH • Multi-level disc abnormalities • LDH material

Modified from Saal JA: Natural history and nonoperative treatment of lumbar disc herniation. Spine 21(24S):7S, 1996.
LDH, Lumbar disc herniation; *SLR*, straight leg raise.

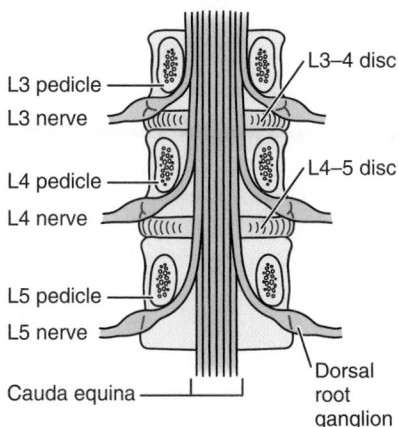

L3 pedicle
L3 nerve
L4 pedicle
L4 nerve
L5 pedicle
L5 nerve
Cauda equina
L3–4 disc
L4–5 disc
Dorsal root ganglion

Figure 9-11 A coronal schematic view of the exiting lumbar spinal nerve roots. Note that the exiting root takes the name of the vertebral body under which it travels into the neural foramen. Because of the way the nerve roots exit, L4–L5 disc pathology usually affects the L5 root rather than the L4 root. (Redrawn from Borenstein DG, Wiesel SW, Boden SD: Low back pain: medical diagnosis and comprehensive management, Philadelphia, 1995, WB Saunders, p. 5.)

changes in the L3 disc with changes in posture. The pressure in the standing position is classified as the norm, and the values given are increases or decreases above or below this norm that occur with the change in posture.

In the lumbar spine, the nerve roots exit through relatively large intervertebral foramina, and as in the thoracic spine, each one is named for the vertebra above it (in the cervical spine, the nerve roots are named for the vertebra below). For example, the L4 nerve root exits between the L4 and L5 vertebrae. Because of the course of the nerve root as it exits, the L4 disc (between L4 and L5) only rarely compresses the L4 nerve root; it is more likely to compress the L5 nerve root (Figure 9-11).

In general, the L5–S1 segment is the most common site of problems in the vertebral column because this level bears more weight than any other vertebral level. The center of gravity passes directly through this vertebra, which is of benefit because it may decrease the shearing stresses to this segment. There is a transition from the mobile segment, L5, to the stable or fixed segment of the sacrum (S1), which can increase the stress on this area. Because the angle between L5 and S1 is greater than those between the other vertebrae, this joint has a greater chance of having stress applied to it. Another factor that increases the amount of stress on this area is the relatively greater amount of movement that occurs at this level compared with other levels of the lumbar spine.

PATIENT HISTORY

Problems of the lumbar spine are difficult to diagnose; in fact, diagnosing pain due to a disc is primarily diagnosis

of exclusion.[23] Most of the examination commonly revolves around differentiating symptoms of a herniated disc (or space occupying lesion), which refers radicular symptoms into the leg from other conditions (e.g., inflammatory reaction, sprains, strains, facet syndrome) more likely to cause localized pain.[24] If there are no radicular symptoms below the knee, it often becomes difficult for the examiner to determine where in the spine the problem is, or for that matter, whether the problem is truly in the lumbar spine or coming from problems in the pelvic joints, primarily the sacroiliac joints, or the hips. Waddell pointed out that in only about 15% of cases can a definitive diagnosis as to the pathology of back pain be made.[3] Hall broke low back pain into four categories—two of which are **back pain dominant** and two of which are **leg pain dominant** (Table 9-2).[25] Pattern 1 suggests disc involvement, whereas pattern 2 suggests facet joint involvement. Pattern 3 suggests nerve root involvement (primarily by a disc or some other space occupying lesion or an injury accompanied by inflammatory swelling), and pattern 4 suggests neurogenic intermittent claudication (pressure on the cauda equina). Thus, only by taking a careful history, followed by a detailed examination, is the examiner able to determine the cause of the problem.[26–28] Even then, some doubt may remain.

In addition to the questions listed under the "Patient History" section in Chapter 1, the examiner should obtain the following information from the patient:

1. *What is the patient's age?*[29] Different conditions affect patients at different ages. For example, disc problems usually occur between the ages of 15 and 40 years, and ankylosing spondylitis is evident between 18 and 45 years. Osteoarthritis and spondylosis are more evident in people older than 45 years of age, and malignancy of the spine is most common in people older than 50 years of age.

2. *What is the patient's occupation?*[3,30] Back pain tends to be more prevalent in people with strenuous occupations,[31] although it has been reported that familial influences have an effect as well as occupation.[32,33] For example, truck drivers (vibration) and warehouse workers have a high incidence of back injury.[34] Patients who have chronic low back pain develop a **deconditioning syndrome,** which compounds the problem as it leads to decreased muscle strength, impaired motor control, and decreased coordination and postural control.[35] How active is the patient at work (usual job, light duties, full time, frequent days off because of back pain, unemployed because of back, retired)?

3. *What is the patient's sex?* Lower back pain has a higher incidence in women. Female patients should be asked about any changes that occur with menstruation, such as altered pain patterns, irregular menses, and swelling of the abdomen or breasts. Has the patient ever been diagnosed with osteoporosis? Knowledge

TABLE **9-2**

Patterns of Back Pain

	Pattern	Where Pain Is Worst	Aggravating Movement	Relieving Movement	Onset	Duration	Probable Cause
Back Dominant Pain/ Mechanical Cause	1	Back/buttocks (>90% back pain) Myotomes seldom affected Dermatomes not affected	Flexion Stiff in morning	Extension	Hours to days	Days to months (sudden or slow)	Disc involvement (minor herniation, spondylosis), sprain, strain
	2	Back/buttocks Myotomes seldom affected Dermatomes not affected	Extension/ Rotation	Flexion	Minutes to hours	Days to weeks (sudden)	Facet joint involvement, strain
Leg Pain Dominant/ Nonmechanical Cause	3	Leg (usually below knee) Myotomes commonly affected (especially in chronic cases) Pain in dermatomes	Flexion	Extension	Hours to Days	Weeks to months	Nerve root irritation (most likely cause—disc hernation)
	4	Leg (usually below knee) (May be bilateral) Myotomes commonly affected (especially in chronic cases) Pain in dermatomes	Walking (extension)	Rest (sitting) and/or postural change	With walking	?	Neurogenic intermittent claudication (stenosis)

Modified from Hall H: A simple approach to back pain management. Patient Care 15:77–91, 1992.

of the date of the most recent pelvic examination is also useful. Ankylosing spondylitis is more common in men.

4. *What was the mechanism of injury?* Was major trauma (e.g., car accident) involved? Lifting commonly causes low back pain (Tables 9-3 and 9-4). This is not surprising when one considers the forces exerted on the lumbar spine and disc. For example, a 77-kg (170-lb) man lifting a 91-kg (200-lb) weight approximately 36 cm (14 inches) from the intervertebral disc exerts a force of 940 kg (2072 lbs) on that disc. The force exerted on the disc can be calculated as roughly ten times the weight being lifted. Pressure on the intervertebral discs varies depending on the position of the spine. Nachemson and colleagues showed that pressure on the disc can be decreased by increasing the supported inclination of the back rest (e.g., an angle of 130° decreases the pressure on the

disc by 50%).[21,22] Using the arms for support can also decrease the pressure on the disc. When one is standing, the disc pressure is approximately 35% of the pressure that occurs in the relaxed sitting position. The examiner should also keep in mind that stress on the lower back tends to be 15% to 20% higher in men than in women because men are taller and their weight is distributed higher in the body.

5. *How long has the problem bothered the patient?* Acute back pain lasts 3 to 4 weeks. Subacute back pain lasts up to 12 weeks. Chronic pain is anything longer than 3 months. Waddell has outlined predictors (yellow flags) of chronicity with back pain patients.[3,36]

6. *Where are the sites and boundaries of pain?* Have the patient point to the location or locations. Note whether the patient indicates a specific joint or whether the pain is more general. The more specific the pain, the easier it is to localize the area of

TABLE **9-3**

Some Implications of Painful Reactions

Activity	Reaction of Pain	Possible Structural and Pathological Implications
Lying sleeping	↓	Decreased compressive forces—low intradiscal pressures Absence of forces produced by muscle activity
	↑	Change of position—noxious mechanical stress Decreased mechanoreceptor input Motor segment "relaxed" into a position compromising affected structure Poor external support (bed) Nonmusculoskeletal cause
First rising (stiffness)	↑	Nocturnal imbibition of fluid, disc volume greatest Mechanical inflammatory component (apophyseal joints) Prolonged stiffness, active inflammatory disease (e.g., ankylosing spondylitis)
Sitting	↑	Compressive forces High intradiscal pressure
With extension	↓	Intradiscal pressure reduced Decreased paraspinal muscle activity
	↑	Greater compromise of structures of lateral and central canals Compressive forces on lower apophyseal joints
With flexion	↓	Little compressive load on lower apophyseal joints Greater volume lateral and central canals Reduced disc bulge posteriorly
	↑	Very high intradiscal pressures Increased compressive loads upper and mid apophyseal joints Mechanical deformation of spine
Prolonged sitting	↑	Gradual creep of tissues
Sitting to standing	↑	Creep, time for reversal, difficulty in straightening up Extension of spine, increase disc bulge posteriorly

Walking	↑	Shock loads greater than body weight
		Compressive loads (vertical creep)
		Leg pain
		    Neurological claudication
		    Vascular claudication

Driving	↑	Sitting: Compressive forces Vibration: Vibro creep repetitive loading, decreased hysteresis loading, decreased hysteresis Increased dural tension sitting with legs extended Short hamstrings: Pull lumbar spine into greater flexion
Coughing, sneezing, straining	↑	Increased pressure subarachnoid space (increased blood flow, Batson plexus, compromises space in lateral and central canal) Increased intradiscal pressure Mechanical "jarring" of sudden uncontrolled movement

From Jull GA: Examination of the lumbar spine. In Grieve GP, editor: Modern manual therapy of the vertebral column, Edinburgh, 1986, Churchill Livingstone, p. 553.

TABLE **9-4**

Some Mechanisms of Musculoskeletal Pain

Behavior of Pain	Possible Mechanisms
Constant ache	Inflammatory process, venous hypertension
Pain on movement	Noxious mechanical stimulus (stretch, pressure, crush)
Pain accumulates with activity	Repeated mechanical stress Inflammatory process Degenerative disc—hysteresis decreased, less protection from repetitive loading
Pain increases with sustained postures	Fatigue of supporting muscles Gradual creep of tissues may stress affected part of motor unit
Latent nerve root pain	Movement has produced an acute and temporary neurapraxia

From Jull GA: Examination of the lumbar spine. In Grieve GP, editor: Modern manual therapy of the vertebral column, Edinburgh, 1986, Churchill Livingstone, p. 553.

Predictors of Chronicity Within the First 6 to 8 Weeks (Yellow Flags)[3]

- Nerve root pain or specific spinal pathology
- Reported severity of pain at the acute stage
- Beliefs about pain being work related
- Psychological distress
- Psychosocial aspects of work
- Compensation
- Time off work
- The longer someone is off work with back pain, the lower the probability that they will return to work

---

pathology. Unilateral pain with no referral below the knee may be caused by injury to muscles (strain) or ligaments (sprain), the facet joint, or, in some cases, the sacroiliac joints. This is called **mechanical low back pain** (in older books it is called "lumbago"). With each of these injuries, there is seldom if ever peripheralization of the symptoms. The symptoms tend to stay centralized in the back. If the muscles and ligaments are affected, movement will decrease and pain will increase with repeated movements. If the pain extends to the hip, the hip must be cleared by examination. With facet joint problems, the range of motion (ROM) remains the same (it may be restricted from the beginning), as does the pain with

repeated movements. Pain on standing that improves with walking and pain on forward flexion with no substantial muscle tenderness suggests disc involvement.[37] The sacroiliac joints will show pain when pain-provoking (stress) tests are used. A minor disc injury (protrusion) may show the same symptoms, but the pain is more likely to be bilateral if it is a central protrusion.[38]

"Mechanical" Low Back Pain[3]

- Pain is usually cyclic
- Low back pain is often referred to the buttocks and thighs
- Morning stiffness or pain is common
- Start pain (i.e., when starting movement) is common
- There is pain on forward flexion and often also on returning to the erect position
- Pain is often produced or aggravated by extension, side flexion, rotation, standing, walking, sitting, and exercise in general
- Pain usually becomes worse over the course of the day
- Pain is relieved by a change of position
- Pain is relieved by lying down, especially in the fetal position

---

7. *Is there any radiation of pain? Is the pain centralizing or peripheralizing* (Figure 9-12)?[39,40] **Centralization** implies the pain is moving toward or is centered in the lumbar spine.[41-43] **Peripheralization** implies the pain is being referred or is moving into the limb. If so, it is helpful for the examiner to remember and correlate this information with dermatome findings when evaluating sensation. The examiner must be careful when looking at the lumbar spine that he or she does not consider every back problem a disc problem. It has been reported that disc problems account for only about 5% of low back pain cases.[44] Some authors feel the only definitive clinical diagnosis of a disc problem is neurological pain extending below the knee.[25] This means that although there may be pain in the back and in the leg, the leg pain is dominant.[3] Pain on the anterolateral aspect of the leg is highly suggestive of L4 disc problems, whereas pain radiating to the posterior aspect of the foot suggests L5 disc problems if the history indicates a disc may be injured.[45] Pain radiating into the leg below the knee is highly suggestive of a disc lesion, but isolated back or buttock pain does not rule out the disc. Minor injuries, such as protrusion of the disc, may result only in back or buttock pain.[45] Such an injury makes diagnoses more difficult because such pain may also result from muscle or ligament injury or from injury or degeneration to the adjacent facet joints.

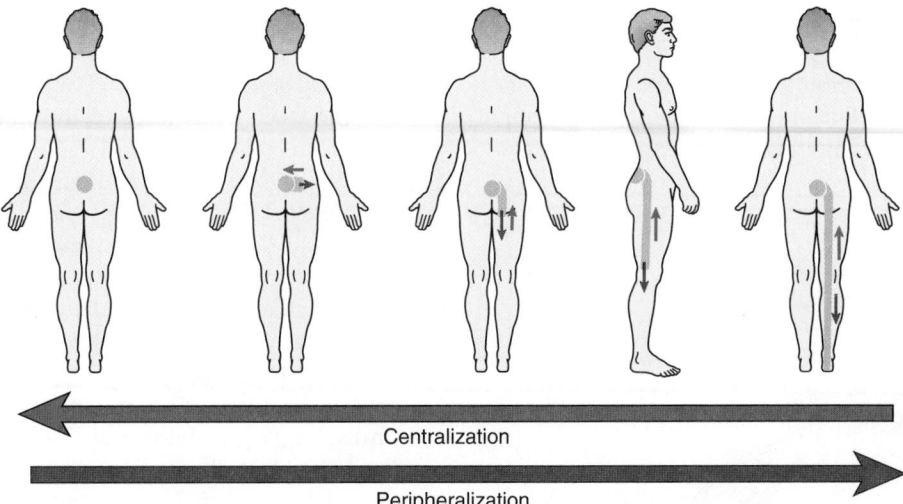

Centralization

Peripheralization

Figure 9-12 Centralization of pain is the progressive retreat of the most distal extent of referred or radicular pain toward the lumbar midline. Peripheralization of pain moves in the opposite direction.

Lumbar and sacroiliac pain tend to be referred to the buttock and posterior leg (and sometimes to the lateral aspect of the leg). Hip pain tends to be in the groin and anterior thigh although it may be referred to the knee (usually medial side). The hip can be ruled out later in the examination by the absence of a hip capsular pattern and a negative sign of the buttock.[46] The examiner must also determine whether the musculoskeletal system is involved or whether the pain is being referred from another structure or system (e.g., abdominal organs). Abnormal signs and symptoms or red flags (see Table 1-1) would lead the examiner to consider causes other than the musculoskeletal system.

8. *Is the pain deep? Superficial? Shooting? Burning? Aching?* Questions related to the depth and type of pain often help to locate the structure injured and the source of pain.

9. *Is the pain improving? Worsening? Staying the same?* The answers to these questions indicate whether the condition is settling down and improving, or they may indicate that the condition is in the inflammation phase (acute) or in the healing phase. Does the patient complain of more pain than the injury would suggest should occur? If so, psychosocial testing may be appropriate.

10. *Is there any increase in pain with coughing? Sneezing? Deep breathing? Laughing?* All of these actions increase the **intrathecal pressure** (the pressure inside the covering of the spinal cord) and would indicate the problem is in the lumbar spine and affecting the neurological tissue.

11. *Are there any postures or actions that specifically increase or decrease the pain or cause difficulty?*[39,47] For example, if sitting increases the pain and other symptoms, the examiner may suspect that sustained flexion

is causing mechanical deformation of the spine or increasing the intradiscal pressure.[48] Classically, disc pathology causes increased pain on sitting, lifting, twisting, and bending.[49] It is the most common space-occupying lesion in the lumbar spine and, therefore, is the most common cause of radiating pain below the knee. If standing increases the pain and other symptoms, the examiner may suspect that extension, especially relaxed standing, is the cause. If walking increases the pain and other symptoms, extension is probably causing the mechanical deformation, because walking accentuates extension. If lying (especially prone lying) increases the pain and other symptoms, extension may be the cause. Persistent pain or progressive increases in pain while the patient is in the supine position may lead the examiner to suspect neurogenic or space-occupying lesions, such as an infection, swelling, or tumor. Remember that pain may radiate to the lumbar spine from pathological conditions in other areas as well as from direct mechanical problems. For example, tumors of the pancreas refer pain to the low back. Stiffness or pain after rest may indicate ankylosing spondylitis or Scheuermann disease. Pain from mechanical breakdown tends to increase with activity and decrease with rest. Discogenic pain increases if the patient maintains a single posture (especially flexion) for a long period. Pain arising from the spine almost always is influenced by posture and movement.

The pelvis is the key to proper back posture. Ideally, an individual should be able to stand with the pelvis in neutral. In this position, the anterior superior iliac spines (ASISs) are one to two finger widths lower than the posterior superior iliac spines (PSISs). For the pelvis to "sit" properly on the femora, the abdominal, hip flexor, hip extensor, and back extensor muscles must be strong, supple, and "balanced" (Figure 9-13). Any deviation in the normal alignment should be noted and recorded. For example, shoe heel height can modify the pelvic angle and lumbar curve, altering the stress on the spine.[50]

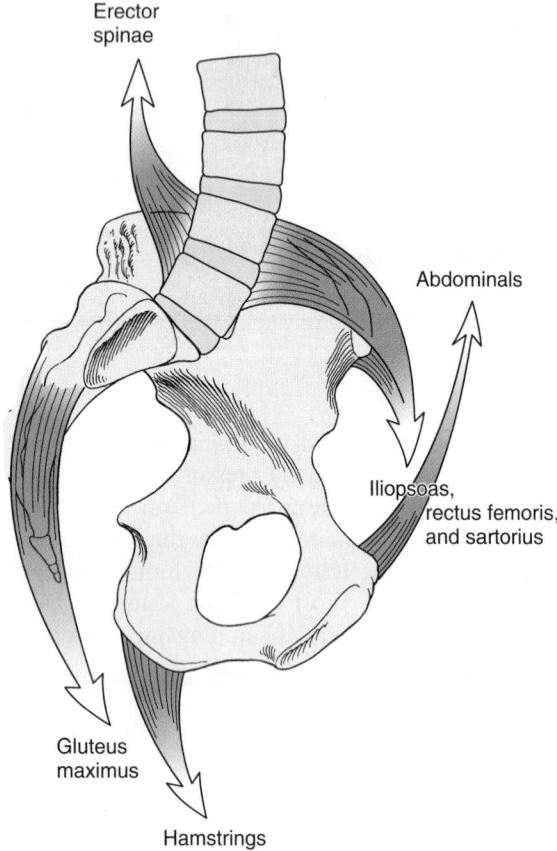

Figure 9-13 Muscles "balancing" the pelvis. (Modified from Dyrek DA, Micheli LJ, Magee DJ: Injuries to the thoracolumbar spine and pelvis. In Zachazewski JE, Magee DJ, WS Quillen, editors: Athletic injuries and rehabilitation, Philadelphia, 1996, WB Saunders, p. 470.)

12. *Is the pain worse in the morning or evening? Does the pain get better or worse as the day progresses? Does the pain wake you up at night?* For example, osteoarthritis of the facet joints leads to morning stiffness, which in turn is relieved by activity.

13. *Which movements hurt? Which movements are stiff?* Table 9-5 demonstrates some of the causes of mechanical low back pain and their symptoms. The examiner must help the patient differentiate between true pain and discomfort that is caused by stretching. **Postural,** or **static, muscles** (e.g., iliopsoas) tend to respond to pathology with tightness in the form of spasm or adaptive shortening; **dynamic,** or **phasic, muscles** (e.g., abdominals) tend to respond with atrophy. Pathology affecting both types of muscles can lead to a pelvic crossed syndrome (discussed later). Does the patient describe a painful arc of movement on forward or side flexion? If so, it may indicate a disc protrusion with a nerve root riding over the bulge or instability in part of the ROM.[47] Patients with lumbar instability or lumbar muscle spasm have trouble moving to the seated position, whereas patients with discogenic pain usually have pain in flexion (e.g., sitting) and the pain may increase the longer they are seated.

14. *Is paresthesia (a "pins and needles" feeling) or anesthesia present?* A patient may experience a sensation or a lack of sensation if there is pressure on a nerve root. Paresthesia occurs if pressure is relieved from a nerve trunk, whereas if the pressure is on the nerve trunk, the patient experiences a numb sensation. Does the patient experience any paresthesia or tingling and numbness in the extremities, perineal (saddle) area, or pelvic area? Abnormal sensations in the perineal area often have associated micturition (urination) problems. These symptoms may indicate a myelopathy and are considered by many to be an emergency

TABLE 9-5

Differential Diagnosis of Mechanical Low Back Pain

	Muscle Strain	Herniated Nucleus Pulposus	Osteoarthritis	Spinal Stenosis	Spondylolisthesis	Scoliosis
Age (year)	20 to 40	30 to 50	>50	>60	20	30
Pain pattern						
Location	Back (unilateral)	Back, leg (unilateral)	Back (unilateral)	Leg (bilateral)	Back	Back
Onset	Acute	Acute (prior episodes)	Insidious	Insidious	Insidious	Insidious
Standing	↑	↓	↑	↑	↑	↑
Sitting	↓	↑	↓	↓	↓	↓
Bending	↑	↑	↓	↓	↑	↑
Straight leg raise	–	+	–	+ (stress)	–	–
Plain x-ray	–	–	+	+	+	+

From Borenstein DG, et al: Low back pain: medical diagnosis and comprehensive management, Philadelphia, 1995, WB Saunders, p. 189.

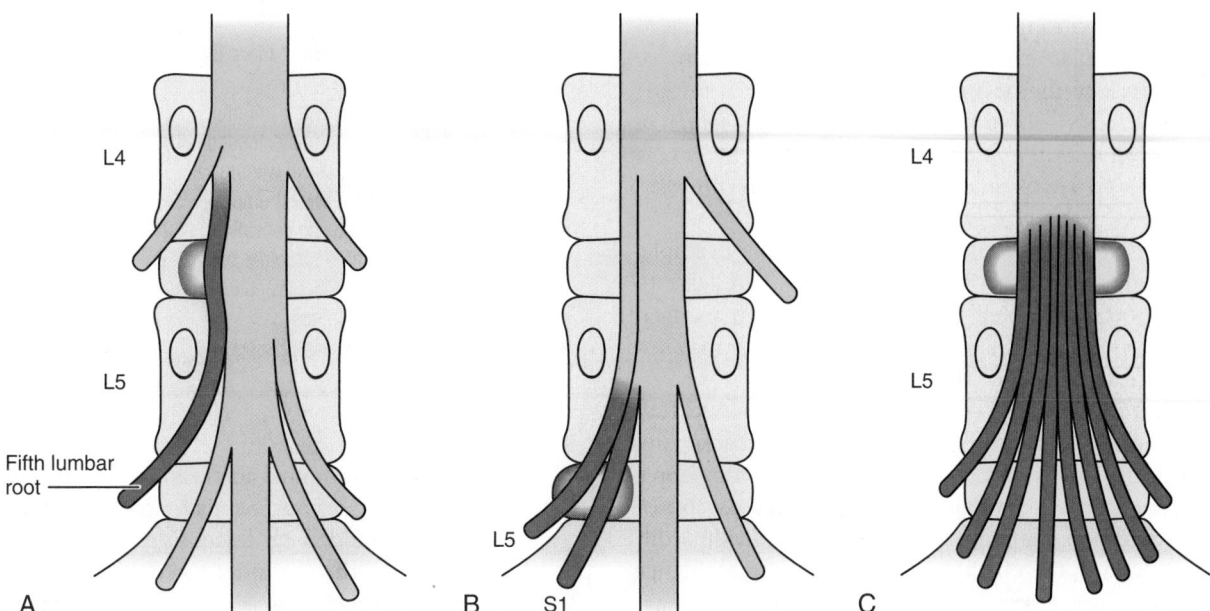

Figure 9-14 Possible effects of disc herniation. A, Herniation of the disc between L4 and L5 compresses the fifth lumbar root. **B,** Large herniation of the L5–S1 disc compromises not only the nerve root crossing it (first sacral nerve root) but also the nerve root emerging through the same foramen (fifth lumbar nerve root). **C,** Massive central sequestration of the disc at the L4–L5 level involves all of the nerve roots in the cauda equina and may result in bowel and bladder paralysis. (Redrawn from MacNab I: Backache, Baltimore, 1977, Williams & Wilkins, pp. 96–97.)

surgical situation because of potential long-term bowel and bladder problems if the pressure on the spinal cord is not relieved as soon as possible.[51,52] The examiner must remember that the adult spinal cord ends at the bottom of the L1 vertebra and becomes the cauda equina within the spinal column. The nerve roots extend in such a way that it is rare for the disc to pinch on the nerve root of the same level. For example, the L5 nerve root is more likely to be compressed by the L4 intervertebral disc than by the L5 intervertebral disc (Figure 9-14). Seldom is the nerve root compressed by the disc at the same level, except when the protrusion is more lateral.

15. *Has the patient noticed any weakness or decrease in strength? Has the patient noticed that his/her legs have become weak while walking or climbing stairs?* This may be the result of an injury to the muscles themselves, their nerve supply, or reflex inhibition caused by pain.[28,53]

16. *What is the patient's usual activity or pastime? Before the injury, did the patient modify or perform any unusual repetitive or high-stress activity?* Such questions help the examiner determine whether the cause of injury was macrotrauma, microtrauma, or a combination of both.

17. *Which activities aggravate the pain? Is there anything in the patient's lifestyle that increases the pain?* Many common positions assumed by patients are similar to those in some of the provocative special tests. For example, getting into and sitting in a car is similar to the slump test and straight leg raise test. Long sitting in bed is a form of straight leg raise. Reaching up into a cupboard can be similar to an upper limb tension test. A word of caution: There can be a 10° to 20° difference in straight leg raise in lying and sitting because of the change in lordosis and position of the pelvis.[3]

18. *Which activities ease the pain?* If there are positions that relieve the pain, the examiner should use an understanding of anatomy to determine which tissues would have stress taken off them in the pain-relieving postures, and these postures may later be used as resting postures during the treatment.

19. *What is the patient's sleeping position? Does the patient have any problems sleeping? What type of mattress does the patient use (hard, soft)?* The best sleeping position is in side lying with the legs bent in a semifetal position. If the patient lies prone, the lumbar spine often falls into extension increasing the stress on the posterior elements of the vertebrae. In supine lying, the spine tends to flatten out, decreasing the stress on the posterior elements.

20. *Does the patient have any difficulty with micturition?* If so, the examiner should proceed with caution, because the condition may involve more than the lumbar spine (e.g., a myelopathy, cauda equina syndrome, tabes dorsalis, tumor, multiple sclerosis). Conversely, these symptoms may result from a disc protrusion or spinal stenosis with minimal or no back pain or sciatica. A disc derangement can cause total

urinary retention; chronic, longstanding partial retention; vesicular irritability; or the loss of desire or awareness of the necessity to void.

21. *Are there any red flags that the examiner should be aware of, such as a history of cancer, sudden weight loss for no apparent reason, immunosuppressive disorder, infection, fever, or bilateral leg weakness?*

22. *Is the patient receiving any medication?* For example, the long-term use of steroid therapy can lead to osteoporosis. Also, if the patient has taken medication just before the assessment, the examiner may not get a true reading of the pain.

23. *Is the patient able to cope during daily activities?* Psychosocial issues often play a role in low back pain, especially if it is chronic.[54–57] It is normal for people suffering prolonged pain to exhibit altered psychosocial behaviors that are subject to wide individual differences and the effects of learning.[58] Fear avoidance questionnaires, especially Waddell, et al.,[59] **Fear-Avoidance Beliefs Questionnaire (FABQ)** (Figure 9-15) and Linton and Hallden's **Acute Low Back Pain Screening Questionnaire**[60] (Figure 9-16), are becoming more commonly used in lumbar examination.[61–67] The **New Zealand Acute Low Back Pain Guide** outlines yellow flags indicating psychosocial barriers for recovery with questions related to attitudes and beliefs about back pain, behavior, compensation issues, diagnosis and treatment, emotions, family and work.[58] These yellow flags should be seen as factors that can be influenced positively to facilitate recovery and reduce work loss and long term disability.[58] Haggman, et al.[68] felt that two questions were particularly significant to ask the patient to screen for depressive symptoms:1) "During the past month, have you often been bothered by feeling down, depressed, or hopeless?" and 2) "During the past month, have you been bothered by little interest or pleasure in doing things?"[37,69] If the answers to these questions are positive, the patient should be monitored closely and if progress does not occur, then further psychological follow-ups should be considered.[70] Does the patient have trouble with work, leisure activities, washing, or dressing? How far can the patient walk before the pain begins?[71] What is the patient's level of disability? Disability implies the effect of the pathology on activity, not pain. Thus, disability testing commonly revolves around activities of daily living (ADLs) and functional activities. Thus, this question may be tied in with the use of the questions in the functional assessment discussed later.

Finally, the examiner must be aware that although in most cases, people who have low back pain have simple mechanical back problems or have nerve root problems involving the disc, there is always the possibility of nonmusculoskeletal causes (e.g.,

> ### Psychosocial Yellow Flag Barriers to Recovery[58]
>
> - Belief that pain and activity are harmful
> - "Sickness behaviors" (such as extended rest)
> - Low or negative moods, social withdrawal
> - Treatment that does not fit best practice
> - Problems with claim and compensation
> - History of back pain, time-off, other claims
> - Problems at work, poor job satisfaction
> - Heavy work, unsociable hours
> - Overprotective family or lack of support

kidney stones, abdominal aortic aneurysm, pancreatic problems) or serious spinal pathology (e.g., tumors).[23,37] Waddell outlined signs and symptoms that would lead the examiner to conclude that more serious pathology is present in the lumbar spine (Table 9-6).[3]

OBSERVATION

The patient must be suitably undressed. Males must wear only shorts, and females must wear only a bra and shorts. When doing the observation, the examiner should note the patient's willingness to move and the pattern of movement. The patient should be observed for the following traits, first in the standing and then in the sitting position.

Body Type

There are three general body types (see Figure 15-24): **ectomorphic**—thin body build, characterized by relative prominence of structures developed from the embryonic ectoderm; **mesomorphic**—muscular or sturdy body build, characterized by relative prominence of structures developed from the embryonic mesoderm; and **endomorphic**—heavy (fat) body build, characterized by relative prominence of structures developed from the embryonic endoderm.

Gait

Does the gait appear to be normal when the patient walks into the examination area, or is it altered in some way? If it is altered, the examiner must take time to find out whether the problem is in the limb or whether the gait is altered to relieve symptoms elsewhere.

Attitude

What is the patient's appearance? Is the patient tense, bored, lethargic, healthy looking, emaciated, overweight?

FEAR AVOIDANCE BELIEFS QUESTIONNAIRE (FABQ)

NAME:_____   DATE:_____/_____/_____
                                                                          MM   DD   YY

Here are some of the things other patients have told us about their pain. For each statement please circle the number from 0 to 6 to indicate how much physical activity such as bending, lifting, walking, or driving affects or would affect your pain.

	Completely Disagree			Unsure			Completely Agree
1. My pain was caused by physical activity.	0	1	2	3	4	5	6
2. Physical activity makes my pain worse.	0	1	2	3	4	5	6
3. Physical activity might harm my _____	0	1	2	3	4	5	6
4. I should not do physical activities that (might) make my pain worse.	0	1	2	3	4	5	6
5. I cannot do physical activities that (might) make my pain worse.	0	1	2	3	4	5	6

The following statements are about how your normal work affects or would affect your pain.

	Completely Disagree			Unsure			Completely Agree
6. My pain was caused by my work or by an accident at work.	0	1	2	3	4	5	6
7. My work aggravated my pain.	0	1	2	3	4	5	6
8. I have a claim for compensation for my pain.	0	1	2	3	4	5	6
9. My work is too heavy for me.	0	1	2	3	4	5	6
10. My work makes or would make my pain worse.	0	1	2	3	4	5	6
11. My work might harm my_____ .	0	1	2	3	4	5	6
12. I **should not** do my regular work with my present pain.	0	1	2	3	4	5	6
13. I **cannot** do my normal work with my present pain.	0	1	2	3	4	5	6
14. I cannot do my normal work until my pain is treated.	0	1	2	3	4	5	6
15. I do not think that I will be back to my normal work within 3 months.	0	1	2	3	4	5	6
16. I do not think that I will ever be able to go back to that work.	0	1	2	3	4	5	6

Figure 9-15 Fear-Avoidance Beliefs Questionnaire (FABQ). (From Waddell G, Newton M, Henderson I, et al: A fear-avoidance beliefs questionnaire [FABQ] and the role of fear-avoidance beliefs in chronic low back pain and disability. Pain 52:157–168, 1993.)

Acute Low Back Pain Screening Questionnaire

(Linton & Halldén, 1996)

Today's Date __/__/__

Name _____   ACC Claim Number _____

Address _____   Telephone (__) _____ (home)

_____   (__) _____ (work)

Job Title (occupation) _____   Date stopped work for this episode __/__/__

These questions and statements apply if you have aches or pains, such as back, shoulder, or neck pain. Please read and answer each question carefully. Do not take too long to answer the questions. However, it is important that you answer every question. There is always a response for your particular situation.

1. What year were you born?   19 _____

2. Are you: ☐ male   ☐ female

3. Were you born in New Zealand?   ☐ yes   ☐ no

4. Where do you have pain? Place a ✓ for all the appropriate sites.   2 X count

   ☐ neck   ☐ shoulders   ☐ upper back   ☐ lower back   ☐ leg

5. How many days of work have you missed because of pain during the past 18 months? Tick (✓) one.

   ☐ 0 days [1]   ☐ 1–2 days [2]   ☐ 3–7 days [3]   ☐ 8–14 days [4]   ☐ 15–30 days [5]

   ☐ 1 month [6]   ☐ 2 months [7]   ☐ 3–6 months [8]   ☐ 6–12 months [9]   ☐ over 1 year [10]

6. How long have you had your current pain problem? Tick (✓) one.

   ☐ 0–1 weeks [1]   ☐ 1–2 weeks [2]   ☐ 3–4 weeks [3]   ☐ 4–5 weeks [4]   ☐ 6–8 weeks [5]

   ☐ 9–11 weeks [6]   ☐ 3–6 months [7]   ☐ 6–9 months [8]   ☐ 9–12 months [9]   ☐ over 1 year [10]

7. Is your work heavy or monotonous? Circle the best alternative.

   0   1   2   3   4   5   6   7   8   9   10
   Not at all   *Extremely*

8. How would you rate the pain that you have had during the past week? Circle one.

   0   1   2   3   4   5   6   7   8   9   10
   No pain   *Pain as bad as it could be*

9. In the past three months, on average, how bad was your pain? Circle one.

   0   1   2   3   4   5   6   7   8   9   10
   No pain   *Pain as bad as it could be*

10. How often would you say that you have experienced pain episodes, on average, during the past 3 months? Circle one.

    0   1   2   3   4   5   6   7   8   9   10
    Never   *Always*

11. Based on all the things you do to cope, or deal with your pain, on an average day, how much are you able to decrease it? Circle one.   10-x

    0   1   2   3   4   5   6   7   8   9   10
    Can't decrease it at all   *Can decrease it completely*

12. How tense or anxious have you felt in the past week? Circle one.

    0   1   2   3   4   5   6   7   8   9   10
    Absolutely calm and relaxed   *As tense and anxious as I've ever felt*

13. How much have you been bothered by feeling depressed in the past week? Circle one.

    0   1   2   3   4   5   6   7   8   9   10
    Not at all   *Extremely*

Figure 9-16 Acute Low Back Pain Screening Questionnaire. (From Linton SJ, Halldén K: Can we screen for problematic back pain? A screening questionnaire for predicting outcome in acute and subacute back pain. Clin J Pain 14[3]:209–215, 1998.)

14. In your view, how large is the risk that your current pain may become persistent? Circle one.

　　0　　1　　2　　3　　4　　5　　6　　7　　8　　9　　10
　　No risk　　　　　　　　　　　　　　　　　　*Very large risk*

15. In your examination, what are the chances that you will be working in 6 months? Circle one.　　10-x

　　0　　1　　2　　3　　4　　5　　6　　7　　8　　9　　10
　　No chance　　　　　　　　　　　　　　　　　*Very large chance*

16. If you take into consideration your work routines, management, salary, promotion possibilities and work mates, how satisfied are you with your job? Circle one.　　10-x

　　0　　1　　2　　3　　4　　5　　6　　7　　8　　9　　10
　　Not at all　　　　　　　　　　　　　　　　　*Completely*
　　satisfied　　　　　　　　　　　　　　　　　　*satisfied*

Here are some of the things which other people have told us about their back pain. For each statement please circle one number from 0 to 10 to say how much physical activities, such as bending, lifting, walking, or driving would affect your back.

17. Physical activity makes my pain worse.

　　0　　1　　2　　3　　4　　5　　6　　7　　8　　9　　10
　　Completely　　　　　　　　　　　　　　　　　*Completely*
　　disagree　　　　　　　　　　　　　　　　　　*agree*

18. An increase in pain is an indication that I should stop what I am doing until the pain decreases.

　　0　　1　　2　　3　　4　　5　　6　　7　　8　　9　　10
　　Completely　　　　　　　　　　　　　　　　　*Completely*
　　disagree　　　　　　　　　　　　　　　　　　*agree*

19. I should not do my normal work with my present pain.

　　0　　1　　2　　3　　4　　5　　6　　7　　8　　9　　10
　　Completely　　　　　　　　　　　　　　　　　*Completely*
　　disagree　　　　　　　　　　　　　　　　　　*agree*

Here is a list of 5 activities. Please circle the one number which best describes your current ability to participate in each of these activities.

20. I can do light work for an hour.　　10-x

　　0　　1　　2　　3　　4　　5　　6　　7　　8　　9　　10
　　Can't do it because　　　　　　　　　　　　*Can do it without pain*
　　of pain problem　　　　　　　　　　　　　　*being a problem*

21. I can walk for an hour.　　10-x

　　0　　1　　2　　3　　4　　5　　6　　7　　8　　9　　10
　　Can't do it because　　　　　　　　　　　　*Can do it without pain*
　　of pain problem　　　　　　　　　　　　　　*being a problem*

22. I can do ordinary household chores.

　　0　　1　　2　　3　　4　　5　　6　　7　　8　　9　　10
　　Can't do it because　　　　　　　　　　　　*Can do it without pain*　　10-x
　　of pain problem　　　　　　　　　　　　　　*being a problem*

23. I can go shopping.

　　0　　1　　2　　3　　4　　5　　6　　7　　8　　9　　10
　　Can't do it because　　　　　　　　　　　　*Can do it without pain*　　10-x
　　of pain problem　　　　　　　　　　　　　　*being a problem*

24. I can sleep at night.

　　0　　1　　2　　3　　4　　5　　6　　7　　8　　9　　10
　　Can't do it because　　　　　　　　　　　　*Can do it without pain*
　　of pain problem　　　　　　　　　　　　　　*being a problem*　　10-x

Score

Scoring Instructions-Acute Pain Screening Questionnaire.

- For Question 4, count the number of pain sites and multiply by 2.

- For Question 6, 7, 8, 9, 10, 12, 13, 14, 17, 18, and 19 the score is the number that has been ticked or circled.

- For Question 11, 15, 16, 20, 21, 22, 23, and 24 the score is 10 minus the number that has been ticked or circled.

- Write the score in the shaded box beside each item-Questions 4 to 24.

- Add them up, and write the sum in the box provided. This is the total score.

Note: the scoring method is built into the questionnaire.

Interpretation of Scores-Acute Pain Screening Questionnaire.

Questionnaire scores greater than 105 indicate that the patient is At Risk.

This score produces:

- 75% correct identification of those not needing modification to ongoing management

- 86% correct identification of those who will have between 1 and 30 days off work

- 83% correct identification of those who will have more than 30 days off work

Figure 9-16, cont'd

▼ TABLE **9-6**

Indications of Serious Spinal Pathology

Red Flags	Cauda Equina Syndrome/Widespread Neurologic Disorder	Inflammatory Disorders (Ankylosing Spondylitis and Related Disorders)
• Presentation age <20 years or onset >55 years • Violent trauma, such as a fall from a height, car accident • Constant, progressive, nonmechanical pain • Thoracic pain • Previous history carcinoma, systemic steroids, drug abuse, HIV • Weight loss (unexpected) • Systematically unwell • Persisting severe restriction of lumbar flexion • Widespread neurology • Structural deformity • Investigations when required sedimentation rate (ESR) >25 plain x-ray: vertebral collapse or bone destruction • Blood in urine or stools	• Difficulty with micturition • Loss of anal sphincter tone or fecal incontinence • Saddle anesthesia about the anus, perineum or genitals • Widespread (> one nerve root) or progressive motor weakness in the legs or gait disturbance • Sensory level	• Gradual onset before age 40 years • Marked morning stiffness • Persisting limitation of spinal movements in all directions • Peripheral joint involvement • Iritis, skin rashes (psoriasis), colitis, urethral discharge • Family history

From Waddell G: The back pain revolution, New York, 1998, Churchill Livingstone, p. 12.
ESR, Erythrocyte sedimentation rate; *HIV,* human immunodeficiency virus.

Total Spinal Posture

The patient should be examined in the habitual relaxed posture (see Chapter 15) that he or she would usually adopt. With acute back pain, the patient presents with some degree of antalgic (painful) posturing. Usually, a loss of lumbar lordosis is present, and there may be a lateral shift or scoliosis. This posturing is involuntary and often cannot be reduced because of the muscle spasm.[72,73]

The patient should be observed anteriorly, laterally, and posteriorly (Figure 9-17). During the observation, the examiner should pay particular attention to whether the patient holds the pelvis "in neutral" naturally; if not, is he or she able to achieve the "neutral pelvis" position in standing (normal lordotic curve with the ASISs being slightly lower [one to two finger widths] than the PSISs). Many people with back pain are unable to maintain a **neutral pelvis** position. Three questions should be considered when looking for a neutral pelvis and whether the pelvis can be stabilized:

1. Can the patient get into the "neutral pelvis" position? If not, what is restricting the movement or what muscles are weak so the position cannot be attained?
2. Can the patient hold (i.e., stabilize) the neutral pelvis statically? If not, what muscles need to be strengthened?
3. Can the patient hold (i.e., stabilize) the neutral pelvis when moving dynamically? If not, which muscles are

weak and/or not functioning correctly (i.e., functioning isometrically, concentrically, eccentrically).

These questions will help the examiner determine if the pelvis (and lumbar spine) can be stabilized during different movements or positions so that other muscles originating from the pelvis can function properly. For example, side lying hip abduction should be able to be performed in the frontal plane with the lower limbs, pelvis, trunk and shoulder aligned in the frontal plane (**active hip abduction test** ☑) (Figure 9-18).[74] If the leg wobbles, the pelvis tips, the shoulders or trunk rotate, the hip flexes or the abducted limb medially rotates, it is an indication of lack of movement control and lack of muscle strength and balance.

Anteriorly, the head should be straight on the shoulders, and the nose should be in line with the manubrium, sternum, and xiphisternum or umbilicus. The shoulders and clavicle should be level and equal, although the dominant side may be slightly lower. The waist angles should be equal. Does the patient show a lateral shift or list (Figure 9-19)? Such a shift may be straight lateral movement or it may be a scoliosis (rotation involved). The straight shift is more likely to be caused by mechanical dysfunction and muscle spasm and is likely to disappear on lying down or hanging.[3,75] True scoliosis commonly has compensating curves and does not change with hanging or lying down. The arbitrary "high" points on both iliac crests should be the same height. If they are

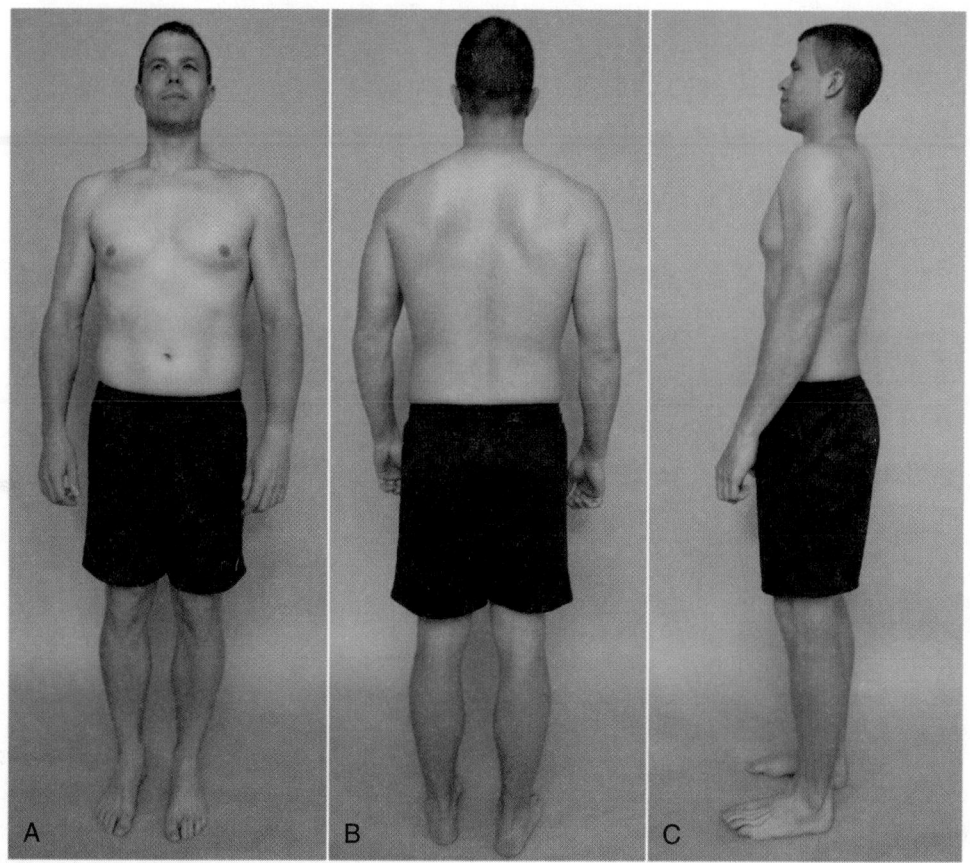

Figure 9-17 Views of the patient in the standing position. A, Anterior view. **B,** Posterior view. **C,** Lateral view.

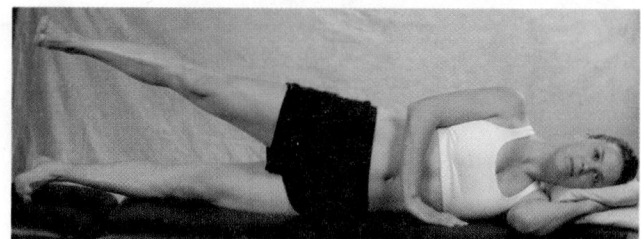

Figure 9-18 Active hip abduction test. Note how shoulders, trunk, pelvis, and lower limbs are all in alignment in a negative test.

not, the possibility of unequal leg length should be considered. The difference in height would indicate a functional limb length discrepancy. This discrepancy could be caused by altered bone length, altered mechanics (e.g., pronated foot on one side), or joint dysfunction (Table 9-7). The ASISs should be level. The patellae should point straight ahead. The lower limbs should be straight and not in genu varum or genu valgum. The heads of the fibulae should be level. The medial malleoli should be level, as should be the lateral malleoli. The medial longitudinal arches of the feet should be evident, and the feet should angle out equally. The arms should be an equal distance from the trunk and equally medially or laterally rotated. Any protrusion or depression of the sternum, ribs, or costicartilage, as well as any bowing of bones,

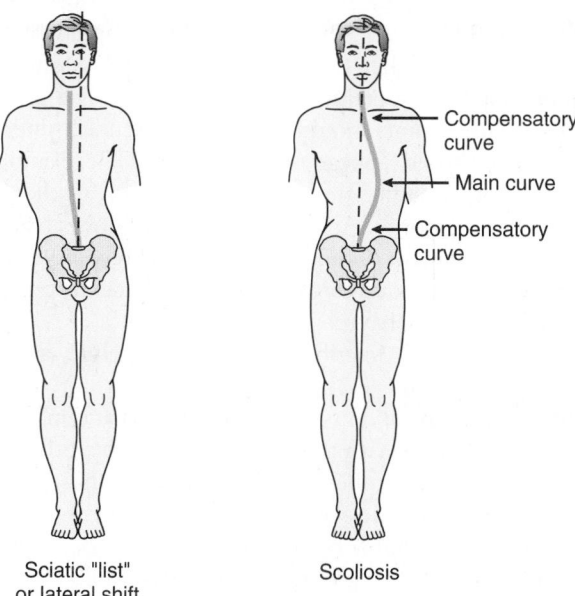

Figure 9-19 Lateral shift or list.

should be noted. The bony or soft-tissue contours should be equal on both sides.

From the side, the examiner should look at the head to ensure that the ear lobe is in line with the tip of the shoulder (acromion process) and the arbitrary highpoint

TABLE **9-7**

Functional Limb Length Difference

Joint	Functional Lengthening	Functional Shortening
Foot	Supination	Pronation
Knee	Extension	Flexion
Hip	Lowering	Lifting
	Extension	Flexion
	Lateral rotation	Medial rotation
Sacroiliac	Anterior rotation	Posterior rotation

From Wallace LA: Lower quarter pain: mechanical evaluation and treatment. In Grieve GP, editor: Modern manual therapy of the vertebral column, Edinburgh, 1986, Churchill Livingstone, p. 467.

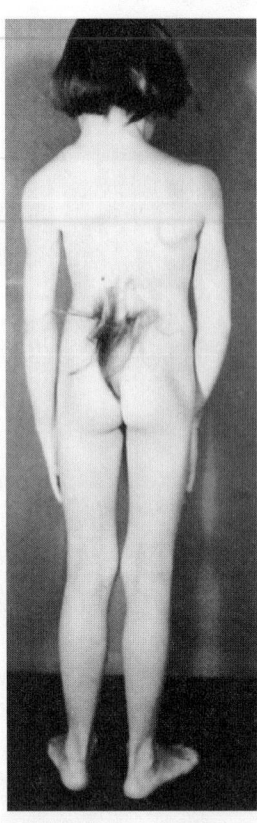

Figure 9-20 Congenital scoliosis and a diastematomyelia in a 9-year-old girl. This type of hairy patch strongly indicates a congenital maldevelopment of the neural axis. (From Rothman RH, Simeone FA: The spine, Philadelphia, 1982, WB Saunders, p. 371.)

of the iliac crest. Each segment of the spine should have a normal curve. Are any of the curves exaggerated or decreased? Is lordosis present? Kyphosis? Do the shoulders droop forward? Normally with a neutral pelvis, the ASISs are slightly lower than the PSISs. Are the knees straight, flexed, or in recurvatum (hyperextended)?

From behind, the examiner should note the level of the shoulders, spines and inferior angles of the scapula, and any deformities (e.g., a Sprengel deformity). Any lateral spinal curve (scoliosis) should be noted (Figure 9-20). If the scoliotic curve is because of a disc herniation, the herniation usually occurs on the convex side of the curve.[76] The waist angles should be equal from the posterior aspect, as they were from the anterior aspect. The PSISs should be level. The examiner should note whether the PSISs are higher or lower than the ASISs and the patient's ability to maintain a neutral pelvis. The gluteal folds and knee joints should be level. The Achilles tendons and heels should appear to be straight. The examiner should note whether there is any protrusion of the ribs or bowing of bones. Any deviation in the normal spinal postural alignment should be noted and recorded. The various possible sources of pathology related to posture are discussed in Chapter 15.

Janda and Jull described a lumbar or **pelvic crossed syndrome** (Figure 9-21) to show the effect of muscle imbalance on the ability of a patient to hold and maintain a neutral pelvis.[77] With this syndrome, they hypothesized that there was a combination of weak, long muscles and short, strong muscles, which resulted in an imbalance pattern leading to low back pain.[78] They felt that only by treating the different groups appropriately could the back pain be relieved. The weak, long inhibited muscles were the abdominals and gluteus maximus, whereas the strong tight (shortened) muscles were the hip flexors (primarily iliopsoas) and the back extensors. The imbalance pattern promotes increased lumbar lordosis because of the forward pelvic tilt and hip flexion contracture and overactivity of the hip flexors compensating for the weak abdominals. The weak gluteals result in increased activity in the

hamstrings and erector spinae as compensation to assist hip extension. Interestingly, although the long spinal extensors show increased activity, the short lumbar muscles (e.g., multifidus, rotatores) show weakness. Also, the hamstrings show tightness as they attempt to pull the pelvis backward to compensate for the anterior rotation caused by the tight hip flexors. Weakness of gluteus medius results in increased activity of the quadratus lumborum and tensor fasciae latae on the same side. This syndrome is often seen in conjunction with **upper crossed syndrome** (see Chapter 3). The two syndromes together are called the *layer syndrome*.[77]

Markings

A "faun's beard" (tuft of hair) may indicate a spina bifida occulta or diastematomyelia (see Figure 9-20).[79] Café au lait spots may indicate neurofibromatosis or collagen disease (Figure 9-22). Unusual skin markings or the presence of skin lesions in the midline may lead the examiner to consider the possibility of underlying neural and mesodermal anomalies. Musculoskeletal anomalies tend to form at the same time embryologically. Thus, if the examiner finds one anomaly, he or she must consider the possibility of other anomalies.

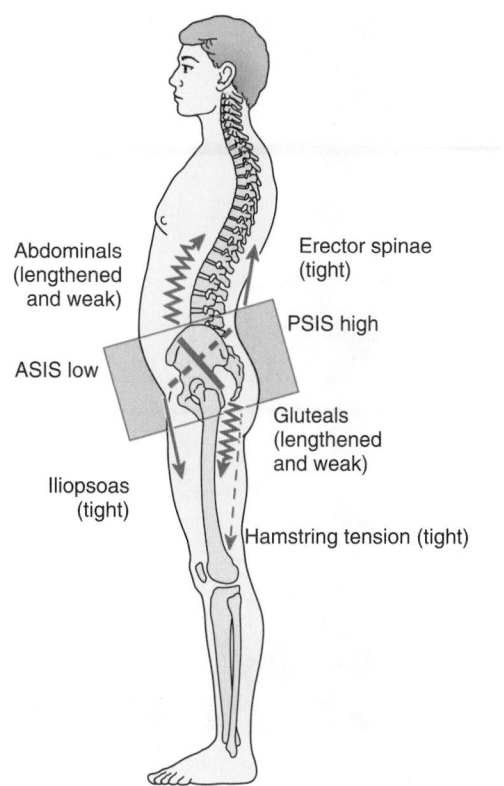

Figure 9-21 **The pelvic crossed syndrome as described by Janda and Jull.**

Abdominals
(lengthened
and weak)

Erector spinae
(tight)

PSIS high

ASIS low

Gluteals
(lengthened
and weak)

Iliopsoas
(tight)

Hamstring tension (tight)

Step Deformity

A step deformity in the lumbar spine may indicate a spondylolisthesis. The "step" occurs because the spinous process of one vertebra becomes prominent when either the vertebra above (for example, spondylitic spondylolisthesis) or the affected vertebra (for example, spondylolytic spondylolisthesis) slips forward on the one below (Figure 9-23).

EXAMINATION

When assessing the lumbar spine, the examiner must remember that referral of symptoms or the presence of neurological symptoms often makes it necessary to "clear" or rule the lower limb pathology. Many of the symptoms that occur in the lower limb may originate in the lumbar spine. Unless there is a history of definitive trauma to a peripheral joint, a screening or scanning examination must accompany assessment of that joint to rule out problems within the lumbar spine referring symptoms to that joint. It is often helpful at this stage to ask the patient to demonstrate the movements that produce or have produced the pain. When asking the patient to do this, the examiner must allow time for symptoms to disappear before completing the examination.

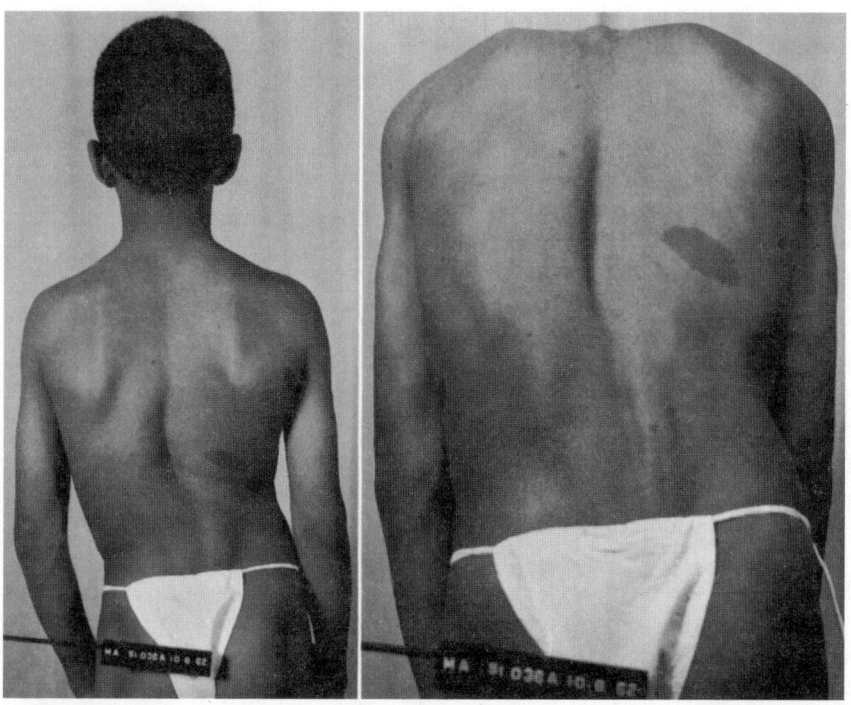

Figure 9-22 **Neurofibromatosis with scoliosis.** Note the café au lait spots on the right side of the trunk. (From Tachdjian MO: Pediatric orthopedics, Philadelphia, 1990, WB Saunders, p. 1290.)

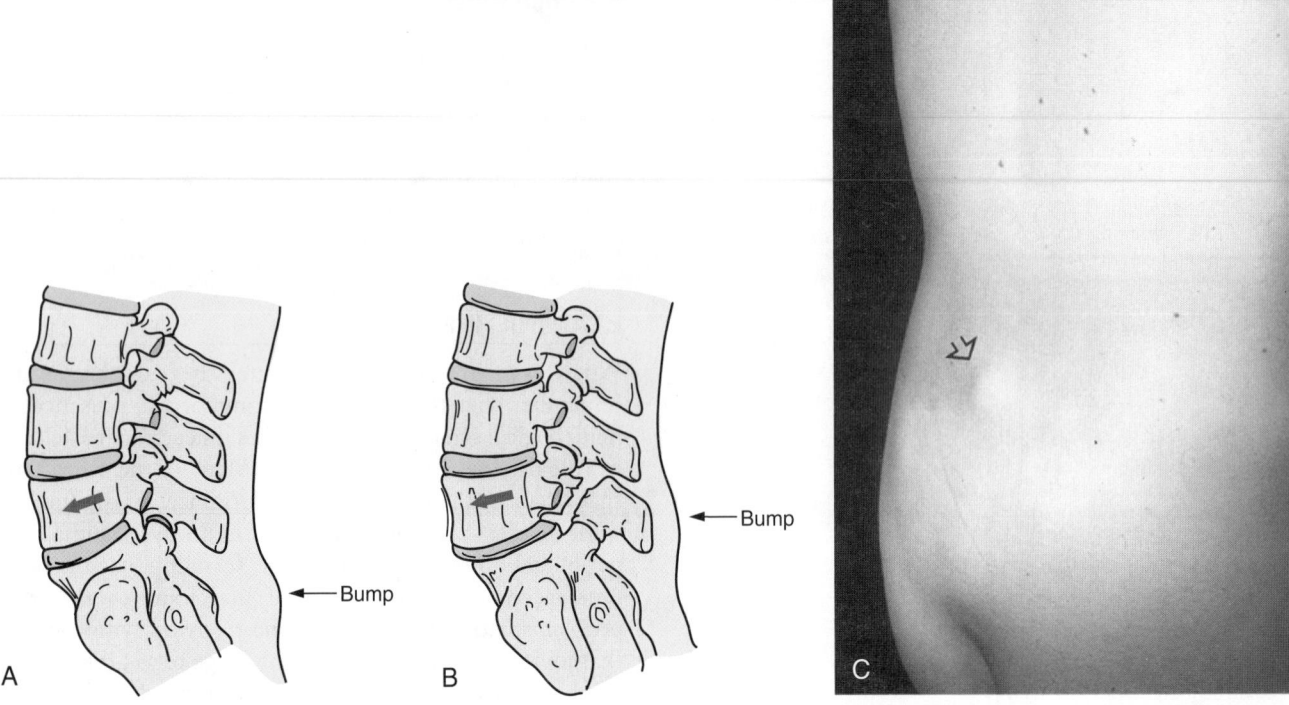

Figure 9-23 Step deformity in the lumbar spine. A, Caused by spondylosis. **B,** Caused by spondylolisthesis. **C,** Spinous process protrusion caused by step deformity.

Active Movements

Active movements are performed with the patient standing (Figure 9-24). The examiner is looking for differences in ROM and the patient's willingness to do the movement. The ROM taking place during the active movement is normally the summation of the movements of the entire lumbar spine, not just movement at one level, along with hip movement. The most painful movements are done last. If the problem is mechanical, at least one or more of the movements will be painful.[27]

While the patient is doing the active movements, the examiner looks for limitation of movement and its possible causes, such as pain, spasm, stiffness, or blocking. As the patient reaches the full range of active movement, passive overpressure may be applied, but only if the active movements appear to be full and pain free. The overpressure must be applied with extreme care, because the upper body weight is already being applied to the lumbar joints by virtue of their position and gravity. If the patient reports that a sustained position increases the symptoms, then the examiner should consider having the patient maintain the position (e.g., flexion) at the end of the ROM for 10 to 20 seconds to see whether symptoms increase. Likewise, if repetitive motion or combined movements have been reported in the history as causing symptoms, these movements should be performed as well, but only after the patient has completed the basic movements.

The greatest motion in the lumbar spine occurs between the L4 and L5 vertebrae and between L5 and S1. There is considerable individual variability in the ROM of the lumbar spine (Figure 9-25).[80-84] In reality, little obvious movement occurs in the lumbar spine especially in the individual segments because of the shape of the facet joints, tightness of the ligaments, presence of the intervertebral discs, and size of the vertebral bodies.

Active Movements of the Lumbar Spine

- Forward flexion (40° to 60°)
- Extension (20° to 35°)
- Side (lateral) flexion, left and right (15° to 20°)
- Rotation, left and right (3° to 18°)
- Sustained postures (if necessary)
- Repetitive motion (if necessary)
- Combined movements (if necessary)

For flexion (forward bending), the maximum ROM in the lumbar spine is normally 40° to 60°. The examiner must differentiate the movement occurring in the lumbar spine from that occurring in the hips or thoracic spine. Some patients can touch their toes by flexing the hips, even if no movement occurs in the spine. On forward

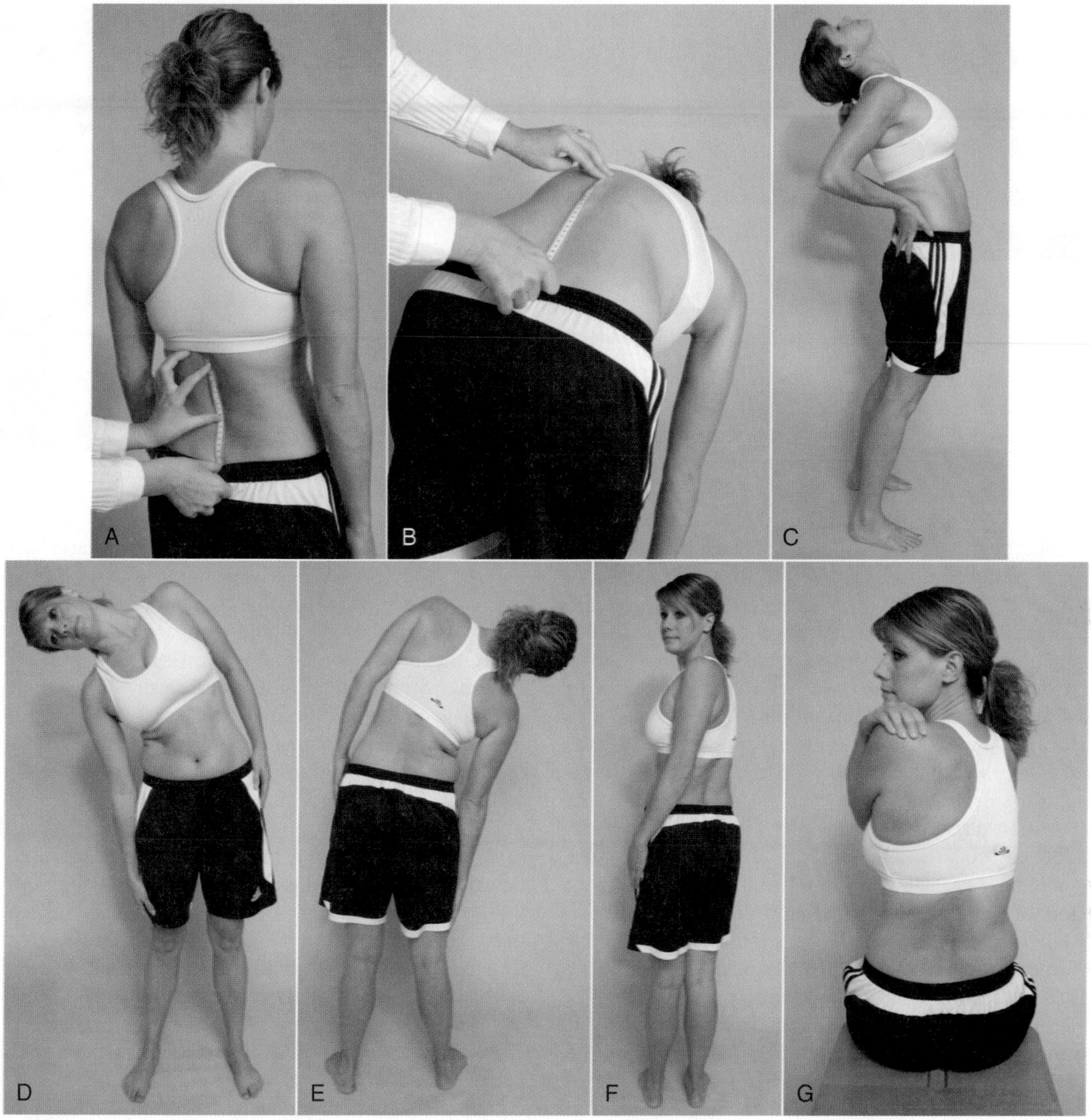

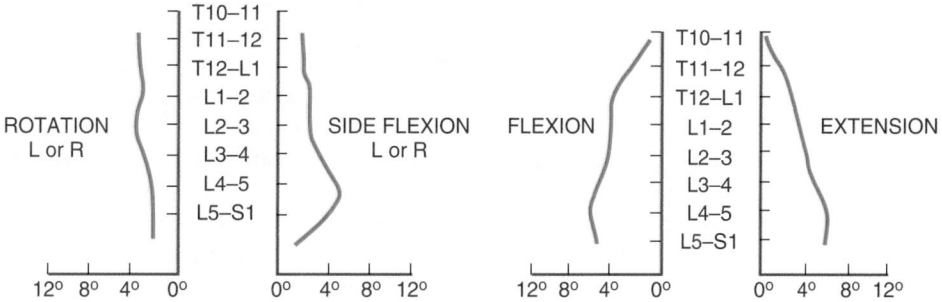

Figure 9-24 Active movements of the lumbar spine. A and **B,** Measuring forward flexion using tape measure. **C,** Extension. **D,** Side flexion (anterior view). **E,** Side flexion (posterior view). **F,** Rotation (standing). **G,** Rotation (sitting).

Figure 9-25 Average range of motion (ROM) in the lumbar spine. (Adapted from Grieve GP: Common vertebral joint problems, Edinburgh, 1981, Churchill Livingstone.)

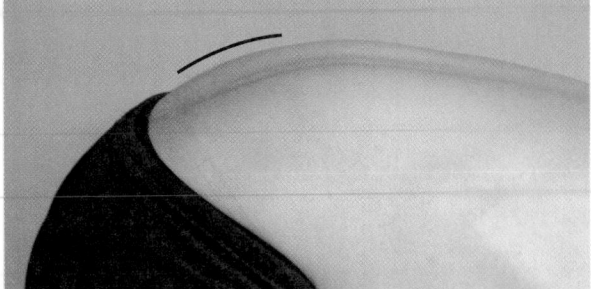

Figure 9-26 On forward flexion, the lumbar curve should normally flatten or go into slight flexion, as shown.

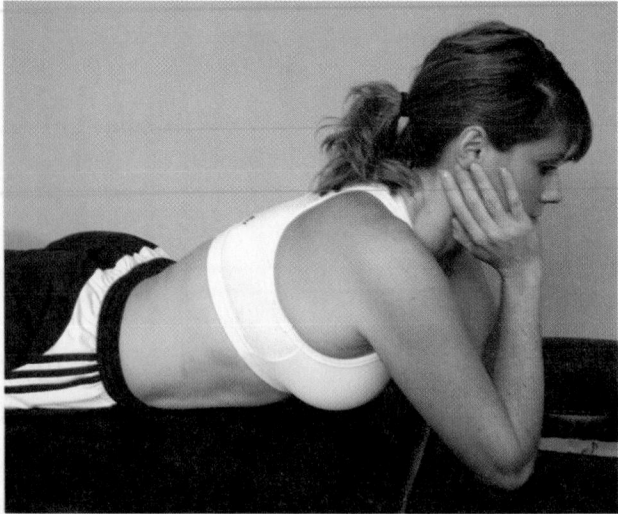

Figure 9-27 The sphinx position.

flexion, the lumbar spine should move from its normal lordotic curvature to at least a straight or slightly flexed curve (Figure 9-26).[85] If this change in the spine does not occur, there is probably some hypomobility in the lumbar spine resulting from either tight structures or muscle spasm. The degree of injury also has an effect. For example, the more severely a disc is injured (for example, if sequestration has occurred rather than a protrusion), the greater the limitation of movement.[86] With disc degeneration, intersegmental motion may increase as disc degeneration increases up to a certain point and follows Kirkaldy-Willis's description of degenerative changes in the disc.[87] He divided the changes into three stages: dysfunctional, unstable, and stable. During the first two phases, intersegmental motion increases in flexion, rotation, and side flexion[88] and then decreases in the final stabilization phase. During the unstable phase, it is often possible to see an instability "jog" during one or more movements, especially flexion, returning to neutral from flexion, or side flexion.[89,90] An **instability jog** is a sudden movement shift or "rippling" of the muscles during active movement, indicating an unstable segment.[85,91] Similarly, muscle twitching during movement or complaints of something "slipping out" during lumbar spine movement may indicate instability.[92] If the patient bends one or both knees on forward flexion, the examiner should watch for nerve root symptoms or tight hamstrings, especially if spinal flexion is decreased when the knees are straight. If tight hamstrings or nerve root symptoms are suspected, the examiner should perform suitable tests (see "Special Tests" section) to determine if the hamstrings or nerve root restriction (see "Knee Flexion Test") are the cause of the problem. When returning to the upright posture from forward flexion, the patient with no back pain first rotates the hips and pelvis to about 45° of flexion; during the last 45° of extension, the low back resumes its lordosis. In patients with back pain, commonly, most movement occurs in the hips, accompanied by knee flexion, and sometimes with hand support working up the thighs.[93] As with the thoracic spine, the examiner may use a tape measure to determine the increase in spacing of the spinous processes on forward flexion. Normally, the measurement should increase 7 to 8 cm (2.8 to 3.1 inches)

if it is taken between the T12 spinous process and S1 (see Figures 9-24, *A* and *B*). The examiner should note how far forward the patient is able to bend (i.e., to midthigh, knees, midtibia, or floor) and compare this finding with the results of straight leg raising tests (see "Special Tests" section). Straight leg raising, especially if bilateral, is essentially the same movement done passively, except that it is a movement occurring from below upward instead of from above downward.

During the active movements, especially during flexion or extension, the examiner should watch for a **painful arc.** The pain seen in a lumbar painful arc tends to be neurologically based (i.e., it is lancinating or lightening-like), but it may also be caused by instability. If it does occur on movement in the lumbar spine, it is likely that a space-occupying lesion (most likely a small herniation of the disc) is pinching the nerve root in part of the range as the nerve root moves with the motion.[75]

Maigne described an active movement flexion maneuver to help confirm lumbar movement and control.[72] In this **happy round maneuver,** the patient bends forward and places the hands on a bed or on the back of a chair. The patient then attempts to arch or hunch the back. Most patients with lumbar pathology are unable to sustain the hunched position.

Extension (backward bending) is normally limited to 20° to 35° in the lumbar spine. While performing the movement, the patient is asked to place the hands in the small of the back to help stabilize the back. Bourdillon and Day have advocated doing this movement in the prone lying position to hyperextend the spine.[94] They called the resulting position the **sphinx position.** The patient hyperextends the spine by resting on the elbows with the hands holding the chin (Figure 9-27) and allows the abdominal wall to relax. The position is held for 10 to 20 seconds to see if symptoms occur or, if present, become worse.

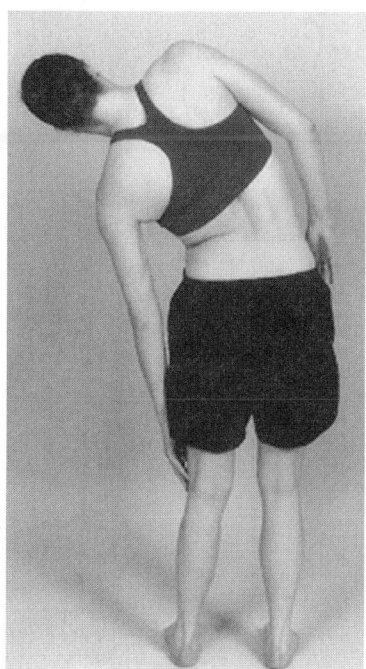

Figure 9-28 Lateral (side) flexion. Note that lower lumbar spine stays straight and upper lumbar and lower thoracic spine side flexes. This finding would indicate hypomobility in the lower lumbar spine.

Side (lateral) flexion or side bending is approximately 15° to 20° in the lumbar spine. The patient is asked to run the hand down the side of the leg and not to bend forward or backward while performing the movement. The examiner can then eyeball the movement and compare it with that of the other side. The distance from the fingertips to the floor on both sides may also be measured, noting any difference. In the spine, the movement of side flexion is a **coupled movement** with rotation. Because of the position of the facet joints, both side flexion and rotation occur together although the amount of movement and direction of movement may not be the same. Table 9-8 shows how different authors interpret the coupled movement in the spine. As the patient side flexes, the examiner should watch the lumbar curve. Normally, the lumbar curve forms a smooth curve on side flexion, and there should be no obvious sharp angulation at only one level. If angulation does occur, it may indicate hypomobility below the level or hypermobility above the level in the lumbar spine (Figure 9-28). Mulvein and Jull advocated having the patient do a lateral shift (Figure 9-29) in addition to side flexion.[95] Their viewpoint is that lateral shift in the lumbar spine focuses the movement more in the lower spine (L4–S1) and helps eliminate the compensating movements in the rest of the spine.

Rotation in the lumbar spine is normally 3° to 18° to the left or right, and it is accomplished by a shearing movement of the lumbar vertebrae on each other. Although the patient is usually in the standing position, rotation may be performed while sitting to eliminate pelvic and hip movement. If the patient stands, the

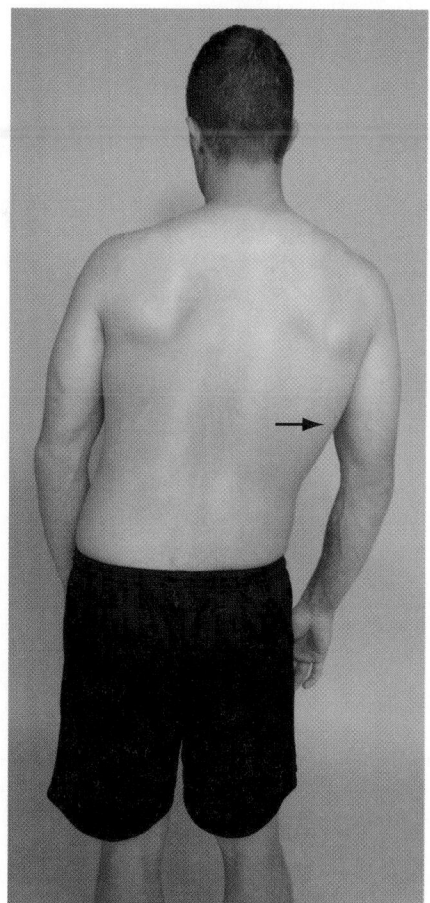

Figure 9-29 Lumbar lateral shift.

TABLE **9-8**

Coupled Movements (Side Flexion and Rotation) Believed to Occur in the Spine in Different Positions (Note the Differences)

Author	In Neutral	In Flexion	In Extension
MacConnaill		Ipsilateral	Contralateral
Farfan		Contralateral	Contralateral
Kaltenborn		Ipsilateral	Ipsilateral
Grieve		Ipsilateral	Contralateral
Fryette	Contralateral	Ipsilateral	Ipsilateral
Pearcy		Ipsilateral (L5–S1) Contralateral (L4, 5)	
Oxland		Ipsilateral (L5–S1)* Contralateral (L5–S1)**	

Ipsilateral implies both movements occur in the same direction, contralateral implies they occur in opposite directions.
*If side flexion is induced first.
**If rotation is induced first.

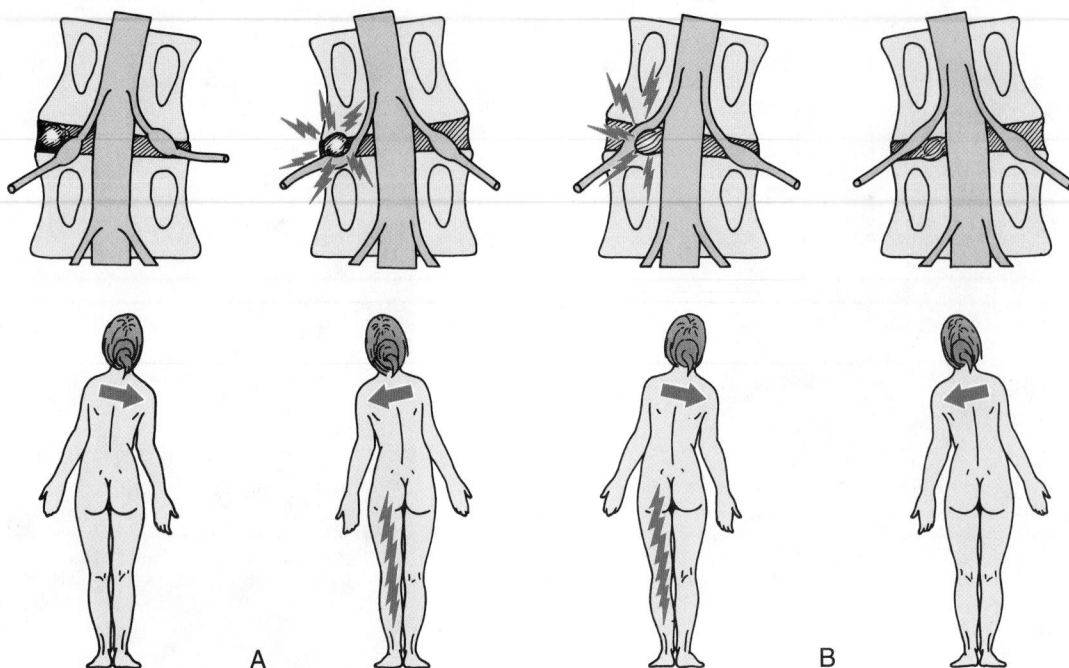

Figure 9-30 Patients with herniated disc problems may sometimes list to one side. This is a voluntary or involuntary mechanism to alleviate nerve root irritation. The list in some patients is toward the side of the sciatica; in others, it is toward the opposite side. A reasonable hypothesis suggests that when the herniation is lateral to the nerve root **(A)**, the list is to the side opposite the sciatica because a list to the same side would elicit pain. Conversely, when the herniation is medial to the nerve root **(B)**, the list is toward the side of the sciatica because tilting away would irritate the root and cause pain. (Redrawn from White AA, Panjabi MM: Clinical biomechanics of the spine, ed 2, Philadelphia, 1990, JB Lippincott, p. 415.) (© Augustus A. White III and MM Panjabi.)

examiner must take care to watch for this accessory movement and try to eliminate it by stabilizing the pelvis.

If a movement such as side flexion toward the painful side increases the symptoms, the lesion is probably intra-articular, because the muscles and ligaments on that side are relaxed. If a disc protrusion is present and lateral to the nerve root, side flexion to the painful side increases the pain and radicular symptoms on that side. If a movement (such as, side flexion away from the painful side) alters the symptoms, the lesion may be articular or muscular in origin, or it may be a disc protrusion medial to the nerve root (Figure 9-30).

McKenzie advocated repeating the active movements, especially flexion and extension, ten times to see whether the movement increases or decreases the symptoms.[39] He also advocated, like Mulvein and Jull,[95] a side gliding movement in which the head and feet remain in position and the patient shifts the pelvis to the left and to the right.

If the examiner finds that side flexion and rotation have been equally limited and extension has been limited to a lesser extent, a capsular pattern may be suspected. A capsular pattern in one lumbar segment, however, is difficult to detect.

Because back injuries rarely occur during a "pure" movement (such as, flexion, extension, side flexion, or rotation), it has been advocated that **combined movements** of the spine should be included in the examination.[96,97] The examiner may want to test the following more habitual combined movements: lateral flexion in flexion, lateral flexion in extension, flexion and rotation, and extension and rotation. These combined movements (Figure 9-31) may cause signs and symptoms different from those produced by single plane movements and are definitely indicated if the patient has shown that a combined movement is what causes the symptoms. For example, if the patient is suffering from a facet syndrome, combined extension and rotation is the movement most likely to exacerbate symptoms.[98] Other symptoms that would indicate facet involvement include absence of radicular signs or neurological deficit, hip and buttock pain, and sometimes leg pain above the knee, no paresthesia, and low back stiffness.[99,100]

While the patient is standing, the examiner may perform a **quick test** of the lower peripheral joints (Figure 9-32), provided the examiner feels the patient has the ability to do the test. The patient squats down as far as possible, bounces two or three times, and returns to the standing position. This action quickly tests the ankles, knees, and hips as well as the sacrum for any pathological condition. If the patient can fully squat and bounce without any signs and symptoms, these joints are probably free of pathology related to the complaint. However, this test should be used only with caution and should not be done with patients suspected of having arthritis or pathology in the lower limb joints, pregnant patients, or older patients who exhibit weakness and

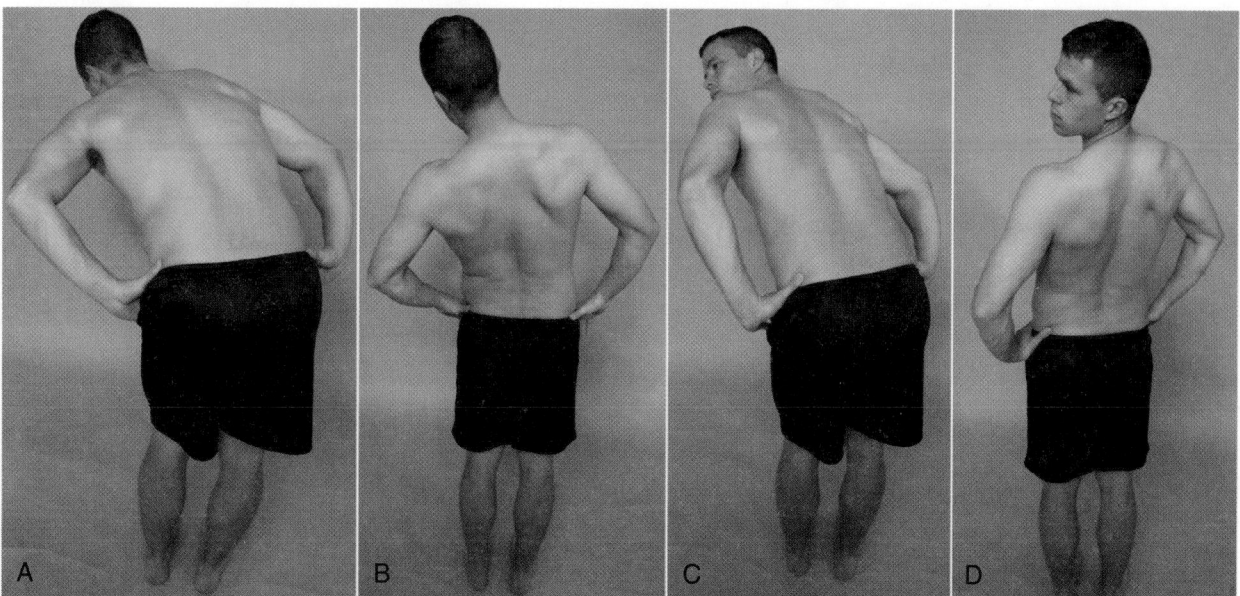

Figure 9-31 Combined active movements. A, Lateral flexion in flexion. **B,** Lateral flexion in extension. **C,** Rotation and flexion. **D,** Rotation and extension.

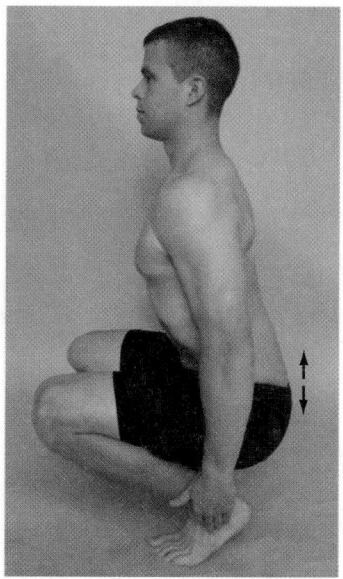

Figure 9-32 **Quick test.**

hypomobility. If this test is negative, there is no need to test the peripheral joints (peripheral joint scan) with the patient in the lying position.

The patient is then asked to balance on one leg and to go up and down on the toes four or five times. This is, in effect, a **modified Trendelenberg test.** While the patient does this, the examiner watches for **Trendelenburg sign** (Figure 9-33). A positive Trendelenburg sign is shown by the nonstance side ilium dropping down instead of elevating as it normally would when standing on the leg. A weak gluteus medius muscle or a coxa vara

(abnormal shaft-neck angle of the femur) on the stance leg side may produce a positive sign. If the patient is unable to complete the movement by going up and down on the toes, the examiner should suspect an S1 nerve root lesion. Both legs are tested.

McKenzie advocated doing flexion movements with the patient in the supine lying position as well.[39] In the standing position, flexion in the spine takes place from above downward, so pain at the end of the ROM indicates that L5–S1 is affected. When the patient is in the supine lying position with the knees being lifted to the chest, flexion takes place from below upward so that pain at the beginning of movement indicates that L5–S1 is affected. Remember that greater stretch is placed on L5–S1 when the patient is in the lying position.

During the observation stage of the assessment, the examiner will have noted any changes in functional limb length (see Table 9-7). Wallace developed a method for measuring **functional leg length.**[101] The patient is first assessed in a relaxed stance. In this position, the examiner palpates the ASISs and the PSISs, noting any asymmetry. The examiner then places the patient in a symmetric stance, ensuring that the subtalar joint is in the neutral position (see Chapter 13), the toes are straight ahead, and the knees are extended. The ASISs and PSISs are again assessed for asymmetry. If differences are still noted, the examiner should check for structural leg length differences (see Chapters 10 and 11), sacroiliac joint dysfunction, or weak gluteus medius or quadratus lumborum (Figure 9-34). The pelvis may also be leveled with the use of calibrated blocks or cards so that the functional length difference can be recorded.

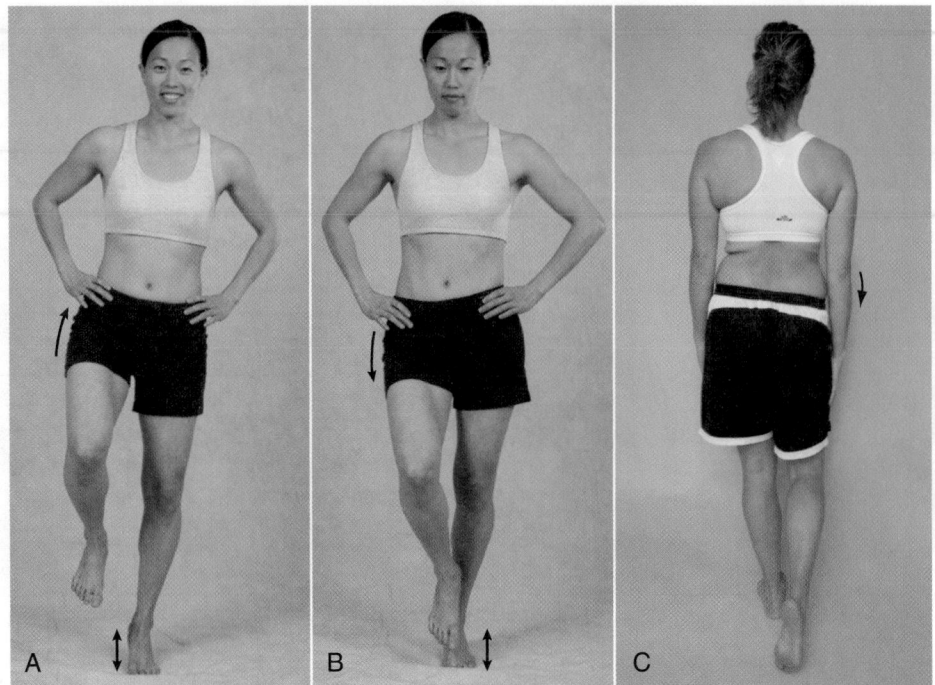

Figure 9-33 Trendelenburg and S1 nerve root test. A, Negative Trendelenburg test (hip hikes) while doing S1 test (up and down on toes). **B,** Positive Trendelenburg test (hip drops) while doing S1 test. If patient cannot go up on toes, it would indicate a positive S1 test. **C,** Posterior view. Positive Trendelenburg test for a weak right gluteus medius.

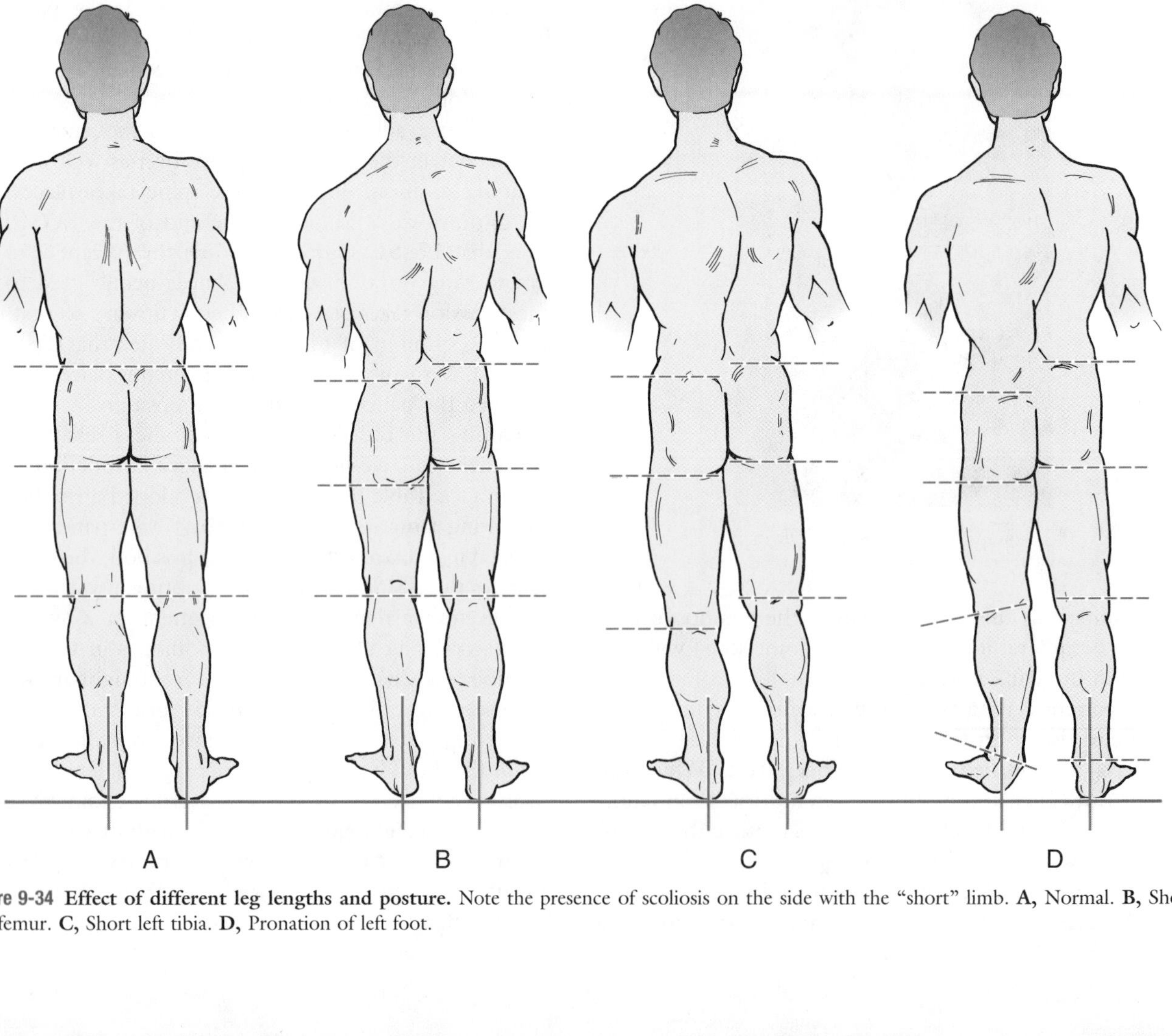

A B C D

Figure 9-34 Effect of different leg lengths and posture. Note the presence of scoliosis on the side with the "short" limb. **A,** Normal. **B,** Short left femur. **C,** Short left tibia. **D,** Pronation of left foot.

Passive Movements

In the lumbar spine, passive movements are difficult to perform because of the weight of the body. If active movements are full and pain free, overpressure can be attempted with care. However, it is safer to check the end feel of the individual vertebrae in the lumbar spine during the assessment of joint play movements. The end feel is the same, but the examiner has better control of the patient and is less likely to overstress the joints.

Passive Movements of the Lumbar Spine and Normal End Feel

- Flexion (tissue stretch)
- Extension (tissue stretch)
- Side flexion (tissue stretch)
- Rotation (tissue stretch)

Resisted Isometric Movements

Resisted isometric muscle strength of the lumbar spine is first tested in the neutral position. The patient is seated. The contraction must be resisted and isometric so that no movement occurs (Figure 9-35). Because of the strength of the trunk muscles, the examiner should say, "Don't let me move you," so that movement is minimized. The examiner tests flexion, extension, side flexion, and rotation. Figure 9-36 shows the axes of movement of the lumbar spine. The lumbar spine should be in a neutral position, and the painful movements should be done last. The examiner should keep in mind that strong abdominal muscles help to reduce the load on the lumbar spine by approximately 30% and on the thoracic spine by

approximately 50%, as a result of the increased intrathoracic and intra-abdominal pressures caused by the contraction of these muscles. Table 9-9 lists the muscles acting on the lumbar vertebrae.

Provided neutral isometric testing is normal or only causes a small amount of pain, the examiner can go on to other tests, which will place greater stress on the muscles. These tests are often dynamic and provide both concentric and eccentric work for the muscles supporting the spine. With all of the following tests, the examiner should ensure that the patient can hold a neutral pelvis. If there is excessive movement of the ASIS (supine) or PSIS (prone) when doing the test, the patient should not be allowed to do them. In normal individuals, the ASIS

TABLE **9-9**

Muscles of the Lumbar Spine: Their Actions and Nerve Root Derivations

Action	Muscles Acting	Nerve Root Derivation
Forward flexion	1. Psoas major	L1–L3
	2. Rectus abdominis	T6–T12
	3. External abdominal oblique	T7–T12
	4. Internal abdominal oblique	T7–T12, L1
	5. Transversus abdominis	T7–T12, L1
	6. Intertransversarii	L1–L5
Extension	1. Latissimus dorsi	Thoracodorsal (C6–C8)
	2. Erector spinae	
	iliocostalis lumborum	L1–L3
	longissimus thoracis	L1–L5
	3. Transversospinalis	L1–L5
	4. Interspinales	L1–L5
	5. Quadratus lumborum	T12, L1–L4
	6. Multifidus	L1–L5
	7. Rotatores	L1–L5
	8. Gluteus maximus	L1–L5
Side flexion	1. Latissimus dorsi	Thoracodorsal (C6–C8)
	2. Erector spinae	
	iliocostalis lumborum	L1–L3
	longissimus thoracis	L1–L5
	3. Transversalis	L1–L5
	4. Intertransversarii	L1–L5
	5. Quadratus lumborum	T12, L1–L4
	6. Psoas major	L1–L3
	7. External abdominal oblique	T7–T12
Rotation*	1. Transversalis	L1–L5
	2. Rotatores	L1–L5
	3. Multifidus	L1–L5

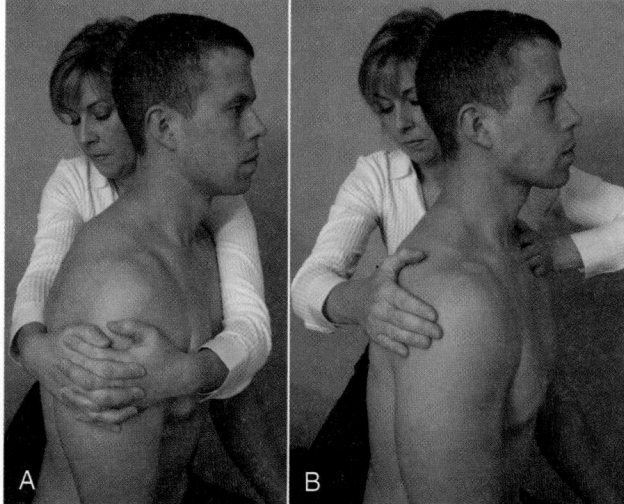

Figure 9-35 Positioning for resisted isometric movements of the lumbar spine. A, Flexion, extension, and side flexion. **B,** Rotation to right.

*Very little rotation occurs in the lumbar spine because of the shape of the facet joints. Any rotation would be a result of shearing movement.

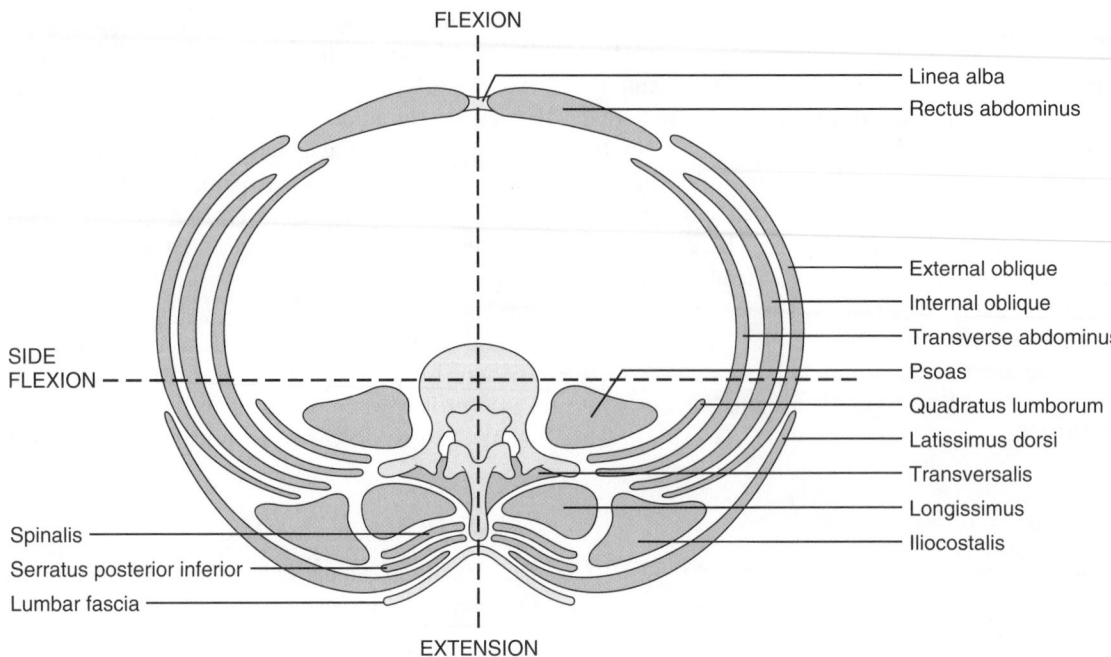

FLEXION

Linea alba
Rectus abdominus

External oblique
Internal oblique
Transverse abdominus
Psoas
Quadratus lumborum
Latissimus dorsi
Transversalis
Longissimus
Iliocostalis

SIDE
FLEXION

Spinalis
Serratus posterior inferior
Lumbar fascia

EXTENSION

Figure 9-36 Diagram of relations of the lumbar spine showing movement.

Resisted Isometric Movements of the Lumbar Spine

- Forward flexion
- Extension
- Side flexion (left and right)
- Rotation (left and right)
- Dynamic abdominal endurance
- Double straight leg lowering
- Dynamic extensor endurance
- Isotonic horizontal side support
- Internal/external abdominal oblique test

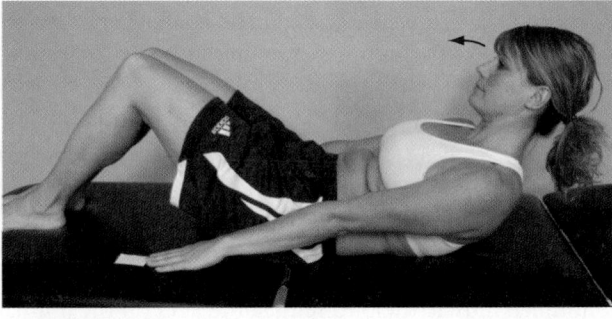

Figure 9-37 Dynamic abdominal endurance test. The patient tucks in the chin and curls up the trunk lifting the trunk off the bed. Ideally, the scapula should clear the bed.

---

or PSIS should not move when doing the tests. Motivation may also affect the results.[102]

Dynamic Abdominal Endurance Test.[103,104] This test checks the endurance of the abdominals. The patient is in supine with the hips at 45° and knees at 90° and hands at sides. A line is drawn 8 cm (for patients over 40 years of age) or 12 cm (for patients under 40 years of age) distal to the fingers. The patient tucks in the chin and curls the trunk to touch the line with the fingers (Figure 9-37) and repeats as many curls as possible using a cadence of twenty-five repetitions per minute. The number of repetitions possible before cheating (holding breath, altered mechanics) or fatigue occurs is recorded as the score. The test may also be done as an isometric test (Figure 9-38) by assuming the end position and holding it. The grading for this **isometric abdominal test** would be as follows[105-107]:

- Normal (5) = Hands behind neck, until scapulae clear table (20 to 30 second hold)

- Good (4) = Arms crossed over chest, until scapulae clear table (15 to 20 second hold)
- Fair (3) = Arms straight, until scapulae clear table (10 to 15 second hold)
- Poor (2) = Arms extended, toward knees, until top of scapulae lift from table (1 to 10 second hold)
- Trace (1) = Unable to raise more than head off table

McGill[108] advocated doing the isometric test by starting with the patient resting against a back rest angled at 60° from the horizontal with the hips and knees flexed to 90° and the arms folded across the chest and the hands on opposite shoulders (Figure 9-39). The patient's feet are held securely and the back rest is lowered away from the patient's back while the patient maintains the 60° position as long as possible.

Dynamic Extensor Endurance Test.[103,109,110] This test is designed to test the strength of iliocostalis lumborum

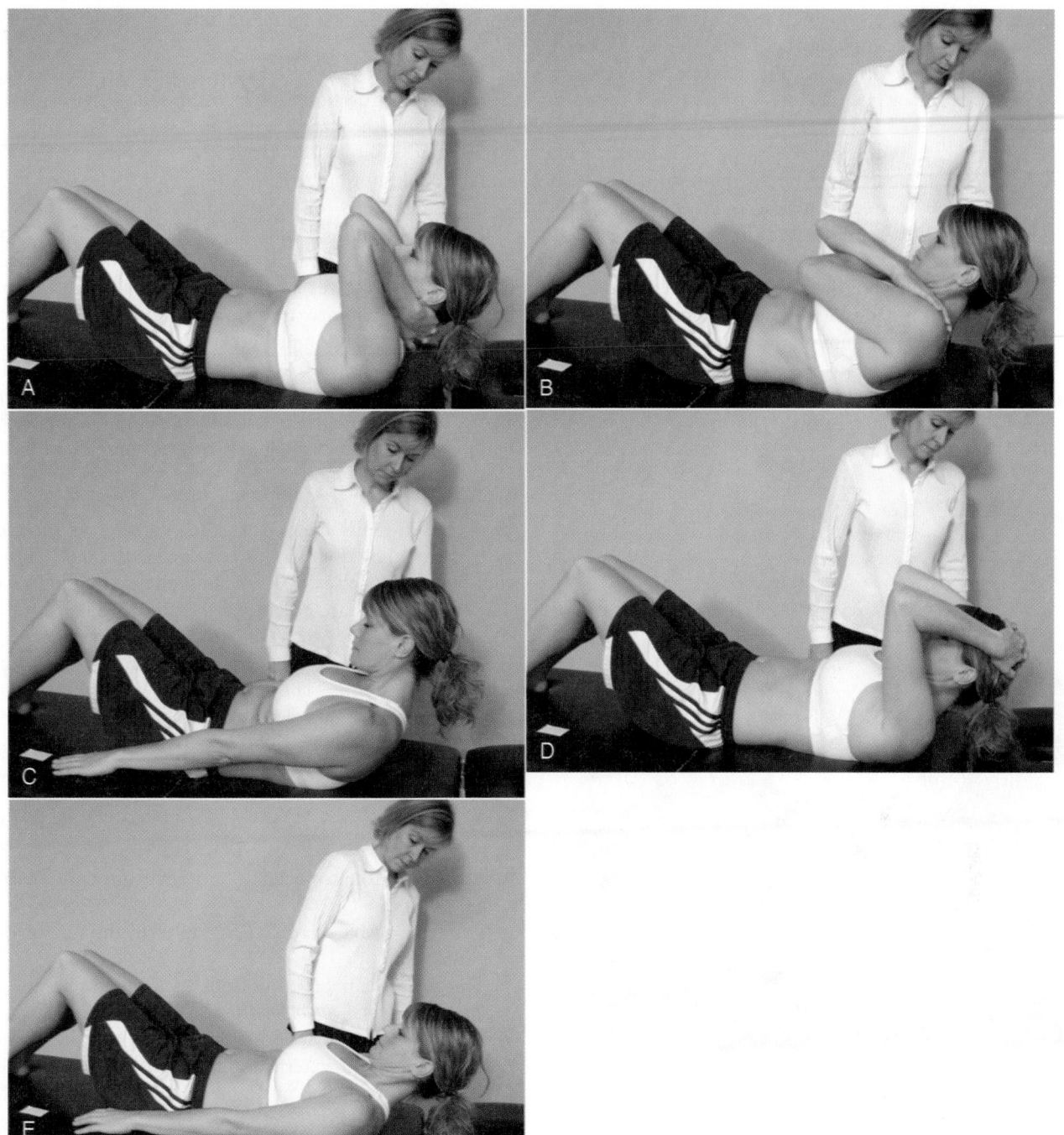

Figure 9-38 Isometric abdominal test. A, Hands behind neck. **B,** Arms crossed over chest, scapulae off table. **C,** Arms straight, scapulae off table. **D,** Hands behind head, top of scapulae off table. **E,** Arms straight, only head off table.

(erector spinae) and multifidus. The patient is placed in prone lying with the hips and iliac crests resting on the end of the examining table and the hips and pelvis stabilized with straps (Figure 9-40). Initially, the patient's hands support the upper body in 30° flexion on a chair or bench (see Figure 9-40, *A*). Keeping the spine straight, the examiner instructs the patient to extend the trunk to neutral and then lower the head to the start position. During the exercise, the patient's arms are crossed at the chest. The cadence is twenty-five repetitions per minute. The number of repetitions possible before cheating (holding breath, altered mechanics) or fatigue occurs is recorded as the score. The test may also be done isometrically, and the examiner times how long the patient can hold the contraction without pelvic or spinal movement. This test may also be done with the patient beginning in prone lying and extending the spine if the preceding test is too hard.[111,112] In this case, the patient can start with the hands by the side, moving the hands in the small of the back, and finally moving the hands behind the head for increasing difficulty. The test, if done isometrically **(isometric extensor test)** (Figure 9-41), would be graded as follows[105–107]:

- Normal (5) = With hands clasped behind the head, extends the lumbar spine, lifting the head, chest, and ribs from the floor (20 to 30 second hold)
- Good (4) = With hands at the side, extends the lumbar spine, lifting the head, chest, and ribs from the floor (15 to 20 second hold)
- Fair (3) = With hands at the side, extends the lumbar spine, lifting the sternum off the floor (10 to 15 second hold)
- Poor (2) = With hands at the side, extends the lumbar spine, lifting the head off the floor (1 to 10 second hold)

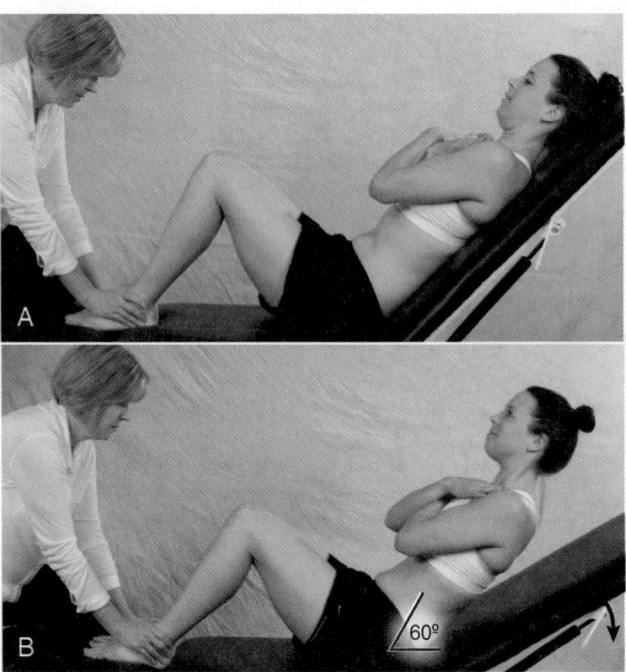

Figure 9-39 **McGill's isometric abdominal test. A,** Start position: back rest at 60°. **B,** Hold position.

- Trace (1) = Only slight contraction of the muscle with no movement

Biering and Sorensen described a similar test **(Biering-Sorensen fatigue test)** in which the subject had arms by the side, and the time the patient was able to hold the straight position before fatigue was recorded (i.e., the patient could not hold the position).[113,114] The start position is the same as for the dynamic test.

Double Straight Leg Lowering Test.[111,112,115] (Note: This test checks the abdominals. It should only be performed if the patient receives a "normal" grade in the dynamic abdominal endurance test or the abdominal isometric test.) This is an abdominal eccentric test that can place a great deal of stress on the spine so the examiner must ensure the patient is able to hold a neutral pelvis before doing the exercise. It also causes greater abdominal activation than curlups.[116] The patient lies supine and flexes the hips to 90° (Figure 9-42, *A*) and then straightens the knees (Figure 9-42, *B*). The patient then positions the pelvis in neutral (i.e., the PSISs are slightly superior to the ASISs) by doing a posterior pelvic tilt and holding the spinous processes tightly against the examining table. The straight legs are eccentrically lowered (Figure 9-42, *C*). As soon as the ASISs start to rotate forward, the test is stopped, the angle measured (plinth to thigh angle), and the knees bent. The test must be done slowly, and the patient must not hold his or her breath. The grading of the test is as follows[106]:

- Normal (5) = Able to reach 0° to 15° from table before pelvis tilts
- Good (4) = Able to reach 16° to 45° from table before pelvis tilts
- Fair (3) = Able to reach 46° to 75° from table before pelvis tilts
- Poor (2) = Able to reach 75° to 90° from table before pelvis tilts
- Trace (1) = Unable to hold pelvis in neutral at all

Internal/External Abdominal Obliques Test.[111,112] This test checks the combined action of the internal oblique muscle of one side and the external oblique muscle on the opposite side. The patient is in supine lying with hands by the

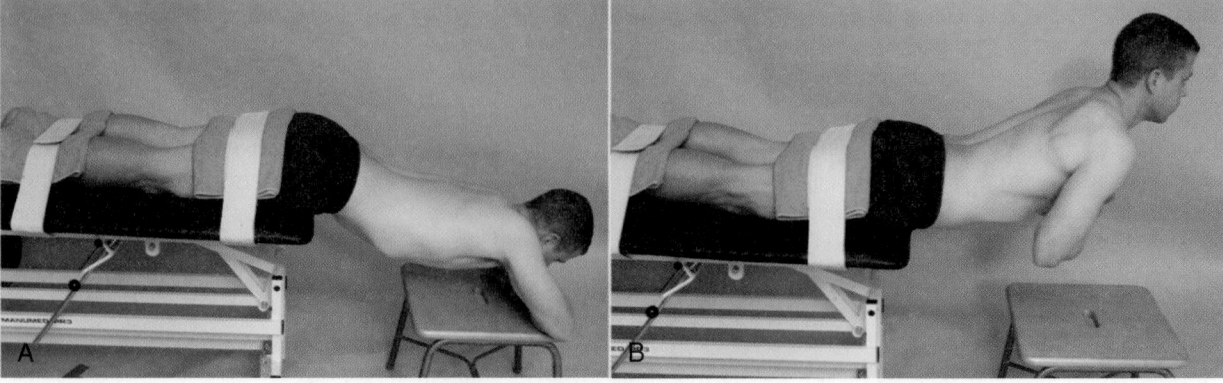

Figure 9-40 **Dynamic extensor endurance test. A,** Starting position. **B,** End position.

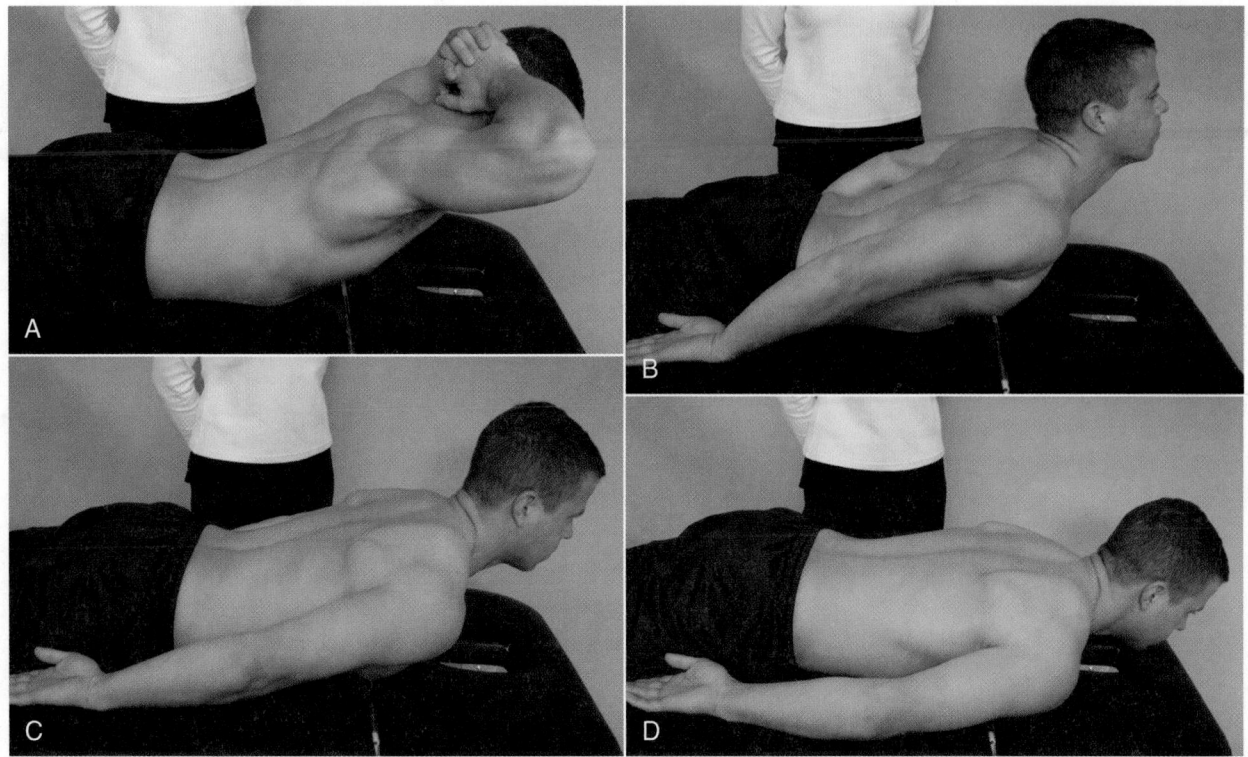

Figure 9-41 **Isometric extensor test.** **A,** Hands behind head, lift head, chest, and ribs off bed. **B,** Hands at side, lift head, chest, and ribs off bed. **C,** Hands at side, lift sternum off bed. **D,** Hands at side, lift head off bed.

side. The patient is asked to lift the head and shoulder on one side and reach over and touch the fingernails of the other hand (Figure 9-43, *A*). The examiner counts the number of repetitions the patient performs. The patient's feet should not be supported and the patient should breathe normally. The test can be made more difficult by asking the patient to put the hands on the opposite shoulders across the chest (Figure 9-43, *B*) and do the test by taking the elbow toward where the fingers would have rested beside the body or, more difficult still, by putting the hands behind the head and taking the elbows toward the position where the fingernails would have rested beside the body (Figure 9-43, *C*). The grading of the test, if done isometrically **(isometric internal/external abdominal oblique test),** would be as follows[106]:

- Normal (5) = Flexes and rotates the lumbar spine fully with hands behind head (20 to 30 second hold)
- Good (4) = Flexes and rotates the lumbar spine fully with hands across chest (15 to 20 second hold)
- Fair (3) = Flexes and rotates the lumbar spine fully with arms reaching forward (10 to 15 second hold)
- Poor (2) = Unable to flex and rotate fully
- Trace (1) = Only slight contraction of the muscle with no movement
- (0) = No contraction of the muscle

Dynamic Horizontal Side Support (Side Bridge) Test.[117] This movement tests the quadratus lumborum muscle. The patient is in a side lying position resting the upper body

on his or her elbow (Figure 9-44, *A*). To begin, the patient side lies with the knees flexed to 90°. The examiner asks the patient to lift the pelvis off the examining table (Figure 9-44, *B*) and straighten the spine. The patient should not roll forward or backward when doing the test. The patient repeats the movement as many times as possible in a dynamic test or holds for as long as possible in an isometric test. In younger, more fit patients, the test can be made more difficult by having the legs straight and asking the patient to lift the knees and pelvis off the examining table with the feet as the base so the whole body is straight (Figure 9-44, *C*). As an isometric test, the test would be graded as follows:

- Normal (5) = Able to lift pelvis off examining table and hold spine straight (10 to 20 second hold)
- Good (4) = Able to lift pelvis off examining table but has difficulty holding spine straight (5 to 10 second hold)
- Fair (3) = Able to lift pelvis off examining table and cannot hold spine straight (less than 5 second hold)
- Poor (2) = Unable to lift pelvis off examining table

McGill reported that the side bridge should be able to be held 65% of the extensor time for men and 39% for women and 99% of the flexor time for men and 79% for women.[118]

Back Rotators/Multifidus Test. This test checks the ability of the lumbar rotators and multifidus to stabilize the

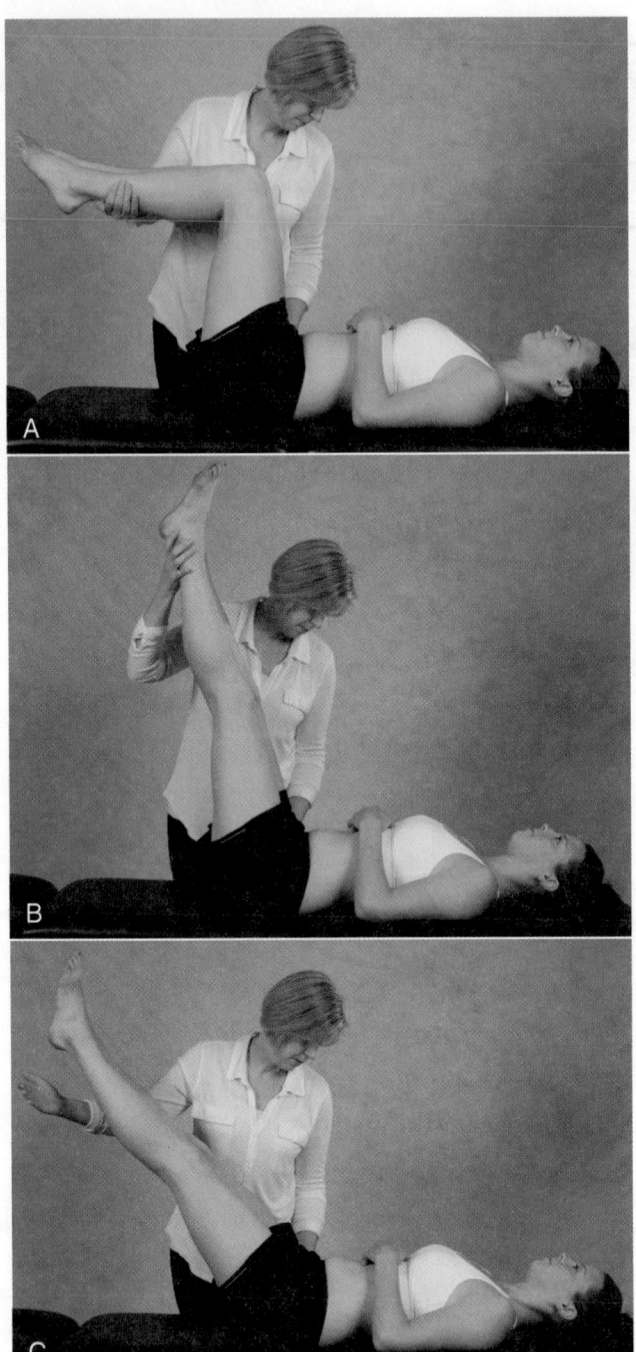

Figure 9-42 Double straight leg lowering test. A, Flexing hips to 90°. **B,** Start position with knees straight. **C,** Example of leg lowering. Note how the examiner is watching for anterior pelvic rotation which would indicate an inability to hold a neutral pelvis.

trunk during dynamic extremity movement. The patient assumes the quadriped position (Figure 9-45, *A*) and is asked to hold the "neutral pelvis" position and breathe normally. The patient is then asked to do the following movements (Figure 9-45, *B–D*):

1. Single straight arm lift and hold
2. Single straight leg lift and hold

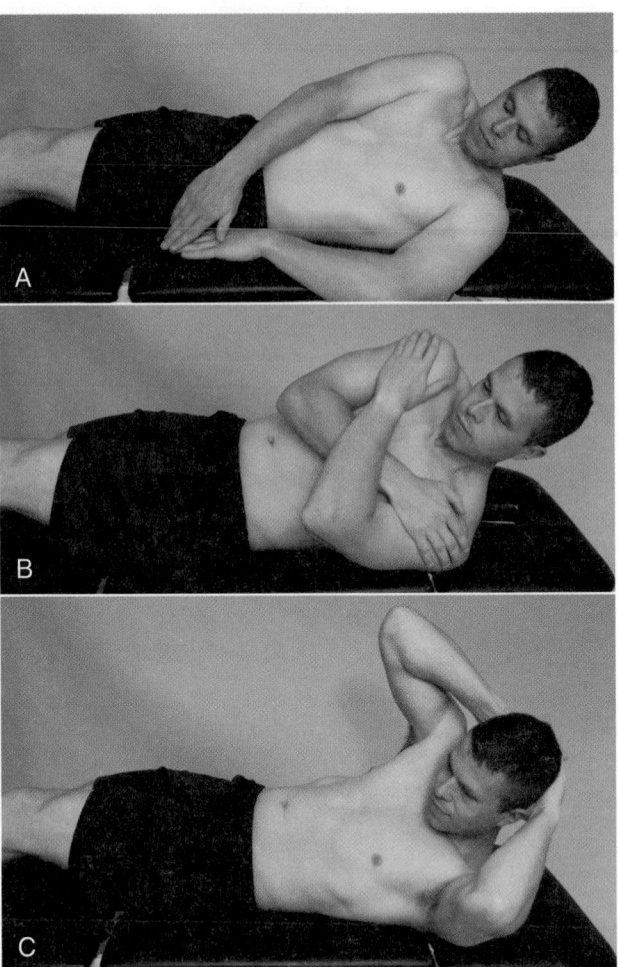

Figure 9-43 Internal/external abdominal oblique test. A, Test position with hands at side. **B,** Test position with hands on shoulders. **C,** Test position with hands behind head.

3. Contralateral straight arm and straight leg lift and hold
   The scoring for the test would be as follows:
- Normal (5) = Able to do contralateral arm and leg, both sides while maintaining neutral pelvis (20 to 30 second hold)
- Good (4) = Able to maintain neutral pelvis while doing single leg lift but not able to hold neutral pelvis when doing contralateral arm and leg (20 second hold)
- Fair (3) = Able to do single arm lift and maintain neutral pelvis (20 second hold)
- Poor (2) = Unable to maintain neutral pelvis while doing single arm lift

If tested isokinetically, the back extensors are stronger than the flexors. Men produce a force equal to approximately 65% of body weight in flexion, whereas women produce approximately 65% to 70% of their body weight in flexion. In extension, men produce approximately 90% to 95% of their body weight, and women produce 80% to 95% of their body weight, depending on the speed tested. In rotation, men produce approximately 55% to 65% of their body weight, whereas women produce

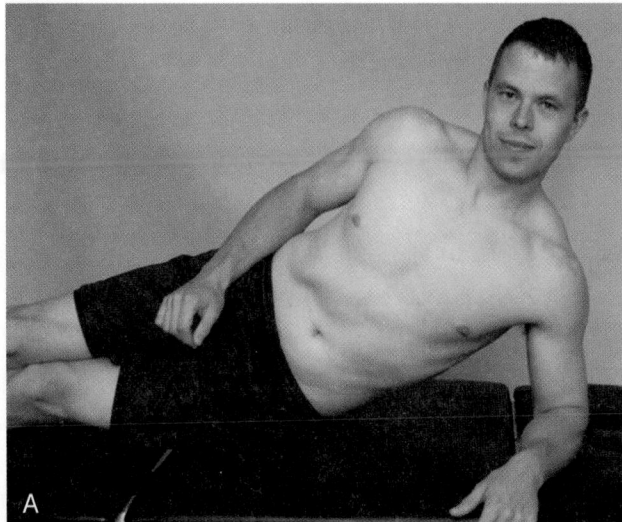

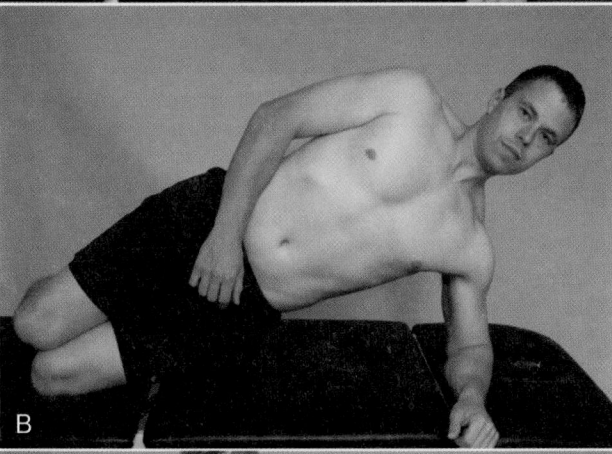

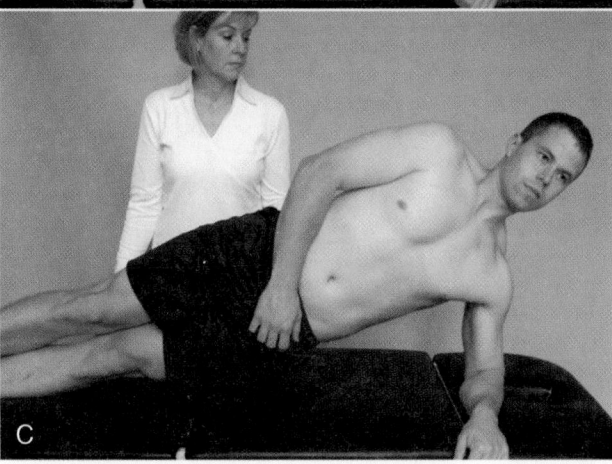

Figure 9-44 Dynamic horizontal side support. A, Start position. **B,** Lifting pelvis off bed using knees as support. **C,** Lifting pelvis off bed using feet and ankles as support.

approximately 40% to 55% of their body weight, depending on the speed tested.[119]

Peripheral Joint Scanning Examination

After the resisted isometric movements of the lumbar spine have been completed, if the examiner did not use the quick test to test the peripheral joints or is unsure of the findings or whether the peripheral joints are involved, the peripheral joints should be quickly scanned to rule out obvious pathology in the extremities. Any deviation from normal should lead the examiner to do a detailed examination of that joint. The following joints are scanned.[120]

Lower Limb Scanning Examination

- Sacroiliac joints
- Hip joints
- Knee joints
- Ankle joints
- Foot joints

Sacroiliac Joints

With the patient standing, the examiner palpates the PSIS on one side with one thumb and one of the sacral spines with the other thumb. The patient then fully flexes the hip on that side, and the examiner notes whether the PSIS drops as it normally should or whether it elevates, indicating fixation of the sacroiliac joint on that side (Figure 9-46). The examiner then compares the other side. The examiner next places one thumb on one of the patient's ischial tuberosities and one thumb on the sacral apex. The patient is then asked to flex the hip on that side again. If the movement is normal, the thumb on the ischial tuberosity moves laterally. If the sacroiliac joint on that side is fixed, the thumb moves up. The other side is then tested for comparison. This test has also been called *Gillet's* or the *sacral fixation test* (see Chapter 10).

Hip Joints

These joints are actively moved through flexion, extension, abduction, adduction, and medial and lateral rotation in as full a ROM as possible. Any pattern of restriction or pain should be noted. As the patient flexes the hip, the examiner may palpate the ilium, sacrum, and lumbar spine to determine when movement begins at the sacroiliac joint on that side and at the lumbar spine during the hip movement. The two sides should be compared.

Knee Joints

The patient actively moves the knee joints through as full a range of flexion and extension as possible. Any restriction of movement or abnormal signs and symptoms should be noted.

Foot and Ankle Joints

Plantar flexion, dorsiflexion, supination, and pronation of the foot and ankle as well as flexion and extension of the toes are actively performed through a full ROM. Again, any alteration in signs and symptoms should be noted.

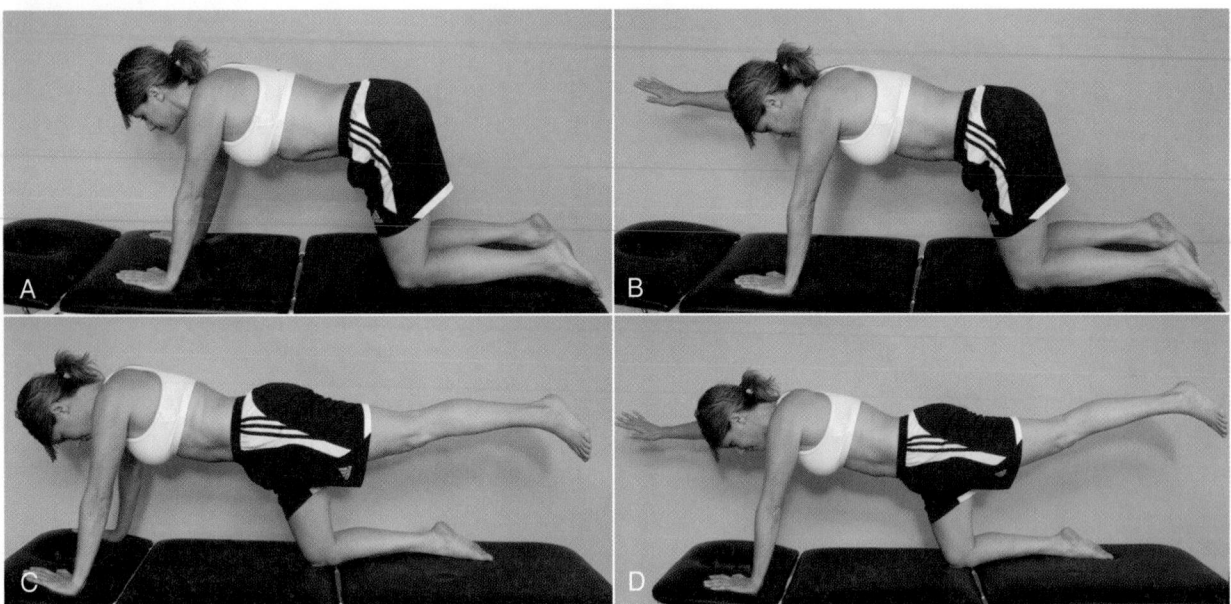

Figure 9-45 Back rotators/multifidus test. A, Start position. **B,** Single straight arm lift. **C,** Single straight leg lift. **D,** Contralateral straight arm and leg lift.

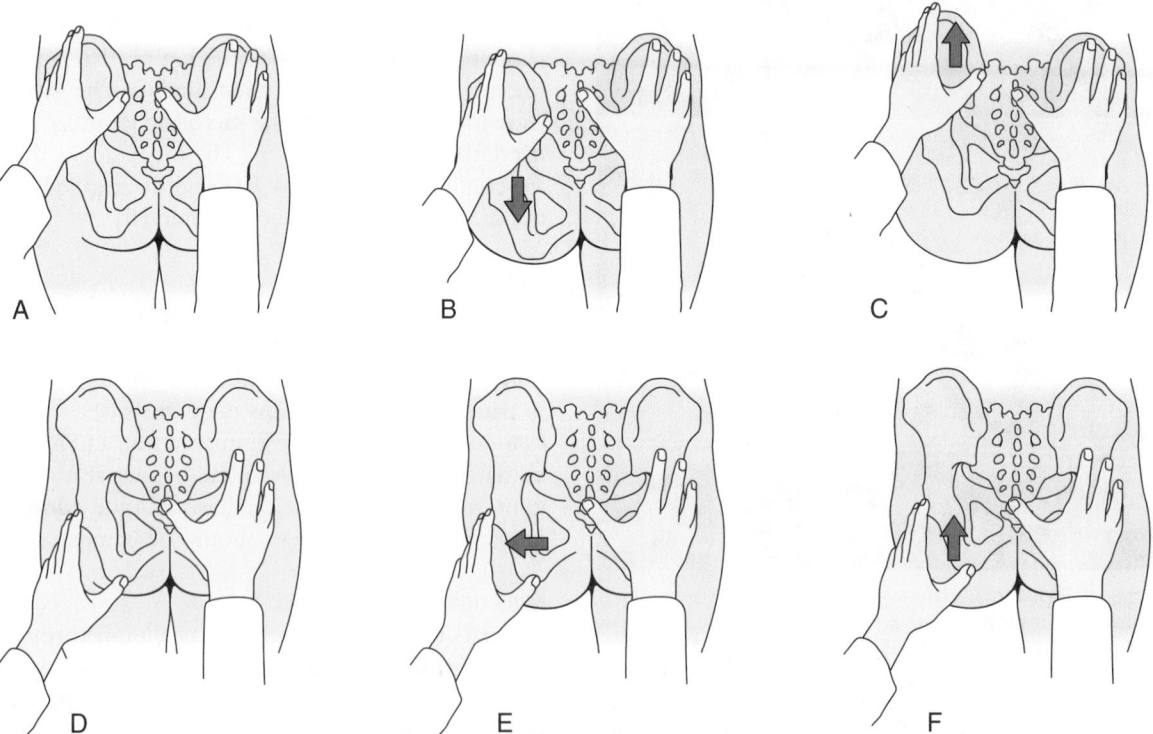

Figure 9-46 Tests to demonstrate left sacroiliac fixation. A, Examiner places the left thumb on the posterior superior iliac spine (PSIS) and the right thumb over one of the sacral spinous processes. **B,** With normal movement, the examiner's left thumb moves downward as the patient raises the left leg with full hip flexion. **C,** If the joint is fixed, the examiner's left thumb moves upward as the patient raises the left leg. **D,** The examiner places the left thumb over the ischial tuberosity and the right thumb over the apex of the sacrum. **E,** With normal movement, the examiner's left thumb moves laterally as the patient raises the left leg with full hip flexion. **F,** If the joint is fixed, the examiner's left thumb moves slightly upward as the patient raises the left leg. (Modified from Kirkaldy-Willis WH: Managing low back pain, New York, 1983, Churchill Livingstone, p. 94.)

TABLE **9-10**

Lumbar Root Syndromes

Root	Dermatome	Muscle Weakness	Reflexes/Special Tests Affected	Paresthesias
L1	Back, over trochanter, groin	None	None	Groin, after holding posture, which causes pain
L2	Back, front of thigh to knee	Psoas, hip adductors	None	Occasionally front of thigh
L3	Back, upper buttock, front of thigh and knee, medial lower leg	Psoas, quadriceps—thigh wasting	Knee jerk sluggish, PKB positive, pain on full SLR	Inner knee, anterior lower leg
L4	Inner buttock, outer thigh, inside of leg, dorsum of foot, big toe	Tibialis anterior, extensor hallucis	SLR limited, neck-flexion pain, weak knee jerk; side flexion limited	Medial aspect of calf and ankle
L5	Buttock, back and side of thigh, lateral aspect of leg, dorsum of foot, inner half of sole and first, second, and third toes	Extensor hallucis, peroneals, gluteus medius, ankle dorsiflexors, hamstrings—calf wasting	SLR limited to one side, neck-flexion pain, ankle jerk decreased, crossed-leg raising—pain	Lateral aspect of leg, medial three toes
S1	Buttock, back of thigh, and lower leg	Calf and hamstrings, wasting of gluteals, peroneals, plantar flexors	SLR limited	Lateral two toes, lateral foot, lateral leg to knee, plantar aspect of foot
S2	Same as S1	Same as S1 except peroneals	Same as S1	Lateral leg, knee, heel
S3	Groin, inner thigh to knee	None	None	None
S4	Perineum, genitals, lower sacrum	Bladder, rectum	None	Saddle area, genitals, anus, impotence

Manipulation and traction are contraindicated if S4 or massive posterior displacement causes bilateral sciatica and S3 pain.
PKB, Prone knee bending; *SLR*, straight leg raising.

Myotomes

Having completed the scanning examination of the peripheral joints, the examiner next tests the patient's muscle power for possible neurological weakness (Table 9-10).[120] With the patient lying supine, the myotomes are assessed individually (Figure 9-47). When testing myotomes (Table 9-11), the examiner should place the test joint or joints in a neutral or resting position and then apply a resisted isometric pressure. The contraction should be held for at least 5 seconds to show any weakness. If feasible, the examiner should test the two sides simultaneously to provide a comparison. The simultaneous bilateral comparison is not possible for movements involving the hip and knee joints because of the weight of the limbs and stress to the low back, so both sides must be done individually. The examiner should not apply pressure over the joints, because this action may mask symptoms.

Remember that the examiner has previously tested the S1 myotome with the patient standing and has tested for a positive Trendelenburg sign (modified Trendelenburg test); these movements are repeated here only if the examiner is unsure of the result and wants to test again. The ankle movements should be tested with the knee flexed approximately 30°, especially if the patient complains of

Myotomes of the Lumbar and Sacral Spines

- L2: Hip flexion
- L3: Knee extension
- L4: Ankle dorsiflexion
- L5: Great toe extension
- S1: Ankle plantar flexion, ankle eversion, hip extension
- S2: Knee flexion

sciatic pain, because full dorsiflexion is considered a provocative maneuver for stretching of neurological tissue. Likewise, the extended knee increases the stretch on the sciatic nerve and may result in false signs, such as weakness that results from pain rather than from pressure on the nerve root. Rainville, et al.[121] have recommended testing the L3 and L4 nerve roots at the same time by doing a **single leg sit-to-stand** test to check for unilateral quadriceps weakness (Figure 9-48). Note that the patient can hold the examiner's hands for balance.

If the patient is in extreme pain, all tests with the patient in the supine position should be completed before the patient is tested in prone. This reduces the amount of movement the patient must do, decreasing the patient's discomfort. Ideally, all tests in the standing position

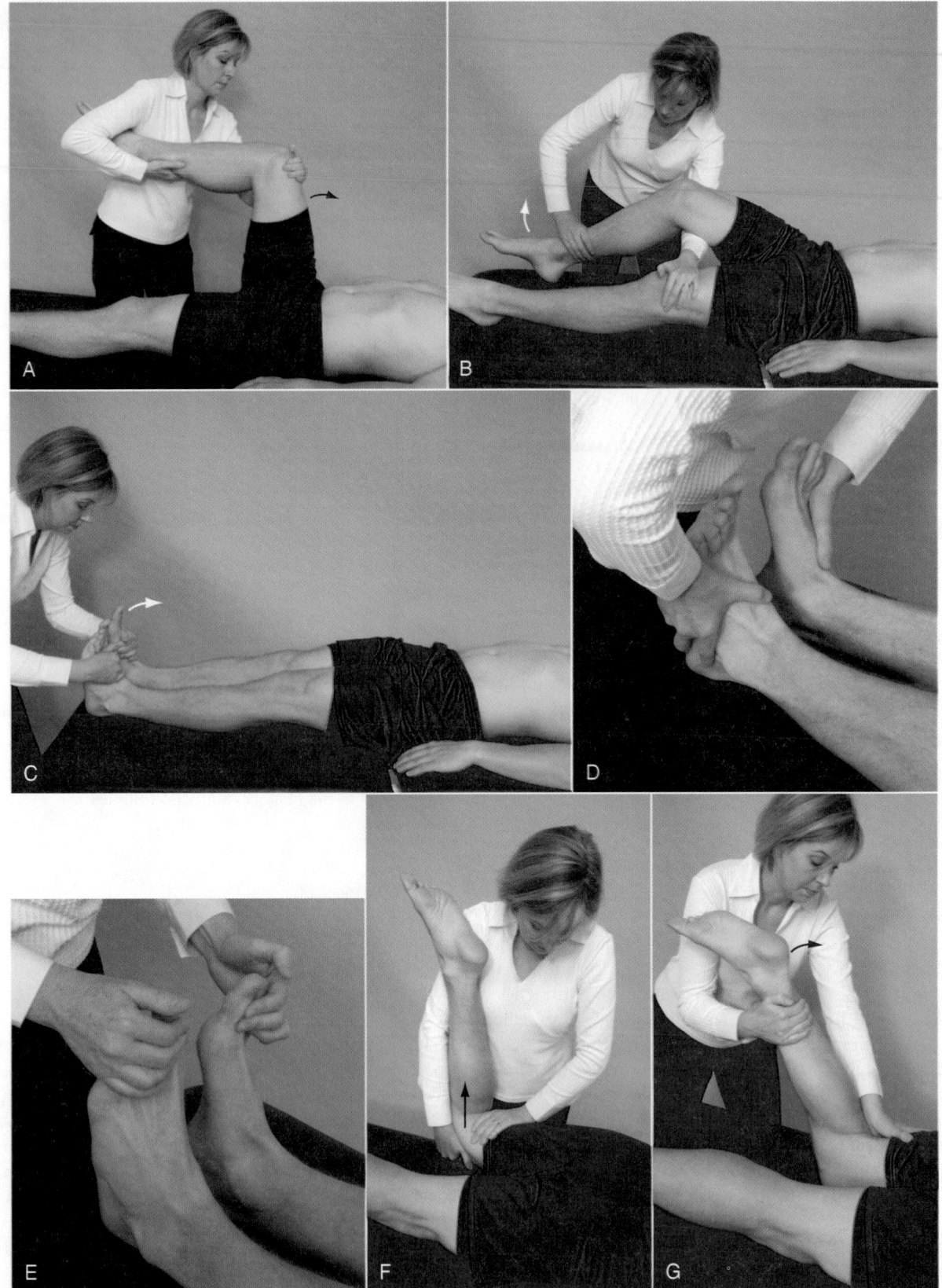

Figure 9-47 Positioning to test myotomes. A, Hip flexion (L2). **B,** Knee extension (L3). **C,** Foot dorsiflexion (L4). **D,** Ankle eversion (S1). **E,** Extension of the big toe (L5). **F,** Hip extension (S1). **G,** Knee flexion (S1–S2).

TABLE **9-11**

Myotomes of the Lower Limb

Nerve Root	Test Action	Muscles
L1–L2	Hip flexion	Psoas, iliacus, sartorius, gracilis, pectineus, adductor longus, adductor brevis
L3	Knee extension	Quadriceps, adductor longus, magnus, and brevis
L4	Ankle dorsiflexion	Tibialis anterior, quadriceps, tensor fasciae latae, adductor magnus, obturator externus, tibialis posterior
L5	Toe extension	Extensor hallucis longus, extensor digitorum longus, gluteus medius and minimus, obturator internus, semimembranosus, semitendinosus, peroneus tertius, popliteus
S1	Ankle plantar flexion Ankle eversion	Gastrocnemius, soleus, gluteus maximus, obturator internus, piriformis, biceps femoris, semitendinosus, popliteus, peroneus longus and brevis, extensor digitorum brevis
S2	Hip extension Knee flexion	Biceps femoris, piriformis, soleus, gastrocnemius, flexor digitorum longus, flexor hallucis longus, intrinsic foot muscles
S3	Knee flexion	Intrinsic foot muscles (except abductor hallucis), flexor hallucis brevis, flexor digitorum brevis, extensor digitorum brevis

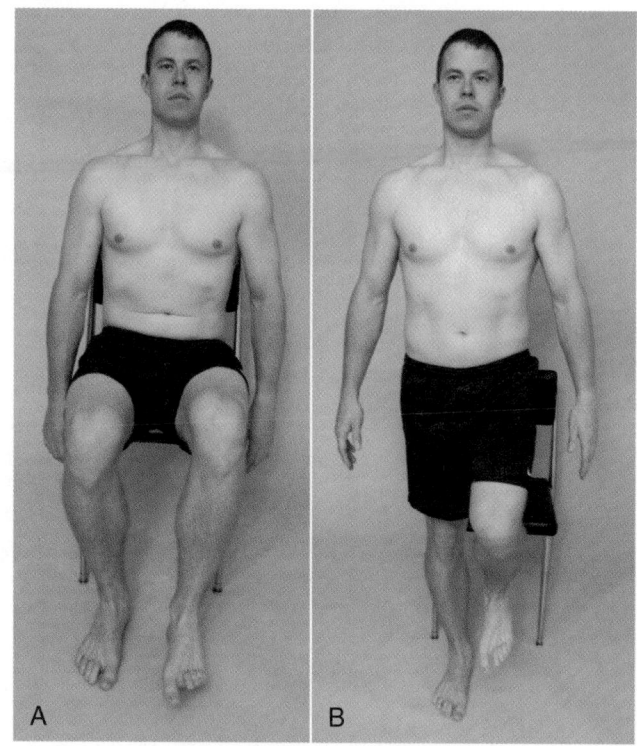

Figure 9-48 Single leg sit-to-stand test.

should be performed first, followed by tests in the sitting, supine, side lying, and prone positions. This procedure is shown in the précis at the end of the chapter.

To test hip flexion (L2 myotome), the examiner flexes the patient's hip to 30° to 40°. The examiner then applies a resisted force into extension proximal to the knee while ensuring that the heel of the patient's foot is not resting on the examining table (see Figure 9-47, *A*). The other side is then tested for comparison. To prevent excessive stress on the lumbar spine, the examiner must ensure that the patient does not increase the lumbar lordosis while doing the test and that only one leg at a time is tested.

To test knee extension or the L3 myotome, the examiner flexes the patient's knee to 25° to 35° and then applies a resisted flexion force at the midshaft of the tibia ensuring the heel is not resting on the examining table (see Figure 9-47, *B*). The other side is tested for comparison.

To test ankle dorsiflexion (L4 myotome), the examiner asks the patient to place the feet at 90° relative to the leg (plantigrade position). The examiner applies a resisted force to the dorsum of each foot and compares the two sides (see Figure 9-47, *C*). Ankle plantar flexion (S1 myotome) is compared in a similar fashion, but the resistance is applied to the sole of the foot. Because of the strength of the plantar flexor muscles, it is better to test this myotome with the patient standing. The patient slowly moves up and down on the toes of each foot (for at least 5 seconds) in turn (**modified Trendelenburg test**), and the examiner compares the differences as previously described. Ankle eversion (S1 myotome) is tested with the patient in the supine lying position, and the examiner applies a force to move the foot into inversion (see Figure 9-47, *D*).

Toe extension (L5 myotome) is tested with the patient holding both big toes in a neutral position. The examiner applies resistance to the nails of both toes and compares the two sides (see Figure 9-47, *E*). It is imperative that the resistance be isometric, so the amount of force in this case is less than that applied during knee extension, for example.

Hip extension (S1 myotome) is tested with the patient lying prone. This test needs to be done only if the patient is unable to do plantar flexion testing in standing or ankle eversion. The knee is flexed to 90°. The examiner then lifts the patient's thigh slightly off the examining table while stabilizing the leg. A downward force is applied to the patient's posterior thigh with one hand while the

Oswestry Disability Index

Section 1 - Pain intensity
☐ I have no pain at the moment.
☐ The pain is very mild at the moment.
☐ The pain is moderate at the moment.
☐ The pain is fairly severe at the moment.
☐ The pain is very severe at the moment.
☐ The pain is the worst imaginable at the moment.

Section 2 - Personal care (washing, dressing, etc.)
☐ I can look after myself normally without causing extra pain.
☐ I can look after myself normally but it is very painful.
☐ It is painful to look after myself and I am slow and careful.
☐ I need some help but manage most of my personal care.
☐ I need help every day in most aspects of self care.
☐ I do not get dressed, wash with difficulty, and stay in bed.

Section 3 - Lifting
☐ I can lift heavy weights without extra pain.
☐ I can lift heavy weights but it gives extra pain.
☐ Pain prevents me from lifting heavy weights off the floor but I can manage if they are conveniently positioned (e.g., on a table).
☐ Pain prevents me from lifting heavy weights but I can manage light to medium weights if they are conveniently positioned.
☐ I can lift only very light weights.
☐ I cannot lift or carry anything at all.

Section 4 - Walking
☐ Pain does not prevent me walking any distance.
☐ Pain prevents me walking more than 1 mile.
☐ Pain prevents me walking more than ¼ of a mile.
☐ Pain prevents me walking more than 100 yards.
☐ I can only walk using a stick or crutches.
☐ I am in bed most of the time and have to crawl to the toilet.

Section 5 - Sitting
☐ I can sit in any chair as long as I like.
☐ I can sit in my favorite chair as long as I like.
☐ Pain prevents me from sitting for more than 1 hour.
☐ Pain prevents me from sitting for more than ½ an hour.
☐ Pain prevents me from sitting for more than 10 minutes.
☐ Pain prevents me from sitting at all.

Section 6 - Standing
☐ I can stand as long as I want without extra pain.
☐ I can stand as long as I want but it gives me extra pain.

☐ Pain prevents me from standing for more than 1 hour.
☐ Pain prevents me from standing for more than ½ an hour.
☐ Pain prevents me from standing for more than 10 minutes.
☐ Pain prevents me from standing at all.

Section 7 - Sleeping
☐ My sleep is never disturbed by pain.
☐ My sleep is occasionally disturbed by pain.
☐ Because of pain I have less than 6 hours sleep.
☐ Because of pain I have less than 4 hours sleep.
☐ Because of pain I have less than 2 hours sleep.
☐ Pain prevents me from sleeping at all.

Section 8 - Sex life (if applicable)
☐ My sex life is normal and causes no extra pain.
☐ My sex life is normal but causes some extra pain.
☐ My sex life is nearly normal but is very painful.
☐ My sex life is severely restricted by pain.
☐ My sex life is nearly absent because of pain.
☐ Pain prevents any sex life at all.

Section 9 - Social life
☐ My social life is normal and causes me no extra pain.
☐ My social life is normal but increases the degree of pain.
☐ Pain has no significant effect on my social life apart from limiting my more energetic interests (e.g., sport).
☐ Pain has restricted my social life and I do not go out as often.
☐ Pain has restricted social life to my home.
☐ I have no social life because of pain.

Section 10 - Traveling
☐ I can travel anywhere without pain.
☐ I can travel anywhere but it gives extra pain.
☐ Pain is bad but I manage journeys of over two hours.
☐ Pain restricts me to journeys of less than one hour.
☐ Pain restricts me to short necessary journeys under 30 minutes.
☐ Pain prevents me from traveling except to receive treatment.

Section 11 - Previous treatment
Over the past three months have you received treatment, tablets, or medicines of any kind for your back or leg pain? Please tick the appropriate box.
☐ No
☐ Yes (if yes, please state the type of treatment you have received)

Figure 9-49 Oswestry Disability Index. (Redrawn from Fairbank JC, Couper J, Davies JB, et al: The Oswestry low back pain disability questionnaire. Physiotherapy 66:271–273, 1980.)

other hand ensures that the patient's thigh is not resting on the table (see Figure 9-47, *F*).

Knee flexion (S1–S2 myotomes) is tested in the same position (prone) with the knee flexed to 90°. An extension isometric force is applied just above the ankle (see Figure 9-47, *G*). Although it is possible to test both knee flexors at the same time, it is not advisable to do this because the stress on the lumbar spine is too great.

Functional Assessment

Injury to the lumbar spine can greatly affect the patient's ability to function. Activities such as standing, walking, bending, lifting, traveling, socializing, dressing, and sexual intercourse can be affected. Numerical scoring tables may be used to determine the degree of pain caused by lumbar spine pathology or disability.

The Quebec Back Pain Disability Scale:

This questionnaire is about the way your back pain is affecting your daily life. People with back problems may find it difficult to perform some of their daily activities. We would like to know if you find it difficult to perform any of the activities listed below, because of your back. For each activity there is a scale of 0 to 5. Please choose one response option for each activity (do not skip any activities) and circle the corresponding number.

Today, do you find it difficult to perform the following activities because of your back?

	Not difficult at all (score: 0)	Minimally difficult (score: 1)	Somewhat difficult (score: 2)	Fairly difficult (score: 3)	Very difficult (score: 4)	Unable to do (score: 5)
1. Get out of bed						
2. Sleep through the night						
3. Turn over in bed						
4. Ride in a car						
5. Stand up for 20–30 minutes						
6. Sit in a chair for several hours						
7. Climb one flight of stairs						
8. Walk a few blocks (300–400 m)						
9. Walk several kilometres						
10. Reach up to high shelves						
11. Throw a ball						
12. Run one block (about 100 m)						
13. Take food out of the refrigerator						
14. Make your bed						
15. Put on socks (pantyhose)						
16. Bend over to clean the bathtub						
17. Move a chair						
18. Pull or push heavy doors						
19. Carry two bags of groceries						
20. Lift and carry a heavy suitcase						

Add the numbers for a total score: _____

Minimum detectable change (90% confidence) 15 points

Figure 9-50 The Quebec Back Pain Disability Scale. (Modified from Kopec JA, Esdaile JM, Abrahamowicz M, et al: The Quebec Back Pain Disability Scale. Measurement properties. Spine 20:341–352, 1995.)

Care must be taken when selecting one of these scales to ensure that it measures the disability from the patient's perspective.[122-125] Examples are the Oswestry Disability Index[126-128] (Figure 9-49), the Quebec Back Pain Disability Scale[129,130] (Figure 9-50), and the Hendler 10-Minute Screening Test for Chronic Back Pain Patients (Figure 9-51).[124,127,131] It has been reported that the Hendler test helps to differentiate organic from functional low back pain.[132] The Oswestry Disability Index is a good functional scale because it deals with ADLs and therefore is based on the patient's response and concerns affecting daily life. It is the most commonly used functional back scale. The disability index is calculated by dividing the total score (each section is worth from 1 to 6 points) by the number of sections answered and multiplying by 100. The Roland-Morris Disability Questionnaire is short and simple, and it is suitable for following up on progress in clinical settings and for combining with other measures of function (e.g., work disability) (Figure 9-52).[133,134] Other numerical back pain scales include the Functional Rating Index,[135,136] the Dallas Pain Questionnaire,[137] the Million Index,[138] the Japanese Orthopedic Association Scale,[139] the Iowa Low Back Rating Scale,[140] the Bournemouth Questionnaire,[141,142] the Scoliosis Research

Hendler 10-Minute Screening Test for Chronic Back Pain Patients

Instructions: Each question is asked by an examiner, and the patient is given points according to the response that he makes. The number of points to be awarded for the various responses is shown in the column at the right. At the end of the test, the examiner calculates the total number of points. The results are interpreted as explained in the Key.

Points

I How did the pain that you now experience occur?

(a) Sudden onset with accident or definable event — 0

(b) Slow, progressive onset without acute exacerbation — 1

(c) Slow, progressive onset with acute exacerbation without accident or event — 2

(d) Sudden onset without an accident or definable event — 3

II Where do you experience the pain?

(a) One site, specific, well-defined, consistent with anatomical distribution — 0

(b) More than one site, each well-defined and consistent with anatomical distribution — 1

(c) One site, inconsistent with anatomical considerations, or not well-defined — 2

(d) Vague description, more than one site, of which one is inconsistent with anatomical considerations, or not well-defined or anatomically explainable — 3

III Do you ever have trouble falling asleep at night, or are you ever awakened from sleep?

If the answer is "no," score 3 points and go to question IV. If the answer is "yes," proceed:

What keeps you from falling asleep, or what awakens you from sleep?

IIIA (a) Trouble falling asleep every night due to pain — 0

(b) Trouble falling asleep due to pain more than three times a week — 1

(c) Trouble falling asleep due to pain less than three times a week — 2

(d) No trouble falling asleep due to pain — 3

(e) Trouble falling asleep which is not related to pain — 4

IIIB (a) Awakened by pain every night — 0

(b) Awakened from sleep by pain more than three times a week — 1

(c) Not awakened from sleep by pain more than twice a week — 2

(d) Not awakened from sleep by pain — 3

(e) Restless sleep, or early morning awakening with or without being able to return to sleep, both unrelated to pain — 4

IV Does weather have any effect on your pain?

(a) The pain is always worse in both cold and damp weather. — 0

(b) The pain is always worse with damp weather or with cold weather. — 1

(c) The pain is occasionally worse with cold or damp weather. — 2

(d) The weather has no effect on the pain. — 3

V How would you describe the type of pain that you have?

(a) Burning; or sharp, shooting pain; or pins and needles; or coldness; or numbness — 0

Points

(b) Dull, aching pain, with occasional sharp, shooting pains not helped by heat; or, the patient is experiencing hyperesthesia — 1

(c) Spasm-type pain, tension-type pain, or numbness over the area, relieved by massage or heat — 2

(d) Nagging or bothersome pain — 3

(e) Excruciating, overwhelming, or unbearable pain, relieved by massage or heat — 4

VI How frequently do you have your pain?

(a) The pain is constant. — 0

(b) The pain is nearly constant, occurring 50%–80% of the time. — 1

(c) The pain is intermittent, occurring 25%–50% of the time. — 2

(d) The pain is only occasionally present, occurring less than 25% of the time. — 3

VII Does movement or position have any effect on the pain?

(a) The pain is unrelieved by position change or rest, and there have been previous operations for the pain. — 0

(b) The pain is worsened by use, standing, or walking; and is relieved by lying down or resting the part. — 1

(c) Position change and use have variable effects on the pain. — 2

(d) The pain is not altered by use or position change, and there have been no previous operations for the pain. — 3

VIII What medications have you used in the past month?

(a) No medications at all — 0

(b) Use of non-narcotic pain relievers; non-benzodiazepine tranquilizers; or use of antidepressants — 1

(c) Less than three-times-a-week use of a narcotic, hypnotic, or benzodiazepine — 2

(d) Greater than four-times-a-week use of a narcotic, hypnotic, or benzodiazepine — 3

IX What hobbies do you have, and can you still participate in them?

(a) Unable to participate in any hobbies that were formerly enjoyed — 0

(b) Reduced number of hobbies or activities relating to a hobby — 1

(c) Still able to participate in hobbies but with some discomfort — 2

(d) Participate in hobbies as before — 3

X How frequently did you have sex and orgasms before the pain, and how frequently do you have sex and orgasms now?

(a^1) Sexual contact, prior to pain, three to four times a week, with no difficulty with orgasm; now sexual contact is 50% or less than previously, and coitus is interrupted by pain — 0

Figure 9-51 Hendler 10-Minute Screening Test for Chronic Back Pain Patients. (Redrawn from Hendler N, Vierstein M, Gucer P, et al: A preoperative screening test for chronic back pain patients. Psychosomatics 20:806–808, 1979. Copyright © Nelson Hendler, MD, 1979.)

Points

(a²) (For people over 45) Sexual contact twice a week, with a 50% reduction in frequency since the pain   0

(a³) (For people over 60) Sexual contact once a week, with a 50% reduction in frequency of coitus since the onset of pain   0

(b) Pre-pain adjustment as defined above (a¹–a³), with no difficulty with orgasm; now loss of interest in sex and/or difficulty with orgasm or erection   1

(c) No change in sexual activity now as opposed to before the onset of pain   2

(d) Unable to have sexual contact since the onset of pain, and difficulty with orgasm or erection prior to the pain   3

(e) No sexual contact prior to the pain, or absence of orgasm prior to the pain   4

XI Are you still working or doing your household chores?

(a) Works every day at the same pre-pain job or same level of household duties   0

(b) Works every day but the job is not the same as pre-pain job, with reduced responsibility or physical activity   1

(c) Works sporadically or does a reduced amount of household chores   2

(d) Not at work, or all household chores are now performed by others   3

XII What is your income now compared with before your injury or the onset of pain, and what are your sources of income?

(a) Any one of the following answers scores   0
  1. Experiencing financial difficulty with family income 50% or less than previously
  2. Was retired and is still retired
  3. Patient is still working and is not having financial difficulties

(b) Experiencing financial difficulty with family income only 50%–75% of the pre-pain income   1

(c) Patient unable to work, and receives some compensation so that the family income is at least 75% of the pre-pain income   2

(d) Patient unable to work and receives no compensation, but the spouse works and

Points

family income is still 75% of the pre-pain income   3

(e) Patient doesn't work, yet the income from disability or other compensation sources is 80% or more of gross pay before the pain; the spouse does not work   4

XIII Are you suing anyone, or is anyone suing you, or do you have an attorney helping you with compensation or disability payments?

(a) No suit pending, and does not have an attorney   0

(b) Litigation is pending, but is not related to the pain   1

(c) The patient is being sued as the result of an accident   2

(d) Litigation is pending or workmen's compensation case with a lawyer involved   3

XIV If you had three wishes for anything in the world, what would you wish for?

(a) "Get rid of the pain" is the only wish   0

(b) "Get rid of the pain" is one of the three wishes   1

(c) Doesn't mention getting rid of the pain, but has specific wishes usually of a personal nature such as for more money, a better relationship with spouse or children, etc.   2

(d) Does not mention pain, but offers general, nonpersonal wishes such as for world peace   3

XV Have you ever been depressed or thought of suicide?

(a) Admits to depression; or has a history of depression secondary to pain and associated with crying spells and thoughts of suicide   0

(b) Admits to depression, guilt, and anger secondary to the pain   1

(c) Prior history of depression before the pain or a financial or personal loss prior to the pain; now admits to some depression   2

(d) Denies depression, crying spells, or "feeling blue"   3

(e) History of a suicide attempt prior to the onset of pain   4

POINT TOTAL

Key to Hendler Screening Test for Chronic Back Pain

A score of 18 points or less suggests that the patient is an objective pain patient and is reporting a normal response to chronic pain. One may proceed surgically if indicated, and usually finds the patient quite willing to participate in all modalities of therapy, including exercise and psychotherapy. Occasionally, a person with conversion reaction or posttraumatic neurosis will score less than 18 points; this is because subjective distress is being experienced on an unconscious level. Persons scoring 14 points or less can be considered objective pain patients with more certainty than those at the upper range (14–18) of this group.

A score of 15–20 points suggests that the patient has features of an objective pain patient as well as of an exaggerating pain patient. This implies that a person with a poor premorbid adjustment has an organic lesion that has produced the normal response to pain; however, because of the person's poor pre-pain adjustment, the chronic pain produces a more extreme response than would otherwise occur.

A score of 19–31 points suggests that the patient is an exaggerating pain patient. Surgical or other interventions may be carried out with caution. This type of patient usually has a premorbid (pre-pain) personality that may increase his likelihood of using or benefiting from the complaint of chronic pain. The patient may show improvement after treatment in a chronic pain treatment center, where the main emphasis is placed on an attitude change toward the chronic pain.

A score of 32 points or more suggests that a psychiatric consultation is needed. These patients freely admit to a great many pre-pain problems, and show considerable difficulty in coping with the chronic pain they now experience. Surgical or other interventions should not be carried out without prior approval of a psychiatric consultant. Severe depression, suicide, and psychosis are potential problems in this group of affective pain patients.

Test copyright 1979 by Nelson Hendler, M.D., M.S.

Figure 9-51, cont'd

Roland and Morris Disability Questionnaire (with instructions)

When your back hurts, you may find it difficult to do some of the things you normally do.

This list contains some sentences that people have used to describe themselves when they have back pain. When you read them, you may find that some stand out because they describe you *today*. As you read the list, think of yourself today. When you read a sentence that describes you today, put a tick against it. If the sentence does not describe you, then leave the space blank and go on to the next one. Remember, only tick the sentence if you are sure that it describes you *today*.

Because of my back or leg pain (sciatica) today:

YES	NO	
		1. I stay at home most of the time because of my back.
		2. I change position frequently to try to get my back comfortable.
		3. I walk more slowly than usual because of my back.
		4. Because of my back, I am not doing any of the jobs that I usually do around the house.
		5. Because of my back, I use a handrail to get upstairs.
		6. Because of my back, I lie down to rest more often.
		7. Because of my back, I have to hold on to something to get out of an easy chair.
		8. Because of my back, I try to get other people to do things for me.
		9. I get dressed more slowly than usual because of my back.
		10. I only stand up for short periods of time because of my back.
		11. Because of my back, I try not to bend or kneel down.
		12. I find it difficult to get out of a chair because of my back.
		13. My back is painful almost all the time.
		14. I find it difficult to turn over in bed because of my back.
		15. My appetite is not very good because of my back pain.
		16. I have trouble putting on my socks (or stockings) because of the pain in my back.
		17. I only walk short distances because of my back pain.
		18. I sleep less well because of my back.
		19. Because of my back pain, I get dressed with help from someone else.
		20. I sit down for most of the day because of my back.
		21. I avoid heavy jobs around the house because of my back.
		22. Because of my back pain, I am more irritable and bad tempered with people than usual.
		23. Because of my back, I go upstairs more slowly than usual.
		24. I stay in bed most of the time because of my back.

Figure 9-52 Roland-Morris disability questionnaire (with instructions). The higher the number of "yes" responses, the greater the disability. (From Roland M, Morris R: A study of the natural history of back pain. Part I: Development of a reliable and sensitive measure of disability in low back pain. Spine 8:144, 1983.)

```
┌─────────────────────────────────────────────────┐
│        FUNCTIONAL RATING SCALE FOR THE LUMBAR SPINE
│
│  A. Physical criteria                        _____
│  B. Patient's perception                     _____
│  C. Physician's perception                   _____
│     TOTAL                                    _____
│
│  A. PHYSICAL CRITERIA (Max: 30)
│     1. Range of motion–Total flexion and    _____
│        extension in degrees
│        Points (1 point for every 10 degrees– _____
│        15 points maximum)
│     2. Trunk strength–Total flexion and extension  _____
│        in kilograms
│        Points (1 point for every 8 kg, male
│        patients–15 points maximum)
│        Points (1 point for every 4 kg, female
│        patients–15 points maximum)
│
│  B. PATIENT'S PERCEPTION (Max: 40)
│     1. Average pain (visual-analog scale)    (15) _____
│     2. How disabled:                              _____
│        No disability, able to work full-time  (10)
│        Able to work full-time but at a lower  (8)
│        level
│        Able to work part-time but at usual    (6)
│        level
│        Able to work only part-time and at     (4)
│        lower level
│        Not able to work at all                (0)
│     3. Activities you can perform–1 point     _____
│        for each Yes answer
│
│  C. PHYSICIAN'S PERCEPTION (Max: 30)
│     1. How much pain would you expect for this _____
│        patient at this time? (visual-analog scale)
│     2. At the present time, what is the degree _____
│        of impairment?
│        None                                   (10)
│        Mild but should not affect most activities (8)
│        Moderate, cannot perform some strenuous
│        activities                             (6)
│        Only light activities, cannot perform any
│        strenuous activities                   (2)
│        Severely limited, cannot perform most light
│        activities or some activities of daily living (0)
│     3. Current drugs and daily doses (quantity): _____
│        Analgesics (occasional) use = less than 5
│        times per week)
│        Major narcotic, regular use            (0)
│        Major narcotic, occasional use         (2)
│        Minor narcotic, regular use            (4)
│        Minor narcotic, occasional use         (6)
│        Nonnarcotic, regular use               (8)
│        Nonnarcotic, occasional use            (10)
│     TOTAL                                     _____
└─────────────────────────────────────────────────┘
```

Figure 9-53 Functional rating scale for the lumbar spine. (Modified from Lehmann TR, Brand RA, German TW: A low back rating scale. Spine 8:309, 1983.)

Society form (SRS-22 for those with spinal deformity),[143-145] the Lumbar Spinal Stenosis Questionnaire,[146] and the Aberdeen Back Pain Scale.[147] Thomas provide a good review of these and other scales.[124] Lehman and colleagues developed a rating scale for lumbar dysfunction (Figure 9-53) that includes assessment criteria,

physician criteria, and, perhaps more importantly, patient criteria for determining the degree of dysfunction.[140] These criteria can be evaluated during the normal assessment for the patient.

Waddell and colleagues developed a series of tests to differentiate between organic and nonorganic back pain.[148] Each test counts +1 if positive or 0 if negative:

1. Superficial skin tenderness to light pinch over wide area of lumbar spine
2. Deep tenderness over wide area, often extending to thoracic spine, sacrum, or pelvis
3. Low back pain on axial loading of spine in standing
4. Straight leg raising test positive when specifically tested, but not when patient is seated with knee extended to test Babinski reflex
5. Abnormal neurological (motor or sensory) patterns
6. Overreaction

Positive findings of +3 or more should be investigated for nonorganic cause; these patients may also have social and psychological components to their complaint.[3,149,150]

Waddell also described a simple clinical functional capacity evaluation (Figure 9-54),[3] which examiners may find useful for testing patients.[151]

Simmonds, et al.[152] came up with several functional tests or physical performance measures that they felt would be useful and discriminate between individuals with and without low back pain:

- **Timed 15 Meter (50 Foot) Walk:** Patient walks 7.5 m (25 ft) as fast as he or she can, turns, and returns to the starting position while being timed.
- **Loaded Reach Test:** Patient stands next to a wall, which has a meter ruler at shoulder height. The patient reaches forward with weight at shoulder height as far as he or she can while keeping the heels on the floor. The weight should not exceed a maximum of 5% of body weight or 4.5 kg (9.9 lbs).
- **Repeated Sit-to-Stand:** This timed test involves the patient starting by sitting in a chair. The patient then stands fully and returns to sitting, repeating the sequence as fast as possible. The average value of two trials is used as the time.
- **Repeated Trunk Flexion**[153]**:** This timed test involves the patient starting in a standing position and then flexing forward as far as possible and returning to the upright posture as fast as tolerable, repeating the motion ten times. The average value of two trials is used as the time.
- **Biering-Sorensen Fatigue Test:** Described previously under "Resisted Isometric Movements."

Special Tests

Special tests should always be considered as an integral part of a much larger examination process.[154] They should never be used in isolation.[155] Many of the special tests in

A Simple Clinical Functional Capacity Evaluation

The test area should be quiet and free of passing people. Put up warning signs for staff and other patients when tests are taking place. The patient should not need to walk a long distance to reach the test area or between the different tests. Ask the patient to wear comfortable shoes and loose clothing.

- **Five minutes of walking.** The distance walked up and down between marks 20 m apart in 5 min. Choose a quiet, empty corridor with a non-slip surface or hard carpet. There should be walls or doors on either side that can be used if necessary for support, but not handrails. Patients should not use walking aids but can use the walls for support or can sit down for a rest. Inform the patient of the time at the end of each lap or every minute if they are slower (mean, 185 m).

- **One minute of stair climbing.** Climbing up and down a straight flight of standard stairs with one handrail and an opposite wall within easy reach. Have a chair available for resting if the patient needs it. Count the number of steps up and down, eg. 20 up and 15 down = 35 steps (mean, 48 steps).

- **One minute of stand-ups.** The number of times the patient can stand up from a chair in 1 min. Use a firm, upright chair with a padded seat and back rest but no arm rests. The seat height should be about 45 cm, or 18 inches. There should not be any wall or other furniture within reach that the patient could use for support (mean, 11 stand-ups).

Standardization of test instructions. The tester should have written instructions. The test should have written instructions. The tester must respond neutrally at all times and maintain a "test" atmosphere. Do not give the patient any advice or encouragement during the tests as feedback influences their performance. Only give information on the time to help patients to pace themselves if they are able. Tell the patient this is a test of current performance. It is a measure of how much they can manage, bearing in mind the journey home after their assessment. These instructions are designed to prevent anxiety and over-exertion.

Figure 9-54 Simple clinical functional capacity evaluation as described by Waddell. (From Waddell G: The back pain revolution, New York, 1998, Churchill Livingstone, p. 41.)

the lumbar spine are purported to have poor diagnostic value.[156] Because these are clinical tests and commonly depend on the skill of the examiner, many of them show low reliability and validity or have not been studied at all.[157-161] Thus, the icons are graded primarily on clinical experience.

For the reader who would like to review them, the reliability, validity, specificity, sensitivity, and odds ratios of some of the special tests used in the lumbar spine are available on the Evolve website.

When the examiner performs special tests in the lumbar assessment, the straight leg raising test, the prone knee bending (PKB) test, and the slump test should always be done, especially if there are neurological symptoms. The other tests need be done only if the examiner believes they are relevant or to confirm a diagnosis.

Key Tests Performed on the Lumbar Spine Depending on Suspected Pathology*

- *For neurological dysfunction:*
  - ☑ Centralization/peripheralization
  - ⚠ Cross straight leg raise test
  - ⚠ Femoral nerve traction test
  - ⚠ Prone knee bending test or variant
  - ☑ Slump test or variant
  - ☑ Straight leg raise or variant
- *For lumbar instability:*
  - ❓ H and I test
  - ☑ Passive lumbar extension test
  - ⚠ Prone segmental instability test
  - ❓ Specific lumbar torsion test
  - ⚠ Test for anterior lumbar spine instability
  - ⚠ Test for posterior lumbar spine instability
- *For joint dysfunction:*
  - ❓ Bilateral straight leg raise test
  - ❓ One-leg standing (stork standing) lumbar extension test
  - ⚠ Quadrant test
- *For muscle tightness:*
  - ☑ 90–90 straight leg raise test
  - ⚠ Ober test
  - ⚠ Rectus femoris test
  - ⚠ Thomas test
- *Other tests:*
  - ❓ Sign of the buttock

*The author recommends these key tests be learned by the clinician to facilitate a diagnosis. See Chapter 1, p. 55, Key for Classifying Special Tests.

Tests for Neurological Dysfunction (Neurodynamic Tests)

Neurodynamic tests check the mechanical movement of the neurological tissues as well as their sensitivity to mechanical stress or compression.[162,163] These neurodynamic tests, along with relevant history and decreased ROM, are considered by some to be the most important physical signs of disc herniation,[164] regardless of the degree of disc injury. Most of the special tests for neurological involvement are progressive or sequential. The patient is positioned, and one maneuver is tried; if no symptoms result, a second provocative, enhancing, or sensitizing maneuver is carried out, and so on, while the examiner watches to see if the patient's symptoms are reproduced. The order in which these maneuvers are done also makes a difference. For example, with straight leg raising, the results are different if the hip is flexed with the knee extended than if the hip is flexed with the knee first flexed and then extended after the hip is in position.

Because of **tension points,** the neurological tissues move in different directions (Figure 9-55) depending on where the stress is applied,[163,165] and the direction of movement varies depending on where movement is initiated. For example, when doing the straight leg raising test, movement is toward the hip; with dorsiflexion as a sensitizing maneuver, the neurological tissue moves toward the ankle. If knee extension is performed in the slump test, the neurological tissue moves toward the knee.[162] This movement in different directions or in convergence toward the joint being moved can produce different symptoms depending on where and in what direction the movement occurs. The neurological tissue

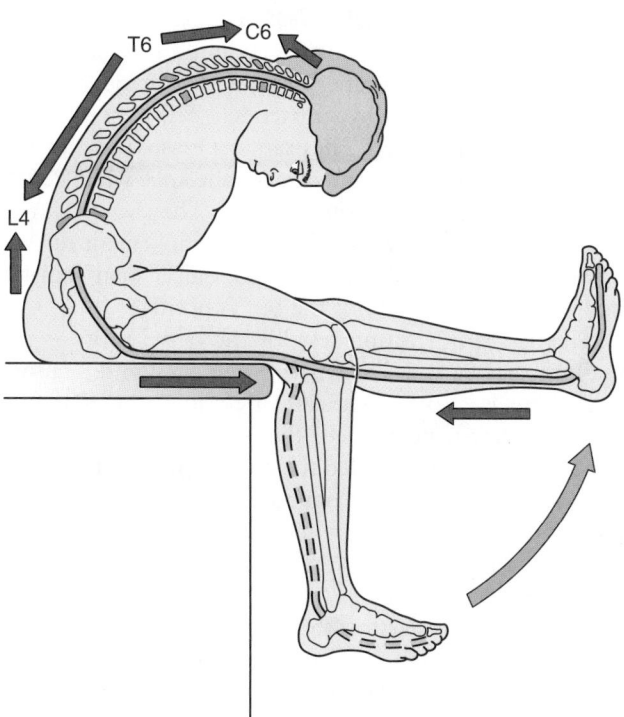

Figure 9-55 Postulated neurobiomechanics that occur with slump movement. The approximate points C6, T6, L4, and the knee are where the neural tissue does not move in relation to the movements of the spinal canal. It is important to understand, however, that movement of neurological tissue is toward the joint where movement was initiated. (Modified from Butler DS: Mobilisation of the nervous system, Melbourne, 1991, Churchill Livingstone, pp. 41–42.)

may move in one direction for one part of the test and in another direction for the next part of the test. Pathology may restrict this normal movement. Tension points are areas where there is minimal movement of the neurological tissue. According to Butler,[163] these areas are C6, the elbow, the shoulder, T6, L4, and the knee. It is important to realize, however, that the amount of tension placed on these points depends on the position of the extremity.

For a neurodynamic test to be positive, it must reproduce the patient's symptoms. Because these are provocative tests designed to put stress on the neurological tissue, they often cause discomfort or pain, which may be bilateral. However, if the patient's symptoms are not reproduced, the test should be considered negative. As a second check for a positive test, the symptoms that have been produced may be increased or decreased by adding or taking away the sensitizing parts (i.e., sensitizing tests such as neck flexion, foot dorsiflexion) of the test.[166,167]

The examiner has no need to do all or most of the neurodynamic tests listed. Some examiners will find one method more effective, others will find other tests more effective. The examiner should develop the skill to do two or three tests effectively and develop an understanding of how the neurological tissue is being stretched and which neurological tissue in particular is demonstrating signs and symptoms.

⚠ *Babinski Test.* The examiner runs a pointed object along the plantar aspect of the patient's foot.[168] A positive Babinski test or reflex suggests an upper motor neuron lesion if present on both sides and may be evident in lower motor neuron lesions if seen only on one side. The reflex is demonstrated by extension of the big toe and abduction (splaying) of the other toes. In an infant up to a few weeks old, a positive test is normal. The test is often performed to determine the presence of the Babinski reflex, which is a pathological reflex.

❓ *"Bowstring" Test (Cram Test or Popliteal Pressure Sign).* The examiner carries out a straight leg raising test, and pain results (Figure 9-56).[18,169] While maintaining the thigh in the same position, the examiner flexes the knee slightly (20°), reducing the symptoms. Thumb or finger pressure is then applied to the popliteal area to reestablish the painful radicular symptoms. The test indicates tension or pressure on the sciatic nerve and is a modification of the straight leg raising test.

The test may also be done in the sitting position with the examiner passively extending the knee to produce pain. The examiner then slightly flexes the knee so that the pain and symptoms disappear. The examiner holds this slightly flexed position by clasping the patient's leg between the examiner's knees. The examiner then presses the fingers of both hands into the popliteal space. Pain resulting from these maneuvers indicates a positive test and pressure or tension on the sciatic nerve. In this case, the test is called the **sciatic tension test** or **Deyerle's sign.**[58,170,171]

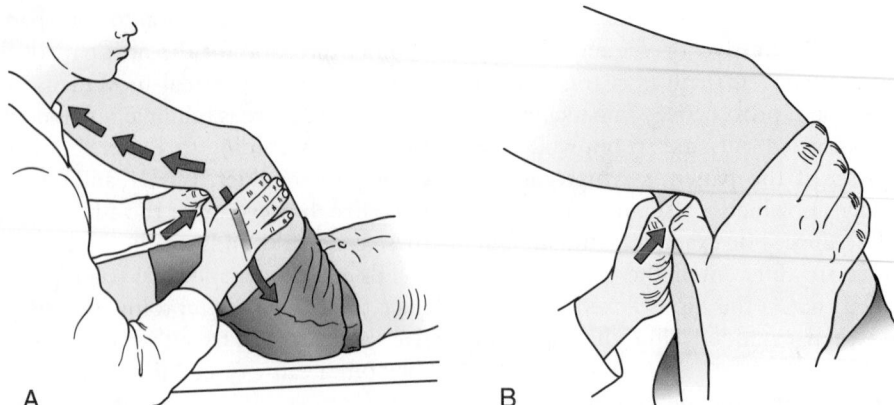

Figure 9-56 Bowstring sign. A, The examiner does a straight leg raise test. If a positive test results, the examiner relieves the pain by flexing the knee slightly. **B,** The examiner then pushes into the popliteal space to increase the stress on the sciatic nerve looking for a return of the same symptoms that present with the straight leg raise test.

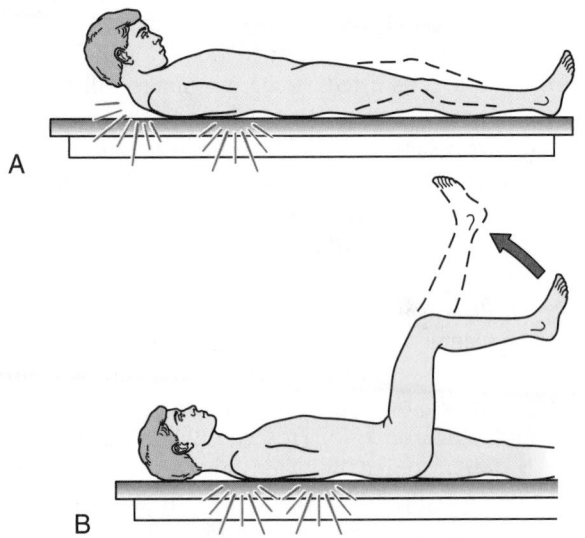

Figure 9-57 Brudzinski-Kernig test. A, In Brudzinki's portion of the test, the patient lies supine and elevates the head from the table. When the head is lifted, the patient complains of neck and low back discomfort and attempts to relieve the meningeal irritation by involuntary flexion of the knees and hips. **B,** In the Kernig portion of the test, the patient lies supine with the hip and knee flexed to 90°. The patient then extends the knee. If the patient complains of pain in the lower back, neck, or head on knee extension, it is suggestive of meningeal irritation. Returning to knee flexion will relieve the pain.

🔘 *Brudzinski-Kernig Test.* The patient is supine with the hands cupped behind the head (Figure 9-57).[170,172–174] The patient is instructed to flex the head onto the chest. The patient raises the extended leg actively by flexing the hip until pain is felt. The patient then flexes the knee, and if the pain disappears, it is considered a positive test. The mechanics of the Brudzinski-Kernig test are similar to those of the straight leg raising test except that the patient performs the movements actively. Pain is a positive sign and may indicate meningeal irritation, nerve root involvement, or dural irritation. Brudzinski originally described the neck flexion aspect of the test, and Kernig described the hip flexion component. The two

parts of the test may be done individually, in which case they are described as the test of the original author.

🔘 *Compression Test.*[75] The patient lies supine with the hips and knees flexed. The hips are flexed until the PSISs start to move backward (usually about 100° hip flexion). The examiner then applies direct pressure against the patient's feet or buttocks applying axial compression to the spine. If radicular pain into the posterior leg is produced, the test is thought to be positive for a possible disc herniation.

⚠️ *Femoral Nerve Traction Test.* The patient lies on the unaffected side with the unaffected limb flexed slightly at the hip and knee (Figure 9-58).[175] The patient's back should be straight, not hyperextended. The patient's head should be slightly flexed. The examiner grasps the patient's affected or painful limb and extends the knee while gently extending the hip approximately 15°. The patient's knee is then flexed on the affected side; this movement further stretches the femoral nerve. Neurological pain radiates down the anterior thigh if the test is positive.

This is also a traction test for the nerve roots at the midlumbar area (L2–L4). As with the straight leg raising test, there is also a contralateral positive test. That is, when the test is performed, the symptoms occur in the opposite limb. This is called the **crossed femoral stretching test.**[176] Pain in the groin and hip that radiates along the anterior medial thigh indicates an L3 nerve root problem; pain extending to the midtibia indicates an L4 nerve root problem.

This test is similar to Ober's test for a tight iliotibial band, so the examiner must be able to differentiate between the two conditions. If the iliotibial band is tight, the test leg does not adduct but remains elevated away from the table as the tight tendon riding over the greater trochanter keeps the leg abducted. Femoral nerve injury presents with a different history, and the referred pain (anteriorly) tends to be stronger.

🔘 *Flip Sign.* While the patient is sitting, the examiner extends the patient's knee and looks for symptoms. The

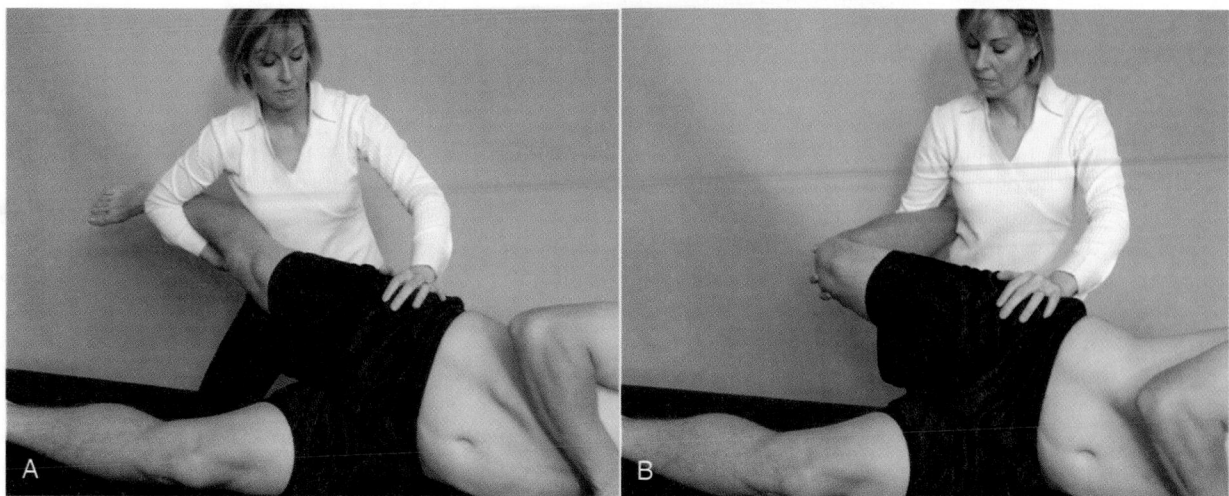

Figure 9-58 **Femoral nerve traction test. A,** The hip and knee are extended. **B,** Then knee is flexed.

patient is then placed supine, and a unilateral straight leg raising test is performed. For the sign to be positive, both tests must cause pain in the sciatic nerve distribution. If only one test is positive, the examiner should suspect problems in the lower lumbar spine. This is a combination of the classic Lasègue test and the sitting root test.

? *Gluteal Skyline Test.* The patient is relaxed in a prone position with the head straight and arms by the sides.[177] The examiner stands at the patient's feet and observes the buttocks from the level of the buttocks. The affected gluteus maximus muscle appears flat as a result of atrophy. The patient is asked to contract the gluteal muscles. The affected side may show less contraction, or it may be atonic and remain flat. If this occurs, the test is positive and may indicate damage to the inferior gluteal nerve or pressure on the L5, S1, or S2 nerve roots.

? *Knee Flexion Test.*[178] The patient, who has complained of sciatica, is in a standing position. The patient is asked to bend forward to touch the toes. If the patient bends the knee on the affected side while forward flexing the spine, the test is positive for sciatic nerve root compression. Likewise, if the patient is not allowed to bend the knee, spinal flexion is decreased.

? *Naffziger Test.* The patient lies supine while the examiner gently compresses the jugular veins (which lie beside the carotid artery) for approximately 10 seconds (Figure 9-59). The patient's face flushes, and then the patient is asked to cough. If coughing causes pain in the low back, the spinal theca is being compressed, leading to an increase in intrathecal pressure. The theca is the covering (pia mater, arachnoid mater, and dura mater) around the spinal cord.

⚠ *Oppenheim Test.* The examiner runs a fingernail along the crest of the patient's tibia.[168] A negative Oppenheim test is indicated by no reaction or no pain. A positive test is indicated by a positive Babinski sign

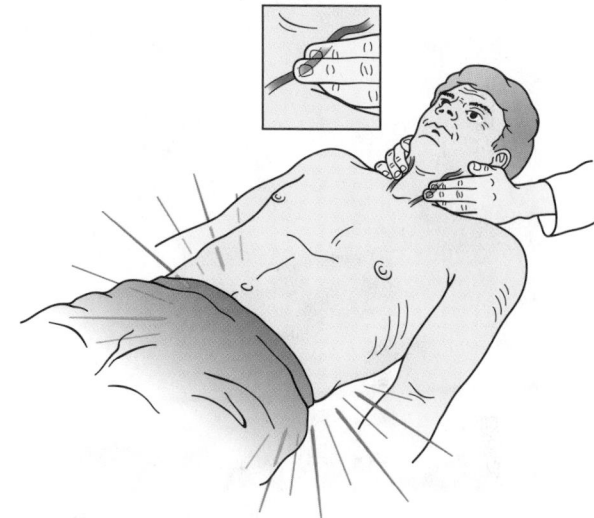

Figure 9-59 **Naffziger test.** This test may be done while the patient is standing or lying down. The examiner applies bilateral compression to the jugular veins, which is hypothesized to increase cerebral spinal fluid pressure. This increased pressure in the subarachnoid space in the root canal may cause back or leg pain by irritating a local mechanical or inflammatory condition.

(positive pathological reflex) and suggests an upper motor neuron lesion.

⚠ *Prone Knee Bending (Nachlas) Test.* The patient lies prone while the examiner passively flexes the knee as far as possible so that the patient's heel rests against the buttock.[179,180] At the same time, the examiner should ensure that the patient's hip is not rotated. If the examiner is unable to flex the patient's knee past 90° because of a pathological condition in the knee, the test may be performed by passive extension of the hip while the knee is flexed as much as possible. Unilateral neurological pain in the lumbar area, buttock, posterior thigh or sometimes the anterior thigh may indicate an L2 or L3 nerve root lesion (Figure 9-60).

This test also stretches the femoral nerve. Pain in the anterior thigh indicates tight quadriceps muscles or stretching of the femoral nerve. A careful history and pain differentiation helps delineate the problem. If the rectus femoris is tight, the examiner should remember that taking the heel to the buttock may cause anterior torsion to the ilium, which could lead to sacroiliac or lumbar pain. The flexed knee position should be maintained for 45 to 60 seconds. Butler has suggested modifications of the PKB test to stress individual peripheral nerves[163] (Table 9-12 and Figure 9-61).

▲ *Sitting Root Test.* This test is a modification of the slump test. The patient sits with a flexed neck. The knee is actively extended while the hip remains flexed at 90°. Increased pain indicates tension on the sciatic nerve. This test is sometimes used to catch the patient unaware. In this case, the examiner passively extends the knee while pretending to examine the foot. Davis, et al.[181] reported that pain should occur before 22° of knee extension remains for the test to be positive if knee extension is the last part of the test performed. Patients with true sciatic pain arch backward and complain of pain into the buttock, posterior thigh, and calf when the leg is straightened, indicating a positive test.[182] The **Bechterewis test** follows a similar pattern.[183] The patient is asked to extend one knee at a time. If no symptoms result, the patient is asked to extend both legs simultaneously. Symptoms in the back or leg indicate a positive response.[184]

✓ *Slump Test.* The slump test has become the most common neurological test for the lower limb. The patient is seated on the edge of the examining table with the legs supported, the hips in neutral position (i.e., no rotation, abduction, or adduction), and the hands behind the back (Figure 9-62). The examination is performed in sequential steps. First, the patient is asked to "slump" the back into thoracic and lumbar flexion. The examiner maintains the patient's chin in the neutral position to prevent neck and head flexion. The examiner then uses one arm to apply overpressure across the shoulders to maintain flexion of the thoracic and lumbar spines. While this position is held, the patient is asked to actively flex the cervical spine and head as far as possible (i.e., chin to chest). The examiner then applies overpressure to maintain flexion of all three parts of the spine (cervical, thoracic, and lumbar) using the hand of the same arm to maintain overpressure in the cervical spine. With the other hand, the examiner then holds the patient's foot in maximum dorsiflexion. While the examiner holds these positions, the patient is asked to actively straighten the knee as much as possible. The test is repeated with the other leg and then with both legs at the same time. If the patient is unable to fully extend the knee because of pain, the examiner releases the overpressure to the cervical spine and the patient

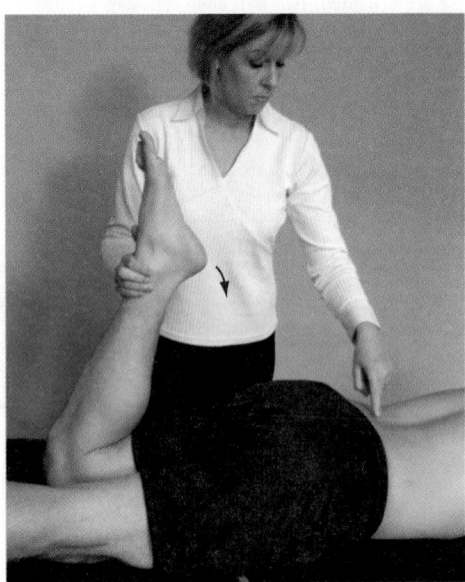

🎞 **Figure 9-60 Basic prone knee bending (PKB1) test,** which stresses the femoral nerve and L2–L4 nerve root. The examiner is pointing to where pain may be expected in the lumbar spine with a positive test.

TABLE **9-12**

Prone Knee Bending Test and Its Modification

	Basic Prone Knee Bending (PKB1)	Prone Knee Bending (PKB2)	Prone Knee Extension (PKE)
Cervical spine	Rotation to test side	Rotation to test side	—
Thoracic and lumbar spine	Neutral	Neutral	Neutral
Hip	Neutral	Extension, adduction	Extension, abduction, lateral rotation
Knee	Flexion	Flexion	Extended
Ankle	—	—	Dorsiflexion
Foot	—	—	Eversion
Toes	—	—	—
Nerve bias	Femoral nerve, L2–L4 nerve root	Lateral femoral cutaneous nerve	Saphenous nerve

Data from Butler DA: Mobilisation of the nervous system, Melbourne, 1991, Churchill Livingstone.

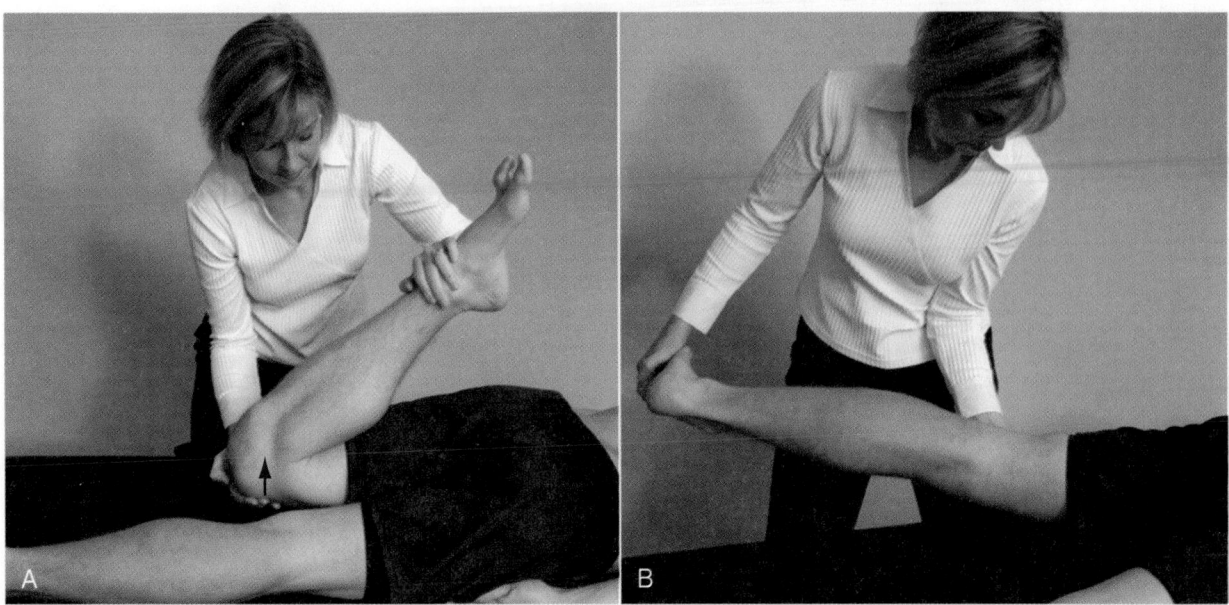

Figure 9-61 Modifications to the prone knee bending (PKB) test to stress specific nerve. **A,** PKB2 (lateral femoral cutaneous nerve). **B,** Prone knee extension (PKE) (saphenous nerve). See Table 9-12 for movements at each joint.

actively extends the neck. If the knee extends further, the symptoms decrease with neck extension, or if the positioning of the patient increases the patient's symptoms, then the test is considered positive for increased tension in the neuromeningeal tract.[185–188] Some clinicians modify the test to make the knee extension of the test passive. Once the patient is positioned with the three parts of the spine in flexion, the examiner first passively extends the knee. If symptoms do not result, then the examiner passively dorsiflexes the foot. A positive test would indicate the same lesion.

Butler advocated doing bilateral knee extension in the slump position.[163] Any asymmetry in the amount of knee extension is easier to note this way. Also, the effect of releasing neck flexion on the patient's symptoms should be noted. Butler has also suggested modifications to the slump test to stress individual nerves[163] (Table 9-13 and Figure 9-63). In hypermobile patients, more hip flexion (more than 90°), as well as hip adduction and medial rotation may be required to elicit a positive response.[163] It is important that if symptoms are produced in any phase of the sequence, the provocative maneuvers are stopped to prevent undue discomfort to the patient.

When doing the slump test, the examiner is looking for reproduction of the patient's pathological symptoms, not just the production of symptoms.[189] The test does place stress on certain tissues, so some discomfort or pain is not necessarily symptomatic for the problem. For example, nonpathological responses include pain or discomfort in the area of T8–T9 (in 50% of normal patients), pain or discomfort behind the extended knee and hamstrings, symmetric restriction of knee extension, symmetric restriction of ankle dorsiflexion, and symmetric increased range of knee extension and ankle dorsiflexion on release of neck flexion.[163]

✓ *Straight Leg Raising Test.* Also known as Lasègue's test, the straight leg raising test (Figure 9-64) is done with the patient completely relaxed.[190–197] It is one of the most common neurological tests of the lower limb. It is a passive test, and each leg is tested individually with the normal leg being tested first. With the patient in the supine position, the hip medially rotated and adducted and the knee extended, the examiner flexes the hip until the patient complains of pain or tightness in the back or back of the leg.[163] If the pain is primarily back pain, it is more likely a disc herniation from pressure on the anterior theca of the spinal cord,[198] or the pathology causing the pressure is more central. "Back pain only" patients who have a disc prolapse have smaller, more central prolapses.[198] If pain is primarily in the leg, it is more likely that the pathology causing the pressure on neurological tissues is more lateral. Disc herniations or pathology causing pressure between the two extremes are more likely to cause pain in both areas.[199] The examiner then slowly and carefully drops the leg back (extends it) slightly until the patient feels no pain or tightness. The patient is then asked to flex the neck so the chin is on the chest, or the examiner may dorsiflex the patient's foot, or both actions may be done simultaneously. Most commonly, foot dorsiflexion is done first. Both of these maneuvers are considered to be provocative or sensitizing tests for neurological tissue. Table 9-14 and Figure 9-65 show modifications of the straight leg raising test that can be used to stress different peripheral nerves to a greater

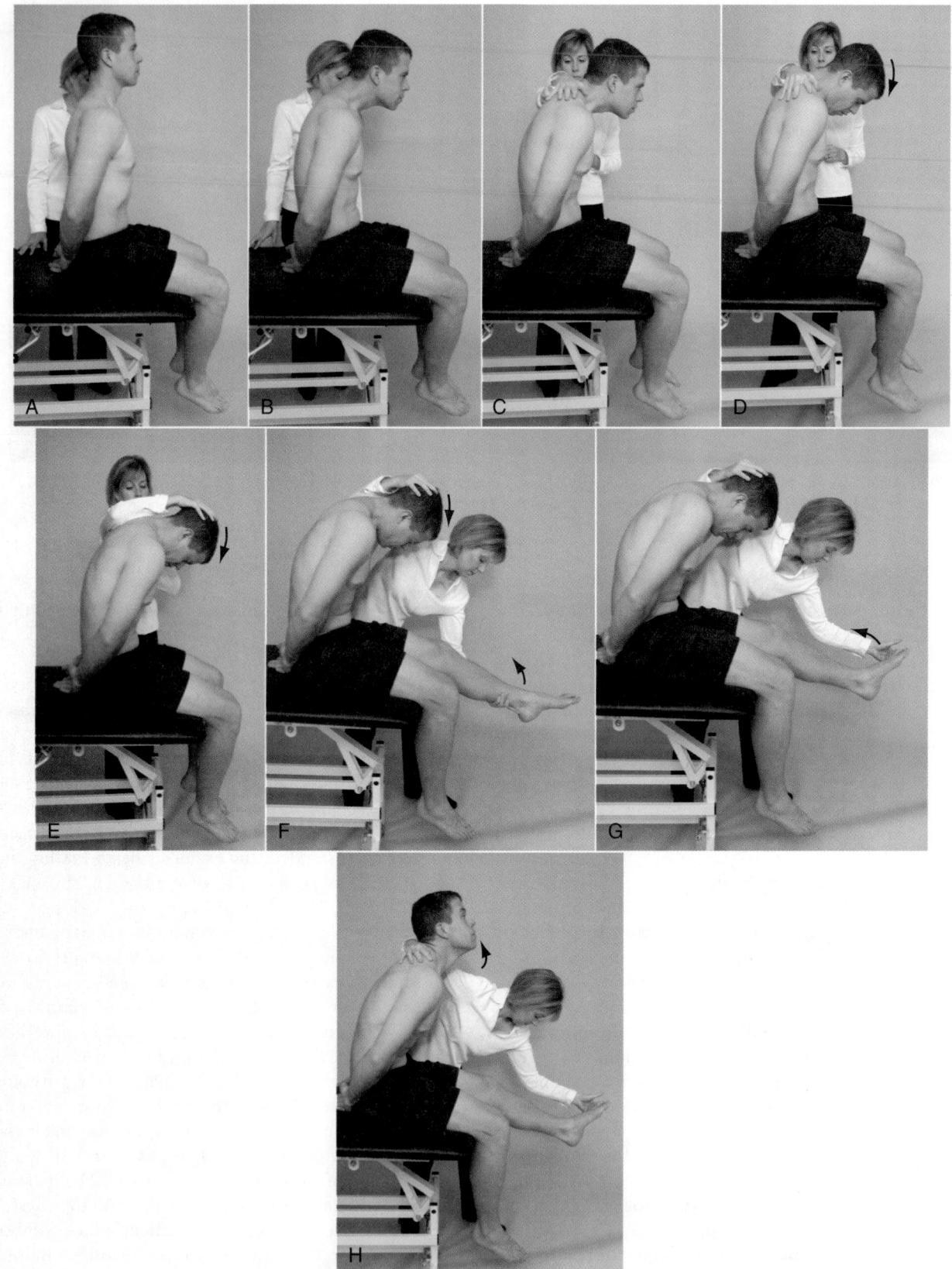

Figure 9-62 Sequence of subject postures in the slump test. A, Patient sits erect with hands behind back. **B,** Patient slumps lumbar and thoracic spine while either patient or examiner keeps the head in neutral. **C,** Examiner pushes down on shoulders while patient holds head in neutral. **D,** Patient flexes head. **E,** Examiner carefully applies overpressure to cervical spine. **F,** Examiner extends patient's knee while holding the cervical spine flexed. **G,** While holding the knee extended and cervical spine flexed, the examiner dorsiflexes the foot. **H,** Patient extends head, which should relieve any symptoms. If symptoms are reproduced at any stage, further sequential movements are not attempted.

TABLE **9-13**

Slump Test and Its Modifications

	Slump Test (ST1)	Slump Test (ST2)	Side Lying Slump Test (ST3)	Long Sitting Slump Test (ST4)
Cervical spine	Flexion	Flexion	Flexion	Flexion, rotation
Thoracic and lumbar spine	Flexion (slump)	Flexion (slump)	Flexion (slump)	Flexion (slump)
Hip	Flexion (90°+)	Flexion (90°+), abduction	Flexion (20°)	Flexion (90°+)
Knee	Extension	Extension	Flexion	Extension
Ankle	Dorsiflexion	Dorsiflexion	Plantar flexion	Dorsiflexion
Foot	—	—	—	—
Toes	—	—	—	—
Nerve bias	Spinal cord, cervical and lumbar nerve roots, sciatic nerve	Obturator nerve	Femoral nerve	Spinal cord, cervical and lumbar nerve roots, sciatic nerve

Data from Butler DA: Mobilisation of the nervous system, Melbourne, 1991, Churchill Livingstone.

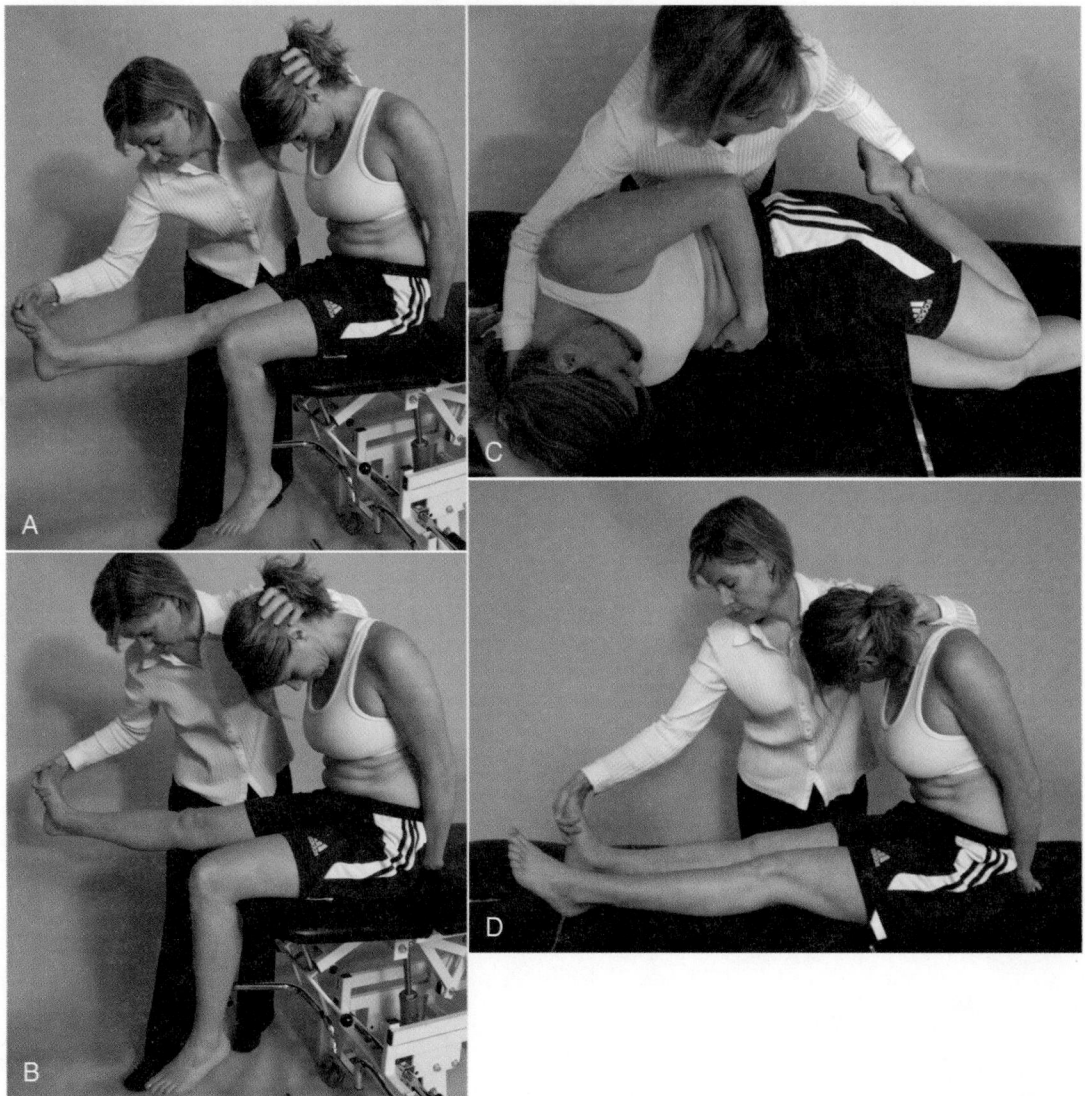

Figure 9-63 Modifications of the slump test (ST) to stress specific nerve. A, Basic ST1 test (spinal cord, nerve roots). **B,** ST2 (obturator nerve). **C,** ST3 (femoral nerve). **D,** ST4 (spinal cord, nerve roots). See Table 9-13 for movements at each joint.

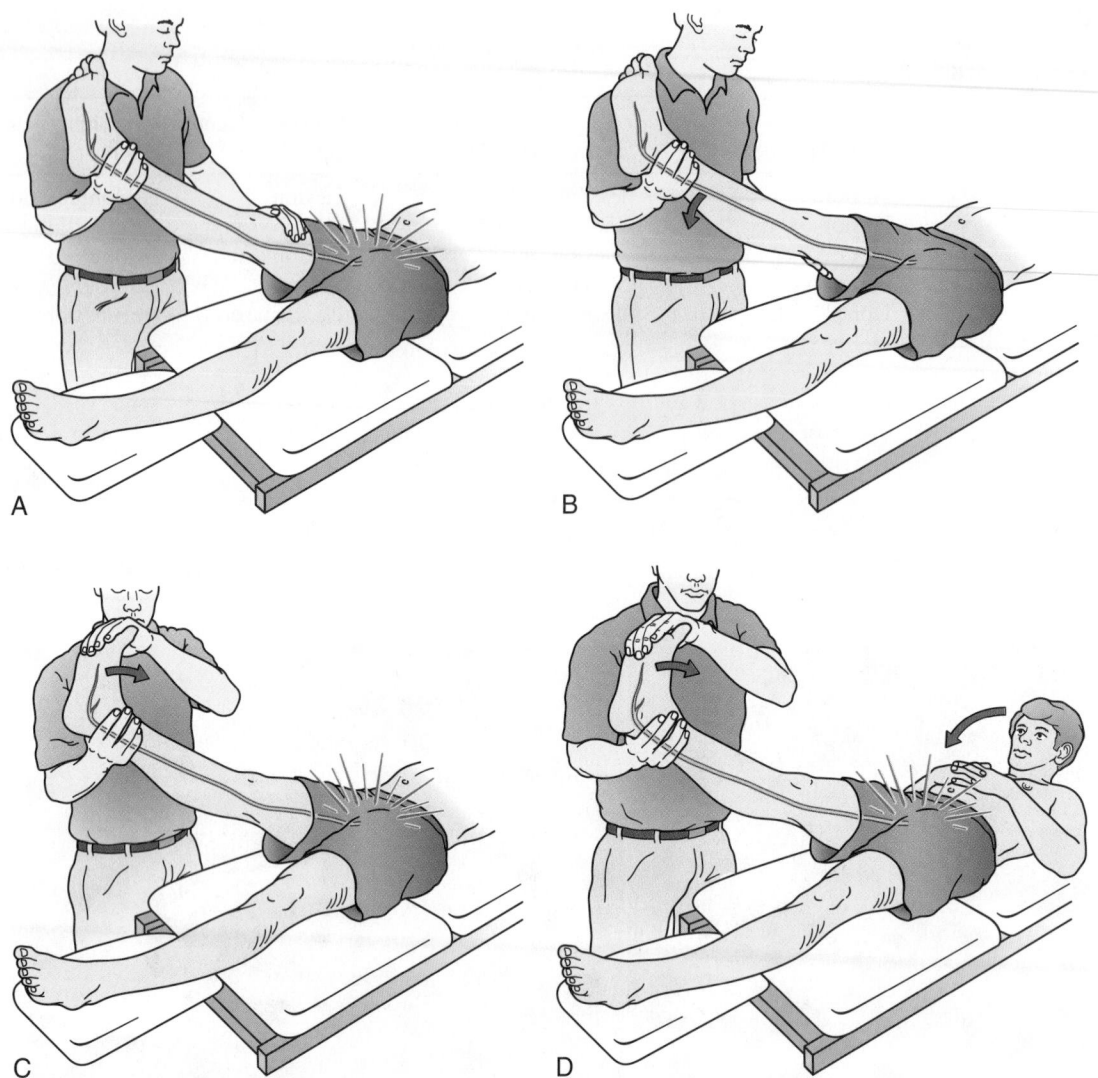

Figure 9-64 Straight leg raising. A, Radicular symptoms are precipitated on the same side with straight leg raising. **B,** The leg is lowered slowly until pain is relieved. **C,** The foot is then dorsiflexed, causing a return of symptoms; this indicates a positive test. **D,** To make the symptoms more provocative, the neck can be flexed by lifting the head at the same time as the foot is dorsiflexed.

TABLE **9-14**

Straight Leg Raising Test and Its Modifications

	SLR (Basic)	SLR2	SLR3	SLR4	Cross (Well Leg) SLR5
Hip	Flexion and adduction	Flexion	Flexion	Flexion and medial rotation	Flexion
Knee	Extension	Extension	Extension	Extension	Extension
Ankle	Dorsiflexion	Dorsiflexion	Dorsiflexion	Plantar flexion	Dorsiflexion
Foot	—	Eversion	Inversion	Inversion	—
Toes	—	Extension	—	—	—
Nerve bias	Sciatic nerve and tibial nerve	Tibial nerve	Sural nerve	Common peroneal nerve	Nerve root (disc prolapse)

Data from Butler, D.A.: Mobilisation of the nervous system. Melbourne, 1991, Churchill Livingstone.
SLR, Straight leg raising.

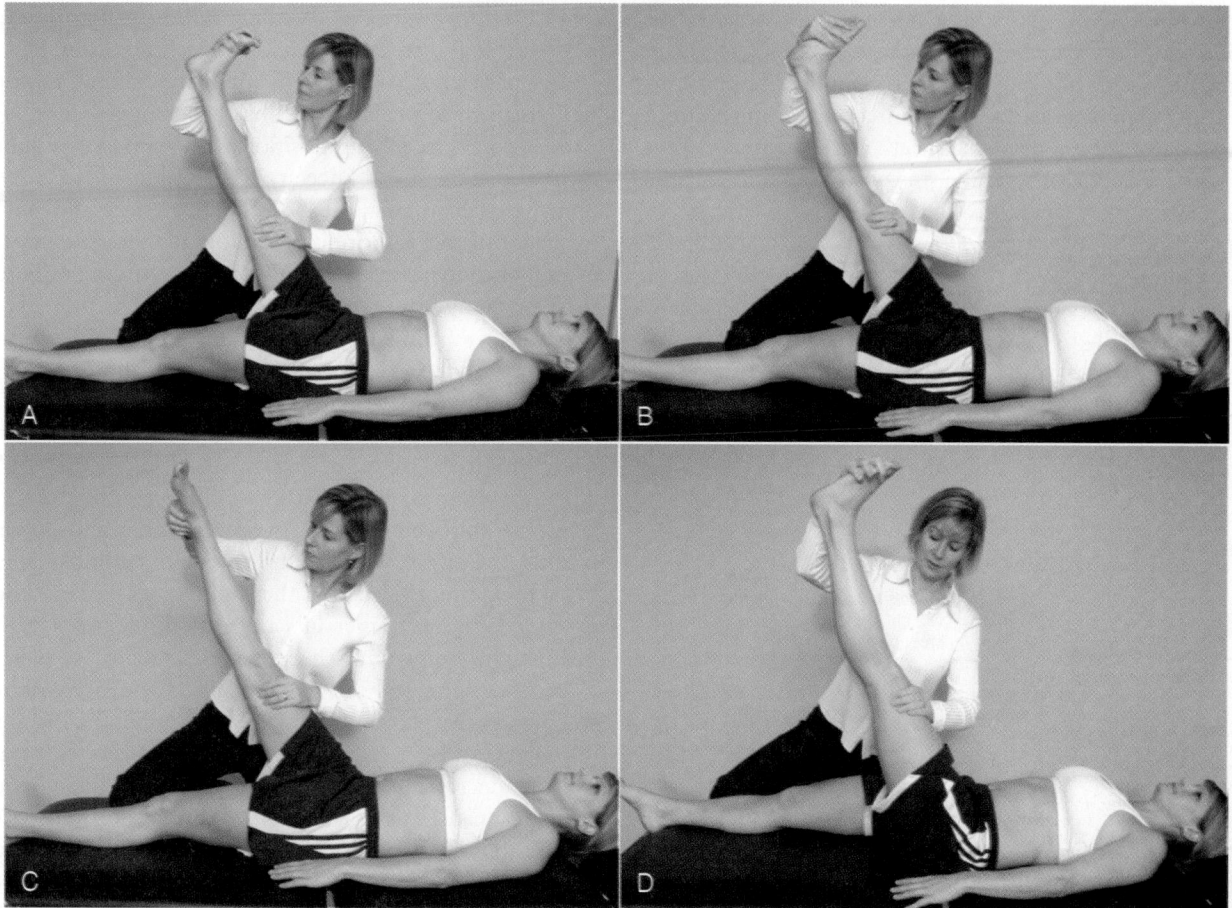

Figure 9-65 Modifications to straight leg raising (SLR) to stress specific nerve. **A,** Basic SLR and SLR2 (sciatic and tibial nerves). **B,** SLR3 (sural nerve). **C,** SLR4 (common peroneal nerve). **D,** SLR5 (intervertebral disc and nerve root). See Table 9-14 for movements at each joint.

degree; these are referred to as straight leg raising tests with a particular nerve bias.

The neck flexion movement has also been called **Hyndman's sign, Brudzinski sign, Linder sign,** and the **Soto-Hall test.** If the examiner desires, neck flexion may be done by itself as a passive movement (passive neck flexion). Tension in the cervicothoracic junction is normal and should not be considered a production of symptoms. If lumbar, leg, or arm symptoms are produced, the neurological tissue is involved. The ankle dorsiflexion movement has also been called the **Bragard's test.** Pain that increases with neck flexion, ankle dorsiflexion, or both indicates stretching of the dura mater of the spinal cord or a lesion within the spinal cord (e.g., disc herniation, tumor, meningitis). Pain that does not increase with neck flexion may indicate a lesion in the hamstring area (tight hamstrings) or in the lumbosacral or sacroiliac joints. **Sicard's test** involves straight leg raising and then extension of the big toe instead of foot dorsiflexion. **Turyn's test** involves only extension of the big toe.[200]

With unilateral straight leg raising, the nerve roots, primarily the L5, S1, and S2 nerve roots (sciatic nerve), are normally completely stretched at 70°, having an excursion of approximately 2 to 6 cm (0.8 to 2.4 inches).[195] Pain after 70° is probably joint pain from the lumbar area (e.g., facet joints) or sacroiliac joints (Figure 9-66). However, if the examiner suspects hamstring tightness, the hamstrings must also be cleared by examination (see Chapter 11). The examiner should compare the two legs for any differences. Although the sciatic nerve roots are commonly stretched at 70° hip flexion, the ROM for straight leg raising and the stress placed on the neurological tissue vary greatly from person to person. For example, patients who are very hypermobile (e.g., gymnasts, synchronized swimmers) may not show a positive straight leg raising test until 110° to 120° of hip flexion, even in the presence of nerve root pathology. It is more important to compare left and right sides for symptoms before deciding whether a lesion is caused by stretching of the neurological tissue or arises from the joints or other soft tissues.

During the unilateral straight leg raising test, tension develops in a sequential manner. It first develops in the greater sciatic foramen, then over the ala of the sacrum, next in the area where the nerve crosses over the pedicle, and finally in the intervertebral foramen. The test causes traction on the sciatic nerve, lumbosacral nerve roots, and dura mater. Adhesions within these areas may result from herniation of the intervertebral disc or extradural or meningeal irritation. Pain comes from the dura mater, nerve root, adventitial sheath of the epidural veins, or synovial facet joints. The test is positive if pain extends from the back down into the leg in the sciatic nerve distribution.

A central protrusion of an intervertebral disc (L4 or L5 disc affecting nerve roots from L4 down to S3) leads to pain primarily in the back with the possibility of bowel and bladder symptoms; a protrusion in the intermediate area causes pain in the posterior aspect of the lower limb and low back; and a lateral protrusion causes pain primarily in the posterior leg with pain below the knee. Having

said this, however, the examiner must realize that the intervertebral disc is only one cause of back pain.

For patients who have difficulty lying supine, a **modified straight leg raising test** has been suggested.[201] The patient is in a side lying position with the test leg uppermost and the hip and knee at 90°. The lumbosacral spine is in neutral but may be positioned in slight flexion or extension if this is more comfortable for the patient. The examiner then passively extends the patient's knee (Figure 9-67), noting pain, resistance, and reproduction of the patient's symptoms for a positive test. The knee position (amount of flexion remaining) on the affected side is compared with that on the good side.

The examiner should then test both legs simultaneously (**bilateral straight leg raising** ❓, Figure 9-68). This test must be done with care, because the examiner is lifting the weight of both lower limbs and thereby placing a large stress on the examiner's lumbar spine. With the patient relaxed in the supine position and knees extended, the examiner lifts both of the legs by flexing the patient's hips until the patient complains of pain or tightness. Because both legs are lifted the pelvis is not stabilized (as it would be by one leg in unilateral straight leg raise), so on hip flexion the pelvis is freer to rotate, thereby decreasing the stress on the neurological tissue. If the test causes pain before 70° of hip flexion, the lesion is probably in the sacroiliac joints; if the test causes pain after 70°, the lesion is probably in the lumbar spine area.

With the unilateral straight leg raising test, 80° to 90° of hip flexion is normal. If one leg is lifted and the patient complains of pain on the opposite side, it is an indication of a space-occupying lesion (e.g., a herniated disc, inflammatory swelling). This finding of pain when the examiner is testing the opposite (good) leg may be called the **well leg raising test of Fajersztajn** (Figure 9-69), a **prostrate leg raising test**, a **sciatic phenomenon**, **Lhermitt's test**, or the **crossover sign** ⚠.[182,195,202] It is typically indicates

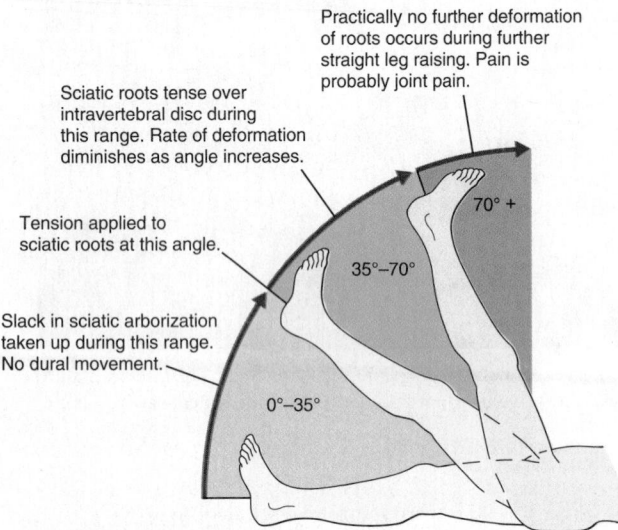

Figure 9-66 Dynamics of single straight leg raising test in most people. (Modified from Fahrni WS: Observations on straight leg raising with special reference to nerve root adhesions. Can J Surg 9:44, 1966.)

Practically no further deformation of roots occurs during further straight leg raising. Pain is probably joint pain.

Sciatic roots tense over intravertebral disc during this range. Rate of deformation diminishes as angle increases.

Tension applied to sciatic roots at this angle.

Slack in sciatic arborization taken up during this range. No dural movement.

70° +

35°–70°

0°–35°

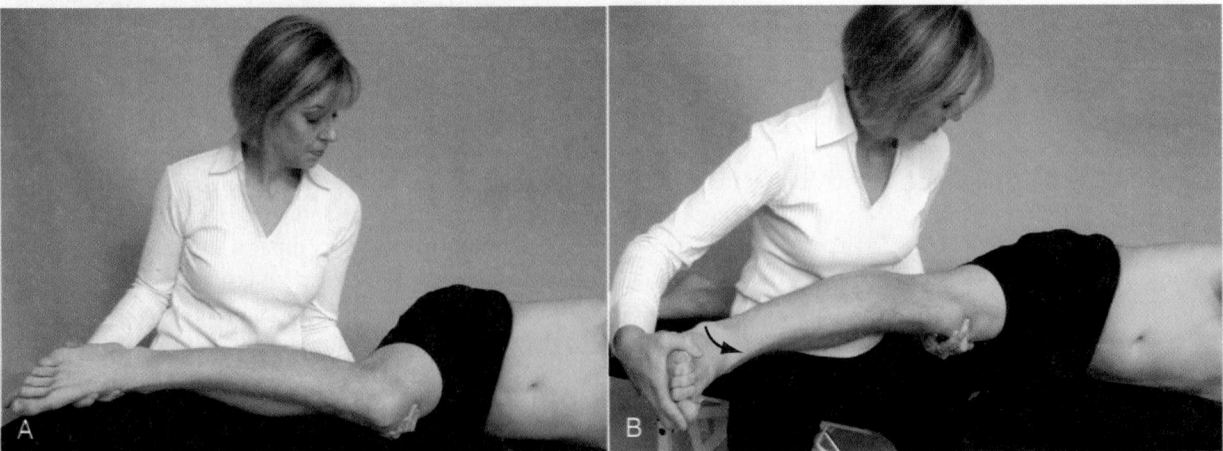

Figure 9-67 Modified straight leg raising for patients who cannot lie supine. A, Starting position with knee flexed to 90°. **B,** Knee is extended as far as possible.

a rather large intervertebral disc protrusion, usually medial to the nerve root (see Figure 9-69), and a poor prognosis for conservative treatment.[197,203] The test causes stretching of the ipsilateral as well as the contralateral nerve root, pulling laterally on the dural sac. A positive Lasègue's and crossover sign can also indicate the degree of disc injury. For example, both are limited to a greater degree if sequestration of the disc occurs.[86] If the examiner finds this test positive, careful questioning about bowel and bladder symptoms is a necessity. Many, but not all, patients with a central protrusion are candidates for surgery, especially if there are bowel and bladder symptoms.

? *Valsalva Maneuver.* The seated patient is asked to take a breath, hold it, and then bear down as if evacuating the bowels (Figure 9-70). If pain increases, it indicates increased intrathecal pressure. The symptoms may

be accentuated by having the patient first flex the hip to a position just short of that causing pain.[195]

Tests for Lumbar Instability

Lumbar instability implies that during movement, the patient loses the ability to control the movement for a brief time (milliseconds), or it may mean the segment is structurally unstable. The brief loss of control often results in a painful catch, apprehension, or an **instability jog** (sudden shift of movement in part of the ROM).[87,204] Pope called this "loss of control in the neutral spine."[205] It commonly occurs with spondylosis owing to degeneration of the disc.[205,206] Structural instability primarily results from spondylolisthesis, and the following tests are designed to test for structural instability.

? *Farfan Torsion Test.*[32,38] This nonspecific test stresses the facet joints, joint capsule, supraspinous and interspinous ligaments, neural arch, the longitudinal ligaments, and the disc. The patient lies prone. The examiner stabilizes the ribs and spine (at about T12) with one hand and places the other hand under the anterior aspect of the ilium. The examiner then pulls the ilium backward (Figure 9-71) causing the spine to be rotated on the opposite side producing torque on the opposite side. The test is said to be positive if it reproduces all or some of the patient's symptoms. The other side is tested for compression.

? *H and I Stability Tests.*[75,92] This set of movements tests for muscle spasm and can be used to detect instability. The H and I monikers relate to the movements that occur (Figure 9-72).

The first part of the test is the "**H**" movement. The patient stands in the normal resting position, which would be considered the center of the "**H**". The pain-free side is tested first. The patient is asked, with guidance from the clinician, to side flex as far as possible (the side of "**H**"). While in this position, the patient is then asked to flex (the front of the "**H**") and then move into extension (the back of the "**H**"). If flexion was more painful than

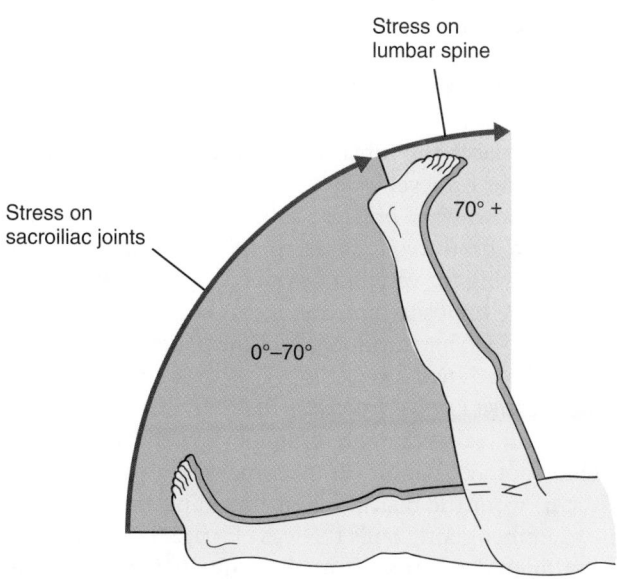

Stress on lumbar spine

Stress on sacroiliac joints

70° +

0°–70°

Figure 9-68 Dynamics of the bilateral straight leg raise.

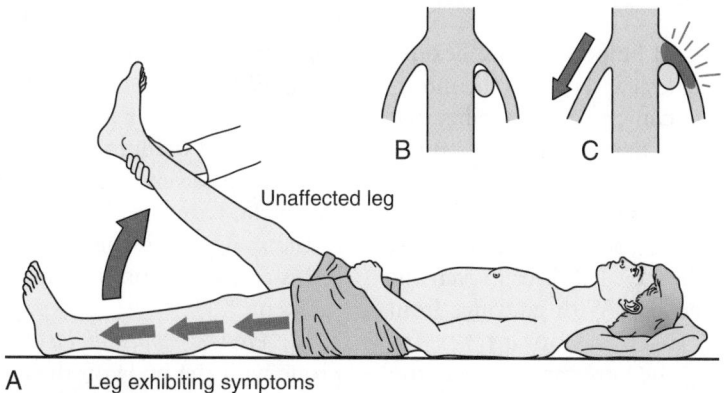

Unaffected leg

B

C

A   Leg exhibiting symptoms

Figure 9-69 Well leg raising test of Fajersztajn. **A,** Movement of nerve roots occurs when the leg on the opposite side is raised. **B,** Position of disc and nerve root before opposite leg is lifted. **C,** When the leg is raised on the unaffected side, the roots on the opposite side slide slightly downward and toward the midline. In the presence of a disc lesion, this movement increases the root tension resulting in radicular signs in the affected leg, which remains on the table. (Modified from DePalma AF, Rothman RH: The intervertebral disc, Philadelphia, 1970, WB Saunders.)

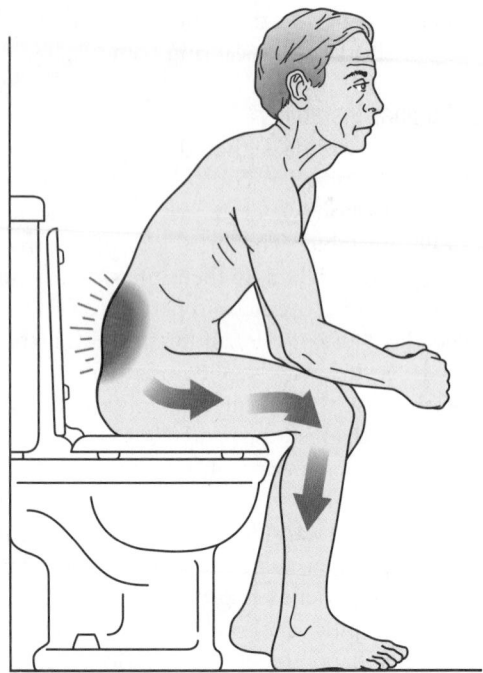

Figure 9-70 The Valsalva maneuver. Increased intrathecal pressure leads to symptoms in the sciatic nerve distribution in a positive test.

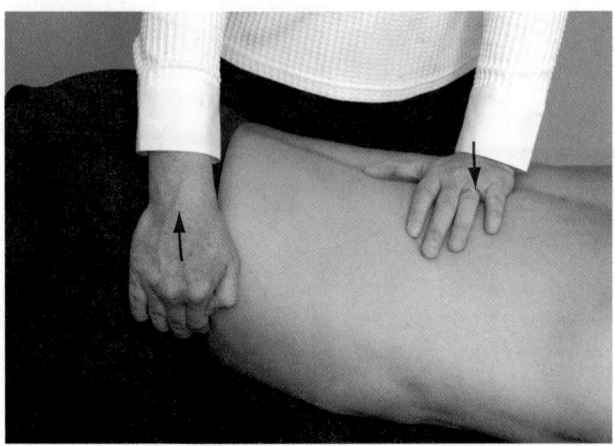

Figure 9-71 Farfan torsion test.

extension, then extension would be done before flexion. The patient then returns to neutral and repeats the movements to the other side. The clinician may stabilize the pelvis with one hand and guide the movement with the other hand on the shoulder.

The second part of the test is the "I" movement. The patient stands in the normal resting position, which would be considered the center of the "I". Pain-free movement (flexion or extension) is tested first. With guidance from the clinician, the patient is asked to forward flex (or extend) the lumbar spine until the hips start to move (top part of "I"). Once in flexion, the patient is guided into side bending (to the pain free side first "I") followed by return to neutral and then side bending to the opposite side. The patient then returns to neutral standing and

does the opposite movement (extension in this case) followed by side bending.

If a hypomobile segment is present, at least two of the movements (the movements into the same quadrant [for example, the top right of the "H" and "I"]) would be limited. If instability is present, one quadrant will again be affected, but only by one of the moves (i.e., by the "H" movement or the "I" movement—not both). For example, if the patient had spondylolisthesis instability in anterior shear (a component of forward flexion) and the "I" is attempted, the shear or slip occurs on forward flexion, and there is little movement during the attempted side bending or flexion. If the "H" is attempted, the side bending is normal, and the following forward flexion is full because the shear occurs in the second phase. So, in this case, the "I" movement is limited but not the "H" movement. This test is primarily for structural instability, but an instability jog may be evident during one of the movements if loss of control occurs. In this case, the end range is commonly normal, but loss of control occurs somewhere in the available ROM.

❓ *Lateral Lumbar Spine Stability Test.*[92] The patient is placed in side lying with the lumbar spine in neutral. The examiner places the forearm over the side of the thorax at about the L3 level as an example. The examiner then applies a downward pressure to the transverse process of L3, which produces a shear to the side on which the patient is lying for vertebra below L3 and a relative lateral shear in the opposite direction to the segments above L3 (Figure 9-73). The production of the patient's symptoms indicates a positive test.

✓ *Passive Lumbar Extension Test.*[207,208] The patient lies prone and relaxed. The examiner passively lifts and extends both extremities at the same time to about 1 foot (30 cm) from the bed. While maintaining the extension, the examiner gently pulls the legs (Figure 9-74). The test is considered positive if, in the extended position, the patient complains of strong pain in the lumbar region, very heavy feeling in the low back, or it feels like the low back is "coming off" and the pain disappears when the legs are lowered to the start position. Numbness or prickling sensation are not positive signs.

❓ *Pheasant Test.* The patient lies prone. With one hand, the examiner gently applies pressure to the posterior aspect of the lumbar spine. With the other hand, the examiner passively flexes the patient's knees until the heels touch the buttocks (Figure 9-75). If this hyperextension of the spine causes the patient to feel pain in the leg, the test is considered positive and indicates an unstable spinal segment.[209]

⚠ *Prone Segmental Instability Test.* The patient lies prone with the body on the examining table and the legs over the edge resting on the floor (Figure 9-76). The examiner applies pressure to the posterior aspect of the lumbar spine while the patient rests in this position. The patient then lifts the legs off the floor, and the examiner

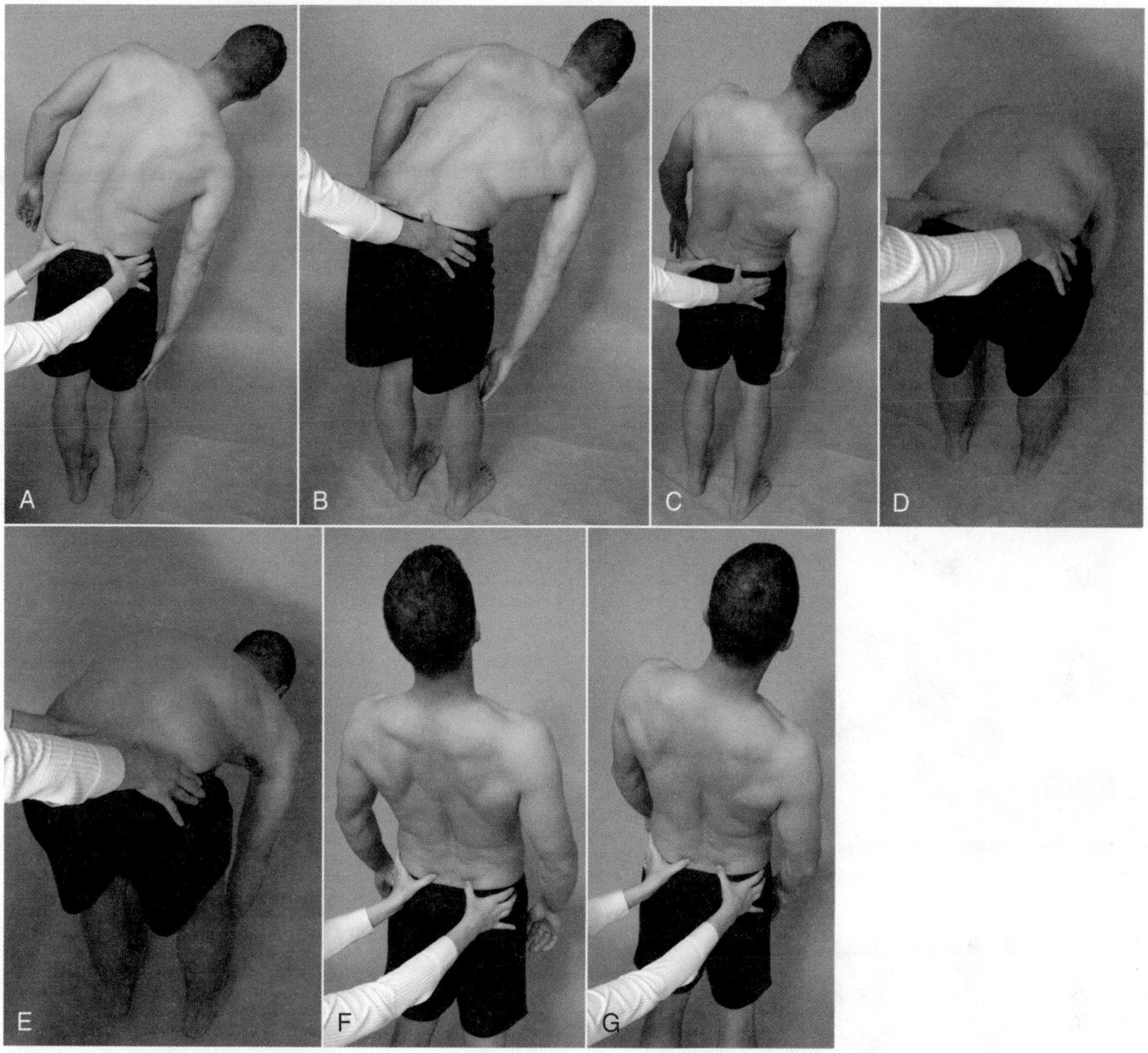

Figure 9-72 H and I stability tests. A, H test—side flexion. **B,** H test—side flexion followed by forward flexion. **C,** H test—side flexion followed by extension. **D,** I test—forward flexion. **E,** I test—forward flexion and side flexion. **F,** I test—extension. **G,** I test—extension and side flexion.

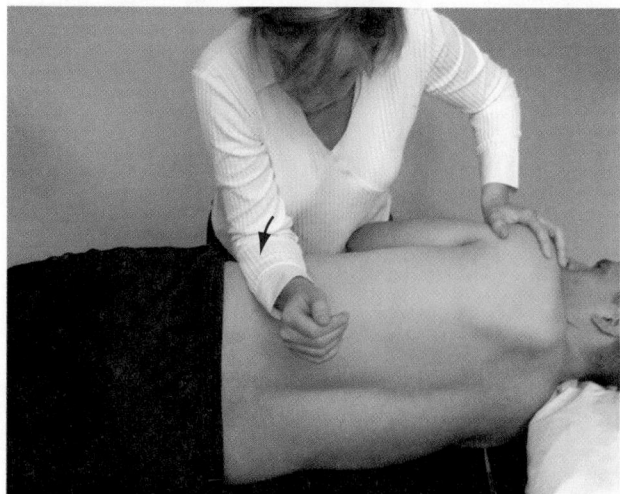

Figure 9-73 Lateral lumbar spine stability test.

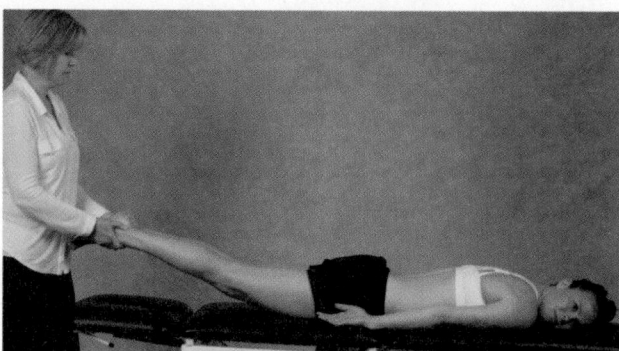

Figure 9-74 Passive lumbar extension test.

again applies posterior compression to the lumbar spine. If pain is elicited in the resting position only, the test is positive, because the muscle action masks the instability.[210,211]

? *Specific Lumbar Spine Torsion Test.*[75,92] This test stresses specific levels of the lumbar spine. To do this, the specific level must be rotated and stressed. An example would be testing the integrity of left rotation on L5 S1. The patient is placed in a right side lying position with the lumbar spine in slight extension (slight lordosis).

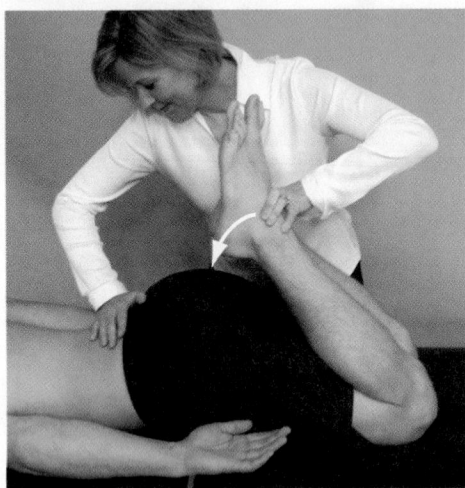

Figure 9-75 Pheasant test.

To achieve rotation and side bending, the examiner grasps the right arm and pulls it upward and forward at a 45° angle until movement is felt at the L5 spinous process. This "locks" all the vertebrae above L5. The examiner then stabilizes the L5 spinous process by holding the left shoulder back with the examiner's elbow while rotating the pelvis and sacrum forward until S1 starts to move (Figure 9-77) with the opposite hand. Minimal movement should occur, and a normal capsular tissue stretch should be felt when L5 S1 is stressed by carefully pushing the shoulder back with the elbow and rotating the pelvis forward with the other arm/hand. This test position is a common position used to manipulate the spine, so the examiner should take care not to overstress the rotation during assessment. In some cases, when doing the test, the examiner may hear a "click" or "pop." This is the same "pop" or "click" that would be heard with a manipulation.

⚠ *Test of Anterior Lumbar Spine Instability.*[92] The patient is placed in side lying with the hips flexed to 70° and knees flexed. The examiner palpates the desired spinous processes (e.g., L4 to L5). By pushing the patient's knees posteriorly with the body along the line of the femur, the examiner can feel the relative movement of the L5 spinous process on L4 (Figure 9-78). Normally, there should be little or no movement. Other levels of the spine may be tested in a similar fashion. A problem with the test is that the examiner should ensure that the posterior ligaments of the spine are relatively loose or relaxed. This can be

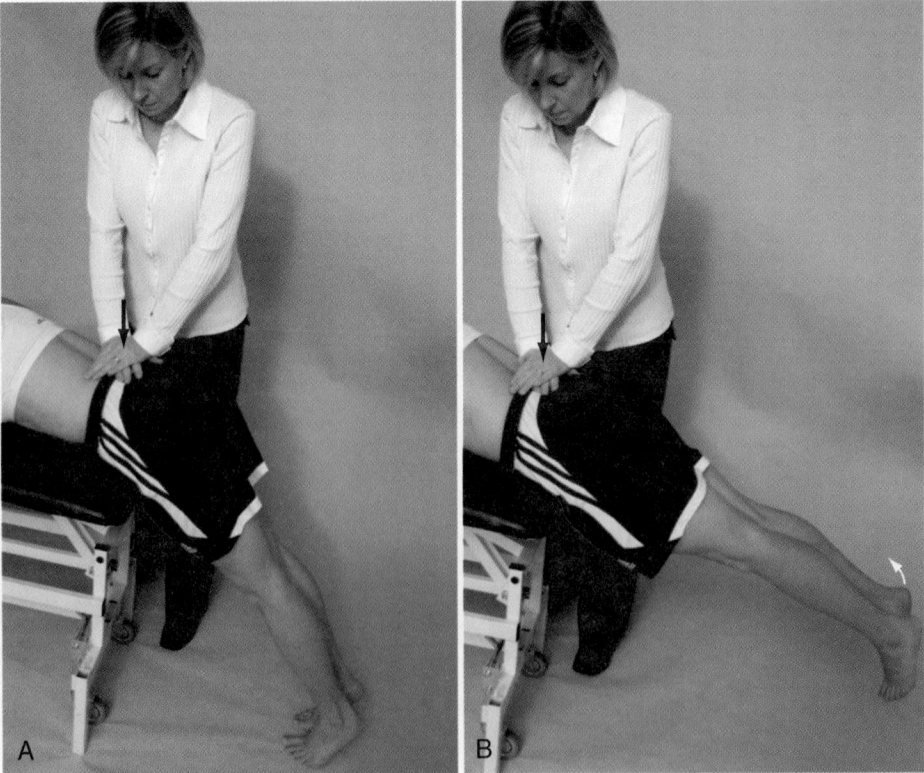

Figure 9-76 Prone segmental instability test. A, Toes on floor. **B,** Feet lifted off floor.

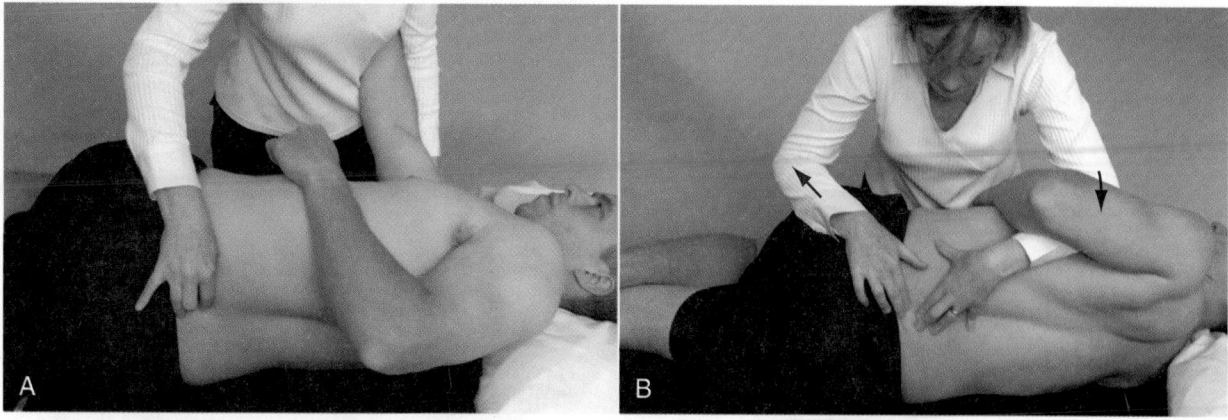

Figure 9-77 Specific lumbar spine torsion test (to L5–S1). **A,** Start position. **B,** Final position.

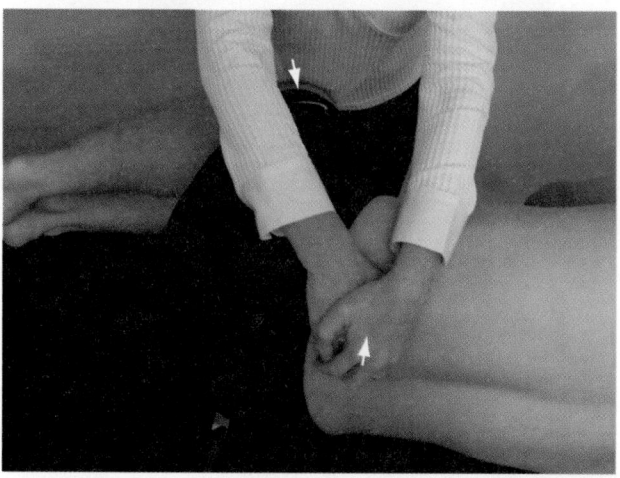

Figure 9-78 Test of anterior lumbar spine stability.

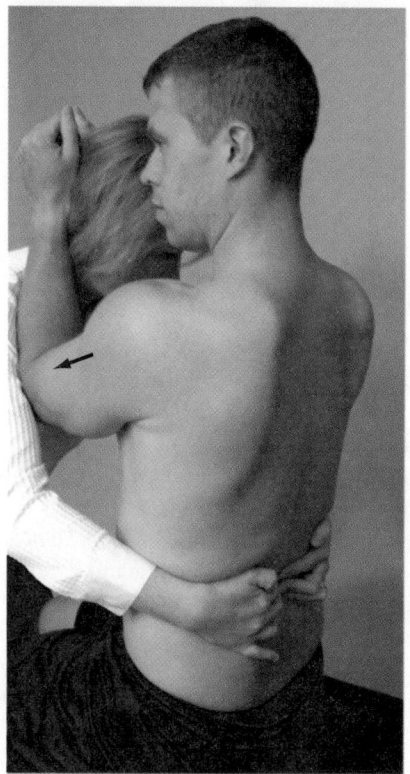

Figure 9-79 Test of posterior lumbar spine instability.

controlled by altering the amount of hip flexion. With greater hip flexion, the posterior ligaments tighten more from the bottom (sacrum) up.

⚠ **Test of Posterior Lumbar Spine Instability.**[92] The patient sits on the edge of the examining table. The examiner stands in front of the patient. The patient places the pronated arms with elbows bent on the anterior aspect of the examiner's shoulders. The examiner puts both hands around the patient so the fingers rest over the lumbar spine and with the heels of the hands gently pull the lumbar spine into full lordosis. To stress L5 on S1, the examiner stabilizes the sacrum with the fingers of both hands and asks the patient to push through the forearm while maintaining the lordotic posture (Figure 9-79). This produces a posterior shear of L5 on S1. Other levels of the spine may be tested in a similar fashion.

Tests for Joint Dysfunction

❓ **McKenzie's Side Glide Test.** The patient stands with the examiner standing to one side. The examiner grasps the patient's pelvis with both hands and places a shoulder

against the patient's lower thorax. Using the shoulder as a block, the examiner pulls the pelvis toward the examiner's body (Figure 9-80). The position is held for 10 to 15 seconds, and then the test is repeated on the opposite side.[39,184] If the patient has an evident scoliosis, the side to which the scoliosis curves should be tested first. A positive test is indicated by increased neurological symptoms on the affected side. It also indicates whether the symptoms are actually causing the scoliosis.

❓ **Milgram's Test.** The patient lies supine and actively lifts both legs simultaneously off the examining table 5 to 10 cm (2 to 4 inches), holding this position for 30

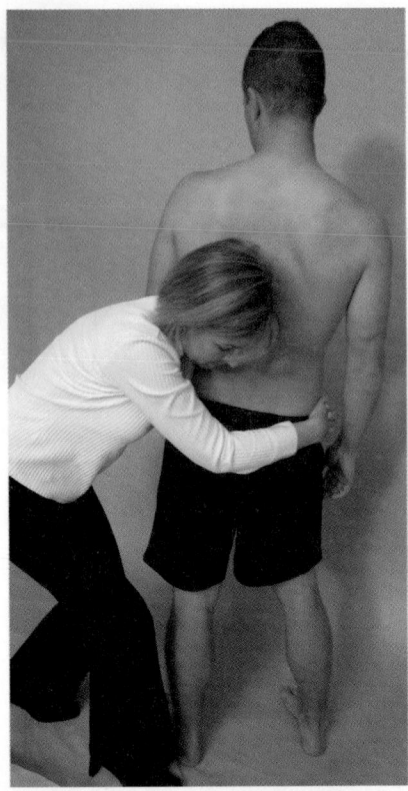

Figure 9-80 McKenzie's side glide test.

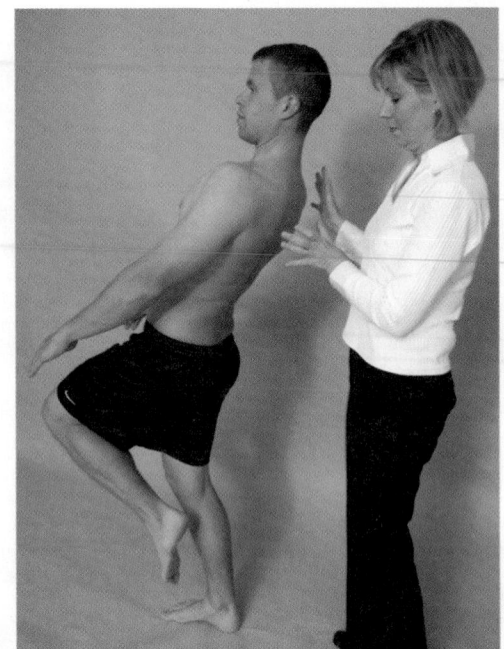

Figure 9-81 One-leg standing lumbar extension test.

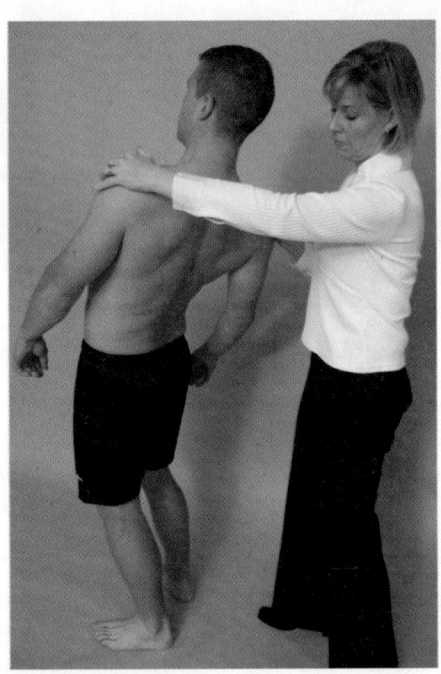

Figure 9-82 Quadrant test for the lumbar spine.

seconds. The test is positive if the limbs or affected limb cannot be held for 30 seconds or if symptoms are reproduced in the affected limb.[183,184] This test should always be performed with caution because of the high stress load placed on the lumbar spine.

❓ One-Leg Standing (Stork Standing) Lumbar Extension Test. The patient stands on one leg and extends the spine while balancing on the leg (Figure 9-81). The test is repeated with the patient standing on the opposite leg. A positive test is indicated by pain in the back and is associated with a pars interarticularis stress fracture (spondylolisthesis). If the stress fracture is unilateral, standing on the ipsilateral leg causes more pain.[212-214] If rotation is combined with extension and pain results, this indicates possible facet joint pathology on the side to which rotation occurs.

❓ Quadrant (Extension Quadrant) Test. The patient stands with the examiner standing behind. The patient extends the spine while the examiner controls the movement by holding the patient's shoulders. The examiner may use his or her shoulders to hold the occiput and take the weight of the head. Overpressure is applied in extension while the patient side flexes and rotates to the side of pain. The movement is continued until the limit of range is reached or until symptoms are produced (Figure 9-82). The position causes maximum narrowing of the intervertebral foramen and stress on the facet joint to the side on which rotation occurs.[215] The test is positive if symptoms are produced.[216] Cipriano described a similar test as **Kemp's test.**[200]

❓ Schober Test. The Schober test may be used to measure the amount of flexion occurring in the lumbar spine. A point is marked midway between the two PSISs ("dimples of the pelvis"), which is the level of S2; then, points 5 cm (2 inches) below and 10 cm (4 inches) above that level are marked. The distance between the three points is measured, the patient is asked to flex forward, and the distance is remeasured. The difference between the two measurements indicates the amount of flexion occurring in the lumbar spine. Little reported a modification of the Schober test to measure extension as well.[217] After completion of the flexion movement, the patient extends the spine, and the distance between the marks is noted. Little also advocated using four marking points (one below the dimples and three above) with 10 cm (4 inches) between them.

? **Yeoman's Test.** The patient lies prone while the examiner stabilizes the pelvis and extends each of the patient's hips in turn with the knees extended. The examiner then extends each of the patient's legs in turn with the knee flexed. In both cases, the patient remains passive. A positive test is indicated by pain in the lumbar spine during both parts of the test.

Tests for Muscle Tightness

✓ **90–90 Straight Leg Raising Test.** See "Tests for Tight Hamstrings" in Chapter 11.

⚠ **Ober Test.** See "Tests for Tight Tensor Fasciae Latae" in Chapter 11.

⚠ **Rectus Femoris Test.** See "Tests for Tight Rectus Femoris" in Chapter 11.

⚠ **Thomas Test.** See "Tests for Tight Iliopsoas" in Chapter 11.

Tests for Muscle Dysfunction

? **Beevor Sign.** The patient lies supine. The patient flexes the head against resistance, coughs, or attempts to sit up with the hands resting behind the head.[183,218] The sign is positive if the umbilicus does not remain in a straight line when the abdominals contract, indicating pathology in the abdominal muscles (i.e., paralysis).

Tests for Intermittent Claudication

Intermittent claudication implies arterial insufficiency to the tissues. It is most commonly evident when activity occurs because of the increased vascular demand of the tissues. There are two types of intermittent claudication—vascular and neurogenic. The vascular type is most commonly the result of arteriosclerosis, arterial embolism, or thrombo-angiitis obliterans and commonly manifests itself with symptoms in the legs. The neurogenic type is sometimes called **pseudoclaudication** or *cauda equina syndrome* and is commonly associated with spinal stenosis and its effect on circulation to the spinal cord and cauda equina.[219-224] The symptoms in this case may be manifested in the back or sciatic nerve distribution.

⚠ **Bicycle Test of van Gelderen.**[225] The patient is seated on an exercise bicycle and is asked to pedal against resistance. The patient starts pedaling while leaning backward to accentuate the lumbar lordosis (Figure 9-83). If pain into the buttock and posterior thigh occurs, followed by tingling in the affected lower extremity, the first part of the test is positive. The patient is then asked to lean forward while continuing to pedal. If the pain subsides over a short period of time, the second part of the test is positive; if the patient sits upright again, the pain returns. The test determines whether the patient has neurogenic intermittent claudication.

? **Stoop Test.** The stoop test is performed to assess neurogenic intermittent claudication to determine whether a relation exists among neurogenic symptoms,

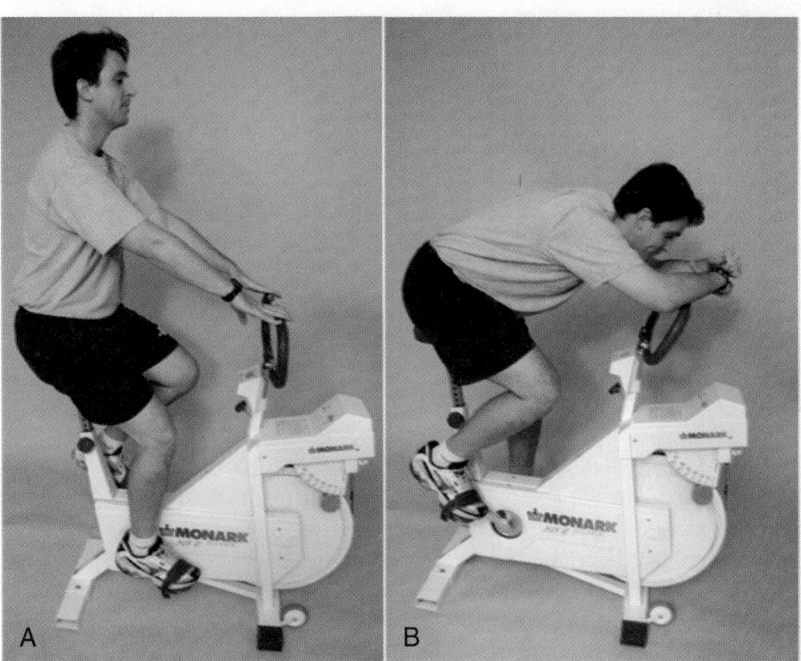

Figure 9-83 Bicycle test of van Gelderen. A, Sitting erect. **B,** Sitting flexed.

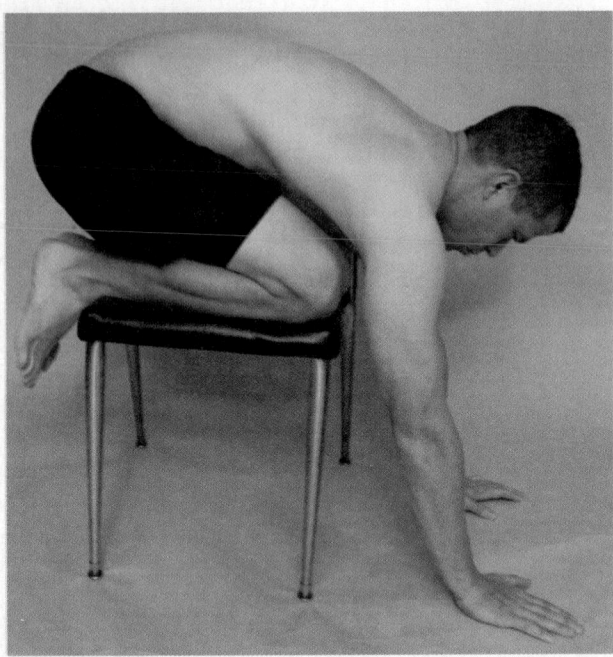

Figure 9-84 Burns test.

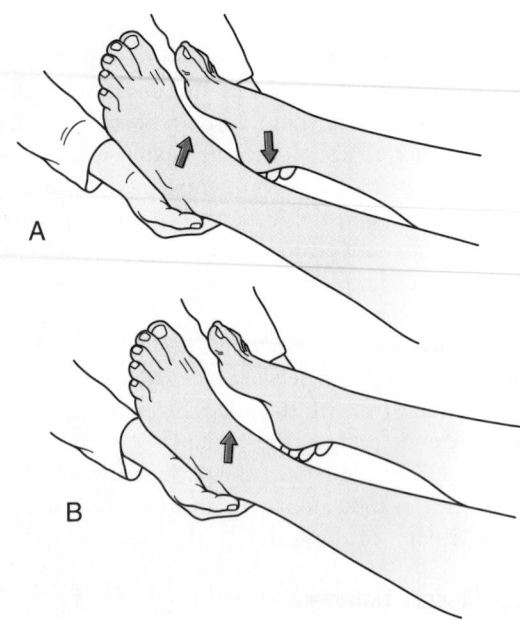

Figure 9-85 The Hoover test. A, Normally, when the patient attempts to elevate one leg, the opposite leg pushes down as a counterbalance. **B,** When the "weak" leg attempts to elevate but the opposite (asymptomatic) leg does not help by pushing down, at least some of the weakness is probably feigned.

posture, and walking.[226] When the patient with neurogenic intermittent claudication walks briskly, pain ensues in the buttock and lower limb within a distance of 50 m (165 feet). To relieve the pain, the patient flexes forward. These symptoms may also be relieved when the patient is sitting and forward flexing. If flexion does not relieve the symptoms, the test is negative. Extension may also be used to bring the symptoms back.

? *Treadmill Test.*[227,228] This test may also be used to determine if the patient has intermittent claudication. Two trials are conducted—one at 1.2 mph and one at the patient's preferred walking speed. The patient walks upright (no leaning forward or holding hand rails is allowed) on the treadmill for 15 minutes or until the onset of severe symptoms (symptoms that would make patient stop walking in usual life situations). Time to first symptoms, total ambulatory time, and precipitating symptoms are recorded.

Tests for Malingering

? *Burns Test.* The patient is asked to kneel on a chair and then bend forward to touch the floor with the fingers (Figure 9-84). The test is positive for malingering if the patient is unable to perform the test or the patient overbalances.[184]

? *Hoover Test.* The patient lies supine. The examiner places one hand under each calcaneus while the patient's legs remain relaxed on the examining table (Figure 9-85).[229–231] The patient is then asked to lift one leg off the table, keeping the knees straight, as for active straight leg raising. If the patient does not lift the leg or the examiner does not feel pressure under the opposite heel, the patient is probably not really trying or may be

a malingerer. If the lifted limb is weaker, however, pressure under the normal heel increases, because of the increased effort to lift the weak leg. The two sides are compared for differences.

Other Tests

? *Sign of the Buttock.* The patient lies supine,[148] and the examiner performs a passive unilateral straight leg raising test. If there is unilateral restriction, the examiner then flexes the knee to see whether hip flexion increases. If the problem is in the lumbar spine or hamstrings, hip flexion increases when the knee is flexed. This finding indicates a negative sign of the buttock test. If hip flexion does not increase when the knee is flexed, it is a positive sign of the buttock test and indicates pathology in the buttock behind the hip joint, such as a bursitis, tumor, or abscess.[232] The patient should also exhibit a noncapsular pattern of the hip.

Reflexes and Cutaneous Distribution

After the special tests, the reflexes should be checked for differences between the two sides (Figure 9-86) if one suspects neurological involvement in the patient's problem.

The deep tendon reflexes are tested with a reflex hammer with the patient's muscles and tendons relaxed. The patellar reflex may be performed with the patient sitting or lying, and the hammer strikes the tendon directly. To test the patellar reflex (C3 to C4), the knee

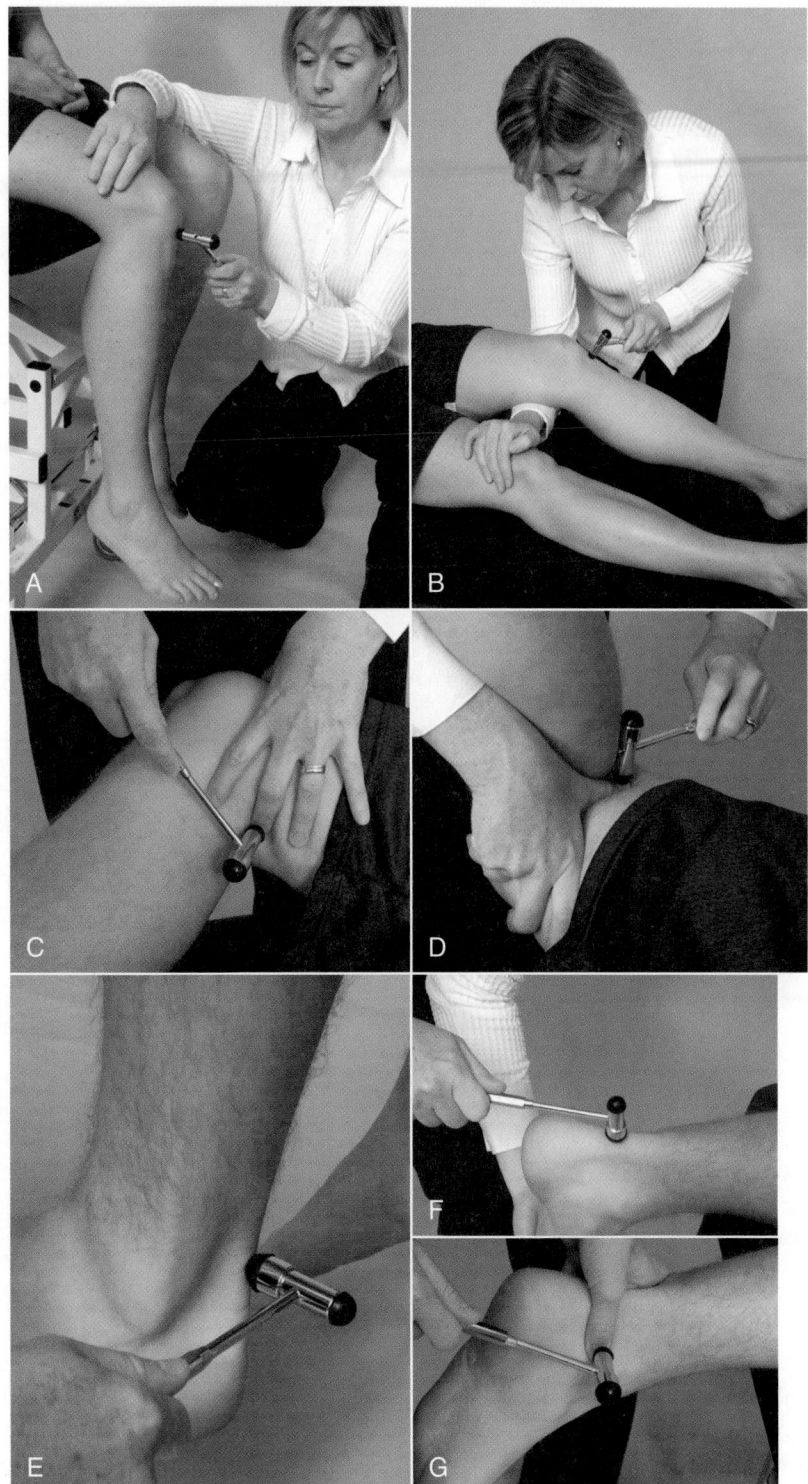

Figure 9-86 Reflexes of the lower limb. A, Patellar (L3) in sitting position. **B,** Patellar (L3) in lying position. **C,** Medial hamstrings (L5) in supine lying position. **D,** Lateral hamstrings (S1, S2) in prone lying position. **E,** Achilles (S1) in sitting position. **F,** Achilles (S1) in kneeling position. **G,** Posterior tibial (L4, L5) in prone lying position.

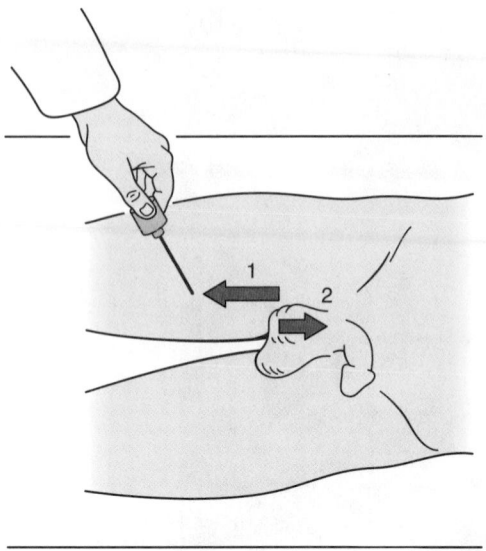

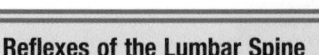

Figure 9-87 Cremasteric reflex. *1,* The examiner runs a sharp object along the inner thigh. *2,* A negative reflex is indicated by the scrotum's rising on that side.

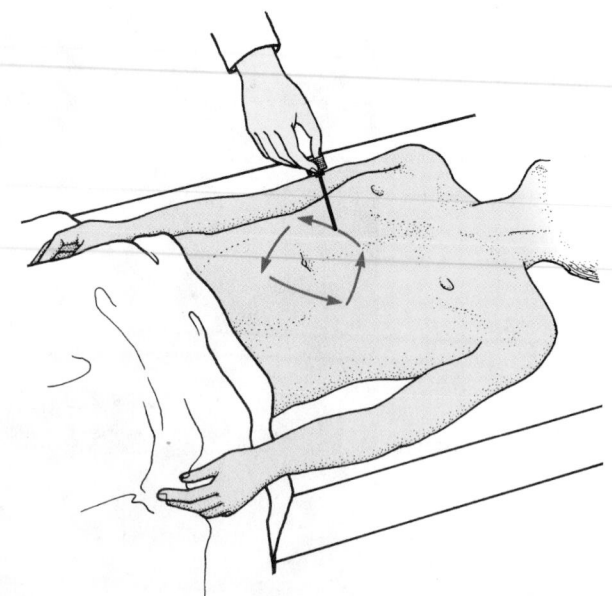

Figure 9-88 Superficial abdominal reflex.

Reflexes of the Lumbar Spine

- Patellar (L3–L4)
- Medial hamstring (L5–S1)
- Lateral hamstring (S1–S2)
- Posterior tibial (L4–L5)
- Achilles (S1–S2)

TABLE **9-15**

Differential Diagnosis of Intermittent Claudication

	Vascular	Neurogenic
Pain	Related to exercise; occurs at various sites simultaneously	Related to exercise; sensations spread from area to area
Pulse	Absent after exercise	Present after exercise
Protein content of cerebrospinal fluid	Normal	Raised
Sensory change	Variable	Follows more specific dermatomes
Reflexes	Normal	Decreased but returns quickly

---

is flexed to 30° (supine lying) or 90° (sitting). The Achilles reflex (S1 to S2) may be tested in prone, sitting, or kneeling position. To test the Achilles reflex, the ankle is at 90° or slightly dorsiflexed. The examiner must ensure that the patient's dorsiflexors are relaxed before doing the test; otherwise, the test will not work. This is done by passively dorsiflexing the foot and feeling for the "springing back" of the foot into plantar flexion. If this does not occur, the dorsiflexors are not relaxed. To test the hamstring reflex (semimembrinosus: L5, S1, and biceps femoris: S1 to S2), the examiner places the thumb over the appropriate tendon and taps the thumbnail to elicit the reflex. Again, the knee should be slightly flexed with the hamstrings relaxed to perform the test.

Neurogenic intermittent claudication may cause the reflexes to be absent soon after exercise (Table 9-15).[233,234] If neurogenic intermittent claudication is suspected, it is necessary to test the reflexes immediately, because reflexes may return within 1 to 3 minutes after stopping the activity.

Another reflex that may be tested is the **superficial cremasteric reflex,** which occurs in males only (Figure 9-87). The patient lies supine while the examiner strokes the inner side of the upper thigh with a pointed object. The test is negative if the scrotal sac on the tested side pulls up. Absence or reduction of the reflex bilaterally suggests an upper motor neuron lesion. A unilateral absence suggests a lower motor neuron lesion between L1 and L2. Absences have increased significance if they are associated with increased deep tendon reflexes.[235]

Two other superficial reflexes are the **superficial abdominal reflex** (Figure 9-88) and the **superficial anal reflex.** To test the superficial abdominal reflex, the examiner uses a pointed object to stroke each quadrant of the abdomen of the supine patient in a triangular fashion

TABLE **9-16**

Peripheral Nerve Lesions

Nerve (Root Derivation)	Sensory Supply	Sensory Loss	Motor Loss	Reflex Change	Lesion
Lateral cutaneous nerve of thigh (L2–L3)	Lateral thigh	Lateral thigh; often intermittent	None	None	Lateral inguinal entrapment
Posterior cutaneous nerve of thigh (S1–S2)	Posterior thigh	Posterior thigh	None (note: Sciatic nerve often involved, too)	None (note: Sciatic nerve often involved, too)	Local (buttock) trauma Pelvic mass Hip fracture
Obturator nerve (L2–L4)	Medial thigh	Often none ± medial thigh	Thigh adduction	None	Pelvic mass
Femoral nerve (L2–L4)	Anteromedial thigh and leg	Anteromedial thigh and leg	Knee extension ± hip flexion	Diminished knee jerk	Retroperitoneal or pelvic mass Femoral artery aneurysm (or puncture) Diabetic mononeuritis
Saphenous branch of femoral nerve (L2–L4)	Anteromedial knee and medial leg	Medial leg	None (note: Positive Tinel sign 5 to 10 cm above medial femoral epicondyle of knee)	None (note: Positive Tinel sign 5 to 10 cm above medial femoral epicondyle of knee)	Local trauma Entrapment above medial femoral condyle
Sciatic nerve (L4–L5, S1)	Anterior and posterior leg Sole and dorsum of foot	Entire foot	Foot dorsiflexion Foot inversion ± plantar flexion ± knee flexion	Diminished ankle jerk	Pelvic mass Hip fracture Piriformis entrapment Misplaced buttock injection
Common peroneal nerve (division of sciatic nerve)	Anterior leg, dorsum of foot	None or dorsal foot	Foot dorsiflexion, inversion, and eversion (note: Positive Tinel sign at lateral fibular neck)	None (note: Positive Tinel sign at lateral fibular neck)	Entrapment pressure at neck of fibula Rarely, diabetes, vasculitis, leprosy

From Reilly BM: Practical strategies in outpatient medicine, Philadelphia, 1991, WB Saunders, p. 928.

around the umbilicus. Absence of the reflex (reflex movement of the skin) indicates an upper motor neuron lesion; unilateral absence indicates a lower motor neuron lesion from T7 to L2, depending on where the absence is noted, as a result of the segmental innervation. The examiner tests the superficial anal reflex by touching the perianal skin. A normal result is shown by contraction of the anal sphincter muscles (S2 to S4).

Finally, the examiner should perform one or more of the pathological reflex tests (see Table 1-33) used to determine upper motor lesions or pyramidal tract disease, such as the Babinski or Oppenheim tests (see "Special Tests"). The presence of these reflexes indicates the possible presence of disease or upper motor neuron lesion, whereas their absence reflects the normal situation.

If neurological symptoms are found, the examiner must check the dermatome patterns of the nerve roots as well as the peripheral sensory distribution of the periph-

eral nerves (Table 9-16 and Figure 9-89). Remember that dermatomes vary from person to person, and the accompanying representations are estimations only. The examiner tests for sensation by running relaxed hands over the back, abdomen, and lower limbs (front, sides, and back), being sure to cover all aspects of the leg and foot. If any difference between the sides is noted during this **sensation scan,** the examiner may then use a pinwheel, pin, cotton ball, or brush to map out the exact area of sensory difference and determine the peripheral nerve or nerve root affected.

Pain may be referred from the lumbar spine to the sacroiliac joint and down the leg as far as the foot. Seldom is pain referred up the spine (Figure 9-90). Pain may be referred to the lumbar spine from the abdominal organs, the lower thoracic spine, and the sacroiliac joints. Muscles may also refer pain to the lumbar area (Table 9-17).[236]

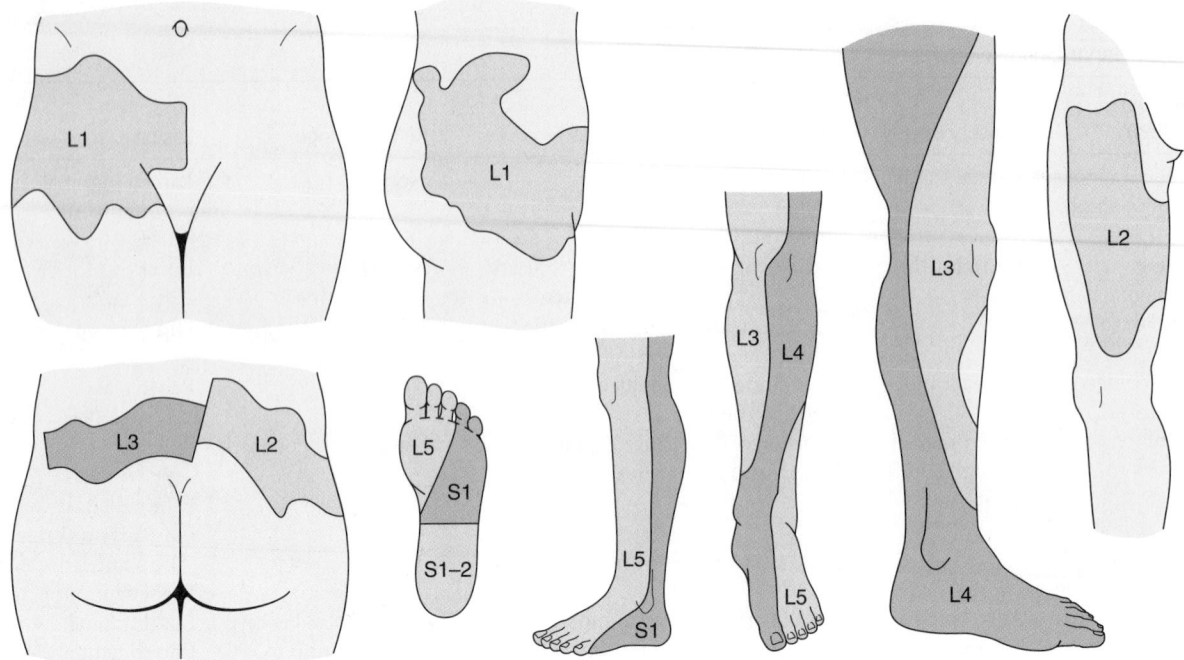

Figure 9-89 Lumbar dermatomes.

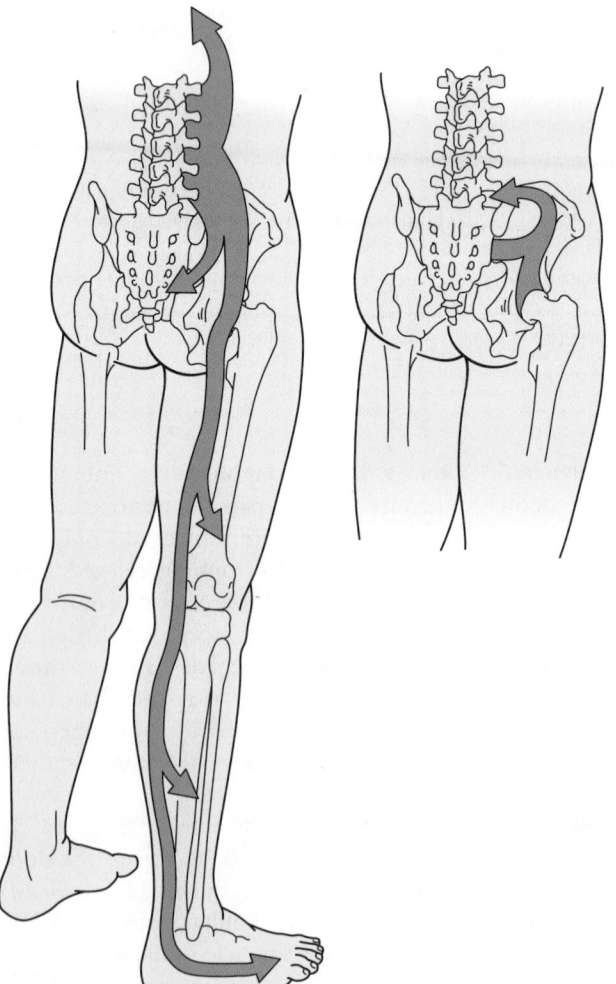

Figure 9-90 Referral of pain from and to the lumbar spine.

TABLE 9-17

Lumbar Muscles and Referral of Pain

Muscle	Referral Pattern
Ilicostalis lumborum	Below T12 ribs lateral to spine down to buttock
Longissimus	Beside spine down to gluteal fold
Multifidus	Lateral to spine, sacrum to gluteal cleft, posterior leg, and lower abdomen
Abdominals	Below xiphisternum and along anterior rib cage down along inguinal ligament to genitals
Serratus posterior inferior	Lateral to spine in T9–T12 posterior rib area

Data from Travell JG, Simons DG: Myofascial pain and dysfunction: the trigger point manual, Baltimore, 1983, Williams & Wilkins.

Peripheral Nerve Injuries of the Lumbar Spine

Lumbosacral Tunnel Syndrome. This syndrome involves compression of the L5 nerve root as it passes under the iliolumbar ligament in the iliolumbar canal (Figure 9-91). The usual cause of compression is trauma (inflammation), osteophytes, or a tumor. Symptoms are primarily sensory (L5 dermatome) and pain. There is minimal or no effect on the L5 myotome.[237]

Joint Play Movements

The joint play movements have special importance in the lumbar spine, because they are used to determine the end

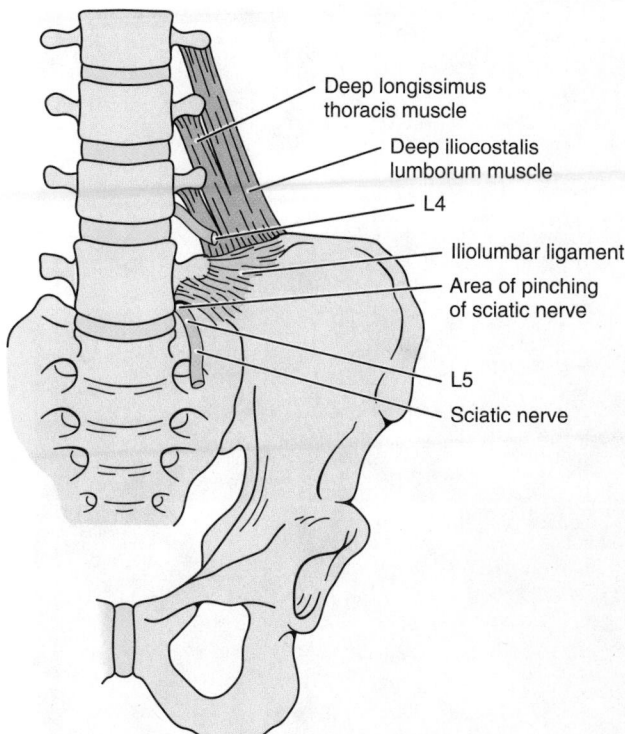

Figure 9-91 Lumbosacral tunnel syndrome. This syndrome involves compression of the L5 nerve root as it passes under the iliolumbar ligament in the iliolumbar canal.

Labels in figure:
Deep longissimus thoracis muscle
Deep iliocostalis lumborum muscle
L4
Iliolumbar ligament
Area of pinching of sciatic nerve
L5
Sciatic nerve

feel of joint movement as well as the presence of joint play. They are often used to replace passive movements in the lumbar spine, which are difficult to perform because of the need to move the heavy trunk or lower limbs. As the joint play movements are performed, the examiner should note any decreased ROM, pain, or difference in end feel.[238]

Joint Play Movements of the Lumbar Spine

- Flexion
- Extension
- Side flexion
- Posteroanterior central vertebral pressure (PACVP)
- Posteroanterior unilateral vertebral pressure (PAUVP)
- Transverse vertebral pressure (TVP)

Flexion, Extension, and Side Flexion

The movements tested during these motions are sometimes called **passive intervertebral movements (PIVMs)**.[239] Flexion is accomplished with the patient in the side lying position. The examiner flexes both of the patient's bent knees toward the chest by flexing the hips (Figure 9-92, *A*). While palpating between the spinous processes of the lumbar vertebrae with one hand (one

finger on the spinous process, one finger above, and one finger below the process), the examiner passively flexes and releases the patient's hips; the examiner's body weight is used to cause the movement. The examiner should feel the spinous processes gap or move apart on flexion. If this gapping does not occur between two spinous processes, or if it is excessive in relation to the other gapping movements, the segment is hypomobile or hypermobile, respectively. The results, however, will depend on the skill of the examiner as interrater reliability studies have shown only average reliability.[239]

Extension (Figure 9-92, *B*) and side flexion (Figure 9-92, *C*) are tested in a similar fashion, except that the movement is passive extension or passive side flexion rather than passive flexion. Side flexion is most easily accomplished by grasping the patient's uppermost leg and rotating the leg upward, which causes side flexion in the lumbar spine by tilting the pelvis. Hip pathology must be ruled out before this is performed.

Central, Unilateral, and Transverse Vertebral Pressure

These movements are sometimes called **passive accessory intervertebral movements (PAIVMs)**. To perform the last three joint play movements, the patient lies prone.[240] The lumbar spinous processes are palpated beginning at L5 and working up to L1. If the examiner plans to test end feel over several occasions, the same examining table should be used to improve reliability.[241] Likewise, the patient should be positioned the same way each time. The greatest movement occurs with the spine in neutral.[242] Interrater reliability of these techniques is often low.[243]

The examiner positions the hands, fingers, and thumbs as shown in Figure 9-92, *D*, to perform **posteroanterior central vertebral pressure (PACVP)**. Pressure is applied through the thumbs, with the vertebrae being pushed anteriorly (see Figure 8-39). The examiner must apply the pressure slowly and carefully so that the feel of the movement can be recognized. In reality, the movement is minimal. This springing test may be repeated several times to determine the quality of the movement through the range available, and the end feel.

To perform **posteroanterior unilateral vertebral pressure (PAUVP)**, the examiner moves the fingers laterally away from the tip of the spinous process about 2.5 to 4.0 cm (1.0 to 1.5 inches) so that the thumbs rest on the muscles overlying the lamina or the transverse process of the lumbar vertebra (Figure 9-92, *E*). The same anterior springing pressure is applied as in the central pressure technique. This springing pressure causes a slight rotation of the vertebra in the opposite direction, which can be confirmed by palpating the spinous process while doing the technique. The two sides should be evaluated and compared.

To perform **transverse vertebral pressure (TVP)**, the examiner's fingers are placed along the side of the

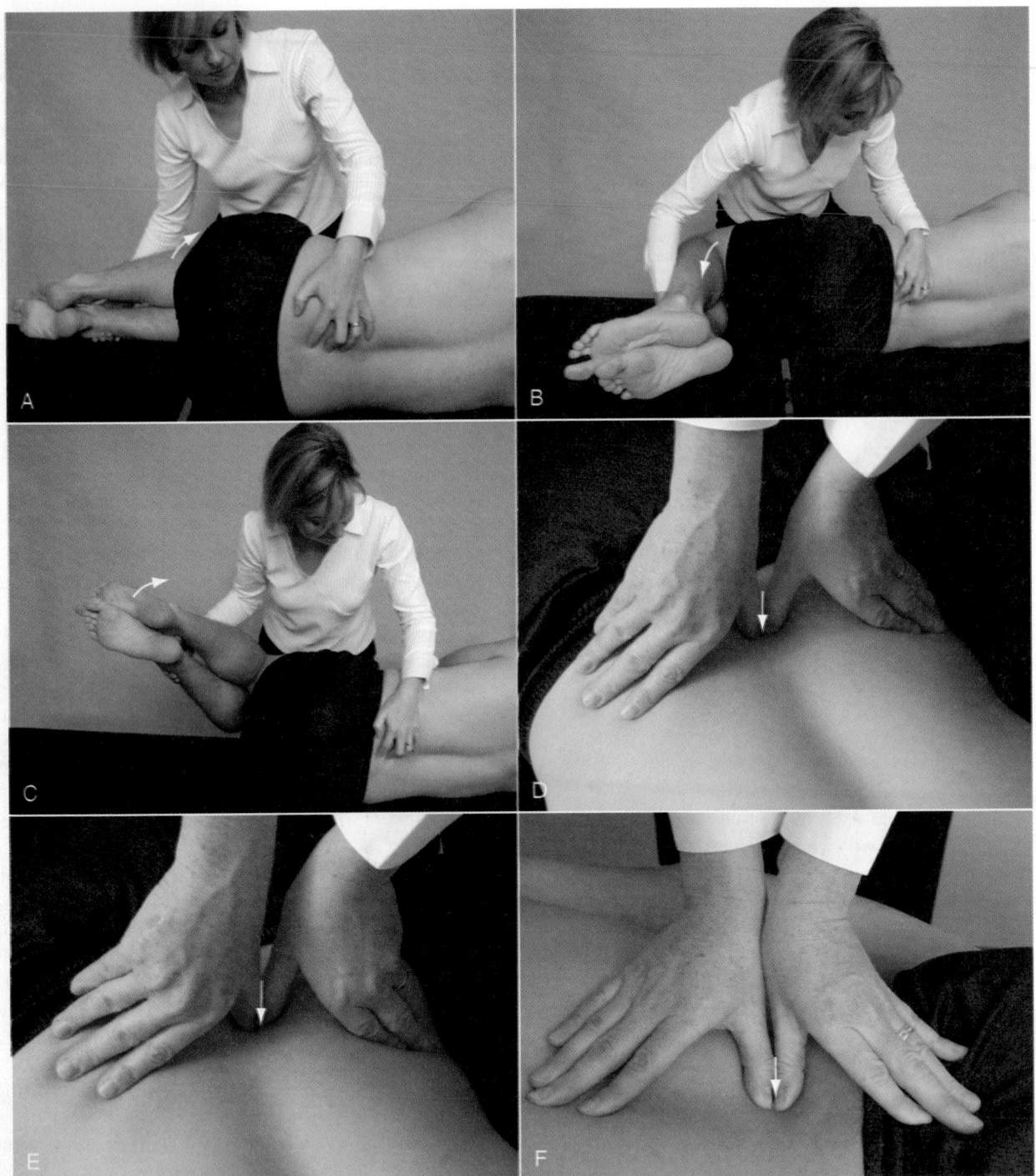

Figure 9-92 Joint play movements of the lumbar spine. A, Flexion. **B,** Extension. **C,** Side flexion. **D,** Posteroanterior central vertebral pressure (PACVP). **E,** Posteroanterior unilateral vertebral pressure (PAUVP). **F,** Transverse vertebral pressure (TVP).

spinous process of the lumbar spine (Figure 9-92, *F*). The examiner then applies a transverse springing pressure to the side of the spinous process, which causes the vertebra to rotate in the direction of the pressure, feeling for the quality of movement. Pressure should be applied to both sides of the spinous process to compare the quality of movement through the range available and the end feel.

Palpation

If the examiner, having completed the examination of the lumbar spine, decides that the problem is in another joint, palpation should not be done until that joint is completely examined. However, when palpating the lumbar spine, any tenderness, altered temperature, muscle spasm, or other signs and symptoms that may indicate the source

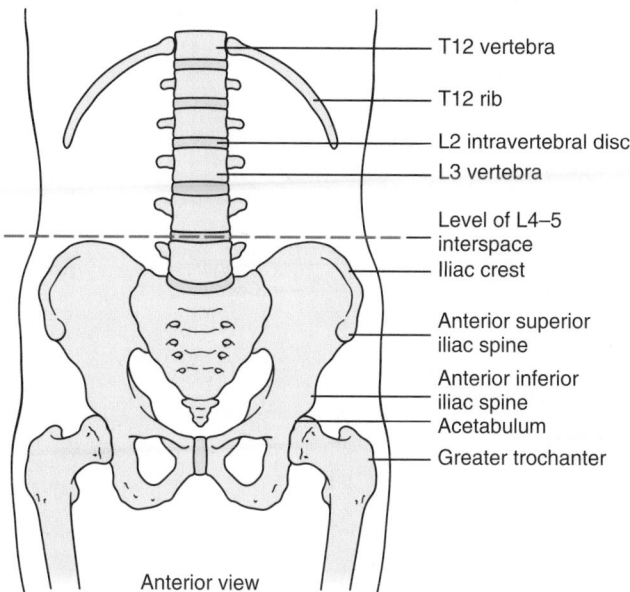

Figure 9-93 **Bony landmarks of the lumbar spine (anterior view).**

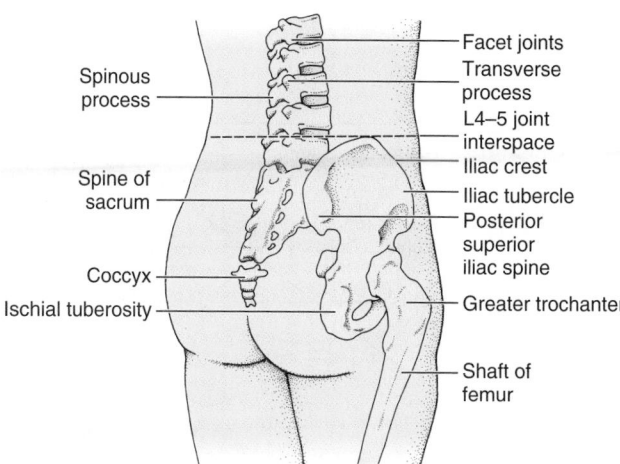

Figure 9-94 **Bony landmarks of the lumbar spine (posterior view).**

of pathology should be noted. If the problem is suspected to be in the lumbar spine area, palpation should be carried out in a systematic fashion, starting on the anterior aspect and working around to the posterior aspect.

Anterior Aspect

With the patient lying supine, the following structures are palpated anteriorly (Figure 9-93).

Umbilicus. The umbilicus lies at the level of the L3–L4 disc space and is the point of intersection of the abdominal quadrants. It is also the point at which the aorta divides into the common iliac arteries. With some patients, the examiner may be able to palpate the anterior aspects of the L4, L5, and S1 vertebrae along with the discs and anterior longitudinal ligament with careful deep palpation. The abdomen may also be carefully palpated for symptoms (e.g., pain, muscle spasm) arising from internal organs. For example, the appendix is palpated in the right lower quadrant and the liver in the right upper quadrant; the kidneys are located in the left and right upper quadrants, and the spleen is found in the left upper quadrant.

Inguinal Area. The inguinal area is located between the ASIS and the symphysis pubis. The examiner should carefully palpate for symptoms of a hernia, abscess, infection (lymph nodes), or other pathological conditions in the area.

Iliac Crest. The examiner palpates the iliac crest from the ASIS, moving posteriorly and looking for any symptoms (e.g., hip pointer or apophysitis).

Symphysis Pubis. The examiner uses both thumbs to palpate the symphysis pubis. Standing at the patient's side, the examiner pushes both thumbs down onto the symphysis pubis so that the thumbs rest on the superior aspect of the pubic bones (see Figure 10-15). In this way, one can ensure that the two pubic bones are level. The

symphysis pubis and pubic bones may also be carefully palpated for any tenderness (e.g., osteitis pubis).

Posterior Aspect

The patient is then asked to lie prone, and the following structures are palpated posteriorly (Figure 9-94).

Spinous Processes of the Lumbar Spine. The examiner palpates a point in the midline, which is on a line joining the high point of the two iliac crests. This point is the L4–L5 interspace. After moving down to the first hard mass, the fingers will be resting on the spinous process of L5. Moving toward the head, the interspaces and spinous processes of the remaining lumbar vertebrae can be palpated. In addition to looking for tenderness, muscle spasm, and other signs of pathology, the examiner should watch for signs of a spondylolisthesis, which is most likely to occur at L4–L5 or L5–S1. A visible or palpable dip or protrusion from one spinous process to another may be evident, depending on the type of spondylolisthesis present. In addition, absence of a spinous process may be seen in a spina bifida. If the examiner moves laterally 2 to 3 cm (0.8 to 1.2 inches) from the spinous processes, the fingers will be resting over the lumbar facet joints. These joints should also be palpated for signs of pathology. Because of the depth of these joints, the examiner may have difficulty palpating them. However, pathology in this area results in spasm of the overlying paraspinal muscles, which can be palpated.

Sacrum, Sacral Hiatus, and Coccyx. If the examiner returns to the spinous process of L5 and moves caudally, the fingers will be resting on the sacrum. Like the lumbar spine, the sacrum has spinous processes, but they are much harder to distinguish because there are no interposing soft-tissue spaces between them. The S2 spinous process is at the level of a line joining the two PSISs ("posterior dimples"). Moving distally, the examiner's fingers may palpate the sacral hiatus, which is the caudal portion of the sacral canal. It has an inverted U shape and lies approximately 5 cm (2 inches) above the tip of the

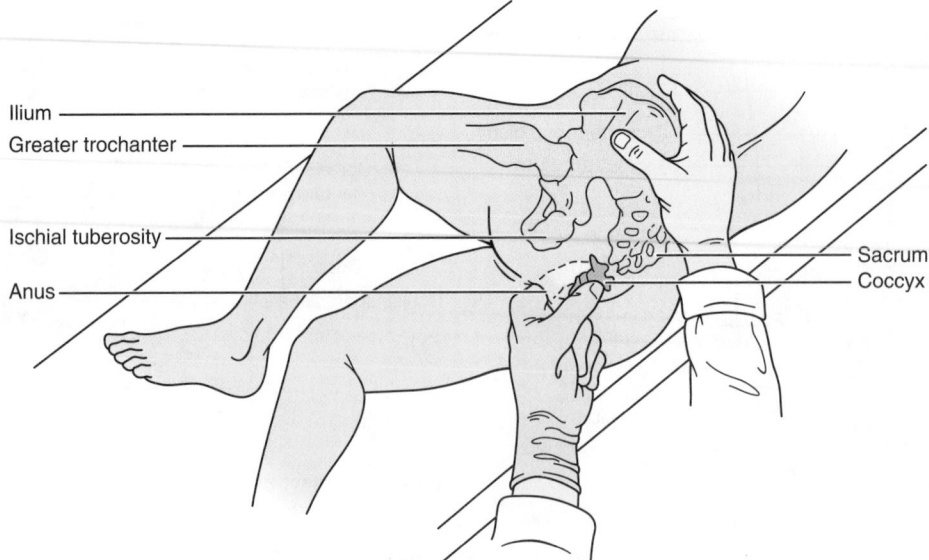

Ilium

Greater trochanter

Ischial tuberosity

Anus

Sacrum

Coccyx

Figure 9-95 Palpation of the coccyx.

coccyx. The two bony prominences on each side of the hiatus are called the **sacral cornua** (see Figure 10-67). As the examiner's fingers move farther distally, they eventually rest on the posterior aspect of the coccyx. Proper palpation of the coccyx requires a rectal examination using a surgical rubber glove (Figure 9-95). The index finger is lubricated and inserted into the anus while the patient's sphincter muscles are relaxed. The finger is inserted as far as possible and then rotated so that the pulpy surface rests against the anterior surface of the coccyx. The examiner then places the thumb of the same hand against the posterior aspect of the sacrum. In this way, the coccyx can be moved back and forth. Any major tenderness (e.g., coccyodynia) should be noted.

Iliac Crest, Ischial Tuberosity, and Sciatic Nerve. Beginning at the PSISs, the examiner moves along the iliac crest, palpating for signs of pathology. Then, moving slightly distally, the examiner palpates the gluteal muscles for spasm, tenderness, or the presence of abnormal nodules. Just under the gluteal folds, the examiner should palpate the ischial tuberosities on both sides for any abnormality. As the examiner moves laterally, the greater trochanter of the femur is palpated. It is often easier to palpate if the hip is flexed to 90°. Midway between the ischial tuberosity and the greater trochanter, the examiner may be able to palpate the path of the sciatic nerve. The nerve itself is not usually palpable. Deep to the gluteal muscles, the piriformis muscle should also be palpated for potential pathology. This muscle is in a line dividing the PSIS of the pelvis and greater trochanter of the femur from the ASIS and ischial tuberosity of the pelvis.

Diagnostic Imaging[244–254]

It is imperative when using diagnostic imaging, to correlate clinical findings with imaging findings, because many anomalies, congenital abnormalities, and aging changes may be present that are not related to the patient's problems and may be seen in asymptomatic individuals.[255,256]

Risk Factors for Vertebral Fractures[256]

- Age 50 years or older
- Significant trauma (external trauma or fall from a height)
- History of osteoporosis
- Corticosteroid use
- Substance abuse (higher rate of trauma)

Plain Film Radiography

Routine plane lumbosacral x-rays are most appropriate when risk factors of a vertebral fracture are present or if patient has not improved after a course of conservative treatment (about 1 month).[256] In adults under 50 years of age with no signs or symptoms of systemic disease, imaging is not required.[257] For patients over 50 years of age, plain x-rays and laboratory tests can rule out most systemic diseases.[257]

Normally, anteroposterior and lateral views are taken.[258] In some cases, two lateral views may be taken, one that shows the whole lumbar spine, and one that focuses on the lower two segments. Oblique views are taken if spondylolysis or spondylolisthesis is suspected.[123]

Anteroposterior View. With this view (Figure 9-96), the examiner should note the following:

1. Shape of the vertebrae.
2. Any wedging of the vertebrae, possibly resulting from fracture (Figure 9-99).
3. Disc spaces. Do they appear normal, or are there height decreases, as occurs in spondylosis?

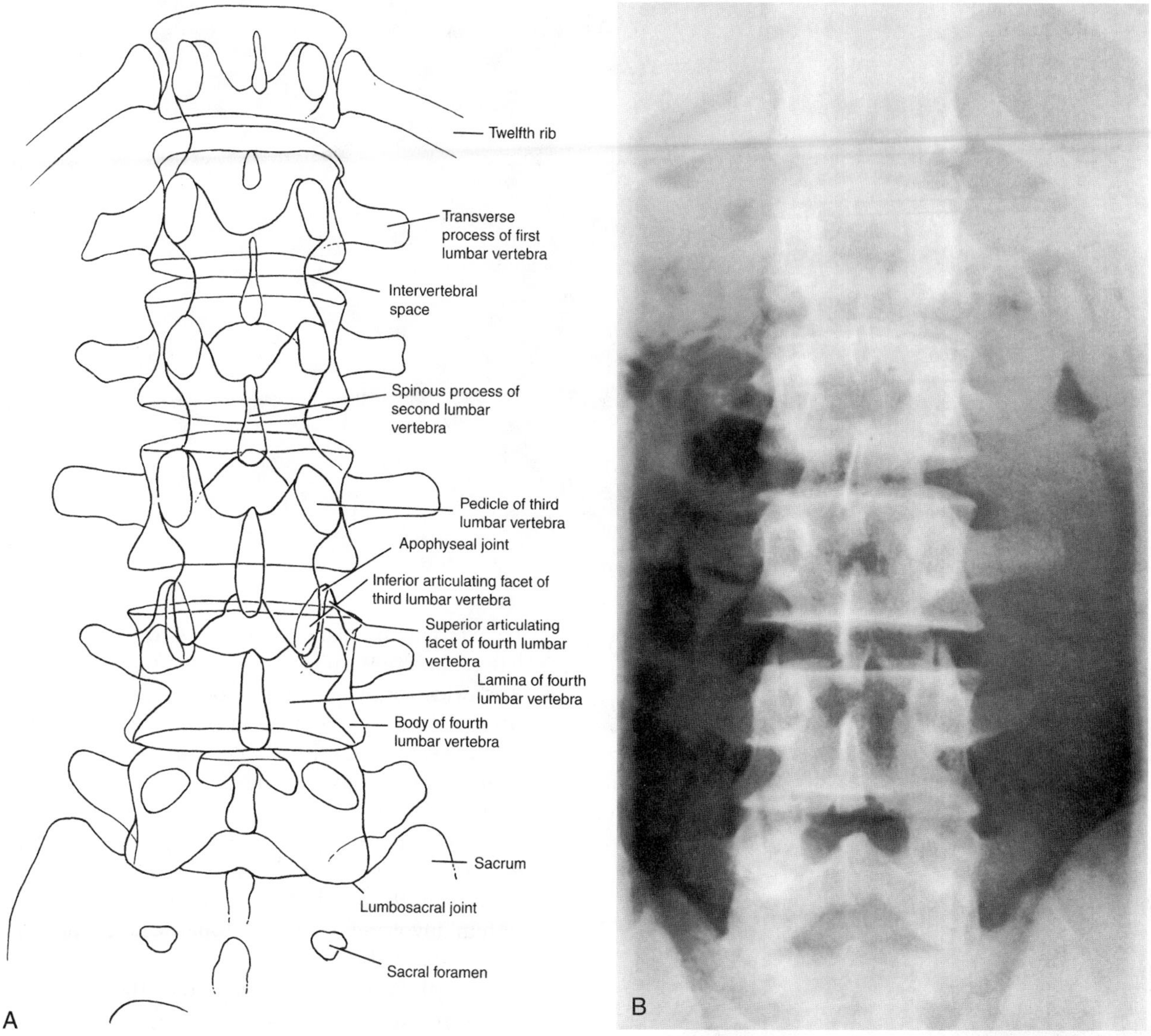

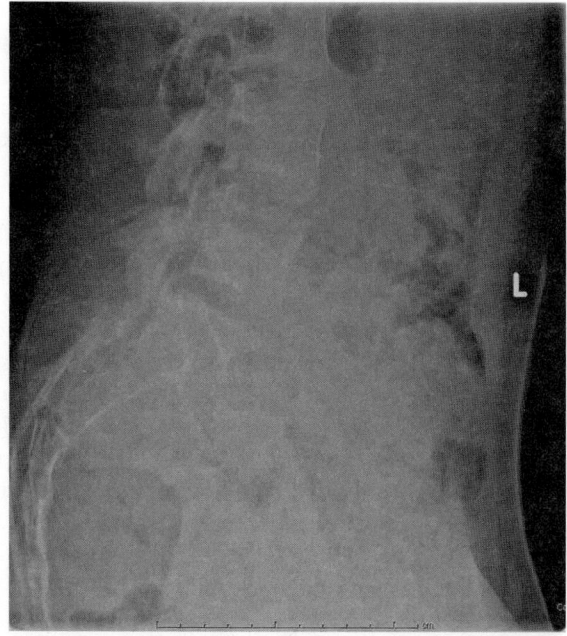

Figure 9-96 **Anteroposterior radiograph of the lumbar spine. A,** Film tracing. **B,** Radiograph. (From Finneson BE: Low back pain, Philadelphia, 1973, JB Lippincott, pp. 52–53.)

— Twelfth rib

Transverse process of first lumbar vertebra

Intervertebral space

Spinous process of second lumbar vertebra

Pedicle of third lumbar vertebra

Apophyseal joint

Inferior articulating facet of third lumbar vertebra

Superior articulating facet of fourth lumbar vertebra

Lamina of fourth lumbar vertebra

Body of fourth lumbar vertebra

Sacrum

Lumbosacral joint

Sacral foramen

A

B

Figure 9-97 **Lateral L5–S1 (coned) view of the lumbar spine.**

Common X-Ray Views of the Lumbar Spine Depending on Pathology

- Anteroposterior view (see Figure 9-96)
- Lateral view (see Figure 9-106)
- Oblique view (spondylosis, spondylolisthesis) (see Figure 9-110)
- Lateral L5–S1 (coned) view (Figure 9-97)
- Anteroposterior axial view
- Lateral view in flexion (Figure 9-98, *A*)
- Lateral view in extension (Figure 9-98, *B*)

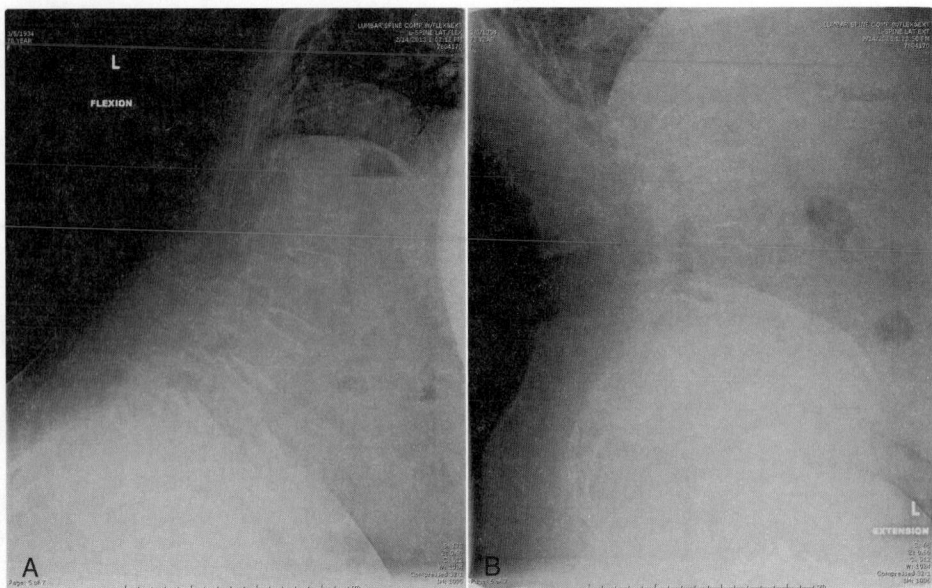

Figure 9-98 Lateral view of the lumbar spine. A, In flexion. **B,** In extension.

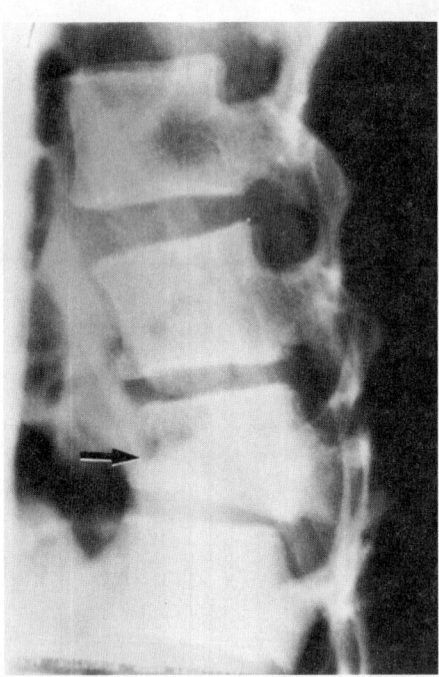

Figure 9-99 Wedging *(arrow)* of a vertebral body. Some wedging may also be seen in the vertebra above.

4. Any vertebral deformity, such as a hemivertebra or other anomalies (Figures 9-100 through 9-103).
5. The presence of a bamboo spine, as seen in ankylosing spondylitis.
6. Any evidence of lumbarization of S1, making S1–S2 the first mobile segment rather than L5–S1. Lumbarization occurs in 2% to 8% of the population (Figure 9-104).
7. Any evidence of sacralization of L5, making the L4–L5 level the first mobile segment rather than L5–S1. This anomaly occurs in 3% to 6% of the population (Figure 9-105).
8. Any evidence of spina bifida occulta, which occurs in 6% to 10% of the population (see Figure 9-102).

Lateral View. With this view (Figure 9-106), the examiner should note the following:

1. Any evidence of spondylosis or spondylolisthesis, which occurs in 2% to 4% of the population (Figure 9-107). The degree of slipping can be graded as shown in Figure 9-108.[259] New grading or classification system involving lateral sacropelvic and spinopelvic balance have also been suggested.[260]
2. A normal lordosis. Do the intervertebral foramina appear normal?
3. Any wedging of the vertebrae.
4. Normal disc spacing.
5. Alignment of the vertebrae should be noted. Disruption of the curve may indicate spinal instability.
6. Any osteophyte formation or traction spurs (Figure 9-109).[251,261] Traction spurs indicate an unstable lumbar intervertebral segment. A traction spur occurs approximately 1 mm from the disc border; an osteophyte occurs at the disc border with the vertebral body.

Oblique View. With the oblique view (Figure 9-110), the examiner should look for any evidence of spondylolisthesis (sometimes referred to as a "Scottie dog decapitated") or spondylolysis (sometimes referred to as a "Scottie dog with a collar;" Figure 9-111).

Motion Views. In some cases, motion views may be used to demonstrate abnormal spinal motion or structural abnormalities. These are usually lateral views showing flexion and extension to demonstrate instability or spondylolisthesis (Figure 9-112), but they may also include anteroposterior views with side bending.[166,262,263]

Text continued on p. 630

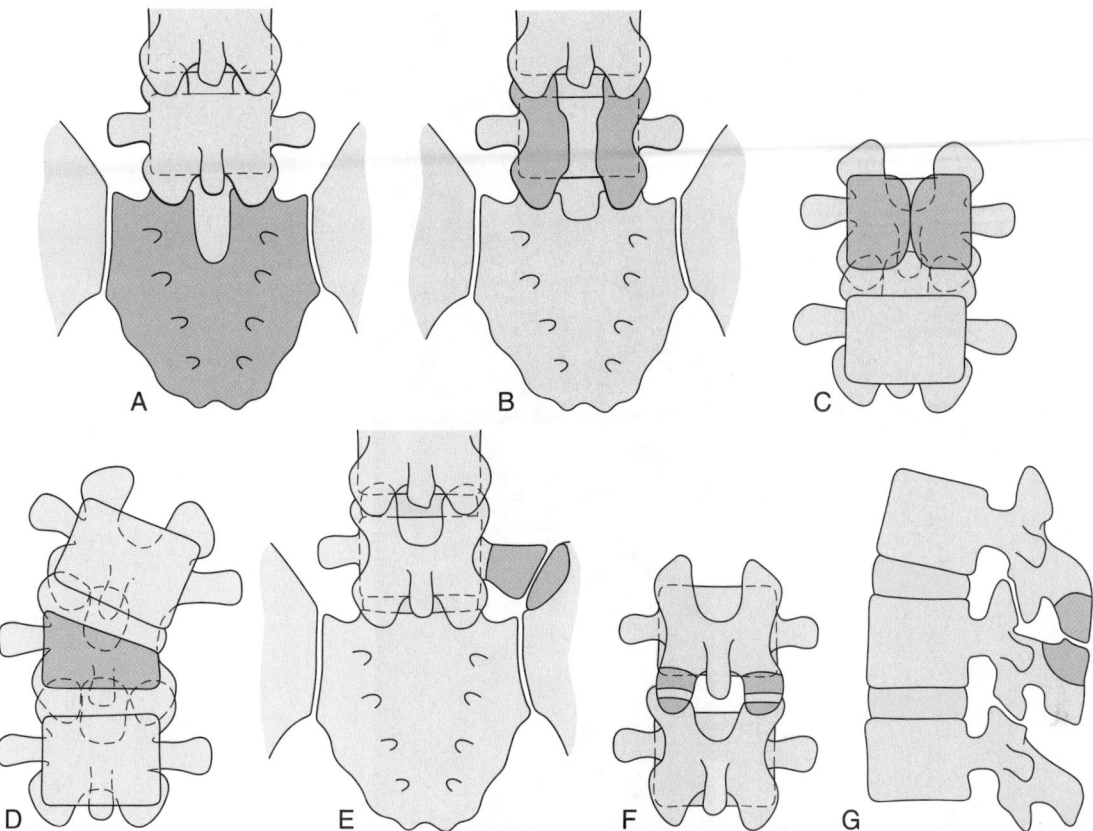

Figure 9-100 Diagrammatic representation of the x-ray appearance of common anatomical anomalies in the lumbosacral spine. **A,** Spina bifida occulta, S1. **B,** Spina bifida, L5. **C,** Anterior spina bifida ("butterfly vertebra"). **D,** Hemivertebra. **E,** Iliotransverse joint (transitional segments). **F,** Ossicles of Oppenheimer. These are free ossicles seen at the tip of the inferior articular facets and are usually found at the level of L3. **G,** "Kissing" spinous processes. (Redrawn from MacNab I: Backache, Baltimore, 1977, Williams & Wilkins, pp. 14–15.)

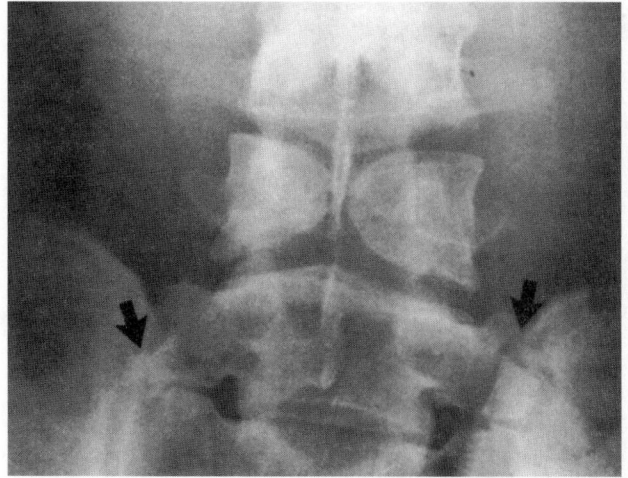

Figure 9-101 Butterfly vertebra. Also note transitional segments *(large arrows)*. (Modified from Jaeger SA: Atlas of radiographic positioning: normal anatomy and developmental variants, Norwalk, CT, 1988, Appleton & Lange, p. 333.)

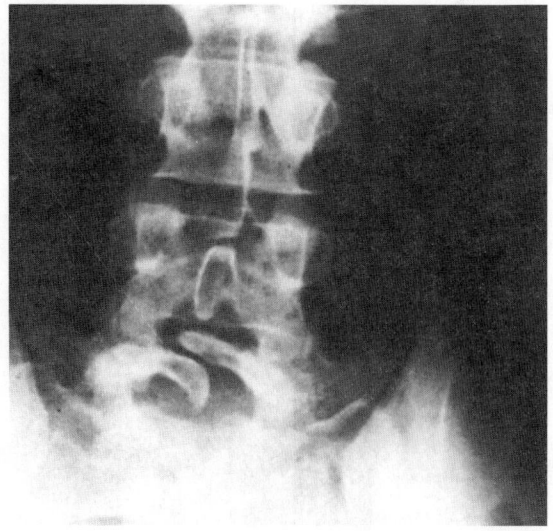

Figure 9-102 Spina bifida occulta. (From Jaeger SA: Atlas of radiographic positioning: normal anatomy and developmental variants, Norwalk, CT, 1988, Appleton & Lange, p. 317.)

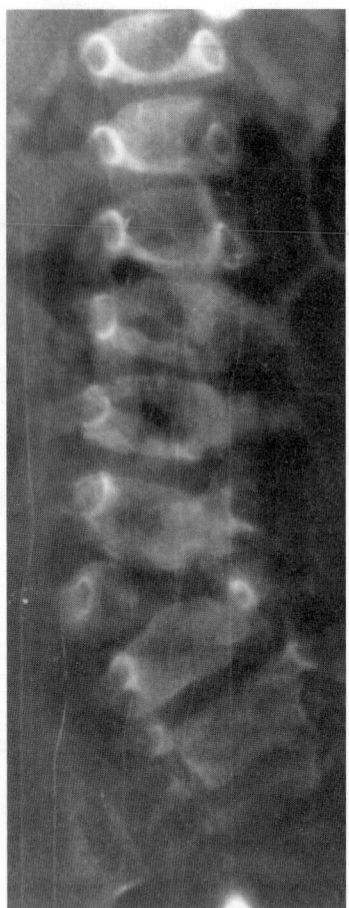

Figure 9-103 Hemivertebra shown on an anteroposterior radiograph.

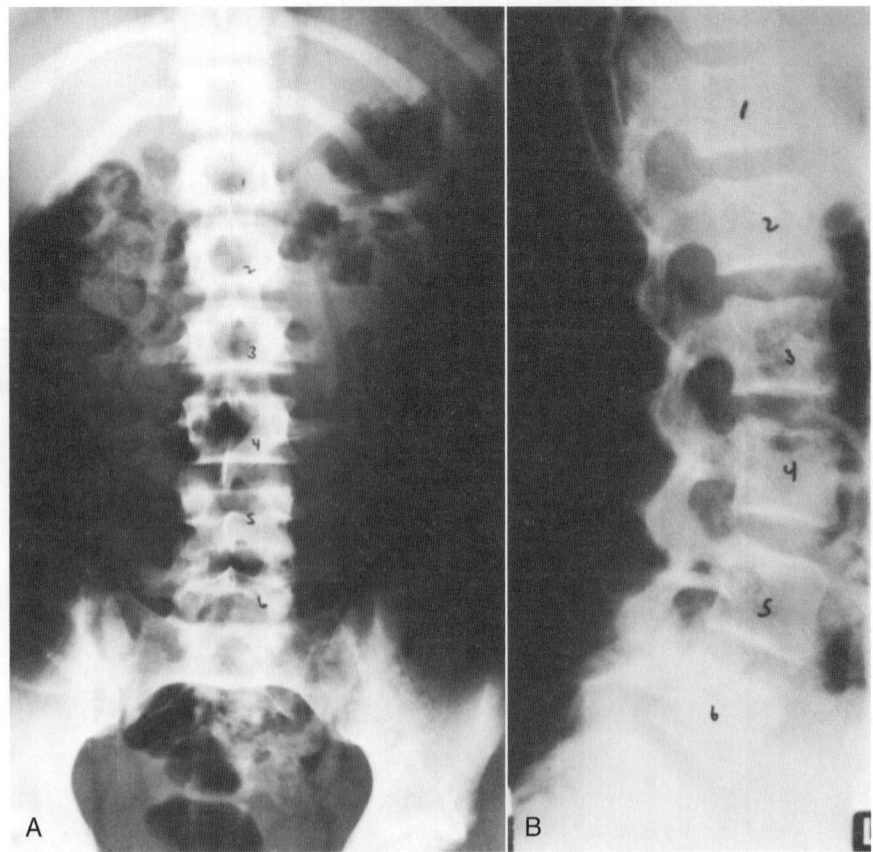

Figure 9-104 Lumbarization of the S1 vertebra seen on anteroposterior (**A**) and lateral (**B**) radiographs.

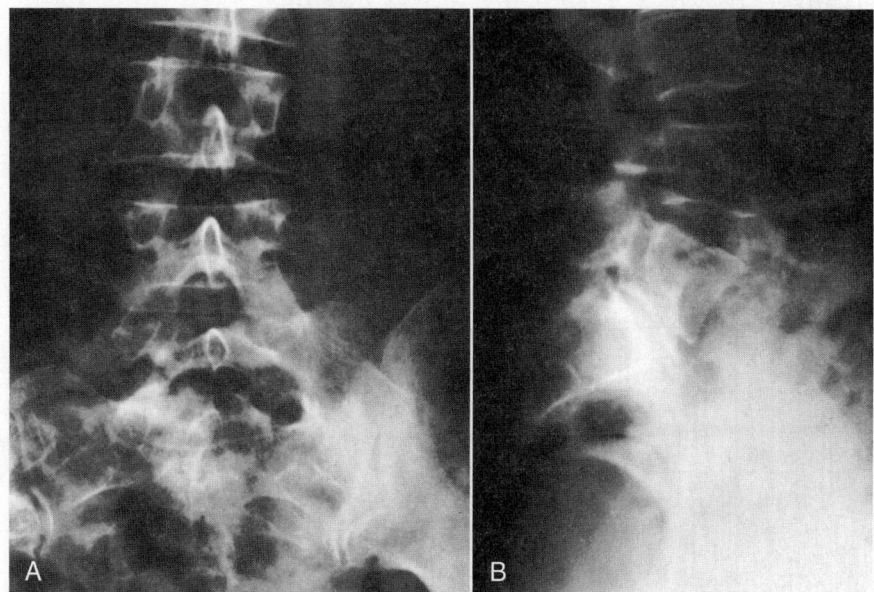

Figure 9-105 Unilateral sacralization of the fifth lumbar vertebra. A, Note the massive formation of sacral ala on the left side with a relatively normal transverse process on the right (anteroposterior view). **B,** Lateral view showing the narrow disc space and the massive arches. (From O'Donoghue DH: Treatment of injuries to athletes, ed 4, Philadelphia, 1984, WB Saunders, p. 403.)

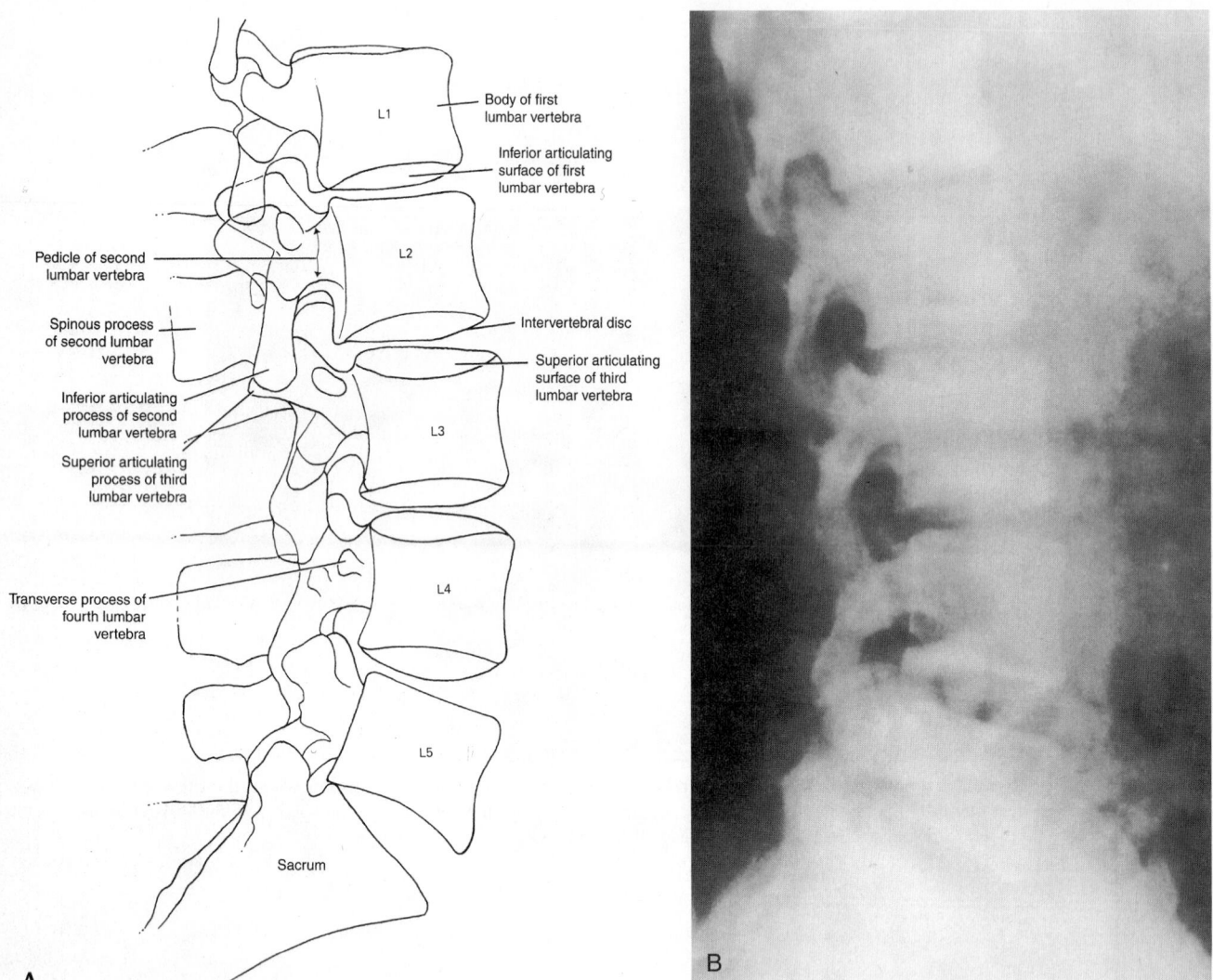

Body of first
lumbar vertebra

Inferior articulating
surface of first
lumbar vertebra

Pedicle of second
lumbar vertebra

Spinous process
of second lumbar
vertebra

Intervertebral disc

Superior articulating
surface of third
lumbar vertebra

Inferior articulating
process of second
lumbar vertebra

Superior articulating
process of third
lumbar vertebra

Transverse process of
fourth lumbar
vertebra

Sacrum

L1
L2
L3
L4
L5

A

B

Figure 9-106 Lateral radiograph of the lumbar spine. A, Film tracing. **B,** Radiograph. (From Finneson BE: Low back pain, Philadelphia, 1973, JB Lippincott, pp. 54–55.)

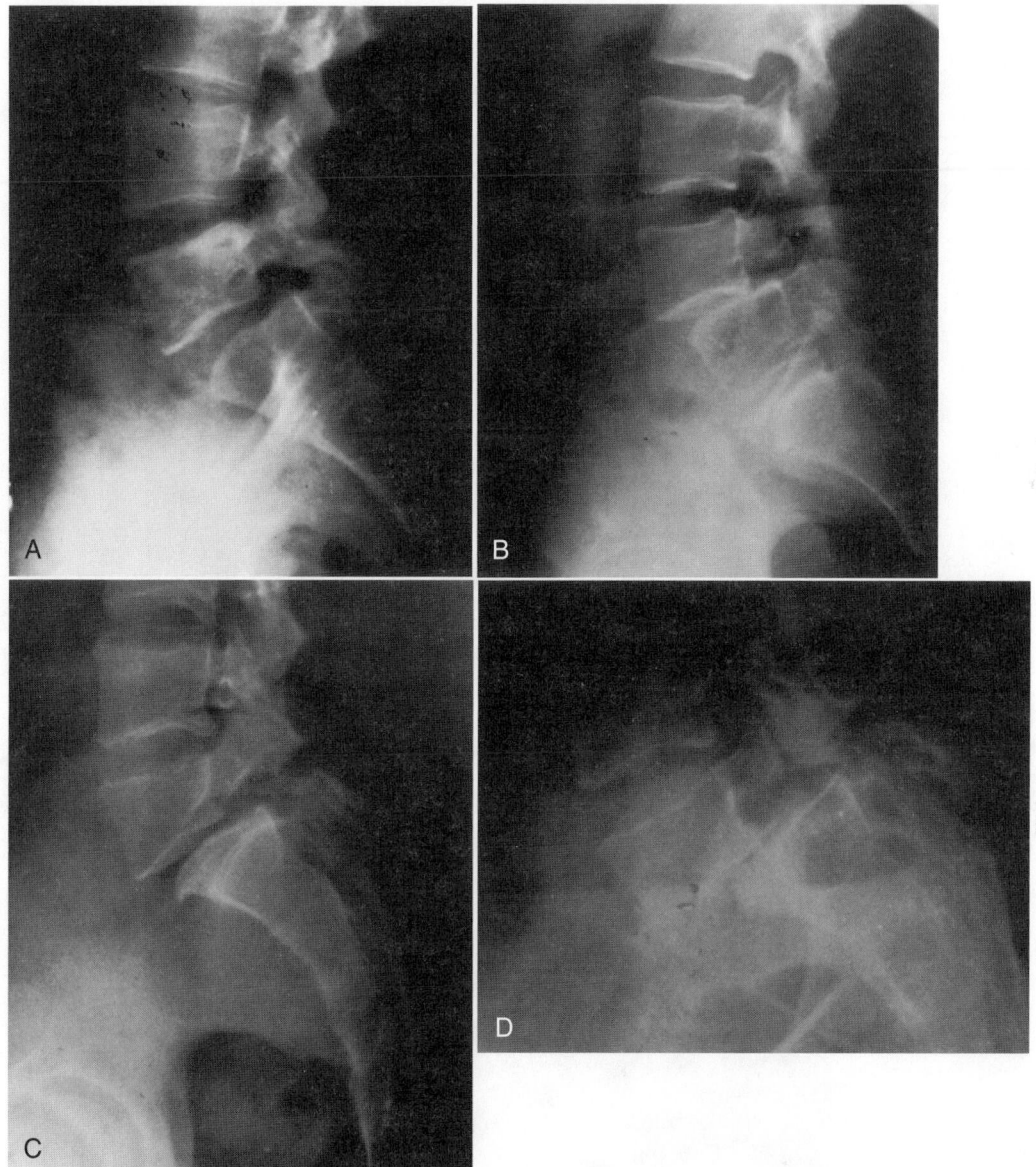

Figure 9-107 Spondylolisthesis. A, Grade 1: Arch defect in L5 with mild forward displacement of L5 on S1; backache but no gross disability. **B,** Grade 2: More forward slipping between L4 and L5 with collapse of the intervertebral disc; definite symptomatic back with restriction of motion, muscle spasm, and curtailment of activities. **C,** Grade 3: More extensive slipping combined with a wide separation at the arch defect and degenerative changes of the disc; grossly symptomatic. **D,** Grade 4: Vertebrae slipped forward more than halfway; severe disability. (From O'Donoghue DH: Treatment of injuries to athletes, ed 4, Philadelphia, 1984, WB Saunders, p. 402.)

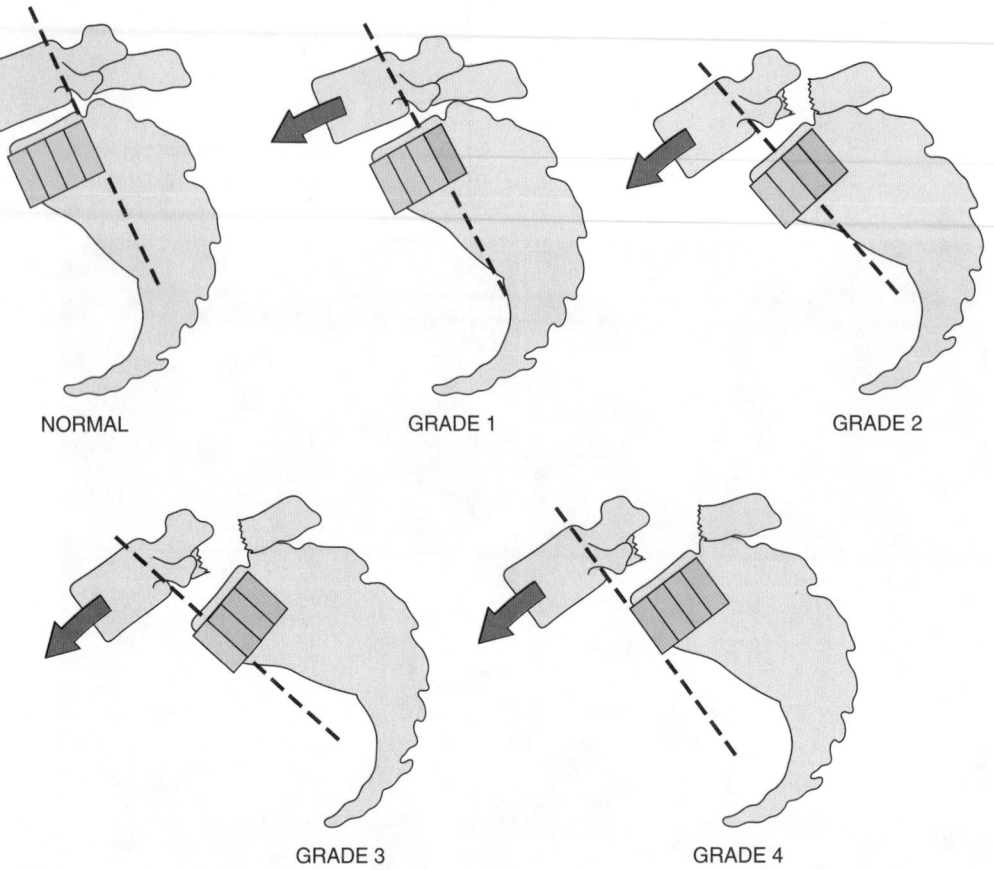

NORMAL GRADE 1 GRADE 2

GRADE 3 GRADE 4

Figure 9-108 Meyerding grading system for slipping in spondylolisthesis.

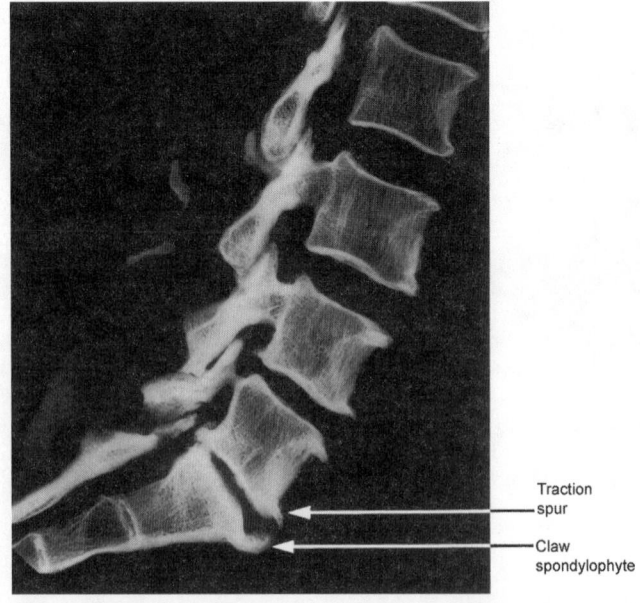

Traction spur

Claw spondylophyte

Figure 9-109 **Lateral radiograph of a thin-slice pathological section of lumbar spine.** Note traction spur and claw spondylophyte. (From Rothman RH, Simeone FA: The spine, Philadelphia, 1982, WB Saunders, p. 512.)

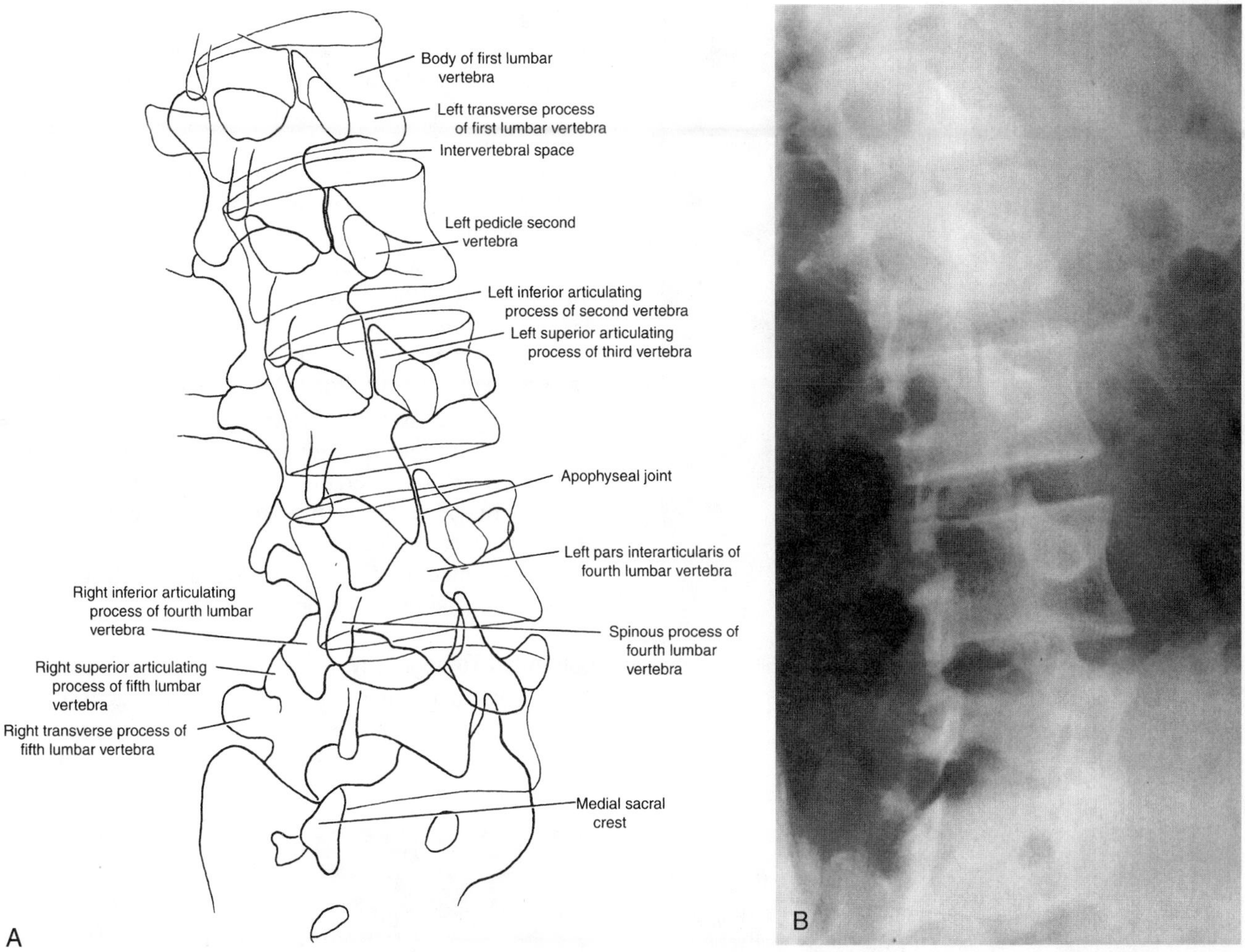

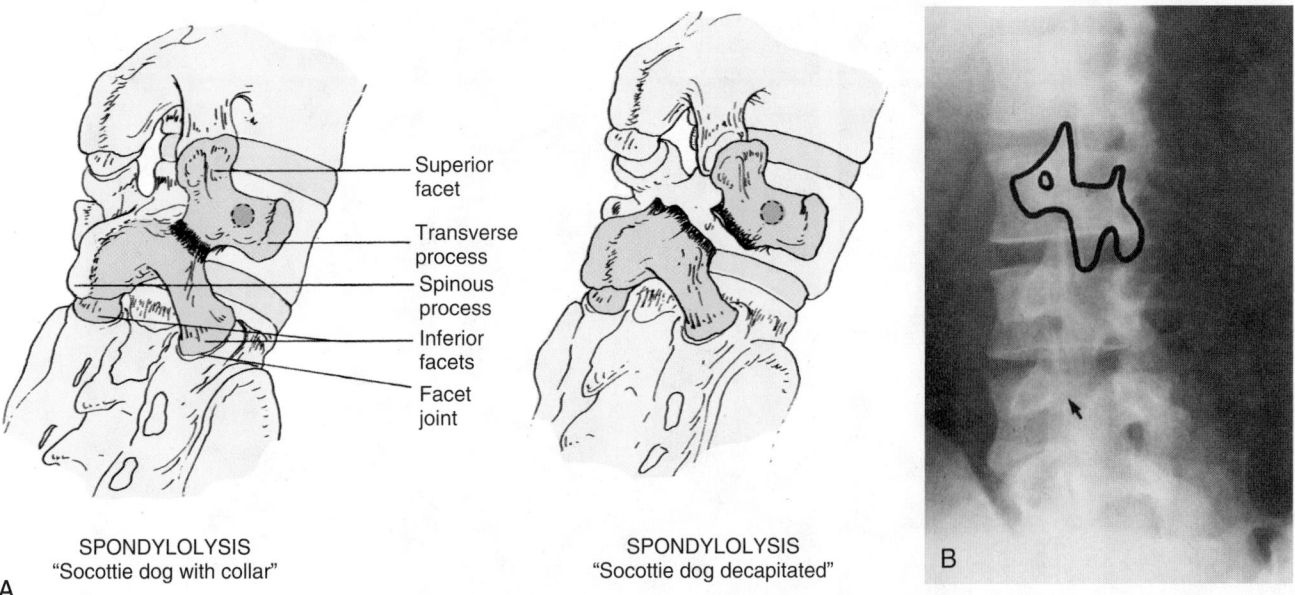

Body of first lumbar vertebra

Left transverse process of first lumbar vertebra

Intervertebral space

Left pedicle second vertebra

Left inferior articulating process of second vertebra

Left superior articulating process of third vertebra

Apophyseal joint

Left pars interarticularis of fourth lumbar vertebra

Right inferior articulating process of fourth lumbar vertebra

Spinous process of fourth lumbar vertebra

Right superior articulating process of fifth lumbar vertebra

Right transverse process of fifth lumbar vertebra

Medial sacral crest

A
B

Figure 9-110 Left posterior oblique radiograph of the lumbar spine. A, Film tracing. **B,** Radiograph. (From Finneson BE: Low back pain, Philadelphia, 1973, JB Lippincott, pp. 56–57.)

Superior facet

Transverse process

Spinous process

Inferior facets

Facet joint

SPONDYLOLYSIS
"Socottie dog with collar"

SPONDYLOLYSIS
"Socottie dog decapitated"

A
B

Figure 9-111 A, Diagrammatic representation (posterior oblique view) of spondylolysis and spondylolisthesis. **B,** Posterior oblique film showing "Scottie dog" at L2. L4 shows Scottie dog with a "collar" *(arrow),* indicating spondylolysis.

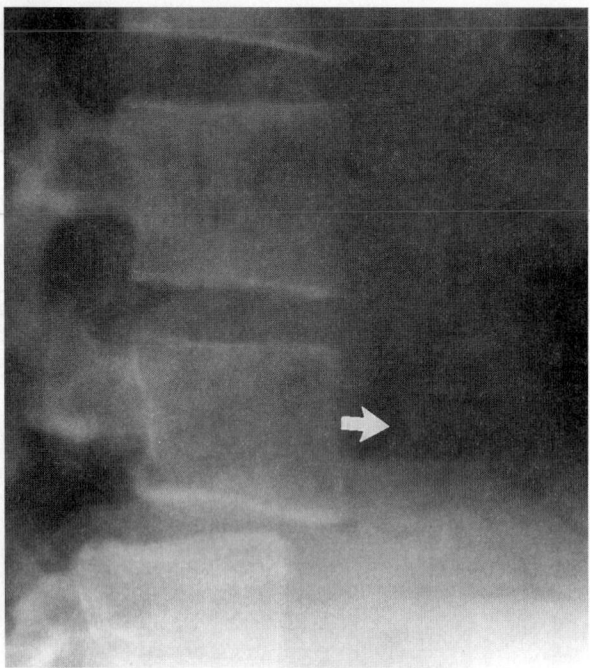

Figure 9-112 Lumbar spine in flexion. Note forward slipping of one vertebra on the one below *(arrow)*.

Myelography

A myelogram, although seldom used today because of its complications and replacement by computed tomography (CT) scans and magnetic resonance imaging (MRI), can confirm the presence of a protruding intervertebral disc, osteophytes, a tumor, or spinal stenosis (Figures 9-113 through 9-115). The examiner must be careful of the side effects of myelograms, which include headache, stiffness, low back pain, cramps, and paresthesia in the lower limbs. Although side effects do occur, no permanent injuries have been noted.

Radionuclide Imaging (Bone Scans)

Bone scans are useful for detecting active bone disease processes and areas of high bone turnover. In children, the epiphyseal and metaphyseal areas of the long bones show increased uptake. In adults, only the metaphyseal area is so affected. Traumatic bone injuries, tumors, metabolic abnormalities (e.g., Paget disease), infection, and arthritis may be detected on bone scan.[124]

Computed Tomography

A CT scan may be used to delineate a fracture or to show the presence of spinal stenosis caused by protrusion

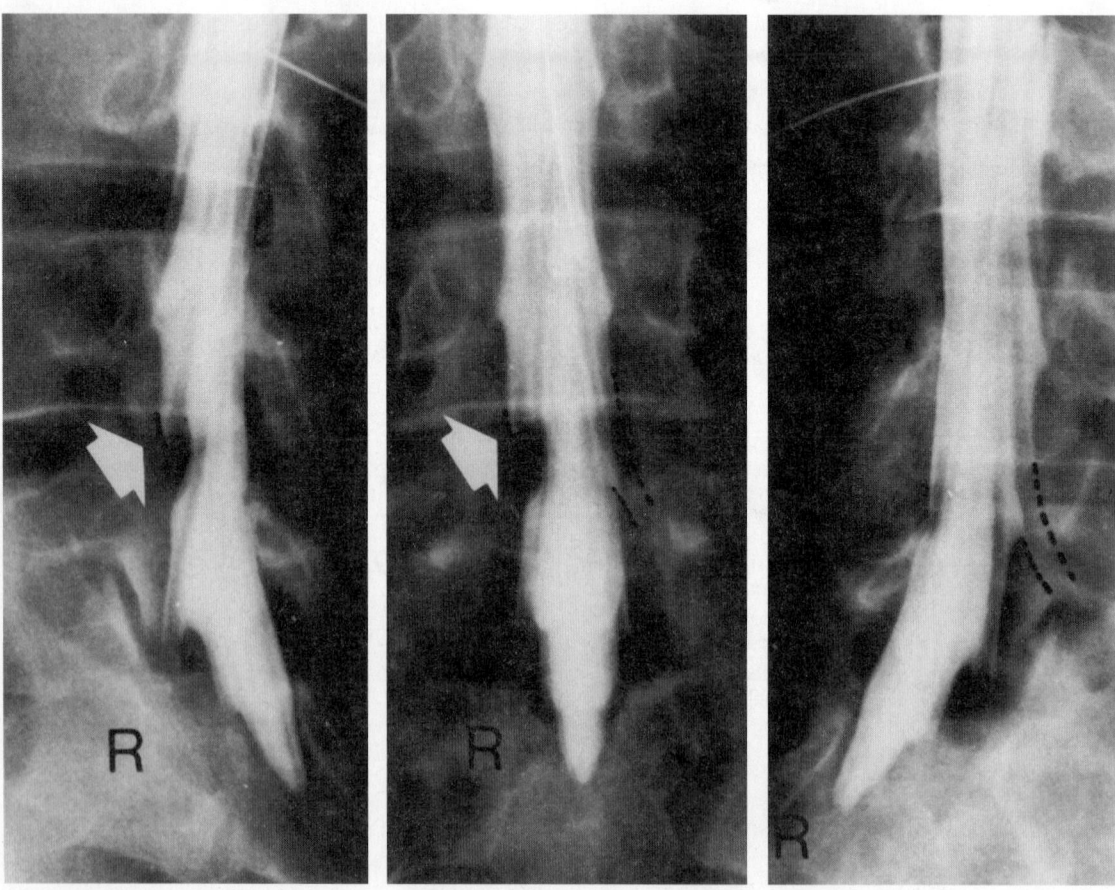

Figure 9-113 Metrizamide myelograms illustrating a herniated disc at L4–L5 on the right. Note lack of filling of the nerve root sleeve and indentation *(arrow)* of the dural sac. (From Rothman RH, Simeone FA: The spine, Philadelphia, 1982, WB Saunders, p. 550.)

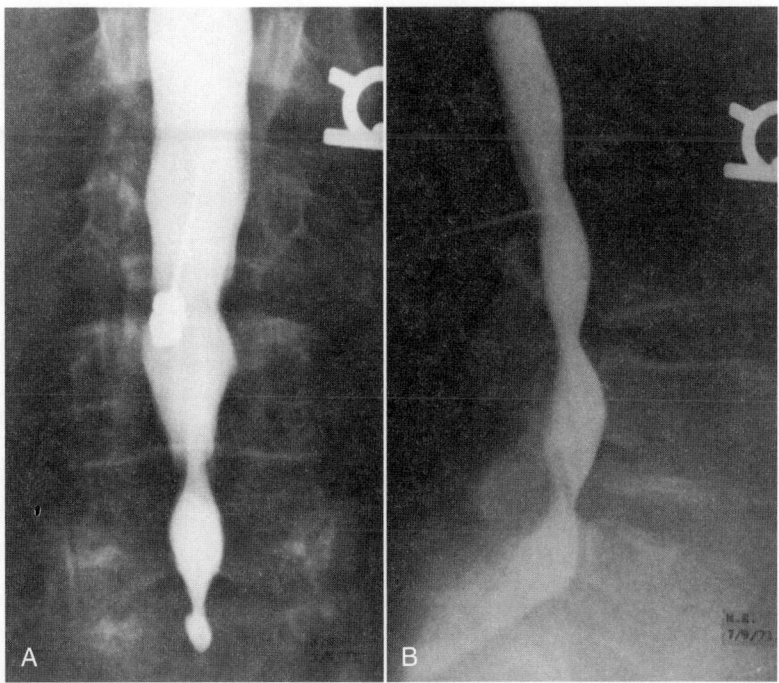

Figure 9-114 Oil myelograms showing the characteristic appearance of chronic disc degeneration and spinal stenosis with diffuse posterior bulging of the annulus and osteophyte formation. **A,** Symmetric wasting of the dye column is shown in the anteroposterior view. Note the hourglass configuration. **B,** Indentation of the dye column of the annulus anteriorly and the buckled ligamentum flavum and facet joints posteriorly (lateral view). (From Rothman RH, Simeone FA: The spine, Philadelphia, 1982, WB Saunders, p. 553.)

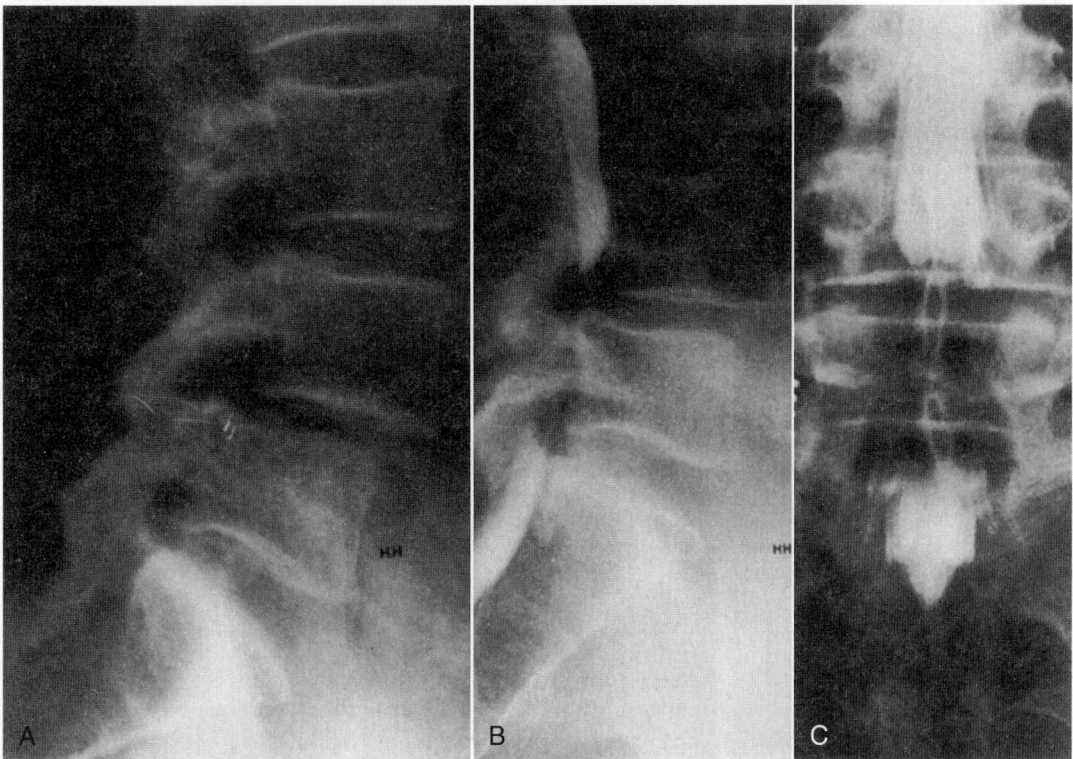

Figure 9-115 Metrizamide myelograms showing stenotic block at the L4–L5 level as a result of degenerative spondylolisthesis and spinal stenosis at the L4–L5 level. **A,** Note the 4-mm anterior migration of L4 on L5 caused by the degenerative spondylolisthesis. **B** and **C,** The extensive block on the myelogram is caused by spinal stenosis. (From Rothman RH, Simeone FA: The spine, Philadelphia, 1982, WB Saunders, p. 553.)

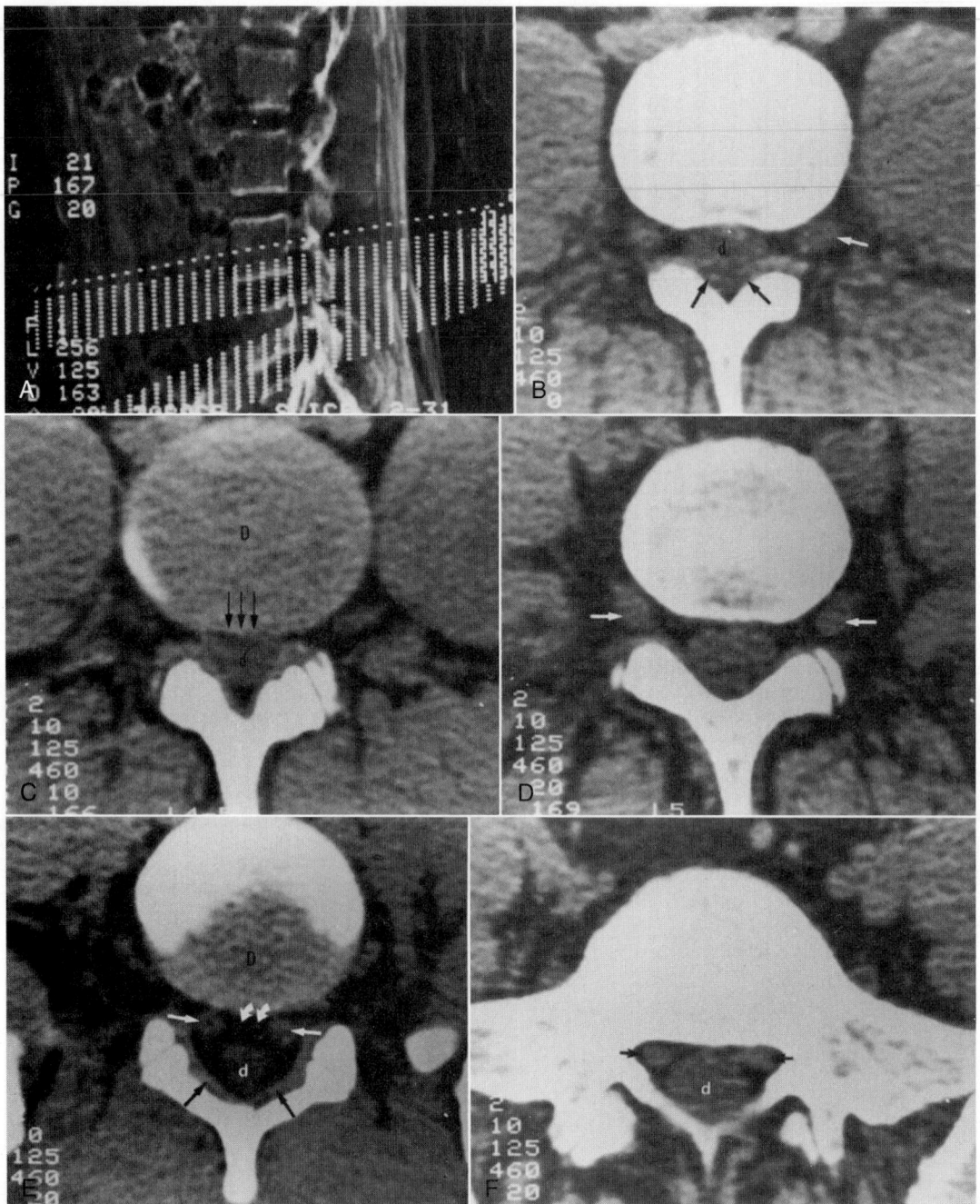

Figure 9-116 Normal disc anatomy on computed tomography (CT). A, Scout view. The chosen sections *(dashed lines)* can be planned and angled along the planes of the discs. **B,** CT scan through the L4 vertebral body shows the neural foramina and the L4 nerve root ganglia *(white arrow indicates left ganglion)*. The dural sac *(d)* and ligamenta flava *(black arrows)* are shown. **C,** CT scan through the L4–L5 disc (labeled *D*) shows very little fat between the posterior margin of the disc *(arrows)* and the dural sac *(d)*. The nerve roots are not clearly shown. **D,** CT scan through the L5 vertebral body and foramina shows the L5 nerve root ganglia *(arrows)*. **E,** CT scan through the L5–S1 disc space (labeled *D*) shows the L5 nerve roots *(straight white arrows)*, the dural sac *(d)*, and the ligamenta flava *(black arrows)*. Small epidural veins are noted *(curved arrows)*. **F,** At the S1 level, the S1 nerve roots *(arrows)* and dural sac *(d)* are clearly visualized. (From Weissman BNW, Sledge CB: Orthopedic radiology, Philadelphia, 1986, WB Saunders, p. 306.)

or a tumor, or if a bony abnormality is suspected[256] (Figures 9-116 through 9-119). As with plain x-rays, results must be correlated with clinical findings, because the anatomical changes seen are often unassociated with the patient's symptoms.[255,264,265] This technique provides an axial projection of the spine, showing the anatomy of not only the spine but also the paravertebral muscles, vascular structures, and organs of the body cavity. In doing so, it shows more precisely the relation among the intervertebral discs, spinal canal, facet joints, and intervertebral foramina. It may be used to evaluate spinal stenosis, the shape of the spinal canal, epidural scarring

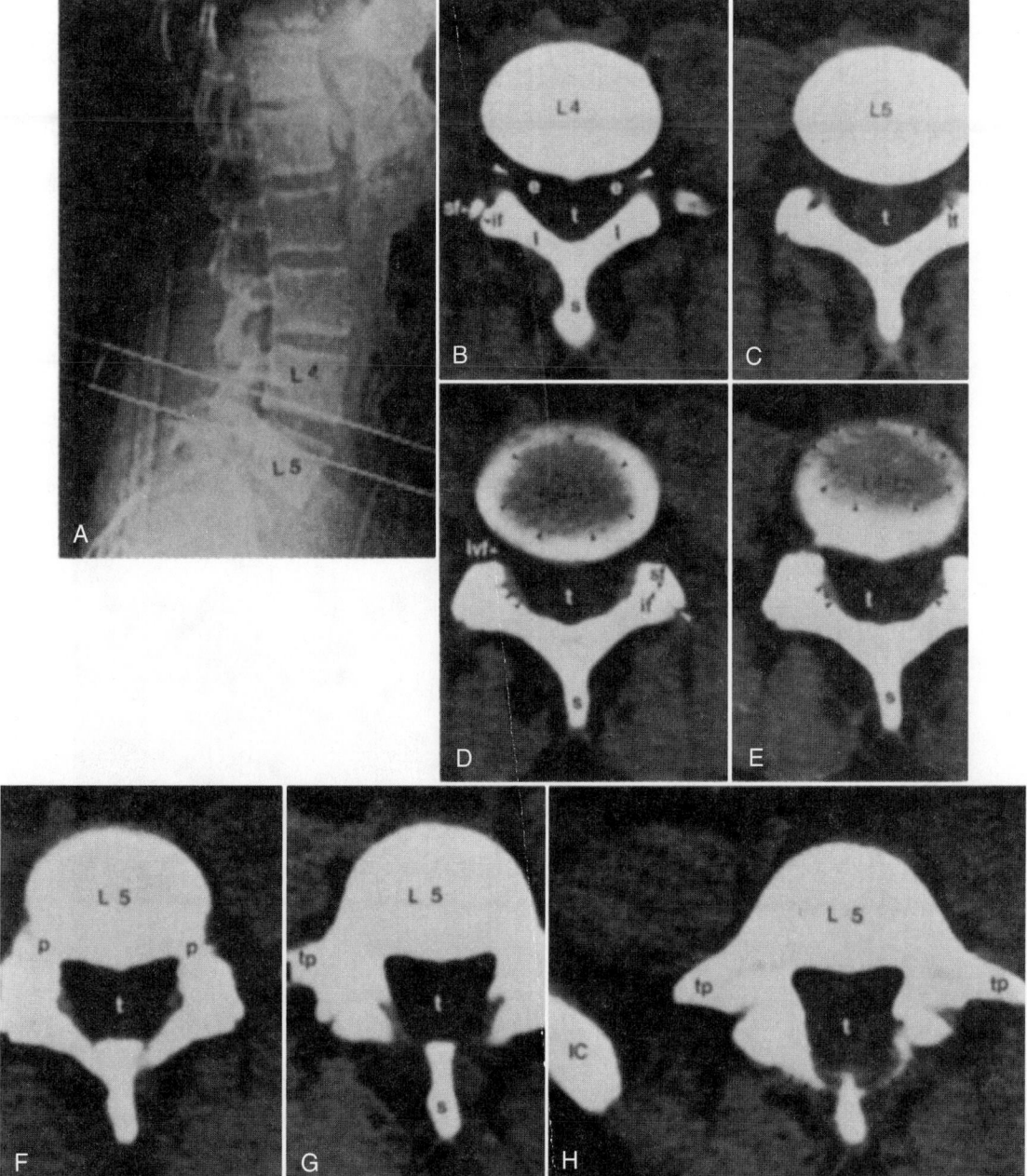

Figure 9-117 Soft-tissue detail of the L4–L5 intervertebral disc space on computed tomography (CT). A, Lateral digital scout view obtained through the lumbosacral spine. The upper and lower scan limits through the L4–L5 region are designated with an electronic cursor. Scan collimation is 5 mm thick; incrementation is 3 mm (2-mm overlap). **B,** Axial CT section of L4. The L4 root ganglia and spinal nerves are seen within the intervertebral foramina *(white arrowheads)* surrounded by abundant epidural fat *(e)*. The thecal sac *(t)* is bounded anterolaterally by fat in the lateral recess. The posterior arch of L4 consists of inferior facets *(if)*, laminae *(l)*, and spinous process *(s)*. The superior facet of L5 *(sf)* is just visible. **C,** The next lower axial section demonstrates the L4–L5 facet articulations. The ligamentum flavum *(lf)* is contiguous with the facet joint capsule. Again, the thecal sac *(t)* is readily apparent; it is slightly higher in density than the adjacent epidural fat. Note that without subarachnoid contrast media, the intrathecal contents cannot be discerned. **D,** Axial CT section of the L4–L5 disc space. The disc *(multiple black arrowheads)* is a region of central hypodensity surrounded by the cortical margin of L4. The posterior arch of L4 projects below the disc level. The intervertebral foramina *(ivf)* have begun to close. The cartilaginous articular surfaces *(white arrowhead)* between superior *(sf)* and inferior *(if)* facets are poorly demonstrated with these window settings. The ligamentum flavum *(double black arrowheads)* is noted medial to the facet joints. *s,* Spinous process; *t,* thecal sac. **E,** The next inferior CT section demonstrates the disc *(multiple arrowheads)* positioned somewhat more anteriorly, marginated posteriorly at this level by the posterosuperior cortical rim of the L5 body. The ligamentum flavum *(double arrowheads)* normally maintains a flat medial surface adjacent to the thecal sac *(t)*. The posterior arch of L4 and its spinous process *(s)* are still in view. **F,** Axial CT section through the L5 body at the level of the pedicles *(p)*. The canal now completely encloses the thecal sac *(t)*. **G,** Immediately below, only the spinous process *(s)* of the posterior arch of L4 is visible. The transverse process *(tp)* of L5 is noted. *t,* Thecal sac. **H,** At the level of the iliac crest *(IC)*, the posterior arch of L5 *(small arrowheads)* has just begun to form. The transverse processes *(tp)* are quite large at this level. *t,* Thecal sac. (From LeMasters DL, Dowart RL: High-resolution, cross-sectional computed tomography of the normal spine. Orthop Clin North Am 16:359, 1985.)

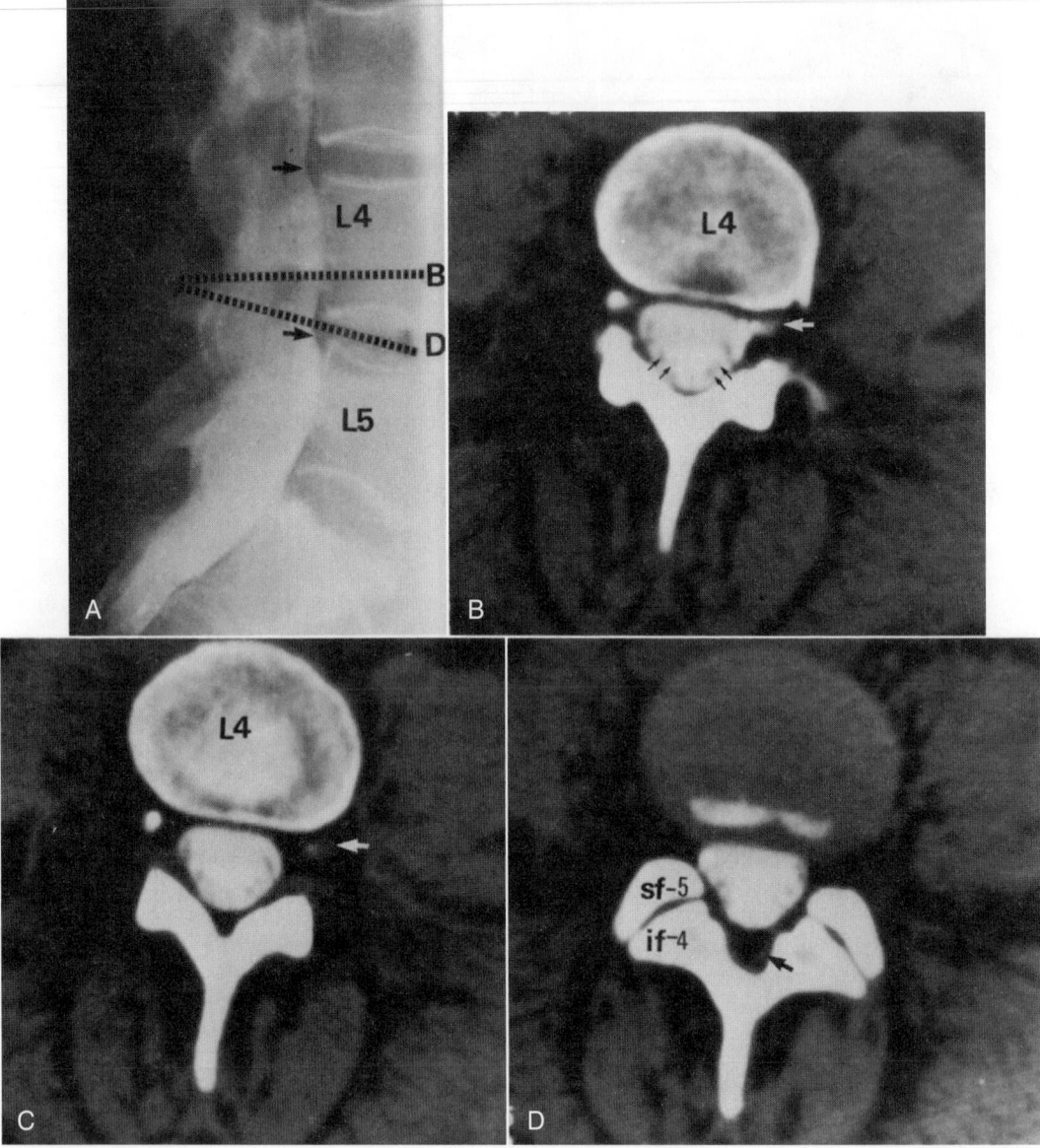

Figure 9-118 Computed tomography (CT) anatomy of L4 nerve roots. A, Lateral view during metrizamide myelography showing indentations on the anterior aspect of the contrast column *(arrows)* at L3–L4 and L4–L5 resulting from bulging intervertebral discs. The levels for subsequent CT sections B and D are marked. **B,** CT section through the L4 vertebra and L4–L5 foramina 1 hour after a metrizamide myelogram. Contrast agent fills the left axillary pouch *(white arrow)* and the right nerve root sleeve. Small arrows indicate the filling defects produced by the remaining nerve roots. **C,** CT section slightly more distal than B shows the L4 nerve root ganglia (left ganglion is indicated by arrow). **D,** Section through the L4–L5 disc and the posterior inferior body of L4 shows an abnormally bulging disc without compression of the subarachnoid space. The ligamentum flavum on the left *(arrow)*, the superior facet of L5 *(sf-5)*, and the inferior facet of L4 *(if-4)* are indicated. (From Weissman BNW, Sledge CB: Orthopedic radiology, Philadelphia, 1986, WB Saunders, p. 284.)

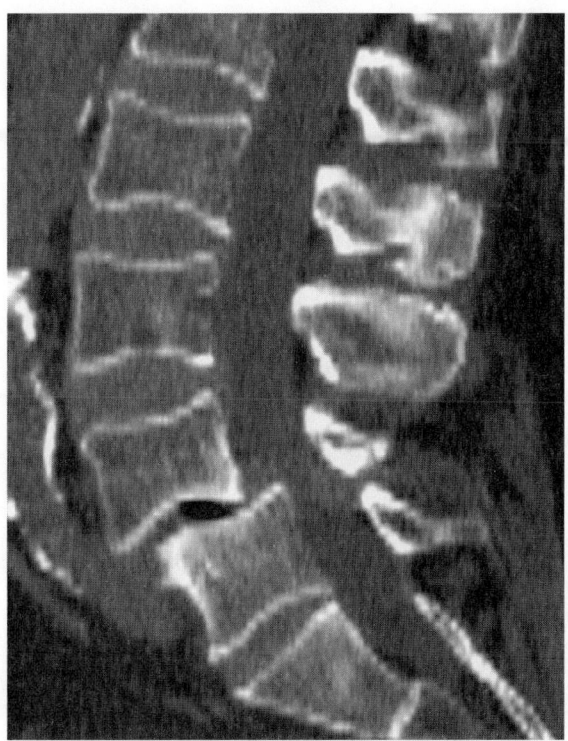

Figure 9-119 Degenerative spondylolisthesis. Sagittal reformatted image derived from transverse CT scans of the lumbar spine shows degeneration at the L4–L5 level with a vacuum phenomenon. A grade II spondylolisthesis at the L4–L5 level results from osteoarthritis of the facet joints. (From Resnick D, Kransdorf MJ: Bone and joint imaging, Philadelphia, 2005, WB Saunders, p. 146.)

(after surgery), facet joint arthritis, tumors, and trauma.[124,266,267] It may be used in conjunction with a water-soluble contrast medium (computer-assisted myelography) to further delineate the structures.

Magnetic Resonance Imaging

MRI is a noninvasive technique that can be used in several planes (transaxial, coronal, or sagittal) to delineate bony and soft tissues. This technique is commonly used to diagnose tumors, to view the spinal cord within the spinal canal, and to assess for syringomyelia, cord infarction, or traumatic injury.[124,268] The delineation of soft tissues is much greater with MRI than with CT.[269] For example, with MRI, the nucleus pulposus and the annulus fibrosis are easier to differentiate because of their different water contents, making it the preferred imaging modality for disc disease and radiculopathy (Figures 9-120 through 9-124).[23,256,270,271] As with other diagnostic imaging techniques, clinical findings must support what is seen before the structural abnormalities can be considered the source of the problem.[255,264,272–274] Up to 30% of asymptomatic patients with no history of low back pain show disc abnormalities.[23,275] Things to look for on MRI are disc height, presence or absence of annular tears, degenerative signs, and end plate changes.[23]

Discography[276]

For discography, radiopaque dye is injected into the nucleus pulposus. It is not a commonly used technique but may be used to see whether injection of dye reproduces the patient's symptoms, making it diagnostic (Figure 9-125).

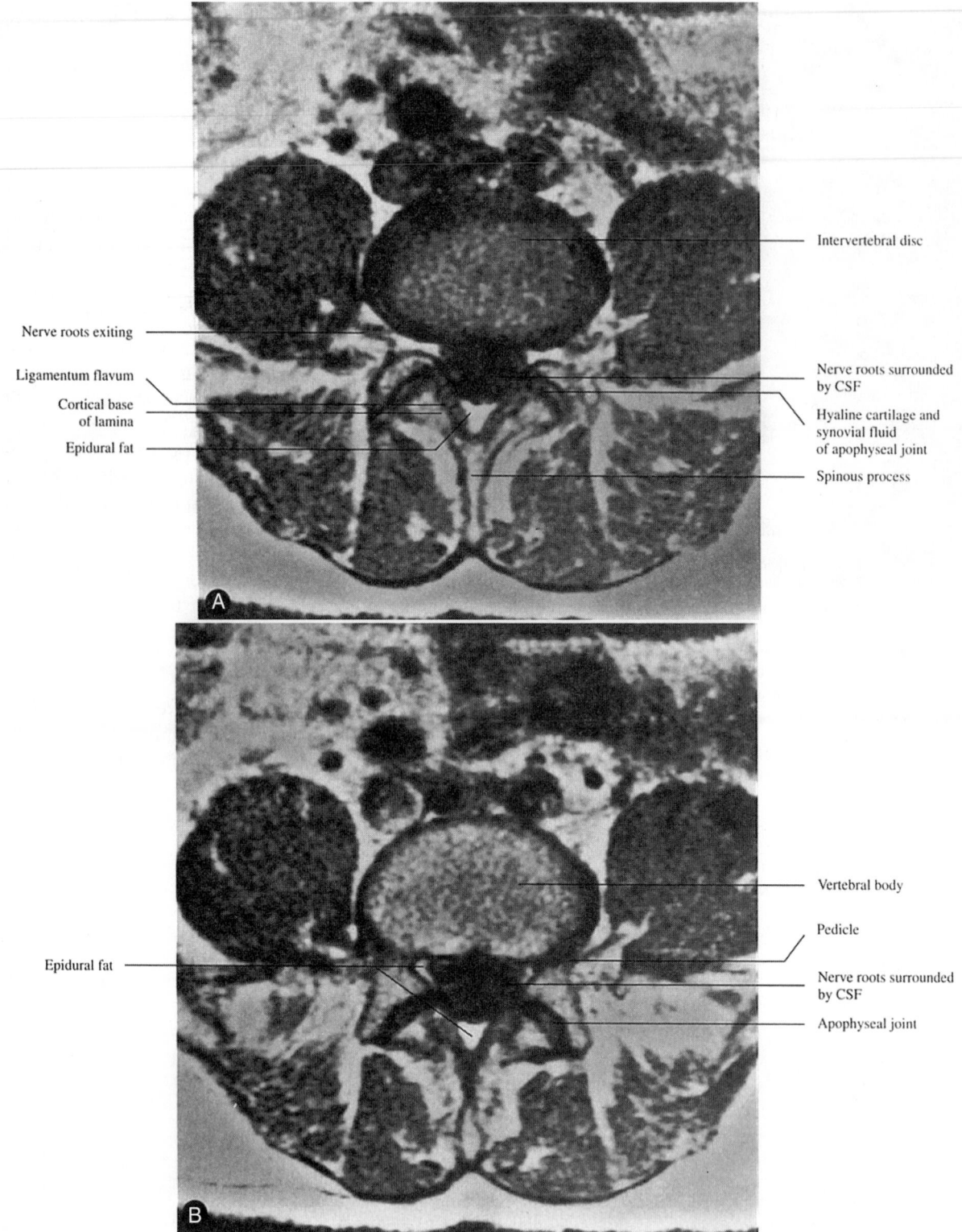

Figure 9-120 Magnetic resonance imaging (MRI) of normal lumbar spine. A, Level of neural canal. **B,** Level of pedicle. *CSF,* Cerebrospinal fluid. (From Bassett LW, Gold RH, Seeger LL: MRI atlas of the musculoskeletal system, London, 1989, Martin Dunitz, p. 40.)

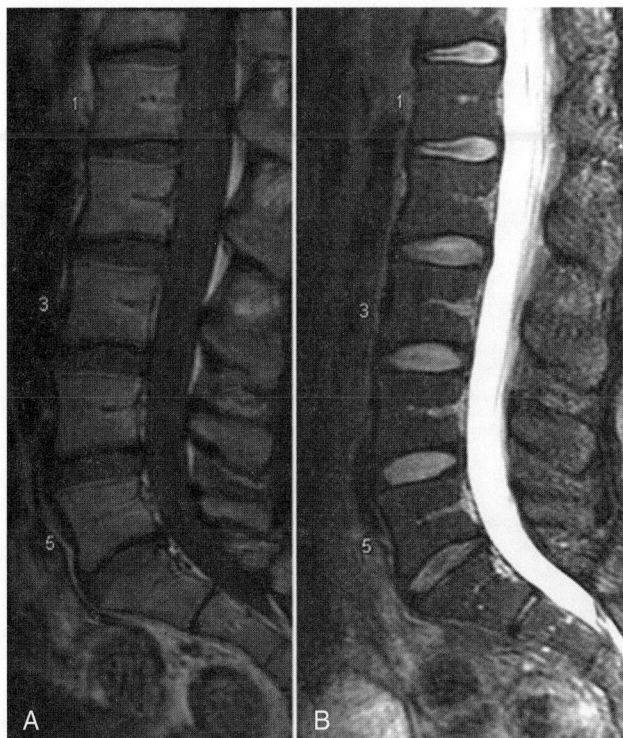

Figure 9-121 Sagittal **(A)** T$_1$-weighted and **(B)** fat-saturated T$_2$-weighted fast spin echo sequences of the lumbar spine, showing normal disc spaces with normal disc and adjacent bone marrow signal. (From Majumdar S, Link TM, Steinbach LS, et al: Diagnostic tools and imaging methods in intervertebral disc degeneration. Orthop Clin North Am 42:503, 2011.)

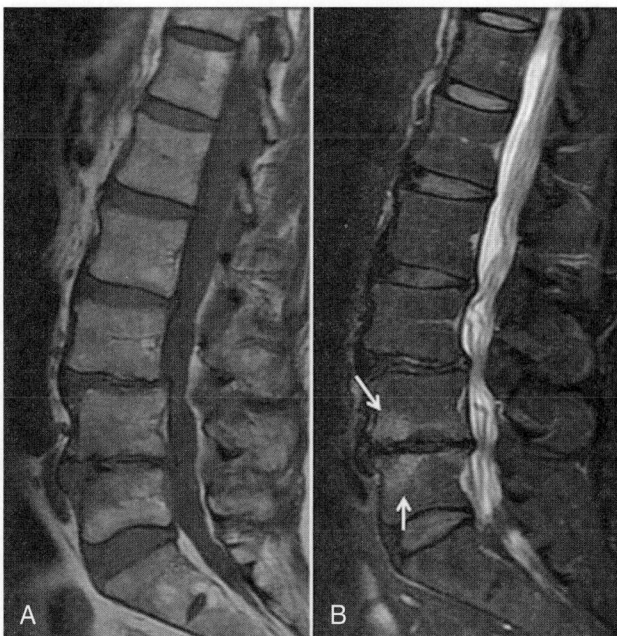

Figure 9-122 Sagittal T$_1$-weighted and fat-saturated **(A)** T$_2$-weighted fast spin echo **(B)** sequences of the lumbar spine demonstrate severe degenerative disc disease at L3/4 and L4/5 with disc height loss, disc desiccation, decreased signal, posterior disc bulges, and Modic type 1 reactive end-plate changes at L4/5 *(arrows)*. Note substantial spinal canal narrowing from L3–S1. (From Majumdar S, Link TM, Steinbach LS, et al: Diagnostic tools and imaging methods in intervertebral disk degeneration. Orthop Clin North Am 42:503, 2011.)

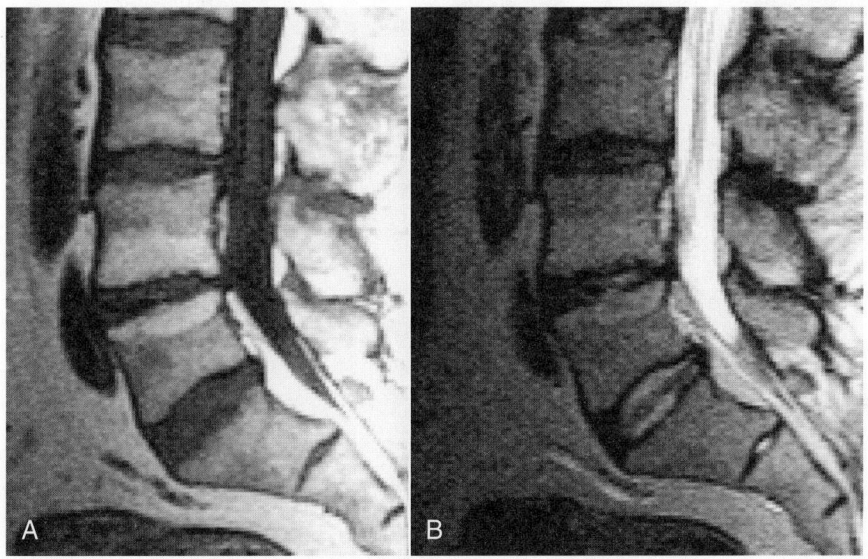

Figure 9-123 Type II vertebral endplates. Sagittal T1-weighted **(A)** and T2-weighted **(B)** spin echo magnetic resonance (MR) images of the lumbar spine show signal intensity changes at the L4–L5 level that are typical of a type II end plate. The signal intensity of subchondral bone at this level is identical to that of fat. There is also evidence of degeneration of the intervertebral disc at this level, with a decrease in disc space height and loss of disc signal on the T2-weighted image. (From Resnick D, Kransdorf MJ: Bone and joint imaging, Philadelphia, 2005, WB Saunders, p. 144.)

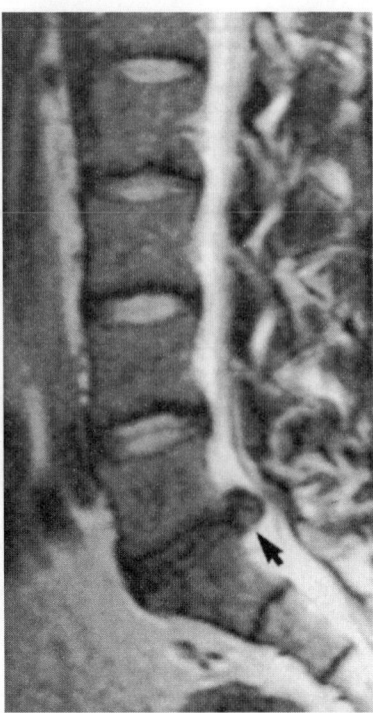

Figure 9-124 Normal and abnormal intervertebral disc: sagittal T2-weighted (TR/TE, 3400/96) spin echo magnetic resonance (MR) imaging technique. In discs that are relatively normal (L1–L2, L3–L4, and L4–L5), a central portion of high signal intensity containing a horizontal line of low signal intensity is evident. In the disc (L2–L3) with mild intervertebral (osteo)chondrosis, minimal loss of signal intensity is shown, particularly in its anterior third. With severe intervertebral (osteo)chondrosis (L5–S1), the disc is of low signal intensity and diminished in height. A large posterior extruded disc *(arrow)* with low signal intensity is also evident. (From Resnick D, Kransdorf MJ: Bone and joint imaging, Philadelphia, 2005, WB Saunders, p. 399.)

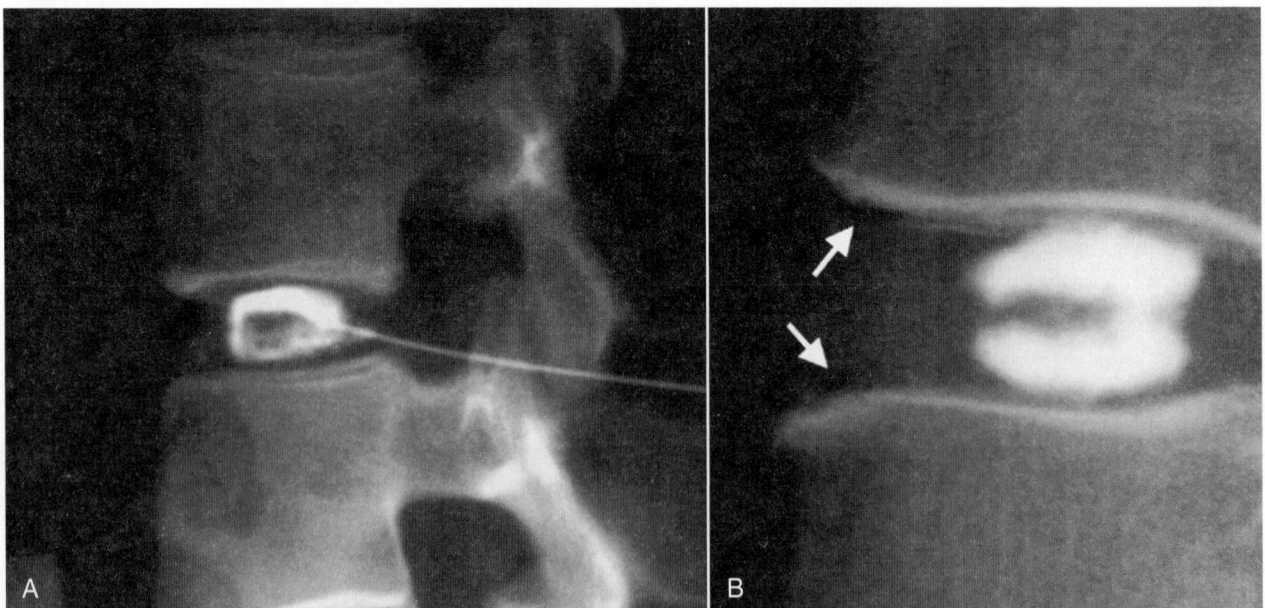

Figure 9-125 Lumbar discography. A, Lateral lumbar spine with discographic needle entry low in the posterior disc margin. Note the normal unilocular appearance of the nucleogram. **B,** Normal bilocular appearance of the nucleogram. The anterior arrows identify anterior vacuum phenomena in the anulus fibrosus, consistent with peripheral annular tears that were asymptomatic at discography. (From Resnick D, Kransdorf MJ: Bone and joint imaging, Philadelphia, 2005, WB Saunders, p. 164.)

PRÉCIS OF THE LUMBAR SPINE ASSESSMENT*

History (sitting)
Observation (standing)
Examination
  Active movements (standing)
    Forward flexion
    Extension
    Side flexion (left and right)
    Rotation (left and right)
    Quick test (if possible)
    Trendelenburg test and S1 nerve root test (modified Trendelenburg test)
  Passive movements (only with care and caution)
  Peripheral joint scan (standing)
    Sacroiliac joints
  Functional assessment
  Special tests (standing)
    For lumbar instability:
      H and I test
    For joint dysfunction:
      One-leg standing (stork standing) lumbar extension test
      Quadrant test
  Resisted isometric movements (sitting)
    Forward flexion
    Extension
    Side flexion (left and right)
    Rotation (left and right)
  Special tests (sitting)
    For neurological dysfunction:
      Slump test or one of its variants
    For lumbar instability:
      Test for anterior lumbar spine instability
      Test for posterior lumbar spine instability
  Resisted isometric movements (supine lying)
    Dynamic abdominal endurance
    Double straight leg lowering
    Internal/external abdominal obliques test
  Peripheral joint scan (supine lying)
    Hip joints (flexion, abduction, adduction, and medial and lateral rotation)
    Knee joints (flexion and extension)
    Ankle joints (dorsiflexion and plantar flexion)
    Foot joints (supination, pronation)
    Toe joints (flexion, extension)
  Myotomes (supine lying)
    Hip flexion (L2)
    Knee extension (L3)
    Ankle dorsiflexion (L4)
    Toe extension (L5)

    Ankle eversion or plantar flexion (S1)
  Special tests (supine lying)
    For neurological dysfunction:
      Straight leg raise test or one of its variants
    For neurological dysfunction:
      90–90 straight leg raise test
      Rectus femoris test
      Thomas test
    Other tests:
      Sign of the buttock
  Reflexes and cutaneous distribution (anterior and side aspects)
  Palpation (supine lying)
  Resisted isometric movements (side lying)
    Horizontal side support
  Special tests (side lying)
    For neurological dysfunction:
      Femoral nerve traction test
    For lumbar instability:
      Specific lumbar torsion test
    For muscle tightness:
      Ober test
  Joint play movements (side lying)
    Flexion
  Peripheral joint scan (prone lying)
    Hip joints (extension, medial and lateral rotation)
  Myotomes (prone lying)
    Hip extension (S1)
    Knee flexion (S1, S2)
  Resisted isometric movements
    Dynamic extension test
  Special tests (prone lying)
    For neurological dysfunction:
      Prone knee bending test or one of its variants
    For lumbar instability:
      Passive lumbar extension test
      Prone segmental instability test
  Reflexes and cutaneous distribution (prone lying) (posterior aspect)
  Joint play movements (prone lying)
    Posteroanterior central vertebral pressure (PACVP)
    Posteroanterior unilateral vertebral pressure (PAUVP)
    Transverse vertebral pressure (TVP)
  Palpation (prone lying)
  Resisted isometric movements (quadriped position)
    Back rotators/multifidus test
  Diagnostic imaging

*The précis is shown in an order that limits the amount of movement that the patient has to do but ensures that all necessary structures are tested. After any examination, the patient should be warned of the possibility that symptoms may exacerbate as a result of the assessment.

CASE STUDIES

When doing these case studies, the examiner should list the appropriate questions to ask and should specify why they are being asked, what to look for and why, and what things should be tested and why. Depending on the patient's answers (and the examiner should consider different responses), several possible causes of the patient's problem may become evident (examples given in parentheses). The examiner should prepare a differential diagnosis chart and then decide how different diagnoses may affect the treatment plan. For example, an 18-year-old female synchronized swimmer was "boosting" another swimmer out of the water and felt a sharp pain in her back. She found that she could no longer swim because of the pain. She demonstrated paresthesia on the dorsum of the foot and lateral aspect of the leg. Describe your assessment plan for this patient (acute disc herniation versus lumbar strain) (Table 9-18).

1. A 23-year-old man comes to you complaining of a low backache. He works as a dishwasher, and although the pain has been present for 5 months, he has not missed any work. The pain gets worse as the day progresses and is relieved by rest. X-rays reveal some sclerosis in the area of the sacroiliac joints. Describe your assessment plan for this patient (ankylosing spondylitis versus lumbar sprain).

2. A 36-year-old woman comes to you complaining of a chronic backache of 6 months' duration. The pain has been gradually increasing in severity and is worse at rest and in the morning on arising from bed. When present, the pain is centered in her low back and radiates into her buttocks and posterior left thigh. Describe your assessment plan for this patient (lumbar stenosis versus lumbar disc lesion).

3. A 13-year-old female gymnast comes to you complaining of low back pain. The pain increases when she extends the spine. Like most gymnasts, she is hypermobile in most of her joints. Describe your assessment plan for this patient (spondylolisthesis versus lumbar sprain).

4. A 56-year-old male steel worker comes to you complaining of low back pain that was brought on when he slipped on ice and twisted his trunk while trying to avoid falling. The injury occurred 2 days earlier, and he has right-sided sciatica. X-rays show some lipping at L4–L5 and L5–S1 with slight narrowing of the L5 disc. He has difficulty bending forward. Describe your assessment plan for this patient (lumbar spondylosis versus acute lumbar disc herniation).

5. A 28-year-old man had a laminectomy for a herniated L5 disc 2 days earlier. He is still an inpatient. Describe your assessment plan for this patient.

6. A 32-year-old man comes to you complaining of back pain and stiffness, especially with activity. He has a desk job and has no history of unusual activity. Describe your assessment plan for this patient (chronic lumbar sprain versus lumbar spina bifida occulta).

7. A 39-year-old male electrician comes to you complaining of back pain after a motor vehicle accident in which he was hit from behind while stopped for a red light. The accident occurred 3 days earlier. Describe your assessment program for this patient (lumbar sprain versus lumbar stenosis).

8. A 26-year-old woman comes to you complaining of low back pain. She appears to have a functional leg length difference. Describe your assessment plan for this patient (lumbar sprain versus congenital anomaly).

TABLE **9-18**

Differential Diagnosis of Lumbar Strain and Posterolateral Lumbar Disc Herniation at L5 to S1

	Lumbar Strain	Lumbar Disc (L5 to S1)
History	Mechanism of injury: flexion, side flexion and/or rotation under load or without control	Quick movement into flexion, rotation, side flexion, or extension (may or may not be under load)
Pain	In lumbar spine, may be referred into buttocks	In lumbar spine with referral into posterior leg to foot (radicular pain)
	May increase with extension (muscle contraction) or flexion (stretch)	Increases with extension
Observation	Scoliosis may be present Muscle spasm	Scoliosis may be present Muscle guarding
Active movement	Pain especially on stretch (flexion, side flexion, and rotation)	Pain especially on extension and flexion
	Pain on unguarded movement Limited ROM	Side flexion and rotation may be affected Limited ROM
Resisted isometric movement	Pain on muscle contraction (often minimal pain) Myotomes normal	Minimal pain unless large protrusion L5–S1 myotomes may be affected
Special tests	Neurological tests negative	SLR and slump test often positive
Sensation	Normal	L5–S1 dermatomes may be affected
Reflexes	Normal	L5–S1 reflexes may be affected
Joint play	Muscle guarding	Muscle guarding

ROM, Range of motion; *SLR,* straight leg raising.

REFERENCES

1. Deyo RA, Phillips WR: Low back pain: a primary care challenge. Spine 21:2826–2832, 1996.
2. Frymoyer JW, Akeson W, Brandt K, et al: Clinical perspectives. In Frymoyer JW, Gordon SL, editors: New perspectives in low back pain, Park Ridge, IL, 1989, American Academy of Orthopedic Surgeons.
3. Waddell G: The back pain revolution, New York, 1998, Churchill Livingstone.
4. Beattie P: Current understanding of lumbar intervertebral disc degeneration: a review with emphasis upon etiology, pathophysiology, and lumbar magnetic resonance imaging findings. J Orthop Sports Phys Ther 38:329–340, 2008.
5. Hu SS, Tribus CB, Diab M, et al: Spondylolisthesis and spondylolysis. J Bone Joint Surg Am 90:656–671, 2008.
6. Taylor JR, Twomey LT: Structure and function of lumbar zygapophyseal (facet) joints. In Boyling JD, Palastanga N, editors: Grieve's modern manual therapy: the vertebral column, ed 2, Edinburgh, 1994, Churchill Livingstone.
7. Iwamoto J, Abe H, Tsukimura Y, et al: Relationship between radiographic abnormalities of lumbar spine and incidence of low back pain in high school and college football players: a prospective study. Am J Sports Med 32:781–786, 2004.
8. Fujiwana A, Tamai K, Yoshida H, et al: Anatomy of the iliolumbar ligament. Clin Orthop Relat Res 380:167–172, 2000.
9. Aihara T, Takahashi K, Yamagata M, et al: Does the iliolumbar ligament prevent anterior displacement of the fifth lumbar vertebra with defects of the pars? J Bone Joint Surg Br 82:846–850, 2000.
10. Kramer J: Intervertebral disk disease: causes, diagnosis, treatment and prophylaxis, Chicago, 1981, Year Book Medical.
11. Farfan HF: Mechanical disorders of the low back, Philadelphia, 1973, Lea & Febiger.
12. Coventry MB, Ghormley RK, Kernohan JW: The intervertebral disc: its microscopic anatomy and pathology. Part I: Anatomy, development and physiology; Part II: Changes in the intervertebral disc concomitant with age; Part III: Pathological changes in the intervertebral disc. J Bone Joint Surg 27:105 (Part I), 233 (Part II), 460 (Part III), 1945.
13. Bogduk N: The innervation of the lumbar spine. Spine 8:286–293, 1983.
14. Edgar MA, Ghadially JA: Innervation of the lumbar spine. Clin Orthop 115:35–41, 1976.
15. Vernon-Roberts B, Moore RJ, Fraser RD: The natural history of age-related disc degeneration—the pathology and sequelae of tears. Spine 32:2797–2804, 2007.
16. Ledsome JR, Lessoway V, Susak LE, et al: Diurnal changes in lumbar intervertebral distance, measured using ultrasound. Spine 21:1671–1675, 1996.
17. Saal JA: Natural history and nonoperative treatment of lumbar disc herniation. Spine 21(24S):2S–9S, 1996.
18. Macnab I: Backache, Baltimore, 1977, Williams & Wilkins.
19. Spector LR, Madigan L, Rhyme A, et al: Cauda equina syndrome. J Am Acad Orthop Surg 16:471–479, 2008.
20. Takahashi K, Shima I, Porter RW: Nerve root pressure in lumbar disc herniation. Spine 24:2003–2006, 1999.
21. Nachemson A, Morris JM: In vivo measurements of intradiscal pressure. J Bone Joint Surg Am 46:1077–1092, 1964.
22. Nachemson A, Elfstrom C: Intravital dynamic pressure measurements in lumbar discs. Scand J Rehabil Med (suppl 1):5–40, 1970.
23. Madigan L, Vaccaro AR, Spector LR, et al: Management of symptomatic lumbar degenerative disc disease. J Am Acad Orthop Surg 17:102–111, 2009.
24. Deyo RA, Rainville J, Kent DL: What can the history and physical examination tell us about low back pain? J Am Med Assoc 268:760–765, 1992.
25. Hall H: A simple approach to back pain management. Patient Care 15:77–91, 1992.
26. Walsh M: Evaluation of orthopedic testing of the low back for nonspecific low back pain. J Manip Physiol Ther 21:232–236, 1998.
27. Leboeuf-Yde C, Kyuik KO: Is it possible to differentiate people with or without low back pain on the basis of tests of lumbopelvic dysfunction? J Manip Physiol Ther 23:160–167, 2000.
28. Vroomen PC, de Krom MC, Knottnerus JA: Consistency of history taking and physical examination in patients with suspected lumbar nerve root involvement. Spine 25:91–97, 2000.
29. Frymoyer JW: Epidemiology. In Frymoyer JW, Gordon SL, editors: New perspectives in low back pain, Park Ridge, IL, 1989, American Academy of Orthopedic Surgeons.
30. White AA: The 1980 symposium and beyond. In Frymoyer JW, Gordon SL, editors: New perspectives in low back pain, Park Ridge, IL, 1989, American Academy of Orthopedic Surgeons.
31. Luoma K, Riihimaki H, Luukkonen R, et al: Low back pain in relation to lumbar disc degeneration. Spine 25:487–492, 2000.
32. Videman T, Battié MC: The influence of occupational on lumbar degeneration. Spine 24:1164–1168, 1999.

33. Richardson JK, Chung T, Schultz JS, et al: A familial predisposition toward lumbar disc injury. Spine 22:1487–1493, 1997.

34. Wilder DG, Pope MH, Frymoyer FW: The biomechanics of lumbar disc herniation and the effect of overload and instability. J Spinal Dis 1:16–32, 1988.

35. Luoto S, Taimela S, Hurri H, et al: Psychomotor speed and postural control in chronic low back pain patients: a controlled follow-up study. Spine 21:2621–2627, 1996.

36. Stewart J, Kempenaar L, Lanchlin D: Rethinking yellow flags. Man Ther 16:196–198, 2011.

37. Brodke DS, Ritter SM: Nonoperative management of low back pain and lumbar disc degeneration. J Bone Joint Surg Am 86:1810–1818, 2004.

38. Young S, Aprill C: Characteristics of a mechanical assessment for chronic lumbar facet joint pain. J Man Manip Ther 8:78–84, 2000.

39. McKenzie RA: The lumbar spine: mechanical diagnosis and therapy, Waikanae, New Zealand, 1981, Spinal Publications.

40. Donelson R, Aprill C, Metcalf R, et al: A prospective study of centralization of lumbar and referred pain: a predictor of symptomatic discs and annular competence. Spine 22:1115–1122, 1997.

41. Long AL: The centralization phenomenon: its usefulness as a predictor of outcome in conservative treatment of chronic low back pain (a pilot study). Spine 20:2513–2521, 1995.

42. Aina A, May S, Clare H: The centralization phenomenon of spinal symptoms: a systematic review. Man Ther 9(3):134–143, 2004.

43. Skyttle L, May S, Petersen P: Centralization: its prognostic value in patients with referred symptoms and sciatica. Spine 30:E293–E299, 2005.

44. Mooney V: Where does the pain come from? Spine 12:754, 1987.

45. Vucetic N, Maattanen H, Svensson O: Pain and pathology in lumbar disc hernia. Clin Orthop Relat Res 320:65–72, 1995.

46. Greenwood MJ, Erhard RE, Jones DL: Differential diagnosis of the hip vs lumbar spine: five case reports. J Orthop Sports Phys Ther 27:308–315, 1998.

47. Stoddard A: Manual of osteopathic practice, New York, 1970, Harper & Row.

48. Lord MJ, Small JM, Dinsay JM, et al: Effects of sitting and standing. Spine 22:2571–2574, 1997.

49. Liss H, D Liss: History and past medical history. In Cole AJ, Herring SA, editors: The low back pain handbook, Philadelphia, 1997, Hanley & Belfus.

50. Bendix T, Sorenson SS, Klausen K: Lumbar curve, trunk muscles, and line of gravity with different heel heights. Spine 9:223–227, 1984.

51. Shapiro S: Medical realities of cauda equina syndrome secondary to lumbar disc herniation. Spine 25:348–352, 2000.

52. Ahn UM, Ahn N, Buchowski JM, et al: Cauda equina syndrome secondary to lumbar disc herniation. Spine 25:1515–1522, 2000.

53. Hides JA, Stokes MH, Saide M, et al: Evidence of lumbar multifidus muscle wasting ipsilateral to symptoms in patients with acute/subacute low back pain. Spine 19:165–172, 1994.

54. Bishop A, Foster NE: Do physical therapists in the United Kingdom recognize psychosocial factors in patients with acute low back pain. Spine 30:1316–1322, 2005.

55. Antony MM, Bieling PJ, Cox BJ, et al: Psychometric properties of the 42-item and 21-item versions of the depression anxiety stress scales in clinical groups and a community sample. Psych Assess 10:176–181, 1998.

56. Brown TA, Chorpita BF, Korotitsch W, et al: Psychometric properties of the depression anxiety stress scales (DASS) in clinical samples. Behav Res Ther 35:79–89, 1997.

57. Lovibond PF, Lovibond SH: The structure of negative emotional states: comparison of the expression anxiety stress scales (DASS) with the Beck depression and anxiety inventories. Behav Res Ther 33:335–343, 1995.

58. Accident Compensation Corp: New Zealand acute low back pain guide, Wellington, New Zealand, 2004, New Zealand Guidelines Groups.

59. Waddell G, Newton M, Henderson I, et al: A fear-avoidance questionnaire (FABQ) and the role of fear avoidance beliefs in chronic low back pain and disability. Pain 52:157–168, 1993.

60. Linton SJ, Hallden K: Can we screen for problematic back pain? A screening questionnaire for predicting outcome in acute and subacute low back pain. Clin J Pain 14(3):209–215, 1998.

61. Vlaeyen JW, Kole-Snijders AM, Boeren RG, et al: Fear of movement/(re)injury in chronic low back pain and its relation to behavioral performance. Pain 62:363–372, 1995.

62. Asmundson GJ, Norton PJ, Norton GR: Beyond pain: the role of fear and avoidance of chronicity. Clin Psych Rev 19:97–119, 1999.

63. McCracken LM, Gross RT, Aikens J, et al: The assessment of anxiety and fear in persons with chronic pain: a comparison of instruments. Behav Res Ther 34:927–933, 1996.

64. Fritz JM, George SZ, Delitto A: The role of fear avoidance beliefs in acute low back: relationships with current and future disability and work status. Pain 94:7–15, 2001.

65. Crombez G, Vlaeyen JW, Heuts PH, et al: Pain-related fear is more disabling than pain itself: evidence on the role of pain related fear in chronic back pain disability. Pain 80:329–359, 1999.

66. Vlaeyen JW, Crombez G: Fear of movement/(re) injury, avoidance and pain disability in chronic low back pain patients. Man Ther 4:187–195, 1999.

67. Walsh DA, Radcliffe JC: Pain beliefs and perceived physical disability of patients with chronic low back pain. Pain 97:23–31, 2002.

68. Haggman S, Maher CG, Refshauge KM: Screening for symptoms of depression by physical therapists managing low back pain. Phys Ther 84:1157–1166, 2004.

69. Kroenke K, Spitzer RL, Williams JB: The patient health questionnaire-2: validity of a two-item depression screener. Med Care 41:1284–1292, 2003.

70. Grotle M, Brox JI, Veierod MB, et al: Clinical course and prognostic factors in acute low back pain: patients consulting primary care for the first time. Spine 30:976–982, 2005.

71. McGregor AH, Doré CJ, McCarthy ID, et al: Are subjective clinical findings and objective clinical tests related to motion characteristics of low back pain subjects? J Orthop Sports Phys Ther 28:370–377, 1998.

72. Maigne R: Diagnosis and treatment of pain of vertebral origin, Baltimore, 1996, Williams & Wilkins.

73. Evans RC: Illustrated essentials in orthopedic physical assessment, St Louis, 1994, Mosby.

74. Nelson-Wong E, Flynn T, Callaghan JP: Development of acute hip abduction as a screening test for identifying occupational low back pain. J Orthop Sports Phys Ther 39:649–657, 2009.

75. Meadows JT: Orthopedic differential diagnosis in physical therapy: a case study approach, New York, 1999, McGraw-Hill.

76. Matsui H, Ohmori K, Kanamori M, et al: Significance of sciatic scoliotic list in operated patients with lumbar disc herniation. Spine 23:338–342, 1998.

77. Jull G, Janda V: Muscles and motor control in low back pain. In Twomey LT, Taylor JR, editors: Physical therapy for the low back, New York, 1987, Churchill Livingstone.

78. Schink, MB: Muscle imbalance patterns associated with low back pain syndromes. In Watkins RG, editor: The spine in sports, St Louis, 1996, Mosby.

79. Matson DD, Woods RP, Campbell JB, et al: Diastematomyelia (congenital clefts of the spinal cord). Pediatrics 6:98–112, 1950.

80. Allbrook D: Movements of the lumbar spinal column. J Bone Joint Surg Br 39:339–345, 1957.

81. Moll JMH, Wright V: Normal range of spinal mobility: an objective clinical study. Ann Rheum Dis 30:381–386, 1971.

82. Moll J, Wright V: Measurement of spinal movement. In Jayson M, editor: The lumbar spine and back pain, New York, 1976, Grune & Stratton.

83. Pennal GF, Conn GS, McDonald G, et al: Motion studies of the lumbar spine. J Bone Joint Surg Br 54:442–452, 1972.

84. Tanz SS: Motion of the lumbar spine: a roentgenologic study. Am J Roentgenol 69:399–412, 1953.

85. Okawa A, Shinomiya K, Komori H, et al: Dynamic motion study of the whole lumbar spine by videofluoroscopy. Spine 23:1743–1749, 1998.

86. Vucetic N, Svensson O: Physical signs in lumbar disc hernia. Clin Orthop Relat Res 333:192–201, 1996.

87. Kirkaldy-Willis WH: Managing low back pain, New York, 1983, Churchill-Livingstone.

88. Fujiwara A, Lim TH, An HS, et al: The effect of disc degeneration and facet joint osteoarthritis on the segmental flexibility of the lumbar spine. Spine 25:3036–3044, 2000.

89. Paris WV: Physical signs of instability. Spine 10:277–279, 1985.

90. Ogon M, Bender BR, Hooper DM, et al: A dynamic approach to spinal instability: part II hesitation and giving-way during interspinal motion. Spine 22:2859–2866, 1997.

91. Schneider G, Pearcy MJ, Bogduk N: Abnormal motion in spondylolytic spondylolisthesis. Spine 30:1159–1164, 2005.

92. Dobbs AC: Evaluation of instabilities of the lumbar spine. Orthop Phys Ther Clin North Am 8:387–400, 1999.

93. Porter JL, Wilkinson A: Lumbar-hip flexion motion: a comparative study between asymptomatic and chronic low back pain in 18 to 36 year old men. Spine 22:1508–1514, 1997.

94. Bourdillon JF, Day EA: Spinal manipulation, London, 1987, Wm Heinemann Medical Books.

95. Mulvein K, Jull G: Kinematic analyses of the lumbar lateral flexion and lumbar lateral shift movement techniques. J Man Manip Ther 3:104–109, 1995.

96. Edwards BC: Clinical assessment: the use of combined movements in assessment and treatment. In Twomey LT, Taylor JR, editors: Physical therapy of the low back: clinics in physical therapy, Edinburgh, 1987, Churchill Livingstone.

97. Brown L: An introduction to the treatment and examination of the spine by combined movements. Physiotherapy 74:347–353, 1988.

98. Watkins RG: Lumbar spine injuries. In Watkins RG, editor: The spine in sports, St Louis, 1996, Mosby.

99. Hourigan CL, Bassett JM: Facet syndrome: clinical signs, symptoms, diagnosis, and treatment. J Manip Physiol Ther 12:293–297, 1989.

100. Lippitt AB: The facet joint and its role in spine pain management with facet joint injections. Spine 9:746–750, 1984.

101. Wallace LA: Limb length difference and back pain. In Grieve GP, editor: Modern manual therapy of the vertebral column, Edinburgh, 1986, Churchill Livingstone.

102. Moreau CE, Green BN, Johnson CD, et al: Isometric back extension endurance tests: a review of the literature. J Manip Physiol Ther 24:110–122, 2001.

103. Moreland J, Finch E, Stratord P, et al: Interrater reliability of six tests of trunk muscle function and endurance. J Orthop Sports Phys Ther 26:200–208, 1997.

104. Ito T, Shirado O, Suzuki H, et al: Lumbar trunk muscle endurance testing: an inexpensive alternative to a machine for evaluation. Arch Phys Med Rehabil 77(1):75–79, 1996.

105. Kendall F: Muscles, testing and function, ed 3, Baltimore, 1983, Williams & Wilkins.

106. Reese NB: Muscle and sensory testing, Philadelphia, 1999, WB Saunders.

107. Jorgensen K, Nicolaisen T: Trunk extensor endurance: determination and relation to low-back trouble. Ergonomics 30:259–267, 1987.

108. McGill S: Low back disorders—evidence-based prevention and rehabilitation, Champaign, 2002, Human Kinetics.

109. Ng JK, Richardson CA, Jull GA: Electromyographic amplitude and frequency changes in the iliocostalis lumborum and multifidus muscles during a trunk holding exercise. Phys Ther 77:954–961, 1987.

110. Moffroid MT: Endurance of trunk muscles in persons with chronic low back pain: assessment, performance, training. J Rehab Res Train 34:440–447, 1997.

111. Clarkson HM: Musculoskeletal assessment, ed 2, Philadelphia, 2000, Lippincott Williams & Wilkins.

112. Reese NB: Muscle and sensory testing, Philadelphia, 1999, WB Saunders.

113. Biering-Sorensen F: Physical measurements as risk indicators for low back trouble over a one-year period. Spine 9:106–109, 1984.

114. Latimer J, Maher CG, Refshauge K, et al: The reliability and validity of the Biering-Sorenson test in asymptomatic subjects and subjects reporting current or previous nonspecific low back pain. Spine 24:2085–2090, 1999.

115. Youdas JW, Garrett TR, Egan KS, et al: Lumbar lordosis and pelvic inclination in adults with chronic low back pain. Phys Ther 80:261–275, 2000.

116. Shields RK, Heiss DG: An electromyographic comparison of abdominal muscle synergies during curl and double straight leg lowering exercises with control of the pelvic position. Spine 22:1873–1879, 1999.

117. McGill SM: Low back exercises: evidence for improving exercise regimes. Phys Ther 78:754–765, 1998.

118. McGill SM, Childs A, Liebenson C: Endurance times for low back stabilization exercises: clinical targets for testing and training from a normal database. Arch Phys Med Rehabil 80:941–944, 1999.

119. Smith SS, Mayer TG, Gatchel RJ, et al: Quantification of lumbar function: isometric and multispeed isokinetic trunk strength measures in sagittal and axial planes in normal subjects. Spine 10:757–764, 1985.

120. Cyriax J: Textbook for orthopaedic medicine, vol. I: diagnosis of soft tissue lesions, London, 1975, Balliere Tindall.

121. Rainville J, Jouve C, Finno M, et al: Comparison of four tests of quadriceps strength in L3 or L4 radiculopathies. Spine 28(21):2466–2471, 2003.

122. Grotle M, Brox JI, Vollestad NK: Functional status and disability questionnaire: what do they assess? A systematic review of back specific outcome questionnaires. Spine 30:130–140, 2004.

123. Mayer, TG: Assessment of lumbar function. Clin Orthop 221:99–109, 1987.

124. Thomas AM: The spine. In Pynsent P, Fairbank J, Carr A, editors: Outcome measures in orthopedics, Oxford, 1994, Butterworth Heinemann.

125. Beurskens AJ, de Vet HC, Koke AJ, et al: Measuring the functional status of patients with low back pain. Spine 20:1018–1028, 1995.

126. Fairbank JC, Pynsent PB: The Oswestry disability index. Spine 25:2940–2953, 2000.

127. Fairbank JC, Cooper J, Davies JB, et al: The Oswestry low back pain disability questionnaire. Physiotherapy 66:271–273, 1980.

128. Frost H, Lamb SE, Stewart-Brown S: Responsiveness of a patient specific outcome measure compared with the Oswestry Disability Index v2.1 and Roland and Morris Disability Questionnaire for patients with subacute and chronic low back pain. Spine 33:2450–2457, 2008.

129. Kopec JA, Esdaile JM, Abrahamowicz M, et al: The Quebec Back Pain Disability Scale: measurement properties. Spine 20(3):341–352, 1995.

130. Davidson M, Keating JL: A comparison of five low back disability questionnaires: reliability and responsiveness. Phys Ther 82(1):8–24, 2002.

131. Borenstein DG, Wiesel SW, Boden SD: Low back pain: medical diagnosis and comprehensive management, Philadelphia, 1995, WB Saunders.

132. Hendler N, Mollett A, Talo S, et al: A comparison between the Minnesota Multiphasic Personality Inventory and the Mensana Clinic Back Pain Test for validating the complaint of chronic back pain. J Occup Med 30:98–102, 1988.

133. Roland M, Fairbank J: The Roland-Morris Disability Questionnaire and the Oswestry Disability Questionnaire. Spine 25:3115–3124, 2000.

134. Stratford PW, Binkley J, Solomon P, et al: Defining the minimum level of detectable change for the Roland-Morris questionnaire. Phys Ther 76:359–365, 1996.

135. Feise RJ, Menke JM: Functional rating index: a new valid and reliable instrument to measure the magnitude of clinical change in spinal conditions. Spine 26:78–87, 2001.

136. Chansirinukor W, Maher CG, Latimer J, et al: Comparison of the Functional Rating Index and the 18-item Roland-Morris Disability Questionnaire: responsiveness and reliability. Spine 30(1):141–145, 2005.

137. Lawlis GF, Cuencas R, Selby D, et al: The development of the Dallas Pain Questionnaire. Spine 14:511–516, 1989.

138. Million R, Hall W, Haavick-Nilsen K, et al: Assessment of the progress of the back pain patient. Spine 7:204–212, 1982.

139. Japanese Orthopedic Association: Assessment of treatment of low back pain. J Jap Orthop Assoc 60:909–911, 1986.

140. Lehmann TR, Brand RA, German TW: A low back rating scale. Spine 8:308–315, 1983.

141. Bolton JE, Breen AC: The Bournemouth questionnaire: a short-form comprehensive outcome measure. I. Psychometric properties in back pain patients. J Manip Physiol Ther 22:503–510, 1999.

142. Larsen K, Leboeuf-Yde C: The Bournemouth questionnaire: can it be used to monitor and predict treatment outcome in chiropractic patients with persistent low back pain? J Manip Physiol Ther 28:219–227, 2005.

143. Berven S, Deviren V, Demir-Deviren S, et al: Studies in the modified Scoliosis Research Society outcomes instrument in adults: validation, reliability and discriminatory capacity. Spine 28:2164–2169, 2004.

144. Haher TR, Group JM, Shin TM, et al: Results of the Scoliosis Research Society instrument for evaluation of surgical outcome in adolescent scoliosis: a multicentre study of 244 patients. Spine 24:1435–1440, 1999.

145. Bridwell KH, Cats-Baril W, Harrast J, et al: The validity of the SRS-22 instrument in an adult spinal deformity population compared with Oswestry and SF12. Spine 30:455–461, 2005.

146. Stucki G, Daltroy L, Lang MH, et al: Measurement properties of a self administered outcome measure in lumbar spinal stenosis. Spine 21:796–803, 1996.

147. Williams NH, Wilkinson C, Russell IT: Extending the Aberdeen back pain scale to include the whole spine: a set of outcome measures for the neck, upper and lower back. Pain 94:261–274, 2001.

148. Waddell G, McCulloch J, Kummel E: Nonorganic physical signs in low back pain. Spine 5:117–125, 1980.

149. Burton AK, Tillotson KM, Main CJ, et al: Psychosocial predictors of outcome in acute and subacute low back trouble. Spine 20:722–728, 1995.

150. Gatchel RJ, Polatin PB, Mayer TG: The dominant role of psychosocial risk factors in the development of chronic low back pain disability. Spine 20:2702–2709, 1995.

151. Harding VR, Williams AC, Richardson PH, et al: The development of a battery of measures for assessing physical functioning of chronic pain patients. Pain 58:367–375, 1994.

152. Simmonds MJ, Olson SL, Jones S, et al: Psychometric characteristics and clinical usefulness of physical performance tests in patients with low back pain. Spine 23:2412–2421, 1998.

153. Marras WS, Wongsamm PE: Flexibility and velocity of normal and impaired lumbar spine. Arch Phys Med Rehabil 67:213–217, 1986.

154. Andersson GB, Deyo RA: History and physical examination in patients with herniated lumbar discs. Spine 21(24S):10S–18S, 1996.

155. Cook C, Hegedus E: Diagnostic utility of clinical tests for spinal dysfunction. Man Ther 16:21–25, 2011.

156. Cook CE, Hegedus EJ: Orthopedic physical examination tests—an evidence based approach, Upper Saddle River, NJ, 2008, Prentice Hall/Pearson.

157. Hestbaek L, Leboeuf-Yde C: Are chiropractic tests for the lumbo-pelvic spine reliable and valid? A systematic critical literature review. J Manip Physiol Ther 23:258–266, 2000.

158. Deville WL, van der Windt DA, Dzaferagic A, et al: The test of Lasègue: systematic review of the accuracy in diagnosing herniated discs. Spine 25:1140–1147, 2000.

159. Strender LE, Sjoblom A, Sundell K, et al: Interexaminer reliability in physical examination of patients with low back pain. Spine 22:814–820, 1997.

160. McCarthy CJ, Gittins M, Roberts C, et al: The reliability of the clinical tests and questions recommended in international guidelines for low back pain. Spine 32:921–926, 2007.

161. Paatelma M, Karvonen E, Heiskanen J: Clinical perspective: how do clinical test results differentiate chronic and subacute low back pain patients from "non-patients"? J Man Manip Ther 17:11–19, 2009.

162. Shacklock M: Neurodynamics. Physiotherapy 81:9–16, 1995.

163. Butler DA: Mobilisation of the nervous system, Melbourne, 1991, Churchill Livingstone.

164. Vucetic N, Astrand P, Guntner P, et al: Diagnosis and prognosis in lumbar disc herniation. Clin Orthop Relat Res 361:116–122, 1999.

165. Slater H, Butler DS, Shacklock MD: The dynamic central nervous system: examination and assessment using tension tests. In Boyling JD, Palastanga N, editors: Grieve's modern manual therapy: the vertebral column, ed 2, Edinburgh, 1994, Churchill Livingstone.

166. Butler D, Gifford L: The concept of adverse mechanical tension in the nervous system. Physiotherapy 75:622–636, 1989.

167. Herrington L, Bendix K, Cornwall C, et al: What is the normal response to structural differentiation within the slump and straight leg raise tests? Man Ther 13:289–294, 2008.

168. Dommisse GF, Grobler L: Arteries and veins of the lumbar nerve roots and cauda equina. Clin Orthop 115:22–29, 1976.

169. Cram RH: A sign of sciatic nerve root pressure. J Bone Joint Surg Br 35:192–195, 1953.

170. Brudzinski J: A new sign of the lower extremities in meningitis of children (neck sign). Arch Neurol 21:217, 1969.

171. Deyerle WM, May VR: Sciatic tension test. South Med J 49:999–1005, 1956.

172. Wartenberg R: The signs of Brudzinski and of Kernig. J Pediatr 37:679–684, 1950.

173. Brody IA, Williams RH: The signs of Kernig and Brudzinski. Arch Neurol 21:215, 1969.

174. Kernig W: Concerning a little noted sign of meningitis. Arch Neurol 21:216, 1969.

175. Dyck P: The femoral nerve traction test with lumbar disc protrusion. Surg Neurol 6:163–166, 1976.

176. Kreitz BG, Coté P, Yong-Hing K: Crossed femoral stretching test: a case report. Spine I 21:1584–1586, 1996.

177. Katznelson A, Nerubay J, Level A: Gluteal skyline (G.S.L.): a search for an objective sign in the diagnosis of disc lesions of the lower lumbar spine. Spine 7:74–75, 1982.

178. Rask M: Knee flexion test and sciatica. Clin Orthop 134:221, 1978.

179. Herron LD, Pheasant HC: Prone knee-flexion provocative testing for lumbar disc protrusion. Spine 5:65–67, 1980.

180. Postacchini F, Cinotti G, Gumina S: The knee flexion test: a new test for lumbosacral root tension. J Bone Joint Surg Br 75:834–835, 1993.

181. Davis DS, Anderson IB, Carson MC, et al: Upper limb neural tension and seated slump tests: the false positive rate among healthy young adults without cervical or lumbar symptoms. J Man Manip Ther 16:136–141, 2008.

182. Spengler DM: Low back pain: assessment and management, Orlando, FL, 1982, Grune & Stratton.

183. Hudgins WR: The crossed-straight-leg raising test. N Engl J Med 297:1127, 1977.

184. Palmer ML, Epler M: Clinical assessment procedures in physical therapy, Philadelphia, 1990, JB Lippincott.

185. Maitland GD: The slump test: examination and treatment. Aust J Physiother 31:215–219, 1985.

186. Philip K, Lew P, Matyas TA: The inter-therapist reliability of the slump test. Aust J Physiother 35:89–94, 1989.

187. Maitland GD: Negative disc exploration: positive canal signs. Aust J Physiother 25:129–134, 1979.

188. Fidel C, Martin E, Dankaerts W, et al: Cervical spine sensitizing maneuvers during the slump test. J Man Manip Ther 4:16–21, 1996.

189. Johnson EK, Chiarello CM: The slump test: the effects of head and lower extremity position on knee extension. J Orthop Sports Phys Ther 26:310–317, 1997.

190. Breig A, Troup JDG: Biomechanical considerations in straight-leg-raising test: cadaveric and clinical studies of the effects of medical hip rotation. Spine 4:242–250, 1979.

191. Charnley J: Orthopedic signs in the diagnosis of disc protrusion with special reference to the straight-leg-raising test. Lancet 1:186–192, 1951.

192. Edgar MA, Park WM: Induced pain patterns on passive straight-leg-raising in lower lumbar disc protrusion. J Bone Joint Surg Br 56:658–667, 1974.

193. Fahrni WH: Observations on straight-leg-raising with special reference to nerve root adhesions. Can J Surg 9:44–48, 1966.

194. Goddard BS, JD Reid: Movements induced by straight-leg-raising in the lumbosacral roots, nerves, and plexus and in the intrapelvic section of the sciatic nerve. J Neurol Neurosurg Psychiatry 28:12–18, 1965.

195. Scham SM, Taylor TKF: Tension signs in lumbar disc prolapse. Clin Orthop 75:195–204, 1971.

196. Urban LM: The straight-leg-raising test: a review. J Orthop Sports Phys Ther 2:117–133, 1981.

197. Wilkins RH, Brody IA: Lasègue's sign. Arch Neurol 21:219–220, 1969.

198. Summers B, Malhan K, Cassar-Pullicino V: Low back pain on passive straight leg raising: the anterior theca as a source of pain. Spine 30:342–345, 2005.

199. Shiqing X, Quanzhi Z, Dehao F: Significance of the straight-leg-raising test in the diagnosis and clinical evaluation of lower lumbar intervertebral disc protrusion. J Bone Joint Surg Am 69:517–522, 1987.

200. Cipriano JJ: Photographic manual of regional orthopedic tests, Baltimore, 1985, Williams & Wilkins.

201. Hall T, Hepburn M, Elvey RL: The effect of lumbosacral posture on a modification of the straight leg raise test. Physiotherapy 79:566–570, 1993.

202. Woodhall R, Hayes GJ: The well-leg-raising test of Fajersztajn in the diagnosis of ruptured lumbar intervertebral disc. J Bone Joint Surg Am 32:786–792, 1950.

203. Khuffash B, Porter RW: Cross leg pain and trunk list. Spine 14:602–603, 1989.

204. Kotilainen K, Valtonen S: Clinical instability of the lumbar spine after microdiscectomy. Acta Neurochir 125:120–126, 1993.

205. Pope MH, Frymoyer JW, Krag MH: Diagnosing instability. Clin Orthop Relat Res 279:60–67, 1992.

206. Fritz JM, Erhard RE, Hagen BF: Segmental instability of the lumbar spine. Phys Ther 78:889–896, 1998.

207. Kasai Y, Morishita K, Kawakita E, et al: A new evaluation method for lumbar spinal instability: passive lumbar extension test. Phys Ther 86:1661–1667, 2006.

208. Alqarni AM, Schneiders AG, Hendrick PA: Clinical tests to diagnose lumbar segmental instability: a systematic review. J Orthop Sports Phys Ther 41:130–140, 2011.

209. Kirkaldy-Willis WH: Managing low back pain, Edinburgh, 1983, Churchill Livingstone.

210. Wadsworth CT, DeFabio RF, Johnson D: The spine. In Wadsworth CT: Manual examination and treatment of the spine and extremities, Baltimore, 1988, Williams & Wilkins.

211. Hicks GE, Fritz JM, Delitto A, et al: Interrater reliability of clinical examination measures for identification of lumbar segmental instability. Arch Phys Med Rehabil 84:1858–1864, 2003.

212. Garrick JG, Webb DR: Sports injuries: diagnosis and management, Philadelphia, 1990, WB Saunders.

213. Jackson DW, Ciullo JV: Injuries of the spine in the skeletally immature athlete. In Nicholas JA, Hershmann EB, editors: The lower extremity and spine in sports medicine, vol 2, St Louis, 1986, Mosby.

214. Jackson DW, Wiltse LL, Dingeman RD, et al: Stress reactions involving the pars interarticularis in young athletes. Am J Sports Med 9:304–312, 1981.

215. Lyle MA, Manes S, McGuinness M, et al: Relationship of physical examination findings and self-reported symptoms severity and physical function in patients with degenerative lumbar conditions. Phys Ther 85:120–133, 2005.

216. Corrigan B, Maitland GD: Practical orthopedic medicine, London, 1985, Butterworths.

217. Little H: The neck and back: the rheumatological physical examination, Orlando, FL, 1986, Grune & Stratton.

218. Post M: Physical examination of the musculoskeletal system, Chicago, 1987, Year Book Medical.

219. Blou JN, Logue V: Intermittent claudication of the cauda equina. Lancet (May):1081–1085, 1961.

220. Dyck P, Pheasant HC, Doyle JB, et al: Intermittent cauda equina compression syndrome. Spine 2:75–81, 1977.

221. Floman Y, Wiesel SW, Rothman RH: Cauda equina syndrome presenting as a herniated lumbar disc. Clin Orthop Relat Res 147:234–237, 1980.

222. Wilson CB, Ehni G, Grollmus J: Neurogenic intermittent claudication. Clin Neurosurg 18:62–85, 1970.

223. Laslett M: Bilateral buttock pain caused by aortic stenosis: a case report of claudication of the buttock. Man Ther 5:227–233, 2000.

224. Kikuchi S, Watanabe E, Hasue M: Spinal intermittent claudication due to cervical and thoracic degenerative spine disease. Spine 21:313–318, 1996.

225. Dyck P, Doyle JB: "Bicycle test" of van Gelderen in diagnosis of intermittent cauda equina compression syndrome. J Neurosurg 46:667–670, 1977.

226. Dyck P: The stoop-test in lumbar entrapment radiculopathy. Spine 4:89–92, 1979.

227. Deen HG, Zimmerman RS, Lyons MK, et al: Use of an exercise treadmill to measure baseline functional status and surgical outcome in patients with severe spinal stenosis. Spine 23:244–248, 1998.

228. Tokuhashi Y, Matsuzaki H, Sano S: Evaluation of clinical lumbar instability using the treadmill. Spine 18:2321–2324, 1993.

229. Archibald KC, Wiechec F: A reappraisal of Hoover's test. Arch Phys Med Rehabil 51:234–238, 1970.

230. Arieff AJ, Tigay EI, Kurtz JF, et al: The Hoover sign: an objective sign of pain and/or weakness in the back or lower extremities. Arch Neurol 5:673–678, 1961.

231. Hoover CF: A new sign for the detection of malingering and functional paresis of the lower extremities. JAMA 51:746–747, 1980.

232. Gurney B, Boissonault WG, Andrews R: Differential diagnosis of a femoral neck/head stress fracture. J Orthop Sports Phys Ther 36:80–88, 2006.

233. Dyck P, Pheasant HC, Doyle JB, et al: Intermittent cauda equina compression syndrome. Spine 2:75–81, 1977.

234. Joffe R, Appleby A, Arjona V: Intermittent ischemia of the cauda equina due to stenosis of the lumbar canal. J Neurol Neurosurg Psychiatry 29:315–318, 1966.

235. Hoppenfeld S: Physical examination of the spine and extremities, New York, 1976, Appleton-Century-Crofts.

236. Travell JG, Simons DG: Myofascial pain and dysfunction: the trigger point manual, Baltimore, 1983, Williams & Wilkins.

237. Pecina MM, Krmpotic-Nemanic J, Markiewitz AD: Tunnel syndromes, Boca Raton, FL, 1991, CRC Press.

238. Haneline MT, Cooperstein R, Young M, et al: Spinal motion palpation: a comparison of studies that assessed intersegmental end feel vs excursion. J Manip Physiol Ther 31:616–626, 2008.

239. Inscoe EL, Witt PL, Gross MT, et al: Reliability in evaluating passive intervertebral motion of the lumbar spine. J Man Manip Ther 3:135–143, 1995.

240. Maitland GD: Examination of the lumbar spine. Aust J Physiother 17:5–11, 1971.

241. Latimer J, Holland M, Lee M, et al: Plinth padding and measures of posteroanterior lumbar stiffness. J Manip Physiol Ther 20:315–319, 1997.

242. Edmonston SJ, Allison GT, Gregg CD, et al: Effect of position on the posteroanterior stiffness of the lumbar spine. Man Ther 3:21–26, 1998.

243. Binkley J, Stratford PW, Gill C: Interrater reliability of lumbar accessory motion mobility testing. Phys Ther 75:786–795, 1995.

244. Fullenlove TM, Williams AJ: Comparative roentgen findings in symptomatic and asymptomatic backs. Radiology 68:572–574, 1957.

245. Gillespie HW: The significance of congenital lumbosacral abnormalities. Br J Radiol 22:270–275, 1949.

246. Magora A, Schwartz A: Relation between the low back pain syndrome and x-ray findings. Scand J Rehabil Med 10:135–145, 1978.

247. Southworth JD, Bersack SR: Anomalies of the lumbosacral vertebrae in five hundred and fifty individuals without symptoms referable to the low back. Am J Roentgenol 64:624–634, 1950.

248. Tulsi RS: Sacral arch defect and low backache. Australas Radiol 18:43–50, 1974.

249. Willis TA: An analysis of vertebral anomalies. Am J Surg 6:163–168, 1929.

250. Willis TA: Lumbosacral anomalies. J Bone Joint Surg Am 41:935–938, 1959.

251. Macnab I: The traction spur: an indicator of segmental instability. J Bone Joint Surg Am 53:663–670, 1971.

252. Friberg O: Functional radiography of the lumbar spine. Ann Med 21:341–346, 1989.

253. Boden SD: The use of radiographic imaging studies in the evaluation of patients who have degenerative disorders of the lumbar spine. J Bone Joint Surg Am 78:114–124, 1996.

254. Kingston RS: Radiology of the spine. In Watkins RG, editor: The spine in sports, St Louis, 1996, Mosby.

255. Boden SD, Wiesel SW: Lumbar spine imaging: role in clinical decision making. J Am Acad Orthop Surg 4:238–248, 1996.

256. Atlas SJ, Nardin RA: Evaluation and treatment of low back pain: an evidence-based approach to clinical care. Muscle Nerve 27:265–284, 2003.

257. Jarvik JG, Deyo RA: Diagnostic evaluation of low back pain with emphasis on imaging. Ann Intern Med 137:586–597, 2002.

258. Deyo RA, Bigos SJ, Maravilla KR: Diagnostic imaging procedures for the lumbar spine. Ann Intern Med 111:865–868, 1989.

259. Timon SJ, Gardner MJ, Wanich T, et al: Not all spondylolisthesis grading instruments are reliable. Clin Orthop Relat Res 434:157–162, 2005.

260. Li Y, Hresko MY: Radiographic analysis of spondylolisthesis and sagittal spinopelvic deformity. J Am Acad Orthop Surg 20(4):194–205, 2012.

261. Pate D, Goobar J, Resnick D, et al: Traction osteophytes of the lumbar spine: radiographic: pathologic correlation. Radiology 166:843–846, 1988.

262. Bigg-Wither G, Kelly P: Diagnostic imaging in musculoskeletal physiotherapy. In Refshauge K, Gass E: Musculoskeletal physiotherapy: clinical science and practice, Oxford, 1995, Butterworth Heinemann.

263. Wood KB, Popp CA, Transfeldt EE, et al: Radiographic evaluation of instability in spondylolisthesis. Spine 19:1697–1703, 1994.

264. Herzog RJ: The radiologic assessment for a lumbar disc herniation. Spine 21(24S):19S–38S, 1996.

265. Forristall RM, Marsh HO, Pay NT: Magnetic resonance imaging and contrast CT of the lumbar spine: comparison of diagnostic methods and correlation with surgical findings. Spine 13:1049–1054, 1988.

266. Lehman RA, Helgeson MD, Keeler KA, et al: Comparison of magnetic resonance imaging and computed tomography in predicting facet arthrosis in the cervical spine. Spine 34:65–68, 2008.

267. Masharawi Y, Kjaer P, Bendix T, et al: The reproducibility of quantitative measurements in lumbar magnetic resonance imaging of children from the general population. Spine 33(9):2094–2100, 2008.

268. Cousins JP, Haughton VM: Magnetic resonance imaging of the spine. J Am Acad Orthop Surg 17:22–30, 2009.

269. Fujiwara A, Tamai K, An HS, et al: The interspinous ligament of the lumbar spine: magnetic resonance images and their clinical significance. Spine 25:358–363, 2000.

270. Milette PC, Fontaine S, Lepanto L, et al: Differentiating lumbar disc protrusions, disc bulges and discs with normal contour but abnormal signal intensity: Magnetic resonance imaging with discographic correlations. Spine 24:44–53, 1999.

271. Saiffudin A, Braithwaite I, White J, et al: The value of lumbar spine magnetic resonance imaging in the demonstration of annular tears. Spine 23:453–457, 1998.

272. Ito M, Incorvaia KM, Yu SF, et al: Predictive signs of discogenic lumbar pain on magnetic resonance imaging with discography correlation. Spine 23:1252–1260, 1998.

273. Beattie PF, Meyers SP: Magnetic resonance imaging in low back pain: general principles and clinical issues. Phys Ther 78:738–753, 1998.

274. Raininko R, Manninen H, Battié MC, et al: Observer variability in the assessment of disc degeneration on magnetic resonance images of the lumbar and thoracic spine. Spine 20:1029–1035, 1995.

275. Boden SD, Davis DO, Dina TS, et al: Abnormal magnetic resonance scans of the lumbar spine in asymptomatic subjects: a prospective investigation. J Bone Joint Surg 72:403–408, 1990.

276. Bogduk N, Modic MT: Controversy: lumbar discography. Spine 21:402–404, 1996.

277. Magnussen L, Strand LI, Lygren H: Reliability and validity of the back performance scale: observing activity limitation in patients with back pain. Spine 29(8):903–907, 2004.

278. Demircan MN: Cramp finding: can it be used as a new diagnostic and prognostic factor in lumbar disc surgery? Eur Spine J 11:47–51, 2002.

279. Hanten WP, Dawson DD, Iwata M, et al: Craniosacral rhythm: reliability and relationships with cardiac and respiratory rates. J Orthop Sports Phys Ther 27(3):213–218, 1998.

280. Gilleard WL, Brown JM: An electromyographic validation of an abdominal muscle test. Arch Phys Med Rehabil 75:1002–1007, 1994.

281. Beattie P, Rothstein JM, Lamb RL: Reliability of the attraction method for measuring lumbar spine backward bending. Phys Ther 67(3):364–369, 1987.

282. Kippers V, Parker AW: Toe-touch test: a measure of its validity. Phys Ther 67(11):1680–1684, 1987.

283. Gross MT, Burns CB, Chapman SW, et al: Reliability and validity of rigid lift and pelvic leveling device method in assessing functional leg length

284. Bayar B, Bayar K, Yakut E, et al: Reliability and validity of the Functional Rating Index in older people with low back pain: preliminary report. Aging Clin Exp Res 16(1):49–52, 2004.

285. Hagg O, Fritzell P, Romberg K, et al: The General Function Score: a useful tool for measurement of physical disability. Validity and reliability Eur Spine J 10(3):203–210, 2001.

286. Holm I, Friis A, Storheim K, et al: Measuring self-reported functional status and pain in patients with chronic low back pain by postal questionnaires: a reliability study. Spine 28(8):828–833, 2003.

287. Hall GL, Hetzler RK, Perrin D, et al: Relationship of timed sit-up tests to isokinetic abdominal strength. Res Q Exerc Sport 63(1):80–84, 1992.

288. Holt AE, Shaw NJ, Shetty A, et al: The reliability of the low back outcome score for back pain. Spine 27(2):206–210, 2002.

289. Razmjou H, Kramer JF, Yamada R: Intertester reliability of the McKenzie evaluation in assessing patients with mechanical low-back pain. J Orthop Sports Phys Ther 30(7):368–389, 2000.

290. Kilpikoski S, Airaksinen O, Kankaanpaa M, et al: Interexaminer reliability of low back pain assessment using the McKenzie method. Spine 27(8):E207–E214, 2002.

291. Clare HA, Adams R, Maher CG: Reliability of McKenzie classification of patients with cervical or lumbar pain. J Manip Physiol Ther 28(2):122–127, 2005.

292. Donahue MS, Riddle DL, Sullivan MS: Intertester reliability of a modified version of McKenzie's lateral shift assessments obtained on patients with low back pain. Phys Ther 76(7):706–716, 1996.

293. John C, Piva SR, Fritz JM: Responsiveness of the numeric pain rating scale in patients with low back pain. Spine 30(11):1331–1334, 2005.

294. Wittink H, Turk DC, Carr DB, et al: Comparison of the redundancy, reliability, and responsiveness to change among SF-36, Oswestry Disability Index, and Multidimensional Pain Inventory. Clin J Pain 20(3):133–142, 2004.

295. Gronblad M, Hupli M, Wennerstrand P, et al: Intercorrelation and test-retest reliability of the Pain Disability Index (PDI) and the Oswestry Disability Questionnaire (ODQ) and their correlation with pain intensity in low back pain patients. Clin J Pain 9(3):189–195, 1993.

296. Fritz JM, Piva SR: Physical Impairment Index: reliability, validity and responsiveness in patients with acute low back pain. Spine 28(11):1189–1194, 2003.

297. Hodges P, Richardson C, Jull G: Evaluation of the relationship between laboratory and clinical test of transversus abdominis function. Physiother Res Int 1(1):30–40, 1996.

298. Alaranta H, Hurri H, Heliovaara M, et al: Non-dynamometric trunk performance tests: reliability and normative data. Scand J Rehab Med 26:211–215, 1994.

299. Stratford PW, Binkley JM, Riddle DL: Development and initial validation of the Back Pain Functional Scale. Spine 25(16):2095–2102, 2000.

300. Brouwer S, Kuijer W, Dijkstra PU, et al: Reliability and stability of the Roland Morris Disability Questionnaire: intra class correlation and limits of agreement. Disabil Rehabil 26(3):162–165, 2004.

301. Riddle DL, Stratford PW, Binkley JM: Sensitivity to change of the Roland-Morris Back Pain questionnaire: part 2. Phys Ther 78(11):1197–1207, 1998.

302. Archenholtz B, Ahlmen M, Bengtsson C, et al: Reliability of articular indices and function tests in a

inequality. J Orthop Sports Phys Ther 27(4):285–294, 1998.

population study of rheumatic disorders. Clin Rheumatol 8(2):215–224, 1989.

303. Williams R, Binkley J, Bloch R, et al: Reliability of the modified-modified Schober and double inclinometer methods for measuring lumbar flexion and extension. Phys Ther 73(1):33–44, 1993.

304. Perret C, Poiraudeau S, Fermanian J, et al: Validity, reliability, and responsiveness of the fingertip-to-floor test. Arch Phys Med Rehabil 82(11):1566–1570, 2001.

305. Potter BK, Freedman BZ, Andersen RC, et al: Correlation of Short Form-36 and disability status with outcomes of arthroscopic acetabular labral debridement. Am J Sports Med 33(6):864–870, 2005.

306. Taylor S, Frost H, Taylor A, et al: Reliability and responsiveness of the shuttle walking test in patients with chronic low back pain. Physiother Res Int 6(3):170–178, 2001.

307. Zwierska I, Nawaz S, Walker RD, et al: Treadmill versus shuttle walk tests of walking ability in intermittent claudication. Med Sci Sports Exerc 36(11):1835–1840, 2004.

308. Gabbe BJ, Bennell KL, Majswelner H, et al: Reliability of common lower extremity musculoskeletal screening tests. Phys Ther Sports 5:90–97, 2004.

309. Vincent-Smith B, Gibbons P: Inter-examiner and intra-examiner reliability of the standing flexion test. Man Ther 4(2):87–93, 1999.

310. van den Hoogen HJ, Koes BW, Deville W, et al: The inter-observer reproducibility of Lasègue's sign in patients with low back pain in general practice. Br J Gen Pract 46(413):727–730, 1996.

311. Kosteljanetz M, Bang F, Schmidt-Olsen S: The clinical significance of straight leg raising (Lasègue's sign) in the diagnosis of prolapsed lumbar disc: interobserver variation and correlation with surgical finding. Spine 13:393–395, 1988.

312. Deen HG Jr, Zimmerman RS, Lyons MK, et al: Test-retest reproducibility of the exercise treadmill examination in lumbar spinal stenosis. Mayo Clin Proc 75(10):1002–1007, 2000.

313. Fritz JM, Erhard RE, Delitto A, et al: Preliminary results of the use of a two-stage treadmill test as a clinical diagnostic tool in the differential diagnosis of lumbar spinal stenosis. J Spinal Disord 10(5):410–416, 1997.

314. Heiss DG, Fitch DS, Fritz JM, et al: The interrater reliability among physical therapists newly training in a classification system for acute low back pain. J Orthop Sports Phys Ther 34:430–439, 2004.

SUGGESTED READINGS

Adams MA, May S, Freeman BJ, et al: Effects of backward bending on lumbar intervertebral discs: relevance to physical therapy treatments for low back pain. Spine 25:431–437, 2000.

Adams MA, Hutton WC: The mechanical function of the lumbar apophyseal joints. Spine 8:327–330, 1983.

Anderson BJ, Ortengren GR, Nachemson AL, et al: The sitting posture: an electromyographic and discometric study. Orthop Clin North Am 6:105–120, 1975.

Andersson GB, Brown MD, Dvorak J, et al: Consensus summary on the diagnosis and treatment of lumbar disc herniation. Spine 21(24S):75S–78S, 1996.

Barasch E, DeMaro R: Typical MRI findings in sports medicine evaluation for degenerative disc disease. J Orthop Sports Phys Ther 10:290–296, 1989.

Bassett LW, Gold RH, Seeger LL: MRI atlas of the musculoskeletal system, London, 1989, Martin Dunitz.

Bellew J: Lumbar facets: an anatomic framework for low back pain. J Man Manip Ther 4:149–156, 1996.

Bogduk N, Twomey LT: Clinical anatomy of the lumbar spine, New York, 1987, Churchill Livingstone.

Bordge JA, Leboeuf-Yde C, Lothe J: Prognostic values for physical examination findings in patients with chronic low back pain treated conservatively: a systematic literature review. J Manip Physiol Ther 24:292–295, 2001.

Braggins S: Back care: a clinical approach, New York, 2000, Churchill Livingstone.

Brown A, Snyder-Mackler L: Diagnosis of mechanical low back pain in a laborer. J Orthop Sports Phys Ther 29:534–539, 1999.

Brown L: Treatment and examination of the spine by combined movements. Physiotherapy 76:66–74, 1990.

Brown MD: Diagnosis of pain syndromes of the spine. Orthop Clin North Am 6:233–248, 1975.

Cacayorin ED, Hockhauser L, Petro GR: Lumbar and thoracic spine pain in the athlete: radiographic evaluation. Clin Sports Med 6:767–783, 1987.

Cameron DM, Bohannon RW, Owen SV: Influence of hip position on measurements of the straight leg raise test. J Orthop Sports Phys Ther 19:168–172, 1994.

Carmichael SW, Buckart SL: Clinical anatomy of the lumbosacral complex. Phys Ther 59:966–968, 1979.

Cavanaugh JM: Neural mechanisms of lumbar pain. Spine 20:1804–1809, 1995.

Chadwick PR: Examination, assessment and treatment of the lumbar spine. Physiotherapy 70:2–7, 1984.

Chernukha KV, Daffner RD, Reigel DH: Lumbar lordosis measurement: a new method versus Cobb technique. Spine 23:74–80, 1998.

Childs JD, Piva SR, Fritz JM: Responsiveness of the numeric pain rating scale in patients with low back pain. Spine 30:1331–1334, 2005.

Cox ME, Asselin S, Gracovetsky SA, et al: Relationship between functional evaluation measures and self-assessment in nonacute low back pain. Spine 25:1817–1826, 2000.

Crock HV: Normal and pathological anatomy of the lumbar spinal nerve root canals. J Bone Joint Surg Br 63:487–490, 1981.

Crock HV, Yoshizawa H: The blood supply of the lumbar vertebral column. Clin Orthop 115:6–21, 1976.

Crouch JE: Functional human anatomy, Philadelphia, 1972, Lea & Febiger.

Crow NE: The "normal" lumbosacral spine. Radiology 72:97, 1959.

Cyriax J: Examination of the spinal column. Physiotherapy 56:2–6, 1970.

Daffner RD, Vaccaro AR: Adult degenerative lumbar scoliosis. Am J Ortho 32:77–82, 2003.

Davies EM: Backache and its treatment by active exercise. Physiotherapy 49:81–84, 1963.

Davis PR: The mechanics and movements of the back in working situations. Physiotherapy 53:44–47, 1967.

Delaney PM, Hubka MJ: The diagnostic utility of McKenzie clinical assessment for lower back pain. J Manip Physio Ther 22:628–629, 1999.

Deyo RA: Comparative validity of the sickness impact profile and shorter scales for functional assessment in low back pain. Spine 11:951–954, 1986.

Deyo RA: Measuring the functional status of patients with low back pain. Arch Phys Med Rehabil 69:1044–1053, 1988.

Deyo RA, Andersson G, Bombardier C, et al: Outcome measures for studying patients with low back pain. Spine 19:2032S–2036S, 1994.

Deyo RA, Haselkorn J, Hoffman R, et al: Designing studies of diagnostic tests for low back pain or radiculopathy. Spine 19:2057S–2065S, 1994.

Dixon A St: Diagnosis of low back pain: sorting the complainers. In Jayson M, editor: The lumbar spine and back pain, New York, 1976, Grune & Stratton.

Dohrmann GJ, Norwack WJ: The upgoing great toe: optimal method of elicitation. Lancet 799:339–341, 1973.

Dommisse GF, Grobler L: Arteries and veins of the nerve roots and cauda equina. Clin Orthop 115:22–29, 1976.

Doug G, Porter RW: Walking and cycling tests in neurogenic and intermittent claudications. Spine 14:965–969, 1989.

Downey BJ, Taylor NF, Niere KR: Manipulative physiotherapists can reliably palpate nominated lumbar spinal levels. Man Ther 4:151–156, 1999.

Dutton M: Orthopedic examination, evaluation and intervention, New York, 2004, McGraw Hill.

Dvorak J: Neurophysiologic tests in diagnosis of nerve root compression caused by disc herniation. Spine 21(24S):39S–44S, 1996.

Edgelow PI: Physical examination of the lumbosacral complex. Phys Ther 59:974–977, 1979.

Evans JH, Kagan A: The development of a functional rating scale to measure the treatment outcome of chronic spinal patients. Spine 11:277–281, 1986.

Evanski PM, Carver D, Nehemkis A, et al: The Burns test in low back pain: correlation with the hysterical personality. Clin Orthop 140:42–44, 1979.

Fairbank JCT, Hall H, van Akkerveeken PF, et al: Diagnoses and neuromechanisms: history taking and physical examination. In Weinstein JN, Wiesel SW, editors: The lumbar spine, Philadelphia, 1990, WB Saunders.

Finneson BE: Low back pain, ed 2, Philadelphia, 1981, JB Lippincott.

Fisk JW: The straight leg raising test: its relevance to possible disc pathology. N Z Med J 81:557–560, 1975.

Floman Y, Wiesel SW, Rothman RH: Cauda equina syndrome presenting as a herniated lumbar disc. Clin Orthop 147:234–237, 1980.

Forrester DM, Brown JC: The radiology of joint disease, Philadelphia, 1987, WB Saunders.

Forst JJ: Contribution to the clinical study of sciatica. Arch Neurol 21:220–221, 1969.

Friberg O: Clinical symptoms and biomechanics of lumbar spine and hip joint in leg length inequality. Spine 8:643–651, 1983.

Frymoyer JW, Nelson RM, Spangford E, et al: Clinical tests applicable to the study of chronic low back disability. Spine 16:681–682, 1991.

Garfin SR, Rydevik B, Lind B, et al: Spinal nerve root compression. Spine 20:1810–1820, 1995.

Gartland JJ: Fundamentals of orthopedics, Philadelphia, 1979, WB Saunders.

Gill K, Krag MH, Johnson GB, et al: Repeatability of four clinical methods for assessment of lumbar spinal motion. Spine 13:50–53, 1988.

Ginsberg GM, Bassett GS: Back pain in children and adolescents: evaluation and differential diagnosis. J Am Acad Orthop Surg 5:67–78, 1997.

Golub BS, Silverman B: Transforaminal ligaments of the lumbar spine. J Bone Joint Surg Am 51:947–956, 1969.

Gould JA: The spine: orthopedic and sports physical therapy, St Louis, 1990, Mosby.

Gregory PL, Batt ME, Kerslake RW, et al: Single photon emission computerized tomography and reverse gantry computerized tomography findings in patients with back pain investigated for spondylolysis. Clin J Sports Med 15:79–86, 2005.

Grieve GP: Common vertebral joint problems, Edinburgh, 1981, Churchill Livingstone.

Grieve GP: Mobilisation of the spine, Edinburgh, 1979, Churchill Livingstone.

Grimes PF, Massie JB, Garfin SR: Anatomic and biomechanical analysis of the lower lumbar foraminal ligaments. Spine 25:2009–2014, 2000.

Gutrecht JA, Espinosa PA, Dyck PJ: Early descriptions of common neurologic signs. Mayo Clin Proc 43:807–814, 1968.

Haas M, Jacobs GE, Raphael D, et al: Low back pain outcome measurement assessment in chiropractic teaching clinics: responsiveness and applicability of two functional disability questionnaires. J Manip Physiol Ther 18:79–87, 1995.

Hall GW: Neurologic signs and their discoveries. JAMA 95:703–707, 1930.

Hall TM, Elvey RL: Nerve trunk pain: physical diagnosis and treatment. Man Ther 4:63–73, 1999.

Harada M, Abumi K, Ito M, et al: Cineradiographic motion analysis of normal lumbar spine during forward and backward flexion. Spine 25:1932–1937, 2000.

Helfet, AJ, Lee DM: Disorders of the lumbar spine, Philadelphia, 1978, JB Lippincott.

Herman MJ, Pizzutillo PD: Spondylolysis and spondylolisthesis in the child and adolescent: a new classification. Clin Orthop Relat Res 434:46–54, 2005.

Hilibrand AS, Rand N: Degenerative lumbar stenosis: diagnosis and management. J Am Acad Orthop Surg 7:239–249, 1999.

Hirsch C, Ingelmark RO, Miller M: The anatomical bases for low back pain. Acta Orthop Scand 33:1–17, 1963.

Hollinshead WH, Jenkins DB: Functional anatomy of the limbs and back, Philadelphia, 1981, WB Saunders.

Jackson HC, Winkelmann RK, Bickel WH: Nerve endings in the human lumbar spinal column and related structures. J Bone Joint Surg Am 48:1272–1281, 1966.

Jaeger SA: Atlas of radiographic positioning: normal anatomy and development variants, Norwalk, CT, 1988, Appleton & Lange.

Jayson M: The lumbar spine and back pain, New York, 1987, Grune & Stratton.

Jenis LG, An HS: Lumbar foraminal stenosis. Spine 25:389–394, 2000.

Jensen GM: Biomechanics of the lumbar intervertebral disk: a review. Phys Ther 60:765–773, 1980.

Johnson TR, Stenbach LS: Essentials of musculoskeletal imaging, Rosemont, IL, 2004, American Academy of Orthopedic Surgeons.

Jonck LM: The mechanical disturbances resulting from lumbar disc space narrowing. J Bone Joint Surg Br 43:362–375, 1961.

Jones DM, Tearse DS, El-Khoury GY, et al: Radiographic abnormalities of the lumbar spine in college football players: a comparative analysis. Am J Sports Med 27:335–338, 1999.

Jull GA: Examination of the lumbar spine. In Grieve GP, editor: Modern manual therapy of the vertebral column, Edinburgh, 1986, Churchill Livingstone.

Kapandji LA: The physiology of joints, vol. 3: the trunk and vertebral column, New York, 1974, Churchill Livingstone.

Kay AG: An extensive literature review of the lumbar multifidus: anatomy. J Man Manip Ther 8:102–114, 2000.

Keim HA: The adolescent spine, New York, 1982, Springer-Verlag.

Keim HA: Low back pain. Clin Symp 26:2–32, 1974.

Kingston RS: Radiology of the spine. In Watkins RG, editor: The Spine in sports, St Louis, 1996, Mosby.

Kirkaldy-Willis WH: Diagnosis and treatment of lumbar spinal stenosis: American Academy of Orthopaedic Surgeons Symposium on the Lumbar Spine, St Louis, 1976, Mosby.

Kirkaldy-Willis WH: Managing low back pain, New York, 1983, Churchill Livingstone.

Kirkaldy-Willis WH: The relationship of structural pathology to the nerve root. Spine 9:49–52, 1984.

Knutson GA, Owens E: Erector spinae and quadratus lumborum muscle endurance tests and supine leg-length alignment asymmetry: an observational study. J Manip Physiol Ther 28:575–581, 2005.

Koreska J, Robertson D, Mills RH, et al: Biomechanics of the lumbar spine and its clinical significance. Orthop Clin North Am 8:121–133, 1977.

Lachacz JG: Management and rehabilitation of athletic lumbar spine injuries. In Canavan PK, editor: Rehabilitation in sports medicine: a comprehensive guide, Stanford, CT, 1998, Appleton-Lange.

Lamb DW: The neurology of spinal pain. Phys Ther 59:971–973, 1979.

Lucas DB: Mechanics of the spine. Hospital for Joint Diseases (New York Bulletin) 31:115–131, 1970.

Luoto S, Heliovaara M, Hurri H, et al: Static back endurance and the risk of low-back pain. Clin Biomech 10:323–324, 1995.

Lyu RK, Chang HS, Tang LM, et al: Thoracic disc herniation mimicking acute lumbar disc disease. Spine 24:416–418, 1999.

Madson TJ, Youdas JW, Suman VJ: Reproducibility of lumbar spine range of motion measurements using the back range of motion device. J Orthop Sports Phys Ther 29:470–477, 1999.

Maffey-Ward L, Jull G, Wellington L: Toward a clinical test of lumbar kinesthesia. J Orthop Sports Phys Ther 24:354–358, 1996.

Maher C, Adams R: Reliability of pain and stiffness assessments in clinical manual lumbar spine examination. Phys Ther 74:801–811, 1994.

Maigne R: Orthopaedic medicine: a new approach to vertebral manipulation, Springfield, IL, 1972, Charles C. Thomas.

Maitland GD: The Maitland concept: assessment, examination, and treatment by passive movement. In Twomey LT, Taylor JR, editors: Physical therapy of the low back, Edinburgh, 1987, Churchill Livingstone.

Manal TJ, Claytor R: The Delitto classification scheme and the management of lumbar spine dysfunction. Athl Ther Today 10:17–25, 2005.

Mayer T, Gatchel R, Keeley J, et al: A male incumbent worker industrial database: lumbar/cervical functional testing. Spine 19:765–770, 1994.

McCall IW: Radiologic assessment of back pain. Semin Orthop 1:71–85, 1986.

McKinnis LN: Fundamentals of musculoskeletal imaging, Philadelphia, 2005, FA Davis.

McLean IP: Tests for lumbar root tension. J Bone Joint Surg Br 76:678, 1994.

McRae R: Clinical orthopaedic examination, New York, 1976, Churchill Livingstone.

Mierau D, Cassidy JD, Yong-Hing K: Low back pain and straight leg raising in children and adolescents. Spine 14:526–528, 1989.

Mitchell FL, Moran PS, Pruzzo NA: An evaluation and treatment manual of osteopathic muscle energy procedures, Valley Park, MO, 1979, Mitchell, Moran & Pruzzo.

Miyasaka K, Ohmori K, Suzuki K, et al: Radiographic analysis of lumbar motion in relation to lumbosacral stability: investigation of moderate to maximum motion. Spine 25:732–737, 2000.

Mooney V, Andersson GB: Trunk strength testing in patient evaluation and treatment. Spine 19:2483–2485, 1994.

Morris JM: Biomechanics of the spine. Arch Surg 107:418–423, 1973.

Murphy RW: Nerve roots and spinal nerves in degenerative disc disease. Clin Orthop 129:46–60, 1977.

Nachemson A: Towards a better understanding of low back pain: a review of the mechanics of the lumbar disc. Rheumatol Rehabil 14:129–143, 1975.

O'Donoghue DH: Treatment of injuries to athletes, ed 4, Philadelphia, 1984, WB Saunders.

Ombregt L, Bisschop B, ter Veer HJ, et al: A system of orthopedic medicine, London, 1995, WB Saunders.

O'Sullivan PB: Lumbar segmental "instability": clinical presentation and specific stabilizing exercise management. Man Ther 5:2–12, 2000.

O'Sullivan PB: Diagnosis and classification of chronic low back pain disorders: maladaptive movement and motor control impairments as underlying mechanism. Man Ther 10:242–255, 2005.

Paris SV: Anatomy as related to function and pain. Orthop Clin North Am 14:475–489, 1983.

Petly NJ, Moore AP: Neuromusculoskeletal examination and assessment, New York, 1987, Churchill Livingstone.

Phillips DR, Twomey LT: A comparison of manual diagnosis with a diagnosis established by a uni-level lumbar spinal block procedure. Man Ther 2:82–87, 1996.

Polly DW, Kilkelly FX, McHale KA, et al: Measurement of lumbar lordosis: evaluation of intraobserver, interobserver and technique variability. Spine 21:1530–1536, 1996.

Porter RW, Miller CG: Back pain and trunk list. Spine 11:596–600, 1986.

Porter RW, Trailescu IF: Diurnal changes in straight leg raising. Spine 15:103–106, 1990.

Porterfield JA, DeRosa C: Mechanical low back pain: perspectives in functional anatomy, Philadelphia, 1991, WB Saunders.

Quick Reference Guide for Physicians: Acute low back problems in adults: assessment and treatment, Rockville, MD, 1994, U.S. Department of Health and Human Services.

Ramsey RH: The anatomy of the ligamentum flava. Clin Orthop 44:129–140, 1966.

Rankine JJ, Fortune DG, Hutchinson CE, et al: Pain drawings in the assessment of nerve root compression: a comparative study with lumbar spine magnetic resonance imaging. Spine 23:1668–1676, 1998.

Rauschnig W, Heithoff KB, Stoller DW, et al: Radiology. In Weinstein JN, Weisel SW, editors: The lumbar spine, Philadelphia, 1990, WB Saunders.

Reilly BM: Practical strategies in outpatient medicine, Philadelphia, 1984, WB Saunders.

Resnick D, MJ Kransdorf: Bone and joint imaging, Philadelphia, 2005, WB Saunders.

Richardson JK, Iglarsh ZA: Clinical orthopedic physical therapy, Philadelphia, 1994, WB Saunders.

Riddle DL: Classification and low back pain: a review of the literature and critical analysis of selected systems. Phys Ther 78:708–737, 1998.

Robinson LR: Role of neurophysiologic evaluation in diagnosis. J Am Acad Orthop Surg 8:190–199, 2000.

Rose K, Balasubramaniam P: Nerve root canals in the lumbar spine. Spine 9:16–18, 1984.

Rothman RH, Simeone FA: The spine, Philadelphia, 1982, WB Saunders.

Rydevik B, Brown MD, Lundberg G: Pathoanatomy and pathophysiology of nerve root compression. Spine 9:7–15, 1984.

Saal JS: The role of inflammation in lumbar pain. Spine 20:1821–1827, 1995.

Saunders HD, Saunders R: Evaluation, treatment and prevention of musculoskeletal disorders, Chaska, MN, 1993, Saunders Group.

Schenk R: A combined approach to lumbar examination. J Man Manip Ther 4:77–80, 1996.

Seimen LP: Low back pain: clinical diagnosis and management, Norwalk, CT, 1983, Appleton-Century-Crofts.

Selby DK: When to operate and what to operate on. Orthop Clin North Am 14:577–588, 1983.

Selim AJ, Fincke G, Ren XS, et al: Patient characteristics and patterns of use for lumbar spine radiographs: results from the veterans health study. Spine 25:2440–2444, 2000.

Shacklock MO, Butler DS, Slater H: The dynamic central nervous system: structure and clinical neurobiomechanics. In Boyling JD, Palastanga N, editors: Grieve's modern manual therapy, Edinburgh, 1994, Churchill Livingstone.

Shaw WS, Pransky G, Patterson W, et al: Early disability risk factors for low back pain assessed at outpatient occupational health clinics. Spine 30:572–580, 2005.

Simmons ED, Guyer RD, Graham-Smith A, et al: Radiographic assessments for patients with low back pain. Spine 20:1839–1841, 1995.

Smith SA, Massie JB, Chesnut R, et al: Straight leg raising: anatomical effects on the spinal nerve root with and without fusion. Spine 18:992–999, 1993.

Snook SH: Low back pain in industry: American Academy of Orthopaedic Surgeons Symposium on Idiopathic Low Back Pain, St Louis, 1982, Mosby, pp. 23–38.

Sorensen FB: Physical measurements as risk indicators for low back trouble over a one year period. Spine 9:106–119, 1984.

Spivak JM: Degenerative lumbar spine stenosis. J Bone Joint Surg Am 80:1053–1066, 1998.

Sullivan MS, Schoaf LD, Riddle DL: The relationship of lumbar flexion to disability in patients with low back pain. Phys Ther 80:240–250, 2000.

Supik LF, Broom MJ: Sciatic tension signs and lumbar disc herniation. Spine 19:1066–1069, 1994.

Tachdjian MO: Pediatric orthopedics, Philadelphia, 1972, WB Saunders.

Tenhula JA, Rose SJ, Delitto A: Association between direction of lateral lumbar shift, movement tests and side of symptoms in patients with low back pain syndrome. Phys Ther 70:480–486, 1990.

Thelander U, Fagerlund M, Friberg S, et al: Straight leg raising test versus radiologic size, shape, and position of lumbar disc hernias. Spine 17:395–399, 1992.

Troyanovich SJ, Harrison DD, Harrison DE: Low back pain and the lumbar intervertebral disc: clinical considerations for the doctor of chiropractic. J Manip Physiol Ther 22:96–104, 1999.

Van Wijmen PM: The use of repeated movements in the McKenzie method of spinal examination. In Boyling JD, Palastanga N, editors: Grieve's modern manual therapy: the vertebral column, ed 2, Edinburgh, 1994, Churchill Livingstone.

Vanharanta H, Sachs BL, Spivey M, et al: A comparison of CT/discography, pain response and radiographic disc height. Spine 13:321–324, 1988.

Vialle R, Levassor N, Rillardon L, et al: Radiographic analysis of the sagittal alignment and balance of the spine in asymptomatic subjects. J Bone Joint Surg Am 87:260–267, 2005.

Waddell G: Clinical assessment of lumbar impairment. Clin Orthop 221:110–120, 1987.

Waddell G, Main CJ: Assessment of severity in low back disorders. Spine 9:204–208, 1984.

Watkins RG: History, physical examination, and diagnostic tests for back and lower extremity problems. In Watkins RG, editor: The spine in sports, St Louis, 1996, Mosby.

Weise MD, Garfin SR, Gelberman RH, et al: Lower extremity sensibility testing in patients with herniated lumbar intervertebral discs. J Bone Joint Surg Am 67:1219–1224, 1985.

Weissman BNW, Sledge CB: Orthopedic radiology, Philadelphia, 1986, WB Saunders.

White AA, Panjabi MM: Clinical biomechanics of the spine, Philadelphia, 1978, JB Lippincott.

Wiesel SW, Bernini P, Rothman RH: The aging lumbar spine, Philadelphia, 1982, WB Saunders.

Williams M, Solomonov M, Zhou BH, et al: Multifidus spasms elicited by prolonged lumbar flexion. Spine 25:2916–2924, 2000.

Williams PL, Warwick R, editors: Gray's anatomy, ed 36, British, Edinburgh, 1980, Churchill Livingstone.

Williams RM, Goldsmith CH, Minuk T: Validity of the double inclinometer method for measuring lumbar flexion. Physiother Can 50:147–152, 1998.

Wittink H, Michel TH, Kulich R, et al: Aerobic fitness testing in patients with chronic low back pain: which test is best? Spine 25:1704–1710, 2000.

Yingling VR, McGill SM: Anterior shear of spinal motion segments: kinematics, kinetics and resultant injuries observed in a porcine model. Spine 24:1882–1889, 1999.

Yong-Hing K, Kirkaldy-Willis WH: The pathophysiology of degenerative disease of the lumbar spine. Orthop Clin North Am 14:491–504, 1983.

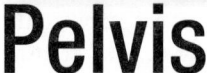

Pelvis

The sacroiliac joints form the "key" of the arch between the two pelvic bones; with the symphysis pubis, they help to transfer the weight from the spine to the lower limbs and provide elasticity to the pelvic ring (Figure 10-1). This triad of joints also acts as a buffer to decrease the force of jars and bumps to the spine and upper body caused by contact of the lower limbs with the ground. Because of this shock-absorbing function, the structure of the sacroiliac and symphysis pubis joints is different from that of most joints that are assessed. Assessment of the sacroiliac joints and symphysis pubis should be included in the examination of the lumbar spine and/or hips if there is no direct trauma to either one of these joints.[1] Normally, a comprehensive examination of the sacroiliac joints is not made until examination of the lumbar spine and/or hip has been completed. If both of these joints are examined and the problem still appears to be present and remains undiagnosed, an examination of the pelvis should be initiated.

APPLIED ANATOMY

The **sacroiliac joints** are part synovial joint and part syndesmosis. A syndesmosis is a type of fibrous joint in which the intervening fibrous connective tissue forms an interosseous membrane or ligament. The synovial portion of the joint is C-shaped, with the convex iliac surface of the C facing anteriorly and inferiorly. Kapandji[2] states that the greater or the more acute the angle of the C, the more stable the joint and the less the likelihood of a lesion to the joint. The sacral surface is slightly concave.

The size, shape, and roughness of the articular surfaces of the sacrum vary greatly among individuals. In the child, these surfaces are smooth. In the adult, they become irregular depressions and elevations that fit into one another; by so doing, they restrict movement at the joint and add strength to the joint for transferring weight from the lower limb to the spine. The articular surface of the ilium is covered with fibrocartilage; the articular surface of the sacrum is covered with hyaline cartilage that is three times thicker than that of the ilium. In older persons, parts of the joint surfaces may be obliterated by adhesions.

Sacroiliac Joint	
Resting position:	Neutral
Capsular pattern:	Pain when joints are stressed
Close pack:	Nutation
Loose pack:	Counternutation

Although the sacroiliac joints are relatively mobile in young people, they become progressively stiffer with age. In some cases, ankylosis results. The movements that occur in the sacroiliac and symphysis pubis joints are slight compared with the movements occurring in the spinal joints.

The sacroiliac joints are supported by several strong ligaments (Figure 10-2)—the long posterior sacroiliac ligaments that limit anterior pelvic rotation[3] or sacral counternutation, the short posterior sacroiliac ligament that limits all pelvic and sacral movement, the posterior interosseous ligament that forms part of the sacroiliac articulation (the syndesmosis), and the anterior sacroiliac ligaments.[4] The sacrotuberous ligament and sacrospinous ligament limit nutation and posterior innominate rotation and provides vertical stability.[4] The iliolumbar ligament stabilizes L5 on the ilium.[4]

The sacroiliac joints and symphysis pubis have no muscles that control their movements directly, although muscles do provide pelvic stability. However, they are influenced by the action of the muscles moving the lumbar spine and hip, because many of these muscles attach to the sacrum and pelvis (Table 10-1).

The muscles that support the pelvic girdle as well as the lumbar spine and hips can be divided into groups.[5–7] The outer group consists of four groupings, which act primarily in crossing or oblique patterns of force couples to stabilize the pelvis. The deep posterior longitudinal system consists of the erector spinae, thoracolumbar fascia, and the hamstring muscles, along with the sacrotuberous ligament (Figure 10-3). The superficial posterior oblique system includes the latissimus dorsi, gluteus maximus, and the intervening thoracolumbar fascia (Figure 10-4, *A*). The anterior oblique system consists of the internal and external obliques, the contralateral adductors, and the abdominal fascia in between (Figure 10-4, *B*). The lateral system consists of gluteus medius and minimus and the contralateral adductors (Figure 10-5). The innermost muscle group consists of the multifidus, transverse abdominus, diaphragm (Figure 10-6), and pelvic floor muscles (Figure 10-7) that can play a role in stabilizing the pelvis and indirectly the lumbar spine. The anterior-posterior superficial group controls the anterior-posterior rotation of the pelvis on the fixed

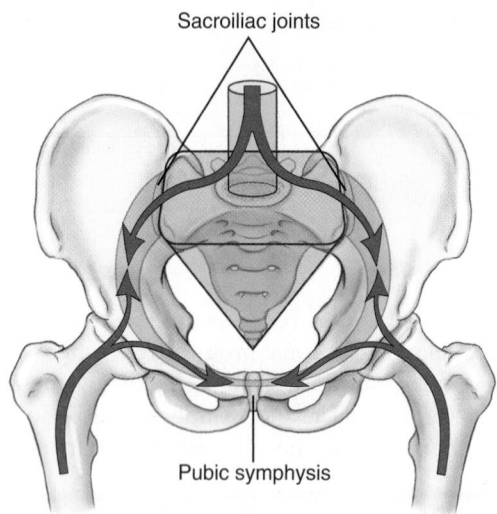

Figure 10-1 The components of the pelvic ring. The *arrows* show the direction of body weight force as it is transferred between the pelvic ring, trunk, and femurs. The keystone of the pelvic ring is the sacrum, which is wedged between the two ilia and secured bilaterally by the sacroiliac joints. (From Neumann DA: Kinesiology of the musculoskeletal system, ed 2, St Louis, 2010, CV Mosby, p. 360. Redrawn after Kapandji IA: The physiology of joints, vol 3, New York, 1974, Churchill Livingstone.)

femur. This group consists of the hamstrings and gluteus maximus, erector spinae, rectus abdominis, internal and external obliques, psoas, rectus femoris and sartorius, and the iliofemoral and sacrotuberous ligaments (Figure 10-8). These muscle systems help to actively stabilize the pelvic joints and contribute significantly to load transfer during gait and pelvic rotational activities.[5]

The **symphysis pubis** is a fibrocartilaginous joint held together by the pubic ligament. There is a disc of fibrocartilage between the two joint surfaces called the **interpubic disc.** This joint does allow limited movement.

The **sacrococcygeal joint** is usually a fused line (symphysis) united by a fibrocartilaginous disc. It is found between the apex of the sacrum and the base of the coccyx. Occasionally, the joint is freely movable and synovial. With advanced age, the joint may fuse and be obliterated.

PATIENT HISTORY

In addition to the questions listed under the "Patient History" section in Chapter 1, the examiner should obtain the following information from the patient:

1. *Was there any known mechanism of injury? Has there been more than one episode?* For example, the sacroiliac joints are commonly injured by a sudden jar caused by inadvertently stepping off a curb, an overzealous kick (either missing the object or hitting the ground), a fall on the buttocks, or a lift and twist maneuver.[8] Has the patient experienced any recent falls, twists, or strains? These movements increase the chance of sacroiliac joint sprains.

2. *Where is the pain, and does it radiate?* With a lesion of the sacroiliac joint, deep, dull, undefined pain tends to be unilateral and can be referred to the posterior thigh, iliac fossa, and buttock on the affected

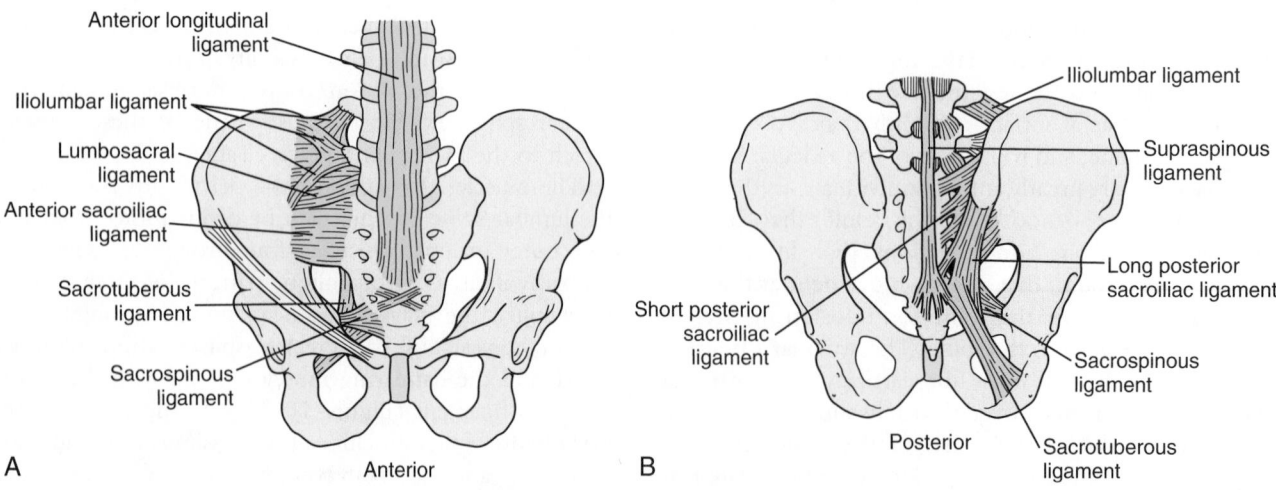

Figure 10-2 Ligaments of the pelvis. A, Anterior view. **B,** Posterior view.

TABLE **10-1**

Muscles Attaching to the Pelvis

Muscles	Nerve Root Derivation
Latissimus dorsi	Thoracodorsal (C6–C8)
Erector spinae	L1–L3
Multifidus	L1–L5
External oblique	T7–T12
Internal oblique	T7–T12, L1
Transverse abdominis	T7–T12, L1
Rectus abdominis	T6–T12
Pyramidalis	Subcostal (T12)
Quadratus lumborum	T12, L1–L4
Psoas minor	L1
Iliacus	Femoral (L2, L3)
Levator ani	S4, inferior rectal nerve/ pudendal nerve
Sphincter ani externus	S2–S4
Superficial transverse perineal ischiocavernous	S2–S4
Coccygeus	S4, S5
Gluteus maximus	Inferior gluteal (L5, S1, S2)
Gluteus medius	Superior gluteal (L5, S1)
Gluteus minimus	Superior gluteal (L5, S1)
Obturator internus	Nerve to obturator internus (L5, S1)
Obturator externus	Obturator (L3, L4)
Piriformis	L5, S1, S2
Interior gemellus	Nerve to quadratus femoris (L5, S1)
Superior gemellus	Nerve to obturator internus (L5, S1)
Pectineus	Femoral (L2, L3)
Semimembranosus	Sciatic (L5, S1, S2)
Semitendinosus	Sciatic (L5, S1, S2)
Biceps femoris	Sciatic (L5, S1, S2)
Tensor fascia lata	Superior gluteal (L4, L5)
Sartorius	Femoral (L2, L3)
Rectus femoris	Femoral (L2–L4)
Gracilis	Obturator (L2, L3)
Adductor magnus	Obturator/sciatic (L2–L4)
Adductor longus	Obturator (L2–L4)
Adductor brevis	Obturator (L2–L4)

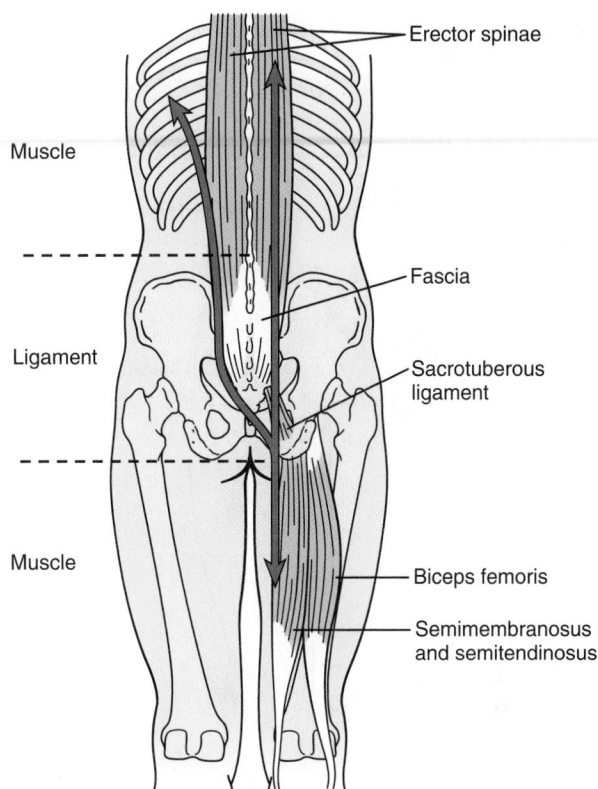

Figure 10-3 The deep longitudinal muscle system of the outer group (includes the erector spinae, deep lamina of the thoracolumbar fascia, sacrotuberous ligament, and biceps femoris muscle).

side. Sacroiliac pain does not commonly extend below the knee.

3. *When does the pain occur? Does the pain keep the patient awake?* Pain that is caused by sacroiliac joint problems is usually felt when turning in bed, getting out of bed, or stepping up with the affected leg. Often, the pain is constant and unrelated to position. Symphysis pubis pain tends to be localized and increases with any movement involving the adductor or rectus abdominus muscles.

4. *What particular movements bother the patient?* Usually transitional type movements (e.g., sit to stand, single

leg squat) cause pain in the sacroiliac joint if it is involved.

5. *What is the patient's habitual working stance? Is a great deal of sitting or twisting involved?* The examiner should look for postures that potentially increase the stress on the sacroiliac joints (e.g., standing, especially on one leg).

6. *What is the patient's usual activity or pastime?* Again, would any of these activities stress the sacroiliac joints?

7. *Is there any particular position or activity that aggravates the condition?* Climbing or descending stairs, walking, and standing from a sitting position all stress the sacroiliac joint (Tables 10-2 and 10-3).

8. *What is the patient's age?* Apophyseal injuries and avulsion fractures of the pelvis can occur in young athletes.[9] Ankylosing spondylitis is found primarily in men between the ages of 15 and 35 years. Hypomobility is likely to be seen in men between 40 and 50 and in women after 50 years of age.[10]

9. *Does the patient have or feel any weakness in the lower limbs?* Neurological deficit in the limbs can be present if the sacroiliac joint is affected.

10. *Has the patient had any difficulty with micturition?* It has been reported that sacroiliac joint dysfunction can lead to urinary problems.[11]

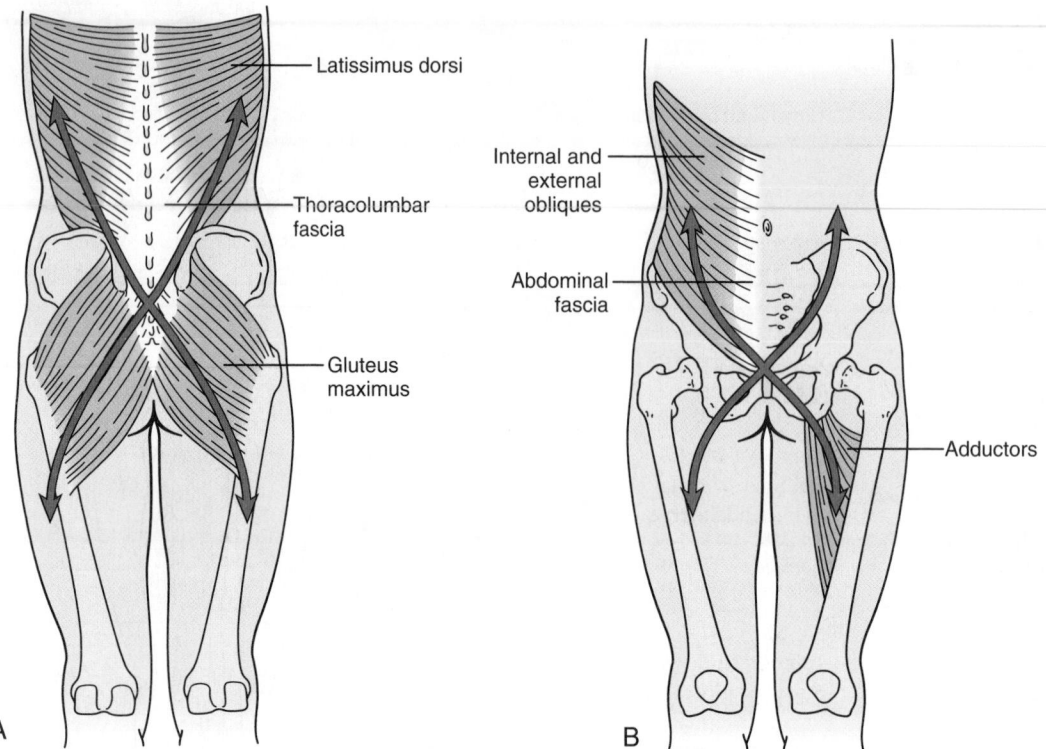

Figure 10-4 A, The posterior oblique muscle system of the outer group (includes the latissimus dorsi, gluteus maximus, and intervening thoracolumbar fascia). **B,** The anterior oblique muscle system of the outer group (includes the external and internal obliques, contralateral adductors of the thigh, and intervening anterior abdominal fascia).

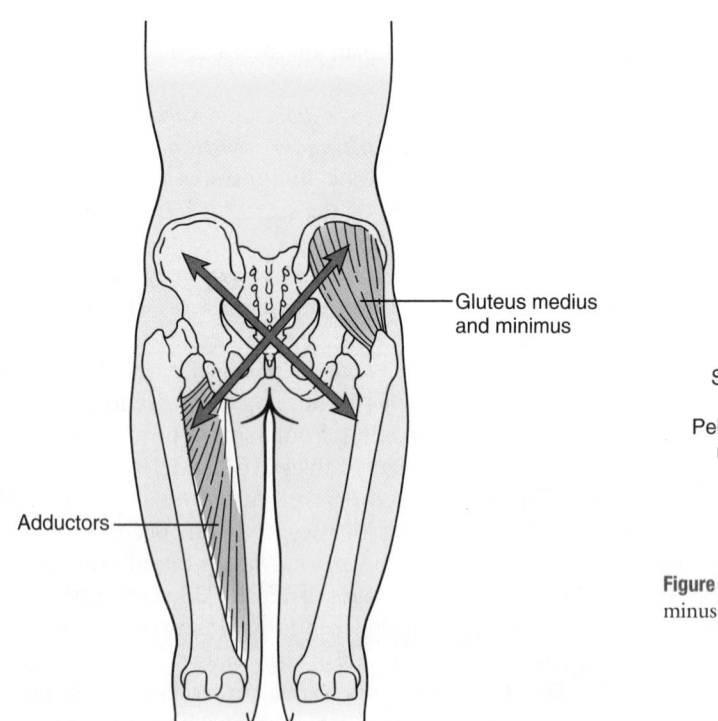

Figure 10-5 The lateral muscle system of the outer group (includes the gluteus medius and minimus and contralateral adductors of the thigh).

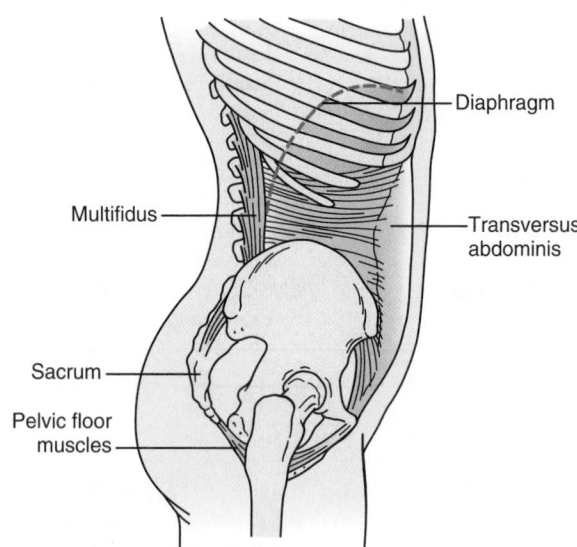

Figure 10-6 The inner muscle unit including multifidus, transverse abdominus, and the pelvis floor muscles.

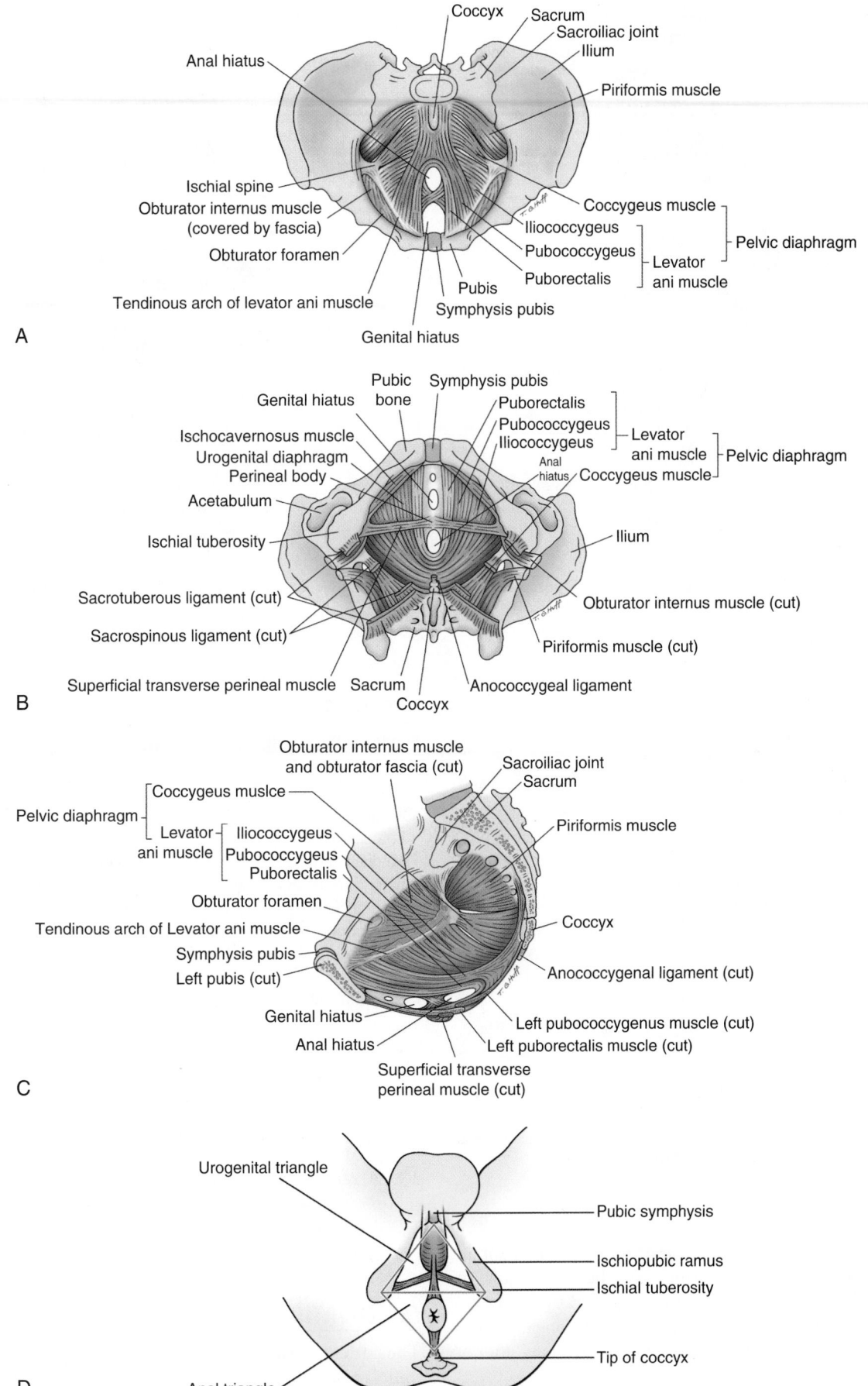

Figure 10-7 Muscles of the pelvic floor. A, Superior view. **B,** Inferior view. **C,** Medial view (female). **D,** Subdivisions of perineum.

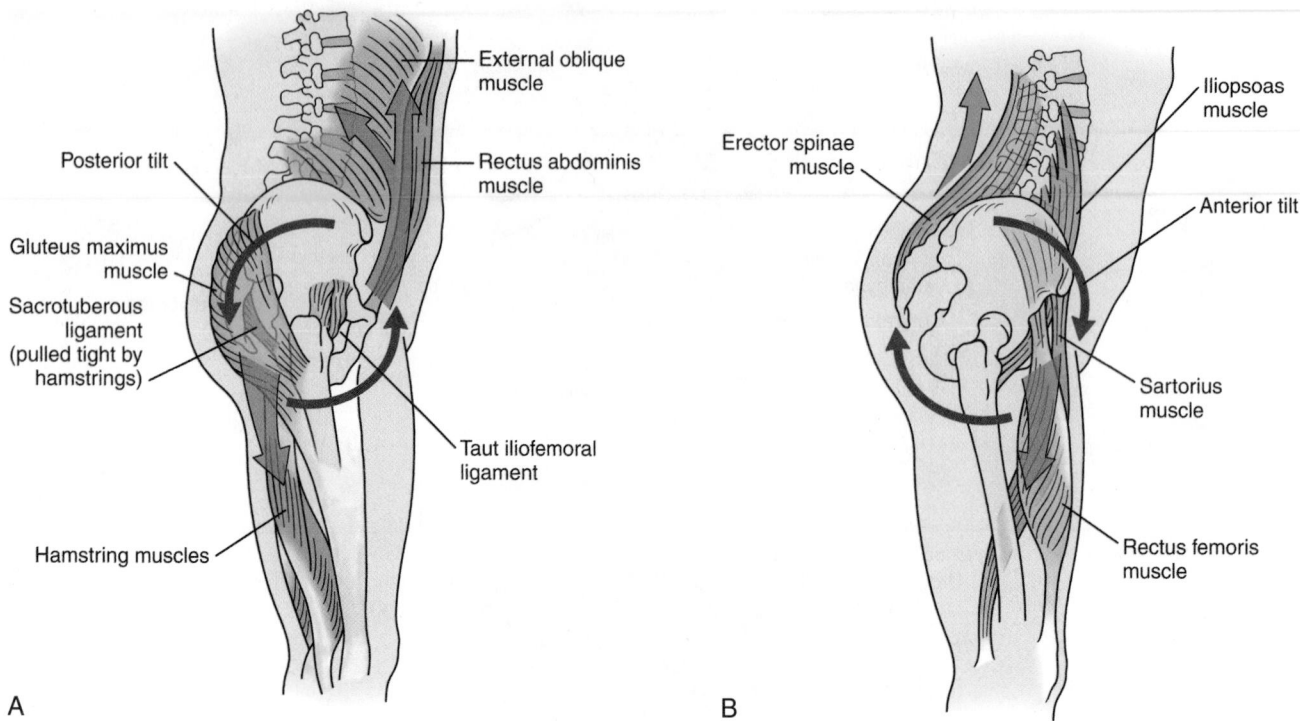

Figure 10-8 **The anterior-posterior superficial muscle group. A,** Muscles and ligaments involved in posterior tilt. **B,** Muscles and ligaments involved in anterior tilt.

TABLE 10-2

Pelvic Motions with Lumbar Spine Movement

Lumbar Spine	Innominate	Sacrum
Flexion	Anterior rotation	Nutation followed by counternutation
Extension	Posterior rotation (slight)	Nutation
Rotation	Same side: posterior rotation Opposite side: anterior rotation	Nutation on same side
Side flexion	Same side: anterior rotation Opposite side: posterior rotation	Side bend

Adapted from Dutton M: Orthopedic examination, evaluation and intervention, ed 3, New York, 2012, McGraw-Hill.

TABLE 10-3

Pelvic Motions with Hip Movement

Hip	Innominate
Flexion	Posterior rotation
Extension	Anterior rotation
Medial rotation	Inflare (medial rotation)
Lateral rotation	Outflare (lateral rotation)
Abduction	Superior glide
Adduction	Inferior glide

Adapted from Dutton M: Orthopedic examination, evaluation and intervention, ed 3, New York, 2012, McGraw-Hill.

11. *Has there been a recent pregnancy?* In females, sprain of the sacroiliac ligaments can be the result of increased laxity of the ligaments caused by hormonal changes. It may take 3 to 4 months or longer for the ligaments to return to their normal state after a pregnancy.

12. *Does the patient have a past history of rheumatoid arthritis, Reiter syndrome, or ankylosing spondylitis?* Each of these conditions can involve the sacroiliac joints.

13. *Are there any psychosocial issues that are relevant in the presence of pathology?* Questions about anxiety, depression, and other psychosocial issues should be addressed if considered important.[12]

OBSERVATION

The patient must be suitably undressed. For the sacroiliac joints to be observed properly, the patient is often required

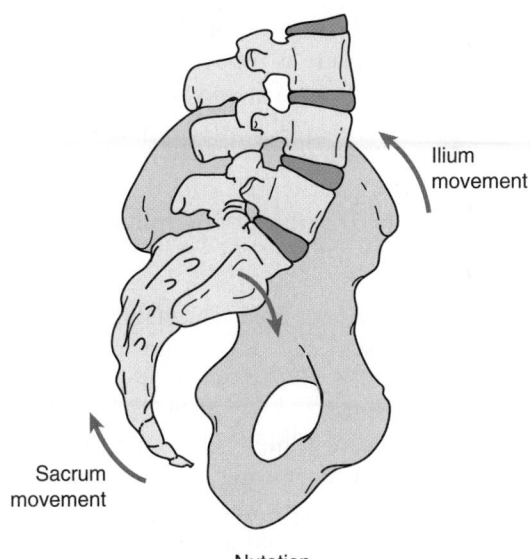

Nutation

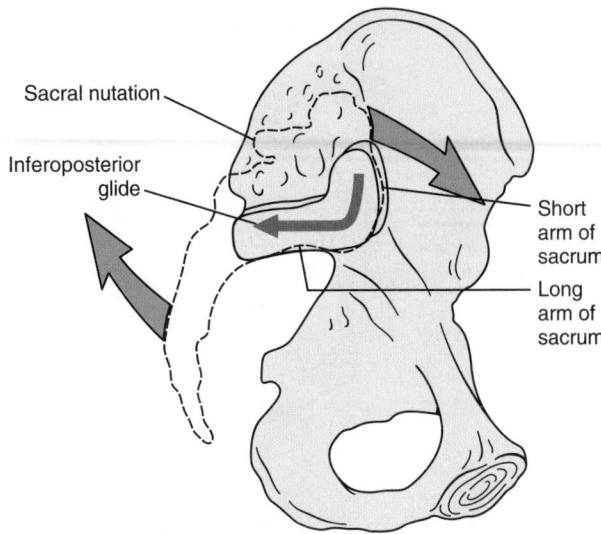

Figure 10-10 When the sacrum nutates, its articular surface glides infero-posteriorly relative to the innominate bones. (Redrawn from Lee D: The pelvic girdle, ed 3, Edinburgh, 2004, Churchill Livingstone, p. 60.)

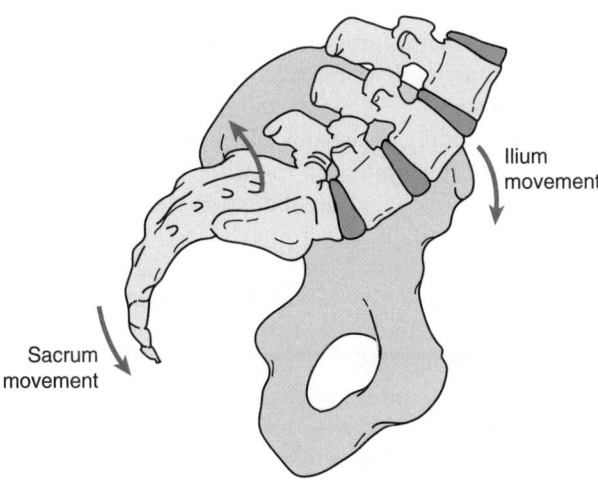

Counternutation

Figure 10-9 Movements of nutation and counternutation occurring at the sacroiliac joint.

to be nude from the middle of the chest to the toes. If he or she wishes to wear shorts, they must be rolled down as far as possible so that the sacroiliac joints are visible. The posterior, superior, and inferior iliac spines must be visible. The patient stands and is viewed from the front, side, and back. The examiner should note the following:

1. Are the posture (see Chapter 15) and gait (see Chapter 14) normal? **Nutation**[5,13] (sacral locking) is the forward motion of the base of the sacrum into the pelvis; it could also be described as the backward rotation of the ilium on the sacrum (Figure 10-9). It is the most stable position of the sacroiliac joint and is an example of **form closure.** When moving from supine lying to standing, the sacrum normally moves bilaterally, just as it does in early movement of trunk

flexion. The ilia move closer together, and the ischial tuberosities move farther apart.[10] Unilaterally, the sacrum normally moves with hip flexion of the lower limb.[5] Pathologically, if nutation occurs only on one side (where it should occur bilaterally), the examiner will find that the anterior superior iliac spine (ASIS) is higher and the posterior superior iliac spine (PSIS) is lower on that side.[13] The result is an apparent or functional short leg on the same side.[14] Nutation is limited by the anterior sacroiliac ligaments, the sacrospinous ligament, and the sacrotuberous ligament and is more stable than counternutation. Nutation occurs when a person assumes a "pelvic tilt" position. During nutation, the sacrum will slide down its short part and then posteriorly along its long part (Figure 10-10).[5]

Counternutation (sacral unlocking), or *contranutation* as it is sometimes called, is the opposite movement to nutation. It indicates an anterior rotation of the ilium on the sacrum or backward motion of the base of the sacrum out of the pelvis.[5] The iliac bones move farther apart, and the ischial tuberosities approximate.[10] Pathologically, if counternutation occurs only on one side as it does during extension of the extremity on that side, the lower limb on that side will probably be medially rotated.[5] Pathological or abnormal counternutation on one side occurs when the ASIS is lower and the PSIS is higher on one side.[13] Counternutation is limited by the posterior sacroiliac ligaments. Counternutation occurs when a person assumes a "lordotic" or "anterior pelvic tilt" position. During counternutation, the sacrum will slide anteriorly along its long arm and then superiorly up its short arm (Figure 10-11).[5] This

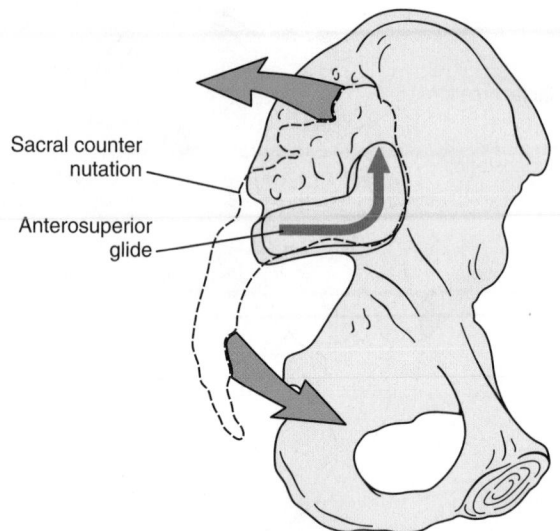

Figure 10-11 When the sacrum counternutates, its articular surface glides anterosuperiorly relative to the innominate bones. (Redrawn from Lee D: The pelvic girdle, ed 3, Edinburgh, 2004, Churchill Livingstone, p. 60.)

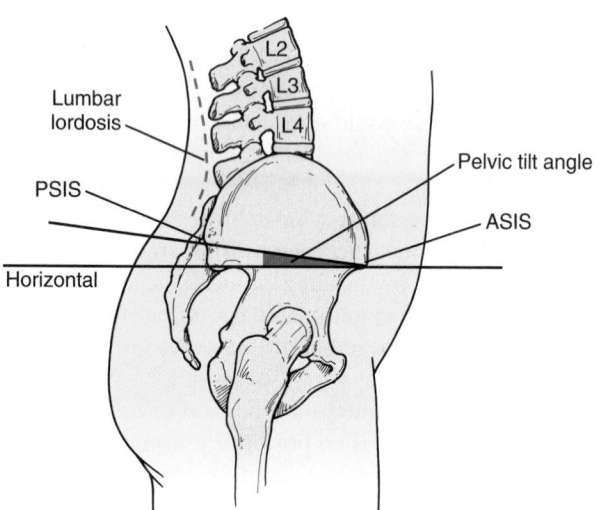

Figure 10-12 Pelvic tilt angle (7° to 15°).

motion is resisted by the long posterior sacroiliac ligament supported by the multifidus (contraction of multifidus causes nutation of the sacrum).[5]

Levine and Whittle[15] found that anterior and posterior pelvic tilt has an effect on lumbar lordosis with an average change of 20° being possible (9° posteriorly and 11° anteriorly). Thus, looking for the "**neutral pelvis**" position becomes important especially for later rehabilitation. Based on their data, a "neutral pelvis" would be somewhere between the two extremes. Pelvic tilt is the angle between a line joining the ASIS and PSIS, and a horizontal line (Figure 10-12). Average pelvic tilt is 11° ± 4°.[15,16]

Ideal pelvic alignment would see the ASIS on the same vertical plane as the symphysis pubis.[17]

Three questions should be considered when looking for a "neutral pelvis" and whether the pelvis can be stabilized:

i. Can the patient get into the "neutral pelvis" position? If not, what is restricting the movement, or what is weak so that the movement does not occur?

ii. Can the patient hold (i.e., stabilize) the "neutral pelvis" statically while moving distal joints dynamically? If not, what muscles need to be strengthened?

iii. Can the patient hold (i.e., stabilize) the "neutral pelvis" when moving it dynamically? If not, which muscles are weak and/or not functioning correctly (i.e., functioning isometrically, concentrically, eccentrically)?

These questions will help the examiner determine if the pelvis (and lumbar spine) can be stabilized during different movements or positions so that other muscles that originate from the pelvis can function properly. The ability to be able to stabilize the pelvis statically or dynamically plays a significant role in proper functioning of the whole kinetic chain. For example, side lying hip abduction should be able to be performed in the frontal plane with the lower limbs, pelvis, trunk and shoulders aligned in the frontal plane (**active hip abduction test** ☑).[18] If the leg wobbles, the pelvis tips, the shoulders or trunk rotate, the hip flexes or the abducted limb medially rotates, it is an indication of lack of movement control, lack of muscle balance and an inability to stabilize the pelvis while doing the movement so that the muscles have a firm base from which to function.

Gait is often affected if the pathology involves the pelvis. If the sacroiliac joints are not free to move, the stride length is decreased and a vertical limp may be present.[8] A painful sacroiliac joint may also cause reflex inhibition of the gluteus medius, leading to a Trendelenburg gait or lurch.

2. Are the ASISs level when viewed anteriorly (Figure 10-13)? On the affected side, the ASIS often tends to be higher and slightly forward. The examiner must remember this difference, if present, when the patient is viewed from behind (Figure 10-14). If the ASIS and PSIS on one side are higher than the ASIS and PSIS on the other side, this indicates an **upslip** of the ilium on the sacrum on the high side, a short leg on the opposite side, or muscle spasm caused by lumbar pathology (e.g., disc lesion).[19-22] If the ASIS is higher on one side and the PSIS is lower at the same time, it indicates an **anterior torsion** of the sacrum (pathological nutation) on that side.[19] This torsion may result in a spinal scoliosis or an altered functional leg

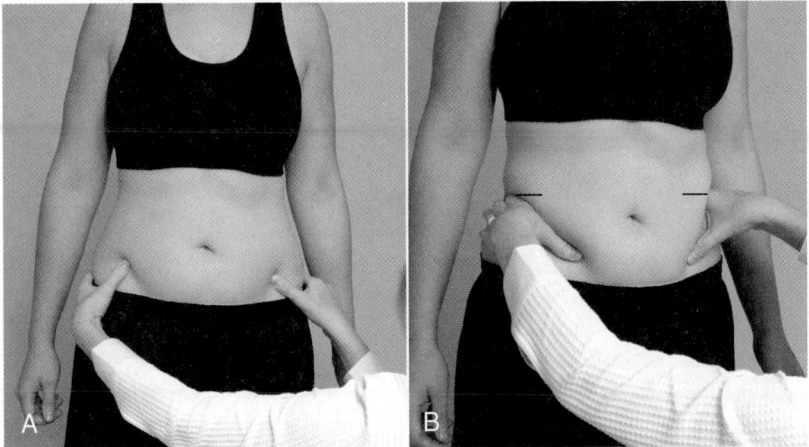

Figure 10-13 Anterior observational view. A, Level of anterior superior iliac spines (ASISs). **B,** Level of iliac crests.

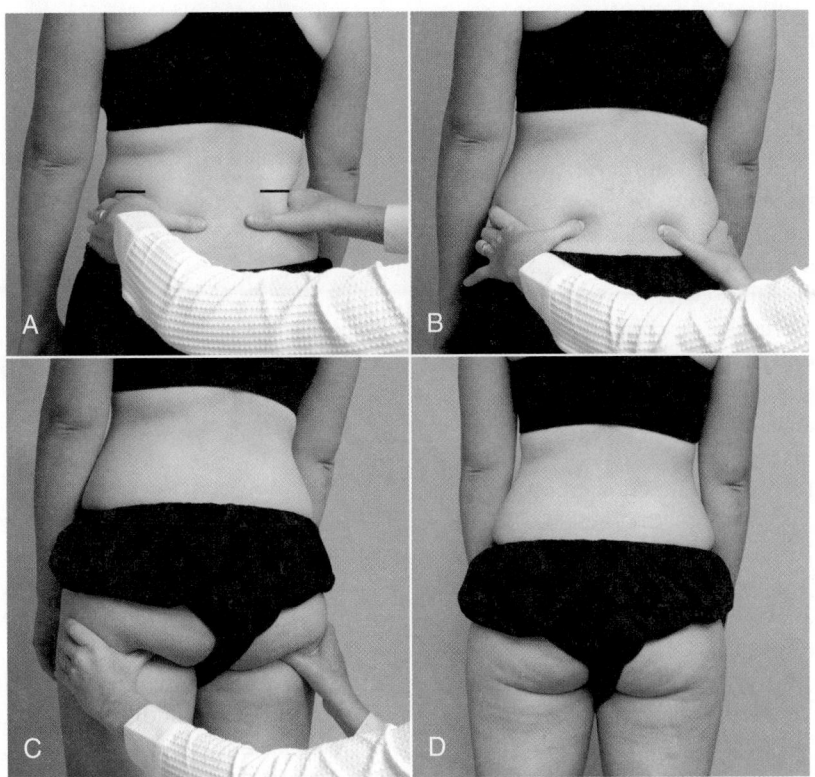

Figure 10-14 Posterior observational view. A, Level of iliac crests. **B,** Level of posterior superior iliac spines (PSISs). **C,** Level of ischial tuberosities. **D,** Level of gluteal folds.

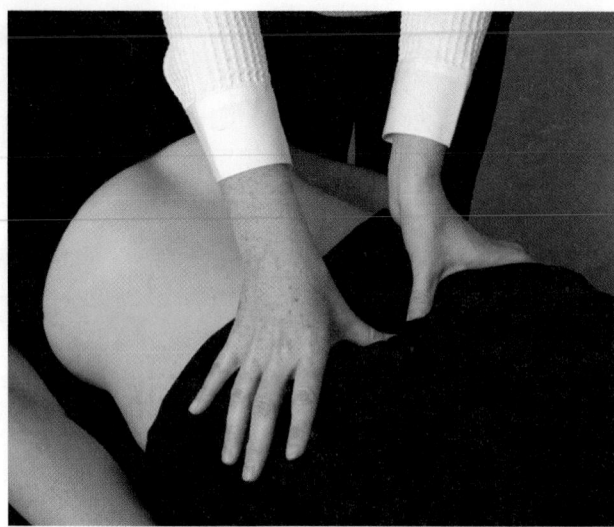

Figure 10-15 Determining level of pubic bones.

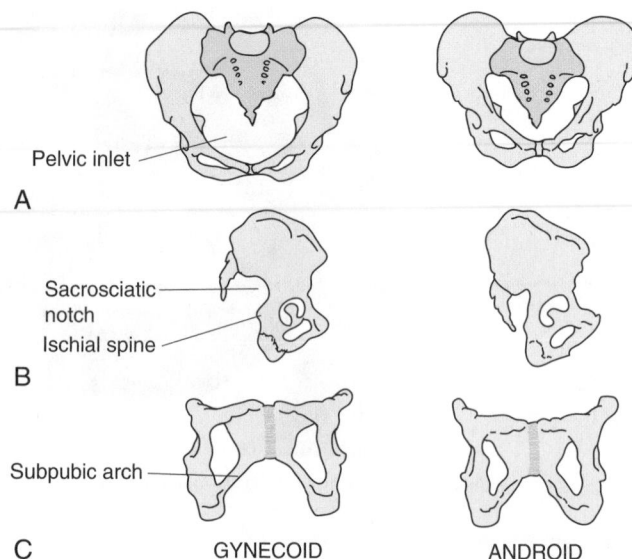

Pelvic inlet

A

Sacrosciatic notch

Ischial spine

B

Subpubic arch

C GYNECOID ANDROID

Figure 10-16 Gynecoid (predominantly female) and android (primarily male) pelvises. **A,** Anterior view. **B,** Lateral view. **C,** Anterior view of the pubis and ischium.

length, or both. Anterior rotational dysfunction is seen most frequently following a posterior horizontal thrust of the femur (dashboard injury), golf or baseball swing, or any forced anterior diagonal pattern.[20] The sacrum is lower on the side of the pelvis that has rotated backward. The most common rotation of the innominate bones is left posterior torsion or rotation (pathological counternutation). The posterior rotational dysfunctions are usually the result of falling on an ischial tuberosity, lifting when forward flexed with the knees straight, repeated standing on one leg, vertical thrusting onto an extended leg, or sustaining hyperflexion and abduction of hips.

3. Are both pubic bones level at the symphysis pubis? The examiner tests for level equality by placing one finger or thumb on the superior aspect of each pubic bone and comparing the heights (Figure 10-15). If the ASIS on one side is higher, the pubic bone on that side is suspected to be higher, and this can be confirmed by this procedure, indicating a backward torsion problem of the ilium on that side. This procedure is usually done with the patient lying supine.

4. Does the patient, when standing, have equal weight on both feet, favor one leg, or have a lateral pelvic tilt? This finding may indicate pathology in the sacroiliac joints, the leg, the spine, or a short leg.

5. Are the ASISs equidistant from the center line of the body?

6. What type of pelvis does the patient have?[23] Gynecoid and android types are the most common (as described in Figure 10-16 and Table 10-4).

7. Are the iliac crests level? Altered leg length may alter their height.

8. Are the PSISs level?

TABLE 10-4

A Comparison of the Two Most Common Types of Pelvis

Feature	Gynecoid	Android
Inlet	Round	Triangular
Sacrosciatic notch	Average size	Narrow
Sacrum	Average	Forward
Subpubic arch	Inclination curved	Inclination straight

9. Are the buttock contours or gluteal folds normal? The painful side is often flatter if there is loss of tone in the gluteus maximus muscle.

10. Is there any unilateral or bilateral spasm of the erector spinae muscles?

11. Are the ischial tuberosities level? If one tuberosity is higher, it may indicate an upslip of the ilium on the sacrum on that side.[19]

12. Is there excessive lumbar lordosis? Forward or backward sacral torsion may increase or decrease the lordosis.

13. Are the PSISs equidistant from the center line of the body?

14. Are the sacral sulci equal? If one is deeper, it may indicate a sacral torsion.

15. Do the feet face forward to the same degree? Often, the affected limb is medially rotated. With spasm of the piriformis muscle, the limb is laterally rotated on the affected side.

EXAMINATION

Before assessing the pelvic joints, the examiner should first assess the lumbar spine and hip, unless the history definitely indicates that one of the pelvic joints is at fault. The lumbar spine and hip can, and frequently do, refer pain to the sacroiliac joint area. Because the sacroiliac joints are in part a syndesmosis, movements at these joints are minimal compared with those of the other peripheral joints. It should also be remembered that any condition that alters the position of the sacrum relative to the ilium causes a corresponding change in the position of the symphysis pubis.

Although many tests and test movements have been described to help determine if there is sacroiliac dysfunction, many of them are imprecise and their reliability has been questioned.[24-30] At the present time, they are the best tests available. It is important for the examiner to consider all aspects of the assessment, including the history and the patient's symptoms along with the various tests and movements, before diagnosing sacroiliac joint problems.[4,5,24,31–33]

Active Movements

Unlike other peripheral joints, the sacroiliac joints do not have muscles that directly control their movement. However, because contraction of the muscles of the other joints may stress these joints or the symphysis pubis, the examiner must be careful during the active or resisted isometric movements of other joints and must be sure to ask the patient about the exact location of the pain on each movement. Table 10-1 outlines the muscles that attach to the pelvis. For example, resisted abduction of the hip can cause pain in the sacroiliac joint on the same side if the joint is injured, because the gluteus medius muscle pulls the ilium away from the sacrum when it contracts strongly. In addition, side flexion to the same side increases the shearing stress to the sacroiliac joint on that side. When doing active movements, the examiner is attempting to reproduce the patient's symptoms rather than just looking for pain.

The sacroiliac joints move in a "nodding" fashion of anteroposterior rotation. Normally, the PSISs approximate when the patient stands and separate when the patient lies prone. When he or she stands on one leg, the pubic bone on the supported side moves forward in relation to the pubic bone on the opposite side as a result of rotation at the sacroiliac joint.

The stability at the sacroiliac joint is determined by three factors—form closure, force closure, and motor control along with psychological aspects.[12,34] **Form closure** refers to the close packed position of the joint where no outside forces are necessary to hold the joint stable. Thus, intrinsic factors such as joint shape, coefficient of friction of the joint surfaces, and integrity of the ligaments contribute to form closure.[5,12,35] **Force closure** would be similar to the loose packed position in that extrinsic factors, primarily the muscles and their neurological control, along with the capsule are needed to maintain stability of the joint as well as the forces applied to the joint.[5,12,35] These two forms of closure and neurological control enable the sacroiliac joints to self lock as they go into close pack and slightly release when the joint unlocks.

During the active movements of the pelvic joints, the examiner looks for unequal movement, loss of or increase in movement (hypomobility or hypermobility), tissue contracture, tenderness, or inflammation.

Active Movements That Stress the Sacroiliac Joints

- Forward flexion of the spine (40° to 60°)
- Extension of the spine (20° to 35°)
- Rotation of the spine, left and right (3° to 18°)
- Side flexion of the spine, left and right (15° to 20°)
- Flexion of the hip (100° to 120°)
- Abduction of the hip (30° to 50°)
- Adduction of the hip (30°)
- Extension of the hip (0° to 15°)
- Medial rotation of the hip (30° to 40°)
- Lateral rotation of the hip (40° to 60°)

The movements of the spine put a stress on the sacroiliac joints as well as on the lumbar and lumbosacral joints. During forward flexion of the trunk, the innominate bones and pelvic girdle as a whole rotate anteriorly as a unit on the femoral heads bilaterally. The same thing occurs when one rises from supine lying to sitting. If one leg is actively extended at the hip, the innominate on that side will unilaterally rotate anteriorly.[5] During the anterior rotation of the innominate bones (counternutation), the innominate slides posteriorly along its long arm and inferiorly down its short arm (Figure 10-17).[5] Initially, the sacrum nutates up to about 60° of forward flexion, but once the deep posterior structures (deep and posterior oblique muscle systems, thoracolumbar fascia, and the sacrotuberous ligament) become tight, the innominates continue to rotate anteriorly on the femoral heads, but the sacrum begins to counternutate.[5] This counternutation causes the sacroiliac joint to be vulnerable to instability as greater muscle action (force closure) is required to maintain stability with counternutation.[7] Thus, the earlier counternutation occurs during forward flexion, the more vulnerable is the sacroiliac joint to instability problems. Excessive counternutation is more likely to occur in patients who have tight hamstrings.[5]

To test forward flexion, the patient stands with weight equally distributed on both legs. The examiner sits behind the patient and palpates both PSISs (Figure 10-18). The patient is asked to bend forward (see Tables 10-2 and 10-3) and the symmetry of movement of the PSIS superiorly is noted. At the same time, the examiner should note the amount of flexion that has occurred when sacral nutation begins. This can be done by having the patient repeat the forward bending motion while the examiner palpates the PSIS (inferior aspect) on one side with one thumb while the other thumb palpates the sacral base so

the thumbs are parallel. In the first 45° of forward flexion, the sacrum will move forward (nutate) (Figure 10-19, *A*), but near 60° (normally), the sacrum will begin to counternutate or move backwards (Figure 10-19, *B*).[5] During the sacral counternutation, the two PSISs should move upward equally in relation to the sacrum and toward each other or approximate. At the same time, the ASIS will tend to flare out.

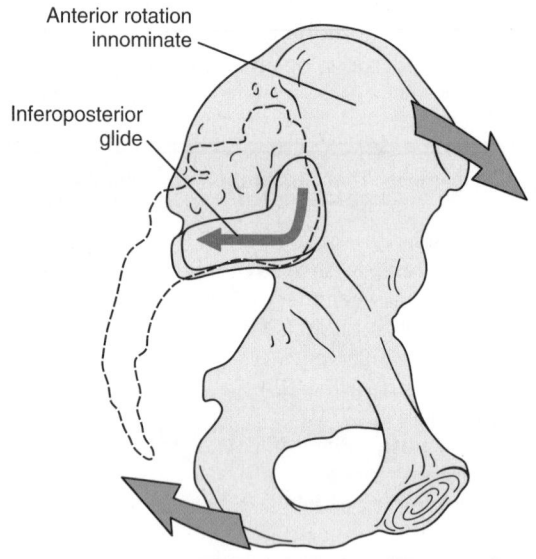

Figure 10-17 When the innominate rotates anteriorly, its articular surface glides inferoposteriorly relative to the sacrum. (Redrawn from Lee D: The pelvic girdle, ed 2, Edinburgh, 1999, Churchill Livingstone, p. 51.)

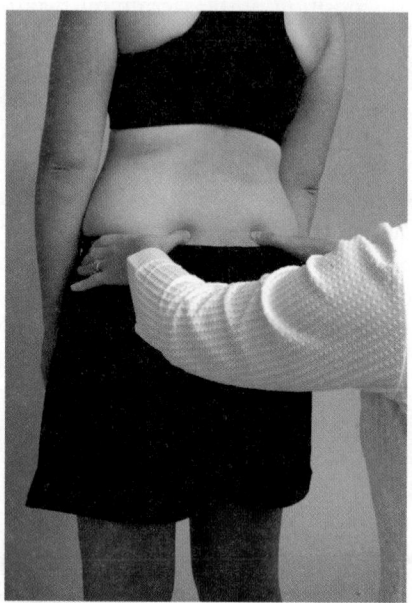

Figure 10-18 Examiner palpating posterior superior iliac spine (PSIS) prior to forward flexion.

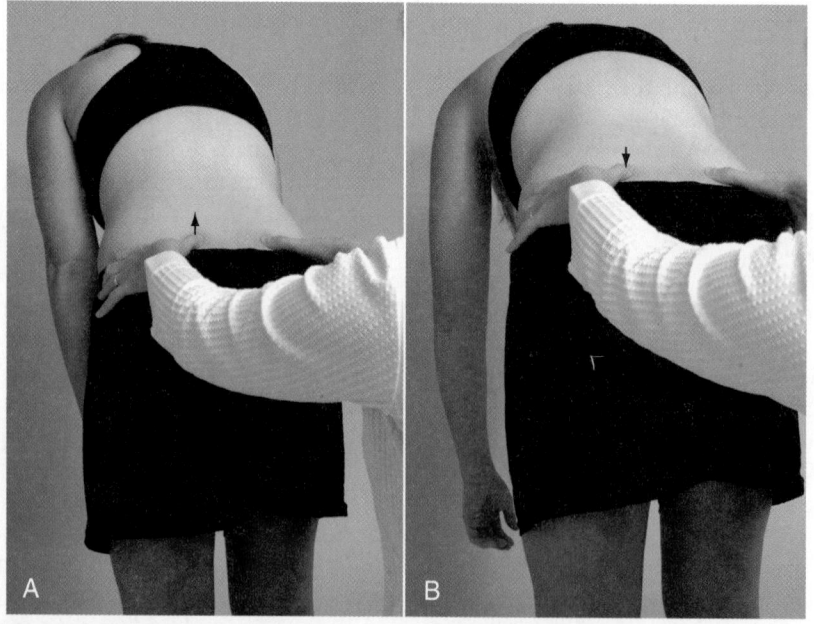

Figure 10-19 Examiner palpating for sacral nutation. One thumb is on the posterior superior iliac spine (PSIS); the other thumb is parallel to it on the sacrum. Examiner is feeling for forward movement (nutation) of the sacrum that occurs early in movement (**A**) and backward movement (counternutation) of the sacrum, which normally occurs around 60° of hip flexion (**B**).

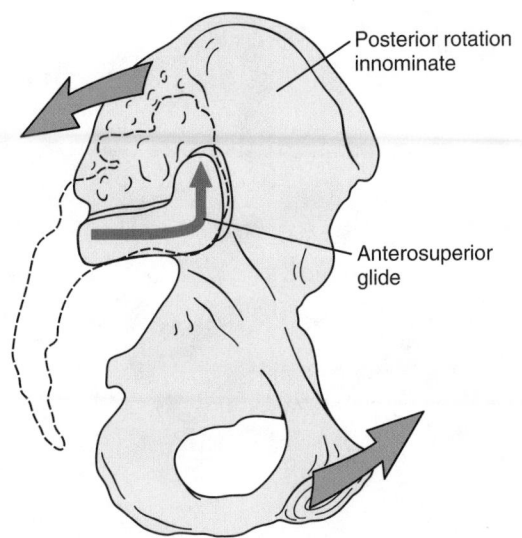

Figure 10-20 When the innominate posteriorly rotates, its articular surface glides anterosuperiorly relative to the sacrum. (Redrawn from Lee D: The pelvic girdle, ed 2, Edinburgh, 1999, Churchill Livingstone, p. 51.)

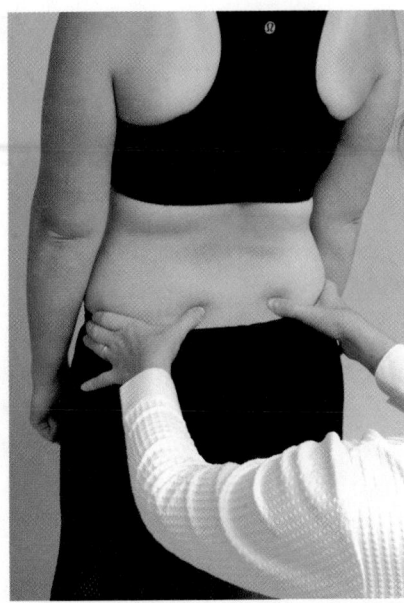

Figure 10-21 Examiner palpating posterior superior iliac spine (PSIS) for asymmetric movement on backward bending.

During extension, the opposite movements occur (see Tables 10-2 and 10-3).[5,8] During extension or backward bending of the trunk, the innominate bones (the pelvic girdle) as a whole unit rotate posteriorly (nutation) on the femoral heads bilaterally. If one leg is actively flexed at the hip, the innominate on that side unilaterally rotates posteriorly.[5] During the posterior rotation of the innominate bones, the innominate slides anteriorly along the long arm and superiorly up the short arm. This movement is the same as sacral nutation (Figure 10-20). With backward bending, both PSISs move inferiorly an equal amount.

To test backward bending, the patient stands with weight equally distributed on both legs. The examiner sits behind the patient and palpates both PSISs. The patient is asked to bend backwards while the examiner notes any asymmetry (Figure 10-21). Normally, the PSISs move inferiorly. During backward bending, the innominate bones and sacrum remain in the same position, so there should be no change in their relationship.[5] The examiner palpates both sides of the sacrum at the level of S1. As the patient extends, the sacrum should normally move forward. This is called the **sacral flexion test.**

Side flexion normally produces a torsion movement between the ilia and the sacrum. As the patient side flexes, the innominate bones bend to the same side and the sacrum rotates slightly in the opposite direction; the thumb of the examiner on the same side (the thumbs are palpating on each side of the sacrum at the level of S1) moves forward. This is called the **sacral rotation test.**[5] If this torsion movement does not occur (e.g., in hypomobility), the patient finds that more effort is required to side flex and it is harder to maintain balance.[8]

During rotation, the pelvic girdle moves in the direction of the rotation causing intrapelvic torsion. The innominate, which is on the side to which rotation is occurring, rotates posteriorly while the opposite innominate rotates anteriorly, pushing the sacrum into rotation in the same direction (i.e., right rotation of the trunk and pelvis causes right rotation of the sacrum). This causes the sacrum to nutate on the side to which rotation occurs and counternutate on the opposite side.[5]

The hip movements performed are also affected by sacroiliac lesions. As the patient flexes each hip maximally, the examiner should observe the ROM present, the pain produced, and the movement of the PSISs. The examiner first notes whether the PSISs are level before the patient flexes the hip. Normally, flexion of the hip with the knee flexed to 90° or more causes the sacroiliac joint on that side to drop or move caudally in relation to the other sacroiliac joint (**Gillet test**). If this drop does not occur, it may indicate hypomobility on the flexed side. The examiner can observe this movement by placing one thumb over the PSIS and the other thumb over the spinous process of S2 (Figure 10-22, *A*). In the patient with a normal sacroiliac joint, the thumb on the PSIS drops (Figure 10-22, *B*). If it is hypomobile, the thumb moves up on hip flexion. The two sides are compared. Sturesson and colleagues[36] have questioned whether much movement occurs at all because the stress of doing the test on one leg causes "force closure" of the sacroiliac joints, thus limiting movement.

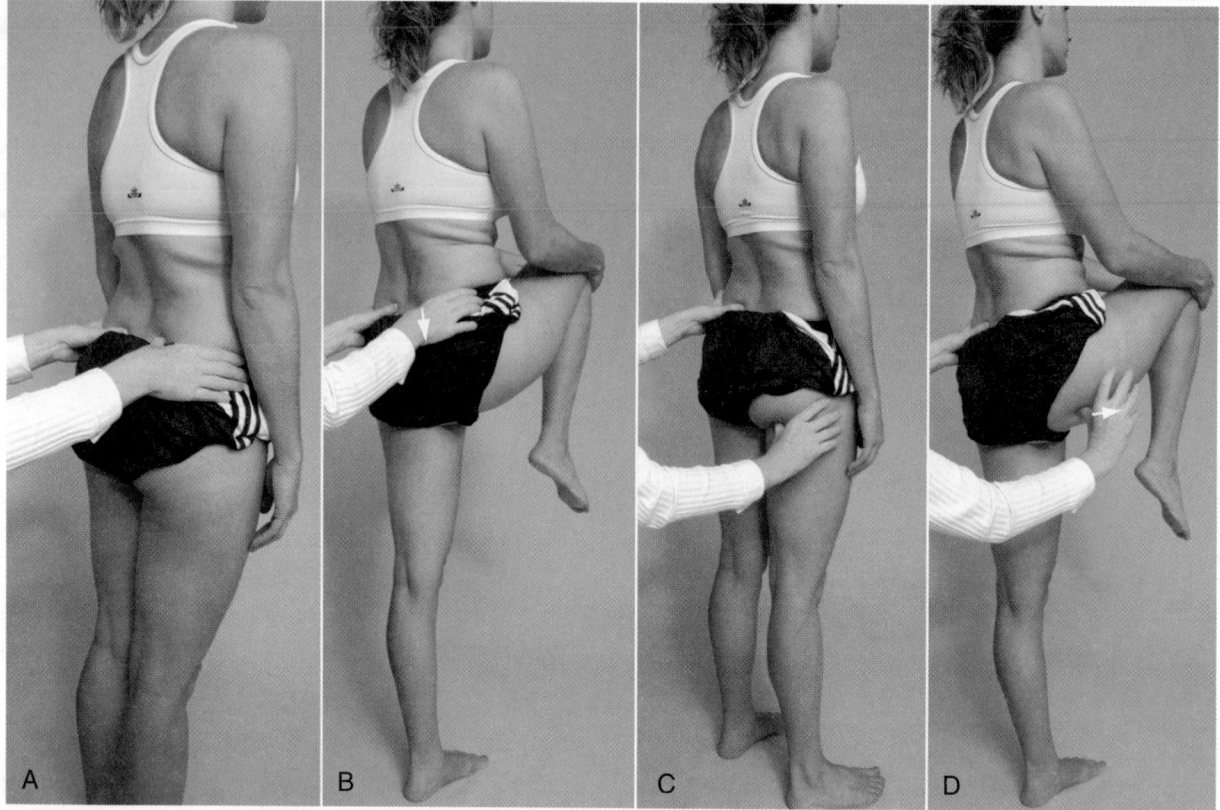

Figure 10-22 Active movements demonstrating how to show hypomobility of the sacroiliac joints. A, Starting position for sacral spine and posterior superior iliac spine (PSIS). **B,** Hip flexion; the ilium drops as it normally should *(arrow)*. **C,** Starting position for sacral spine and ischial tuberosity. **D,** Hip flexion. Ischial tuberosity moves laterally *(arrow),* as expected.

The examiner then leaves the one thumb over the sacral spinous process and moves the other thumb over the ischial tuberosity (Figure 10-22, *C*). The patient is again asked to flex the hip as far as possible. Normally, the thumb over the ischial tuberosity moves laterally (Figure 10-22, *D*). With a fixed or hypomobile joint, the thumb moves superiorly or toward the head. Again, the two sides are compared.

The examiner then sits in front of the standing patient and palpates the ASIS. Testing one leg at a time, the patient pivots the leg on the heel into medial and lateral rotation. When doing these movements, the ASIS should move medially and laterally. Both sides are compared.[5]

The position of the sacrum can then be determined. To do this, the examiner tests the patient in two positions—sitting and prone—doing three movements: flexion, staying in neutral, and extension. Before testing, the examiner palpates the base of the sacrum and the inferior lateral angle (near apex) of the sacrum on both sides (Figure 10-23). Normally, the sacral bone and the inferior lateral angle of the sacrum are level (i.e., one is not more anterior or posterior than the other). The first test involves the patient sitting with the feet supported and the spine fully flexed. The examiner palpates the four

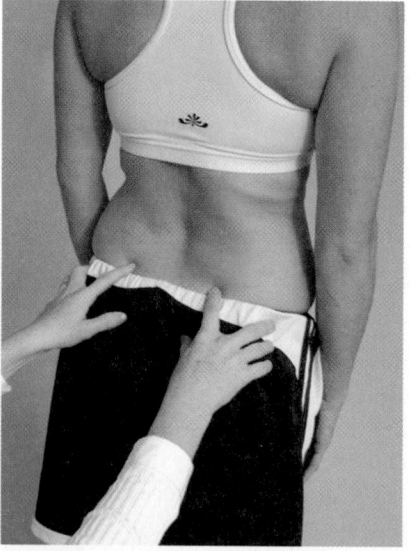

Figure 10-23 Examiner palpating base of sacrum and inferior lateral angle of the sacrum for anteroposterior symmetry.

points (Figure 10-24) and determines their relationship to one another. The patient is then put in prone lying with the spine in neutral and the relationship of the four points determined. The examiner then asks the patient to fully extend the spine and then determines the relationship of the four points. In any of the positions tested, if the examiner found, for example, an anterior left sacral base along with a posterior right inferior lateral angle, it would indicate a left rotated sacrum.[5]

The final active movements of the pelvis that the examiner may observe is the action of the pelvic floor muscles

(Table 10-5). If the pelvis has been found to be unstable or the patient is suffering from incontinence, the examiner can ask the patient to contract the muscles by asking the patient to squeeze the muscles tight by trying to stop peeing and hold the contraction. With strong pelvic floor muscles, the patient should have little trouble holding the contraction for at least 30 seconds.

Passive Movements

The passive movements of the pelvic joints involve stressing of the ligaments and the joints themselves. They are not true passive movements, like those done at other joints, but are in reality stress or provocative tests. It should be noted, however, that the effectiveness of these tests in confirming sacroiliac joint problems has been questioned even when combined in a clinical prediction rule.[31,37] Lee[12] feels these passive movements or tests should be used to determine symmetry or asymmetry of stiffness rather than normal, hypermobile, or hypomobile. It is her contention that asymmetry at the two sacroiliac joints is the problem, not the amount of movement. Laslett, et al.[38] and van der Wurff, et al.[39] felt that individually the sacroiliac provocative tests were not reliable enough to make a diagnosis, but a combination of the tests were. They felt that if two of four tests were positive (see box on the next page), these tests were the best predictors of an intra-articular sacroiliac joint block. If all six tests were negative, sacroiliac joint pathology could be ruled out.[40] Doing the passive movement is more likely to eliminate muscle tension effects that cause compression and increased stiffness.[12] Because of their anatomic

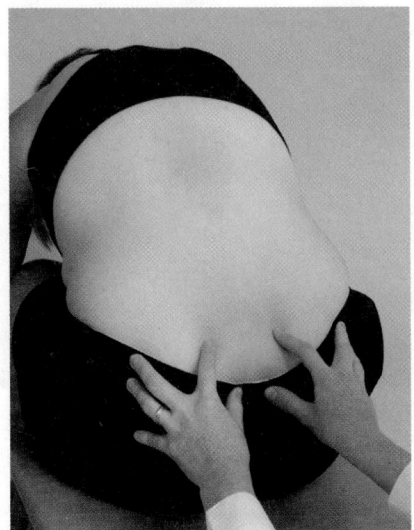

Figure 10-24 Examiner palpating position of sacrum in flexed sitting.

TABLE **10-5**

Muscles of the Pelvic Floor, Their Actions, and Nerve Root Derivation

Muscles	Action	Nerve Root Derivation
Obturator internus	Rotates thigh laterally Abducts flexed thigh at hip	Nerve to obturator internus
Piriformis	Rotates thigh laterally Abducts flexed thigh Stabilizes hip	Ventral rami of S1, S2
Gluteus maximus	Extends thigh Rotates pelvis back on femur Laterally rotates thigh Abducts thigh	Inferior gluteal nerve, L5, S1, S2
Levator ani*†	Supports pelvic viscera Raises pelvic floor	Ventral rami of S3, S4 Perineal nerve
Coccygeus† (also called *ischiococcygeus*)	Supports pelvic viscera Draws coccyx forward	Ventral rami of S4, S5
Superficial transverse perineal (transverse peroneal profundus)	Supports pelvic viscera	Pudendal nerve, S2, S3, S4

*Made up of three muscles: iliococcygeus, pubococcygeus and puborectalis depending on origin and insertion.
†These two muscles make up the pelvic or urogenital diaphragm.

makeup, the pelvic joints do not move to the same degree or in the same fashion as other joints of the body. When doing these provocative passive movements/tests, the examiner is looking for the **reproduction of the patient's symptoms,** not just pain or discomfort.[33,41]

Key Stress Tests (Passive Movements) of the Sacroiliac Joints*

⚠ Approximation test
✓ Gapping test
❓ Ipsilateral prone kinetic test
✓ Knee-to-shoulder test
❓ Passive extension and medial rotation of ilium on sacrum
❓ Passive flexion and lateral rotation of ilium on sacrum
⚠ Prone gapping test
⚠ Sacral thrust test
✓ Thigh thrust test

*See Chapter 1, p. 55, Key for Classifying Special Tests.

Laslet et al's Clinical Prediction Rule for Sacroiliac Involvement[38,39]

SACROILIAC PROVOCATION TESTS:
1. ⚠ Approximation test (compression provocation test)
2. ✓ Gapping test (distraction provocation test)
*3. ⚠ Sacral thrust test
4. ✓ Thigh thrust test
5. ✓ Gaenslen's test (see "Special Tests")
6. ⚠ Pain on palpation of sacral sulcus medial to posterior superior iliac spine (PSIS)

Note: If two of the first four tests or three or more of the six tests are positive, then the sacroiliac joint pathology is present.

⚠ *Approximation (Transverse Posterior Stress) Test.*[5,38] The patient is in the side lying position, and the examiner's hands are placed over the upper part of the iliac crest, pressing toward the floor (Figure 10-25). The movement causes forward pressure on the sacrum. An increased feeling of pressure in the sacroiliac joints indicates a possible sacroiliac lesion and/or a sprain of the posterior sacroiliac ligaments.

❓ *Femoral Shear Test.* The patient lies in the supine position. The examiner slightly flexes, abducts, and laterally rotates the patient's thigh at approximately 45° from the midline. The examiner then applies a graded force through the long axis of the femur, which causes an anterior-to-posterior shear stress to the sacroiliac joint on the same side (Figure 10-26).[42]

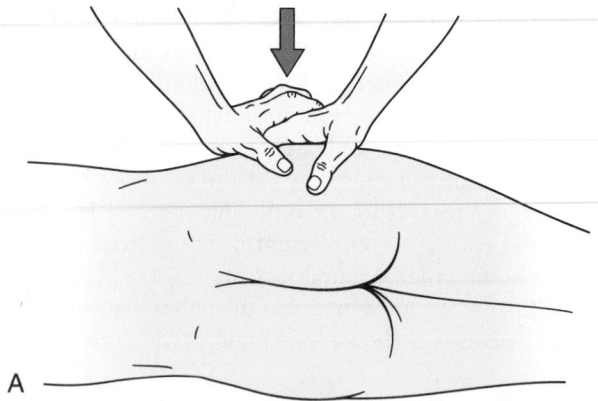

A

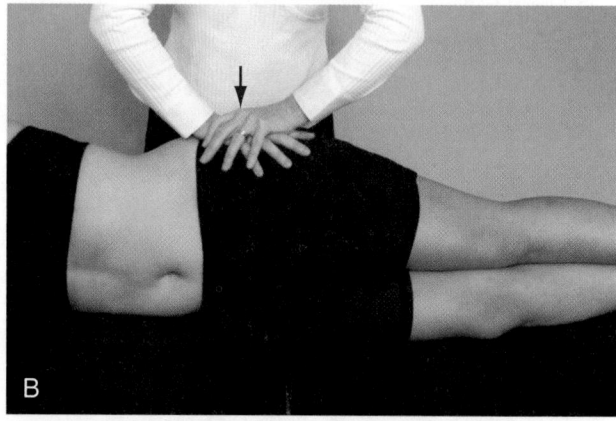

B

Figure 10-25 Approximation test. A, Diagram of posterior view. **B,** Anterior view.

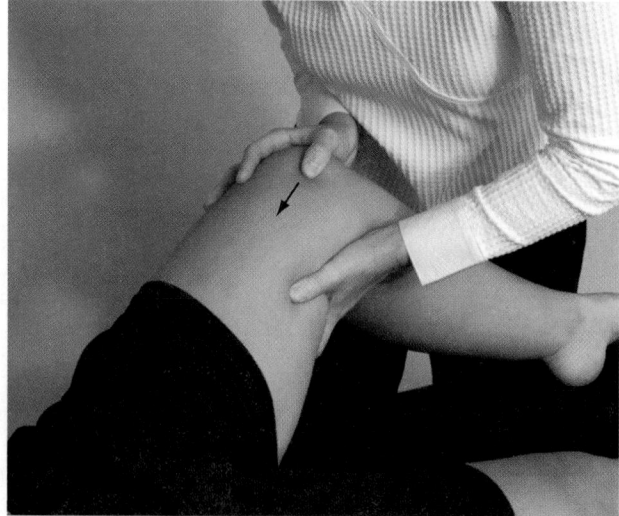

Figure 10-26 Femoral shear test.

✓ *Gapping (Transverse Anterior Stress or Distraction Provocation) Test.*[5,38] The patient lies supine while the examiner applies crossed-arm pressure to the ASIS (Figure 10-27, *A*) (some examiners prefer not to cross arms, Figure 10-27, *B*). The examiner pushes down and out with the arms. The test is positive only if unilateral gluteal or

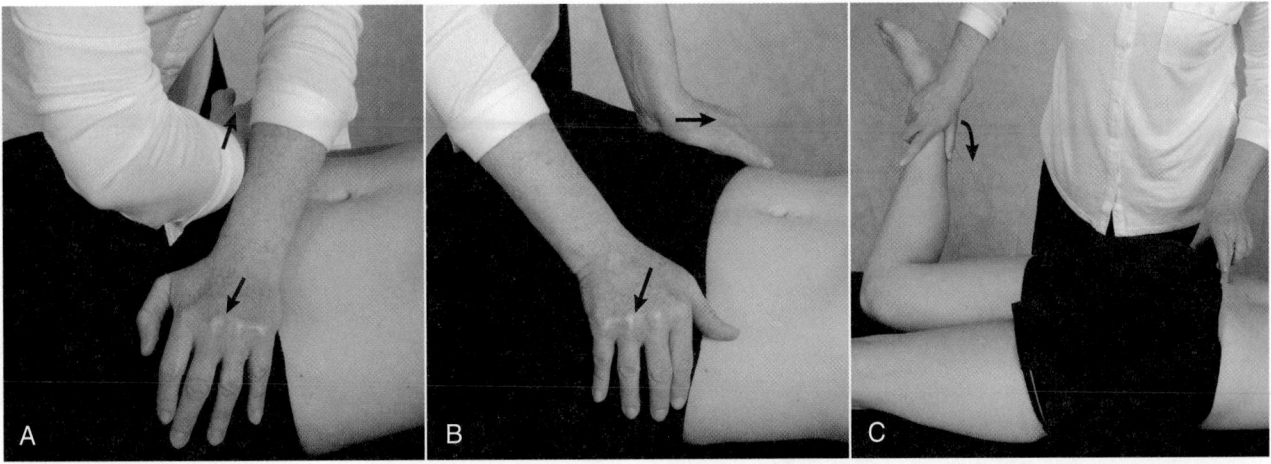

Figure 10-27 Gapping test. A, In supine—crossed arms. **B**, In supine—arms not crossed. **C**, In prone—using hip medial rotation.

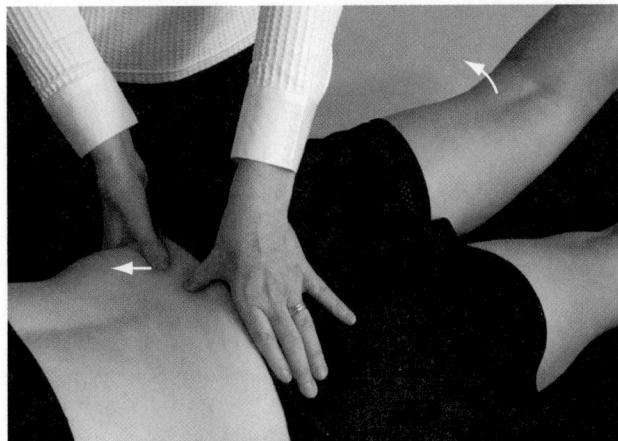

Figure 10-28 Ipsilateral prone kinetic test. On extension, the posterior superior iliac spine (PSIS) and sacral crest move superiorly and laterally.

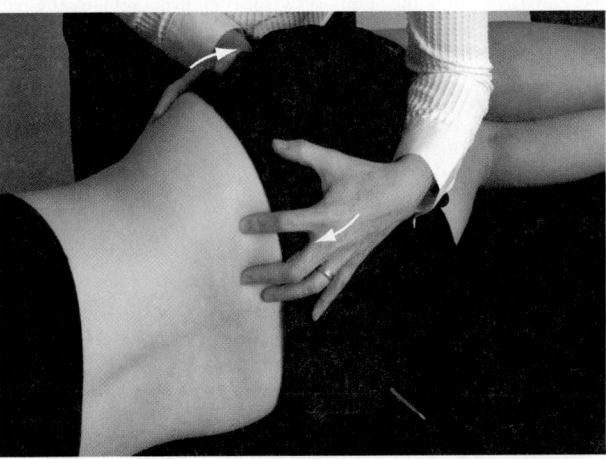

Figure 10-29 Passive extension and medial rotation of the ilium on the sacrum. The innominate bone is held in extension and medial rotation. The examiner palpates the sacrum and ilium with the fingers while rotating the ilium forward. With hypomobility, the relative movement is less than on the unaffected side, indicating an outflare.

posterior leg pain is produced, indicating a sprain of the anterior sacroiliac ligaments. Care must be taken when performing this test. The examiner's hands pushing against the ASIS can elicit pain, because the soft tissue is being compressed between the examiner's hands and the patient's pelvis.

Ipsilateral Prone Kinetic Test.[5,8] This test is designed to assess the ability of the ilium to flex and to rotate laterally or posteriorly. The patient lies prone while the examiner places one thumb on the PSIS and the other thumb parallel to it on the sacrum. The patient is then asked to actively extend the leg on the same side (Figure 10-28). Normally, the PSIS should move superiorly and laterally. If it does not, it indicates hypomobility with a posterior rotated ilium, or **outflare.**

Passive Extension and Medial Rotation of Ilium on Sacrum.[5,8] The patient is in side lying position on the side that is not being tested. The examiner places one hand over the ASIS area of the anterior ilium. The other hand is placed over the PSIS in such a way that the fingers of the hand palpate the posterior ilium and sacrum. The examiner then pulls the ilium forward with the hand over the ASIS and pushes the posterior ilium forward with the other hand while feeling the relative movement of the ilium on the sacrum (Figure 10-29). The unaffected side is then tested for comparison. If the affected side moves less, it indicates hypomobility and a posterior rotated ilium, or outflare.

Passive Flexion and Lateral Rotation of Ilium on Sacrum. The patient is positioned as for the previously mentioned test. In this case, the examiner pushes the anterior ilium backward with the anterior hand, and the posterior hand and arm pull the ilium posteriorly while palpating the relative movement (Figure 10-30). The unaffected side is then tested for comparison. If the

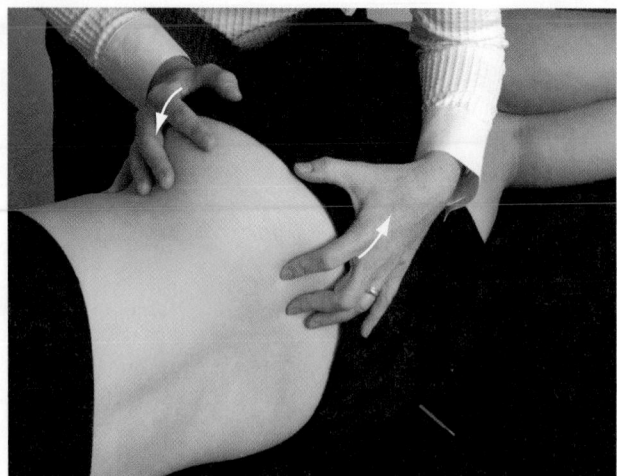

Figure 10-30 **Passive flexion and lateral rotation of the ilium on the sacrum.** The innominate bone is held in flexion and lateral rotation. The examiner palpates the sacrum and ilium with the left fingers while rotating the ilium backward. With hypomobility, the relative movement is less than on the unaffected side, indicating an inflare.

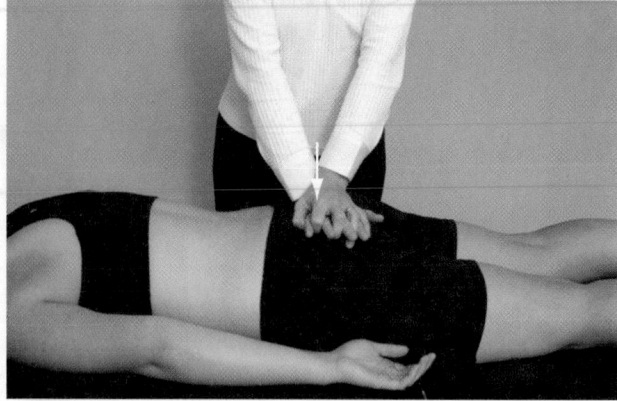

Figure 10-31 **Sacral apex pressure test.** Patient is lying prone.

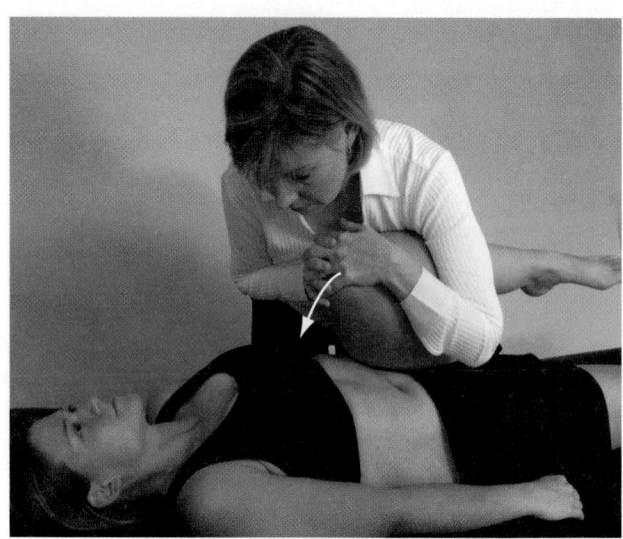

Figure 10-32 **Sacroiliac rocking (knee-to-shoulder) test.**

affected side moves less, it is a sign of hypomobility and an anterior rotated ilium, or **inflare.**

If both this test and the previously mentioned one are positive, it means an upslip has occurred to the ilium relative to the sacrum.

Passive Lateral Rotation of the Hip. The patient lies supine. The examiner flexes the hip and knee to 90° and then laterally rotates the hip. This movement, provided the hip is normal, stresses the sacroiliac joint on the test side.[10]

Prone Gapping (Hibb's) Test. The posterior sacroiliac ligaments may be stressed with the patient in the prone position (Figure 10-27, *C*). To perform the test, the patient's hips must have full ROM and be pathology free. The patient lies prone, and the examiner stabilizes the pelvis with his or her chest. The patient's knee is flexed to 90° or greater, and the hip is medially rotated as far as possible. While pushing the hip into the very end of medial rotation, the examiner palpates the sacroiliac joint on the same side. The test is repeated on the other side, with the examiner comparing the degree of opening and the quality of the movement at each sacroiliac joint as well as stressing the posterior sacroiliac ligaments.

Sacral Apex Pressure (Prone Springing or Sacral Thrust) Test.[38] The patient lies in a prone position on a firm surface while the examiner places the base of his or her hand at the apex of the patient's sacrum (Figure 10-31). Pressure is then applied to the apex of the sacrum, causing a shear of the sacrum on the ilium. The test may indicate a sacroiliac joint problem if pain is produced over the joint. The test causes a rotational shift of the sacroiliac joints.

Sacroiliac Rocking (Knee-to-Shoulder) Test. This test is also called the **sacrotuberous ligament stress test.** The

patient is in a supine position (Figure 10-32). The examiner flexes the patient's knee and hip fully and then adducts the hip. To perform the test properly, both the hip and knee must demonstrate no pathology and have full range of motion (ROM). The sacroiliac joint is "rocked" by flexion and adduction of the patient's hip. To do the test properly, the knee is moved toward the patient's opposite shoulder. Some authors[5,42] believe that the hip should be medially rotated as it is flexed and adducted to increase the stress on the sacroiliac joint. Simultaneously, the sacrotuberous ligament may be palpated (see Figure 10-2 for location) for tenderness. Pain in the sacroiliac joints indicates a positive test. Care must be taken, because the test places a great deal of stress on the hip and sacroiliac joints. If a longitudinal force is applied through the hip in a slow, steady manner (for 15 to 20 seconds) in an oblique and lateral direction, further stress is applied to the sacrotuberous ligament.[5] While performing the test, the examiner may palpate the

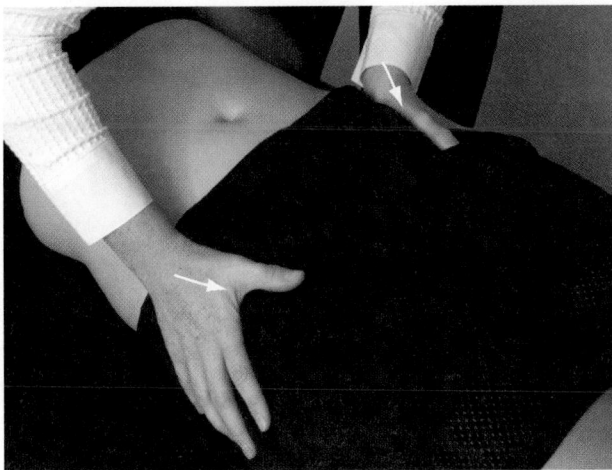

Figure 10-33 "Squish" test.

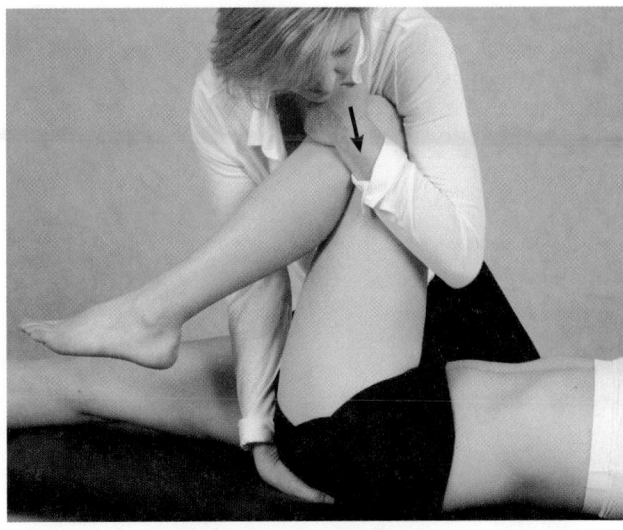

Figure 10-35 Thigh thrust test.

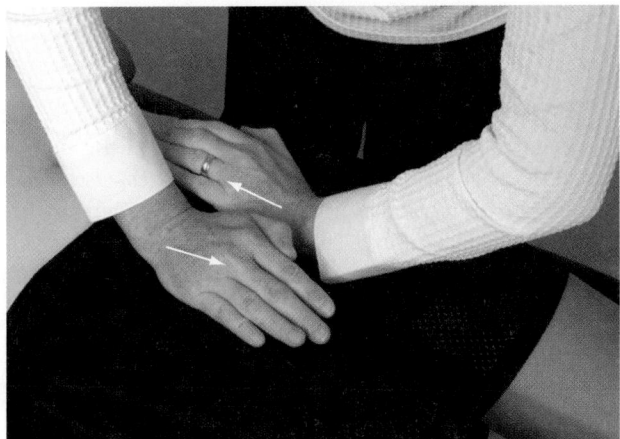

Figure 10-34 **Superoinferior symphysis pubis stress test.** Patient is lying supine.

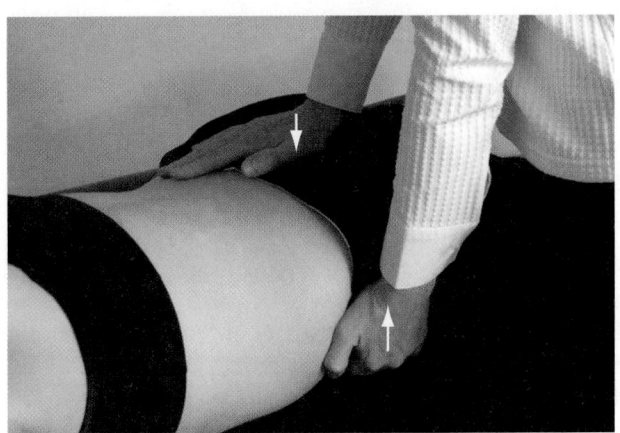

Figure 10-36 **Torsion stress test.** Patient is lying prone.

sacroiliac joint on the test side to feel for the slight amount of movement that normally is present.

"Squish" Test. With the patient in the supine position, the examiner places both hands on the patient's ASISs and iliac crests and pushes down and in at a 45° angle (Figure 10-33). This movement tests the posterior sacroiliac ligaments. A positive test is indicated by pain.

Superoinferior Symphysis Pubis Stress Test.[5,8] The patient lies supine. The examiner places the heel of one hand over the superior pubic ramus of one pubic bone and the heel of the other hand over the inferior pubic ramus of the other pubic bone. The examiner then squeezes the hands together, applying a shearing force to the symphysis pubis (Figure 10-34). Production of pain in the symphysis pubis is considered a positive test.

Thigh Thrust Test (Also Called Oostagard, 4P, Sacrotuberous Stress, or POSH [Posterior Shear] Test).[38] The patient lies supine while the examiner passively flexes the hip on the test side to 90°. Using one hand to palpate the

sacroiliac joint, the examiner thrusts down through the knee and hip on the text side (Figure 10-35). Pain in the sacroiliac joint on thrusting is a positive test.

Torsion Stress Test.[5] The patient lies prone. The examiner palpates the spinous process of L5 with one thumb holding it stable. The examiner's other hand is placed around the anterior ilium on the opposite side and lifts the contralateral ilium up (Figure 10-36). This rotational movement stresses the lumbosacral junction, the iliolumbar ligament, the anterior sacroiliac ligament, and the sacroiliac joint.

Resisted Isometric Movements

As previously stated, there are no specific muscles acting directly on the sacroiliac joints and symphysis pubis. However, contraction of adjacent muscles can stress these joints and cause force closure.[35] The examiner performs these movements with the patient supine and attempts to reproduce the patient's symptoms.

Resisted Isometric Movements Stressing the Sacroiliac Joints

- Forward flexion of spine (the abdominals stress the symphysis pubis)
- Flexion of hip (the iliacus stresses the sacroiliac joint)
- Abduction of hip (the gluteus medius stresses the sacroiliac joint)
- Adduction of the hip (the adductors stress the symphysis pubis)
- Extension of hip (the gluteus maximus and erector spinae cause force closure)
- Pelvic floor muscles—transverse abdominus/multifidus force couple causes force closure
- Abdominal obliques cause force closure
- Latissimus dorsi causes force closure

Key Tests Performed on the Sacroiliac Joints Depending on Suspected Pathology*[44,45]

- **For neurological involvement:**
  - ☑ Prone active straight leg raise test (three parts)
  - ☑ Straight leg raise test
  - ☑ Supine active straight leg raise test (three parts)
- **For sacroiliac joint involvement:**
  - ☑ Flamingo test
  - ☑ Gaenslen's test
  - ⚠ Gillet's test
- **For limb length:**
  - ☑ Leg length measurement
- **For muscle dysfunction:**
  - ☑ 90–90 Straight leg raise test
  - ☑ Patrick test
  - ☑ Trendelenburg test

*The author recommends these key tests be learned by the clinician to facilitate a diagnosis. See Chapter 1, p. 55, Key for Classifying Special Tests.

Functional Assessment

Functional assessment of the pelvic joints by themselves is very difficult because these joints do not work in isolation. Functionally, they should be considered part of the lumbar spine or part of the hip joint, depending on the area that the presenting pathology most affects.

Special Tests

The examiner should use only those special tests that are considered necessary to confirm the diagnosis. Few special tests that accurately diagnose sacroiliac joint pathology have been validated.[35] Dreyfuss, et al.[31,43] showed that the sacral sulcus (the area of soft tissue just medial to the PSIS) was tender in 89% of sacroiliac joint patients. When performing these tests, especially the stress or provocative tests, the examiner is attempting to reproduce the patient's symptoms.

For the reader who would like to review them, the reliability, validity, specificity, sensitivity, and odds ratios of some of the special tests used in the pelvis are available on the Evolve website.

If muscle tightness is suspected as part of the problem, muscle should be tested for length.

Tests for Neurological Involvement

❓ Prone Knee Bending (Nachlas) Test. Normally, this is used to test for a tight rectus femoris, an upper lumbar joint lesion, an upper spine nerve root lesion, or a hypomobile sacroiliac joint. The patient lies prone, and the examiner flexes the knee so that the heel is brought to the buttocks. If pain is felt in the front of the thigh before full range is reached, the problem is in the rectus femoris muscle. If the pain is in the lumbar spine, the problem is in the lumbar spine, usually the L3 nerve root, especially if these are radicular symptoms. If the problem is a hypomobile sacroiliac joint, the ipsilateral pelvic rim (ASIS) rotates forward, usually before the knee reaches 90° flexion.[42,46]

☑ Straight Leg Raising (Lasègue's) Test. Although the Lasègue sign is primarily considered a test of the neurological tissue around the lumbar spine, this test also places a stress on the sacroiliac joints. With the patient in the supine position (Figure 10-37), the examiner passively flexes the patient's hip with the knee extended. Pain occurring after 70° is usually indicative of joint pain. However, in hypermobile persons, joint pain is often not experienced until after 120° of hip flexion. Therefore, it is more important to watch for the production of the patient's symptoms than for the actual ROM. In addition, the ROM obtained should be compared with the unaffected side. If the examiner then does a passive bilateral straight leg raising (SLR) test in a similar fashion, pain occurring before 70° is usually indicative of sacroiliac joint problems. DonTigny[47] has reported that the straight leg raise can be affected by sacroiliac problems. If, when doing SLR, the pain in the sacroiliac joint is unaltered or decreases, the examiner may suspect an anterior torsion. If the pain increases in the sacroiliac joint, a posterior torsion is possible. If pain increases on the opposite side, an anterior torsion on the opposite side should be suspected.

Lee[5] advocated several modifications to the straight leg test (Figure 10-38, A) if sacroiliac joint problems are suspected. These tests are called **active SLR tests** and were originally designed to test for postpartum pelvic problems.[48–50] In the first modification, Lee recommends that the test be done actively by the patient in supine (**supine active straight leg raise test ☑**).[12,48–50] As the patient actively lifts the leg, the examiner asks whether the patient notes any "effort differences" between the two sides. The examiner then stabilizes and compresses the pelvis while the patient actively does the straight leg raise providing form closure of the joints by squeezing the

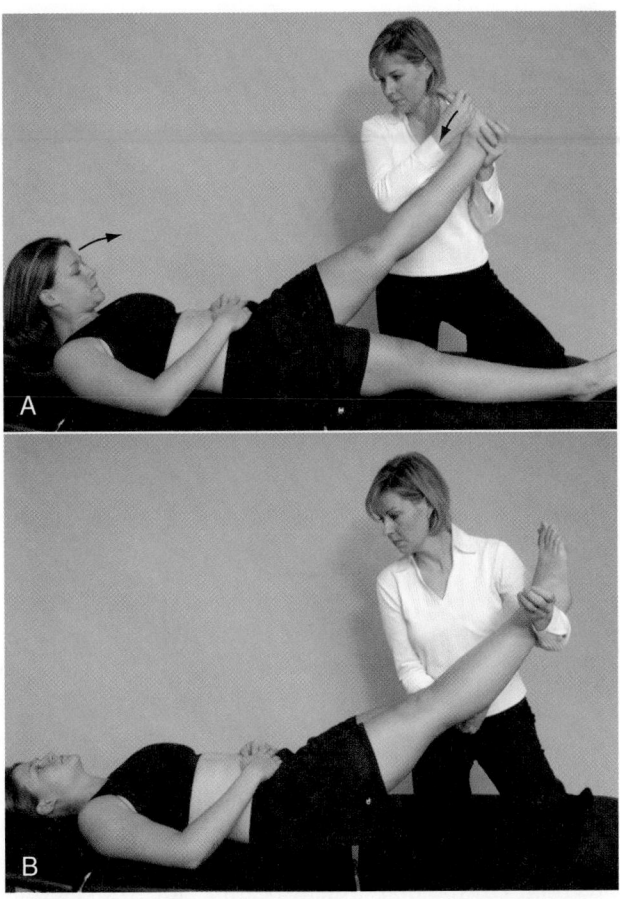

Figure 10-37 Straight leg raising (SLR) test. A, Unilateral (head may be flexed, ankle may be dorsiflexed, or both). **B,** Bilateral.

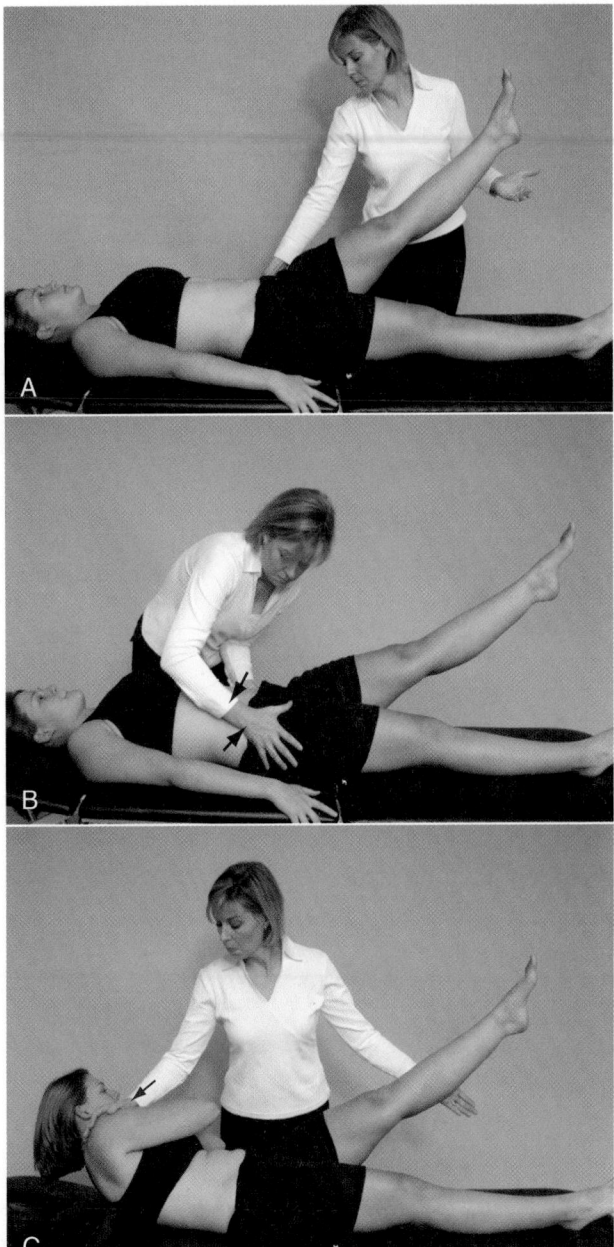

Figure 10-38 Functional test of supine-active straight leg raise. A, Patient actively does straight leg raise to provide comparison with ease of doing test in other two positions. **B,** With form closure augmented (compression of innominate bones). **C,** With force closure augmented (resisted muscle action).

innominate bones together anteriorly (Figure 10-38, *B*). If the pain decreases or the SLR is easier to do with form closure (with no increased neurological signs), the test is considered positive for possible sacroiliac joint problems. At the same time, the examiner can check the contraction of the pelvic floor/transverse abdominus/multifidus force couple by palpating medial to the ASIS bilaterally. If the force couple functions properly, tension is felt symmetrically and the abdomen moves inward. If superficial tension is felt, it means the internal obliques are contracting, and there is a force-couple imbalance.[12] Multifidus may be palpated close to the spinous process, and it should contract when the pelvic floor contracts. Another modification tests force closure at the sacroiliac joints.[5] The patient is asked to flex and rotate the trunk toward the side that the SLR is actively being performed. The trunk motion is resisted by the examiner (Figure 10-38, *C*). The two sides are compared for any difference. Force closure tests the ability of the muscles to stabilize the sacroiliac joints during movement.

Lee[5] also advocates doing active hip extension **(active prone hip extension test)** with the leg straight under three conditions **(prone active straight leg raise test** ✓). The first condition is hip extension (Figure 10-39, *A*). The second condition includes the same movement as the first with the examiner applying manual compression to the innominate bones (form closure) (Figure 10-39, *B*). The third condition has the examiner resisting extension of the contralateral medially rotated arm (force closure) as the patient extends the straight leg (Figure 10-39, *C*). If function improves when force closure stabilization is used, exercise will probably benefit the patient.

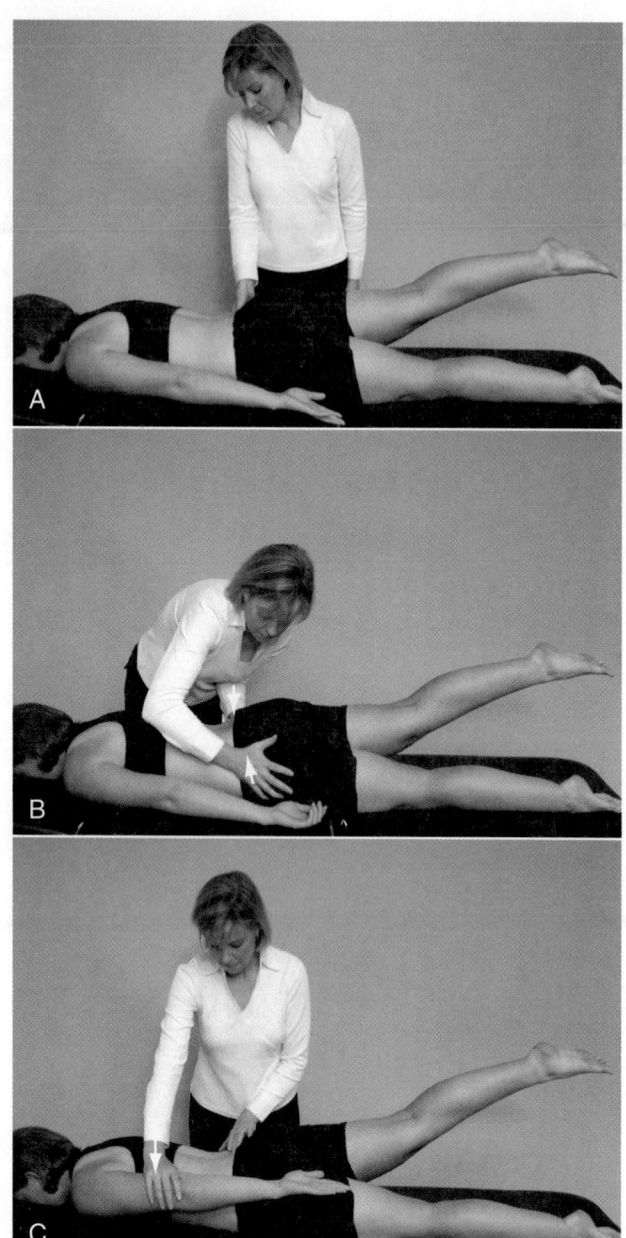

Figure 10-39 Functional test of prone-active straight leg raise. **A,** Patient actively extends straight leg to provide comparison with ease of doing test in other two positions. **B,** With form closure augmented (compression of innominate bones). **C,** With force closure augmented (resisted muscle action).

A more detailed description of the SLR test is given in Chapter 9.

Tests for Sacroiliac Joint Involvement

Lee[12] has reported that active mobility tests should not be used to test the passive mobility of the sacroiliac joints. She felt passive movements used to look for asymmetry were more effective.

✓ **Flamingo Test or Maneuver.** The patient is asked to stand on one leg (Figure 10-40). When the patient

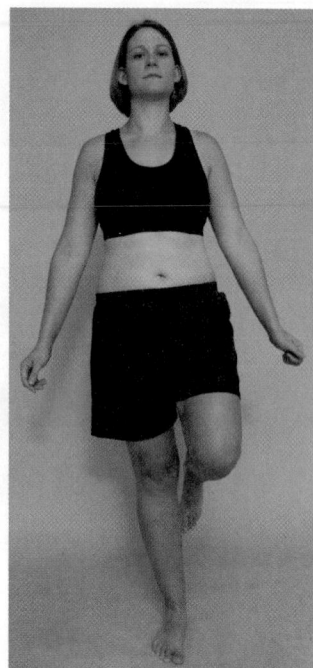

Figure 10-40 Flamingo test.

is standing on one leg, the weight of the trunk causes the sacrum to shift forward and distally (caudally) with forward rotation. The ilium moves in the opposite direction. On the non–weight-bearing side, the opposite occurs, but the stress is greatest on the stance side.[10] Pain in the symphysis pubis or sacroiliac joint indicates a positive test for lesions in whichever structure is painful. The stress may be increased by having the patient hop on one leg. This position is also used to take a stress x-ray of the symphysis pubis.

✓ **Gaenslen's Test.** The patient lies on the side with the upper leg (test leg) hyperextended at the hip (Figure 10-41, *A*). The patient holds the lower leg flexed against the chest. The examiner stabilizes the pelvis while extending the hip of the uppermost leg. Pain indicates a positive test. The pain may be caused by an ipsilateral sacroiliac joint lesion, hip pathology, or an L4 nerve root lesion.

Gaenslen's test is sometimes done with the patient supine (Figure 10-41, *B*), but this position may limit the amount of hyperextension available. The patient is positioned so that the test hip extends beyond the edge of the table. The patient draws both legs up onto the chest and then slowly lowers the test leg into extension. The other leg is tested in a similar fashion for comparison. Pain in the sacroiliac joints is indicative of a positive test.

⚠ **Gillet's (Sacral Fixation) Test.**[20] This test is also called the *ipsilateral posterior rotation test*. While the patient stands, the sitting examiner palpates the PSISs with one thumb and the other thumb parallel with the first thumb on the sacrum. The patient is then asked to stand on one leg while pulling the opposite knee up toward the chest. This causes the innominate bone on the same side to

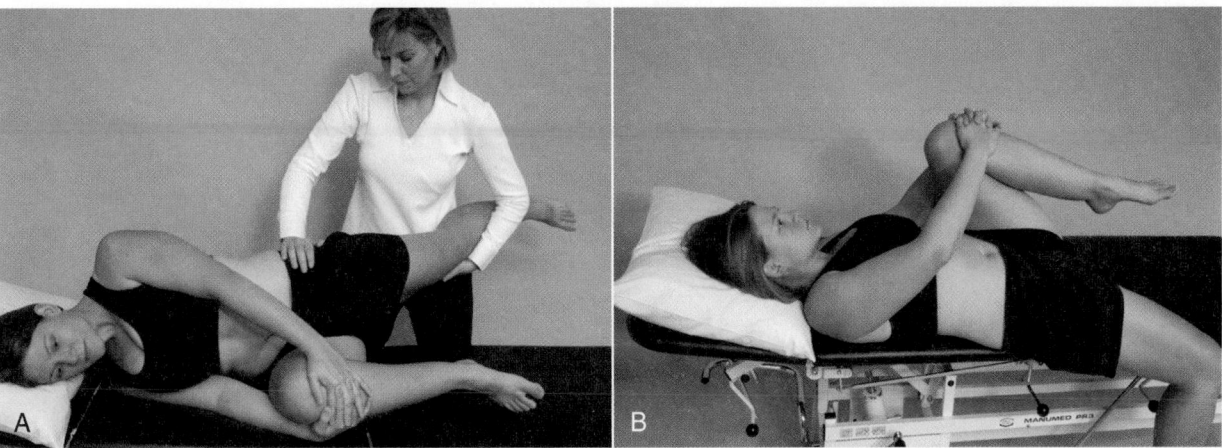

Figure 10-41 Gaenslen's test. A, With patient in side lying position, examiner extends test leg. **B,** With patient supine, test leg is extended over edge of table.

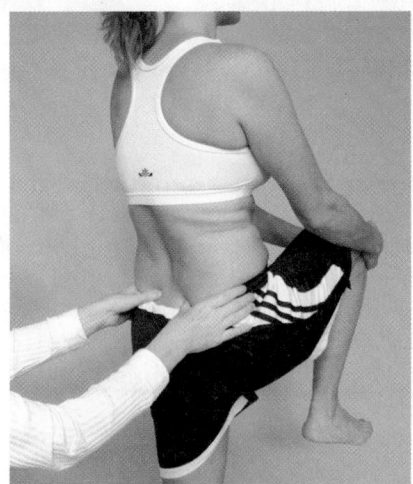

Figure 10-42 Gillet's (sacral fixation) test.

rotate posteriorly. The test is repeated with the other leg palpating the other PSIS. If the sacroiliac joint on the side on which the knee is flexed (i.e., the ipsilateral side) moves minimally or up, the joint is said to be hypomobile, or "blocked," indicating a positive test.[30] On the normal side, the test PSIS moves down or inferiorly (Figure 10-42). This test is similar to the test performed during hip flexion in active movement; the only difference is the points of palpation during the movement.

Jackson[4] has suggested a modification to the test. After completing the Gillet's test, he suggests that the examiner palpate the same PSIS and sacrum and ask the patient to do a repeat of the Gillet test using the other leg, which causes the opposite innominate bone to rotate posteriorly. As the patient flexes the hip and knee, the lumbar spine begins to flex, causing the sacrum to move inferiorly and resulting in the test innominate (side opposite to the leg being flexed) to rotate anteriorly.

Goldthwait's Test. The patient lies supine. The examiner places one hand under the lumbar spine so that each finger is in an interspinous space (i.e., L5–S1, L4–L5, L3–L4, and L2–L3 interspaces). The examiner uses the other hand to perform SLR. If pain is elicited before movement occurs at the interspaces, the problem is in the sacroiliac joint. Pain during interspace movement indicates a lumbar spine dysfunction. As with the SLR test, pain may be referred along the course of the sciatic nerve if there is neurological (e.g., nerve root) involvement.[46]

Ipsilateral Anterior Rotation Test.[5] The patient stands with weight equally distributed on both feet. The examiner sits behind the patient and palpates one PSIS with one thumb and the sacrum on a parallel line with the other thumb. The patient is asked to extend the ipsilateral leg. Normally, the PSIS should move superiorly and laterally (Figure 10-43). The other side is tested for comparison. This test determines the ability of the innominate on the test side to rotate anteriorly while the sacrum rotates to the opposite side.[5]

Laguere's Sign. The patient lies supine (Figure 10-44). To test the left sacroiliac joint, the examiner flexes, abducts, and laterally rotates the patient's left hip, applying an overpressure at the end of the ROM. The examiner must stabilize the pelvis on the opposite side by holding the opposite ASIS down. Pain in the left sacroiliac joint constitutes a positive test. The other side is tested for comparison. This test should be performed with caution for patients with hip pathology, because hip pain may ensue.

Mazion's Pelvic Maneuver (Standing Lunge Test).[51] The patient stands in a straddle position with the limb on the unaffected side forward so that the feet are 0.5 to 1 meter (2 to 3 feet) apart. The patient bends forward, trying to touch the floor, until the heel of the back leg lifts off the floor. If pain is produced in the lower trunk on the affected side, it is considered a positive test for unilateral forward displacement of the ilium relative to the sacrum.

Patrick Test. See Chapter 11.

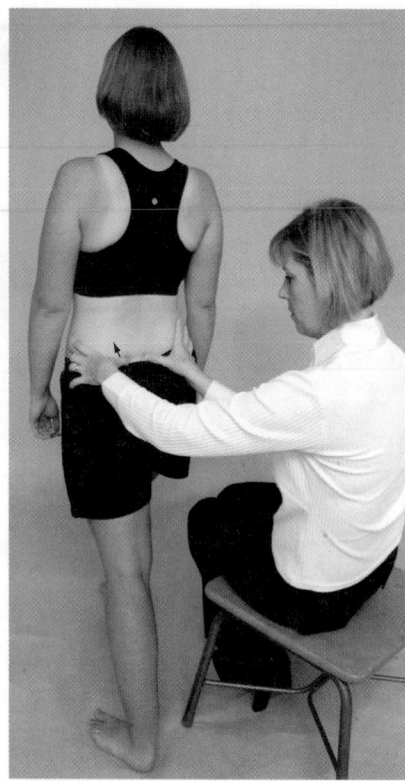

Figure 10-43 Ipsilateral anterior rotation test.

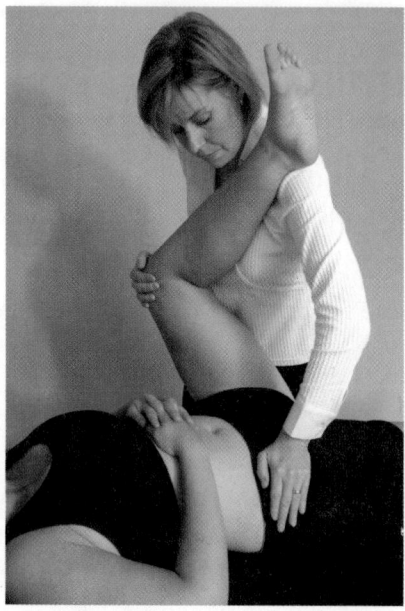

Figure 10-44 Laguere's sign.

▲ *Piedallu's Sign.* The patient is asked to sit on a hard, flat surface (Figure 10-45). This position keeps the muscles (e.g., hamstrings) from affecting the pelvic flexion symmetry and increases the stability of the ilia. In effect, it is a test of the sacrum on the ilia. The examiner palpates the PSISs and compares their heights. If one PSIS, usually

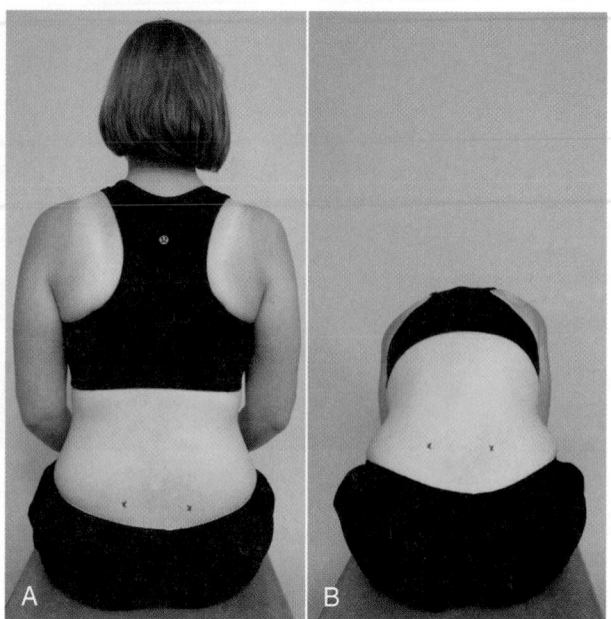

Figure 10-45 Piedallu's sign. **A,** Starting position. **B,** Test position.

the painful one, is lower than the other, the patient is asked to forward flex while remaining seated. If the lower PSIS becomes the higher one on forward flexion, the test is positive; it is that side that is affected. Because the affected joint does not move properly and is hypomobile, it goes from a low to a high position. This is believed to indicate an abnormality in the torsion movement at the sacroiliac joint.

▲ *Supine-to-Sit (Long Sitting) Test.* The patient lies supine with the legs straight. The examiner ensures that the medial malleoli are level. The patient is asked to sit up, and the examiner observes whether one leg moves up (proximally) farther than the other (Figures 10-46 and 10-47). If so, it is believed that there is a functional leg length difference resulting from a pelvic dysfunction caused by pelvic torsion or rotation.[42,52,53] It may also be caused by spasm of the lumbar muscles in the presence of lumbar pathology.

✓ *Yeoman's Test.* The patient lies prone. The examiner flexes the patient's knee to 90° and extends the hip (Figure 10-48). Pain localized to the sacroiliac joint indicates pathology in the anterior sacroiliac ligaments. Lumbar pain indicates lumbar involvement.[46] Anterior thigh paresthesia may indicate a femoral nerve stretch.

Tests for Limb Length

❓ *Functional Limb Length Test.*[54] The patient stands relaxed while the examiner palpates the ASISs and PSISs, noting any asymmetry. The patient is then placed in the "correct" stance (subtalar joints neutral, knees fully extended, and toes facing straight ahead), and the ASISs and PSISs are palpated with the examiner noting whether the asymmetry has been corrected. If the asymmetry has

Chapter 10 Pelvis   **673**

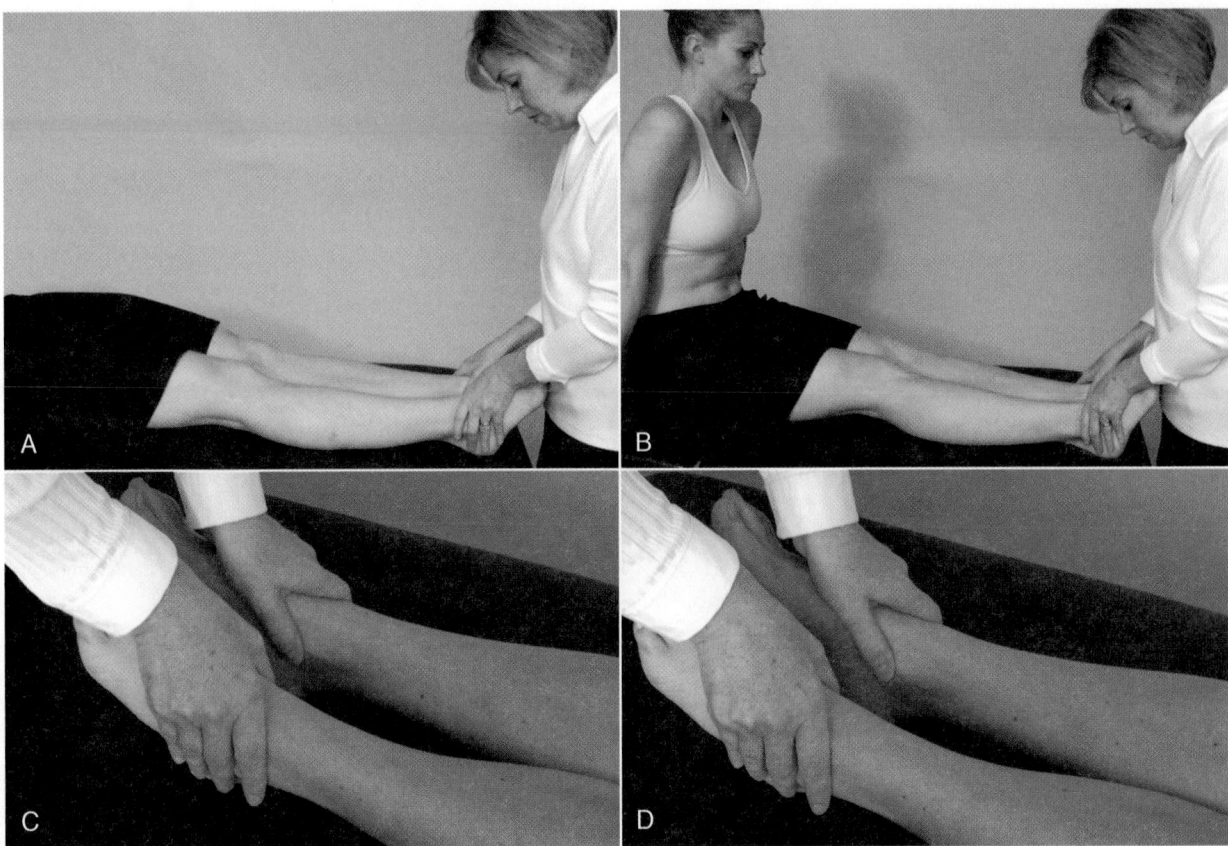

Figure 10-46 Supine-to-sit test for functional leg length discrepancy. A, Initial position. **B,** Final position. **C,** Symmetric leg lengths. **D,** Asymmetric leg lengths.

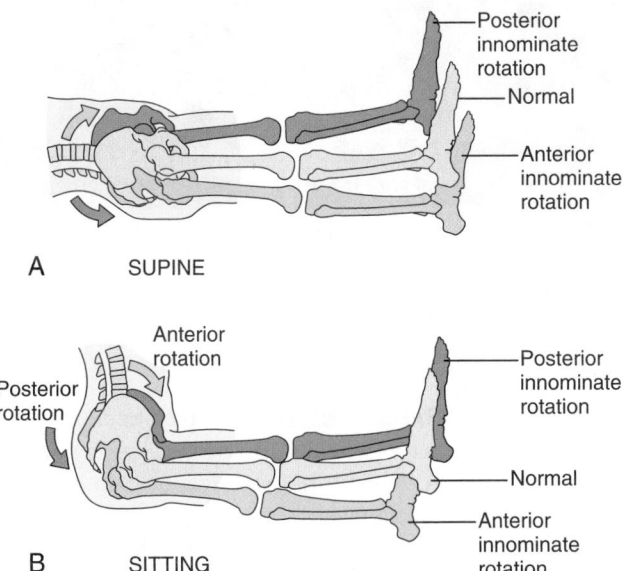

Figure 10-47 Supine-to-sit test. Leg length reversal; supine **(A)** versus sitting **(B)**. If the lower limb on the affected side appears longer when a patient lies supine but shorter when sitting, the test is positive, implicating anterior innominate rotation of the affected side. (Redrawn from Wadsworth CT, editor: Manual examination and treatment of the spine and extremities, Baltimore, 1988, Williams & Wilkins, p. 82.)

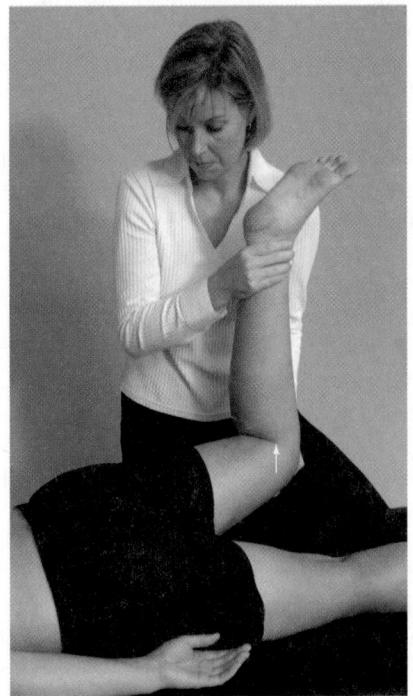

Figure 10-48 Yeoman's test.

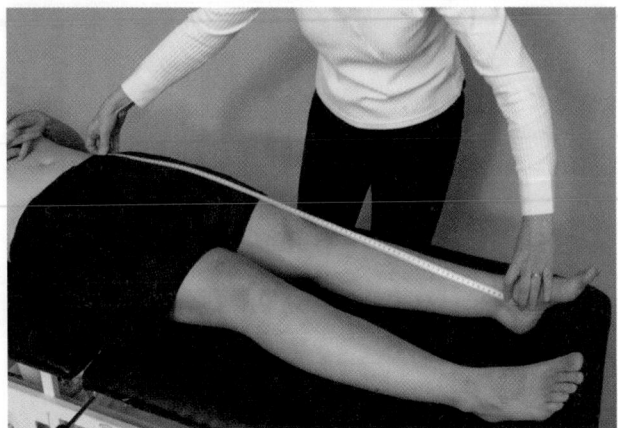

Figure 10-49 Measuring leg length (anterior superior iliac spine [ASIS] to medial malleolus).

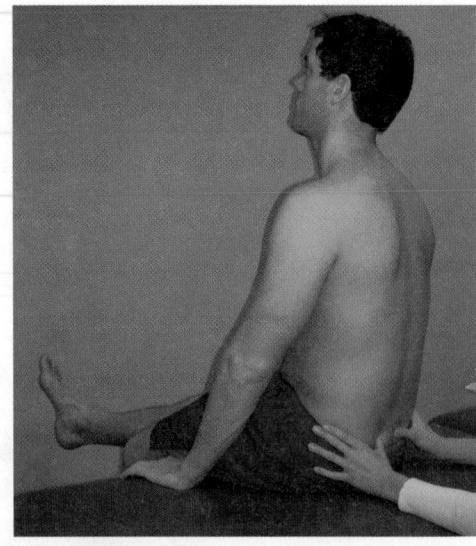

Figure 10-50 Test of functional length of hamstrings and the sacrotuberous ligament.

been corrected by "correct" positioning of the limb, the leg is structurally normal (i.e., the bones have proper length), but abnormal joint mechanics (functional deficit) are producing a functional leg length difference. Therefore, if the asymmetry is corrected by proper positioning, the test is positive for a functional leg length difference.

✓ *Leg Length Test.* The leg length test, described in detail in Chapter 11, should always be performed if the examiner suspects a sacroiliac joint lesion. Nutation (backward rotation) of the ilium on the sacrum results in a decrease in leg length—as does counternutation (anterior rotation) on the opposite side. If the iliac bone on one side is lower, the leg on that side is usually longer.[47] True leg length is measured by placing the patient in a supine position with the ASISs level and the patient's lower limbs perpendicular to the line joining the ASISs (Figure 10-49). Using a flexible tape measure, the examiner obtains the distance from the ASIS to the medial or lateral malleolus on the same side. The measurement is repeated on the other side, and the results are compared. A difference of 1 to 1.3 cm (0.5 to 1 inch) is considered normal. It should be remembered, however, that leg length differences within this range may also be pathological if symptoms result.[55]

Other Tests

❓ *Functional Hamstring Length.*[5] The patient sits on the examining table with the knees flexed to 90°, no weight on feet, and spine in neutral. The examiner sits behind the patient and palpates the PSIS with one thumb while the other thumb rests parallel on the sacrum. The patient is asked to actively extend the knee (Figure 10-50). Normally, full knee extension is possible without posterior rotation of the pelvis or flexion of the lumbar spine. Tight hamstrings would cause the pelvis to rotate posteriorly and/or the spine to flex.

✓ *90–90 SLR Test for Hamstring Tightness.* See Chapters 11 and 12.

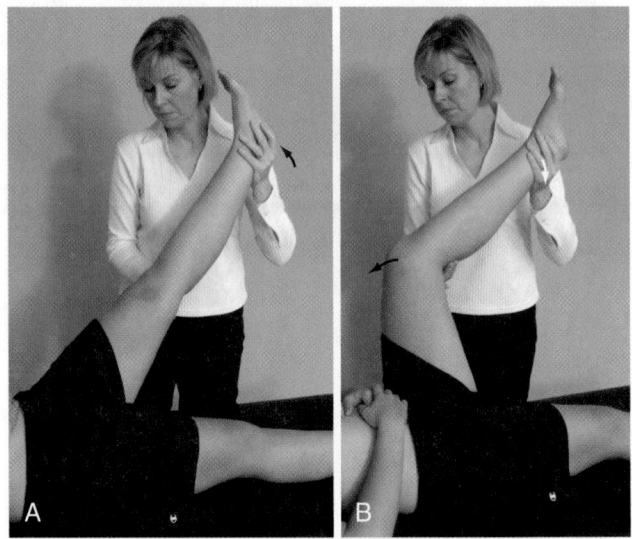

Figure 10-51 Sign of the buttock test. A, Hip is flexed with knee straight until resistance or pain is felt. **B,** The knee is then flexed to see whether further hip flexion can be achieved. If further hip flexion can be achieved, the test is negative.

❓ *Sign of the Buttock Test.* With the patient supine, the examiner performs a passive unilateral SLR test as done previously (Figure 10-51). If restriction or pain is found on one side, the examiner flexes the patient's knee while holding the patient's thigh in the same position. Once the knee is flexed, the examiner tries to flex the hip further. If the problem is in the lumbar spine or hamstrings, hip flexion increases. This finding indicates a negative sign of the buttock test. If hip flexion does not increase when the knee is flexed, it is a positive sign of the buttock test and indicates pathology in the buttock, such as a bursitis, tumor, or abscess. The patient with

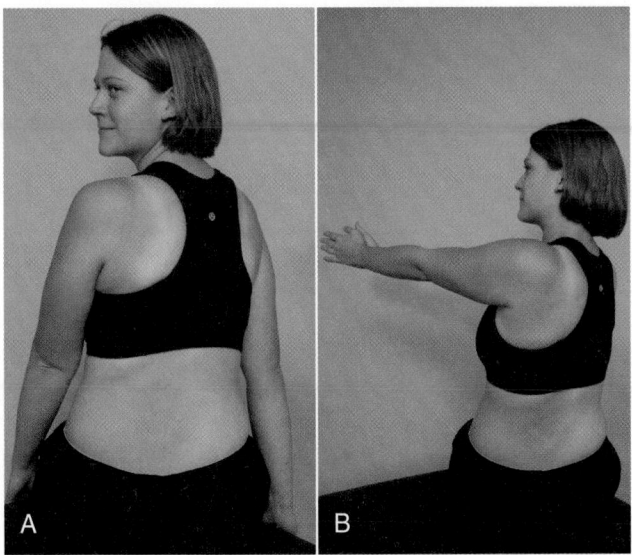

Figure 10-52 Test of functional length of the thoracolumbar fascia and the latissimus dorsi muscle. A, Test without stretch. **B,** Test with muscle and fascia under stretch.

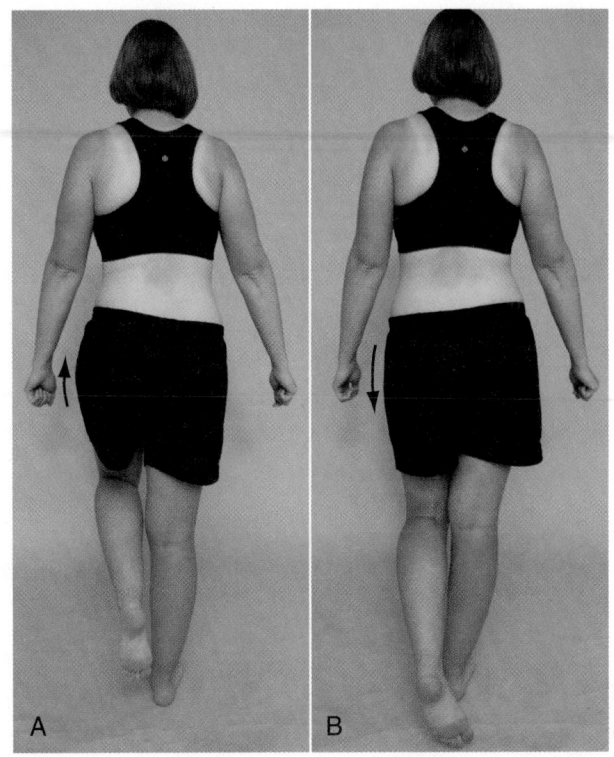

Figure 10-53 Trendelenburg sign. A, Negative test. **B,** Positive test.

this pathology would also exhibit a noncapsular pattern of the hip.

? *Thoracolumbar Fascia Length.*[5] The patient sits on the examining table with the knees bent to 90° and a neutral spine. The examiner stands behind the patient. The patient is asked to rotate left and right fully and the examiner notes the ROM available (Figure 10-52, *A*). The patient is then asked to forward flex the arms to 90° and laterally rotate and adduct the arms so the little fingers touch each other and palms face up (Figure 10-52, *B*). Holding this arm position, the patient is again asked to rotate left and right as far as possible. The motion will be restricted in the second set of rotations if the thoracolumbar fascia or latissimus dorsi are tight.

✓ *Trendelenburg Test or Sign.* The patient is asked to stand or balance first on one leg and then on the other (Figure 10-53). While the patient is balancing on one leg, the examiner watches the movement of the pelvis. If the pelvis on the side of the non-stance leg rises, the test is considered negative, because the gluteus medius muscle on the opposite (stance) side lifts it up as it normally does in one-legged stance. If the pelvis on the side of the non-stance leg falls, the test is considered positive and is an indication of weakness or instability of the hip abductor muscles, primarily the gluteus medius on the stance side. Therefore, although the examiner is watching what happens on the non-stance side, it is the stance side that is being tested.

Reflexes and Cutaneous Distribution

There are no reflexes to test for the pelvic joints. However, the examiner must be aware of the dermatomes from the

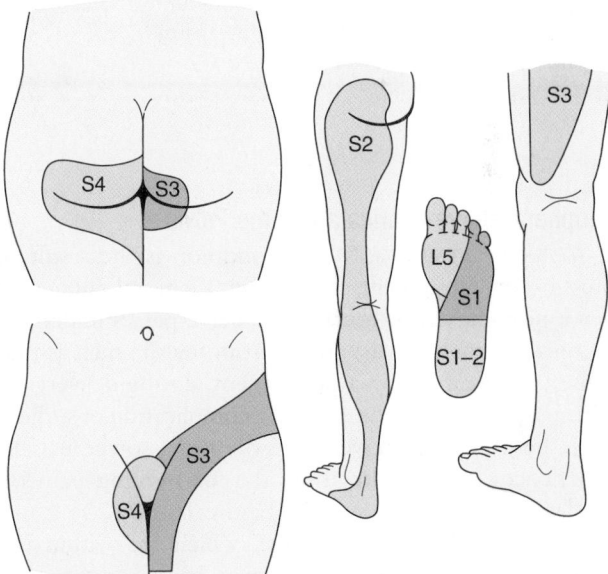

Figure 10-54 Posterior sacral dermatomes. Representation in the lower left is an anterior view.

sacral nerve roots (Figure 10-54). Pain may be referred to the sacroiliac joints from the lumbar spine and the hip (Figure 10-55). In addition, the sacroiliac joint may refer pain to these same structures or along the courses of the superior gluteal and obturator nerves. The muscles of the spine may also refer pain to the sacral area (Table 10-6).

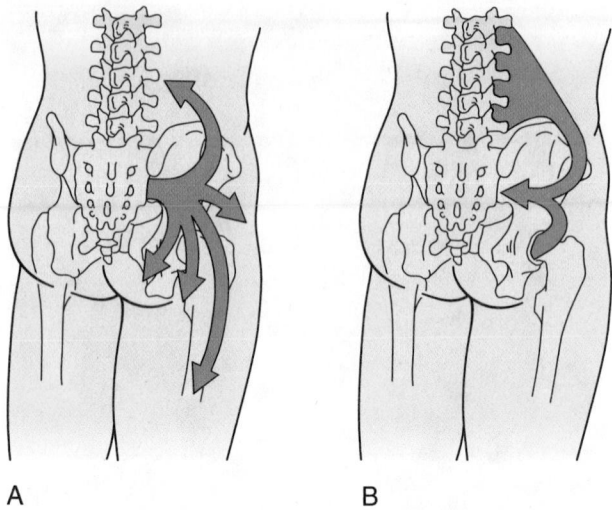

A   B

Figure 10-55 Referred pain from sacroiliac joint (**A**) and to sacroiliac joint (**B**).

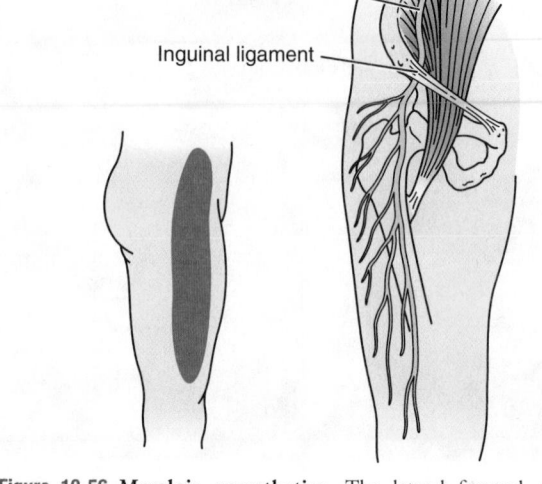

Figure 10-56 Meralgia paresthetica. The lateral femoral cutaneous nerve supplies the skin of the lateral thigh. An area from the inguinal ligament to the knee may be affected.

TABLE 10-6

Muscles and Referral of Pain to Pelvic Area

Muscle	Referral Pattern
Longissimus thoracis	From lower thoracic spine to posterior iliac crest and gluteal area
Iliocostalis lumborum	From area lateral to lumbar spine to sacral and gluteal area
Multifidus	Sacral area

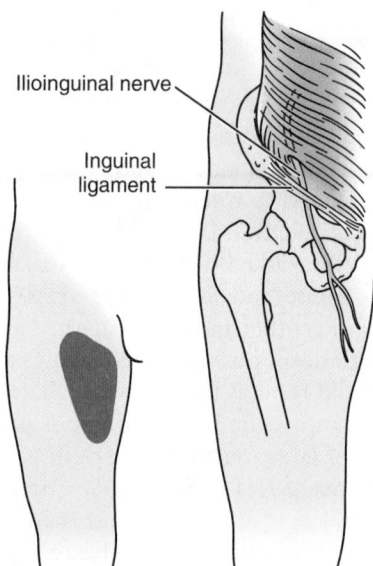

Figure 10-57 Ilioinguinal syndrome. The ilioinguinal nerve lies within the transversus abdominis and emerges below the inguinal ligament. An area of skin on the medial thigh near the genitalia is affected.

Peripheral Nerve Injuries about the Pelvis

Meralgia Paresthetica.[56] This condition is the result of pressure or entrapment of the lateral femoral cutaneous nerve near the ASIS, because the nerve passes under the inguinal ligament. It may result from trauma such as that caused by a seat belt in a car accident, during delivery (in stirrups), by tight clothing, or as a complication of surgery (e.g., hernia). This nerve is sensory only, so the patient experiences sensory alteration and/or burning pain on the lateral aspect of the thigh (Figure 10-56).

Ilioinguinal Nerve.[57] This nerve, which lies within the transverse abdominus muscle, may be compressed by spasm of the muscle (Figure 10-57). The nerve is sensory only, and the sensory alteration and/or pain occurs in the superior aspect of the anterior thigh (in the L1 dermatome area), as well as in the scrotum or labia. There have been reports in the literature[58-61] that this nerve may be entrapped with injury to the external oblique muscle aponeurosis (hockey player's syndrome). The patient feels pain especially on ipsilateral hip extension and contralateral torso rotation. The pain may radiate to the groin, scrotum, hip, and back.

Joint Play Movements

The joint play movements (Figure 10-58) are minimal for the sacroiliac joints and are similar to the passive movements in that they are stress or provocative tests.

To test each of these movements, the patient is in the prone position. For the first joint play movement, the examiner places the heel of one hand over the iliac crest and the heel of the other hand over the apex of the sacrum. The ilium is pushed down or caudally with one hand while the sacrum is pushed up or cephalad with the

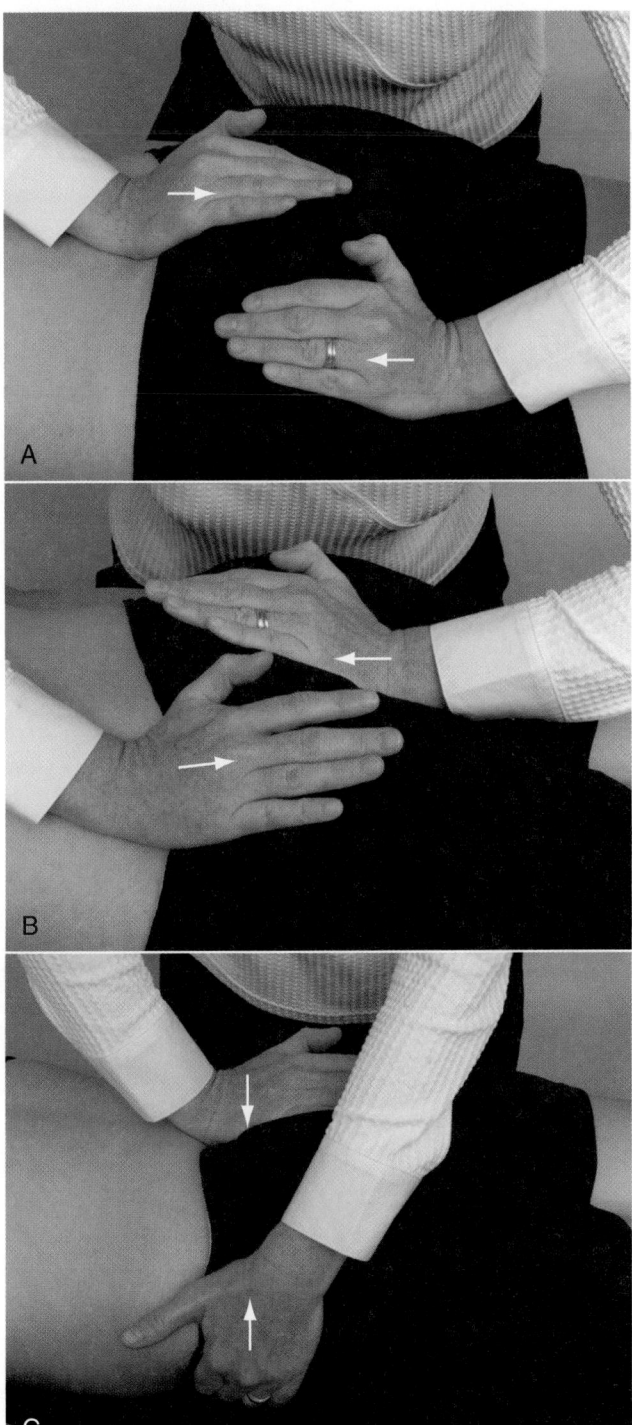

Figure 10-58 Joint play movements of the sacroiliac joints. A, Cephalad movement of sacrum with caudal movement of ilium. **B,** Cephalad movement of ilium with caudal movement of sacrum. **C,** Anterior movement of sacrum on ilium (left side demonstrated).

other hand. The test is repeated for the other ilium (see Figure 10-58, *A*). The examiner should feel only minimal movement, and there should be no pain in the joint if the joint is normal. In an affected sacroiliac joint, there is usually pain over the joint and little or no movement.

> **Joint Play Movements of the Sacroiliac Joints**
>
> • Cephalad movement of the sacrum with caudal movement of the ilium (left and right)
> • Cephalad movement of the ilium with caudal movement of the sacrum (left and right)
> • Anterior movement of the sacrum on the ilium
> • Anteroposterior translation of ilium on sacrum
> • Superoinferior translation of ilium on sacrum
> • Inferoposterior translation of ilium on sacrum
> • Superoanterior translation of ilium on sacrum

This positioning tests for cephalad movement of the sacrum and caudal movement of the ilium.

To test caudal movement of the sacrum and cephalad movement of the ilium, the examiner places the heel of one hand over the base of the sacrum and the heel of the other hand over the ischial tuberosity (see Figure 10-58, *B*). The examiner then pushes the pelvis cephalad and the sacrum caudally. The test is repeated with the other half of the pelvis being moved. The movement and amount of pain are compared.

The anterior movement of the sacrum on the ilium is tested with the patient lying prone (see Figure 10-58, *C*). The examiner places the heel of one hand over the sacrum and places the other hand under the iliac crest in the area of the ASIS on one side. The hand is then pushed down on the sacrum while the other hand lifts up. The process is repeated on the other side, and the results are compared. Similarly, with the patient supine, a wedge may be used against the sacrum with the patient's body weight acting to push the sacrum forward.

Lee[5,62] has advocated a way to test other translations at the sacroiliac joint. The patient lies supine with the hips and knees in the resting position. The examiner palpates the sacral sulcus just medial to the PSIS with the middle and ring fingers of one hand, and the lumbosacral junction with the index finger of the same hand (Figure 10-59). The middle and ring fingers monitor movement between the sacrum and innominate (ilium) bone while the index finger notes movement between the sacrum and L5.

To test anteroposterior translation of the ilium on the sacrum, the examiner, using the other hand, applies pressure through the iliac crest and ASIS. Posterior movement of the ilium should be noted and end range is achieved at the sacroiliac joint when the pelvis is felt to rotate or move at L5–S1 (Figure 10-60). The motion is compared with the other side.

To test superoinferior translation of the innominate (ilium) bone on the sacrum, the examiner applies a superior force through the ischial tuberosity (Figure 10-61). The end of motion is reached when the pelvic girdle is felt to laterally bend beneath L5–S1. The motion is compared with the opposite side.

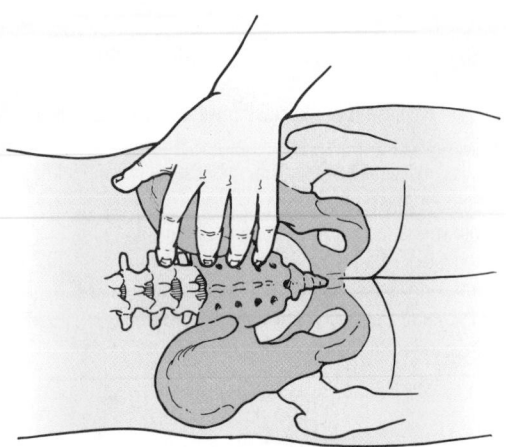

Figure 10-59 Position of the posterior hand for palpation during mobility and stability testing of the sacroiliac joint.

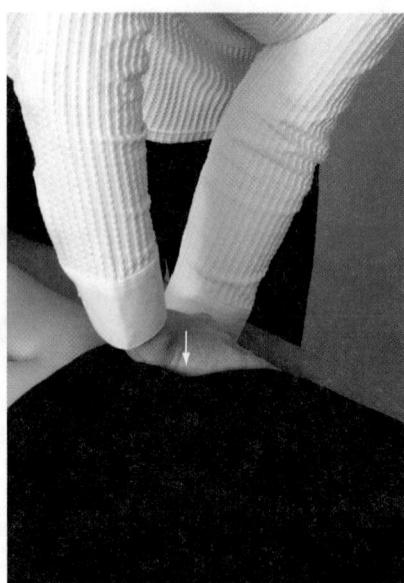

Figure 10-60 Anteroposterior translation of the ilium on the sacrum.

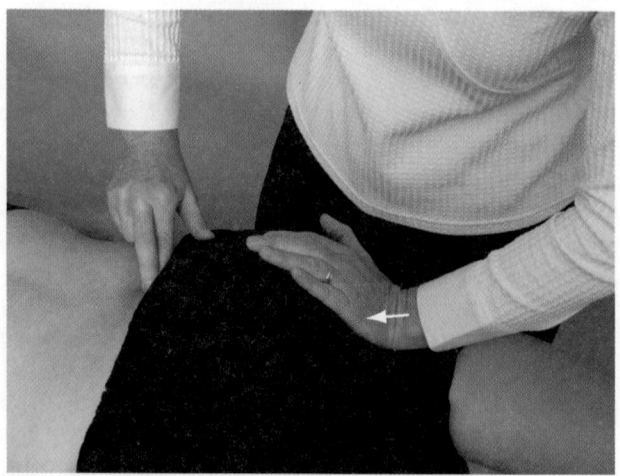

Figure 10-61 Superoinferior translation of the ilium on the sacrum.

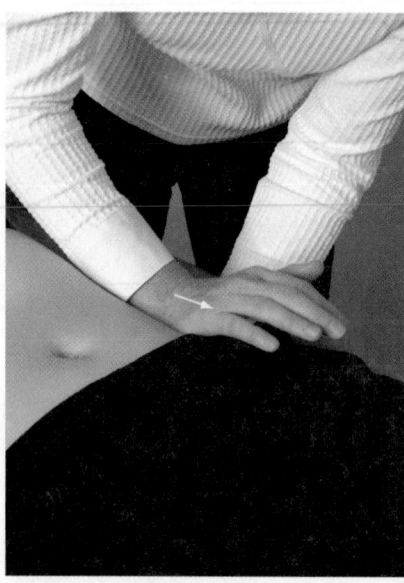

Figure 10-62 Anterior rotation of the innominate requires an infero-posterior glide at the sacroiliac joint.

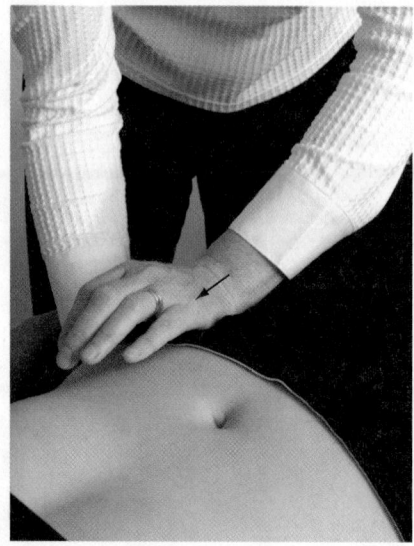

Figure 10-63 Posterior rotation of the innominate requires a supero-anterior glide at the sacroiliac joint.

To test inferoposterior translation of the innominate on the sacrum, the examiner, using the heel of the other hand, applies an anterior rotation force to the ipsilateral ASIS and iliac crest (Figure 10-62). This produces an inferoposterior glide at the sacroiliac joint and is associated with nutation of the sacrum.

To test superoanterior translation of the innominate on the sacrum, the examiner, using the heel of the other hand, applies a posteriorly rotating force to the ipsilateral ASISs and iliac crest (Figure 10-63). This produces a superoanterior glide at the sacroiliac joint and is associated with counternutation of the sacrum.

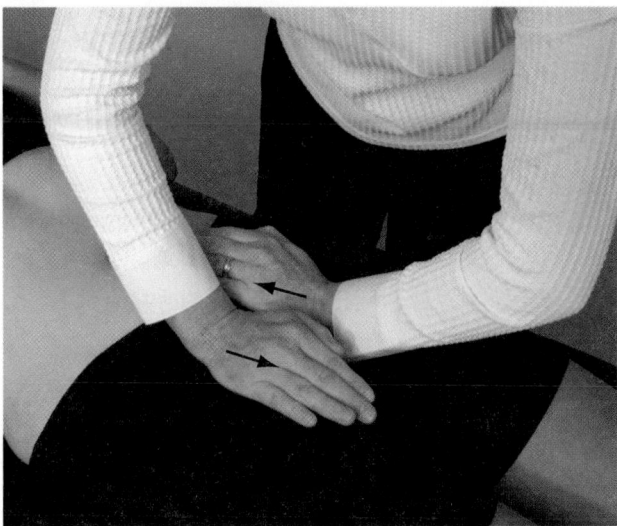

Figure 10-64 Superoinferior translation of one pubic bone on the other.

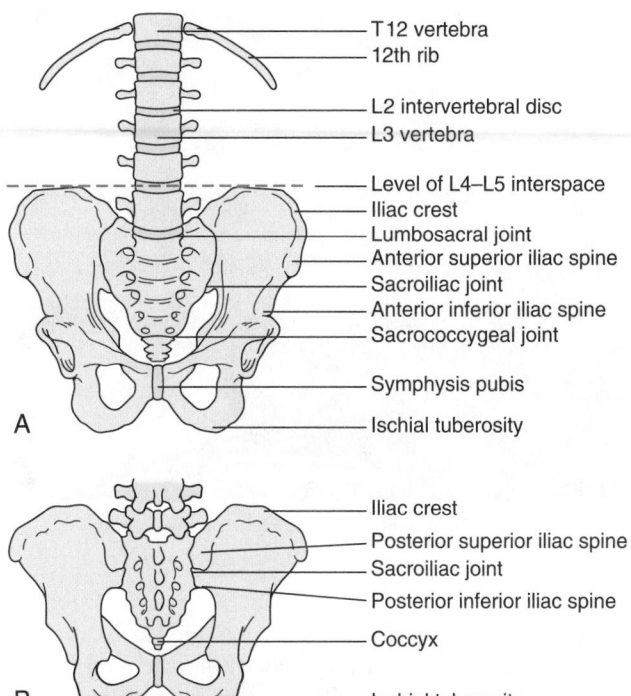

Figure 10-65 Landmarks of the sacroiliac joints and symphysis pubis. **A,** Anterior view. **B,** Posterior view.

An unstable sacroiliac joint has a softer end feel, increased translation, and possible production of symptoms.[62]

***Superoinferior Translation of Symphysis Pubis.*[5]** The patient lies supine. The examiner places the heel of one hand on the superior aspect of the superior ramus of one pubic bone and the heel of the other hand on the inferior aspect of the superior ramus of the opposite pelvic bone. A slow steady inferior force is applied with the uppermost hand while a superior force is applied with the lower hand (Figure 10-64). The examiner is testing the end feel and looking for the production of symptoms.

Palpation[63]

Because many structures are included in the assessment of the pelvic joints, palpation of this area may be extensive, beginning on the anterior aspect and concluding posteriorly. While palpating, the examiner should note any tenderness, muscle spasm, or other signs that may indicate the source of pathology.

Anterior Aspect

The following structures should be carefully and thoroughly palpated (Figure 10-65).

Iliac Crest and Anterior Superior Iliac Spine. The palpating fingers are placed on the iliac crests on both sides and gently moved anteriorly until each ASIS is reached. "Hip pointers" (crushing or contusion of abdominal muscles that insert into iliac crest) may result in tenderness or pain on palpation of the iliac crest—as may undisplaced fractures. The inguinal ligament attaches to the ASIS and runs downward and medially to the symphysis pubis.

McBurney's Point and Baer's Point. The examiner may then draw an imaginary line from the right ASIS to the umbilicus. **McBurney's point** lies along this line approximately one third of the distance from the ASIS and is especially tender in the presence of acute appendicitis. **Baer's point** is located in the right iliac fossa anterior to the right sacroiliac joint and slightly medial to McBurney's point. It is tender in the presence of infection or when there are sprains of the right sacroiliac ligament and indicates spasm and tenderness of the iliacus muscle.

Lymph Nodes, Symphysis Pubis (Pubic Tubercles), Greater Trochanter of the Femur, Trochanteric Bursa, Femoral Triangle, and Surrounding Musculature. The examiner returns to the ASIS and gently palpates the length of the inguinal ligament, feeling for any tenderness or swelling of the lymph nodes or possible inguinal hernia. At the distal end of the inguinal ligament, the examiner comes to the pubic tubercles and symphysis pubis,[64] which should be palpated for tenderness or signs of pathology.

The examiner then places the thumbs over the pubic tubercles and moves the fingers laterally until the bony greater trochanter of the femur is felt. The trochanters are usually level. The trochanteric bursa lies over the greater trochanter and is palpable only if it is swollen.

Returning to the ASIS, the examiner can move on to palpate the **femoral triangle,** which has as its boundaries the inguinal ligament superiorly, the adductor longus muscle medially, and the sartorius muscle laterally. It is in the superior aspect of the triangle that the examiner palpates for swollen lymph nodes. The **femoral pulse** can be palpated deeper in the triangle. Although almost impossible to palpate, the femoral nerve lies lateral to the

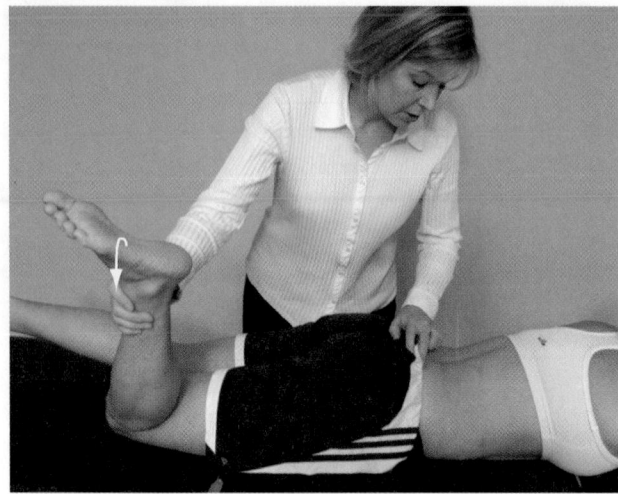

Figure 10-66 Palpation of the right sacroiliac joint.

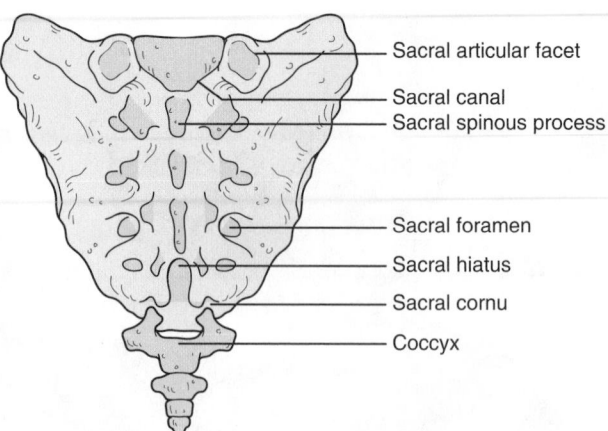

Figure 10-67 Posterior view of the sacrum and coccyx.

artery, whereas the femoral vein lies medial to it. The psoas bursa may also be palpated within the femoral triangle, but only if it is swollen. Before moving on to the posterior structures, the examiner should determine whether the adjacent musculature—the abductor, flexor, and adductor muscles—shows any indication of pathology (e.g., muscle spasm, pain).

Posterior Aspect

To complete the posterior palpation, the patient lies in the prone position, and the following structures are palpated.

Iliac Crest and Posterior Superior Iliac Spine. Again, the examiner places the fingers on the iliac crest and moves posteriorly until they rest on the PSIS, which is at the level of the S2 spinous process. On many patients, dimples indicate the position of the PSIS.

Ischial Tuberosity. If the examiner then moves distally from the PSIS and down to the level of the gluteal folds, the ischial tuberosities may be palpated. It is important that they be palpated, because the hamstring muscles attach here and the bony prominences are what one "sits on."

Sacral Sulcus and Sacroiliac Joints. Returning to the PSIS as a starting point, the examiner should palpate slightly below it on the sacrum adjacent to the ilium. (This area is sometimes referred to as the *sacral sulcus.*) The depth on the right side should be compared with that on the left side. If one side is deeper than the other, sacral torsion or rotation on the ilium around the horizontal plane may be indicated.

If the examiner then moves slightly medially and distal to the PSIS, the fingers rest adjacent to the sacroiliac joints. To palpate these joints, the patient's knee is flexed to 90° or greater, and the hip is passively medially rotated while the examiner palpates the sacroiliac joint on the same side (Figure 10-66). This procedure is identical to the prone gapping test previously described in the "Passive

Movements" section. The procedure is repeated on the other side, and the two results are compared.

Sacrum, Lumbosacral Joint, Coccyx, Sacral Hiatus, Sacral Cornua, and Sacrotuberous and Sacrospinous Ligaments. The examiner again returns to the PSIS and moves to the midline of the sacrum, where the S2 spinous process can be palpated.

Moving superiorly over two spinous processes, the fingers now rest on the spinous process of L5. As a check, the examiner may look to see if the fingers rest just below a horizontal line drawn from the high point of the iliac crests. This horizontal line normally passes through the interspace between L4 and L5. Having found the L5 spinous process, the examiner then palpates between the spinous processes of L5 and S1, feeling for signs of pathology at the lumbosacral joint. Moving laterally approximately 2 to 3 cm (0.8 to 1.2 inches), the fingers lie over the lumbosacral facet joints, which are not palpable. However, the overlying structures may be palpated for tenderness or spasm, which may indicate pathology of these joints or related structures. In a similar fashion, the spinous processes and facet joints of the other lumbar spines and intervening structures can be palpated.

The examiner then returns to the S2 spinous process or tubercle. Carefully palpating farther distally (just before the coccyx), the examiner may be able to palpate the sacral hiatus lying in the midline. If the fingers are moved slightly laterally, the sacral cornua, which constitute the distal aspect of the sacrum, may be palpated (Figure 10-67).

To palpate the coccyx properly, the examiner performs a rectal examination (Figure 10-68). A rubber glove is put on, and the index finger is lubricated. The index finger is then carefully pushed into the rectum as the patient relaxes the sphincter muscles. The index finger then palpates the anterior surface of the coccyx while the thumb of the same hand palpates its posterior aspect. While holding the coccyx between the finger and thumb, the examiner is able to move it back and forth, rocking

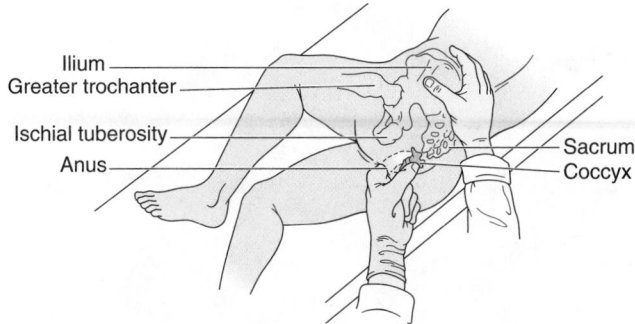

Figure 10-68 Palpation of the coccyx.

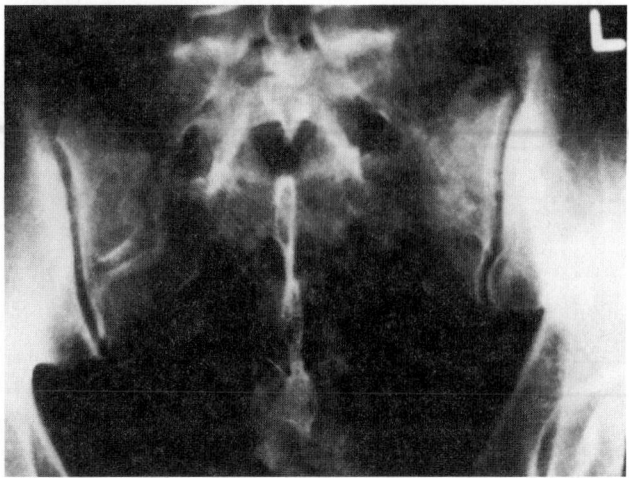

Figure 10-69 Anteroposterior radiograph of the sacroiliac joint.

it at the sacrococcygeal joint. Normally, this action should not cause pain.

The examiner then returns to the PSIS. Moving straight down or distally from the PSIS, the fingers follow the path of the **sacrotuberous ligament,** which should be palpated for tenderness. Slightly more than halfway between the PSIS and ischial tuberosity and slightly medially, the fingers pass over the **sacrospinous ligament,** which is deep to the sacrotuberous ligament. Tenderness in this area may indicate pathology of this ligament.

Diagnostic Imaging[65]

Plain Film Radiography

The following box shows x-rays that may be commonly taken in the pelvic area if pathology is suspected.

On plain film radiography, anteroposterior views (bilateral and single stance) (Figures 10-69 through 10-71), the examiner should look for or note the following:

1. Ankylosis of sacroiliac joints (e.g., ankylosing spondylitis; Figure 10-72).
2. Displacement of one sacroiliac joint and/or the symphysis pubis (Figure 10-73).[66]
3. Demineralization, sclerosis, or periosteal reaction of one or both pubic bones at the symphysis pubis (e.g., osteitis pubis; Figure 10-74).

4. Any fracture.
5. Relation of the sacrum to the ilium.
6. Single leg stance (Flamingo) x-rays can show up to 5 mm of movement at the symphysis pubis in asymptomatic subject comparing alternate leg views.[67,68]
7. Ferguson's angle (also called *lumbosacral angle, sacral base angle,* or *sacral slope*)[69] is formed by a line along the top of the sacral base and a horizontal line (normal: 41°) (Figure 10-75).

Common X-Ray Views of the Pelvic Area

- Anteroposterior view (see Figure 10-73)
- Judet view of the hip and pelvis (Figure 10-76)
- Sacroiliac joints—Ferguson view (30° cephalid angulated anteroposterior) (Figure 10-77)
- Pelvis—pelvic inlet/outlet views (for pelvic ring fracture) (Figure 10-78)

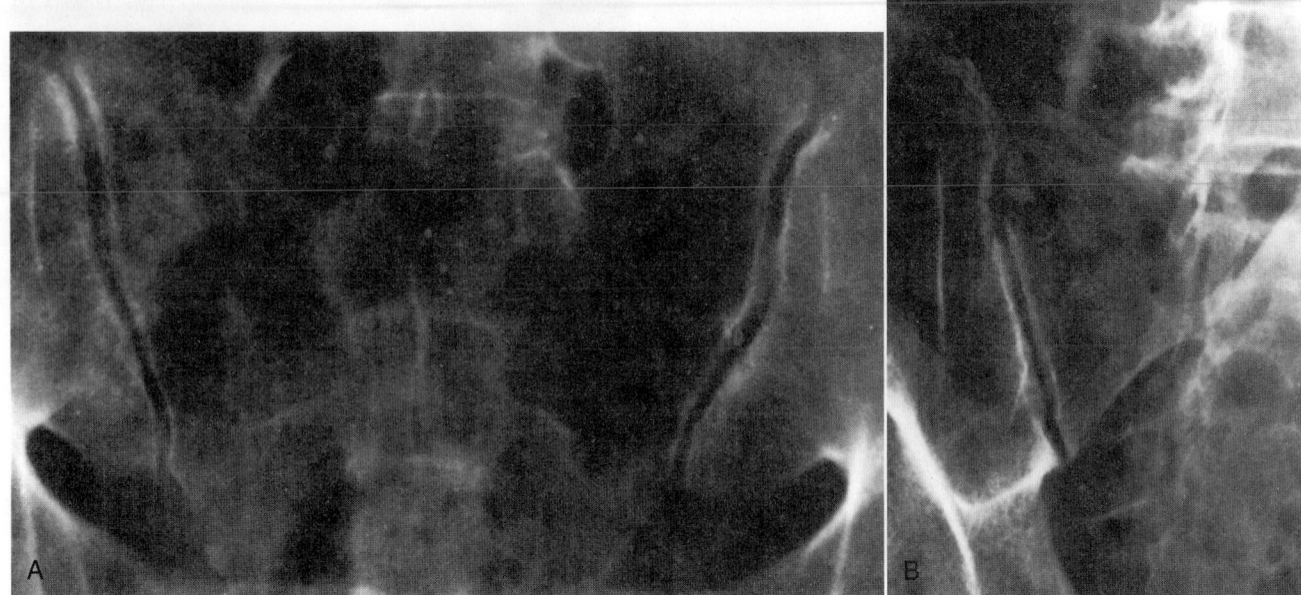

Figure 10-70 Normal sacroiliac joints. Angled (**A**) and oblique (**B**) anteroposterior views show normally maintained cortices and cartilage spaces. (From Weissman BNW, Sledge CB: Orthopedic radiology, Philadelphia, 1986, WB Saunders, p. 347.)

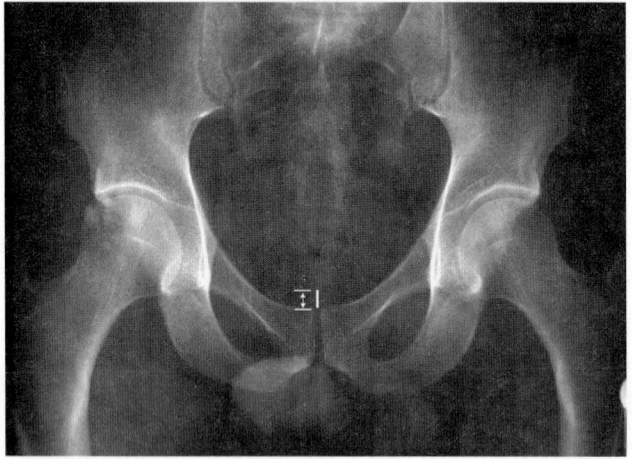

Figure 10-71 A properly centered anteroposterior radiograph must be controlled for rotation and tilt. Proper rotation is confirmed by alignment of the coccyx over the symphysis pubic *(vertical line)*. Propertilt is controlled by maintaining the distance between the tip of the coccyx and the superior border of the symphysis pubis at 1 to 2 cm. (From Byrd JWT: Arthroscopic management of femoroacetabular impingement. Op Tech Sports Med 19:81–94, 2011.)

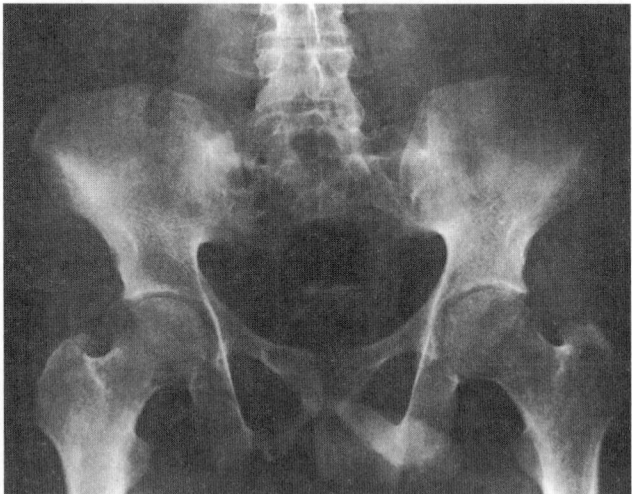

Figure 10-72 Fusion of sacroiliac joint spaces in the late stage of sacroiliitis of ankylosing spondylitis (anteroposterior view). The sclerosis has resorbed, and there is slight narrowing of the left hip joint. (From Rothman RH, Simeone FA: The spine, Philadelphia, 1982, WB Saunders, p. 921.)

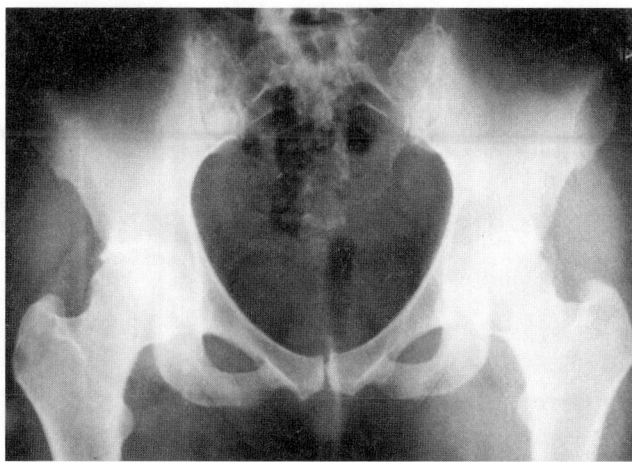

Figure 10-73 Anteroposterior radiograph of the pelvis. Note higher left pubic bone.

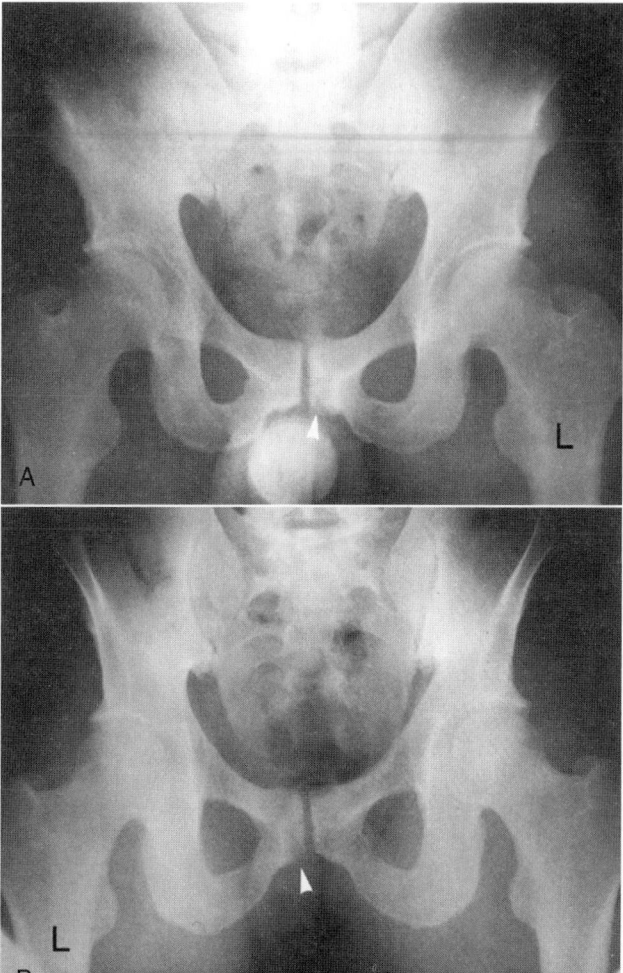

Figure 10-74 Osteitis pubis. A, Anteroposterior view of pelvis showing well-concealed bony lesion at inferior corner of left pubis at the symphysis *(arrowhead)*. **B,** Posterior view of same pelvis; bony fragment is well delineated in this view. (From Wiley JJ: Traumatic osteitis pubis: the gracilis syndrome. Am J Sports Med 11:361, 1983.)

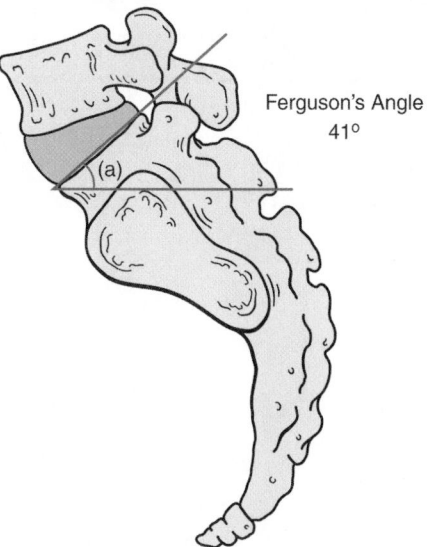

Figure 10-75 Ferguson's angle (normal is approximately 41°).

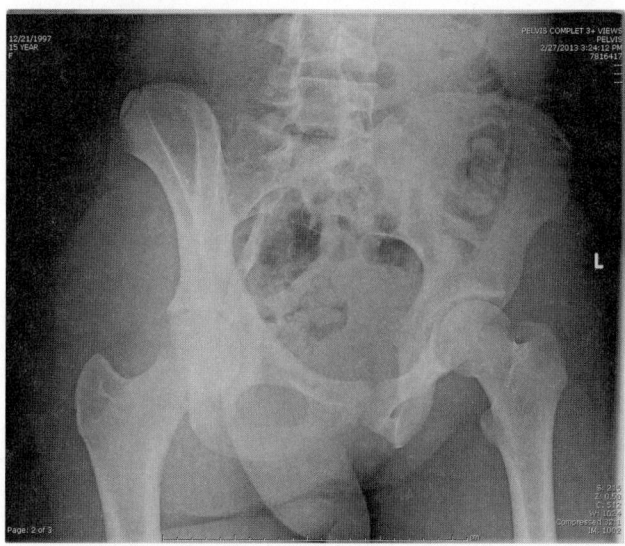

Figure 10-76 Judet view of the left hip and pelvis.

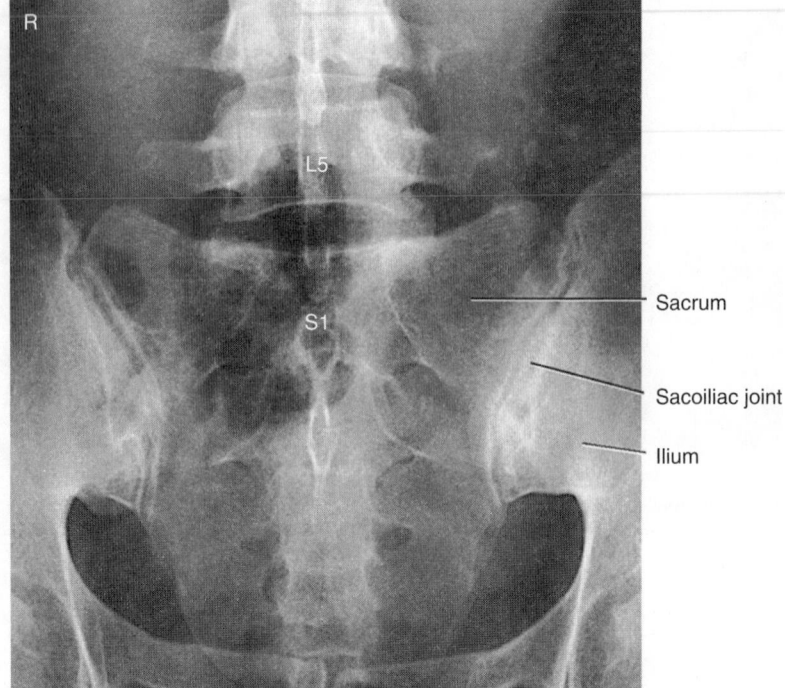

Figure 10-77 Ferguson view (30° cephalid angulated anteroposterior) of the lumbosacral junction and sacroiliac joints (From Frank ED, et al: Merrill's atlas of radiographic positioning and procedures: 3-volume set, ed 12, St Louis, 2012, Mosby.)

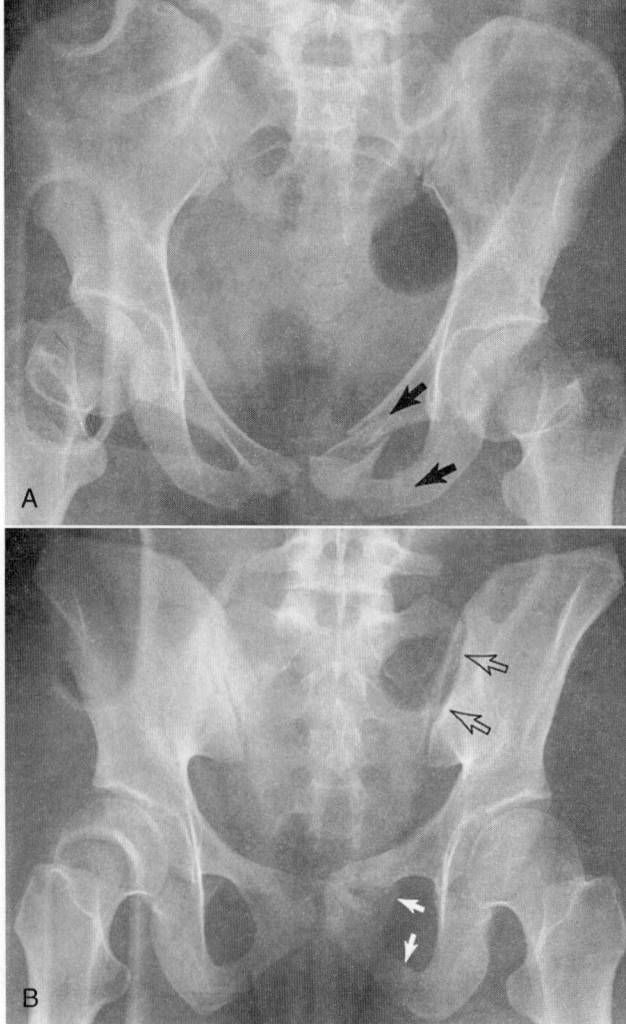

Figure 10-78 A, An anteroposterior inlet projection of a 22-year-old man who suffered a Type III Malgaigne fracture-dislocation reveals minimally displaced vertical fractures *(arrows)* of both the left superior pubic ramus and the left ischiopubic ramus. On this view, the sacrum, ilium, and sacroiliac joints appear normal. **B,** On the anteroposterior outlet view, the diastasis of the left sacroiliac joint becomes obvious *(open arrows)*. (From Taylor JA, et al: Skeletal imaging, ed 2, St Louis, 2010, WB Saunders.)

PRÉCIS OF THE PELVIS ASSESSMENT*

History (sitting)
Observation (standing)
Examination
  Active movements (standing)
    Flexion of the spine
    Extension of the spine
    Rotation of the spine (left and right)
    Side flexion of the spine (left and right)
    Flexion of the hip
    Abduction of the hip
    Adduction of the hip
    Extension of the hip
    Medial rotation of the hip
    Lateral rotation of the hip
  Special tests (standing)
    Flamingo test
    Gillet's test
    Trendelenburg test
  Special tests (sitting)
  Passive movements (supine)
    Gapping test
    Rocking (knee-to-shoulder) test
    Sacral apex pressure test
    Sacral thrust test
    Thigh thrust test
  Resisted isometric movements (supine)†
    Forward flexion of the spine
    Flexion of the hip
    Abduction of the hip
    Adduction of the hip
    Extension of the hip
  Special tests (supine)
    Leg length measurement
    90–90 straight leg raise

    Patrick test
    Straight leg raise test
    Supine active straight leg raise test
  Passive movements (side lying)
    Approximation test
    Passive extension and medial rotation of ilium on
      sacrum
    Passive flexion and lateral rotation of ilium on sacrum
  Special tests (side lying)
    Gaenslen's test
  Reflexes and cutaneous distribution (supine, then prone)
  Passive movements (prone)
    Ipsilateral prone kinetic test
    Sacral apex pressure test
  Special tests (prone)
    Prone active straight leg raise test
  Joint play movements (prone)
    Cephalad movement of the sacrum with caudal
      movement of the ilium
    Cephalad movement of the ilium with caudal
      movement of the sacrum
  Palpation (prone, then supine)
  Diagnostic imaging
    As previously stated, assessment of the sacroiliac joints and symphysis pubis is done only after an assessment of the lumbar spine and hips, unless there has been specific trauma to the sacroiliac joints or symphysis pubis. Completion of the examination of the sacroiliac joints and symphysis pubis, therefore, may involve only passive movements, special tests, joint play movements, and palpation, because the other tests would have been completed when assessing the other joints.
    After any examination, the patient should be warned of the possibility of exacerbation of symptoms as a result of the assessment.

*The précis is shown in an order that will limit the amount of moving or changing position that the patient has to do and yet ensure that all necessary structures are tested.
†If not done in standing.

CASE STUDIES

When doing these case studies, the examiner should list the appropriate questions to be asked and why they are being asked, what to look for and why, and what things should be tested and why. Depending on the answers of the patient (and the examiner should consider different responses), several possible causes of the patient's problem may become evident (examples are given in parentheses). A differential diagnosis chart (Table 10-7) should be made up. The examiner can then decide how different diagnoses may affect the treatment plan.

1. A 26-year-old male soccer player complains of lower abdominal pain that is referred into the right groin. Sit-ups are painful, and he experiences pain when he kicks the ball. Describe your assessment plan for this patient (abdominal strain versus osteitis pubis).
2. A 35-year-old man complains of "back pain." He complains that his back is stiff and sore when he gets up in the morning and that the stiffness remains for most of the day. Sclerosis of the sacroiliac is evident on x-ray. Describe your assessment plan for this patient (ankylosing spondylitis versus osteoarthritis of the sacroiliac joints).
3. An 18-year-old female figure skater complains of back pain that increases when she is skating; the pain is prominent on one leg. The ASIS and PSIS are higher on the right side. Describe your assessment plan for this patient (sacroiliac dysfunction versus short leg syndrome).

TABLE **10-7**

Differential Diagnosis Between Ankylosing Spondylitis and Sacroiliac Arthritis

	Ankylosing Spondylitis	Sacroiliac Arthritis
History	Bilateral sacroiliac pain that may refer to posterior thigh Morning stiffness Male predominance	Bilateral sacroiliac pain referring to gluteal area (S1–S2 dermatomes) Morning stiffness (prolonged) Coughing painful
Observation	Stiff, controlled movement of pelvis	Controlled movement of pelvis
Active Movement	Decreased	Side flexion and extension full Slight limitation of flexion
Passive Movement	Decreased	Normal
Resisted Isometric Movement	Pain and weakness, especially if sacroiliac joints are stressed	Pain, especially if sacroiliac joints are stressed
Special Tests	Sacral stress tests probably positive	Sacral stress tests probably positive
Sensation and Reflexes	Normal	Normal
Palpation	Tender over sacroiliac joints	Tender over sacroiliac joints
Diagnostic Imaging	X-rays diagnostic	X-rays diagnostic
Lab Tests	Erythrocyte sedimentation rate increased human leukocyte antigen (HLA)—B27 HLA present in 80%	Normal

REFERENCES

1. Schwarzer AC, Aprill CN, Bogduk N: The sacroiliac joint in chronic low back pain. Spine 20:31–37, 1995.
2. Kapandji LA: The physiology of the joints, vol. 3: The trunk and vertebral column, New York, 1974, Churchill Livingstone.
3. Vleeming A, Pool-Goudzwaard AL, Hammudoghu D, et al: The function of the long dorsal sacroiliac ligament-its implication for understanding low back pain. Spine 21:556–562, 1996.
4. Jackson R: Diagnosis and treatment of pelvic girdle dysfunction. Orthop Phys Ther Clin North Am 7:413–445, 1998.
5. Lee D: The pelvic girdle, ed 2, Edinburgh, 1999, Churchill Livingstone.
6. Vleeming A, Pool-Goudzwaard AL, Hammudoghu D, et al: The posterior layer of the thoracolumbar fascia: Its function in load transfer from spine to legs. Spine 20:753–758, 1995.
7. Vleeming A, Snidjers CJ, Stoeckart R, et al: The role of the sacroiliac joints in coupling between spine, pelvis, legs and arms. In Vleeming A, Mooney V, Dorman T, et al, editors: Movement, stability and low back pain, Edinburgh, 1997, Churchill Livingstone.
8. Lee DG: Clinical manifestations of pelvic girdle dysfunction. In Boyling JD, Palastanga N, editors: Grieve's modern manual therapy: the vertebral column, ed 2, Edinburgh, 1994, Churchill Livingstone.
9. Patella GA, Andrish JT: Injuries about the hip and pelvis in the young athlete. Clin Sports Med 14:591–628, 1995.
10. Ombregt L, Bisschop B, ter Veer HJ, et al: A system of orthopedic medicine, London, 1995, WB Saunders.
11. Dangaria TR: A case report of sacroiliac joint dysfunction with urinary symptoms. Man Ther 3:220–221, 1998.
12. Lee D: The pelvic girdle. In Magee DJ, Zachazewski JE, Quillen WS, editors: Musculoskeletal rehabilitation—pathology and intervention, Philadelphia, 2007, Elsevier.
13. Maigne R: Orthopaedic medicine: a new approach to vertebral manipulation, Springfield, IL, 1972, Charles C Thomas.
14. Maigne R: Diagnosis and treatment of pain of vertebral origin, Baltimore, 1996, Williams & Wilkins.
15. Levine D, Whittle MW: The effects of pelvic movement on lumbar lordosis in the standing position. J Orthop Sports Phys Ther 24:130–135, 1996.
16. Hagins M, Brown M, Cook C, et al: Intratester and intertester reliability of the palpation meter (PALM) in measuring the pelvic position. J Man Manip Ther 6:130–136, 1998.
17. Kendall FP, McCreary EK, Provance PG: Muscles: testing and function, Baltimore, 1993, Williams & Wilkins.
18. Nelson-Wong E, Flynn T, Callaghan JP: Development of acute hip abduction as a screening test for identifying occupational low back pain. J Orthop Sports Phys Ther 39:649–657, 2009.
19. Mitchell FL, Moran PS, Pruzzo NA: An evaluation and treatment manual of osteopathic muscle energy procedures, Valley Park, MO, 1979, Mitchell, Moran & Pruzzo.
20. Woerman AL: Evaluation and treatment of dysfunction in the lumbar-pelvic-hip complex. In Donatelli R, Wooden MJ, editors: Orthopedic physical therapy, Edinburgh, 1989, Churchill Livingstone.
21. Levangie PK: The association between static pelvic asymmetry and low back pain. Spine 24:1234–1242, 1999.
22. Greenman PE: Innominate shear dysfunction in the sacroiliac syndrome. Man Med 2:114–121, 1986.
23. Bookhout MM, Boissonnault JS: Musculoskeletal dysfunction in the female pelvis. Orthop Phys Ther Clin North Am 5:23–45, 1996.
24. Oldrieve WL: A critical review of the literature on tests of the sacroiliac joint. J Man Manip Ther 3:157–161, 1995.
25. Levangie PK: Four clinical tests of sacroiliac joint dysfunction: the association of test results with innominate torsion among patients with and without low back pain. Phys Ther 79:1043–1057, 1999.
26. Freburger JK, Riddle DL: Measurement of sacroiliac joint dysfunction: a multicenter intertester reliability study. Phys Ther 79:1135–1141, 1999.
27. van der Wurff P, Hagmeijer RH, Meijne W: Clinical tests of the sacroiliac joint—a systematic methodological review. Part 1—reliability. Man Ther 5:30–36, 2000.
28. van der Wurff P, Meijne W, Hagmeijer RH: Clinical tests of the sacroiliac joint—a systematic methodological review, Part 2—validity. Man Ther 5:89–96, 2000.
29. Cibulka MT, Koldehoff R: Clinical usefulness of a cluster of sacroiliac joint tests in patients with and without low back pain. J Orthop Sports Phys Ther 29:83–92, 1999.
30. Meijne W, van Neerbos K, Aufdemkampe G, et al: Intraexaminer and interexaminer reliability of the Gillet test. J Manip Physiol Ther 22:4–9, 1999.
31. Dreyfuss P, Michaelsen M, Pauza K, et al: The value of medical history and physical examination in diagnosing sacroiliac joint pain. Spine 21:2594–2602, 1996.
32. Dreyfuss P, Dreyer S, Griffin J, et al: Positive sacroiliac screening tests in asymptomatic adults. Spine 10:1138–1143, 1994.
33. Laslett M, Williams M: The reliability of selected pain provocation tests for sacroiliac joint pathology. Spine 19:1243–1249, 1994.
34. Arumagam A, Milosavljevic S, Woodley S, et al: Effects of external pelvic compression on form closure, force closure and neuromotor control of the lumbopelvic spine—a systematic review. Manual Therapy 17:275–284, 2012.
35. Pool-Goudzwaard AL, Vleeming A, Stoeckart R, et al: Insufficient lumbopelvic stability: a clinical, anatomical and biomechanical approach to "a-specific" low back pain. Man Ther 3(1):12–20, 1998.

36. Sturesson B, Udeu A, Vleeming A: A radiostereometric analysis of movements of the sacroiliac joints during the standing hip flexion test. Spine 25:364–368, 2000.

37. Ozgocmen S, Bozgeyik Z, Kalcik M, et al: The value of sacroiliac pain provocative tests in early active sacroiliitis. Clin Rheum 27:1275–1282, 2008.

38. Laslett M, Aprill CN, McDonald B, et al: Diagnosis of sacroiliac joint pain: validity of individual provocation tests and composites of tests. Manual Therapy 10:207–218, 2005.

39. van der Wurff P, Buijs EJ, Groen GJ: A multitest regimen of pain provocation tests as an aid to reducing unnecessary minimally invasive sacroiliac joint procedures. Phys Med Rehabil 87:10–14, 2006.

40. Szadek KM, van der Wurff P, Tulder MW, et al: Diagnostic validity of criteria for sacroiliac joint pain: a systematic review. J Pain 10:354–368, 2009.

41. Dreyfus P, Dreyer S, Griffin J, et al: Positive sacroiliac screening tests in asymptomatic adults. Spine 19:1138–1143, 1994.

42. Porterfield JA, DeRosa C: Mechanical low back pain: perspectives in functional anatomy, Philadelphia, 1991, WB Saunders.

43. Dreyfuss P, Deyer SJ, Cole A, et al: Sacroiliac joint pain. J Am Acad Ortho Surg 12:255–265, 2004.

44. Cook CE, Hegedus EJ: Orthopedic physical examination tests—an evidence based approach, Upper Saddle River, NJ, 2008, Prentice Hall/Pearson.

45. Cleland JA, Koppenhaver S: Netter's Orthopedic clinical examination—an evidence based approach, ed 2, Philadelphia, 2011, Saunders.

46. Cipriano JJ: Photographic manual of regional orthopedic tests, Baltimore, 1985, Williams & Wilkins.

47. DonTigny RL: Dysfunction of the sacroiliac joint and its treatment. J Orthop Sports Phys Ther 1:23–35, 1979.

48. Mens JM, Vleeming A, Snijders CJ, et al: The active straight leg raising test and mobility of the pelvic joints. Eur Spine 8:468–473, 1999.

49. Mens JM, Vleeming A, Snijders CJ, et al: Reliability and validity of the active straight leg raise test in posterior pelvic pain since pregnancy. Spine 26:1167–1171, 2001.

50. Mens JM, Vleeming A, Snijders CJ, et al: Validity of the active straight leg raise test for measuring disease severity in patients with posterior pelvic pain after pregnancy. Spine 27:196–200, 2002.

51. Evans RC: Illustrated essentials in orthopedic physical assessment, St Louis, 1994, CV Mosby.

52. Palmer MC, Epler M: Clinical assessment procedures in physical therapy, Philadelphia, 1990, JB Lippincott.

53. Bemis T, Daniel M: Validation of the long sitting test on subjects with iliosacral dysfunction. J Orthop Sports Phys Ther 8:336–345, 1987.

54. Wallace LA: Limb length difference and back pain. In Grieve GP, editor: Modern manual therapy of the vertebral column, Edinburgh, 1986, Churchill Livingstone.

55. Fischer P: Clinical measurement and significance of leg length and iliac crest height discrepancies. J Man Manip Ther 5:57–60, 1997.

56. Pecina MM, Krmpotic-Nemanic J, Markiewitz AD: Tunnel syndromes, Boca Raton, FL, 1991, CRC Press.

57. Borenstein DG, Wiesel SW, Boden SD: Low back pain: medical diagnosis and comprehensive management, Philadelphia, 1995, WB Saunders.

58. Lacroix VJ: Lower abdominal pain syndrome in National Hockey League players: a report of 11 cases. Clin J Sports Med 8:5–9, 1998.

59. Lacroix VJ: A complete approach to groin pain. Phys Sportsmed 28(1):66–86, 2000.

60. Simonet WT, Saylor HL, Sim L: Abdominal wall muscle tears in hockey players. Int J Sports Med 16:126–128, 1995.

61. Taylor DC, Meyers WC, Moylan JA, et al: Abdominal musculature abnormalities as a cause of groin pain in athletes-inguinal hernias and pubalgia. Am J Sports Med 19:239–242, 1991.

62. Lee D: Instability of the sacroiliac joint and the consequences to gait. J Man Manip Ther 4:22–29, 1996.

63. O'Haire C, Gibbons P: Inter-examiner and intra-examiner agreement for assessing sacroiliac anatomical landmarks using palpation and observation: pilot study. Man Ther 5:13–20, 2000.

64. Williams PR, Thomas DP, Downes EM: Osteitis pubis and instability of the pubic symphysis—when nonoperative measures fail. Am J Sports Med 28:350–355, 2000.

65. Ebraheim NA, Mekhail AO, Wiley WF, et al: Yeasting: radiology of the sacroiliac joint. Spine 22:869–876, 1997.

66. Rodriguez C, Miguel A, Lima H, et al: Osteitis pubis syndrome in the professionals soccer athlete: a case report. J Athl Train 36:437–440, 2001.

67. Garras DN, Carothers JT, Olson SA: Single-leg-stance (flamingo) radiographs to assess pelvic stability: how much motion is normal. J Bone Joint Surg Am 90:2114–2118, 2008.

68. Siegel J, Templeman DC, Tornetta P: Single-leg-stance radiographs in the diagnosis of pelvic instability. J Bone Joint Surg Am 90:2119–2125, 2008.

69. Hellems HK, Keats TE: Measurement of the normal lumbosacral angle. Am J Radiol 113:642–645, 1971.

70. Leboeuf C: The sensitivity and specificity of seven lumbo-pelvic orthopedic tests and the arm-fossa test. J Manip Physiol Ther 13(3):138–143, 1990.

71. Kokmeyer DJ, Van der Wurff P, Aufdemkampe G, et al: The reliability of multitest regimens with sacroiliac pain provocation tests. J Manip Physiol Ther 25(1):42–48, 2002.

72. Laslett M, Aprill CN, McDonald B, et al: Diagnosis of sacroiliac joint pain: validity of individual provocation tests and composites of tests. Man Ther 10(3):207–218, 2005.

73. Levin U, Stenstrom CH: Force and time recording for validating the sacroiliac distraction test. Clin Biomech 18:821–826, 2003.

74. Meijne W, van Neerbos K, Aufdemkampe G, et al: Intraexaminer and interexaminer reliability of the Gillet test. J Manip Physiol Ther 22(1):4–9, 1999.

75. Carmichael JP: Inter and intra examiner reliability of palpation for sacroiliac joint dysfunction. J Manip Physiol Ther 10(4):164–171, 1987.

76. O'Haire C, Gibbons P: Inter-examiner and intra-examiner agreement for assessing sacroiliac anatomical landmarks using palpation and observation: pilot study. Man Ther 5(1):13–20, 2000.

77. Riddle DL, Freburger JK: Evaluation of the presence of sacroiliac joint region dysfunction using a combination of tests: a multicenter intertester reliability study. Phys Ther 82(8):772–781, 2002.

SUGGESTED READINGS

Alderink GJ: The sacroiliac joint: Review of anatomy, mechanics, and function. J Orthop Sports Phys Ther 13:71–84, 1991.

Arab AM, Abdollahi I, Joghataei MT, et al: Inter- and intra-rater reliability of single and composites of selected motion palpation and pain provocation tests for sacroiliac joint. Manual Therapy 14:213–221, 2009.

Bourdillon JF: Spinal manipulation, ed 3, New York, 1982, Appleton-Century-Crofts.

Bowen V, Cassidy JD: Macroscopic and microscopic anatomy of the sacroiliac joint from embryonic life until the eighth decade. Spine 6:620–628, 1981.

Brooke R: The sacro-iliac joint. J Anat 58:299–305, 1924.

Carmichael JP: Inter- and intra-examination reliability of palpation for sacroiliac joint dysfunction. J Manip Physiol Ther 10:164–171, 1987.

Cassidy JD: The pathoanatomy and clinical significance of the sacroiliac joints. J Manip Physiol Ther 15:41–42, 1992.

Cohen AS, McNeill JM, Calkins E, et al: The "normal" sacroiliac joint: analysis of 88 sacroiliac roentgenograms. Am J Roentgenol 100:559–563, 1967.

Cyriax J: Textbook of orthopaedic medicine, vol. 1: diagnosis of soft tissue lesions, London, 1975, Bailliere Tindall.

DeMann LE: Sacroiliac dysfunction in dancers with low back pain. Man Ther 2:2–10, 1997.

DeRosa C, Porterfield JA: Lumbar spine and pelvis. In Richardson JK, Iglarsh ZA, editors: Clinical orthopedic physical therapy, Philadelphia, 1994, WB Saunders.

Dietrichs E: Anatomy of the pelvic joints: a review. Scand J Rheumatol Suppl 88:4–6, 1991.

Dykstra PF: Radiology of the normal SI joint. J Man Manip Ther 1:87–94, 1993.

Dyrek DA, Micheli LJ, Magee DJ: Injuries to the thoracolumbar spine and pelvis. In Zachazewski JE, Magee DJ, Quillen WS, editors: Athletic injuries and rehabilitation, Philadelphia, 1996, WB Saunders.

Fickel TE: "Snapping hip" and sacroiliac sprain: example of a cause-effect relationship. J Manip Physiol Ther 12:390–392, 1989.

Finneson BE: Low back pain, Philadelphia, 1981, JB Lippincott.

Forrester DM, Brown JC: The radiology of joint disease, Philadelphia, 1987, WB Saunders.

Frigerio NA, Stowe RR, Howe JW: Movement of the sacroiliac joint. Clin Orthop 100:370–377, 1974.

Gajdosik RL, Alberta CR, Mitman JJ: Influence of hamstring length on the standing position and flexion range of motion of the pelvic angle, lumbar angle, and thoracic angle. J Orthop Sports Phys Ther 20:213–219, 1994.

Gajdosik R, Simpson R, Smith R, et al: Pelvic tilt: intratester reliability of measuring the standing position and range of motion. Phys Ther 65:169–174, 1985.

Gamble JG, Simmons SC, Freedman M: The symphysis pubis: anatomic and pathologic considerations. Clin Orthop 203:261–272, 1986.

Gilliam J, Brunt D, MacMillan M, et al: Relationship of the pelvic angle to the sacral angle: measurement of clinical reliability and validity. J Orthop Sports Phys Ther 20:193–199, 1994.

Gitelman R: A chiropractic approach to biomechanical disorders of the lumbar spine and pelvis. In Haldeman S, editor: Modern developments in the principles and practice of chiropractic, New York, 1980, Appleton-Century-Crofts.

Gray H: Sacro-iliac joint pain: the finer anatomy. N Internat Clin 2:54–64, 1938.

Grieve GP: Common vertebral joint problems, Edinburgh, 1981, Churchill Livingstone.

Grieve GP: Mobilisation of the spine, Edinburgh, 1979, Churchill Livingstone.

Grieve GP: The sacro-iliac joint. Physiotherapy 62:384–400, 1976.

Gross ML, Nasser S, Finerman GA: Hip and pelvis. In DeLee JC, Drez D, editors: Orthopedic sports medicine, Philadelphia, 1994, WB Saunders.

Hanson PG, Angevine M, Juhl JH: Osteitis pubis in sports activities. Phys Sportsmed 6:111–114, 1978.

Harrison DE, Harrison DD, Troyanovich SJ: The sacroiliac joint: a review of anatomy and biomechanics with clinical implications. J Manip Physiol Ther 20:607–617, 1997.

Hollinshead WH, Jenkins DR: Functional anatomy of the limbs and the trunk and vertebral column, New York, 1991, Churchill Livingstone.

Kirkaldy-Willis WH: Managing low back pain, New York, 1983, Churchill Livingstone.

Klinefelter FW: Osteitis pubis. Am J Roentgenol 63:368–371, 1950.

Lazennac JY, Ramare S, Arafati N, et al: Sagittal aligment in lumbosacral fusion: relations between radiological parameters and pain. Eur Spine J 9:47–55, 2000.

Lee DG: Kinematics of the pelvic joints. In Boyling JD, Palastanga N, editors: Grieve's modern manual therapy: the vertebral column, ed 2, Edinburgh, 1994, Churchill Livingstone.

Legaye J, Duval-Beaupre G, Jacquet J, et al: Pelvic evidence: a fundamental pelvic parameter for 3-dimensional regulation of spinal sagittal curves. Eur Spine J 7:99–103, 1998.

Lewitt K, Rosina A: Why yet another diagnostic sign of sacroiliac movement restriction? J Manip Physiol Ther 22:154–160, 1999.

Mac-Thiong JM, Berthonnaud E, Dimar JR, et al: Sagittal alignment of the spine and pelvis during growth. Spine 29:1642–1647, 2004.

Mac-Thiong JM, Wang Z, de Guise JA, et al: Postural model of sagittal spino-pelvic alignment and its relevance for lumbosacral developmental spondylolisthesis. Spine 33:2316–2325, 2008.

Macnab I: Backache, Baltimore, 1977, Williams & Wilkins.

McGillivray D: The pelvic girdle. In Little H, editor: Rheumatological physical examination, Orlando, 1986, Grune & Stratton.

McRae R: Clinical orthopedic examination, New York, 1976, Churchill Livingstone.

Nicholas JA: Football injuries. In Nicholas JA, Hershsmann EB, editors: The lower extremity and spine in sports medicine, vol 2, St Louis, 1986, CV Mosby.

Oldreive WL: A classification of and a critical review of the literature on syndromes of the sacroiliac joint. J Man Manip Ther 6:24–30, 1998.

Oldreive WL: A critical review of the literature on the anatomy and biomechanics of the sacroiliac joint. J Man Manip Ther 4:157–165, 1996.

Oldreive WL: A critical review of the literature on tests of the sacroiliac joint. J Man Manip Ther 3:157–161, 1995.

Osterbauer PJ, De Boer KF, Widmaier A, et al: Treatment and biomechanical assessment of patients with chronic sacroiliac joint syndrome. J Manip Physiol Ther 15:82–90, 1993.

Pitkin HC, Pheasant HC: Sacrathrogenetic telalgia: a study of referred pain. J Bone Joint Surg 18:111–133, 1936.

Porterfield JA, DeRosa C: The sacroiliac joint. In Gould JA, editor: Orthopedic and sports physical therapy, St Louis, 1990, CV Mosby.

Post M: Examination of the thoracic and lumbar spine. In Post M, editor: Physical examination of the musculoskeletal system, Chicago, 1987, Year Book Medical Publishers.

Reilly BM: Practical strategies in outpatient medicine, Philadelphia, 1984, WB Saunders.

Resnick D, Kransdorf MJ: Bone and joint imaging, Philadelphia, 2005, WB Saunders.

Rothman RH, Simeone FA: The spine, Philadelphia, 1982, WB Saunders.

Rudge SR, Swannell AJ, Rose DH, et al: The clinical assessment of sacro-iliac joint involvement in ankylosing spondylitis. Rheumatol Rehabil 21:15–20, 1982.

Schwarzer AC, Aprill CN, Bogduk N: The sacroiliac joint in chronic low back pain. Spine 20:31–37, 1995.

Slipman CW, Sterenfeld EB, Chou LH, et al: The value of radionuclide imaging in the diagnosis of sacroiliac joint syndrome. Spine 21:2251–2254, 1996.

Stoddard A: Manual of osteopathic practice, New York, 1970, Harper & Row.

Stoddard A: Manual of osteopathic technique, Atlantic Highlands, NJ, 1969, Humanities Press.

Sturesson B, Selvik G, Uden A: Movements of the sacroiliac joints—a roentgen stereophotogrammetric analysis. Spine 14:162–165, 1989.

Timm KE: Sacroiliac joint dysfunction in elite rowers. J Orthop Sports Phys Ther 25:288–293, 1999.

Toomey M: The pelvis, hip, and thigh. In Zuluaga M, Briggs C, Carlisle J, et al, editors: Sports physiotherapy: applied science and practice, Melbourne, 1995, Churchill Livingstone.

Toussaint R, Gawlik CS, Rehder U, et al: Sacroiliac dysfunction in construction workers. J Manip Physiol Ther 22:134–138, 1999.

Travell JG, Simons DG: Myofascial pain and dysfunction: the trigger point manual, Baltimore, 1983, Williams & Wilkins.

Vaz G, Roussouly P, Berthonnaud E, et al: Sagittal morphology and equilibrium of pelvis and spine. Eur Spine J 11:80–87, 2002.

Wadsworth CT, DeFabio RP, Johnson D: The spine. In Wadsworth CT, editor: Manual examination and treatment of the spine and extremities, Baltimore, 1988, Williams & Wilkins.

Walheim GG, Olerud S, Ribbe T: Motion of the pelvic symphysis in pelvic instability. Scand J Rehabil Med 16:163–169, 1984.

Walker JM: The sacroiliac joint: a critical review. Phys Ther 72:903–916, 1992.

Weissman BNW, Sledge CB: Orthopedic radiology, Philadelphia, 1986, WB Saunders.

Wells PE: The examination of the pelvic joints. In Grieve GP, editor: Modern manual therapy of the vertebral column, Edinburgh, 1986, Churchill Livingstone.

Wiley JJ: Traumatic osteitis pubis: the gracilis syndrome. Am J Sports Med 11:360–363, 1983.

Williams PL, Warwick R, editors: Gray's anatomy, ed 36, British, Edinburgh, 1980, Churchill Livingstone.

Willis TA: Lumbosacral anomalies. J Bone Joint Surg Am 41:935–938, 1959.

Woerman AL: Evaluation and treatment of pelvic girdle dysfunction. In Saunders HD, Saunders RS, editors: Evaluation, treatment, and prevention of musculoskeletal disorders, Chaska, MN, 1995, Saunders Group.

CHAPTER 11

Hip

The hip joint is one of the largest and most stable joints in the body. If it is injured or exhibits pathology, the lesion is usually immediately perceptible during walking. Because pain from the hip can be referred to the sacroiliac joints or the lumbar spine, it is imperative—unless there is evidence of direct trauma to the hip—that these joints be examined along with the hip.

APPLIED ANATOMY

The hip joint is a multiaxial ball-and-socket joint that has maximum stability because of the deep insertion of the head of the femur into the acetabulum (Figure 11-1). The femoral head is much more stable in the acetabulum for the hip than the humerus is in the glenoid for the shoulder. To allow sufficient movement and proper alignment to occur at the hip joint, the femur has a longer neck than the humerus and is anteverted (Figure 11-2).

Hip Joint	
Resting position:	30° flexion, 30° abduction, slight lateral rotation
Close packed position:	Full extension, medial rotation, and abduction
Capsular pattern:	Flexion, abduction, medial rotation (but in some cases, medial rotation is limited)

In addition, the hip, like the shoulder, has a labrum, which helps to deepen and stabilize the joint.[1,2] The acetabular labrum increases the articular surface area of the acetabulum and volume, and it creates a seal for the central compartment, which is part of the intra-articular hip joint. The seal resists distraction of the femoral head from the socket by maintaining a negative pressure and resists fluid flow that enhances nutrition of the hip articular cartilage, which in turn provides a smooth gliding surface.[3,4] The joint has a strong capsule and very strong muscles that control its actions (Figure 11-3). The acetabulum is formed by fusion of part of the ilium, ischium, and pubis, which taken as a group are sometimes called the *innominate bone* or *pelvis*. The acetabulum opens outward, forward, and downward. It is half of a sphere, and the femoral head is two thirds of a sphere. The hip, already a stable joint because of its bony configuration, is supported by three strong ligaments: the iliofemoral, the ischiofemoral, and the pubofemoral ligaments (Figure 11-4). The iliofemoral ligament (Y ligament of Bigelow) is considered to be the strongest ligament in the body. It is positioned to prevent excessive extension and plays a significant role in stabilizing and in maintaining upright posture at the hip while limiting anterior translation. The acetabular labrum plays a secondary role in stabilizing the hip during lateral rotation while preventing anterior translation.[5] The ischiofemoral ligament, the weakest of these three strong ligaments, winds tightly on extension, helping to stabilize the hip in extension. The pubofemoral ligament prevents excessive abduction of the femur and limits extension. All three ligaments also limit medial rotation of the femur. A fourth ligament of the hip that sometimes is injured is the ligamentum teres or "ligament of the head," which provides a physical attachment of the head of the femur to the acetabulum.[6]

Under low loads, the joint surfaces are incongruous; under heavy loads, they become congruous, providing maximum surface contact. The maximum contact brings the load per unit area down to a tolerable level. Depending on the activity, the forces exerted on the hip will vary.[7]

Forces on the Hip	
Standing:	0.3 times the body weight
Standing on one limb:	2.4 to 2.6 times the body weight
Walking:	1.3 to 5.8 times the body weight
Walking up stairs:	3 times the body weight
Running:	4.5+ times the body weight

When considering movement or kinematics at the hip joint, one must consider whether the pelvis is moving on stationary femur (weight-bearing) or the femur (non–weight-bearing) is moving on the pelvis (Figure 11-5).

PATIENT HISTORY

In addition to the questions listed under the "Patient History" section in Chapter 1, the examiner should obtain the following information from the patient:
1. *What is the age of the patient?* Different conditions occur in different age groups, and range of motion

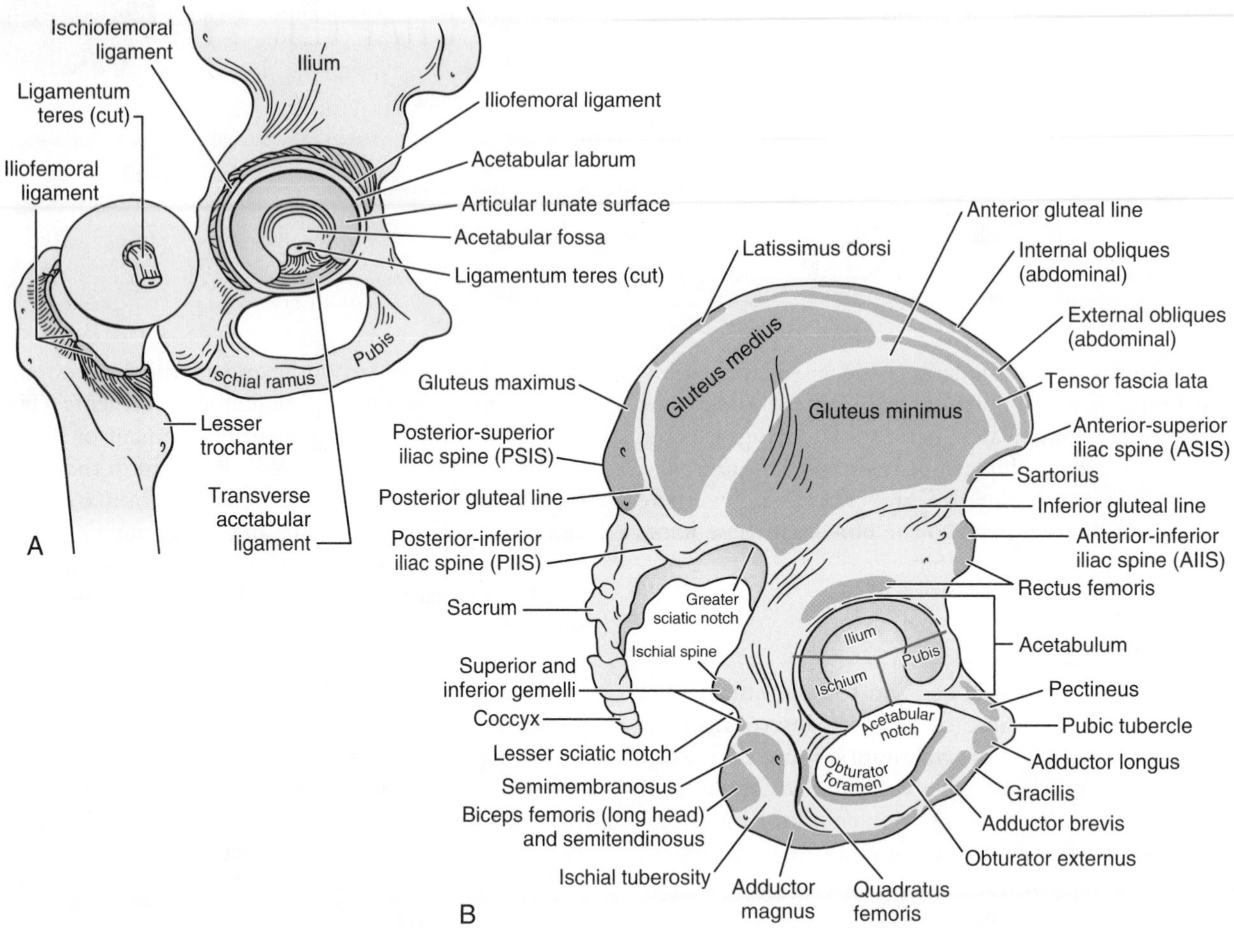

Ischiofemoral ligament

Ligamentum teres (cut)

Iliofemoral ligament

Ilium

Iliofemoral ligament

Acetabular labrum

Articular lunate surface

Acetabular fossa

Ligamentum teres (cut)

Ischial ramus

Pubis

Lesser trochanter

Transverse acctabular ligament

A

Latissimus dorsi

Gluteus medius

Gluteus minimus

Anterior gluteal line

Internal obliques (abdominal)

External obliques (abdominal)

Tensor fascia lata

Anterior-superior iliac spine (ASIS)

Sartorius

Inferior gluteal line

Anterior-inferior iliac spine (AIIS)

Rectus femoris

Acetabulum

Gluteus maximus

Posterior-superior iliac spine (PSIS)

Posterior gluteal line

Posterior-inferior iliac spine (PIIS)

Sacrum

Superior and inferior gemelli

Coccyx

Lesser sciatic notch

Semimembranosus

Biceps femoris (long head) and semitendinosus

Ischial tuberosity

Greater sciatic notch

Ischial spine

Ilium

Ischium

Pubis

Acetabular notch

Obturator foramen

Pectineus

Pubic tubercle

Adductor longus

Gracilis

Adductor brevis

Obturator externus

Adductor magnus

Quadratus femoris

B

Figure 11-1 Anatomy of the hip. A, The right hip opened to show its internal components. **B,** Side view of right innominate bone (pelvis) showing muscle attachments. (Modified from Neumann DA: Kinesiology of the musculoskeletal system—foundations for physical rehabilitation, St Louis, 2002, CV Mosby, pp. 388, 397.)

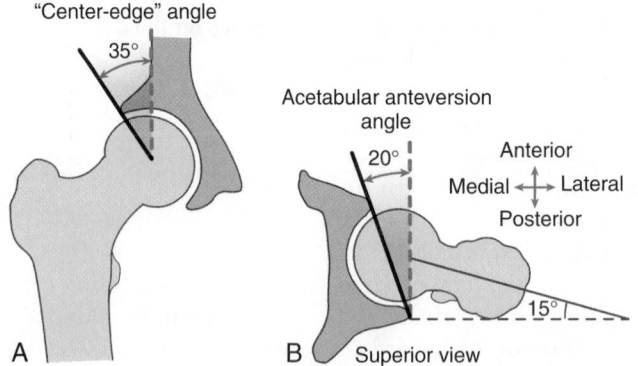

"Center-edge" angle

35°

Acetabular anteversion angle

20°

Anterior

Medial ↔ Lateral

Posterior

15°

A

B   Superior view

Figure 11-2 A, The center-edge angle measures the fixed orientation of the acetabulum within the frontal plane, relative to the pelvis. This measurement defines the extent to which the acetabulum covers the top of the femoral head. The center-edge angle is measured as the intersection of a vertical, fixed reference line *(stippled)* with the acetabular reference line *(bold solid line)* that connects the upper lateral edge of the acetabulum with the center of the femoral head. A more vertical acetabular reference line results in a smaller center-edge angle, providing less superior coverage of the femoral head. **B,** The acetabular anteversion angle measures the fixed orientation of the acetabulum within the horizontal plane, relative to the pelvis. This measurement indicates the extent to which the acetabulum covers the front of the femoral head. The angle is formed by the intersection of a fixed anterior-posterior reference line *(stippled)* with an acetabular reference line *(bold solid line)* that connects the anterior and posterior rim of the acetabulum. A larger acetabular anteversion angle creates less acetabular containment of the anterior side of the femoral head. (A normal femoral anteversion of 15° is also shown.) (From Neumann DA: Kinesiology of the musculoskeletal system—foundations for physical rehabilitation, St Louis, 2010, Mosby, p. 474.)

(ROM) decreases with age. For example, congenital hip dysplasia is seen in infancy, primarily in girls; Legg-Calvé-Perthes disease is more common in boys 3 to 12 years old; and elderly women are more prone to osteoporotic femoral neck fractures.

2. *If trauma was involved, what was the mechanism of injury?* Did the patient land on the outside of the hip (e.g., trochanteric bursitis) or land on or hit the knee, thus jarring the hip (e.g., subluxation, acetabular labral tear)? Was the patient involved in repetitive loading activity (e.g., femoral stress fracture) or osteoporotic (insufficiency injury)?[8] A careful determination of the mechanism of injury often leads to a diagnosis of the problem. Mechanical hip problems are reported as symptoms getting worse with activity, twisting movements are painful, sitting is uncomfortable (hip flexion), getting up from sitting may cause catching, ascending and descending stairs are difficult as is getting in and out of an automobile, and the patient may have difficulty putting on shoes and/or socks.[9,10]

3. *What are the details of the present pain and other symptoms* (Table 11-1)?[11] Hip intra-articular pain, including labral tears and anterior impingement, is felt mainly in the groin and along the front or medial side of the thigh to the knee,[1,12] whereas buttock pain is associated with posterior labral tears and lumbar spine problems.[1,13] Adductor pain may be the result of over-active adductors caused by pelvic instability.[14] Pain may also be referred to the hip area from several structures (Figure 11-6). Pain from the lumbar spine may commonly be referred to the back or lateral aspect of the hip.

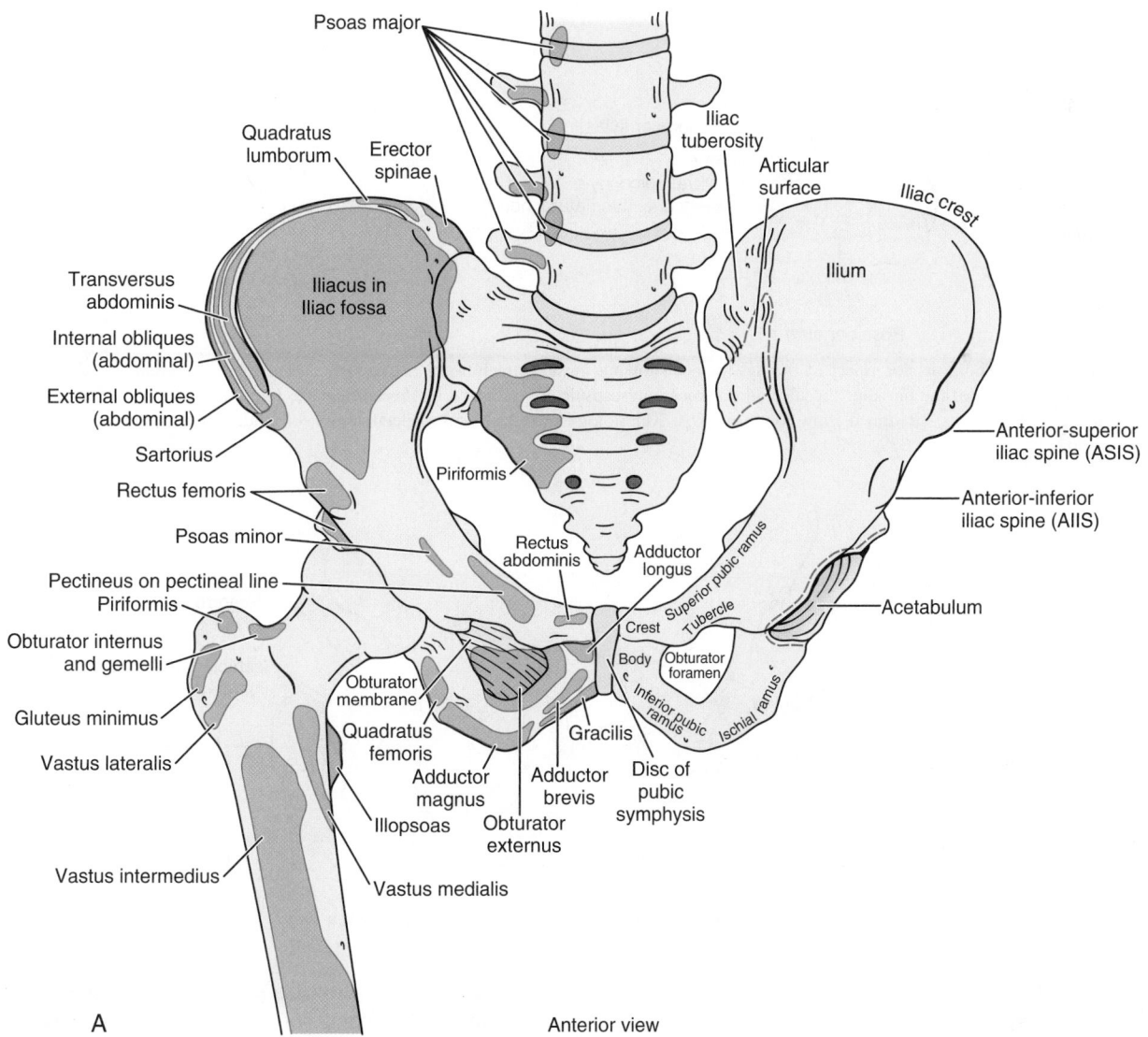

Figure 11-3 A, The anterior aspect of the pelvis, sacrum, and right proximal femur showing muscle attachments *(origins are shown in red, insertions are shown in blue).* A section of the left side of the sacrum is removed to expose the articular surface of the sacroiliac joint. The pelvic attachments of the capsule around the sacroiliac joint are indicated by *dashed lines.*   *Continued*

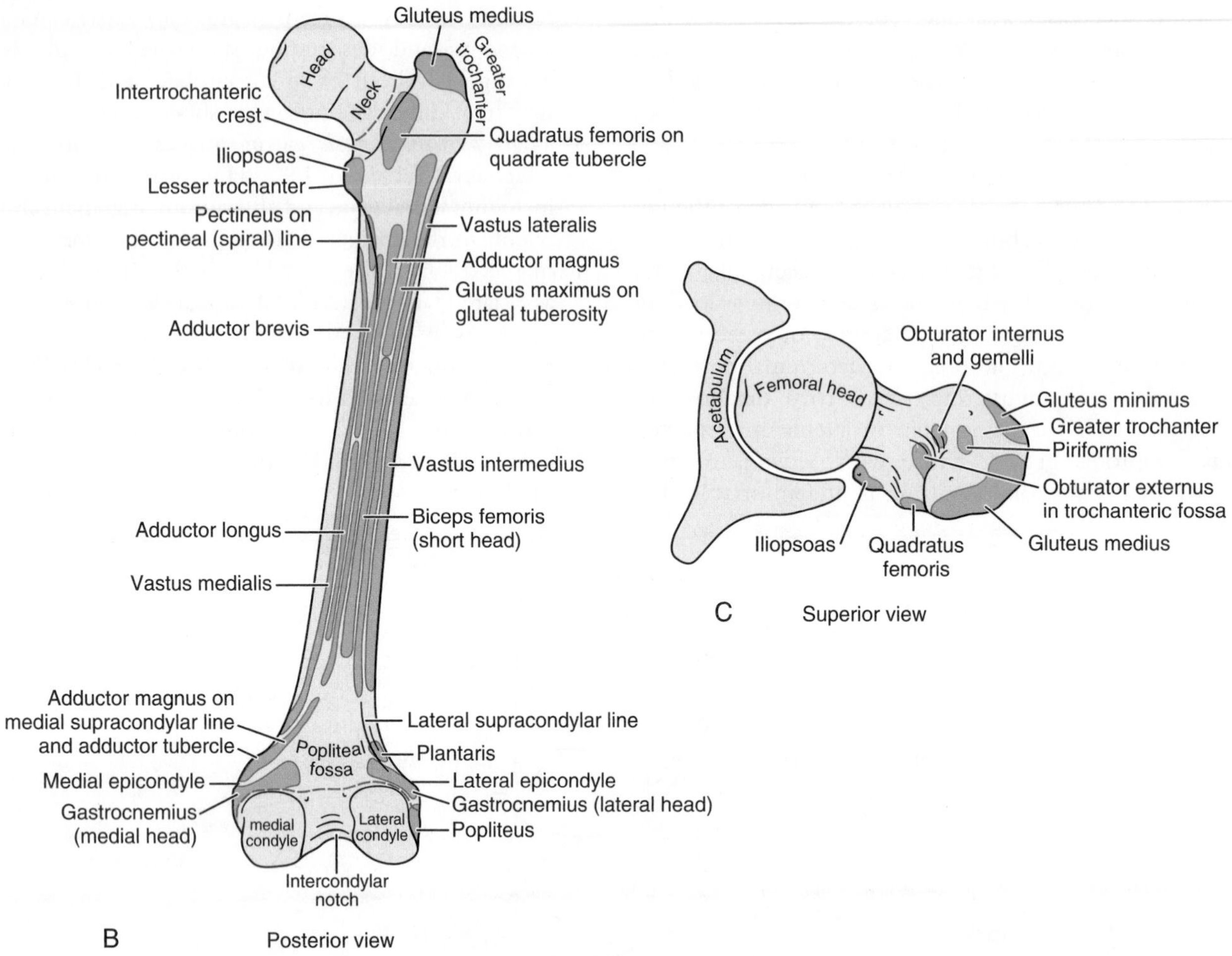

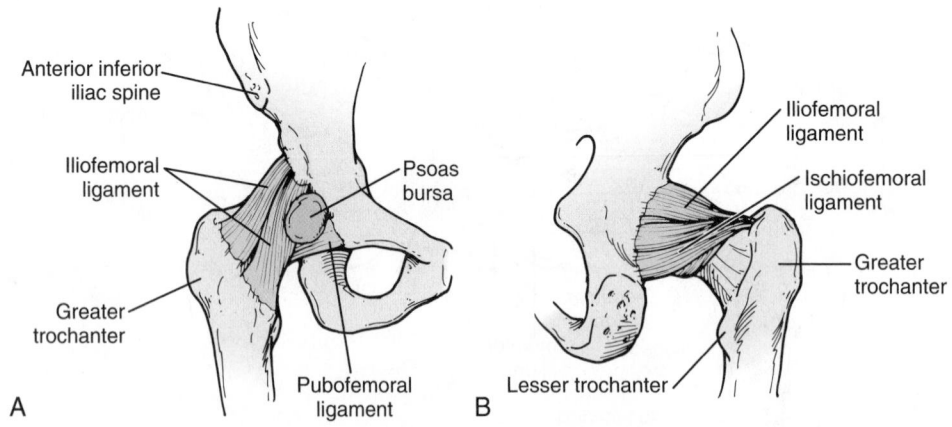

Figure 11-3, cont'd B, The posterior aspect of the right femur showing muscle attachments *(origins are shown in red, insertions are shown in blue).* The femoral attachments of the hip joint capsule and the knee joint capsule are indicated by *dashed lines.* **C,** The superior aspect of the right femur showing muscle attachments. (Redrawn from Neumann DA: Kinesiology of the musculoskeletal system—foundations for physical rehabilitation, St Louis, 2002, CV Mosby, pp. 389, 393.)

Figure 11-4 Ligaments of the hip. A, Anterior view. **B,** Posterior view.

A **sports hernia,** which is commonly caused by a deficient inguinal canal posterior wall, nerve entrapment or adductor tendonopathies, may have an insidious onset of unilateral dull, aching pain in the groin that may be sharp or burning and may radiate into the proximal thigh, low back, lower abdominal muscles, perineum and/or scrotum. The symptoms are aggravated by sudden acceleration, cutting, or kicking.[15–18]

Lateral hip pain may be due to a trochanteric bursitis or tear of the gluteus medius tendon, most

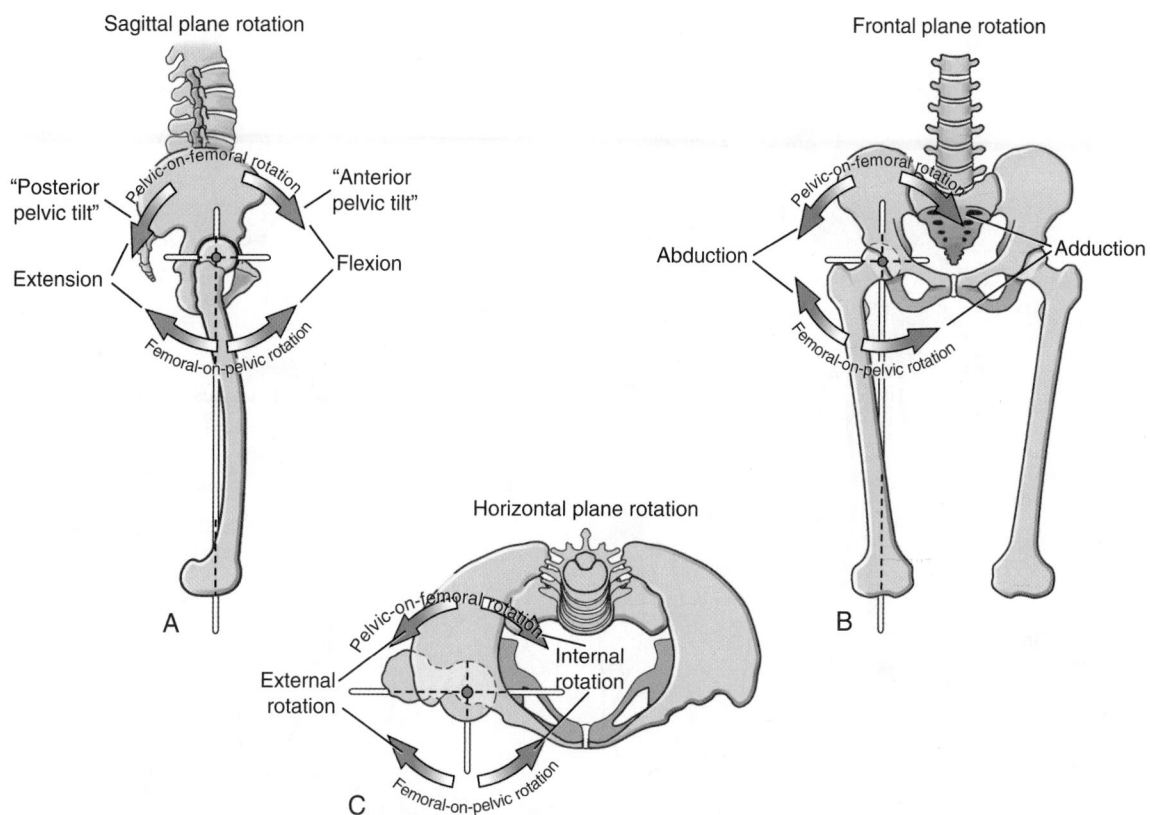

Figure 11-5 The osteokinematics of the right hip joint. Femoral-on-pelvic and pelvic-on-femoral rotations occur in three planes. The axis of rotation for each plane of movement is shown as a *colored dot,* located at the center of the femoral head. **A,** Side view shows sagittal plane rotations around a medial-lateral axis of rotation. **B,** Front view shows frontal plane rotations around an anterior-posterior axis of rotation. **C,** Top view shows horizontal plane rotations around a longitudinal, or vertical, axis of rotation. (From Neumann DA: Kinesiology of the musculoskeletal system— foundations for physical rehabilitation, St Louis, 2010, Mosby, p. 477.)

TABLE 11-1

Diagnostic Clues in Hip Pain

Type of Pain	Possible Causes
Dull, deep, aching	Arthritis, Paget disease
Sharp, intense, sudden, associated with weight bearing	Fracture
Tingling that radiates	Radiculopathy, spinal stenosis, meralgia paresthetica
Increased pain while sitting with the affected leg crossed	Trochanteric bursitis
Pain at sitting, legs not crossed	Ischiogluteal bursitis
Pain after standing, walking	Hip arthrosis
Pain on attempted weight bearing	Occult fracture, severe arthrosis
Unremitting, long duration	Paget disease, metastatic carcinoma, severe arthrosis (occasionally)

From Schon L, Zuckerman JD: Hip pain in the elderly: evaluation and diagnosis. Geriatrics 43:58, 1988.

commonly in older patients.[19] Lateral hip pain may also simulate L4 nerve root pain; therefore, assessment of the back should also be considered for lateral or posterior symptoms. Hip pain may also be referred to the knee or back and may increase on walking. **Clicking** is common with labral tears.[20,21] **Snapping** in and around the hip (coxa saltans) has many causes (Table 11-2). First and most commonly, it may be caused by slipping of the iliopsoas tendon over the osseous ridge of the lesser trochanter or anterior acetabulum, or the iliofemoral ligament may be riding over the femoral head.[22–24] Some call this **internal snapping.** If due to the iliopsoas tendon or iliofemoral ligament, the snapping often occurs at approximately 45° of flexion when the hip is moving from flexion to extension, especially with the hip abducted and laterally rotated (**snapping hip sign** or **extension test**).[25] The snap, which may be accompanied by pain or a jerk, is palpated anteriorly in the inguinal region.[25,26] Second, the snapping may be caused by a tight iliotibial band or gluteus maximus tendon riding over the greater trochanter of the femur.[22,23] This is sometimes called **external snapping.** This snapping or popping, which tends to be felt more lateral, occurs during hip flexion and

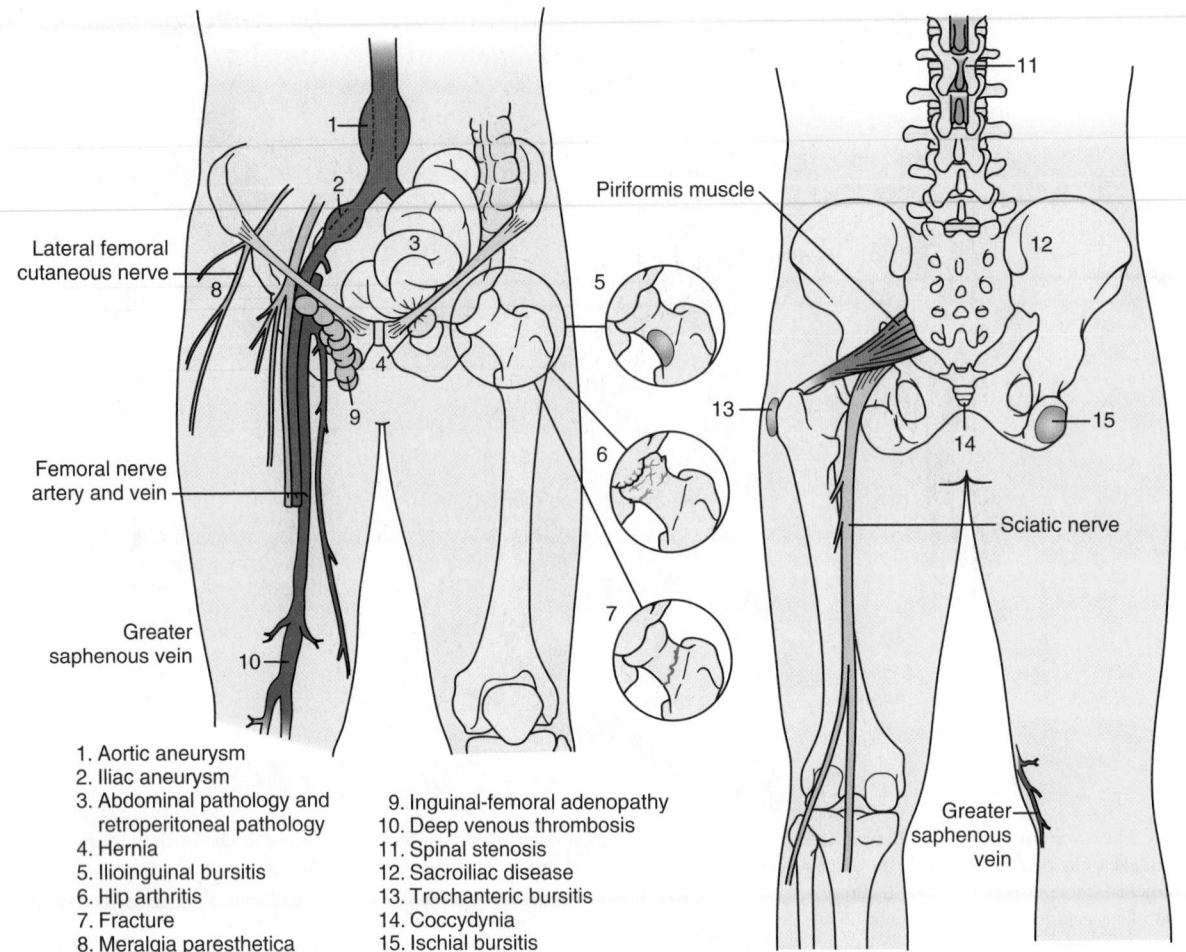

Piriformis muscle

Lateral femoral
cutaneous nerve

Femoral nerve
artery and vein

Greater
saphenous vein

Sciatic nerve

Greater
saphenous
vein

1. Aortic aneurysm
2. Iliac aneurysm
3. Abdominal pathology and
   retroperitoneal pathology
4. Hernia
5. Ilioinguinal bursitis
6. Hip arthritis
7. Fracture
8. Meralgia paresthetica

9. Inguinal-femoral adenopathy
10. Deep venous thrombosis
11. Spinal stenosis
12. Sacroiliac disease
13. Trochanteric bursitis
14. Coccydynia
15. Ischial bursitis

Figure 11-6 Pain in the region of the hip can represent different musculoskeletal and non-musculoskeletal problems. (Redrawn from Schon L, Zuckerman JD: Hip pain in the elderly: evaluation and diagnosis. Geriatrics 43:52, 1988.)

TABLE 11-2

Causes of Snapping Hip (Coxa Saltans) Symptoms

External	Internal	Intra-Articular
• Posterior iliotibial band	• Iliopsoas tendon snapping	• Labral or ligamentum tears
• Anterior gluteus maximus	• Iliofemoral ligament snapping	• Loose bodies
• Trochanteric bursitis	• Hamstring syndrome	• Synovial chondromatosis
	• Iliopsoas bursal/capsular thickening	• Displaced fractures
		• Capsular instability

From Wahl CJ, Warren RF, Adler RS, et al: Internal coxa saltans (snapping hip) as a result of overtraining. Am J Sports Med 32:1303, 2004.

extension, especially if the hip is held in medial rotation, and may be made worse if the trochanteric bursa is inflamed.[26] The third cause of a snapping hip is acetabular labral tears or loose bodies, which may be the result of trauma or degeneration.[23,27–29] This is sometimes referred to as **intra-articular snapping.** In this case, the patient (commonly between 20 to 40 years) complains of a sharp pain into the groin and anterior thigh, especially on pivoting movements.

Passively, clicking may be felt and heard when the extended hip is adducted and laterally rotated.[23,26] Each of these conditions may be referred to as **snapping hip syndrome.**

4. *Is the condition improving? Worsening? Staying the same?* Such a question gives the examiner some idea of the present state of the joint and pathology. Table 11-3 outlines criteria for osteoarthritis in patients with hip pain.[30]

TABLE **11-3**

Classification Criteria for Osteoarthritis of the Hip

Clinical (history, physical examination, laboratory) classification criteria for osteoarthritis of the hip, classification tree format*	**1.** Hip pain, and **2a.** Hip internal rotation < 15°, and **2b.** ESR ≤ 45 mm/hour (if ESR not available, substitute hip flexion ≤ 115°), or **3a.** Hip internal rotation ≥ 15°, and **3b.** Pain on hip internal rotation, and **3c.** Morning stiffness of the hip ≥ 60 minutes, and **3d.** Age > 50 years
Combined clinical (history, physical examination, laboratory) and radiographic classification criteria for osteoarthritis of the hip, traditional format**	Hip pain, and at least two of the following three features: • ESR < 20 mm/hour • Radiographic femoral or acetabular osteophytes • Radiographic joint space narrowing (superior, axial, and/or medial)

Modified from Altman R, Alarcon G, Appelrouth D, et al.: The American College of Rheumatology criteria for the classification and reporting of osteoarthritis of the hip. Arth Rheum 34:511–512, 1991.
ESR, Erythrocyte sedimentation rate (Westergren).
*This classification method yields a sensitivity of 86% and a specificity of 75%.
**This classification method yields a sensitivity of 89% and a specificity of 91%.

5. *Does any type of activity ease the pain or make it worse?* For example, trochanteric bursitis often results from abnormal running mechanics with the feet crossing midline (increased adduction), wide pelvis and genu valgum, or running on tracks with no banking.[26]

6. *Are there any movements that the patient feels are weak or abnormal?* For example, in **piriformis syndrome,** the sciatic nerve may be compressed, the piriformis muscle is tender, and hip abduction and lateral rotation are weak.

7. *What is the patient's usual activity or pastime?* By listening to the patient, the examiner should be able to tell whether repetitive or sustained positions have contributed to the problem. Also, the examiner can develop some idea of the functional impairment felt by the patient.

8. *Is there any past medical and/or surgical history, such as developmental disorders (e.g., hip dysplasia, Legg-Calvé-Perthes disease), systemic illnesses, metabolic, or inflammatory disorders?*[12] A history of alcohol, steroid or tobacco use can increase the risk of osteonecrosis.[12]

OBSERVATION

As the patient comes into the assessment area, the gait should be observed. If the hip is affected, the weight is lowered carefully on the affected side and the knee bends slightly to absorb the shock. The length of the step on the affected side is shorter so that weight can be taken off the leg quickly. If the hip is stiff, the entire trunk and affected leg swing forward together. It is also important to watch for "balance" of the pelvis on the hip. In standing, the patient commonly has the hip slightly flexed if there is pain in the hip.

Pathology in the hip region can lead to tight adductors, iliopsoas, piriformis, tensor fasciae latae, rectus femoris, and hamstrings while, at the same time, the gluteus maximus, medius, and minimus become weak.[31,32] Weak abductors can lead to a Trendelenburg gait or an "abductor lurch." Internal hip pathology or a flexion contracture may lead to a "pelvic wink." This is excessive rotation in the axial plane (more than 40°) toward the affected hip in an attempt by the patient to obtain terminal hip extension.[33] If there is an imbalance of the flexors or extensors in the sagittal plane, the forward–backward motion of the trunk is altered to help maintain balance. For example, a bilateral hip flexion contracture causes the lumbar spine to extend to a greater degree (increased lordosis) as a compensating mechanism. Weak extensors cause the patient to move the trunk backward to maintain balance and avoid falling as a result of the unopposed action of the flexors. If the lateral rotators are significantly stronger than the medial rotators, as is normally the case, excessive toe-out can result. In addition, the patellae may have a "frog eyes" appearance (turn-out). Contracture of either of the rotators may lead to a pivoting at the hip during gait.[34] The different types of gait are discussed in greater detail in Chapter 14.

If the patient uses a cane, it should be held in the hand opposite the affected side to negate some of the force of gravity on the affected hip.[35] The use of a cane can decrease the load on the hip by as much as 40%.[35,36]

The patient should be standing and suitably undressed for the examiner to perform a proper observation. The following aspects are noted from the front, side, and behind:

1. Posture: The examiner should watch for pelvic obliquity caused by, for example, unequal leg length, muscle contractures, or scoliosis (see Chapter 15 for more details). It must be remembered that injury to iliopsoas may also affect the spine. Therefore, when asking patients to do movements involving these muscles, the examiner must watch the effect on the spine and spinal movement (see the "Thomas Test" section later in this chapter). Tightness of the iliopsoas can cause deviation of the spine to the same side.[37]

2. Whether the patient can or will stand on both legs: Two bathroom scales may be used to check symmetry of weight bearing.

3. Balance: It is important to check the patient's proprioceptive control in the joints being assessed. This control may be evaluated by asking the patient to balance first on one leg (the good one) and then the other leg—first with the eyes open, and then with the eyes closed. Differences should be noted through comparison. Loss of proprioceptive control is especially obvious when the patient's eyes are closed. The use of the **stork standing test**[34] (Figure 11-7) has also been advocated for testing proprioception. This test may also test stability at the sacroiliac joints, the knee, and the ankle and foot. With both methods, the examiner should watch for a positive Trendelenburg sign, which would negate the proprioceptive tests.

4. Whether the limb positions are equal and symmetric: The position of the limb may indicate the type of injury. With traumatic posterior hip dislocation, the limb is shortened, adducted, and medially rotated, and the greater trochanter is prominent. With an anterior hip dislocation, the limb is abducted and laterally rotated and may appear cyanotic or swollen owing to pressure in the femoral triangle. With intertrochanteric fractures, the limb is shortened and laterally rotated.

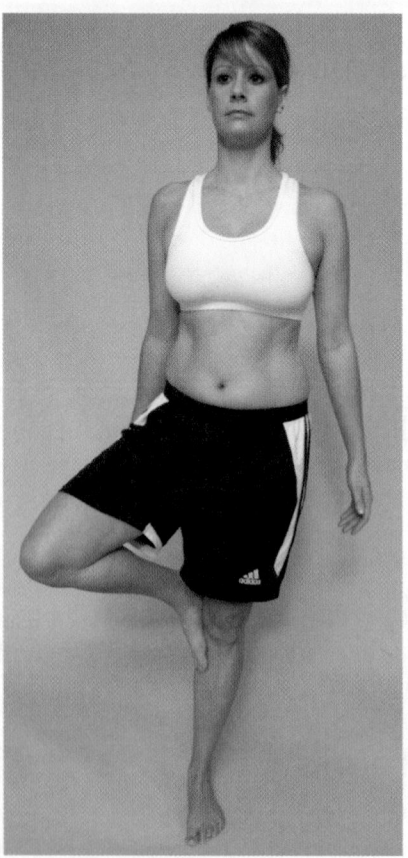

Figure 11-7 Stork standing test.

5. Any obvious shortening of a leg: Shortening of the leg may be demonstrated by a spinal scoliosis if the shortening is present in only one lower limb. Shortening may be structural or functional. Structural changes at the hip that may lead to altered limb length include hip angulation deformity, congenital hypoplasia, femoral growth plate problems and developmental disorders.[12] If the hips are unstable (e.g., bilateral unreduced congenital dislocation of the hip [CDH]), an increased lumbar lordosis may be evident because the head of the femur usually rests above and behind the acetabulum, causing the patient to have an increased lordosis to maintain the center of gravity.

6. Color and texture of the skin

7. Any scars or sinuses

8. The patient's willingness to move: If the hip is painful, the patient has an antalgic gait (see Chapter 14) and does not want to move the hip. If the hip is unstable, the patient has more difficulty controlling its movement.

Anterior View

The examiner should note any abnormality of the bony and soft-tissue contours. With many patients, differences in these contours are difficult to detect because of muscle bulk and other soft-tissue deposition around the hips. The examiner must, therefore, look closely. The same is true for swelling. Swelling in the hip joint itself is virtually impossible to detect by observation, and swelling resulting from a psoas or trochanteric bursitis can easily be missed if the examiner is not carefully observant.

Lateral View

While the patient is viewed from the side, the contour of the buttock should be observed for any abnormality (gluteus maximus atrophy or atonia). In addition, a hip flexion deformity is best observed from this position. The examiner should take the time to compare the two sides and note any subtle differences.

Posterior View

The position of the hip and the effect, if any, of this position on the spine should be noted. For example, a hip flexion contracture may lead to an increased lumbar lordosis. Any differences in bony and soft-tissue contours should again be noted.

EXAMINATION

When doing an examination of the hip, the examiner must keep in mind that pain may be referred to the hip from the sacroiliac joints or the lumbar spine, and vice versa. Therefore, the examination may be an extensive one. If there is any doubt as to the location of the lesion, an assessment of the lumbar spine and sacroiliac joints should be performed along with the hip. It is only through a careful examination of the three areas, especially if there has been no history of trauma, that the examiner can discern the location of the lesion.

As with any examination, the examiner should compare one side of the body with the other, noting any differences. This comparison is necessary because of the individual differences among normal people.

Active Movements

The active movements (Figure 11-8) are done in such a way that the most painful ones are done last. To keep movement of the patient to a minimum, some movements are tested with the patient in the supine position, and others are tested in the prone position. For ease of

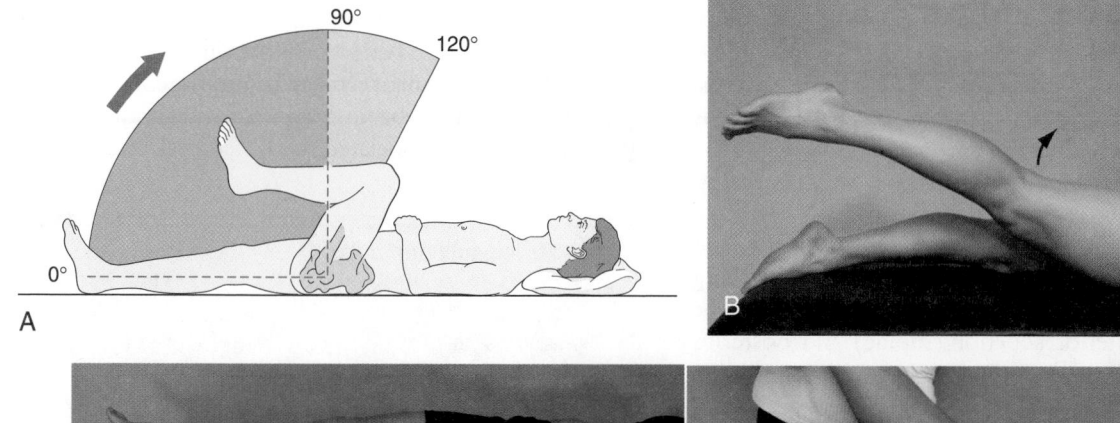

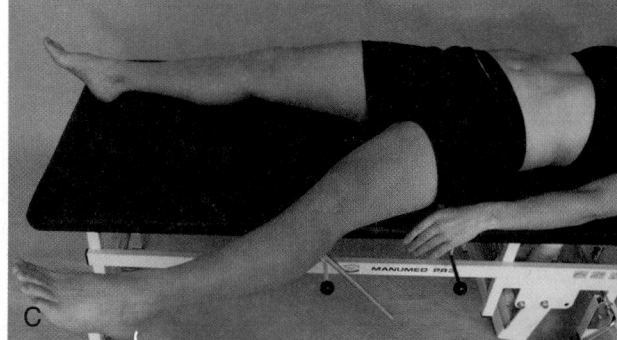

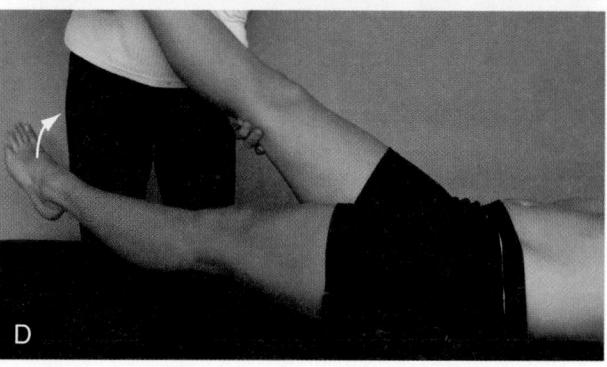

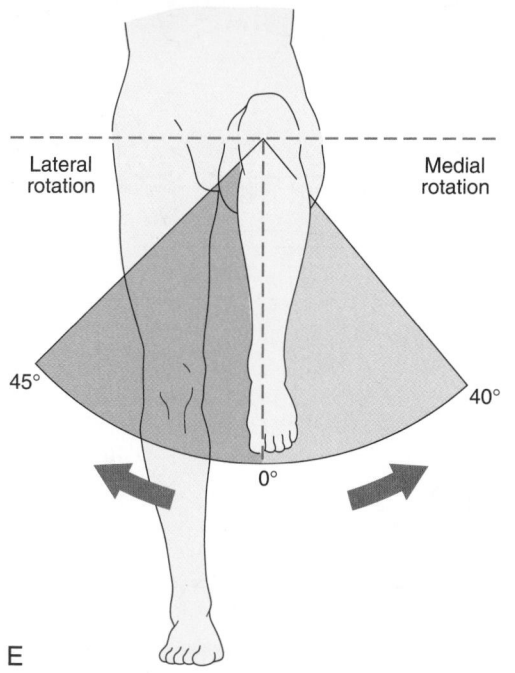

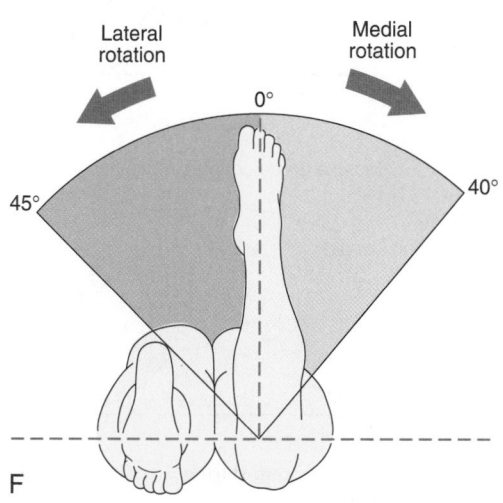

Figure 11-8 Active movements of the hip. A, Flexion. **B,** Extension. **C,** Abduction. **D,** Adduction. **E,** Rotation in the supine position. **F,** Rotation in the prone position. (**A, E,** and **F,** Redrawn from Beetham WP, Polley HF, Slocumb CH, et al: Physical examination of the joints, Philadelphia, 1965, WB Saunders, pp. 134, 137, and 138, respectively.)

description, the movements are described together. The examiner should follow the order as stated in the précis at the end of the chapter when examining the patient. If the history has indicated that repetitive movements, sustained postures, or combined movements have caused symptoms, the examiner should ensure that these movements are tested as well. For example, sustained extension of the hip may provoke gluteal pain in the presence of claudication in the common or internal iliac artery.[38] During the active movements, the examiner should always watch for the possibility of muscle or force-couple imbalances that lead to abnormal muscle recruitment patterns. For example, during extension, the normal pattern is contraction of the gluteus maximus followed by the erector spinae on the opposite side and the hamstrings (depending on the load being extended). If the erector spinae contract first, the pelvis rotates anteriorly and hyperextension of the lumbar spine occurs. When doing the active movements, the examiner should watch the pelvis and the anterior superior (supine) and posterior superior (prone) iliac spines. During hip movement, if the pelvic force-couples are normal, the pelvis and anterior superior iliac spine (ASIS)/posterior superior iliac spine (PSIS) will not move. If they do, it may be an indication of muscle imbalance (Figure 11-9).

Flexion of the hip is tested in the supine position and normally ranges from 110° to 120° with the knee flexed.

If the ASIS begins to move, the movement is stopped because pelvic rotation is occurring rather than hip flexion. The patient's knee is flexed during the test to prevent limitation of movement caused by hamstring tightness. If sharp anterior groin pain that may refer to the gluteal or trochanteric region is elicited on full flexion, adduction and medial rotation, the pain may be the result of **anterior impingement** of the femoral neck against the acetabular rim.[39-45] The pain is made worse by certain movements (e.g., pivoting, movement into extreme rotation) or long periods of sitting, standing or walking.[46] This **femoroacetabular impingement (FAI)** (Figure 11-10) may be cam type or pincer type. Both types are usually associated with femoral head (e.g.,

---

Active Movements of the Hip

- Flexion (110° to 120°)
- Extension (10° to 15°)
- Abduction (30° to 50°)
- Adduction (30°)
- Lateral rotation (40° to 60°)
- Medial rotation (30° to 40°)
- Sustained postures (if necessary)
- Repetitive movements (if necessary)
- Combined movements (if necessary)

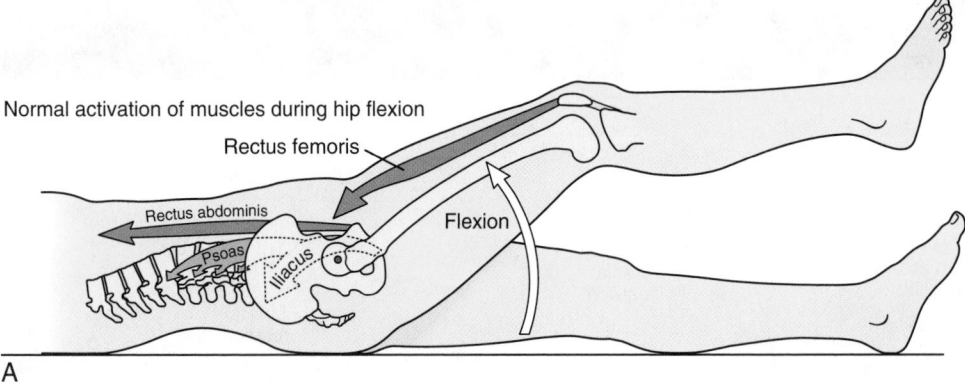

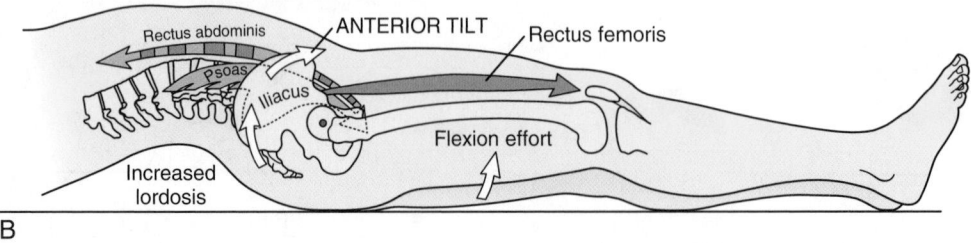

Figure 11-9 Force-couple action during a unilateral straight leg raise. A, With normal activation of the rectus abdominis and the hip flexors (psoas and rectus femoris), the pelvis is stabilized and prevented from anterior tilting by the pull of the hip flexor muscles. **B,** With reduced activation of the rectus abdominis, contraction of the hip flexor muscles causes a marked anterior tilt of the pelvis. Note the increase in lumbar lordosis that accompanies the anterior tilt of the pelvis. (Modified from Neumann DA: Kinesiology of the musculoskeletal system—foundations for physical rehabilitation, St Louis, 2002, CV Mosby, p. 413.)

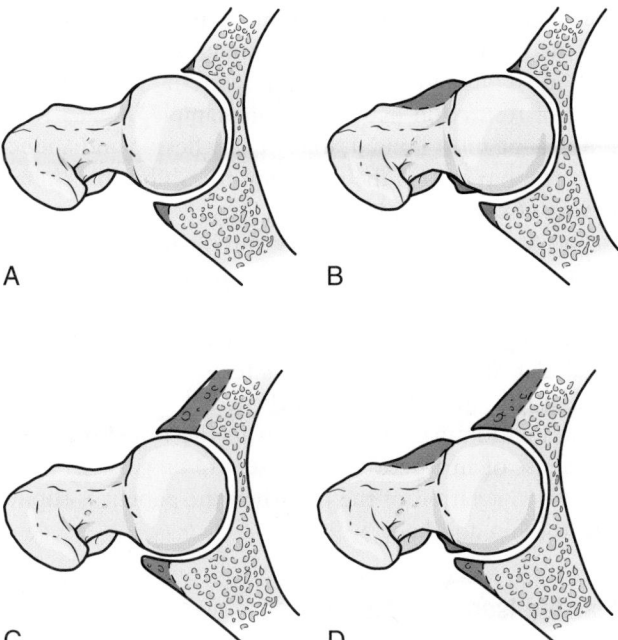

Figure 11-10 Femoroacetabular impingement (FAI) (hip impingement). **A,** Normal hip. **B,** Reduced femoral head-neck offset (cam-type impingement). **C,** Excessive overcoverage of the femoral head (pincer-type impingement). **D,** Combination of cam and pincer types of impingement.

Legg-Calvé-Perthes disease, slipped capital femoral epiphysis) or acetabular dysplasia.[47–52] The cam type impingement (see Figure 11-10, *B*) is commonly due to impingement of a large aspherical femoral head in a tight acetabulum. The deformed (flattened) head (pistol grip deformity or head tilt deformity) leads to shearing of the labrum and acetabular cartilage.[53] The cam type impingement may also lead to increased stress at the symphysis pubis and may be a precursor to athletic pubalgia.[54] Pincer type impingement (see Figure 11-10, *C*) is due to over coverage of the humeral head by a prominent acetabular rim (i.e., the acetabulum overhangs the femoral head due to acetabular dysplasia, acetabular retroversion, or coxa profunda) leading to pinching of the femoral neck against the labrum with the same ultimate result as the cam type degeneration of the labrum and adjacent cartilage.[55–57] In the presence of acetabular retroversion or decreased femoral anteversion, hip flexion in the neutral line is limited to as little as 90° but full range is accomplished if the hip is allowed to laterally rotate and abduct. Lateral rotation may exceed 60° with medial rotation limited.[49,58] The examiner should palpate the ASIS when testing hip movements. In the presence of FSI, the ASIS moves early due to limited hip flexion as the lumbar spine flexes to allow more movement.[59] If medial rotation is measured at 90° flexion, medial rotation in the FSI patient will be limited.[59] During the movement, if the abdominals are weak, the pelvis rotates anteriorly (see Figure 11-8). If the hip flexors are weak, the pelvis rotates posteriorly.

Extension of the hip normally ranges from 0° to 15°. The patient is in the prone position, and the examiner must differentiate between hip extension and spinal extension. Patients often have a tendency to extend the lumbar spine at the same time that they are extending the hip, giving the appearance of increased hip extension. Elevation of the pelvis or superior movement of the PSIS indicates the patient has passed the end of hip extension.

Hip abduction normally ranges from 30° to 50° and is tested with the patient in the supine position. Before asking the patient to do the abduction or adduction movement, the examiner should ensure that the patient's pelvis is "balanced" or level, with the ASISs being level and the legs being perpendicular to a line joining the two ASISs. The patient is then asked to abduct one leg at a time. Abduction is stopped when the pelvis begins to move. Normally, the patient should be able to do hip abduction while the lower extremities, pelvis, trunk and shoulders remain aligned in the frontal plane.[60] Pelvic motion is detected by palpation of the ASIS and by telling the patient to stop the movement as soon as the ASIS on either side starts to move. Normally, the ASIS on the movement side elevates while the opposite ASIS may drop or elevate. When the patient abducts the leg, the opposite ASIS tends to move first; with an **adduction contracture,** this occurs earlier in the range of movement.

If, during abduction, lateral rotation and slight flexion occurs early in the movement, the tensor fascia lata may be stronger and gluteus medius/minimus weak. If lateral rotation occurs later in the ROM, the iliopsoas or piriformis may be overactive. If the pelvis tilts up at the beginning of movement, the quadratus lumborum is overactive. All of these movements demonstrate imbalance patterns.

Hip adduction is normally 30° and is measured from the same starting position as abduction. The patient is asked to adduct one leg over the other while the examiner ensures that the pelvis does not move. An alternative method is for the patient to flex the opposite hip and knee and hold the limb in flexion with the arms; the patient then adducts the test leg under the other leg. This method is useful only for thin patients. When the patient adducts the leg, the ASIS on the same side moves first. This movement occurs earlier in the ROM if there is an **abduction contracture.** Adduction may also be measured by asking the patient to abduct one leg and leave it abducted; the other leg is then tested for the amount of adduction present. The advantage of this method is that the test leg does not have to be flexed to clear the other leg before doing the adduction movement.

Rotation movements may be performed with the patient supine, prone, or sitting. Medial rotation normally ranges from 30° to 40°, and lateral rotation from 40° to 60°. In the supine position, the patient simply rotates the straight leg on a balanced pelvis. Turning the foot or leg outward tests lateral rotation; turning the foot or leg inward tests medial rotation. In another supine test (see Figure 11-8, *E*), the patient is asked to flex both the hip and knee to 90° as the patient would do when being tested in sitting.[61] When using this method, it must be recognized that having the patient rotate the leg outward tests medial rotation, whereas having the patient rotate the leg inward tests lateral rotation. With the patient prone, the pelvis is balanced by aligning the legs at right angles to a line joining the PSISs. The patient then flexes the knee to 90°. Again, medial rotation is being tested when the leg is rotated outward, and lateral rotation is being tested when the leg is rotated inward (see Figure 11-8, *F*). Usually, one of these last two methods (sitting or prone) is used to measure hip rotation, because it is easier to measure the angle when performing the test. However, in prone, the measurement is done on a straight leg, whereas in sitting or supine, rotation is measured with the hip flexed to 90°. It has been found that there is a difference in the amount of lateral rotation between the flexed (less) and straight position, whereas medial rotation shows little difference when measured in the two positions.[61]

Passive Movements

If the range of movement was not full and the examiner was unable to test end feel during the active movements, passive movements should be performed to determine the end feel and passive range of motion (PROM). The passive movements performed are the same as the active movements. All the movements except extension can be tested with the patient in the supine lying position.

Passive Movements of the Hip and Normal End Feel

- Flexion (tissue approximation or tissue stretch)
- Extension (tissue stretch)
- Abduction (tissue stretch)
- Adduction (tissue approximation or tissue stretch)
- Medial rotation (tissue stretch)
- Lateral rotation (tissue stretch)

Sutlive et al.[62] have developed a clinical prediction rule for hip osteoarthritis involving active and passive movement. If four of the five variables are positive, there is a high probability of hip osteoarthritis, and diagnostic imaging should be ordered to confirm the diagnosis.

Clinical Prediction Rule for Hip Osteoarthritis*[62]

- Limited active hip flexion with lateral hip pain
- Active hip extension causes pain
- Limited passive hip medial rotation (25° or less)
- Squatting limited and painful
- Scour test with adduction causes lateral hip or groin pain

---

*Four out of five variables must be positive.

The capsular pattern of the hip is flexion, abduction, and medial rotation. These movements are always the ones most limited in a capsular pattern, although the order of restriction may vary. For example, medial rotation may be most limited, followed by flexion and abduction. The hip joint is the only joint to exhibit this altered pattern of the same movements.

The pelvis should not move during hip movements. Groin discomfort and a limited ROM on medial rotation are good indications of hip problems. Passive hip flexion, adduction, and medial rotation, if painful, may indicate acetabular rim problems or labral tears, especially if clicking and pain into the groin is elicited.[63]

Intra-abdominal inflammation in the lower pelvis, as in the case of an abscess, may cause pain on passive medial and lateral rotation of the hip when the patient is supine with the hip and knee at 90°.

Resisted Isometric Movements

The resisted isometric movements are performed with the patient in the supine position (Figure 11-11). The muscles of the hip play a very significant role in stabilizing the pelvis, so they must be included in any assessment dealing with issues of pelvic control. The examiner should note whether the muscles are weak or strong and tight, and whether the muscle force-couples are acting correctly.[64] When dealing with these muscles and the back and abdominal muscles, the examiner must be able to answer the following three questions in the affirmative to ensure pelvic control is present:

1. Can the patient actively position the pelvis in neutral?
2. Can the patient hold the neutral position statically? (This may include distal movement.)
3. Can the patient control dynamic movement of the pelvis?

Because the hip muscles are very strong and there are many of them (Figure 11-12; Table 11-4), the examiner should position the patient's hip properly and say to the patient, "Don't let me move your hip," to ensure that the movement is isometric. Delahunt et al.[66] advocate testing the adductors with the hip flexed to 45° as the optimal test position (**thigh adductor squeeze test**). By carefully noting which movements cause pain or show weakness when the tests are done isometrically, the examiner should be able to determine which muscle, if any, is at fault (see Table 11-4). For example, the gluteus maximus is the only muscle that is involved in all of the following movements: extension, adduction, and lateral rotation. Therefore, if pain resulted from only these three movements, the examiner would suspect the gluteus maximus muscle. As with active movements, the most painful movements are performed last.

Resisted isometric flexion and extension of the knee must also be performed, because there are two joint muscles (hamstrings and rectus femoris) that act over the

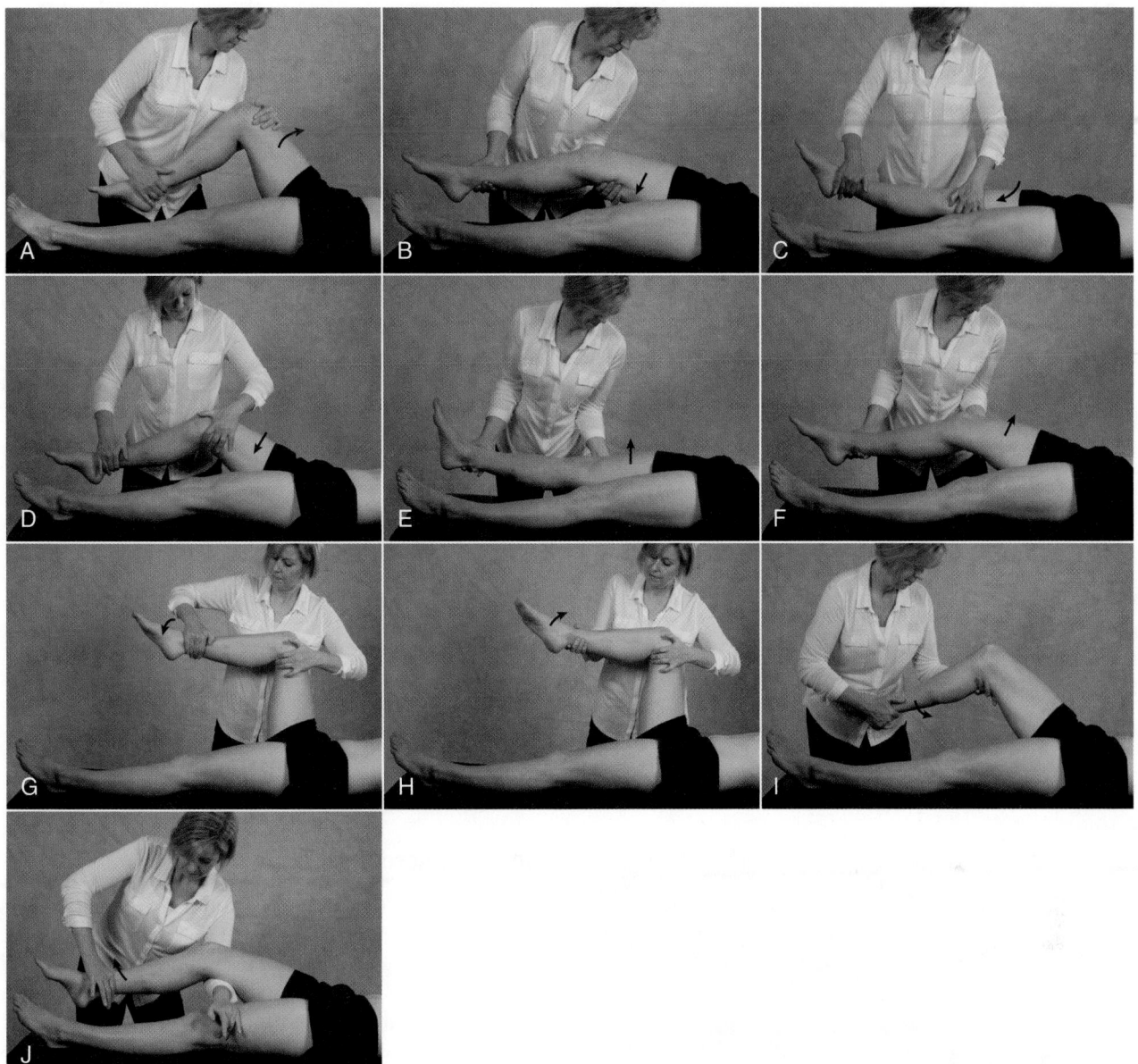

Figure 11-11 Resisted isometric movements around the hip. A, Flexion. **B**, Extension. **C**, Adduction (knee straight). **D**, Adduction (knee bent). **E**, Abduction (knee straight). **F**, Abduction (knee bent). **G**, Medial rotation. **H**, Lateral rotation. **I**, Knee flexion. **J**, Knee extension.

knee as well as the hip. If the history has indicated that concentric, eccentric, or econcentric movement causes symptoms, these movements should also be tested, but only after the isometric tests have been completed. For example, strength of the hamstrings may be determined by doing a **supine plank test** in which the patient is in crook lying, resting on his or her elbows (Figure 11-13).[67] The patient then lifts the buttocks off the table while maintaining the body weight on the elbows and heels. The patient then alternately lifts the injured leg and then the good leg. If pain occurs at the ischial origin or in the hamstrings musculature, or if pelvic "collapse" or rotation occurs, the test is positive for weak hamstrings.

Resisted Isometric Movements of the Hip

- Flexion of the hip
- Extension of the hip
- Abduction of the hip
- Adduction of the hip
- Medial rotation of the hip
- Lateral rotation of the hip
- Flexion of the knee
- Extension of the knee

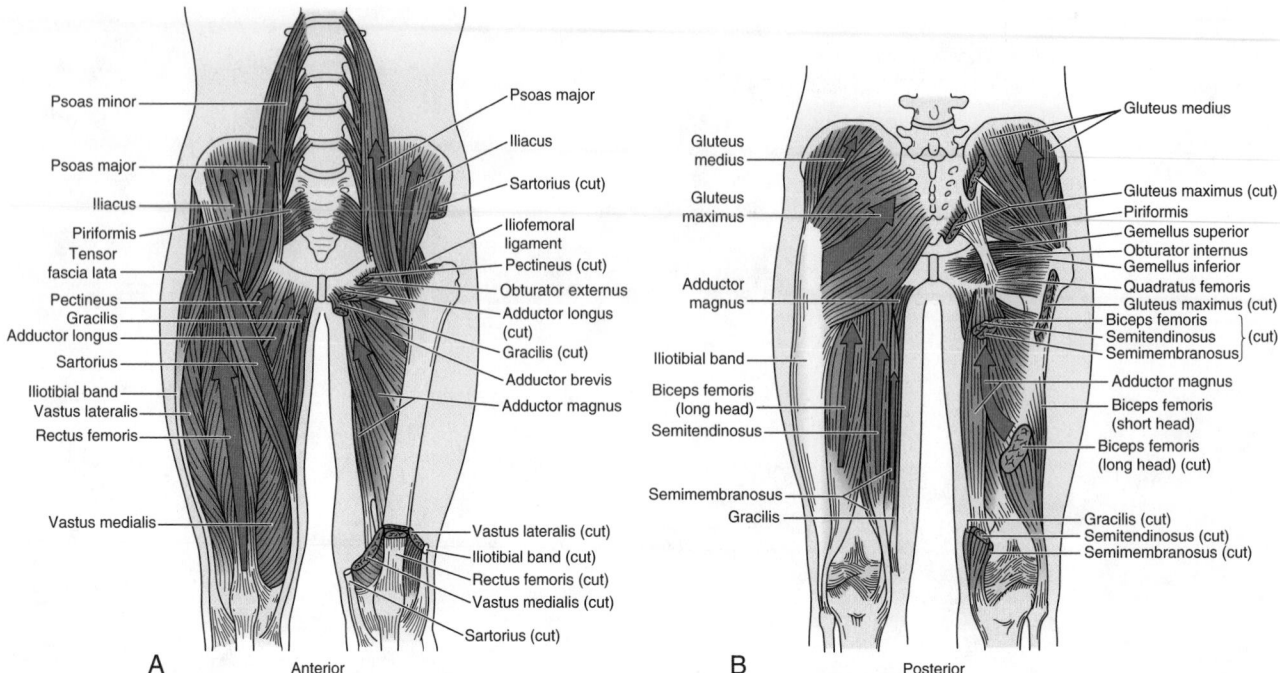

A Anterior

B Posterior

Figure 11-12 Muscles of the hip region. A, Anterior view. The right side shows the primary flexors and adductor muscles of the hip. Many muscles on the left side are cut to expose the adductor brevis and adductor magnus. **B,** Posterior view. The left side highlights the gluteus maximus and hamstring muscles (long head of biceps femoris, semitendinosis, and semimembranosus). The right side shows the hamstring muscles cut to expose the adductor magnus and short head of the biceps femoris. The right side shows the gluteus medius and five of the six short external rotators (i.e., piriformis, gemellus superior and inferior, obturator internus, and quadratus femoris). (Redrawn from Neumann DA: Kinesiology of the musculoskeletal system—foundations for physical rehabilitation, St Louis, 2002, CV Mosby, pp. 411, 419.)

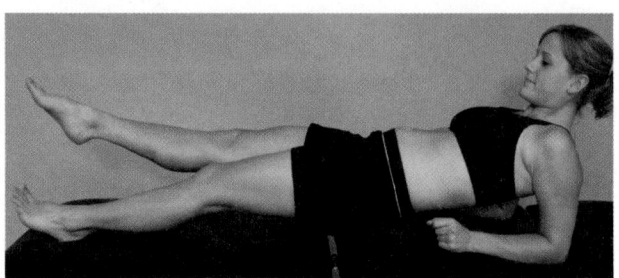

Figure 11-13 The supine plank test is used to assess hamstring strength. The patient elevates the pelvis while keeping the body weight on the elbows and heels. The legs are alternately lifted, starting with lifting the injured leg. (This tests the good leg first.) Pelvic collapse or rotation or pain at the hamstring origin as the contralateral leg is lifted indicates hamstring weakness.

The examiner must be aware that intra-abdominal inflammation in the area of the psoas muscle may cause pain on resisted hip flexion. Intra-abdominal inflammation may also result in a rigid abdominal wall. It has been reported that hip flexors and hip extensors are almost equal in strength[68] and that the adductors are 2.5 times as strong as the abductors.[69] These ratios may vary depending on whether the movement is tested isometrically or isokinetically.

Functional Assessment

Hip motion is necessary for more activities than just ambulation. In fact, more hip ROM is required for activities of daily living (ADLs) than is required for gait; activities such as shoe tying, sitting, getting up from a chair, and picking up things from the floor all require a greater ROM. Table 11-5 illustrates the ranges of motion necessary for various activities. Ideally, the patient should have functional ranges of 120° of flexion, 20° of abduction, and 20° of lateral rotation.

Functional Tests of the Hip

- Squatting
- Going up and down stairs one at a time
- Crossing the legs so that the ankle of one foot rests on the knee of the opposite leg
- Going up and down stairs two or more at a time
- Running straight ahead
- Running and decelerating
- Running and twisting
- One-legged hop (time, distance, crossover)
- Jumping

TABLE **11-4**

Muscles of the Hip: Their Actions, Innervation, and Nerve Root Derivation[65]

Action	Muscles Acting	Innervation	Nerve Root Deviation
Flexion of hip	1. Psoas	L1–L3	L1–L3
	2. Iliacus	Femoral	L2, L3
	3. Rectus femoris	Femoral	L2–L4
	4. Sartorius	Femoral	L2, L3
	5. Tensor fasciae latae	Superior gluteal	L5, S1, S2
	6. Pectineus	Femoral	L2, L3
	7. Adductor longus	Obturator	L2–L4
	8. Adductor brevis	Obturator	L2, L3, L5
	9. Gracilis	Obturator	L2, L3
	10. Gluteus medius (anterior fibers)	Superior gluteal	L5, S1
Extension of hip	1. Biceps femoris (long head)	Sciatic	L5, S1, S2
	2. Semimembranosus	Sciatic	L5, S1, S2
	3. Semitendinosus	Sciatic	L5, S1, S2
	4. Gluteus maximus	Inferior gluteal	L5, S1, S2
	5. Gluteus medius (middle and posterior part)	Superior gluteal	L5, S1
	6. Adductor magnus (ischiocondylar part)	Sciatic	L2–L4
Abduction of hip	1. Tensor fasciae latae	Superior gluteal	L4, L5
	2. Gluteus minimus	Superior gluteal	L5, S1
	3. Gluteus medius	Superior gluteal	L5, S1
	4. Gluteus maximus	Inferior gluteal	L5, S1, S2
	5. Sartorius	Femoral	L2, L3
	6. Piriformis	L5, S1, S2	L5, S1, S2
	7. Rectus femoris	Femoral	L2–L4
Adduction of hip	1. Adductor longus	Obturator	L2–L4
	2. Adductor brevis	Obturator	L2–L4
	3. Adductor magnus (ischiofemoral part)	Obturator	L2–L4
	4. Gracilis	Obturator	L2, L3
	5. Pectineus	Femoral	L2, L3
	6. Biceps femoris (long head)	Sciatic	L5, S1, S2
	7. Gluteus maximus (posterior fibers)	Inferior gluteal	L5, S1, S2
	8. Quadratus femoris	N. to quadratus femoris	L5, S1
	9. Obturator externus	Obturator	L3, L4
Medial rotation of hip	1. Adductor longus	Obturator	L2–L4
	2. Adductor brevis	Obturator	L2–L4
	3. Adductor magnus (posterior head)	Obturator and sciatic	L2–L4
	4. Gluteus medius (anterior part)	Superior gluteal	L5, S1
	5. Gluteus minimus (anterior part)	Superior gluteal	L5, S1
	6. Tensor fasciae latae	Superior gluteal	L4, L5
	7. Pectineus	Femoral	L2, L3
	8. Gracilis	Obturator	L2, L3
Lateral rotation of hip	1. Gluteus maximus	Inferior gluteal	L5, S1, S2
	2. Obturator internus	N. to obturator internus	L5, S1
	3. Obturator externus	Obturator	L3, L4
	4. Quadratus femoris	N. to quadratus femoris	L5, S1
	5. Piriformis	L5, S1–S2	L5, S1, S2
	6. Gemellus superior	N. to obturator internus	L5, S1
	7. Gemellus inferior	N. to quadratus femoris	L5, S1
	8. Sartorius	Femoral	L2, L3
	9. Gluteus medius (posterior part)	Superior gluteal	L5, S1
	10. Gluteus minimus (posterior part)	Superior gluteal	L5, S1
	11. Biceps femoris (long head)	Sciatic	L5, S1, S2

N, nerve.

There are several numerical rating scales with which to rate hip function.[70-76] These rating methods are based primarily on pain, mobility, and gait. Tables 11-6 through 11-8 and Figures 11-14 and 11-15 illustrate three different rating scales. D'Aubigné and Postel[70] (see Tables 11-6 through 11-8) developed one of the first hip rating scales based on pain, mobility, and ability to walk.[71] The Harris hip function scale[72] (see Figure 11-14) is useful for rating hips before and after surgery. This scale is most often used because it emphasizes pain and function. The Western Ontario and McMaster Universities Osteoarthritis Index (WOMAC)[77-82] and the Lower Extremity Function Scale (LEFS) (Figure 11-16)[83-86] were developed to evaluate clinically important and patient-relevant changes in health status primarily with arthroplasties of the hip and knee. The WOMAC scale is made up of three sections with scores ranging from one (none) to five (extreme). The sum of three scores is called the *index* or *global score*. The higher the score, the greater the disability. The SF-36 questionnaire is also sometimes used as a functional assessment tool in arthroplasty cases.[82,87] The Iowa scale (see Figure 11-15) provides a single rating value. The Mayo hip score[73] for hip arthroplasty makes use of greater patient (functional) input and radiographic input (to predict long-term results). This score correlates well with the Harris scale.[71,73] Johanson and colleagues[74] developed a numerical scale that is related to what patients are able to do functionally after total hip replacement. Its value comes from its focus on the outcome from the patient's perspective (Figure 11-17). As Burton and co-workers[75] pointed out, the notion of expectations is more important than the notion of success. Table 11-9 gives a functional strength and endurance testing scheme for the hip.

Several **walking tests** have been developed, especially for the elderly, to give an indication of musculoskeletal functional impairment of the lower limb and may be included in any assessment involving injury to the low limb joints.[88] These include the **Timed "Up and Go" test (TUG test),**[88-91] 13-metre walk test,[88] 6-minute walk test (6MWT),[88,92-96] self-paced walk test,[91,97-99] 2-minute walk test,[92] 10-metre walk test, 12-minute walk test[92] and sit to stand.[91]

If the patient is able to perform normal active movements with little difficulty, the examiner may use a series of functional tests to determine whether increased intensity of activity produces pain or other symptoms. These tests must be geared to the individual patient.[100] Older persons should not be expected to perform the last six activities unless they have been doing these movements or similar ones in the recent past.

TABLE 11-5

Range of Motion Necessary at the Hip for Selected Activities

Activity	Average Range of Motion Necessary
Shoe tying	120° of flexion
Sitting (average seat height)	112° of flexion
Stooping	125° of flexion
Squatting	115° of flexion/20° of abduction/20° of medial rotation
Ascending stairs (average stair height)	67° of flexion
Descending stairs (average stair height)	36° of flexion
Putting foot on opposite thigh	120° of flexion/20° of abduction/20° of lateral rotation
Putting on trousers	90° of flexion

TABLE 11-6

Method of Grading Functional Value of Hip*

Grade	Pain	Mobility	Ability to Walk
0	Pain is intense and permanent	Ankylosis with bad position of the hip	None
1	Pain is severe, even at night	No movement; pain or slight deformity	Only with crutches
2	Pain is severe when walking; prevents any activity	Flexion less than 40°	Only with canes
3	Pain is tolerable with limited activity	Flexion between 40° and 60°	With one cane, for less than 1 hour; very difficult without a cane
4	Pain is mild when walking; it disappears with rest	Flexion between 60° and 80°; patient can reach own foot	A long time with a cane; a short time without cane and with limp
5	Pain is mild and inconstant; normal activity	Flexion between 80° and 90°; abduction at least 15°	Without cane but with slight limp
6	No pain	Flexion more than 90°; abduction to 30°	Normal

From D'Aubigné, RM, Postel M: Functional results of hip arthroplasty with acrylic prosthesis. J Bone Joint Surg Am 36:459, 1954.
*Values used in conjunction with Table 11-7.

TABLE **11-7**

D'Aubigné and Postel Scale for Functional Grading of the Hip

Pain (P)	Ability to Walk (W)	Mobility Normal or Nearly Normal	Grade
		Very Good	**P+ W= 11 or 12**
6	6	Walk without cane, with no pain and no limp	
6	5	Walk without cane, with no pain but slight limp	
5	6	Walk without cane, with no limp but slight pain when starting	
		Good	**P+ W= 10**
5	5	Walk without cane, with slight pain and slight limp	
4	6	Walk without cane, with pain but no limp	
6	4*	Walk without cane, without pain; a cane used to go outdoors	
		Medium	**P+ W= 9**
5	4	Slight pain; a cane is used outdoors	
4	5	Pain after walking some minutes; no cane is used, but there is a slight limp	
6	3†	No pain; a cane used all the time	
		Fair	**P+ W= 8**
5	3	Slight pain; a cane is used all the time	
4	4	Pain after walking; a cane is used outdoors	
≤3	≤3	**Poor**	**P+ W= 7 or less**

Adapted from D'Aubigné, RM, Postel M: Functional results of hip arthroplasty with acrylic prosthesis. J Bone Joint Surg Am 36:460, 1954.
*If the mobility is reduced to 4, the result is classified one grade lower.
†If the mobility is reduced to 3 or less, the result is classified two grades lower.

TABLE **11-8**

Method of Evaluating Improvement Brought About by Operation in Problems of the Hip (Relative Result)

	Preoperative Grading	Postoperative Grading	Difference	Improvement
Pain	3	5	$2 \times 2 = 4$	
Mobility	2	5	$3 = 3$	= 9
Ability to walk	3	4	$1 \times 2 = 2$	

From D'Aubigné RM, Postel M: Functional results of hip arthroplasty with acrylic prosthesis. J Bone Joint Surg Am 36:461, 1954.
Very great improvement = 12 or more, great improvement = 7 to 11, fair improvement = 3 to 7, failure = less than 3.

Special Tests

Only those tests that the examiner believes are necessary should be performed when assessing the hip. Most tests are done primarily to confirm a diagnosis or to determine pathology and should not be used as "stand alone" tests when considering a diagnosis.[101] As with all special tests, if the test is positive, it is highly suggestive that the problem exists, but if it is negative, it does not necessarily rule out the problem. Therefore, special tests should not be taken in isolation but should be used to support the history, observation, and clinical examination.

For the reader who would like to review them, the reliability, validity, specificity, sensitivity, and odds ratios of some of the special tests used in the hip are available on the Evolve website.

Tests for Hip Pathology

❓ *Bryant's Triangle.* With the patient lying supine, the examiner drops an imaginary perpendicular line from the ASIS of the pelvis to the examining table.[104] A second imaginary line is projected up from the tip of the greater trochanter of the femur to meet the first line at a right angle (Figure 11-18). This line is measured, and the two sides are compared. Differences may indicate conditions, such as coxa vara or CDH. This measurement can be done with radiographs, in which case the lines may be drawn on the radiograph.

Text continued on p. 710

Harris Hip Function Scale

(Circle one in each group)

Pain (44 points maximum)

None/ignores	44
Slight, occasional, no compromise in activity	40
Mild, no effect on ordinary activity, pain after unusual activity, uses aspirin	30
Moderate, tolerable, makes concessions, occasional codeine	20
Marked, serious limitations	10
Totally disabled	0

Function (47 points maximum)

Gait (walking maximum distance) (33 points maximum)

1. Limp:
None	11
Slight	8
Moderate	5
Unable to walk	0
2. Support:
None	11
Cane, long walks	7
Cane, full time	5
Crutch	4
Two canes	2
Two crutches	0
Unable to walk	0
3. Distance walked:
Unlimited	11
Six blocks	8
Two to three blocks	5
Indoors only	2
Bed and chair	0

Functional Activities (14 points maximum)

1. Stairs:
Normally	4
Normally with banister	2
Any method	1
Not able	0
2. Socks and tie shoes:
With ease	4
With difficulty	2
Unable	0
3. Sitting:
Any chair, 1 hour	5
High chair, ½ hour	3
Unable to sit ½ hour any chair	0
4. Enter public transport
Able to use public transportation	1
Not able to use public transportation	0

Absence of Deformity (requires all four) (4 points maximum)

1. Fixed adduction <10°   4
2. Fixed internal rotation in extension <10°   0
3. Leg length discrepancy less than 1¼"
4. Pelvic flexion contracture <30°

Range of Motion (5 points maximum)

Instructions

Record 10° of fixed adduction as "—10° abduction, adduction to 10°"

Similarly, 10° of fixed external rotation as "—10° internal rotation, external rotation to 10°"

Similarly, 10° of fixed external rotation with 10° further external rotation as "—10° internal rotation, external rotation to 20°"

Permanent flexion
(1) _____ °

	Range	Index Factor	Index Value*
A. Flexion to _____ °			
(0°–45°)		1.0	
(45°–90°)		0.6	
(90°–120°)		0.3	
(120°–140°)		0.0	
B. Abduction to _____ °			
(0°–15°)		0.8	
(15°–30°)		0.3	
(30°–60°)		0.0	
C. Adduction to _____ °			
(0°–15°)		0.2	
(15°–60°)		0.0	
D. External rotation in extension to _____ °			
(0°–30°)		0.4	
(30°–60°)		0.0	
E. Internal rotation in extension to _____ °			
(0°–60°)		0.0	

*Index Value = Range × Index Factor

Total index value (A + B + C + D + E) _____

Total range of motion points
(multiply total index value × 0.05) _____

Pain points: _____
Function points: _____
Absence of Deformity points: _____
Range of Motion points: _____
  Total points _____
  (100 points maximum)
Comments:

Figure 11-14 Harris hip function scale. (Modified from Harris WH: Traumatic arthritis of the hip after dislocation and acetabular fractures: treatment by mold arthroplasty. An end result study using a new method of result evaluation. J Bone Joint Surg Am 51:737–755, 1969.)

Iowa Functional Hip Evaluation

Chart 1	Chart 2

Chart 1

Date _____

Name _____   Age _____

100-Point Scale for Hip Evaluation

Total points _____

Function (35 points)

Does most of housework or job that
   requires moving about 5

Dresses unaided (includes tying shoes and
   putting on socks) 5

Walks enough to be independent 5

Sits with difficulty at table or toilet 4

Picks up objects from floor by squatting 3

Bathes without help 3

Negotiates stairs foot over foot......................... 3

Carries objects comparable to suitcase.................. 2

Gets into car or public conveyance unaided and rides
   comfortably.. 2

Drives a car 1

Freedom From Pain (35 points) (circle 1 only)

No pain... 35

Pain only with fatigue 30

Pain only with weight-bearing........................ 20

Pain at rest but not with weight-bearing................ 15

Pain sitting or in bed 10

Continuous pain..................................... 0

Gait (10 points) (circle 1 only)

No limp; no support 10

No limp using cane.................................... 8

Abductor limp 8

Short leg limp.. 8

Needs two canes 6

Needs two crutches.................................... 4

Cannot walk 0

Absence of Deformity (10 points)

No fixed flexion over 30°............................. 3

No fixed adduction over 10°........................... 3

No fixed rotation over 10°............................ 2

Not over 1″ shortening (ASIS-MM)*.................... 2

Range of Motion (10 points)

Flexion-extension (normal 140°) .... _____°

Abduction-adduction (normal 80°) .... _____°

External-internal rotation (normal 80°) .... _____°

        Total degrees........................... _____°

        Points (1 point/30°) .... _____°

Muscle Strength (no points)

Straight leg raising:

  Less than gravity _____Gravity _____

  Gravity + resistance _____

Abduction:

  Less than gravity _____Gravity _____

  Gravity + resistance _____

Extension:

  Less than gravity _____Gravity _____

  Gravity + resistance _____

        TOTAL (100 points maximum) _____

Chart 2

Name _____ Diagnosis _____

Age _____ Sex _____ Date of operation _____

Date of follow-up _____

Previous surgery: Date _____ Type _____

Subsequent surgery: Date _____ Type _____

Pain   40%

None 40

Pain with fatigue 35

Pain with weight-bearing:

  Mild... 30

  Moderate 20

  Severe....................................... 10

  Persistence with non–weight-bearing....... 10 (less than above)

  Continuous pain......................... 0

Ability to Function   30%

Work and household duties:

  Full day, usual occupation 10

  Modified work or duties 6

  Severe restriction of work or duties 2

Walking tolerances:

  Long distances 10

  Short distances........................... 6

  Two blocks or less....................... 1

Self-reliance:

  Dresses self unaided 3

  Help with shoes and socks 2

  Sit at table and toilet 3

Stairs:

  Normal 2

  One at a time 1

  Gets into car or public conveyance without
    difficulty.............................. 2

Gait   15%

No limp, no support 15

No limp, with cane....................... 12

Limp, mild, without cane 12

Limp, mild, with cane 9

Limp, moderate, without cane or crutch....... 9

Limp, moderate, with cane or crutch.......... 6

Limp, severe, without cane or crutch.......... 3

Limp, severe, with cane or crutch............. 2

Two canes or crutches 1

Anatomic Assessment   15%

A. Motion:

  Flexion—up to 80° in range 0°–100° × 0.1 ... 8

  Abduction—up to 20° in range 0°–30° × 0.1.. 2

B. Shortening:

  None—½″................................. 3

  ½″–1″ 2

  1″–2″................................... 1

C. Trendelenburg—absent.................... 2

        100%

Figure 11-15 Iowa functional hip evaluation form. *ASIS-MM,* Anterior superior iliac spine to medial malleolus. (Modified from Larson CB: Rating scale for hip disabilities. Clin Orthop 31:86, 1963.)

LOWER EXTREMITY FUNCTION SCALE

We are interested in knowing whether you are having any difficulty at all with the activities listed below *because of your lower limb* problem for which you are currently seeking attention. Please provide an answer for each activity.

Today, *do you or would you* have any difficulty at all with:
(Circle one number on each line)

ACTIVITIES	Extreme Difficulty or Unable to Perform Activity	Quite a Bit of Difficulty	Moderate Difficulty	A Little Bit of Difficulty	No Difficulty
a. Any of your usual work, housework of school activities.	0	1	2	3	4
b. Your usual hobbies, recreational, or sporting activities.	0	1	2	3	4
c. Getting into or out of the bath.	0	1	2	3	4
d. Walking between rooms.	0	1	2	3	4
e. Putting on your shoes or socks.	0	1	2	3	4
f. Squatting.	0	1	2	3	4
g. Lifting an object, like a bag of groceries from the floor.	0	1	2	3	4
h. Performing light activities around your home.	0	1	2	3	4
i. Performing heavy activities around your home.	0	1	2	3	4
j. Getting into or out of a car.	0	1	2	3	4
k. Walking 2 blocks.	0	1	2	3	4
l. Walking a mile.	0	1	2	3	4
m. Going up or down 10 stairs (about 1 flight of stairs).	0	1	2	3	4
n. Standing for 1 hour.	0	1	2	3	4
o. Sitting for 1 hour.	0	1	2	3	4
p. Running on even ground.	0	1	2	3	4
q. Running on uneven ground.	0	1	2	3	4
r. Making sharp turns while running fast.	0	1	2	3	4
s. Hopping.	0	1	2	3	4
t. Rolling over in bed.	0	1	2	3	4
Column Totals:					

Score variation ± 6 LEFS points
MDC & MCID = 9 LEFS points

Score: _____ / 80

Figure 11-16 Lower Extremity Function Scale (LEFS). (From Stratford PW, et al: Validation of the LEFS on patients with total joint arthroplasty. Physiother Can 52:105, 2000.)

A SELF-ADMINISTERED HIP-RATING QUESTIONNAIRE

Which hip is affected by arthritis? (circle one)

Left   Right   Both

Please answer the following questions about the hip(s) you have just indicated.

1. Considering all of the ways that your hip arthritis affects you, mark (X) on the scale for how well you are doing.

0	25	50	75	100
very well	well	fair	poor	very poor

   Circle one response for each question. (The score here is determined by subtraction of the number marked from 100, with the number being interpolated, if necessary, if the mark is between printed numbers. The result is divided by 4, and the answer then rounded off to the nearest integer. The maximum is 25 points.)

2. During the past month, how would you describe the usual arthritis pain in your hip? (maximum, 10 points)
   a. Very severe (2 points)
   b. Severe (4 points)
   c. Moderate (6 points)
   d. Mild (8 points)
   e. None (10 points)

3. During the past month, how often have you had to take medication for your arthritis? (maximum, 5 points)
   a. Always (1 point)
   b. Very often (2 points)
   c. Fairly often (3 points)
   d. Sometimes (4 points)
   e. Never (5 points)

4. During the past month, how often have you had severe arthritis pain in your hip? (maximum, 5 points)
   a. Every day (1 point)
   b. Several days per week (2 points)
   c. One day per week (3 points)
   d. One day per month (4 points)
   e. Never (5 points)

5. How often have you had hip arthritis pain at rest, either sitting or lying down? (maximum, 5 points)
   a. Every day (1 point)
   b. Several days per week (2 points)
   c. One day per week (3 points)
   d. One day per month (4 points)
   e. Never (5 points)

6. How far can you walk without resting because of your hip arthritis pain? (maximum, 15 points)
   a. Unable to walk (3 points)
   b. Less than one city block (6 points)
   c. 1 to <10 city blocks (9 points)
   d. 10 to 20 city blocks (12 points)
   e. Unlimited (15 points)

7. How much assistance do you need for walking? (maximum, 10 points)
   a. Unable to walk (1 point)
   b. Walk only with someone's help (2 points)
   c. Two crutches or walker every day (3 points)
   d. Two crutches or walker several days per week (4 points)
   e. Two crutches or walker once per week or less (5 points)
   f. Cane or one crutch every day (6 points)
   g. Cane or one crutch several days per week (7 points)
   h. Cane or one crutch once per week (8 points)
   i. Cane or one crutch once per month (9 points)
   j. No assistance (10 points)

8. How much difficulty do you have going up or down one flight of stairs because of your hip arthritis? (maximum, 5 points)
   a. Unable (1 point)
   b. Require someone's assistance (2 points)
   c. Require crutch or cane (3 points)
   d. Require banister (4 points)
   e. No difficulty (5 points)

9. How much difficulty do you have putting on your shoes and socks because of your hip arthritis? (maximum, 5 points)
   a. Unable (1 point)
   b. Require someone's assistance (2 points)
   c. Require long shoehorn and reacher (3 points)
   d. Some difficulty, but no devices required (4 points)
   e. No difficulty (5 points)

10. Are you able to use public transportation? (maximum, 3 points)
    a. No, because of my hip arthritis (1 point)
    b. No, for some other reason (2 points)
    c. Yes (3 points)

11. When you bathe—either a sponge bath or in a tub or shower—how much help do you need? (maximum, 3 points)
    a. No help at all (3 points)
    b. Help with bathing one part of my body, like back or leg (2 points)
    c. Help with bathing more than one part of my body (1 point)

12. If you had the necessary transportation, under what circumstances could you go shopping for groceries or clothes? (maximum, 3 points)
    a. Without help (taking care of all shopping needs myself) (3 points)
    b. With some help (need someone to go with me to help on all shopping trips) (2 points)
    c. Completely unable to do any shopping (1 point)

13. If you had household tools and appliances (vacuum, mops, and so on) could you do your own housework? (maximum, 3 points)
    a. Without help (can clean floors, windows, refrigerator, and so on) (3 points)
    b. With some help (can do light housework, but need help with some heavy work) (2 points)
    c. Completely unable to do any housework (1 point)

14. How well are you able to move around? (maximum, 3 points)
    a. Able to get in and out of bed or chair without the help of another person (3 points)
    b. Need the help of another person to get in and out of bed or chair (2 points)
    c. Not able to get out of bed (1 point)

This is the end of the Hip-Rating Questionnaire. Thank you for your cooperation.

Figure 11-17 A self-administered hip-rating questionnaire. The maximum score is 100 points, and the minimum is 16 points. The point values of the answers are not shown in the questionnaire that is administered to patients. (From Johanson NA, Charlson ME, Szatrowski TP, et al: A self-administered hip-rating questionnaire for the assessment of outcome after total hip replacement. J Bone Joint Surg Am 74:589, 1992.)

TABLE 11-9

Functional Testing of the Hip

Starting Position	Action	Functional Test
Standing	Lift foot onto 20-cm step and return (hip flexion-extension)	5 to 6 Repetitions: Functional 3 to 4 Repetitions: Functionally fair 1 to 2 Repetitions: Functionally poor 0 Repetitions: Nonfunctional
Standing	Sit in chair and return to standing (hip extension-flexion)	5 to 6 Repetitions: Functional 3 to 4 Repetitions: Functionally fair 1 to 2 Repetitions: Functionally poor 0 Repetitions: Nonfunctional
Standing	Lift leg to balance on one leg keeping pelvis straight (hip abduction)	Hold 1 to 1.5 minutes: Functional Hold 30 to 59 seconds: Functionally fair Hold 1 to 29 seconds: Functionally poor Cannot hold: Nonfunctional
Standing	Walk sideways 6 m (hip adduction/abduction)	6 to 8 m one way: Functional 3 to 6 m one way: Functionally fair 1 to 3 m one way: Functionally poor 0 m: Nonfunctional
Standing	Test leg off floor (patient may hold onto something for balance) medially rotate non–weight-bearing hip	10 to 12 Repetitions: Functional 5 to 9 Repetitions: Functionally fair 1 to 4 Repetitions: Functionally poor 0 Repetitions: Nonfunctional
Standing	Test leg off floor (patient may hold onto something for balance) laterally rotate non–weight-bearing hip	10 to 12 Repetitions: Functional 5 to 9 Repetitions: Functionally fair 1 to 4 Repetitions: Functionally poor 0 Repetitions: Nonfunctional

Data from Palmer ML, Epler M: Clinical assessment procedures in physical therapy, Philadelphia, 1990, JB Lippincott, pp. 251–254.

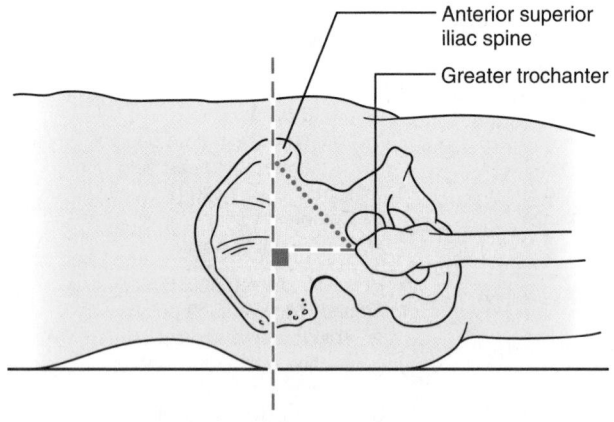

Anterior superior iliac spine

Greater trochanter

Figure 11-18 Bryant's triangle.

? *Craig's Test.* Craig's test measures femoral **anteversion** or forward torsion of the femoral neck (Figure 11-19). Anteversion of the hip is measured by the angle made by the femoral neck with the femoral condyles (Figure 11-20). It is the degree of forward projection of the femoral neck from the coronal plane of the shaft (Figure 11-21), and it decreases during the growing period. At birth, the mean angle is approximately 30°; in the adult, the mean angle is 8° to 15° (Figure 11-22). Increased anteversion leads to squinting patellae and toeing-in (Figure 11-23).[105] Excessive anteversion is twice as common in girls as in boys. A common clinical finding of excessive anteversion is excessive medial hip rotation (more than 60°) and decreased lateral rotation in extension.[105] Gelberman et al.[106] pointed out, however, that rotation should be viewed both in neutral (as in the Craig's test) and with 90° of hip flexion, because rotation shows greater variability in flexion. They felt that greater medial rotation than lateral rotation in both positions was a better indicator of increased femoral anteversion. In retroversion, the plane of the femoral neck rotates backward in relation to the coronal condylar plane (see Figure 11-23) or the acetabulum itself may be retroverted.[49,104,106–109]

For Craig's test, which has been found to correlate well with x-rays (within 4°) in children,[110] the patient lies prone with the knee flexed to 90°. The examiner palpates the posterior aspect of the greater trochanter of the femur. The hip is then passively rotated medially and laterally until the greater trochanter is parallel with the examining table or reaches its most lateral position. The degree of

*The author recommends these key tests be learned by the clinician to facilitate a diagnosis. See Chapter 1, p. 55, Key for Classifying Special Tests.

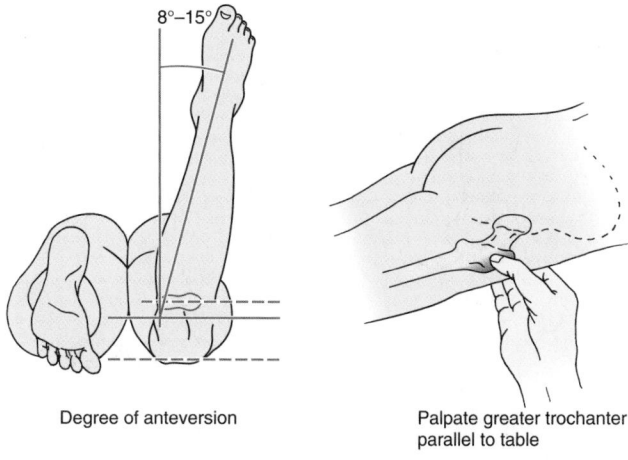

Figure 11-19 Craig's test to measure femoral anteversion.

8°–15°

Degree of anteversion

Palpate greater trochanter parallel to table

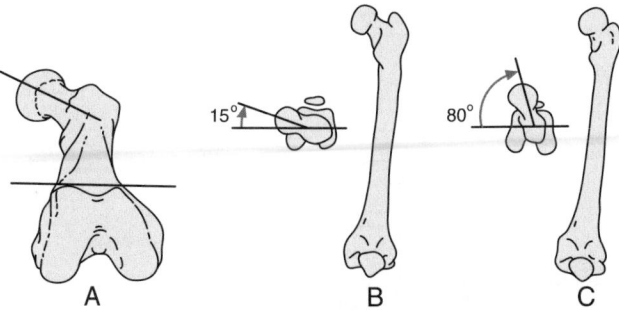

15°   80°

A   B   C

Figure 11-20 Anteversion of the hip. A, Femoral anteversion angle. **B,** Normal angle. **C,** Excessive angle. (**A,** Redrawn from the American Orthopaedic Association: Manual of Orthopaedic Surgery, Chicago, 1979, AOA, p. 45.)

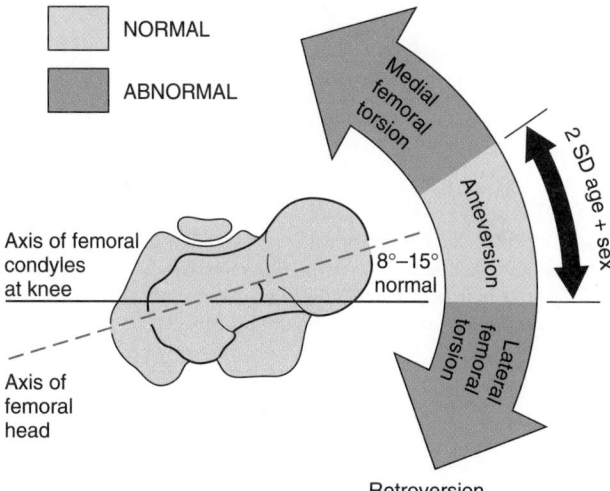

NORMAL

ABNORMAL

Medial femoral torsion

2 SD age + sex

Axis of femoral condyles at knee

8°–15° normal

Anteversion

Lateral femoral torsion

Axis of femoral head

Retroversion

Figure 11-21 Axial view of right femur showing approximately normal angle of anteversion and torsional deformity beyond. (Redrawn from Staheli LT: Medial femoral torsion. Orthop Clin North Am 11:40, 1980.)

anteversion can then be estimated, based on the angle of the lower leg with the vertical.[111] The test is also called the **Ryder method** for measuring anteversion or retroversion.

❓ *Dial Test of the Hip.*[112] The patient lies supine with the hips in neutral (i.e., no rotation). The examiner medially rotates the limb and then releases it allowing the leg to go into lateral rotation. If the patient's leg passively rotates greater than 45° from vertical in the axial plane and if, on testing, there is no mechanical end point, the test is positive for hip instability (Figure 11-24). Both limbs are compared starting with the unaffected side.

⚠ *Flexion-Adduction Test.*[113] This test is used in older children and young adults as a test for hip disease. The patient lies supine while the examiner flexes the patient's hip to at least 90° with the knee flexed (Figure 11-25). The examiner then adducts the flexed leg. Normally, the knee will pass over the opposite hip without rolling the pelvis. In pathological hips, adduction is limited and accompanied by pain or discomfort.

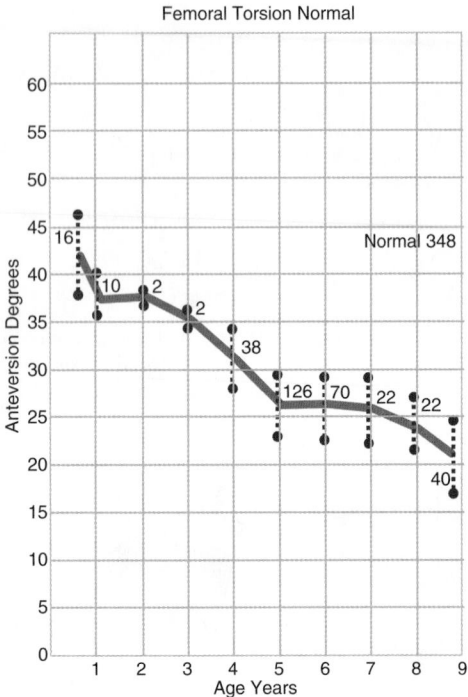

Figure 11-22 The degree of normal femoral torsion in relation to age. *Solid lines* represent the mean; *vertical lines* represent the standard deviation. (Redrawn from Crane L: Femoral torsion and its relation to toeing-in and toeing-out. J Bone Joint Surg Am 41:423, 1959.)

? *Foveal Distraction Test.*[12] The patient is in supine. The examiner abducts the hip to 30° and applies an axial traction to the leg which reduces intra-articular pressure (Figure 11-26). Relief of pain indicates the pain is intra-articular.

✓ *Hip Scour Test.* Maitland[114] called the flexion-adduction test the *quadrant* or *scouring test*. He felt the test stressed or compressed the femoral neck against the acetabulum, or pinched adductor longus, pectineus, iliopsoas, sartorius or tensor fascia lata. The patient lies supine. The examiner flexes and adducts the patient's hip so that the hip faces the patient's opposite shoulder and resistance to the movement is felt (Figure 11-27). As slight resistance is maintained, the patient's hip is taken into abduction while maintaining flexion in an arc of movement. As the movement is performed, the examiner should look for any irregularity in the movement (e.g., "bumps"), pain, or patient apprehension, which may give an indication of where the pathology is occurring in the hip.[114] This motion also causes impingement of the femoral neck against the acetabular rim and pinches the adductor longus, pectineus, iliopsoas, sartorius, and/or tensor fascia lata. Therefore, it should be performed with care.[39-41]

? *Log Roll Test.* The patient lies supine with both lower extremities extended. The examiner passively

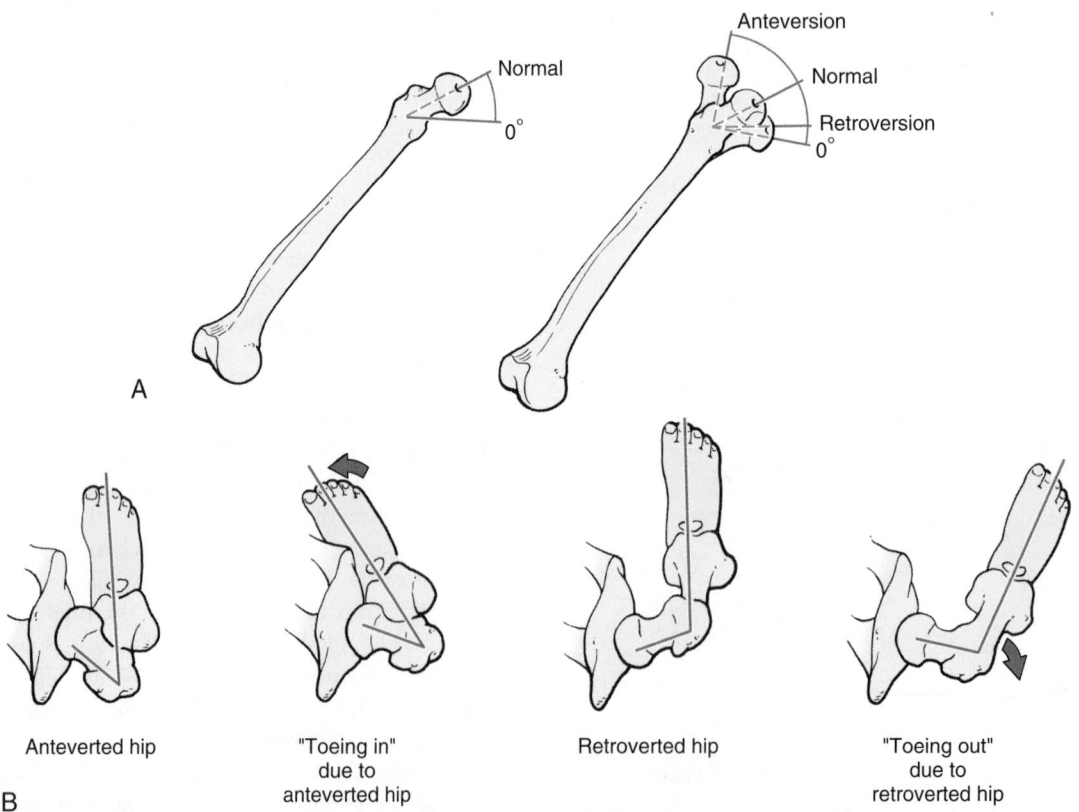

Figure 11-23 Torsion angles of the hip. A, Positions of femoral neck. **B,** Different foot positions with anteversion and retroversion at the hip (coronal views). (Redrawn from Echternach J, editor: *Physical therapy of the hip,* New York, 1990, Churchill Livingstone, p. 25.)

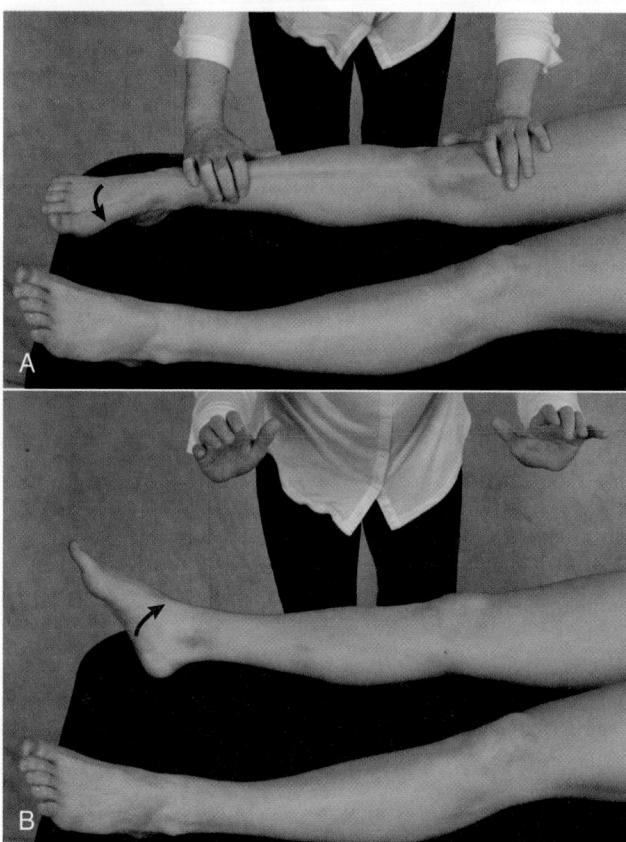

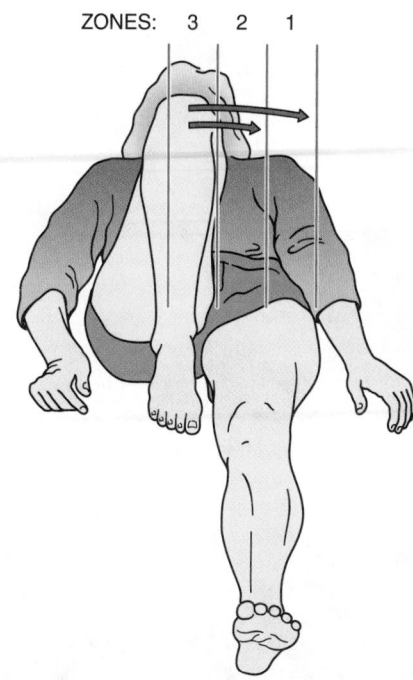

Figure 11-24 Dial test of the hip. A, The examiner medially rotates the hip. **B,** The examiner releases the medial rotation and watches the hip roll into lateral rotation.

Figure 11-25 The normal hip permits the ipsilateral knee to move convincingly across the midline of the body without rolling the pelvis. The knee should enter zone 1 by overlapping the opposite hip and, in the youthful or supple patient, reaches a position lateral to the thigh. Progressive pathologic changes in the hip limit adduction to zones 2 and 3 with the production of pain by this maneuver. (Redrawn from Woods D, Macnicol M: The flexion-adduction test: an early sign of hip disease. J Pediatr Orthop 10:181, 2001.)

medially and laterally rotates the femur to end range comparing both hips (Figure 11-28). If a click is present, it may indicate a labral tear. The maneuver also shows hip rotational mobility, and if restricted or painful, indicates hip pathology.[10,115,116]

⚠ *McCarthy Hip Extension Sign.*[10,117,118] The patient lies supine on the bed with both hips flexed. The examiner then takes the good hip and extends it from the flexed position, first with the hip in lateral rotation, and then repeats the test with the hip in medial rotation. The non-test leg is kept in flexion. The test is repeated with the affected hip. A positive test would be the reproduction of the patient's pain. The test is designed to simulate normal walking and creates a force double the patient's body weight across the hip.[12] McCarthy et al.[117] believed there were three positive tests that would help to predict labral pathology: 1) pain with the McCarthy hip extension test (Figure 11-29), 2) painful impingement with hip flexion abduction and lateral rotation (the anterior labial tear test), and 3) inguinal pain on resisted straight leg raise (Stinchfield resisted hip flexion test).

❓ *Nélaton's Line.* Nélaton's line is an imaginary line drawn from the ischial tuberosity of the pelvis to the ASIS of the pelvis on the same side (Figure 11-30).[107] If the greater trochanter of the femur is palpated well above the

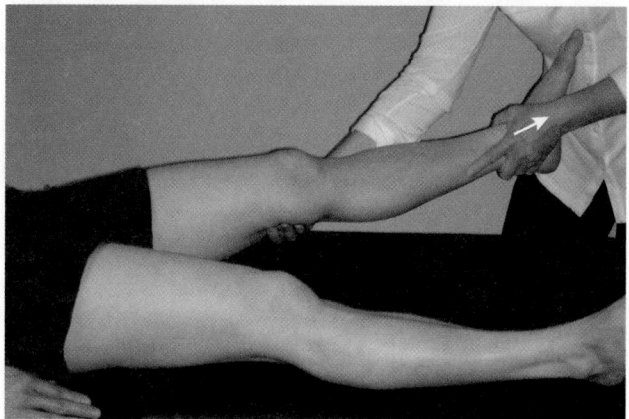

Figure 11-26 Foveal distraction test of the hip.

line, it is an indication of a dislocated hip or coxa vara. The two sides should be compared.

✓ *Patrick's Test (FABER or Figure-4 Test).* The patient lies supine, and the examiner places the patient's test leg so that the foot of the test leg is on top of the knee of the opposite leg (Figure 11-31). The examiner then slowly lowers the knee of the test leg toward the examining table. A negative test is indicated by the test leg's knee falling to the table or at least being parallel with the opposite leg. A positive test is indicated by the test leg's knee remaining above the opposite straight leg. If

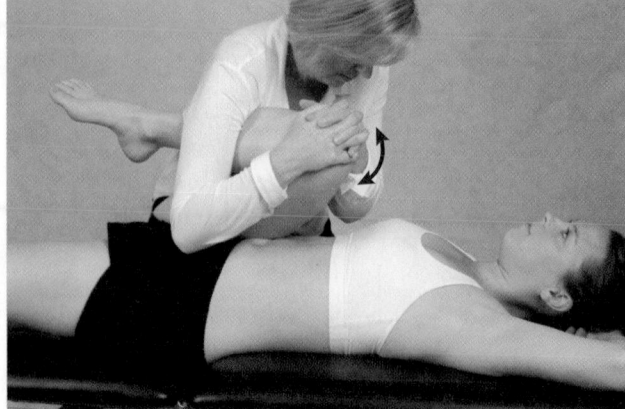

Figure 11-27 Hip scour test.

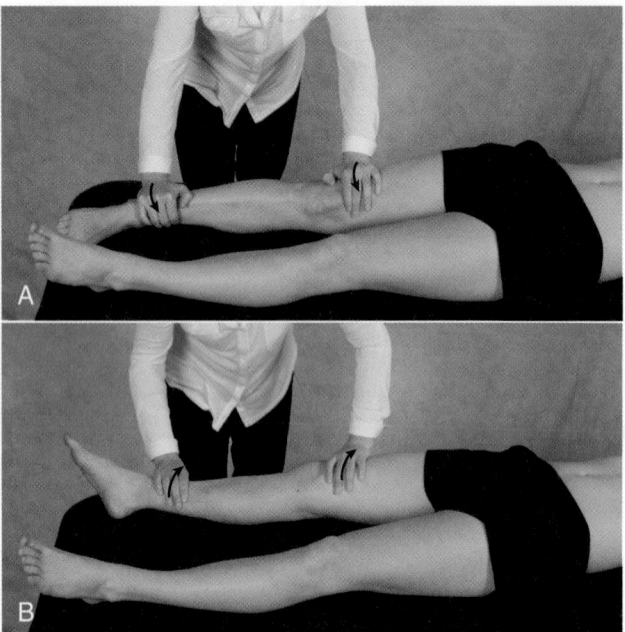

Figure 11-28 Log roll test. **A,** Medial rotation. **B,** Lateral rotation.

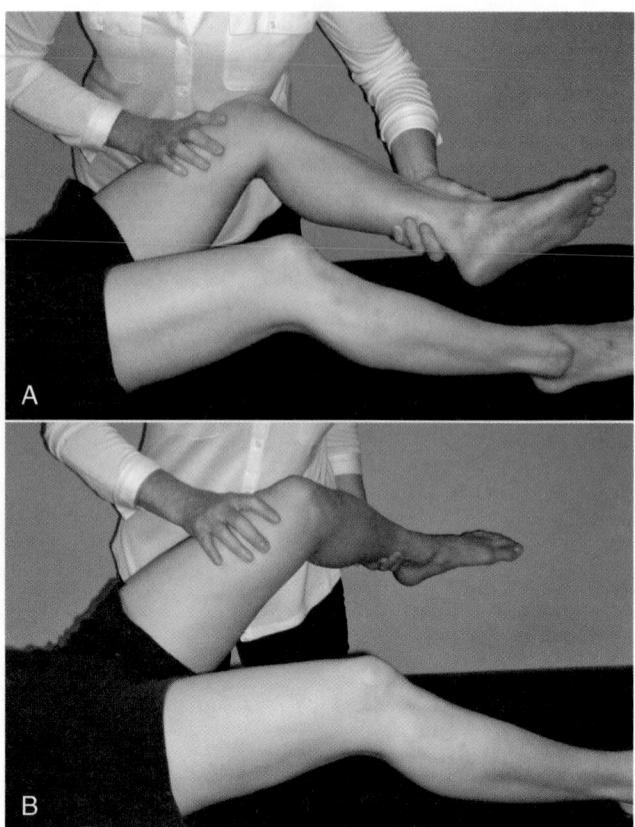

Figure 11-29 **McCarthy hip extension sign. A,** Medial rotation. **B,** Lateral rotation.

positive, the test indicates that the hip joint may be affected, that there may be iliopsoas spasm, or that the sacroiliac joint may be affected. **Flexion, abduction, and external rotation (FABER)** is the position of the hip at which the patient begins the test. The test is sometimes referred to as **Jansen's test.**[119]

Rotational Deformities. Rotational deformities can occur anywhere between the hip and the foot (Table 11-10). Many of these deformities are hereditary. The patient lies supine with the lower limbs straight while the examiner looks at the patellae.[108] If the patellae face in (squinting patellae), it is a possible indication of medial rotation of the femur or the tibia. If the patellae face up, out, and away from each other ("frog eyes" or "grasshopper eyes"), it is a possible indication of lateral rotation of the femur or the tibia. If the tibia is affected, the feet face in ("pigeon toes") for medial rotation and face out more than 10° for excessive lateral rotation of the tibia (Figure 11-32) while

the patellae face straight ahead. Normally, the feet angle out 5° to 10° (**Fick angle**) for better balance.

? *Stinchfield Resisted Hip Flexion Test.*[120–122] The patient lies supine and then actively elevates the straight leg (i.e., flexes the hip) to about 20° to 30° while the examiner applies gentle resistance. In a positive test, pain may be referred into the sensory distribution of the femoral, obturator, or sciatic nerves. A positive test indicates intra-articular pathology, which may include a labral tear, synovitis, arthritis, occult femoral neck fractures, iliopsoas tendinitis/bursitis, and prosthetic failure or loosening.[123]

? *Torque Test.* The patient lies supine close to the edge of the examining table with the femur of the test leg extended over the edge of the table (Figure 11-33). The test leg is extended until the pelvis (i.e., the ASIS) begins to move. The examiner uses one hand to medially rotate the femur to the end of range and the other hand to apply a slow posterolateral pressure along the line of the neck of the femur for 20 seconds to stress the capsular ligaments and test the stability of the hip joint.[124]

Tests for Impingement

? *Anteroposterior Impingement Test.*[47,51] This test is a test for hip dysplasia (e.g., acetabular retroversion), slipped capital femoral epiphysis, and femoroacetabular impingement.[59] The patient lies supine with the hip flexed to 90°. The examiner then medially rotates and adducts the hip which leads to impingement of femoral neck against the acetabular rim (Figure 11-34, *A*). Forced medial rotation can lead to a labral lesion, chondral lesion, or both. Pain is a positive sign. The hip is similarly tested in different degrees of flexion (45° to 120°) with pain increasing with increased flexion.[59]

? *Posteroinferior Impingement Test.*[47,51,112] This test is a test for global acetabular over coverage (e.g., coxa profunda, coxa protrusio), global femoral neck offset

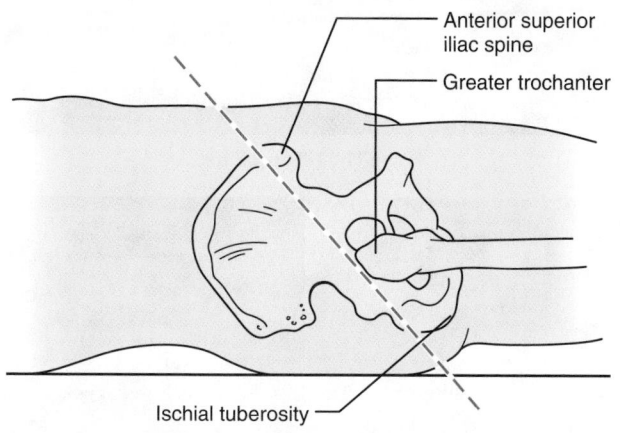

Figure 11-30 Nélaton's line.

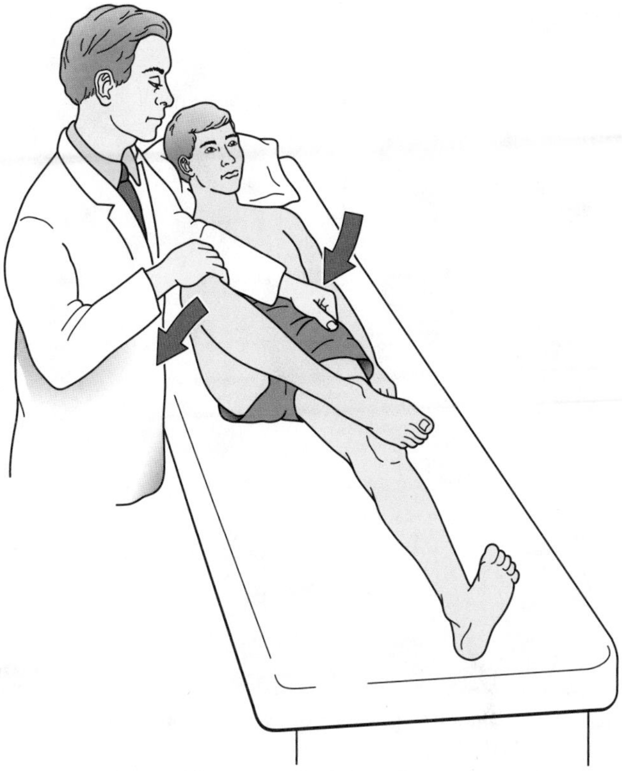

Figure labels: Anterior superior iliac spine; Greater trochanter; Ischial tuberosity

Figure 11-31 Patrick's test (**FABER or Figure-4 test**) for the detection of limitation of motion in the hip. (Redrawn from Beetham WP, et al: Physical examination of the joints, Philadelphia: 1965, WB Saunders, p. 139.)

TABLE **11-10**

Hip Malalignment

Malalignment	Related Posture	Possible Compensating Postures
Excessive anteversion	Toeing-in Subtalar pronation Lateral patellar subluxation Medial tibial torsion Medial femoral torsion	Lateral tibial torsion Lateral rotation at knee Lateral rotation of tibia, femur, and/or pelvis Lumbar rotation on same side
Excessive retroversion	Toeing-out Subtalar supination Lateral tibial torsion Lateral femoral torsion	Medial rotation at knee Medial rotation of tibia, femur, and/or pelvis Lumbar rotation on opposite side
Coxa vara	Pronated subtalar joint Medial rotation of leg Short ipsilateral leg Anterior pelvic rotation	Ipsilateral subtalar supination Contralateral subtalar pronation Ipsilateral plantar flexion Contralateral genu recurvatum Contralateral hip and/or knee flexion Ipsilateral posterior pelvic rotation and ipsilateral lumbar rotation
Coxa valga	Supinated subtalar joint Lateral rotation of leg Long ipsilateral leg Posterior pelvic tilt	Ipsilateral subtalar pronation Contralateral subtalar supination Contralateral plantar flexion Ipsilateral genu recurvatum Ipsilateral hip and/or knee flexion Ipsilateral anterior pelvic rotation and contralateral lumbar rotation

Adapted from Reigger-Krugh C, Keysor, JJ: Skeletal malalignments of the lower quarter: correlated and compensatory motions and postures. J Orthop Sports Phys Ther 23:166–167, 1996.

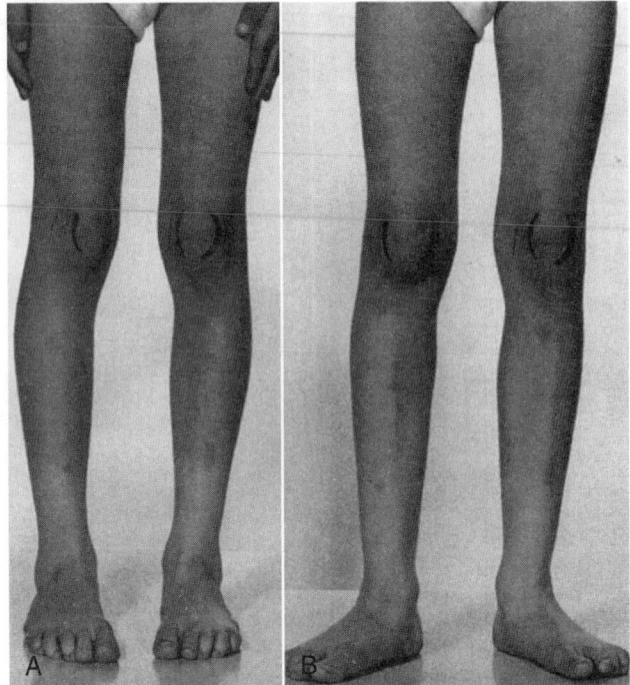

Figure 11-32 Clinical appearance of excessive femoral torsion in a girl. A, With the knees in full extension and the feet aligned (pointing straight forward), the legs appear bowed and the patellae face inward (squinting patella). **B,** On lateral rotation of the hips so that the patellae are facing to the front, the feet and legs point outward and the bowleg appearance is corrected. (From Tachdjian MO: Pediatric orthopedics, Philadelphia, 1990, WB Saunders, p. 2802.)

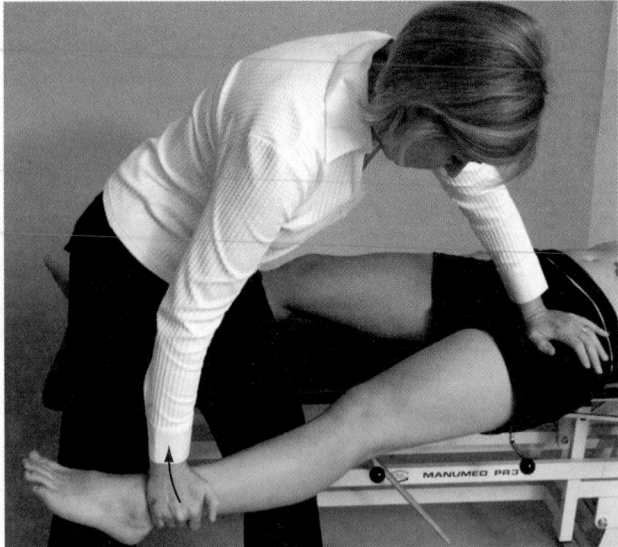

Figure 11-33 Torque test.

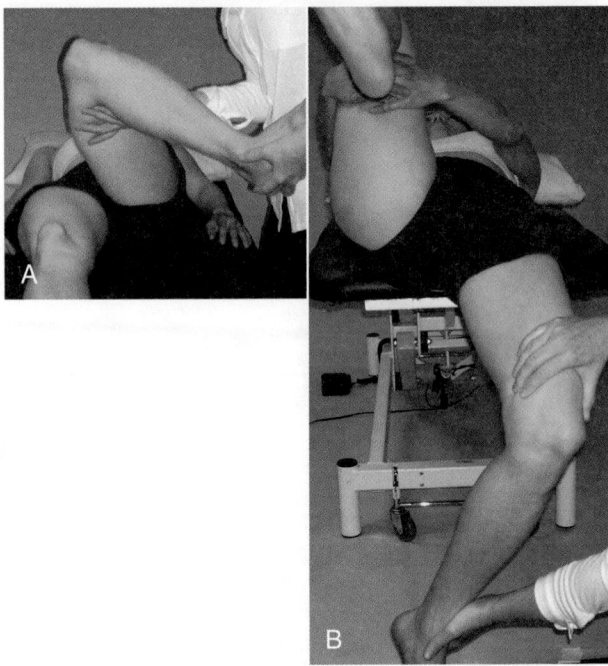

Figure 11-34 **A,** Anteroposterior impingement test. **B,** Posteroinferior impingement test.

abnormalities, and posterior acetabular cartilage damage. The test is also positive in people who place the hip in extremes of ROM (e.g., ballet dancers, martial artists, hockey goal tenders, mountain climbers, yoga practitioners, long striding runners).[59] The patient lies supine with the legs hanging free over the edge of the bed to ensure maximum hip extension. The examiner then laterally rotates the hip quickly (Figure 11-34, *B*). Deep seated groin or buttock pain is an indication of posteroinferior impingement.[47,51,59]

The **dynamic internal (medial) rotation impingement (DIRI) test** ▲ and the **dynamic external (lateral) rotation impingement test (DEXRIT)** ▲ are modifications of the previous two tests that are commonly used in arthroscopies of the hip.[12] In both cases, the patient is in supine lying. The examiner takes the test hip into 90° of flexion. For the DIRI test, the hip is passively moved through a wide arc of adduction and medial rotation while for DEXRIT, the hip is passively moved through a wide arc of abduction and lateral rotation. Pain is a positive test.

Tests for Labral Lesions

Acetabular labral tears rarely occur without some structural osseous abnormality often accompanied by a history of the patient repeatedly going into extreme ranges of motion especially rotation.[46] These tears may be accompanied by damage to the acetabular cartilage.[46,125]

✓ *Anterior Labral Tear Test (Flexion, Adduction, and Internal Rotation [FADDIR] Test).*[10,27,33,51,126] This test, also called the **anterior apprehension test,**[127] is used to test for anterior–superior impingement syndrome, anterior labial tear, and iliopsoas tendinitis. The patient is placed in supine position. The examiner takes the hip into full flexion, lateral rotation, and full abduction as a starting position. The examiner then extends the hip combined with medial rotation and adduction (Figure 11-35). A positive test is indicated by the production of pain, the reproduction of the patient's symptoms with or

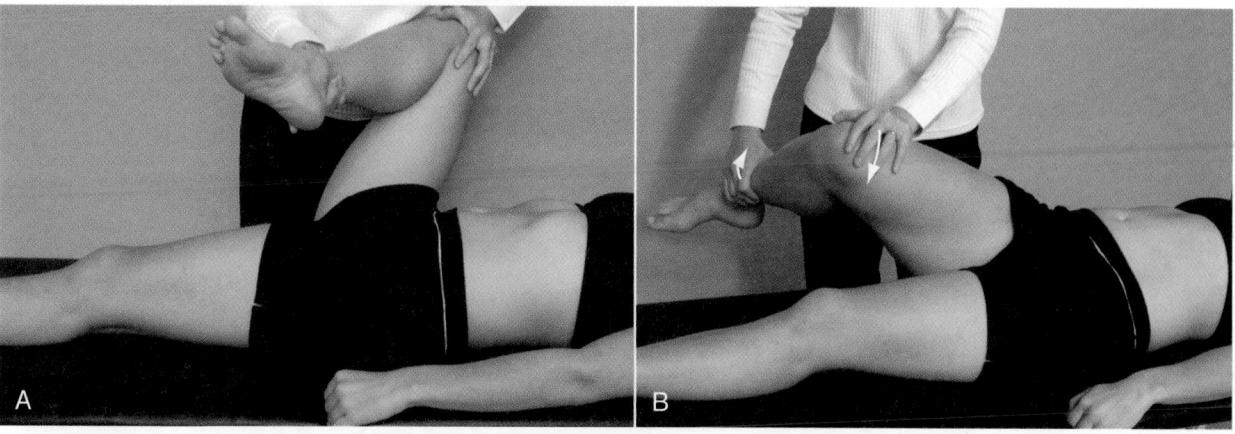

Figure 11-35 Anterior labral tear test. A, Starting position. **B,** End position.

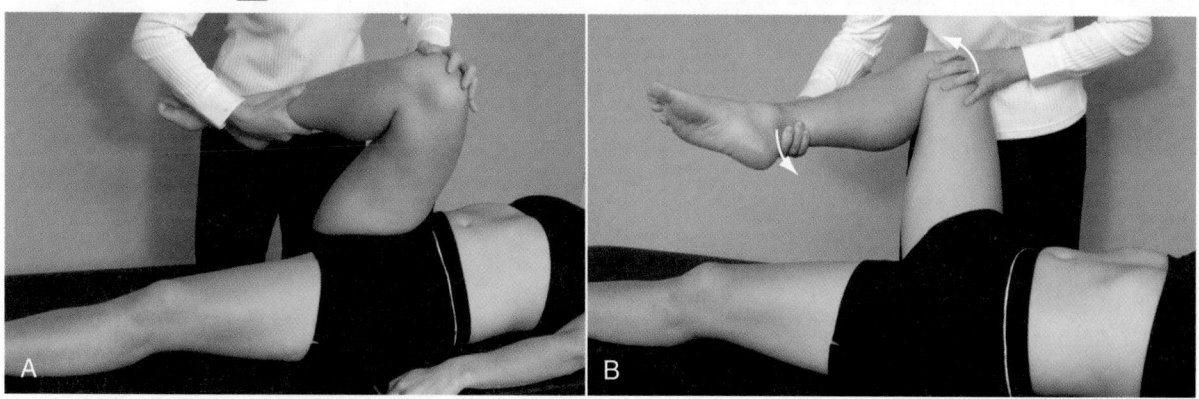

Figure 11-36 Posterior labral tear test. A, Starting position. **B,** End position.

without a click, or apprehension. The test places the greatest strain on the anterolateral labrum, and the examiner should be careful to equate any findings with the patient's symptoms.[10,116]

⚠ *Posterior Labral Tear Test.*[27,51] The patient is placed in supine position. The examiner takes the hip into full flexion, adduction, and medial rotation as a starting position. The examiner then takes the hip into extension combined with abduction and lateral rotation (Figure 11-36). A positive test is indicated by the production of groin pain, patient apprehension, or the reproduction of the patient's symptoms, with or without a click. A positive test is an indication of a labral tear, anterior hip instability, or posterior–inferior impingement. The test is sometimes called the **posterior apprehension test** if apprehension occurs toward the end of ROM when doing the test.

Tests for Femoral Neck Stress Fractures

❓ *Fulcrum Test of the Hip.* The fulcrum test[128] is used to assess for possible stress fracture of the femoral shaft. The patient sits with the knees bent over the end of the bed with feet dangling. The examiner places an arm under the patient's thigh to act as a fulcrum (Figure 11-37). The fulcrum arm is moved from distal to proximal along the thigh as gentle pressure is applied to the dorsum of the knee with the examiner's opposite hand.

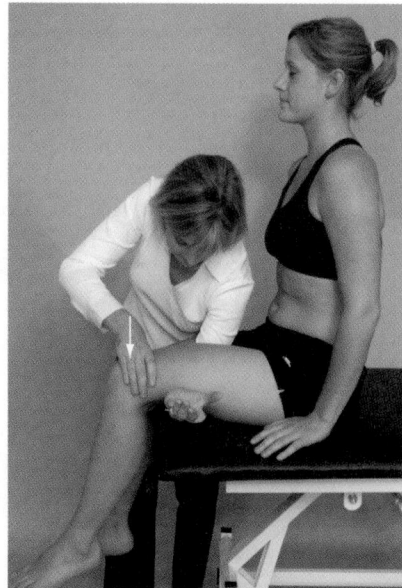

Figure 11-37 Fulcrum test of the hip. Examiner places arm under femur and carefully applies a downward force at the knee.

If a stress fracture is present, the patient complains of a sharp pain and expresses apprehension when the fulcrum arm is under the fracture site. A bone scan confirms the diagnosis.

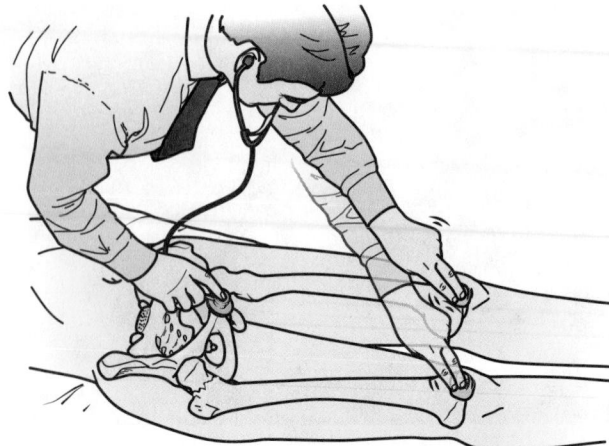

Figure 11-38 Patellar-pubic percussion sign.

⚠ **Heel Strike Test.**[12] The patient is lying supine. The examiner firmly strikes the heel to stimulate heel strike during walking. Pain in the groin may be suggestive of a femoral neck stress fracture. A **single leg hop** (see Chapter 12) would have the same effect with a positive test showing pain in the groin.

⚠ **Patellar-Pubic Percussion Sign.**[101,129] The patient lies supine with the legs extended. The examiner places the bell of the stethoscope over the symphysis pubis. The examiner then percusses each patella with a finger starting with the uninvolved side. Both sides are compared for differences in pitch and loudness. Normally, the sounds are equal. If bone pathology is present (e.g., hip fracture) the affected side has a duller sound (Figure 11-38).

Pediatric Tests for Hip Pathology

Orthopedic tests are commonly performed in newborns to detect problems, especially CDH or developmental dysplasia of the hip (DDH) that covers more than congenital problems, which may be amenable to conservative treatment if caught early.[130–132]

⚠ **Abduction Test (Harts' Sign).**[133] If CDH is not diagnosed early or there is DDH, parents often note that when they change the child's diapers, one leg does not abduct as far as the other one.[131] This is the basis for this test. The child lies supine with the hips and knees flexed to 90°. The examiner then passively abducts both legs, noting any asymmetry or limitation of movement. In addition, if one hip is dislocated, the child often demonstrates asymmetry of fat folds in the gluteal and upper leg area because of the "riding up" of the femur on the affected side.

✓ **Barlow's Test.** Barlow's test is a modification of Ortolani's test[108] (Figure 11-39) used for DDH.[131] The infant lies supine with the legs facing the examiner. The hips are flexed to 90°, and the knees are fully flexed. Each hip is evaluated individually while the examiner's other hand steadies the opposite femur and the pelvis. The examiner's middle finger of each hand is placed over the

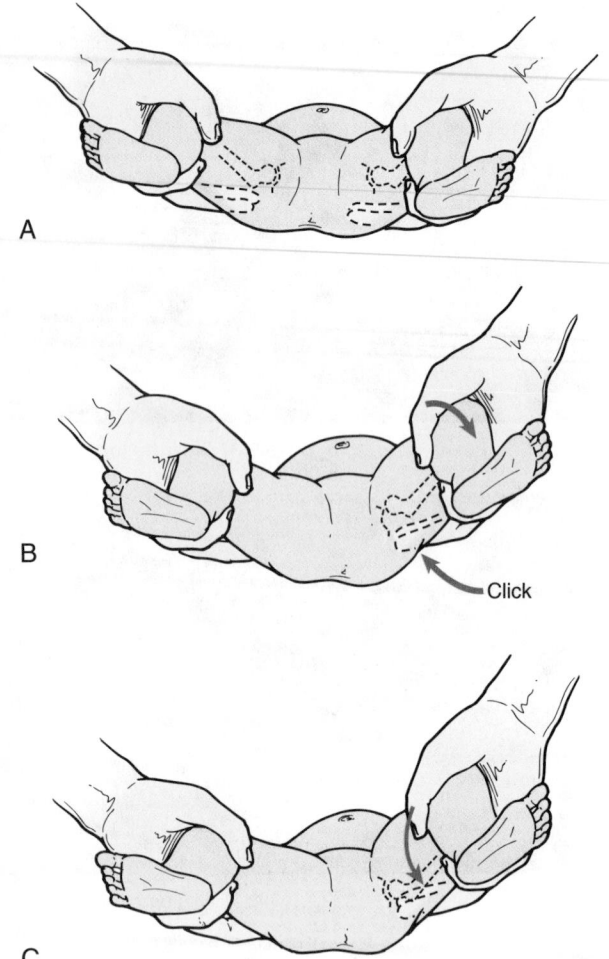

Figure 11-39 Ortolani's sign and Barlow's test. **A,** In the newborn, the two hips can be equally flexed, abducted, and laterally rotated without producing a "click." **B,** Ortolani's sign or first part of Barlow's test. **C,** Second part of Barlow's test.

greater trochanter, and the thumb is placed adjacent to the inner side of the knee and thigh opposite the lesser trochanter. The hip is taken into abduction while the examiner's middle finger applies forward pressure behind the greater trochanter. If the femoral head slips forward into the acetabulum with a click, clunk, or jerk, the test is positive, indicating that the hip was dislocated. This part of the test is identical to Ortolani's test. The examiner then uses the thumb to apply pressure backward and outward on the inner thigh. If the femoral head slips out over the posterior lip of the acetabulum and then reduces again when pressure is removed, the hip is classified as unstable. The hip is not dislocated but is dislocatable. The procedure is repeated for the other hip.

This test may be used for infants up to 6 months of age. It should not be repeated too often, because it may result in a dislocated hip as well as articular damage to the head of the femur.[134]

⚠ **Galeazzi Sign (Allis or Galeazzi Test).** The Galeazzi test is good only for assessing unilateral CDH or

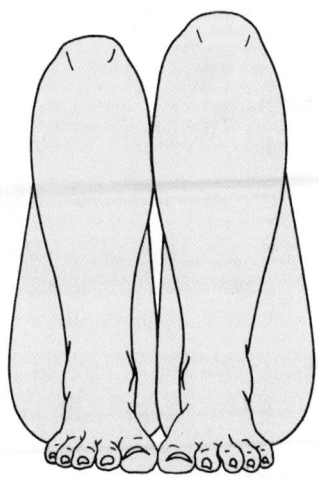

Figure 11-40 Galeazzi sign (Allis test).

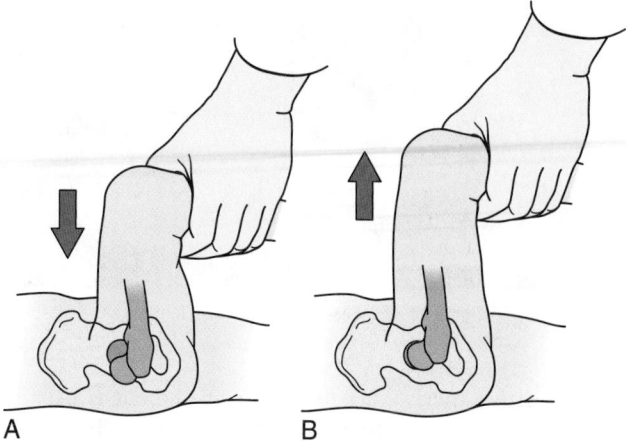

Figure 11-41 **Telescoping of the hip.** Because hip is not fixed in acetabulum, it moves down (**A**) and up (**B**).

unilateral DDH and may be used in children from 3 to 18 months of age.[122] The child lies supine with the knees flexed and the hips flexed to 90°. A positive test is indicated if one knee is higher than the other (Figure 11-40).

✓ *Ortolani's Sign.* Ortolani's test can determine whether an infant has a CDH (see Figures 11-39, *A* and *B*).[106] With the infant supine, the examiner flexes the hips and grasps the legs so that the examiner's thumbs are against the insides of the knees and thighs, and the fingers are placed along the outsides of the thighs to the buttocks. With gentle traction, the thighs are abducted and pressure is applied against the greater trochanters of the femora. Resistance to abduction and lateral rotation begins to be felt at approximately 30° to 40°. The examiner may feel a click, clunk, or jerk, which indicates a positive test and that the hip has reduced; in addition, increased abduction of the hip is obtained. The femoral head has slipped over the acetabular ridge into the acetabulum, and normal abduction of 70° to 90° can be obtained.

This test is valid only for the first few weeks after birth and only for dislocated and lax hips, not for dislocations that are difficult to reduce. The examiner should take care to feel the quality of the click. Soft clicks may occur without dislocation and are thought to be caused by the iliofemoral ligament's clicking over the anterior surface of the head of the femur as it is laterally rotated. Soft clicking usually occurs without the prior resistance that is seen with dislocations. By repeated rotation of the hip, the exact location of the click can be palpated. However, Ortolani's test should not be repeated too often because it could lead to damage of the articular cartilage of the femoral head. As with all clinical tests, if the test is positive, it is highly suggestive that the problem (i.e., CDH) exists, but if it is negative, it does not necessarily rule out the problem.

⚠ *Telescoping Sign (Piston or Dupuytren's Test).*[133] The telescoping sign is evident in a child with a dislocated hip. The child lies in the supine position. The examiner flexes

the knee and hip to 90°. The femur is pushed down onto the examining table. The femur and leg are then lifted up and away from the table (Figure 11-41). With the normal hip, little movement occurs with this action. With the dislocated hip, however, there is a lot of relative movement. This excessive movement is called **telescoping,** or **pistoning.**

Tests for Leg Length

There are two types of leg length discrepancy. The first, called **true leg length discrepancy** or **true shortening,** is caused by an anatomic or structural change in the lower leg resulting from congenital maldevelopment (e.g., adolescent coxa vara, congenital hip dysplasia, bony abnormality) or trauma (e.g., fracture). Because an anatomic short leg results, the spine and pelvis are often affected, leading to lateral pelvic tilt and scoliosis.[135,136]

The second type of leg length discrepancy is called **functional leg length discrepancy** or **functional shortening,** and it is the result of compensation for a change that may have occurred because of positioning rather than structure. For example, a functional leg length discrepancy could occur because of unilateral foot pronation or spinal scoliosis.[135,136]

⚠ *True Leg Length.* Before any measuring is done, the examiner must set the pelvis square, level, or in balance with the lower limbs.[137–139] The legs should be 15 to 20 cm (4 to 8 inches) apart and parallel to each other (Figure 11-42). If the legs are not placed in proper relation to the pelvis, apparent shortening of the limb may occur. The lower limbs must be placed in comparable positions relative to the pelvis, because abduction of the hip brings the medial malleolus closer to the ASIS on the same side and adduction of the hip takes the medial malleolus farther from the ASIS on the same side. If one hip is fixed in abduction or adduction as a result of contracture or some other cause, the normal hip should be adducted or abducted an equal amount to ensure accurate leg length measurement.

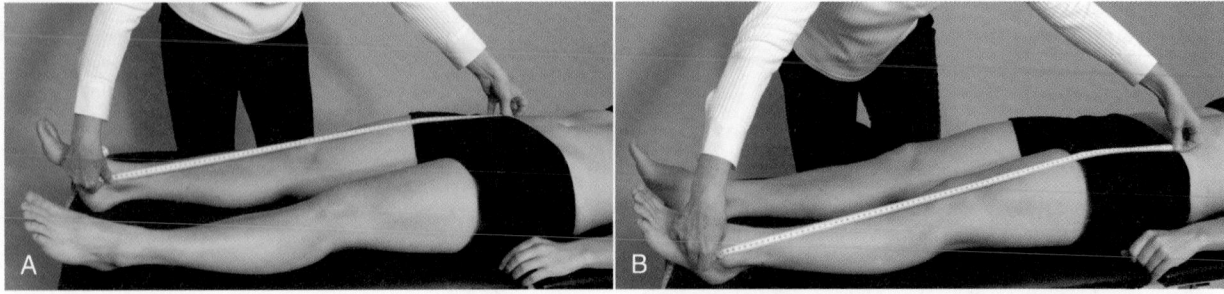

Figure 11-42 **Measuring true leg length. A,** Measuring to the medial malleolus. **B,** Measuring to the lateral malleolus.

In North America, leg length measurement is usually taken from the ASIS to the medial malleolus; however, these values may be altered by muscle wasting or obesity. Measuring to the lateral malleolus is less likely to be affected by the muscle bulk. To obtain the leg length, the examiner measures from the ASIS to the lateral or medial malleolus. The flat metal end of the tape measure is placed immediately distal to the ASIS and pushed up against it. The thumb then presses the tape end firmly against the bone, rigidly fixing the tape measure against the bone. The index finger of the other hand is placed immediately distal to the lateral or medial malleolus and pushed against it. The thumbnail is brought down against the tip of the index finger so that the tape measure is pinched between them. A slight difference (as much as 1 to 1.5 cm) in leg length is considered normal; however, this difference can still cause symptoms.

The **Weber-Barstow maneuver** (visual method) ⚠ may also be used to measure leg length asymmetry. The patient lies supine with the hips and knees flexed (Figure 11-43). The examiner stands at the patient's feet and palpates the distal aspect of the medial malleoli with the thumbs. The patient then lifts the pelvis from the examining table and returns to the starting position. Next, the examiner passively extends the patient's legs and compares the positions of the malleoli using the borders of the thumbs. Different levels indicate asymmetry.[140]

If one leg is shorter than the other (Figure 11-44), the examiner can determine where the difference is by measuring the following:

1. From the iliac crest to the greater trochanter of the femur (for coxa vara or coxa valga): The neck-shaft angle of the femur (Figure 11-45) is normally 150° to 160° at birth and decreases to between 120° and 135° in the adult (Figure 11-46). If this angle is less than 120° in an adult, it is known as **coxa vara;** if it is more than 135° in the adult, it is known as **coxa valga.**
2. From the greater trochanter of the femur to the knee joint line on the lateral aspect (for femoral shaft shortening)
3. From the knee joint line on the medial side to the medial malleolus (for tibial shaft shortening)

The relative length of the tibia may also be examined with the patient lying prone. The examiner places the

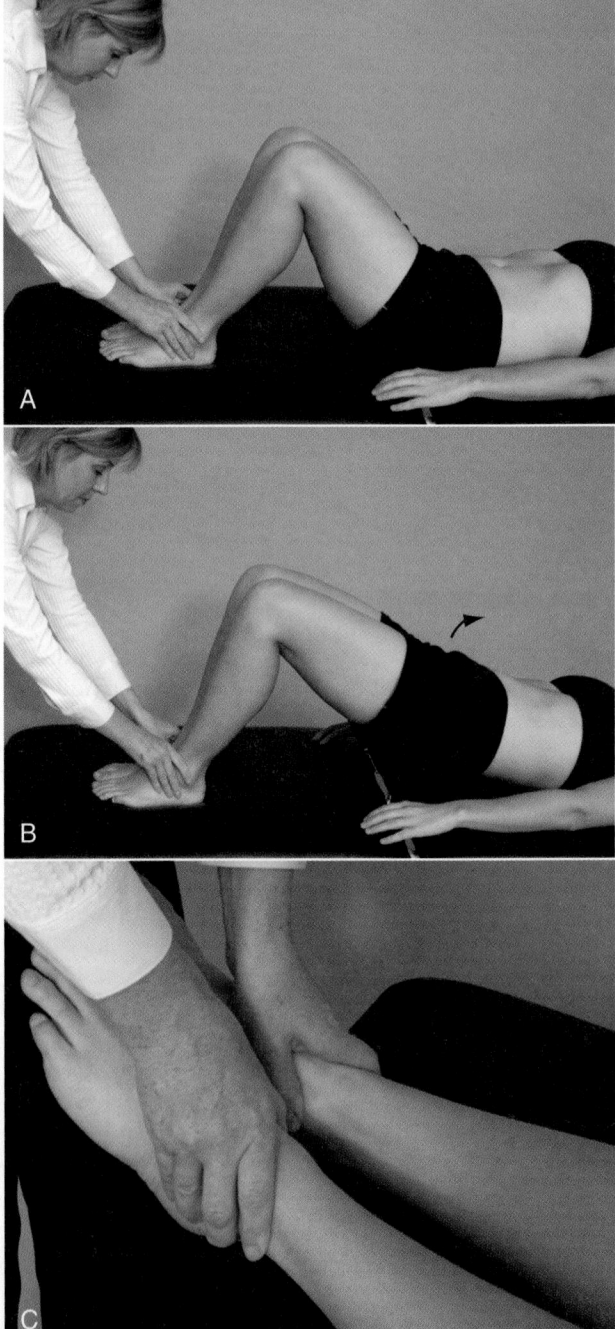

Figure 11-43 **Weber-Barstow maneuver for leg length asymmetry. A,** Starting position. **B,** Patient lifts hips off bed. **C,** Comparing height of medial malleoli with the legs extended.

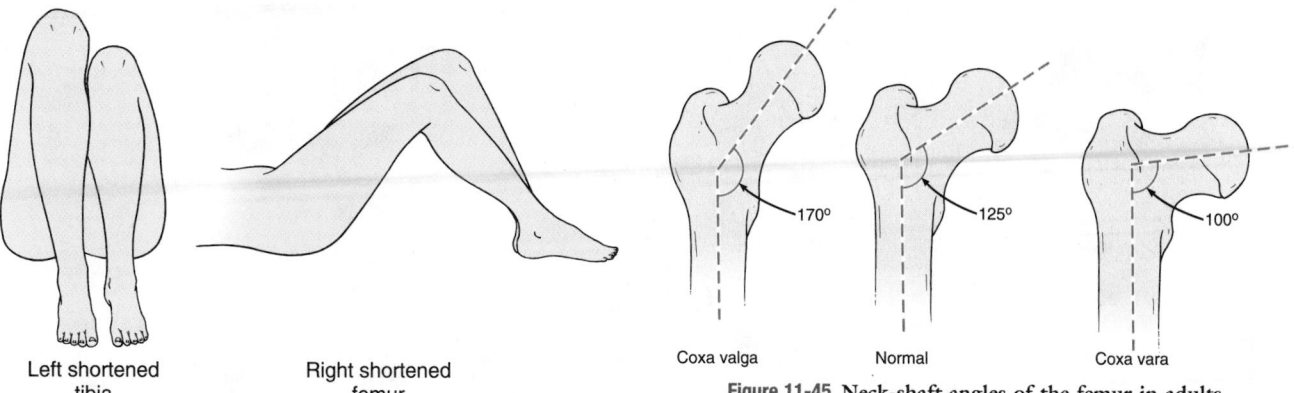

| Left shortened tibia | Right shortened femur |

Figure 11-44 Leg length discrepancy.

Figure 11-45 Neck-shaft angles of the femur in adults.

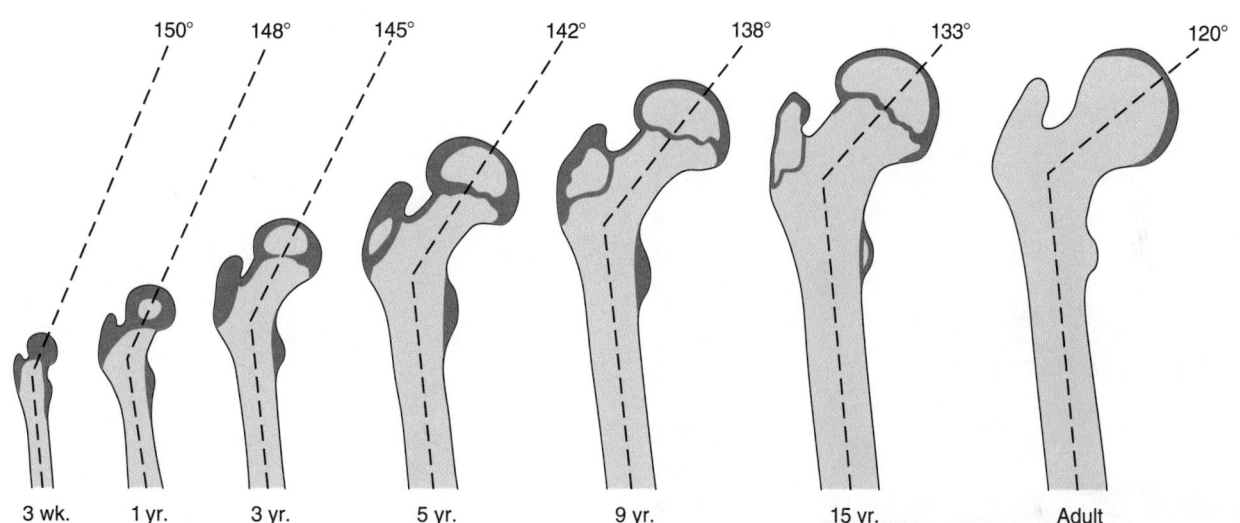

Figure 11-46 Mean angle of the femoral neck shaft in different age groups. *Red area* indicates cartilage. (Modified from von Lanz T, Wachsmuth W: Praktische anatomie, Berlin, 1938, Julius Springer, p. 143.)

thumbs transversely across the soles of the feet just in front of the heels. The knees are flexed 90°, and the relative heights of the thumbs are noted. Care must be taken to ensure that the legs are perpendicular to the examining table (Figure 11-47).[140]

Similarly, the femoral lengths can be compared by having the patient lie supine with the hips and knees flexed to 90°. If one femur is longer than the other, its height will be higher (Figure 11-48).[136]

Apparent shortening, or functional shortening, (Figure 11-49) of the leg is evident if the patient has a lateral pelvic tilt when the measurement is taken. Apparent or functional shortening of the limb is the result of adaptations the patient has made in response to pathology or contracture somewhere in the spine, pelvis, or lower limbs. In reality, there is no structural or anatomic difference in bone lengths. If there were, it would be called true shortening of the limb. When measuring the apparent leg length shortening, the examiner obtains the distance from the tip of the xiphisternum or umbilicus to the medial malleolus (Figure 11-50). If true leg length is

normal but the umbilicus-to-malleolus measurements are different, a functional leg length discrepancy is present.[136] Values obtained by these measurements may be affected by muscle wasting, obesity, asymmetric position of the xiphisternum or umbilicus, or asymmetric positioning of the lower limbs.

⚠ *Standing (Functional) Leg Length.* The patient is first assessed while in a relaxed stance. In this position, the examiner palpates the ASIS and the PSIS, noting any asymmetry. The examiner then places the patient in a symmetric stance, ensuring that the subtalar joint is in neutral position (see Chapter 13), the toes are facing straight ahead, and the knees are extended. The ASIS and PSIS are again assessed for asymmetry. If differences are still noted, the examiner should check for structural leg length differences, sacroiliac joint dysfunction, or weak gluteus medius or quadratus lumborum muscles.

Tests for Muscle Tightness or Pathology

⚠ *Abduction Contracture Test.* This test is used to test the length of the abductor muscles (gluteus medius and

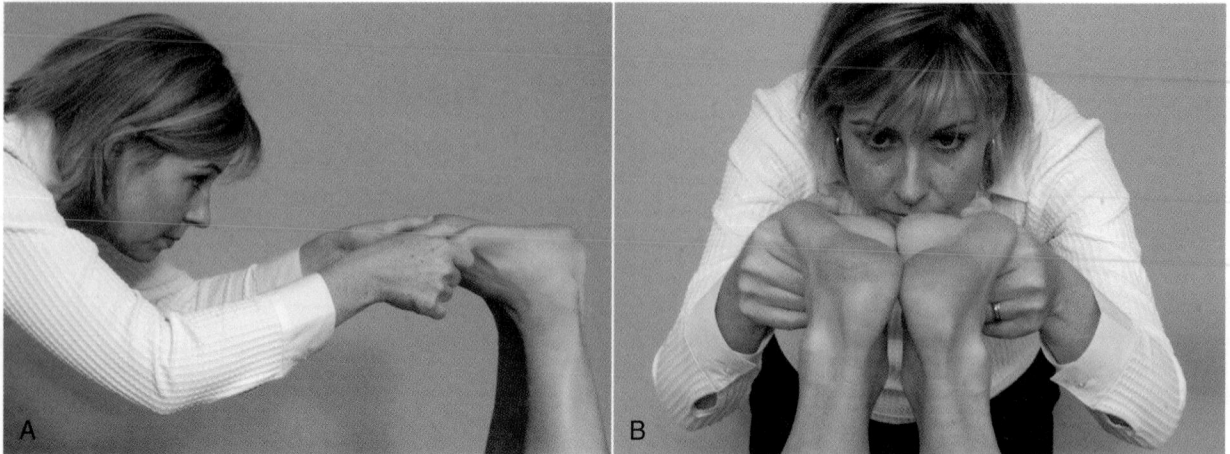

Figure 11-47 Prone knee flexion test for tibial shortening. The prone knee flexion test is completed as the examiner **(A)** passively flexes the patient's knees to 90° and **(B)** sights through the plane of the heel pads to see whether a difference in height is noticeable.

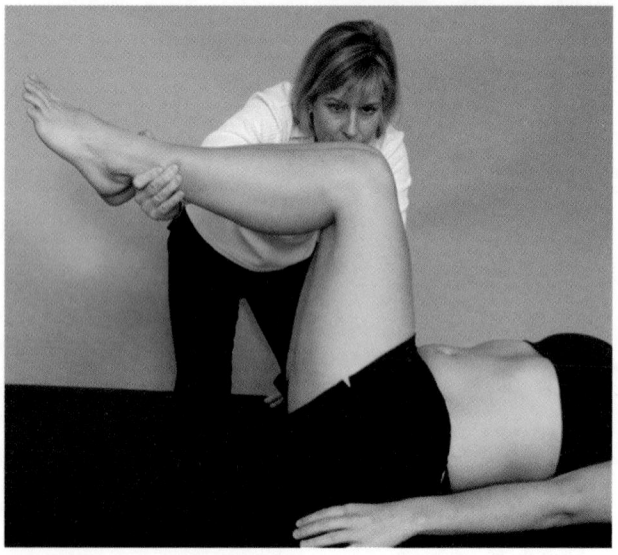

Figure 11-48 Hip flexion test for femoral shortening.

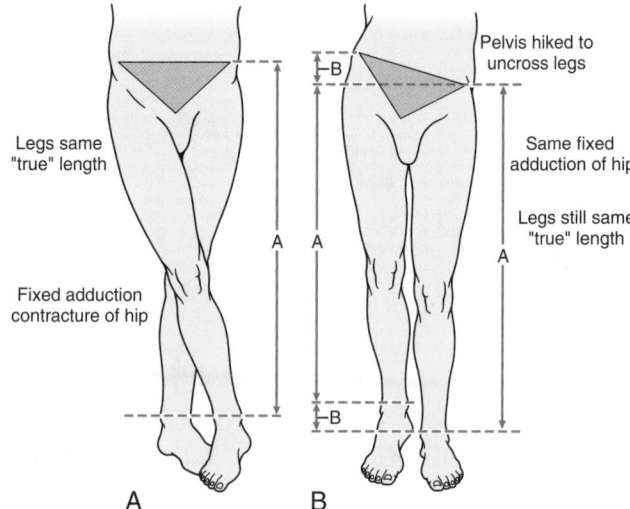

Figure 11-49 Functional shortening due to adduction contracture. **A,** Legs crossed. **B,** Legs uncrossed. Note that uncrossing causes pelvis to elevate on one side, but true leg length is equal on both sides. (Redrawn from the American Orthopaedic Association: Manual of orthopaedic surgery, Chicago, 1972, AOA, p. 45.)

minimus) of the hip. The patient lies supine with the ASISs level. If a contracture is present, the affected leg forms an angle of more than 90° with a line joining each ASIS. If the examiner then attempts to balance the lower limb with the pelvis, the pelvis (i.e., the ASIS) shifts down on the affected side or up on the unaffected side, and balancing is not possible. Normally, hip adduction should be about 30° before the ASIS moves. If the ASIS moves before this, the abductors are tight if a muscle stretch end feel is felt. This type of contracture can lead to **functional lengthening** of the limb rather than true lengthening.

⚠ *Adduction Contracture Test.* This test is designed to test the length of the adductor muscles (adductor longus, brevis and magnus, and pectineus) of the hip. The patient lies supine with the ASISs level. Normally, the examiner can easily "balance" the pelvis on the legs. This "balancing" implies a line joining the ASIS is perpendicular to

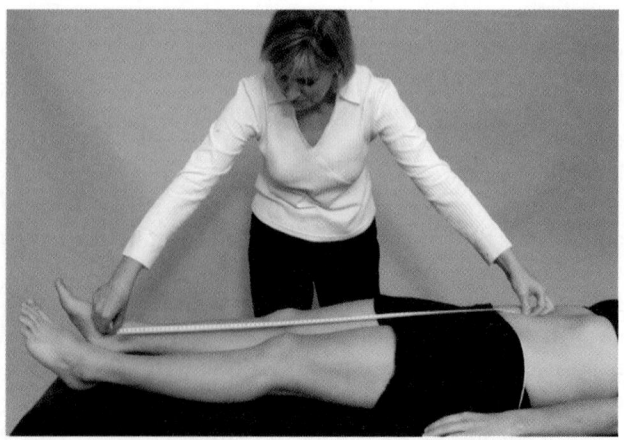

Figure 11-50 Measuring functional leg length.

the two lines formed by the straight legs (Figure 11-51). If a contracture is present, the affected leg forms an angle of less than 90° with the line joining the two ASISs. If the examiner then attempts to "balance" the lower limb with the pelvis, the pelvis (i.e., ASIS) shifts up on the affected side or down on the unaffected side, and balancing is not possible. Normally, hip abduction should be 30° to 50° before the ASIS moves. If the ASIS moves before this, the adductors are tight if a muscle stretch end feel is felt. This type of contracture can lead to functional shortening of the limb rather than true shortening (see Figure 11-49).

Patients, especially children, with adductor spasticity may also be tested by abduction. The patient is supine. The examiner then quickly abducts the leg. If there is a "grab" or "kicking in" of the stretch reflex at less than 30°, the test for adductor spasticity is considered positive. The test should be repeated with the knee flexed to rule out medial hamstring contracture.[141]

Bent-Knee Stretch Test for Proximal Hamstrings.[67] The patient lies supine while the examiner flexes the hip and knee of the test leg maximally (Figure 11-52, *A*). The examiner then slowly extends the knee (Figure 11-52, *B*). Pain in the hamstrings at the ischial origin indicates a positive test. It should be noted that neurological tissues must also be cleared before the test would be considered positive.

Ely's Test (Tight Rectus Femoris, Method 2). The patient lies prone, and the examiner passively flexes the patient's knee (Figure 11-53).[142] On flexion of the knee, the patient's hip on the same side spontaneously flexes, indicating that the rectus femoris muscle is tight on that side and that the test is positive. The two sides should be tested and compared.

Hamstrings Contracture Test (Method 2). The patient is instructed to sit with one knee flexed against the chest to stabilize the pelvis and the other knee extended (Figure 11-54). The patient then attempts to flex the trunk and touch the toes of the extended lower limb (test leg) with the fingers. The test is repeated on the other side. A comparison is made between the two sides. Normally, the patient should be able to at least touch the toes while keeping the knee extended. If he or she is unable to do so, it is an indication of tight hamstrings on the straight leg.

Lateral Step Down Maneuver (Pelvis Drop Test).[143] A 20-cm (8-inch) stool or step is placed in front of the patient. The patient is asked to place one foot on the stool and stand up straight on the stool on one foot. The patient then slowly lowers the non–weight-bearing leg to the floor. This should normally be accomplished with the

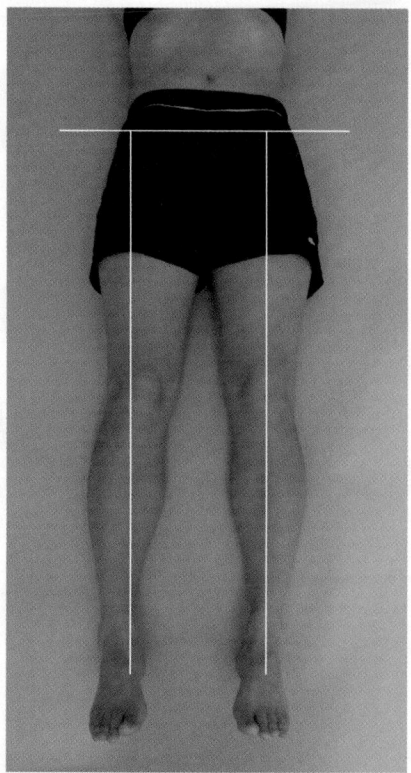

Figure 11-51 Balancing the pelvis on the legs (femora).

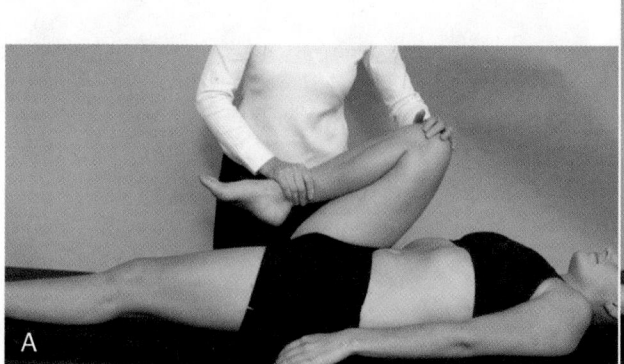
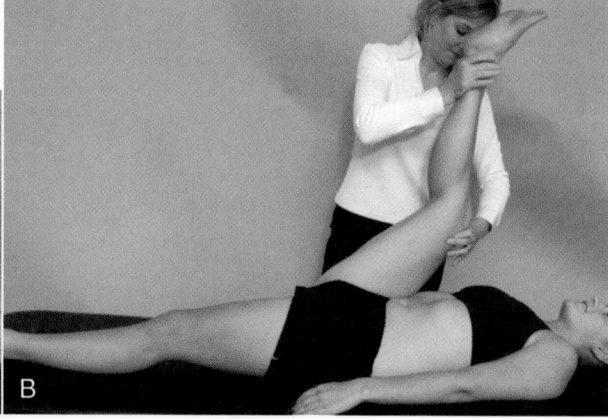

Figure 11-52 The bent-knee stretch test for proximal hamstring tightness is performed with the patient supine. The hip and knee of the test leg are maximally flexed **(A)**, and then the examiner slowly straightens the knee **(B)**.

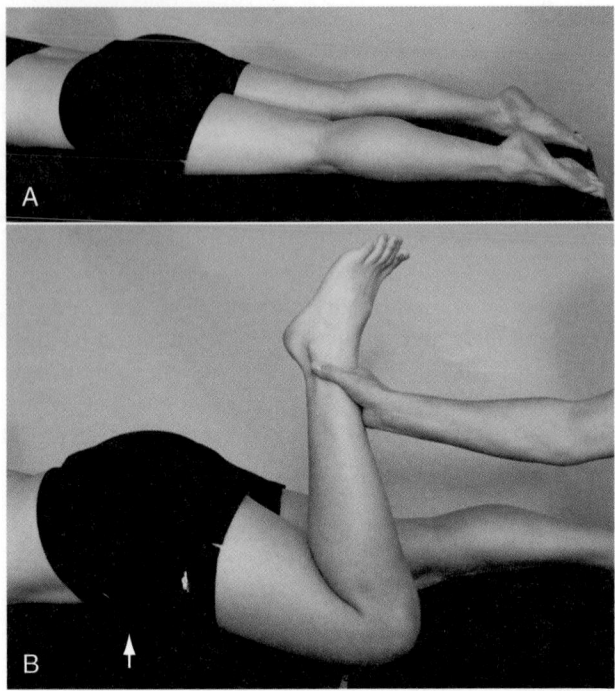

Figure 11-53 Ely's test for a tight rectus femoris. A, Position for the test. **B,** Posture test shown by hip flexion when the knee is flexed.

arms by the side and the trunk relatively erect and no hip adduction or medial rotation (Figure 11-55). If, however, on lowering, the arms abduct, the trunk inclines forward, the weight-bearing hip adducts or medially rotates, and/or the pelvis flexes forward or rotates backwards, it is an indication of an unstable hip or weak lateral rotators.

☑ *90–90 Straight Leg Raising Test (Hamstrings Contracture, Method 1).* The supine patient flexes both hips to 90° while the knees are bent. The patient may grasp behind the knees with both hands to stabilize the hips at 90° of flexion. The patient actively extends each knee in turn as much as possible. For normal flexibility in the hamstrings, knee extension should be within 20° of full extension (Figure 11-56).[34,144] Kuo et al.[145] called this angle the *popliteal angle* (the angle between two lines—one line along the shaft of femur and one line along the line of the tibia). They reported this angle to be 180° from birth to 2 years of age, which then decreased to about 155° by age 6 and remained fairly constant after that. If the angle is less than 125°, the hamstrings were considered to be tight. Normally, or if the hamstrings are tight, the end feel is muscle stretch. Nerve root symptoms may also result, because this positioning is similar to the slump test done in supine lying instead of sitting.

A modification of this test may also be used to test the length of gluteus maximus. The patient assumes the same starting position. While the examiner palpates the ASIS on the same side, the examiner flexes the hip with the knee flexed (Figure 11-57). If the thigh flexes 110° to 120° before the ASIS moves up, gluteus maximus length

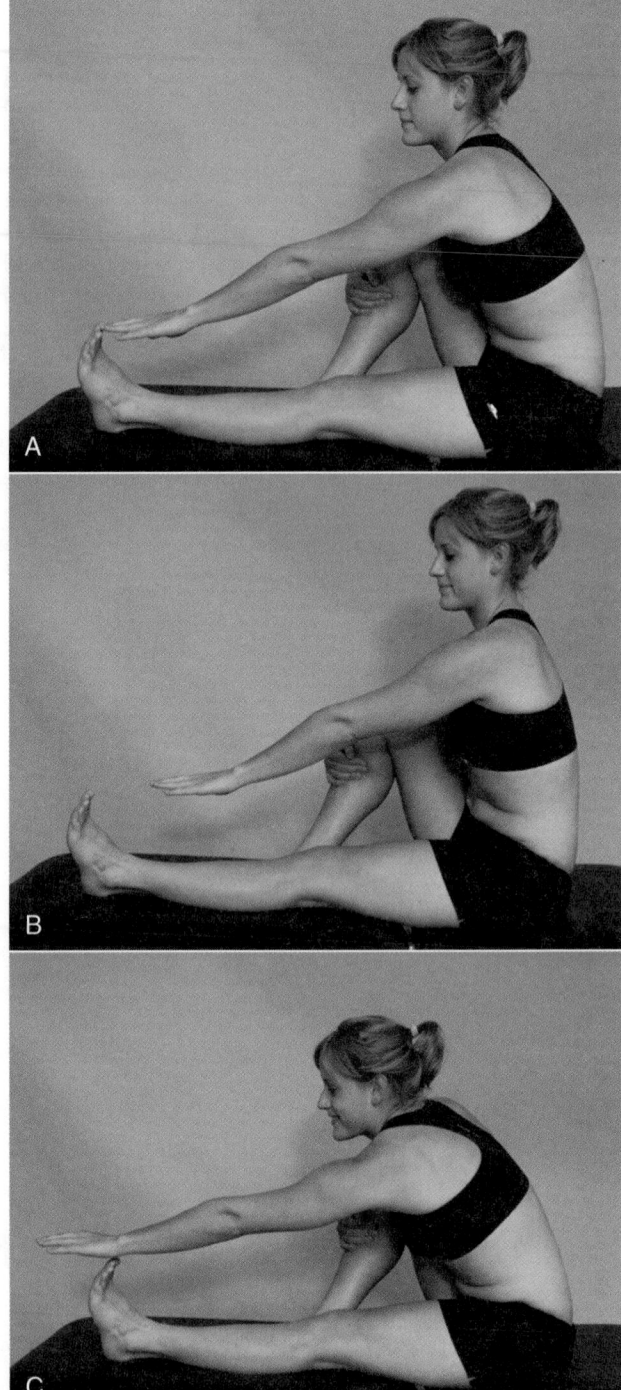

Figure 11-54 Test for hamstring tightness (method 2). A, Negative test. **B,** Positive test. **C,** Hypermobility of hamstrings.

is normal. If the ASIS moves up before the thigh reaches the trunk, gluteus maximus is tight. Both sides should be compared.

Janda[31,32] has reported that the gluteus maximus, medius, and minimus are more likely to be weak than tight. To test gluteus maximus strength, the patient is placed in prone with the hip straight and the knee flexed to 90°. The patient is asked to extend the hip, keeping

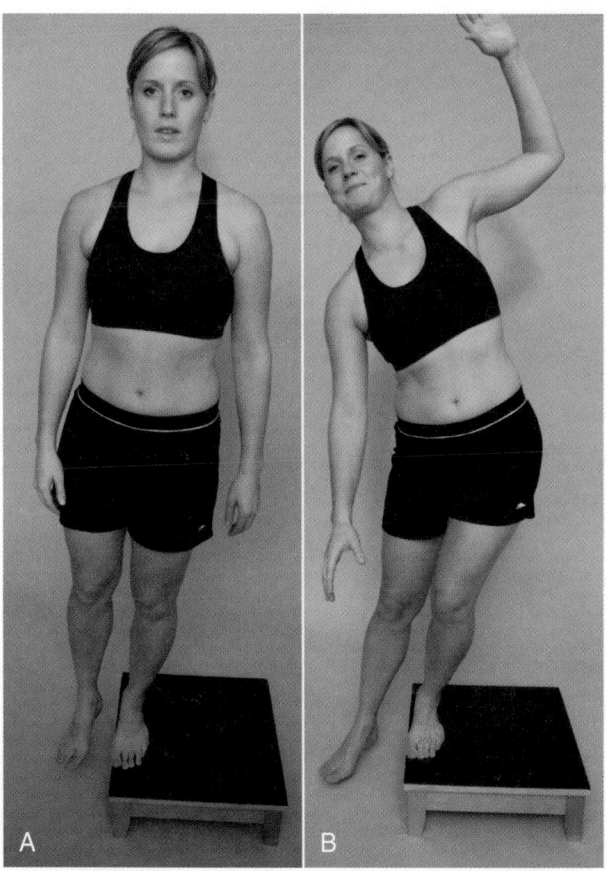

Figure 11-55 Lateral step down maneuver (pelvic drop test). **A,** Normal (negative test). **B,** Positive test.

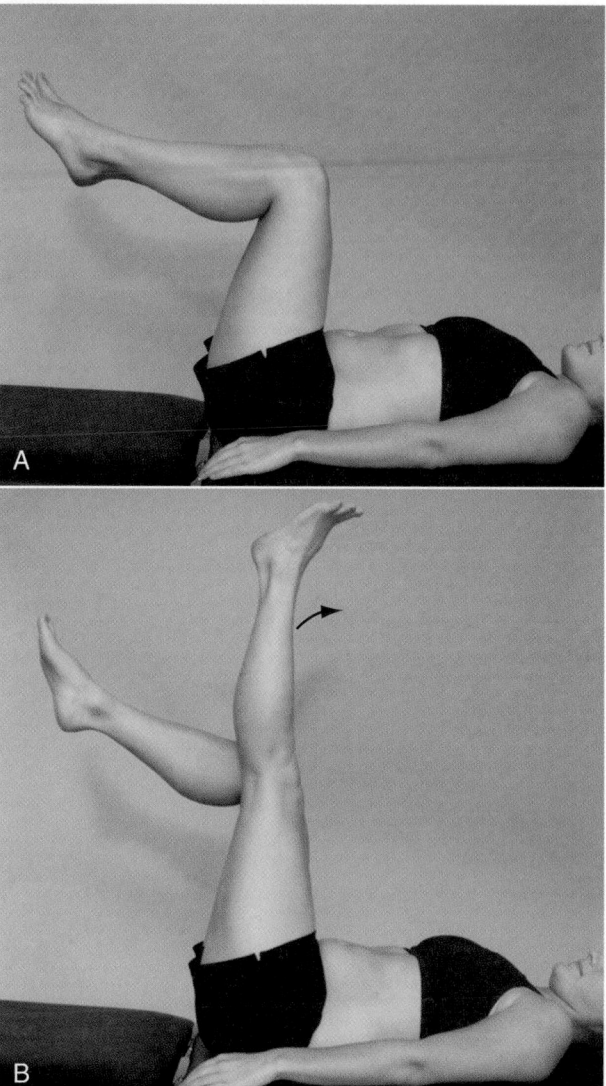

Figure 11-56 The 90–90 straight leg raising test. A, Start position. **B,** End position. Knee angle is measured to show any limitation.

the knee flexed while the examiner applies an anterior force to the posterior thigh. Both legs are tested (good side first) and compared. If the patient attempts to further flex the knee when doing the test, it indicates greater use of hamstrings is occurring. To test the strength of gluteus medius and minimus, the patient is positioned in side lying. The examiner stabilizes the pelvis and asks the patient to abduct the leg against the examiner's resistance applied to the lateral aspect of the thigh (Figure 11-58). Both legs are tested (good side first) and compared.

Noble Compression Test. This test is used to determine whether iliotibial band friction syndrome exists near the knee (Figure 11-59).[146] This syndrome is a chronic inflammation of the iliotibial band near its insertion, adjacent to the femoral condyle. The patient lies supine, and the knee is flexed to 90° accompanied by hip flexion. The examiner then applies pressure with the thumb to the lateral femoral epicondyle or 1 to 2 cm (0.4 to 0.8 inch) proximal to it. While the pressure is maintained, the patient slowly extends the knee. At approximately 30° of flexion (0° being a straight leg), if the patient complains of severe pain over the lateral femoral condyle, a positive test is indicated. The patient usually says it is the same pain that accompanies the patient's activity (e.g., running).

Ober's Test. Ober's test assesses the tensor fasciae latae (iliotibial band) for contracture (Figure 11-60).[147,148] The patient is in the side lying position with the lower leg flexed at the hip and knee for stability. The examiner then passively abducts and extends the patient's upper leg with the knee straight or flexed to 90°. The examiner slowly lowers the upper limb; if a contracture is present, the leg remains abducted and does not fall to the table. When doing this test, it is important to extend the hip slightly so that the iliotibial band passes over the greater trochanter of the femur. To do this, the examiner stabilizes the pelvis at the same time to stop the pelvis from "falling backward." Ober[147] originally described the test with the knee flexed. However, the iliotibial band has a greater stretch placed on it when the knee is extended. Also, when the knee is flexed during the test, greater stress is placed on the femoral nerve. If neurological

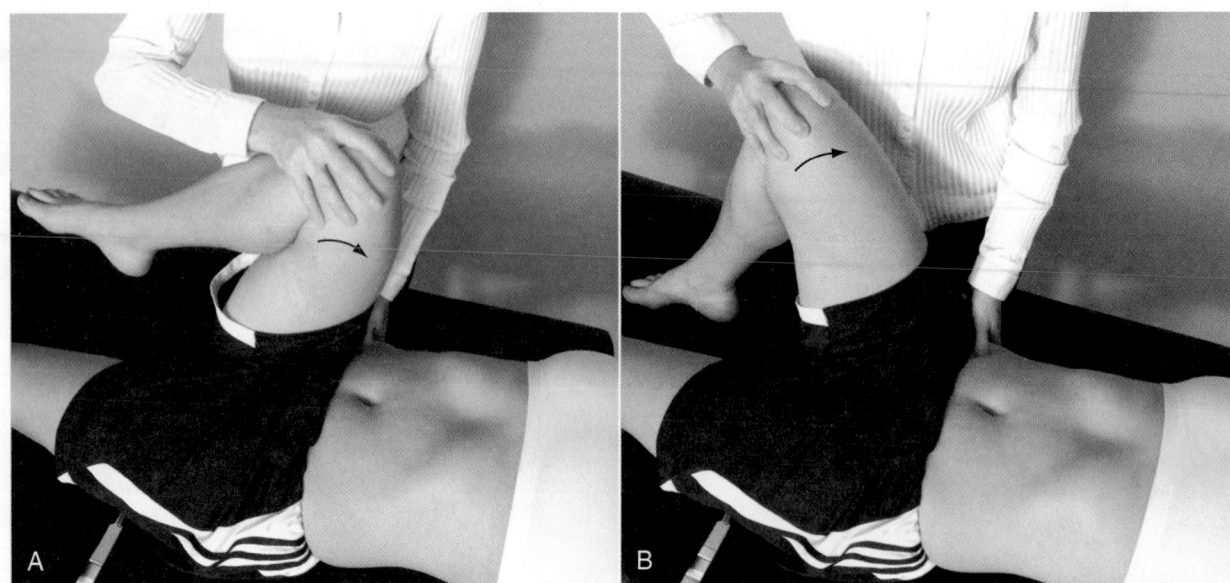

Figure 11-57 Testing for length of gluteus maximus. A, Negative test. **B,** Positive test.

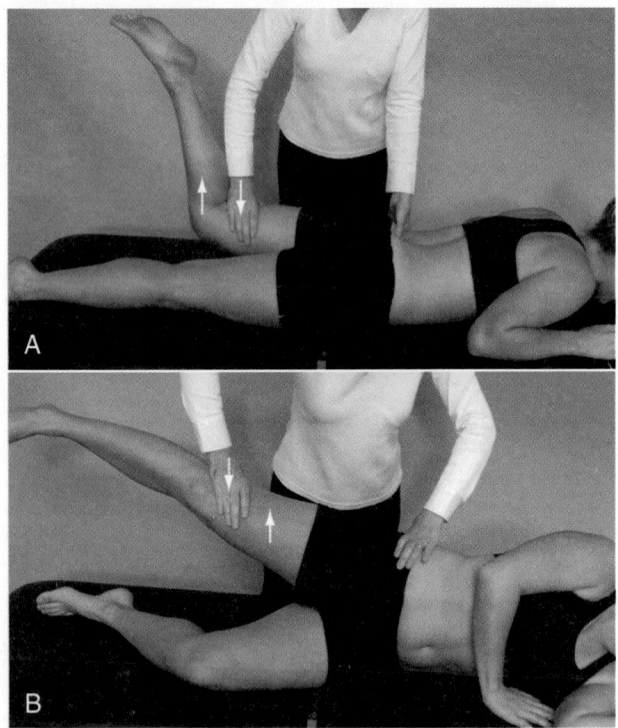

Figure 11-58 Testing for weakness. A, Gluteus maximus. Note examiner is palpating iliac crest (posterior superior iliac spine [PSIS]) to ensure no movement. **B,** Gluteus medius and minimus. Note examiner is palpating iliac crest to ensure no movement.

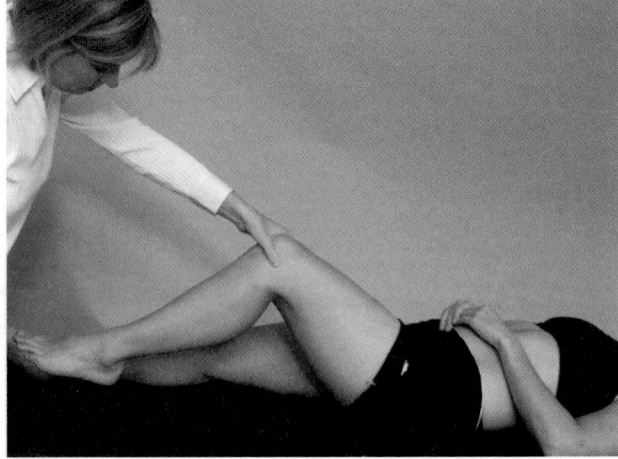

Figure 11-59 Noble compression test for iliotibial band friction syndrome. The patient extends the knee. The examiner is indicating where pain is felt at about 30° of flexion.

signs (i.e., pain, paresthesia) occur during the test, the examiner should consider pathology affecting the femoral nerve. Likewise, tenderness over the greater trochanter should lead the examiner to consider trochanteric bursitis.

Phelps' Test.[119] The patient lies prone with the knees extended. The examiner passively abducts both of the patient's legs as far as possible. The knees are then flexed to 90° (Figure 11-61), and the examiner tries to abduct the hips further. If abduction increases, the test is considered positive for contracture of the gracilis muscle.

Piriformis Test. In about 15% of the population, the sciatic nerve, all or in part, passes through the piriformis muscle rather than below it (Figures 11-62 and 11-63).[26] These people are more likely to suffer from this relatively rare condition, piriformis syndrome.[149] The patient is in the side lying position with the test leg uppermost. The patient flexes the test hip to 60° with the knee flexed. The examiner stabilizes the hip with one hand and applies a downward pressure to the knee (Figure 11-64). If the piriformis muscle is tight, pain is elicited in the muscle. If the piriformis muscle is pinching the sciatic nerve, pain results in the buttock and sciatica may be experienced by

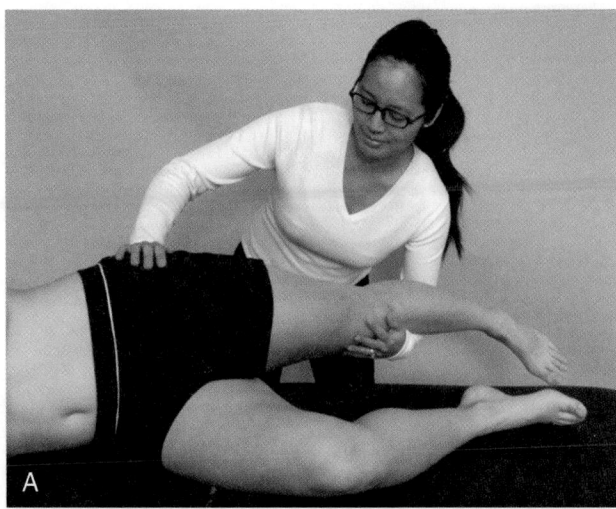

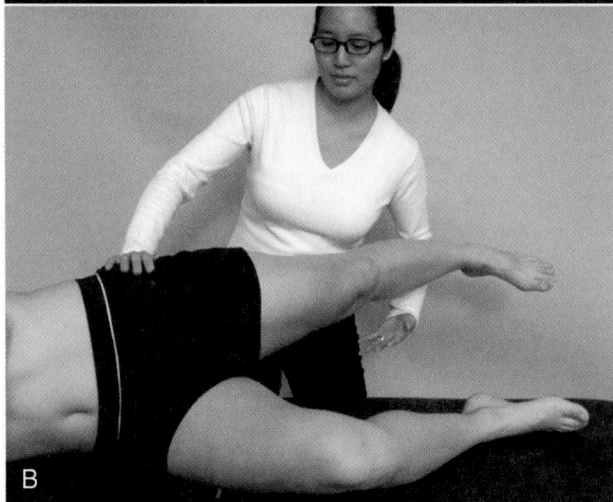

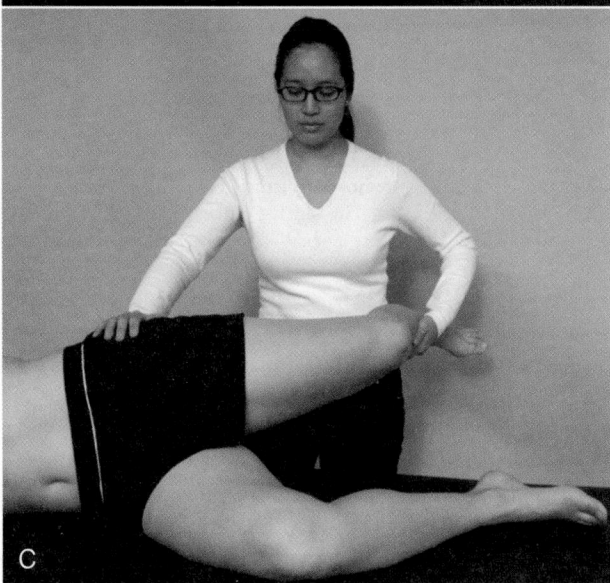

Figure 11-60 Ober's test. A, Knee straight. **B,** The hip is passively extended by the examiner to ensure that the tensor fasciae latae runs over the greater trochanter. A positive test is indicated when the leg remains abducted while the patient's muscles are relaxed. **C,** Test done with the knee flexed.

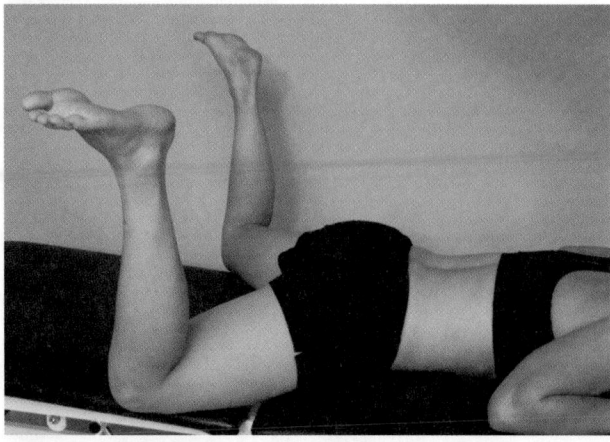

Figure 11-61 Phelps' test. Hips are abducted and knees are flexed to 90°. If abduction increases with knee flexion, the test is positive.

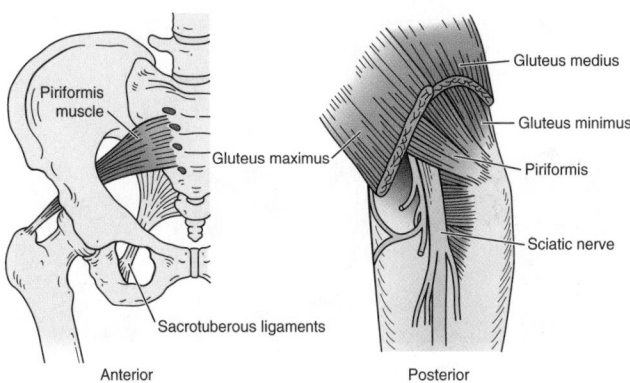

Figure 11-62 Position of the piriformis muscle. (Redrawn from Norris C: Sports injuries: diagnosis and management, ed 3, London, 2004, Butterworth-Heinemann, p. 205.)

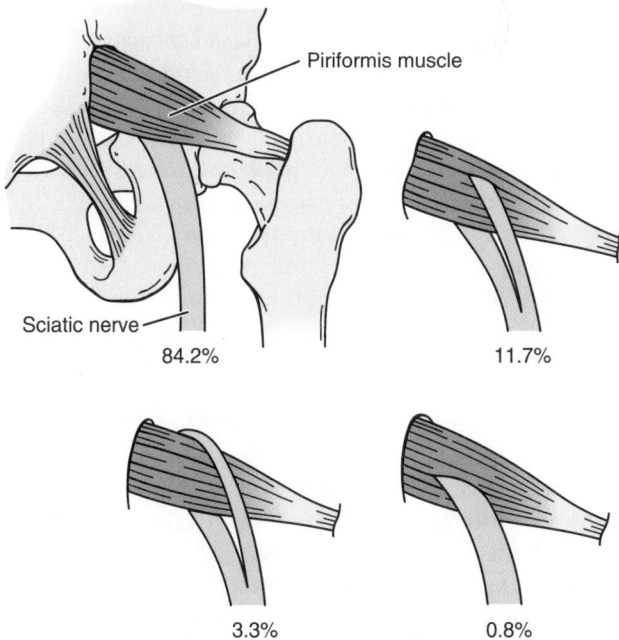

Figure 11-63 Sciatic nerve: Variations in its relationship with the piriformis muscle. (Redrawn from Levin P: Hip dislocations. In Browner BD, et al, editors: Skeletal trauma, Philadelphia, 1992, WB Saunders, p. 1333.)

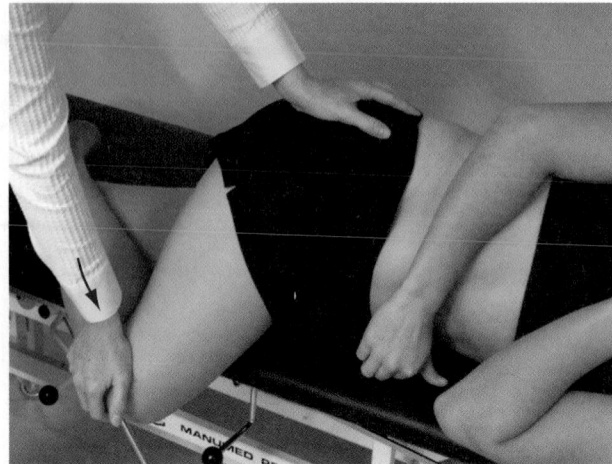

Figure 11-64 Piriformis test.

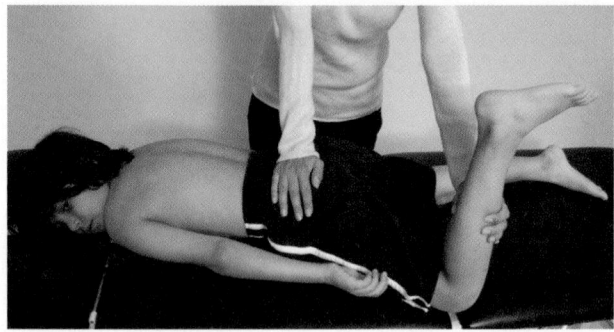

Figure 11-65 Prone lying test for iliotibial band contracture.

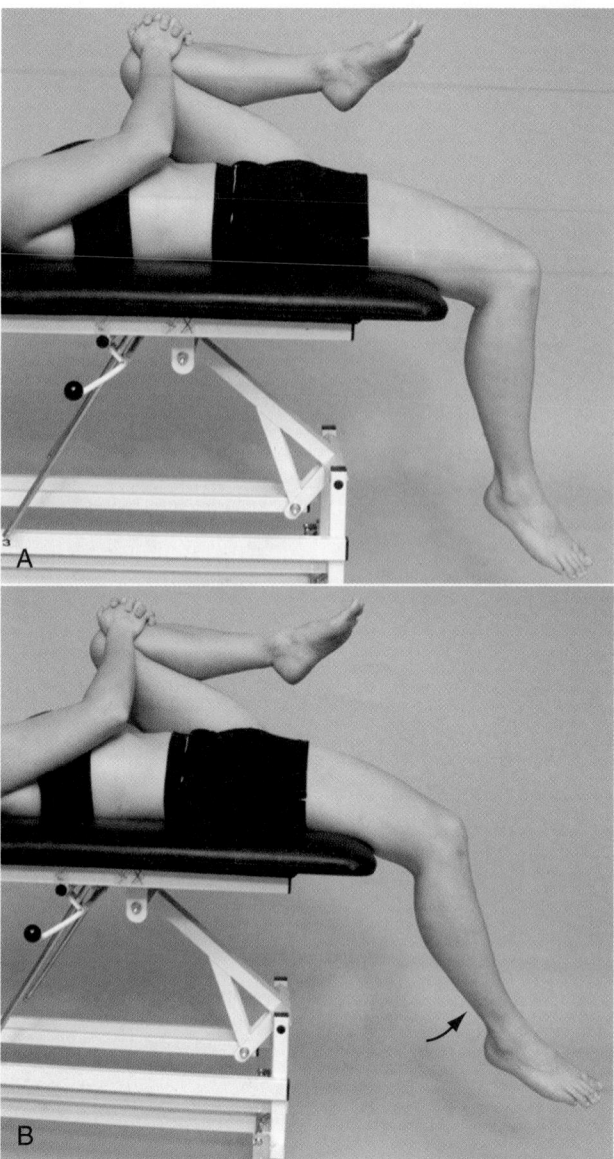

Figure 11-66 Rectus femoris contracture. **A,** The movement leg is brought to the chest. The test leg remains bent over the end of the examining table, indicating a negative test. **B,** The test knee extends, indicating a positive test.

the patient.[34,124] Resisted lateral rotation with the muscle on stretch (hip medially rotated) can cause the same sciatica.[150]

? *Prone Lying Test for Iliotibial Band Contracture.*[151] The patient lies prone while the examiner stands on the opposite side to the leg being tested. The examiner holds the ankle of the test leg and maximally abducts it at the hip, while the other hand applies pressure to the buttock on the same side as the test leg to flatten the pelvis and correct any hip flexion deformity (Figure 11-65). While maintaining the hip in neutral rotation and the knee flexed to 90°, the examiner then adducts the hip until there is a firm end feel. The angle is measured relative to the body's vertical axis and compared with the other side.[151] This test is more commonly done in children.

⚠ *Rectus Femoris Contracture Test (Kendall Test, Method 1).* The patient lies supine with the knees bent over the end or edge of the examining table. The patient flexes one knee onto the chest and holds it (Figure 11-66). The angle of the test knee should remain at 90° when the opposite knee is flexed to the chest. If it does not (i.e., the test knee extends slightly), a contracture is probably present. The examiner may attempt to passively flex the knee to see whether it remains at 90° of its own volition. The examiner should always palpate for muscle tightness when doing any contracture test. If there is no palpable

tightness, the probable cause of restriction is tight joint structures (e.g., the capsule) and the end feel will be different (muscle stretch versus capsular). The two sides should be tested and compared.

? *Sign of the Buttock.* The patient lies supine, and the examiner performs a straight leg raising test. If there is limitation on straight leg raising, the examiner flexes the patient's knee to see whether further hip flexion can be obtained. If hip flexion does not increase, the lesion is in the buttock or the hip, not the sciatic nerve or hamstring muscles. There may also be some limited trunk flexion. Causes of a positive test include ischial bursitis, a neoplasm, an abscess in the buttock, fracture, or hip pathology.

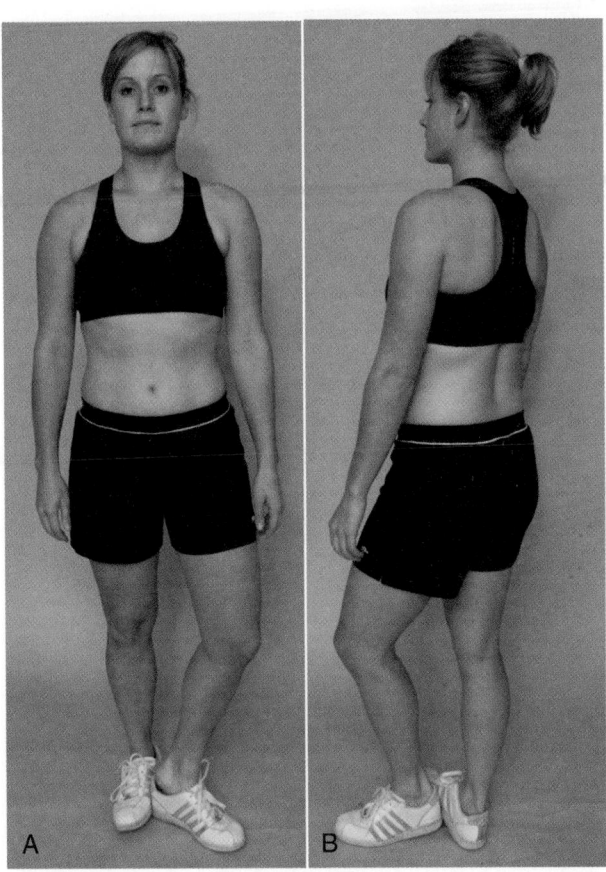

Figure 11-67 Patient doing the "taking off the shoe" test (TOST) test while standing. **A,** Anterior view. **B,** Posterior view.

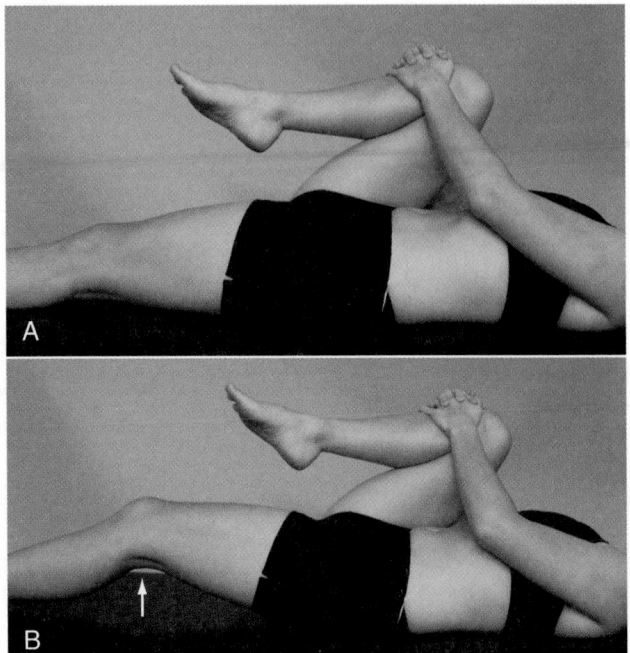

Figure 11-68 Thomas test. **A,** Negative test. **B,** Positive test.

❓ **_"Taking Off the Shoe" Test._**[152] For the "taking off the shoe" test (TOST), the patient stands wearing shoes. The patient is asked to remove the shoe on the affected side with the help of the shoe on the opposite side (Figure 11-67) by putting the heel of the affected side into the medial longitudinal arch of the stance (good) leg to pry the shoe off. In this position, the affected hip is laterally rotated about 90° with 20° to 25° flexion at the knee, leading to contraction of the biceps femoris on the affected side. If a sharp pain is felt in the biceps femoris, it indicates a 1° or 2° muscle strain.

⚠ **_Thomas Test._** The Thomas test is used to assess a hip flexion contracture, the most common contracture of the hip. The patient lies supine while the examiner checks for excessive lordosis, which is usually present with tight hip flexors. The examiner flexes one of the patient's hips, bringing the knee to the chest to flatten out the lumbar spine and to stabilize the pelvis. The patient holds the flexed hip against the chest. If there is no flexion contracture, the hip being tested (the straight leg) remains on the examining table. If a contracture is present, the patient's straight leg rises off the table and a muscle stretch end feel will be felt (Figure 11-68). The angle of contracture can be measured. If the lower limb is pushed down onto the table, the patient may exhibit an increased lordosis; again, this result indicates a positive test. When doing the test, if measurements are taken, the examiner must be sure the restriction is in the hip and not the pelvis or lumbar spine.[153] If the leg does not lift off the table but abducts as the other leg is flexed to the chest, it is called the **"J" sign** or **stroke** and is indicative of a tight iliotibial band on the extended leg side.

⚠ **_Tightness of Hip Rotators._** The medial and lateral hip rotators can be tested by placing the patient in supine lying with the hip and knee flexed to 90°. To test for tightness of the lateral rotators, the patient is asked to medially rotate the hip by rotating the leg outward (Figure 11-69, _A_). If the lateral rotators are tight, medial rotation is less than 30° to 40°, and the end feel is muscle stretch rather than tissue (capsular) stretch. To test for tightness of the medial rotators, the patient is asked to laterally rotate the hip by rotating the leg inward (Figure 11-69, _B_). If the medial rotators are tight, lateral rotation is less than 40° to 60°, and the end feel is muscle stretch rather than tissue (capsular) stretch.

✓ **_Trendelenburg Sign._**[154] This test assesses the stability of the hip and the ability of the hip abductors to stabilize the pelvis on the femur. The patient is asked to stand on one lower limb. Normally, the pelvis on the opposite side should rise; this finding indicates a negative test (Figure 11-70). If the pelvis on the opposite side (non-stance side) drops when the patient stands on the affected leg, a positive test is indicated. The test should always be performed on the normal side first so that the patient understands what to do. If the pelvis drops on the opposite side, it indicates a weak gluteus medius or an unstable hip (e.g., as a result of hip dislocation) on the affected or

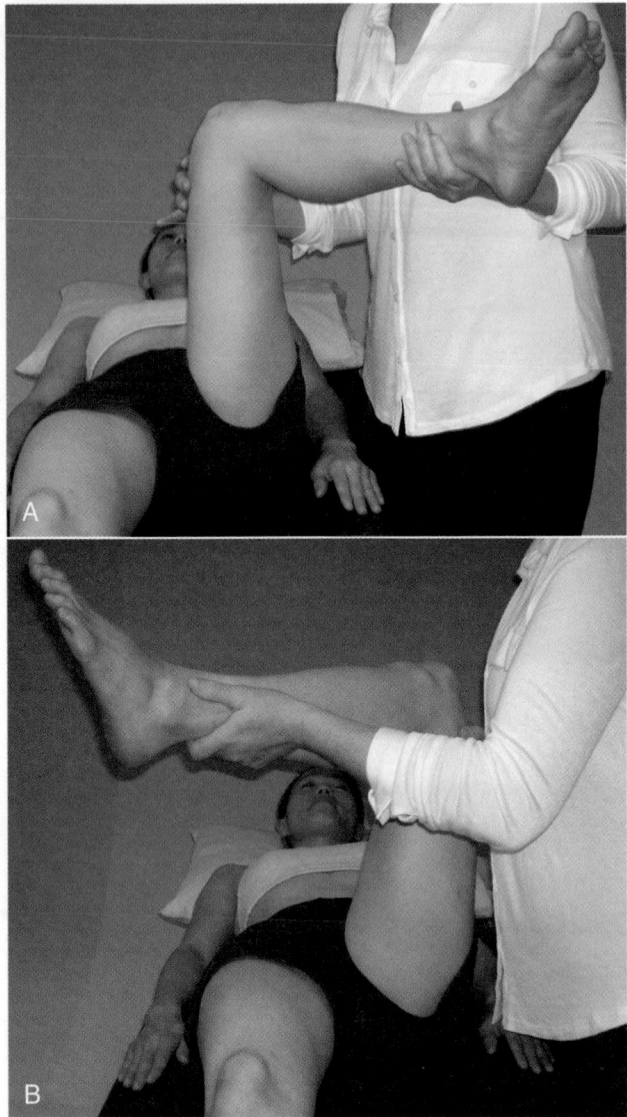

Figure 11-69 A, Testing for tightness of the lateral rotators. **B,** Testing for tightness of the medial rotators.

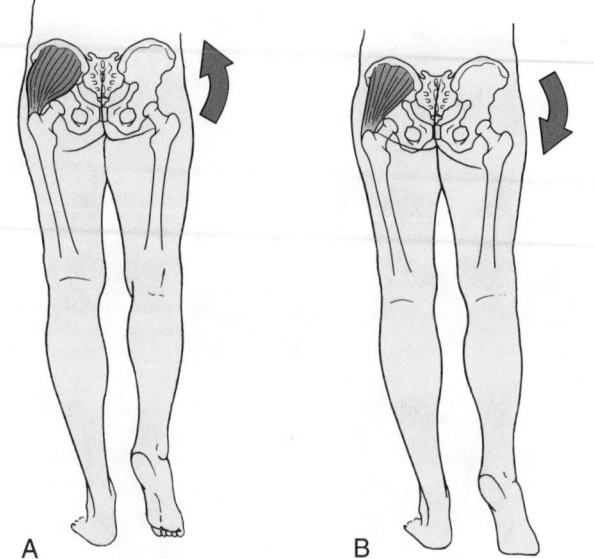

Figure 11-70 Trendelenburg sign. A, Negative test. **B,** Positive test.

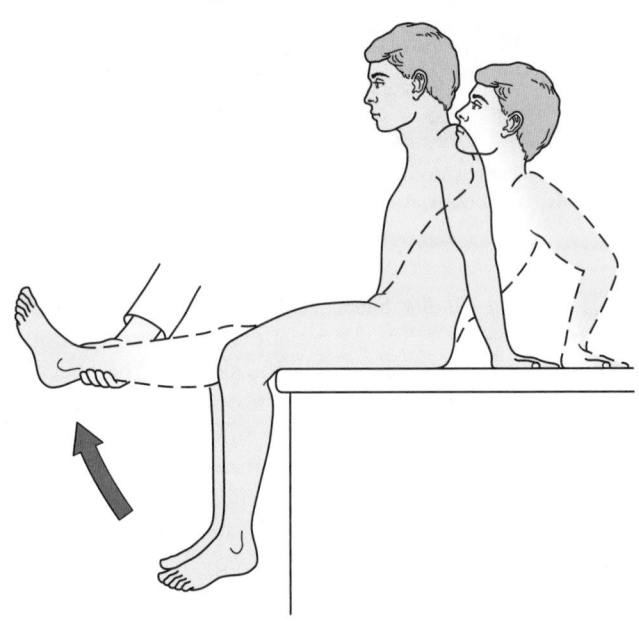

Figure 11-71 Tripod sign.

stance side. To add difficulty to the test and to test overall stability of the hip and pelvis, the patient may be asked to do a **single leg squat.** The normal result should be the same as a negative Trendelenburg test.[155]

🔹 *Tripod Sign (Hamstrings Contracture, Method 3).* The patient is seated with both knees flexed to 90° over the edge of the examining table (Figure 11-71).[156] The examiner then passively extends one knee. If the hamstring muscles on that side are tight, the patient extends the trunk to relieve the tension in the hamstring muscles. The leg is returned to its starting position, and the other leg is tested and compared with the first side. Extension of the spine is indicative of a positive test. The examiner must be aware that nerve root problems (stretching of the sciatic nerve) can cause a similar positive sign, although the symptoms will be slightly different.

Other Tests

⚠️ *Timed "Up and Go" Test.* For the TUG test, the patient sits in an armchair (seat height: 45 cm/17.7 inches). From this position, the patient is asked to rise on the command "ready-go" and walks 3 meters (9.8 feet) to a line on the floor, turns and returns to the same seated position while the examiner times the movement with a stopwatch. If the patient takes more than 24 seconds to complete the task, the test is considered positive as a predictor for falls within 6 months of a hip fracture surgery.[157]

Reflexes and Cutaneous Distribution

There are no reflexes around the hip that can be evaluated easily. However, the examiner should assess the normal dermatome patterns of the nerve roots (Figure 11-72) as well as the sensory distribution of the peripheral nerves (Figure 11-73). Because dermatomes vary from person to person, the accompanying diagrams are estimations only. Testing for altered sensation is performed by running the relaxed hands and fingers of the examiner over the pelvis and legs anteriorly, posteriorly, and laterally in a sensation scanning assessment. Any difference in sensation should be noted and can be mapped out more precisely using a pinwheel, pin, cotton batten, and/or small brush.

True hip pain is usually referred to the groin, but it may also be referred to the ankle, knee, lumbar spine, and sacroiliac joints (Figure 11-74). In children with hip problems (e.g., slipped capital femoral epiphysis, Legg-Calvé-Perthes disease), sensory symptoms may be manifested only in the knee. Similarly, the knee, sacroiliac joints, and lumbar spine may refer pain to the hip. Table 11-11 illustrates muscles of the hip and their referral pattern if injured.

Peripheral Nerve Injuries about the Hip

Sciatic Nerve (L4 to S3). The sciatic nerve (Figure 11-75 and Table 11-12) may be injured anywhere along its path from the lumbosacral spine down the back of the leg to the knee. It is the most commonly injured nerve in the hip region.[158–160] If it is injured in the pelvis or upper femur area (e.g., posterior hip dislocation), the hamstrings and all muscles below the knee can be affected. The result is a high steppage gait with an inability to stand on the heel or toes. There is sensory alteration in the entire foot except the instep and medial malleolus, along with muscle atrophy. Usually, the symptoms are primarily in the common peroneal branch of the sciatic nerve. In the hip region, the sciatic nerve may be compressed by the piriformis muscle (piriformis syndrome) (see Figure 11-63).[161] If piriformis is affected, there is pain and weakness on abduction and lateral rotation of the hip (**sign of Pace and Nagel**). The pain on passive medial rotation of the extended hip (**Freiberg sign**) is also elicited, because this action stretches the piriformis.[162] Burning pain and hyperesthesia may be felt in the sacral and/or gluteal region as well as in the sciatic nerve distribution. Medial rotation with flexion of the hip accentuates the problem.

Superior Gluteal Nerve (L4 to S1). The superior gluteal nerve may be compressed as it passes between the piriformis and inferior border of the gluteus minimus muscle. It may also be injured during hip surgery.[159] The patient complains of acute gluteal pain that increases with ambulation. The hip is often medially rotated, and there is weakness of the hip abductors, resulting in a Trendelenburg gait. Tenderness may be palpated just lateral to the greater sciatic notch.

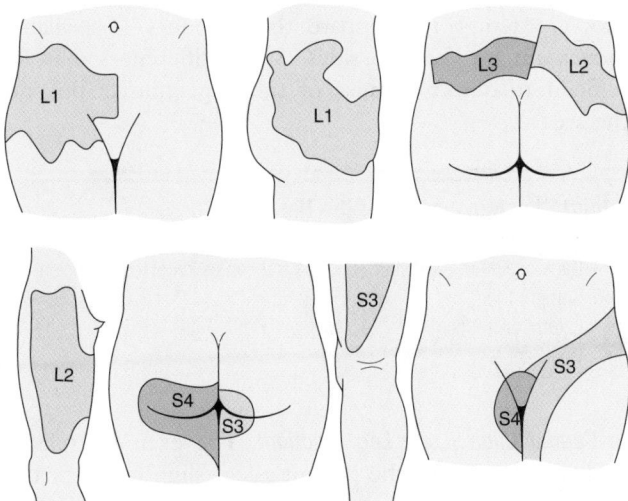

Figure 11-72 Dermatomes around the hip. Only one side is illustrated.

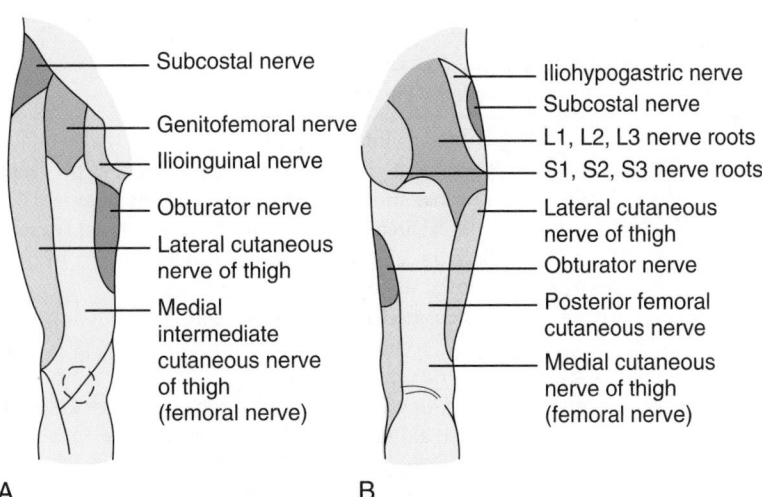

A   B

Figure 11-73 Sensory distribution of peripheral nerves around the hip. A, Anterior view. **B,** Posterior view.

Femoral Nerve (L2 to L4). The femoral nerve (Figure 11-76), although not commonly injured, may be compressed during childbirth or with anterior dislocation of the femur or may be traumatized during hernia surgery, stripping of varicose veins, hip surgery, or fractures.[159] The patient is not able to flex the thigh on the trunk or extend the knee. The deep tendon knee reflex is also lost. Wasting of the quadriceps is most evident. Sensory loss includes the medial aspect of the distal thigh (**anterior femoral cutaneous nerve**) and the medial aspect of the leg and foot (**saphenous nerve**).

Obturator Nerve (L2 to L4). The obturator nerve (Figure 11-77) may be compressed as it leaves the pelvis and enters the leg in the obturator tunnel. Injury to the nerve may be caused by pelvic or hip surgery, pregnancy (obstetric palsy), fractures, or tumors and has been reported as a cause of groin pain in athletes.[159,161,163] Because the obturator nerve controls primarily the adductors, hip adduction is affected, as are knee flexion (gracilis) and hip lateral rotation (obturator externus). Sensory deficit is small, involving a small area in the middle medial part of the thigh, although the patient may complain of pain from the symphysis pubis to the medial aspect of the knee.

Joint Play Movements

The joint play movements (Figure 11-78) are completed with the patient in the supine position. The examiner should attempt to compare the amounts of available movement on the two sides. Small differences may be difficult to detect because of the large muscle bulk in the area.

Joint Play Movements of the Hip

- Caudal glide of the femur (long leg traction or long-axis extension)
- Compression
- Lateral distraction
- Quadrant test

Caudal Glide (Long Leg Traction). The examiner places both hands around the patient's leg, slightly above the

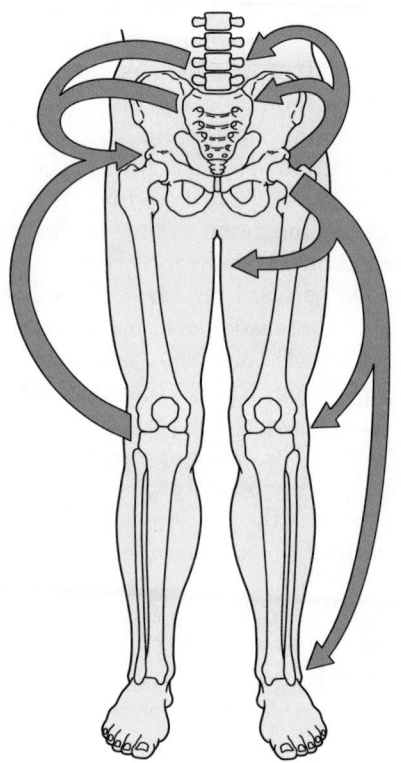

Figure 11-74 Referred pain around the hip. Right side demonstrates referral to the hip. Left side shows referral from hip.

TABLE **11-11**

Hip Muscles and Referral of Pain

Muscle	Referral Pattern
Iliopsoas	Lateral to lumbar spine, anterior thigh
Gluteus maximus	Sacral and gluteal area to lateral aspect of pelvis and posterosuperior thigh
Gluteus medius	Lumbar and sacral gluteal area to lateral aspect of pelvis and upper thigh
Gluteus minimus	Gluteal area to area below iliac crest down lateral aspect of thigh and leg
Piriformis	Sacrum, gluteal area down posterior aspect of thigh
Tensor fasciae latae	Lateral thigh
Sartorius	Anteromedial thigh (along course of muscle)
Pectineus	Groin to upper medial thigh
Rectus femoris	Anterior thigh to knee
Adductor longus and brevis	Anterior thigh to medial thigh to anterior knee to anteromedial leg to ankle
Adductor magnus	Groin along medial thigh to above knee
Gracilis	Anteromedial thigh to knee
Hamstrings	Gluteal area along posterior thigh to knee and posteromedial calf

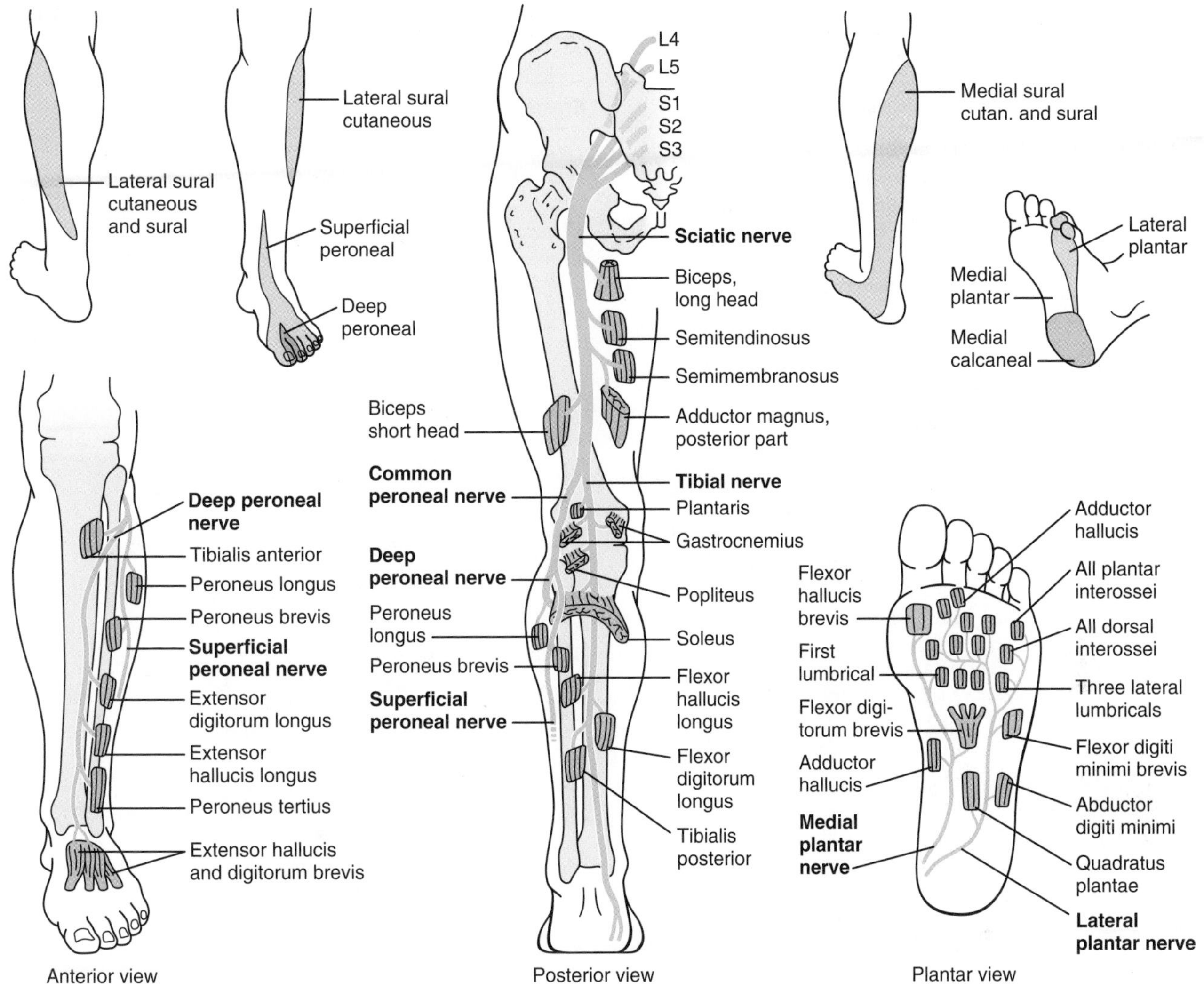
Lateral sural cutaneous and sural
Lateral sural cutaneous
Superficial peroneal
Deep peroneal
L4
L5
S1
S2
S3
Sciatic nerve
Biceps, long head
Semitendinosus
Semimembranosus
Adductor magnus, posterior part
Biceps short head
Common peroneal nerve
Tibial nerve
Plantaris
Gastrocnemius
Deep peroneal nerve
Popliteus
Peroneus longus
Soleus
Peroneus brevis
Superficial peroneal nerve
Flexor hallucis longus
Flexor digitorum longus
Tibialis posterior
Medial sural cutan. and sural
Lateral plantar
Medial plantar
Medial calcaneal
Deep peroneal nerve
Tibialis anterior
Peroneus longus
Peroneus brevis
Superficial peroneal nerve
Extensor digitorum longus
Extensor hallucis longus
Peroneus tertius
Extensor hallucis and digitorum brevis
Flexor hallucis brevis
First lumbrical
Flexor digi-torum brevis
Adductor hallucis
Medial plantar nerve
Adductor hallucis
All plantar interossei
All dorsal interossei
Three lateral lumbricals
Flexor digiti minimi brevis
Abductor digiti minimi
Quadratus plantae
Lateral plantar nerve
Anterior view
Posterior view
Plantar view

Figure 11-75 Sciatic nerve.

ankle. The examiner then leans back, applying a long-axis extension (traction) to the entire lower limb. Part of the movement occurs in the knee. If one suspects some pathology in the knee or the knee is stiff, both hands should be placed around the thigh just proximal to the knee, and traction force should again be applied (see Figure 11-78, *A*). The first method enables the examiner to apply a greater force. During the movement, any telescoping or excessive movement occurring in the hip should be noted, since it may indicate an unstable joint.

Compression. The examiner places the patient's knee in the resting position and then applies a compressive force to the hip through the longitudinal axis of the femur by pushing through the femoral condyles (see Figure 11-78, *B*).

Lateral Distraction. The examiner applies a lateral distraction force to the hip by placing a wide strap around the leg as high up in the groin as possible. The strap is then wrapped around the examiner's buttocks. The examiner leans back, using the buttocks to apply the distraction force to the hip. The proximal hand is used to palpate the hip or greater trochanter movement, while the distal hand prevents abduction of the leg, and, hence, torque to the hip (see Figure 11-78, *C*).

Palpation

During palpation of the hip and associated muscles, the examiner should note any tenderness, temperature, muscle spasm, or other signs and symptoms that may indicate the source of pathology. Intra-articular pain in the hip is rarely palpable.[164]

Anterior Aspect

The following structures should be palpated anteriorly, as shown in Figure 11-79.

Iliac Crest, Greater Trochanter, and Anterior Superior Iliac Spine. The iliac crests are easily palpated and should be level. The crest should be palpated for any tenderness because several muscles insert into this structure. In athletes, a condition called a **"hip pointer"** may be located on the iliac crest. This occurs from a strain or contusion

TABLE **11-12**

Peripheral Nerve Injuries (Neuropathy) About the Hip

	Muscle Weakness	Sensory Alteration	Reflexes Affected
Sciatic nerve (L4 through S3)	Hamstrings Tibialis anterior Extensor digitorum longus Extensor digitorum brevis Extensor hallucis longus Peroneus tertius Peroneus longus Peroneus brevis Gastrocnemius Soleus Plantaris Tibialis posterior Flexor digitorum longus Flexor hallucis longus Flexor accessorius (quadratus plantae) Abductor digiti minimi Flexor digiti minimi Lumbricales Interossei Adductor hallucis Abductor hallucis Flexor digitorum brevis Flexor hallucis brevis	Posterior thigh and leg Whole foot except instep and medial malleolus	Medial hamstrings (L5–S1) Lateral hamstrings (S1–S2) Achilles (S1–S2) Tibialis posterior (L4–L5)
Superior gluteal nerve	Gluteus medius Gluteus minimus Tensor fasciae latae	None	None
Femoral nerve (L2 through L4)	Iliacus Psoas Sartorius Pectineus Quadriceps	Medial side of thigh and leg	Patellar (L3–L4)
Obturator nerve (L2 through L4)	Adductor brevis Adductor magnus Adductor longus Obturator externus Gracilis	Middle thigh on anterior aspect	None

of the muscles that insert into the crest. The iliac tubercle is felt during palpation along the lateral aspect of the crest. The examiner then moves anteriorly to the ASIS. The greater trochanter, located approximately 10 cm (4 inches) distal to the iliac tubercle of the iliac crest, is palpated next. If the examiner's thumbs are placed over each ASIS, the fingers will naturally lie along the lateral aspect of each thigh and the greater trochanter can be felt with the fingers on each side. If the trochanteric bursa is swollen, it may also be palpated over the greater trochanter.

Inguinal Ligament, Femoral Triangle, Hip Joint, and Symphysis Pubis. The examiner's fingers are placed on the ASIS. Palpation gently continues along the inguinal ligament to the pelvic tubercles (symphysis pubis) with the examiner noting any signs of pathology. The psoas bursa, if swollen, is usually palpable under the inguinal ligament at its midpoint. Moving distal to the inguinal ligament, the examiner palpates the femoral triangle, the boundaries of which are the inguinal ligament superiorly, the sartorius muscle laterally, and the adductor longus muscle medially (Figure 11-80). Within the femoral triangle, the examiner may palpate swollen lymph glands (Figure 11-81) and the femoral artery. The femoral nerve lies lateral to the artery and the femoral vein lies medial to it, but neither of these structures is easily palpated. At this stage, the examiner may decide to palpate for an inguinal hernia in the male. The head of the femur is then palpated. Although the hip joint is deep and not easily palpable, the surrounding structures may show signs of pathology. The head of the femur is 1 to 2 cm (0.4 to 0.8 inch) below the middle third of the inguinal ligament and is found on a

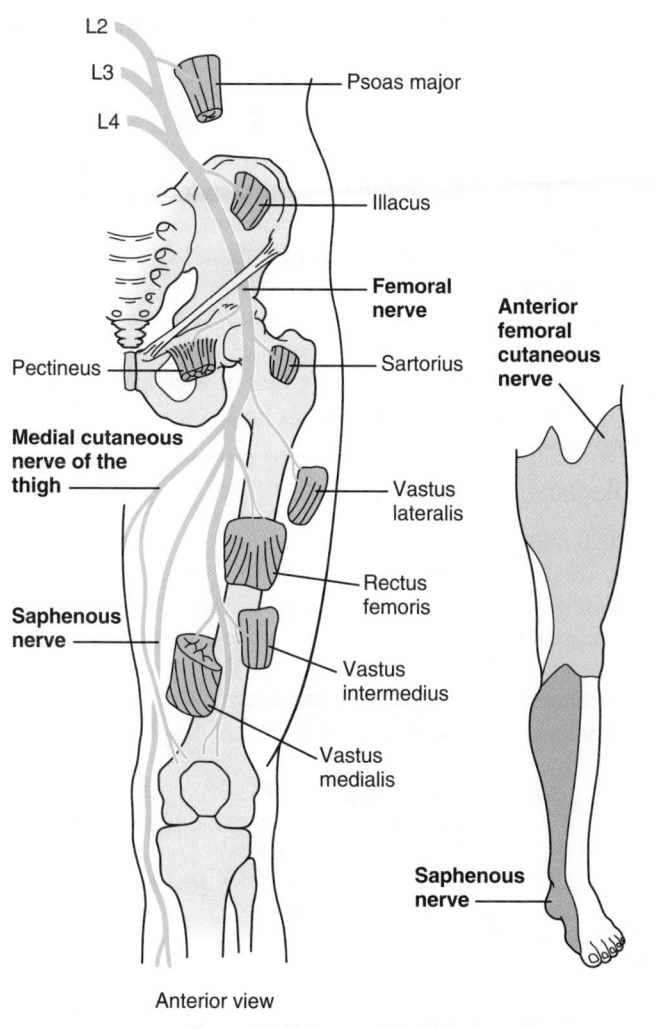

Figure 11-76 Femoral nerve.

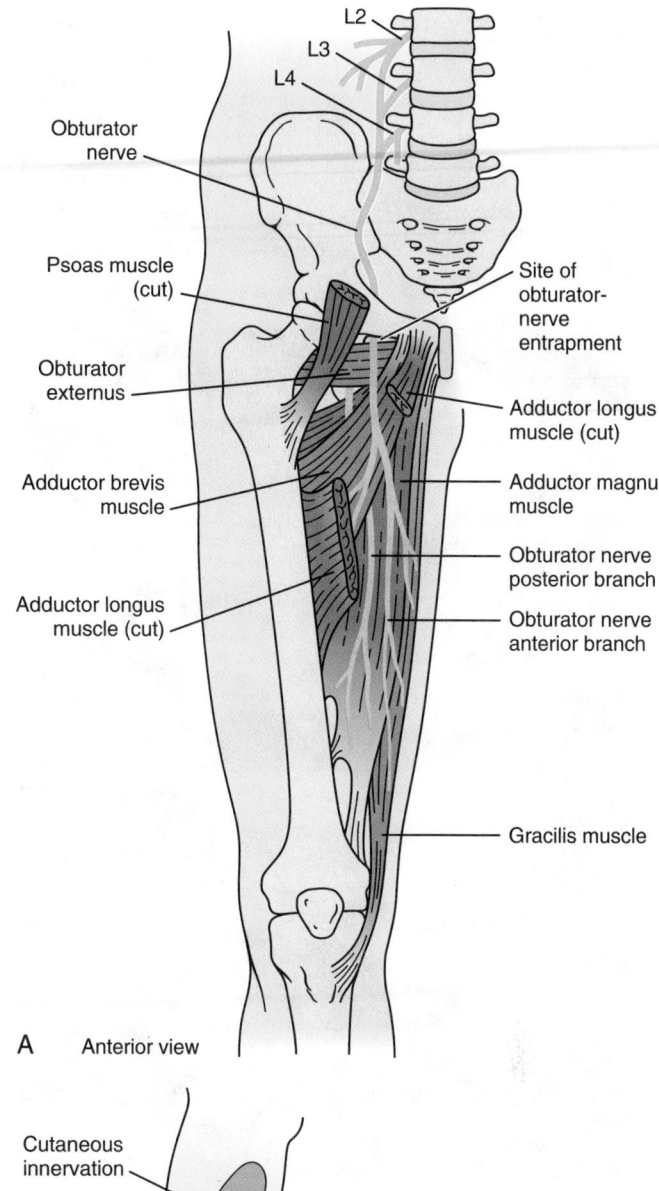

horizontal line running halfway between the pubic tubercle and the greater trochanter.

The examiner concludes the anterior palpation by palpating the hip flexor, adductor, and abductor muscles for signs of pathology.

Posterior Aspect

The patient is then asked to lie in the prone position so that the following structures can be palpated posteriorly.

Iliac Crest, Posterior Superior Iliac Spine, Ischial Tuberosity, and Greater Trochanter. The examiner begins posterior palpation by following the iliac crests, which are easily palpable, posteriorly to the PSIS. On most patients, each PSIS is evident by the presence of overlying skin dimples. As the examiner moves caudally, the ischial tuberosities, which are approximately at the level of the gluteal folds, may be felt. If the ischial bursa is swollen, it is sometimes palpable over the ischial tuberosities. The tuberosities should also be palpated for possible tenderness of the hamstring muscle insertions. Laterally, the posterior

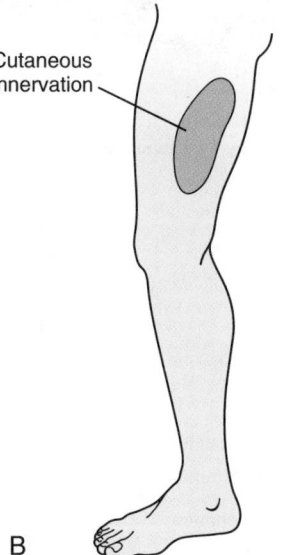

Figure 11-77 Obturator nerve. A, Anatomy of the obturator nerve. **B,** Cutaneous sensory distribution of the anterior branch of the obturator nerve.

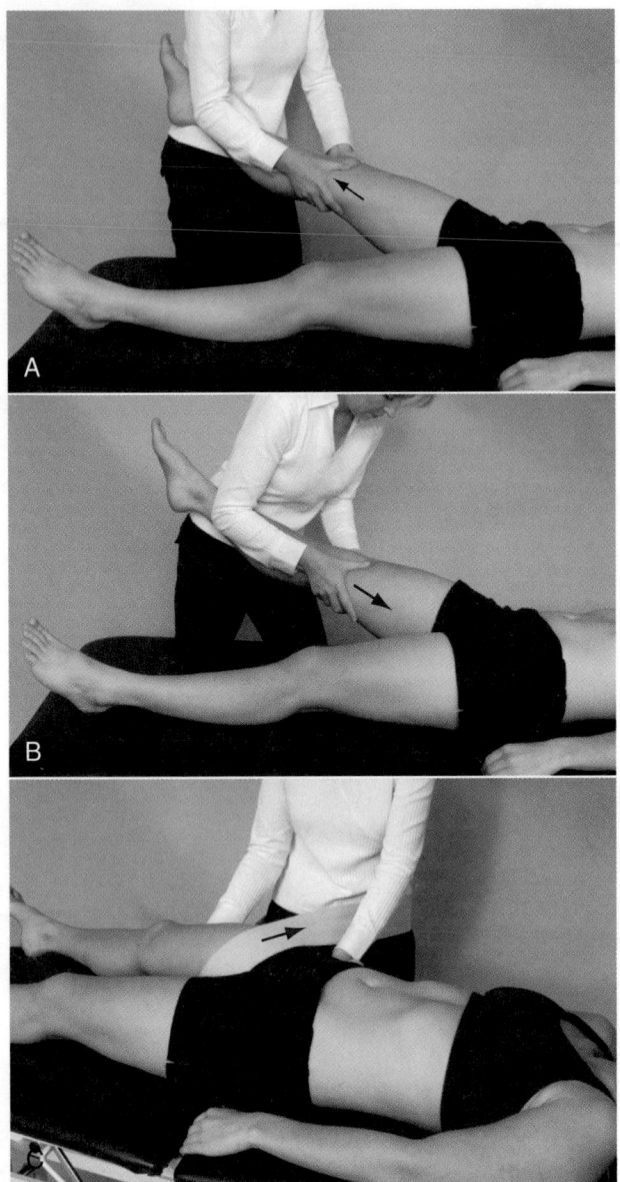

Figure 11-78 Joint play movements of the hip. A, Long leg traction (applied above the knee). **B,** Compression. **C,** Lateral distraction.

aspect of the greater trochanter is felt. If the distance between the ischial tuberosity and greater trochanter is divided in half, the fingers lie over the sciatic nerve as it enters the lower limb. Normally, the nerve is not palpable. The examiner then palpates upward from the midpoint to determine whether there is any tenderness of the hip lateral rotators, especially the piriformis muscle. In addition, the gluteal and hamstring muscle bellies should be palpated for signs of pathology.

Sacroiliac, Lumbosacral, and Sacrococcygeal Joints. If the examiner suspects pathology in these joints, they should be palpated. Detailed descriptions of their palpation are given in Chapters 9 and 10.

Diagnostic Imaging

Plain Film Radiography[165]

Normally, the standard views of the hip include anteroposterior views and axial or frog-leg views. The following box shows common x-rays views used for the hip.

Common X-Ray Views of the Hip Depending on Pathology

- Anteroposterior view of the hip (Figure 11-82)
- Lateral view (cross table, only affected hip) (see Figure 11-114)
- Lateral axial ("frog-leg") view (see Figure 11-117)
- Anteroposterior view of both hips and pelvis (see Figure 11-86)
- Anteroposterior oblique view (Figure 11-83)
- Anteroposterior internal (medial) rotation view

Anteroposterior View. The examiner should compare the two hips, noting the following features:

1. Neck-shaft angle, femoral head uncovering and head-tear drop distance (Figure 11-84): Abnormal head-neck offset (i.e., flattening of superior femoral head so that it is aspherical and flattening of the normal concave surface of the lateral femoral neck[166]) is called a **pistol grip deformity** (Figure 11-85;

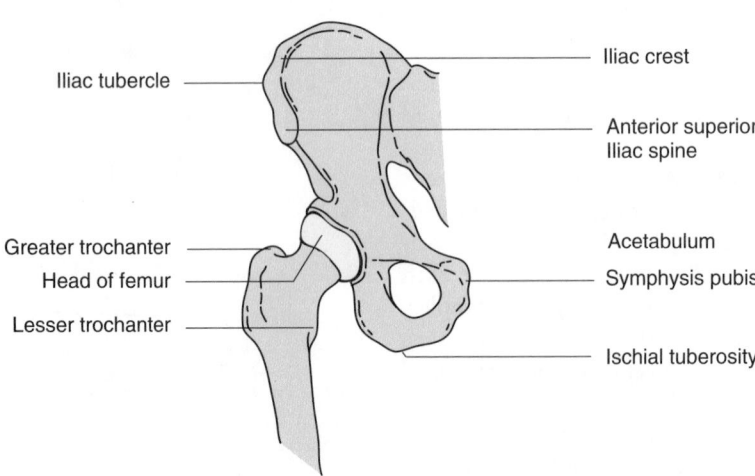

Figure 11-79 Landmarks of the hip (anterior view).

Iliac tubercle
Iliac crest
Anterior superior Iliac spine
Greater trochanter
Head of femur
Lesser trochanter
Acetabulum
Symphysis pubis
Ischial tuberosity

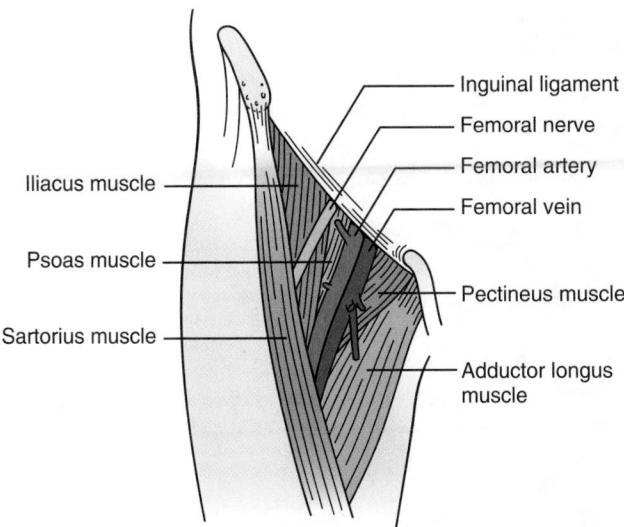

Figure 11-80 Femoral triangle containing the femoral artery, vein, and nerve. Note the inguinal ligament above, iliacus and psoas laterally, and adductors medially. The sartorius attaches to the anterosuperior spine, whereas the adductor muscles attach along the pubic ramus. (Modified from Anson BJ: *Atlas of human anatomy*, Philadelphia, 1963, WB Saunders, p. 583.)

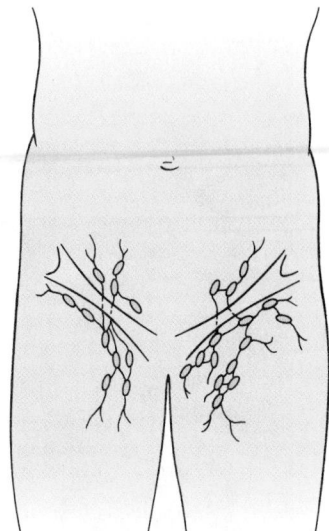

Figure 11-81 Lymph glands in the groin area.

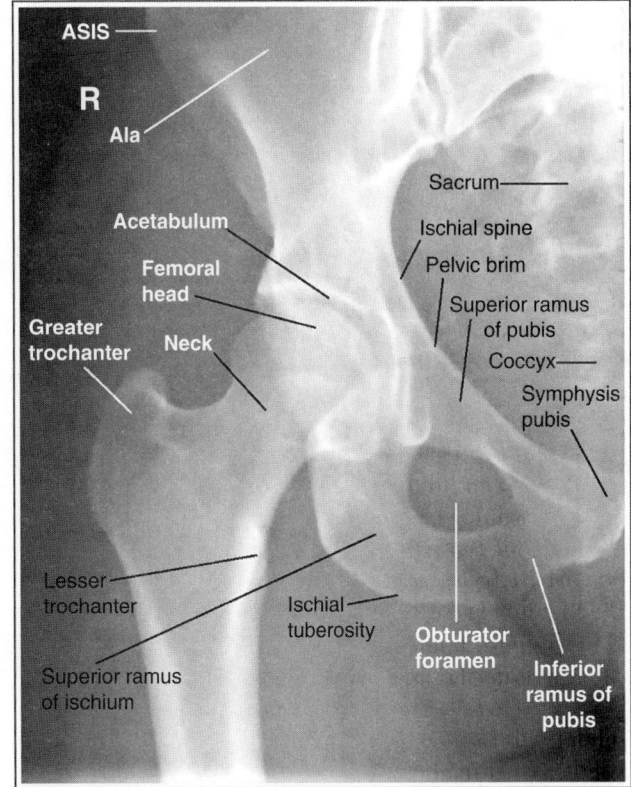

Figure 11-82 Anteroposterior view of the hip. (From McQuillen Martensen K: *Radiographic image analysis*, ed 3, St Louis, 2011, Saunders/Elsevier, p. 397.)

see Figure 11-103) and may be seen in femoroacetabular impingement, femoral head dysplasia, slipped capital femoral epiphysis, and Legg-Calvé-Perthes disease.[50,166]

2. Joint spaces and pelvic lines and other landmarks (Figures 11-86 and 11-87).
3. Is there any bone disease (i.e., Legg-Calvé-Perthes disease, bony cysts, or tumors; Figure 11-88)?
4. What is the neck-shaft angle?[167] The examiner should note whether the angle is normal or whether the patient exhibits a coxa vara or coxa valga (Figures 11-89 and 11-90).
5. What is the shape of the femoral head?[168] The femoral head is normally spherical but can show changes with DDH, Legg-Calvé-Perthes disease, slipped capital femoral epiphysis, and FAI.
6. The obturator foramen should be symmetrical.[165]
7. The distance from the symphysis pubis to the tip of the coccyx should be 1 to 3 cm (0.4 to 1.2 inches) (see Figure 10-71).[165]
8. Is coxa profunda (acetabular overcoverage) present (Figure 11-91)?
9. Is protrusio acetabuli, which occurs if the medial aspect of the femoral head is medial to the ilioschial line, present (Figure 11-92)?
10. Is the acetabulum anteverted (normal) or retroverted (see Figure 11-2, *B*)? A retroverted acetabulum is indicated by the "crossover sign" (Figure 11-93). Normally, the anterior wall should cover less of the femoral head than the posterior wall, which should be at the level of the center of the femoral head or lateral to it[59] (posterior wall sign). The crossover sign

or figure-eight sign occurs because the anterior aspect of the acetabular rim is more lateral than the posterior aspect of the acetabulum[56] (Figure 11-94). The posterior wall sign occurs when the posterior aspect of the acetabular rim is more medial than the center of the hip joint, and so there is less posterior coverage of the femoral head.[56]

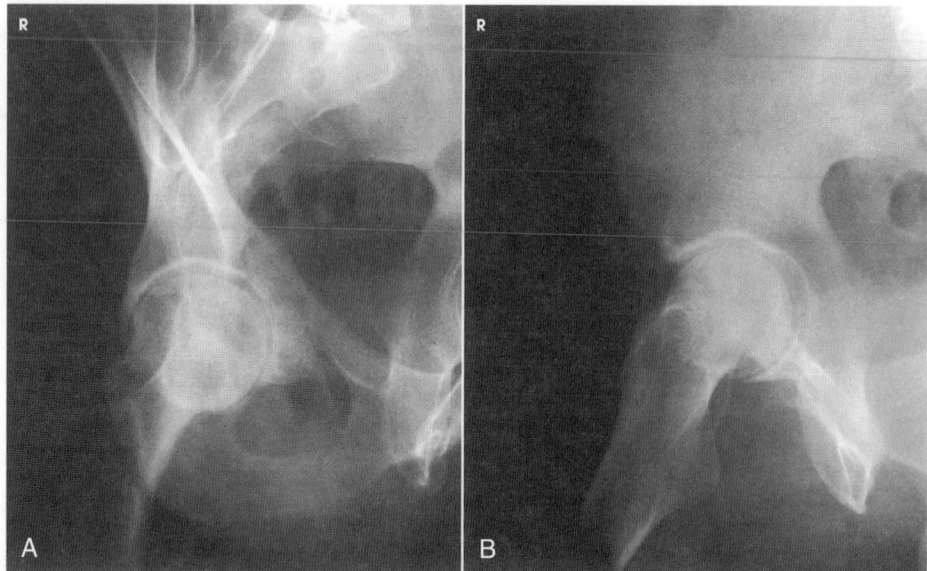

Figure 11-83 Anteroposterior oblique view of the hip (Judet method). A, Left posterior oblique. **B,** Right posterior oblique. (From Long BW, Rafert JA: Orthopedic radiography, Philadelphia, 1995, Saunders.)

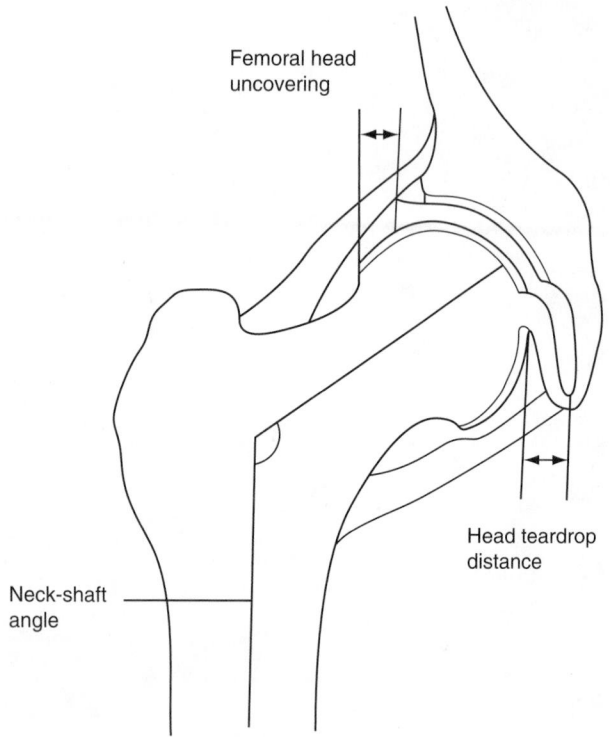

Figure 11-84 Three radiologic measurements of the hip. (From Richardson JK, Iglarsh ZA: Clinical orthopedic physical therapy, Philadelphia, 1994, WB Saunders, p. 358.)

11. Is the femoral head in the normal position? The distance from the femoral head to the ilioischeal line should be less than 10 mm (Figure 11-95).

12. Are the femoral head and acetabulum congruent (Figure 11-96)?

13. Are the femoral head and acetabulum normal on both sides? In development dysplasia of the hip, both structures may show dysplasia, and the **acetabular index** (Tonnis angle) on the affected side may be more than the normal 30° in the newborn (20° in 2-year olds). The acetabular index is determined by first drawing Hilgenreiner's line. An intersecting line is drawn from the lateral to the medial edge of the acetabulum, and the angle formed by the two lines is called the *acetabular index,* or **Hilgenreiner's angle** (Table 11-13). The greater the slope angle, the less stable the femoral head in the acetabulum. Figure 11-97 shows measurements that may be taken with DDH.

14. What is the femoral head extrusion index? Normal is about 25% (Figure 11-98).

15. Are there any osteophytes or arthritis (Figure 11-99)? Kellgren and Lawrence[169] have developed a radiographic grading scale for hip osteoarthritis (Table 11-14).

16. Whether **Shenton's line** is normal: Normally, Shenton's line is curved, drawn along the medial curved edge of the femur and continuing upward in a smooth arc along the inferior edge of the pubis (Figure 11-100). If the head of the femur is dislocated or fractured, two lines form two separate arcs, indicating a broken line. A broken Shenton's line is diagnostic of pathology.

17. The acetabular (Tonnis) angle or index should be between 0° and 10° in adults (Figure 11-101).

18. The lateral central edge angle is normally less than 25° (Figure 11-102): If the angle is less than 25°, it could indicate insufficient coverage of the femoral head.

19. Is there evidence of femoroacetabular impingement (Table 11-15; Figure 11-103)?

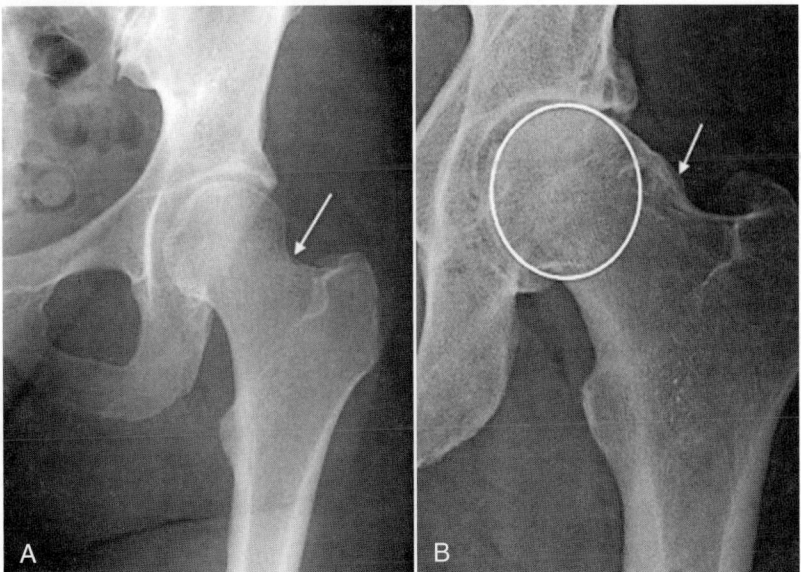

Figure 11-85 A, Normal frontal radiograph of hip shows concavity of femoral head and neck *(arrow).* **B,** Pistol grip deformity with abnormal extension of epiphyseal scar in a patient with cam impingement. (From Patel K, Wallace R, Busconi BD: Radiology. Clin Sports Med 30:254, 2011.)

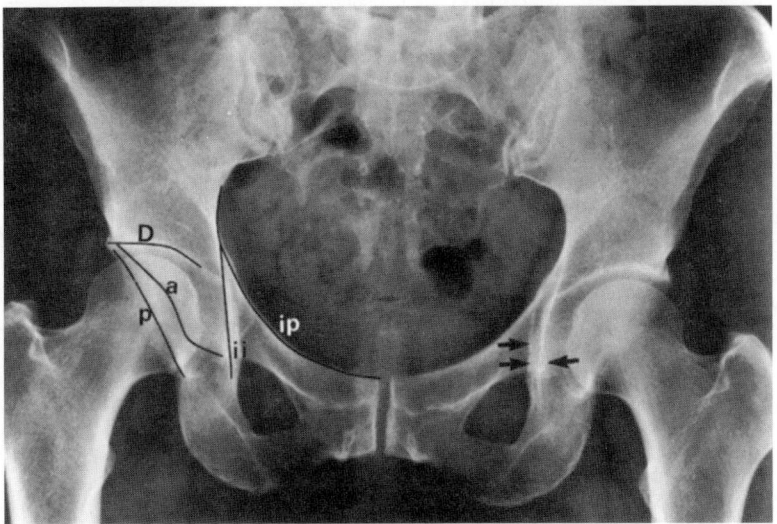

Figure 11-86 Pelvic lines. The iliopubic *(ip)* and ilioischial *(ii)* lines help in assessing the anterior and posterior columns. The acetabular dome *(D)* and anterior *(a)* and posterior *(p)* lips *(rims)* of the acetabulum are seen. The teardrop figure *(arrows)* is a composite shadow made up laterally of the anterior aspect of the acetabular fossa and medially of the quadrilateral surface of the ilium. The more posterior aspect of the quadrilateral surface *(represented by the ilioischial line)* is superimposed on the teardrop in this nonrotated view. (From Weissman BNW, Sledge CB: Orthopedic radiology, Philadelphia, 1986, WB Saunders, p. 343.)

20. Is there any evidence of fracture or dislocation (Figures 11-104 and 11-105)? Is the pelvic ring intact, or has it been disrupted? Disruption of the pelvic ring indicates a severe injury.
21. Is there evidence of pelvic distortion?
22. Are Hilgenreiner's and Perkins' lines within normal limits?[170] **Hilgenreiner's line** is horizontal, drawn between the inferior parts of the ilium. **Perkins' line** is vertical, drawn through the upper outer point of the acetabulum (Figure 11-106). Normally, the developing femoral head or ossification center of the femoral head lies in the inner distal quadrant formed by the two lines. If the ossification center lies in the upper outer quadrant, the finding is indicative of a dislocation or DDH.[131] In the newborn, the ossification center is not visible (Figure 11-107).

23. **"Sagging rope" sign:** With Legg-Calvé-Perthes disease, only the head of the femur is affected. If avascular necrosis of a developing femoral head occurs, the "sagging rope" sign may be seen (Figure 11-108). The sign indicates damage to the growth plate with marked metaphyseal reaction. Its presence indicates a severe disease process.

Text continued on p. 746

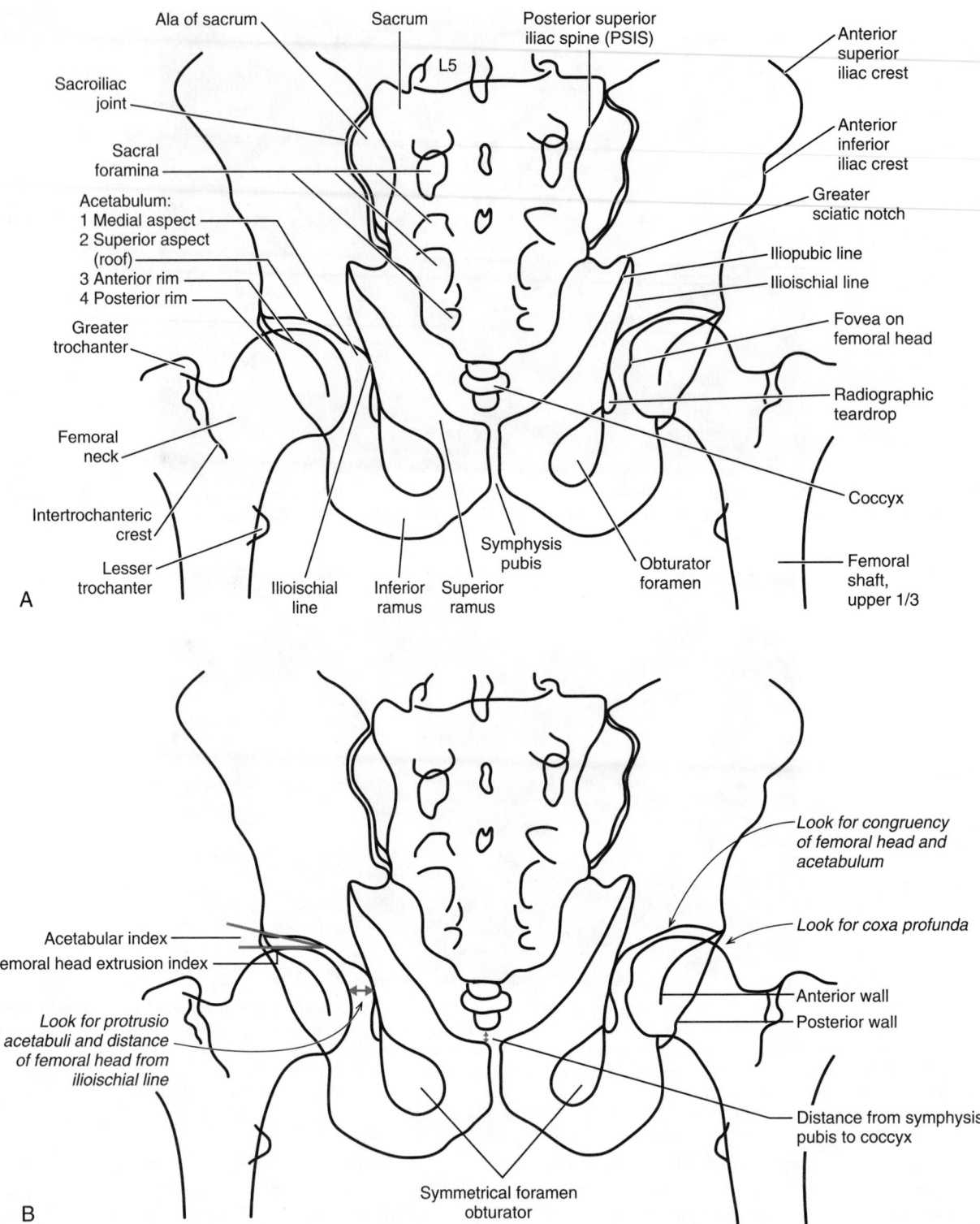

Figure 11-87 A, Tracing of anteroposterior radiograph of the pelvis. **B,** Measurements and things to look for on an anteroposterior radiograph. (Redrawn and modified from McKinnis LN: Fundamentals of musculoskeletal imaging, Philadelphia, 2005, FA Davis, p. 297.)

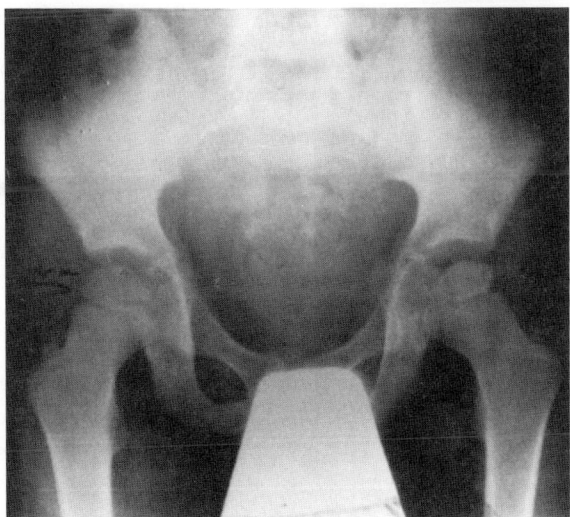

Figure 11-88 Legg-Calvé-Perthes disease of the left hip.

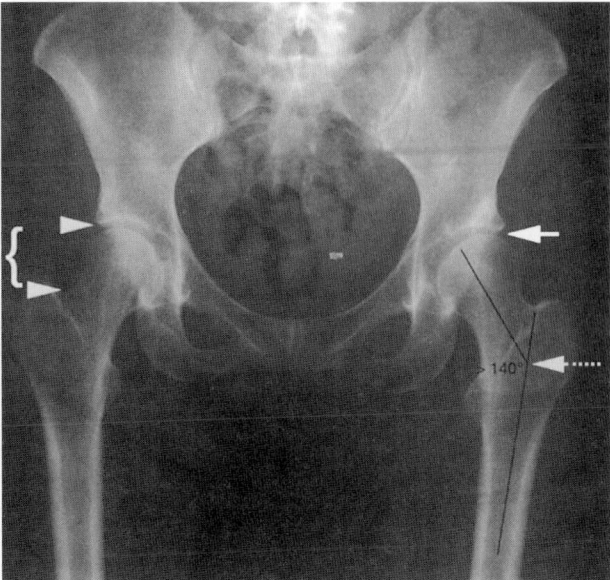

Figure 11-90 Anteroposterior view of an adult patient with a valgus alignment at the hip joint shows a neck-shaft angle that exceeds 140° *(white dotted arrow)*. Note also the increased portion of the articular aspect of the femoral head that is uncovered *(white arrow)*. This attribute becomes even more important if the superior aspect of the weight-bearing surface of the acetabulum is smaller than normal. In this patient, the trochanteric acetabular distance (the distance from a line drawn parallel to the superior aspect of the weight-bearing surface of the dome to a line parallel to the superior aspect of the tip of the greater trochanter) exceeds 2.5 cm *(arrowheads)*. Normally, the trochanteric acetabular distance in adults averages about 2.2 cm. (From Johnson TR, Steinbach LS: Essentials of musculoskeletal imaging, Rosemont, IL, 2004, American Academy of Orthopedic Surgeons, p. 457.)

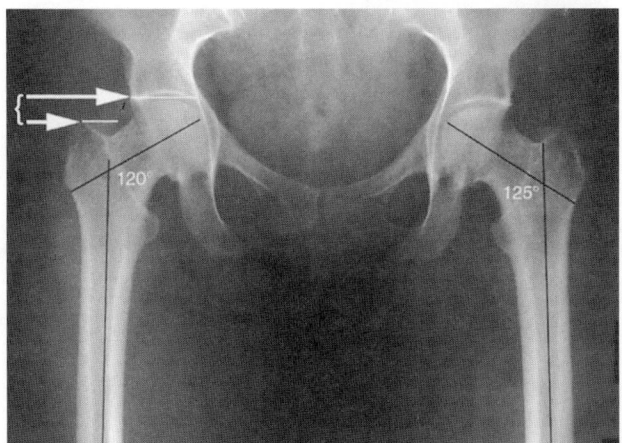

Figure 11-89 Anteroposterior view of the pelvis in an adult patient with coxa vara of the hip joint shows a neck-shaft angle of less than 125° and a decreased trochanteric acetabular distance *(white arrows)*. This configuration contributes to the potential for abnormal joint reaction forces with an increased risk of a medial osteoarthritis developing at the hip joint. In this patient, the loss of the medial joint space and/or early arthrokatadysis or medial migration of the femoral heads can be seen, as can early development of osteophytes at the acetabulum and femoral head. (From Johnson TR, Steinbach LS: Essentials of musculoskeletal imaging, Rosemont, IL, 2004, American Academy of Orthopedic Surgeons, p. 458.)

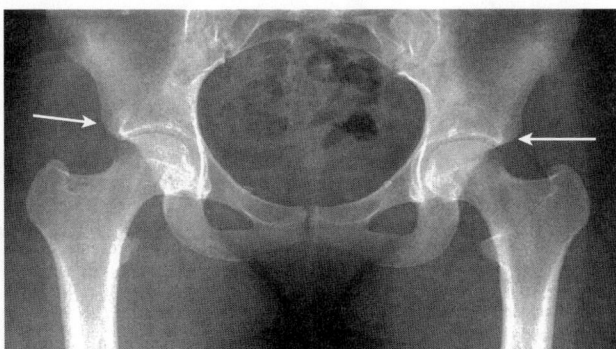

Figure 11-91 Anteroposterior radiograph demonstrating global acetabular overcoverage (i.e., coxa profunda), which may lead to cam type femoroacetabular impingement (FAI). (From Sierra RJ, et al: Hip disease in the young active patient: evaluation and nonarthroplasty surgical options. J Am Acad Orthop Surg 16:693, 2008.)

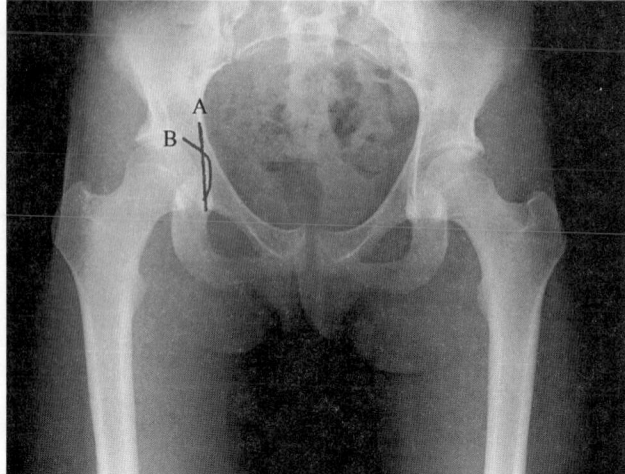

Figure 11-92 The radiograph appearance of protrusio acetabuli on an anteroposterior pelvic view. *Line A* represents the ilioischial line, and *line B* represents the floor of the acetabular fossa, which is medial to *line A*. A similar pathologic condition can also be seen on the radiograph of the patient's left hip. (From Clohisy JC, Carlisle JC, Beaulé PE, et al: A systematic approach to the plain radiographic evaluation of the young adult hip. J Bone Joint Surg Am 90:53, 2008).

TABLE **11-13**

Average Values of Hilgenreiner's Angle (Acetabular Index)

	Newborn	6 Months Old	1 Year Old
Male	26°	20°	20°
Female	28°	22°	20°

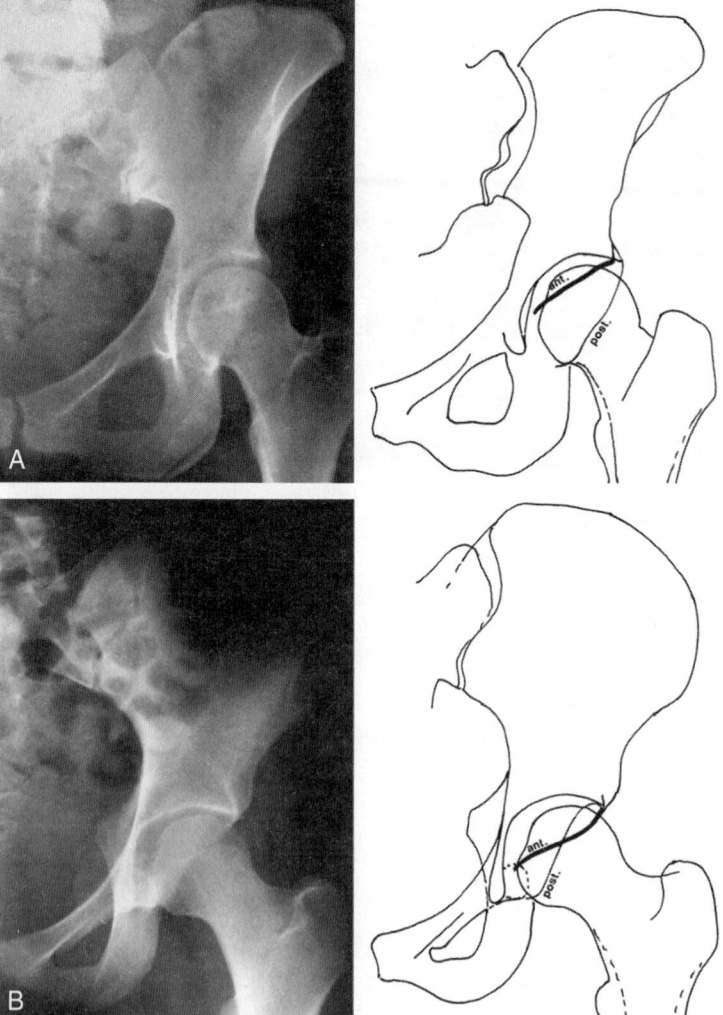

Figure 11-93 A, Radiograph and tracing of the normal (anteverted) acetabulum. The posture of this pelvis is flexed more at the lumbosacral junction than in the case described in **B.** The outline of the obturator foramen is more circular and the ischial spine is obscured. In such a flexed pelvis the anteverted attitude of the acetabulum is seen at a maximum. When an acetabulum is retroverted adoption of a similar posture minimizes the appearance of retroversion. The line of the edge of the posterior wall is located at or even lateral to the center of the femoral head. **B,** Radiograph and tracing showing acetabular retroversion and the "cross-over" or figure-eight sign. Compare with **A.** The line of the posterior wall is shown thin, that of the anterior wall thick. The line of the edge of the posterior wall is located well medial to the center of the femoral head. (From Reynolds D: Retroversion of the acetabulum: a cause of hip pain. J Bone Joint Surg Br 81:285, 1999.)

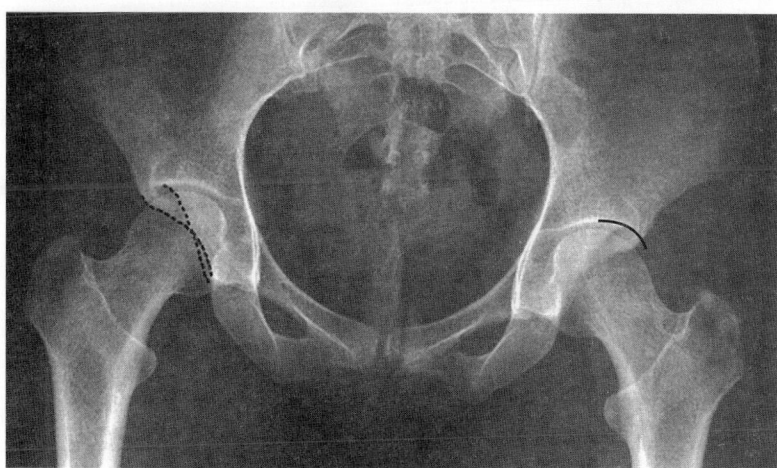

Figure 11-94 Anteroposterior radiograph of the pelvis of a 22-year-old woman who presented with groin pain. Clinical examination strongly suggested femoroacetabular impingement (FAI). The radiograph demonstrates bilateral acetabular retroversion as determined by crossover of the anterior and posterior acetabular walls *(dotted lines)* (crossover sign) on the right hip. The left hip demonstrates a pistol grip deformity. (From Parvizi J, Leunig M, Ganz R: Femoroacetabular impingement. J Am Acad Orthop Surg 15[9]:561–570, 2007.)

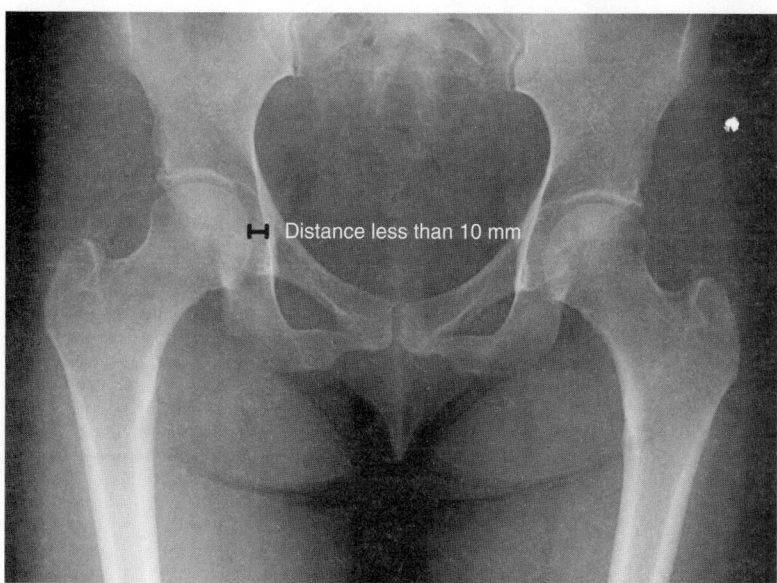

Distance less than 10 mm

Figure 11-95 Normal position of the femoral head in the acetabulum. (From Clohisy JC, Carlisle JC, Beaulé PE, et al: A systematic approach to the plain radiographic evaluation of the young adult hip. J Bone Joint Surg Am 90:59, 2008.)

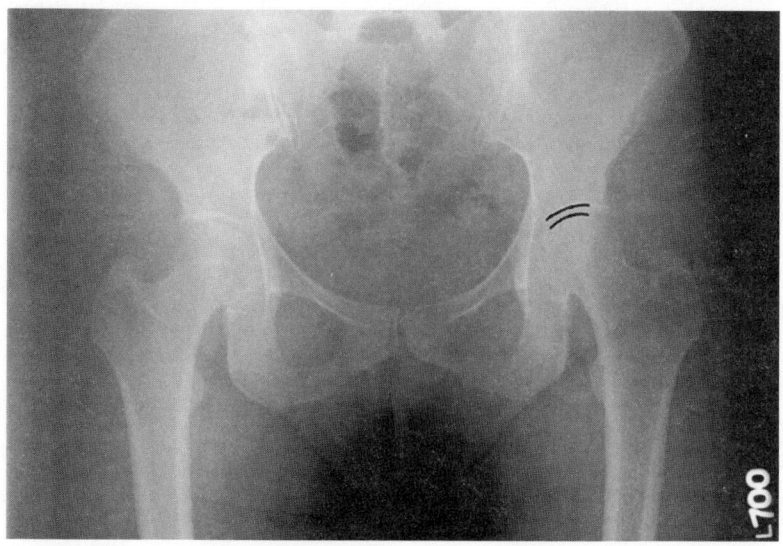

Figure 11-96 Congruency of the femoral head and the acetabulum. (From Clohisy JC, Carlisle JC, Beaulé PE, et al: A systematic approach to the plain radiographic evaluation of the young adult hip. J Bone Joint Surg Am 90:62, 2008.)

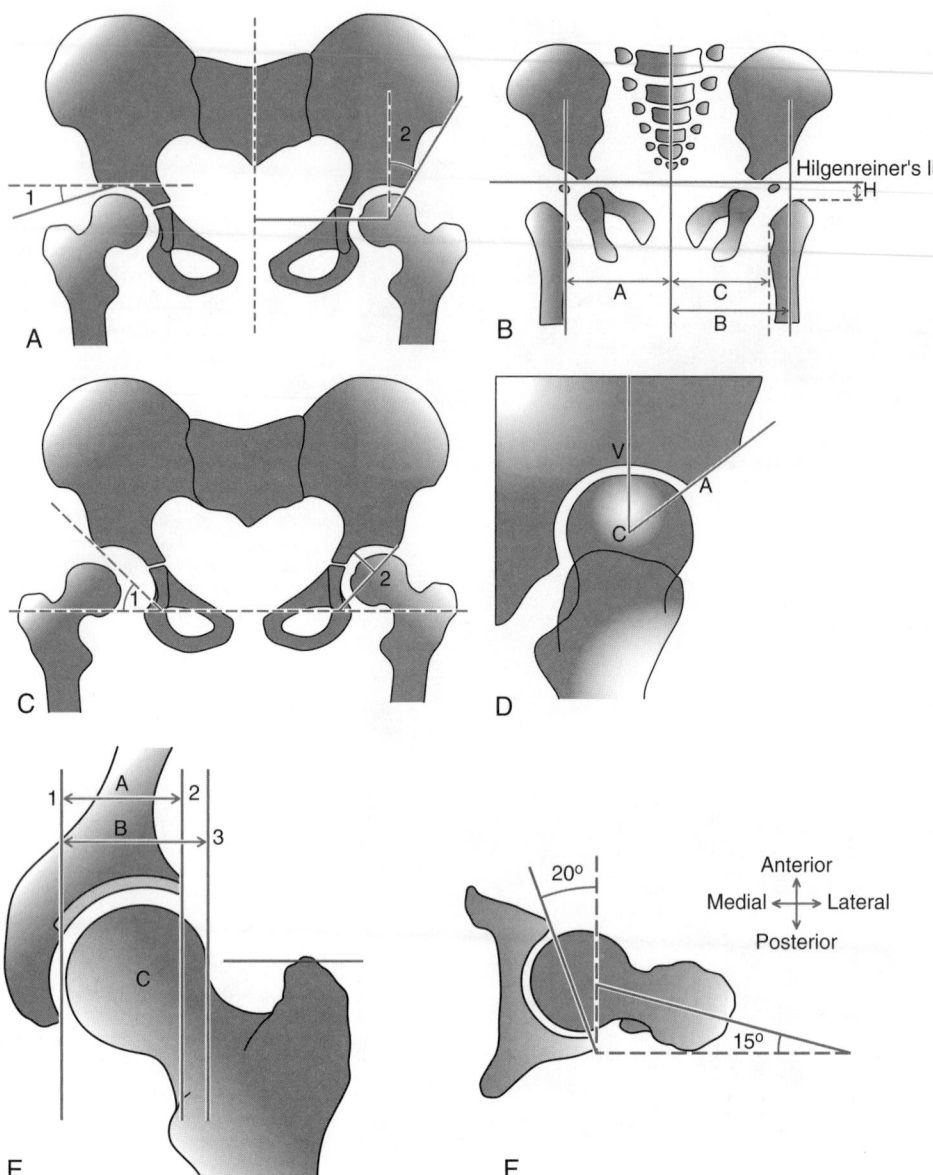

Figure 11-97 Additional measurements performed on conventional radiographs in patients with developmental dysplasia of the hip (DDH). **A,** *1:* Slope of the lateral edge of the acetabulum. The angle formed between a line that is parallel to Hilgenreiner's line and tangent to the roof of the acetabulum and a line that is parallel to the lateral edge of the acetabulum is termed the slope. The normal acetabulum has a slope of the lateral edge that is defined as positive. *2:* Center-edge *(CE)* angle. This angle lies between a line drawn from the center of the femoral head, perpendicular to the line connecting the centers of each femoral head, and a line drawn from the center of the head to the superolateral ossified edge of the acetabulum. The CE angle has a negative value. **B,** *Right hip:* The pelvic midline is drawn vertically through the centers of the sacrum and the symphysis pubis. The lateral displacement of each femoral head is indicated by the length of a line *(A)* drawn horizontally from the pelvic midline to the center of the femoral head. *Left hip:* The C/B ratio compared *C,* the distance from the pelvic midline to the medial beak of the femoral metaphysis, and *B,* the distance from the pelvic midline to the lateral acetabular edge. **C,** *1:* The angle that lies between a line connecting the teardrops on the inferior margin of the acetabula and a line drawn from the most superolateral ossified edge of the acetabulum to the teardrop constitutes the adult acetabular index or angle. *2:* The greatest perpendicular distance between the medial articular surface of the acetabulum and a line drawn from the teardrop to the superolateral ossified edge of the acetabulum is the acetabular depth. **D,** Vertical center-edge angle, drawn on a false profile view. It is defined as the angle subtended by a line *(V–C)* drawn from the center of the femoral head extending vertically upward and a line *(C–A)* drawn from the center of the femoral head obliquely to the anterior edge of the acetabulum. The angle lies between the two lines. **E,** Percentage of the femoral head covered by the acetabulum. This represents the relative width of the weight-bearing surface of the acetabulum *(A),* represented by line *1–2,* and that of the femoral head, represented by line *1–3.* Normal acetabular coverage is 75% or above when the ratio of *1–2:1–3* is determined. **F,** The acetabular anteversion angle describes the extent to which the acetabulum surrounds the femoral head within the horizontal plane. Measured from above, this angle is normally about 20°. As shown, the angle is formed by the intersection of an anterior-posterior reference line *(stippled)* and a line across the rim of the acetabulum. The 15° of normal anteversion of the proximal femur is also indicated. **(A–D,** Redrawn from Restrick D, Kransdorf MJ: Bone and joint imaging, Philadelphia, 2005, Elsevier, p. 1286; Courtesy of N. Lektakul, MD, Bangkok, Thailand. **E,** Redrawn from Delaunay S, Dussault RG, Kaplan PA, et al: Radiographic measurements of dysplastic adult hips. Skeletal Radiol 26:75, 1997. **F,** Redrawn from Neumann DA: Kinesiology of the musculoskeletal system—foundations for physical rehabilitation, St Louis, 2002, CV Mosby, p. 398.)

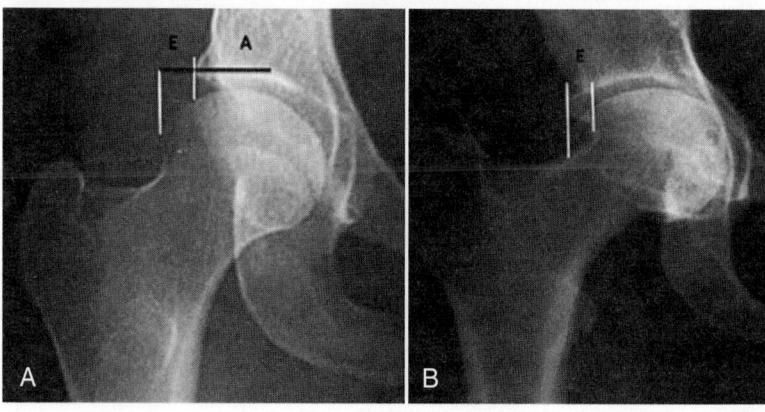

Figure 11-98 Femoral head extrusion index [E/A+E].
Normal extrusion index (**A**) is about 25%. In coxa profunda and protrusio acetabuli (**B**) more femoral head is covered and the index is 0 or negative. (From Patel K, Wallace R, Busconi BD: Radiology. Clin Sports Med 30:257, 2011.)

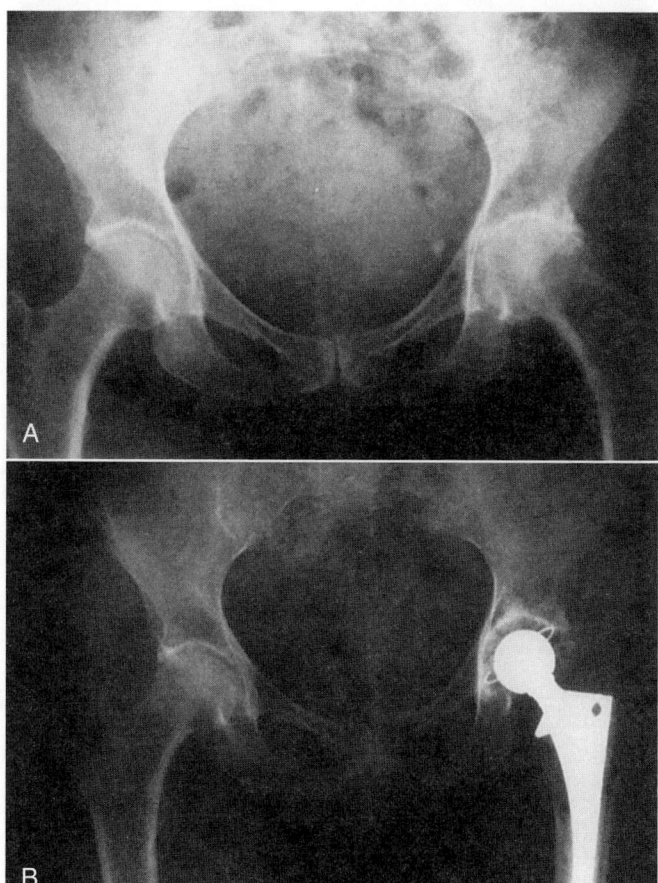

Figure 11-99 Arthritis of the left hip. A, Before surgery. Note decreased joint space and unevenness of femoral head. **B,** After total hip surgery.

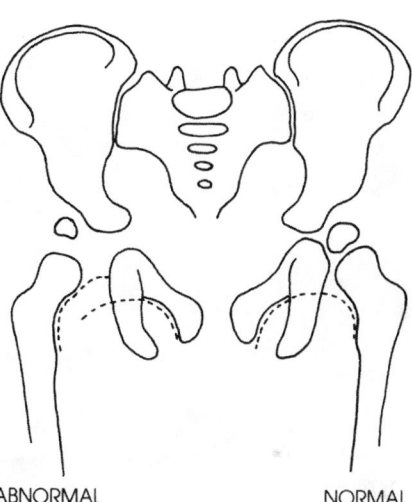

Figure 11-100 Shenton's line.

TABLE **11-14**

Kellgren and Lawrence Grading Scale for Hip Osteoarthritis

Grade	Radiographic Findings
0	No evidence of joint space narrowing, osteophyte formation, or sclerosis (normal radiograph)
1	Possible narrowing of the joint space medially and possible osteophytes around the femoral head
2	Definite narrowing of the joint space, definite osteophytes, and slight sclerosis
3	Marked narrowing of the joint space, slight osteophytes, some sclerosis, and cyst formation, and deformity of the femoral head and acetabulum
4	Gross loss of joint space with sclerosis and cysts, marked deformity of femoral head and acetabulum, large osteophytes

Modified from Kellgren JH, Lawrence JS: Radiological assessment of osteo-arthrosis. Ann Rheum Dis 16:494–502, 1957.

TABLE **11-15**

Key Radiographic Features of Dysplasia and Femoroacetabular Impingement

| | Dysplasia | FEMOROACETABULAR IMPINGEMENT | |
		Pincer Type	Cam Type
Anteroposterior pelvic/hip radiograph	Center-edge angle < 25°, Tonnis angle > 10°	Crossover and/or posterior wall sign, ischial sign, coxa profunda	Pistol-grip deformity
Lateral radiograph	—	—	Alpha angle > 50.5°, offset ratio < 0.15
False-profile radiograph	Anterior center-edge angle < 25°	Narrowing of posterior articular surface	—

From Beaulé PE, O'Neill M, Rakhra K: Acetabular labral tears. J Bone Joint Surg Am 91:705, 2009.

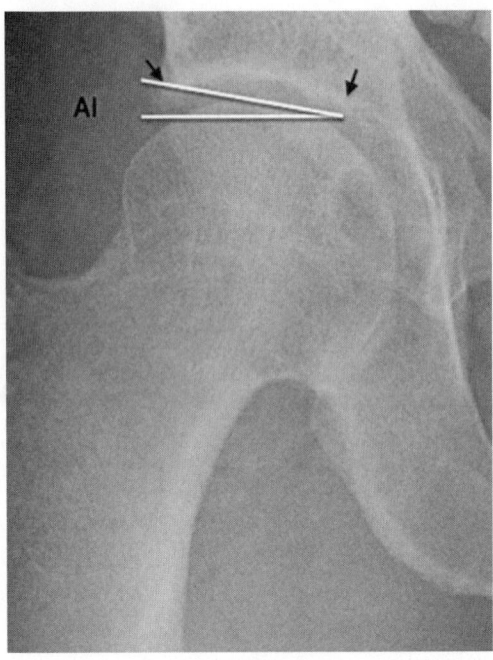

Figure 11-101 Acetabular index is an angle formed by a horizontal line and a line connecting the medial point of the sclerotic zone *(small black arrow)* with the lateral center of the acetabulum. Normal acetabular index is positive while in coxa profunda and protrusio acetabuli acetabular index is 0 or negative. (From Patel K, Wallace R, Busconi BD: Radiology. Clin Sports Med 30:256, 2011.)

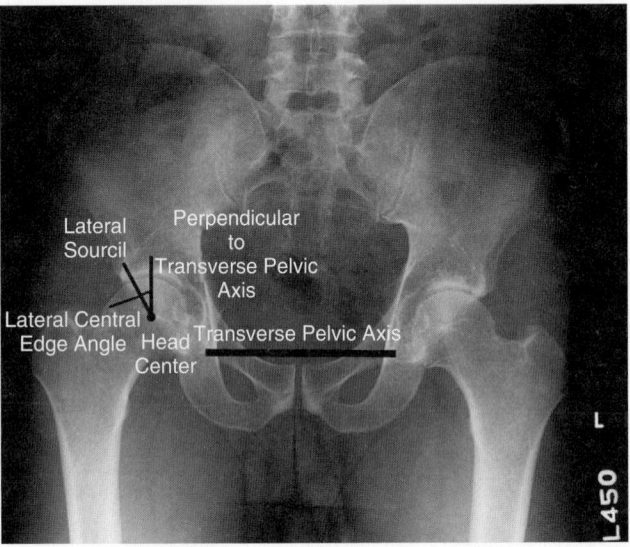

Figure 11-102 Lateral central edge angle. (Modified from Clohisy JC, Carlisle JC, Beaulé PE, et al: A systematic approach to the plain radiographic evaluation of the young adult hip. J Bone Joint Surg Am 90:55, 2008.)

24. **"Teardrop" sign:** Migration of the femoral head upward in relation to the pelvis, caused by degeneration as seen in osteoarthritis, may be detected by the "teardrop" sign (Figure 11-109). The teardrop is visible at the base of the pubic bone, extending vertically downward to terminate in a round teardrop, or head. The x-ray beam must be centered relative to the pelvis. A line is drawn between the two teardrops and extended to the femoral heads on both sides. The examiner can then measure from the teardrop to the femoral head. A difference of more than 10 mm between the two sides indicates significant migration of the head of the femur. Serial films or films taken over time often show a progression of the migration.

25. **"Head-at-risk" signs:** With Legg-Calvé-Perthes disease, the examiner should note the following radiologic "head-at-risk" signs on an anteroposterior film:
    a. Cage's sign, a small osteoporotic segment on the lateral side of the epiphysis that appears to be translucent (Figure 11-110)
    b. Calcification lateral to the epiphysis (if collapse is occurring)
    c. Lateral subluxation of the head (an increase in the inferomedial joint space)

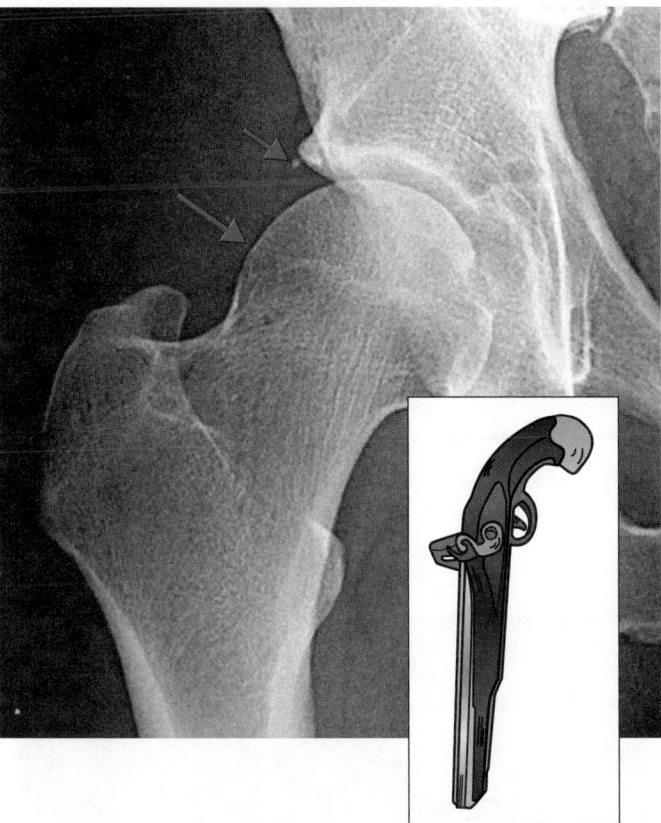

Figure 11-103 A 36-year-old male with cam-type femoroacetabular impingement (FAI). Anteroposterior view of the right hip demonstrates the pistol grip deformity of the lateral femoral head-neck junction *(long arrow)*. Note the calcifications of the labrum *(short arrow)*. (Modified from Zaragoza EJ, Beaulé PE: Imaging of the painful non-arthritic hip: a practical approach to surgical relevancy. Oper Tech Orthop 14:44, 2004.)

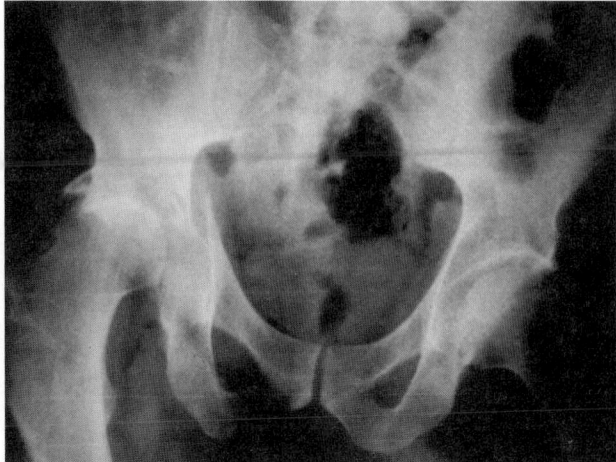

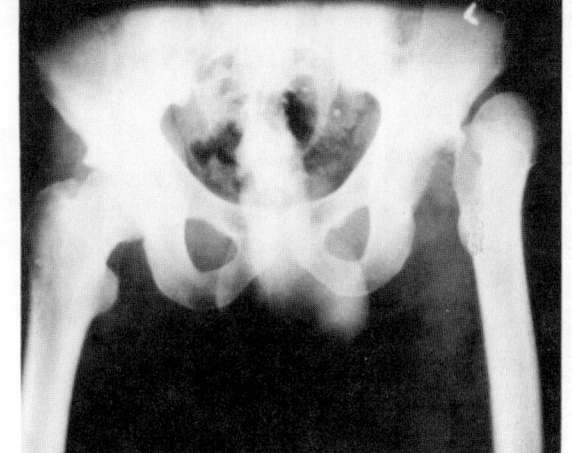

Figure 11-104 Trauma to the hip. A, Fractured right acetabulum. **B,** Dislocated left femur.

d. Angle of the epiphyseal line (horizontal, in this case)
e. Metaphyseal reaction
   Patients who exhibit three or more "head-at-risk" signs have a poor prognosis, and surgery is usually performed.
26. Signs of a **slipped capital femoral epiphysis**[171]: With a slipped capital femoral epiphysis (Figure 11-111), the following x-ray signs may be noted:
   a. The epiphyseal line may widen.
   b. Lipping or stepping may be seen, as occurs on lateral films.
   c. The superior femoral neck line does not transect the overhanging ossified epiphysis as it does in the normal hip.
   d. Shenton's line does not describe a continuous arc. (The line is also broken if the hip is dislocated or subluxed.)

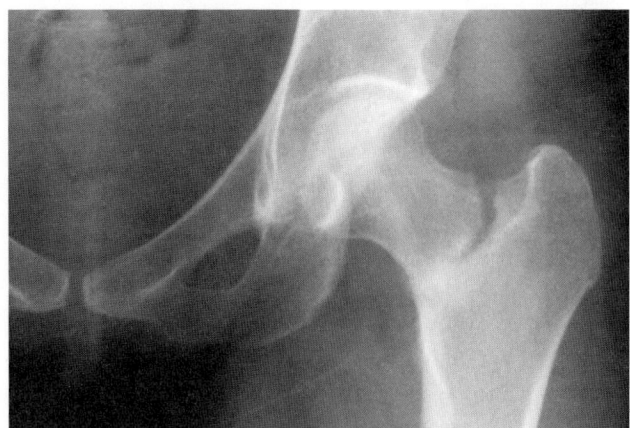

Figure 11-105 Stress fracture of the femoral neck.

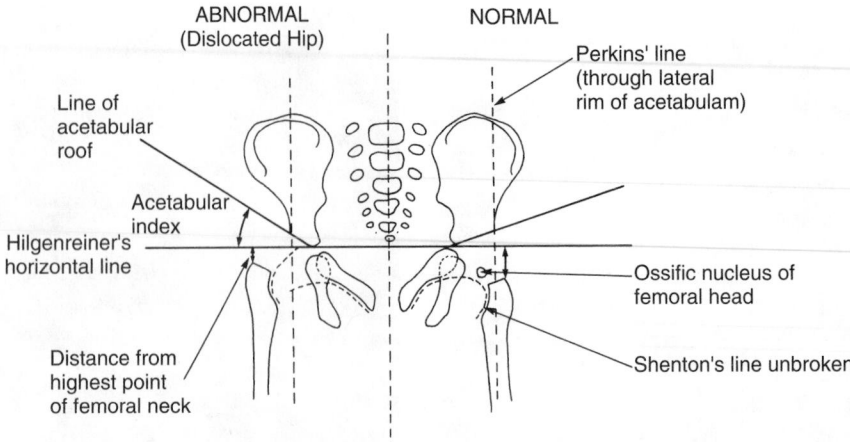

Figure 11-106 Radiological findings in congenital dislocation of the hip (CDH) compared with normal findings in a 12- to 15-month-old child. Acetabular index: Normal = 30°, in newborn = 27.5°. If the ossific nucleus of the femoral head is present, it should sit in the inner lower quadrant.

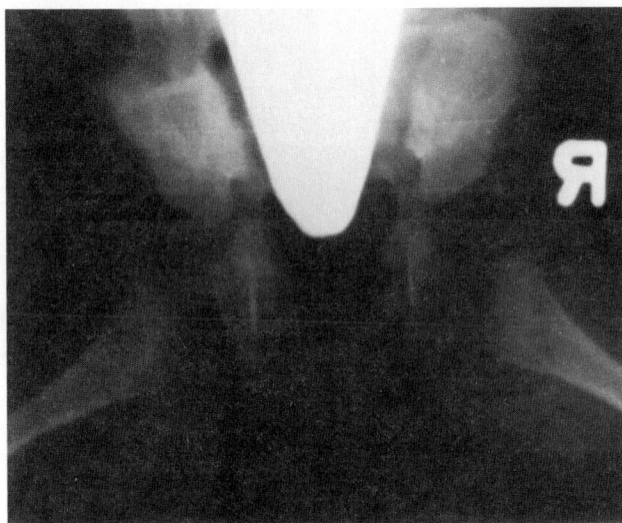

Figure 11-107 Radiograph of the hip in the newborn. Ossification of the femoral head has not yet developed.

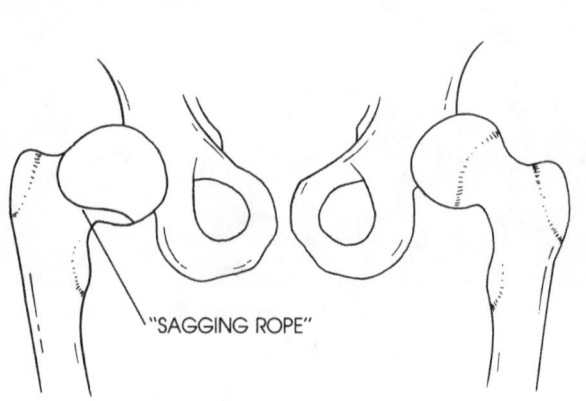

Figure 11-108 Sagging rope sign.

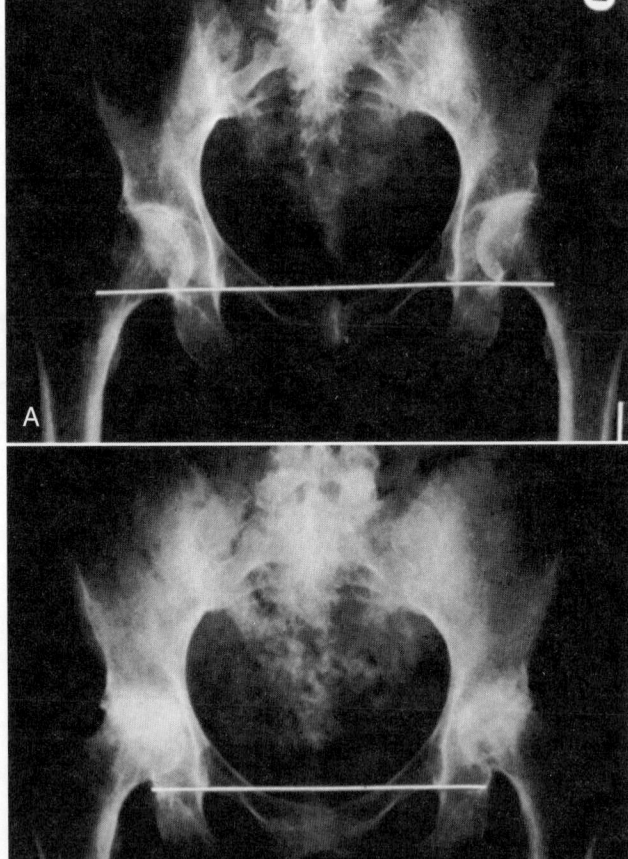

Figure 11-109 Teardrop sign. A, A line has been drawn between the tips of the two "teardrops" and extended into the femoral neck. Osteoarthritis of both hip joints appears to be equal, with equivalent narrowing of the joint space, but the left hip is already at a slightly higher level than the right in relation to the line. **B,** Later, both hips have gradually moved upward as a result of loss of the bone at the apex of each femoral head. The left hip is now at a higher level than the right, confirming the original observation that the process of destruction in the left hip was more advanced. (From Greubel-Lee DM: Disorders of the hip, Philadelphia, 1983, JB Lippincott, pp. 61, 146.)

In addition to a slipped capital femoral epiphysis causing a coxa vara, fractures, or congenital malformations can lead to the same deformity (Figures 11-112 and 11-113).

Cross Table Lateral View. This view (Figure 11-114) can be used to measure the head-neck offset ratio (Figure 11-115). This ratio is used when femoroacetabular impingement (cam type) is suspected. If the ratio is less than 0.17, a cam deformity may be present.[165]

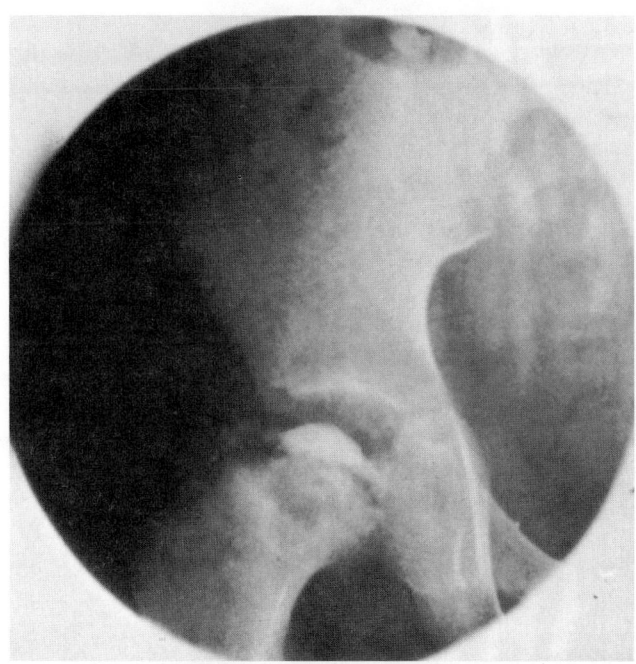

Figure 11-110 All of the **signs of the "head-at-risk"** are present: lateral subluxation, abnormal direction of the growth plates, Cage's sign, lateral calcification, and irregularity of the epiphysis. (From Greubel-Lee DM: Disorders of the hip, Philadelphia, 1983, JB Lippincott, p. 146.)

False-Profile Hip Radiograph.[165] This view is used to calculate the anterior center-edge angle. A vertical line is drawn through the center of the femoral head. A second line is drawn from the most anterior point of the acetabular "eyebrow" (sourcil) to the vertical line. The angle created is the anterior center edge angle (Figure 11-116; see Figure 11-2, *A*). Structural instability is indicated if the angle is less than 20°.

Lateral (Axial "Frog-Leg") View. For this view, the patient is supine with the hips in flexion, abduction, and lateral rotation. This view provides a true lateral view of the femoral head and neck (Figure 11-117).[172] The examiner looks for any pelvic distortion or any slipping of the femoral head, as may be seen in slipped capital femoral epiphysis. The lateral view is the first in which slipping may be seen. This view will also show head-neck offset deformity.[165]

Arthrography

Although arthrograms are not routinely done on the hip, they may be done if the hip cannot be reduced following a dislocation (Figure 11-118). The arthrogram may indicate a possible inverted limbus (infolding of a meniscus-like structure) or an hourglass configuration from a contracted capsule. It is also useful in CDH to show where the unossified femoral head lies relative to the labrum. A normal hip arthrogram is shown in Figure 11-119.

Computed Tomography

Computed tomography scanning is useful in assessing abnormalities of the hip, especially bony ones.[110] For example, it can be used to measure anteversion and retroversion, and it can show the size and shape of the acetabulum and femoral head as well as the congruity and

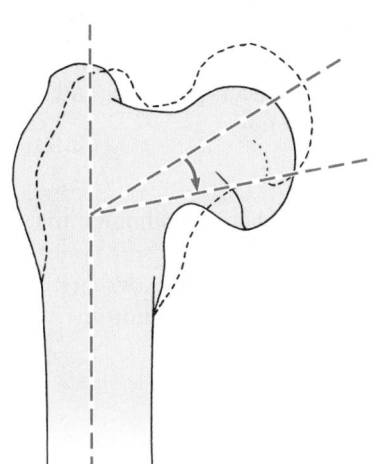

Congenital

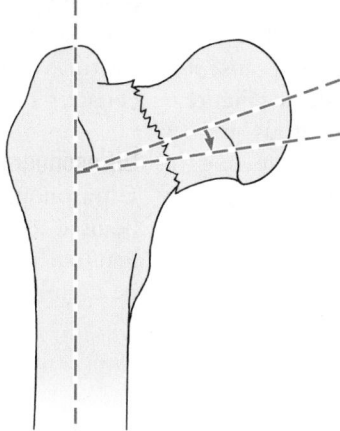

Fracture

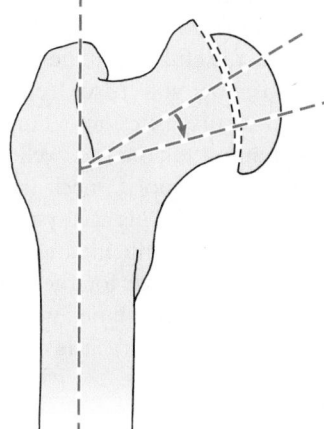

Slipped capital femoral epiphysis

Figure 11-111 Some causes of coxa vara.

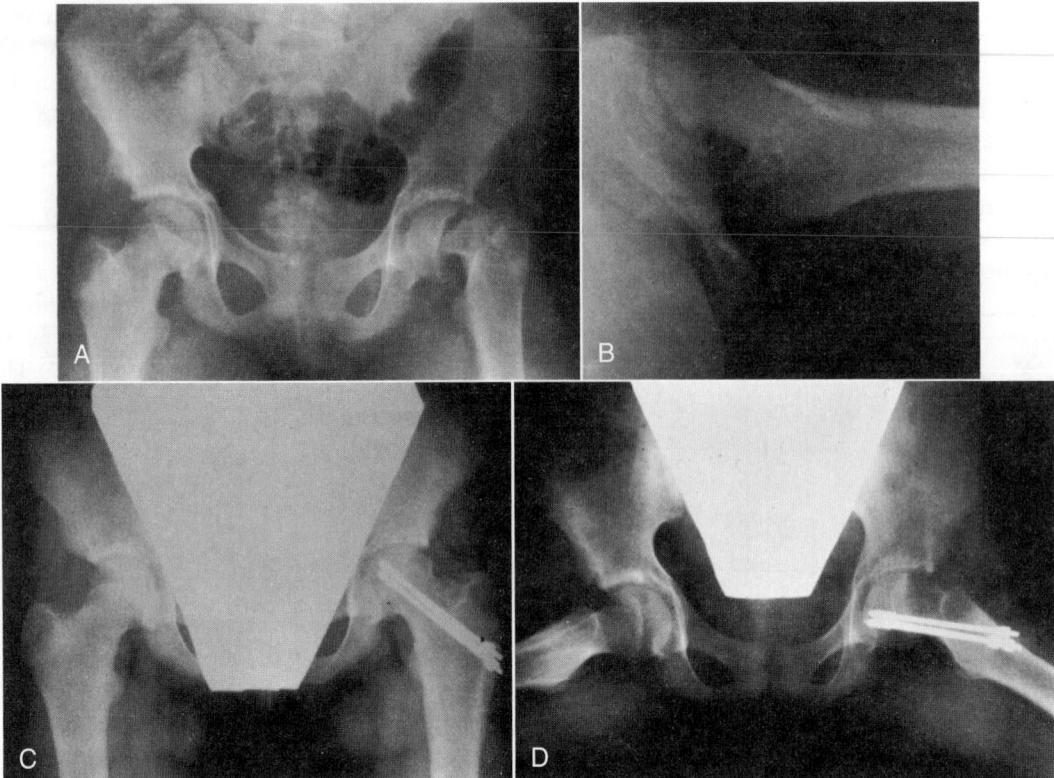

Figure 11-112 Acute slipped femoral epiphysis in a 14-year-old boy. After a fall, the patient complained of severe pain in the left groin and anterior thigh and was unable to bear weight on the left lower limb. **A** and **B,** Preoperative radiographs show the severe slip on the left. The patient was placed in bilateral split Russell traction with medial rotation straps on the left thigh and leg. Gradually, within a period of 3 to 4 days, the slip was reduced. **C** and **D,** Postoperative radiographs approximately 6 months later show closure of epiphyseal plate and normal position of femoral head. The hip had full range of motion (ROM). (From Tachdjian MO: Pediatric orthopedics, Philadelphia, 1972, WB Saunders, p. 470.)

position of the femoral head relative to the acetabulum (Figures 11-120 and 11-121) and can be used to assess femoroacetabular impingement.[173] In newborns, the lack of ossification limits its use.

Magnetic Resonance Imaging[174]

Magnetic resonance imaging (MRI) (Figures 11-122 and 11-123) is a useful technique to study the hip because it is able to show soft tissue (e.g., labral lesions [Figure 11-124], cartilage lesions, bursitis, ligamentous teres lesions, tendon lesions) as well as osseous tissue (e.g., osteonecrosis, femoral neck stress fractures) (Figure 11-125).[8,125,175,176] This ability makes it an excellent technique to use for congenital abnormalities. It is also the examination of choice for the evaluation of unexplained hip pain.[164] When combined with arthrography (magnetic resonance arthrograph), it is often more sensitive to hip

lesions but also produces more false positives.[177] Signs seen on MRI should always be correlated with clinical findings as abnormal hip findings are common in asymptomatic patients.[178]

Scintigraphy (Bone Scan)

Bone scans may be used in the hip to help diagnose stress fractures (especially of femoral neck), necrosis, and tumors (Figures 11-126 and 11-127).

Ultrasonography

Ultrasonography is a non-irradiation technique that may be used to detect hip abnormalities and soft-tissue problems such as swelling.[164,179-181] Dynamic sonography may be useful for diagnosing snapping hip syndrome.[175]

Text continued on p. 758

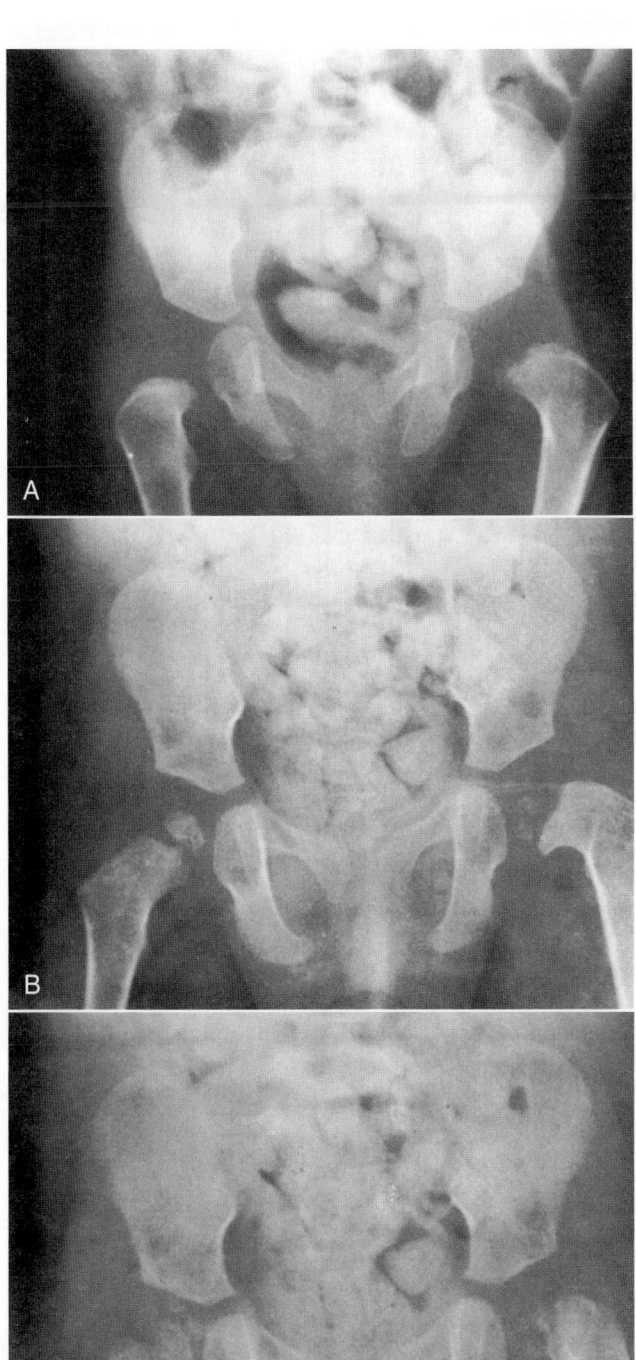

Figure 11-113 Congenital coxa vara of the left hip in an infant.
A, Anteroposterior radiographs of both hips at 3 months of age, taken
because of limited abduction of left hip and suspicion of congenital hip
dislocation. It was interpreted to be normal. **B** and **C,** Radiographs
of the hips of same patient at 1 year of age when he started walking
with a painless gluteus medius lurch on the left. Varus deformity of
the left hip is evident. (From Tachdjian MO: Pediatric orthopedics,
Philadelphia, 1972, WB Saunders, p. 587.)

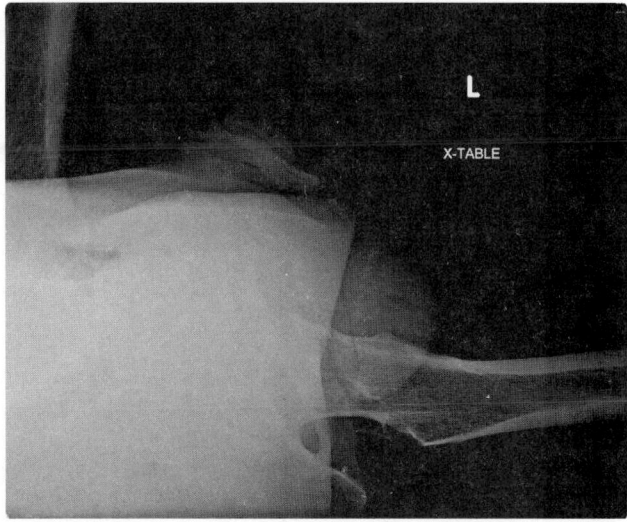

Figure 11-114 Cross table lateral view of the hip used to measure
head-neck offset ratio.

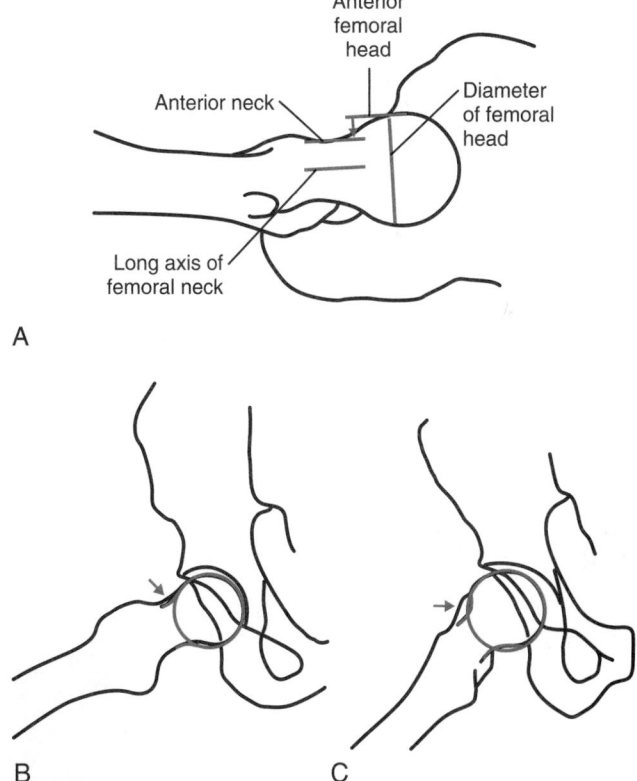

Figure 11-115 A, Tracing to show technique for calculating the head-
neck offset ratio. Three parallel lines are drawn with *line 1* drawn
through the center of the long axis of the femoral neck, *line 2* drawn
through the anteriormost aspect of the femoral neck, and *line 3*
drawn through the anterior most aspect of the femoral head. The head-
neck offset ratio is calculated by measuring the distance between *lines
2* and *3,* and dividing by the diameter of the femoral head. **B,** Moderate
head-neck offset and/or mild cam impingement. **C,** Anterolateral head-
neck offset reduced.[165]

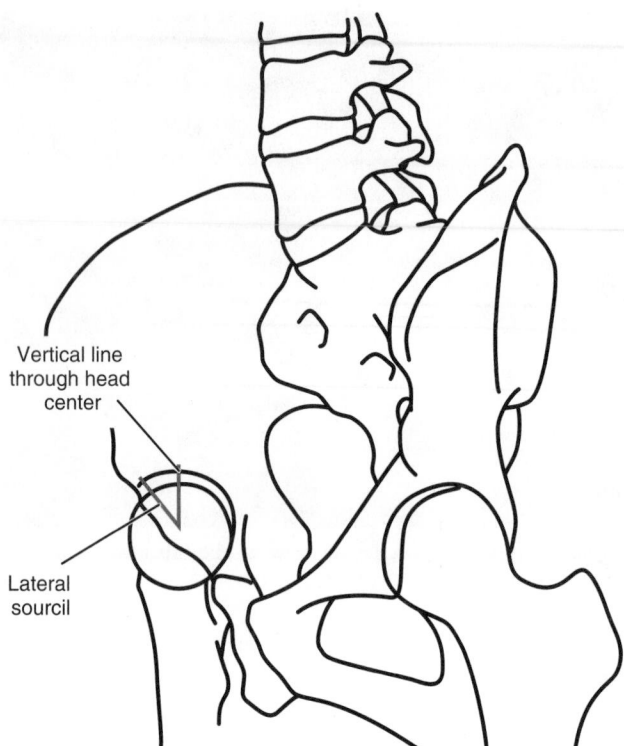

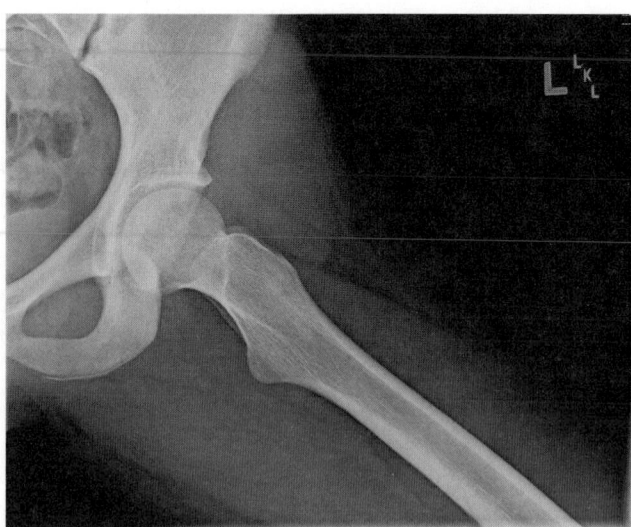

Figure 11-117 Lateral (axial "frog-leg") view.

Figure 11-116 Tracing to show technique for calculating the anterior center-edge angle on a false-profile radiograph. A vertical line is drawn through the center of the femoral head. A second line is drawn through the center of the femoral head, passing through the most anterior point of the acetabular sourcil. The angle created by the intersection of these two lines is the anterior center-edge angle. Values of less than 20° can be indicative of structural instability.[165]

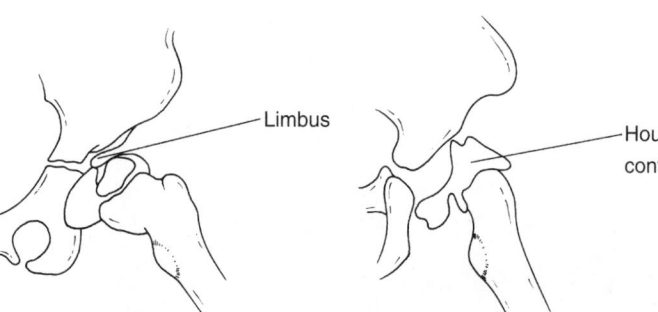

Figure 11-118 Tracings of arthrograms in congenital dislocation of the hip (CDH).

Figure 11-119 Normal hip arthrogram. Normal examination after intra-articular injection of approximately 6 mL of contrast medium. **A,** Anteroposterior view. **B,** Frog lateral views. *c,* Contrast agent outlining articular cartilage (recess capitis); *i,* inferior articular recess; *ir,* recess colli inferior; *l,* acetabular labrum; *lt,* defect on contrast from transverse ligament; *s,* superior articular recess; *sr,* recess colli superior; *z,* zona orbicularis (impression on the intra-articular contrast by the iliofemoral ischiofemoral ligaments of the hip joint capsule). (From Weissman BNW, Sledge CB: Orthopedic radiology, Philadelphia, 1986, WB Saunders, p. 396.)

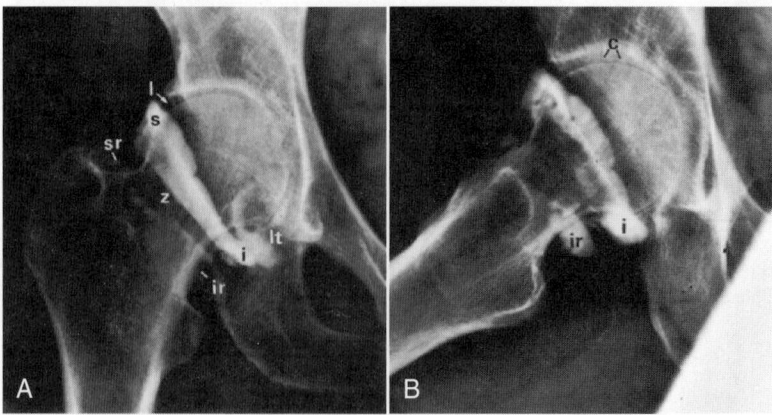

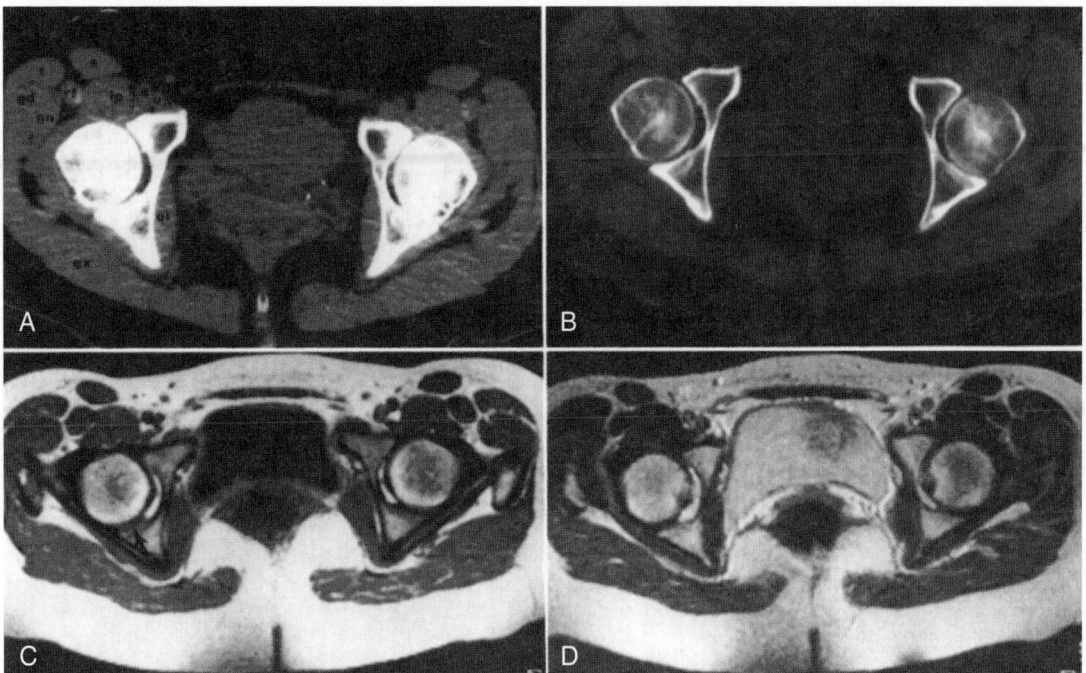

Figure 11-120 A, Normal computed tomography (CT) image at the level of the midacetabulum obtained with soft-tissue window settings, showing the homogenous, intermediate signal of musculature. Common femoral artery; *gd,* gluteus medius; *gn,* gluteus minimus; *gx,* gluteus maximus; *ip,* iliopsoas; *oi,* obturator internus; *ra,* rectus abdominis; *rf,* rectus femoris; *s,* sartorius; *t,* tensor fasciae latae; *v,* common femoral vein. **B,** Axial CT at bone window settings reveals improved delineation of cortical and medullary osseous details. Note anterior and posterior semilunar acetabular articular surfaces and the central nonarticular acetabular fossa. **C,** Normal midacetabular T1-weighted axial 0.4-T MRI (TR, 600 msec; TE, 20 msec) of a different patient shows a normal, high-signal-intensity image of muscle and absence of signal in the cortical bone. The thin articular hyaline cartilage is of intermediate signal intensity *(arrow).* **D,** T2-weighted MRI (TR, 2000 msec; TE, 80 msec) shows decreasing high-signal intensity in fatty marrow and subcutaneous tissue with increased signal intensity in the fluid-filled urinary bladder. (From Pitt MJ, Lund PJ, Speer DP: Imaging of the pelvis and hip. Orthop Clin North Am 21:553, 1990.)

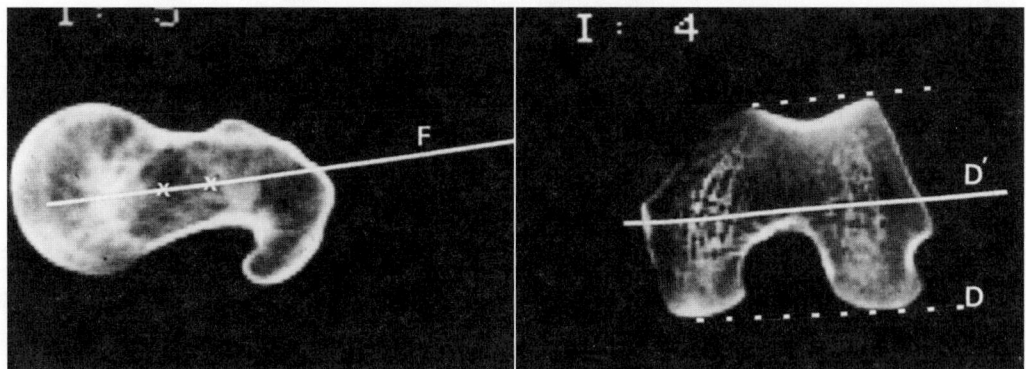

Figure 11-121 Computed tomography for determining femoral anteversion (using a femoral specimen). The diacondylar line *(D)* is drawn along the condyles, although Hernandez and co-workers construct it *(D')* midway between the anterior and posterior femoral surfaces *(dashed lines).* The axis of the femoral neck *(F)* is shown. The angle between the femoral neck axis *(F)* and the diacondylar line is the angle of anteversion. In this case, there is 2° of retroversion. (From Weissman BNW, Sledge CB: Orthopedic radiology, Philadelphia, 1986, WB Saunders, p. 399.)

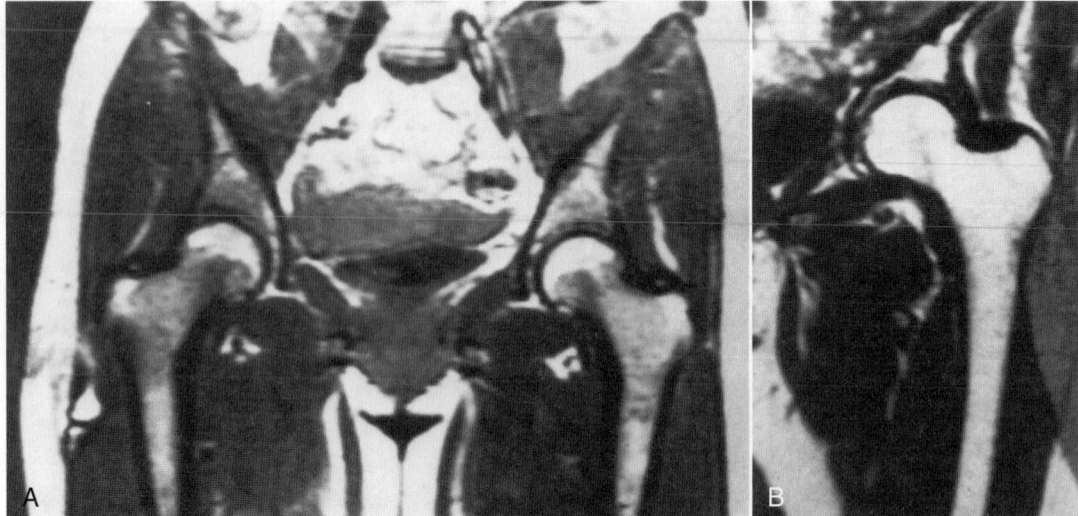

Figure 11-122 A, Normal MRI scan of a young adult. Spin-echo T1-weighted image (600/25). Note the bright signal of fat in the region of the femoral epiphysis and the greater trochanter. The intermediate signal intensity in the femoral neck represents hemopoietic marrow. **B,** Normal elderly woman with same imaging sequence shows replacement of hemopoietic marrow in the femoral neck by fatty marrow. (From Dalinka MK, Neustadter LM: Radiology of the hip. In Steinberg ME, editor: The hip and its disorders, Philadelphia, 1991, WB Saunders, p. 68.)

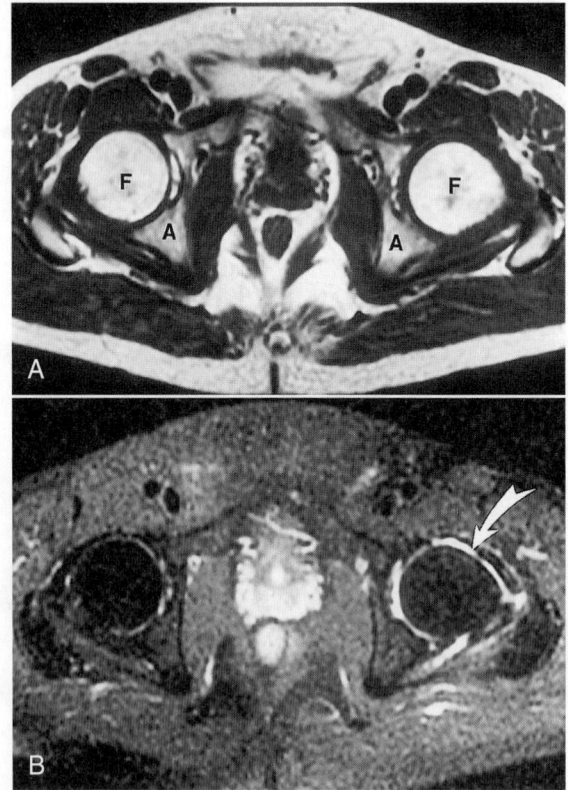

Figure 11-123 Normal adult bone marrow. A, Transaxial T1-weighted (TR/TE, 600/8) spin echo MR image of the pelvis. Yellow marrow within the femoral heads *(F)* is isointense to subcutaneous fat. Red marrow within the acetabula *(A)* has signal intensity between that of muscle and fat. **B,** Transaxial fat-suppressed T2-weighted (TR/TEeff, 4000/60) fast spin echo magnetic resonance (MR) image. The signal intensity of both yellow and red marrow decreases. A small effusion is seen in the left hip *(arrow)*. (From Resnick D, Kransdorf MJ: Bone and joint imaging, Philadelphia, 2005, Elsevier, p. 119.)

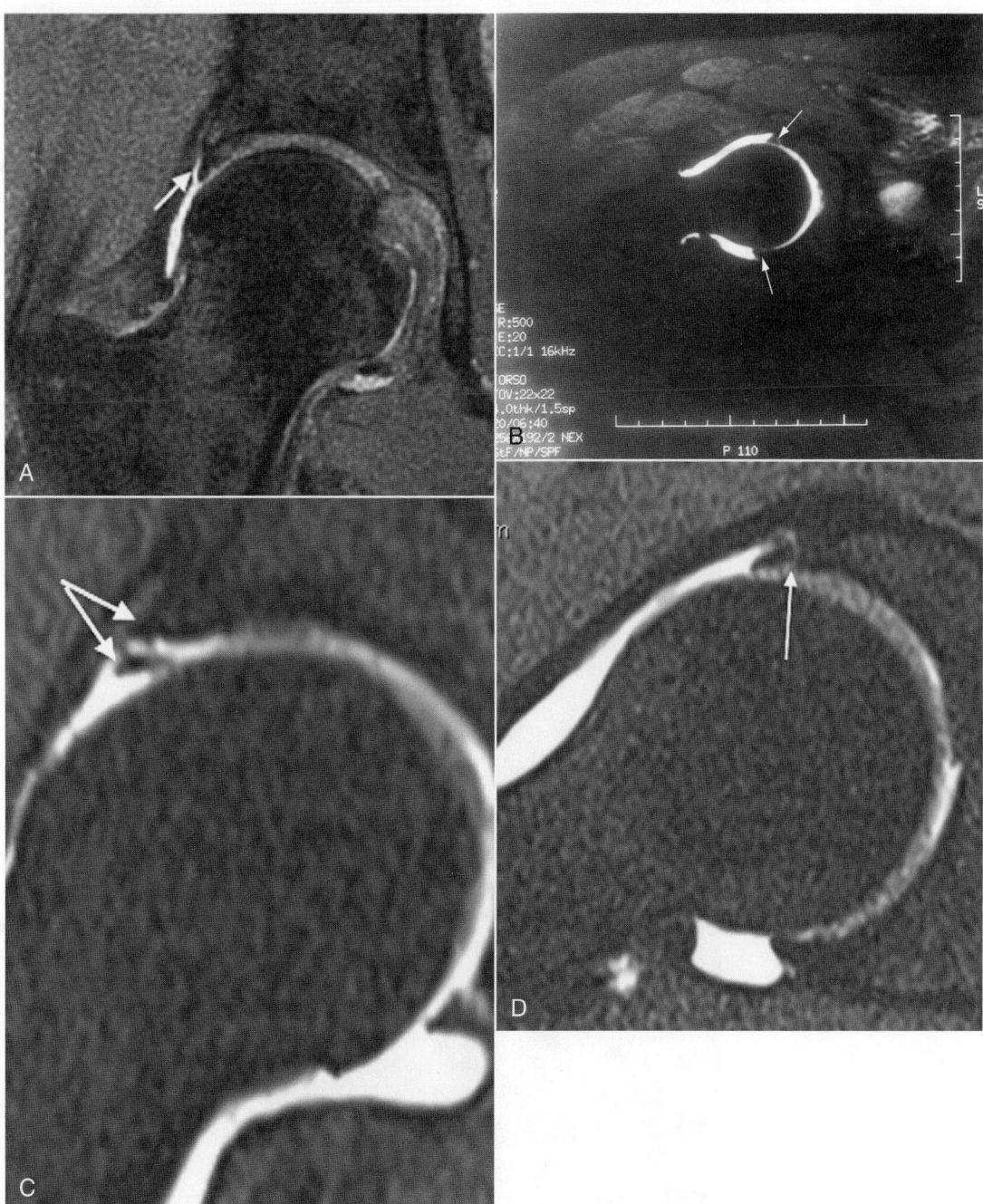

Figure 11-124 Acetabular labral tears. A, Normal hip. Arrow indicates the normal space (perilabral sulcus) between the capsule, lateral acetabular rim and labrum. **B,** Acetabular labral tear *(arrow).* **C,** Corneal T1 F5-weighted image shows longitudinal bucket handle type tear with labral fragments *(arrow).* **D,** Oblique axial T1 F5-weighted image showing detachment *(arrow)* of the anterior labrum. (**A, C,** and **D,** From Patel K, Wallace R, Busconi BD, et al: Radiology. Clin Sports Med 30:241,247, 2011. **B,** From DeLee J, et al: DeLee and Drez's orthopaedic sports medicine, ed 2, Philadelphia, 2003, WB Saunders.)

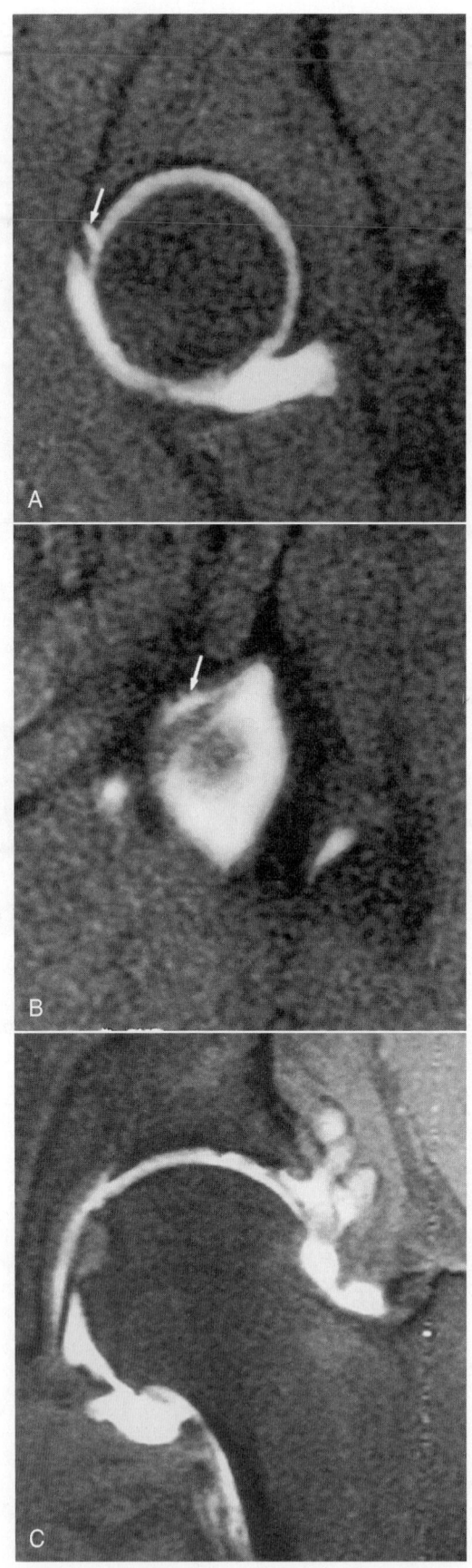

Figure 11-125 Acetabular labrum: tear and cystic degeneration. A and **B,** Partial detachment of the anterosuperior portion of the labrum *(arrows)* is seen on fat-suppressed sagittal **(A)** and coronal **(B)** T1-weighted (TR/TE, 600/16) spin echo magnetic resonance (MR) arthrographic images. **C,** In a different patient, a fat-suppressed coronal T1-weighted (TR/TE, 700/12) spin echo MR arthrographic image demonstrates a massive superior labral tear with a perilabral ganglion cyst. (From Resnick D, Kransdorf MJ: Bone and joint imaging, Philadelphia, 2005, Elsevier. **A** and **B,** Courtesy J. Tomanek, MD, Johnson City, TN.)

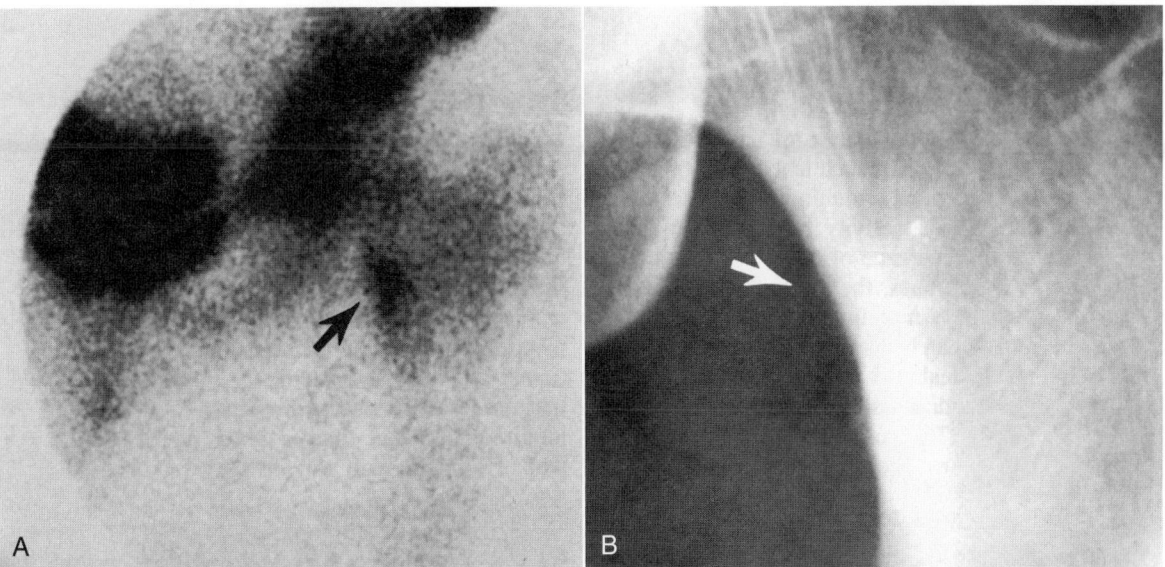

Figure 11-126 Stress fracture. This athletic young woman complained of a persistent hip pain aggravated by activity. **A,** Radionuclide examination reveals a focal, sharply marginated area of increased activity in the femoral neck *(arrow)*. **B,** Radiograph of the hip delineates a minimal amount of indistinct new bone formation along the medial aspect of the femoral neck *(arrow)*. (From Resnick D, Kransdorf MJ: Bone and joint imaging, Philadelphia, 2005, Elsevier, p. 797.)

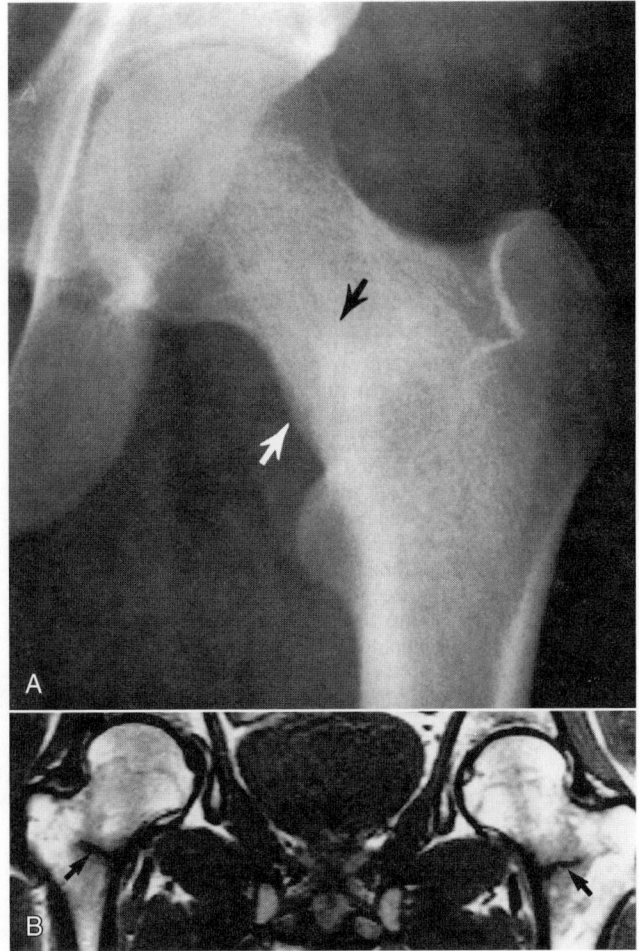

Figure 11-127 Femoral neck stress fracture. A, In the medial portion of the femoral neck, observe the presence of buttressing and sclerosis *(arrows)*. **B,** Coronal intermediate-weighted (TR/TE, 2000/20) spin echo magnetic resonance (MR) image reveals bilateral fatigue fractures *(arrows)* in the medial portion of the femoral neck. The fracture itself and the surrounding marrow edema are of low signal intensity. (From Resnick D, Kransdorf MJ: Bone and joint imaging, Philadelphia, 2005, Elsevier, p. 800.)

PRÉCIS OF THE HIP ASSESSMENT*

History
Observation
Examination
   Functional assessment
   Special tests (standing)
      Trendelenburg test
   Active movements (supine)
      Hip flexion
      Hip abduction
      Hip adduction
      Hip lateral rotation
      Hip medial rotation
   Passive movements (supine) as in active movements (if
      necessary)
   Resisted isometric movements (supine)
      Hip flexion
      Hip extension
      Hip adduction
      Hip abduction
      Hip medial rotation
      Hip lateral rotation
      Knee flexion
      Knee extension
   Special tests (supine)
      Abduction/adduction tests
      Anterior labral tear test
      Anteroposterior impingement test
      Flexion-adduction test
      Heel strike test
      Hip rotator tightness
      Hip scour test
      Leg length tests
      90–90 straight leg raise test
      Noble compression test
      Patellar-pubic percussion sign

      Patrick test
      Posterior labral tear test
      Posteroinferior impingement test
      Rectus femoris test
      Thomas test
   Reflexes and cutaneous distribution (supine)
      Reflexes
      Sensory scan
      Peripheral nerves
   Joint play movements (supine)
      Caudal glide
      Compression
      Lateral distraction
      Quadrant test
   Palpation (supine)
   Special tests (side lying)
      Ober test
   Active movement (prone)
      Hip extension
   Passive movement (prone)
      Hip extension
   Resisted isometric movements (prone)
      Hip medial rotation (if not previously done)
      Hip lateral rotation (if not previously done)
      Knee flexion (if not previously done)
      Knee extension (if not previously done)
   Reflexes and cutaneous distribution (prone)
   Palpation (prone)
   Diagnostic imaging
After the rest of the examination is completed, the
   examiner can ask the patient to perform any
   appropriate additional functional tests.
After any examination, the patient should be warned of
   the possibility of exacerbation of symptoms as a result
   of the assessment.

*The précis is shown in an order that limits the amount of moving that the patient must do but ensures that all necessary structures are tested.

CASE STUDIES

When doing these case studies, the examiner should list the appropriate questions to be asked and why they are being asked, what to look for and why, and what things should be tested and why. Depending on the answers of the patient (and the examiner should consider different responses), several possible causes of the patient's problem may become evident (examples are given in parentheses). A differential diagnosis chart (Table 11-16) should be made up. The examiner can then decide how different diagnoses may affect the treatment plan.

1. A 14-year-old boy was well until he fell from a chair onto his buttocks. He did not appear hurt, but 1 week later his parents brought him in for assessment because of a limp and pain in his right thigh and knee. The teenager is a tall, thin boy who prefers to walk with the right foot laterally rotated. Design your assessment plan for this patient (slipped capital femoral epiphysis versus ischial bursitis).

2. A 71-year-old woman had an Austin Moore prosthesis inserted into the left hip 1 day ago. The prosthesis has relieved the pain she had in her hip. X-rays reveal that the prosthesis is solid. The surgeon has asked you to get the patient up and moving. Before doing this, however, you must do a bedside assessment. Outline how you would do the assessment.

3. A 7-year-old boy is brought by his parents for assessment. He walks with a limp and has done so during the past 5 weeks at irregular times, the limp becoming more pronounced when the boy becomes tired. The boy also complains of a painful

CASE STUDIES—cont'd

left knee. Describe your assessment plan for this patient (Legg-Calvé-Perthes disease versus slipped capital femoral epiphysis).

4. A 3-week-old girl is referred to you to be fitted with a Pavlik harness for CDH. Before you can fit the harness, you must do an assessment. Design your assessment plan for this patient.

5. A 55-year-old man complains of hip and back pain. There is some sciatica with pain into the groin. The pain is especially bad when he walks. He has a desk job but has been very active throughout his life. Describe your assessment plan for this patient (piriformis syndrome versus lumbar spondylosis).

6. A 35-year-old woman complains of lateral hip pain. She states that she was in a motor vehicle accident 2 weeks ago in which she was hit from

the passenger side (she was driving) and her car was pushed against a telephone pole. She was wearing a seat belt. Describe your assessment plan for this patient (trochanteric bursitis versus muscle contusion).

7. An 18-year-old man was surfing when he was thrown by a wave and hurt his hip. The hip is medially rotated and shortened. He has some sciatic pain. Describe your assessment plan for this patient (posterior hip dislocation versus trochanteric fracture).

8. A 23-year-old female diver comes to you complaining of hip pain. She says it bothers her when she does any quick flexion of the hip. Describe your assessment plan for this patient (psoas bursitis versus psoas strain).

TABLE **11-16**

Differential Diagnosis of Slipped Capital Femoral Epiphysis and Ischial Bursitis

	Slipped Capital Femoral Epiphysis	Ischial Bursitis
History	Trauma may or may not be a factor Growth spurt may be involved More common on boys May be acute or chronic Pain into hip, groin, thigh to knee	Usually results from trauma (fall) Usually acute but can become chronic Pain over ischial tuberosity and sometimes into hamstrings
Observation	Lurching gait	Gait generally normal although may be antalgic
Active movement	Abduction, medial rotation, and flexion limited	Flexion limited
Passive movement	Capsular pattern	Noncapsular pattern
Resisted isometric movement	Normal but stress may cause pain	Hamstrings contraction sometimes painful
Special tests	True leg length difference Trendelenburg test positive	Leg lengths equal Trendelenburg test negative
Sensation	Normal	Normal
Reflexes	Normal	Normal
Joint play movements	May cause pain or relief	Normal
Diagnostic imaging	Diagnostic	Negative

REFERENCES

1. Lewis CL, Sahrmann SA: Acetabular labral tears. Phys Ther 86:110–121, 2006.
2. Huffman GR, Safran M: Tears of the acetabular labrum in athletes: diagnosis and treatment. Sports Med Arthro Rev 10:141–150, 2002.
3. Safran MR: The acetabular labrum: anatomic and functional characteristics and rationale for surgical intervention. J Am Acad Orthop Surg 18:338–345, 2010.
4. Frechill MT, Safran MR: The labrum of the hip: diagnosis and rationale for surgical correction. Clin Sports Med 30(2):293–315, 2011.
5. Myers CA, Register BC, Lertwanich P, et al: Role of the acetabular labrum and the iliofemoral ligament in hip stability. Am J Sports Med 39(suppl 1):S85–S91, 2011.
6. Botser IB, Martin DE, Stout CE, et al: Tears of the ligamentum teres—prevalence in hip arthroscopy using two classification systems. Am J Sports Med 39(suppl 1):S117–S125, 2011.
7. Van Den Bogert AJ, Read L, Nigg BM: An analysis of hip joint loading during walking, running and skiing. Med Sci Sports Exer 31:131–142, 1999.
8. Gurney B, Boissonault WG, Andrews R: Differential diagnosis of a femoral neck/head stress fracture. J Orthop Sports Phys Ther 36:80–88, 2006.
9. Byrd JW: Physical examination. In Byrd JW, editor: Operative hip arthroscopy, ed 2, New York, 2005, Springer.
10. Domb BG, Brooks AG, Byrd JW: Clinical examination of the hip joint in athletes. J Sports Rehabil 18:3–23, 2009.
11. Schon L, Zuckerman JD: Hip pain in the elderly: evaluation and diagnosis. Geriatrics 43:48–62, 1988.
12. Plante M, Wallace R, Busconi BD: Clinical diagnosis of hip pain. Clin Sports Med 30:225–238, 2011.
13. Hase T, Ueo T: Acetabular labral tear: arthroscopic diagnosis and treatment. Arthroscopy 15:138–141, 1999.
14. Mens J, Inklaar H, Koes BW, et al: A new view on adduction-related groin pain. Clin J Sports Med 16:15–19, 2006.
15. Minnich JM, Hanks JB, Muschaweck U, et al: Sports hernia—diagnosis and treatment highlighting a minimal repair surgical technique. Am J Sports Med 39:1341–1349, 2011.
16. Morales-Conde S, Socas M, Barranco A: Sportsman hernia: what do we know? Hernia 14:5–15, 2010.
17. Garvey JF, Read JW, Turner A: Sportsman hernia: what can we do? Hernia 14:17–25, 2010.
18. Litwin DE, Sneider EB, McEnaney PM, et al: Athletic pubalgia (sports hernia). Clin Sports Med 30:417–434, 2011.
19. Kagan A: Rotator cuff tears of the hip. Clin Orthop Relat Res 368:135–140, 1999.
20. Narvani AA, Tsiridis E, Kendall S, et al: A preliminary report on prevalence of acetabular labrum tears in sports patients with groin pain. Knee Surg Sports Traumatol Arthrosc 11:403–408, 2003.
21. Safran MR, Giordano G, Lindsey DP, et al: Strains across the acetabular labrum during hip motion—a cadaveric model. Am J Sports Med 39(suppl 1):S92–S102, 2011.
22. Reid DC: Sports injury assessment and rehabilitation, New York, 1992, Churchill Livingstone.
23. Allen WC: Coxa saltans: the snapping hip revisited. J Am Acad Orthop Surg 3:303–308, 1995.
24. Wahl CJ, Warren RF, Adler RS, et al: Internal coxa saltans (snapping hip) as a result of overtraining. Am J Sports Med 32:1302–1309, 2004.
25. Johnston CA, Wiley JP, Lindsay DM, et al: Iliopsoas bursitis and tendinitis: a review. Sports Med 25:271–283, 1998.
26. Mellman MR, McPherson EJ, Dorr LD, et al: Differential diagnosis of back and lower extremity problems. In Watkins RG, editor: The spine in sport, St Louis, 1996, CV Mosby.
27. Fitzgerald RH: Acetabular labrum tears—diagnosis and treatment. Clin Orthop Relat Res 311:60–68, 1995.
28. Dorrell JH, Catterall A: The torn acetabular labrum. J Bone Joint Surg Br 68:400–403, 1986.
29. Rashleigh-Belcher HJ, Cannon SR: Recurrent dislocation of the hip with a "Bankart type" lesion. J Bone Joint Surg Br 68:398–399, 1986.
30. Altman R, Alarcon G, Appelrouth D, et al: The American College of Rheumatology criteria for the classification and reporting of osteoarthritis of the hip. Arth Rheum 34:505–514, 1991.
31. Janda V: On the concept of postural muscles and posture in man. Aust J Physiother 29:83–85, 1983.
32. Jull JA, Janda V: Muscles and motor control in low back pain: Assessment and management. In Twomey LT, Taylor JR, editors: Physical therapy of the low back, New York, 1987, Churchill Livingstone.
33. Braly BA, Beall DP, Martin HD: Clinical examination of the athletic hip. Clin Sports Med 25:199–210, 2006.
34. Saudek CE: The hip. In Gould JA, editor: Orthopedic and sports physical therapy, St Louis, 1990, CV Mosby.
35. Krebs DE, Robbins CE, Lavine L, et al: Hip biomechanics during gait. J Orthop Sports Phys Ther 28:51–59, 1998.
36. Brand RA, Crowninshield RD: The effect of cane use on hip contact force. Clin Orthop 147:181–184, 1980.
37. Aspinall W: Clinical implications of iliopsoas dysfunction. J Man Manip Ther 1:41–46, 1993.
38. Ombregt L, Bissehop P, ter Veer HJ, et al: A system of orthopedic medicine, London, 1995, WB Saunders.
39. Ito K, Minka MA, Leung M, et al: Femoroacetabular impingement and the cam-effect—a MRI-based quantitative anatomical study of the femoral head-neck offset. J Bone Joint Surg Br 83:171–176, 2001.
40. Leunig M, Werlen S, Ungersbock A, et al: Evaluation of the acetabular labrum by MR arthrography. J Bone Joint Surg Br 79:230–234, 1997.
41. Klaue K, Durnin CW, Ganz R: The acetabular rim syndrome-a clinical presentation of dysplasia of the hip. J Bone Joint Surg Br 73:423–429, 1991.
42. Crawford JR, Villar RN: Current concepts in the management of femoroacetabular impingement. J Bone Joint Surg Br 87:1459–1462, 2005.
43. Ferguson TA, Matta J: Anterior femoroacetabular impingement: a clinical presentation. Sports Med Arthro Rev 10:134–140, 2002.
44. Santori N, Villar RN: Acetabular labral tears: result of arthroscopic partial limbectomy. Arthroscopy 16:11–15, 2000.
45. Philippon MJ, Maxwell RB, Johnson TL, et al: Clinical presentation of femoroacetabular impingement. Knee Surg Sports Traumatol Arthrosc 15:1041–1047, 2007.
46. Beaulé PE, O'Neill M, Rakhra K: Acetabular labral tears. J Bone Joint Surg Am 91:701–710, 2009.
47. Ganz R, Parvizi J, Beck M, et al: Femoroacetabular impingement—a case for osteoarthritis of the hip. Clin Orthop Relat Res 417:112–120, 2003.
48. Zaragoza EJ, Beaulé PE: Imaging of the painful non-arthritic hip: a practical approach to surgical relevancy. Oper Tech Orthop 14:42–48, 2004.
49. Reynolds D, Lucas J, Klaue K: Retroversion of the acetabulum. J Bone Joint Surg Br 81:281–288, 1999.
50. Beck M, Kalhor M, Leung M, et al: Hip morphology influences the pattern of damage to the acetabular cartilage—femoroacetabular impingement as a cause of early osteoarthritis of the hip. J Bone Joint Surg Br 87:1012–1018, 2005.
51. Parvizi J, Leung M, Ganz R: Femoroacetabular impingement. J Am Acad Orthop Surg 15:561–570, 2007.
52. Ejnisman L, Philippon MJ, Lertwanich P: Femoroacetabular impingement: the femoral side. Clin Sports Med 30:369–377, 2011.
53. Allen D, Beaulé PE, Ramadan D, et al: Prevalence of associated deformities and hip pain with cam-type femoroacetabular impingement. J Bone Joint Surg Br 91:589–594, 2009.
54. Birmingham PM, Kelly BT, Jacobs R, et al: The effect of dynamic femoroacetabular impingement on pubic symphysis motion—a cadaveric study. Am J Sports Med 40:1113–1118, 2012.
55. Beaulé PE, Allen DJ, Clohisy JC, et al: The young adult with hip impingement: deciding on the optimal intervention. J Bone Joint Surg Am 91:210–221, 2009.
56. Siebenrock KA, Schoeniger R, Ganz R: Anterior femoro-acetabular impingement due to acetabular retroversion—treatment with periacetabular osteotomy. J Bone Joint Surg Am 85:278–286, 2003.
57. Byrd JW, Jones KS: Arthroscopic management of femoroacetabular impingement in athletes. Am J Sports Med 39(suppl 1):S7–S13, 2011.
58. Audenaert EA, Peeters I, Vigneron L, et al: Hip morphology characteristics and range of internal rotation in femoroacetabular impingement. Am J Sports Med 40:1329–1336, 2012.
59. Sierra RJ, Trousdale RT, Ganz R, et al: Hip disease in the young active patient: evaluation and nonarthroplasty surgical options. J Am Acad Orthop Surg 16:689–703, 2008.
60. Davis AM, Bridge P, Miller J, et al: Interrater and intrarater reliability of the active hip abduction test. J Orthop Sports Phys Ther 41:953–960, 2011.
61. Simoneau GG, Hoenig KJ, Lepley JE, et al: Influence of hip position and gender on active hip internal and external rotation. J Orthop Sports Phys Ther 28:158–164, 1998.
62. Sutlive TG, Lopez HP, Schnitker DE, et al: Development of a clinical prediction rule for diagnosing hip osteoarthritis in individuals with unilateral hip pain. J Orthop Sports Phys Ther 38:542–550, 2008.
63. Klaue K, Durnin CW, Ganz R: The acetabular rim syndrome: a clinical presentation of dysplasia of the hip. J Bone Joint Surg Br 73:423–429, 1991.
64. Ward SR, Winters TM, Blemken SS: The architectural design of the gluteal muscle group: implications for movement and rehabilitation. J Orthop Sports Phys Ther 40:95–102, 2010.
65. Neuman DA: Kinesiology of the hip: a focus on muscular actions. J Orthop Sports Phys Ther 40:83–94, 2010.
66. Delahunt E, Kennelly C, McEntee BL, et al: The high adductor squeeze test: 45° of hip flexion as the optimal test position for eliciting adductor muscle activity and maximum pressure values. Manual Therapy 16:476–480, 2011.

67. Fredericson M, Moore W, Guillet M, et al: High hamstring tendinopathy in runners. Phys Sportsmed 33:32–43, 2005.

68. Tis LL, Perrin DH, Snead DB, et al: Isokinetic strength of the trunk and hip in female runners. Isok Exerc Sci 1:22–25, 1991.

69. Donatelli R, Catlin PA, Backer GS, et al: Isokinetic hip abductor to adductor torque ratio in normals. Isok Exerc Sci 1:103–111, 1991.

70. D'Aubigné RM, Postel M: Functional results of hip arthroplasty with acrylic prosthesis. J Bone Joint Surg Am 36:451–475, 1954.

71. Murray D: The hip. In Pynsent P, Fairbank J, Carr A, editors: Outcome measures in orthopedics, Oxford, 1994, Butterworth Heinemann.

72. Harris WH: Traumatic arthritis of the hip after dislocation and acetabular fractures: treatment by mold arthroplasty. An end result study using a new method of result evaluation. J Bone Joint Surg Am 51:737–755, 1969.

73. Kavanagh BF, Fitzgerald RH: Clinical and roentgenographic assessment of total hip arthroplasty: a new hip score. Clin Orthop 193:133–140, 1985.

74. Johanson NA, Charlson ME, Szatrowski TP, et al: A self-administered hip-rating questionnaire for the assessment of outcome after total hip replacement. J Bone Joint Surg Am 74:587–597, 1992.

75. Burton KE, Wright V, Richards J: Patients' expectations in relation to outcome of total hip replacement surgery. Ann Rheum Dis 38:471–474, 1979.

76. Jaglal S, Lakhani Z, Schatzker J: Reliability, validity, and responsiveness of the lower extremity measure for patients with a hip fracture. J Bone Joint Surg Am 82:955–962, 2000.

77. Jogi P, Spaulding SJ, Zecevic AA, et al: Comparison of the original and reduced versions of the Berg Balance Scale and the Western Ontario and McMaster Universities Osteoarthritis Index in patients following hip or knee arthroplasty. Physiother Can 63:107–114, 2011.

78. McConnell S, Kolopack P, Park AM: The Western Ontario and McMaster Universities Osteoarthritis Index (WOMAC): a review of its utility and measurement properties. Arth Rheum 45:453–461, 2001.

79. Jogi P, Kraemer JF, Birmingham T: Comparison of the Western Ontario and McMaster Universities Osteoarthritis Index (WOMAC) and the Lower Extremity Functional Scale (LEFS) questionnaires in patients awaiting or having undergone total knee arthroplasty. Physiother Can 57:208–216, 2005.

80. Jones CA, Voaklander DC, Johnston DW, et al: The effect of age on pain, function, and quality of life after total hip and knee arthroplasty. Arch Intern Med 161(3):454–460, 2001.

81. Bellamy N, Buchanan WW, Goldsmith CH, et al: Validation study of WOMAC: a health status instrument for measuring clinically important patient relevant outcomes to antirheumatic drug therapy in patients with osteoarthritis of the hip or knee. J Rheumatol 15(12):1833–1840, 1988.

82. Jones CA, Voaklander DC, Johnston DW, et al: Health related quality of life outcomes after total hip and knee arthroplasties in a community based population. J Rheumatol 27:1745–1752, 2000.

83. Stratford PW, Binkley JM, Watson J, et al: Validation of the LEFS on patients with total joint arthroplasty. Physiother Can 52:97–105, 2000.

84. Binkley JM, Stratford PW, Lott SA, et al: The lower extremity functional scale (LEFS): scale development, measurement properties, and clinical application. Physical Therapy 79:371–383, 1999.

85. Yeung TS, Wessel J, Stratford P, et al: Reliability, validity and responsiveness of the lower extremity functional scale for inpatients of an orthopedic rehabilitation ward. J Orthop Sports Phys Ther 39:468–477, 2009.

86. Lin CW, Moseley AM, Refshauge KM, et al: The lower extremity functional scale has good clinimetric properties in people with ankle fracture. Physical Therapy 89:580–588, 2009.

87. Ritter MA, Albohm MJ, Keating M, et al: Comparative outcomes of total joint arthroplasty. J Arthroplasty 10:737–741, 1995.

88. Mori B, Lundon K, Kreder HJ: 13-metre walk test applied to the elderly with musculoskeletal impairment: validity study. Physiother Can 57:217–224, 2005.

89. Nordin E, Rosendahl E, Lundin-Olsson L: Time "up and go" test: reliability in older people dependent in activities of daily living—focus on cognitive state. Phys Ther 86:646–655, 2006.

90. Yeung TS, Wessel J, Stratford P, et al: The timed up and go test for use on an inpatient orthopedic rehabilitation ward. J Orthop Sports Phys Ther 38:410–417, 2008.

91. Wright AA, Cook CE, Baxter GD, et al: A comparison of 3 methodological approaches to defining major clinically important improvement of 4 performance measures in patients with hip osteoarthritis. J Orthop Sports Phys Ther 41(5):319–327, 2011.

92. Butland RJ, Pang J, Gross ER, et al: Two-, six- and 12-minutes walking tests in respiratory disease. Br Med J 284:1607–1608, 1982.

93. Peel C, Ballard D: Reproducibility of the 6-minute walk test in older women. J Aging Phys Act 9:184–193, 2001.

94. Rikli RE, Jones CJ: The reliability of validity of a 6-minute walk test as a measure of physical endurance in older adults. J Aging Phys Act 6:363–375, 1998.

95. Harada ND, Chin V, Stewart AL: Mobility-related function in older adults: assessment with a 6-minute walk test. Arch Phys Med Rehabil 80:837–841, 1999.

96. Segura-Orti E, Martinez-Olmos FJ: Test-retest reliability and minimal detectable change scores for sit to stand to sit tests, the six minute walk test, the one leg heel rise test and handgrip strength in people undergoing hemodialysis. Physical Therapy 91(8):1244–1252, 2011.

97. Ekblom B, Day WC, Hartley LH, et al: Reproducibility of exercise prescribed by pace description. Scand J Sports Sci 1:16–19, 1979.

98. Cunningham DA, Rechnitzer PA, Pearce ME, et al: Determinates of self-selected walking pace across ages 19 to 66. J Gerontol 37:560–564, 1982.

99. Bassey J, Fentem PH, MacDonald IC, et al: Self-paced walking as a method for exercise testing in elderly and young men. Clin Sci Mol Med 51:609–612, 1976.

100. Tinetti ME: Performance-oriented assessment of mobility problems in elderly patients. J Am Geriatr Soc 34:119–126, 1986.

101. Reiman MP, Goode AP, Hegedus EJ, et al: Diagnostic accuracy of clinical tests of the hip: a systematic review with meta-analysis. Br J Sports Med 10:1–11, 2012.

102. Cook CE, Hegedus EJ: Orthopedic physical examination tests—an evidence based approach, Upper Saddle River, NJ, 2008, Prentice Hall/Pearson.

103. Cleland JA, Koppenhaver S: Netter's orthopedic clinical examination—an evidence based approach, ed 2, Philadelphia, 2011, Saunders/Elsevier.

104. Crane L: Femoral torsion and its relation to toeing-in and toeing-out. J Bone Joint Surg Am 41:421–428, 1959.

105. Tonnis D, Heinecke A: Acetabular and femoral anteversion: relationship with osteoarthritis of the hip. J Bone Joint Surg Am 81:1747–1770, 1999.

106. Gelberman RH, Cohen MS, Desai SS, et al: Femoral anteversion: a clinical assessment of idiopathic intoeing gait in children. J Bone Joint Surg Br 69(1): 75–79, 1987.

107. Adams MC: Outline of orthopaedics, London, 1968, E & S Livingstone.

108. Tachdjian MO: Pediatric orthopedics, Philadelphia, 1972, W.B. Saunders.

109. Staheli LT: Medial femoral torsion. Orthop Clin North Am 11:39–50, 1980.

110. Ruwe PA, Gage JR, Ozonoff MB, DeLuca PA: Clinical determination of femoral anteversion. J Bone Joint Surg Am 74:820–830, 1992.

111. Souza RB, Powers CM: Concurrent criterion-related validity and reliability of a clinical test to measure femoral anteversion. J Orthop Sports Phys Ther 39:586–592, 2009.

112. Boykin RE, Anz AW, Bushnell BD, et al: Hip instability. J Am Acad Orthop Surg 19(6):340–348, 2011.

113. Woods D, Macnicol M: The flexion-adduction test: an early sign of hip disease. J Pediatr Orthop 10:180–185, 2001.

114. Maitland GD: The peripheral joints: examination and recording guide, Adelaide, Australia, 1973, Virgo Press.

115. Austin AB, Souza RB, Meyer JL, et al: Identification of abnormal hip motion associated with acetabular labral pathology. J Orthop Sports Phys Ther 38:558–565, 2008.

116. Martin RL, Enseki KR, Draovitch P, et al: Acetabular labral tears of the hip: examination and diagnostic challenges. J Orthop Sports Phys Ther 36:503–515, 2006.

117. McCarthy JC, Lee J-O: Hip arthroscopy: indications, outcomes, and complications. J Bone Joint Surg Am 87: 1138–1145, 2005.

118. Fagerson T: Hip and thigh. In Magee DJ, Zachazewski JE, Quillen WS, editors: Pathology and intervention in musculoskeletal rehabilitation, Philadelphia, 2009, Elsevier.

119. Evans RC: Illustrated essentials in orthopedic physical assessment, St Louis, 1994, CV Mosby.

120. McGrory BJ: Stinchfield resisted hip flexion test. Hosp Physician 35:41–42, 1999.

121. McCarthy JC, Noble PC, Schuck MR, et al: The role of labral lesions to development of early degenerative hip disease. Clin Orthop Relat Res 393:25–37, 2001.

122. McGrory BJ: Stinchfield resisted inflection test. Hosp Phys 35:41–42, 1999.

123. Callaghan JJ: Examination of the hip. In Clarke CR, Bonfiglio M, editors: Orthopedics: essentials of diagnosis and treatment, New York, 1994, Churchill Livingstone.

124. Lee D: The pelvic girdle, Edinburgh, 1989, Churchill Livingstone.

125. Burgess RM, Rushton A, Wright C, et al: The validity and accuracy of clinical diagnostic tests used to detect labral pathology of the hip: a systematic review. Manual Therapy 16:318–326, 2011.

126. Suenaga E, Noguchi Y, Jingushi S, et al: Relationship between the maximum flexion-internal rotation test and the torn acetabulum labrum of a dysplastic hip. J Orthop Sci 7:26–32, 2002.

127. Shu B, Safran MR: Hip instability: anatomic and clinical considerations of traumatic and atraumatic instability. Clin Sports Med 30:349–367, 2011.

128. Johnson AW, Weiss CB, Wheeler DL: Stress fractures of the femoral shaft in athletes—more common than expected: a new clinical test. Am J Sports Med 22:248–256, 1994.

129. Adams SL, Yarnold PR: Clinical use of the patellar-pubic percussion sign in hip trauma. Am J Emerg Med 15:173–175, 1997.

130. Darmonov AV: Clinical screening for congenital dislocation of the hip. J Bone Joint Surg Am 78:383–388, 1996.

131. Guille JT, Pizzutillo PD, MacEwan GD: Developmental dysplasia of the hip from birth to six months. J Am Acad Orthop Surg 8:232–242, 2000.

132. Mahan ST, Katz JN, Kim YJ: To screen or not to screen? A decision analysis of utility of screening for developmental dysplasia of the hip. J Bone Joint Surg Am 91:1705–1719, 2009.

133. LeVeau B: Hip. In Richardson JK, Iglarsh ZA, editors: Clinical orthopedic physical therapy, Philadelphia, 1994, WB Saunders.

134. Moore FH: Examining infants' hips: can it do harm? J Bone Joint Surg Br 71:4–5, 1989.

135. Bolz S, Davies GJ: Leg length differences and correlation with total leg strength. J Orthop Sports Phys Ther 6:123–129, 1984.

136. Reider B: The orthopedic physical examination, Philadelphia, 1999, WB Saunders.

137. Clarke GR: Unequal leg length: an accurate method of detection and some clinical results. Rheumatol Phys Med 11:385–390, 1972.

138. Fisk JW, Balgent ML: Clinical and radiological assessment of leg length. N Z Med J 81:477–480, 1975.

139. Woerman AL, Binder-Macleod SA: Leg-length discrepancy assessment: accuracy and precision in five clinical methods of evaluation. J Orthop Sports Phys Ther 5:230–239, 1984.

140. Woerman AL: Evaluation and treatment of dysfunction in the lumbar-pelvic-hip complex. In Donatelli R, Wooden MJ, editors: Orthopedic physical therapy, Edinburgh, 1989, Churchill Livingstone.

141. Crawford AH: Neurologic disorders. In Steinberg ME, editor: The hip and its disorders, Philadelphia, 1991, WB Saunders.

142. Gruebel-Lee DM: Disorders of the hip, Philadelphia, 1983, JB Lippincott.

143. Zimney NJ: Clinical reasoning in the evaluation and management of undiagnosed chronic hip pain in a young adult. Phys Ther 78:62–73, 1998.

144. Palmar ML, Epler M: Clinical assessment procedures in physical therapy, Philadelphia, 1990, JB Lippincott.

145. Kuo L, Chung W, Bates E, et al: The hamstring index. J Pediatr Ortho 17:78–88, 1997.

146. Noble HB, Hajek MR, Porter M: Diagnosis and treatment of iliotibial band tightness in runners. Phys Sportsmed 10:67–68, 71–72, 74, 1982.

147. Ober FB: The role of the iliotibial and fascia lata as a factor in the causation of low-back disabilities and sciatica. J Bone Joint Surg 18:105–110, 1936.

148. Strauss EJ, Kim S, Calcei JG, et al: Iliotibial band syndrome: evaluation and management. J Am Acad Orthop Surg 19:728–736, 2011.

149. Tonley JC, Yun SM, Kochevar RJ, et al: Treatment of an individual with piriformis syndrome focusing on hip muscle strengthening and movement re-education: a case report. J Orthop Sports Phys Ther 40:103–111, 2010.

150. Garrick JG, Webb DR: Sports injuries: diagnosis and treatment, Philadelphia, 1990, WB Saunders.

151. Gautam VK, Anand S: A new test for estimating iliotibial band contracture. J Bone Joint Surg Br 80:474–475, 1998.

152. Zeren B, Oztekin HH: A new self-diagnostic test for biceps femoris muscle strains. Clin J Sports Med 16:166–169, 2006.

153. Thurston A: Assessment of fixed flexion deformity of the hip. Clin Orthop 169:186–189, 1982.

154. Trendelenburg F: Trendelenburg's test (1895). Clin Orthop Relat Res 355:3–7, 1998.

155. Crossley KM, Zhang W-J, Schache AG, et al: Performance on the single-leg squat task indicates hip abductor muscle function. Am J Sports Med 39:866–873, 2011.

156. American Orthopaedic Association: Manual of orthopaedic surgery, Chicago, 1972, AOA.

157. Kristensen MT, Foss NB, Kehlet H: Timed "up and go" test as a predictor of falls within 6 months after hip fracture surgery. Physical Therapy 87:24–30, 2007.

158. Cornwall R, Radomisli TE: Nerve injury in traumatic dislocation of the hip. Clin Orthop Relat Res 377:84–91, 2000.

159. Dettart MM, Riley LH: Nerve injuries in total hip arthroplasty. J Am Acad Orthop Surg 7:101–111, 1999.

160. Giannoudis PV, DaCosta AA, Raman R, et al: Double-crush syndrome after acetabular fractures—a sign of poor prognosis. J Bone Joint Surg Br 87:401–407, 2005.

161. Pecina MM, Krmpotic-Nemanic J, Markiewitz AD: Tunnel syndromes, Boca Raton, Florida, 1991, CRC Press.

162. Vandertop WP, Bosman NJ: The piriformis syndrome—a case report. J Bone Joint Surg Am 73:1095–1096, 1991.

163. Bradshaw C, Bell S, Brukner P: Obturator nerve entrapment—a cause of groin pain in athletes. Am J Sports Med 25:402–408, 1997.

164. Kelly BT, Williams RJ, Philippon MJ: Hip arthroscopy: current indications, treatment options, and management issues. Am J Sports Med 31:1020–1037, 2003.

165. Clohisy JC, Carlisle JC, Beaulé PE, et al: A systematic approach to the plain radiographic evaluation of the young adult hip. J Bone Joint Surg Am 90:47–66, 2008.

166. Harris WH: Etiology of osteoarthritis of the hip. Clin Orthop Relat Res 213:20–33, 1986.

167. Oh CW, Thacker MM, Mackenzie WG, et al: Cox vara—a novel measurement technique in skeletal dysplasias. Clin Orthop Relat Res 147:125–131, 2006.

168. Sugano N, Kubo T, Takaoka K, et al: Diagnostic criteria for non-traumatic osteonecrosis of the femoral head. J Bone Joint Surg Br 81:590–599, 1999.

169. Kellgren JH, Lawrence JS: Radiological assessment of osteo-arthrosis. Ann Rheum Dis 16:494–502, 1957.

170. Perkins G: Signs by which to diagnose congenital dislocation of the hip. Clin Orthop 274:3–5, 1992.

171. Loder RT, Aronsson DD, Dobbs MB, et al: Slipped capital femoral epiphysis. J Bone Joint Surg Am 82:1170–1188, 2000.

172. Bigg-Wither G, Kelly P: Diagnostic imaging in musculoskeletal physiotherapy. In Refshauge K, Gass E, editors: Musculoskeletal physiotherapy, Oxford, 1995, Butterworth Heinemann.

173. Kang AC, Gooding AJ, Coates MH, et al: Computed tomography assessment of hip joints in asymptomatic individuals in relation to femoroacetabular impingement. Am J Sports Med 38:1160–1165, 2010.

174. Edwards DJ, Lomas D, Villar RN: Diagnosis of the painful hip by magnetic resonance imaging and arthroscopy. J Bone Joint Surg Br 77:374–376, 1995.

175. Guanch CA: MR imaging of the hip. Sports Med Arthrosc Rev 17:49–55, 2009.

176. Mitchell B, McCrory P, Brukner P, et al: Hip joint pathology: clinical presentation and correlation between magnetic resonance arthrography, ultrasound and arthroscopic findings in 25 consecutive cases. Clin J Sports Med 13:152–156, 2003.

177. Byrd JW, Jones KS: Diagnostic accuracy of clinical assessment, magnetic resonance imaging, magnetic resonance arthrography, and intra-articular injection in hip arthroscopy patients. Am J Sports Med 32(7):1668–1674, 2004.

178. Register B, Pennock AT, Ho CP, et al: Prevalence of abnormal hip findings in asymptomatic participants—a prospective, blended study. Am J Sports Med 40:2720–2724, 2012.

179. Harke HT, Kumar SJ: The role of ultrasound in the diagnosis and management of congenital and dysplasia of the hip. J Bone Joint Surg Br 73:622–628, 1991.

180. Holen KJ, Tegnander A, Eik-Nes SH, et al: The use of ultrasound in determining the initiation of treatment in instability of the hip in neonates. J Bone Joint Surg Br 81:846–851, 1999.

181. Falliner A, Schwinzer D, Hahne HJ, et al: Comparing ultrasound measurements of neonatal hips using the method of Graf and Terjesen. J Bone Joint Surg Br 88:104–106, 2006.

182. Jonson SR, Gross MT: Intraexaminer reliability, interexaminer reliability, and mean values for nine lower extremity skeletal measures in healthy naval midshipmen. J Orthop Sports Phys Ther 25:253–263, 1997.

183. Salen BA, Spangfort EV, Nygren AL, et al: The Disability Rating Index: an instrument for the assessment of disability in clinical settings. J Clin Epidemiol 47:1423–1434, 1994.

184. Cliborne AV, Waineer RS, Rhon DI, et al: Clinical hip tests and a functional squat test in patients with knee osteoarthritis: reliability, prevalence of positive test findings, and short-term response to hip mobilization. J Orthop Sports Phys Ther 34:676–685, 2004.

185. Cibulka MT, White DM, Woehrle J, et al: Hip pain and mobility deficits—hip osteoarthritis: clinical practice guidelines. J Orthop Sports Phys Ther 39(4):A1–A25, 2009.

186. Ross MD, Nordeen MH, Barido M: Test-retest reliability of Patrick's hip range of motion test in healthy college-aged men. J Strength Cond Res 17(1):156–161, 2003.

187. Remy F, Chantelot C, Fontaine C, et al: Inter- and intra-observer reproducibility in radiographics diagnosis and classification of femoral trochlear dysplasia. Surg Radiol Anat 20:285–289, 1998.

188. Hinson R, Brown SH: Supine leg length differential estimation: an inter- and intra-examiner reliability study. Chiropr Res J 5(1):17–22, 1998.

SUGGESTED READINGS

Andersson G: Hip assessment: a comparison of nine different methods. J Bone Joint Surg Br 54:621–625, 1972.

Bassett LW, Gold RH, Seeger LL: MRI atlas of the musculoskeletal system, London, 1989, Martin Dunitz.

Beck M, Sledge JB, Gautier E, et al: The anatomy and function of the gluteus minimus muscle. J Bone Joint Surg Br 82:358–363, 2000.

Beetham WP, Polley HF, Slocumb CH, et al: Physical examination of the joints, Philadelphia, 1965, WB Saunders.

Bertol P, Macnicol MF, Mitchell GP: Radiographic features of neonatal congenital dislocation of the hip. J Bone Joint Surg Br 64:176–179, 1982.

Bos CFA, Bloem JL, Obermann WR, et al: Magnetic resonance imaging in congenital dislocation of the hip. J Bone Joint Surg Br 70:174–178, 1988.

Brignall CG, Stainky GD: The snapping hip. J Bone Joint Surg Br 73:253–254, 1991.

Broughton NS, Brougham DI, Cole WG, et al: Reliability of radiological measurements in the assessment of the child's hip. J Bone Joint Surg Br 71:6–8, 1989.

Bryant MJ, Kernehan WG, Nixon JR, et al: A statistical analysis of hip scores. J Bone Joint Surg Br 75:705–709, 1993.

Bunker TD, Esler CN, Leach WJ: Rotator cuff tear of the hip. J Bone Joint Surg Br 79:618–620, 1997.

Caborn DN, Grollman LJ, Nyland JA, et al: Running. In Fu FH, Stone DA, editors: Sports injuries: mechanisms, prevention, treatment, Baltimore, 1994, Williams & Wilkins.

Callaghan JJ, Dysart SH, Savory CF, et al: Assessing the results of hip replacement: a comparison of five different rating systems. J Bone Joint Surg Br 72:1008–1009, 1990.

Cameron DM, Bohannon RW: Relationship between active knee extension and active straight leg raise test measurements. J Orthop Sports Phys Ther 17:257–259, 1993.

Campbell JD: Injuries to the pelvis, hip, and thigh. In Orthopedic knowledge update: sports medicine, Rosemont, IL, 1994, American Academy of Orthopaedic Surgeons.

Chung SMK: Hip disorders in infants and children, Philadelphia, 1981, Lea & Febiger.

Clarke GR: Unequal leg length: an accurate method of detection and some clinical results. Rheumatol Phys Med 11:385–390, 1972.

Clarkson HM: Musculoskeletal assessment: joint range of motion and manual muscle strength, ed 2, Baltimore, 2000, Williams & Wilkins.

Crock HV: An atlas of the arterial supply of the head and neck of the femur in man. Clin Orthop 152:17–27, 1980.

Crouch JE: Functional human anatomy, Philadelphia, 1973, Lea & Febiger.

Cyriax J: Textbook of orthopaedic medicine, vol. 1: diagnosis of soft tissue lesions, London, 1975, Bailliere Tindall.

Dalinka MK, Neustadter LM: Radiology of the hip. In Steinberg ME, editor: The hip and its disorders, Philadelphia, 1991, WB Saunders.

Danbert RJ: Clinical assessment and treatment of leg length inequalities. J Manip Physiol Ther 11:290–295, 1988.

Debrunner HN: Orthopaedic diagnosis, London, 1973, E & S Longman Group.

D'Souza L, Hynes D, McManus F: Radiological screening for congenital hip dislocation in the infant "at risk," J Bone Joint Surg Br 78:319–320, 1996.

Dutton M: Orthopedic examination, evaluation and intervention, New York, 2004, McGraw-Hill.

Edelson R, Stevens P: Meralgia paresthetica in children. J Bone Joint Surg Am 76:1993–1999, 1994.

Ekstrand J, Wiktorsson M, Oberg P, et al: Lower extremity goniometric measurements: a study to determine their reliability. Arch Phys Med Rehabil 663:171–175, 1982.

Fickel TE: "Snapping hip" and sacroiliac sprain: example of a cause-effect relationship. J Manip Physiol Ther 12:390–392, 1989.

Fisk JW, Bargent ML: Clinical and radiological assessment of leg length. N Z Med J 81:477–480, 1975.

Forrester DM, Brown JC: The radiology of joint disease, Philadelphia, 1987, WB Saunders.

Friberg O: Clinical symptoms and biomechanics of lumbar spine and hip joint in leg length inequality. Spine 8:643–651, 1983.

Gajdosik RL, Rieck MA, Sullivan DK, et al: Comparison of four clinical tests for assessing hamstring muscle length. J Orthop Sports Phys Ther 18:614–618, 1993.

Gelberman RH, Cohen MS, Shaw BA, et al: The association of femoral retroversion with slipped capital femoral epiphysis. J Bone Joint Surg Am 68:1000–1007, 1986.

Gerberg LF: Nontraumatic hip pain in active children: a critical differential. Phys Sportsmed 24:69–74, 1996.

Goddard NJ, Gosling PT: Intra-articular fluid pressure and pain in osteoarthritis of the hip. J Bone Joint Surg Br 70:52–55, 1988.

Gogia PP, Braatz JH: Validity and reliability of leg length measurements. J Orthop Sports Phys Ther 8:185–188, 1986.

Greenwood MJ, Erhard RE, Jones DL: Differential diagnosis of the hip vs lumbar spine: five case reports. J Orthop Sports Phys Ther 27:308–315, 1998.

Grieve GP: The hip. Physiotherapy 57:212–219, 1971.

Guidera KJ, Einbecker ME, Berman CG, et al: Magnetic resonance imaging evaluation of congenital dislocation of the hips. Clin Orthop 261:96–101, 1990.

Harcke HT, Kumar SJ: The role of ultrasound in the diagnosis and management of congenital dislocation and dysplasia of the hip. J Bone Joint Surg Am 73:622–628, 1991.

Hardcastle P, Nade S: The significance of the Trendelenburg test. J Bone Joint Surg Br 67:741–746, 1985.

Hernandez RJ, Poznanski AK: CT evaluation of pediatric hip disorders. Orthop Clin North Am 16:513–541, 1985.

Hicklin SP, DePretis MC: Lower extremity: Hip. In Myers RS, editor: Saunders manual of physical therapy practice, Philadelphia, 1995, WB Saunders.

Hoaglund FT, Low WD: Anatomy of the femoral neck and head, with comparative data from Caucasians and Hong Kong Chinese. Clin Orthop 152:10–16, 1980.

Hoaglund FT, Yau AC, Wong WL: Osteoarthritis of the hip and other joints in southern Chinese in Hong Kong. J Bone Joint Surg Am 55:545–557, 1973.

Hollinshead WH, Jenkins DB: Functional anatomy of the limbs and back, Philadelphia, 1981, WB Saunders.

Hoppenfeld S: Physical examination of the spine and extremities, New York, 1976, Appleton-Century-Crofts.

Hunt GC, Fromherz WA, Danoff J, et al: Femoral transverse torque: an assessment method. J Orthop Sports Phys Ther 7:319–324, 1986.

Johanson NA, Liang MH, Daltroy L, et al: American Academy of Orthopedic Surgeons lower limb outcomes assessment instruments—reliability, validity and sensitivity to change. J Bone Joint Surg Am 86:902–909, 2004.

Johnson TR, Steinbach LS: Essentials of musculoskeletal imaging, Rosemont, IL, 2004, American Academy of Orthopedic Surgeons.

Jones DA: Neonatal hip stability and the Barlow test. J Bone Joint Surg Br 73:216–218, 1991.

Judge RD, Zuidema GD, Fitzgerald FT: Clinical diagnosis: a physiological approach, Boston, 1982, Little, Brown.

Kallio PE, Mah ET, Foster BK, et al: Slipped capital femoral epiphysis: incidence and clinical assessment of physical instability. J Bone Joint Surg Br 77:752–755, 1995.

Kaltenborn FM: Mobilization of the extremity, Oslo, 1980, Olaf Norlis Bokhandel.

Kane TJ, Henry G, Furry D: A simple roentgenographic measurement of femoral anteversion. J Bone Joint Surg Am 74:1540–1542, 1992.

Kapandji IA: The physiology of the joints, vol. 2: lower limb, New York, 1970, Churchill Livingstone.

Kernohan WG, Nugent GE, Haugh PE, et al: Sensitivity of manual palpation in testing the neonatal hip. Clin Orthop 294:211–215, 1993.

Kim VT, Azuma H: The nerve endings of the acetabular labrum. Clin Orthop 320:176–181, 1995.

Kopell HP, Thompson WA: Peripheral entrapment neuropathies of the lower extremity. N Engl J Med 262:56–60, 1960.

Landon GC, Galante JO: Physical examination of the hip joint. In Post M, edtior: Physical examination of the musculoskeletal system, Chicago, 1987, Year Book Medical Publishers.

Larson CB: Rating scale for hip disabilities. Clin Orthop 31:85–93, 1963.

Lausten GS, Jorgensen F, Boesen J: Measurement of anteversion of the femoral neck: ultrasound and computerized tomography compared. J Bone Joint Surg Br 71:237–239, 1989.

Lerangic PK, Norkin CC: Joint structure and function—a comprehensive analysis, Philadelphia, 2005, FA Davis.

Maeda R: Diagnosis and management of hip disorders. Orthop Phys Ther Clin North Am 7:397–412, 1998.

Mansour ES, Steingard MA: Anterior hip pain in the adult: an algorithmic approach to diagnosis. JAOA 97:32–38, 1997.

McGann WA: History and physical examination. In Steinberg ME, editor: The hip and its disorders, Philadelphia, 1991, WB Saunders.

McGrory BJ, Burke DW, Moran SJ: Posterior instability of the hip in the adult. Clin Orthop Relat Res 341:151–154, 1997.

McKinnis LN: Fundamentals of musculoskeletal imaging, Philadelphia, 2005, FA Davis.

McRae R: Clinical orthopaedic examination, New York, 1976, Churchill Livingstone.

Milch H: The measurement of hip motion in the sagittal and coronal planes. J Bone Joint Surg Am 41:731–736, 1959.

Montgomery WH, Pink M, Perry J: Electromyographic analysis of hip and knee musculature during running. Am J Sports Med 22:272–278, 1994.

Morelli V, Smith V: Groin injuries in athletes. Am Fam Physician 64:1405–1415, 2001.

Morscher E, Figner G: Measurement of leg length. Prog Orthop Surg 1:21–27, 1977.

Moseley CF: The biomechanics of the pediatric hip. Orthop Clin North Am 11:3–16, 1980.

Murphy SB, Simon SR, Kijewski PK, et al: Femoral anteversion. J Bone Joint Surg Am 69:1169–1176, 1987.

Neumann DA: Kinesiology of the musculoskeletal system—foundations for physical rehabilitation, St Louis, 2002, CV Mosby.

Nichols PJR, Bailey NTJ: The accuracy of measuring leg length differences: an "observer error" experiment. Br Med J 2:1247–1248, 1955.

Noesberger B, Eichenberger AR: Overuse injuries of the hip and snapping hip syndrome. Oper Tech Sports Med 5:138–142, 1997.

O'Donoghue DH: Treatment of injuries to athletes, ed 4, Philadelphia, 1984, WB Saunders.

Patel K, Wallace R, Busconi BD: Radiology. Clin Sports Med 30:239–283, 2011.

Pavlov H: Roentgen examination of groin and hip pain in the athlete. Clin Sports Med 6:829–843, 1987.

Pearrsal AW: Assessing acute hip injury: examination, diagnosis and triage. Phys Sportsmed 23:36–48, 1995.

Pellecchia GL, Lugo-Larcheveque N, DeLuca PA: Differential diagnosis in physical therapy evaluation of thigh pain in an adolescent boy. J Orthop Sports Phys Ther 23:51–55, 1996.

Peterson HA, Klassen RA, McLeod RA, et al: The use of computerized tomography in dislocation of the hip and femoral neck anteversion in children. J Bone Joint Surg Br 63:198–208, 1981.

Petty NJ, Moore AP: Neuromusculoskeletal examination and assessment—a handbook for therapists, London, 1998, Churchill Livingstone.

Pitt MJ, Lund PJ, Speer DP: Imaging of the pelvis and hip. Orthop Clin North Am 21:545–559, 1990.

Poggi JJ, Callahan JJ, Spritzer CE, et al: Changes on magnetic resonance images after traumatic hip dislocation. Clin Orthop 319:249–259, 1995.

Quarrier NF, Wightman AB: A ballet dancer with chronic hip pain due to a lesser trochanter bony avulsion: the challenge of a differential diagnosis. J Orthop Sports Phys Ther 28:168–173, 1998.

Radin EL: Biomechanics of the hip. Clin Orthop 152:28–34, 1980.

Rask MR: Superior gluteal nerve entrapment syndrome. Muscle Nerve 3:304–307, 1980.

Reigger-Krugh C, Keysor JJ: Skeletal malalignments of the lower quarter: correlated and compensatory motions and postures. J Orthop Sports Phys Ther 23:164–170, 1996.

Resnick D, Kransdorf MJ: Bone and joint imaging, Philadelphia, 2005, Elsevier.

Roach KE, Miles TP: Normal hip and knee active range of motion: the relationship to age. Phys Ther 71:656–665, 1991.

Rydell N: Biomechanics of the hip. Clin Orthop 92:6–15, 1973.

Sanders B, Nemeth WC: Hip and thigh injuries. In Zachazewski JE, Magee DJ, Quillen WS, editors: Athletic injuries and rehabilitation, Philadelphia, 1996, WB Saunders.

Schaberg JE, Harper MC, Allen WC: The snapping hip syndrome. Am J Sports Med 12:361–365, 1984.

Schmalzried TP, Amstutz HC, Dorey FJ: Nerve palsy associated with total hip replacement. J Bone Joint Surg Am 73:1074–1080, 1991.

Siffert RS: Lower limb-length discrepancy. J Bone Joint Surg Am 69:1100–1106, 1987.

Sims K: Assessment and treatment of hip osteoarthritis. Man Ther 4:136–144, 1999.

Solomon L: Patterns of osteoarthritis of the hip. J Bone Joint Surg Br 58:176–183, 1976.

Spiera H: Osteoarthritis as a misdiagnosis in elderly patients. Geriatrics 42:37–42, 1987.

Staheli LT: Torsional deformity. Pediatr Clin North Am 33:1373–1383, 1986.

Starkey C, Ryan J: Evaluation of orthopedic and athletic injuries, Philadelphia, 1996, FA Davis.

Swain R, Snodgrass S: Managing groin pain: even when the cause is not obvious. Phys Sportsmed 23:55–66, 1995.

Tomberlin JP, Saunders HD: Evaluation, treatment, and prevention of musculoskeletal disorders, Chaska, MN, 1994, The Saunders Group.

Tonnis D, Heinecke A: Acetabular and femoral anteversion: relationship with osteoarthritis of the hip. J Bone Joint Surg Am 81:1747–1770, 1999.

Wadsworth CT: Manual examination and treatment of the spine and extremities, Baltimore, 1988, Williams & Wilkins.

Waters PM, Mills MB: Hip and pelvic injuries in the young athlete. In Stanitski CL, DeLee JC, and Drez D, editors: Pediatric and adolescent sports medicine, Philadelphia, 1994, WB Saunders.

Wiessman BNW, Sledge CB: Orthopedic radiology, Philadelphia, 1986, WB Saunders.

Williams PL, Warwick P, editors: Gray's anatomy, ed 36, British, Edinburgh, 1980, Churchill Livingstone.

Yoshioka Y, Cooke TD: Femoral anteversion: assessment based on functional axes. J Orthop Res 5:86–91, 1987.

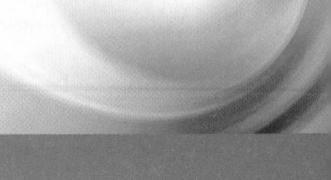

CHAPTER 12

Knee

The knee joint is particularly susceptible to traumatic injury because it is located at the ends of two long lever arms, the tibia and the femur. In addition, because the joint connects one long bone "sitting" on another long bone, it depends on the ligaments and muscles that surround it for its strength and stability, not on its bony configuration.[1]

Because the knee joint depends on its ligaments to such a great extent, it is imperative that the ligaments be tested during the examination of the knee. Therefore the ligamentous tests are not included under the "Special Tests" section but instead are listed in a separate section to ensure that they are always included in the examination of the knee.

Because of its anatomical arrangement, the knee is a complicated area to assess, and the examiner must take time to ensure that all relevant structures are tested. It must also be remembered that the lumbar spine, hip, and ankle may refer pain to the knee, and these joints must be assessed if it appears that joints other than the knee may be involved. For example, a slipped capital femoral epiphysis at the hip commonly refers pain to the knee, and this knee pain may predominate.

APPLIED ANATOMY

The **tibiofemoral joint** is the largest joint in the body. It is a modified hinge joint having 2° of freedom. The synovium around the joint is extensive; it communicates with many of the bursae and pouches around the knee joint. Although the synovial membrane "encapsulates" the entire knee joint, its distribution within the knee is such that the cruciate ligaments, which run from the middle of the tibial plateau to the intercondylar area of the femur, are extrasynovial. (*Cruciate* means that the ligaments cross each other.)

The articular surfaces of the tibia and femur are not congruent, which enables the two bones to move different amounts, guided by the muscles and ligaments. The two bones approach congruency in full extension, which is the close packed position. Kaltenborn[2] has stated that the close packed position includes full lateral rotation of the tibia. The lateral femoral condyle projects anteriorly more than the medial femoral condyle to help prevent lateral dislocation of the patella. In females, this enlargement is important because of the female's broader pelvis and increased inward angle of the femur, which allow the femoral condyles to be parallel with the ground (Figure 12-1). The resting position of the joint is approximately 25° of flexion, and the capsular pattern is flexion more limited than extension.

The space between the tibia and femur is partially filled by two menisci that are attached to the tibia to add congruency. The **medial meniscus** is a small part of a large circle (i.e., C shaped) and is thicker posteriorly than anteriorly. The **lateral meniscus** is a large part of a small circle (i.e., O shaped) and is generally of equal thickness throughout. Both menisci are thicker along the periphery and thinner along the inner margin.

During the movement from extension to flexion, both menisci move posteriorly, the lateral meniscus being displaced more than the medial meniscus. The lateral meniscus has an excursion of 10 mm, and the medial meniscus has an excursion of 2 mm. The menisci are avascular in their cartilaginous inner two thirds and are partly vascular and fibrous in their outer one third.[3] They are held in place by the coronary ligaments attaching to the tibia.

The menisci serve several functions in the knee. They aid in lubrication and nutrition of the joint and act as shock absorbers (a meniscectomy can reduce shock absorption capacity at the knee by 20%),[4] spreading the stress over the articular cartilage and decreasing cartilage wear. They make the joint surfaces more congruent and improve weight distribution by increasing the area of contact between the condyles. The menisci reduce friction during movement and aid the ligaments and capsule in preventing hyperextension. The menisci prevent the joint capsule from entering the joint and participate in the "locking" mechanism of the joint into close pack by directing the movement of the femoral articular condyles. Because more recent literature indicates that removal of

Tibiofemoral Joint	
Resting position:	25° flexion
Close packed position:	Full extension, lateral rotation of tibia
Capsular pattern:	Flexion, extension

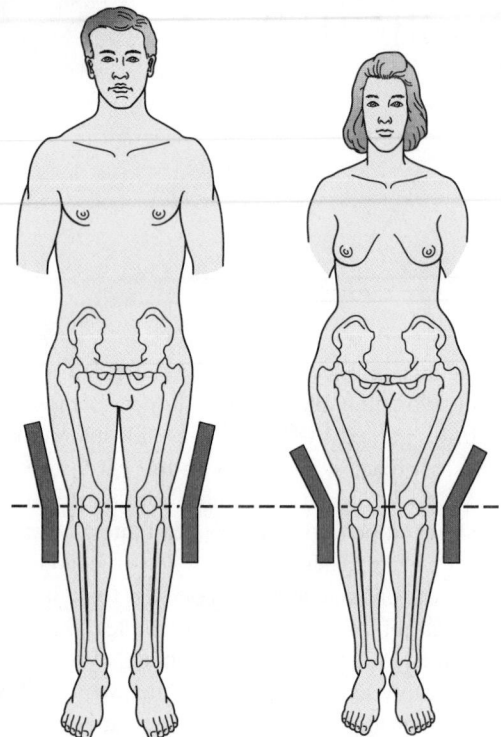

Figure 12-1 Q-angle differences in males and females. Because of the broader pelvis in the female, it is necessary for the femur to come inward at an increased angle to make the distal end of the condyles parallel with the ground. The quadriceps, patella, and patellar tendon form an angle centered at the patella. As the quadriceps contracts, the angle tends to straighten, which forces the patella laterally. (Redrawn from O'Donoghue D: Treatment of injuries to athletes, ed 4, Philadelphia, 1984, WB Saunders, p. 522.)

the entire meniscus can lead to early degeneration of the joint,[5,6] most surgeons today remove only the torn portion of the meniscus, or, if the tear is in the outer one third where there is sufficient circulation to aid healing, the surgeon may attempt to surgically repair (suture) the meniscus.

It is generally believed that the meniscus possesses minimal innervation so there is minimal or no pain when it is damaged unless the coronary ligaments have been damaged as well. Gray[7] has reported, however, that the menisci possess innervation in their outer two thirds with the anterior and posterior horns being well innervated. Because the menisci are primarily avascular, especially in the inner two thirds, there is seldom bloody effusion in injury; however, there may be synovial effusion. Their poor blood supply, especially in the inner two thirds, gives the menisci a low regeneration potential.

The lateral meniscus is not as firmly attached to the tibia as the medial meniscus and therefore is less prone to injury. The coronary ligaments, also referred to as the *meniscotibial ligaments,* tend to be longer on the lateral aspect, and the horns of the lateral meniscus are closer together.

The **patellofemoral joint** is a modified plane joint, the lateral articular surface of the patella being wider. The patella contains the thickest layer of cartilage in the body and, in reality, is a sesamoid bone found within the patellar tendon. It has five facets, or ridges: superior, inferior, lateral, medial, and odd. It is the odd facet that is most frequently the first part of the patella to be affected in chondromalacia patellae (i.e., premature degeneration of the patellar cartilage) or patellofemoral syndrome.

During the movement from flexion to extension, different parts of the patella articulate with the femoral condyles (Figure 12-2).[8,9] The odd facet does not come into contact with the femoral condyles until at least 135° of flexion is reached. Incorrect alignment or malalignment of the patellar movement over the femoral condyles can lead to patellofemoral arthralgia. The capsule of this joint is continuous with the capsule of the tibiofemoral joint.

The **patella** improves the efficiency of extension during the last 30° of extension (i.e., 30° to 0° of extension with the straight leg being 0°), because it holds the quadriceps tendon away from the axis of movement. The patella also functions as a guide for the quadriceps or patellar tendon, decreases friction of the quadriceps mechanism, controls capsular tension in the knee, acts as a bony shield for the cartilage of the femoral condyles, and improves the aesthetic appearance of the knee (Figure 12-3).

Patellar Loading with Activity	
Walking:	0.3 times the body weight
Climbing stairs:	2.5 times the body weight
Descending stairs:	3.5 times the body weight
Squatting:	7 times the body weight

The **superior tibiofibular joint** is a plane synovial joint between the tibia and the head of the fibula. It is supported by anterior and posterior ligaments of the same name. Movement occurs in this joint with any activity involving the ankle. Hypomobility at this joint can lead to pain in the knee area on activity, because the fibula can bear up to one sixth of the body weight. In approximately 10% of the population, the capsule of this joint is continuous with that of the tibiofemoral joint.

PATIENT HISTORY

In addition to the questions listed under the "Patient History" section in Chapter 1, the examiner should obtain the following information from the patient:

1. *How did the accident occur, or what was the mechanism of injury?*[10,11] The primary mechanisms of injury in the knee are a valgus force (with or without

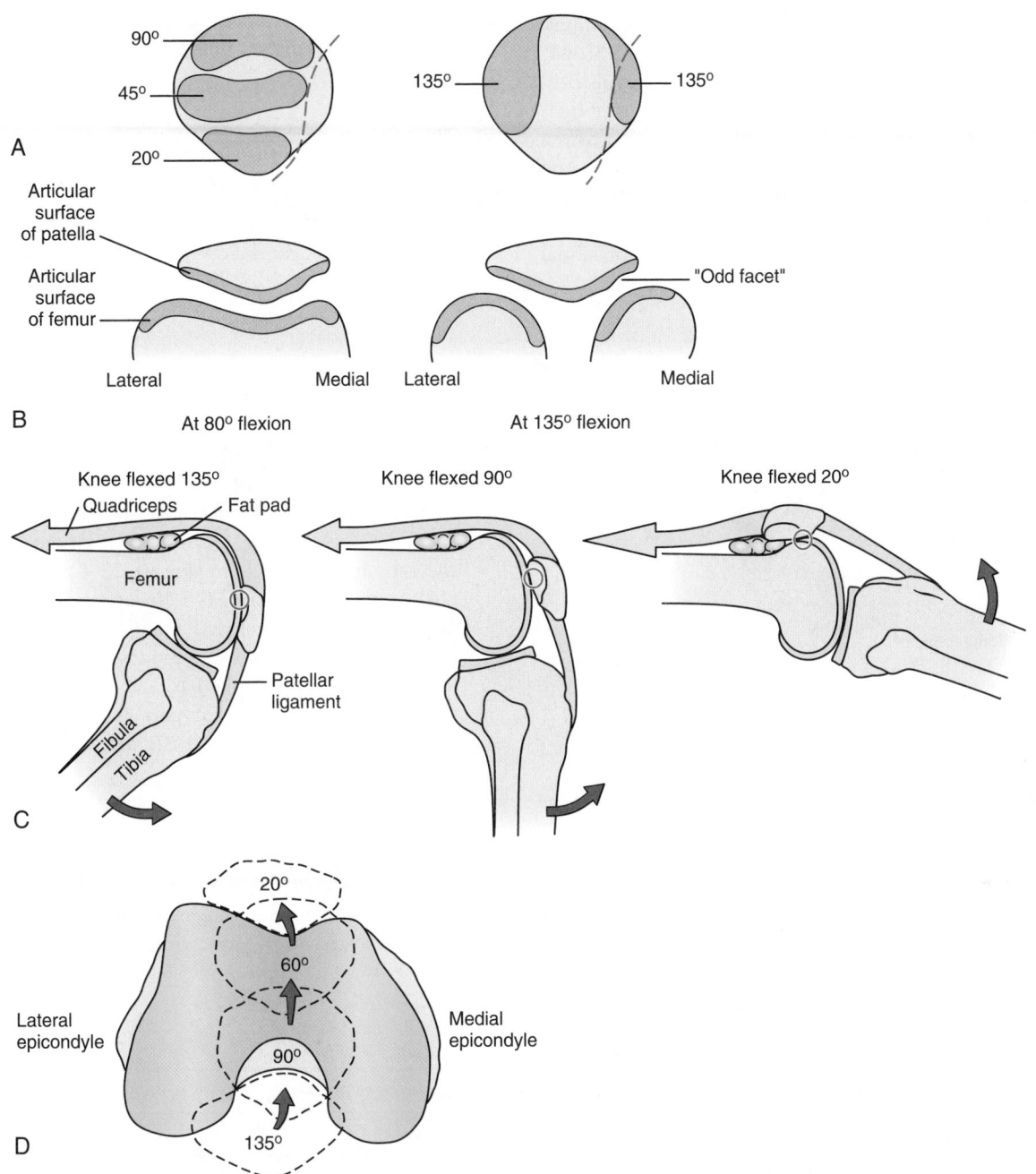

Figure 12-2 A, Area of contact of the patella during different degrees of flexion. **B,** Articulation between patella and femur. **C,** The circles depicted on the patella indicate the point of maximal contact between the patella and the femur. As the knee is extended, the contact point on the patella migrates from superior to inferior pole. Note the suprapatellar fat pad deep to the quadriceps. **D,** The path and contact areas of the patella on the intercondylar groove of the femur. The degree values 135, 90, 60, and 20 indicate flexed positions of the knee. (**C** and **D,** Redrawn from Neumann DA: Kinesiology of the musculoskeletal system—foundations for physical rehabilitation, St Louis, 2002, Mosby, p. 448.)

rotation), hyperextension, flexion with posterior translation, and a varus force.[12] The first often results in injury to the medial collateral ligament, frequently accompanied by injury to the posteromedial capsule, medial meniscus, and anterior cruciate ("terrible triad"). The second leads to anterior cruciate injuries, often associated with meniscus tears. The third mechanism of injury often involves the posterior cruciate ligament, and the fourth mechanism involves the lateral collateral ligament, the posterolateral capsule, and the posterior cruciate ligament. Was the injury the result of trauma, such as a direct or an indirect blow? Bauer, et al.[13] developed a clinical prediction rule for determining whether a fracture was present in an acute knee injury (see the box on the next page). Was the patient bearing weight at the time of injury? From which direction did the injuring force come? For example, meniscal injuries, especially those on the medial side, occur as a result of a torsion injury that combines compression and rotation. Slowly developing forces tend to cause bony avulsions, whereas rapidly developing forces tend to tear ligaments. In young children, injuries to the growth plate or physis may occur instead of injury to the ligaments, especially during a rapid growth spurt when the physis is weaker than the ligaments. Injuries may occur to the distal femoral physis, the proximal

Bauer's Clinical Prediction Rule for Acute Knee Fracture*[13]

- Severe joint line tenderness
- Severe localized swelling with effusion and ecchymosis
- Flexion less than 90°
- Inability to bear weight

*The presence of these signs would indicate that an x-ray assessment is warranted.

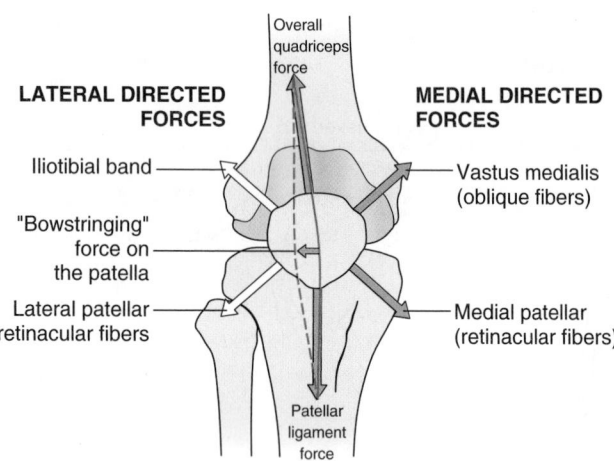

Figure 12-3 The major guiding forces acting on the patella are shown as it moves through the intercondylar groove of the femur. Each structure has a natural tendency to pull the patella laterally or medially. In most cases, the opposing forces counteract one another so that the patella moves optimally during flexion and extension. (Redrawn from Neumann DA: Kinesiology of the musculoskeletal system—foundations for physical rehabilitation, St Louis, 2002, Mosby, p. 463.)

tibial physis, and the tibial tubercle apophysis (traction epiphysis).[14,15] Injury to this last structure is called *Osgood-Schlatter disease*. Table 12-1 lists typical mechanisms of injury to the knee and the structures injured. The lower limb may be viewed as an open (foot off the ground) or a closed (foot on the ground) kinetic chain (Figure 12-4). There is less chance of injury when the lower limb is an open kinetic chain. As a closed kinetic chain, the lower limb is an encapsulated system in which all parts work in concert. Forces applied to one part of the chain must be absorbed by that part as well as by other parts of the closed chain. If the forces are too great, injury results.

2. *Has the knee been injured before, or does it have any feeling of weakness?*
3. *What is the patient able or unable to do functionally? Is there disability on running, cutting, pivoting, twisting, climbing, or descending stairs?* Positive responses to these questions should alert the

TABLE 12-1

Mechanisms of Injury to the Knee and Possible Structures Injured

Mechanism of Injury	Structure Possibly Injured
Varus or valgus contact without rotation	1. Collateral ligament 2. Epiphyseal fracture 3. Patellar dislocation or subluxation
Varus or valgus contact with rotation	1. Collateral and cruciate ligaments 2. Collateral ligaments and patellar dislocation or subluxation 3. Meniscus tear
Blow to patellofemoral joint, or fall on flexed knee, foot dorsiflexed	1. Patellar articular injury or osteochondral fracture
Blow to tibial tubercle, or fall on flexed knee, foot plantar flexed	1. Posterior cruciate ligament
Anterior blow to tibia, resulting in knee hyperextension (contact hypertension)	1. Anterior cruciate ligament 2. Anterior and posterior cruciate ligament
Noncontact hyperextension	1. Anterior cruciate ligament 2. Posterior capsule
Noncontact deceleration	1. Anterior cruciate ligament
Noncontact deceleration, with tibial medial rotation or femoral lateral rotation on fixed tibia	1. Anterior cruciate ligament

TABLE **12-1**

Mechanisms of Injury to the Knee and Possible Structures Injured—cont'd

Mechanism of Injury	Structure Possibly Injured
Noncontact, quickly turning one way with tibia rotated in opposite direction	1. Patellar dislocation or subluxation
Noncontact, rotation with varus or valgus loading	1. Meniscus injury
Noncontact, compressive rotation	1. Meniscus injury 2. Osteochondral fracture
Hyperflexion	1. Meniscus (posterior horn) 2. Anterior cruciate ligament
Forced medial rotation	1. Meniscus injury (lateral meniscus)
Forced lateral rotation	1. Meniscus injury (medial meniscus) 2. Medial collateral ligament and possibly anterior cruciate ligament 3. Patellar dislocation
Flexion-varus-medial rotation	1. Anterolateral instability
Flexion-valgus-lateral rotation	1. Anteromedial instability
Dashboard injury	1. Isolated posterior cruciate ligament 2. Posterior cruciate ligament and posterior capsule 3. Posterolateral instability 4. Posteromedial instability 5. Patellar fracture 6. Tibial fracture (proximal) 7. Tibial plateau fracture 8. Acetabular and pelvic fracture

Adapted from Clancy W: Evaluation of acute knee injuries. In American Association of Orthopaedic Surgeons, Symposium on Sports Medicine: The knee, St Louis, 1985, Mosby; Strobel M, Stedtfeld HW: Diagnostic evaluation of the knee, Berlin, 1990, Springer-Verlag.

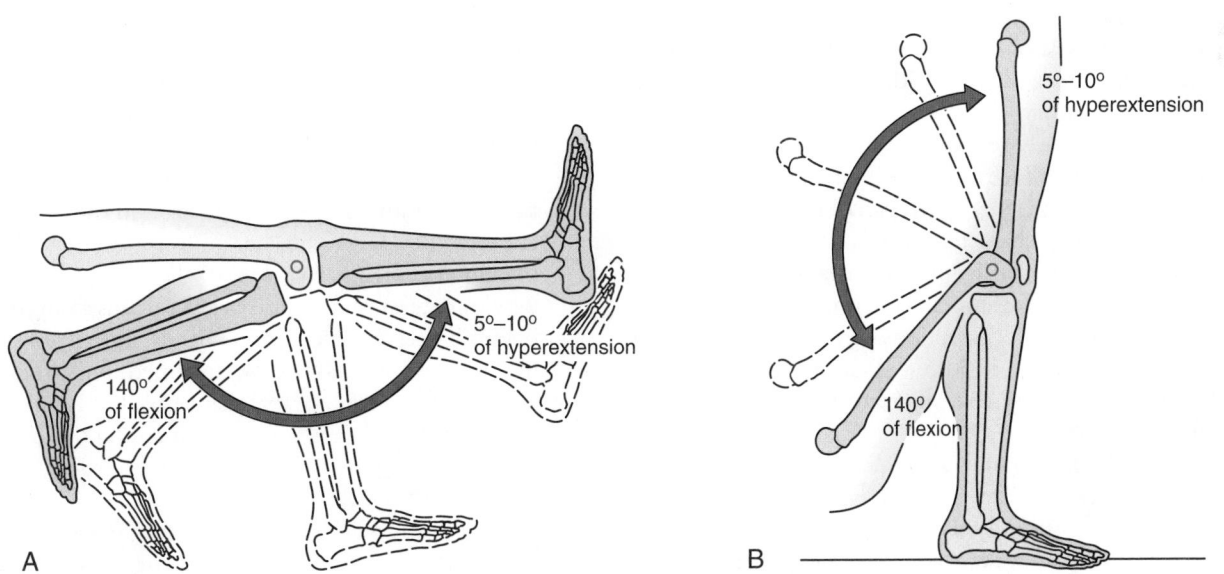

Figure 12-4 Sagittal plane motion at the knee. A, Tibial-on-femoral perspective (open kinetic chain). **B,** Femoral-on-tibial perspective (closed kinetic chain). (Modified from Neumann DA: Kinesiology of the musculoskeletal system—foundations for physical rehabilitation, St Louis, 2002, Mosby, p. 444.)

examiner to instability caused by injured ligaments, muscle dysfunction, joint articular problems, or meniscus problems.[16]

4. *Is there any "clicking," or was there a "pop" when the injury occurred?* A distinct pop may indicate an anterior cruciate ligament tear or osteochondral fracture. Popping on the lateral aspect of the knee may be due to the popliteus tendon snapping over the lateral femoral inferoposterior tubercle within 2 cm of the muscle's attachment into the femur.[17]

5. *Did the injury occur during acceleration, during deceleration, or when the patient was moving at a constant speed?* Acceleration and twisting injuries may involve the meniscus. Deceleration injuries often involve the cruciate ligaments. Constant speed with cutting may involve the anterior cruciate ligament.

6. *Is there any pain? If so, where? What type is it? Retropatellar? Does the patient point to one spot with one finger or a more general area indicating the problem is more diffuse, aching?* Aching pain may indicate degenerative changes, whereas sharp, "catching" pain usually indicates a mechanical problem. Arthritic pain is more likely to be associated with stiffness in the morning and eases with activity. Anterior knee pain may be due to patellofemoral problems, bursa (prepatellar, infrapatellar) pathology, fat pad pathology, tendinosis, or Osgood-Schlatter disease.[18,19] Patellofemoral pain tends to be insidious and occurs spontaneously, often from overuse, which makes establishing the source of the problem important.[20,21] Pain at rest is not usually mechanical in origin. Pain during activity is usually seen in structural abnormalities, such as subluxation or patellar tracking disorders. Pain after activity or with overuse is characteristic of inflammatory disorders, such as synovial plica irritation or early tendinosis or paratenonitis leading to jumper's knee or Sinding-Larsen-Johansson syndrome.[22-27] Generalized pain in the area of the knee is usually characteristic of contusions or partial tears of muscles or ligaments. Instability rather than pain tends to be the major presenting factor in complex ligament disruptions or muscle dysfunction (e.g., quadriceps rupture). Pain in the knee on ankle movements may implicate the superior tibiofibular joint.

7. *Do certain positions or activities have an increased or decreased effect on the pain? Which activities produce pain? How much activity is needed to produce pain? Which positions or activities ease the pain? Does the pain go away when activity ceases?* The examiner must take note of constant pain that is unrelated to activity, time, or posture, because it usually indicates serious pathology, such as a tumor. Does the patient have confidence in the knee? Such a question gives the examiner some idea of the functional impairment from the patient's perspective.[28]

8. *Does the knee "give way?"*[28] This finding usually indicates instability in the knee, meniscus pathology, patellar subluxation (if present when rotation or stopping is involved), undisplaced osteochondritis dissecans, patellofemoral syndrome, plica, or loose body. Giving way when walking uphill or downhill is more likely the result of a retropatellar lesion.[16,29] If the patient complains that the patella "slips out of place," it may be because of patellar subluxation or a pathological plica.[30]

9. *Has the knee ever locked?* True locking of the knee is rare. Loose bodies may cause recurrent locking. Locking must be differentiated from catching, which is momentary locking or giving way as a result of reflex inhibition or pain.[30] **Locking** in the knee usually means that the knee cannot fully extend with flexion often being normal, and it is related to meniscus pathology. Hamstring muscle spasm may also limit extension and is sometimes referred to as **spasm locking.**

10. *On movement, is there any grating or clicking in the knee?* Grating or clicking may be caused by degeneration or by one structure's snapping over another.

11. *Is the joint swollen? Does the swelling occur with activity or several hours after activity, or does the joint feel tight at rest?* Swelling with activity may be caused by instability, and tightness at rest may be caused by arthritic changes or patellofemoral dysfunction. Is the swelling recurrent? If so, what activity causes it? Swelling with pivoting or twisting may be a result of meniscus problems or instability at the tibiofemoral joint. Recurrent swelling caused by climbing or descending slopes or stairs may be related to patellofemoral dysfunction.[30] Often there is no swelling in the knee after severe injury, because the fluid extravasates into the soft tissues surrounding the joint and because a number of structures around the knee joint are avascular and can be injured without bloody swelling occurring. Synovial swelling may occur 8 to 24 hours after the injury; swelling caused by blood begins to occur almost immediately. Localized swelling may be caused by an inflamed bursa (Figure 12-5).[31] The deep infrapatellar bursa has been noted as a source of anterior knee pain and could be misdiagnosed as patellofemoral arthralgia or Osgood-Schlatter disease.[32,33]

12. *Is the gait normal? Does the patient put weight on the limb? Can the patient extend the knee while walking? Is the stride length altered on the affected limb?* All these questions give an indication of the patient's functional disability and how much the knee is bothering the patient.

13. *What type of shoes does the patient wear?* Shoes with negative heels (e.g., "earth shoes") can increase the incidence of patellofemoral syndrome.

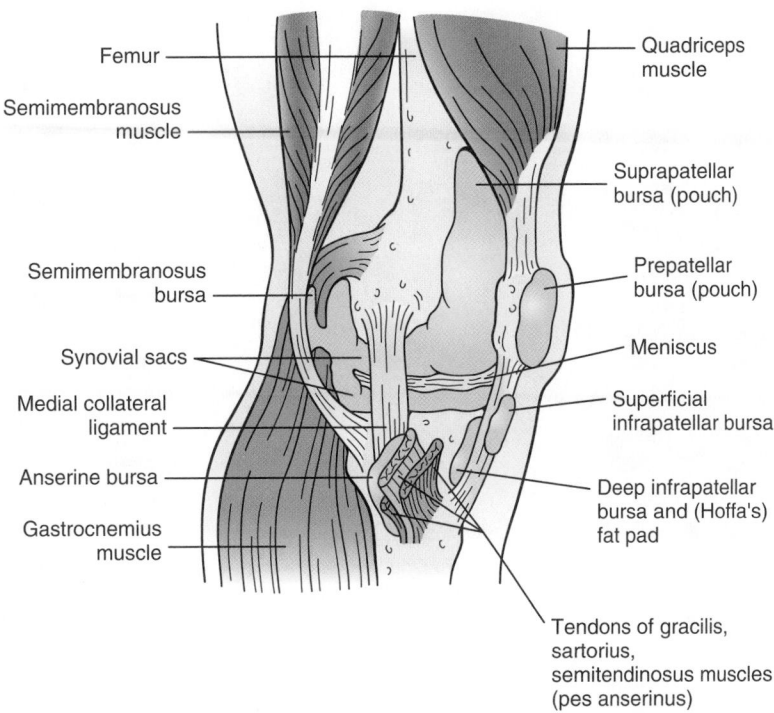

Femur

Semimembranosus muscle

Semimembranosus bursa

Synovial sacs

Medial collateral ligament

Anserine bursa

Gastrocnemius muscle

Quadriceps muscle

Suprapatellar bursa (pouch)

Prepatellar bursa (pouch)

Meniscus

Superficial infrapatellar bursa

Deep infrapatellar bursa and (Hoffa's) fat pad

Tendons of gracilis, sartorius, semitendinosus muscles (pes anserinus)

Figure 12-5 The bursae around the knee (medial aspect).

OBSERVATION

For a proper observation, the patient must be suitably undressed so that the examiner can observe the posture of the spine as well as the hips, knees, and ankles. Initially, the examiner should note whether the patient puts weight on the affected limb or stands with only a slight amount of weight on the affected side. In addition to the common observational items mentioned in Chapter 1, the examiner should look for the following alterations around the knee.

Anterior View, Standing

From the anterior aspect (Figure 12-6), the examiner should note any malalignment, including **genu varum** (bowleg) or **genu valgum** (knock-knee) deformity (Figure 12-7). Any observable malalignment may lead to or be the result of malalignment elsewhere (Table 12-2).[34] These deformities may be unilateral or bilateral. Although in adults the legs should be relatively straight, in the child, the normal development of the knee is from genu varum to straight, to genu valgum, and then to straight. Initially, a child's lower limbs are in genu varum until 18 or 19 months, when they straighten. The knee then goes into genu valgum until about 3 to 4 years of age (Figure 12-8). The limbs should be almost straight by age 6 years and should remain that way. In the adult, the knee is normally in approximately 6° of valgus.

To observe genu varum and genu valgum, the patient is positioned so that the patellae face forward and the

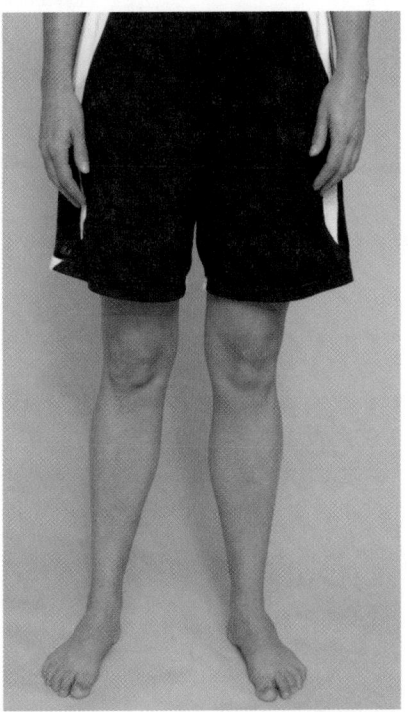

Figure 12-6 Anterior view of the lower limbs. Note the wider than normal base width.

medial aspects of the knees and medial malleoli of both limbs are as close together as possible. If the knees touch and the ankles do not, the patient has a genu valgum. A distance of 9 to 10 cm (3.5 to 4 inches) between the ankles is considered excessive. If two or more fingers

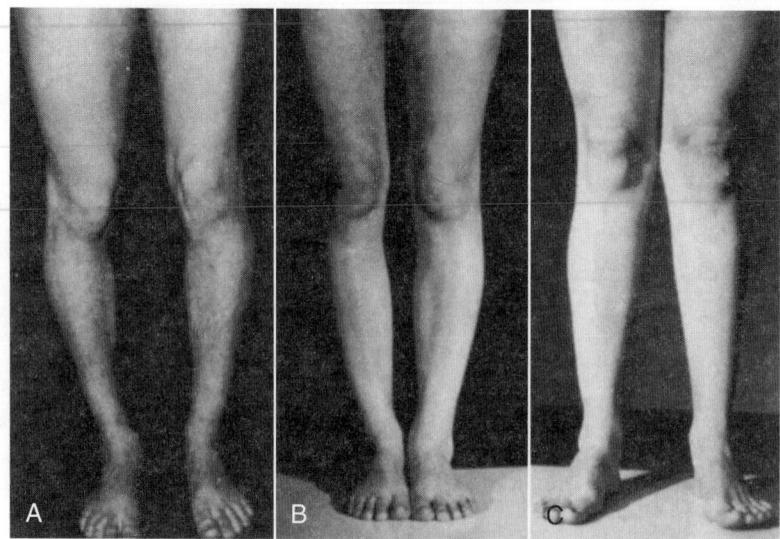

Figure 12-7 Genu varum and genu valgum. A, Tibia vara of proximal third. Genu varum deformity located mainly in proximal tibia. Along with lateral tibial torsion and medial femoral torsion, this gives a "bandy-legged" appearance. **B,** Genu varum of entire lower extremities. **C,** Genu valgum deformity of both lower extremities. (From Hughston JC, Walsh WM, Puddu G: Patellar subluxation and dislocation, Philadelphia, 1984, WB Saunders, p. 221.)

TABLE 12-2

Malalignment About the Knee and Possible Correlated and Compensatory Motions or Postures

Malalignment	Possible Correlated Motions or Postures	Possible Compensatory Motions or Postures
Genu valgum	Pes planus Excessive subtalar pronation Lateral tibial torsion Lateral patellar subluxation Excessive hip adduction Ipsilateral hip excessive medial rotation Lumbar spine contralateral rotation	Forefoot varus Excessive subtalar supination to allow the lateral heel to contact the ground In-toeing to decrease lateral pelvic sway during gait Ipsilateral pelvic lateral rotation
Genu varum	Excessive lateral angulation of the tibia in the frontal plane; tibial varum Medial tibial torsion Ipsilateral hip lateral rotation Excessive hip abduction	Forefoot valgus Excessive subtalar pronation to allow the medial heel to contact the ground Ipsilateral pelvic medial rotation
Genu recurvatum	Ankle plantar flexion Excessive anterior pelvic tilt	Posterior pelvic tilt Flexed trunk posture Excessive thoracic kyphosis
Lateral tibial torsion	Out-toeing Excessive subtalar supination with related rotation along the lower quarter	Functional forefoot varus Excessive subtalar pronation with relaxed rotation along the lower quarter
Medial tibial torsion	In-toeing Metatarsus adductus Excessive subtalar pronation with related rotation along the lower quarter	Functional forefoot valgus Excessive subtalar supination with relaxed rotation along the lower quarter
Excessive tibial retroversion (posterior slant of tibial plateaus)	Genu recurvatum	
Inadequate tibial retrotorsion (posterior deflection of proximal tibia due to hamstrings pull)	Flexed knee posture	
Inadequate tibial retroflexion (bowing of the tibia)	Altered alignment of Achilles tendon causing altered associated joint motion	
Bowleg deformity of the tibia (tibial varum)	Medial tibial torsion	Forefoot valgus Excessive subtalar pronation

From Riegger-Krugh C, Keysor JJ: Skeletal malalignments of the lower quarter: correlated and compensatory motions and postures. J Orthop Sports Phys Ther 23:166–167, 1996.

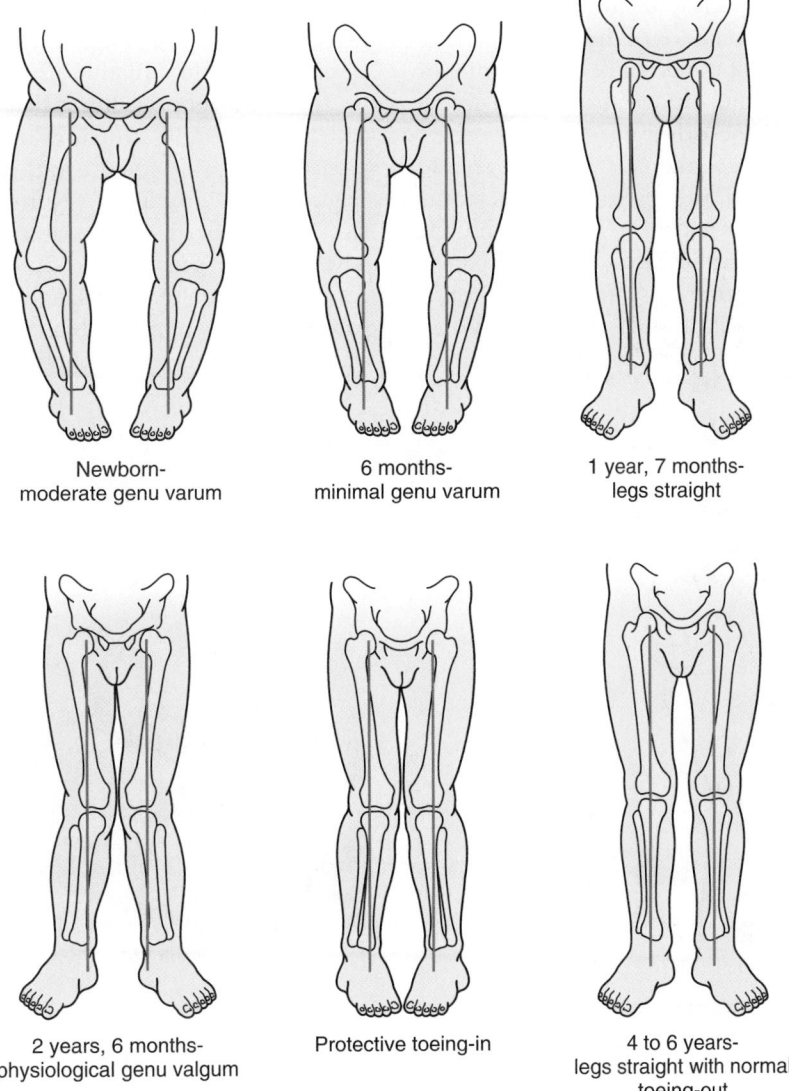

Newborn-
moderate genu varum

6 months-
minimal genu varum

1 year, 7 months-
legs straight

2 years, 6 months-
physiological genu valgum

Protective toeing-in

4 to 6 years-
legs straight with normal
toeing-out

Figure 12-8 Physiological evolution of lower limb alignment at various ages in infancy and childhood. (Redrawn from Tachdjian MO: Pediatric orthopedics, Philadelphia, 1972, WB Saunders, p. 1463.)

(4 cm [1.6 inch]) fit between the knees when the ankles are together, the patient has a varus deformity or genu varum.[35] On x-ray studies, the normal **tibiofemoral shaft angle** is approximately 6° (Figure 12-9).

Alignment is often different between males and females.[36] Some of these misalignments, if excessive, can lead to patellofemoral symptoms or instability.[37] These excessive differences are sometimes referred to as **miserable malalignment syndrome** and can include anterior pelvic tilt, increased hip anteversion, decreased tibiofemoral angle, genu recurvatum, navicular drop, and increased foot pronation (Figure 12-10).[38]

The patient is asked to extend the knees to see whether the movement can be performed and what effect it has on the knee. Both knees should extend equally. If not, something must be limiting the movement (swelling, loose body, or meniscus). Normally, a person does not

stand with the knees fully extended. If, however, the patient has an excessive lordosis, the knees are often hyperextended to maintain the center of gravity. This change can lead to posterior knee pain.

Is there any apparent swelling or ecchymosis in or around the knees (see Figure 1-10)? If there is intracapsular swelling, or at least sufficient swelling, the knee assumes a position of 15° to 25° of flexion, which provides the synovial cavity with the maximum capacity to hold fluid. This position is also called the **resting position** of the knee. Is the swelling intracapsular or extracapsular? Intracapsular swelling is evident over the entire joint; extracapsular swelling tends to be more localized. An example of extracapsular swelling is shown in Figure 12-11, which illustrates **prepatellar bursitis.**

The examiner should ask the patient to contract the quadriceps muscles to see whether there is any visible wasting of the muscles, especially of the vastus medialis obliquus (VMO). The prominence of the vastus medialis results from the obliquity of the distal fibers, the inferior position of its insertion, and the thinness of the fascial covering compared with the other quadriceps muscles. Muscle defects (third-degree strain or rupture) should also be watched for when the patient contracts the muscles. Third-degree strains may be indicated by muscle "bunching," abnormal mechanics (e.g., unilateral patella alta with patella tendon rupture), or a palpable defect.[30]

The position of the patella should be noted. When viewing the patellae, the examiner should note whether they face straight ahead, tilt outward ("grasshopper eyes" patellae), tilt inward ("squinting" patellae), or are rotated ("spin") in or out[39] (Figure 12-12). Rotation and tilt may be caused by tight structures that alter the position of the patella. These tight structures may include muscles (e.g., rectus femoris, iliotibial band, gastrocnemius) or fascia (e.g., lateral retinaculum). Normally, the patellae should face straight ahead with no lateral tilt or rotation. If these deviations are seen in the observation phase, they are considered static problems, and the examiner should test patellar movement passively and watch the patellae during active movements to see whether it is a dynamic problem

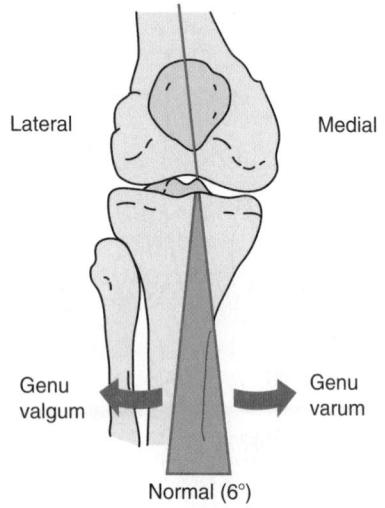

Figure 12-9 Normal tibiofemoral shaft angle.

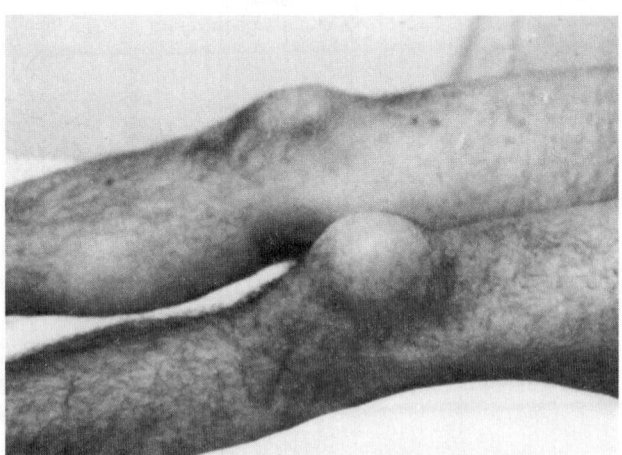

Figure 12-11 Prepatellar bursitis.

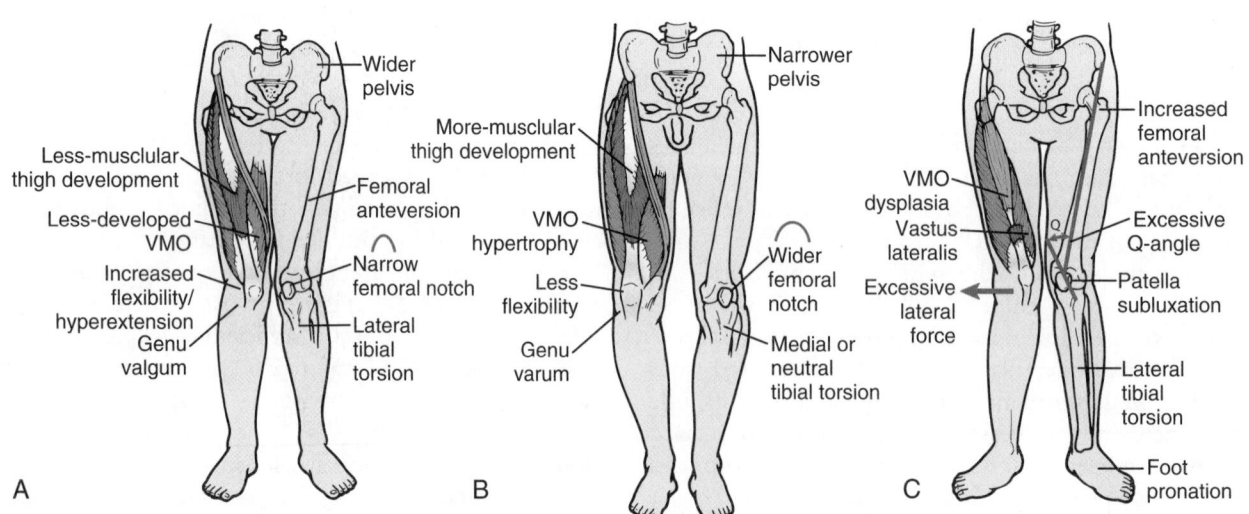

Figure 12-10 A, Normal female alignment with wider pelvis, femoral anteversion, genu valgum, hyperflexibility, lateral tibial torsion, and narrow notch. **B,** Normal male alignment demonstrates a narrower pelvis, more developed musculature, genu varum, medial or neutral tibial torsion, and wider notch. **C,** Miserable malalignment syndrome is a term coined to describe patients who have increased femoral anteversion, genu valgum, vastus medialis obliquus (VMO) dysplasia, lateral tibial torsion, and forefoot pronation. These factors create excessive lateral forces and contribute to patellofemoral dysfunction. (From Griffin LY, editor: Rehabilitation of the injured knee, St Louis, 1995, Mosby, pp. 298–299.)

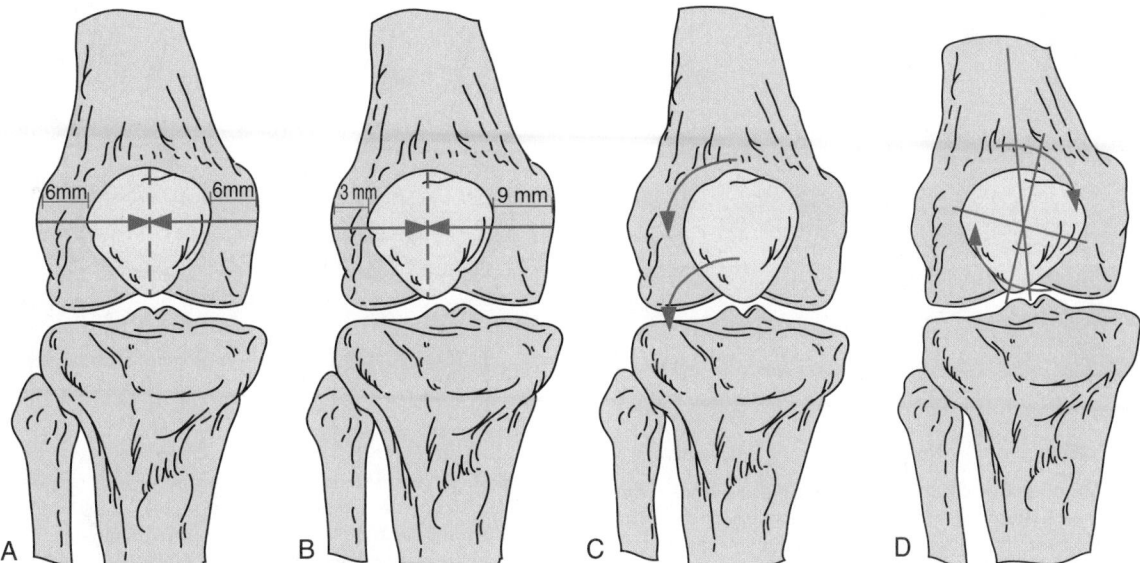

Figure 12-12 Assessment of the patellar glide component. Ideally, the patella should be centered on the superior portion of the femoral articular surface at 20° flexion. **A,** Ideal alignment. **B,** Lateral glide of the patella. **C,** Lateral tilt of the patella. **D,** Lateral rotation ("spin") of inferior pole of patella. (From McConnell J, Fulkerson J: The knee: patellofemoral and soft tissue injuries. In Zachazewski JE, et al, editors: Athletic injuries and rehabilitation, Philadelphia, 1996, WB Saunders, pp. 711–712.)

as well.[40] A squinting or rotated patella may indicate medial femoral or lateral tibial torsion (Figure 12-13). Patients with abnormal torsion are prone to patellofemoral instability.

Any bruising or discoloration around the knee should also be noted, as well as any scars or signs indicating recent injury or surgery.

Lateral View, Standing

The examiner then views the patient from both sides for comparison. It should be noted whether **genu recurvatum** (hyperextended knee)[41] is present and whether one or both patellae are higher **(patella alta)** or lower **(patella baja** or **patella infera)**[42] than normal (Figure 12-14). For example, patella alta can increase the patellofemoral contact force during flexion, which may contribute to anterior knee pain.[43] With an abnormally high patella, a **"camel sign"** may be present (Figure 12-15); because of the high patella (one "hump"), the infrapatellar fat pad (second hump) or an inflamed infrapatellar bursa (just anterior to the fat pad) becomes more prominent. This finding is especially noticeable in females. In this position, the examiner should also note (Figure 12-16) whether the inferior pole of the patella is tilted in (inferior tilt). Ideally, the plane of the patella and that of the femoral condyles should be the same. If the inferior pole tilts in, fat pad irritation may occur.[44] Habitual genu recurvatum may make a patient prone to posterior cruciate tears because of the stretching of the posterior oblique

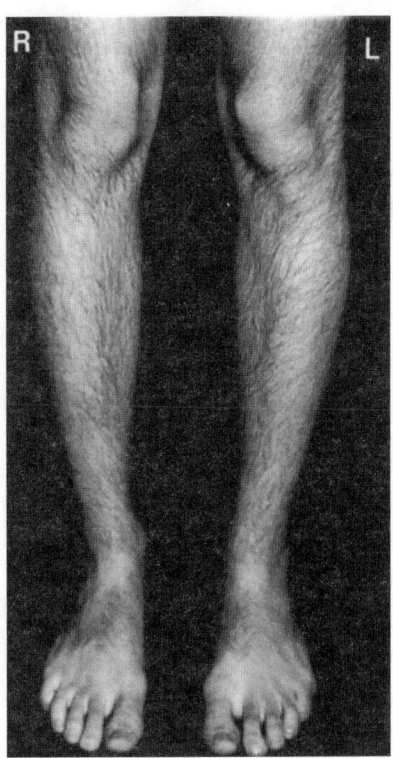

Figure 12-13 "Squinting" patellae, especially prominent on the patient's left knee. Both patellae point inward in a medial fashion, a sign of excessive femoral anteversion or increased medial femoral torsion. (From Carson WG Jr, James SL, Larsen RL, et al: Patellofemoral disorders: physical and radiographic evaluation. I. Physical examination. Clin Orthop 185:169, 1984.)

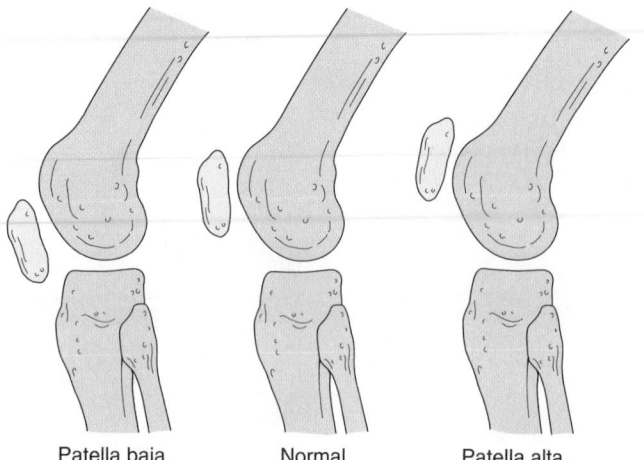

Patella baja   Normal   Patella alta

Figure 12-14 The normal patellar posture for exerting deceleration forces in the functional position of 45° of knee flexion places the patellar articular surface squarely against the anterior femur. A lower posture represents patella baja. A higher posture represents patella alta. Patella alta makes the patella less efficient in exerting normal forces. (Redrawn from Hughston JC, Walsh WM, Puddu G: Patellar subluxation and dislocation, Philadelphia, 1984, WB Saunders, p. 8.)

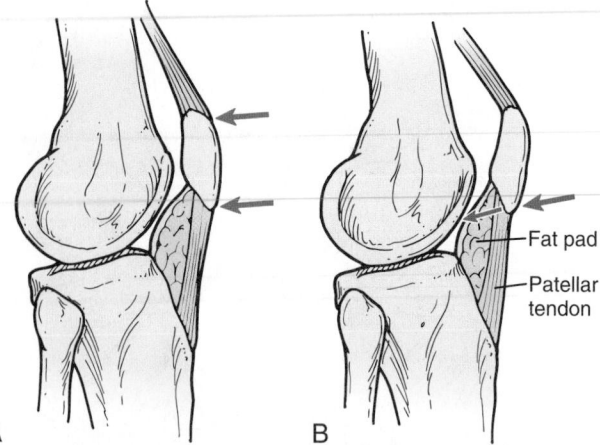

A   B

Figure 12-16 Assessment of the anteroposterior component of the patella. Ideally, the superior and inferior poles of the patella should be parallel in the sagittal plane of the knee, **A.** Commonly, in individuals with patellar malalignment, the inferior patellar pole pushes posteriorly into the infrapatellar fat pad, **B.** This may irritate the fat pad. (Redrawn from McConnell J, Fulkerson J: The knee: patellofemoral and soft tissue injuries. In Zachazewski JE, et al, editors: Athletic injuries and rehabilitation, Philadelphia, 1996, WB Saunders, p. 712.)

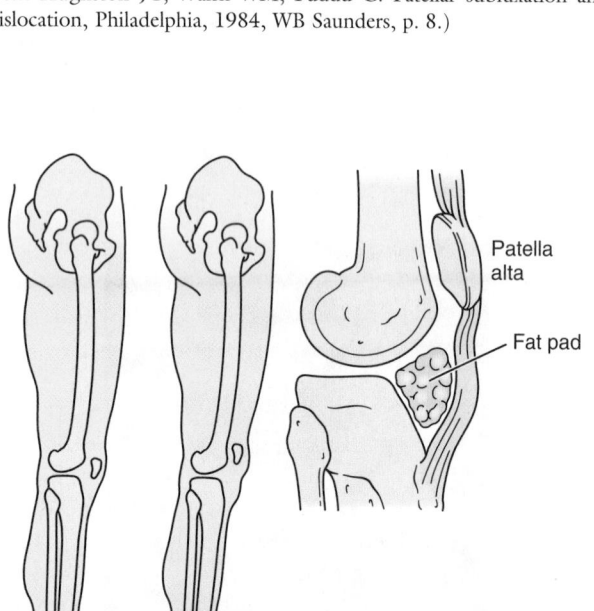

Normal   Patella alta

Figure 12-15 Camel sign. Double hump seen from side caused by high-riding patella and uncovered infrapatellar fat pad. (Modified from Hughston JC, Walsh WM, Puddu G: Patellar subluxation and dislocation, Philadelphia, 1984, WB Saunders, p. 22.)

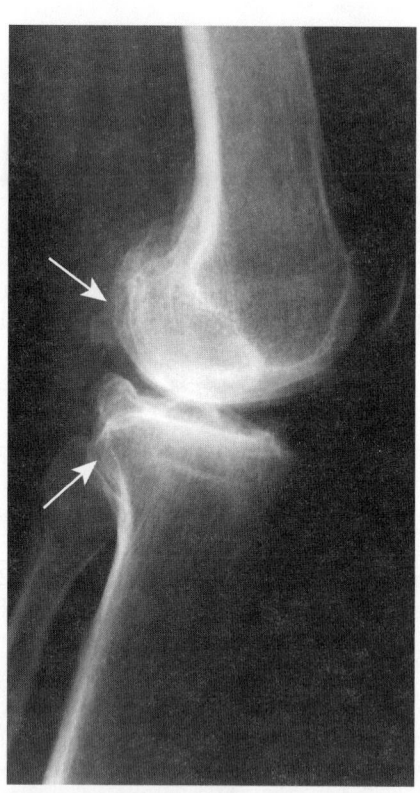

Figure 12-17 Osteophytic lipping *(arrows)* in posterior knee limits flexion and produces a bone-to-bone end feel.

ligament.[30] If one knee (normal) hyperextends and the other one (injured) does not, it may indicate meniscus pathology that is limiting extension. Osteoarthritic lipping (Figure 12-17) or synovial hypertrophy (rheumatoid arthritis) may also limit movement.

Posterior View, Standing

Next, the examiner views the patient from behind, looking for findings similar to those from the anterior aspect. In addition, the examiner looks for abnormal swellings, such as a popliteal (Baker's) cyst, which is caused by herniation

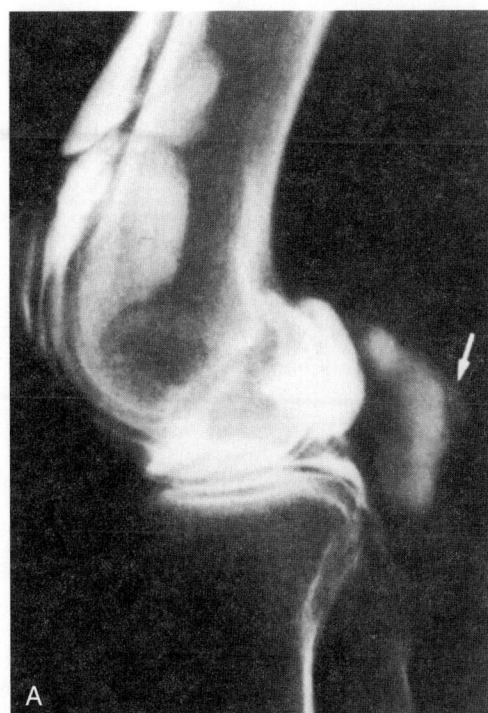
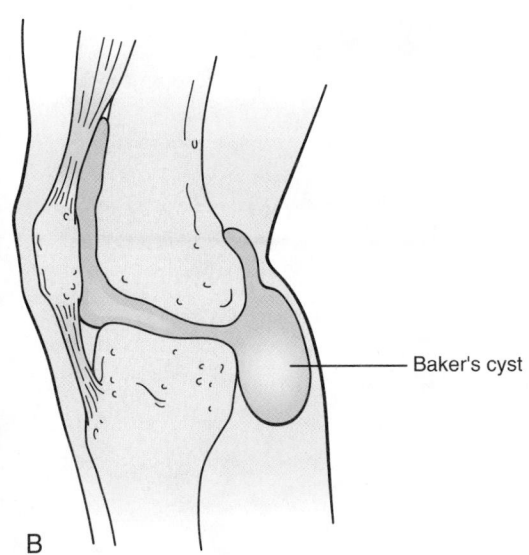

Baker's cyst

Figure 12-18 Popliteal (Baker's) cysts. A, This 74-year-old man presented with the acute onset of calf pain and swelling without knee pain. The initial suspected diagnosis was popliteal thrombosis. A venogram was normal. The arthrogram revealed a collection of dye posterior to the joint space—a popliteal cyst *(arrow)*. **B,** Schematic diagram of Baker's cyst. (**A,** From Reilly BM: Practical strategies in outpatient medicine, Philadelphia, 1991, WB Saunders, p. 1179.)

of synovial tissue through a weakening in the posterior capsule wall (Figure 12-18).

Anterior and Lateral Views, Sitting

For the final part of the observation, the patient sits with the knee flexed to 90° and the feet either partially bearing weight (on a stool) or dangling free. The patient is observed from the front and from the side. In this position, the patella should face forward and should rest on the distal end of the femur. With patella alta, the patella becomes more aligned with the anterior surface of the femur (angled upward). If the patella is laterally displaced or laterally displaced with a patella alta, the patellae take on the appearance of "frog eyes" or "grasshopper eyes" (Figure 12-19), meaning that the patellae face upward and outward, away from each other. Patella alta sometimes causes a concavity proximal to the patella in thin patients.[30] Any bony enlargements, such as those seen in Osgood-Schlatter disease (i.e., an enlarged tibial tubercle), should be noted (Figure 12-20), as should abnormal swelling. Swelling of the pes anserine bursa and a meniscal cyst (Figure 12-21) are best visualized in the seated position.[30,45] Meniscal cysts may also present as isolated medial or lateral swelling.[29]

In the same position, any **tibial torsion** should be noted (Figure 12-22).[44,46] If there is tibial torsion, it is medial torsion that is associated with genu varum; genu valgum is associated with lateral tibial torsion. Normally, the patella faces straight ahead while the foot faces slightly laterally (Fick angle). With medial tibial torsion, the feet point toward each other, resulting in a "pigeon-toed" foot deformity. These deformities can be exacerbated by habitual postures. The positions illustrated in Figures 12-23, 12-24, *A,* and 12-25 cause problems only if they are used habitually. Excessive tibial torsion can contribute to conditions such as chondromalacia patellae, patellofemoral instability, and fat pad entrapment. When standing, most people exhibit a lateral tibial torsion, the Fick angle (see Figure 13-13), which increases as the child grows. This angle is approximately 5° in babies and as much as 18° in adults. To test for tibial torsion, the examiner aligns the patient's straight legs (knees extended) so that the patellae face straight ahead. The examiner then looks at the feet to determine their angle relative to the shaft of the tibia.

Femoral torsion, or anteversion (discussed in Chapter 11), can also affect the position of the patella relative to the femur and tibia.

Gait

The examiner should also observe the patient's gait (see Chapter 14), noting any differences in stride length, walking speed, cadence, or linear and angular displacement. In addition, the examiner should watch for

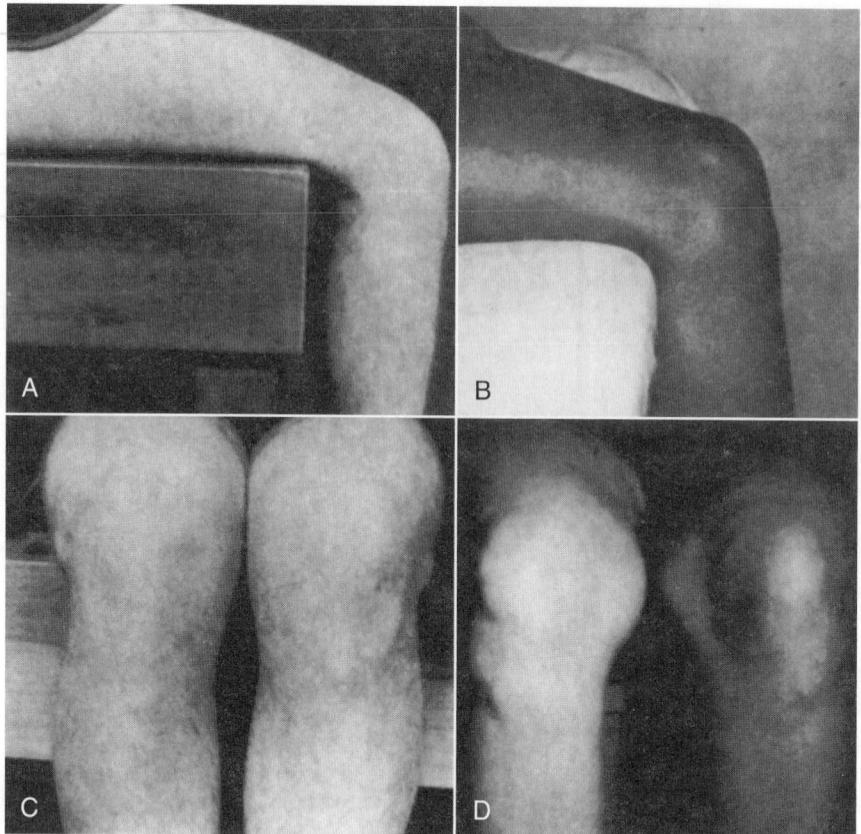

Figure 12-19 A, Normal knee seen from side; patella faces straight ahead in line with femur. **B,** Patella alta seen from side; patella points toward ceiling. **C,** Normal patellae seen from front; patellae centered in outline of knees. **D,** High and lateral posturing of patellae seen from front, giving "grasshopper eyes" or "frog eyes" appearance. (From Hughston JC, Walsh WM, Puddu G: Patellar subluxation and dislocation, Philadelphia, 1984, WB Saunders, p. 23.)

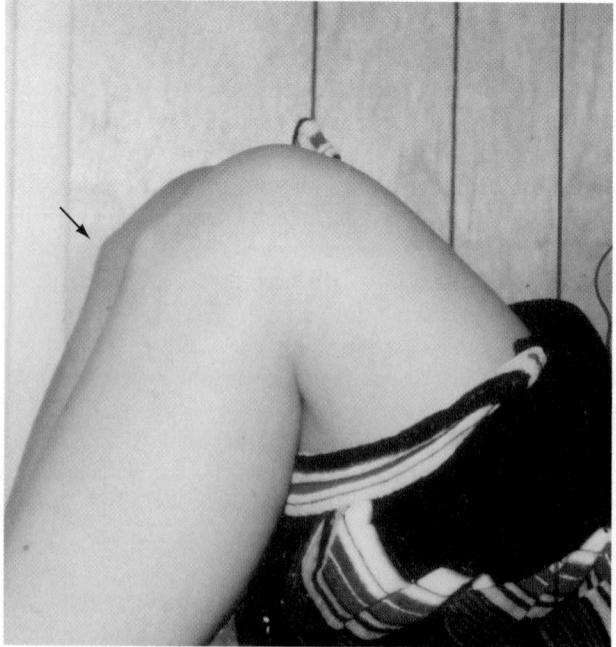

Figure 12-20 Osgood-Schlatter disease with enlarged tibial tuberosity (*arrow*).

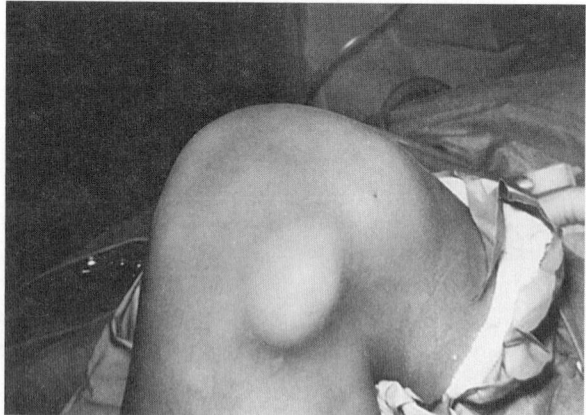

Figure 12-21 Lateral meniscus cyst. (From Reider B: The orthopedic physical examination, Philadelphia, 1999, WB Saunders, p. 209.)

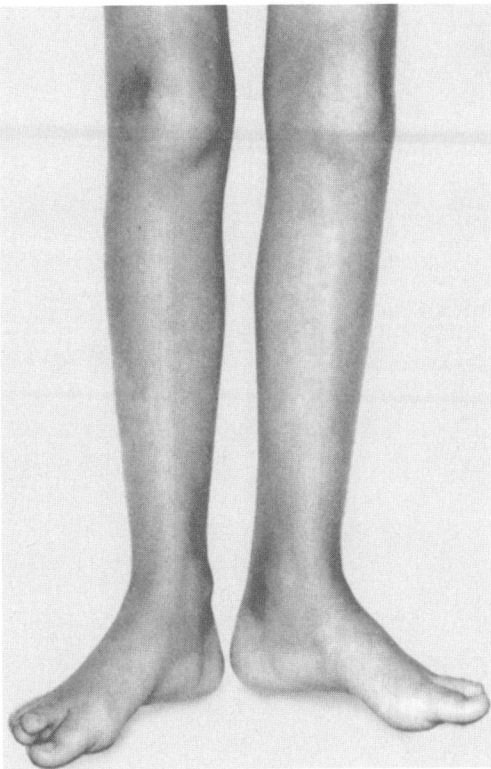

Figure 12-22 Exaggerated lateral tibial torsion. In stance, with the patellae facing straight forward, the feet point outward. (From Tachdjian MO: Pediatric orthopedics, Philadelphia, 1990, WB Saunders, p. 2816.)

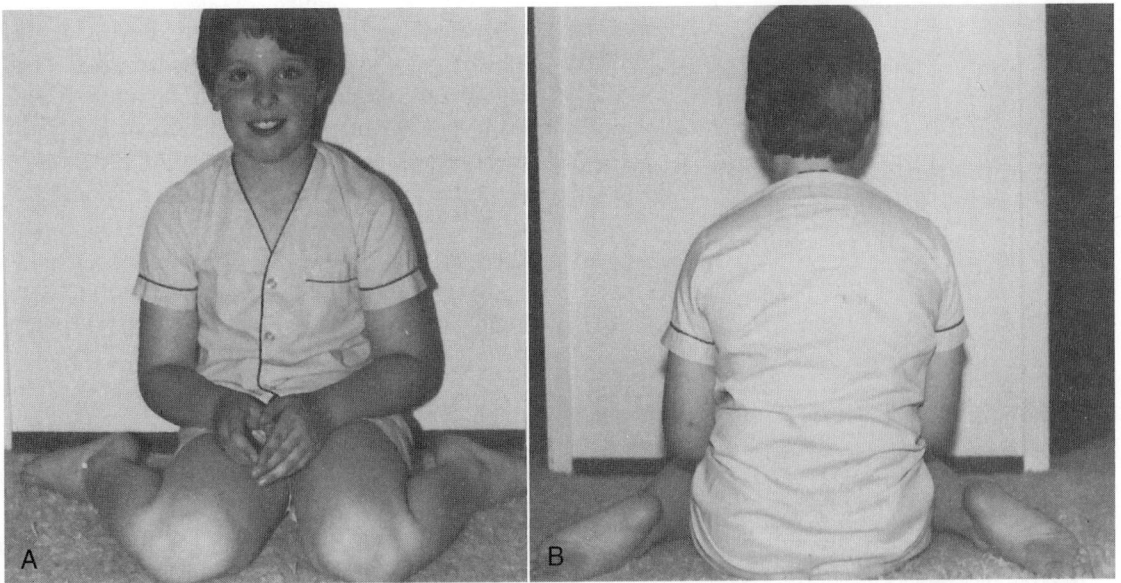

Figure 12-23 "Television" or "W" sitting position may lead to excessive lateral tibial torsion. **A,** Anterior view. **B,** Posterior view.

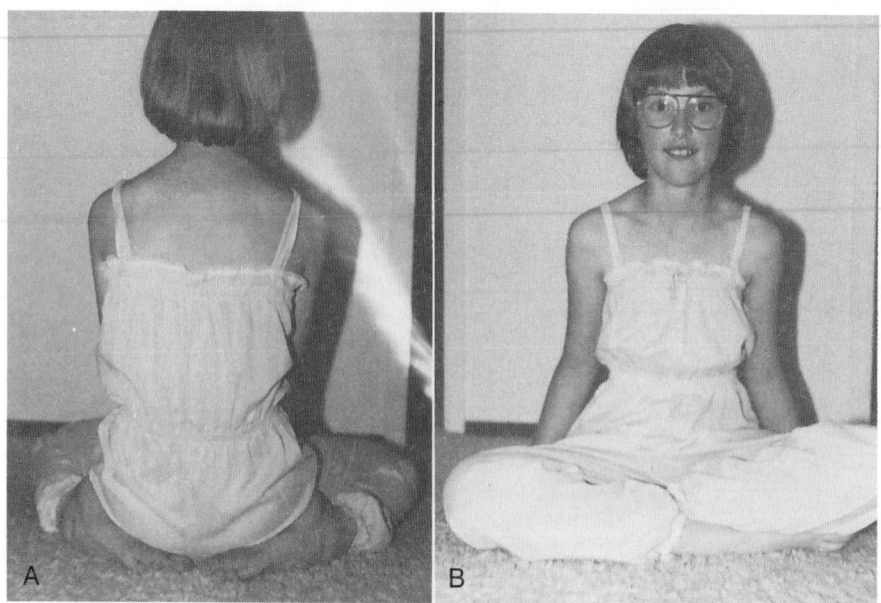

Figure 12-24 Medial tibial torsion. A, Position to be avoided to prevent excessive medial tibial torsion. **B,** Tailor position maintains normal medial tibial torsion.

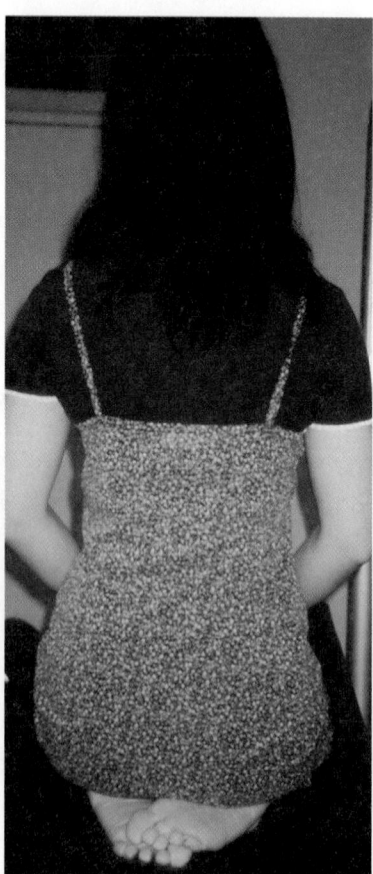

Figure 12-25 Traditional Japanese kneeling requires full knee flexion, often accompanied by medial tibial rotation.

abnormal patellar movement, indicating possible patellar tracking problems, and abnormal motion of the tibia relative to the femur, indicating possible instability problems.

Movement at the pelvis, hip, and ankle should also be observed. For example, weak hip abductors (positive Trendelenburg sign) may lead to increased stress on the knee. If this is combined with medial tibial torsion, patellofemoral syndromes may result.[30,47] Tight heel cords may result in gait with the knee flexed, which can put extra pressure on the patellofemoral joint. Similarly, pronation of the foot and lateral tibial torsion may lead to patellofemoral pathology or anteromedial joint pain.[30] Tight hamstrings result in increased knee flexion, which can lead to the need for more ankle dorsiflexion. If no further dorsiflexion is possible, the foot pronates to compensate, thus increasing the **dynamic Q-angle.**[48]

EXAMINATION

Although the examination focuses primarily on the knee, the examiner must keep in mind that knee pathology may be the result of biomechanical (e.g., alignment, asymmetry) and pathological (e.g., hypomobility, hypermobility, muscle weakness, instability) issues in other joints in the kinetic chain, including the lumbar spine, pelvis, hips, ankles, and feet. Thus the examination, like the history and observation, may be extensive to rule out other kinetic chain contributors.[49-54] For example, Dutton[55]

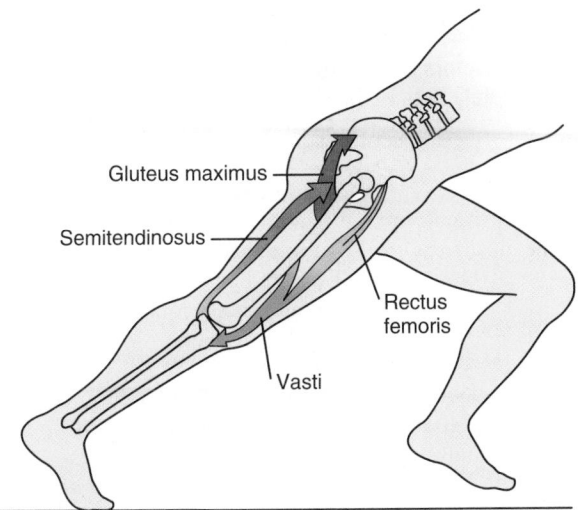

Figure 12-26 The action of several 1 joint and 2 joint muscles is depicted during the hip-and-knee extension phase of running. Observe that the vasti extend the knee, which then stretches the distal end of the semi-tendinosus. The gluteus maximus extends the hip, which then stretches the proximal end of the rectus femoris. The stretch placed on the active biarticular muscles reduces the rate and amount of their overall contraction. (Redrawn from Neumann D: Kinesiology of the musculoskeletal system—foundations for physical rehabilitation, St Louis, 2002, Mosby, p. 468.)

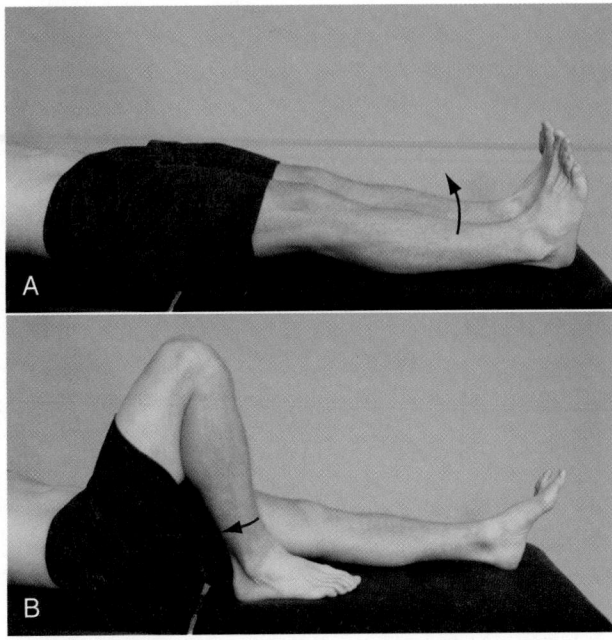

Figure 12-27 Active movements of the knee. A, Extension. **B,** Flexion.

Active Movements of the Knee Complex

- Flexion (0° to 135°)
- Extension (0° to 15°)
- Medial rotation of the tibia on the femur (20° to 30°)
- Lateral rotation of the tibia on the femur (30° to 40°)
- Repetitive movements (if necessary)
- Sustained postures (if necessary)
- Combined movements (if necessary)

---

believed the gracilis and adductor longus and magnus play a significant role along with the iliotibial band in knee stability. Also, several muscles that are two joint muscles acting over the hip and knee (e.g., rectus femoris, hamstrings, sartorius, gracilis) and knee and ankle (gastrocnemius) should be tested for functional mobility, because their action at one joint can affect the other joint (Figure 12-26).

Active Movements

The examination is performed initially with the patient sitting and then with the patient in lying position. During the active movements, the examiner should observe 1) the excursion of the patella to ensure that it tracks freely and smoothly; 2) the range of motion (ROM) available; 3) whether pain occurs during the movement, and if so, where; and 4) what appears to be limiting the movement. The active movements may be done in the sitting or supine position, and, as always, the most painful movements should be done last (Figure 12-27).

Full knee flexion is 135° (0° being straight knee). As the patient moves the knee through flexion and extension, the examiner should watch the movement of the patella as it "tracks" along the femoral trochlea. The examiner should note whether the movement is smooth from beginning to end or whether there is a lag or abrupt jump of the patella as it attempts to center in the groove.[56] The patella does not follow a straight path as the knee moves from extension to flexion. Normally, it follows a

curved pattern moving medially in early flexion and then laterally (Figure 12-28).[57] In the presence of pathological patellar tracking and patellar instability, an inverted **"J" sign** may be noted.[58,59] During the initiation of flexion (e.g., going in to a squat), the laterally located patella moves suddenly medially to enter the trochlea. The key to the J sign is the sudden movement medially instead of the normal smooth movement pattern. As in the observation phase, the examiner should note whether dynamic movement causes lateral tilt, anteroposterior tilt, or rotation of the patella during movement.[48,57]

Active knee extension is approximately 0° but may be −15°, especially in women, who are more likely to have hyperextended knees (genu recurvatum). The knee extensor muscles develop the greatest force near 60°, and the knee flexor muscles develop their greatest force at 45° to 10°. To complete the last 15° of knee extension, a 60% increase in force of the quadriceps muscles is required. The examiner should also watch for evidence of **quadriceps lag,** which means the quadriceps muscles are not

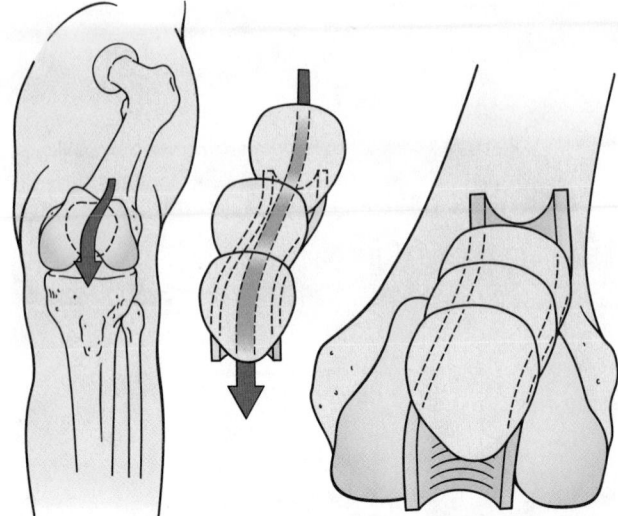

Figure 12-28 Multiplanar patellar path during knee flexion. (Redrawn from Stanitski CL, DeLee JC, Drez D, editors: Pediatric and adolescent sports medicine, Philadelphia, 1994, WB Saunders, p. 307.)

strong enough to fully extend the knee. The lag results from loss of mechanical advantage, muscle atrophy, decreasing power of the muscle as it shortens, adhesion formation, effusion, or reflex inhibition (Table 12-3). In non–weight-bearing, active medial rotation of the tibia on the femur should be 20° to 30°, whereas active lateral rotation should be 30° to 40° at 90° flexion in non–weight-bearing (Figure 12-29, A). In weight bearing (closed kinetic chain), the femur rotates on the tibia (Figure 12-29, B).

If, during the history, the patient has complained that repetitive or combined movements or sustained postures have resulted in symptoms, these movements should also be tested.

Passive Movements

If, on active movements, the ROM is full, overpressure may gently be applied to test the end feel of the various movements in the tibiofemoral joint. This action would preclude the need to do passive movements to the tibiofemoral joint. However, the examiner must do movements of the patella passively (Figure 12-30).

Passive Movements of the Knee Complex and Normal End Feel

- Flexion (tissue approximation)
- Extension (tissue stretch)
- Medial rotation of tibia on femur (tissue stretch)
- Lateral rotation of tibia on femur (tissue stretch)
- Patellar movement (tissue stretch—all directions)

TABLE 12-3

Selected Factors That Contribute to the Inability to Completely Extend the Knee

Factor	Clinical Examples
Reduced force production from the quadriceps	Disuse atrophy of quadriceps following trauma and/or prolonged immobilization
	Lacerated femoral nerve
	Herniated disc compressing L3 or L4 nerve roots
	Severe pain
	Excessive swelling in the knee
Excessive resistance from connective tissues	Excessive tightness in hamstring or other knee flexor muscles
	Excessive stiffness in the anterior cruciate ligament, posterior capsule, or collateral ligaments
	Scarring of the skin in the popliteal fossa
	Excessive swelling in the knee
Faulty arthrokinematics	Lack of "screw-home" rotation mechanics
	Lack of anterior slide of the tibia*
	Meniscal block or other derangement
	Lack of superior slide of the patella*

From Neumann DA: Kinesiology of the musculoskeletal system— foundations for physical rehabilitation, St Louis, 2002, Mosby, p. 460.
*Assume tibial-on-femoral knee extension.

At the tibiofemoral joint, the end feel of flexion is tissue approximation; the end feel of extension and of medial and lateral rotation of the tibia on the femur is tissue stretch. During passive movement, the examiner is also looking for a capsular pattern of the tibiofemoral joint.[60] This pattern is more limitation of flexion than of extension. Passive medial rotation of the tibia on the femur should be approximately 30° when the knee is flexed to 90°. Passive lateral rotation of the tibia on the femur at 90° of knee flexion should be 40°.

Although full knee extension is usually preferable for everyday activities (e.g., standing, walking), full flexion (135°) is often not necessary except where people kneel back on their heels. However, approximately 117° of flexion is necessary for activities, such as squatting to tie a shoelace or to pull on a sock. Sitting in a chair requires approximately 90° of flexion, and climbing stairs (average height) requires approximately 80° of flexion.

Lancaster, et al.[61] advocated doing a **motion palpation test** when assessing the knee for articular damage when the damage is severe. The patient sits on the edge of the examining table with the knees flexed to about 90°. The examiner passively moves the patient's knee between 100° and 0° flexion three to four times at about 30°/sec.

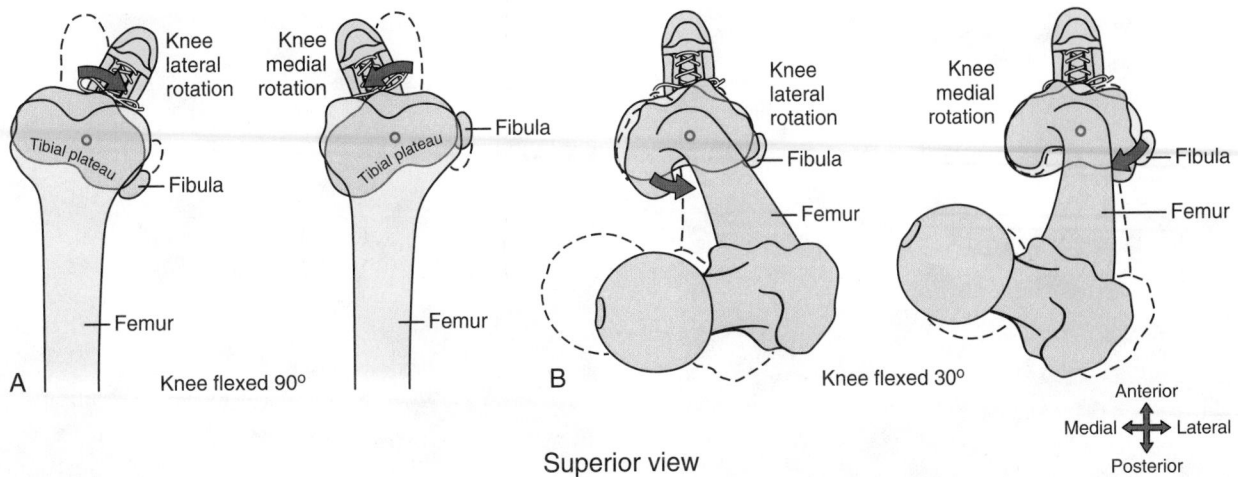

Figure 12-29 **Horizontal plane (axial) rotation at the knee. A,** Tibial-on-femoral rotation at 90° flexion (open kinetic chain). **B,** Femoral-on-tibial rotation (closed kinetic chain). (Redrawn from Neumann DA: Kinesiology of the musculoskeletal system—foundations for physical rehabilitation, St Louis, 2002, Mosby, p. 445.)

While doing this movement with one hand, the examiner applies about 2.3 kg (5 lbs) compression over the patellofemoral joint while the index finger of the same hand palpates immediately distal to the inferior pole of the patella (Figure 12-31). The examiner is palpating for joint crepitus and location, and severity of any discomfort that would indicate positive signs or possible articular damage.

Passive medial and lateral movement of the patella is also carried out to determine its mobility and to compare it with the unaffected side. Normally, the patella should move up to half its width medially and laterally in extension (Figure 12-32). When the patella is pushed medially or laterally, the examiner should note whether it stays parallel to the femoral condyles or whether it tilts or rotates.[40] For example, if pushed medially when the medial structures are tight, the lateral border of the patella tilts up. Likewise, tight lateral structures cause the medial border to tilt up. If the lateral structures are tight superiorly, the inferior pole of the patella medially rotates. These are examples of dynamic tilt and rotation problems of the patella. The side-to-side passive motion of the patella should also be tested in 45° of flexion, which is a more functional position and gives a better indication of functional instability of the patella.[62] The end feel of these movements is tissue stretch. Lateral displacement must be performed with care, especially in patients who have experienced a dislocated patella.

The examiner must also ensure full and normal flexibility of the quadriceps, hamstring, iliotibial band, and abductor and adductor muscles of the thigh, as well as the gastrocnemius muscles (Figure 12-33). Tightness of any of these structures or of the lateral retinaculum can alter gait and postural mechanics, which may lead to pathology. For example, tight hamstrings can contribute to patellofemoral pathology because of increased knee

flexion at heel strike and during stance phase.[48] Limitation of hip rotation in extension can lead to patellofemoral pathology as well.[30] If the rectus femoris is tight, full excursion of the patella in the trochlea is not possible, especially if the hip is extended. A tight iliotibial band can lead to lateral tracking of the patella.[48,63] Tests for the hamstring, abductor, adductor, and rectus femoris muscles have been described in Chapter 11. A functional test for the quadriceps (described under the "Special Tests" section in this chapter) is also a passive movement test (heel to buttock) for the femoral nerve. To test the gastrocnemius muscle, the examiner extends the patient's knee and, while holding it straight, dorsiflexes the patient's ankle. The examiner should be able to reach at least 90° (plantigrade), although 10° to 15° of dorsiflexion is more common.

Resisted Isometric Movements

For a proper test of the muscles, resisted isometric movements must be performed. In some cases (e.g., patellofemoral pain syndrome [PFPS]), hip strength should also be tested as hip abductors and lateral rotators have been found to be weak in PFPS patients.[64] The patient should be tested in the supine position (Figure 12-34).

Resisted Isometric Movements of the Knee Complex

- Flexion of the knee
- Extension of the knee
- Ankle plantar flexion
- Ankle dorsiflexion
- Hip abductors (in alignment cases)
- Hip lateral rotators (in alignment cases)

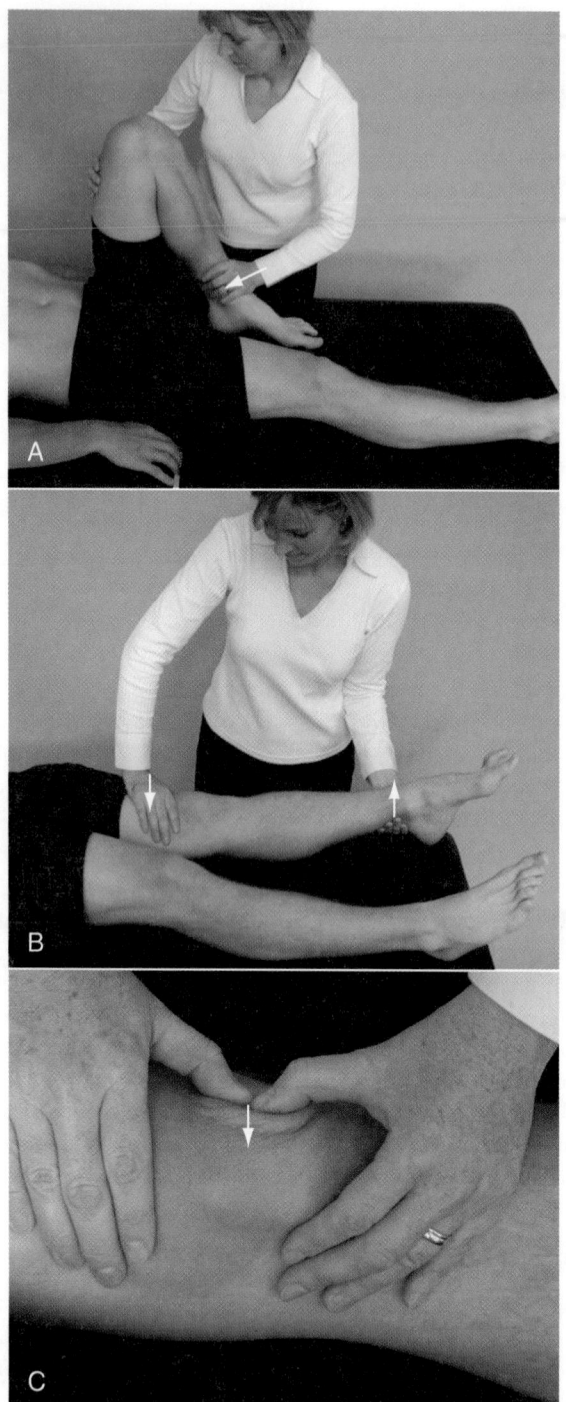

Figure 12-30 Passive movements of the knee. A, Flexion. **B,** Extension. **C,** Medial glide of patella.

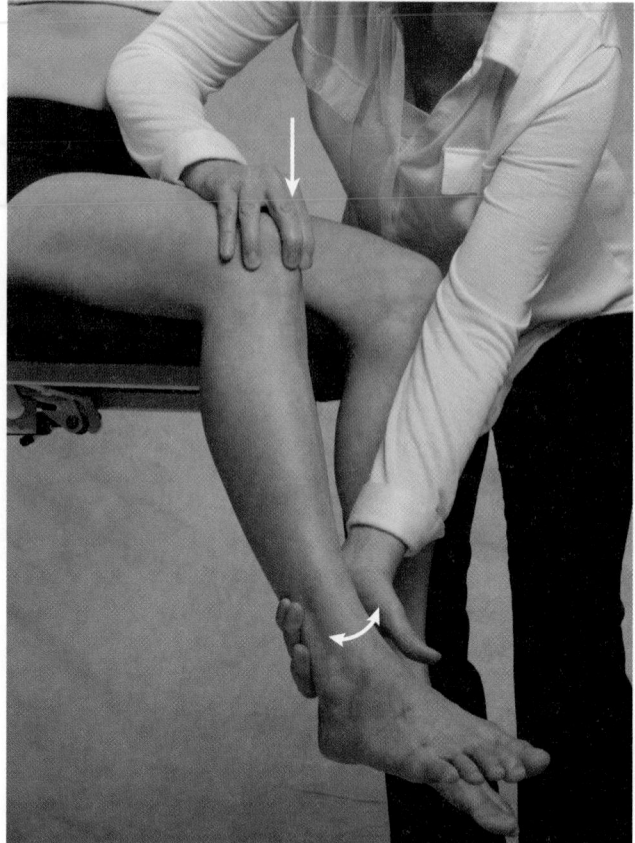

Figure 12-31 Motion palpation test of the patellofemoral joint.

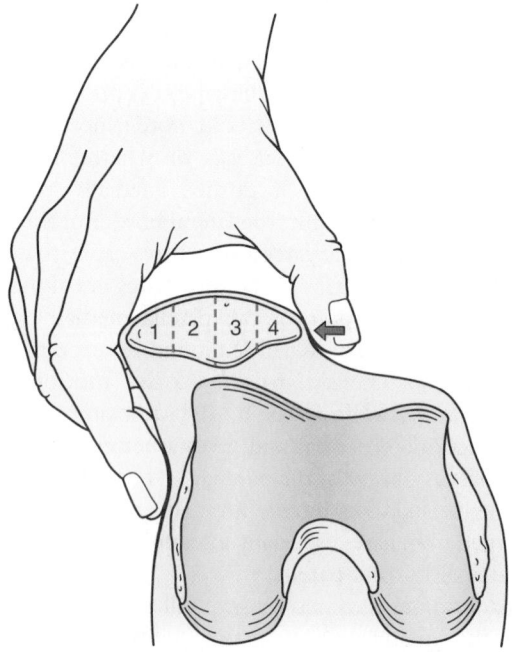

Figure 12-32 Passive lateral glide test demonstrating a patella being subluxated laterally to its second quadrant. Decreased patellar mobility (hypomobile) is manifested by less than one quadrant of medial and lateral glide; movement of more than two quadrants (one half of patellar width) is considered hypermobile. (Redrawn from Jackson DW, editor: The anterior cruciate ligament: current and future concepts, New York, 1993, Raven Press, p. 358.)

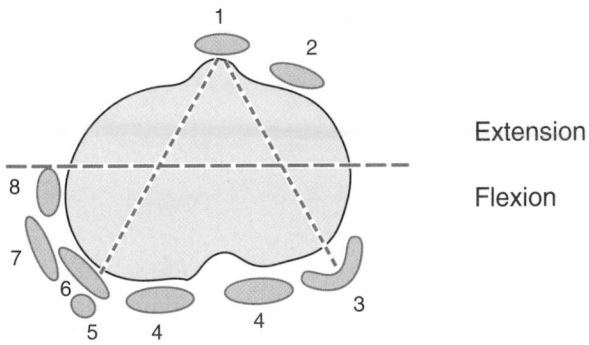

Figure 12-33 Movement diagram of the knee showing quadriceps hamstrings tripod. *1,* Patellar tendon (quadriceps); *2,* iliotibial band; *3,* biceps femoris; *4,* gastrocnemius; *5,* semitendinosus; *6,* semimembranosus; *7,* gracilis; *8,* sartorius.

Ideally, these resisted isometric movements are performed with the joint in its resting position. Segal and Jacob[65] suggest testing the quadriceps muscle at 0°, 30°, 60°, and 90° while observing any abnormal tibial movement (e.g., ligament instability) or excessive pain from patellar compression (e.g., patellofemoral syndrome). Figure 12-35 shows the quadriceps complex components and their angle of pull. Table 12-4 lists the muscles acting at the knee.

Although these movements are tested with the patient in the supine-lying position, the hamstrings are often tested with the patient prone. If the knee is flexed to 90° and the heel is turned out, the greatest stretch is placed on the lateral hamstring muscle (biceps femoris). If the heel is turned in, the greatest stretch is placed on the medial hamstring (semimembranosus and semitendinosus) muscles.

Ankle movements are tested because the gastrocnemius muscle crosses the posterior knee and both plantar and dorsiflexion movements cause movement of the fibula. Dorsiflexion causes the fibula to move up and increases the stress being applied to the ligaments supporting the superior tibiofibular joint. Plantar flexion decreases the stress on these ligaments and also brings the gastrocnemius into play, supporting the posterior knee and assisting knee flexion.

If the history has indicated concentric, eccentric, or econcentric movements have caused symptoms, these types of contractions should be tested as well, but only after isometric testing has been performed.

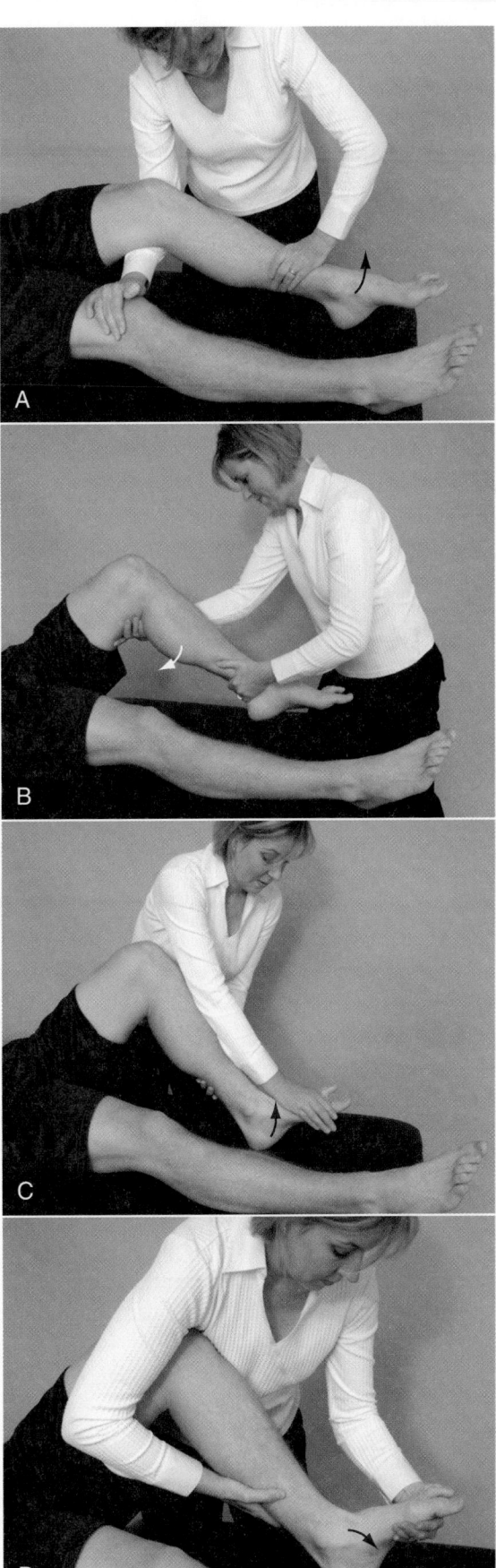

Figure 12-34 Resisted isometric movements of the knee. A, Knee extension. **B,** Knee flexion. **C,** Ankle dorsiflexion. **D,** Ankle plantar flexion.

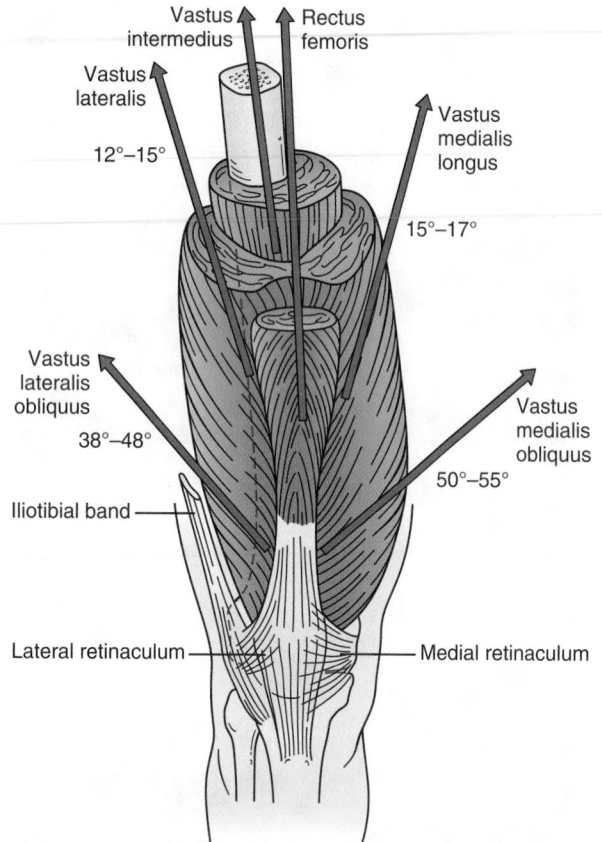

Vastus
intermedius

Rectus
femoris

Vastus
lateralis

12°–15°

Vastus
medialis
longus

15°–17°

Vastus
lateralis
obliquus

38°–48°

Vastus
medialis
obliquus

50°–55°

Iliotibial band

Lateral retinaculum

Medial retinaculum

Figure 12-35 Components of the quadriceps femoris complex. Note the angle of insertion of the various components of the complex. The orientation of the muscle fibers dictates the line of action and pull on the patella. (Redrawn from McConnell J, Fulkerson J: The knee: patellofemoral and soft tissue injuries. In Zachazewski JE, et al, editors: Athletic injuries and rehabilitation, Philadelphia, 1996, WB Saunders, p. 697.)

Kannus and colleagues[66] developed a scoring scale for measuring isokinetic and isometric strength (Figure 12-36). The scale can be used to show improvement in strength over time. When using isokinetic values, different test parameters may be used. It is important to realize, however, that most knee isokinetic tests are not done with the knee in a functional position.

Isokinetic Test Parameters Commonly Used for the Knee

- Left/right peak torque ratio
- Left/right average (mean) torque ratio
- Ratio of peak torque to body weight
- Torque curve analysis
- Bilateral total work comparison
- Hamstrings/quadriceps ratio (left and right)
- Ratio of average power to body weight
- Time ratio to torque development
- Time to 50% peak torque
- Endurance (fatigue) ratio (first to last repetition)

Depending on the speed, the hamstring/quadriceps ratio is normally between 50% and 60%.[67] As the speed of isokinetic testing increases, however, the ratio approaches 1:1, or 100%.[68,69]

Functional Assessment

Instabilities produced on the examining table are easily produced functionally, especially in athletes who participate in activities, such as vigorous cutting and jumping or rapid deceleration, which produce high physiological joint loads. Functional tests and numerous numerical knee rating systems have been developed for the knee, many of them for specific populations (e.g., athletes) or to assess outcomes after surgery or for specific conditions. The examiner must pick the appropriate test or scale, realizing that each has advantages and disadvantages.[70–73]

Clinical Screening Criteria for Doing a Functional Performance Screening Test of the Lower Limb*

- No pain
- No effusion
- No crepitus
- Full active range of motion (ROM) with terminal knee extension
- Symmetrical gait including climbing and descending stairs
- Good muscle strength in muscles around joint being tested (80% of normal or grade ≥ 4)
- One repetition maximum leg press ≥ 125% relative strength index with controlled concentric and eccentric phases
- Balance: Single leg stance ≥ 45 seconds (eyes open and closed)
- Single leg quarter squat ≥ 45 seconds (eyes open and closed)
- Single leg half squat ≥ 45 seconds (eyes open and closed)

Modified from Clark NC: Functional performance testing following knee ligament injury. Phys Ther Sport 2:101, 2001.

*Note: These criteria may be used for any lower limb injury.

If the active, passive, and resisted isometric movements are performed with little difficulty, the examiner may put the patient through a series of **functional tests** to see whether these sequential activities produce pain or other symptoms. These tests may be scored by the time taken to do the test or by the distance or height attained when doing the test. If the results are so measured, three measurements should be taken and averaged. In some cases, the results of different tests may be combined. Fonseca and coworkers[74] found that the time ratio of figure-eight running to straight running was one of the most effective ways of differentiating patients with anterior cruciate ligament deficiencies from normal patients (Figure 12-37). Some of these tests may involve walking (e.g., Timed "Up and Go" test [TUG test], sit-to-stand test). These walking tests may be used when any lower limb joint is affected but are primarily designed for elderly people.[75] Boonstra

TABLE **12-4**

Muscles of the Knee: Their Actions, Nerve Supply, and Nerve Root Derivation

Action	Muscles Acting	Nerve Supply	Nerve Root Derivation
Flexion of knee	1. Biceps femoris	Sciatic	L5, S1, S2
	2. Semimembranosus	Sciatic	L5, S1, S2
	3. Semitendinosus	Sciatic	L5, S1, S2
	4. Gracilis	Obturator	L2, L3
	5. Sartorius	Femoral	L2, L3
	6. Popliteus	Tibial	L4, L5, S1
	7. Gastrocnemius	Tibial	S1, S2
	8. Tensor fasciae latae (in 45° to 145° of flexion)	Superior gluteal	L4, L5
	9. Plantaris	Tibial	S1, S2
Extension of knee	1. Rectus femoris	Femoral	L2–L4
	2. Vastus medialis	Femoral	L2–L4
	3. Vastus intermedius	Femoral	L2–L4
	4. Vastus lateralis	Femoral	L2–L4
	5. Tensor fasciae latae (in 0° to 30° of flexion)	Superior gluteal	L4, L5
Medial rotation of flexed leg (non–weight-bearing)	1. Popliteus	Tibial	L4, L5
	2. Semimembranosus	Sciatic	L5, S1, S2
	3. Semitendinosus	Sciatic	L5, S1, S2
	4. Sartorius	Femoral	L2, L3
	5. Gracilis	Obturator	L2, L3
Lateral rotation of flexed leg (non–weight-bearing)	1. Biceps femoris	Sciatic	L5, S1, S2

Scoring Scale for Isokinetic and Isometric Strength Measurements of the Knee Joint

	Peak Torque		Difference		Score[†]
	Uninjured	*Injured*	*Absolute*	*Percent*	
Isokinetic					
Extension 60°/sec	_____	_____	_____	_____	_____
Flexion 60°/sec	_____	_____	_____	_____	_____
Extension 180°/sec	_____	_____	_____	_____	_____
Flexion 180°/sec	_____	_____	_____	_____	_____
Isometric					
Extension 60°	_____	_____	_____	_____	_____
Flexion 60°	_____	_____	_____	_____	_____
Total score (maximum 100 points)					_____

[†]Scoring System
Isometric
17 points = percent difference (uninjured – injured): ≤2%
15 points = percent difference (uninjured – injured): 3% to 5%
13 points = percent difference (uninjured – injured): 6% to 10%
9 points = percent difference (uninjured – injured): 11% to 25%
5 points = percent difference (uninjured – injured): 26% to 49%
0 points = percent difference (uninjured – injured): ≥50%

Isometric
16 points = percent difference (uninjured – injured): ≤2%
14 points = percent difference (uninjured – injured): 3% to 5%
12 points = percent difference (uninjured – injured): 6% to 10%
8 points = percent difference (uninjured – injured): 11% to 25%
4 points = percent difference (uninjured – injured): 26% to 49%
0 points = percent difference (uninjured – injured): ≥50%

Figure 12-36 Scoring scale for isokinetic and isometric strength measurements of the knee joint. (Modified from Kannus P, Jarvineaa M, Latvala K: Knee strength evaluation. Scand J Sport Sci 9:9, 1987.)

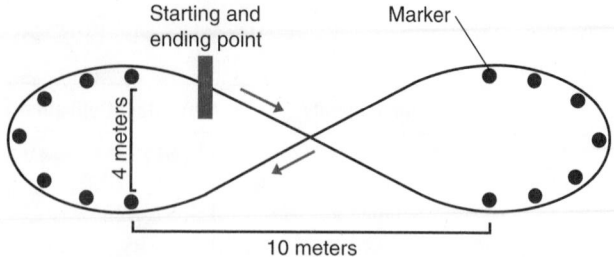

Figure 12-37 **Figure-eight running track.** (Redrawn from Fonseca ST, Magee DJ, Wessel J, et al: Validation of a performance test for outcome evaluation of knee function. Clin J Sport Med 2:253, 1992.)

et al.[75] felt the TUG test could be used as a global functional test following total knee arthroplasty while the sit-to-stand was a more biomechanical function test.

Sequential Functional Tests for the Knee

- Walking
- Ascending and descending stairs (walking → running)
- Squatting (both knees should flex symmetrically)
- Squatting and then bouncing at the end of the squat (again, the two knees should act symmetrically)
- Running straight ahead
- Running straight ahead and stopping on command
- Vertical jump
- Running and twisting (figure-eight running, carioca)
- Jumping and going into a full squat
- Hard cuts, twists, pivots

These functional activities, which are provided as examples, must be geared to the individual patient, and in some cases, to specific pathology.[76] Paxton et al.[77] recommended doing knee-specific, activity-specific, and general health questionnaires to provide a more accurate assessment of outcomes. Squatting reveals limitations of flexion and may cause impingement with meniscal lesions. Duck waddle, if attempted, can demonstrate increased symptoms in meniscal and ligamentous lesions. Older patients should not be expected to accomplish the last five or six (see earlier) movements unless they have been doing these or similar activities in the recent past. Daniel and coworkers[78] outlined different functional and intensity levels that are useful especially for getting an indication of functional activities from a patient's perspective (Table 12-5). Functional strength tests for sedentary individuals are shown in Table 12-6.

Strobel and Stedtfeld[79] put forward the **one-leg hop test.** The patient stands and does a "long jump" hop on one leg while landing on the same leg. This is a **single-leg hop for distance** (Figure 12-38, *A*).[80-83] Noyes and

---

TABLE 12-5

Patient Activity Scale

Functional Levels

Level I: Activities of daily living

Level II: Straight running; sports that do not involve lower-limb agility activities; occupations involving heavy lifting

Level III: Activities that require lower-limb agility but not involving jumping, hard cutting, or pivoting

Level IV: Activities involving jumping, hard cutting, or pivoting

Intensity

W: Work-related or occupational
LR: Light recreational
VR: Vigorous recreational
C: Competitive

Exposure

Number of hours per year of participation at any given functional level and intensity

From Daniel D, et al, editors: Knee ligaments: structure, injury and repair, New York, 1990, Raven Press, p. 522.

TABLE 12-6

Functional Testing of the Knee

Starting Position	Action	Functional Test
Standing	1. Walking backward 2. Running forward 20° (knee flexion)	6–8 m: Functional 3–6 m: Functionally fair 1–3 m: Functionally poor 0 m: Nonfunctional
Standing	1. Squat 20° to 30° 2. Jump, lifting body off floor	5 to 6 Repetitions: Functional 3 to 4 Repetitions: Functionally fair 1 to 2 Repetitions: Functionally poor 0 Repetitions: Nonfunctional

Data from Palmar ML, Epler M: Clinical assessment procedures in physical therapy, Philadelphia, 1990, JB Lippincott, pp. 275–276.

associates[80] considered symmetry of less than 85% between the legs to be abnormal. The test is repeated three times alternately with each leg. If instability is evident, the distance for the affected leg is less than that for the normal leg. Any functional deficit between the two limbs has been called the **limb symmetry index (LSI).**[84] Juris et al.[85] advocated doing a **maximal controlled leap** in

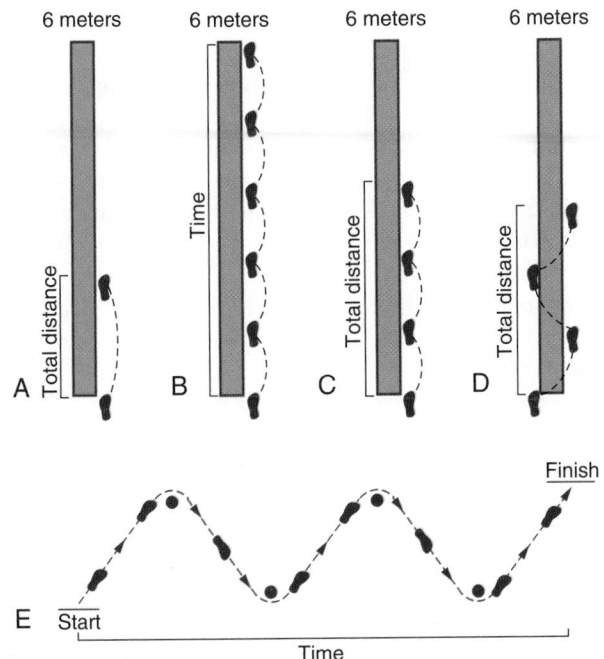

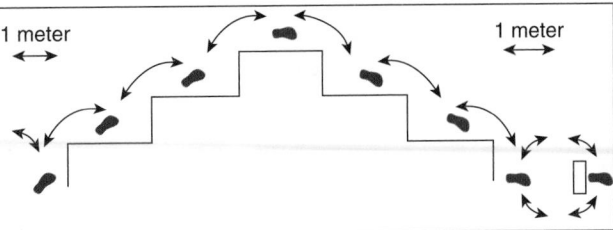

Figure 12-39 Stair hop test. (Modified from Hopper DM, Goh SC, Wentworth LA, et al: Test-retest reliability of knee rating scales and functional hop tests one year following anterior cruciate ligament reconstruction. *Phys Ther Sport* 3:10–18, 2002.)

Figure 12-38 Hop tests. A, Single hop for distance. **B,** Timed hop. **C,** Triple hop for distance. **D,** Crossover hop for distance. **E,** 30-m agility hop test.

addition to the one-leg hop test. For this test, which is said to test force absorption, the patient stands on one foot and "leaps forward" to land on the opposite foot. Patients should be instructed to maintain the flexed hip/knee position during takeoff and extend the leg for landing. Patients must "stick" on landing with no movement of the landing foot and must be upright with hands on hips within 1 second. The distance is measured and the test repeated with the opposite start leg.

Since the advent of the single-leg hop, modifications have been developed.[86] Each test is usually repeated three times, and the average of the three scores is used as the measured value. These modifications include the following:

1. **Single-leg hop for time:** With this test, the patient is assessed for the time taken to hop 6 m (20 ft) on one leg (Figure 12-38, *B*). The good leg is tested first, followed by the injured leg.[80,81,87]
2. **Triple hop:** With this test, the patient is asked to hop as far as possible, taking three hops. The distance for the good leg is compared with that for the injured leg (Figure 12-38, *C*).[80,81,87]
3. **Crossover hop:** A straight line is marked on the floor. The patient is asked to take three consecutive hops on one foot, crossing over the straight line each time (Figure 12-38, *D*). The good limb is tested, followed by the injured limb, and the average distances attained with each leg are compared.[80] Risberg and Ekeland[88] modified this test and called it the **side jump test.** For

this test, two 6-meter parallel lines are placed 30 cm (12 inches) apart on the floor. Outside one line, ten marks are made at 60-cm (24-inch) intervals. Outside the other line, marks are made at 60-cm (24-inch) intervals but starting at 30 cm (12 inches) so that the marks are staggered from one side to the other. The patient is asked to hop from marker to marker on each line. The good leg is timed, followed by the injured leg.

4. **Agility hop:** This hop test requires a space of 30 m (100 ft). Cones are placed 6 m (20 ft) apart (see Figure 12-38, *E*). The patient is then timed as he or she hops through the cones. The good limb is tested, followed by the injured limb, and the average times attained with each leg are compared.[87]
5. **Stairs hop test (stairs hopple test)[88]:** The patient is timed as he or she hops up and down several steps (20 to 25 steps recommended), first on the good leg and then on the injured leg. Hopper et al.[84] recommended a different stair hop test. For this test, patients are asked to hop up and then down a three-step platform, then turn about a marker fixed 1 meter from the platform, and then hop back up and down the step (Figure 12-39).

These functional tests are for active persons and can be quite demanding; however, they have been shown to have high test-retest reliability.[84] Losee[89] mentioned several additional tests. For example, in the **deceleration test,** the patient is asked to run at full speed and to stop suddenly on command.[28] The test is positive for rotary instability if the patient stops without using the quadriceps or decelerates in a crouched position (more than 30° flexion of the knee). The effect of the test can be accentuated by having the patient turn away from the affected leg just as he or she is about to stop.[90] As the patient does the test, the examiner should watch to ensure that the patient uses the affected leg to help stop. With instability problems, the patient uses only the good leg to stop, "hopping through" with the injured leg.

For the **"disco test,"** the patient stands on one leg with the knee flexed 10° to 20°. The patient is asked to rotate or twist left and right while holding the flexed

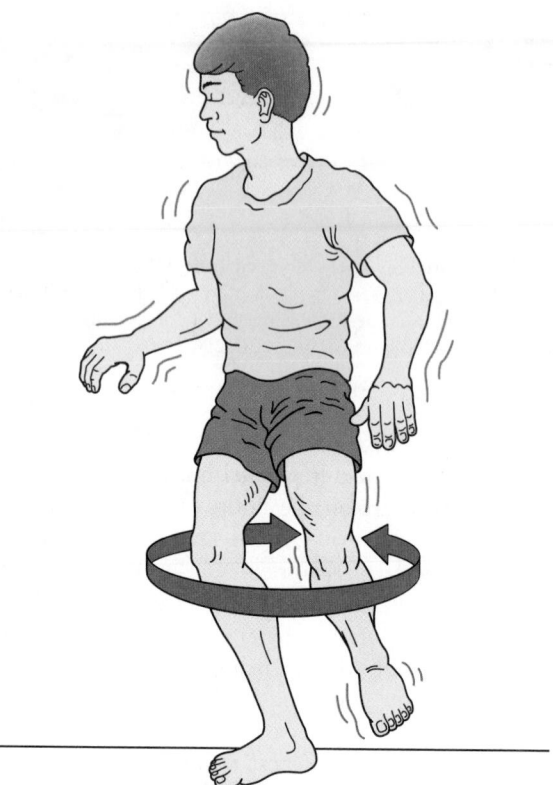

Figure 12-40 Losee disco test. Flexion, compression, and rotation may lead to shift of femur on tibia, causing rotary instability.

position (Figure 12-40).[28] Apprehension during the test or refusal to do the test is a positive sign for rotary instability. If pain is felt on the joint line, it may indicate meniscus pathology, in which case it is called **Merke's sign.**[79] Pain on medial rotation along the joint line implies medial meniscus pathology, and pain on lateral rotation implies lateral meniscus pathology.

Larson[91] advocated the **leaning hop test.** For this test, the patient hops up and down on one leg while abducting the opposite leg. A positive test is apprehension during the test or refusal to do the test and is a positive sign for rotary instability.

Numerical rating systems are commonly done to determine the state of the knee. Most of these measures combine clinical (e.g., ROM) and functional (e.g., stair climbing) measures. Many of these scoring systems have not been tested on normal subjects and show possible interviewer bias, nor are the values given to each measure explained. In addition, there may be male and female differences.[92,93]

Noyes and colleagues[94–97] developed the Cincinnati Knee Rating System (Figure 12-41), which deals with pain, swelling, stability, and activity level and is a good functional rating system for active persons. Irrgang and associates[98] use two scales, an Activities of Daily Living

Scale[99] and a Sports Activity Scale (Figures 12-42 and 12-43), to detect clinically significant changes over time. The Knee Society[100] also has a rating scale (Figure 12-44). The Knee Society advocates keeping knee rating and functional assessment separate. This knee-rating scale deals first with pain, ROM, and stability, giving positive points up to 100 and grouping deductions that can take away from the overall value. Function is dealt with separately on the scale.

Lysholm and Gillquist[101] developed a frequently used scale primarily designed to score clinical instability that may also be used for chondral lesions of the knee (Table 12-7).[102–106] The **International Knee Documentation Committee** has also developed a number of assessment forms, three of which are included here (Figures 12-45 to 12-47).[97,107–112] The **Tegner Activity Scale**[102,106,113] (Figure 12-48) is useful in determining the patient's current level of activity relative to his or her previous level and can also be used as a guide for rehabilitation and the level of activity the patient hopes to achieve. Table 12-8 and the **Kajula Score Questionnaire** (Figure 12-49) show examples of a patellofemoral joint evaluation scale that can be used to assess functional levels in patients with patellofemoral syndrome after surgery or nonsurgery.[114,115] Similar scales used to measure patellofemoral dysfunction also exist.[116–119] Other scales, such as the Western Ontario and McMaster University Osteoarthritis Index (WOMAC), Knee Injury and Osteoarthritis Outcome Score (KOOS),[103,112,120] and Lequesne Index, have been developed to determine the outcome of arthroplasties in osteoarthritis (see Chapter 11).[121–131] Each of these knee-rating scales is slightly different. The scale that works best for the examiner and the examiner's clientele should be used. Other knee-rating scales are also available.[101,132–137]

Ligament Stability

Because the knee, more than any other joint in the body, depends on its ligaments to maintain its integrity, it is imperative that the ligaments be tested. The ligaments of the knee joint act as primary stabilizers and guide the movement of the bones in proper relation to one another. Depending on the motion being tested, the ligaments act as primary or secondary restraints (Table 12-9). For example, the anterior cruciate ligament is the primary restraint to anterior tibial displacement and a secondary restraint to varus-valgus motion in full extension and rotation.[98,138] If the primary restraint is injured, pathological motion occurs. If the secondary restraint is injured but the primary restraint is not, pathological motion in that direction does not occur. If both primary and secondary restraints are injured, the pathological motion is greater.[98] There are several ligaments around the knee, but four deserve special mention (Figure 12-50).

Text continued on p. 805

Cincinnati Knee Rating System

Symptoms (50 points):

Left	Right		
□	□	20	**1. Pain**
□	□	20	No pain, normal knee, performs 100%.
□	□	16	Occasional pain with strenuous sports or heavy work, knee not entirely normal, some limitations, but minor and tolerable.
□	□	12	Occasional pain with light recreational sports or moderate work activities, frequently brought on by vigorous activities, running, heavy labor, strenuous sports.
□	□	8	Pain, usually brought on by sports, light recreational activities, or moderate work. Occasionally occurs with walking, standing, or light work.
□	□	4	Pain is a significant problem with activities as simple as walking. Relieved by rest. Unable to do sports.
□	□	0	Pain present all the time, occurs with walking, standing, and at nighttime. Not relieved with rest.
□	□		I do not know what my pain level is. I have not tested my knee.

Intensity of pain:
□ Mild □ Moderate □ Severe
Frequency: □ Intermittent □ Constant

Left	Right	
□	□	*Location of pain:* Medial (inner side)
□	□	Anterior-patellar (front/knee cap)
□	□	Posterior (back of knee)
□	□	Diffuse (all over)
□	□	*Pain occurs on:* Stairs
□	□	Sitting
□	□	Kneeling
□	□	Standing
□	□	*Type of pain:* Sharp
□	□	Aching
□	□	Throbbing
□	□	Burning

Left	Right		
□	□	10	**2. Swelling** No swelling, normal knee, 100% activity.
□	□	8	Occasional swelling with strenuous sports or heavy work. Some limitations but minor and tolerable.
□	□	6	Occasional swelling with light recreational sports or moderate work activities, frequently brought on by vigorous activities, running, heavy labor, or strenuous sports.
□	□	4	Swelling limits sports and moderate work. Occurs infrequently with simple walking activities or light work (about 3 times/year).
□	□	2	Swelling brought on by simple walking activities and light work. Relieved with rest.
□	□	0	Severe problem all of the time, with simple walking activities.
□	□		I do not know what my swelling level is. I have not tested my knee.

If swelling occurs, it is: (check one box on each line)
Intensity: □ Mild □ Moderate □ Severe
Frequency: □ Intermittent □ Constant

Left	Right		
□	□	20	**3. Giving-way.** No giving-way, normal knee, performs 100%.
□	□	16	Occasional giving-way with strenuous sports or heavy work. Can participate in all sports but some guarding or limitations are still present.
□	□	12	Occasional giving-way with light recreational activities or moderate work. Able to compensate, limits vigorous activities; sports or heavy work; not able to cut or twist suddenly.
□	□	8	Giving-way limits sports and moderate work; occurs infrequently with walking or light work (about 3 times/year).
□	□	4	Giving-way with simple walking activities and light work. Occurs once per month. Requires guarding.
□	□	0	Severe problem with simple walking activities; cannot turn or twist while walking without giving-way.
□	□		I do not know my level of giving-way. I have not tested my knee.

4. Other Symptoms (unscored)

Left	Right	Knee stiffness			Kneecap grinding			Knee locking
□	□	None	□	□	None	□	□	None
□	□	Occasional	□	□	Mild	□	□	Occasional
□	□	Frequent	□	□	Moderate	□	□	Frequent
			□	□	Severe			

Figure 12-41 Cincinnati Knee Rating System. (From Noyes FR, McGinniss GH, Mooar LA: Functional disability in the anterior cruciate insufficient knee syndrome. Sports Med 1:287–288, 1984.)

Continued

Cincinnati Knee Rating System (*Continued*)

Function (50 points):

			5. Overall activity level
☐	☐	20	No limitation, normal knee, able to do everything including strenuous sports or heavy labor.
☐	☐	16	Perform sports including vigorous activities, but at a lower performance level, involves guarding or some limits to heavy labor.
☐	☐	12	Light recreational activities possible with rare symptoms, more strenuous activities cause problems. Active but in different sports, limited to moderate work.
☐	☐	8	No sports or recreational activities possible. Walking activities possible with rare symptoms, limited to light work.
☐	☐	4	Walking, activities of daily living cause moderate symptoms, frequent limitation.
☐	☐	0	Walking, activities of daily living cause severe problems, persistent symptoms.
☐	☐		I do not know what my real activity level is, I have not tested my knee, or I have given up strenuous sports.

			6. Walking
☐	☐	10	Normal, unlimited.
☐	☐	8	Slight/mild problem.
☐	☐	6	Moderate problem: smooth surface possible up to 800 m.
☐	☐	4	Severe problem: only 2–3 blocks possible.
☐	☐	2	Severe problem: requires cane, crutches.

			7. Stairs
☐	☐	10	Normal, unlimited.
☐	☐	8	Slight/mild problem.
☐	☐	6	Moderate problem: only 10–15 steps possible.
☐	☐	4	Severe problem: requires bannister, support.
☐	☐	2	Severe problem: only 1–5 steps possible.

			8. Running activity
☐	☐	5	Normal, unlimited: fully competitive, strenuous.
☐	☐	4	Slight/mild problem: run half-speed.
☐	☐	3	Moderate problem: only 2–4 km possible.
☐	☐	2	Severe problem: only 1–2 blocks possible.
☐	☐	1	Severe problem: only a few steps.

			9. Jumping or twisting activities
☐	☐	5	Normal, unlimited, fully competitive, strenuous.
☐	☐	4	Slight/mild problem: some guarding, but sports possible.
☐	☐	3	Moderate problem: gave up strenuous sports; recreational sports possible.
☐	☐	2	Severe problem: affects all sports, must constantly guard.
☐	☐	1	Severe problem: only light activity possible (golf, swimming).

Total: Left [   ]   *Right* [   ]   (Maximum: 100 points)

Figure 12-41, cont'd

Activities of Daily Living Scale of the Knee Outcome Survey

Instructions:
The following questionnaire is designed to determine the symptoms and limitations that you experience because of your knee while you perform your usual *daily activities*. Please answer each question by **checking the statement that best describes you over the last 1 to 2 days.** For a given question, more than one of the statements may describe you, but please mark ONLY the statement that best describes you during your usual daily activities.

Symptoms

1. To what degree does pain in your knee affect your daily activity level?
   ___ I never have pain in my knee.
   ___ I have pain in my knee, but it does not affect my daily activity.
   ___ Pain affects my activity slightly.
   ___ Pain affects my activity moderately.
   ___ Pain affects my activity severely.
   ___ Pain in my knee prevents me from performing all daily activities.

2. To what degree does grinding or grating of your knee affect your daily activity level?
   ___ I never have grinding or grating in my knee.
   ___ I have grinding or grating in my knee, but it does not affect my daily activity.
   ___ Grinding or grating affects my activity slightly.
   ___ Grinding or grating affects my activity moderately.
   ___ Grinding or grating affects my activity severely.
   ___ Grinding or grating in my knee prevents me from performing all daily activities.

3. To what degree does stiffness in your knee affect your daily activity level?
   ___ I never have stiffness in my knee.
   ___ I have stiffness in my knee, but it does not affect my daily activity.
   ___ Stiffness affects my activity slightly.
   ___ Stiffness affects my activity moderately.
   ___ Stiffness affects my activity severely.
   ___ Stiffness in my knee prevents me from performing all daily activities.

4. To what degree does swelling in your knee affect your daily activity level?
   ___ I never have swelling in my knee.
   ___ I have swelling in my knee, but it does not affect my daily activity.
   ___ Swelling affects my activity slightly.
   ___ Swelling affects my activity moderately.
   ___ Swelling affects my activity severely.
   ___ Swelling in my knee prevents me from performing all daily activities.

5. To what degree does slipping of your knee affect your daily activity level?
   ___ I never have slipping of my knee.
   ___ I have slipping of my knee, but it does not affect my daily activity.
   ___ Slipping of my knee affects my activity slightly.
   ___ Slipping of my knee affects my activity moderately.
   ___ Slipping of my knee affects my activity severely.
   ___ Slipping of my knee prevents me from performing all daily activities.

6. To what degree does buckling of your knee affect your daily activity level?
   ___ I never have buckling of my knee.
   ___ I have buckling of my knee, but it does not affect my daily activity level.
   ___ Buckling of my knee affects my activity slightly.
   ___ Buckling of my knee affects my activity moderately.
   ___ Buckling of my knee affects my activity severely.
   ___ Buckling of my knee prevents me from performing all daily activities.

7. To what degree does weakness or lack of strength of your leg affect your daily activity level?
   ___ My leg never feels weak.
   ___ My leg feels weak, but it does not affect my daily activity.
   ___ Weakness affects my activity slightly.
   ___ Weakness affects my activity moderately.
   ___ Weakness affects my activity severely.
   ___ Weakness of my leg prevents me from performing all daily activities.

Functional Disability with Activities of Daily Living

8. How does your knee affect your ability to walk?
   ___ My knee does not affect my ability to walk.
   ___ I have pain in my knee when walking, but it does not limit my ability to walk.
   ___ My knee prevents me from walking more than 1 mile.
   ___ My knee prevents me from walking more than 1/2 mile.
   ___ My knee prevents me from walking more than 1 block.
   ___ My knee prevents me from walking.

9. Because of your knee, do you walk with crutches or a cane?
   ___ I can walk without crutches or a cane.
   ___ My knee causes me to walk with one crutch or a cane.
   ___ My knee causes me to walk with two crutches.
   ___ Because of my knee, I cannot walk, even with crutches.

10. Does your knee cause you to limp when you walk?
    ___ I can walk without a limp.
    ___ Sometimes my knee causes me to walk with a limp.
    ___ Because of my knee, I cannot walk without a limp.

11. How does your knee affect your ability to go up stairs?
    ___ My knee does not affect my ability to go up stairs.
    ___ I have pain in my knee when going up stairs, but it does not limit my ability to go up stairs.
    ___ I am able to go up stairs normally, but I need to rely on use of a railing.
    ___ I am able to go up stairs one step at a time with the use of a railing.
    ___ I have to use crutches or a cane to go up stairs.
    ___ I cannot go up stairs.

Figure 12-42 Activities of Daily Living Scale of the Knee Outcome Survey. (From Irrgang JJ, et al: Ligamentous and meniscal injuries. In Zachazewski JE, et al, editors: Athletic injuries and rehabilitation, Philadelphia, 1996, WB Saunders, pp 683–684.)   *Continued*

Activities of Daily Living Scale of the Knee Outcome Survey (Continued)

12. How does your knee affect your ability to go down stairs?
    - ____ My knee does not affect my ability to go down stairs.
    - ____ I have pain in my knee when going down stairs, but it does not limit my ability to go down stairs.
    - ____ I am able to go down stairs normally, but I need to rely on use of a railing.
    - ____ I am able to go down stairs one step at a time with the use of a railing.
    - ____ I have to use crutches or a cane to go down stairs.
    - ____ I cannot go down stairs.

13. How does your knee affect your ability to stand?
    - ____ My knee does not affect my ability to stand. I can stand for unlimited amounts of time.
    - ____ I have pain in my knee when standing, but it does not limit my ability to stand.
    - ____ Because of my knee, I cannot stand for more than 1 hour.
    - ____ Because of my knee, I cannot stand for more than 1/2 hour.
    - ____ Because of my knee, I cannot stand for more than 10 minutes.
    - ____ I cannot stand because of my knee.

14. How does your knee affect your ability to kneel on the front of your knee?
    - ____ My knee does not affect my ability to kneel on the front of my knee. I can kneel for unlimited amounts of time.
    - ____ I have pain when kneeling on the front of my knee, but it does not limit my ability to kneel.
    - ____ I cannot kneel on the front of my knee for more than 1 hour.
    - ____ I cannot kneel on the front of my knee for more than 1/2 hour.
    - ____ I cannot kneel on the front of my knee for more than 10 minutes.
    - ____ I cannot kneel on the front of my knee.

15. How does your knee affect your ability to squat?
    - ____ My knee does not affect my ability to squat. I can squat all the way down.
    - ____ I have pain when squatting, but I can still squat all the way down.
    - ____ I cannot squat more than 3/4 of the way down.
    - ____ I cannot squat more than halfway down.
    - ____ I cannot squat more than 1/4 of the way down.
    - ____ I cannot squat at all.

16. How does your knee affect your ability to sit with your knee bent?
    - ____ My knee does not affect my ability to sit with my knee bent. I can sit for unlimited amounts of time.
    - ____ I have pain when sitting with my knee bent, but it does not limit my ability to sit.
    - ____ I cannot sit with my knee bent for more than 1 hour.
    - ____ I cannot sit with my knee bent for more than 1/2 hour.
    - ____ I cannot sit with my knee bent for more than 10 minutes.
    - ____ I cannot sit with my knee bent.

17. How does your knee affect your ability to rise from a chair?
    - ____ My knee does not affect my ability to rise from a chair.
    - ____ I have pain when rising from the seated position, but it does not affect my ability to rise from the seated position.
    - ____ Because of my knee, I can only rise from a chair if I use my hands and arms to assist.
    - ____ Because of my knee, I cannot rise from a chair.

18. How would you rate your current level of knee function during your *usual daily activities* on a scale from 0 to 100, with 100 being your level of knee function prior to your injury?

    _____

19. How would you rate the *overall function* of your knee during your *usual daily activities*?
    - _____ normal
    - _____ nearly normal
    - _____ abnormal
    - _____ severely abnormal

20. As a result of your knee injury, how would you rate your *current level of daily activity*?
    - _____ normal
    - _____ nearly normal
    - _____ abnormal
    - _____ severely abnormal

21. Since initiation of treatment for your knee, how would you describe your progress?
    - _____ greatly improved
    - _____ somewhat improved
    - _____ neither improved/worsened
    - _____ somewhat worse
    - _____ greatly worse

Changes in Daily Activity Level

Please use the following scale to answer questions A–C below.

1 = I was able to perform *unlimited physical work,* which included lifting and climbing.
2 = I was able to perform *limited physical work,* which included lifting and climbing.
3 = I was able to perform *unlimited light activities,* which included walking on level surfaces and stairs.
4 = I was able to perform *limited light activities,* which included walking on level surfaces and stairs.
5 = I was *unable to perform light activities,* which included walking on level surfaces and stairs.

A. ____ *Prior to your knee injury,* how would you describe your usual daily activity? Please indicate only the **HIGHEST** level of activity that described you before your knee injury.

B. ____ *Prior to surgery or treatment* of your knee, how would you describe your usual daily activity? Please indicate only the **HIGHEST** level of activity that described you prior to surgery or treatment to your knee.

C. ____ How would you describe your *current level* of daily activity? Please indicate only the **HIGHEST** level of activity that describes you over the last 1 to 2 days.

Figure 12-42, cont'd

Sports Activity Scale of the Knee Outcome Survey

Instructions:

The following questionnaire is designed to determine the symptoms and limitations that you experience because of your knee while you participate in sports activities. Please answer each question by checking the statement that best describes you over the last 1 to 2 days. For a given question, more than one of the statements may describe you, but please mark ONLY the statement which best describes you when you participate in sports activities.

Symptoms

1. To what degree does pain in your knee affect your sports activity level?
   ___ I never have pain in my knee.
   ___ Knee pain does not affect my activity.
   ___ Slightly.
   ___ Moderately.
   ___ Severely.
   ___ Prevents me from performing all sports activities.

2. To what degree does grinding or grating of your knee affect your sports activity level?
   ___ I never have grinding or grating in my knee.
   ___ Grinding/grating does not affect my activity.
   ___ Slightly.
   ___ Moderately.
   ___ Severely.
   ___ Prevents me from performing all sports activities.

3. To what degree does stiffness in your knee affect your sports activity level?
   ___ I never have stiffness in my knee.
   ___ Knee stiffness does not affect my activity.
   ___ Slightly.
   ___ Moderately.
   ___ Severely.
   ___ Prevents me from performing all sports activities.

4. To what degree does swelling in your knee affect your sports activity level?
   ___ I never have swelling in my knee.
   ___ Knee swelling does not affect my activity.
   ___ Slightly.
   ___ Moderately.
   ___ Severely.
   ___ Prevents me from performing all sports activities.

5. To what degree does partial giving way or slipping of your knee affect your sports activity level?
   ___ I never have partial giving way or slipping of my knee.
   ___ Partial giving way does not affect my activity.
   ___ Slightly.
   ___ Moderately.
   ___ Severely.
   ___ Prevents me from performing all sports activities.

6. To what degree does complete giving way or buckling of your knee affect your sports activity level?
   ___ I never have complete giving way or buckling in my knee.
   ___ Knee buckling does not affect my activity.
   ___ Slightly.
   ___ Moderately.
   ___ Severely.
   ___ Prevents me from performing all sports activities.

Functional Disability with Sports Activities

1. How does your knee affect your ability to run straight ahead?
   ___ I am able to run straight ahead full speed without limitations.
   ___ I have pain in my knee, but it does not affect my ability.
   ___ Slightly.
   ___ Moderately.
   ___ Severely.
   ___ Prevents me from running.

2. How does your knee affect your ability to jump and land on your involved leg?
   ___ I am able to jump and land on my involved leg without limitations.
   ___ I have pain in my knee, but it does not affect my ability.
   ___ Slightly.
   ___ Moderately.
   ___ Severely.
   ___ Prevents me from jumping and landing.

3. How does your knee affect your ability to stop and start quickly?
   ___ I am able to start and stop quickly without limitations.
   ___ I have pain in my knee, but it does not affect my ability.
   ___ Slightly.
   ___ Moderately.
   ___ Severely.
   ___ Prevents me from stopping and starting quickly.

4. How does your knee affect your ability to cut and pivot on your involved leg?
   ___ I am able to cut and pivot on my involved leg without limitations.
   ___ I have pain in my knee, but it does not affect my ability.
   ___ Slightly.
   ___ Moderately.
   ___ Severely.
   ___ Prevents me from jumping and landing.

Figure 12-43 Sports Activity Scale of the Knee Outcome Survey. (From Irrgang JJ, et al: Ligamentous and meniscal injuries. In Zachazewski JE, et al, editors: Athletic injuries and rehabilitation, Philadelphia, 1996, WB Saunders, pp 683–685.)

Knee Society Knee Score

Patient category
A. Unilateral or bilateral (opposite knee successfully replaced)
B. Unilateral, other knee symptomatic
C. Multiple arthritis or medical infirmity

Pain	Points	Function	Points
None	50	Walking	50
Mild or occasional	45	Unlimited	40
Stairs only	40	>10 blocks	30
Walking and stairs	30	5–10 blocks	20
Moderate		<5 blocks	10
Occasional	20	Housebound	0
Continual	10	Unable	
Severe	0	Stairs	
		Normal up and down	50
Range of Motion		Normal up; down with rail	40
(5° = 1 point)	25	Up and down with rail	30
		Up with rail; unable down	15
Stability (maximum		Unable	0
movement in any position)			
		Subtotal	
Anteroposterior			
<5 mm	10	Deductions (minus)	
5–10 mm	5	Cane	5
10 mm	0	Two canes	10
Mediolateral		Crutches or walker	20
<5°	15		
6°–9°	10	**Total deductions**	
10°–14°	5		
15°	0	**Function score**	

Subtotal

Deductions (minus)

Flexion contracture
  5°–10°   2
  10°–15°   5
  16°–20°   10
  >20°   15
Extension lag
  <10°   5
  10°–20°   10
  >20°   15
Alignment
  5°–10°   0
  0°–4°   3 points each degree
  11°–15°   3 points each degree
  Other   20

Total deductions

Pain score
(if total is a minus number,
score is 0)

Figure 12-44 Knee Society knee score. (From Insall JN, Dorr LD, Scott RD, et al: Rationale of the Knee Society clinical rating system. Clin Orthop 248:14, 1989.)

TABLE 12-7

Lysholm Scoring Scale

	Points
Limp (5 points)	
None	5
Slight or periodic	3
Severe and constant	0
Support (5 points)	
Full support	5
Stick or crutch	3
Weight bearing impossible	0
Stair climbing (10 points)	
No problems	10
Slightly impaired	6
One step at a time	2
Unable	0
Squatting (5 points)	
No problems	5
Slightly impaired	4
Not past 90°	2
Unable	0
Walking running and jumping (70 points)	
Instability	
Never giving way	30
Rarely during athletic or other severe exertion	25
Frequently during athletic or other severe exertion (or unable to participate)	20
Occasionally in daily activities	10
Often in daily activities	5
Every step	0
Pain	
None	30
Inconstant and slight during severe exertion	25
Marked on giving way	20
Marked during severe exertion	15
Marked on or after walking more than 2 km	10
Marked on or after walking less than 2 km	5
Constant and severe	0
Swelling	
None	10
With giving way	7
On severe exertion	5
On ordinary exertion	2
Constant	0
Atrophy of thigh (5 points)	
None	5
1 to 2 cm	3
More than 2 cm	0
Total Score	**100**

Modified from Lysholm, J, Gillquist J: Evaluation of knee ligament surgery results with special emphasis on use of a scoring scale. Am J Sports Med 10:150–154, 1982.

TABLE 12-8

Patellofemoral Joint Evaluation Scale*

	Points
Limp	
None	5
Slight or episodie	3
Severe	0
Assistive devices	
None	5
Cane or brace	3
Unable to bear weight	0
Stair climbing	
No problem	20
Slight impairment	25
Very slowly	10
One step at a time, always same leg first	5
Unable	0
Crepitation	
None	5
Annoying	3
Limits activities	2
Severe	0
Inability, "Giving Way"	
Never	20
Occasionally with vigorous activities	10
Frequently with vigorous activities	8
Occasionally with daily activities	5
Frequently with daily activities	2
Every day	0
Swelling	
None	10
After vigorous activities only	5
After walking or mild activities	2
Constant	0
Pain	
None	35
Occasionally with vigorous activities	30
Marked with vigorous activities	20
Marked with walking 1 mile or mild to moderate rest pain	15
Marked with walking less than 1 mile	10
Constant and severe	0

From Karlsson J, et al: Eleven year follow up of patellofemoral pain syndromes. Clin J Sport Med 6:23, 1996.
*Functional results were assessed according to the patellofemoral scoring scale. Excellent results equal 90 to 100 points, good equals 80 to 89 points, fair equals 60 to 79 points, and poor equals less than 60 points.

2000 IKDC SUBJECTIVE KNEE EVALUATION FORM

Your Full Name _____

Today's Date: _____/_____/_____   Date of Injury: _____/_____/_____
　　　　　　　Day　Month　Year　　　　　　　　　　　　　Day　Month　Year

SYMPTOMS*:

*Grade symptoms at the highest activity level at which you think you could function without significant symptoms, even if you are not actually performing activities at this level.

1. What is the highest level of activity that you can perform without significant knee pain?

　　　　❏Very strenuous activities like jumping or pivoting as in basketball or soccer
　　　　❏Strenuous activities like heavy physical work, skiing, or tennis
　　　　❏Moderate activities like moderate physical work, running, or jogging
　　　　❏Light activities like walking, housework, or yard work
　　　　❏Unable to perform any of the above activities due to knee pain

2. During the past 4 weeks, or since your injury, how often have you had pain?

	0	1	2	3	4	5	6	7	8	9	10	
Never	❏	❏	❏	❏	❏	❏	❏	❏	❏	❏	❏	Constant

3. If you have pain, how severe is it?

	0	1	2	3	4	5	6	7	8	9	10	
No pain	❏	❏	❏	❏	❏	❏	❏	❏	❏	❏	❏	Worst pain imaginable

4. During the past 4 weeks, or since your injury, how stiff or swollen was your knee?

　　　　❏Not at all
　　　　❏Mildly
　　　　❏Moderately
　　　　❏Very
　　　　❏Extremely

5. What is the highest level of activity you can perform without significant swelling in your knee?

　　　　❏Very strenuous activities like jumping or pivoting as in basketball or soccer
　　　　❏Strenuous activities like heavy physical work, skiing, or tennis
　　　　❏Moderate activities like moderate physical work, running, or jogging
　　　　❏Light activities like walking, housework, or yard work
　　　　❏Unable to perform any of the above activities due to knee swelling

6. During the past 4 weeks, or since your injury, did your knee lock or catch?

　　　　❏Yes　❏No

7. What is the highest level of activity you can perform without significant giving wat in your knee?

　　　　❏Very strenuous activities like jumping or pivoting as in basketball or soccer
　　　　❏Strenuous activities like heavy physical work, skiing, or tennis
　　　　❏Moderate activities like moderate physical work, running, or jogging
　　　　❏Light activities like walking, housework, or yard work
　　　　❏Unable to perform any of the above activities due to giving way of the knee

Figures 12-45 2000 IKDC Subjective Knee Evaluation score. (Developed by the International Knee Documentation Committee [IKDC].)

page 2 – 2000 IKDC SUBJECTIVE KNEE EVALUATION FORM

SPORTS ACTIVITIES:

8. What is the highest level of activity you can participate in on a regular basis?

   ❑ Very strenuous activities like jumping or pivoting as in basketball or soccer
   ❑ Strenuous activities like heavy physical work, skiing, or tennis
   ❑ Moderate activities like moderate physical work, running, or jogging
   ❑ Light activities like walking, housework, or yard work
   ❑ Unable to perform any of the above activities due to knee

9. How does your knee affect your ability to:

		Not difficult at all	Minimally difficult	Moderately difficult	Extremely difficult	Unable to do
a.	Go up stairs	❑	❑	❑	❑	❑
b.	Go down stairs	❑	❑	❑	❑	❑
c.	Kneel on the front of your knee	❑	❑	❑	❑	❑
d.	Squat	❑	❑	❑	❑	❑
e.	Sit with your knee bent	❑	❑	❑	❑	❑
f.	Rise from a chair	❑	❑	❑	❑	❑
g.	Run straight ahead	❑	❑	❑	❑	❑
h.	Jump and land on your involved leg	❑	❑	❑	❑	❑
i.	Stop and start quickly	❑	❑	❑	❑	❑

FUNCTION:

10. How would you rate the function of your knee on a scale of 0 to 10 with 10 being normal, excellent function, and 0 being the inability to perform any of your usual daily activities that may include sports?

FUNCTION PRIOR TO YOUR KNEE INJURY:

Cannot perform daily activities	0	1	2	3	4	5	6	7	8	9	10	No limitation in daily activities
	❑	❑	❑	❑	❑	❑	❑	❑	❑	❑	❑	

CURRENT FUNCTION OF YOUR KNEE:

Cannot perform daily activities	0	1	2	3	4	5	6	7	8	9	10	No limitation in daily activities
	❑	❑	❑	❑	❑	❑	❑	❑	❑	❑	❑	

Figures 12-45, cont'd

Continued

Scoring Instructions for the 2000 IKDC SUBJECTIVE KNEE EVALUATION FORM

Several methods of scoring the IKDC Subjective Knee Evaluation Form were investigated. The results indicate the sum of the scores for each item performed as well as more sophisticated scoring methods.

The responses to each item are scored using an ordinal method such that a score of 1 is given to responses that represent the lowest level of function or highest level of symptoms, For example, item 1, which is related to the highest level of activity without significant pain is scored by assigning a score of 1 to the response "Unable to perform any of the above activities due to knee" and a score of 5 to the response "Very strenuous activities like jumping or pivoting as in basketball or soccer." For item 2, which is related to the frequency of pain over the past 4 weeks, the response "Constant" is assigned a score of 1 and "Never" is assigned a score of 11.

The IKDC Subjective Knee Evaluation Form is scored by summing the scores for the individual items and then transforming the score to a scale that ranges form 0 to 100. **Note:** The response to item 10 "Function Prior to Knee Injury" is not included in the overall score. The steps to score the IKDC Subjective Knee Evaluation Form are as follows:

1. Assign a score to the individual's response for each item, such that lowest score represents the lowest level of function or highest level of symptoms.
2. Calculate the raw score by summing the responses to all items with the exception of the response to item 10, "Function Prior to Your Knee Injury"
3. Transform the raw score to a 0 to 100 scale as follows:

$$\text{IKDC Score} = \left[\frac{\text{Raw Score} - \text{Lowest Possible Score}}{\text{Range of Scores}} \right] \times 100$$

Where the lowest possible score is 18 and the range of possible scores is 87. Thus, if the sum of scores for the 18 items is 60, the IKDC Score would be calculated as follows:

$$\text{IKDC Score} = \left[\frac{60 - 18}{87} \right] \times 100$$

$$\text{IKDC Score} = 48.3$$

The transformed score is interpreted as a measure of function such that higher scores represent higher levels of function and lower levels of symptoms. A score of 100 is interpreted to mean no limitation with activities of daily living or sports activities and the absence of symptoms.

The IKDC Subjective Knee Score can still be calculated if there are missing data, as long as there are responses to at least 90% of the items (i.e., responses have been provided for at least 16 items). To calculate the raw IKDC score when there are missing data, substitute the average score of the items that have been answered for the missing item score(s). Once the raw IKDC score has been calculated, it is transformed to the IKDC Subjective Knee Score as described above.

Figures 12-45, cont'd

2000 IKDC KNEE HISTORY FORM

Patient Name _____   Birthdate _____/_____/_____
                                                                                Day   Month   Year

Date of Injury _____/_____/_____   Date of Initial Exam _____/_____/_____   Today's Date _____/_____/_____
                Day   Month   Year   Day   Month   Year   Day   Month   Year

Involved Knee: ❑Right   ❑Left

Contralateral: ❑Normal   ❑Nearly Normal   ❑Abnormal   ❑Severely abnormal

Onset of Symptoms: (date)_____/_____/_____
                                   Day   Month   Year
Chief Complaint: _____

Activity at Injury: ❑ADL   ❑Sports   ❑Traffic   ❑Work

Mechanism of Injury:

❑Non-traumatic gradual onset   ❑Traumatic non-contact onset
❑Non-traumatic sudden onset   ❑Traumatic contact onset

Previous Surgery:

Type of Surgery: (check all that apply)

Meniscal Surgery

❑Medial meniscectomy   ❑Lateral meniscectomy
❑Medial meniscal repair   ❑Lateral meniscal repair
❑Medial meniscal transplant   ❑Lateral meniscal transplant

Ligament Surgery

❑ACL Repair   ❑Intraarticular ACL reconstruction   ❑Extraarticular ACL reconstruction
❑PCL Repair   ❑Intraarticular PCL reconstruction   ❑Posterolateral corner reconstruction
❑Medial collateral ligament repair/reconstruction
❑Lateral collateral ligament repair/reconstruction

Type of Graft   ❑Ipsilateral   ❑Contralateral
    Patella tendon graft
    ❑Single hamstring graft
    ❑2 Bundle hamstring graft
    ❑4 Bundle hamstring graft
    ❑Quadriceps tendon graft
    ❑Allograft
    ❑Other

Figures 12-46 2000 IKDC Knee History Form. (Developed by the International Knee Documentation Committee [IKDC].)

Continued

Page 2 – 2000 IKDC KNEE HISTORY FORM

Extensor Mechanism Surgery

       ❏Patella tendon repair   ❏Quadriceps tendon repair

Patellofemoral Surgery

       ❏Extensor Mechanism Realignment

        Soft Tissue Realignment

          ❏Medial imbrication   ❏Lateral release

        Bone Realignment

          Movement of the tibial tubercle
            ❏Proximal   ❏Distal   ❏Medial   ❏Lateral   ❏Anterior

       ❏Trochleoplasty

       ❏Patellectomy

Osteoarthritis Surgery

       ❏Osteotomy

       ❏Articular Surface Surgery   ❏Shaving   ❏Abrasion   ❏Drilling   ❏Microfracture
       ❏Cell therapy   ❏Osteochondral autograft transfer/mosaic-plasty   ❏Other

      Total number of previous surgeries_____

Imaging Studies:

      ❏Structural   ❏MRI   ❏CT   ❏Arthrogram

      ❏Metabolic (bone scan)

      Findings:

        Ligament _____

        Meniscus _____

        Articular Cartilage _____

        Bone _____

Figures 12-46, cont'd

2000 IKDC KNEE EXAMINATION FORM

Patient Name:_____   **Date of Birth:**_____/_____/_____
                                                                          Day   Month   Year

Gender: ? F   ? M   **Age:**_____   **Date of Examination:**_____/_____/_____
                                                                                        Day   Month   Year

Generalized Laxity: ? tight   ? normal   ? lax

Alignment: ? obvious varus   ? normal   ? obvious varus

Patella Position: ? obvious baja   ? normal   ? obvious alta

Patella Subluxation/Dislocation: ? centered   ? subluxable   ? subluxed   ? dislocated

Range of Motion (Ext/Flex):   Index Side: passive_____/_____/_____   active_____/_____/_____
                                                     Opposite Side: passive_____/_____/_____   active_____/_____/_____

SEVEN GROUPS	FOUR GRADES				*Group Grade			
	A Normal	B Nearly Normal	C Abnormal	D Severely Abnormal	A	B	C	D
1. Effusion	? None	? Mild	? Moderate	? Severe	?	?	?	?
2. Passive Motion Deficit								
ΔLack of extension	? <3°	? 3 to 5°	? 6 to 10°	? >0°				
ΔLack of flexion	? 0 to 5°	? 6 to 15°	? 16 to 25°	? >25°	?	?	?	?
3. Ligament Examination								
(manual, instrumented, x-ray)								
ΔLachman(25° flex) (134N)	? −1 to 2mm	? 3 to 5mm(1$^+$)	? 6 to 10mm(2$^+$)	? >10mm(3$^+$)				
		? <−1 to −3	? <−3 stiff					
ΔLachman(25° flex) manual max	? −1 to 2mm	? 3 to 5mm	? 6 to 10mm	? >10mm				
Anterior endpoint:	? firm		? soft					
ΔTotal AP Translation (25° flex)	? 0 to 2mm	? 3 to 5mm	? 6 to 10mm	? >10mm				
ΔTotal AP Translation (70° flex)	? 0 to 2mm	? 3 to 5mm	? 6 to 10mm	? >10mm				
ΔPosterior Drawer Test (70° flex)	? 0 to 2mm	? 3 to 5mm	? 6 to 10mm	? >10mm				
ΔMed Joint Opening (20° flex/valgus rot)	? 0 to 2mm	? 3 to 5mm	? 6 to 10mm	? >10mm				
ΔLat Joint Opening (20° flex/varus rot)	? 0 to 2mm	? 3 to 5mm	? 6 to 10mm	? >10mm				
ΔExternal Rotation Test (30° flex prone)	? <5°	? 6 to 10°	? 11 to 19°	? >20°				
ΔExternal Rotation Test (90° flex prone)	? <5°	? 6 to 10°	? 11 to 19°	? >20°				
ΔPivot Shift	? equal	? +glide	? ++(clunk)	? +++(gross)				
ΔReverse Pivot Shift	? equal	? glide	? gross	? marked	?	?	?	?
4. Compartment Findings		crepitation with						
ΔCrepitus Ant. Compartment	? none	? moderate	? mild pain	? >mild pain				
ΔCrepitus Med. Compartment	? none	? moderate	? mild pain	? >mild pain				
ΔCrepitus Lat. Compartment	? none	? moderate	? mild pain	? >mild pain				
5. Harvest Site Pathology	? none	? mild	? moderate	? severe				
6. X-ray Findings								
Med. Joint Space	? none	? mild	? moderate	? severe				
Lat. Joint Space	? none	? mild	? moderate	? severe				
Patellofemoral	? none	? mild	? moderate	? severe				
Ant. Joint Space (sagittal)	? none	? mild	? moderate	? severe				
Post. Joint Space (sagittal)	? none	? mild	? moderate	? severe				
7. Functional Test								
One Leg Hop (% of opposite side)	? ≥90%	? 89 to 76%	? 75 to 50%	? <50%				
** Final Evaluation					?	?	?	?

*   Group grade: The lowest grade within a group determines the group grade

** Final evaluation: the worst group grade determines the final evaluation for acute and subacute patients. For chronic patients compare preoperative and postoperative evaluations. In a final evaluation only the first 3 groups are evaluated but all groups must be documented. Δ Difference in involved knee compared to normal or what is assumed to be normal.

IKDC COMMITTEE AOSSM: Anderson, A., Bergfeld, J., Boland, A. Dye, S., Feagin, J., Harner , C. Mohtadi, N. Richmond, J. Shelbourne, D., Terry, G. ESSKA: Staubli, H., Hefti, F., Hoher, J., Jacob, R., Mueller, W., Neyret, P. APOSSM: Chan, K., Kurosaka, M.

Figures 12-47 2000 IKDC Knee Examination Form. (Developed by the International Knee Documentation Committee [IKDC].)

Continued

INSTRUCTIONS FOR THE 2000 IKDC KNEE EXAMINATION FORM

The Knee Examination Form contains items that fall into one of seven measurement domains. However, only the first three of these domains are graded. The seven domains assessed by the Knee Examination Form are:

1. *Effusion*

    An effusion is assessed by ballotting the knee. A fluid wave (less than 25 cc) is graded mild, easily ballotteable fluid – moderate (25-60 cc), and a tense knee secondary to effucion (greater than 60 cc) is rated severe.

2. *Passive Motion Deficit*

    Passive range of motion is measured with a gonimeter and recorded on the form for the index side and opposite or normal side. Record values for zero point/hyperextension/flexion (e.g., 10 degrees of hyperextension, 150 degrees of flexion = 10/0/150; 10 degrees of flexion to 150 degrees of flexion = 0/10/150). Extension is compared to that of the normal knee.

3. *Ligament Examination*

    The Lachman test, total AP translation at 70 degrees, and medial and lateral joint opening may be assessed with manual, instrumented or stress x-ray examination. Only one should be graded, preferably a "measured displacement." A force of 134 N (30 lbs) and the maximum manual are recorded in instrumented examination of both knees. Only the measured displacement at the standard force of 134 N is used for grading. The numerical values for the side to side difference are rounded off, and the appropriate box is marked.

    The end point is assessed in the Lachman test. The end point affects the grading when the index knee has 3-5 mm more anterior laxity then the normal knee. In this case, a soft end point results in an abnormal grade rather than a nearly normal grade.

    The 70-degree posterior sag is estimated by comparing the profile of the injured knee to the normal knee and palpating the medial femoral tibial stepoff. It may be confirmed by noting that contraction of the quadriceps pulls the tibia anteriorly.

    The external rotation tests are performed with the patient prone and the knee flexed 30° and 70°. Equal external rotational torque is applied to both feet and the degree of external rotation is recorded.

    The pivot shift and reverse pivot shift are performed with the patient supine, with the hip in 10-20 degrees of abduction and the tibia in neutral rotation using either the losee, Noyes, or Jakob techniques. The greatest subluxation, compared to the normal knee, should be recorded.

4. *Compartment Findings*

    Patellofemoral crepitation is elicited by extension against slight resistance. Medial and lateral compartment crepitation is elicited by extending the knee from a flexed position with a varus stress and then a valgus stress (i.e., McMurray test). Grading is based on intensity and pain.

5. *Harvest Site Pathology*

    Note tenderness, irritation or numbness at the autograft harvest site.

6. *X-ray Findings*

    A bilateral, double leg PA weightbearing roentgenogram at 35-45 degrees of flexion (tunnel view) is used to evaluate narrowing of the medial and lateral joint spaces. The Merchant view at 45 degrees is used to document patellofemoral narrowing. A mild grade indicates minimal change (i.e., small osteophytes, slight sclerosis or flattening of the femoral condyle) and narrowing of the joint space which is just detectable. A moderate grade may have those changes and joint space narrowing (e.g., a joint space of 2-4 mm side or up to 50% joint space narrowing). Severe changes include a joint space of less than 2 mm or greater than 50% joint space narrowing.

7. *Functional Test*

    The patient is asked to perform a one leg hop for distance on the index and normal side. Three trials for each leg are recorded and averaged. A ratio of the index to normal knee is calculated.

Figures 12-47, cont'd

TEGNER ACTIVITY LEVEL SCALE

Please indicate in the spaces below the HIGHEST level of activity that you participated in BEFORE YOUR INJURY and the highest level you are able to participate in CURRENTLY.

BEFORE INJURY: Level_____   CURRENT: Level_____

Level 10	Competitive sports-soccer, football, rugby (national elite)
Level 9	Competitive sports-soccer, football, rugby (lower divisions), ice hockey, wrestling, gymnastics, basketball
Level 8	Competitive sports-racquetball or bandy, squash or badminton, track and field athletics (jumping, etc.), down-hill skiing
Level 7	Competitive sports-tennis, running, motorcars speedway, handball Recreational sports-soccer, football, rugby, bandy, ice hockey, basketball, squash, racquetball, running
Level 6	Recreational sports-tennis and badminton, handball, racquetball, down-hill skiing, jogging at least 5 times per week
Level 5	Work-heavy labor (construction, etc.) Competitive sports-cycling, cross-country skiing Recreational sports-jogging on uneven ground at least twice weekly
Level 4	Work-moderately heavy labor (e.g., truck driving, etc.)
Level 3	Work-light labor (nursing, etc.)
Level 2	Work-light labor Walking on uneven ground possible, but impossible to back pack or hike
Level 1	Work-sedentary (secretarial, etc.)
Level 0	Sick leave or disability pension because of knee problems

SURGICAL HISTORY

Have you had any additional surgeries to your knee other than those performed by Dr. Stone?

Yes/No

If Yes:

What procedure(s) were performed? _____

When was the surgery performed? _____

Who performed the surgery? _____

Figures 12-48 Tegner Activity Level Scale. (Modified from Tegner Y, Lysholm J: Rating systems in the evaluation of knee ligament injuries. Clin Orthop Relat Res 198: 43-49, 1985; and Tegner Y, Lysholm J, Odensten M, et al: Evaluation of cruciate ligament injuries. Acta Orthop Scand 59:336–341, 1988.)

Collateral and Cruciate Ligaments

Collateral Ligaments. The **medial (tibial) collateral ligament** lies more posteriorly than anteriorly on the medial aspect of the tibiofemoral joint. It is made up of two layers, one superficial and one deep. The deep layer is a thickening of the joint capsule that blends with the medial meniscus; it is sometimes called the *medial capsular ligament.* The superficial layer is a strong, broad triangular strap. It starts distal to the adductor tubercle and extends to the medial surface of the tibia, approximately 6 cm (2.4 inches) below the joint line. It blends with the posterior capsule and is separated from the capsule and the medial meniscus by a bursa.

The entire medial collateral ligament is tight throughout the full ROM, although there is varying stress placed on different parts of the ligament as it moves through the full range because of the shape of the femoral condyles. All of its fibers are taut on full extension. In flexion, the anterior fibers are the most taut; in mid range, the posterior fibers are the most taut.[139]

The **lateral (fibular) collateral ligament** is round and lies under the tendon of the biceps femoris muscle. It runs from the lateral epicondyle of the femur to the fibular head. It also lies more posteriorly than anteriorly. This ligament is tight in extension and loosens in flexion, especially after 30° flexion. As the knee flexes, it provides protection to the lateral aspect of the knee. It is not attached to the lateral meniscus but rather is separated from it by a small fat pad.[139]

Cruciate Ligaments. The cruciate ligaments cross each other and are the primary rotary stabilizers of the knee.[140] These strong ligaments are named in relation to their attachment to the tibia and are intracapsular but extrasynovial. Each ligament has an anteromedial and a posterolateral portion. The anterior cruciate ligament has, in addition, an intermediate portion.

The **anterior cruciate ligament** extends superiorly, posteriorly, and laterally, twisting on itself as it extends from the tibia to the femur. Its main functions are to prevent anterior movement of the tibia on the femur, to check lateral rotation of the tibia in flexion, and, to a lesser extent, to check extension and hyperextension at the knee. It also helps to control the normal rolling and gliding movement of the knee. The anteromedial bundle is tight in both flexion and extension, limits anterior translation and helps stabilize medial and lateral rotation,[141,142] whereas the posterolateral bundle is tight in low flexion angles (closer to extension) and medial rotation. It limits

KUJALA SCORE QUESTIONNAIRE

Anterior Knee Pain Questionnaire

Which knee is affected?   Left   Right   Both

How long have you had the problem? _____ Years _____ Months

For each question, circle the letter that best corresponds to the problems you have with your knee:

1. Limp
   A. None (5)
   B. Slight/Occasional (3)
   C. Constant (0)
2. Taking weight on your leg
   A. Full weight on leg without pain (5)
   B. Painful on weight bearing (3)
   C. Unable to fully weight bear on leg (0)
3. Walking
   A. Unlimited (5)
   B. More than one mile (3)
   C. Between ½ to 1 mile (2)
   D. Unable to walk any distance (0)
4. Stairs
   A. No problems (10)
   B. Slight pain going down (7)
   C. Pain going up and down (3)
   D. Unable to go up or down stairs
      without pain (0)
5. Squatting
   A. No difficulty (5)
   B. Repeated squatting is painful (4)
   C. Painful each time (3)
   D. Possible, but not taking full weight (2)
   E. Unable to squat (0)
6. Running
   A. No problems (10)
   B. Pain after greater than 1 mile (8)
   C. Slight pain from the start,
      but able to run (6)
   D. Painful to run (3)
   E. Unable to run (0)
7. Jumping
   A. No difficulty (10)
   B. Slight discomfort (7)
   C. Constant pain (3)
   D. Unable to jump (0)

8. Prolonged sitting with knee bent
   A. No problems (10)
   B. Pain/stiffness after exercises (8)
   C. Constantly painful (6)
   D. Pain forces you to regularly straighten knee (4)
   E. Unable to sit with knee bent (0)
9. Pain
   A. None (10)
   B. Slight and occasional (8)
   C. Interferes with sleep (6)
   D. Occasionally severe (3)
   E. Constant and severe (0)
10. Swelling
    A. None (10)
    B. After severe exertion (8)
    C. After daily activities (6)
    D. Every evening (4)
    E. Constantly present (0)
11. Feeling of instability giving way in the knee cap.
    A. None (10)
    B. Occasionally with sporting or
       high load activities (6)
    C. Occasionally in daily activities (4)
    D. At least 1 dislocation of knee cap (2)
    E. More than 1 dislocation (0)
12. Wasting of thigh muscles
    A. None (5)
    B. Noticeable compared to other leg (3)
    C. Greatly reduced thigh muscle size
       compared to the other leg (0)
13. Loss of knee bend
    A. None (5)
    B. Slight at the end of movement (3)
    C. Severe limitation of movement (0)

Score = _____/100
Note: 1 km = 0.62 miles

Figure 12-49 Kujala score questionnaire. (From Herrington L, Al-Sherhi A: A controlled trial of weight-bearing versus non–weight-bearing exercises for patellofemoral pain. J Orthop Sports Phys Ther 37[4]:160, 2007.)

TABLE 12-9

Primary and Secondary Restraints of the Knee

Tibial Motion	Primary Restraints	Secondary Restraints
Anterior translation	ACL	MCL, LCL; middle third of mediolateral capsule; popliteus corner, semimembranosus corner, iliotibial band
Posterior translation	PCL	MCL, LCL; posterior third of mediolateral capsule; popliteus tendon; anterior and posterior meniscofemoral ligaments
Valgus rotation (medial gapping)	MCL	ACL, PCL; posterior capsule when knee fully extended, semimembranosus corner
Varus rotation (lateral gapping)	LCL	ACL, PCL; posterior capsule when knee fully extended, popliteus corner
Lateral rotation	MCL, LCL	Popliteus corner
Medial rotation	ACL, PCL	Anteroposterior meniscofemoral ligaments, semimembranosus corner

Modified from Zachazewski JE, et al, editors: Athletic injuries and rehabilitation, Philadelphia, 1996, WB Saunders, p 627.
ACL, Anterior cruciate ligament; *LCL,* lateral collateral ligament; *MCL,* medial collateral ligament; *PCL,* posterior cruciate ligament.

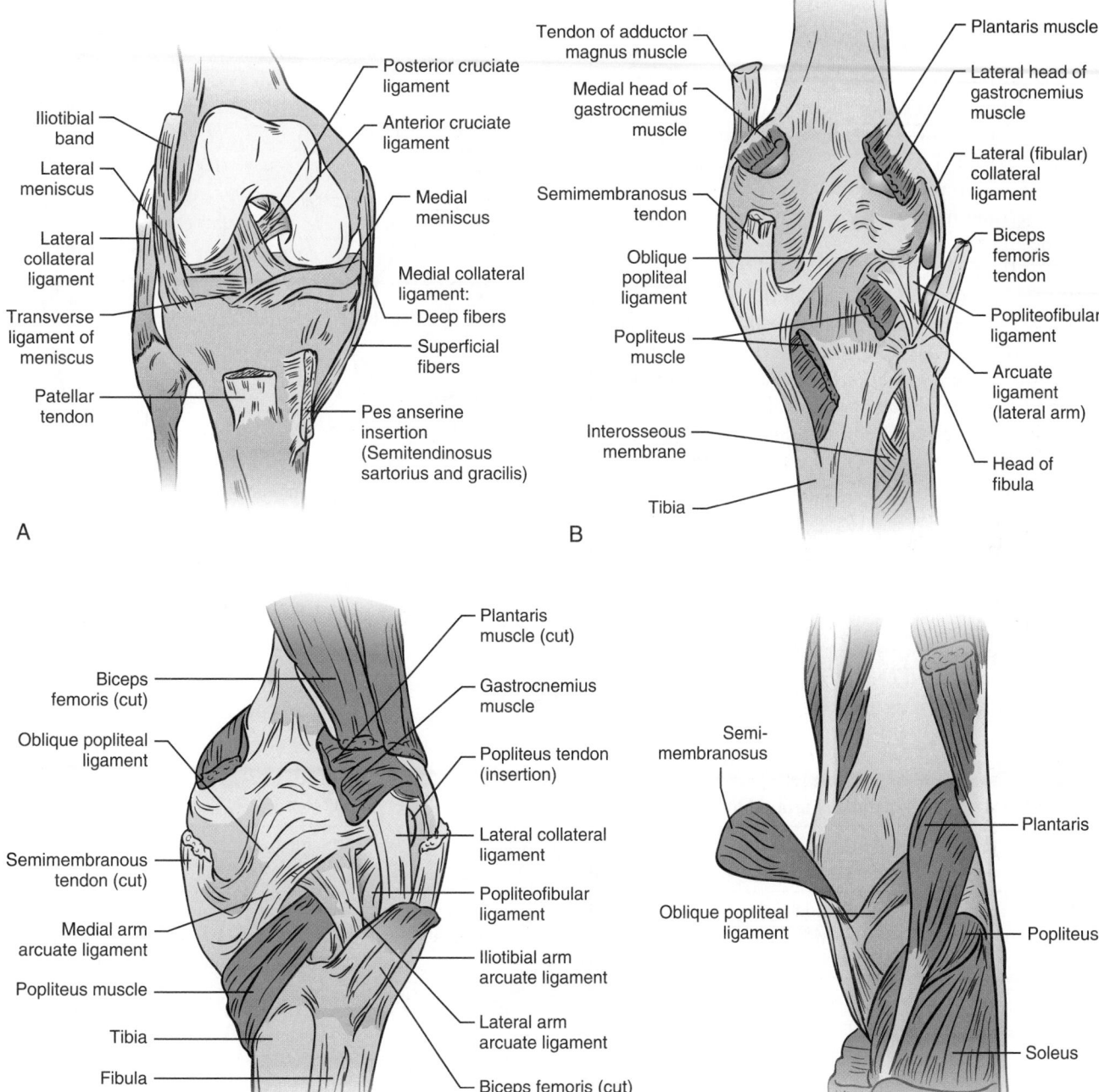

Figure 12-50 Anterior and posterior views of knee. A, Anterior view. The patellar tendon is removed, and the knee is flexed. Note that the cruciate ligament rises in front of the anterior tibial spine, not from it. Note also that the medial meniscus is firmly attached to the medial collateral ligament. **B,** Posterior view with the knee extended and the posterior ligament removed. The two layers of the medial collateral ligament are shown, as is the tibial portion of the lateral collateral ligament. The posterior cruciate ligament rises behind the tibia, not on its upper surface. Note the femoral attachment of the anterior cruciate ligament on the back of the notch. **C,** Posterior oblique view showing superficial structures of posterolateral corner. **D,** Posterior oblique view showing deeper structures including popliteus.

anterior translation, hyperextension, and rotation.[141] As a whole, the ligament has the least amount of stress on it between 30° and 60° flexion.[139,140,143,144]

The **posterior cruciate ligament** extends superiorly, anteriorly, and medially from the tibia to the femur. This

strong, fan-shaped ligament, the stoutest ligament in the knee, is a primary stabilizer of the knee against posterior movement of the tibia on the femur, and it checks extension and hyperextension. In addition, the ligament helps to maintain rotary stability and functions as the knee's central axis of rotation. Along with the anterior cruciate ligament, it acts as a rotary guide to the "screwing home" mechanism of the knee.[139,144] For the posterior cruciate ligament, the bulk of the fibers are tight at 30° flexion, but the posterolateral fibers are loose in early flexion.

With lateral rotation of the tibia, both collateral ligaments become more taut, and the cruciate ligaments become relaxed (Figure 12-51). With medial rotation of the tibia, the reverse action occurs: the collateral ligaments become more relaxed, and the cruciate ligaments become tighter.[139,145]

LaPrade et al.[146] have stressed the importance of the popliteus in controlling rotation of the tibia on the femur by contributing to lateral rotation stability. They felt the muscle, in fact, acts like a dynamic ligament to help stabilize the knee (see Figure 12-50). Morgan et al.[147] reported that the oblique popliteal ligament, which is an expansion of the semimembranosus tendon (see Figure 12-50), was the primary structure preventing hyperextension of the knee.

Testing of Ligaments

When testing the ligaments of the knee, the examiner must watch for four one-plane instabilities and four rotational instabilities (Table 12-10 and Figure 12-52).

There are a number of tests for each type of instability. The examiner should use the one or two tests that he or

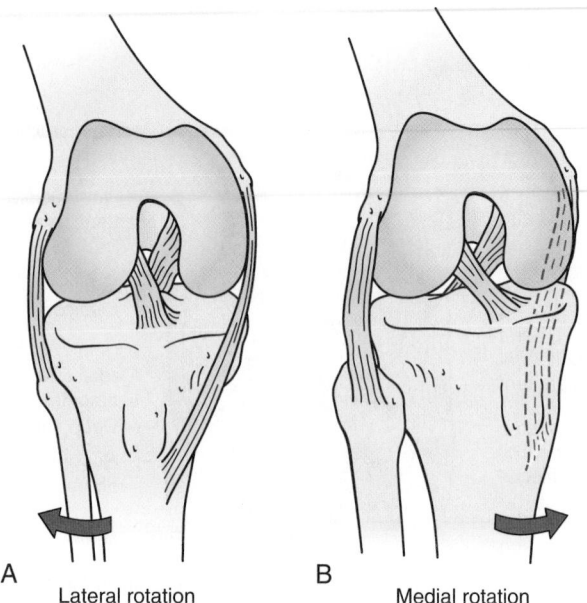

A Lateral rotation   **B** Medial rotation

Figure 12-51 Effect of tibial rotation on cruciate and collateral ligaments. A, The collateral ligament is taut; the cruciate ligament is lax. **B,** The collateral ligament is lax; the cruciate ligament is taut.

TABLE 12-10

Tests for Ligamentous Instability around the Knee

Instability	Tests Used to Determine Instability	Structures Injured to Some Degree If Test Positive*	Notes
One-plane medial (straight medial)	1. Abduction (valgus) stress with knee in **full extension**	1. Medial collateral ligament (superficial and deep fibers) 2. Posterior oblique ligament 3. Posteromedial capsule 4. Anterior cruciate ligament 5. Posterior cruciate ligament 6. Medial quadriceps expansion 7. Semimembranosus muscle	1. If either cruciate ligament is torn (third-degree sprain) or stretched, rotary instability will also be evident 2. Order of injury is usually medial collateral ligament, then posteromedial corner, posterior capsule, anterior cruciate ligament, and finally posterior cruciate ligament
	2. Abduction (valgus) stress with knee **slightly flexed (20° to 30°)**	1. Medial collateral ligament (superficial and deep fibers) 2. Posterior oblique ligament 3. Posterior cruciate ligament	1. Depending on degree of pain, opening and end feel, primarily signifies medial collateral ligament sprain (first, second, or third degree) 2. If posterior cruciate ligament is torn (third-degree sprain), rotary instability will also be evident 3. Opening of 12° to 15° signifies injury to posterior cruciate ligament 4. If tibia is laterally rotated, stress is taken off posterior cruciate ligament 5. If tibia is medially rotated, stress is increased on cruciate ligaments while medial collateral ligament relaxes

TABLE **12-10**

Tests for Ligamentous Instability around the Knee—cont'd

Instability	Tests Used to Determine Instability	Structures Injured to Some Degree If Test Positive*	Notes
One-plane lateral (straight lateral)	1. Adduction (varus) stress with knee in **full extension**	1. Lateral collateral ligament 2. Posterolateral capsule 3. Arcuate-popliteus complex 4. Biceps femoris tendon 5. Anterior cruciate ligament 6. Posterior cruciate ligament 7. Lateral gastrocnemius muscle	1. If either cruciate ligament is torn (third-degree sprain) or stretched, rotary instability will also be evident 2. Order of injury is lateral collateral ligament, arcuate-popliteus complex, anterior cruciate ligament, posterior cruciate ligament 3. With severe injury (third degree), common peroneal nerve and circulation may be affected
	2. Adduction (varus) stress with knee **slightly flexed** (20° to 30°) and tibia laterally rotated	1. Lateral collateral ligament 2. Posterolateral capsule 3. Arcuate-popliteus complex 4. Iliotibial band 5. Biceps femoris tendon	1. Depending on degree of pain, opening and end feel, primarily signifies lateral collateral ligament sprain (first, second, or third degree) 2. If tibia is not laterally rotated, maximum stress will not be placed on lateral collateral ligament 3. Lateral rotation of tibia results in relaxation of both cruciate ligaments 4. With flexion, the iliotibial band lies over the center of the lateral joint line 5. If tibia is medially rotated, stress is increased on both cruciate ligaments while lateral collateral ligament relaxes 6. Order of injury is lateral collateral ligament, arcuate-popliteus complex, and iliotibial band and/or biceps femoris
One-plane anterior	1. Lachman test (**20° to 30° knee flexion**) or its modifications	1. Anterior cruciate ligament 2. Posterior oblique ligament 3. Arcuate-popliteus complex	1. Medial collateral ligament and iliotibial band lax in this position 2. Tests primarily posterolateral bundle of anterior cruciate ligament 3. Primarily tests anterior cruciate ligament but with severe injury (third-degree), structures in posteromedial and posterolateral corners may also be injured
	2. Anterior drawer sign (**90° knee flexion**) 3. Active drawer test (**90° knee flexion**)	1. Anterior cruciate ligament 2. Posterolateral capsule 3. Posteromedial capsule 4. Medial collateral ligament 5. Iliotibial band 6. Posterior oblique ligament 7. Arcuate-popliteus complex	1. Tests primarily anteromedial bundle of anterior cruciate ligament 2. If anterior cruciate ligament and medial or lateral structures are torn (third-degree sprain) or stretched, rotary instability will also be evident 3. Be sure posterior cruciate has not been injured, giving possible false-positive test
One-plane posterior	1. Posterior drawer sign (**90° knee flexion**) 2. Posterior sag sign 3. Active drawer test 4. Godfrey test 5. Reverse Lachman test (**20° to 30° knee flexion**)	1. Posterior cruciate ligament 2. Arcuate-popliteus complex 3. Posterior oblique ligament 4. Anterior cruciate ligament	1. If posterior cruciate ligament and medial or lateral structures are torn (third-degree sprain) or stretched, rotary instability will also be evident 2. With severe injury (third-degree), collateral ligaments may also be injured

Continued

TABLE **12-10**

Tests for Ligamentous Instability around the Knee—cont'd

Instability	Tests Used to Determine Instability	Structures Injured to Some Degree If Test Positive*	Notes
Anteromedial rotary	1. Slocum test (foot laterally rotated 15°) 2. Lemaire's anteromedial jolt test 3. Dejour test	1. Medial collateral ligament (superficial and deep fibers) 2. Posterior oblique ligament 3. Posteromedial capsule 4. Anterior cruciate ligament	1. Test must not be done in extreme lateral rotation of tibia because passive stabilizing will result from "coiling" to maximum rotation
Anterolateral rotary	1. Slocum test (foot medially rotated 30°) 2. Losee test 3. Jerk test of Hughston 4. Active pivot shift 5. Nakajima test	1. Anterior cruciate ligament 2. Posterolateral capsule 3. Arcuate-popliteus complex 4. Lateral collateral ligament 5. Iliotibial band	1. **Tests go from flexion to extension** 2. Tests bring about anterior subluxation of the tibia on femur, causing patient to experience "giving way" sensation 3. Slocum test must not be done in extreme medial rotation of tibia because passive stabilization will result from "coiling" to maximum rotation 4. Shift may be "slip" (second degree) or "jerk" (third degree), depending on degree of sprain or injury
	1. Lateral pivot shift test of Macintosh 2. Slocum ALRI test 3. Crossover test 4. Flexion-rotation drawer test 5. Flexion-extension valgus test 6. Martens test	1. Anterior cruciate ligament 2. Posterolateral capsule 3. Arcuate-popliteus complex 4. Iliotibial band	1. **Tests go from extension to flexion** 2. Tests cause reduction of anterior subluxed tibia on femur 3. Shift may be "slip" (second degree) or "jerk" (third degree), depending on degree of sprain or injury
Posteromedial rotary	1. Hughston's posteromedial drawer sign 2. Posteromedial pivot shift test	1. Posterior cruciate ligament 2. Posterior oblique ligament 3. Medial collateral ligament (superficial and deep fibers) 4. Semimembranosus muscle 5. Posteromedial capsule 6. Anterior cruciate ligament	1. Watch for changing position of tibial tubercle relative to femoral condyles
Posterolateral rotary	1. Hughston's posterolateral drawer sign 2. Jakob test (reverse pivot shift maneuver) 3. External rotational recurvatum test 4. Dynamic posterior shift test 5. Loomer's test 6. Active posterolateral drawer sign	1. Posterior cruciate ligament 2. Arcuate-popliteus ligament 3. Lateral collateral ligament 4. Biceps femoris tendon 5. Posterolateral capsule 6. Anterior cruciate ligament	1. Watch for changing position of tibial tubercle relative to femoral condyles

ALRI, Anterolateral rotary instability.

*The amount of displacement gives an indication of how badly and how much of the structures are injured (i.e., first-, second-, or third-degree sprain).

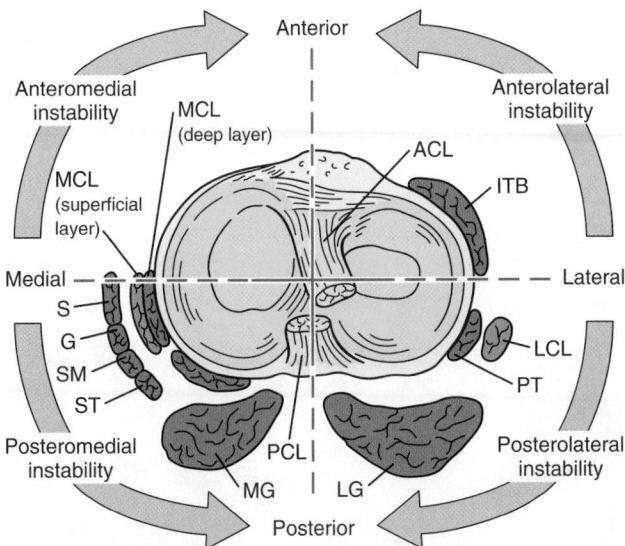

Figure 12-52 Instabilities about the knee. *ACL,* Anterior cruciate ligament; *G,* gracilis; *ITB,* iliotibial band; *LCL,* lateral collateral ligament; *LG,* lateral gastrocnemius, *MCL,* medial collateral ligament; *MG,* medial gastrocnemius; *PCL,* posterior cruciate ligament; *POL,* posterior oblique ligament; *PT,* popliteal tendon; *S,* sartorius; *SM,* semimembranosus; *ST,* semitendinosus.

she believes gives the best results. It is not essential to do all of the tests discussed. The techniques chosen must be practiced diligently so that the examiner becomes proficient at doing them; only with practice will the examiner be able to determine which structures are injured. It is also important to understand that the direction of instability does not imply that only structures in that direction are injured. For example, with anterolateral rotary instability (ALRI), it is not necessarily structures on the anterolateral side of the knee that are injured. In fact, posterior structures are often commonly injured as well. With ALRI, the posterolateral capsule and the arcuate-popliteus complex may also be injured.[28]

Instabilities About the Knee

- One-plane medial instability
- One-plane lateral instability
- One-plane anterior instability
- One-plane posterior instability
- Anteromedial rotary instability
- Anterolateral rotary instability
- Posteromedial rotary instability
- Posterolateral rotary instability

When testing for ligament stability of the knee, the examiner should keep the following points in mind:

1. The normal knee is tested first to establish a baseline and to show the patient what to expect. This action helps to gain the patient's confidence by showing what the test involves.

2. When one is comparing the normal and injured limbs, the test must be the same for both limbs. The examiner must use the same initial starting position and the same amount of force, apply the same force at the same point or throughout the range, and note the position at which the displacement occurs.[148]

3. The muscles must be relaxed if the tests are to be valid. Maximum laxity would be demonstrated with the patient under anesthesia.

4. The appropriate stress should be applied gently.

5. The stress is repeated several times and increased to the point of pain to demonstrate maximum laxity without causing muscle spasm.

6. It is not only the degree of opening but also the quality of the opening (i.e., the end feel) that is of concern. Left-right differences of 3 mm or more are classified as pathological.[148]

7. If the ligament is intact, there should be an abrupt stop or end feel when the ligament is stressed. A soft or indistinct end feel usually signifies ligamentous injury.[149]

8. Ligaments of the knee tend to act in concert to maintain stability, and individual ligaments are difficult to isolate in terms of their function. Therefore more than one test may be found to be positive when assessing for the different instabilities. For example, a patient may exhibit a one-plane medial and one-plane anterior instability as well as an anteromedial rotary instability and/or ALRI, depending on the severity of the injury to the various ligamentous structures.

9. Tests for ligament instability are more accurate for assessment of a chronic injury than for assessment of an acute injury in the unanesthetized knee because of the presence of muscle spasm and swelling in the acutely injured knee.

10. For the tests involving rotary instability in which the tibia is moved in relation to the femur, if the movement is into extension, subluxation of the tibia relative to the femur occurs in a positive test. If the movement is into flexion, reduction of the tibia relative to the femur occurs in a positive test.

11. Positive rotational tests should not be repeated too frequently because they may lead to articular cartilage damage, further meniscal tearing, or further damage to injured ligaments.

12. Because the ligamentous tests are subjective tests, the more experience the examiner has in doing them, the more accurate will be the interpretation of the test. The examiner should select only one or two from each group of tests and learn to do them well rather than learn all of the tests and risk doing them poorly.

Tests for One-Plane Medial Instability

The **abduction (valgus stress) test** ☑ is an assessment for one-plane (straight) medial instability, which means

Key Ligamentous Tests Performed on the Knee*†150

- *For one-plane medial instability:*
  - ✓ Hughston's valgus stress at 0° and 30°
  - ✓ Valgus stress at 0° and 30°
- *For one-plane lateral instability:*
  - ✓ Hughston's varus stress at 0° and 30°
  - ✓ Varus stress at 0° and 30°
- *For one-plane anterior instability:*
  - ⚠ Active drawer test
  - ✓ Drawer test
  - ✓ Lachman test or its modifications
- *For one-plane posterior instability:*
  - ✓ Active drawer test
  - ✓ Drawer test
  - ⚠ Godfrey test
  - ✓ Posterior sag
- *For anteromedial rotary instability:*
  - ⚠ Slocum test
- *For anterolateral rotary instability (ALRI):*
  - ⚠ Crossover test
  - ✓ Jerk test of Hughston
  - ✓ Losee test
  - ⚠ Noyes flexion-rotation drawer test
  - ✓ Pivot shift test
  - ⚠ Slocum ARLI test
- *For posteromedial rotary instability:*
  - ⚠ Hughston's posteromedial drawer test
  - ⚠ Posteromedial pivot shift test
- *For posterolateral rotary instability:*
  - ⚠ External rotation recurvatum
  - ⚠ Hughston's posterolateral drawer test
  - ⚠ Jakob test
  - ⚠ Loomer's posterolateral rotary instability test
  - ⚠ Tibial external rotation (dial) test

*See Chapter 1, p. 55, Key for Classifying Special Tests.
†If the pathology indicates a ligamentous problem, the clinician should have the ability to do at least one test well from each type of instability.

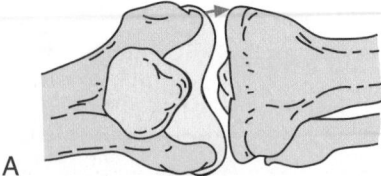

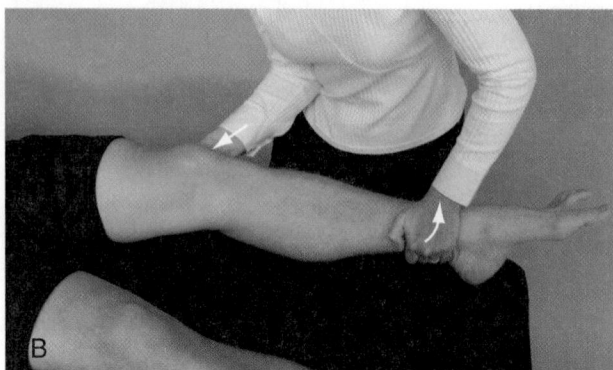

Figure 12-53 **Abduction (valgus stress) test. A,** "Gapping" on the medial aspect of the knee. **B,** Positioning for testing the medial collateral ligament (extended knee).

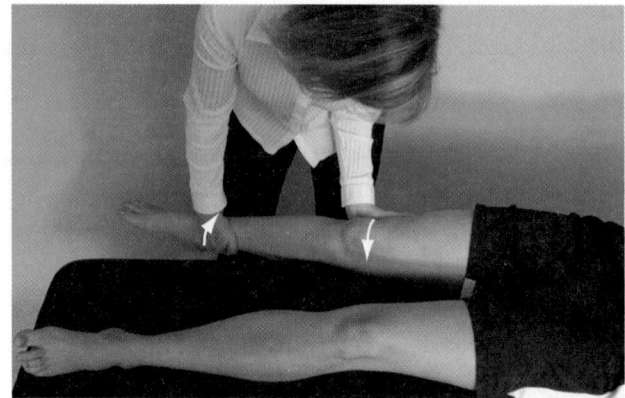

Figure 12-54 Applying a valgus stress with thigh supported on examining table.

that the tibia moves away from the femur (i.e., gaps) on the medial side (Figure 12-53). The examiner applies a valgus stress (pushes the knee medially) at the knee while the ankle is stabilized in slight lateral rotation either with the hand or with the leg held between the examiner's arm and trunk. The knee is first in full extension, and then it is slightly flexed (20° to 30°) so that it is "unlocked."[86]

It has been advocated that resting the test thigh on the examining table enables the patient to relax more and is easier for the examiner. The knee rests on the edge of the table; the lower leg is controlled by the examiner's stabilizing the thigh on the table, and the lower leg is abducted, applying a valgus stress to the knee (Figure 12-54).[30] Similarly, a varus stress may be applied to stress the lateral structures.

Hughston[30] advocates a third way to do this test (**Hughston's valgus stress test** ✓). The patient is positioned as described earlier, and the examiner faces the patient's foot, placing his or her body against the patient's thigh to help stabilize the upper leg in combination with one hand, which can also palpate the joint line. With the other hand, the examiner grasps the patient's big toe and applies a valgus stress, allowing any natural rotation of the tibia (Figure 12-55). Similarly, a varus stress may be applied to test the lateral structures, but in this case, the examiner grasps the lateral aspect of the foot near the fifth and fourth toes. A varus stress is then applied to the knee. Doing the test in this fashion often allows the patient to relax more and is less likely to lead to muscle spasm limiting movement.

If the test is positive (i.e., the tibia moves away from the femur an excessive amount when a valgus stress is applied) when the knee is *in extension,* the following structures may have been injured to some degree:
1. Medial collateral ligament (superficial and deep fibers)
2. Posterior oblique ligament

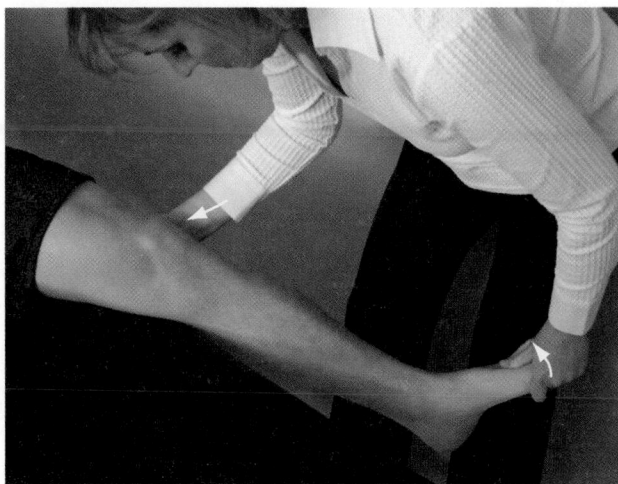

Figure 12-55 Hughston's valgus stress test.

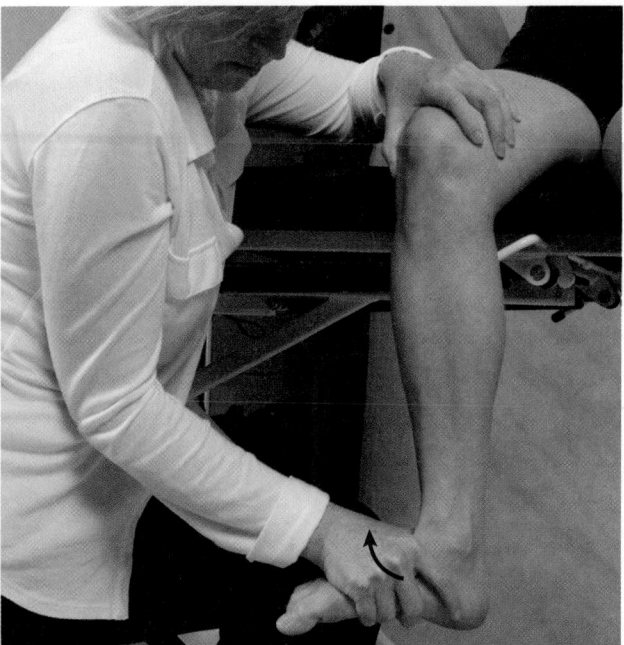

Figure 12-56 **Swain test.** Pain along the medial side of the knee indicates medial collateral ligament complex injury.

3. Posteromedial capsule
4. Anterior cruciate ligament
5. Posterior cruciate ligament
6. Medial quadriceps expansion
7. Semimembranosus muscle

A positive finding on full extension is classified as a major disruption of the knee. The examiner usually finds that one or more of the rotary tests are also positive. If the examiner applies lateral rotation to the foot when performing the test in extension and finds excessive lateral rotation on the affected side, it is a sign of possible antero-medial rotary instability.

If the test is positive when the knee is *flexed* to 20° to 30°, the following structures may have been injured to some degree:
1. Medial collateral ligament
2. Posterior oblique ligament
3. Posterior cruciate ligament
4. Posteromedial capsule

This flexed part of the valgus stress test would be classified as the true test for one-plane medial instability.

Lonergan and Taylor[151] advocated doing the **Swain test** ⚠ for the knee. For this test, the patient is seated with the knees flexed to 90° over the edge of the examining table. The examiner then passively laterally rotates the tibia on the femur of the good leg followed by the injured leg. A positive test is indicated by pain along the medial side of the joint indicating injury to the medial collateral ligament complex, because with the knee flexed to 90° the cruciates are lax, whereas the collateral ligaments are tight. Post surgery, pain on the medial joint line may indicate inadequate healing; or, in the chronic medial side laxity, joint line pain may be medial or posteromedial (Figure 12-56).[152]

If a stress radiograph is taken when the test is performed in full extension, a 5-mm opening indicates a grade 1 injury; up to 10 mm, a grade 2 injury; and more than 10 mm, a grade 3 injury.[139,153] Both limbs should be viewed for differences.[154]

Tests for One-Plane Lateral Instability

The **adduction (varus stress) test** ☑ is an assessment for one-plane lateral instability (i.e., the tibia moves away from the femur an excessive amount on the lateral aspect of the leg). The examiner applies a varus stress (pushes the knee laterally) at the knee while the ankle is stabilized (Figure 12-57). The test is first done with the knee in full extension and then with the knee in 20° to 30° of flexion. If the tibia is laterally rotated in full extension before the test, the cruciate ligaments are uncoiled, and maximum stress is placed on the collateral ligaments.

As previously mentioned (see the "Tests for One-Plane Medial Instability" section), **Hughston's varus stress test** ☑ may be used. In this case, the examiner grasps the fifth and fourth toes and applies a varus stress to the knee in extension and slightly (20° to 30°) flexed.

If the test is positive (i.e., the tibia moves away from the femur when a varus stress is applied) *in extension*, the following structures may have been injured to some degree:
1. Fibular or lateral collateral ligament
2. Posterolateral capsule
3. Arcuate-popliteus complex
4. Biceps femoris tendon
5. Posterior cruciate ligament
6. Anterior cruciate ligament
7. Lateral gastrocnemius muscle
8. Iliotibial band

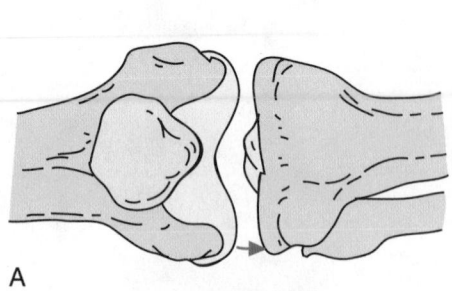 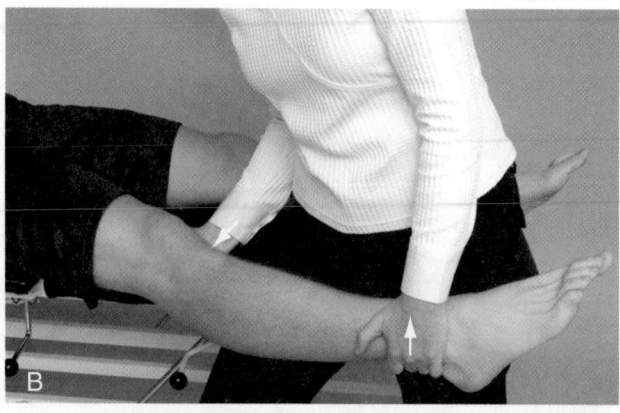

Figure 12-57 Adduction (varus stress) test. A, One-plane lateral instability "gapping" on the lateral aspect. **B,** Positioning for testing lateral collateral ligament in extension.

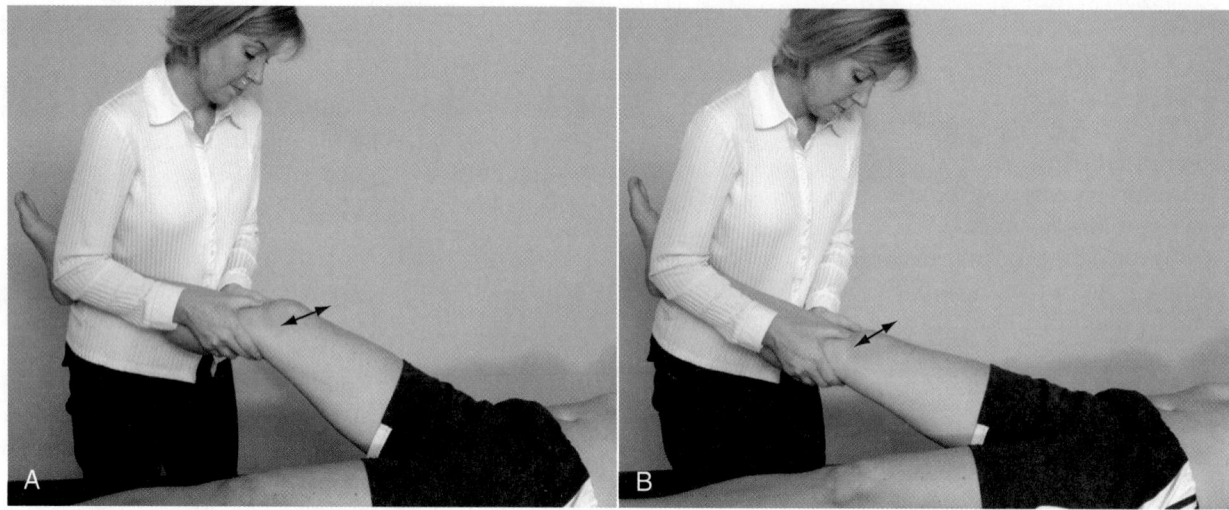

Figure 12-58 Varus-valgus test. A, Knee flexed. **B,** Knee extended.

The examiner usually finds that one or more rotary instability tests are also positive. A positive test indicates major instability of the knee.

If the test is positive when the knee is *flexed* 20° to 30° with lateral rotation of the tibia, the following structures may have been injured to some degree:
1. Lateral collateral ligament
2. Posterolateral capsule
3. Arcuate-popliteus complex
4. Iliotibial band
5. Biceps femoris tendon

This flexed part of the varus stress test is classified as the true test for one-plane lateral instability.

If a stress radiograph is taken when the test is performed in full extension, a 5-mm opening indicates a grade 1 injury; up to 8 mm, a grade 2 injury; and more than 8 mm, a grade 3 injury to the lateral ligaments of the knee.[139,153]

Both varus and valgus stress testing (**varus-valgus test**) can be performed at the same time while the examiner palpates the joint line. The examiner holds the ankle between the examiner's waist and forearm while the patient lies supine with the knee extended and then flexed. At the same time, the examiner palpates the medial and lateral joint lines with the fingers. Varus and valgus stresses are applied with the heels of the examiner's hands (Figure 12-58).[79]

Tests for One-Plane Anterior Instability

Some clinicians[28,30] believe that the posterior cruciate ligament should be tested (see the "Tests for One-Plane Posterior Instability" section) or observed for a posterior sag before the anterior cruciate ligament is tested to rule out false-positive tests for anterior translation. In either case, the examiner should be aware that a torn posterior cruciate can lead to a false-positive anterior translation test if the patient is tested in supine position with the knee flexed, because gravity causes the tibia to sag posteriorly.

Active Drawer Test. For the anterior drawer test (also called the **quadriceps active test**), the patient is positioned as for the normal drawer test. The examiner

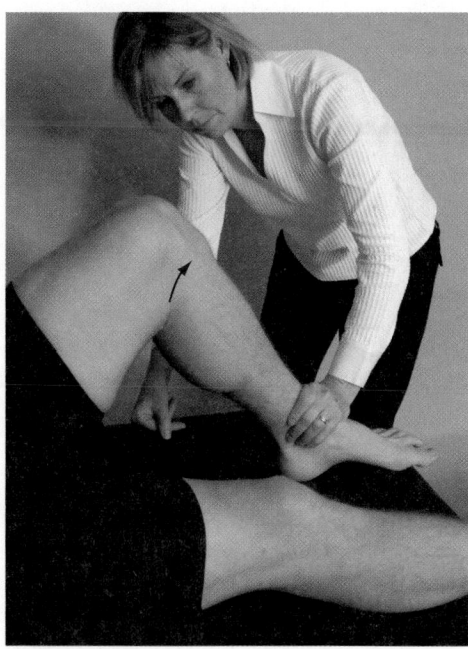

Figure 12-59 Active anterior drawer test. Examiner watches for excessive anterior shift.

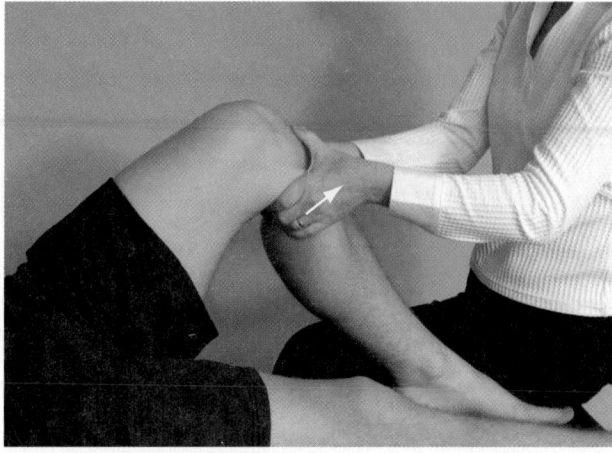

Figure 12-60 Position for drawer sign.

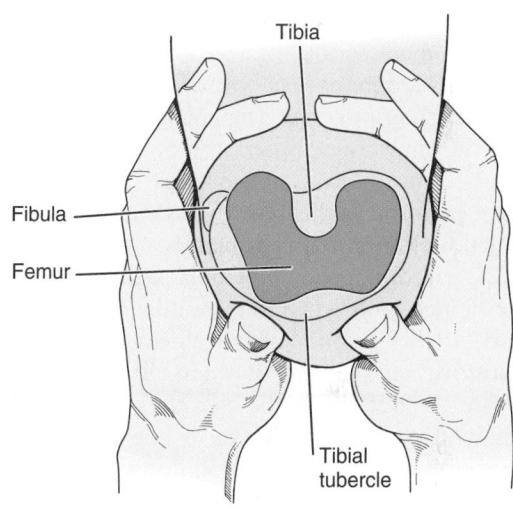

Figure 12-61 This view of the knee from above shows the inside of the knee joint during performance of the anterior drawer test in flexion. The hands are in place, and the overlay of the femur on the tibia demonstrates that the anterior and posterior motions are normal. The index fingers are ensuring that the hamstrings are relaxed. If, on pulling or pushing tibia, rotation of tibial plateau occurs, the examiner should check for rotary instabilities. (Redrawn from Hughston JC: Knee ligaments: injury and repair, St Louis, 1993, Mosby, p. 111.)

holds the patient's foot down. The patient is asked to try to straighten the leg, and the examiner prevents the patient from doing so (isometric test). Muller[139] advocated allowing the foot to be free and noting when the foot is lifted off the table, which occurs only after the tibia has shifted forward and stabilized. If the anterior cruciate ligament or posterior cruciate ligament is torn, the anterior contour of the knee changes as the tibia is drawn forward. If the posterior cruciate ligament is torn, a posterior sag is evident before the patient contracts the quadriceps. Contraction of the quadriceps causes the tibia to shift forward to its normal position, indicating a positive test for a torn posterior cruciate ligament.[155,156] If there is no posterior sag present and if the tibia shifts forward more on the injured side than the noninjured side, it is a positive test for anterior cruciate ligament disruption (Figure 12-59).[155] A second part of the test may be instituted by having the patient contract the hamstrings isometrically so that the tibial plateau moves posteriorly. This part of the test accentuates the posterior sag for posterior cruciate insufficiency, if present, and ensures maximum movement for anterior cruciate insufficiency if a quadriceps contraction is tried a second time.[79] The active drawer test is a better expression of posterior cruciate insufficiency than of anterior cruciate insufficiency.[157]

With the drawer sign or test, if the anterior or posterior cruciate ligament is torn (third-degree sprain), some rotary instability is evident when the appropriate ligamentous tests are performed.

✓ *Drawer Sign.* The drawer sign is a test for one-plane anterior and one-plane posterior instabilities.[158] The

difficulty with this test is in determining the neutral starting position if the ligaments have been injured. The patient's knee is flexed to 90°, and the hip is flexed to 45°. In this position, the anterior cruciate ligament is almost parallel with the tibial plateau. The patient's foot is held on the table by the examiner's body with the examiner sitting on the patient's forefoot and the foot in neutral rotation. The examiner's hands are placed around the tibia to ensure that the hamstring muscles are relaxed (Figures 12-60 and 12-61). The tibia is then drawn forward on the femur **(anterior drawer test).** The normal amount of movement that should be present is approximately 6 mm. This part of the test assesses one-plane anterior instability. If the test is positive (i.e., the tibia moves forward more than 6 mm on the femur), the following structures may have been injured to some degree:

1. Anterior cruciate ligament (especially the anteromedial bundle)
2. Posterolateral capsule
3. Posteromedial capsule
4. Medial collateral ligament (deep fibers)
5. Iliotibial band
6. Posterior oblique ligament
7. Arcuate-popliteus complex

If only the anterior cruciate ligament is torn, the test is negative, because other structures (posterior capsule and posterolateral and posteromedial structures) limit movement. In addition, hemarthrosis, a torn medial meniscus (posterior horn) wedged against the medial femoral condyle, or hamstring spasm may result in a false-negative test. Hughston[30] points out that tearing of the coronary or meniscotibial ligament can allow the tibia to translate forward more than normal, even in the presence of an intact anterior cruciate ligament. In this case, when the anterior drawer test is performed, anteromedial rotation (subluxation) of the tibia occurs.

When performing this test, the examiner must ensure that the posterior cruciate ligament is not torn or injured. If it has been torn, it allows the tibia to drop or slide back on the femur, and when the examiner pulls the tibia forward, a large amount of movement occurs, giving a false-positive sign (see the "Posterior Sag Sign" section). Therefore the test should be considered positive only if it is shown that the posterior sag is not present.

Weatherwax[159] described a modified way of testing the anterior drawer (**90–90 anterior drawer**). The patient lies supine. The examiner flexes the patient's hip and knee to 90° and supports the lower leg between the examiner's trunk and forearm. The examiner places the hands around the tibia, as with the standard test, and applies sufficient force to slowly lift the patient's buttock off the table (Figure 12-62).

If, when doing the anterior drawer test, there is an audible snap or palpable jerk (**Finochietto jumping sign**) when the tibia is pulled forward and the tibia moves forward excessively, a meniscus lesion is probably accompanying the torn anterior cruciate ligament.[79]

After the anterior movement of the tibia on the femur, the posterior movement of the tibia on the femur should be completed (**posterior drawer test**). In this part of the test, the tibia is pushed back on the femur. This phase is a test for one-plane posterior instability. If the test is positive or a posterior sag is evident, the following structures may have been injured to some degree:

1. Posterior cruciate ligament
2. Arcuate-popliteus complex
3. Posterior oblique ligament
4. Anterior cruciate ligament

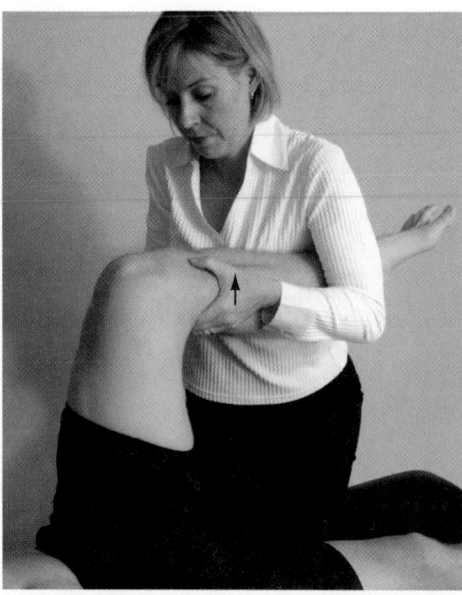

Figure 12-62 Anterior drawer test in 90° flexion with the hip flexed 90°.

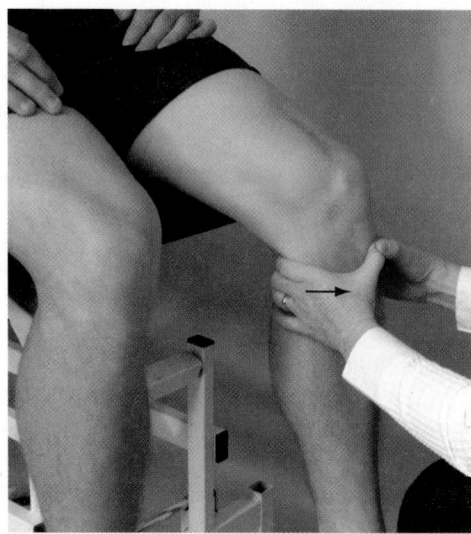

Figure 12-63 Anterior drawer test in sitting position. Examiner feels anterior shift with thumbs.

If the arcuate-popliteus complex remains intact, a positive posterior drawer sign may not be elicited.[160] If, when the tibia is pushed backward, the examiner forcefully rotates the tibia laterally and excessive movement occurs, the test is positive for posterolateral instability. Warren[161] calls this maneuver the **arcuate spin test**.

Feagin[162] advocated doing the drawer test with the patient sitting with the leg hanging relaxed over the end of the examining table (**sitting anterior drawer test**). The examiner places the hands as with the standardized test and slowly draws the tibia first forward and then backward to test the anterior and posterior drawer (Figure 12-63). The examiner uses the thumbs to palpate the

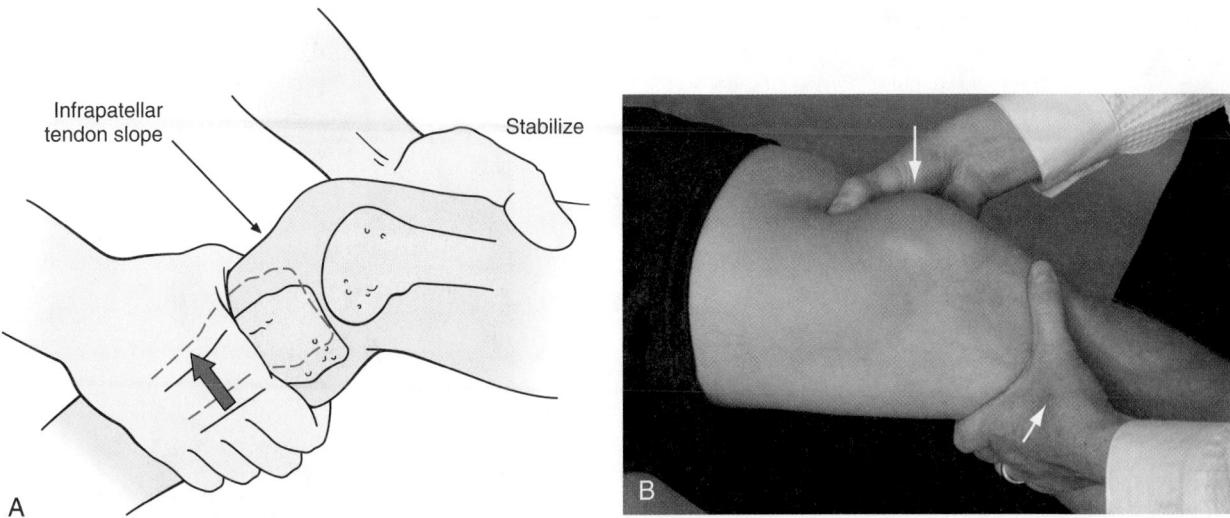

Figure 12-64 Hand position for classic Lachman test.

tibial plateau movement relative to the femur. The examiner may also note any rotational deformity. The advantage of doing the test this way is that the posterior sag is eliminated because the effect of gravity is eliminated.

☑ *Lachman Test.* The Lachman test, which may also be referred to as the **Ritchie, Trillat, or Lachman-Trillat test,** is the best indicator of injury to the anterior cruciate ligament, especially the posterolateral band,[163–168] although this has been questioned.[169] It is a test for one-plane anterior instability.[86,170] The patient lies supine with the involved leg beside the examiner. The examiner holds the patient's knee between full extension and 30° of flexion. This position is close to the functional position of the knee, in which the anterior cruciate ligament plays a major role. The patient's femur is stabilized with one of the examiner's hands (the "outside" hand) while the proximal aspect of the tibia is moved forward with the other ("inside") hand (Figure 12-64). Frank[171] reported that to achieve the best results, the tibia should be slightly laterally rotated and the anterior tibial translation force should be applied from the posteromedial aspect. Therefore the hand on the tibia should apply the translation force. A positive sign is indicated by a "mushy" or soft end feel when the tibia is moved forward on the femur (increased anterior translation with medial rotation of the tibia) and disappearance of the infrapatellar tendon slope.[168] A false-negative test may occur if the femur is not properly stabilized, if a meniscus lesion blocks translation, or if the tibia is medially rotated.[171] A positive sign indicates that the following structures may have been injured to some degree:

1. Anterior cruciate ligament (especially the posterolateral bundle)
2. Posterior oblique ligament
3. Arcuate-popliteus complex

Other ways of doing the Lachman test have also been advocated. The method that works for the examiner and

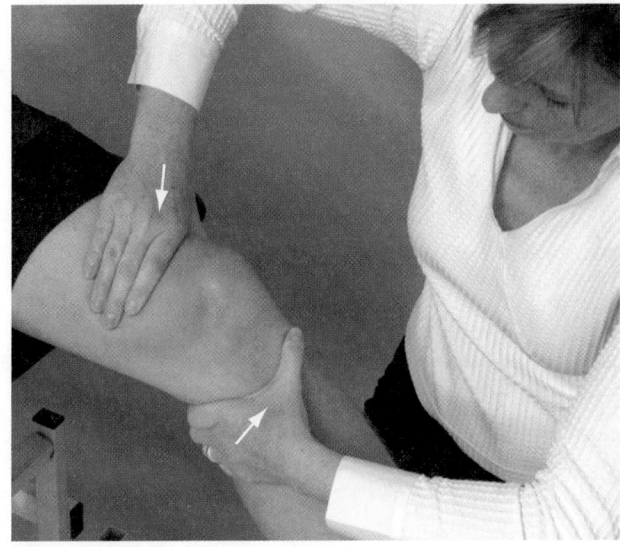

Figure 12-65 Lachman test (modification 1).

that the examiner can use competently should be selected. Another method (**modification 1**) has the patient sitting with the leg over the edge of the examining table. The examiner sits facing the patient and supports the foot of the test leg on the examiner's thigh so that the patient's knee is flexed 30°. The examiner stabilizes the thigh with one hand and pulls the tibia forward with the other hand (Figure 12-65). Abnormal forward motion is considered to be a positive test.[172]

For examiners with small hands, the **stable Lachman test (modification 2)** is recommended. The patient lies supine with the knee resting on the examiner's knee (Figure 12-66). One of the examiner's hands stabilizes the femur against the examiner's thigh, and the other hand applies an anterior stress.[79,173] Adler and associates[174] described a modification of this method, which they called the **drop leg Lachman test (modification 3).** The

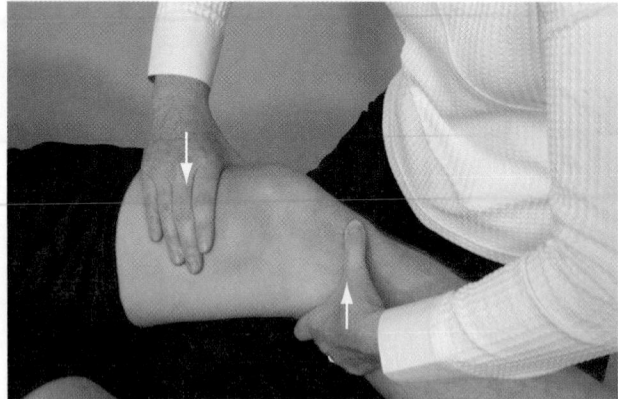

Figure 12-66 Stable Lachman test (modification 2).

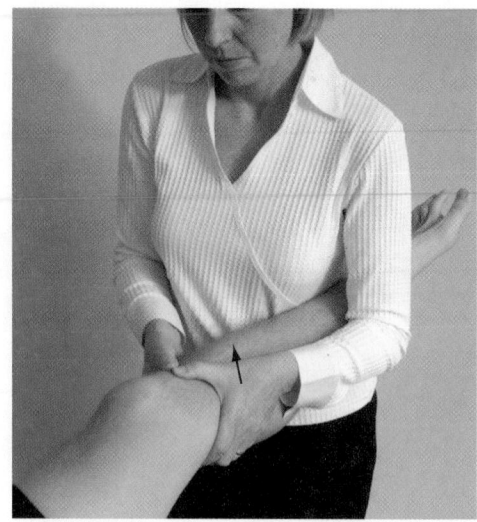

Figure 12-68 Lachman test (modification 4).

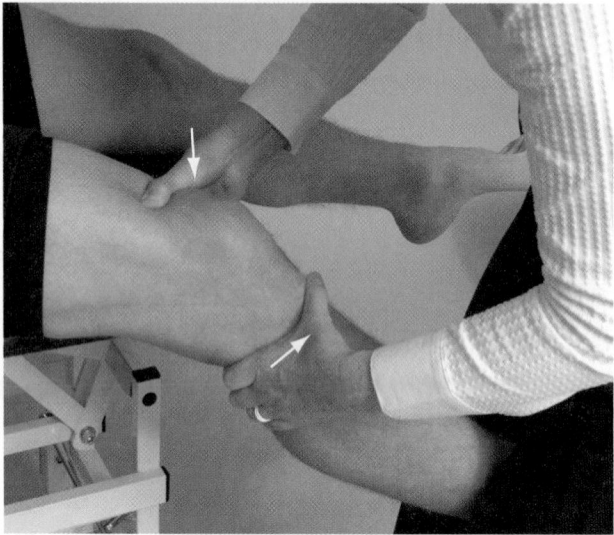

Figure 12-67 Drop leg Lachman test (modification 3).

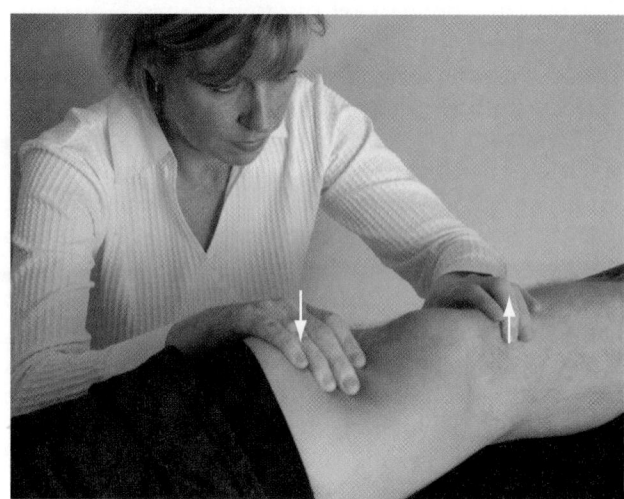

Figure 12-69 Lachman test (modification 5).

patient lies supine, and the leg to be examined is abducted off the side of the examining table and the knee is flexed to 25°. One of the examiner's hands stabilizes the femur against the table while the patient's foot is held between the examiner's knees. The examiner's other hand is then free to apply the anterior translation force (Figure 12-67). They found there was greater anterior laxity demonstrated when doing the test this way than when doing it the classical way.[174]

Modification 4 has the patient lying supine while the examiner stabilizes the foot between the examiner's thorax and arm. Both hands are placed around the tibia, the knee is flexed 20° to 30°, and an anterior drawer movement is performed.[79] This technique allows gravity to control movement of the femur, which may not be sufficient to show a good positive test (Figure 12-68).

Another way of doing the test **(modification 5)** is for the patient to lie supine while the examiner stands beside the leg to be tested with the eyes level with the knee. The examiner grasps the femur with one hand and the tibia

with the other hand.[79] The tibia is pulled forward, and any abnormal motion is noted (Figure 12-69). As with the regular Lachman test, the examiner may have difficulty stabilizing the femur if the examiner has small hands.

To perform the **prone Lachman test (modification 6)**,[162,175,176] the patient lies prone, and the examiner stabilizes the foot between the examiner's thorax and arm and places one hand around the tibia. The other hand stabilizes the femur (Figure 12-70). Gravity assists anterior movement with this method, but it is more difficult to determine the quality of the end feel.

For the **active (no touch) Lachman test (modification 7)**,[79,177,178] the patient lies supine with the knee over the examiner's forearm so that the knee is flexed approximately 30° (Figure 12-71, *A*). The patient is asked to actively extend the knee, and the examiner watches for anterior displacement of the tibia relative to the unaffected side. The test may also be carried out with the foot held down on the table to increase the pull of the quadriceps. In this case, the test has been called the **maximum quadriceps test (modification 8)** (Figure 12-71, *B*).[79] The examiner must be certain that there is no posterior sag before performing the test.

The Lachman test may be graded with a stress radiograph: a 3- to 6-mm anterior movement of the tibia relative to the femur is classified as a grade 1 injury; 6 to 9 mm, grade 2; 10 to 16 mm, grade 3; and 16 to 20 mm, grade 4.[79]

Tests for One-Plane Posterior Instability[179,180]

One-plane posterior instability implies injury to the posterior cruciate ligament. It has been pointed out, however, that isolated posterior cruciate injuries are rare, and if a posterior cruciate ligament injury is suspected, it is important to complete a full knee examination looking at all the ligaments, especially those involving the posterolateral corner.[181]

⚠ *Active Drawer Test.* This test has been described previously.

✓ *Drawer Sign or Test.* This test has been described previously. Veltri and Warren[156] report that the posterior drawer test is one of the most effective means of clinically diagnosing posterior cruciate and posterolateral (popliteus) corner injuries.

⚠ *Godfrey (Gravity) Test.*[79] The patient lies supine, and the examiner holds both legs while flexing the patient's hips and knees to 90° (Figure 12-72). If there is posterior instability, a posterior sag of the tibia is seen. If manual posterior pressure is applied to the tibia, posterior displacement may increase.

✓ *Posterior Sag Sign (Gravity Drawer Test).*[86] The patient lies supine with the hip flexed to 45° and the knee flexed to 90°. In this position, the tibia "drops back," or sags back, on the femur because of gravity if the posterior cruciate ligament is torn (Figure 12-73). Posterior tibial displacement is more noticeable when the knee is flexed 90° to 110° than when the knee is only slightly flexed. It is a test for one-plane posterior instability. Normally, the medial tibial plateau extends 1 cm anteriorly beyond the femoral condyle when the knee is flexed 90°. If this "step" is lost, which is what occurs with a positive posterior sag caused by a torn posterior cruciate ligament, this **step-off test** or **thumb sign** is considered positive.[35,47,157,179] The examiner must be careful because the position could result in a false-positive anterior drawer test for the anterior cruciate ligament if the sag remains unnoticed. If there is minimal or no swelling, the sag is evident because of an obvious concavity distal to the patella. If the posterior sag sign is present, the following structures may have been injured to some degree:

1. Posterior cruciate ligament
2. Arcuate-popliteus complex

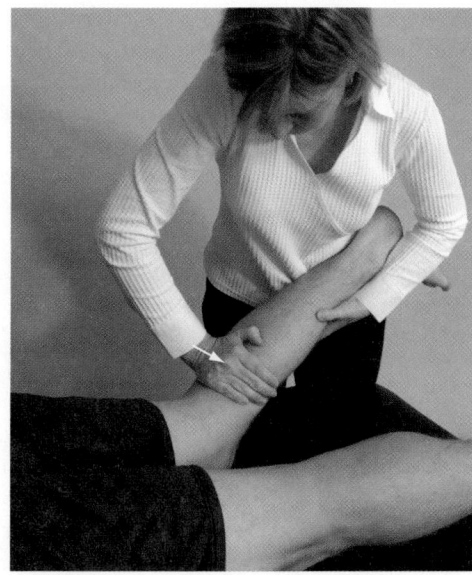

Figure 12-70 Prone Lachman test (modification 6).

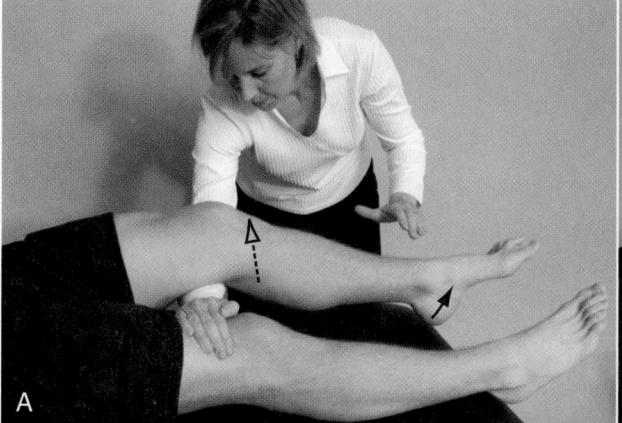
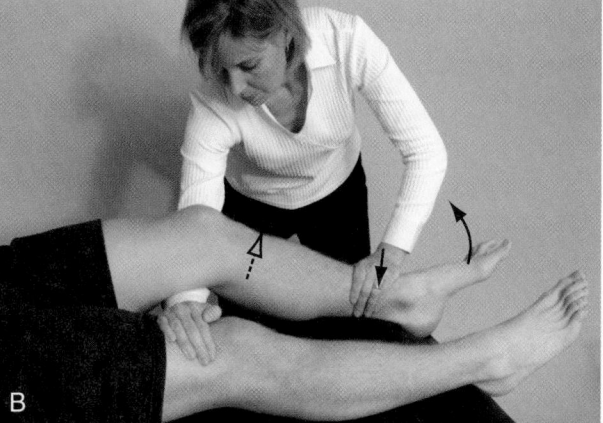

Figure 12-71 A, No-touch Lachman test (**modification 7**). Open arrow shows where the examiner watches for shift. **B, Active Lachman (maximum quadriceps) test (modification 8).**

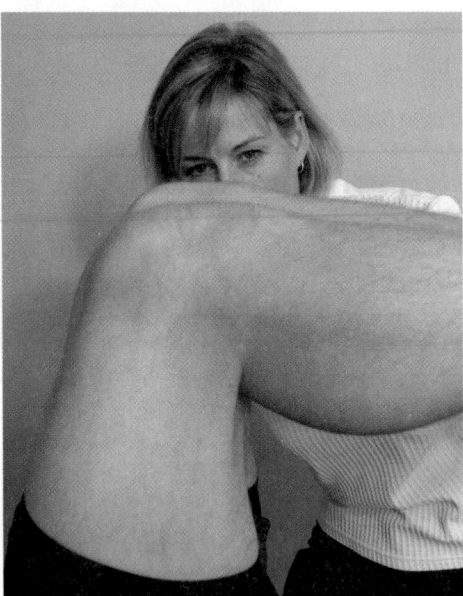

Figure 12-72 **Godfrey test.** Examiner watches for posterior shift, which is not evident in this case.

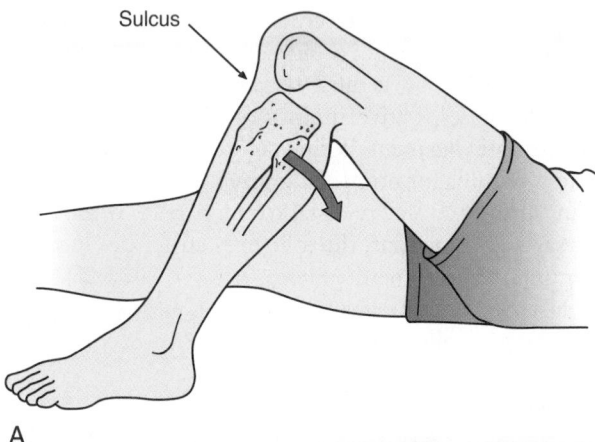

A

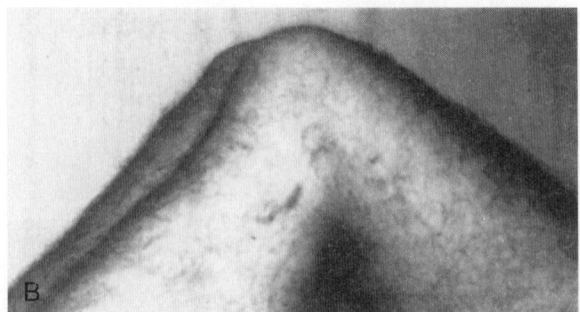

Figure 12-73 **Sag sign. A,** Illustration of posterior sag sign. **B,** Note profile of two knees; the left (nearer) sags backward compared with the normal right knee, indicating posterior cruciate defect. (From O'Donoghue DH: Treatment of injuries to athletes, ed 4, Philadelphia, 1984, WB Saunders, p. 450.)

3. Posterior oblique ligament
4. Anterior cruciate ligament

If it appears that the patient has a positive posterior sag sign, the patient should carefully extend the knee while the examiner holds the hip in 90° to 100° of flexion. This action is sometimes called the **voluntary anterior drawer sign,** and the results are similar to those of the active anterior drawer test. As the patient does this slowly, the tibial plateau moves or shifts forward to its normal position, indicating that the tibia was previously posteriorly subluxated (posterior cruciate tear) on the femur.

⚠ *Reverse Lachman Test.*[79] The patient lies prone with the knee flexed to 30°, and the examiner grasps the tibia with one hand while fixing the femur with the other hand (Figure 12-74). The examiner ensures that the hamstring muscles are relaxed. The examiner then pulls the tibia up (posteriorly), noting the amount of movement and the quality of the end feel. It is a test for the posterior cruciate ligament. The examiner should be wary of a false-positive test if the anterior cruciate ligament has been torn, because gravity may cause an anterior shift. This test is not as accurate for the posterior cruciate ligament as the posterior drawer test, because when the posterior cruciate ligament is torn, the greatest posterior displacement is at 90°.

Tests for Anteromedial Rotary Instability

For these rotary tests, the examiner is watching for abnormal tibial motion. In this case, the examiner watches the medial side of the tibia to see if it rotates anteriorly more than the uninjured side.

❓ *Dejour Test.*[28] The patient lies supine. The examiner holds the patient's leg with one arm against the body and the hand under the calf to lift the tibia while applying a valgus stress. The other hand pushes the femur down (Figure 12-75). In extension, this action causes anteromedial subluxation in the pathological knee. If the knee is then flexed, the tibial plateau reduces suddenly,

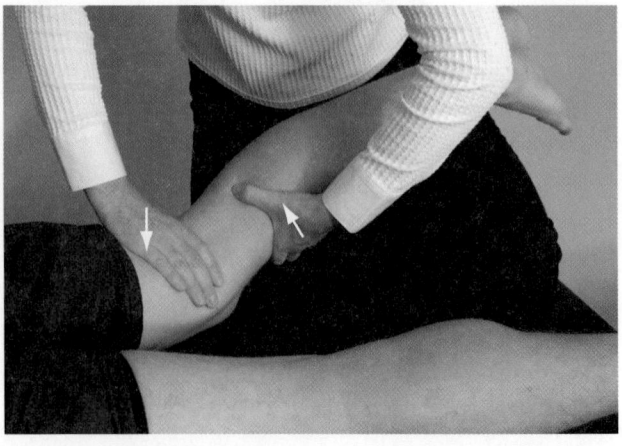

Figure 12-74 Reverse Lachman test.

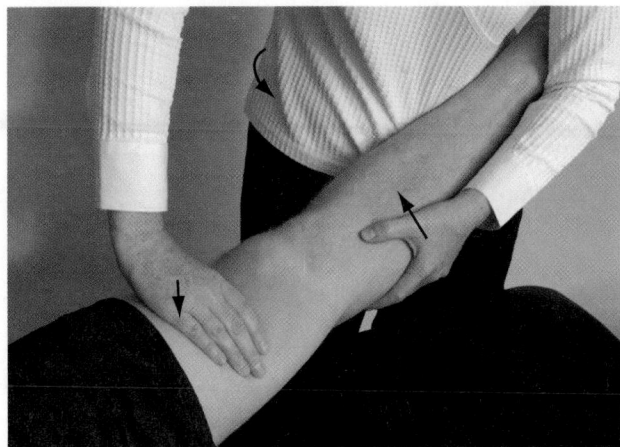

Figure 12-75 Dejour test.

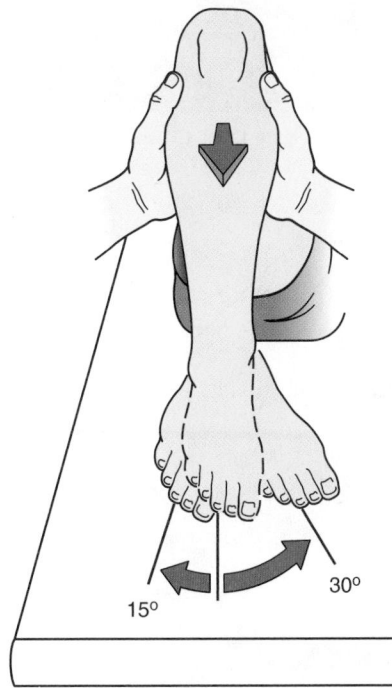

Figure 12-76 Slocum test in supine lying.

indicating a positive test. If the jolt is painful, it indicates that the medial meniscus has been injured. If it is not painful, the posteromedial corner has been injured.

Slocum Test. The Slocum test assesses both anterior rotary instabilities.[182] The patient's knee is flexed to 80° or 90°, and the hip is flexed to 45°. The foot is first placed in 30° medial rotation (Figure 12-76). The examiner then sits on the patient's forefoot to hold the foot in position and draws the tibia forward; if the test is positive, movement occurs primarily on the lateral side of the knee. This movement is excessive relative to the unaffected side and indicates ALRI. It also indicates that the following structures may have been injured to some degree:
1. Anterior cruciate ligament
2. Posterolateral capsule

3. Arcuate-popliteus complex
4. Lateral collateral ligament
5. Posterior cruciate ligament
6. Iliotibial band

If the examiner finds anterolateral instability during this first position of the Slocum test, the second part of the test, which assesses anteromedial rotary instability in this position, is of less value.[183]

In the second part of the test, the foot is placed in 15° of lateral rotation, and the tibia is drawn forward by the examiner. This part of the test is sometimes referred to as **Lemaire's T drawer test.** If the test is positive, the movement occurs primarily on the medial side of the knee. This movement is excessive relative to the unaffected side and indicates anteromedial rotary instability. It also indicates that the following structures may have been injured to some degree:
1. Medial collateral ligament (especially the superficial fibers, although the deep fibers may also be affected)
2. Posterior oblique ligament
3. Posteromedial capsule
4. Anterior cruciate ligament

For the Slocum test, it is imperative that the examiner medially or laterally rotate the foot to the degrees shown. If the examiner rotates the tibia as far as it will go, the test will be negative for movement, because this action tightens all of the remaining structures.

If a stress radiograph is taken during the test, minimal or no movement indicates a negative test; 1 mm or less, a grade 1 injury; 1 to 2 mm, a grade 2 injury; and more than 2 mm, a grade 3 injury.[153]

The test may also be performed with the patient sitting with the knees flexed over the edge of the examining table (Figure 12-77).[139] The examiner applies an anterior or a posterior force while holding the foot medially or laterally rotated. If this procedure is used, the examiner must remember that use of the anterior force tests for anterior rotary instability, whereas use of the posterior force tests for posterior rotary instability (see "Hughston's Postero-medial and Posterolateral Drawer Sign" in later sections). The examiner should note whether the movement is excessive on the medial or on the lateral side of the knee relative to the normal knee. Excessive movement indicates a positive test.

Tests for Anterolateral Rotary Instability

When performing these tests, the examiner is looking for abnormal (excessive) anterior rotation of the tibia on the lateral side relative to the femur.

Active Pivot Shift Test.[184] The patient sits with the foot on the floor in neutral rotation and the knee flexed 80° to 90°. The patient is asked to isometrically contract the quadriceps while the examiner stabilizes the foot. A positive test is indicated by anterolateral subluxation of the lateral tibial plateau and is indicative of anterolateral instability (Figure 12-78).

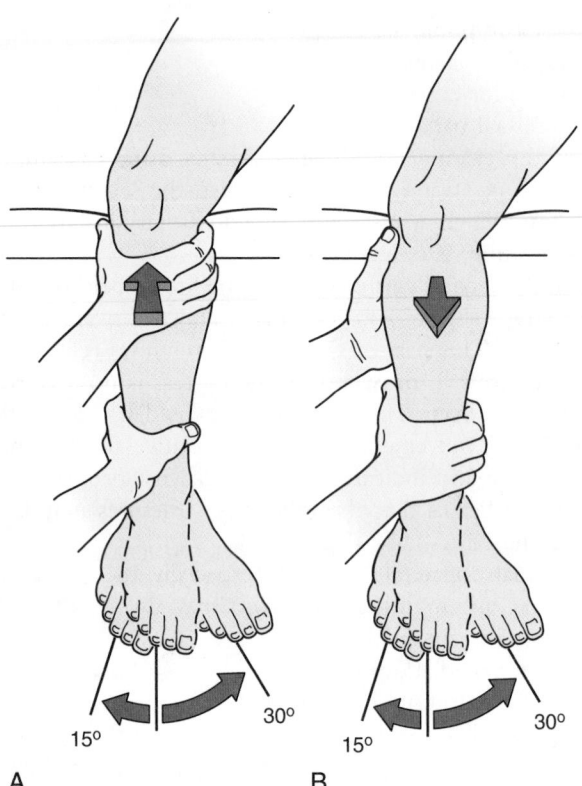

A   B

Figure 12-77 Slocum test with the patient in the sitting position. Examiner rotates foot one way (i.e., medially or laterally) and then pushes the tibia backwards (**A**) or pulls it forward (**B**), comparing the amount of rotation and anterior and posterior movement in each knee.

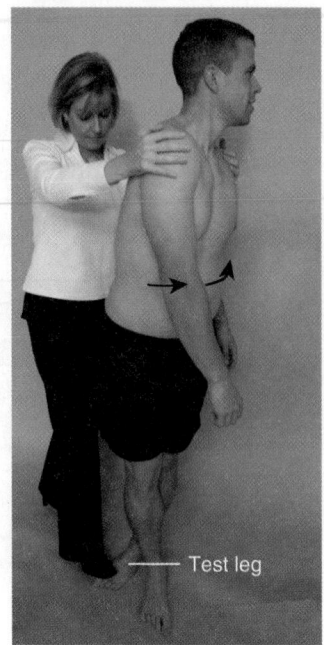

Figure 12-79 Crossover test.

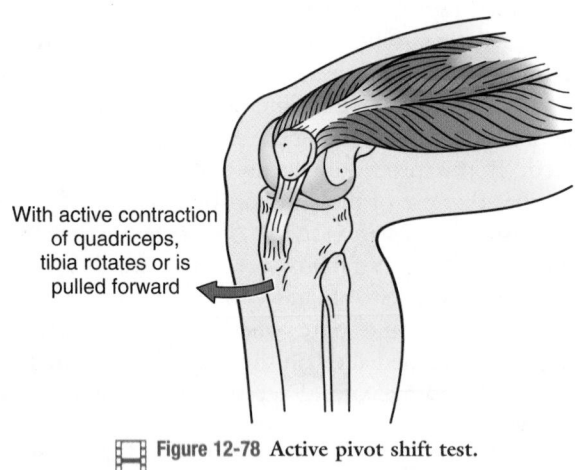

With active contraction of quadriceps, tibia rotates or is pulled forward

Figure 12-78 Active pivot shift test.

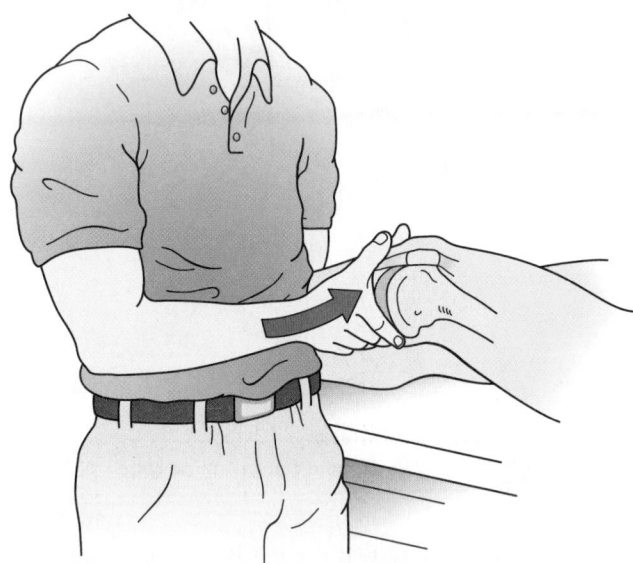

Figure 12-80 Flexion-extension valgus test. *Arrow* shows compression. (Redrawn from Hanks GA, Joyner DM, Kalenak A: Anterolateral instability of the knee. J Sports Med 9:226, 1981.)

Crossover Test of Arnold. The patient is asked to cross the uninvolved leg in front of the involved leg (Figure 12-79). The examiner then carefully steps on the patient's involved foot to stabilize it and instructs the patient to rotate the upper torso away from the injured leg approximately 90° from the fixed foot. When this position is achieved, the patient contracts the quadriceps muscles, producing the same symptoms and testing the same structures as in the lateral pivot shift test.

Flexion-Extension Valgus Test. The patient lies supine, and the examiner holds the patient's leg as in the Noyes test. The examiner palpates the joint line with the thumb and fingers of both hands, and a valgus stress and axial compression are applied while the knee is flexed and extended (Figure 12-80). If the anterior cruciate ligament is torn, the examiner feels the reduction and subluxation. The tibia is not rotated, so the subluxation is easily felt.[185]

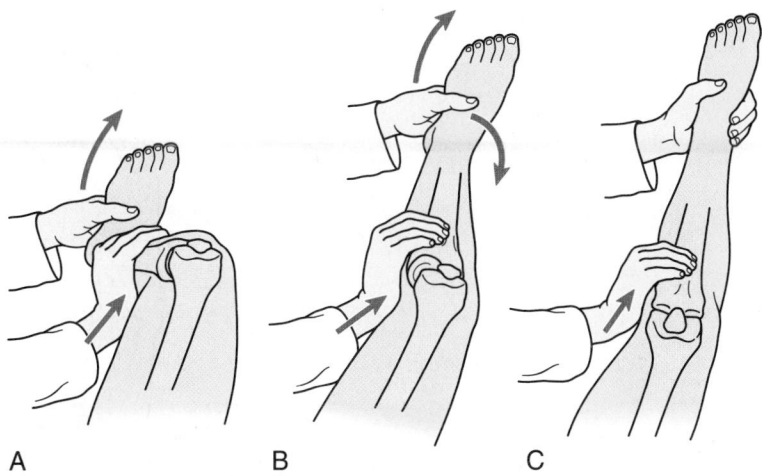

A   B   C

Figure 12-81 Jerk test of Hughston. A, The knee is flexed to 90°, and the heel of one hand is placed behind the fibular head to produce medial rotation of the tibia. **B,** At 20° to 30°, the lateral tibial plateau subluxates anteriorly. **C,** At full extension, the lateral tibial plateau is reduced. (Redrawn from Irrgang JJ, et al: The knee: ligamentous and meniscal injuries. In Zachazewski JE, et al, editors: Athletic injuries and rehabilitation, Philadelphia, 1996, WB Saunders, pp. 683–644.)

☑ **Jerk Test of Hughston.**[186] This test is similar to the pivot shift maneuver. The positioning of the patient and the examiner is the same, except that the patient's hip is flexed to 45°. With this test, the knee is first flexed to 90°. The leg is then extended, maintaining medial rotation and a valgus stress (Figure 12-81). At approximately 20° to 30° of flexion, the tibia shifts forward, causing a subluxation of the lateral tibial plateau with a jerk if the test is positive. If the leg is carried into further extension, it spontaneously reduces. A positive jerk test indicates that the same structures are injured as indicated by a positive pivot shift maneuver and assesses ALRI. According to the literature,[139] this test is not as sensitive as the pivot shift test.

☑ **Lateral Pivot Shift Maneuver (Test of MacIntosh).** This is the primary test used to assess ALRI of the knee and is an excellent test for ruptures (third-degree sprains) of the anterior cruciate ligament.[187-190] Like most provocative tests, it does have a disadvantage, however. In the apprehensive patient, because of the forces applied during the test, protective muscle contraction may lead to a false-negative test.[28] Lane et al.[191] stated that the pivot shift test closely correlates with patient outcomes. The presence of a pivot shift post surgery often precludes return to sports, is associated with continuation of symptoms, correlates with decreased patient satisfaction, and increases the likelihood of osteoarthrosis. During this test, the tibia moves away from the femur on the lateral side (but rotates medially) and moves anteriorly in relation to the femur (Figure 12-82). Table 12-11 outlines the effect of some soft tissue changes that can affect the pivot shift test.

Normally, the knee's center of rotation changes constantly through its ROM as a result of the shape of the femoral condyles, ligamentous restraint, and muscle tension. The path of movement of the tibia on the femur

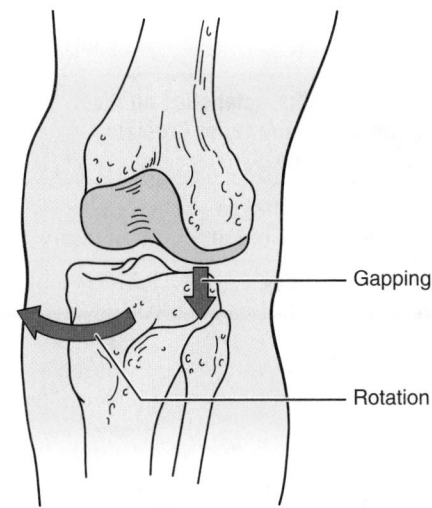

Gapping

Rotation

Figure 12-82 Anterolateral rotary instability (ALRI).

is described as a combination of rolling and sliding with rolling predominating when the instant center is near the joint line and sliding predominating when the instant center shifts distally from the contact area. The MacIntosh test is a duplication of the anterior subluxation-reduction phenomenon that occurs during the normal gait cycle when the anterior cruciate ligament is torn. Therefore it illustrates a **dynamic subluxation.** This shift occurs between 20° and 40° of flexion (0° being full extension). It is this phenomenon that gives the patient the clinical description of feeling the knee "give way" (Figure 12-83).

The patient lies supine with the hip both flexed and abducted 30° and relaxed in slight medial rotation (20°). The examiner holds the patient's foot with one hand while the other hand is placed at the knee, holding the

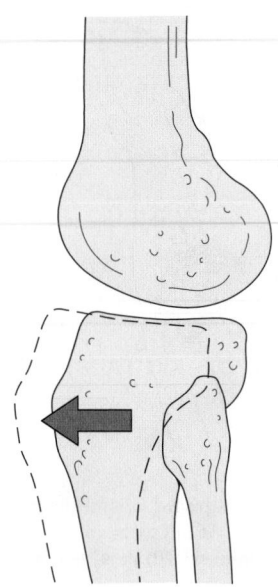

Figure 12-83 Anterior shift of the tibia during the lateral pivot shift test.

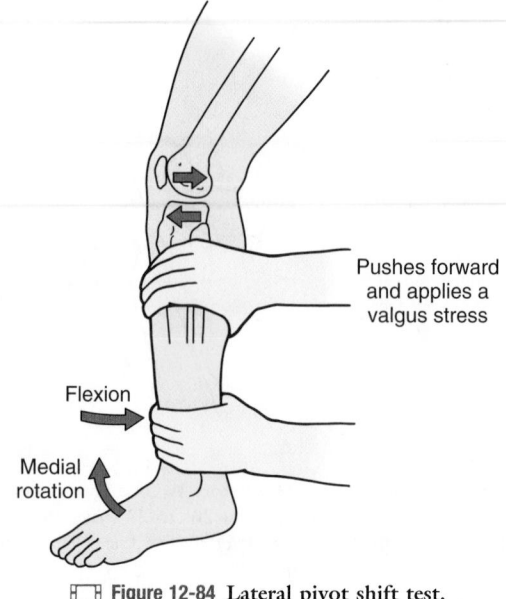

Pushes forward and applies a valgus stress

Flexion

Medial rotation

Figure 12-84 Lateral pivot shift test.

TABLE **12-11**

Effect of Soft-Tissue Characteristics on Pivot Shift Examination in the Anterior Cruciate Ligament–Deficient Knee

Soft-Tissue Factors	Effect on Pivot Shift	Mechanism
ITB tightness	Decreases	Restricts subluxation
ITB tightness	Decreases	Allows internal rotation throughout ROM so that there is no shift
MCL laxity	Decreases	Limits compression of lateral compartment with valgus stress
PLC	Increases	Increases external rotation
Medial meniscectomy	Increases	Increases anterior translation
Bucket-handle meniscus tear	Decreases	Blocks extension
Flexion contracture	Decreases	Prevents extension

From Lane CG, Warren R, Pearle AD: The pivot shift. J Am Acad Orthop Surg 16:686, 2008.
ITB, Iliotibial band; *MCL,* medial collateral ligament; *PLC,* posterolateral corner; *ROM,* range of motion.

leg in slight medial rotation. This is done by placing the heel of the hand behind the fibula and over the lateral head of the gastrocnemius muscle with the tibia medially rotated, causing the tibia to subluxate anteriorly as the knee is taken into extension (Figure 12-84). Bach and colleagues[192] modified the position to slight lateral rotation, because they believed that lateral tibial rotation gives a more pronounced pivot shift when the test is positive. In slight flexion, the secondary restraints (i.e., hamstrings, lateral femoral condyle, lateral meniscus) are less efficient than in full flexion. It is important to realize that in full extension subluxation does not occur, because of the "locking home" of the tibia on the femur.[28] With slight flexion, however, the secondary restraints are less restrictive, and subluxation occurs. The examiner then applies a valgus stress to the knee while maintaining a medial rotation torque on the tibia at the ankle. Kurosaka, et al.[193] recommend applying an axial (compression) load to the knee while doing the test. If a click occurred during the test, they related the click to meniscus pathology. The leg is then flexed, and at approximately 30° to 40° the tibia reduces or "jogs" backward. The patient says that that is what the "giving way" feels like, indicating a positive test. The reduction of the tibia on the femur is caused by the change in position of the iliotibial band when it switches from an extensor function to a flexor function, pulling the tibia back into its normal position (Figure 12-85). The test involves two phases: first subluxation and then reduction. The iliotibial band must be intact for the test to work. In cases of anterolateral instability in which the iliotibial band has also been torn, the test does not work (the subluxation will be evident, but the "jog" will not occur). In addition, if either meniscus has been torn, it may limit or prevent the subluxation reduction motion seen in the test.

If the patient is tense or apprehensive, the test can be modified; this is called the **soft pivot shift test** ⚠ (Figure 12-86). The patient lies supine, and the examiner supports the test foot with one hand while placing the other hand over the calf muscle 10 to 20 cm (4 to 8 inches) distal to the knee joint. The examiner flexes and extends

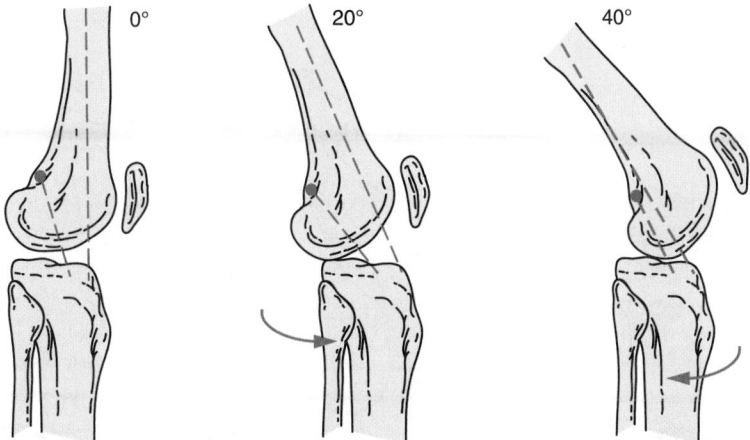

Figure 12-85 Biomechanics of the pivot shift. Three phases occur during the pivot shift maneuver. Under load transmission in the lateral compartment, the tibia rolls from a reduced position in neutral rotation to anterior subluxation and some medial rotation. Under increasing flexion to 20°, the condyle becomes jammed behind the posterior slope of the lateral plateau. The iliotibial band, especially the femorotibial portion, becomes tight until, at 30° to 40°, it is gliding behind the flexion axis, initiating reduction in more flexion and some lateral rotation.

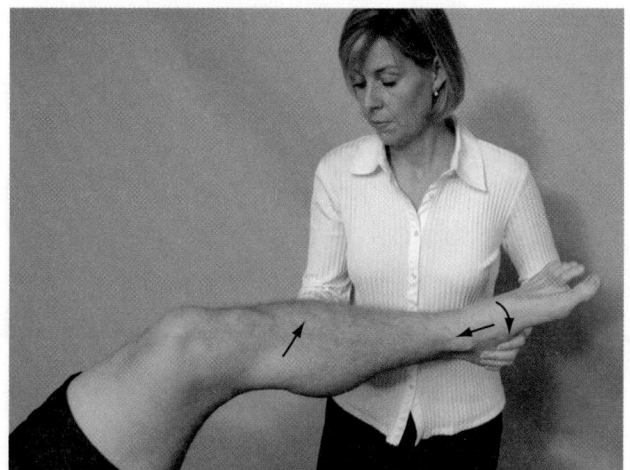

Figure 12-86 Soft pivot shift test. Examiner watches for anterior shift.

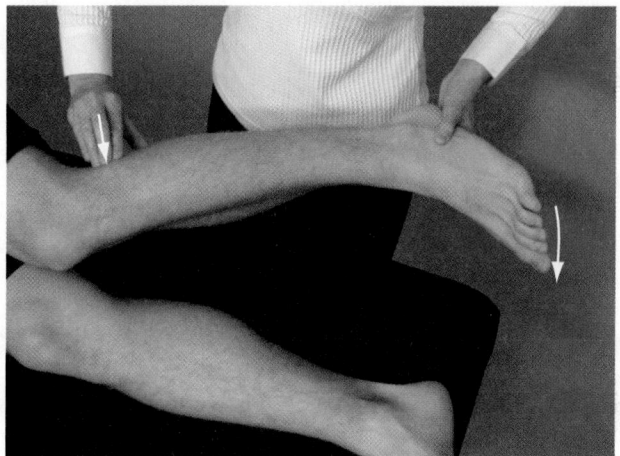

Figure 12-87 Lemaire's jolt test for anterolateral rotary instability (ALRI).

the knee slowly and gently to relax the patient. After three to five cycles, the examiner applies axial compression while the other hand over the calf exerts an anterior pressure. In a positive test, the tibia subluxates and reduces, but not with the same apprehensive, jerky feeling.[79] Kennedy[153] advocated pushing on the fibular head with the thumb when performing this maneuver. Because hip abduction and adduction have an effect on the iliotibial band, hip position plays an important role in the test. Subluxation is most obvious when the hip is abducted and least obvious when it is adducted. In addition, lateral rotation of the tibia allows greater subluxation because, like abduction, it decreases the stress on the iliotibial band.[79] If the test is positive, the following structures have probably been injured to some degree:

1. Anterior cruciate ligament
2. Posterolateral capsule
3. Arcuate-popliteus complex
4. Lateral collateral ligament
5. Iliotibial band

Lemaire's Jolt Test.[28] The patient is in side-lying position with the test leg uppermost. For the test to work, the patient must be relaxed. With one hand, the examiner medially rotates the tibia by grasping the foot and medially rotating it with the knee in extension. The back of the other hand pushes lightly against the biceps tendon and head of the fibula while the hand on the foot flexes and extends the knee (Figure 12-87). In a positive test, at about 15° to 20° of flexion, a "jolt" occurs with displacement of the tibia, indicating a positive test for anterolateral instability.

Losee Test. This test is a clinical duplication of the ALRI mechanism of injury. The patient lies supine while relaxed.[194] The examiner holds the patient's ankle and

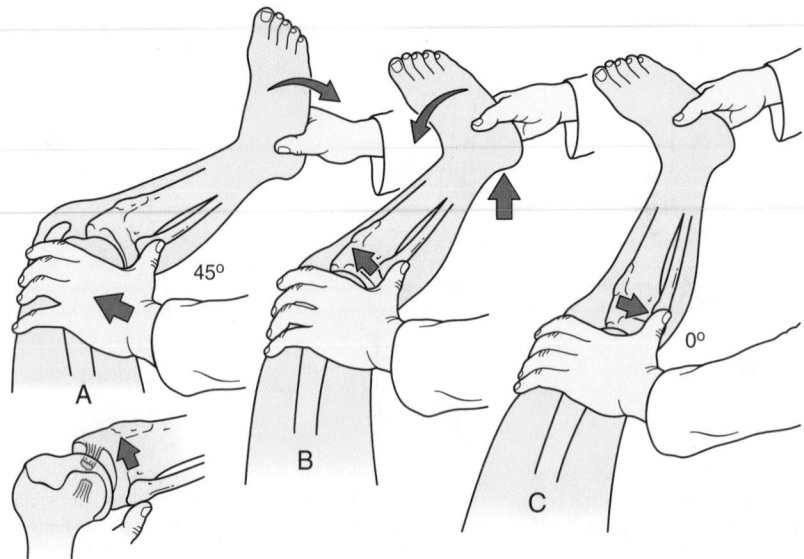

Figure 12-88 The **Losee test** begins with the knee in flexion and the tibia in lateral rotation and valgus stress (**A**). As the knee is extended (**B**), the foot is allowed to medially rotate, and the previously reduced *(A)* tibia subluxes as the knee approaches full extension (**C**). A palpable "clunk" correlates with anterior cruciate ligament tear. (Redrawn from Scott WN, editor: Ligament and extensor mechanism injuries of the knee: diagnosis and treatment, St Louis, 1991, Mosby, p. 96.)

foot so that the leg is laterally rotated. The knee is then flexed to 30°, and the examiner ensures that the hamstring muscles are relaxed (Figure 12-88). The lateral rotation ensures that the subluxation of the knee is reduced at the beginning of the test. With the examiner's other hand positioned so that the fingers lie over the patella and the thumb is hooked behind the fibular head, a valgus force is applied to the knee; the examiner can use the abdomen as a fulcrum while extending the patient's knee and applying forward pressure behind the fibular head with the thumb. The valgus stress compresses the structures in the lateral compartment and makes the anterior subluxation, if present, more noticeable. At the same time, the foot and ankle are allowed to drift into medial rotation. If the foot and ankle are not allowed to rotate medially, the anterior subluxation of the lateral tibial plateau may be prevented. Just before full extension of the knee, there is a "clunk" forward if the test is positive, and the patient must recognize the movement as the instability that was previously experienced. This clunk means that the tibia has subluxated anteriorly and indicates injury to the same structures as those indicated by a positive pivot shift maneuver. Kocher et al.[195] reported that the test could be used as a good check of functional instability after surgical reconstruction.

Martens Test.[79] The patient and examiner are positioned as for the Noyes test. The examiner grips the patient's leg distal to the knee joint with one hand and pushes the femur posteriorly with the other hand. A valgus stress is applied to the knee as the knee is flexed until the tibia reduces, indicating a positive test (Figure 12-89).

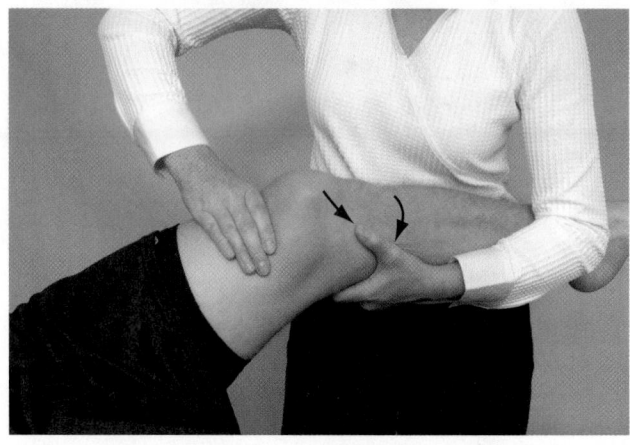

Figure 12-89 Martens test.

Nakajima Test.[79] The patient lies supine, and the examiner stands on the side of the test leg. The patient's foot is held with one hand, which medially rotates the tibia. The knee is flexed to 90°. The examiner's other hand is placed over the lateral femoral condyle with the thumb behind the head of the fibula, pushing it forward. The examiner slowly extends the knee while pushing the head of the fibula forward, noting whether subluxation occurs, which indicates a positive test.

Noyes Flexion-Rotation Drawer Test. Described by Noyes et al.,[196] this test is a modification of the pivot shift maneuver. It can be used in the acutely injured knee and is felt by some[12] to be more sensitive than the other ALRI tests. The patient lies supine, and the examiner holds the patient's ankle between the examiner's trunk and arm

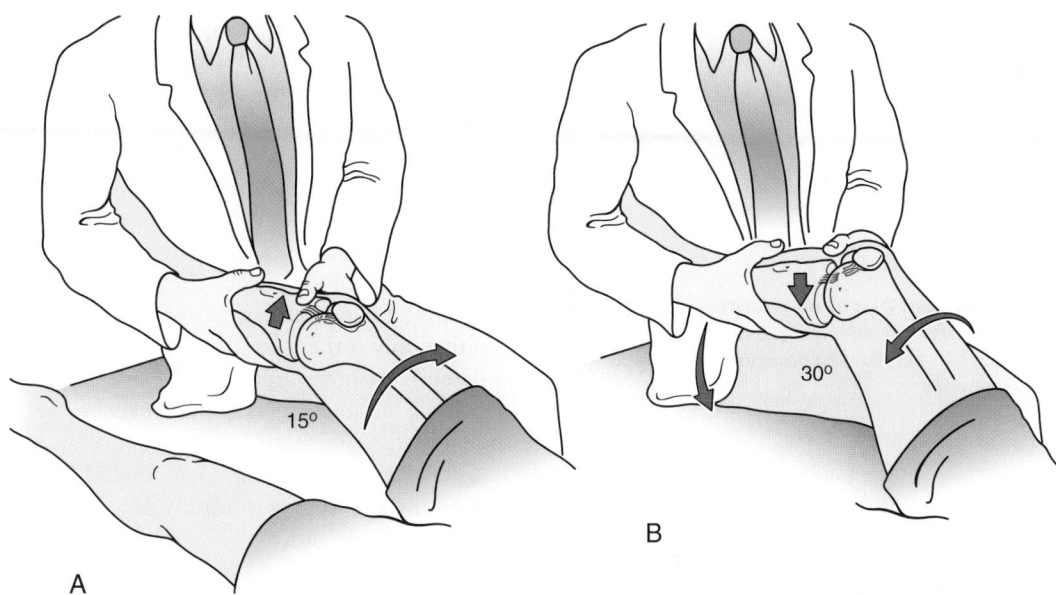

Figure 12-90 **Flexion-rotation drawer test combines elements of Lachman test and lateral pivot shift.** Flexion from **A** to **B** results in posterior reduction of subluxated tibia and medial rotation of femur. Positive test results correlate with anterior cruciate ligament disruption. (Redrawn from Scott WN, editor: Ligament and extensor mechanism injuries of the knee: diagnosis and treatment, St Louis, 1991, Mosby, p. 94.)

with the hands around the tibia (Figure 12-90). The examiner flexes the patient's knee to 20° to 30° while maintaining the tibia in neutral rotation. The tibia is then pushed posteriorly, as in a posterior drawer test. This posterior movement reduces the subluxation of the tibia, indicating a positive test for ALRI. If the tibia is alternately pushed posteriorly and released and the femur is allowed to rotate freely, the reduction and subluxation are seen and felt as the femur rotates medially and laterally.

⚠ *Slocum Test.* This test has been described previously.

⚠ *Slocum Anterolateral Rotary Instability Test.* ALRI is also assessed by the Slocum ALRI test.[139,183] The patient is in the side-lying position (approximately 30° from supine). The bottom leg is the uninvolved leg. The knee of the uninvolved leg is flexed to add stability (Figure 12-91). The foot of the involved leg rests and is stabilized on the examining table with the patient's foot in medial rotation and the knee in extension and valgus. This position helps to eliminate hip rotation during the test. The examiner applies a valgus stress to the knee while flexing the knee. The subluxation of the knee reduces at between 25° and 45° of flexion if the test is positive. A positive test indicates injury to the same structures as indicated in the pivot shift maneuver. The main advantage of this test is that it aids in relaxation of the patient's hamstring muscles and is easier to perform on heavy or tense patients.

Tests for Posteromedial Rotary Instability[197–200]

When performing these tests, the examiner is looking for abnormal (excessive) posterior rotation of the medial side

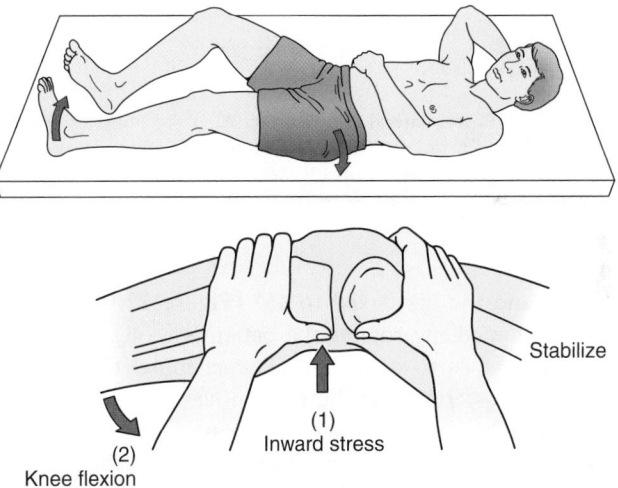

Figure 12-91 Slocum anterolateral rotary instability (ALRI) test.

of the tibia relative to the femur. A note of caution: if the leg is positioned so that gravity may affect the relation of the tibia to the femur (e.g., supine-lying position, hip at 45°, knee at 90°), the medial side of the tibia may "drop back" into excessive posterior rotation just by positioning. In this case, if the examiner is not aware of this abnormal position, a false-positive test for anteromedial rotary instability may occur if testing for anteromedial rotary instability when in fact the real problem is posteromedial rotation instability.

⚠ *Hughston's Posteromedial and Posterolateral Drawer Sign.* The patient lies supine with the knee flexed to 80°

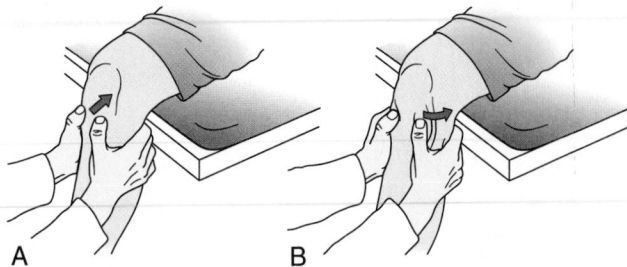

Figure 12-92 Posteromedial and posterolateral drawer test, anterior view. A, Starting position for posterolateral drawer test. **B,** Positive posterolateral drawer test with posterior and lateral rotation of the lateral tibial condyle.

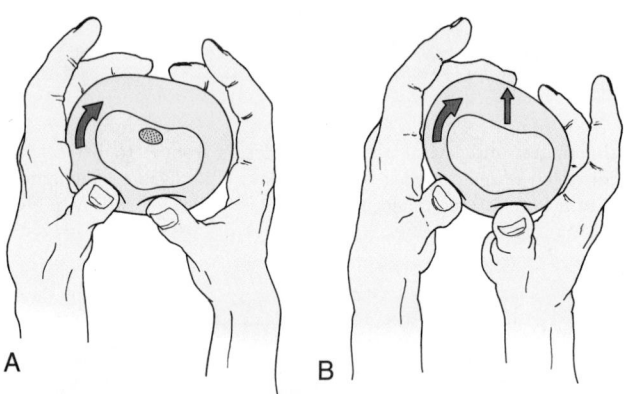

Figure 12-93 Posterolateral drawer test. A, If the posterior cruciate ligament is intact, the tibia rotates posterolaterally. **B,** If the posterior cruciate ligament is torn, the tibia rotates posterolaterally and subluxates posteriorly.

to 90° and the hip flexed to 45° (Figure 12-92).[201] The examiner medially rotates the patient's foot slightly and sits on the foot to stabilize it. The examiner then pushes the tibia posteriorly. If the tibia moves or rotates posteriorly on the medial aspect an excessive amount relative to the normal knee, the test is positive and indicates posteromedial rotary instability. A positive test indicates that the following structures have probably been injured to some degree:

1. Posterior cruciate ligament
2. Posterior oblique ligament
3. Medial collateral ligament (superficial and deep fibers)
4. Semimembranosus tendon
5. Posteromedial capsule
6. Anterior cruciate ligament
7. Medial meniscus

The medial tubercle rotates posteriorly around the posterior cruciate ligament when the tibia is in mild medial rotation. If the posterior cruciate ligament is also torn, the posteromedial movement is greater, and the tibia subluxates posteriorly (Figure 12-93).

The test may also be done with the patient sitting with the knee flexed over the edge of the examining table. The

examiner pushes posteriorly while holding the patient's leg in medial rotation, watching for the same excessive movement.

Posterolateral rotary instability may be tested in a similar fashion.[201] The patient and examiner are in the same position, but the patient's foot is slightly laterally rotated. If the tibia rotates posteriorly on the lateral side an excessive amount relative to the uninvolved leg when the examiner pushes the tibia posteriorly, the test is positive for posterolateral rotary instability. The test is positive only if the posterior cruciate ligament and lateral collateral ligaments are torn.[202] The examiner may palpate the fibula while doing the movement to feel for excessive movement.

Ⓐ *Posteromedial Pivot Shift Test.*[203] The patient lies relaxed in the supine position. The examiner passively flexes the knee more than 45° while applying a varus stress, compression, and medial rotation of the tibia; in a "positive" knee, these movements cause subluxation of the medial tibial plateau posteriorly (Figure 12-94, *A*). The examiner then takes the knee into extension. At about 20° to 40° of flexion, the tibia shifts into the reduced position (Figure 12-94, *B*). A positive test indicates that the following structures are injured:

1. Posterior cruciate ligament
2. Medial collateral ligament
3. Posterior oblique ligament

Tests for Posterolateral Rotary Instability[202,204–208]

The examiner is looking for abnormal (excessive) posterior rotation of the lateral side of the tibia when performing these tests. As with the posteromedial rotation, the examiner must always be aware that positioning the leg (gravity may cause the lateral tibia to "drop back") may lead to a false-positive ALRI when, in fact, the problem is actually a posterolateral instability problem.

Ⓐ *Active Posterolateral Drawer Sign.*[209] The patient sits with the foot on the floor in neutral rotation. The knee is flexed to 80° to 90°. The patient is asked to isometrically contract the hamstrings, primarily the lateral one (biceps femoris), while the examiner stabilizes the foot. A positive test for posterolateral instability is posterior subluxation of the lateral tibial plateau (Figure 12-95).

Ⓐ *Dynamic Posterior Shift Test.*[210] The patient lies supine, and the examiner flexes the hip and knee of the test leg to 90° with the femur in neutral rotation. One hand of the examiner stabilizes the anterior thigh while the other hand extends the knee. If the test is positive, the tibia reduces anteriorly with a clunk as extension is reached. The test is positive for posterior and posterolateral instabilities. If the knee is painful before extension is accomplished, the hip flexion may be decreased, but the hamstrings must be kept tight (Figure 12-96).

⚠ *External Rotation Recurvatum Test.* There are two methods for performing this test. In the first method, the patient lies in the supine position with the lower limbs

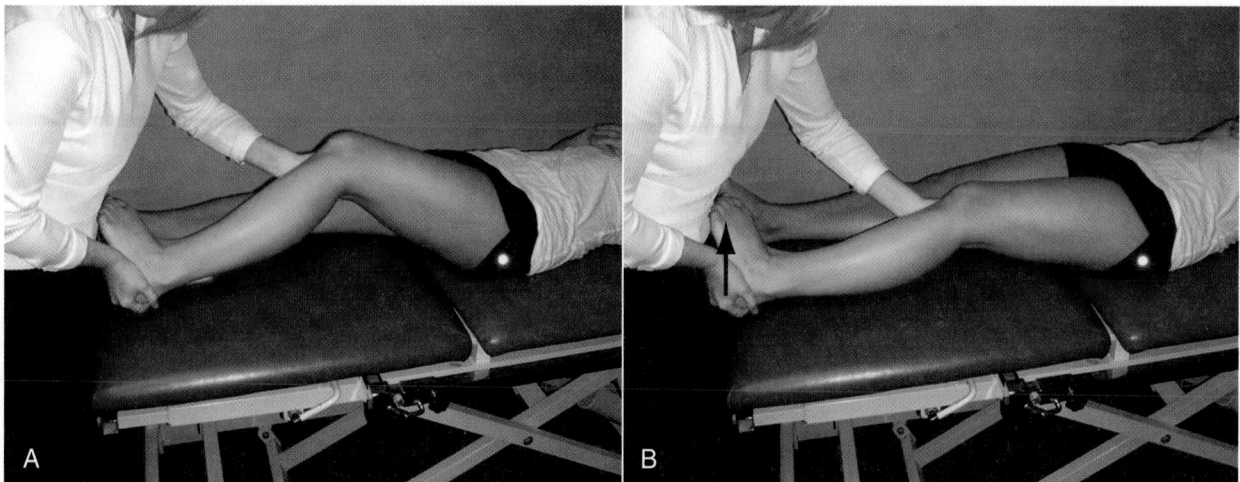

Figure 12-94 Posteromedial pivot shift test. A, Starting position. **B,** In a positive test, the tibia will jog into reduction at between 20° and 40° of flexion as the knee is extended.

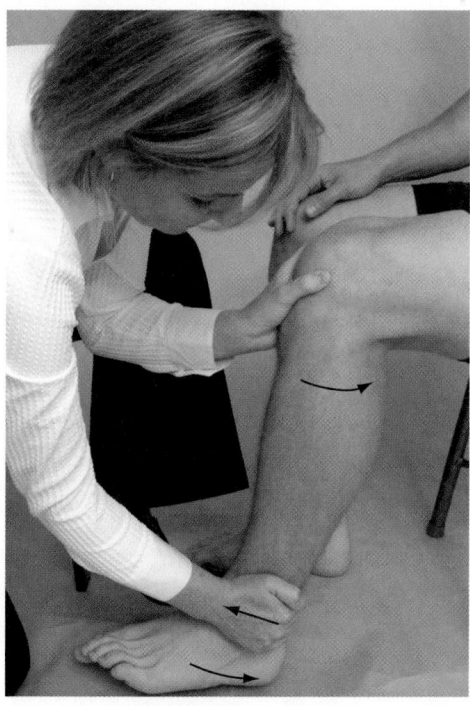

Figure 12-95 Active posterolateral drawer sign or test. Examiner watches for posterolateral shift of tibia.

relaxed. The examiner gently grasps the big toe of each foot and lifts both feet off the examining table (Figure 12-97, *A*).[201,204,211] The patient is told to keep the quadriceps muscles relaxed (i.e., it is a passive test). While elevating the legs, the examiner watches the tibial tuberosities. LaPrade et al.[212] suggest one of the examiner's hands should hold the toes while the other hand gently holds the distal thigh near the knee to prevent the thigh lifting off the table. In this case, the tibia will sublux anteriorly (Figure 12-97, *B*) and the affected leg will show

a higher heel height indicating injury to the posterolateral structures. With a positive test, the affected knee goes into relative hyperextension on the lateral aspect because of the force of gravity with the tibia and tibial tuberosity rotating laterally. The affected knee has the appearance of a relative genu varum. It is a test for posterolateral rotary instability in extension and injury to the anterior cruciate ligament (ACL).[212]

In the second method, the patient lies supine, and the examiner's hand holds the patient's heel or foot and flexes the knee to 30° to 40° (Figure 12-98).[201] The examiner's other hand holds the posterolateral aspect of the patient's knee and slowly extends it. With the hand on the knee, the examiner feels the relative hyperextension and lateral rotation occurring in the injured limb compared with the uninjured limb.

⚠ *Hughston's Posteromedial and Posterolateral Drawer Sign.* This test has been described previously. For posterolateral instability to occur, the following structures must have been injured to some degree:
1. Posterior cruciate ligament
2. Arcuate-popliteus complex
3. Lateral collateral ligament
4. Biceps femoris tendon
5. Posterolateral capsule
6. Anterior cruciate ligament

⚠ *Jakob Test (Reverse Pivot Shift Maneuver).* This is a test for posterolateral rotary instability,[139,213] and it can be performed in two ways. In the first method, the patient stands and leans against a wall with the uninjured side adjacent to the wall and the body weight distributed equally between the two feet (Figure 12-99). The examiner's hands are placed above and below the involved knee, and a valgus stress is exerted while flexion of the patient's knee is initiated. If there is a jerk in the knee or the tibia shifts posteriorly and the "giving way"

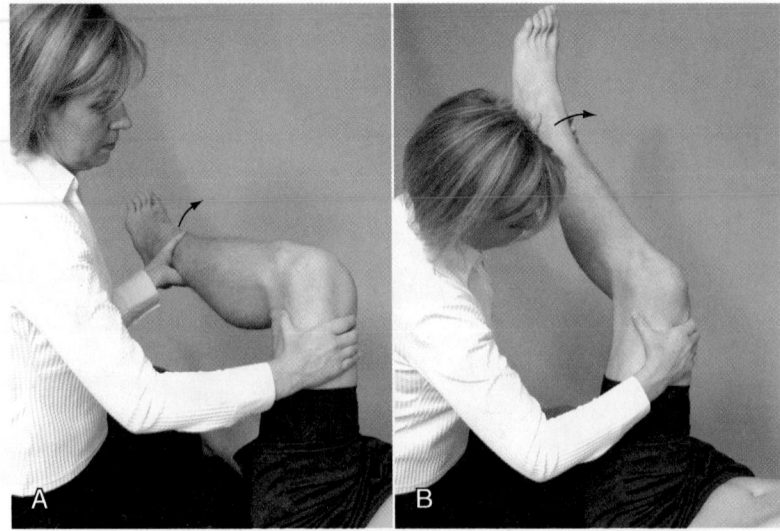

Figure 12-96 Dynamic posterior shift test. A, Starting position in flexion. **B,** Extended position in which posterior shift occurs.

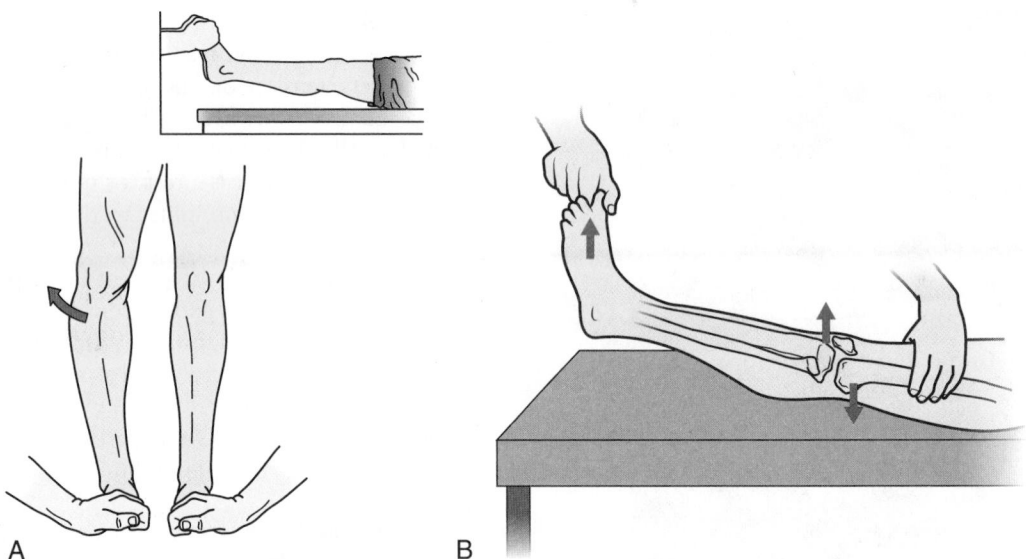

Figure 12-97 External rotational recurvatum test. A, Method 1, the examiner grasps the big toe of each foot. **B,** Method 2, the examiner grasps the big toe with one hand while the other gently holds the distal thigh near the knee to prevent the thigh from lifting off the table. In a positive test, differences in heel height from the table are demonstrated.

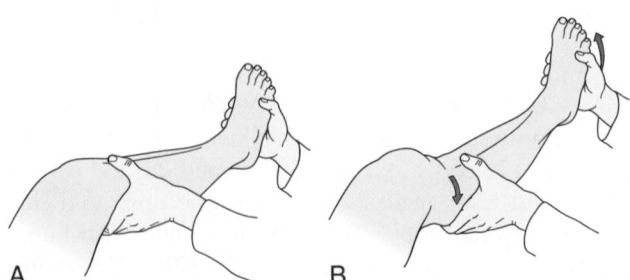

Figure 12-98 External rotation recurvatum test (method 2). The test is begun by holding the knee in flexion (left). As the knee is slowly extended, the hand at the knee feels the lateral rotation and recurvatum at the posterolateral aspect of the knee.

phenomenon occurs during this maneuver, it indicates injury to the lateral collateral ligament, arcuate-popliteus complex, and mid third of the lateral capsule.[202]

In the second method, the patient lies in the supine position with the hamstring muscles relaxed. The examiner faces the patient, lifts the patient's leg, and supports the leg against the examiner's pelvis. The examiner's other hand supports the lateral side of the calf with the palm on the proximal fibula. The knee is flexed to 70° to 80° of flexion, and the foot is laterally rotated, causing the lateral tibial plateau to subluxate posteriorly (Figure 12-100, *A*). The knee is taken into extension by its own weight while the examiner leans on the foot to impart a valgus stress to the knee through the leg. As the knee approaches 20° of flexion, the lateral tibial tubercle shifts forward or anteriorly into the neutral rotation and reduces the subluxation, indicating a positive test (Figure 12-100, B). The leg is then flexed again, and the foot falls back into lateral rotation and posterior subluxation.

▲ *Loomer's Posterolateral Rotary Instability Test.*[211,214] The patient lies supine and flexes both hips and both knees to 90°. The examiner then grasps the feet and maximally laterally rotates both tibias (Figure 12-101). The test is considered positive if the injured tibia laterally rotates

excessively and there is a posterior sag of the affected tibial tubercle; both signs must be present for a positive test. This test is similar to the **Bousquet external hypermobility test.**[28]

Veltri and associates[215–218] describe a modification of Loomer's test that is called the **tibial lateral rotation test** or **dial test of the knee** ▲ (Figure 12-102). This test is designed to show loss of the posterolateral support structures of the knee. Griffith, et al. reported that this test could also test medial knee joint structures.[219] The patient may be placed supine or prone. The examiner places one hand behind the posterior proximal tibia to support the tibia and maintain it in the reduced (normal) position.[218] The examiner then flexes the knee to 30°, extends the foot over the side of the examining table, and stabilizes the femur on the table.[220] The examiner then laterally rotates the tibia on the femur and compares the amount of rotation with that on the good side. If the test is done in supine position, the examiner can observe the amount of tibial tubercle movement and compare. The test is then repeated with the knee flexed to 90° and the thigh still

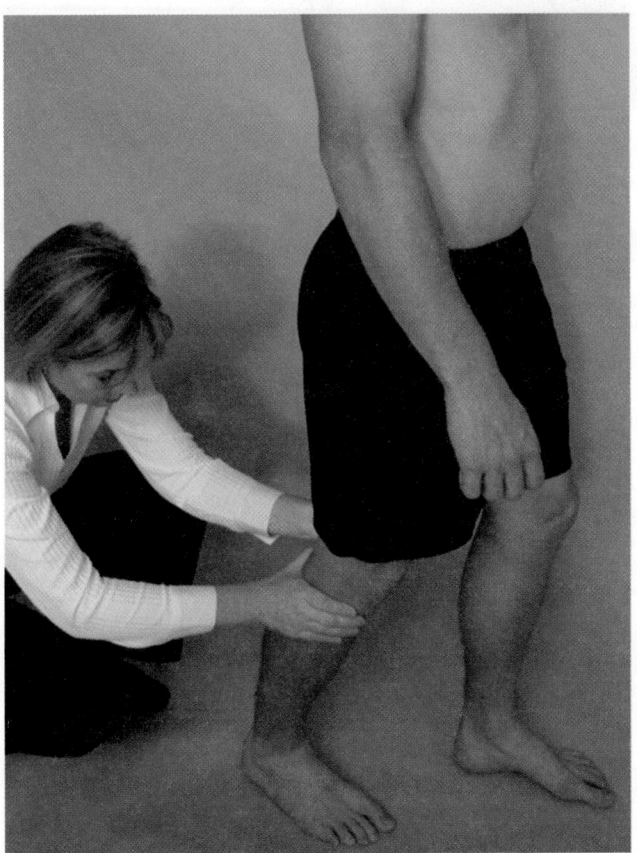

Figure 12-99 Jakob test (method 1, showing valgus stress and flexion).

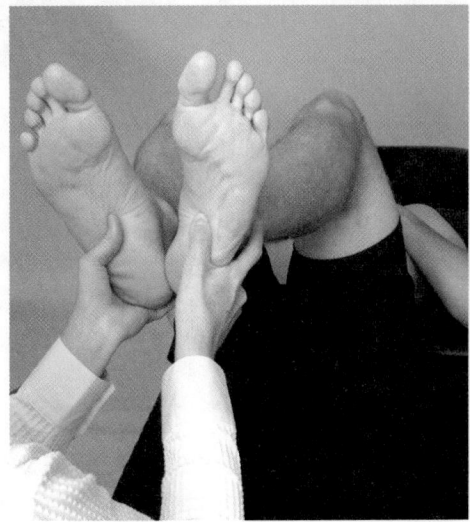

Figure 12-101 Loomer's test for posterolateral rotary instability.

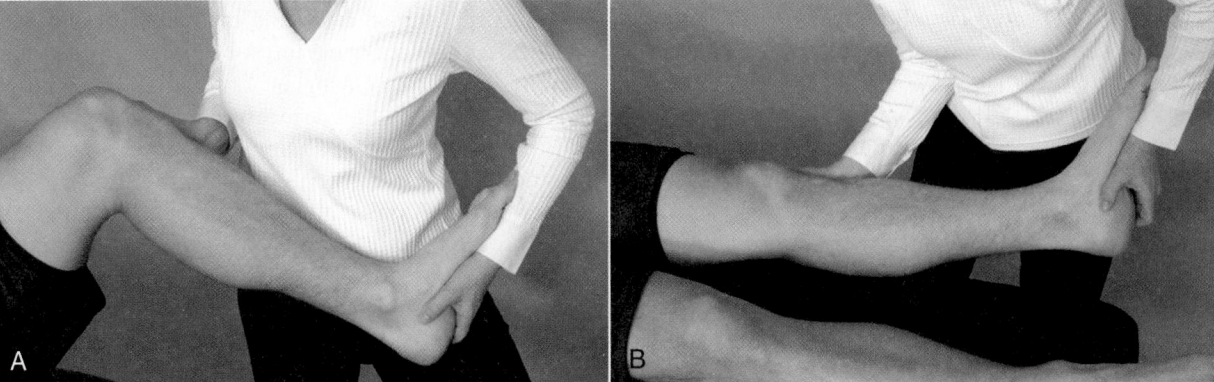

Figure 12-100 Reverse pivot shift test, method 2. **A,** Flexed position with lateral rotation causes lateral tibial tubercle to subluxate. **B,** As the extended position is approached, the lateral tibial tubercle reduces.

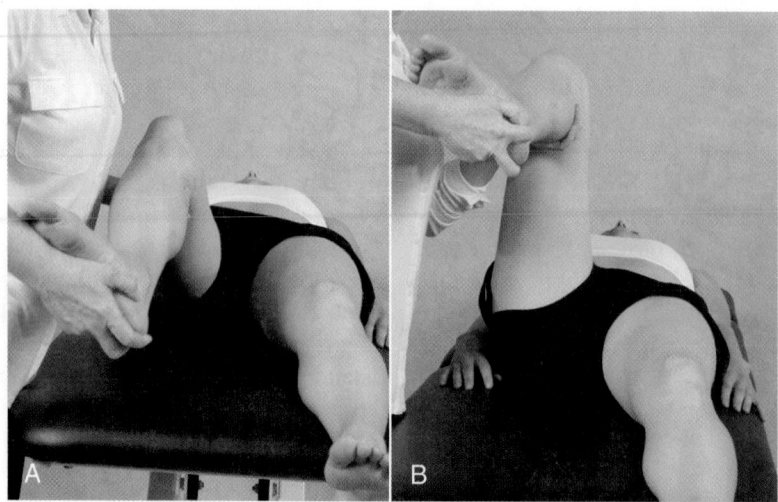

Figure 12-102 Tibial lateral rotation test or dial test in supine position. A, At 30° flexion. **B,** At 90° flexion. The examiner watches for increased lateral rotation on the affected side, which may occur at 30° or 90° (see text).

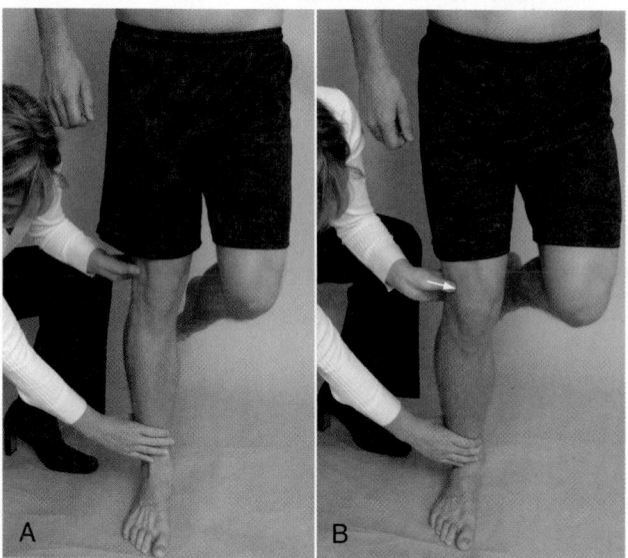

Figure 12-103 Standing apprehension test for posterolateral instability. A, Starting position. **B,** With knee flexed.

on the examining table. If the tibia rotates less at 90° than at 30°, an isolated posterolateral (popliteus corner) injury is more likely. If the knee rotates more at 90°, injury to both the popliteus corner and posterior cruciate injury are more likely.[156,202,204–206] If the pain is on the medial joint line, a positive test may indicate injury to the medial ligament complex[151,152] (see Swain test).

? *Standing Apprehension Test.*[221] The patient stands on the affected knee. The examiner then pushes anteriorly and medially on the anterolateral part of the lateral femoral condyle crossing the joint line. The patient is then asked to slightly flex the knee while the examiner pushes with the thumb (Figure 12-103). Condylar movement and a "giving way" sensation are considered positive signs for posterolateral instability.

Ligament Testing Devices

Ligament testing devices for the knee have been developed to help quantify the displacement occurring in the knee and how this displacement is modified when ligaments are injured. Most commonly, these devices test anteroposterior displacement, although more expensive ones may test other displacements. These devices are used primarily to assist in diagnosing ligament injuries (third-degree sprains) by detecting abnormal (pathological) motion, to provide a quantified measurement of motion, and to measure the amount of motion after surgery (e.g., whether normal motion limits were reestablished).[222–225]

The most commonly used ligament testing devices are the KT-1000 arthrometer (most common), the Genucom, the Stryker knee laxity tester, the Rolimeter and the Telos device. The KT-1000 and Rolimeter are reported to be best for anterior laxity, whereas the Telos device is best for posterior laxity.[226] Other units have been developed but are not commonly used.[28,227–230] These devices should be considered adjuncts to clinical assessment and should be used primarily to confirm a clinical diagnosis.[30]

Each of these devices works on the principle of positioning the limb in a specific manner, applying a force that causes displacement, and subsequently measuring the amount of displacement or translation caused by the applied force.[222,231,232] The measurements obtained depend on the experience and ability of the examiner, the joint position, muscle activity or inactivity, the constraints present in the joint and those imposed by the testing systems, the amount of displacing force, and the measurement system used.[222] The greatest sources of error when using the arthrometer are the inability to stabilize the patellar sensor pad and lack of muscle relaxation.[233]

Because the KT-1000 arthrometer is the most commonly used testing device for anteroposterior displacement, it is briefly described here. More detailed

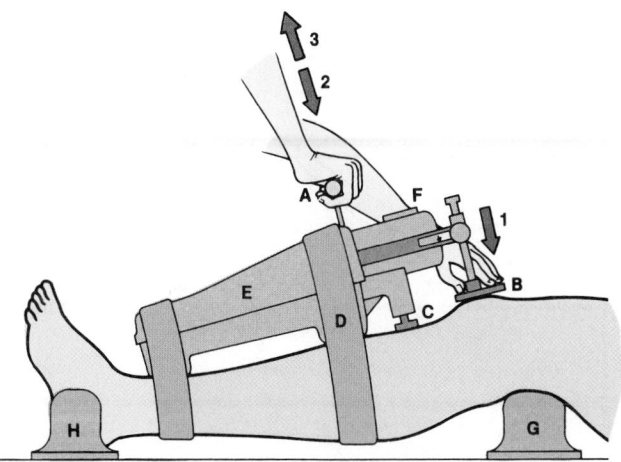

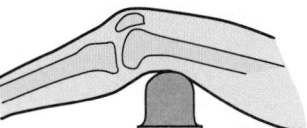

Flex knee (20°–30°) to engage
patella in femoral trochlea

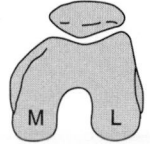

Support thigh to place
patella facing up

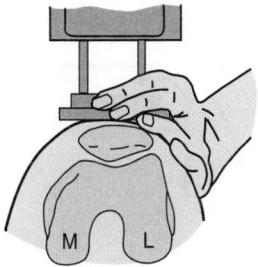

Apply pressure to
stabilize patella

Figure 12-104 KT-1000 arthrometer. A posterior *(2)* or anterior *(3)* force is applied. A constant force *(1)* is applied to stabilize the patellar sensor pad. **A,** Force handle; **B,** patellar sensor pad; **C,** tibial sensor pad; **D,** Velcro straps; **E,** arthrometer body; **F,** displacement dial; **G,** thigh support; **H,** foot support. (From Daniel D, Akeson W, O'Conner J, editors: Knee ligaments: structure, injury and repair, New York, 1990, Raven Press, p. 428.)

Figure 12-105 The knee is supported in a flexed position to engage the patella in the femoral trochlea. In some patients, the thigh support must be raised an additional 3 to 6 cm to provide sufficient knee flexion to engage the patella in the femoral trochlea. This may be done by placing a board under the thigh support. The thigh should be supported so that the patella is facing up. Occasionally, a thigh strap is used to accomplish this task. The examiner stabilizes the patellar sensor with manual pressure. The stabilizing hand should rest against the lateral thigh and should apply 1 to 2.25 kg (2 to 5 lbs) of pressure on the patellar sensor pad. The hand position, patellar sensor position, and patellar sensor pressure must remain constant throughout the test. Variation of the pressure on the patellar sensor pad and rotation of the pad is a common cause of measurement error. (From Daniel D, et al, editors: Knee ligaments: structure, injury and repair, New York, 1990, Raven Press, p. 428.)

descriptions of its use are found elsewhere[98,231–233] and should be consulted if the examiner plans to use this device. The arthrometer is placed on the anterior aspect of the tibia and is held in place with two Velcro straps (Figures 12-104 and 12-105). A thigh support and foot support help to hold the leg in proper alignment with straps if necessary. There are two sensor pads, one on the tibial tubercle and one on the patella. Because the patella is one of the sensor points, knees that are swollen and demonstrate a ballotable patella should not be tested unless the knee is aspirated to minimize false-positive readings.[234] These pads detect relative movement. Forces to translate the tibia are applied through a force-sensing handle.

After the device is properly positioned and the leg is properly relaxed, several tests may be performed, first on the good knee and then on the injured knee.

Quadriceps Neutral Test. The patient's knee is flexed to 90°, and the arthrometer is positioned on the leg. A 9-kg (20-lb) posterior force is applied through the apparatus to establish a reference position. The patient is then asked to perform an isolated quadriceps contraction. If the tibia shifts forward, the knee angle is altered until there is no movement of the tibia when the quadriceps contracts. This position is called the **quadriceps neutral angle** or **quadriceps active position,** and it usually occurs at about 70° flexion (see Figure 12-135). This position is found on the good knee and is used as a reference or starting position for the injured knee. If, when the injured knee is tested in this position, the anterior displacement is greater than 1 mm, the translation is abnormal and probably indicates a posterior cruciate ligament sprain.[222,233]

Test in Quadriceps Active Position. With the patient's leg positioned at the quadriceps neutral angle, the examiner applies a 9-kg (20-lb) anterior force, followed by a 9-kg (20-lb) posterior force. The results for the good and injured knee are compared.[222,233]

Test in 30° Flexion. With the patient's leg positioned as shown in Figure 12-104, five tests are performed:
1. 9-kg (20-lb) posterior displacement
2. 7-kg (15-lb) anterior (Lachman) displacement
3. 9-kg (20-lb) anterior (Lachman) displacement
4. Maximum anterior (Lachman) displacement, usually 14 to 18 kg (30 to 40 lb)
5. Quadriceps active anterior displacement

The difference between the 7-kg and the 9-kg anterior displacement tests is called the **compliance index.** For the maximum anterior displacement test, the examiner manually pulls or translates the tibia forward on the femur, using a pull of approximately 14 to 18 kg (30 to 40 lb). For the quadriceps active test, the patient is asked to lift the heel slowly off the table; displacement as the heel leaves the table is noted. Differences of more than 3 mm between the good and injured legs are con-

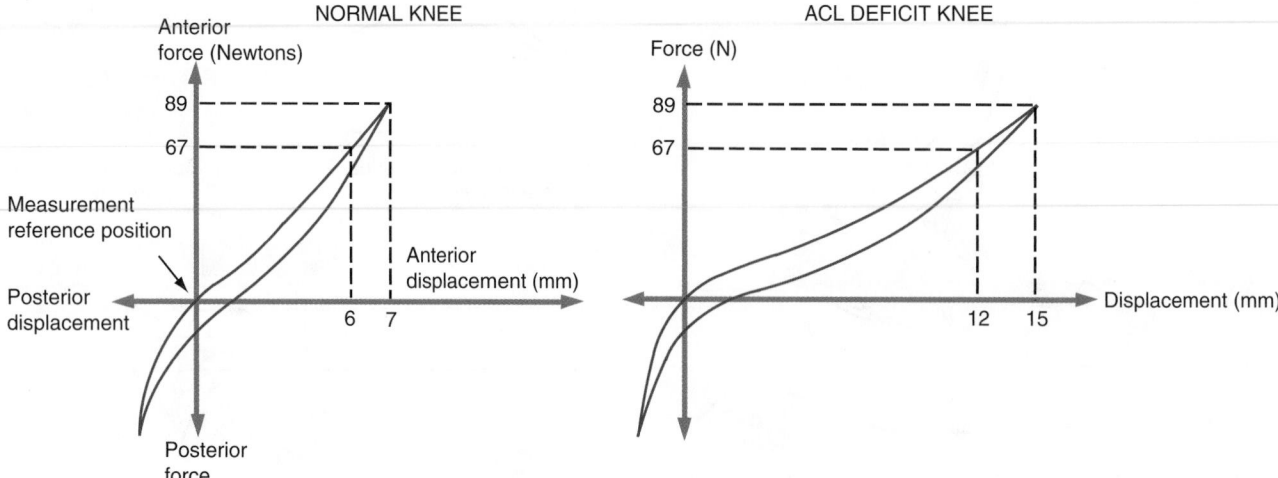

Figure 12-106 Force-displacement curves for normal knees and for knees with anterior cruciate ligament (ACL) deficit. The compliance index is obtained by measuring the displacement between the 67- and 89-N anterior-force levels. On this curve, the compliance index for the normal knee is 1 mm; for the knee with an ACL deficit, it is 3 mm. (From Daniel D, et al, editors: Knee ligaments: structure, injury and repair, New York, 1990, Raven Press, p. 433.)

sidered diagnostic for injury to the anterior cruciate or posterior cruciate.[222,233] Force displacement curves (Figure 12-106) and frequency distribution curves (Figure 12-107) demonstrate differences between the normal and pathological knees. Tests involving larger translation forces have been found to be more responsive to translation differences.[235]

It is important to realize that the accuracy of the readings for these devices depends very much on positioning, muscle relaxation, and the experience of the operator. Reliability of any of these measuring devices may be greatly affected if these factors are not controlled.[222,227,228,232,236–243]

Special Tests

Although most special tests on the knee are done only if the examiner suspects certain pathologies and wants to do a confirming test, tests for swelling should always be performed.

For the reader who would like to review them, the reliability, validity, specificity, sensitivity, and odds ratios of some of the special tests used on the knee are available on the Evolve website.

Tests for Meniscus Injury

Although there are several tests for a meniscus injury, none can be considered definitive without considerable experience on the part of the examiner. Even with experience, the examiner must do a thorough history and examination, because a positive test is more likely to be found if one suspects the condition is present.[244,245] Because the menisci are avascular and have no nerve supply on their inner two thirds, an injury to the meniscus can result in

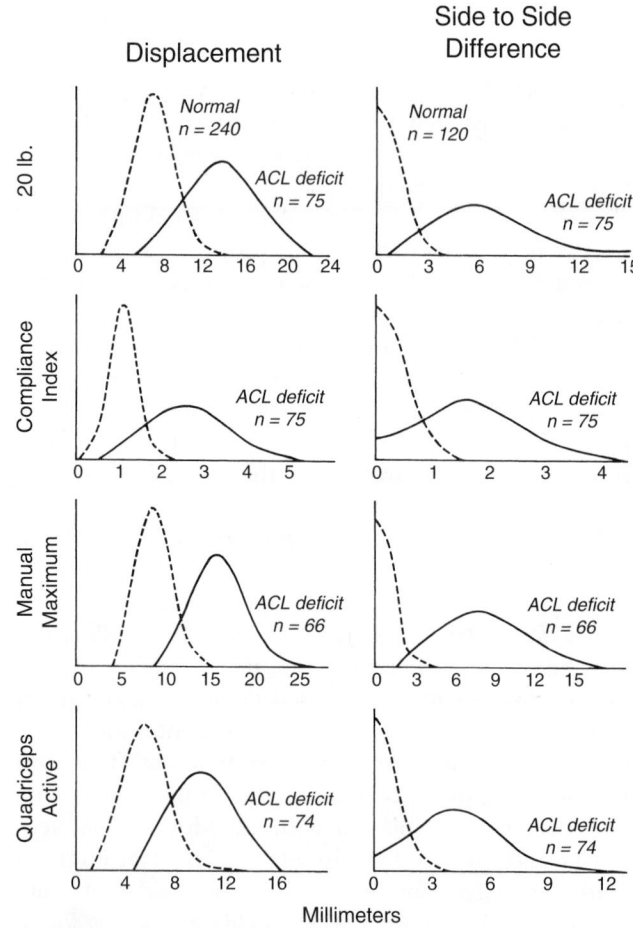

Figure 12-107 Frequency distribution curves of anterior laxity in normal knee in 30° of flexion and in knees with unilateral chronic anterior cruciate ligament disruption. (From Daniel DM, Stone ML: Diagnosis of knee ligament injury: test and measurements of joint laxity. In Feagin JA, editor: The crucial ligaments, New York, 1988, Churchill Livingstone, p. 298.)

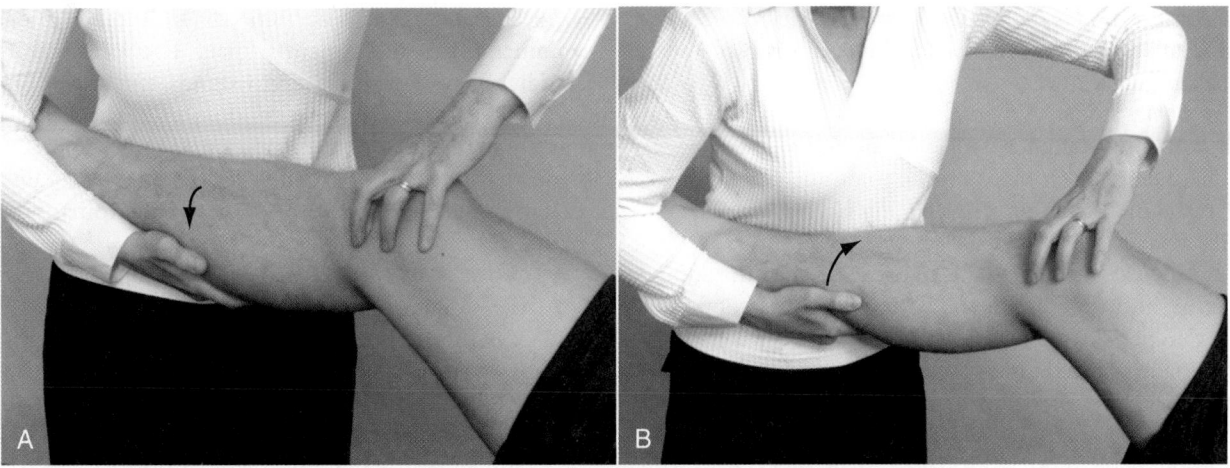

Figure 12-108 Anderson medial-lateral grind test. A, Flexion and valgus stress. **B,** Extension and varus stress.

little or no pain or swelling, making diagnosis even more difficult. Often, a combination of tests and clinical signs is needed to have a high level of suspicion of meniscus injury.[246,247] In some cases, however, joint line pain or tenderness, if the ligaments have been ruled out as causes of the pain, is the result of meniscus pathology. It has been found, however, that only about 50% of meniscus injuries have joint line pain or tenderness, especially with anterior cruciate tears, so this finding should not be used in isolation for diagnosis.[248]

❓ *Anderson Medial-Lateral Grind Test.*[249] The patient lies supine. The examiner holds the test leg between the trunk and the arm while the index finger and thumb of the opposite hand are placed over the anterior joint line (Figure 12-108). A valgus stress is applied to the knee as it is passively flexed to 45°; then a varus stress is applied to the knee as it is passively extended, producing a circular motion to the knee. The motion is repeated, increasing the varus and valgus stresses with each rotation. A distinct grinding is felt on the joint line if there is meniscus pathology. The test may also show a pivot shift if the anterior cruciate ligament has been torn.

☑ *Apley's Test.*[250] The patient lies in the prone position with the knee flexed to 90°. The patient's thigh is then anchored to the examining table with the examiner's knee (Figure 12-109). The examiner medially and laterally rotates the tibia, combined first with distraction, while noting any restriction, excessive movement, or discomfort. Then the process is repeated using compression instead of distraction. If rotation plus distraction is more painful or shows increased rotation relative to the normal side, the lesion is probably ligamentous. If the rotation plus compression is more painful or shows decreased rotation relative to the normal side, the lesion is probably a meniscus injury.

❷ Bohler's Sign. The patient lies in the supine position, and the examiner applies varus and valgus stresses to the knee. Pain in the opposite joint line (valgus stress for lateral meniscus) on stress testing is a positive sign for meniscus pathology.[79]

⚠ "Bounce Home" Test. The patient lies in the supine position, and the heel of the patient's foot is cupped in the examiner's hand (Figure 12-110). The patient's knee is completely flexed, and the knee is passively allowed to extend. If extension is not complete or has a rubbery end feel ("springy block"), there is something blocking full extension. The most likely cause of a block is a torn meniscus. Oni[251] reported that if the knee is allowed to quickly extend in one movement or jerk and the patient experiences a sharp pain on the joint line, which may radiate up or down the leg, the test is positive for a meniscus lesion.

❷ Bragard's Sign. The patient lies supine, and the examiner flexes the patient's knee. The examiner then laterally rotates the tibia and extends the knee (Figure 12-111). Pain and tenderness on the medial joint line indicate medial meniscus pathology. If the examiner then medially rotates the tibia and flexes the knee, the pain and tenderness decrease.[79] Both of these symptoms indicate medial meniscus pathology.

❷ Cabot's Popliteal Sign.[79] The patient lies supine, and the examiner positions the test leg in the figure-four position. The examiner palpates the joint line with the thumb and forefinger of one hand and places the other hand proximal to the ankle of the test leg. The patient is asked to isometrically straighten the knee while the examiner resists the movement. A positive test, signifying a meniscus lesion, is indicated by pain on the joint (Figure 12-112).

⚠ Childress' Sign. The patient squats and performs a "duck waddle."[79] Pain, snapping, or a click is considered positive for a posterior horn lesion of the meniscus.

⚠ Dynamic Knee Test. The patient lies supine with the hip flexed, abducted to 60° and laterally rotated 45° with the knee in 90° flexion so that the lateral border of the foot of the test leg rests on the examining table (Figure 12-113, *A*). The examiner palpates the lateral joint line while adducting the hip (knee still in 90° flexion) (Figure

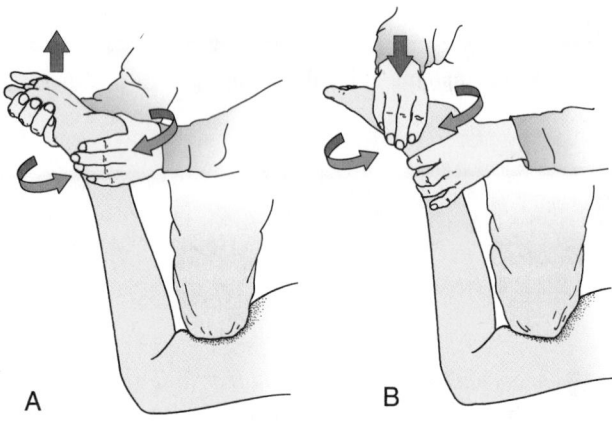

Figure 12-109 Apley's test. A, Distraction (ligaments). **B,** Compression (meniscus).

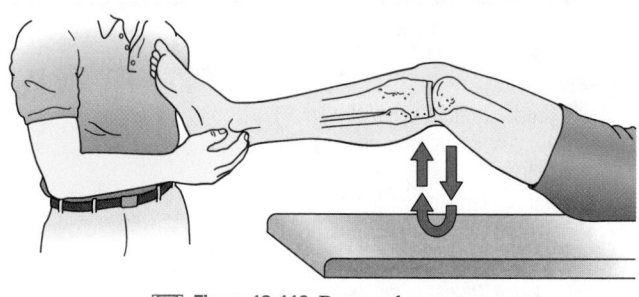

Figure 12-110 Bounce home test.

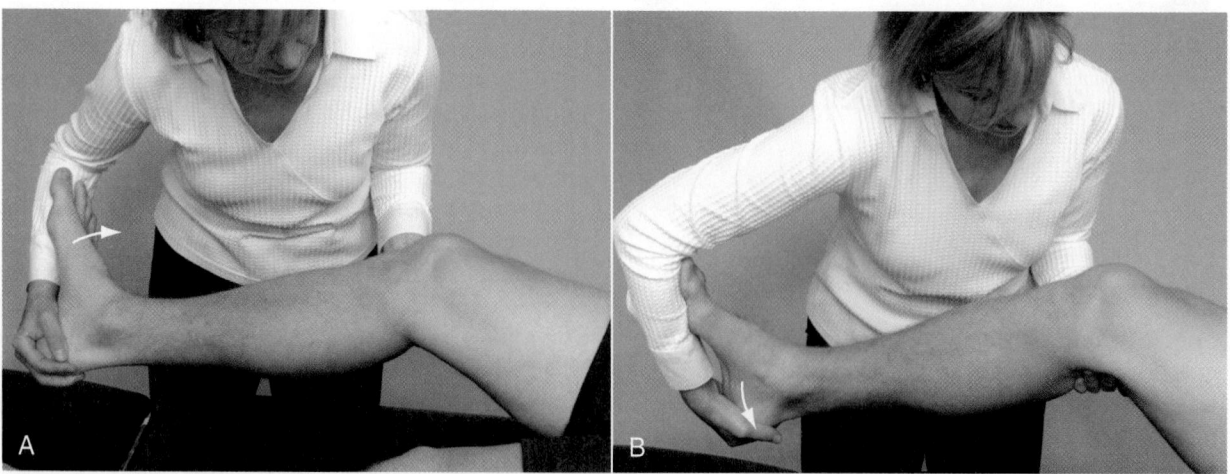

Figure 12-111 Bragard's sign for a meniscus lesion. A, Medial meniscus test. **B,** Lateral meniscus test.

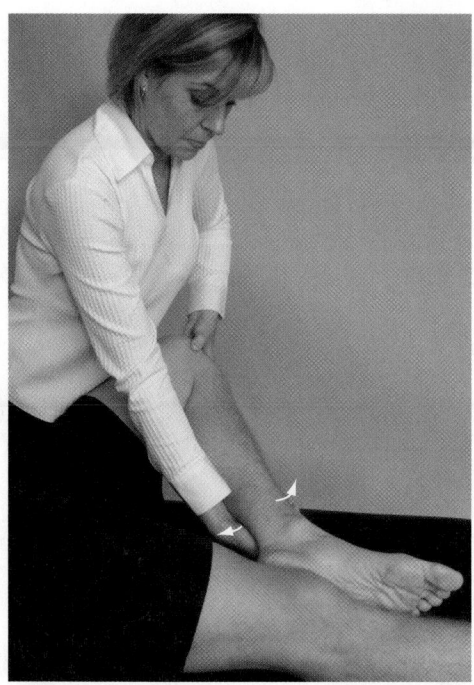

Figure 12-112 Cabot's popliteal sign for a meniscus lesion.

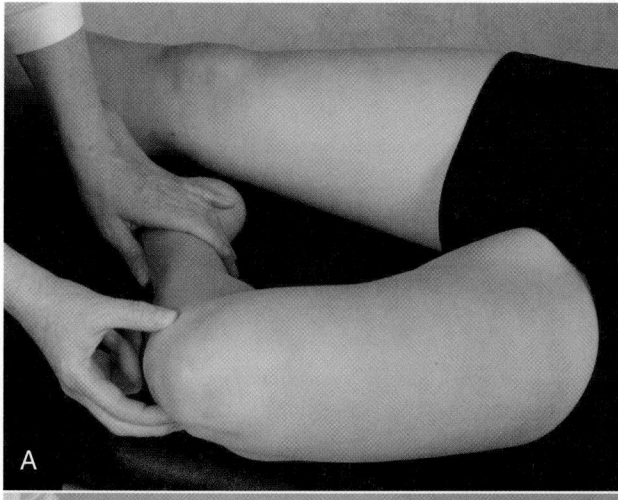
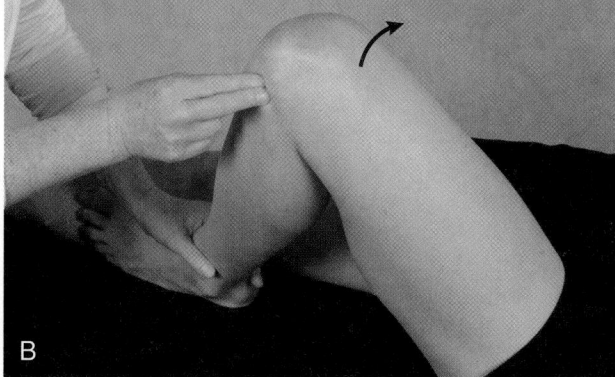

Figure 12-113 Dynamic knee test. A, Starting position. Hip flexed and abducted, knee at 90°. **B,** The examiner then adducts the flexed hip while palpating the lateral joint line.

12-113, *B*). If there is increased pain on joint line or a sharp pain at end of adduction, the test is considered positive for a lateral meniscus tear.

☑ *Ege's Test.* This test has been described as a weight-bearing McMurray's Test.[252] The patient stands with the knees in extension and the feet 30 to 40 cm (11 to 15 inches) away from each other. To test the medial meniscus, the patient laterally rotates each tibia maximally and squats causing the distance between the knees and lateral rotation to increase. The patient then stands slowly while leaving the feet laterally rotated (Figure 12-114, *A* and *B*). To test the lateral meniscus, both tibias are medially rotated maximally while the patient squats and then stands up (Figure 12-114, *C* and *D*). A full squat in medial rotation is very difficult even in healthy individuals. Both tests are considered positive if pain and/or a click is felt by the patient along the joint line or heard by the examiner. The pain or click may be heard when squatting or coming out of the squat. It was reported that anterior tears are more likely to occur in earlier knee flexion while posterior horn tears cause the click or pain in more flexion. The test may not be as useful in acute cases (less than 6 weeks). It is purported to be as or more accurate than joint line pain.

❓ *Kromer's Sign.* This test is similar to Bohler's sign except that the knee is flexed and extended while the varus and valgus stresses are applied.[79] A positive test is indicated by the same pain on the opposite joint line.

☑ *McMurray Test.* The McMurray test is the grandfather of meniscus tests of the knee. However, the reliability and sensitivity of the test has been found to be low.[253] The patient lies in the supine position with the knee completely flexed (the heel to the buttock).[254,255] The examiner then medially rotates the tibia and extends the knee (Figure 12-115). If there is a loose fragment of the lateral meniscus, this action causes a snap or click that is often accompanied by pain. By repeatedly changing the amount of flexion and then applying the medial rotation to the tibia followed by extension, the examiner can test the entire posterior aspect of the meniscus from the posterior horn to the middle segment. The anterior half of the meniscus is not as easily tested because the pressure on the meniscus is not as great. To test the medial meniscus, the examiner performs the same procedure with the knee laterally rotated. Kim and colleagues[256] reported that meniscus lesions may be found on the medial side with medial rotation and on the lateral side with lateral rotation.

The test may be modified by medially rotating the tibia, extending the knee, and moving through the full ROM to test the lateral meniscus. The process is repeated several times. The tibia is then laterally rotated, and the process is repeated to test the medial meniscus. Both methods are described by McMurray.[254]

❓ *Modified Helfet Test.*[257] In the normal knee, the tibial tuberosity is in line with the midline of the patella when

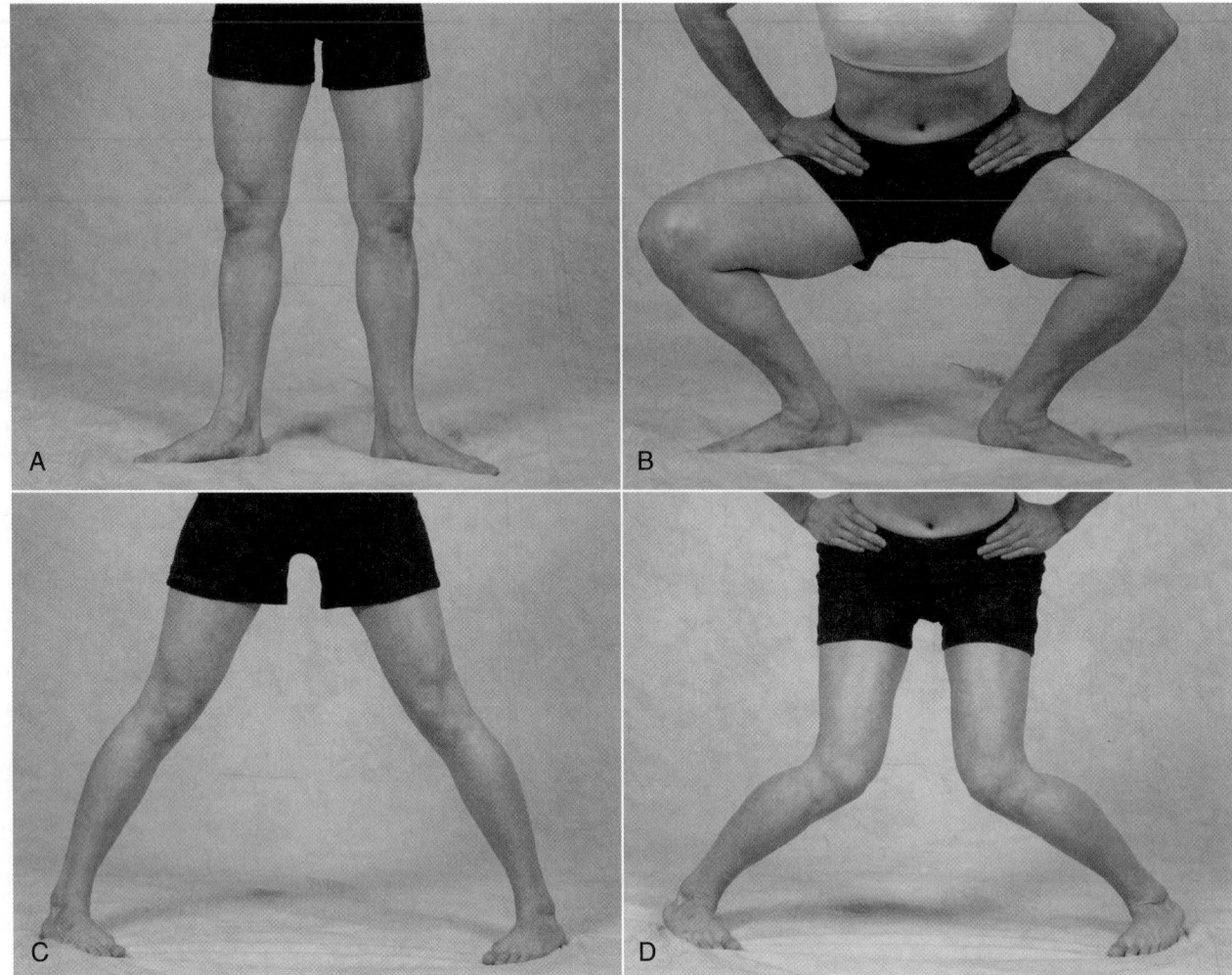

Figure 12-114 Ege's test. The patient is weight bearing. To detect a medial meniscal tear, both lower extremities are first held in maximum lateral rotation (**A**). The patient then squats while maintaining the lateral rotation (**B**). For lateral meniscal tears, both lower extremities are held in maximum medial rotation (**C**). Maximum medial rotations of both lower extremities are preserved during squatting (**D**).

the knee is flexed to 90°. When the knee is extended, however, the tibial tubercle is in line with the lateral border of the patella (Figure 12-116). If this change does not occur with the change in movement, rotation is blocked, indicating that there is injury to the meniscus, there is a possible cruciate injury, or the quadriceps muscles have insufficient strength to "screw home" the knee.

O'Donohue's Test. If a patient experiences pain along the joint line, the patient is asked to lie in the supine position. The examiner flexes the knee to 90°, rotates it medially and laterally twice, and then fully flexes and rotates it both ways again. A positive sign is indicated by increased pain on rotation in either or both positions and is indicative of capsular irritation or a meniscus tear.

Passler Rotational Grind Test.[79] The patient sits with the test knee extended and held at the ankle between the examiner's legs proximal to the examiner's knees. The examiner places both thumbs over the medial joint line

and moves the knee in a circular fashion, medially and laterally rotating the tibia while the knee is rotated through various flexion angles. Simultaneously, the examiner applies a varus or a valgus stress (Figure 12-117). Pain elicited on the joint line indicates a meniscus lesion.

Payr's Test. The patient lies supine with the test leg in the figure-four position (Figure 12-118). If pain is elicited on the medial joint line, the test is considered positive for a meniscus lesion, primarily in the middle or posterior part of the meniscus.[79]

Steinman's Tenderness Displacement Test. Steinman's sign is indicated by point tenderness and pain on the joint line that appears to move anteriorly when the knee is extended and moves posteriorly when the knee is flexed. It indicates a possible meniscus tear. Medial pain is elicited on lateral rotation, and lateral pain is elicited on medial rotation.

Test for Retreating or Retracting Meniscus. The patient sits on the edge of the examining table or lies in the

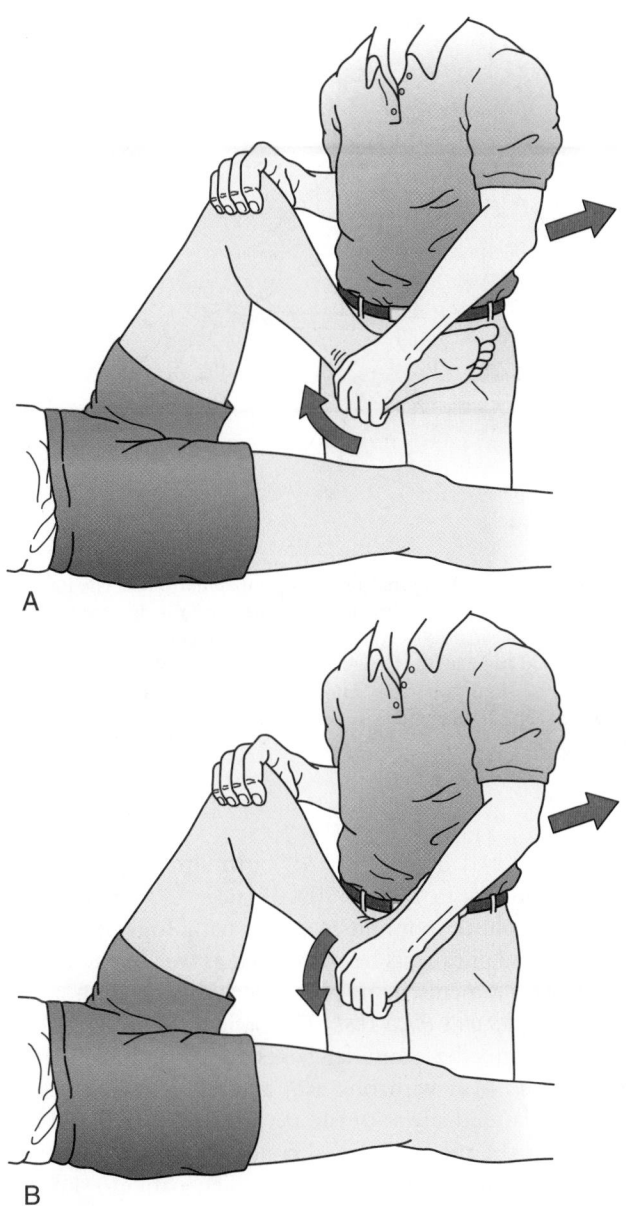

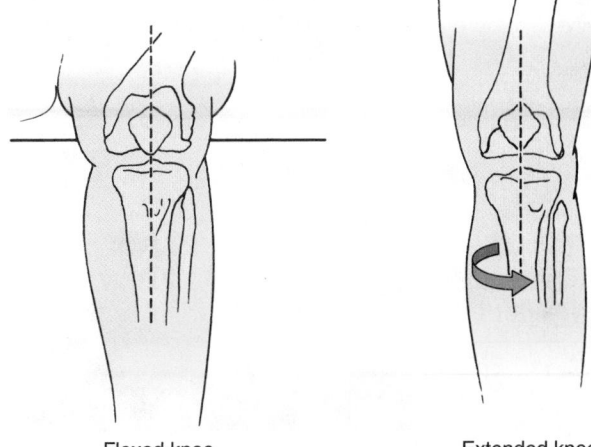

Flexed knee   Extended knee

Figure 12-116 Modified Helfet test (negative test shown).

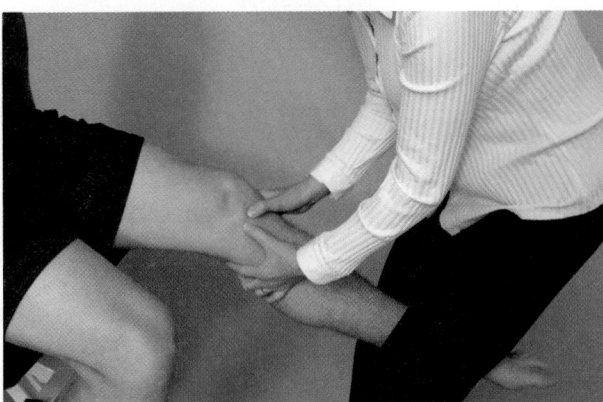

Figure 12-117 Passler rotational grind test for meniscus pathology.

Figure 12-115 McMurray test. A, For medial meniscus test. **B,** For lateral meniscus test.

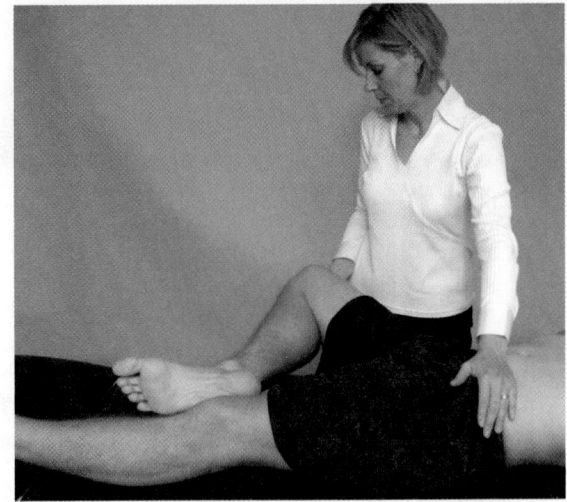

Figure 12-118 Payr's sign for a meniscus lesion.

supine position with the knee flexed to 90°.[257] The examiner places one finger over the joint line of the patient's knee anterior to the medial collateral ligament, where the curved margin of the medial femoral condyle approaches the tibial tuberosity (Figure 12-119). The patient's leg and foot are then passively laterally rotated, and the meniscus normally disappears. The leg is medially and laterally rotated several times with the meniscus appearing and disappearing. The knee must be flexed and the muscles relaxed to do the test. If the meniscus does not appear, a torn meniscus is indicated because rotation of the tibia is not occurring. The examiner must palpate carefully, because a distinct structure is difficult to palpate. If the examiner medially and laterally rotates

the unaffected leg several times first, the meniscus can be felt pushing against the finger on medial rotation, and it disappears on lateral rotation.

✓ *Thessaly Test.*[258] The patient stands flat footed on one leg while the examiner provides his or her hands for

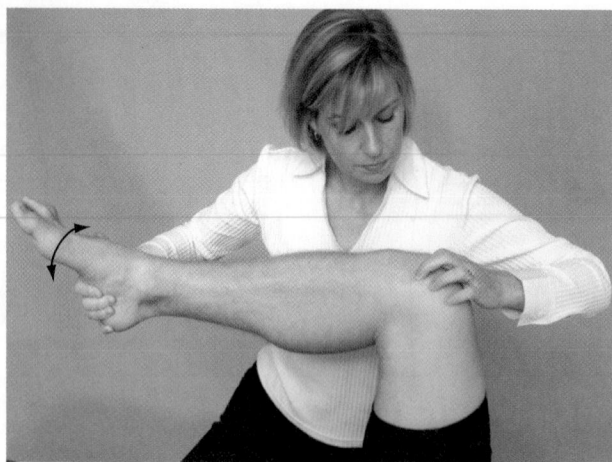

Figure 12-119 Test for a retreating meniscus.

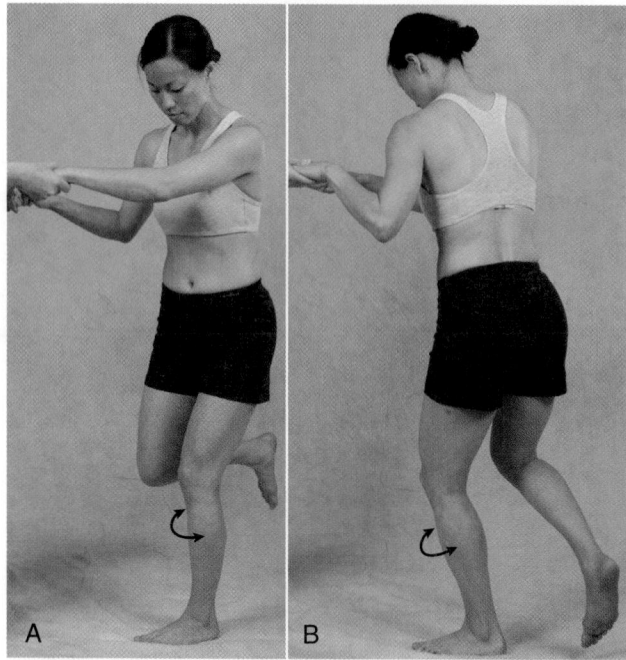

Figure 12-120 Thessaly test. Patient stands on test leg. **A,** In 5° flexion with rotation. **B,** In 20° flexion with rotation.

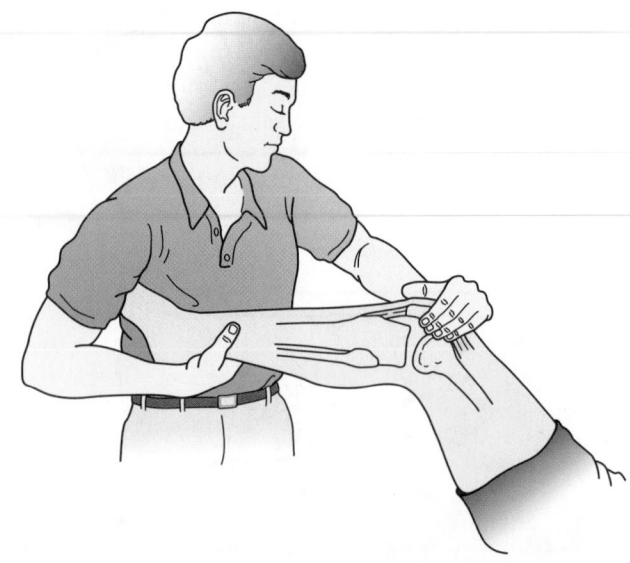

Figure 12-121 Examination for suprapatellar plica. The foot and tibia are held in medial rotation. The patella is displaced slightly medially with the fingers over the course of the plica. The knee is passively flexed and extended, eliciting a "pop" of the plica and associated tenderness. (Redrawn from Hughston JC, Walsh WM, Puddu G: Patellar subluxation and dislocation, Philadelphia, 1984, WB Saunders, p. 29.)

balance. The patient then flexes the knee to 5° and rotates the femur on the tibia medially and laterally three times while maintaining the 5° flexion (Figure 12-120, *A*). The good leg is tested first, and then the injured leg. The test is then repeated at 20° flexion (Figure 12-120, *B*). The test is considered positive for a meniscus tear if the patient experiences medial or lateral joint line discomfort. The patient may also have a sense of locking or catching in the knee.

Tests for Plica Lesions

In the knee, plica are embryological remnants that have remained in some people after birth.[259–261] Normally, they are reabsorbed by the time of birth although remnants may be present in 20% to 50% of knees.[262–264] Because an abnormal plica can mimic meniscus pathology, it is essential that the plica tests be performed as well as the meniscus tests if a meniscus or plica injury is suspected.

⚠ *Hughston's Plica Test.* The patient lies in the supine position, and the examiner flexes the knee and medially rotates the tibia with one arm and hand while pressing the patella medially with the heel of the other hand and palpating the medial femoral condyle with the fingers of the same hand (Figure 12-121). The patient's knee is passively flexed and extended while the examiner feels for "popping" of the plica band under the fingers. The popping indicates a positive test.[186]

⚠ *Mediopatellar Plica Test (Mital-Hayden Test or Medial Plica Shelf Test).* The patient lies in the supine position with the affected knee flexed to 30° resting on a support or the examiner's arm (Figure 12-122). The examiner then pushes the patella medially with the thumb. If the patient complains of pain or a click, it indicates a positive test caused by pinching of the edge of the plica between the medial femoral condyle and the patella. The pain may indicate a mediopatellar plica.[265]

⚠ *Patellar Bowstring Test.*[55] The patient lies on his or her side with the test leg uppermost. Using the heel of one hand, the examiner pushes the patella medially and holds it there. The examiner then flexes the patient's knee and medially rotates the tibia with the other hand. The patient's knee is then extended (Figure 12-123) while the examiner feels for any sounds.

⚠️ *Plica "Stutter" Test.* The patient is seated on the edge of the examining table with both knees flexed to 90°. The examiner places a finger over one patella to palpate during movement. The patient is then instructed to slowly extend the knee. If the test is positive, the patella stutters or jumps somewhere between 60° and 45° of flexion (0° being straight leg) during an otherwise smooth movement. The test is effective only if there is no joint swelling.

Tests for Swelling

When assessing swelling, the examiner must determine the type and amount of swelling that are present. Although

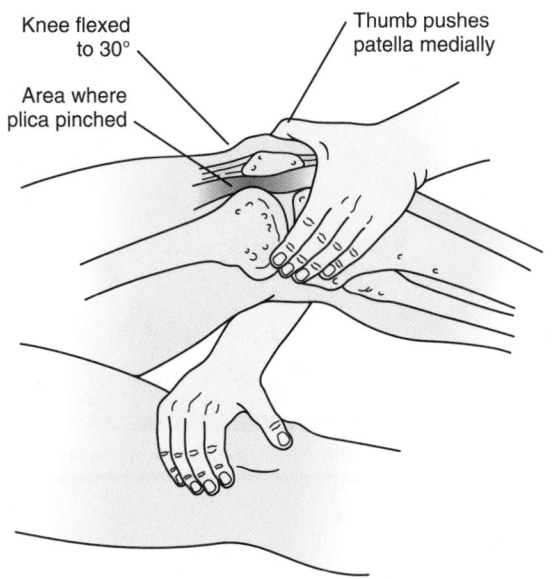

Knee flexed to 30°

Area where plica pinched

Thumb pushes patella medially

🎞 **Figure 12-122** Positioning for mediopatellar plica test.

the tests for swelling are listed under the "Special Tests" section, the examiner should always be testing for swelling when examining the knee. In addition, the examiner must differentiate between swelling and synovial thickening. With swelling, the knee assumes its resting position of 15° to 25° of flexion, which allows the synovial cavity the maximum capacity for holding fluid. If the injury is sufficiently severe, the fluid extravasates into the soft tissue surrounding the joint as a result of torn structures (i.e., ligaments, capsule, synovium). Therefore lack of effusion should not lull the examiner into thinking the injury is a minor one.

If the swelling consists of blood that results in a hemarthrosis (within the joint), it may be caused by a ligament tear, osteochondral fracture, or peripheral meniscus tear. "Blood" swelling comes on very quickly (within 1 to 2 hours), and the skin becomes very taut. On palpation, it has a "doughy" feeling and is relatively hard to the touch. The joint surface feels warm. Usually, excess blood should be aspirated, or osteoarthritis may result from irritation of the cartilage. Blood swelling in the form of ecchymosis may also be seen around the knee, but commonly this blood will begin to "track" down the leg because of gravity as it becomes visible (see Figure 1-10).

Normally, synovial fluid swelling caused by joint irritation occurs in 8 to 24 hours. The feeling within the joint is a fluctuating or "boggy" feeling. The joint surface feels warm and tender. Swelling usually occurs with activity and disappears after a few days of inactivity.

The third type of joint swelling is purulent or pus swelling, in which the joint surface is hot to the touch. Often it is red, and the patient has general signs of infection or pyrexia.

✅ *Brush, Stroke, or Bulge Test.* Also called the *wipe test,* this test assesses minimal effusion. The examiner

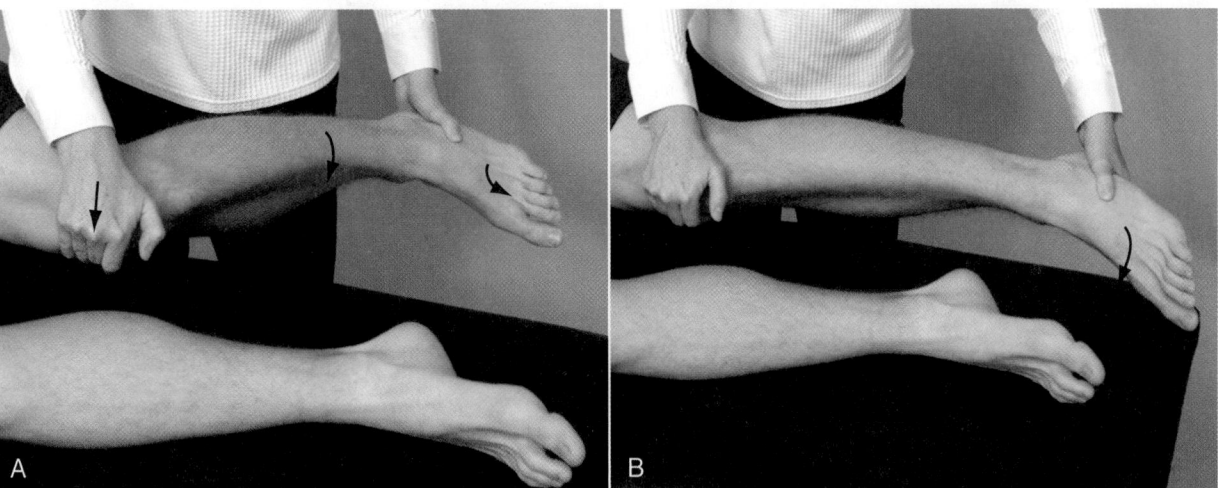

Figure 12-123 Bowstring test for plica. **A,** Using the heel of one hand, the examiner pushes the patella medially and holds it there. The examiner then flexes the patient's knee and medially rotates the tibia with the other hand. **B,** The patient's knee is then extended while the examiner feels for any sounds.

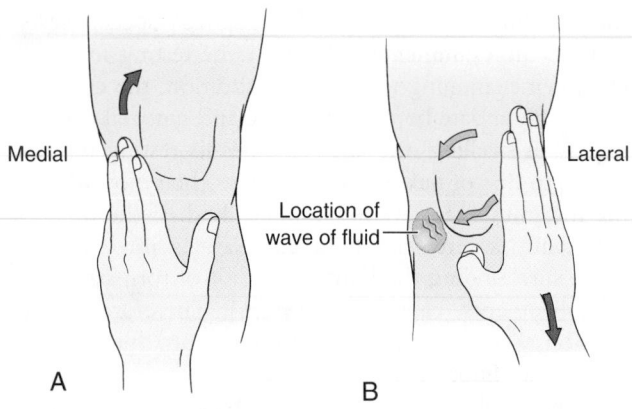

Medial

Location of wave of fluid

Lateral

A   B

Figure 12-124 Brush test for swelling. A, Hand strokes up. **B,** Hand strokes down.

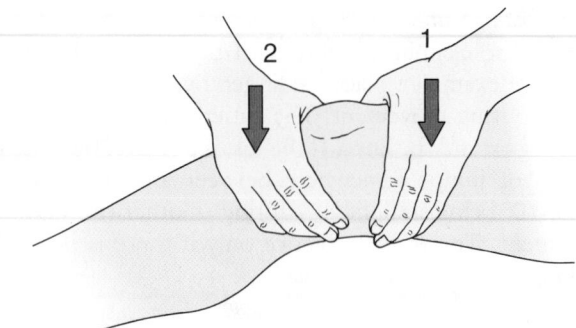

2   1

Figure 12-125 Hand positioning for fluctuation test. First one hand is pushed down *(arrow 1);* then the other hand is pushed down *(arrow 2).* The examiner will feel fluid shifting back and forth under one hand and then the other.

TABLE 12-12

Effusion Grading Scale of the Knee Joint Based on the Stroke Test

Grade	Test Result
Zero	No wave produced on downstroke
Trace	Small wave on medial side with downstroke
1+	Larger bulge on medial side with downstroke
2+	Effusion spontaneously returns to medial side after upstroke (no downstroke necessary)
3+	So much fluid that it is not possible to move the effusion out of the medial aspect of the knee

From Sturgill LP, et al: Interrater reliability of a clinical scale to assess knee joint effusion. J Orthop Sports Phys Ther 39:846, 2009.

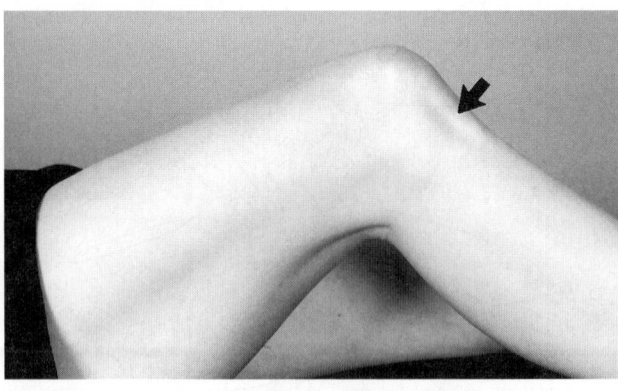

Figure 12-126 Indentation test. *Arrow* indicates where to watch for filling of indentation.

commences just below the joint line on the medial side of the patella, stroking proximally toward the patient's hip as far as the suprapatellar pouch two or three times with the palm and fingers (Figure 12-124). With the opposite hand, the examiner strokes down the lateral side of the patella. A wave of fluid passes to the medial side of the joint and bulges just below the medial distal portion or border of the patella. The wave of fluid may take up to 2 seconds to appear. Normally, the knee contains 1 to 7 mL of synovial fluid. This test shows as little as 4 to 8 mL of extra fluid within the knee. Sturgill, et al.[266] developed an effusion grading scale based on the stroke test (Table 12-12).[86]

Fluctuation Test. The examiner places the palm of one hand over the suprapatellar pouch and the palm of the other hand anterior to the joint with the thumb and index finger just beyond the margins of the patella (Figure 12-125). By pressing down with one hand and then the other, the examiner may feel the synovial fluid fluctuate under the hands and move from one hand to the other, indicating significant effusion.

Indentation Test.[267] The patient lies supine. The examiner passively flexes the good leg, noting an indentation on the lateral side of the patellar tendon (Figure 12-126). The good knee is fully flexed, and the indentation remains. The injured knee is then slowly flexed while the examiner watches for the disappearance of the indentation. At that point, knee flexion is stopped. The disappearance of the indentation is caused by swelling and indicates a positive test. The angle at which the indentation disappears depends on the amount of swelling. The greater the swelling, the sooner the indentation disappears. If the thumb and finger are placed on each side of the patellar tendon, the fluid can be made to fluctuate back and forth. This method, like the brush test, can detect minimal levels of swelling.

Patellar Tap Test ("Ballotable Patella"). With the patient's knee extended or flexed to discomfort, the examiner applies a slight tap or pressure over the patella (Figure 12-127). When this is done, a floating of the patella should be felt. This is sometimes called the **"dancing patella"** sign. A modification of this test calls

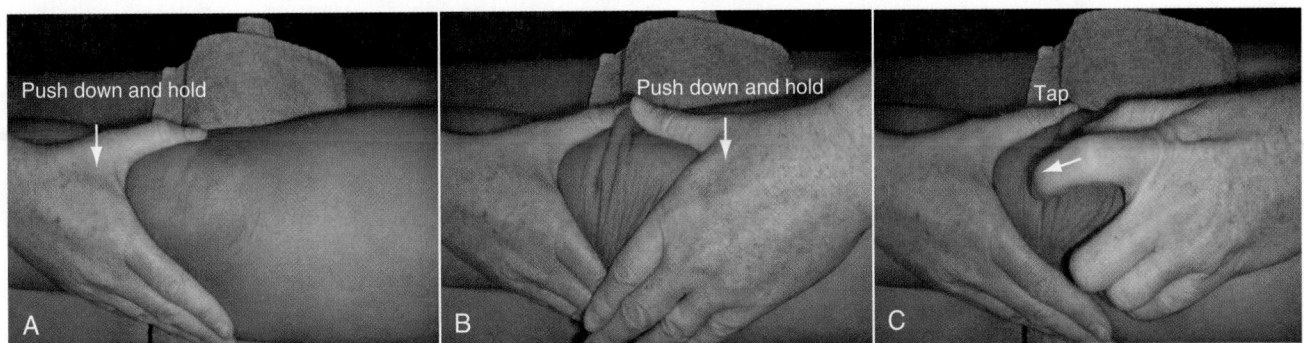

Figure 12-127 Patellar tap test ("ballotable patella"). A, Step 1. **B,** Step 2. **C,** Step 3.

for the examiner to apply the thumb and forefinger of one hand lightly on both sides of the patella. The examiner then strokes down on the suprapatellar pouch with the other hand.[79] A positive test is indicated by separation of the thumb and forefinger. This test can detect a large amount of swelling (40 to 50 mL) in the knee, which can also be noted by observation.

❓ *Peripatellar Swelling Test*.[268] The patient lies supine with the knee extended. The examiner carefully milks fluid from the suprapatellar pouch distally. With the opposite hand, the examiner palpates adjacent to the patellar tendon (usually on the medial side) for fluid accumulation or a wave of fluid passing under the fingers. Reider[45] calls this a **palpable fluid wave.** If less swelling is evident, Reider[45] suggests the **visible fluid wave.** The examiner strokes the fluid into the suprapatellar pouch. With one hand, the examiner then squeezes or pushes down on the suprapatellar pouch while watching the hollows on each side of the patella for a wave of fluid to pass. This test is similar to the brush test.

Tests for Patellofemoral Dysfunction

Patellofemoral dysfunction, or PFPS, implies there is some pathology affecting the patellofemoral joint.[58,269] This pathology may be the result of biomechanical factors or pathophysiological processes or loss of tissue homeostasis resulting in synovitis and an inflamed fat pad.[270] Commonly, patients with patellofemoral problems experience pain when climbing or descending stairs, when stepping up or down, with prolonged sitting (movie sign), when squatting, or when getting up from a chair. The examiner should consider assessing the whole lower kinetic chain and its effect on the patellofemoral joint when PFPS is suspected.[49–54,271,272] For example, it has been found that hip abductors and external rotators are weak and the iliotibial band is tight in PFPS patients.[64,273,274] In some cases, the pain may cause reflex inhibition, resulting in buckling or giving way of the knee.[275]

Nijs et al.[276] reported that the vastus medialis coordination test, the patellar apprehension test, and the eccentric step test had the most positive likelihood ratio in patients with patellofemoral pain syndrome.

Risk Factors That May Contribute to Patellofemoral Pain Syndrome*

- Patellar dysplasia (e.g., patella alta or baja)
- Tight patellar retinaculum (especially lateral)
- Abnormal patellar tracking
- Abnormal patellar tilt or rotation
- Abnormal patellar alignment relative to the femur (e.g., Q-angle outside the normal 13° to 18°)
- Crossover gait
- Excessive genu valgum/varum
- Muscle weakness (e.g., vastus medialis obliquus [VMO], hip abductor and lateral rotators, ankle dorsiflexors)
- Muscle imbalance (e.g., quadriceps/hamstrings ratio)
- Excessive tibial torsion (especially medial)
- Foot malalignment (e.g., rearfoot varus or valgus, excessive pronation/supination of the foot)
- Muscle hypomobility (e.g., quadriceps, hamstrings, gastrocnemius, iliotibial band, hip adductors)
- Trauma to patella (e.g., dislocation, direct blow)
- Abnormal repetitive stress to patella (e.g., running on the same side of road or sidewalk continually [camber of road or sidewalk affects foot-knee mechanics])
- Training shoes worn (e.g., control shoe versus cushioning shoe, shoes "broken down")
- Excessive pelvic tilt (anterior/posterior, medial/lateral)

*Patellofemoral pain syndrome may be the result of any or all of the above. In reality, the definitive cause of patellofemoral pain syndrome is unknown.

❓ *Active Patellar Grind Test*.[45] The patient sits on the examining table with the knee flexed 90° over the edge of the table. While the patient slowly straightens the knee, the examiner places a hand over the patella to feel for crepitus. Where in the ROM that pain occurs gives an indication of what part of the patella is demonstrating pathology (see Figure 12-2). Greater force can be applied through the patella by asking the patient to step up and step down on a small stool while the examiner gently palpates the patella for crepitus and pain (**step up–step down test**).[45]

⚠ *Clarke's Sign (Patellar Grind Test)*. This test assesses the presence of a problem with the articulation between the articular surface of the patella and the articular surfaces of the femoral condyles, but it is not specific to one pathology, and the validity of the test has been questioned.[277] The examiner presses down slightly proximal to the upper pole or base of the patella with the web of the hand as the patient lies relaxed with the knee extended (Figure 12-128). Reider[45] recommends pushing down on the patella directly. The patient is then asked to contract the quadriceps muscles while the examiner pushes down. If the patient can complete and maintain the contraction without pain, the test is considered negative. If the test causes retropatellar pain and the patient cannot hold a contraction, the test is considered positive. Because the examiner can achieve a positive test on anyone if sufficient pressure is applied to the patella, the amount of pressure that is applied must be carefully controlled. The best way to do this is to repeat the procedure several times, increasing the pressure each time and comparing the results with those of the unaffected side. To test different parts of the

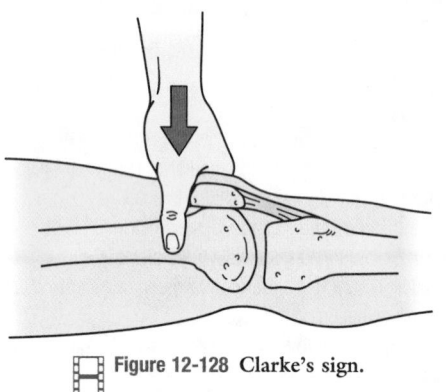

Figure 12-128 Clarke's sign.

patella, the knee should be tested in 30°, 60°, and 90° of flexion as well as in full extension.

Eccentric Step Test.[135,136,276] The patient stands on a 15-cm (6 inch)–high step or stool while keeping the hands on the hips. The patient steps down, first leading with the injured leg (this tests the good leg first) as slowly and smoothly as he or she can (Figure 12-129, *B*). The test is considered positive if pain is felt by the patient during the test.

Frund's Sign. The patient is in the sitting position. The examiner percusses the patella in various positions of knee flexion. Pain indicates a positive test and may signify chondromalacia patellae.

Lateral Pull Test. The patient lies supine with the leg extended. The patient contracts the quadriceps while the examiner watches the movement of the patella.[278] Normally, the patella moves superiorly, or superiorly and laterally in equal proportions (Figure 12-130). If lateral movement is excessive, the test is positive for lateral overpull of the quadriceps, resulting in a patellofemoral arthralgia. Watson, et al.[279] have questioned the reliability of this test especially when performed by inexperienced examiners.

McConnell Test for Chondromalacia Patellae. The patient is sitting with the femur laterally rotated. The patient performs isometric quadriceps contractions at 120°, 90°, 60°, 30°, and 0° with each contraction held for 10 seconds (Figure 12-131). If pain is produced during any of the contractions, the patient's leg is passively returned to full extension by the examiner. The patient's leg is then fully supported on the examiner's knee, and the examiner pushes the patella medially. The

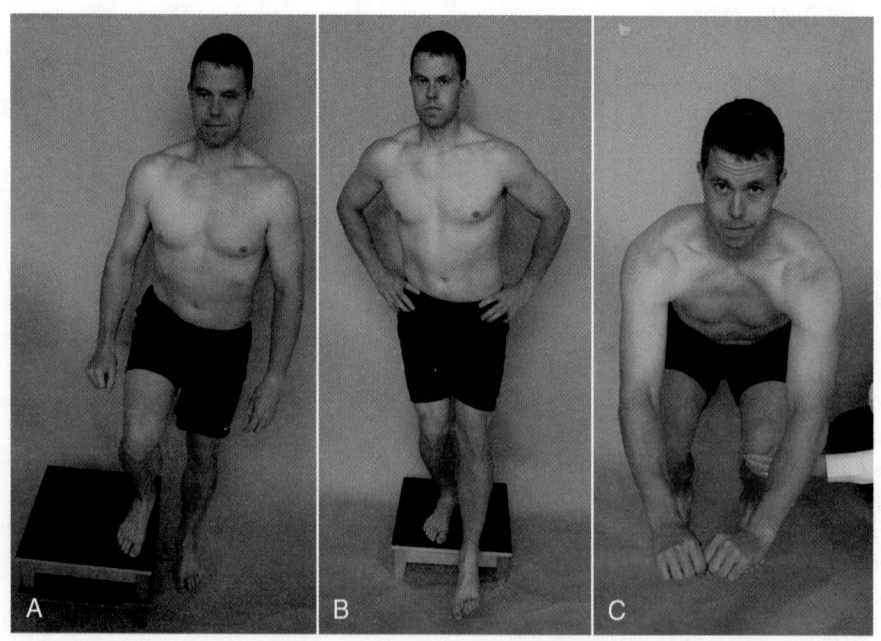

Figure 12-129 Step tests. **A,** Step up test. **B,** Eccentric step test. **C,** Waldron test.

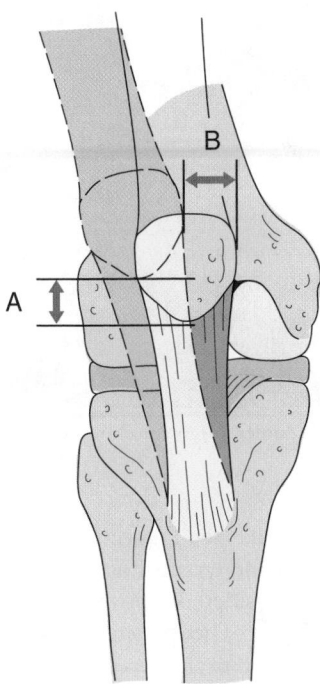

Figure 12-130 **Lateral pull test.** Normally, A > B or A = B; with lateral overpull of the quadriceps, B > A. (From Kolowich PA, Paulos LE, Rosenberg TD, et al: Lateral release of the patella: indications and contraindications. Am J Sports Med 18:361, 1990.)

medial glide is maintained while the knee is returned to the painful angle, and the patient performs an isometric contraction, again with the patella held medially. If the pain is decreased, the pain is patellofemoral in origin. Each angle is tested in a similar fashion.[280]

⍰ *Passive Patellar Tilt Test.* The patient lies supine with the knee extended and the quadriceps relaxed. The examiner stands at the end of the examining table and lifts the lateral edge of the patella away from the lateral femoral condyle. The patella should not be pushed medially or laterally but rather should remain in the femoral trochlea.[278] The normal angle is 15°, although males may have an angle 5° less than that of females (Figure 12-132). Patients with angles less than this are prone to patellofemoral syndrome. Watson, et al.[279] have questioned the reliability of this test, especially when performed by inexperienced examiners.

⚠ *Step Up Test.*[275] The patient stands beside a stool that is 25 cm (10 inches) high. The examiner asks the patient to step up sideways onto the stool using the good leg. The test is repeated with the other leg. Normally, the patient should have no difficulty doing the test and have no pain. Inability to do the test may indicate patellofemoral arthralgia, weak quadriceps, or an inability to stabilize the pelvis (Figure 12-129, *A*).

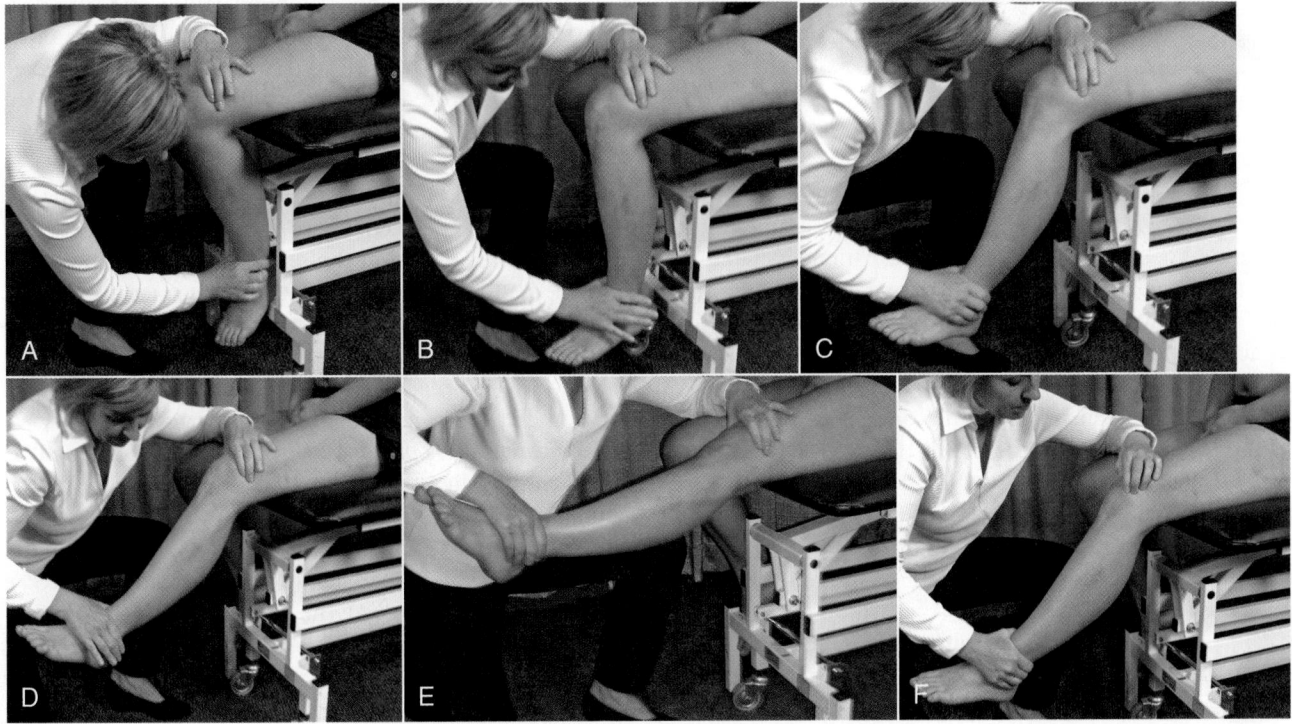

Figure 12-131 **McConnell test for chondromalacia patellae. A,** 120°. **B,** 90°. **C,** 60°. **D,** 30°. **E,** 0°. **F,** Testing at 60°, holding patella medially.

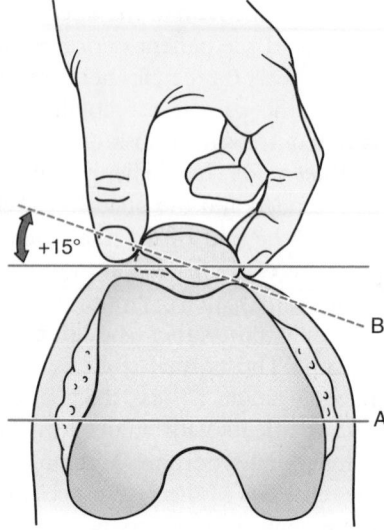

Figure 12-132 Passive patellar tilt test. (Redrawn from Kolowich PA, Paulos LE, Rosenberg TD, et al: Lateral release of the patella: indications and contraindications. Am J Sports Med 18:361, 1990.)

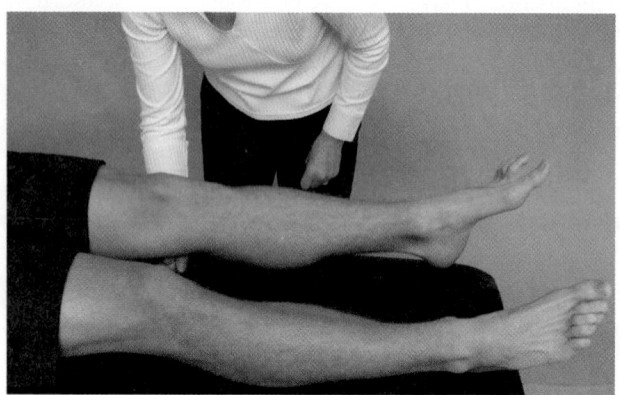

Figure 12-133 Vastus medialis coordination test.

(?) *Vastus Medialis Coordination Test.*[276,281] The patient lies supine while the examiner places a fist under the patient's knee (Figure 12-133). The patient is asked to slowly extend the knee without pressing into the examiner's fist or lifting the leg away from the fist while trying to achieve full extension. The test is considered positive if the patient cannot fully extend the knee or has difficulty achieving full extension smoothly or tries to use the hip flexors or extensors to accomplish the task.

(?) *Waldron Test.* This test also assesses the presence of patellofemoral syndrome and functions in a similar fashion to the step up test and the eccentric step test.[46] The examiner palpates the patella while the patient performs several slow deep knee bends (these may be unilateral squats or bilateral for easier comparison) (Figure 12-129, C). As the patient goes through the ROM, the examiner should note the amount of crepitus (significant only if accompanied by pain), where it occurs in the ROM, the amount of pain, and whether there is "catching" or poor

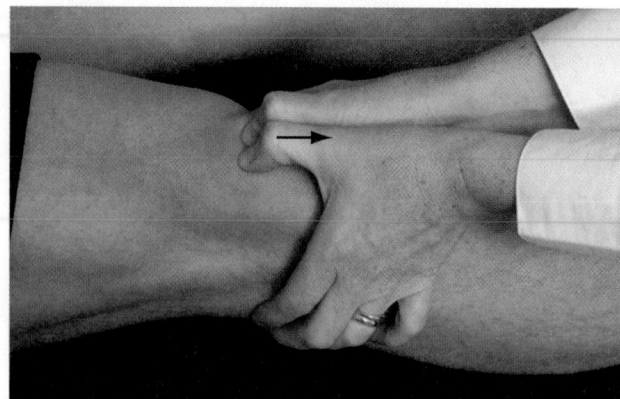

Figure 12-134 Zohler's sign for chondromalacia patellae.

tracking of the patella (see Figure 12-28) throughout the movement. If pain and crepitus occur together during the movement, it is considered a positive sign.[46]

(?) *Zohler's Sign.*[79] The patient lies supine with the knees extended. The examiner pulls the patella distally and holds it in this position. The patient is asked to contract the quadriceps (Figure 12-134). Pain indicates a positive test for chondromalacia patellae. However, the test may be positive (false positive) in a large proportion of the normal population.

Other Tests

(?) *Daniel's Quadriceps Neutral Angle Test.*[282] The patient lies supine, and the unaffected leg is tested first. The patient's hip is flexed to 45°, and the knee is flexed to 90° with the foot flat on the examining table. The patient is asked to extend the knee isometrically while the examiner holds down the foot. If tibial displacement is noted, knee flexion is decreased (posterior tibial displacement) or increased (anterior tibial displacement). The process is repeated until the angle at which there is no tibial displacement is reached (Figure 12-135). This angle, the quadriceps neutral angle, averages 70° (range, 60° to 90°). The injured knee is placed in the same neutral angle position, and the patient is asked to contract the quadriceps. Any anterior displacement indicates posterior cruciate ligament insufficiency. The quadriceps neutral angle is primarily used for machine testing of laxity (e.g., KT-1000 arthrometer, Stryker knee laxity test apparatus).

(✓) *Fairbank's Apprehension Test.* This is a test for **dislocation of the patella.**[186,283] The patient lies in the supine position with the quadriceps muscles relaxed and the knee flexed to 30° while the examiner carefully and slowly pushes the patella laterally (Figure 12-136). Tanner, et al.[284] believed the patella should be pushed laterally and distally to make the test more sensitive. If the patient feels the patella is going to dislocate, the patient contracts the quadriceps muscles to bring the patella back "into line." This action indicates a positive test. The patient will also have an apprehensive look.

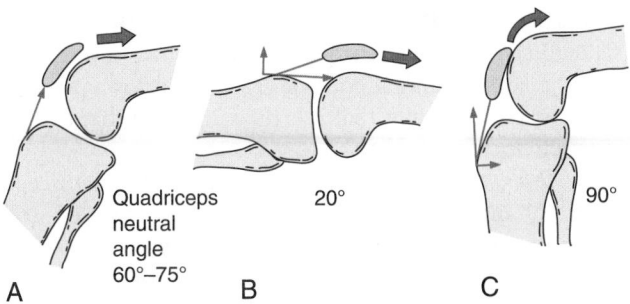

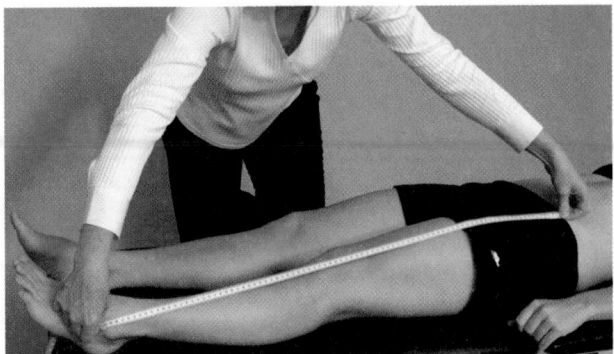

Figure 12-137 Measuring leg length (to the lateral malleolus).

Figure 12-135 During open chain knee extension, tibial translation is a function of the shear force produced by the patellar tendon. **A,** Quadriceps neutral position. The patellar tendon force is perpendicular to the tibial plateaus and results in compression of the joint surfaces without shear force. **B,** At flexion angles less than the angle of the quadriceps neutral position, orientation of the patellar tendon produces anterior shear of the tibia. **C,** At angles greater than the angle of the quadriceps neutral position, patellar tendon force causes a posterior shear of the tibia. (From Daniel DM, Stone ML, Barnett P, et al: Use of the quadriceps active test to diagnose posterior cruciate ligament disruption and measure posterior laxity of the knee. J Bone Joint Surg Am 70:386–391, 1988.)

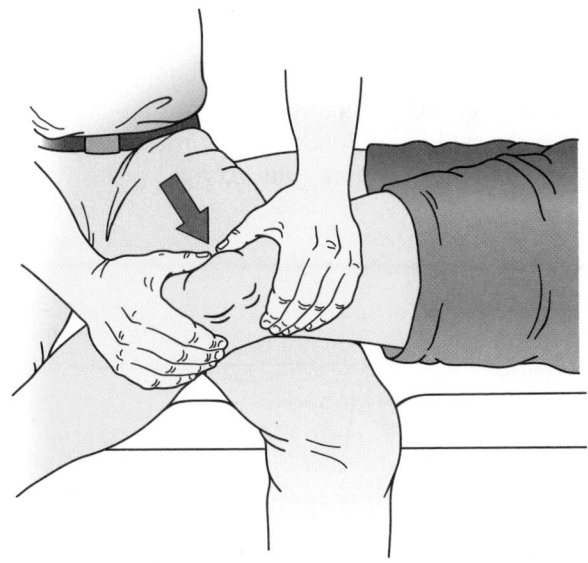

Figure 12-136 Apprehension test. (Redrawn from Hughston JC, Walsh WM, Puddu G: Patellar subluxation and dislocation, Philadelphia, 1984, WB Saunders, p. 29.)

Functional Leg Length. The patient stands in the normal relaxed stance. The examiner palpates the anterior superior iliac spines (ASISs) and then the posterior superior iliac spines (PSISs) and notes any differences. The examiner then positions the patient so that the patient's subtalar joints are in neutral while bearing weight (see Chapter 13). While the patient holds this position with the toes straight ahead and the knee straight, the examiner repalpates the ASISs and the PSISs. If the previously noted differences remain, the pelvis and sacroiliac joints should be evaluated further. If the previously noted

differences disappear, the examiner should suspect a functional leg length difference caused by hip, knee, ankle, or foot problems—primarily ankle or foot problems.

? ***Functional Test for Quadriceps Contusion.*** The patient lies in the prone position while the examiner passively flexes the knee as much as possible. If passive knee flexion is 90° or more, it is only a mild contusion. If passive knee flexion is less than 90°, the contusion is moderate to severe, and the patient should not be allowed to bear weight. Normally, the heel-to-buttock distance should not exceed 10 cm (4 inches) in men and 5 cm (2 inches) in women. This test may also be used to test tightness of the quadriceps (vasti) muscles. If the range is limited and the end feel is muscle stretch, the vastus medialis, lateralis, and/or intermedius is tight. Testing for a tight rectus femoris is described in Chapter 11.

✓ ***Measurement of Leg Length.*** The patient lies in the supine position with the legs at a right angle to a line joining the two ASISs. With a tape measure, the examiner obtains the distance from one ASIS to the lateral or medial malleolus on that side, placing the metal end of the tape measure immediately distal to and up against the ASIS (Figure 12-137). The tape is stretched so that the other hand pushes the tape against the distal aspect of the medial (or lateral) malleolus, and the reading on the tape measure is noted. The other side is tested similarly. A difference between the two sides of as much as 1.0 to 1.5 cm is considered normal. However, the examiner must remember that even this difference may result in pathological symptoms. If there is a difference, the examiner can determine its site of occurrence by measuring from the high point on the iliac crest to the greater trochanter (for coxa vara), from the greater trochanter to the lateral knee joint line (for femoral shaft length), and from the medial knee joint line to the medial malleolus (for tibial length). The two legs are then compared. The examiner must also remember that torsion deformities to the femur or tibia can alter leg length.

? ***Measurement of Muscle Bulk (Anthropometric Measurements for Effusion and Atrophy).*** The examiner selects areas where muscle bulk or swelling is greatest and measures the circumference of the leg. It is important to note on the patient's chart how far above or below the apex or base of the patella one is measuring and whether the tape measure is placed above or below that mark. The following are common measurement points:

1. 15 cm (6 inches) below the apex of the patella
2. Apex of the patella or joint line
3. 5 cm (2 inches) above the base of the patella
4. 10 cm (4 inches) above the base of the patella
5. 15 cm (6 inches) above the base of the patella
6. 23 cm (9 inches) above the base of the patella

Hughston[47] advocated using the lateral joint line rather than the patella for the beginning point of measurement; he believed that the joint line was more constant. The examiner must also note, if possible, whether swelling or muscle bulk is being measured and remember that there is no correlation between muscle bulk and strength.

⚠ *Moving Patellar Apprehension Test for Lateral Patellar Instability.*[285] For the moving patellar apprehension test (MPAT), the patient lies supine with the thigh on the examining table and the examiner holding the leg in full extension off the table. The examiner then translates the patella laterally using the examiner's thumb, and the patella is held laterally while the examiner flexes the knee to 90° and then returns the leg to full extension (step 1). If there is patient apprehension or contraction of the quadriceps, the test is considered positive. If the patella is then translated medially and the knee flexed, there will be no apprehension or protective quadriceps contraction (step 2) as the patella most commonly subluxes or dislocates laterally. For the test to be positive, both step 1 (apprehension) and step 2 (no apprehension) must occur.

⚠ *Noble Compression Test.* This is a test for **iliotibial band friction syndrome.**[286] The patient lies in the supine position, and the examiner flexes the patient's knee to 90°, accompanied by hip flexion (Figure 12-138). Pressure is then applied to the lateral femoral epicondyle, or 1 to 2 cm (0.4 to 0.8 inch) proximal to it, with the thumb. While the pressure is maintained, the patient's knee is passively extended. At approximately 30° of flexion (0° being straight leg), the patient experiences severe pain over the lateral femoral condyle. Pain indicates a positive test. The patient states that it is the same pain that occurs with activity.

⚠ *Q-Angle or Patellofemoral Angle.* The quadriceps angle (Q-angle) is defined as the angle between the quadriceps muscles (primarily the rectus femoris) and the patellar tendon and represents the angle of quadriceps muscle force (Figure 12-139).[287–290] The angle is obtained by first ensuring that the lower limbs are at a right angle to the line joining the two ASISs. A line is then drawn from the ASIS to the midpoint of the patella on the same side and from the tibial tubercle to the midpoint of the patella. The angle formed by the crossing of these two lines is called the *Q-angle.* The foot should be placed in a neutral position in regard to supination and pronation and the hip in a neutral position in regard to medial and lateral rotation, because it has been found that different foot and hip positions alter the Q-angle.[291]

Normally, the Q-angle is 13° for males and 18° for females when the knee is straight (Figure 12-140), although Grelsamer, et al.[292] reported male and female values are similar when patient height is considered. Any angle less than 13° may be associated with chondromalacia patellae or patella alta. An angle greater than 18° is often associated with chondromalacia patellae, subluxing patella, increased femoral anteversion, genu valgum,

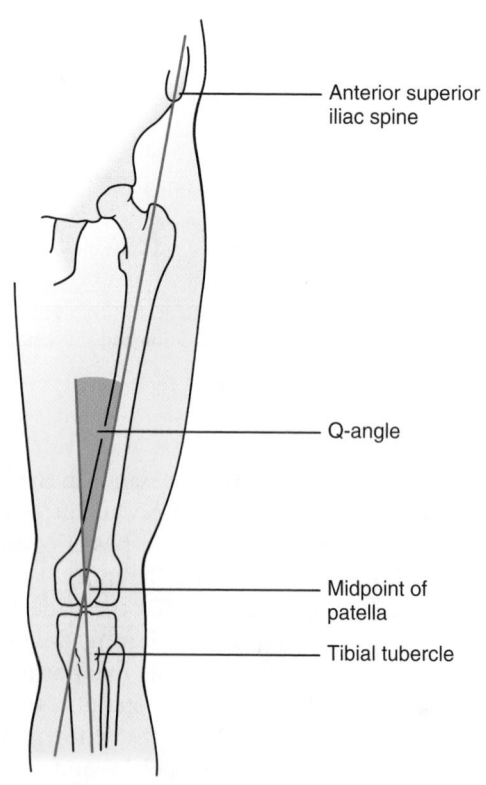

Figure 12-138 Noble compression test for iliotibial band friction syndrome.

Figure 12-139 Quadriceps angle (Q-angle).

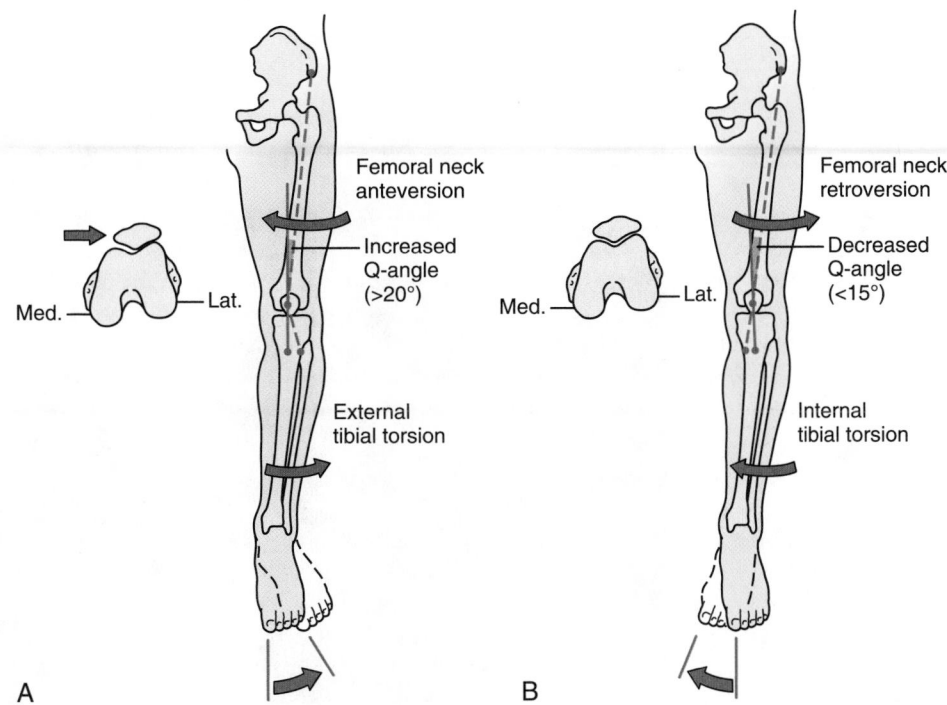

Figure 12-140 A, Femoral neck anteversion and lateral tibial torsion increase the Q-angle and lead to lateral tracking of the patella on the femoral sulcus. **B,** Femoral neck retroversion and medial tibial torsion decrease the Q-angle and tend to centralize the tracking of the patella. (Redrawn from Tria AJ, Palumbo RC: Conservative treatment of patellofemoral pain. Semin Orthop 5:116–117, 1990.)

lateral displacement of tibial tubercle, or increased lateral tibial torsion. During the test, which may be done either with radiographs or physically on the patient, the quadriceps should be relaxed. If measured with the patient in the sitting position, the Q-angle should be 0° (Figure 12-141). While the patient is in a sitting position, the presence of the **"bayonet sign,"** which indicates an abnormal alignment of the quadriceps musculature, patellar tendon, or tibial shaft, should be noted (Figure 12-142).

Hughston et al.[186] advocate doing the test with the quadriceps contracted. If measured with the quadriceps contracted and the knee fully extended, the Q-angle should be 8° to 10°. Any angle greater than 10° is considered abnormal. The examiner must ensure that a standardized measurement procedure is used to ensure consistent values.[293]

? *Radulescu Sign.*[294,295] The patient lies prone with the knee flexed to 90°. The examiner stabilizes the patient's thigh with one hand while medially rotating the tibia with the other hand to try to sublux the fibular head anteriorly (Figure 12-143). A positive test is indicated by pain, subluxation of the fibular head, and/or apprehension.

Tests for Hamstring Tightness. These tests are described in Chapter 11.

⚠ *Test for Knee Extension Contracture (Heel Height Difference).*[296] The patient lies prone with the thighs supported and the legs relaxed. The examiner measures the difference in heel height (Figure 12-144). One centimeter of

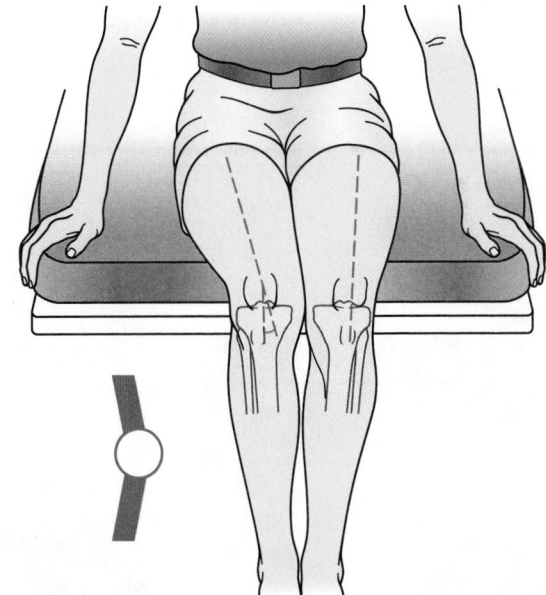

Figure 12-141 Q-angle in flexed position. Exaggerated Q-angle in the patient's right knee is seen as residual positive Q-angle with the knee flexed. Normally, the Q-angle in flexion should be 0°. (Redrawn from Hughston JC, Walsh WM, Puddu G: Patellar subluxation and dislocation, Philadelphia, 1984, WB Saunders, p. 24.)

difference approximates 1°, depending on leg length. The test, along with the accompanying end feel, would be used to test for joint contracture (tissue stretch) and possibly tight hamstrings (muscle stretch). Swelling may also cause a positive test.

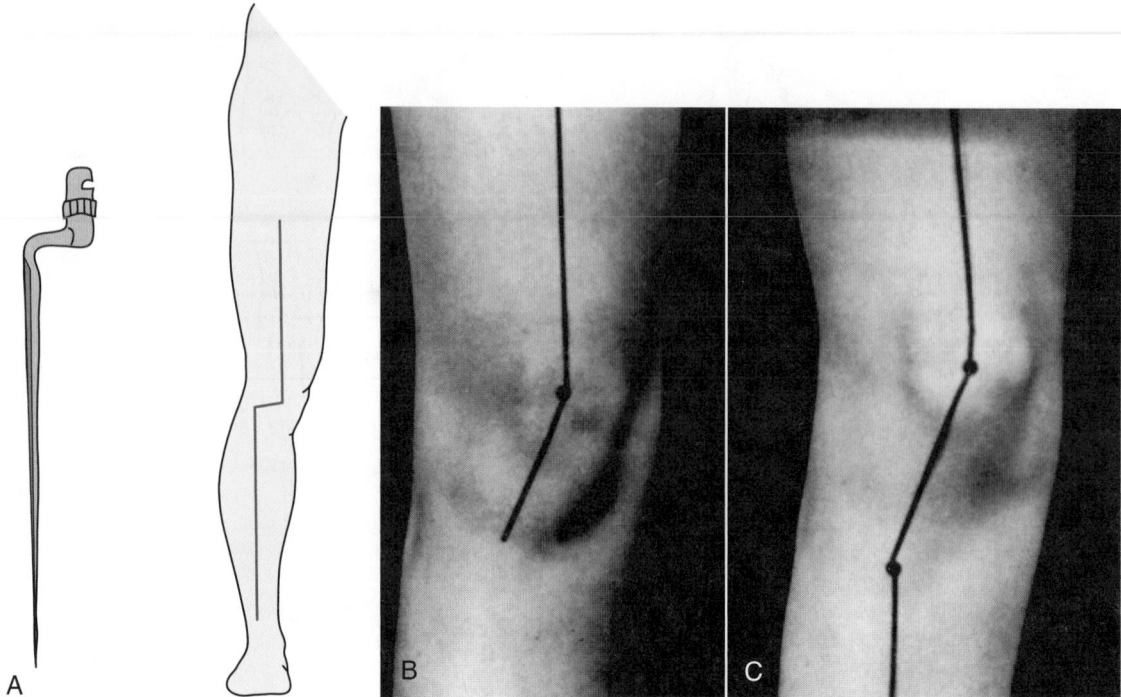

Figure 12-142 Increased Q-angle. A, Bayonet sign. Tibia vara of proximal third causes a markedly increased Q-angle. Alignment of the quadriceps, patellar tendon, and tibial shaft resembles a French bayonet. **B,** Q-angle with the knee in full extension is only slightly increased over normal. **C,** However, with the knee flexed at 30°, there is failure of the tibia to derotate normally and failure of the patellar tendon to line up with the anterior crest of the tibia. This is not an infrequent finding in patients with patellofemoral arthralgia. Increased medial femoral torsion (anteversion) combined with increased lateral tibial torsion causes the same bayonet sign. (**A,** From Hughston JC, et al: Patellar subluxation and dislocation, Philadelphia, 1984, WB Saunders, p 26; **B** and **C,** From Ficat RP, Hungerford DS: Disorders of the patello-femoral joint, Baltimore, 1977, Williams & Wilkins, p. 117.)

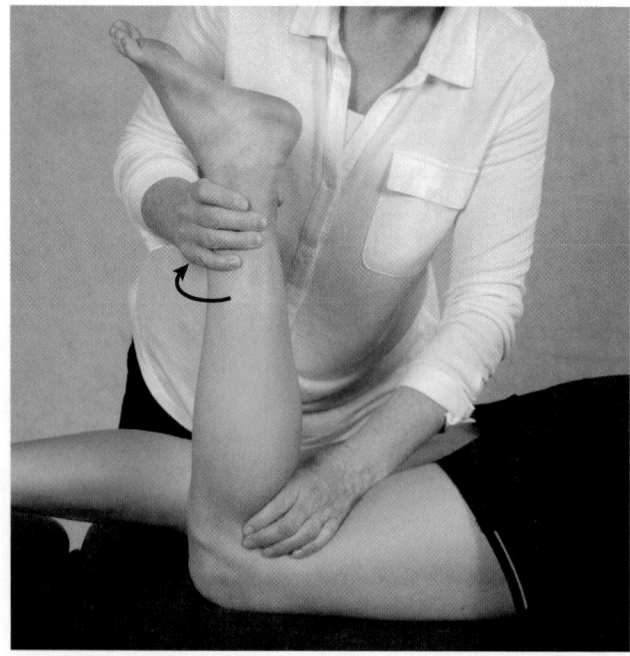

Figure 12-143 Radulescu test for unstable fibular head.

⚠ *Tubercle Sulcus Angle (Q-Angle at 90°).*[30,280] This measurement is also used to measure the angle of quadriceps pull. A vertical line is drawn from the center of the patella to the center of the tibial tubercle. A second horizontal line is drawn through the femoral epicondyle (Figure 12-145). Normally the lines are perpendicular. Angles greater than 10° from the perpendicular are considered abnormal. Lateral patellar subluxation may affect the results.

Another measurement, which is similar to the Q-angle, is the **A-angle,** which measures the relation of the patella to the tibial tubercle. This measurement, which is not as commonly used as the Q-angle, consists of a vertical line that divides the patella into two halves and a line drawn from the tibial tubercle to the apex of the inferior pole of the patella. The resulting angle is called the *A-angle* (Figure 12-146).[297,298] Some have questioned the reliability of this measurement because of the difficulty in consistently finding appropriate landmarks.[299]

❓ *Wilson Test.* This is a test for **osteochondritis dissecans.**[300] The patient sits with the knee flexed over the examining table. The knee is then actively extended with the tibia medially rotated. At approximately 30° of flexion (0° being straight leg), the pain in the knee increases, and the patient is asked to stop the flexion movement. The

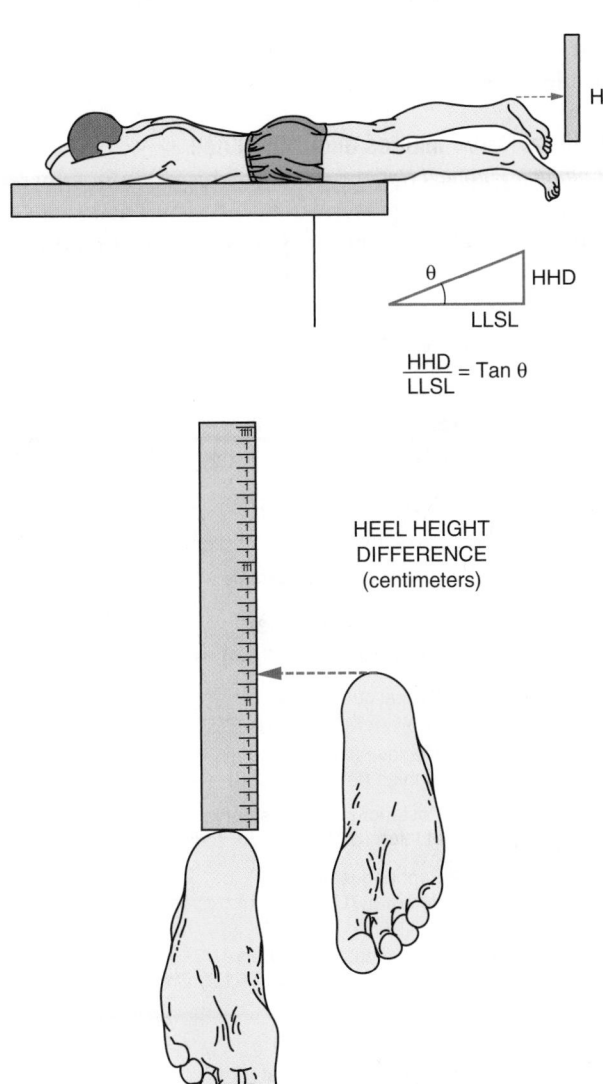

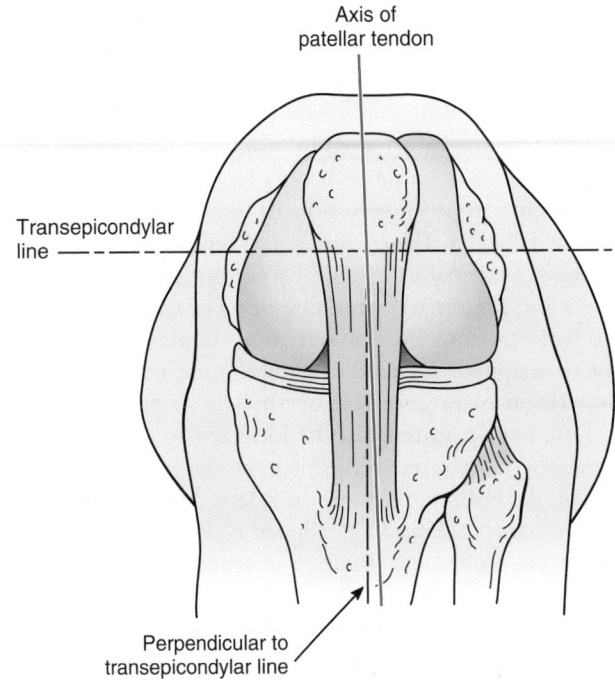

Figure 12-145 Tubercle sulcus angle of 90°. With the knee flexed to 90°, the transepicondylar line is assessed. The axis of the patellar tendon is compared with a perpendicular to the transepicondylar line. (Modified from Kolowich PA, Paulos LE, Rosenberg TD, et al: Lateral release of the patella: indications and contraindications. Am J Sports Med 18:361, 1990.)

Figure 12-144 Heel height difference (HHD). The patient lies prone on the examining table with the lower limbs supported by the thighs. The difference in heel height is measured. The conversion of HHD to degrees of extension lost depends on the leg length. The tangent of angle q is the HHD divided by the lower-leg segment length (LLSL). The LLSL is proportional to patient height. (From Daniel D, Akeson W, O'Conner J, editors: Knee ligaments: structure, injury and repair, New York, 1990, Raven Press, p. 32.)

patient is then asked to rotate the tibia laterally, and the pain disappears. This finding means a positive test, which is indicative of osteochondritis dissecans of the femoral condyle. The test is positive only if the lesion is at the classic site for osteochondritis dissecans of the knee, namely, the medial femoral condyle near the intercondylar notch (Figure 12-147).

Reflexes and Cutaneous Distribution

Having completed the ligamentous and other tests of the knee, if a scanning examination has not been carried out, the examiner next determines whether the reflexes around

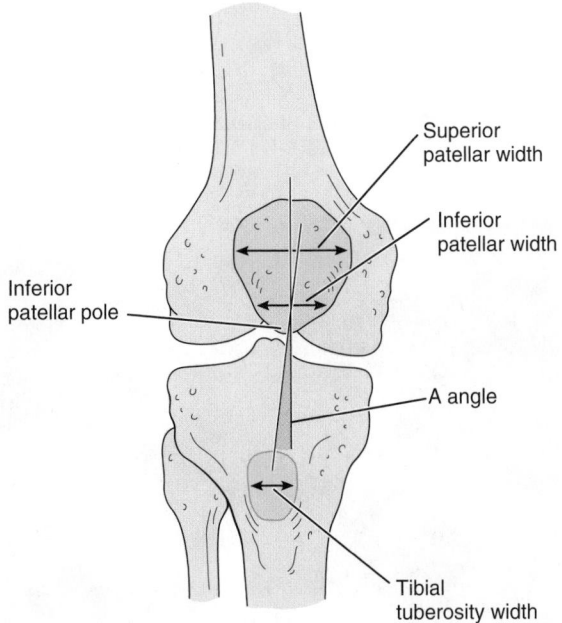

Figure 12-146 Location of landmarks of the A-angle. (Redrawn from Ehrat M, Edwards J, Hastings D, et al: Reliability of assessing patellar alignment: the A-angle. J Orthop Sports Phys Ther 19:23, 1994.)

the knee joint are normal, especially if neurological involvement is suspected (Figure 12-148). The patellar (L3–L4) and medial hamstring (L5–S1) reflexes should be checked for differences between the two sides.

The examiner must keep in mind the dermatome patterns of the various nerve roots (Figure 12-149) as well as the cutaneous distribution of the peripheral nerves (Figure 12-150). To test for altered sensation, a sensation scanning examination should be performed using relaxed hands and fingers to cover all aspects of the thigh, knee, and leg. Any differences in sensation should be noted and can be mapped out further with the use of a pinwheel, pin, cotton batting, or soft brush.

True knee pain tends to be localized to the knee, but it may also be referred to the hip or ankle (Figure 12-151). In a similar fashion, pain may be referred to the knee from the lumbar spine, hip (e.g., slipped capital femoral epiphysis in children), and ankle. Sometimes a lesion of the medial meniscus leads to irritation of the infrapatellar branch of the saphenous nerve. The result is a hyperaesthetic area the size of a quarter on the medial side of the knee. This finding is called **Turner's sign.**[79] Muscles

about the knee and their pain referral pattern are shown in Table 12-13.

Peripheral Nerve Injuries about the Knee

Common Peroneal Nerve (L4 to S2). This nerve is vulnerable to injury in the posterolateral knee and as it winds around the head of the fibula. It has also been reported that the nerve may be stretched as a result of pulling on

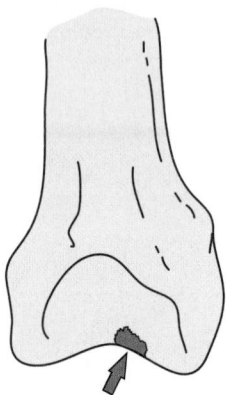

Figure 12-147 Classic site of osteochondritis dissecans.

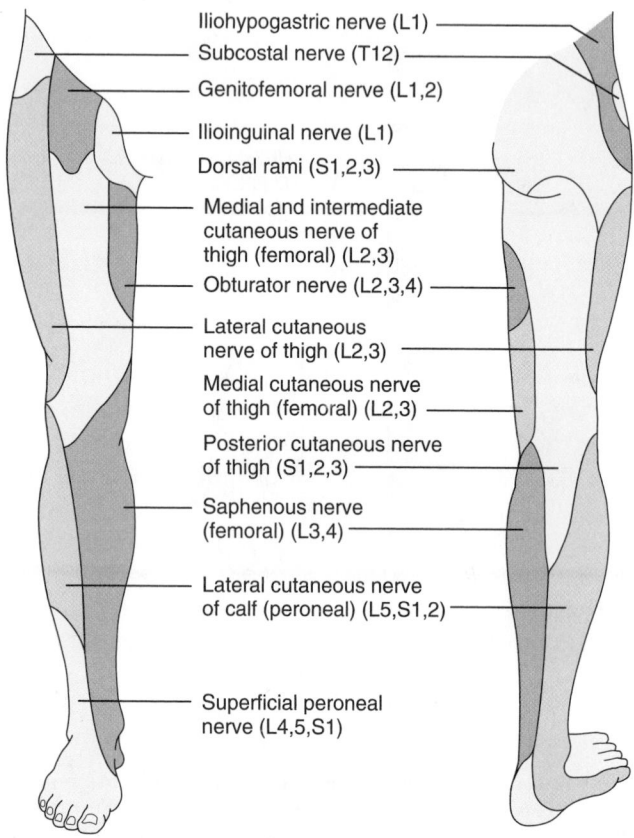

Iliohypogastric nerve (L1)
Subcostal nerve (T12)
Genitofemoral nerve (L1,2)
Ilioinguinal nerve (L1)
Dorsal rami (S1,2,3)
Medial and intermediate cutaneous nerve of thigh (femoral) (L2,3)
Obturator nerve (L2,3,4)
Lateral cutaneous nerve of thigh (L2,3)
Medial cutaneous nerve of thigh (femoral) (L2,3)
Posterior cutaneous nerve of thigh (S1,2,3)
Saphenous nerve (femoral) (L3,4)
Lateral cutaneous nerve of calf (peroneal) (L5,S1,2)
Superficial peroneal nerve (L4,5,S1)

Figure 12-149 Peripheral nerve sensory distribution about the knee.

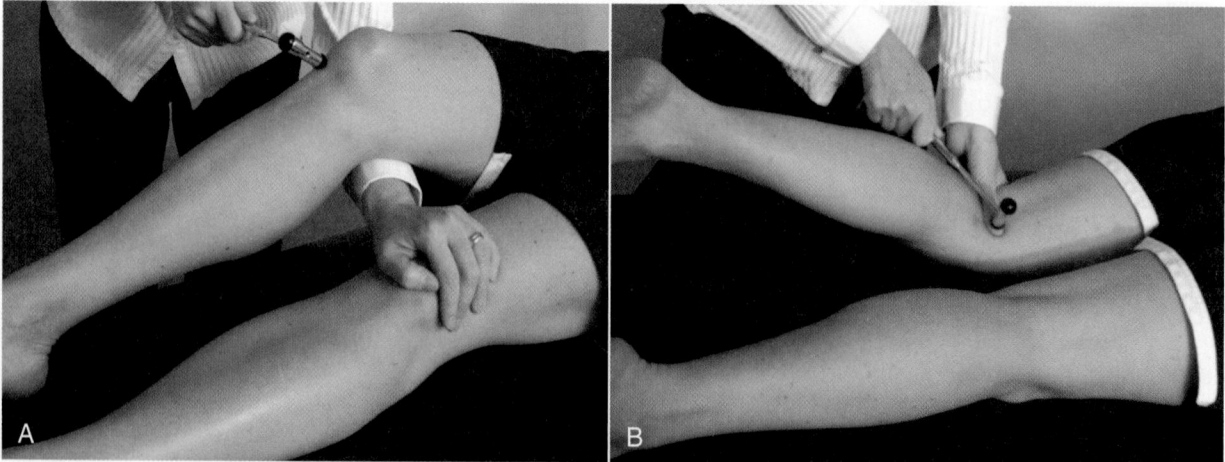

Figure 12-148 Reflexes of the knee. **A,** Patellar (L3). **B,** Medial hamstrings (L5).

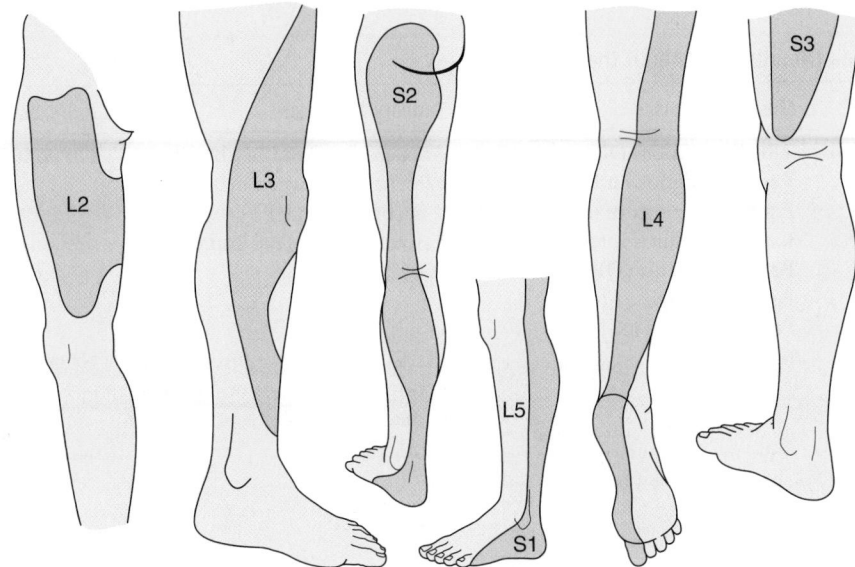

Figure 12-150 Dermatomes about the knee.

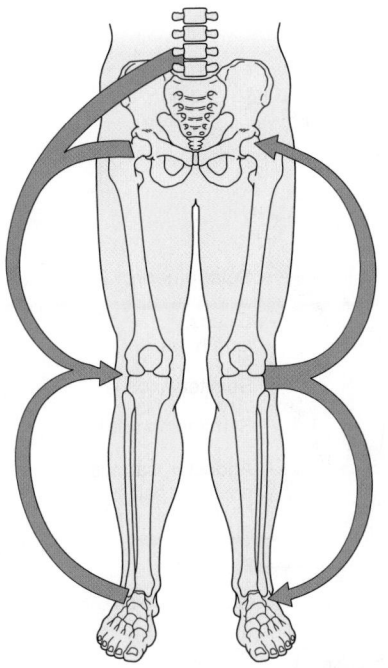

Figure 12-151 Patterns of referred pain to and from the knee.

TABLE **12-13**

Knee Muscles and Referral of Pain

Muscle	Referral Pattern
Tensor fasciae latae	Lateral aspect of thigh
Sartorius	Over course of muscle (anterior thigh)
Quadriceps	Anterior thigh, patella, lateral thigh and knee (vastus lateralis)
Adductor longus and brevis	Superior anterolateral thigh, anterior thigh, proximal to patella and sometimes down anteromedial leg
Adductor magnus	Medial thigh from groin to adductor tubercle
Gracilis	Medial thigh (primarily the midportion)
Semimembranosus and semitendinosus	Ischial tuberosity, posterior thigh, and posteromedial calf
Biceps femoris	Posterior knee up posterior thigh
Popliteus	Posterior knee
Gastrocnemius	Posterior knee, posterolateral calf, and posteromedial calf to foot instep
Plantaris	Posterior knee and calf

the peroneus longus muscle in a lateral ankle sprain,[296,301,302] direct trauma, injury to the posterolateral corner, or a varus stress to the knee.[30,207] The result is weakness or paralysis of muscles supplied by the deep and superficial peroneal nerves, the two branches of the common peroneal nerve (Table 12-14). This causes an inability to dorsiflex the foot (drop foot), resulting in a steppage gait and an inability to evert the foot. Sensory loss is as shown in Figure 12-152.

Saphenous Nerve (L2 to L4). The saphenous nerve is a sensory branch of the femoral nerve that arises near the inguinal ligament and passes down the leg to supply the skin on the medial side of the knee and calf. The nerve is sometimes injured during surgery or trauma, or it may be entrapped as it passes between the vastus medialis and adductor magnus muscles. Entrapment may lead to medial knee pain (burning) that is aggravated by walking, standing, and quadriceps exercises.[303–305] Sensory loss after surgery or trauma is shown in Figure 12-149.

TABLE **12-14**

Peripheral Nerve Injuries (Neuropathy) About the Knee

Nerve	Muscle Weakness	Sensory Alteration	Reflexes Affected
Common peroneal nerve	Tibialis anterior (DP) Extensor digitorum brevis (DP) Extensor digitorum longus (DP) Extensor hallucis longus (DP) Peroneus tertius (DP) Peroneus longus (SP) Peroneus brevis (SP)	Area around head of fibula Web space between first and second toes (DP) Lateral aspect of leg and dorsum of foot (SP)	No common reflexes affected
Saphenous nerve	None	Medial side of knee, may extend down medial side of leg to medial malleolus	None

DP, Deep peroneal branch; *SP*, superficial peroneal branch.

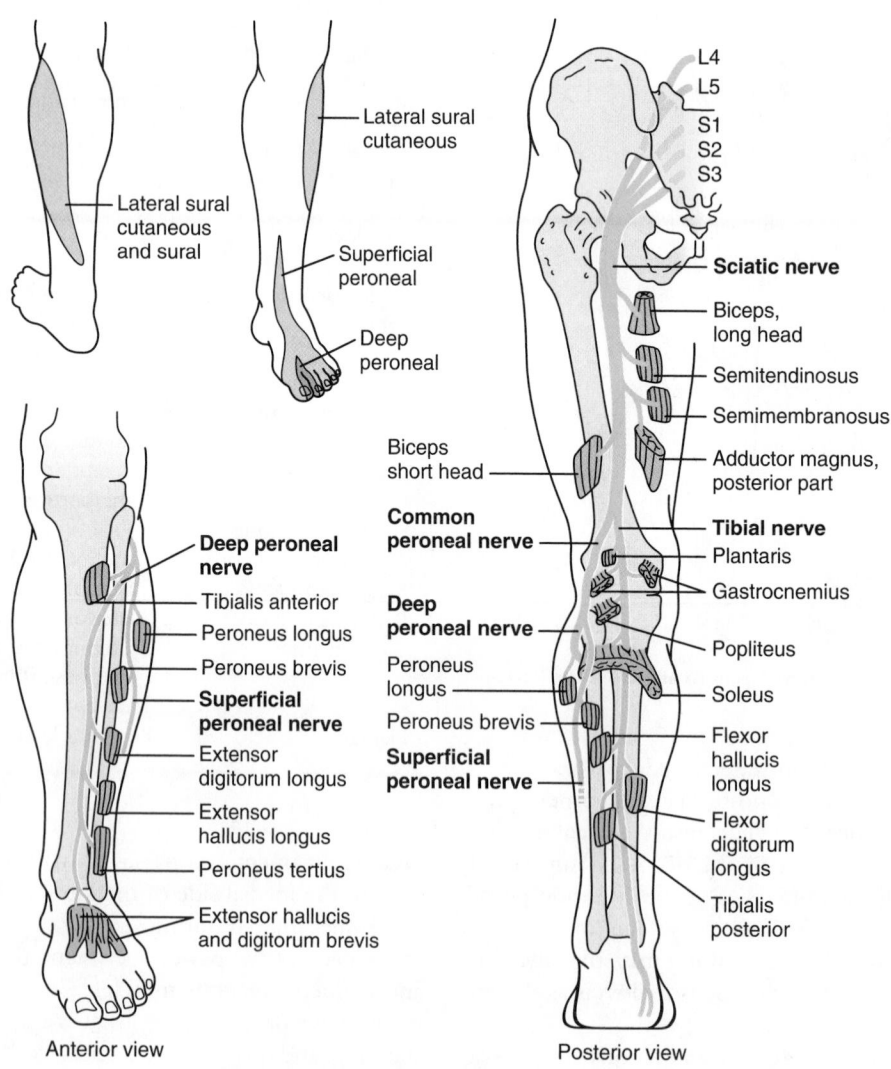

Figure 12-152 Common peroneal nerve.

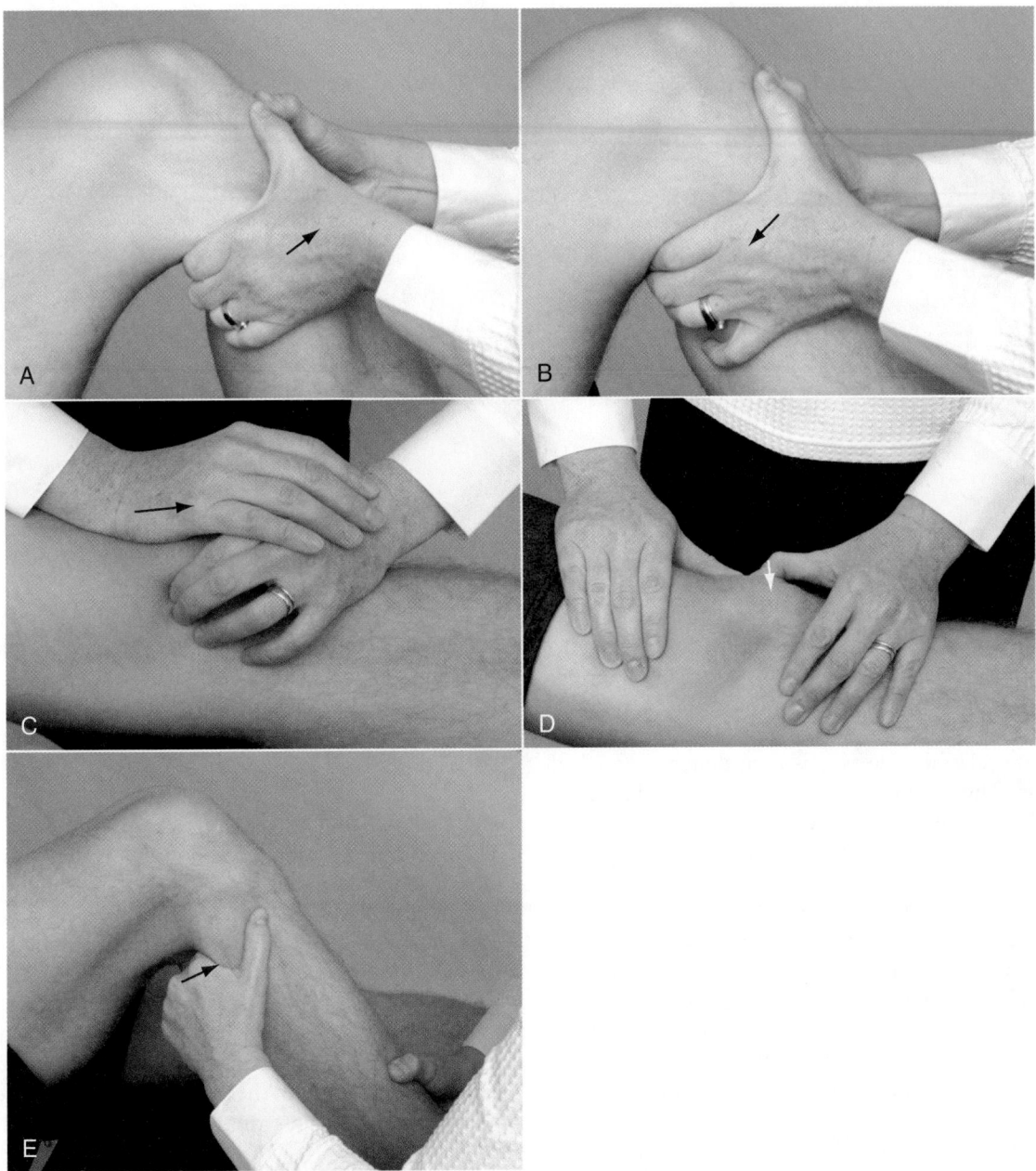

Figure 12-153 Joint play movements of the knee. A, Anterior movement of the tibia on the femur. **B,** Posterior movement of the tibia on the femur. **C,** Patellar movement, distally. **D,** Patellar movement, medially. **E,** Anterior movement of the superior tibiofibular joint.

Joint Play Movements

For joint play movements on the knee, the patient is placed in the supine position (Figure 12-153). The movement on the affected side is compared with that on the normal side.

Backward and Forward Movements of Tibia on Femur

The patient is asked to lie in the supine position with the test knee flexed to 90° and the hip flexed to 45°. The examiner then places the heel of the hand over the tibial

> **Joint Play Movements of the Knee Complex**
>
> - Backward glide of tibia on femur
> - Forward glide of tibia on femur
> - Medial translation of tibia on femur
> - Lateral translation of tibia on femur
> - Medial displacement of patella
> - Lateral displacement of patella
> - Depression of patella
> - Anteroposterior movement of fibula on tibia

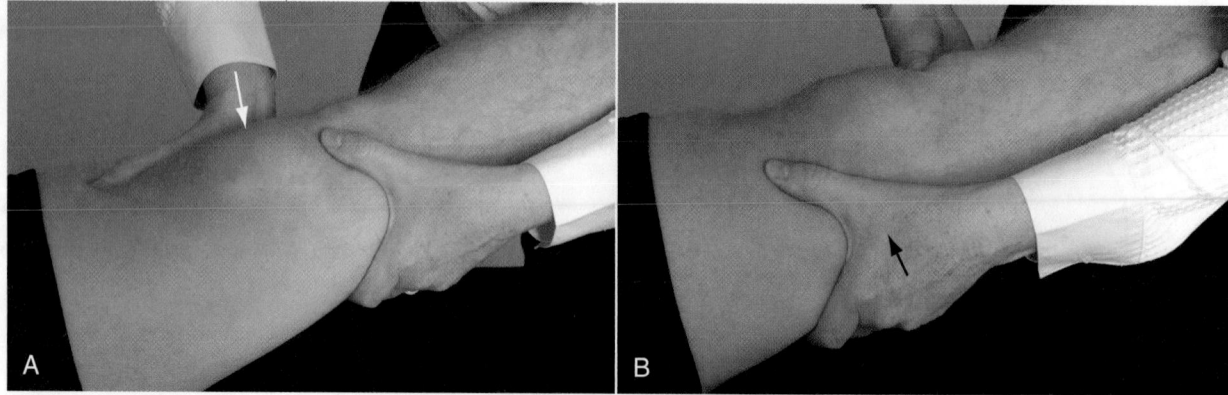

Figure 12-154 Medial and lateral shift of tibia on femur. A, Medial translation for anterior cruciate pathology. **B,** Lateral translation for posterior cruciate pathology.

tuberosity while stabilizing the patient's limb with the other hand and pushing backward with the heel of the hand. The end feel of the movement is normally tissue stretch. To perform the forward movement, the examiner places both hands around the posterior aspect of the tibia. Before performing the joint play movement, the examiner must ensure that the hamstrings and gastrocnemius muscles are relaxed. The tibia is then drawn forward on the femur. The examiner feels the quality of the movement, which normally is tissue stretch. These joint play movements are similar to those used in the anterior and posterior drawer tests for ligamentous stability.

Medial and Lateral Translation of Tibia on Femur

The patient lies supine, and the patient's leg is held between the examiner's trunk and arm. To test medial translation, the examiner puts one hand on the lateral side of the tibia and one hand on the medial side of the femur. The tibia is then pushed or translated medially on the femur. Excessive movement may indicate a torn anterior cruciate ligament (Figure 12-154). To test lateral translation, the examiner puts one hand on the medial side of the tibia and one hand on the lateral side of the femur. The tibia is then pushed or translated laterally on the femur. Excessive movement may indicate a torn posterior cruciate ligament. The normal end feel of each movement is tissue stretch.[79] Liorzou[28] reports that Galway did a similar test with the knee flexed to 90° and the foot on the examining table. If the tibial plateau bulges laterally, Wrisberg's ligament or the lateral meniscus may be injured.

Medial and Lateral Displacements of Patella

The patient is in the supine position with the knee slightly flexed on a pillow or over the examiner's knee (30° flexion). The examiner's thumbs are placed against the medial or lateral edge of the patella, and a force is applied to the side of the patella with the fingers used for stabilization. The process is then repeated with pressure applied to the other side of the patella. The other knee is tested as a comparison.

This joint play is similar to the passive movements of the patella; as in the passive test, the patella can be displaced by approximately half of its width medially and laterally. The examiner must do the movements slowly and carefully to ensure that the patella is not prone to dislocation.

Depression (Distal Movement) of Patella

The patient is in a supine position with the knee slightly flexed. The examiner then places one hand over the patient's patella so that the pisiform bone rests over the base of the patella. The other hand is placed so that the finger and thumb can grasp the medial and lateral edges of the patella to direct its movement. The examiner then rests the first hand over the second hand and applies a caudal force to the base of the patella, directing the caudal movement with the second hand so that the patella does not grind against the femoral condyles.

Anteroposterior Movement of Fibula on Tibia

The patient is supine with the knee flexed to 90° and the hip to 45°. The examiner then sits on the patient's foot and places one hand around the patient's knee to stabilize the knee and leg. The mobilizing hand is placed around the head of the fibula. The fibula is drawn forward on the tibia, and the movement and end feel are tested. The fibula then slides back to its resting position of its own accord. The movement is tested several times and compared with that of the other side. Care must be taken when performing this test because the common peroneal nerve, which winds around the head of the fibula, may be easily compressed, causing pain. If the superior tibiofibular joint is stiff or hypomobile, the test itself will cause discomfort. In most cases, foot dorsiflexion will cause lateral knee pain if the superior tibiofibular joint is hypomobile.

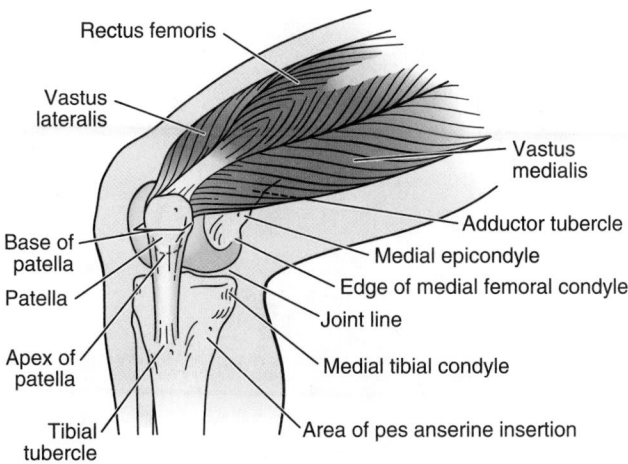

Figure 12-155 Landmarks of the knee.

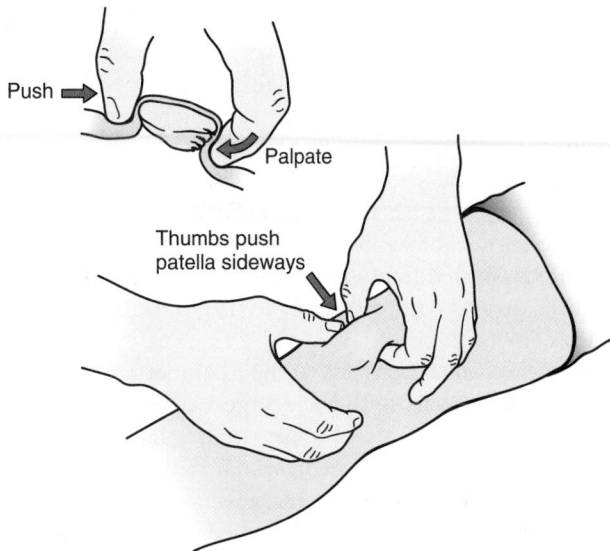

Figure 12-156 **Checking for patellar medial and lateral facet tenderness.** Note that tenderness may be related to structures other than patellar surfaces beneath the examining finger. (Redrawn from Hughston JC, Walsh WM, Puddu G: Patellar subluxation and dislocation, Philadelphia, 1984, WB Saunders, p. 28.)

Palpation

The patient lies supine with the knee slightly flexed. It is wise to put the knee in several positions during palpation. For example, meniscal cysts are best palpated at 45°, whereas the joint line is easiest to palpate at 90°. When palpating, the examiner looks for abnormal tenderness, swelling, nodules, or abnormal temperature. The following structures should be palpated (Figure 12-155).

Anterior Palpation with Knee Extended

Patella, Patellar Tendon, Patellar Retinaculum, Associated Bursa, Cartilaginous Surface of the Patella, and Plica. The patella can easily be palpated over the anterior aspect of the knee. The base of the patella lies superiorly, and the apex lies distally. After palpating the apex of the patella (for possible jumper's knee), the examiner moves distally, palpating the patellar tendon (for paratenonitis or tendinosis) and the overlying infrapatellar bursa (for Parson's knee) as well as the fat pad that lies behind the tendon. When the knee is extended, the fat pad often extends beyond the sides of the tendon. Moving distally, the examiner comes to the tibial tuberosity, which should be palpated for enlargement (possible Osgood-Schlatter disease).

Returning to the patella, the examiner can palpate the skin lying over the patella for pathology (prepatellar bursitis or housemaid's knee) and then extend medially and laterally to palpate the patellar retinaculum on both sides of the patella. With the examiner pushing down on the lateral aspect of the patella, the medial retinaculum can be brought under tension and then palpated for tender areas. The lateral retinaculum can be palpated in a similar fashion with the examiner pushing down on the medial aspect of the patella. By stressing the retinaculum, the examiner is separating the retinaculum from the underlying tissue.

With the quadriceps muscles relaxed, the articular facets of the patella are palpated for tenderness (possible

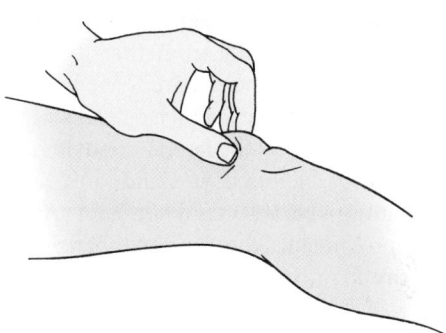

Figure 12-157 Palpation of the suprapatellar pouch.

chondromalacia patellae), as shown in Figure 12-156. This palpation is often facilitated by carefully pushing the patella medially to palpate the medial facets and laterally to palpate the lateral facet.

As the medial edge of the patella is palpated, the examiner should carefully feel for the presence of a mediopatellar plica. The plica, if pathological, may be palpated as a thickened ridge medial to the patella. To help confirm the presence of the plica, the examiner flexes the patient's knee to 30° and pushes the patella medially. If the plica is present and pathological, this maneuver often causes pain.

Suprapatellar Pouch. Returning to the anterior surface of the patella and moving proximally beyond the base of the patella, the examiner's fingers lie over the suprapatellar pouch. The examiner then lifts the skin and underlying tissue between the thumb and fingers (Figure 12-157). In this way, the synovial membrane of the suprapatellar pouch, which is continuous with that of the knee joint, can be palpated as a very slippery surface normally. The examiner should feel for any thickness, tenderness, or nodules, the presence of which may indicate pathology.

Quadriceps Muscles (Vastus Medialis, Vastus Intermedius, Vastus Lateralis, Rectus Femoris) and Sartorius. After palpating the suprapatellar pouch, the examiner palpates the quadriceps for tenderness (possible first- or second-degree strain), defects (third-degree strain), atonia, or hard masses (myositis ossificans).

Medial Collateral Ligament. If the examiner moves medially from the patella so that the fingers lie over the medial aspect of the tibiofemoral joint, the fingers will lie over the medial collateral ligament, which should be palpated along its entire length for tenderness (possible sprain) or other pathology (e.g., Pellegrini-Stieda syndrome—bone development in the medial collateral ligament).

Pes Anserinus. Medial and slightly distal to the tibial tuberosity, the examiner may palpate the pes anserinus (the common aponeurosis of the tendons of gracilis, semitendinosus, and sartorius muscles) for tenderness. Any associated swelling may indicate pes anserine bursitis.

Tensor Fascia Lata (Iliotibial Band and Head of Fibula). As the examiner moves laterally from the tibial tuberosity, the head of the fibula can be palpated. Medial and slightly superior to the fibula, the examiner palpates the insertion of the iliotibial band into the lateral condyle of the tibia. When the knee is extended, it stands out as a strong, visible ridge anterolateral to the knee joint. As the examiner moves proximally, the iliotibial band is palpated along its entire length.

Anterior Palpation with Knee Flexed

Tibiofemoral Joint Line and Meniscus. The patient's knee is flexed at 45°, and the examiner palpates the joint line, especially the anterior half of each meniscus. Medial rotation of the tibia makes the medial edge of the medial meniscus easier to palpate, whereas lateral rotation allows easier palpation of the lateral meniscus. The meniscus is palpated for tenderness (possible meniscal tear), swelling (possible meniscal cyst), or other pathology.[306,307] Joint line tenderness for lateral meniscus tears is more accurate (96%), sensitive (89%) and specific (97%) than for medial meniscus tears (accuracy 74%; sensitivity 86%; and, specificity 67%).[308]

Tibiofemoral Joint Line, Tibial Plateau, Femoral Condyles, and Adductor Muscles. The patient's knee is flexed to 90°. If the examiner returns to the patella, palpates the apex of the patella, and moves medially or laterally, the fingers lie on the tibiofemoral joint line, which should be palpated along its entire length. As the joint line is palpated, the examiner should also palpate the tibial plateau (for possible coronary ligament sprain) medially and laterally, as well as the femoral condyles.

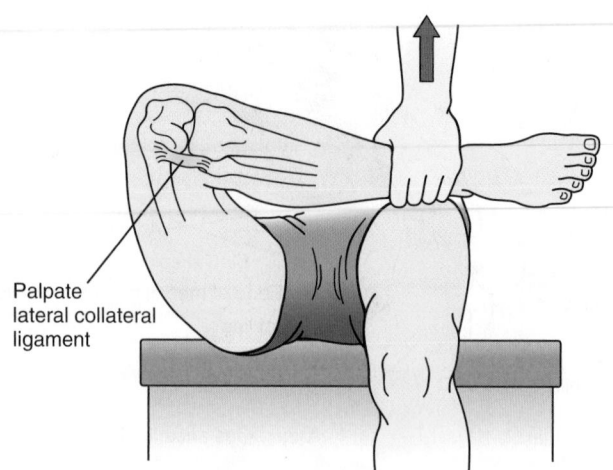

Palpate lateral collateral ligament

Figure 12-158 Palpation of the lateral (fibular) collateral ligament.

Both condyles should be palpated carefully for any tenderness (e.g., osteochondritis dissecans). Beginning at the superior aspect of the femoral condyles, the examiner should note that the lateral condyle extends farther anteriorly (i.e., higher) than the medial condyle. The trochlear groove between the two condyles can then be palpated. As the medial condyle is palpated, a sharp edge appears on the condyle medially. If the edge is followed posteriorly, the adductor tubercle can be palpated on the posteromedial portion of the medial femoral condyle. After palpating the adductor tubercle, the examiner moves proximally, palpating the adductor muscles of the hip for tenderness or other signs of pathology.

Anterior Palpation with Foot of Test Leg Resting on Opposite Knee

Kennedy[153] has advocated palpation of the lateral collateral ligament by having the patient in the sitting or lying position (Figure 12-158). The patient's knee is flexed to 90°, and the hip is laterally rotated so that the ankle of the test leg rests on the knee of the other leg (figure-four position). The examiner then places the knee into a varus position, and the ropelike ligament stands out if the ligament is intact.

Posterior Palpation with the Knee Slightly Flexed

Posterior Aspect of Knee Joint. The soft tissue on the posterior aspect of the knee should be palpated for tenderness or swelling (e.g., Baker's cyst). In some patients, the popliteal artery (pulse) may be palpated by running the hand down the center of the posterior knee.

Posterolateral Aspect of Knee Joint. The posterolateral corner of the knee is sometimes called the *popliteus corner.* The examiner should attempt to palpate the arcuate-popliteus complex, the lateral gastrocnemius muscle, the biceps femoris muscle, and possibly the lateral meniscus in this area. A sesamoid bone is sometimes found inserted in the tendon of the lateral head of the gastrocnemius muscle. This bone, referred to as the **fabella,** may be interpreted as a loose body in the posterolateral aspect of the knee by an unwary examiner (see Figure 12-174).

Posteromedial Aspect of Knee Joint. The posteromedial corner of the knee joint is sometimes referred to as the **semimembranosus corner.** The examiner should attempt to palpate the posterior oblique ligament, the semimembranosus muscle, the medial gastrocnemius muscle, and possibly the medial meniscus in this area for tenderness or pathology.

Hamstring and Gastrocnemius Muscles. After the various parts of the posterior aspect of the knee have been palpated, the tendons and muscle bellies of the hamstring muscle group (biceps femoris, semitendinosus, semimembranosus) proximally and of the gastrocnemius muscle distally should be palpated for tenderness, swelling, or other signs of pathology.

Diagnostic Imaging

Plain Film Radiography

For evaluation of knee injuries, anteroposterior and lateral views are most commonly obtained. Depending on the suspected pathology, other views may be taken as well (see the following box). Usually, the anteroposterior view is taken with the patient bearing weight. Imaging should not be used indiscriminately but should be considered an adjunct to examination; it is used primarily to confirm a diagnosis obtained by careful assessment.[309–311] Stiell and associates[312] have developed the **Ottawa knee rules** for the use of radiography in acute knee injuries.[180,313] They believed knee radiography was only necessary in acute knee injuries if the patient is 55 years of age or older or had isolated tenderness of the patella, tenderness at the head of the fibula, inability to flex the knee to 90°, or an inability to walk four steps (bearing weight). The use of the Ottawa knee rules in children is supported by some[314,315] and questioned by others.[316] Seaburg and Jackson[317] developed the **Pittsburgh Knee Rules.** They felt patients should undergo radiography if there was blunt trauma or a fall as a mechanism of injury, plus either the patient was younger than 12 or older than 50, or the patient had an inability to walk four weightbearing steps. Many clinicians combine both knee rules when making a decision about radiographs of the knee.[318]

Anteroposterior View. When looking at radiographs of the knee (Figure 12-159), the examiner should note any possible fractures (e.g., osteochondral, fibular head), diminished joint space (possible osteoarthritis; Figures 12-160 and 12-161), epiphyseal damage, lipping (see Figure 12-161), loose bodies, alterations in bone texture, abnormal calcification, ossification (e.g., Pellegrini-Stieda syndrome; Figure 12-162) or tumors, accessory ossification centers, varus or valgus deformity, patellar position, patella alta (Figures 12-163 and 12-164) or baja, and

---

Common X-Ray Views of the Knee Depending on Pathology

- Anteroposterior view* (see Figure 12-159, *A*)
- Lateral view—90° flexion (note if fabella present posteriorly) (see Figure 12-169)
- Lateral view—30° flexion* (see Figure 12-159, *B*)
- Intercondylar notch (tunnel) view (AP 45° flexion) (see Figure 12-159, *C*)
- Axial (skyline/sunrise) view of patellofemoral joint (see Figure 12-159, *D*)
- Standing AP (both knees) (see Figure 12-188)
- Standing PA—30° flexion (Figure 12-189)
- Merchant view (patient supine, knee flexed 45°, x-ray beam directed caudally through patella at 60° from vertical) (patellar subluxation, patellofemoral arthritis) (Figure 12-190)
- Tunnel view (see Figure 12-161)

*Should be weightbearing for arthritis.[190]

AP, Anteroposterior; *PA,* posteroanterior.

Ottawa Knee Rules for Radiographs of Acute Knee Injuries[309]

- Patient age younger than 55 or older than 18 years
- Fibular head tenderness
- Patellar tenderness
- Inability to flex knee to 90°
- Inability to bear weight and walk four steps when examined and at time of injury

---

Pittsburgh Knee Rules[314]

- Blunt trauma or fall
- Patient age younger than 12 years or older than 50 years
- Inability to walk four weightbearing steps on affected leg

---

asymmetry of femoral condyles.[319,320] Weight-bearing radiographs of knees in 30° flexion are recommended for cases of suspected arthritis or degeneration.[321] Stress, non–weight-bearing radiographs of this view illustrate excessive gapping medially or laterally, indicating ligamentous instability (Figure 12-165). The examiner should also remember the possible presence of the fabella, which is seen in 20% of the population. Epiphyseal fractures (Figure 12-166) and osteochondritis dissecans (Figure 12-167) may also be seen in this view.[322,323] The presence of the **Segund sign** or **lateral capsular sign,** which is an avulsion fracture, often indicates severe lateral capsular injury and probably anterior cruciate ligament disruption (Figure 12-168).[12,324–326]

Lateral View. With this view,[186,319,327] the examiner should note the same structures as seen with the

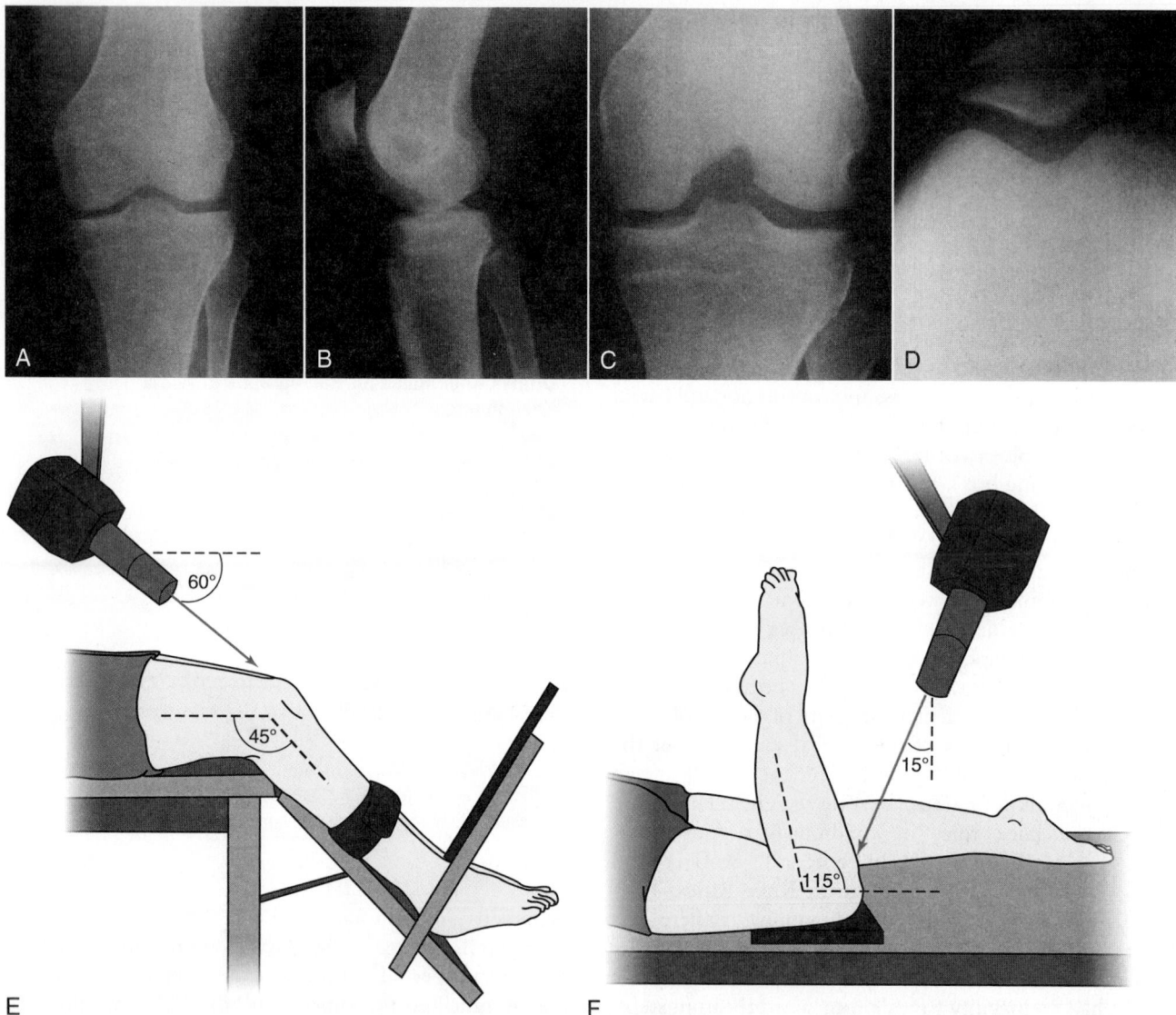

Figure 12-159 Normal radiographs of the knee. A, Anteroposterior view. **B,** Lateral view. **C,** Tunnel view. **D,** Patellofemoral joint skyline (merchant) view. **E,** Positioning for merchant view of patellofemoral joint (supine). **F,** Positioning for prone view of patellofemoral joint. (**A–D,** From Reilly BM: Practical strategies in outpatient medicine, Philadelphia, 1991, WB Saunders, p. 1188.)

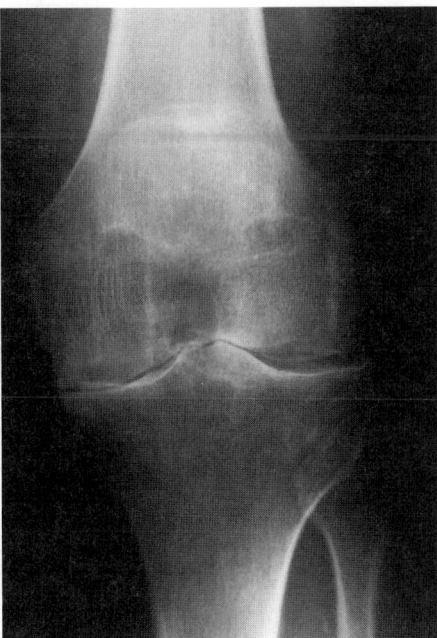

Figure 12-160 Anteroposterior x-ray showing degenerative arthritis of the knee. Note the loss of joint space caused by loss of cartilage (both sides) and meniscus (on medial side).

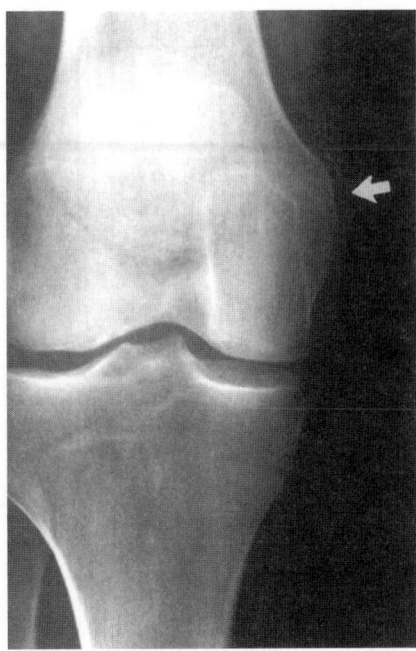

Figure 12-162 Pellegrini-Stieda syndrome. Note calcium formation within the substance of the medial collateral ligament *(arrow)*.

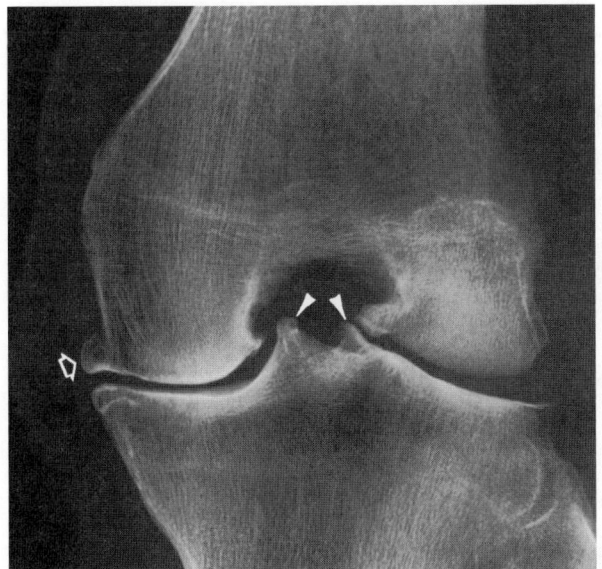

Figure 12-161 Tunnel view: osteoarthritis of the knee—femorotibial compartment abnormalities. Radiograph of a coronal section of a cadaveric knee indicates osteoarthritis changes that are more prominent in the medial femorotibial compartment. Findings include joint space narrowing related to cartilage erosion, subchondral bony sclerosis, osteophytosis *(open arrow),* and sharpening of the tibial spines *(arrowheads).* Degeneration of both the medial meniscus and the lateral meniscus is evident. View may also be used to look for osteochondritis dissecans. (From Resnick D, Kransdorf MJ: Bone and joint imaging, Philadelphia, 2005, WB Saunders, p. 386.)

anteroposterior view (Figures 12-169 to 12-171). This view is usually done in side-lying position with the knee flexed to 45°.[328] To determine the normal positioning of the patella, the standing, weight-bearing lateral view is used to determine the ratio of patellar length to patellar tendon length (Figure 12-172); several methods are possible.[329–332] Berg and associates[333] reported that the Blackburne-Peel method was the most consistent. This view also illustrates Osgood-Schlatter disease (Figure 12-173), the presence of the fabella (Figure 12-174), the arcuate sign (avulsion fracture of the arcuate complex leading to posterolateral instability; Figure 12-175),[207,334] myositis ossificans (Figures 12-176 and 12-177), and avulsion of the anterior cruciate insertion (Figure 12-178). Stress radiographs of this view in kneeling can be used to show complete tears (8 mm or more) of the posterior cruciate ligament.[335,336]

Intercondylar Notch (Tunnel View X-Ray). With this view (patient prone, knee flexed from 45° to 90°) (Figure 12-179), the tibia and intercondylar attachments of the cruciate ligaments can be examined as well as the width of the intercondylar notch, which is less in women.[337] This narrower notch can put the anterior cruciate at greater risk of tearing.[337] Also, any loose bodies or possibility of osteochondritis dissecans, subluxation, trochlear dysplasia, patellar tilt (lateral or medial), or dislocation should be noted.[338]

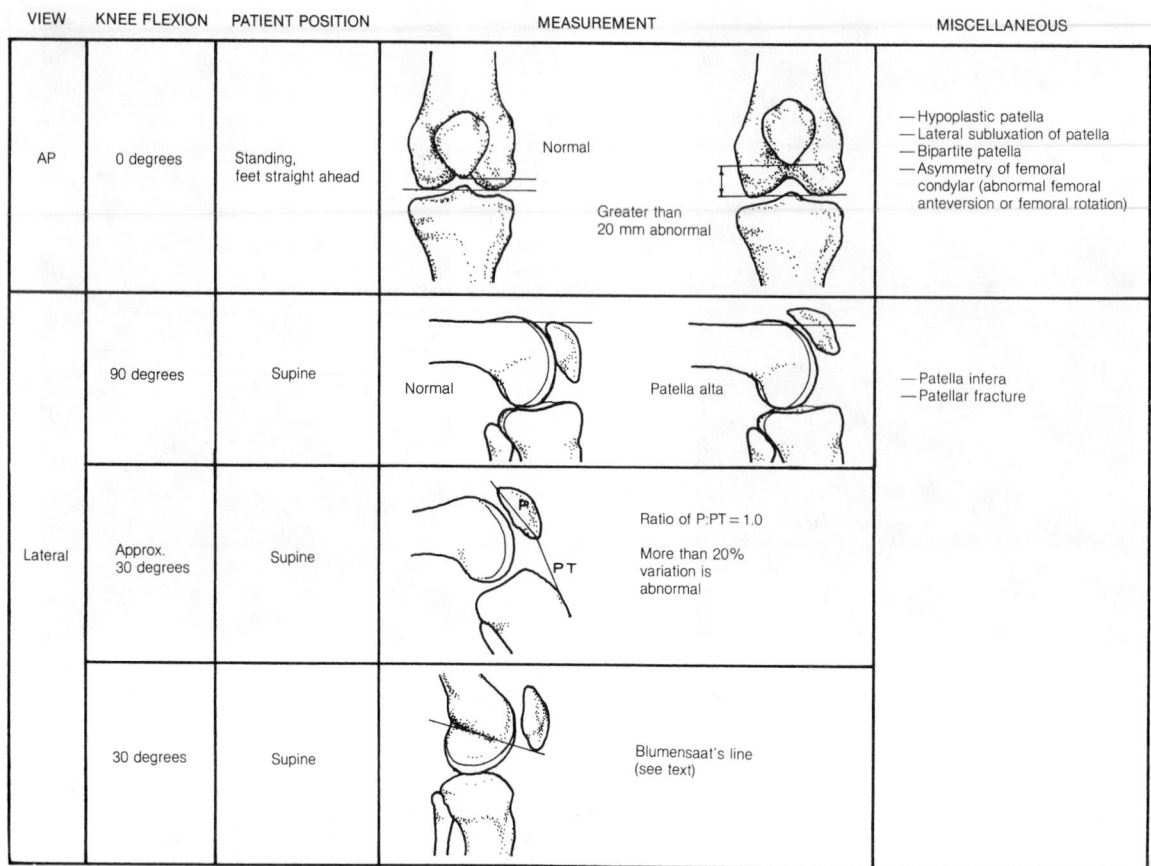

VIEW	KNEE FLEXION	PATIENT POSITION	MEASUREMENT	MISCELLANEOUS
AP	0 degrees	Standing, feet straight ahead	Normal — Greater than 20 mm abnormal	— Hypoplastic patella — Lateral subluxation of patella — Bipartite patella — Asymmetry of femoral condylar (abnormal femoral anteversion or femoral rotation)
Lateral	90 degrees	Supine	Normal — Patella alta	— Patella infera — Patellar fracture
	Approx. 30 degrees	Supine	Ratio of P:PT = 1.0 More than 20% variation is abnormal	
	30 degrees	Supine	Blumensaat's line (see text)	

Figure 12-163 Summary of radiographic findings in patella alta. (From Carson WG Jr, James SL, Larson RL, et al: Patellofemoral disorders: physical and radiographic evaluation. I. Physical examination. Clin Orthop 185:179, 1984.)

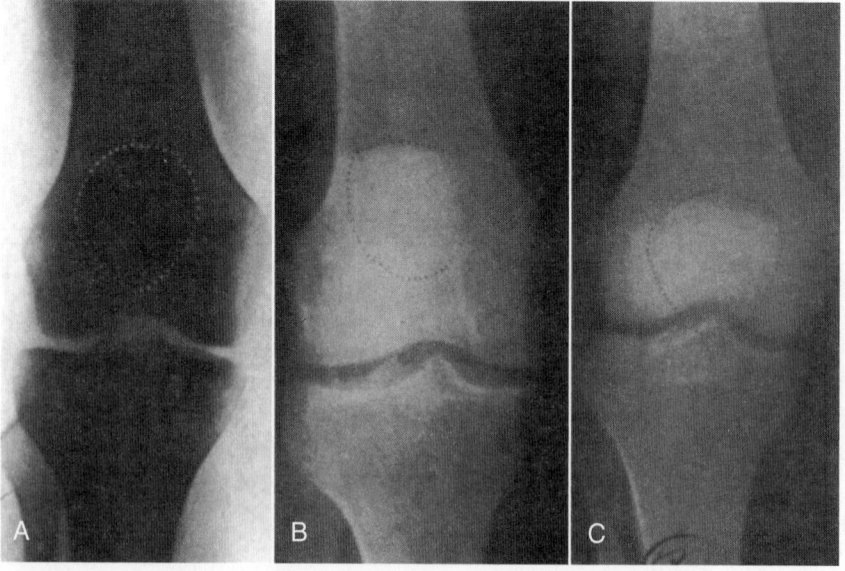

Figure 12-164 Anteroposterior view of the knee. A, Normal patellar position. **B,** Patella alta. **C,** Patella baja. (From Hughston JC et al: Patellar subluxation and dislocation, Philadelphia, 1984, WB Saunders, p. 50.)

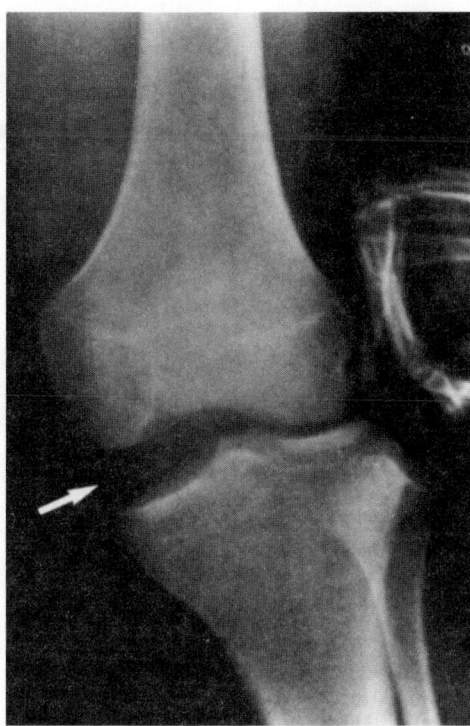

Figure 12-165 This valgus stress radiograph shows the patient's knee in full extension. Note the gapping on the medial side (*arrow*) caused by the stress applied by the examiner's hand (bones to right of knee). (From Mital MA, Karlin LI: Diagnostic arthroscopy in sports injuries. Orthop Clin North Am 11:775, 1980.)

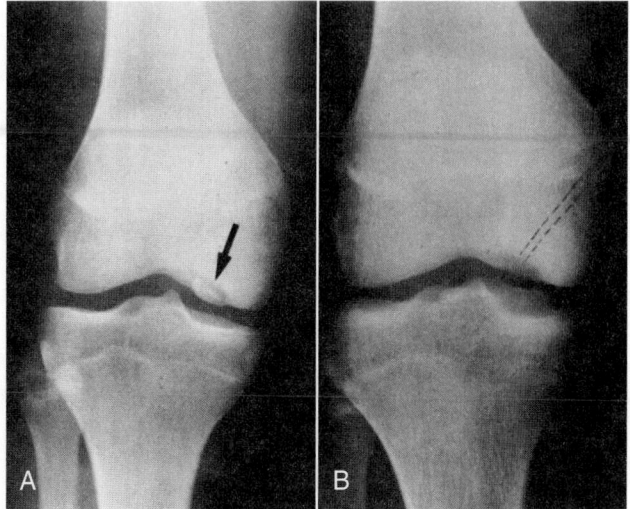

Figure 12-167 A, Osteochondritis dissecans—actually an osteochondral fracture (*arrow*) of the femoral condyle—with almost the entire femoral attachment of the posterior cruciate ligament remaining attached to the fragment. **B,** Three months after repair of posterior cruciate to femur. Excellent function is restored. Complete filling in of this defect is unlikely at this age. (From O'Donoghue DH: Treatment of injuries to athletes, ed 4, Philadelphia, 1984, WB Saunders, p. 575.)

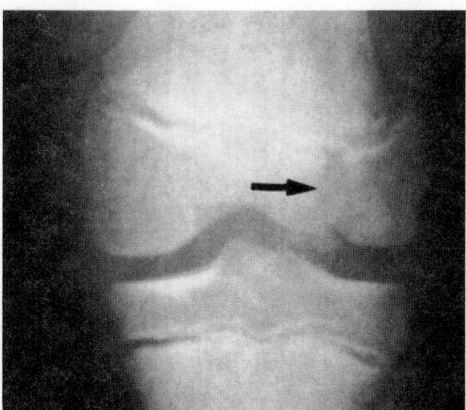

Figure 12-166 A Salter-Harris type III injury (*arrow*) of the growth plate and epiphysis. Main attention should be directed toward restitution of the joint surface. (From Ehrlich MG, Strain RE: Epiphyseal injuries about the knee. Orthop Clin North Am 10:93, 1979.)

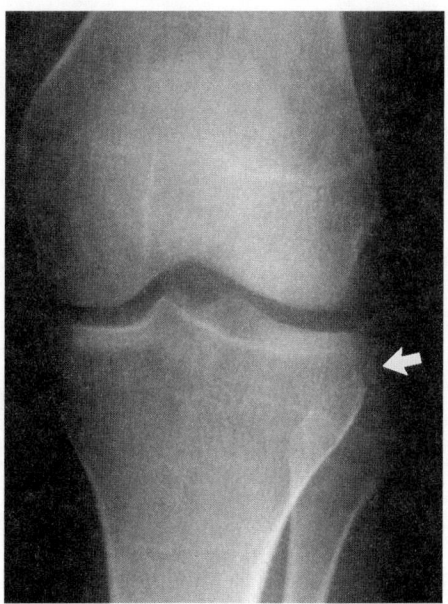

Figure 12-168 Segund sign. Note avulsion fracture adjacent to lateral tibial plateau (*arrow*). This lateral capsular injury often signifies an anterior cruciate ligament tear.

Axial (Skyline) View. This 30° tangential view (Figure 12-180) is primarily used for suspected patellar problems, such as patellar subluxation and dysplasia (Figure 12-181).[51,320,327,339,340] It may be taken at different angles, as shown in Figures 12-182 to 12-184, or it may be used to determine the type of patella present, as shown in Figure 12-185. Figure 12-186 illustrates abnormal patellar forms. Other patellofemoral measurements include lateral patellar displacement (see Figure 12-183) and the lateral/medial trochlear ratio or sulcus angle (see Figure 12-184).[327,341]

Fixed Flexion Posteroanterior View (10° to 30° Knee Flexion). This view is best for determining narrowing of the joint space (Figure 12-187).

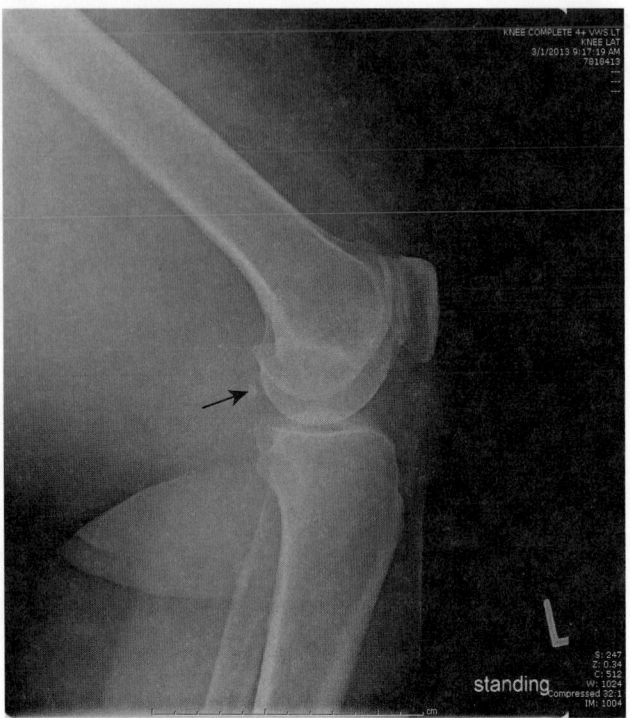

Figure 12-169 Lateral view of the knee – 90° flexion. Note fabella (sesamoid bone) posteriorly (*arrow*).

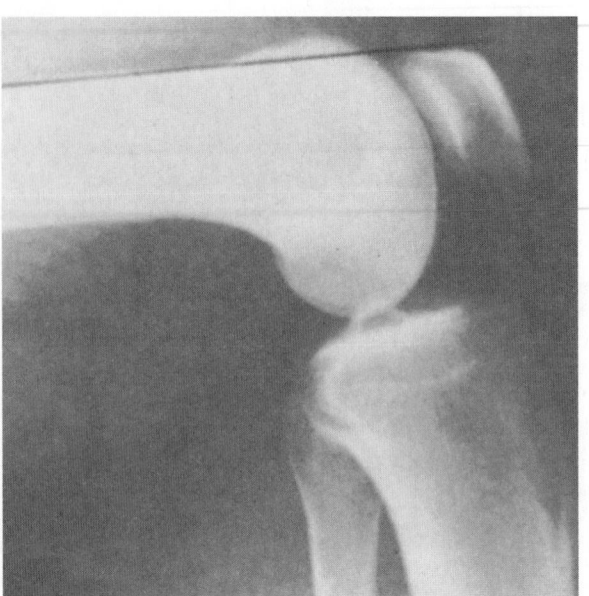

Figure 12-170 Lateral view at 90° shows the normal position of the patella. (From Hughston JC et al: Patellar subluxation and dislocation, Philadelphia, 1984, WB Saunders, p. 52.)

Figure 12-171 Lateral view of the patella at 45°. A, Normal patellar position in relation to the intercondylar notch. B, Patella alta. (From Hughston JC et al: Patellar subluxation and dislocation, Philadelphia, 1984, WB Saunders, p. 52.)

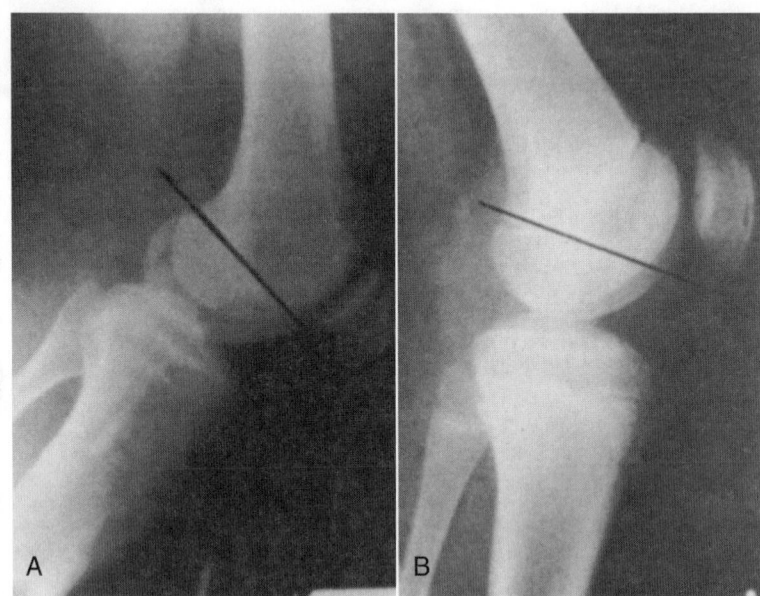

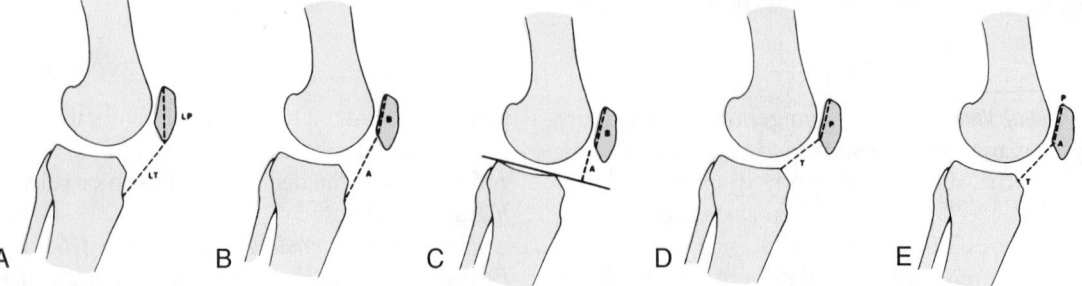

Figure 12-172 Indices for measurement of patellar height. A, Insall-Salvati. **B**, Modified Insall-Salvati. **C**, Blackburne. **D**, de Carvalho. **E**, Caton. (From Grelsamer RP, Meadows S: The modified Insall-Salvati ratio for assessment of patellar height. Clin Orthop 282:172, 1992.)

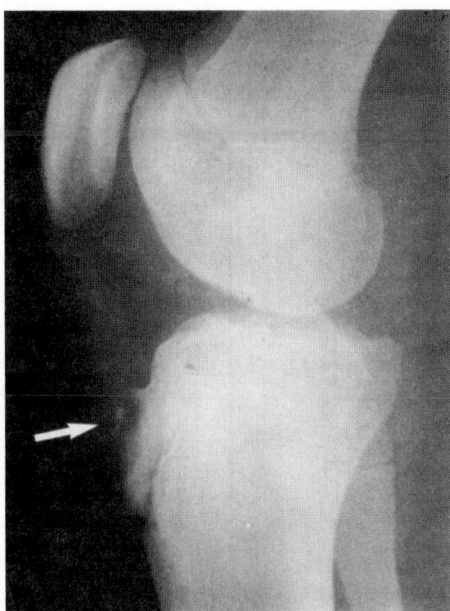

Figure 12-173 Osgood-Schlatter disease, showing epiphysitis of the entire epiphysis (*arrow*), with irregularity of the epiphyseal line. Because this epiphyseal cartilage is continuous with that of the upper tibia, it should not be disturbed. If surgery is used, exposure should be superficial to the epiphyseal cartilage. (From O'Donoghue DH: Treatment of injuries to athletes, ed 4, Philadelphia, 1984, WB Saunders, p. 574.)

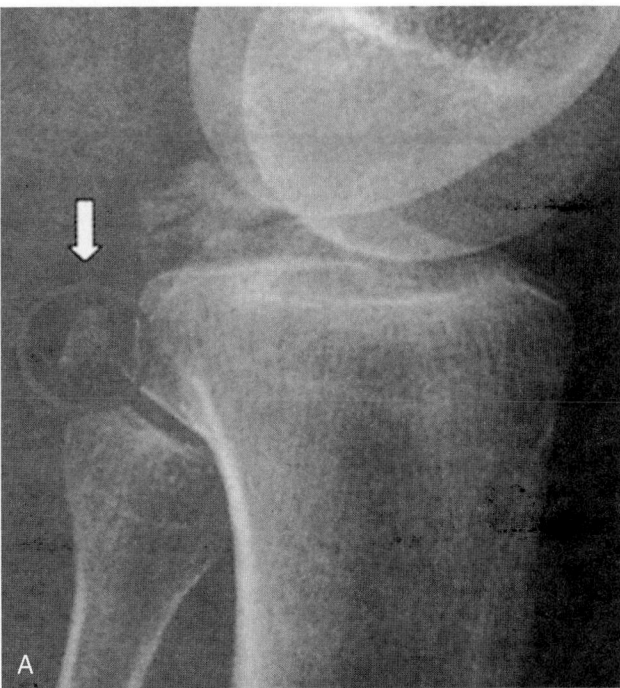

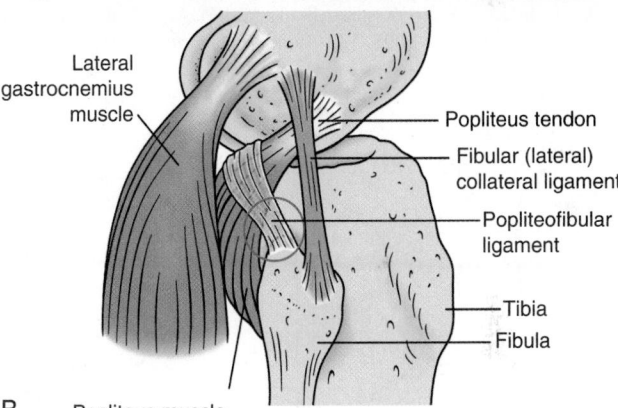

Figure 12-175 Arcuate sign or fibular styloid fracture on lateral radiograph, **A**, with comparative diagram, **B**. The arcuate sign is pathognomonic of posterolateral corner injuries. It is an avulsion fracture of the arcuate complex. The fracture (*denoted by arrow*) is small and posteriorly located with minimal displacement. Circles denote the insertions of the arcuate complex. (From Bahk MS, Cosgarea AJ: Physical examination and imaging of the lateral collateral ligament and posterolateral corner of the knee. Sports Med Arthrosc Rev 14:16, 2006.)

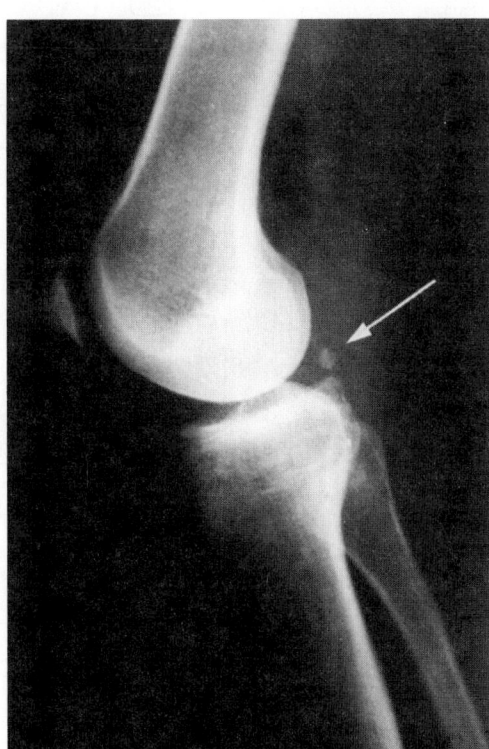

Figure 12-174 Sesamoid bone (fabella) in the gastrocnemius muscle.

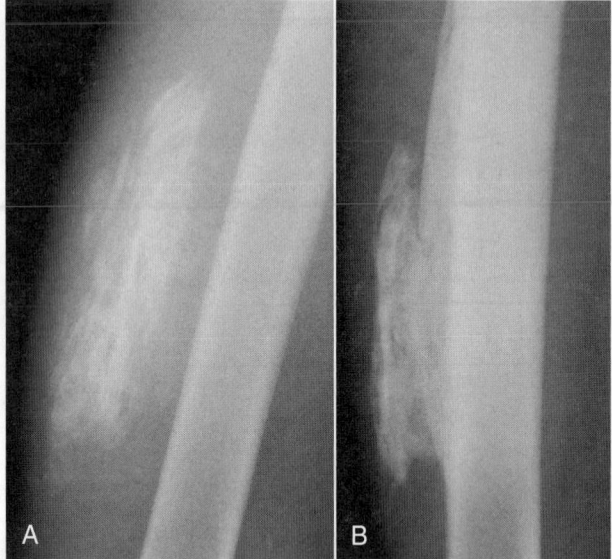

Figure 12-176 Myositis ossificans traumatica: maturing ossification. In this 11-year-old boy who fell from the steps of a swimming pool, lateral radiographs of the femur 1 month, **A**, and 5 months, **B**, after the injury show maturation of the ossifying process. Initially separated from the bone, the process subsequently merged with the anterior femoral surface. (From Resnick D, Kransdorf MJ: Bone and joint imaging, Philadelphia, 2005, WB Saunders. Courtesy of G Greenway, MD, Dallas, p. 1361.)

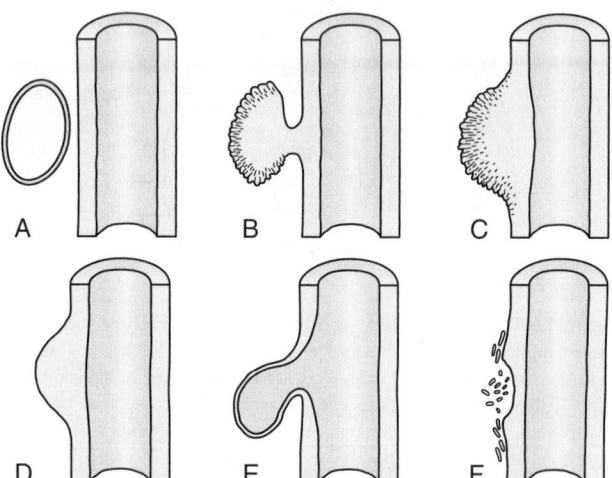

Figure 12-177 Myositis ossificans traumatica: differential diagnosis. **A,** Myositis ossificans traumatica. The shell-like configuration of the ossification, with a clear zone between it and the underlying bone, is typical of this condition. In some cases, there may be a cortical bridge. **B,** Parosteal osteosarcoma. These lesions appear as central ossifying foci with irregular outlines and may be connected to the underlying bone by a stalk. **C,** Periosteal osteosarcoma. These tumors arise in the cortex of the diaphysis of a tubular bone and produce cortical thickening and speculated osteoid matrix. **D,** Osteoma. Characteristic of this lesion is a localized excrescence that produces bulging of the cortical contour. **E,** Osteochondroma. An exostosis protrudes from the cortical surface. Its medullary and cortical bone is continuous with that of the underlying osseous structure. **F,** Juxtacortical (periosteal) chondroma. These periosteal lesions produce localized excavation of the cortex, with periostitis. They may contain calcification. (Redrawn from Resnick D, Kransdorf MJ: Bone and joint imaging, Philadelphia, 2005, WB Saunders, p. 1361.)

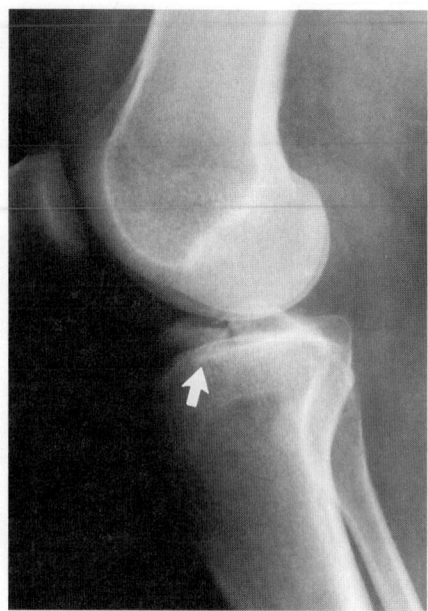

Figure 12-178 Avulsion fracture of the tibial insertion of the anterior cruciate ligament.

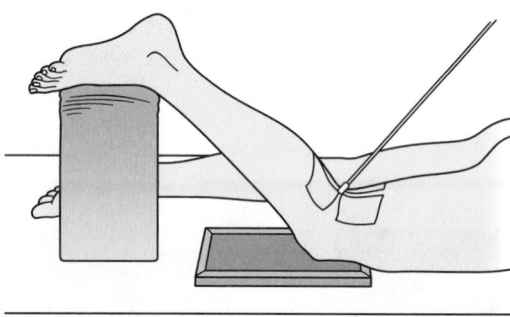

Figure 12-179 Position for intercondylar notch view. (Redrawn from Larson RL, Grana WA, editors: The knee: form, function, pathology and treatment, Philadelphia, 1993, WB Saunders, p. 106.)

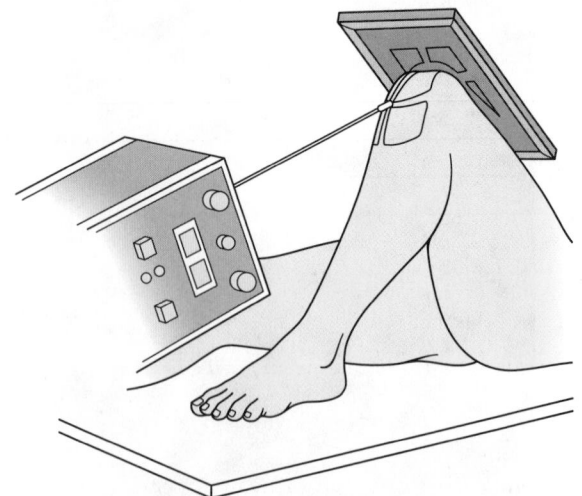

Figure 12-180 Positioning for the patellofemoral (skyline) view. (Redrawn from Larson RL, Grana WA, editors: The knee: form, function, pathology and treatment, Philadelphia, 1993, WB Saunders, p. 107.)

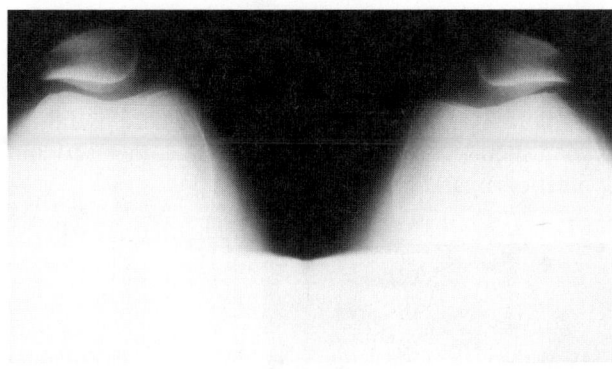

Figure 12-181 Skyline (sunrise) view of patellofemoral joints. Note the lateral displacement of both patellae and shallow trochlea (trochlear dysplasia), especially the one on the right. Note also the alpine hunter's cap shape of patella.

TANGENTIAL VIEW	KNEE FLEXION	TECHNIQUE AND POSITION	MEASUREMENTS	MISCELLANEOUS

Hughston	55 degrees	Prone position. Beam directed cephalad and inferior, 45 degrees from vertical.	1) Sulcus (trochlear) angle: 118°
			
			2) Patella index:
			$$\frac{AB}{XB - XA}$$
			NL: Male 15
			Female 17
				—Patellar dislocation
				—Osteochondral fracture
				—Soft tissue calcification (old dislocated patella or fracture)
				—Patellar subluxation
				  Patellar tilt
				  Increased medial joint space
				  Apex of patella lateral to apex of femoral sulcus
				  Lateral patella edge lateral to femoral condyle
				  Hypoplastic lateral femoral condyle (usually proximal)
				—Patellofemoral osteophytes
				—Subchondral trabeculae orientation (increase or decrease)
				—Patellar configuration (Wiberg-Baugartl)

Merchant	45 degrees	Supine position. Beam directed caudal and inferior, 30 degrees from vertical.	1) Sulcus (trochlear) angle: 138° (normally <145 degrees) 2) Congruence angle: Med. -6° Lat. − +	
Laurin	20 degrees	Sitting position. Beam directed cephaled and superior, 160 degrees from vertical.	1) Lateral patellofemoral angle: LAT. NL: ABNL: ABNL: 2) Patellofemoral index: Ratio A/B Med. Lat. Normal = 1.6 or less	

Figure 12-182 Summary of radiographic findings, tangential view. (From Carson WG Jr, James SL, Larson RL, et al: Patellofemoral disorders: physical and radiographic evaluation. I. Physical examination. Clin Orthop 185:182, 1984.)

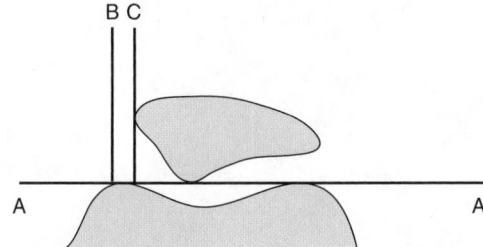

Figure 12-183 Lateral patellar displacement. A line is drawn through the highest points of the medial and lateral femoral condyles *(AA)*. A perpendicular to that line, at the medial edge of the medial femoral condyle *(B)*, normally lies 1 mm or less medial to the patella *(line C)*. (From Laurin CA, Dussault R, Levesque HP: The tangential x-ray investigation of the patellofemoral joint. Clin Orthop 144:16, 1979.)

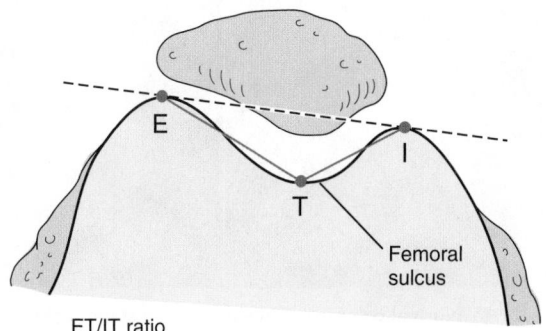

Figure 12-184 The lateral/medial trochlear ratio is the ratio between the external and internal segments *(ET* and *IT)* joining the highest points of the femoral condyles to the deepest point of the trochlear groove. It measures the dysplasia of the medial aspect of the trochlea. (Redrawn from Beaconsfield T, Pintore E, Maffulli N, et al: Radiographic measurements in patellofemoral disorders. Clin Orthop 308:22, 1994.)

Standing Anteroposterior View. This view is best for knee alignment (Figure 12-188).

Arthrography

Arthrograms of the knee are used primarily to diagnose tears in the menisci (Figure 12-191) and plica (Figure 12-192) although their use is being replaced by arthroscopy. Double-contrast arthrograms are also used (Figure 12-193). Arthrograms combined with computed tomography (CT) scans (CT arthrograms) are useful for assessing meniscus tears, articular cartilage, meniscal and popliteal cysts, and synovial plica.[342]

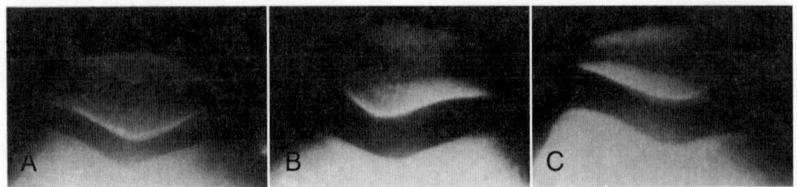

Figure 12-185 **Examples of patellar variations. A,** Wilberg type I. **B,** Wilberg type II. **C,** Wilberg type III. Trochlea of femur also show variations. (From Ficat RP, Hungerford DS: Disorders of the patello-femoral joint, Baltimore, 1977, Williams & Wilkins, p. 53.)

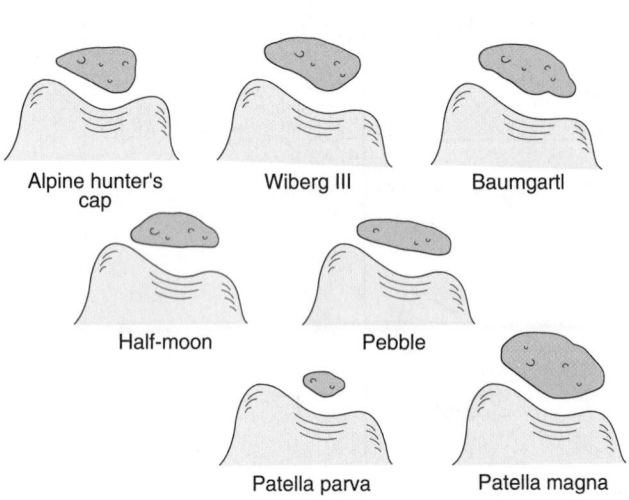

Alpine hunter's cap   Wiberg III   Baumgartl

Half-moon   Pebble

Patella parva   Patella magna

Figure 12-186 Variations in patellar form that are considered dysplastic. (Redrawn from Ficat RP, Hungerford DS: Disorders of the patello-femoral joint, Baltimore, 1977, Williams & Wilkins, p. 55.)

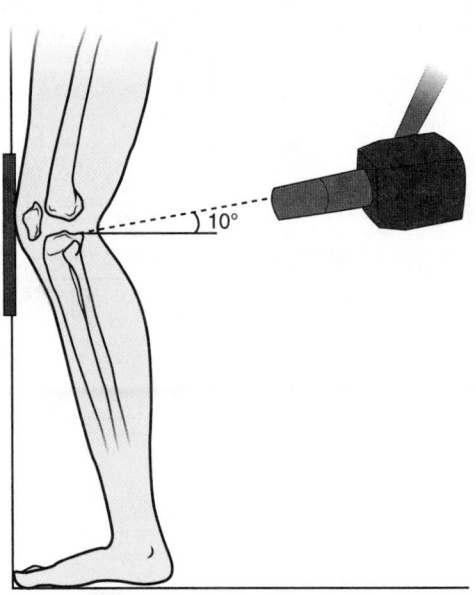

Figure 12-187 **Patient positioning for fixed flexion posteroanterior (PA) view.**

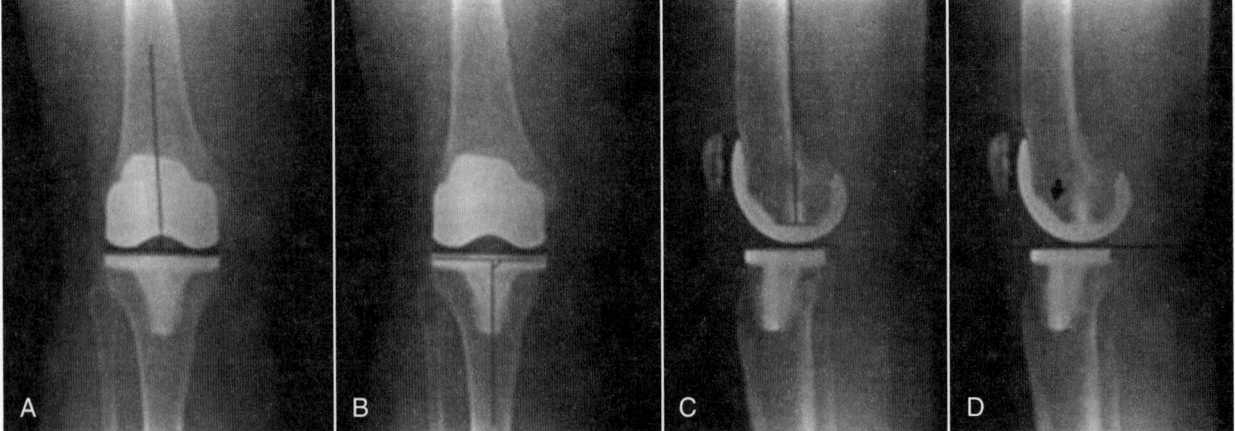

Figure 12-188 **Normal component positioning on standing knee radiographs. A,** Anteroposterior (AP) view of the knee demonstrates the method of measuring femoral component alignment. **B,** The tibial tray should be 90° to the long axis of the tibial shaft. **C,** Lateral radiographs show the femoral component parallel to the femoral shaft. **D,** The tibial tray is at approximately 90° to the tibial shaft. Osteopenia *(arrow)* is seen about the femoral component, consistent with stress shielding. (From Scott WN: Insall & Scott Surgery of the knee, ed 5, Philadelphia, 2011, Churchill Livingstone.)

Arthroscopy

The arthroscope is being used increasingly to diagnose lesions of the knee and to repair many of them surgically.[343–345] By using various approaches (portals) to the knee, the surgeon is able to view all of the structures to determine whether they have been injured (Figure 12-194).

Computed Tomography

CT scans are often used to view soft tissue as well as bone (Figure 12-195).

Magnetic Resonance Imaging

Magnetic resonance imaging (MRI) is advantageous because of its ability to show soft tissue as well as bone

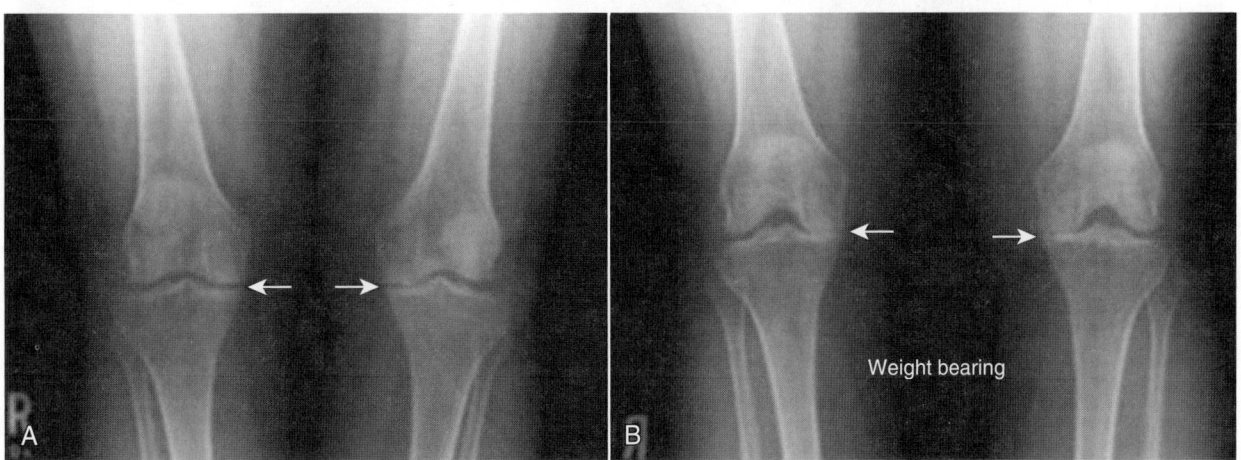

Figure 12-189 The flexed weight-bearing posteroanterior (PA) view. A, Routine standing anteroposterior (AP) film demonstrates moderate bilateral medial compartment joint space narrowing with proliferative changes *(arrows).* **B,** PA flexion view demonstrates the findings to be more severe with marked narrowing of bilateral medial joint compartments, complete loss of the joint space, and bone-on-bone apposition *(arrows).* (From Scott WN: Insall & Scott Surgery of the knee, ed 5, Philadelphia, 2011, Churchill Livingstone.)

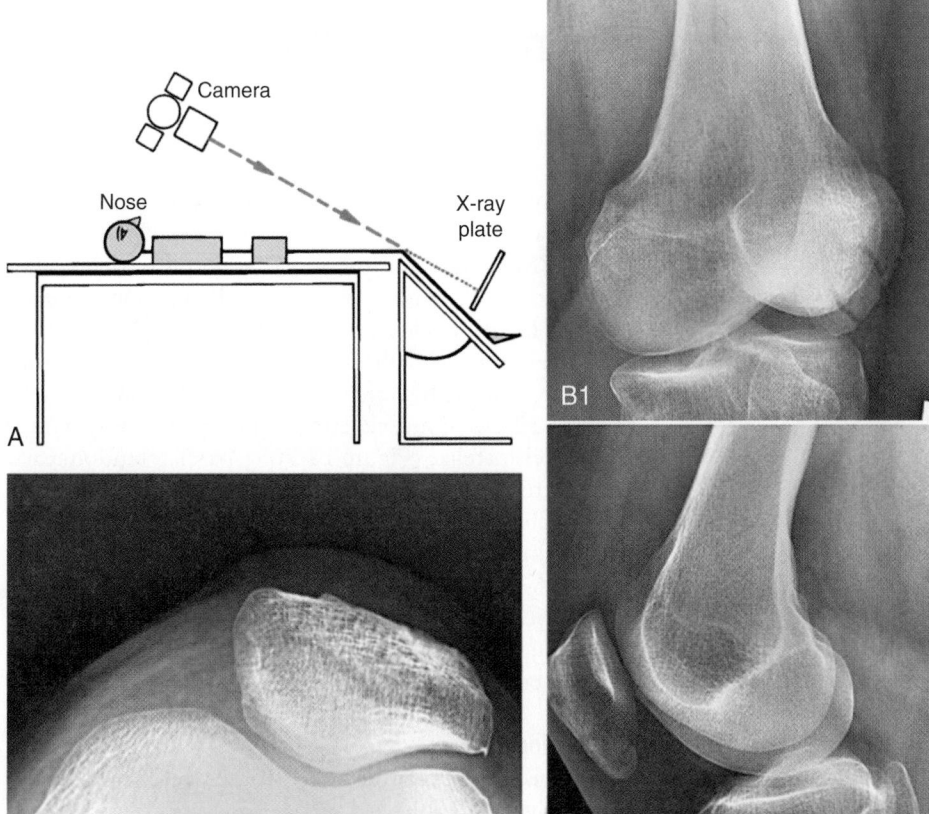

Figure 12-190 A, Merchant tangential view of the patella is made with the knee flexed 45° and the radiograph exposed as shown. **B,** Patellar fracture of the middle and inferior pole is best seen on the oblique view *(B1). B2,* Lateral view. *B3,* Merchant (sunrise) view. (From Johnson GA, et al: Atlas of emergency radiology, St Louis, 2001, WB Saunders; and, Resnick D, Niwayama G: Diagnosis of bone and joint disorders, ed 2, Philadelphia, 1988, WB Saunders.)

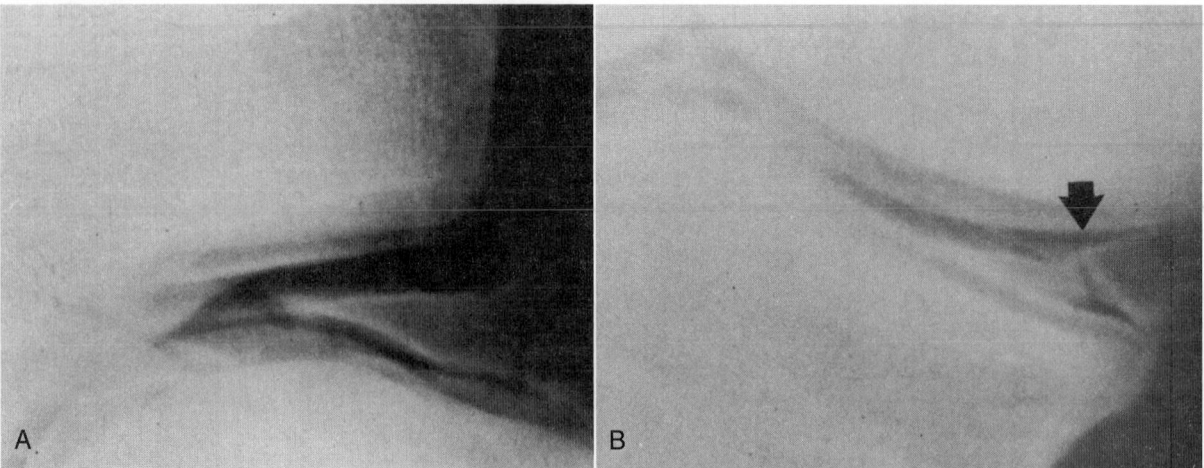

Figure 12-191 Arthrogram demonstrating a torn meniscus. The normal meniscus on the lateral side **(A)** is compared with the easily demonstrated tear in the medial meniscus *(arrow)* in the same patient, **B.** (From Reilly BM: Practical strategies in outpatient medicine, Philadelphia, 1991, WB Saunders, p. 1198.)

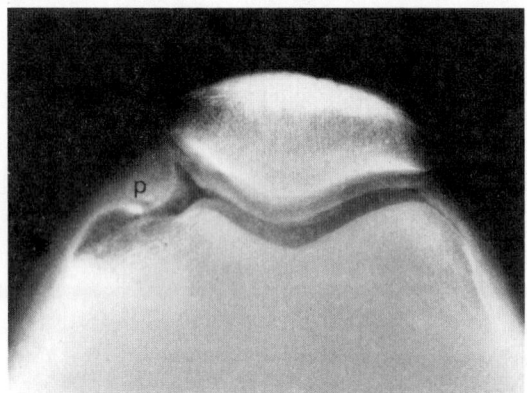

Figure 12-192 Tangential patellar view after arthrography, showing thinning and slight roughening of the patellar cartilage, especially medially. The mediopatellar plica *(p)* is markedly thickened. (From Weissman BNW, Sledge CB: Orthopedic radiology, Philadelphia, 1986, WB Saunders, p. 536.)

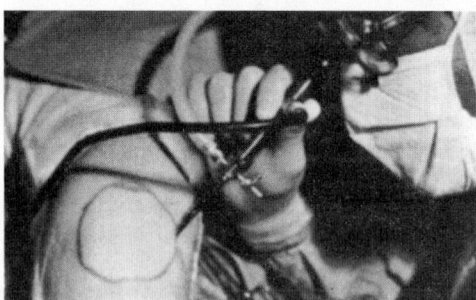

Figure 12-194 Arthroscopy of the knee. (From Patel D: Superior lateral-medial approach to arthroscopic meniscectomy. Orthop Clin North Am 13:301, 1982.)

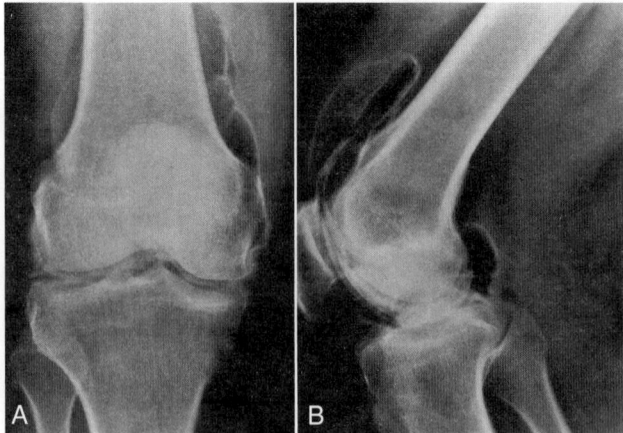

Figure 12-193 Double-contrast arthrogram. A, The anteroposterior view demonstrates the menisci and articular cartilage. **B,** The lateral projection illustrates the extent of the joint space. (From Forrester DM, Brown JC: The radiology of joint disease, ed 3, Philadelphia, 1987, WB Saunders, p. 200.)

tissue while providing no exposure to ionizing radiation.[346] It has largely replaced CT scans for evaluation of the knee.[347] MRI has been found to be useful in diagnosing lesions of the tendon (Figure 12-196), bone bruises (Figure 12-197), menisci (Figures 12-198 and 12-199), plica (Figure 12-200), collateral ligaments (Figure 12-201), cruciate ligaments (Figure 12-202), Baker's cyst (Figure 12-203), muscle strains (Figure 12-204), chondromalacia patellae (Figure 12-205), patellar tendon tears, and fractures, but it should be used only to confirm or clarify a clinical diagnosis.[90,326,348–362] Sagittal proton density magnetic resonance (MR) imaging and other MRI techniques for cartilage (e.g., 3T imaging, T2 mapping, T1-delayed gadolinium-enhanced MRI) are also becoming more common.[360,363] Sanders and Miller[350] provide a good overview of the use of MRI about the knee.

Xeroradiography

Xeroradiography may be used to delineate the edge of bone (Figure 12-206).

Text continued on p. 876

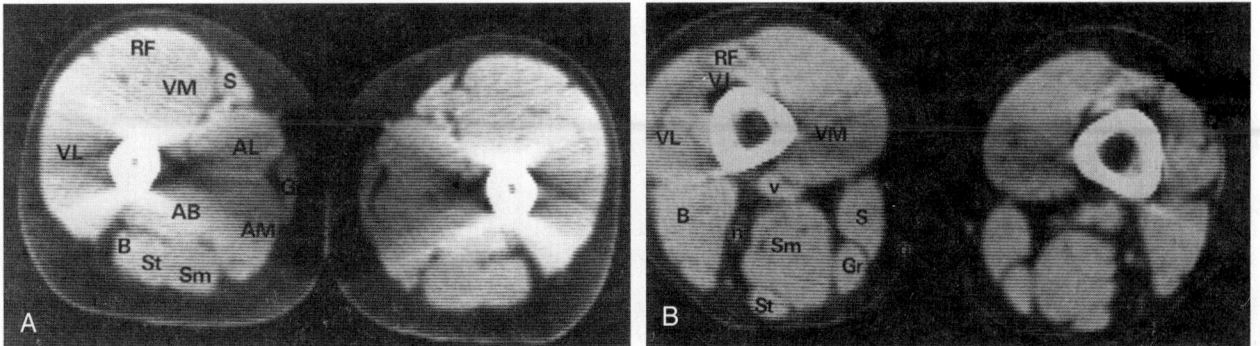

Figure 12-195 Muscular anatomy as shown on computed tomography (CT) scan; images through the upper femur **(A)** and lower third of femur **(B)** are shown. *AB*, Adductor brevis; *AL*, adductor longus; *AM*, adductor magnus; *B*, biceps femoris; *Gr*, gracilis; *n*, tibial and common peroneal nerves; *RF*, rectus femoris; *S*, sartorius; *Sm*, semimembranosus; *St*, semitendinosus; *V*, deep femoral vein and artery; *VI*, vastus intermedius; *VL*, vastus lateralis; *VM*, vastus medialis. (From Weissman BNW, Sledge CB: Orthopedic radiology, Philadelphia, 1986, WB Saunders, p. 504.)

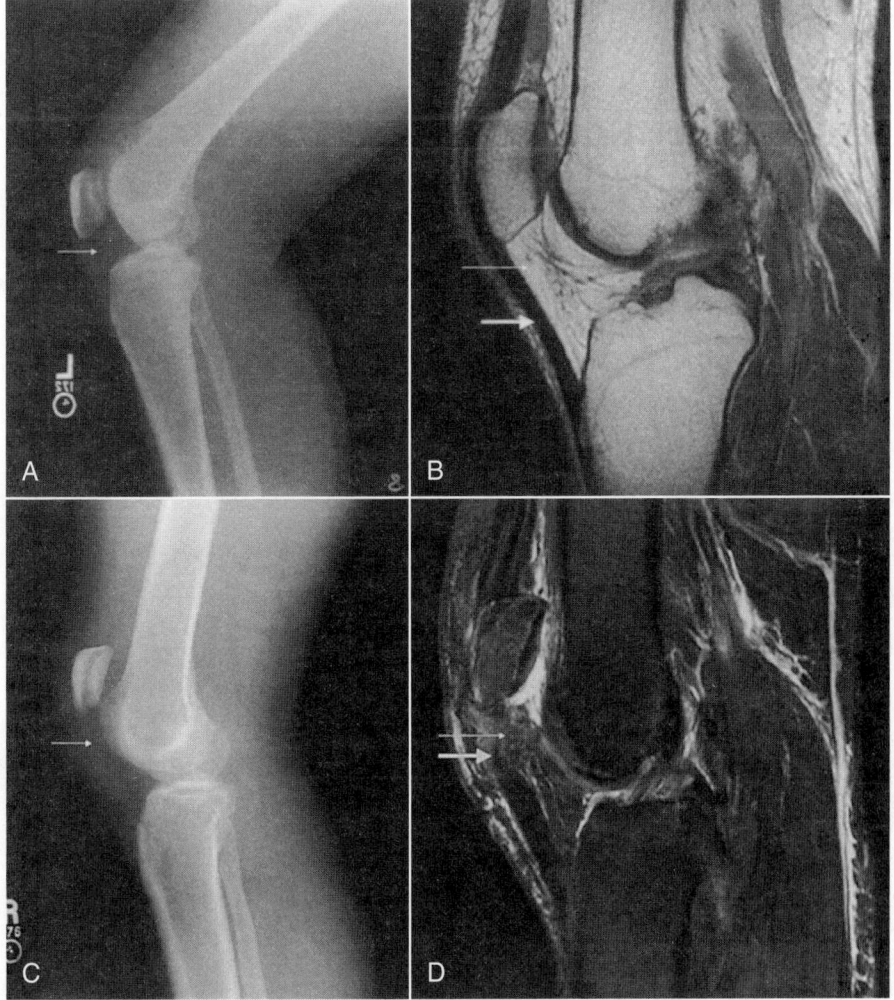

Figure 12-196 A, A lateral plain radiograph and **(B)** a T1-weighted MRI scan of an injured knee show a normal contour of the intact patella tendon *(broad arrow)* and infrapatellar fat pad *(narrow arrow)*. **C,** A lateral plain radiograph and **(D)** a T2-weighted MRI scan of an injured knee show disruption of the patella tendon *(broad arrow)* and infrapatellar fat pad *(narrow arrow)* at the inferior pole with associated patella alta. (From Chin KR, Sodl JF: Infrapatellar fat pad disruption—a radiographic sign of patellar tendon rupture. Clin Orthop Relat Res 440:224–225, 2005.)

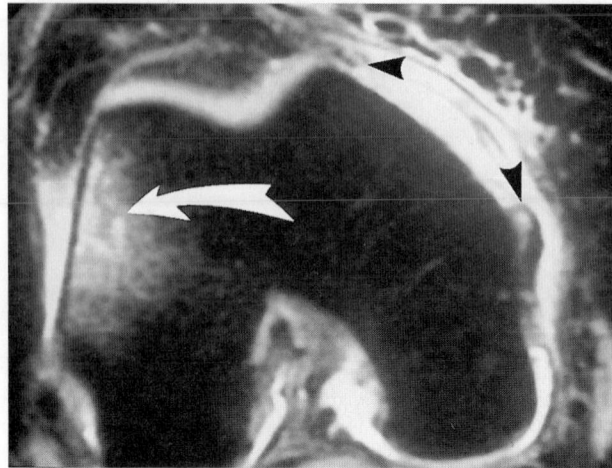

Figure 12-197 Bone bruise from patellar dislocation-relocation injury. Transverse fat-suppressed intermediate-weighted (TR/TEeff, 3500/12) fast spin echo magnetic resonance (MR) image. A high-signal-intensity contusion *(arrow)* is apparent in the lateral femoral condyle. Also note the torn medial patellofemoral ligament *(arrowheads)*. (From Resnick D, Kransdorf MJ: Bone and joint imaging, Philadelphia, 2005, WB Saunders, p. 121.)

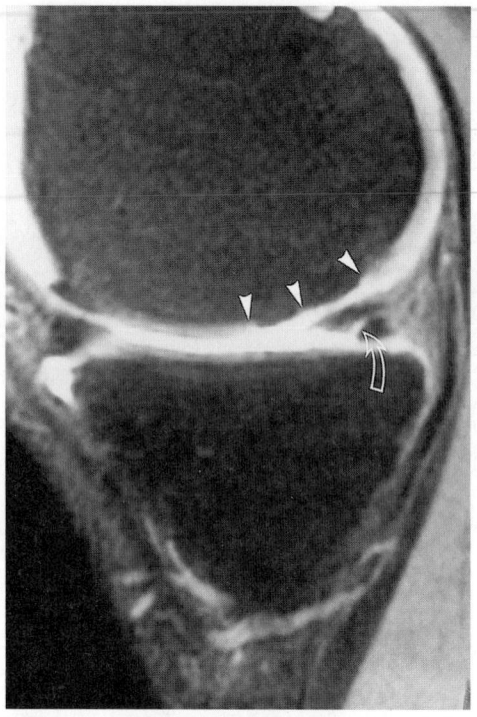

Figure 12-198 Recurrent meniscal tear after partial medial meniscectomy. Sagittal fat-suppressed T1-weighted (TR/TE, 800/15) spin echo magnetic resonance (MR) image after a knee arthrogram performed with a dilute gadolinium mixture. Injected contrast enters the substance of a new meniscal tear *(arrow)* in the remnant of the posterior horn. Also note the degenerative cartilage loss along the medial femoral surface *(arrowheads)*. (From Resnick D, Kransdorf MJ: Bone and joint imaging, Philadelphia, 2005, WB Saunders, p. 126.)

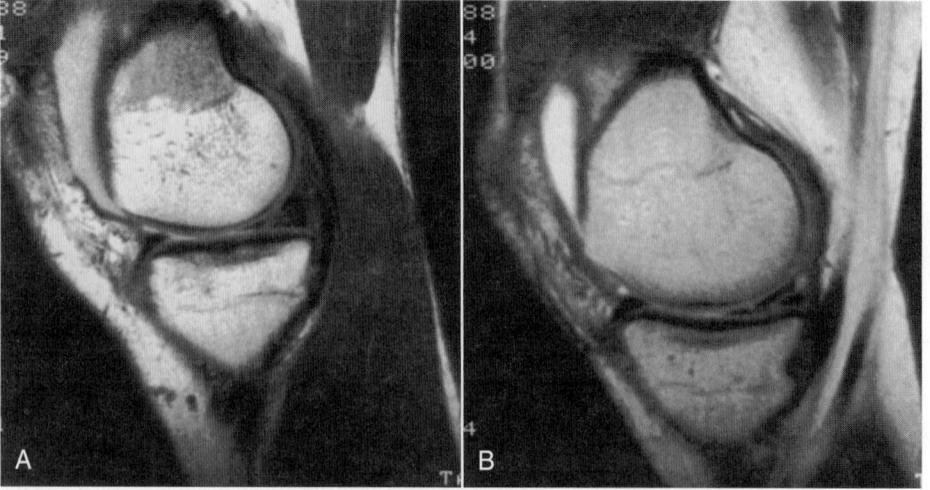

Figure 12-199 Magnetic resonance image (MRI) showing lesion of the posterior horn of the medial meniscus, A. In some cases, contrast can be enhanced by the intra-articular injection of gadolinium diethylenetriamene penta-acetic acid (DTPA). **B,** Inferior longitudinal tear with an associated horizontal tear. (From Strobel M, Stedtfeld HW: Diagnostic evaluation of the knee, Berlin, 1990, Springer-Verlag, p. 240.)

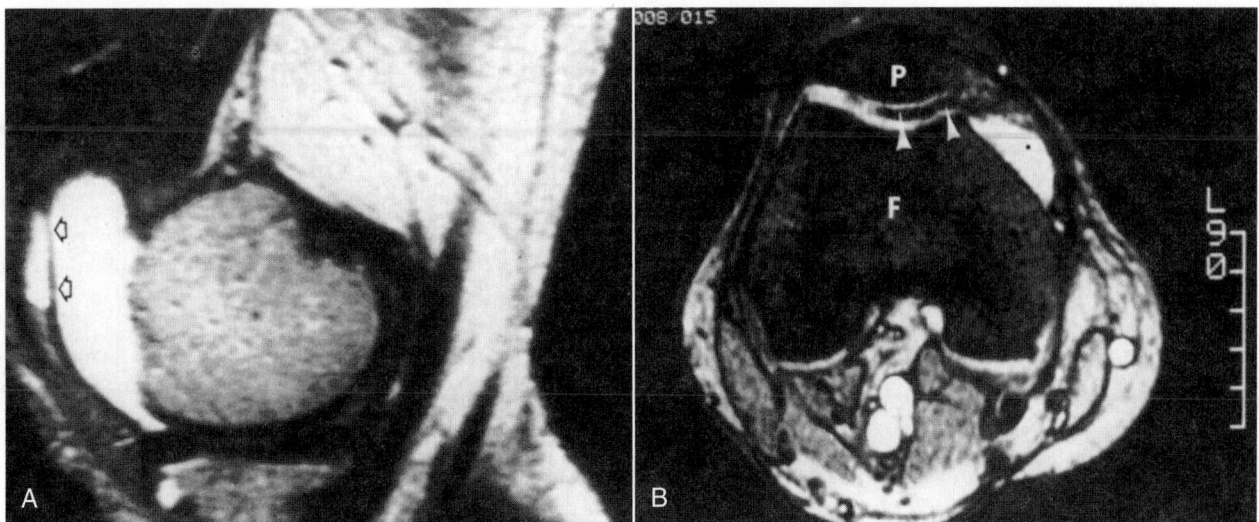

Figure 12-200 Magnetic resonance image (MRI) of mediopatellar plica. A, Sagittal, T2-weighted image located medial to the patella demonstrates an effusion present within the knee joint that appears white. The vertical linear band seen within the joint *(open arrows)* represents the medial plica. **B,** Transaxial STIR image through the patellofemoral joint again demonstrates the effusion *(arrowheads),* which appears bright and surrounds a tonguelike extension of tissue arising from the medial joint line and located between the patella *(P)* and the femur *(F).* This tissue represents a medial plica. In this location, plicae can become hypertrophied and lead to symptoms and signs of internal derangement. (From Kursunoglu-Brahme S, Resnick D: Magnetic resonance imaging of the knee. Orthop Clin North Am 21:571, 1990.)

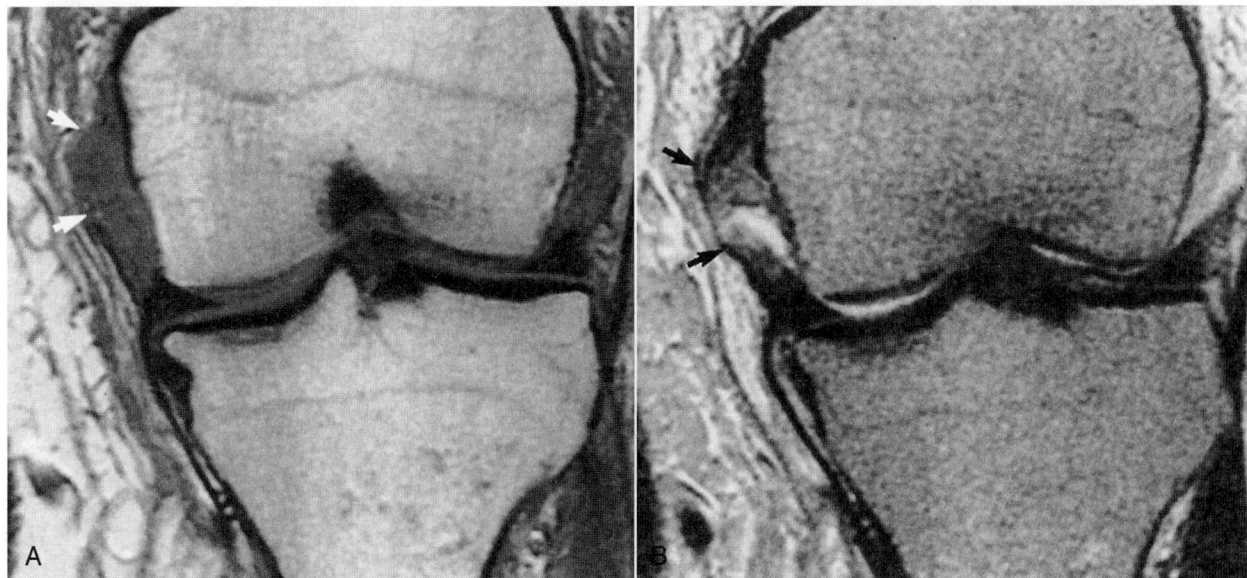

Figure 12-201 Injuries of the medial collateral ligament: complete tear. Coronal intermediate-weighted (TR/TE, 1500/12) **(A)** and T2-weighted (TR/TE, 1500/80) **(B)** spin echo magnetic resonance (MR) images show complete disruption *(arrows)* of the fibers of the medial collateral liga- ment. Note the increase in signal intensity in the ligament and soft tissues in **B.** A joint effusion is present. Additional injuries in this patient included tears of the lateral meniscus and anterior cruciate ligament. (From Resnick D, Kransdorf MJ: Bone and joint imaging, Philadelphia, 2005, WB Saunders, p. 959. Courtesy of V. Chandnani, MD, Pittsburgh.)

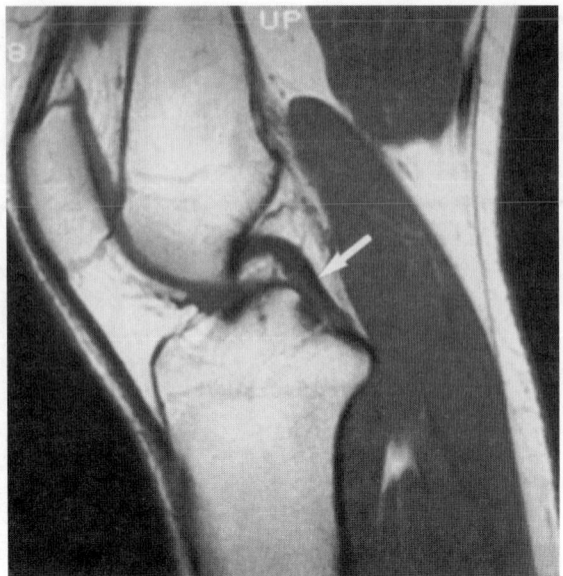

Figure 12-202 Magnetic resonance (MR) image showing intact posterior cruciate ligament *(arrow)*. (From Strobel M, Stedtfeld HW: Diagnostic evaluation of the knee, Berlin, 1990, Springer-Verlag, p. 243.)

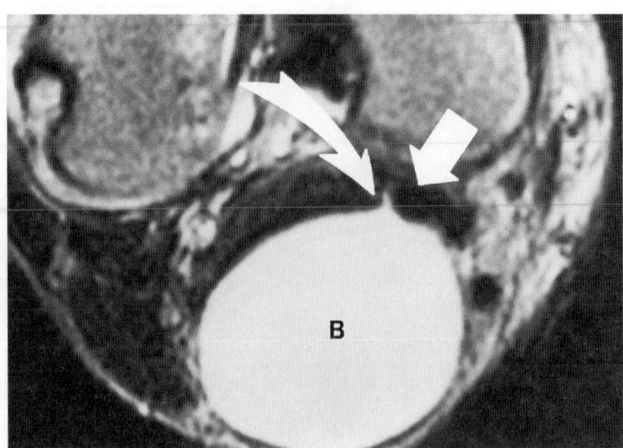

Figure 12-203 Baker's cyst. Transverse T2-weighted (TR/TE, 2500/80) spin echo magnetic resonance (MR) image of the knee. Fluid distends the semimembranosus-gastrocnemius recess *(B)*. The neck of the popliteal cyst is located between the tendons of the medial gastrocnemius *(curved arrow)* and semimembranosus *(straight arrow)* tendons. (From Resnick D, Kransdorf MJ: Bone and joint imaging, Philadelphia, 2005, WB Saunders, p. 124.)

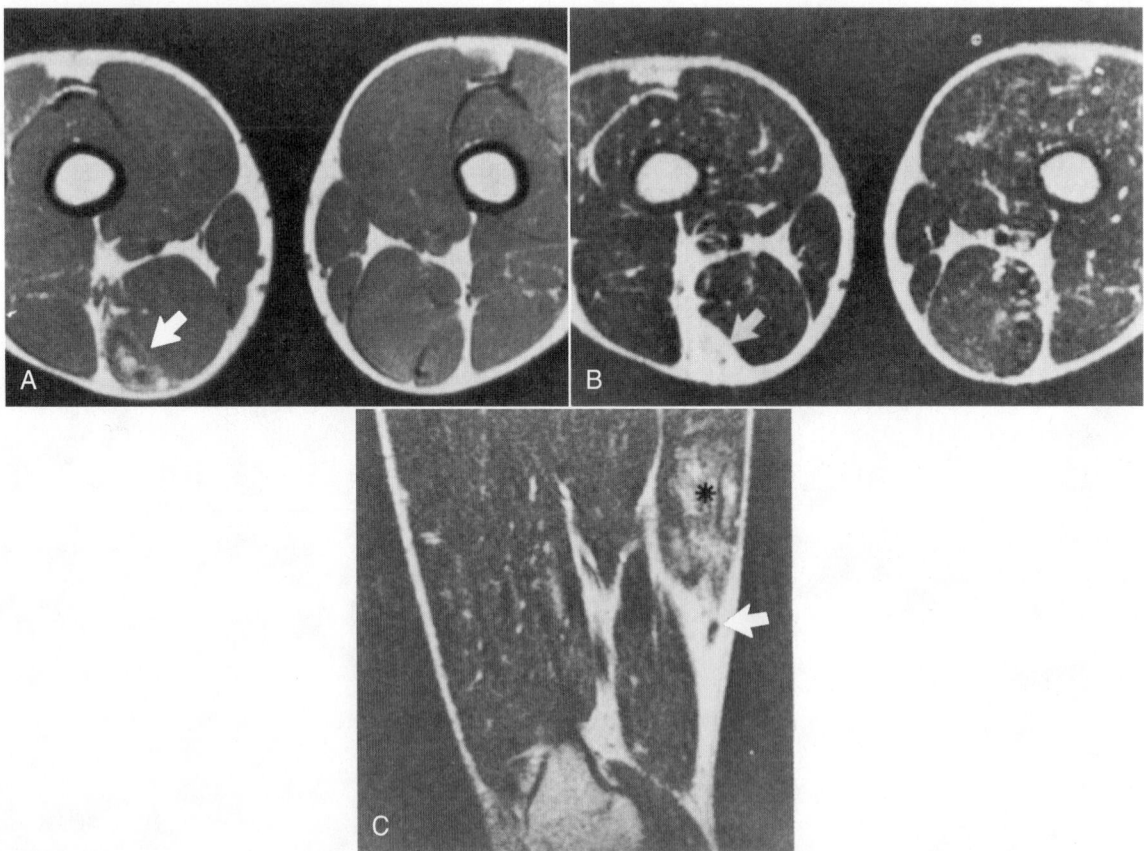

Figure 12-204 Magnetic resonance (MR) images showing tendon rupture in a 22-year-old athlete who pulled his hamstring on two occasions and was unable to run. Seven centimeters above the patella **(A)** axial T1-weighted (TR, 600 msec; TE, 20 msec) and **(B)** T2-weighted (TR, 2000 msec; TE, 85 msec) MR images show abnormally high signal intensity of the right semitendinosus muscle *(arrows)* compared with the normal left side. **C,** Sagittal T2-weighted MR image (TR, 2000 msec; TE, 85 msec) discloses that retracted semitendinosus muscle (asterisk) has an abnormally high signal intensity. The *arrow* indicates a torn musculotendinous junction. (From Bassett LW, Gold RH: Magnetic resonance imaging of the musculoskeletal system: an overview. Clin Orthop 244:20, 1989.)

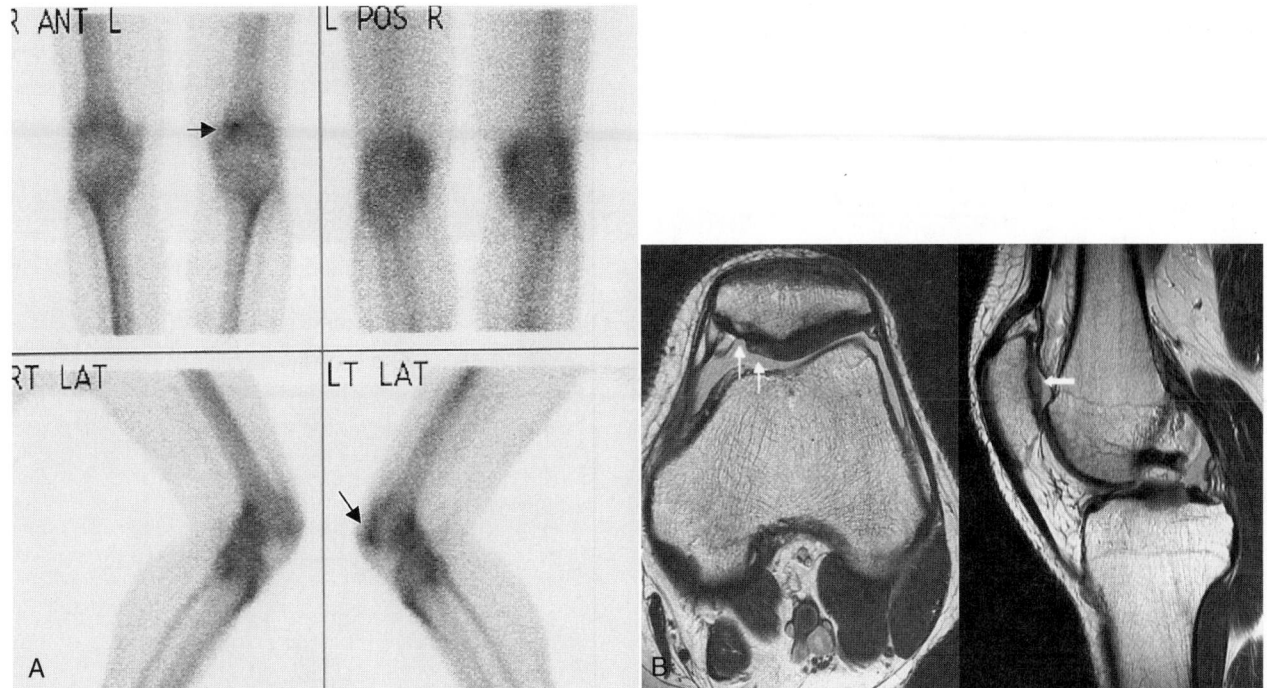

Figure 12-205 Chondromalacia patellae. A, Bone scan shows a focal area of increased uptake in the medial aspect of the left patellofemoral joint *(arrows).* **B,** Intermediate-weighted spin echo magnetic resonance (MR) image shows abnormal signal and erosion in the medial aspect of the patellar cartilage *(arrows).* (From Resnick D, Kransdorf MJ: Bone and joint imaging, Philadelphia, 2005, WB Saunders, p. 112.)

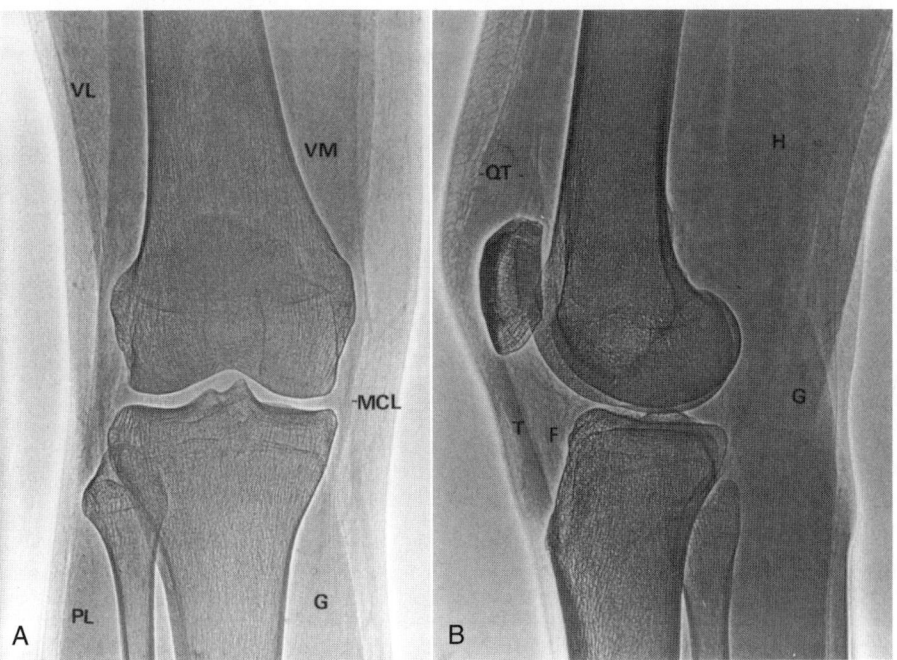

Figure 12-206 Xeroradiography of the knee. A, Anteroposterior view. **B,** Lateral view. *F,* Infrapatellar fat pad; *G,* gastrocnemius; *H,* hamstrings; *MCL,* medial collateral ligament; *PL,* peroneus longus; *QT,* quadriceps tendon; *T,* patellar tendon; *VL,* vastus lateralis; *VM,* vastus medialis. (From Weissman BNW, Sledge CB: Orthopedic radiology, Philadelphia, 1986, WB Saunders, p. 504.)

PRÉCIS OF THE KNEE ASSESSMENT*

History
Observation
Examination
    Active movements (sitting or supine lying)
        Knee flexion
        Knee extension
        Medial rotation of the tibia on the femur
        Lateral rotation of the tibia on the femur
    Passive movements (as in active movements) (sitting or supine lying)
    Resisted isometric movements (sitting or supine lying)
        Knee flexion
        Knee extension
        Ankle plantar flexion
        Ankle dorsiflexion
    Tests for ligament stability (sitting or supine lying)
        For one-plane medial instability:
            Hughston's valgus stress at 0° and 30°
            Valgus stress at 0° and 30°
        For one-plane lateral instability:
            Hughston's varus stress at 0° and 30°
            Varus stress at 0° and 30°
        For one-plane anterior instability:
            Active drawer test
            Drawer test
            Lachman test or its modifications
        For one-plane posterior instability:
            Active drawer test
            Drawer test
            Godfrey test
            Posterior sag
        For anteromedial rotary instability:
            Slocum test
        For anterolateral rotary instability:
            Jerk test of Hughston
            Losee test
            Noyes flexion-rotation drawer test
            Pivot shift test
            Slocum ARLI test
        For posteromedial rotary instability:
            Hughston's posteromedial drawer test
            Posteromedial pivot shift test
        For posterolateral rotary instability:
            External rotation recurvatum
            Hughston's posterolateral drawer test
            Loomer's posterolateral rotary instability test
            Tibial external rotation (Dial) test
    Functional assessment
    Special tests (sitting or supine lying)
        For meniscus lesions:
            McMurray test

        For plica lesions:
            Hughston's plica test
            Mediopatellar plica test
            Plica "stutter" test
        For swelling:
            Brush test (minimal swelling)
            Fluctuation test (moderate swelling)
            Indentation test
            Patellar tap test (moderate swelling)
        For patellofemoral syndrome:
            Clarke's sign
            McConnell test
        For quadriceps pull:
            Q-angle
            Tubercle sulcus test
        For patellar instability:
            Fairbank's apprehension test
            Moving patellar apprehension test (MPAT)
        For iliotibial band friction syndrome:
            Noble compression test
    Reflexes and cutaneous distribution
    Joint play movements (supine)
        Backward and forward movements of the tibia on the femur
        Medial and lateral translation of the tibia on the femur
        Medial and lateral displacements of the patella
        Depression of the patella
        Anteroposterior movement of the fibula on the tibia
    Palpation (supine)
    Tests for ligament stability (prone lying)
        For one-plane anterior instability:
            Lachman test modification 6
    Special tests (prone lying)
        For meniscus lesions:
            Apley's test
    Tests for ligament stability (standing)
        For anterolateral rotary instability:
            Crossover test
        For posterolateral rotary instability:
            Jakob test
    Special tests (standing)
        For meniscus lesions:
            Ege's test
            Thessaly test
        For patellofemoral syndrome:
            Step up test
    Diagnostic imaging
After any examination, the patient should be warned of the possibility of exacerbation of symptoms as a result of the assessment.

*Although examination of the knee may be carried out with the patient in the supine position, some of the tests may require the patient to move to other positions (e.g., standing, lying, prone, sitting). When these tests are used, the examination should be planned in such a way that the movement and, therefore, the discomfort experienced by the patient are kept to a minimum. The sequence should be from standing to sitting, to supine lying, to side lying, and finally, to prone lying.

CASE STUDIES

When doing these case studies, the examiner should list the appropriate questions to be asked and why they are being asked, what to look for and why, and what things should be tested and why. Depending on the answers of the patient (and the examiner should consider different responses), several possible causes of the patient's problem may become evident (examples are given in parentheses). A differential diagnosis chart should be made. The examiner can then decide how different diagnoses may affect the treatment plan. For example, a 16-year-old female volleyball player comes to you with knee pain (Table 12-15). Her knee is painful when she plays, and she sometimes feels a clicking when going up and down stairs. Describe your assessment plan for this patient (meniscus pathology versus plica syndrome).

1. A 59-year-old man presents to you with moderate pain and swelling of 4 months' duration in his right knee. There is no history of trauma. The pain and swelling have become worse during the past month. Describe your assessment plan for this patient (osteoarthritis versus meniscus pathology).

2. A 24-year-old male football player is referred to you for treatment after a surgical repair to the anterior cruciate and medial collateral ligaments of the right knee. He is still in a splint, but the surgeon says the splint can be removed for treatment. Describe your assessment plan for this patient.

3. A 54-year-old man comes to you for treatment. He has difficulty walking and pain in the left hamstrings that is referred into the area of the gluteal fold. There is ecchymosis evident in the posterior knee and a small amount in the superior calf area. Describe your assessment plan for this patient (hamstring strain versus sciatica).

4. An 18-year-old woman presents to your clinic with anterior knee pain. Design your assessment plan for this patient (chondromalacia patellae versus plica syndrome).

5. A 17-year-old male soccer player comes to you saying that his knee feels unstable. He says he was playing soccer, twisted to challenge a player, and felt a pop in his knee. Describe your assessment plan for this patient (osteochondral fracture versus anterior cruciate sprain).

6. A 10-year-old boy is brought to you by his parents. He is experiencing anterior knee pain. Describe your assessment plan for this patient (Osgood-Schlatter syndrome versus chondromalacia patellae).

7. A 20-year-old female rugby player comes to you with lateral knee pain that is sometimes referred down the leg. The knee hurts when she walks. She vaguely remembers being kicked in the knee while playing rugby 10 days earlier. Describe your assessment plan for this patient (superior tibiofibular joint subluxation versus common peroneal nerve neuropraxia).

8. An 18-year-old female swimmer presents to you with medial knee pain. She has just increased her training to 10,000 m per day. Describe your assessment plan for this patient (medial collateral ligament sprain versus chondromalacia patellae).

TABLE 12-15

Differential Diagnosis of Meniscus and Medial Patellar Plica Syndrome

	Medial Meniscus	Medial Patellar Plica Syndrome
History	Mechanism of injury: rotation, flexion, and valgus stress (may be acute or insidious) while weightbearing	Mechanism of injury: flexion, rotation (usually insidious onset)
Pain	Joint line	May be joint line but also superomedial to joint line
Swelling	May be present	May be present
Locking or giving way	Locking more likely	Giving way more likely
Active movement	May be limited	Usually full but extremes of motion may be painful, catching may occur on movement
Passive movement	Pain at extremes	Pain possible at extreme of flexion
Resisted isometric movement	Normal	Normal unless pinching causes pain and reflex inhibition
Ligament tests	Negative	Negative
Special tests	McMurray may be positive; Apley's test may be positive	Mediopatellar plica test positive, plica "stutter" test positive, Hughston plica test positive
Palpation	Joint line tenderness	Plica may demonstrate thickening and be bandlike

REFERENCES

1. Muller W: Form and function of the knee—its relation to high performance and to sports. Am J Sports Med 24:S104–S106, 1996.
2. Kaltenborn F: Mobilization of the extremity joints, Oslo, 1980, Olaf Norles Bokhandel.
3. Arnoczsky S: The blood supply of the meniscus and its role in healing and repair. In American Association of Orthopaedic Surgeons, Symposium on Sports Medicine: the knee, St Louis, 1985, Mosby.
4. Volashin AS, Wosk J: Shock absorption of meniscectomized and painful knees: a comparative in vivo study. J Biomech Eng 5:157–193, 1983.
5. Radin EL, de Lamotte R, Maquet P: Role of the menisci in the distribution of stress in the knee. Clin Orthop 185:290–294, 1984.
6. Seedhom BB: Loadbearing function of the menisci. Physiotherapy 62:223–226, 1976.
7. Gray JC: Neural and vascular anatomy of the menisci of the human knee. J Orthop Sports Phys Ther 29:23–30, 1999.
8. Ficat RP, Hungerford DS: The patello-femoral joint, Baltimore, 1977, Williams & Wilkins.
9. Goodfellow J, Hungerford DS, Zindel M: Patello-femoral joint mechanics and pathology: functional anatomy of the patellofemoral joint. J Bone Joint Surg Br 58:287–290, 1976.
10. Delfico AJ, Garrett WE: Mechanisms of injury of the anterior cruciate ligament in soccer players. Clin Sports Med 17:779–785, 1998.
11. Levine JW, Kiapour AM, Quatman CE, et al: Clinically relevant injury patterns after an anterior cruciate ligament injury provide insight into injury mechanisms. Am J Sports Med 41:385–395, 2013.
12. Tria AJ, Hosea TM: Diagnosis of knee ligament injuries: clinical. In Scott WN, editor: Ligament and extensor mechanism injuries of the knee: diagnosis and treatment, St Louis, 1991, Mosby.
13. Bauer SJ, Hollander JE, Fuchs SH, et al: A clinical decision rule in the evaluation of acute knee injuries. J Emerg Med 13:611–615, 1995.
14. Edwards PH, Grana WA: Physeal fractures about the knee. J Am Acad Orthop Surg 3:63–69, 1995.
15. Veenema KR: Valgus knee instability in an adolescent-ligament sprain or physeal injury. Phys Sportsmed 27:62–75, 1999.
16. Levy M, Smith AD: Diagnosing meniscus injuries: focus on the office exam. Phys Sportsmed 22:47–54, 1994.
17. Cooper DE: Snapping popliteus syndrome—a cause of mechanical knee popping in athletes. Am J Sports Med 27:671–674, 1999.
18. Cutbill JW, Ladly KO, Bray RC, et al: Anterior knee pain: a review. Clin J Sports Med 7:40–45, 1997.
19. Biedert RM, Sanchis-Alfonso V: Sources of anterior knee pain. Clin Sports Med 21:335–347, 2002.
20. Fulkerson JP: Diagnosis and treatment of patients with patellofemoral pain. Am J Sports Med 30:447–456, 2002.
21. Post WR, Fulkerson J: Knee pain diagrams: correlation with physical examination findings in patients with anterior knee pain. Arthroscopy 10:618–623, 1994.
22. Khan KM, Cook JL, Bonar F, et al: Histopathology of common tendinopathies—update and implications for clinical management. Sports Med 27:393–408, 1999.
23. Bassett FH, Soucacous PN, Carr WA: Jumper's knee: patellar tendinitis and patellar tendon rupture. In American Academy of Orthopedic Surgeons: Symposium on the athlete's knee, St Louis, 1980, Mosby.

24. Medlar RC, Lyne ED: Sinding-Larsen-Johansson disease. J Bone Joint Surg Am 60:1113–1116, 1978.
25. Khan KM, Maffulli N, Coleman BD, et al: Patellar tendinopathy: some aspects of basic science and clinical management. Br J Sports Med 32:346–355, 1998.
26. DePalma MJ, Perkins RH: Patellar tendinosis—acute patellar tendon rupture and jumper's knee. Phys Sportsmed 32(5):41–45, 2004.
27. Hale SA: Etiology of patellar tendinopathy in athletes. J Sports Rehab 14:258–272, 2005.
28. Liorzou G: Knee ligaments: clinical examination, Berlin, 1991, Springer-Verlag.
29. Grelsamer RP: Patellar malalignment. J Bone Joint Surg Am 82:1639–1650, 2000.
30. Hughston JC: Knee ligaments: injury and repair, St Louis, 1993, Mosby.
31. McFarland EG, Mamanee P, Queale WS, et al: Olecranon and prepatellar bursitis. Phys Sportsmed 28(3):40–52, 2000.
32. LaPrade RF: The anatomy of the deep infrapatellar bursa of the knee. Am J Sports Med 26:129–132, 1998.
33. Fulkerson RP, Hungerford DS: Evaluation and rehabilitation of nonarthritic anterior knee pain. In Fulkerson JP, Hungerford DS, editors: Disorders of the patellofemoral joint, Baltimore, 1990, Williams & Wilkins.
34. Riegger-Krugh C, Keysor JJ: Skeletal malalignments of the lower quarter: correlated and compensatory motions and postures. J Orthop Sports Phys Ther 23:164–170, 1996.
35. Hawkins RJ: Musculoskeletal examination, St Louis, 1995, Mosby.
36. Fulkerson JP, Arendt EA: Anterior knee pain in females. Clin Orthop Relat Res 372:69–73, 2000.
37. Boden BP, Pearsall AW, Garrett WE, et al: Patellofemoral instability: evaluation and management. J Am Acad Orthop Surg 5:47–57, 1997.
38. Shultz SJ, Nguyen AD, Levine BJ: The relationship between lower extremity alignment characteristics and anterior knee joint laxity. Sports Health 1:54–60, 2009.
39. Post WR, Teitge R, Amis A: Patellofemoral malalignment: looking beyond the view box. Clin Sports Med 21:521–546, 2002.
40. McConnell J: Management of patellofemoral problems. Man Ther 1:60–66, 1996.
41. Loudon JK, Goist HL, Loudon KL: Genu recurvatum syndrome. J Orthop Sports Phys Ther 27:361–367, 1998.
42. Grelsamer RP: Patellar nomenclature—the Tower of Babel revisited. Clin Orthop Relat Res 436:60–65, 2005.
43. Luyckx T, Didden K, Vandenneucker H, et al: Is there a biomechanical explanation for anterior knee pain in patients with patella alta? J Bone Joint Surg Br 91:344–350, 2009.
44. Staheli LT, Engel GM: Tibial torsion: a method of assessment and a survey of normal children. Clin Orthop 86:183–186, 1972.
45. Reider B: The orthopedic physical examination, Philadelphia, 1999, WB Saunders.
46. Waldron VD: A test for chondromalacia patellae. Orthop Rev 12:103, 1983.
47. Hughston JC: Extensor mechanism examination. In Fox JM, Del Pizzo W, editors: The patellofemoral joint, New York, 1993, McGraw-Hill.
48. McConnell J, Fulkerson J: The knee: patellofemoral and soft tissue injuries. In Zachazewski JE, Magee

DJ, Quillen WS, editors: Athletic injuries and rehabilitation, Philadelphia, 1996, WB Saunders.
49. Earl JE, Hertel J, Denegar CR: Patterns of dynamic malalignment, muscle activation, joint motion, and patellofemoral pain syndrome. J Sports Rehab 14:215–233, 2005.
50. Arendt E: Anatomy and malalignment of the patellofemoral joint: its relation to patellofemoral arthrosis. Clin Orthop Relat Res 436:71–75, 2005.
51. Shibanuma N, Sheehan FT, Stanhope SJ: Limb positioning is critical for defining patellofemoral alignment and femoral shape. Clin Orthop Relat Res 434:198–206, 2005.
52. Post WR: Anterior knee pain: diagnosis and treatment. J Am Acad Orthop Surg 13:534–543, 2005.
53. Tyler TF, Nicholas SJ, Mullaney MJ, et al: The role of hip muscle function in the treatment of patellofemoral pain syndrome. Am J Sports Med 34:630–636, 2006.
54. Gibulka MT, Threlkeld-Watkins J: Patellofemoral pain and asymmetrical hip rotation. Phys Ther 85:1201–1207, 2005.
55. Dutton M: Orthopedic examination, evaluation and intervention, New York, 2004, McGraw Hill.
56. Fulkerson JP: Patellofemoral pain disorders: evaluation and management. J Am Acad Orthop Surg 2:124–132, 1994.
57. Katchburian MV, Ball AM, Shih YF, et al: Measurement of patellar tracking: assessment and analysis of the literature. Clin Orthop Relat Res 412:241–259, 2003.
58. Post WR: Clinical evaluation of patients with patellofemoral disorders. Arthroscopy 15:841–851, 1999.
59. Nissen CW, Cullen MC, Hewett TE, et al: Physical and arthroscopic examination techniques of the patellofemoral joint. J Orthop Sports Phys Ther 26:277–285, 1998.
60. Fritz JM, Delitto A, Erhard RE, et al: An examination of the selective tissue tension scheme, with evidence for the concept of a capsular pattern of the knee. Phys Ther 78:1046–1061, 1998.
61. Lancaster AR, Nyland J, Roberts CS: The validity of the motion palpation test for determining patellofemoral joint articular cartilage damage. Phys Ther Sport 8:59–65, 2007.
62. Jacobson KE, Flandry FC: Diagnosis of anterior knee pain. Clin Sports Med 8:179–195, 1989.
63. Rouse SJ: The role of the iliotibial tract in patellofemoral pain and iliotibial band friction syndromes. Physiotherapy 82:199–202, 1996.
64. Cichanowski HR, Schmitt JS, Johnson RJ, et al: Hip strength in collegiate female athletes with patellofemoral pain. Med Sci Sports Exerc 39:1227–1232, 2007.
65. Segal P, Jacob M: The knee, Chicago, 1983, Year Book Medical.
66. Kannus P, Jarvineaa M, Latvala K: Knee strength evaluation. Scand J Sport Sci 9:9, 1987.
67. Goslin BR, Charteris J: Isokinetic dynamometry: normative data for clinical use in lower extremity (knee) cases. Scand J Rehab Med 11:105–109, 1979.
68. Stafford MG, Grana WA: Hamstring/quadriceps ratios in college football players: a high velocity evaluation. Am J Sports Med 12:209–211, 1984.
69. Aagaard P, Simonsen EB, Magnusson SP, et al: A new concept for isokinetic hamstring: quadriceps muscle strength ratio. Am J Sports Med 26:231–237, 1998.
70. Sgaglione NA, Del Pizzo W, Fox JM, et al: Critical analysis of knee ligament rating systems. Am J Sports Med 23:660–667, 1995.

71. Borsa PA, Lephart SM, Irrgang JJ: Sport-specificity of knee scoring systems to assess disability in anterior cruciate ligament-deficient athletes. J Sports Rehab 7:44–60, 1998.

72. Wright RW: Knee injury outcomes measures. J Am Acad Orthop Surg 17:31–39, 2009.

73. Clark NC: Functional performance testing following knee ligament injury. Phys Ther Sport 2:91–105, 2001.

74. Fonseca ST, Magee DJ, Wessel J, et al: Validation of a performance test for outcome evaluation of knee function. Clin J Sport Med 2:251–256, 1992.

75. Boonstra MC, deWaal Malefijt MC, Verdonschot N: How to quantify knee function after total knee arthroplasty? The Knee 15:390–395, 2008.

76. Garratt AM, Brealey S, Gillespie WJ: Patient-assessed health instruments of the knee: a structured review. Rheumatology 43:1414–1423, 2003.

77. Paxton EW, Fithian DC, Stone ML, et al: The reliability and validity of knee specific: general health instruments in assessing acute patellar dislocation outcomes. Am J Sports Med 31:487–492, 2003.

78. Daniel DM, Stone ML, Riehl B: Ligament surgery: the evaluation of results. In Daniel D, Akeson W, O'Conner J, editors: Knee ligaments: structure, injury and repair, New York, 1990, Raven Press.

79. Strobel M, Stedtfeld HW: Diagnostic evaluation of the knee, Berlin, 1990, Springer-Verlag.

80. Noyes FR, Barber SD, Mangine RE: Abnormal lower limb symmetry determined by functional hop tests after anterior cruciate rupture. Am J Sports Med 19:513–518, 1991.

81. Barber SD, Noyes FR, Mangine RE, et al: Quantitative assessment of functional limitations in normal and anterior cruciate ligament-deficient knees. Clin Orthop 255:204–214, 1990.

82. Grindem H, Logerstedt D, Eitzen I, et al: Single-legged hip tests as predictors of self-reported knee function in nonoperatively treated individuals with anterior cruciate ligament injury. Am J Sports Med 39:2347–2354, 2011.

83. O'Donnell SO, Thomas SG, Marks P: Improving the sensitivity of the hop index in patients with an ACL deficient knee by transforming the hop distance scores. BMC Musculoskelet Disord 7:9–14, 2006.

84. Hopper DM, Goh SC, Wentworth LA, et al: Test-retest reliability of knee rating scales and functional hop tests one year following anterior cruciate ligament reconstruction. Phys Ther Sport 3:10–18, 2002.

85. Juris PM, Phillips EM, Dalpe C, et al: A dynamic test of lower extremity function following anterior cruciate ligament reconstruction and rehabilitation. J Orthop Sports Phys Ther 26:184–191, 1997.

86. Logerstedt DS, Snyder-Mackler L, Ritter RC, et al: Knee stability and movement coordination impairments: knee ligament sprain. J Orthop Sports Phys Ther 40:A1–A37, 2010.

87. Booher LD, Hench KM, Worrell TW, et al: Reliability of three single-leg hop tests. J Sports Rehab 2:165–170, 1993.

88. Risberg MA, Ekeland A: Assessment of functional tests after anterior cruciate ligament surgery. J Orthop Sports Phys Ther 19:212–217, 1994.

89. Losee RE: Diagnosis of chronic injury to the anterior cruciate ligament. Orthop Clin North Am 16:83–97, 1985.

90. Jackson DW, Jennings LD, Maywoods RM, et al: Magnetic resonance imaging of the knee. Am J Sports Med 16:29–37, 1988.

91. Larson RL: Physical examination in the diagnosis of rotary instability. Clin Orthop 172:38–44, 1983.

92. Demirdjian AM, Petrie SG, Guanche CA, et al: The outcomes of two knee scoring questionnaires in a normal population. Am J Sports Med 26:46–51, 1998.

93. Hoher J, Bach T, Munster A, et al: Does the mode of data collection change results in a subjective knee score? Self administration vs. interview. Am J Sports Med 25:642–647, 1997.

94. Noyes FR, McGinniss GH, Mooar LA: Functional disability in the anterior cruciate insufficient knee syndrome: review of knee rating systems and projected risk factors in determining treatment. Sports Med 1:278–302, 1984.

95. Noyes FR, Barber SD, Mooar LA: A rationale for assessing sports activity levels and limitations in knee disorders. Clin Orthop 246:238–249, 1989.

96. Barber-Westin SD, Noyes FR, McCloskey JW: Rigorous statistical reliability, validity and responsiveness testing on the Cincinnati knee rating system in 350 subjects with uninjured, injured, or anterior cruciate ligament-reconstructed knees. Am J Sports Med 27:402–416, 1999.

97. Agel J, LaPrade RF: Assessment of differences between the modified Cincinnati and International Knee Documentation Committee patient outcome scores—a prospective study. Am J Sports Med 37:2151–2157, 2009.

98. Irrgang JC, Safran MC, Fu FH: The knee: ligamentous and meniscal injuries. In Zachazewski JE, Magee DJ, Quillen WS, editors: Athletic injuries and rehabilitation, Philadelphia, 1996, WB Saunders.

99. Irrgang JJ, Snyder-Mackler L, Wainner RS, et al: Development of a patient-reported measure of function of the knee. J Bone Joint Surg Am 80:1132–1145, 1998.

100. Insall JN, Dorr LD, Scott RD, et al: Rationale of the Knee Society clinical rating system. Clin Orthop 248:13–14, 1989.

101. Lysholm J, Gillquist J: Evaluation of knee ligament surgery results with special emphasis on use of a scoring scale. Am J Sports Med 10:150–154, 1982.

102. Briggs KK, Lysholm J, Tegner Y, et al: The reliability, validity and responsiveness of the Lysholm Score and Tegner Activity Scale for anterior cruciate injuries of the knee. Am J Sports Med 37:890–897, 2009.

103. Heintjes EM, Bierma-Zeinstra SM, Berger MY, et al: Lysholm scale and WOMAC index were responsive in prospective cohort of young general practice patients. J Clin Epidemiol 61:481–488, 2008.

104. Smith HJ, Richardson JB, Tennant A: Modification and validation of the Lysholm knee scale to assess articular cartilage damage. Osteoarthritis Cartilage 17:53–58, 2009.

105. Kocher MS, Steadman JR, Briggs KK, et al: Reliability, validity and responsiveness of the Lysholm knee scale for various chondral disorders of the knee. J Bone Joint Surg Am 86:1139–1145, 2004.

106. Briggs KK, Steadman JR, Hay CJ, et al: Lysholm Score and Tegner Activity Level in individuals with normal knees. Am J Sports Med 37:898–901, 2009.

107. Hefti F, Mullen W, Jakob RP, et al: Evaluation of knee ligament injuries with the IKDC form. Knee Surg Sports Traumatol Arthrosc 1:226–234, 1993.

108. Anderson AF, Irrgang JJ, Kocher MS, et al: The international knee documentation committee subjective knee evaluation form—normative data. Am J Sports Med 34:128–135, 2006.

109. Kocher MS, Smith JT, Iverson MD, et al: Reliability, validity and responsiveness of a modified international knee documentation committee subjective knee form (Pedi-IKDC) in children with knee disorders. Am J Sports Med 39:933–939, 2011.

110. Schmitt LC, Paterno MV, Huang S: Validity and internal consistency of the International Knee Documentation Committee subjective knee evaluation form in children and adolescents. Am J Sports Med 38:2443–2447, 2010.

111. Greco NJ, Anderson AF, Mann BJ, et al: Responsiveness of the International Knee Documentation Committee subjective knee form in comparison to the Western Ontario and McMaster Universities Osteoarthritis Index, Modified Cincinnati knee rating system and short form 36 in patients with focal articular cartilage defects. Am J Sports Med 38:891–902, 2010.

112. Hambly K, Griva K: IKDC or KOOS—which one captures symptoms and disabilities most important to patients who have undergone initial anterior cruciate ligament reconstruction. Am J Sports Med 38:1395–1404, 2010.

113. Tegner Y, Lysholm J, Odensten M, et al: Evaluation of cruciate ligament injuries. Acta Orthop Scand 59:336–341, 1988.

114. Shea KP, Fulkerson JP: Preoperative computed tomography scanning and arthroscopy in predicting outcome after lateral retinacular release. Arthroscopy 8:327–334, 1992.

115. Karlsson J, Thomeé R, Sward L: Eleven year follow up of patellofemoral pain syndromes. Clin J Sport Med 6:22–26, 1996.

116. Kujala UM, Jaakkola LH, Koskinen SK, et al: Scoring of patellofemoral disorders. Arthroscopy 9:159–163, 1993.

117. Bennell K, Bartam S, Crossley K, et al: Outcome measures in patellofemoral pain syndrome: test retest reliability and inter-relationships. Phys Ther Sport 1:31–41, 2000.

118. Eng J, Pierrynowski MR: Evaluation of soft shoe orthotics in the treatment of patellofemoral pain syndrome. Phys Ther 73:62–68, 1993.

119. Flandry F, Hunt J, Terry G, et al: Analysis of subjective knee complaints using visual analog scales. Am J Sports Med 19:112–118, 1991.

120. Jinks C, Jordan K, Croft P: Measuring the population impact of knee pain and disability with the Western Ontario and McMaster Universities Osteoarthritis Index (WOMAC). Pain 100:55–64, 2002.

121. Brazier JE, Harper R, Munro J, et al: Generic and condition-specific outcome measures for people with osteoarthritis of the knee. Rheumatology 38:870–877, 1999.

122. Anderson JG, Wixson RL, Tsai D, et al: Functional outcome and patient satisfaction in total knee patients over the age of 75. J Arthroplasty 11:831–840, 1996.

123. Kreibich DN, Vaz M, Bourne RB, et al: What is the best way of assessing outcome after total knee replacement? Clin Orthop Relat Res 331:221–225, 1996.

124. Kantz ME, Harris WJ, Levitsky K, et al: Methods for assessing condition-specific and generic functional status outcomes after total knee replacement. Med Care 30(5):MS240–MS252, 1992.

125. Bombardier C, Melfi CA, Paul J, et al: Comparison of a generic and a disease-specific measure of pain and physical function after knee replacement surgery. Med Care 33:AS131–AS144, 1995.

126. Hartley RC, Barton-Hanson NG, Finley R, et al: Early patient outcomes after primary and revision total knee arthroplasty—a prospective study. J Bone Joint Surg Br 84:994–999, 2002.

127. Faucher M, Poiraudeau S, Lefevre-Colan MM, et al: Assessment of the test-retest reliability and construct validity of a modified Lequesne Index in knee osteoarthritis. Joint Bone Spine 70:520–525, 2003.

128. Faucher M, Poiraudeau S, Lefevre-Colan MM, et al: Algo-functional assessment of knee osteoarthritis: comparison of the test-retest reliability and

construct validity of the WOMAN and Lequesne Indexes. Osteoarthritis Cartilage 10:602–610, 2002.

129. Roos EM, Roos HP, Lohmander LS, et al: Knee injury and osteoarthritis outcome score (KOOS) development of a self-administered outcome measure. J Orthop Sports Phys Ther 78:88–96, 1998.

130. Roos EM, Toksvig-Larsen S: Knee injury and Osteoarthritis Outcome Score (KOOS)—validation and comparison to the WOMAN in total knee replacements. Health Qual Life Outcomes 1:17–27, 2003.

131. Rejeski WJ, Ettinger WH, Schumaker S, et al: Assessing performance-related disability in patients with knee osteoarthritis. Osteoarthritis Cartilage 3:157–167, 1995.

132. Kettlekamp DB, Thompson C: Development of a knee scoring scale. Clin Orthop 107:93–99, 1975.

133. Aichroth P, Freeman MA, Smillie IS, et al: A knee function assessment chart. J Bone Joint Surg Br 60:308–309, 1978.

134. Larson R: Rating sheet for knee function. In Smillie I, editor: Diseases of the knee joint, Edinburgh, 1974, Churchill Livingstone.

135. Selfe J, Harper L, Pederson I, et al: Four outcome measures for patellofemoral joint problems. 1. development and validity. Physiotherapy 87:507–515, 2001.

136. Selfe J, Harper L, Pederson I, et al: Four outcome measures for patellofemoral joint problems. 2. reliability and clinical sensitivity. Physiotherapy 87:516–522, 2001.

137. Garratt AM, Brealey S, Robling M, et al: Development of the knee quality of life (KQual-26) 26-item questionnaire: data quality, reliability, validity and responsiveness. Health Quality Life Outcomes 6:48–59, 2008.

138. Shoemaker SC, Daniel DM: The limits of knee motion: in vitro studies. In Daniel D, Akeson W, O'Conner J, editors: Knee ligaments: structure, injury and repair, New York, 1990, Raven Press.

139. Muller W: The knee: form, function and ligament reconstruction, New York, 1983, Springer-Verlag.

140. Detenbeck LC: Function of the cruciate ligaments in knee stability. Am J Sports Med 2:217–221, 1974.

141. DeFranco MJ, Bach BR: A comprehensive review of partial anterior cruciate ligament tears. J Bone Joint Surg Am 91:198–208, 2009.

142. Wu JL, Seon JK, Gadikota HR, et al: In situ forces in the anteromedial and posterolateral bundles of the anterior cruciate ligament under simulated functional loading conditions. Am J Sports Med 38:558–563, 2010.

143. Furman W, Marshall JL, Girgis FG: The anterior cruciate ligament: a functional analysis based on postmortem studies. J Bone Joint Surg Am 58:179–185, 1976.

144. Girgis FG, Marshall JL, Al Monajem ARS: The cruciate ligaments of the knee joint: anatomical, functional and experimental analysis. Clin Orthop 106:216–231, 1975.

145. Baker CL, Norwood LA, Hughston JC: Acute combined posterior and posterolateral instability of the knee. Am J Sports Med 12:204–208, 1984.

146. LaPrade RF, Wozniczka JK, Stellmaker MP, et al: Analysis of the static function of the popliteus tendon and evaluation of an anatomic reconstruction—the "fifth ligament" of the knee. Am J Sports Med 38:543–549, 2010.

147. Morgan PM, LaPrade RF, Wentorf FA, et al: The role of the oblique popliteal ligament and other structures in preventing knee hyperextension. Am J Sports Med 38:550–557, 2010.

148. Daniel DM: Diagnosis of a ligament injury. In Daniel D, Akeson W, O'Conner J, editors: Knee ligaments: structure, injury and repair, New York, 1990, Raven Press.

149. Marshall JL, Baugher WH: Stability examination of the knee: a single anatomic approach. Clin Orthop 146:78–83, 1980.

150. Cleland JA, Koppenhaver S: Netter's orthopedic clinical examination—an evidence based approach, ed 2, Philadelphia, 2011, Saunders/Elsevier.

151. Lonergon KT, Taylor DC: Medial collateral ligament injuries of the knee: an evolution of surgical reconstruction. Tech Knee Surg 1(2):137–145 2002.

152. Marchant MH, Tibor LM, Sekiya JK, et al: Management of medial-sided knee injuries, part 1: medial collateral ligament. Am J Sports Med 39:1102–1113, 2011.

153. Kennedy JC: The injured adolescent knee, Baltimore, 1979, Williams & Wilkins.

154. LaPrade RF, Bernhardson AS, Griffith CJ, et al: Correlation of valgus stress radiographs with medial knee ligament injuries—an in vitro biomechanical study. Am J Sports Med 38:330–338, 2010.

155. Daniel DM, Stone ML, Barnett P, et al: Use of the quadriceps active test to diagnose posterior cruciate ligament disruption and measure posterior laxity of the knee. J Bone Joint Surg Am 70:386–391, 1988.

156. Veltri DM, Warren RF: Isolated and combined posterior cruciate ligament injuries. J Am Acad Orthop Surg 1:67–75, 1993.

157. De Lee JC: Ligamentous injury of the knee. In Stanitski CL, DeLee JC, Drez D, editors: Pediatric and adolescent sports medicine, Philadelphia, 1994, WB Saunders.

158. Butler DL, Noyes FR, Grood ES: Ligamentous restraints to anterior-posterior drawer in the human knee. J Bone Joint Surg Am 62:259–270, 1980.

159. Weatherwax RJ: Anterior drawer sign. Clin Orthop 154:318–319, 1981.

160. Hughston JC: The absent posterior drawer test in some acute posterior cruciate ligament tears of the knee. Am J Sports Med 16:39–43, 1988.

161. Warren RF: Physical diagnosis of the knee. In Post M, editor: Physical examination of the musculoskeletal system, Chicago, 1987, Year Book Medical.

162. Feagin JA: The crucial ligaments, Edinburgh, 1988, Churchill Livingstone.

163. Jonsson T, Althoff B, Peterson L, et al: Clinical diagnosis of ruptures of the anterior cruciate ligament: a comparative study of the Lachman test and the anterior drawer sign. Am J Sports Med 10:100–102, 1982.

164. Paessler HH, Michel D: How new is the Lachman test? Am J Sports Med 20:95–98, 1992.

165. Torg JS, Conrad W, Allen V: Clinical diagnosis of anterior cruciate ligament instability in the athlete. Am J Sports Med 4:84–93, 1976.

166. Jackson R: The torn ACL: natural history of untreated lesions and rationale for selective treatment. In Feagin JA, editor: The crucial ligaments, Edinburgh, 1988, Churchill Livingstone.

167. Rosenberg TD, Rasmussen GL: The function of the anterior cruciate ligament during anterior drawer and Lachman's testing. Am J Sports Med 12:318–322, 1984.

168. Logan MC, Williams A, Lavelle J, et al: What really happens during the Lachman test—a dynamic MRI analysis of tibiofemoral motion. Am J Sports Med 32:369–375, 2004.

169. Cooperman JM, Riddle DL, Rothstein JM: Reliability and validity of judgments of the integrity of the anterior cruciate ligament of the knee using the Lachman's test. Phys Ther 70:225–233, 1990.

170. Johnson DS, Ryan WG, Smith RB: Does the Lachman testing method affect the reliability of the International Knee Documentation Committee (IKDC) Form?

Knee Surg Sports Traumatol Arthrosc 12(3):225–228, 2004.

171. Frank C: Accurate interpretation of the Lachman test. Clin Orthop 213:163–166, 1986.

172. Bechtel SL, Ellman BR, Jordon JL: Skier's knee: the cruciate connection. Phys Sports Med 12:50–54, 1984.

173. Wroble RR, Lindenfeld TN: The stabilized Lachman test. Clin Orthop 237:209–212, 1988.

174. Adler GG, Hockman RA, Beach DM: Drop leg Lachman test—a new test of anterior knee laxity. Am J Sports Med 23:320–323, 1995.

175. Rebman LW: Lachman's test: an alternative method. J Orthop Sports Phys Ther 9:381–382, 1988.

176. Mulligan EP, Harwell JL, Robertson WJ: Reliability and diagnostic accuracy of the Lachman test performed in the prone position. J Orthop Sports Phys Ther 41:749–757, 2011.

177. Cross MJ, Crichton KJ: Clinical examination of the injured knee, Baltimore, 1987, Williams & Wilkins.

178. Cross MJ, Schmidt DR, Mackie IG: A no-touch test for the anterior cruciate ligament. J Bone Joint Surg Br 69:300, 1987.

179. Wind WM, Bergfeld JA, Parker RD: Evaluation and treatment of posterior cruciate ligament injuries revisited. Am J Sports Med 32:1765–1775, 2004.

180. Emparanza JI, Aginaga JR: Validation of the Ottawa knee rules. Ann Emerg Med 38:364–368, 2001.

181. Voos JE, Mauro CS, Wente T, et al: Posterior cruciate ligament—anatomy, biomechanics and outcomes. Am J Sports Med 40:222–231, 2012.

182. Slocum DB, Larson RL: Rotary instability of the knee. J Bone Joint Surg Am 50:211–225, 1968.

183. Slocum DB, James SL, Larson RL, et al: A clinical test for anterolateral rotary instability of the knee. Clin Orthop 118:63–69, 1976.

184. Peterson L, Pitman MI, Gold J: The active pivot shift: the role of the popliteus muscle. Am J Sports Med 12:313–317, 1984.

185. Hanks GA, Joyner DM, Kalenak A: Anterolateral instability of the knee. Am J Sports Med 9:225–231, 1981.

186. Hughston JC, Walsh WM, Puddu G: Patellar subluxation and dislocation, Philadelphia, 1984, WB Saunders.

187. Fetto JF, Marshall JL: Injury to the anterior cruciate ligament producing the pivot shift sign: an experimental study on cadaver specimens. J Bone Joint Surg Am 61:710–714, 1979.

188. Galway HR, MacIntosh DL: The lateral pivot shift: a symptom and sign of anterior cruciate ligament insufficiency. Clin Orthop 147:45–50, 1980.

189. Tamea CD, Henning CE: Pathomechanics of the pivot shift maneuver. Am J Sports Med 9:31–37, 1981.

190. Katz JW, Fingeroth RF: The diagnostic accuracy of ruptures of the anterior cruciate ligament comparing the Lachman test, the anterior drawer sign and the pivot shift test in acute and chronic knee injuries. Am J Sports Med 14:88–91, 1986.

191. Lane CG, Warren R, Pearle AD: The pivot shift. J Am Acad Orthop Surg 16:679–688, 2008.

192. Bach BR, Warren RF, Wickiewitz TL: The pivot shift phenomenon: results and description of a modified clinical test for anterior cruciate ligament insufficiency. Am J Sports Med 16:571–576, 1988.

193. Kurosaka M, Yagi M, Yoshiya S, et al: Efficacy of the axially loaded pivot shift test for the diagnosis of a meniscal tear. Int Orthop 23:271–274, 1999.

194. Losee RE, Ennis TRJ, Southwick WO: Anterior subluxation of the lateral tibial plateau: a diagnostic test and operative review. J Bone Joint Surg Am 60:1015–1030, 1978.

195. Kocher MS, Steadman JR, Briggs KK, et al: Relationships between objective assessment of ligament stability and subjective assessment of symptoms and function after anterior cruciate ligament reconstruction. Am J Sports Med 32:629–634, 2004.

196. Noyes FR, Butler DL, Grood ES, et al: Clinical paradoxes of anterior cruciate instability and a new test to detect its instability. Orthop Trans 2:36, 1978.

197. Sims WF, Jacobson KE: The posterolateral corner of the knee–medial-sided injury patterns revisited. Am J Sports Med 32:337–345, 2004.

198. Jacobson KE, Chi FS: Evaluation and treatment of medial collateral ligament and medial-sided injuries of the knee. Sports Med Arthrosc Rev 14:58–66, 2006.

199. Kurzweil PR, Kelley ST: Physical examination and imaging of the medial collateral ligament and posteromedial corner of the knee. Sports Med Arthrosc Rev 14:67–73, 2006.

200. Tibor LM, Marchant MH, Taylor DC, et al: Management of medial-sided knee injuries, part 2. Am J Sports Med 39:1332–1340, 2011.

201. Hughston JC, Norwood LA: The posterolateral drawer test and external rotational recurvatum test for posterolateral rotary instability of the knee. Clin Orthop 147:82–87, 1980.

202. LaPrade RF, Terry GC: Injuries to the posterolateral aspect of the knee–association of anatomic injury patterns with clinical instability. Am J Sports Med 25:433–438, 1997.

203. Owens TC: Posteromedial pivot shift of the knee: a new test for rupture of the posterior cruciate ligament. J Bone Joint Surg Am 76:532–539, 1994.

204. Chen FS, Rokito AS, Pitman MI: Acute and chronic posterolateral rotary instability of the knee. J Am Acad Orthop Surg 8:97–110, 2000.

205. Ferrari JD, Bach BR: Posterolateral instability of the knee: diagnosis and treatment of acute and chronic instability. Sports Med Arthrosc Rev 7:273–288, 1999.

206. Covey DC: Injuries of the posterolateral corner of the knee. J Bone Joint Surg Am 83:106–117, 2001.

207. Bahk MS, Cosgarea AJ: Physical examination and imaging of the lateral collateral ligament and posterolateral corner of the knee. Sports Med Arthrosc Rev 14:12–19, 2006.

208. Lunden JB, Bzdusek PJ, Monson JK, et al: Current concepts in the recognition and treatment of the posterolateral corner injuries of the knee. J Orthop Sports Phys Ther 40(8):502–515, 2010.

209. Shino K, Horibe S, Ono K: The voluntary evoked posterolateral drawer sign in the knee with posterolateral instability. Clin Orthop 215:179–186, 1987.

210. Shelbourne KD, Benedict F, McCarroll JR, et al: Dynamic posterior shift test: an adjuvant in evaluation of posterior tibial subluxation. Am J Sports Med 17:275–277, 1989.

211. Swain RA, Wilson FD: Diagnosing posterolateral rotary knee instability: two clinical tests hold key. Phys Sportsmed 21:95–102, 1993.

212. LaPrade RF, Ly TV, Griffith C: The external rotation recurvatum test revisited—reevaluation of the sagittal plane tibiofemoral relationship. Am J Sports Med 709–712, 2008.

213. Jakob RP, Hassler H, Staeubli HU: Observations on rotary instability of the lateral compartment of the knee. Acta Orthop Scand 52(suppl 191):1–32, 1981.

214. Loomer RL: A test for knee posterolateral rotary instability. Clin Orthop 264:235–238, 1991.

215. Veltri DM, Warren RF: Posterolateral instability of the knee. J Bone Joint Surg Am 76:460–472, 1994.

216. Veltri DM, Warren RF: Anatomy, biomechanics and physical findings in posterolateral knee instability. Clin Sports Med 13:599–614, 1994.

217. Veltri DM, Deng XH, Torzilli PA, et al: The role of the cruciate and posterolateral ligaments instability of the knee—a biomechanical study. Am J Sports Med 23:436–443, 1995.

218. Ranawat A, Baker CL, Henry S, et al: Posterolateral corner injury of the knee: evaluation and management. J Am Acad Orthop Surg 16:506–518, 2008.

219. Griffith CJ, LaPrade RF, Johansen S, et al: Part 1: static function of the individual components of the main medial knee structures. Am J Sports Med 37:1762–1770, 2009.

220. LaPrade RF, Wentorf F: Acute knee injuries—on the field and sideline evaluation. Phys Sportsmed 27:55–61, 1999.

221. Ferrari DA, Ferrari JD, Coumas J: Posterolateral instability of the knee. J Bone Joint Surg Am 76:187–192, 1994

222. Daniel DM, Stone ML: Instrumented measurement of knee motion. In Daniel D, Akeson W, O'Conner J, editors: Knee ligaments: structure, function, injury and repair, New York, 1990, Raven Press.

223. Harter RA, Osternig LR, Singer KM: Instrumented Lachman tests for the evaluation of anterior laxity after reconstruction of the anterior cruciate ligament. J Bone Joint Surg Am 71:975–983, 1989.

224. Daniel DM, Malcolm LL, Losse G, et al: Instrumented measurement of anterior laxity of the knee. J Bone Joint Surg Am 67:720–726, 1985.

225. Tyler TF, McHugh MP, Gleim GW, et al: Association of KT-1000 measurements with clinical tests of the knee stability 1 year following anterior cruciate ligament reconstruction. J Orthop Sports Phys Ther 29:540–545, 1999.

226. Pugh L, Mascarenhas R, Arneja S, et al: Current concepts in instrumented knee laxity testing. Am J Sports Med 37:199–210, 2009.

227. Edixhoven P, Huiskes R, De Graff R, et al: Accuracy and reproducibility of instrumented knee drawer tests. J Orthop Res 5:378–387, 1987.

228. Andersson C, Gillquist J: Instrumented testing for evaluation of sagittal knee laxity. Clin Orthop 256:178–184, 1990.

229. Markolf KL, Amstutz HC: The clinical relevance of instrumented testing for ACL insufficiency: experience with the UCLA clinical knee testing apparatus. Clin Orthop 223:198–207, 1987.

230. Anderson AF, Snyder RB, Federspiel CF, et al: Instrumented evaluation of knee laxity: a comparison of five arthrometers. Am J Sports Med 20:135–140, 1992.

231. Daniel DM, Stone ML: Diagnosis of knee ligament injury: tests and measurements of joint laxity. In Feagin JA, editor: The crucial ligaments, Edinburgh, 1988, Churchill Livingstone.

232. Bach BR, Johnson JC: Ligament testing devices. In Scott WN, editor: Ligament and extensor mechanism injuries of the knee: diagnosis and treatment, St Louis, 1991, Mosby Year Book.

233. Daniel DM, Stone ML: KT-1000 anterior-posterior displacement measurements. In Daniel D, Akeson W, O'Conner J, editors: Knee ligaments: structure, function, injury and repair, New York, 1990, Raven Press.

234. Wright RW, Luhmann SJ: The effect of knee effusions on KT-1000 arthrometry—a cadaver study. Am J Sports Med 26:571–574, 1998.

235. Stratford PW, Miseferi D, Ogilvie R, et al: Assessing the responsiveness of five KT 1000 knee arthrometer measures used to evaluate anterior laxity at the knee joint. Clin J Sport Med 1:225–228, 1991.

236. Wroble RR, Grood ES, Noyes FR, et al: Reproducibility of genucom knee analysis system testing. Am J Sports Med 18:387–395, 1990.

237. Wroble RR, Van Ginkel LA, Grood ES, et al: Repeatability of the KT-1000 arthrometer in a normal population. Am J Sports Med 18:396–399, 1990.

238. Highgenboten CL, Jackson A, Meske NB: Genucom, KT-1000 and Stryker knee laxity measuring device comparisons: device reproducibility and interdevice comparison in asymptomatic subjects. Am J Sports Med 17:743–746, 1989.

239. McQuade KJ, Sidles JA, Larson KV: Reliability of the genucom knee analysis system. Clin Orthop 245:216–219, 1989.

240. Highgenboten CL, Jackson AW, Jansson KA, et al: KT-1000 arthrometer: conscious and unconscious test results using 15, 20 and 30 pounds of force. Am J Sports Med 20:450–454, 1992.

241. Kowalk DL, Wojtys EM, Disher J, et al: Quantitative analysis of the measuring capabilities of the KT-1000 knee ligament arthrometer. Am J Sports Med 21:744–747, 1993.

242. Forster IW, Warren-Smith CD, Tew M: Is the KT-1000 knee ligament arthrometer reliable? J Bone Joint Surg Br 71:843–847, 1989.

243. Huber FE, Irgang JJ, Harner C, et al: Intratester and intertester reliability of the KT-1000 arthrometer in the assessment of posterior laxity of the knee. Am J Sports Med 25:479–485, 1997.

244. Stratford PW, Binkley J: A review of the McMurray test: definition, interpretation and clinical usefulness. J Orthop Sports Phys Ther 22:116–120, 1995.

245. Bernstein J: Meniscal tears of the knee—diagnosis and individualized treatment. Phys Sportsmed 28:83–90, 2000.

246. Metcalf MH, Barrett GR: Prospective evaluation of 1485 meniscal tear patterns in patients with stable knees. Am J Sports Med 32:675–680, 2004.

247. Hegedus EJ, Cook C, Hasselbald V, et al: Physical examination tests for assessing a torn meniscus in the knee: a systematic review with meta-analysis. J Orthop Sports Phys Ther 37:541–550, 2007.

248. Shelbourne KD, Martini DJ, McCarrell JR, et al: Correlation of joint line tenderness and meniscal lesions in patients with acute anterior cruciate ligament tears. Am J Sports Med 23:166–169, 1995.

249. Anderson AF, Lipscomb AB: Clinical diagnosis of meniscal tears: description of a new manipulative test. Am J Sports Med 14:291–293, 1988.

250. Apley AG: The diagnosis of meniscus injuries: some new clinical methods. J Bone Joint Surg Br 29:78–84, 1947.

251. Oni O: The knee jerk test for diagnosis of torn meniscus. Clin Orthop 193:309, 1985.

252. Akseki D, Ozcan O, Boya H, et al: A new weight bearing meniscal test and a comparison with McMurray's test and joint line tenderness. Arthroscopy 20:951–958, 2004.

253. Hing W, White S, Reid D, et al: Validity of the McMurray's test and modified versions of the test: a systematic literature review. J Man Manip Ther 17:22–35, 2009.

254. McMurray TP: The semilunar cartilages. Br J Surg 29:407–414, 1942.

255. Evans PJ, Bell GD, Frank C: Prospective evaluation of the McMurray test. Am J Sports Med 21:604–608, 1993.

256. Kim SJ, Min BH, Han DY: Paradoxical phenomena of the McMurray test: an arthroscopic examination. Am J Sports Med 24:83–87, 1996.

257. Helfet A: Disorders of the knee, Philadelphia, 1974, JB Lippincott.

258. Karachalios T, Hantes M, Zibis AH, et al: Diagnostic accuracy of a new clinical test (the Thessaly Test) for early detection of meniscal tears. J Bone Joint Surg Am 87:955–962, 2005.

259. Johnson DP, Eastwood DM, Witherow PJ: Symptomatic synovial plica of the knee. J Bone Joint Surg Am 75:1485–1496, 1993.

260. Gray DJ, Gardner E: Prenatal development of the human knee and superior tibiofibular joints. Am J Anat 56:235–287, 1950.

261. Ogata S, Uhthoff HK: The development of synovial plica in human knee joints: an embryologic study. Arthroscopy 6:315–321, 1990.

262. Hardaker WG, Shipple TL, Bassett FH: Diagnosis and treatment of the plica syndrome of the knee. J Bone Joint Surg Am 62:221–225, 1980.

263. Zanoli S, Piazzai E: The synovial plica syndrome of the knee—pathology, differential diagnosis and treatment. Ital J Orthop Traumatol 9:241–250, 1983.

264. Jackson RW, Marshall DJ, Fujisawa Y: The pathologic medial shelf. Orthop Clin North Am 13:307–312, 1982.

265. Mital MA, Hayden J: Pain in the knee in children: the medial plica shelf syndrome. Orthop Clin North Am 10:713–722, 1979.

266. Sturgill LP, Snyder-Mackler L, Manal TJ, et al: Interrater reliability of a clinical scale to assess knee joint effusion. J Orthop Sports Phys Ther 39:845–849, 2009.

267. Mann G, Finsterbush A, Frankel U, et al: A method of diagnosing small amounts of fluid in the knee. J Bone Joint Surg Br 73:346–347, 1991.

268. Sibley MB, Fu FH: Knee injuries. In Fu FH, Stone DA, editors: Sports injuries: mechanisms, prevention, treatment, Baltimore, 1994, Williams & Wilkins.

269. Boling MC, Padua DA, Marshall SW, et al: A prospective investigation of biomechanical risk factors for patellofemoral pain syndrome. Am J Sports Med 37:2108–2116, 2009.

270. Dye SF: The pathophysiology of patellofemoral pain. Clin Orthop Relat Res 436:100–110, 2005.

271. LaBotz M: Patellofemoral syndrome—diagnostic pointers and individualized treatment. Phys Sportsmed 32:22–31, 2004.

272. Witvroux E, Lysons R, Bellemans J, et al: Intrinsic risk factors for the development of anterior knee pain in an athletic population—a 2 year prospective study. Am J Sports Med 28:480–489, 2000.

273. Souza RB, Powers CM: Predictors of hip internal rotation during running—an evaluation of hip strength and femoral structure in women with and without patellofemoral pain. Am J Sports Med 37:579–587, 2009.

274. Hudson Z, Darthuy E: Iliotibial band tightness and patellofemoral pain syndrome: a case control study. Manual Therapy 14:147–151, 2009.

275. Muller K, Snyder-Mackler L: Diagnosis of patellofemoral pain after arthroscopic meniscectomy. J Orthop Sports Phys Ther 30:138–142, 2000.

276. Nijs J, VanGeel C, Vanderauwera C, et al: Diagnostic value of five clinical tests in patellofemoral syndrome. Man Ther 11:69–77, 2006.

277. Doberstein ST, Romeyn RL, Reinke DM: The diagnostic value of the Clarke sign in assessing chondromalacia patella. J Athl Train 43:190–196, 2008.

278. Kolowich PA, Paulos LE, Rosenberg TD, et al: Lateral release of the patella: indications and contraindications. Am J Sports Med 18:359–365, 1990.

279. Watson CJ, Leddy HM, Dynjan TD, et al: Reliability of the lateral pull test and tilt test to assess patellar alignment in subjects with symptomatic knees: student raters. J Orthop Sports Phys Ther 3:368–374, 2001.

280. McConnell J: The management of chondromalacia patellae: a long term solution. Aust J Physiother 32:215–223, 1986.

281. Souza TA: The knee. In Hyde TE, Gengenbach MS, editors: Conservative management of sport injuries, Baltimore, 1997, Williams & Wilkins.

282. Daniel DM, Stone ML, Barnett P, et al: Use of the quadriceps active test to diagnose posterior cruciate ligament disruption and measure posterior laxity of the knee. J Bone Joint Surg Am 70:386–391, 1988.

283. Fairbank HAT: Internal derangement of the knee in children and adolescents. Proc R Soc Med 30:427–432, 1937.

284. Tanner SM, Garth WP, Soileau R, et al: A modified test for patellar instability—the biomechanical basis. Clin J Sports Med 13:327–338, 2003.

285. Ahmed CS, McCarthy M, Gomez JA, et al: The moving patellar apprehension test for lateral patellar instability. Am J Sports Med 37:791–796, 2009.

286. Noble HB, Hajek MR, Porter M: Diagnosis and treatment of iliotibial band tightness in runners. Phys Sportsmed 10:67–74, 1982.

287. Schulthies SS, Francis RS, Fisher AG, et al: Does the Q-angle reflect the force on the patella in the frontal plane. Phys Ther 75:24–30, 1995.

288. Herrington L, Nester C: Q-angle undervalued? The relationship between Q-angle and medio-lateral position of the patella. Clin Biomech 19:1070–1073, 2004.

289. Smith TO, Hunt NJ, Donell ST: The reliability and validity of the Q-angle: a systematic review. Knee Surg Sports Traumatol Arthrosc 16:1068–1079, 2008.

290. Insall J, Falvo KA, Wise DW: Chondromalacia patellae: a prospective study. J Bone Joint Surg Am 58:1–8, 1976.

291. Olerud C, Berg P: The variation of the Q angle with different positions of the foot. Clin Orthop 191:162–165, 1984.

292. Grelsamer RP, Dubey A, Weinstein CH: Men and women have similar Q-angles—a clinical and trigonometric evaluation. J Bone Joint Surg Br 87:1498–1501, 2005.

293. Guerra JP, Arnold MJ, Gajdosik RL: Q-angle: effects of isometric quadriceps contraction and body position. J Orthop Sports Phys Ther 19:200–204, 1994.

294. Cook CE, Hegedus EJ: Orthopedic physical examination tests—an evidence based approach, Upper Saddle River, NJ, 2008, Prentice-Hall/Pearson.

295. Baciu CC, Tudor A, Olaru I: Recurrent luxation of the superior tibio-fibular jointin the adult. Acta Orthop Scand 45:772–777, 1974.

296. Daniel DM, Stone ML: Case studies. In Daniel D, Akeson W, O'Conner J, editors: Knee ligaments: structure, injury and repair, New York, 1990, Raven Press.

297. Arno S: The A-angle: a quantitative measurement of patella alignment and realignment. J Orthop Sports Phys Ther 12:237–242, 1990.

298. DiVeta JA, Vogelbach WD: The clinical efficacy of the A-angle in measuring patellar alignment. J Orthop Sports Phys Ther 16:136–139, 1992.

299. Ehrat M, Edwards J, Hastings D, et al: Reliability of assessing patellar alignment: the A-angle. J Orthop Sports Phys Ther 19:22–27, 1994.

300. Crawford DC, Safran MR: Osteochondritis dissecans of the knee. J Am Acad Orthop Surg 14:90–100, 2006.

301. Hyslop GH: Injuries of the deep and superficial peroneal nerves complicating ankle sprain. Am J Surg 51:436–438, 1941.

302. Sidey J: Weak ankles: a study of common peroneal entrapment neuropathy. Br Med J 56:623–626, 1969.

303. Pecina MM, Krmpotic-Nemanic J, Markiewitz AD: Tunnel syndromes, Boca Raton, FL, 1991, CRC Press.

304. Worth RM, Kettlekamp DB, Defalque RJ, et al: Saphenous nerve entrapment: a cause of medial nerve pain. Am J Sports Med 12:80–81, 1984.

305. Cox JS, Blanda JB: Periarticular pathologies. In DeLee JC, Drez D, editors: Orthopedic sports medicine, Philadelphia, 1994, WB Saunders.

306. Lin J, Chang C: A medial soft tissue mass of the knee. Phys Sportsmed 27:87–90, 1999.

307. Malanga GA, Andrus S, Nadler SF, et al: Physical examination of the knee: a review of common orthopaedic tests. Arch Phys Med Rehabil 84:592–603, 2003.

308. Eren OT: The accuracy of joint line tenderness by physical examination in the diagnosis of meniscal tears. Arthroscopy 19(8):850–854, 2003.

309. O'Shea KJ, Murphy KP, Heekin D, et al: The diagnostic accuracy of history, physical examination and radiographs in the evaluation of traumatic knee disorders. Am J Sports Med 24:164–167, 1996.

310. Gelb HJ, Glasgow SG, Sapega AA, et al: Magnetic resonance imaging of knee disorders: clinical value and cost-effectiveness in a sports medicine practice. Am J Sports Med 24:99–103, 1996.

311. Luhmann SJ, Schootman M, Gordon JE, et al: Magnetic resonance imaging of the knee in children and adolescents. J Bone Joint Surg Am 87:497–502, 2005.

312. Stiell IG, Wells GA, Hoag RH: Implementation of the Ottawa knee rules for the use of radiography in acute knee injuries. JAMA 278:2075–2079, 1997.

313. Nugent P: The Ottawa knee rule—avoiding unnecessary radiographs in sports. Phys Sportsmed 32(5):26–32, 2004.

314. Cohen DM, Jasser JW, Kean JR, et al: Clinical criteria for using radiography for children with acute knee injuries. Ped Emerg Care 14:185–187, 1998.

315. Bulloch B, Neto G, Plint A, et al: Validation of the Ottawa knee rule in children: a multicentre study. Ann Emerg Med 42:48–55, 2003.

316. Khine H, Dorfman DH, Avner JR: Applicability of Ottawa knee rule for knee injury in children. Ped Emerg Care 17:401–404, 2001.

317. Seaberg DC, Jackson R: Clinical decision rule for knee radiographs. Am J Emerg Med 12(5):541–543, 1994.

318. Tandeter HB, Shvartzman P, Stevens MA: Acute knee injuries: use of decision rules for radiograph ordering. Am Fam Physician 60(9):2599–2608, 1999.

319. Carson WG Jr, James SL, Larson RL, et al: Patellofemoral disorders: physical and radiographic evaluation. I. Physical examination. Clin Orthop 185:178–186, 1984.

320. Merchant AC: Extensor mechanism injuries: classification and diagnosis. In Scott WN, editor: Ligament and extensor mechanism injuries of the knee: diagnosis and treatment, St Louis, 1991, Mosby.

321. Davies AP, Calder DA, Marshall T, et al: Plain radiography in the degenerate knee. J Bone Joint Surg Br 81:632–635, 1999.

322. Tatum R: Osteochondritis dissecans of the knee: a radiology case report. J Manip Physiol Ther 23:347–351, 2000.

323. Schenck RC, Goodnight JM: Osteochondritis dissecans—current concepts review. J Bone Joint Surg Am 78:439–456, 1996.

324. Woods GW, Stanley RF, Tullos HS: Lateral capsular sign: x-ray clue to a significant knee instability. Am J Sports Med 7:27–33, 1979.

325. Altchek DW: Diagnosing acute knee injuries: the office exam. Phys Sportsmed 21:85–96, 1993.

326. Schils JP, Resnick D, Sartoris DJ: Diagnostic imaging of ligamentous injuries of the knee. In

Daniel D, Akeson W, O'Conner J, editors: Knee ligaments: structure, injury and repair, New York, 1990, Raven Press.

327. Beaconsfield T, Pintore E, Maffulli N, et al: Radiographic measurements in patellofemoral disorders. Clin Orthop 308:18–28, 1994.

328. Grana WA: Diagnostic evaluation. In Larson RL, Grana WA, editors: The knee: form, function, pathology and treatment, Philadelphia, 1993, WB Saunders.

329. Grelsamer RP, Meadows S: The modified Insall-Salvati ratio for assessment of patellar height. Clin Orthop 282:170–176, 1992.

330. Haas SB, Scuderi GR: Examination and radiographic assessment of the patellofemoral joint. Semin Orthop 5:108–114, 1990.

331. Grelsamer RP, Proctor CS, Brazos AN: Evaluation of patellar shape in the sagittal plane: a clinical analysis. Am J Sports Med 22:61–66, 1994.

332. Phillips CL, Silver DA, Schranz PJ, et al: The measurement of patellar height—a review of the methods of imaging. J Bone Joint Surg Br 92:1045–1053, 2010.

333. Berg EE, Mason SL, Zucas MJ: Patellar height ratios: a comparison of four measurement methods. Am J Sports Med 24:218–221, 1996.

334. LaPrade RF, Ly TV, Wentorf FA, et al: The posterolateral attachments of the knee: a qualitative and quantitative morphologic analysis of the fibular collateral ligament, popliteus tendon, popliteofibular ligament and lateral gastrocnemius tendon. Am J Sports Med 31:854–860, 2003.

335. Hewett TE, Noyes FR, Lee MD: Diagnosis of complete and partial posterior cruciate ligament ruptures—stress radiography compared with KT-1000 and posterior drawer testing. Am J Sports Med 25:648–655, 1997.

336. Jackman T, LaPrade RF, Pontinen T, et al: Intraobserver and interobserver reliability of the kneeling technique of stress radiography for the evaluation of posterior knee laxity. Am J Sports Med 36:1571–1576, 2008.

337. Shelbourne KD, Davis TJ, Klootwyk TE: The relationship between intercondylar notch width of the femur and the incidence of anterior cruciate ligament tears–a prospective study. Am J Sports Med 26:402–408, 1998.

338. Bollier M, Fulkerson JP: The role of trochlear dysplasia in patellofemoral instability. J Am Acad Orthop Surg 19:8–16, 2011.

339. Speakman HB, Weisberg J: The vastus medialis controversy. Physiotherapy 63:249–254, 1977.

340. Murray TF, Dupont JY, Fulkerson JP: Axial and lateral radiographs in evaluating patellofemoral malalignment. Am J Sports Med 27:580–584, 1999.

341. Davies AP, Costa ML, Donnell ST, et al: The sulcus angle and malalignment of the extensor mechanisms of the knee. J Bone Joint Surg Br 82:1162–1166, 2000.

342. Ghelman B, Schraft S: Arthrography of the knee. In Scott WN, editor: Ligament and extensor mechanism injuries of the knee: diagnosis and treatment, St Louis, 1991, Mosby.

343. Mital MA, Karlin LI: Diagnostic arthroscopy in sports injuries. Orthop Clin North Am 11:771–785, 1980.

344. McClelland CJ: Arthroscopy and arthroscopic surgery of the knee. Physiotherapy 70:154–156, 1984.

345. Noyes FR, Bassett RW, Grood ES, et al: Arthroscopy in acute traumatic hemarthrosis of the knee. J Bone Joint Surg Am 62:687–695, 757, 1980.

346. LaPrade RF, Gilbert TJ, Bollom TS, et al: The magnetic resonance imaging appearance of individual structures of the posterolateral knee—a prospective study of normal knees and knees with surgically verified grade III injuries. Am J Sports Med 28:191–199, 2000.

347. Potter HG: Imaging of the multiple-ligament-injured knee. Clin Sports Med 19:425–441, 2000.

348. Cross TM, Gibbs N, Houang MT, et al: Acute quadriceps muscle strains—magnetic resonance imaging features and prognosis. Am J Sports Med 32:710–719, 2004.

349. Chin KR, Sodl JF: Infrapatellar fat pad disruption—a radiographic sign of patellar tendon rupture. Clin Orthop Relat Res 440:222–225, 2005.

350. Sanders TG, Miller MD: A systematic approach to magnetic resonance imaging interpretation of sports medicine injuries of the knee. Am J Sports Med 33:131–148, 2005.

351. Glashow JL, Friedman MJ: Diagnosis of knee ligament injuries: magnetic resonance imaging. In Scott WN, editor: Ligament and extensor mechanism injuries of the knee: diagnosis and treatment, St Louis, 1991, Mosby.

352. Arendt EA: Assessment of the athlete with an acutely injured knee. In Griffin LY, editor: Rehabilitation of the injured knee, St Louis, 1995, Mosby.

353. Gelb HJ, Glasgow SG, Sapega AA, et al: Magnetic resonance imaging of knee disorders: clinical value and cost effectiveness in a sports medicine practice. Am J Sports Med 24:99–103, 1996.

354. Adalberth T, Roos H, Lauren M, et al: Magnetic resonance imaging, scintigraphy and arthroscopic evaluation of traumatic hemarthrosis of the knee. Am J Sports Med 25:231–237, 1997.

355. Munshi M, Davidson M, MacDonald PB, et al: The efficacy of magnetic resonance imaging in acute knee injuries. Clin J Sports Med 10:34–39, 2000.

356. Potter HG, Linklater JM, Allen AA, et al: Magnetic resonance imaging of articular cartilage of the knee. J Bone Joint Surg Am 80:1276–1284, 1998.

357. Ross G, Chapman AW, Newberg AR, et al: Magnetic resonance imaging for the evaluation of acute posterolateral complex injuries of the knee. Am J Sports Med 25:444–448, 1997.

358. Schneider-Kolsky ME, Hoving JL, Warren P, et al: A comparison between clinical assessment and magnetic resonance imaging of acute hamstring injuries. Am J Sports Med 34:1008–1015, 2006.

359. Ben-Galim P, Steinberg EL, Amir H, et al: Accuracy of magnetic resonance imaging of the knee and justified surgery. Clin Orthop Relat Res 447:100–104, 2006.

360. Miller TT: Imaging of the knee. Sports Med Arthrosc Rev 17:56–67, 2008.

361. Quatman CE, Hettrich CM, Schmitt LC, et al: The clinical utility and diagnostic performance of magnetic resonance imaging for identification of early and advanced knee osteoarthritis—a systematic review. Am J Sports Med 39:1557–1568, 2011.

362. Krampla W, Roesel M, Svoboda K, et al: MRI of the knee: how do field strength and radiologist's experience influence diagnostic accuracy and interobserver correlation in assessing chondral and meniscal lesions and the integrity of the anterior cruciate ligament. Eur Radiol 19:1519–1528, 2009.

363. Black BR, Chong LR, Potter HG: Cartilage imaging in sports medicine. Sports Med Arthrosc Rev 17:68–80, 2008.

364. Augustsson J, Thomeé R, Karlsson J: Ability of a new hop test to determine functional deficits after anterior cruciate ligament reconstruction. Knee Surg Sports Traumatol Arthrosc 12:350–356, 2004.

365. McCarthy CJ, Oldham JA: The reliability, validity and responsiveness of an aggregated locomotor function (ALF) score in patients with osteoarthritis of the knee. Rheumatology 43:514–517, 2004.

366. Irrgang JJ, Anderson AF, Boland AL, et al, International Knee Documentation Committee: Responsiveness of the International Knee Documentation Committee subjective knee form. Am J Sports Med 34(10):1567–1573, 2006.

367. Liow RYL, Walker K, Wajid MA, et al: The reliability of the American Knee Society Score. Acta Orthop Scand 71(6):603–608, 2000.

368. Kim S, Lee D, Kim T: The relationship between the MPP test and arthroscopically found medial patellar plica pathology. J Arthrosc Relat Surg 23(12):1303–1308, 2007.

369. Boeree NR, Ackroyd CE: Assessment of the menisci and cruciate ligaments: an audit of clinical practice. Injury 22:291–294, 1991.

370. Bomberg BC, McGinty JB: Acute hemarthrosis of the knee: indications for diagnostic arthroscopy. Arthroscopy 6:221–225, 1990.

371. Braunstein EM: Anterior cruciate ligament injuries: a comparison of arthrographic and physical diagnosis. Am J Roentgenol 138:423–425, 1982.

372. Hughston JC, Andrews JR, Cross MJ, et al: Classification of knee ligament instabilities. I. The medial compartment and cruciate ligaments. J Bone Joint Surg Am 58:159–172, 1976.

373. Lee LK, Yao L, Phelps CT, et al: Anterior cruciate ligament tears: MR imaging compared with arthroscopy and clinical tests. Radiology 166:861–864, 1988.

374. Noyes FR, Paulos L, Mooar LA, et al: Knee sprains and acute knee hemarthrosis: misdiagnosis of anterior cruciate ligament tears. Phys Ther 60:1596–1601, 1980.

375. Rubinstein RA, Shelbourne KD, McCarroll JR, et al: The accuracy of the clinical examination in the setting of posterior cruciate ligament injuries. Am J Sports Med 22:550–557, 1994.

376. Sandberg R, Balkfors B, Henricson A, et al: Stability tests in knee ligament injuries. Arch Orthop Trauma Surg 106:5–7, 1986.

377. Warren RF, Marshall JL: Injuries of the anterior cruciate and medial collateral ligaments of the knee: a retrospective analysis of clinical records. I. Clin Orthop Relat Res 136:191–197, 1978.

378. Jonsson T, Althoff B, Peterson L, et al: Clinical diagnosis of ruptures of the anterior cruciate ligament: a comparative study of the Lachman test and the anterior drawer sign. Am J Sports Med 10:100–102, 1982.

379. Benjaminse A, Gokeler A, van der Schans CP: Clinical diagnosis of an anterior cruciate ligament rupture: a meta-analysis. J Orthop Sports Phys Ther 36:267–288, 2006.

380. Davis E: Clinical examination of the knee following trauma: an evidence-based perspective. Trauma 4:135–145, 2002.

381. Scholten RJ, Opstelten W, Van der Plas CG, et al: Accuracy of physical diagnostic tests for assessing ruptures of the anterior cruciate ligament: a meta-analysis. J Fam Pract 52(9):689–694, 2003.

382. Smith C: Evaluating the painful knee: a hands-on approach to acute ligamentous and meniscal injuries. Sports Med 4(7):362–370, 2004.

383. Anderson AF, Lipscomb AB: Preoperative instrumented testing of anterior and posterior knee laxity. Am J Sports Med 17:1299–1306, 1986.

384. DeHaven KE: Diagnosis of acute knee injuries with hemarthrosis. Am J Sports Med 8:9–14, 1980.

385. Donaldson WF, Warren RF, Wickiewicz T: A comparison of acute anterior cruciate ligament examinations: initial vs examination under anesthesia. Am J Sports Med 13:5–9, 1985.

386. Hardaker WT, Garrett WE, Bassett FH: Evaluation of acute traumatic hemarthrosis of the knee joint. South Med J 83:640–644, 1990.

387. Liu SH, Osti L, Henry M, et al: The diagnosis of acute complete tears of the anterior cruciate ligament: comparison of MRI, arthrometry and clinical examination. J Bone Joint Surg Br 77:586–588, 1995.

388. Kim SJ, Kim HK: Reliability of the anterior drawer test, the pivot shift test, and the Lachman test. Clin Orthop Relat Res 317:237–242, 1995.

389. Harilainen A: Evaluation of knee instability in acute ligamentous injuries. Am Chir Gynaecol 76:269–273, 1987.

390. Mitsou A, Vallianatos P: Clinical diagnosis of ruptures of the anterior cruciate ligament: a comparison between the Lachman test and the anterior drawer sign. Injury 19:427–428, 1988.

391. Solomon DH, Simel DL, Bates DW, et al: Does this patient have a torn meniscus or ligament of the knee? Value of the physical examination. JAMA 286(13):1610–1620, 2001.

392. Watson CJ, Propps M, Ratner J, et al: Reliability and responsiveness of the lower extremity functional scale and the anterior knee pain scale in patients with anterior knee pain. J Orthop Sports Phys Ther 35:136–146, 2005.

393. Fowler PJ, Lubliner JA: The predictive value of five clinical signs in the evaluation of meniscal pathology. Arthroscopy 5:1846, 1989.

394. Scholten RJ, Devilli WL, Opsteuten W, et al: The accuracy of physical diagnostic tests for assessing meniscal lesions of the knee: a meta-analysis. J Fam Pract 50(11):938–944, 2001.

395. Haim A, Yaniv M, Dekel S, et al: Patellofemoral pain syndrome: validity of clinical and radiological features. Clin Orthop Relat Res 451:223–228, 2006.

396. Muellner T, Weinstabl R, Schabus R, et al: The diagnosis of meniscal tears in athletes: a comparison of clinical and magnetic resonance imaging investigations. Am J Sports Med 25(1):7–12, 1997.

397. Sole G, Hamren J, Milosavljevic S, et al: Test-retest reliability of isokinetic knee extension and flexion. Arch Phys Med Rehabil 88(5):626–631, 2007.

398. Clark NC, Gumbrell CJ, Rana S, et al: Intratester reliability and measurement error of the adapted crossover hop for distance. Phys Ther Sport 3:143–151, 2002.

399. Bolgla LA, Keskula DR: Reliability of lower extremity functional performance test. J Orthop Sports Phys Ther 26:138–142, 1997.

400. Ross MD, Langford B, Wheland PJ: Test-retest reliability of 4 single leg horizontal hop tests. J Strength Cond Res 16:617–622, 2002.

401. Bandy WD, Rusche KR, Tekulve FY: Reliability and limb symmetry for five unilateral functional tests for the lower extremities. Isokinetics Exerc Sci 4:108–111, 1994.

402. Reid A, Birmingham TB, Stratford PW, et al: Hop testing provides a reliable and valid outcome measure during rehabilitation after anterior cruciate ligament reconstruction. Physical Therapy 87(3):337–349, 2007.

403. Impellizzeri FM, Bizzini M, Rampinini E, et al: Reliability of isokinetic strength imbalance ratios measured using Cybex NORM dynamometer. Clin Physiol Funct Imaging 28:113–119, 2008.

404. Mokkink LB, Terwee CB, Van Lummel RC, et al: Construct validity of the Dynaport knee test: a comparison with observations of physical therapists. Osteoarthr Cartilage 13:738–743, 2005.

405. Hayes KW, Petersen CM: Reliability of assessing end-feel and pain and resistance sequence in subjects with painful shoulders and knees. J Orthop Sports Phys Ther 31:432–445, 2001.

406. Crossley KM, Bennell KL, Cowan SM, et al: Analysis of outcome measurement for persons with patellofemoral pain: which are reliable and valid? Arch Phys Med Rehabil 85:815–822, 2004.

407. Harrison E, Quinney H, Magee DJ, et al: Analysis of outcome measured used in the study of patellofemoral pain syndrome. Physiother Can 47:264–272, 1995.

408. Anderson AF, Rennirt GW, Standeffer WC: Clinical analysis of the pivot shift tests: description of the pivot drawer test. Am J Knee Surg 13:19–23, 2000.

409. Alkjaer T, Henriksen M, Dyhre-Poulsen P, et al: Forward lunge as a functional performance test in ACL deficient subjects: test-retest reliability. The Knee 16(3):176–182, 2009.

410. Smith TO, Davies L, O'Driscoll M, et al: An evaluation of the clinical tests and outcome measures used to assess patellar instability. The Knee 15:255–262, 2008.

411. Loudon JK, Wiesner D, Goist-Foley HL, et al: Intra-rater reliability of functional performance tests for subjects with patellofemoral pain syndrome. J Athl Train 37:256–261, 2003.

412. Bremander AB, Dahl LL, Roos EM: Validity and reliability of functional performance tests in meniscotomized patients with or without knee osteoarthritis. Scand J Med Sci Sports 17:120–127, 2007.

413. Piva SR, Fitzgerald GK, Irrgang JJ, et al: Get up and go test in patients with knee osteoarthritis. Arch Phys Med Rehabil 85:284–289, 2004.

414. Terwee CB, Mokkink LB, Steultjens MPM, et al: Performance-based methods for measuring the physical function of patients with osteoarthritis of the hip or knee: a systematic review of measurement properties. Rheumatol 45:890–902, 2006.

415. Johanson NA, Liang MH, Daltroy L, et al: American Academy of Orthopaedic Surgeons lower limb outcomes assessment instruments: reliability, validity, and sensitivity to change. J Bone Joint Surg Am 86:902–909, 2004.

416. Bennell KL, Hinman RS, Crossley KM, et al: Is the human activity profile a useful measure in people with knee osteoarthritis? J Rehabil Res Dev 41(4):621–630, 2004.

417. Mehta VM, Paxton LW, Fornalski SX, et al: Reliability of the International Knee Documentation Committee radiographic grading system. Am J Sports Med 35:933–935, 2007.

418. Munich H, Cipriani D, Hall C, et al: The test-retest reliability of an inclined squat strength test protocol. J Orthop Sports Phys Ther 26:209–213, 1997.

419. Sanfridson J, Ryd L, Svahn S: Radiographic measurement of femoral rotation in weight-bearing. Acta Radiol 42:207–217, 2001.

420. Hartmann A, Knols R, Murer K, et al: Reproducibility of an isokinetic strength-testing protocol of the knee and ankle in older adults. Gerontology 55: 259–268, 2009.

421. Meserve BB, Cleland JA, Boucher TR: A meta-analysis examining clinical test utilities for assessing meniscal injury. Clin Rehabil 22:143–161, 2008.

422. Stillman BC, McMeeken JM: The role of weightbearing in the clinical assessment of knee joint position sense. Austr J Phyiother 47:247–253, 2001.

423. Lingard EA, Katz JN, Wright J, et al, Kinemax Outcomes Group: Validity and responsiveness of the knee society clinical rating system in comparison with the SF-36 and WOMAC. J Bone Joint Surg 83:1856–1864, 2001.

424. Kessler S, Käfer W: Comparative assessment of outcome in osteoarthritis: the utility of the knee. Acta Chir Orthop Traumatol Cech 74(5):332–335, 2007.

425. Berry J, Kramer K, Binkley J, et al: Error estimates in novice and expert raters for the KT-1000 arthrometer. J Orthop Sports Phys Ther 29:49–55, 1999.

426. Denti M, Monteleone M, Trevisan C, et al: Instrumental lachman test: comparison between two arthrometers. Intraoperator and interoperator reproducibility in subjects asymptomatic and subjects operated for reconstruction of the anterior cruciate ligament. J Sports Traumatol Rel Res 15(1):29–36, 1993.

427. Robnett NJ, Riddle DL, Kues JM: Intertester reliability of measurements obtained with the KT-1000 on patients with reconstructed anterior cruciate ligaments. J Orthop Sports Phys Ther 21(2):113–119, 1995.

428. Ballantyne BT, French AK, Heimsoth SL, et al: Influence of examiner experience and gender on interrater reliability of KT-1000 arthrometer measurements. Phys Ther 75(10):898–906, 1995.

429. Brosky JA, Nitz AJ, Malone TR, et al: Intrarater reliability of selected clinical outcome measures following anterior cruciate ligament reconstruction. J Orthop Sports Phys Ther 29(1):39–48, 1999.

430. Sernet N, Kartus J, Kohler K, et al: Evaluation of the reproducibility of the KT-1000 arthrometer. Scand J Med Sci Sports 11:120–125, 2001.

431. Wiertsema SH, van Hooff HJA, Migchelsen LAA, et al: Reliability of the KT1000 arthrometer and the Lachman test in patients with an ACL rupture. The Knee 15:107–110, 2008.

432. Steiner ME, Brown C, Zarins B, et al: Measurement of anterior-posterior displacement of the knee. J Bone Joint Surg Am 72(9):1307–1315, 1990.

433. Leamouth DJ: Incidence and diagnosis of anterior cruciate injuries in the accident and emergency department. Injury 22:287–290, 1991.

434. Katz JW, Fingeroth RJ: The diagnostic accuracy of ruptures of the anterior cruciate ligament comparing the Lachman test, the anterior drawer sign, and the pivot shift test in acute and chronic knee injuries. Am J Sports Med 14:88–91, 1986.

435. Dahlstedt LJ, Dalen N: Knee laxity in cruciate ligament injury: value of examination under anesthesia. Acta Orthop Scand 60:181–184, 1989.

436. Cook JL, Khan KM, Kiss ZS, et al: Reproducibility and clinical utility of tendon palpation to detect patellar tendinopathy in young basketball players. Br J Sports Med 35(1):65, 2001.

437. Stratford PW, Binkley JM, Watson J, et al: Validation of the LEFS on patient with total joint arthroplasty. Physiother Can 52:97–105, 2000.

438. Bengtsson J, Mollborg J, Werner S: A study for testing the sensitivity and reliability of the Lysholm knee scoring scale. Knee Surg Sports Traumatol Arthrosc 4:27–31, 1996.

439. Briggs KK, Kocher MS, Rodkey WG, et al: Reliability, validity, and responsiveness of the Lysholm knee score and Tegner activity scale for patients with meniscal injury of the knee. J Bone Joint Surg Am 88(4):698–705, 2006.

440. Risberg MA, Holm I, Steen H, et al: Sensitivity to changes over time for the IKDC form, the Lysholm score, and the Cincinnati knee score: a prospective study of 120 CL reconstructed patients with a 2-year follow-up. Knee Surg Sports Traumatol Arthrosc 7:152–159, 1999.

441. Lee SY, Jee W, Kim J: Radial tear of the medial meniscal root: reliability and accuracy of MRI for diagnosis. Am J Roentgenol 7:81–85, 2008.

442. Raynauld JP, Kauffmann C, Beaudoin G, et al: Reliability of a quantification imaging system using magnetic resonance images to measure cartilage thickness and volume in human normal and

443. Winters K, Tregonning R: Reliability of magnetic resonance imaging for traumatic injury of the knee. NZ Med J 118(1209):U1301, 2005.

444. Thomas S, Pullagura M, Robinson E, et al: The value of magnetic resonance imaging in our current management of ACL and meniscal injuries. Knee Surg Sports Traumatol Arthrosc 15:533–536, 2007.

445. Watson CJ, Prepps M, Galt W, et al: Reliability of McConnell's classification of patellar orientation in symptomatic and asymptomatic subjects. J Orthop Sports Phys Ther 29:378–385, 1999.

446. Herrington LC: The inter-tester reliability of a clinical measurement used to determine the medial/lateral orientation of the patella. Man Ther 7(3):163–167, 2000.

447. Corea JR, Moussa M, Othman AA: McMurray's test tested. Knee Surg Sports Traumatol Arthrosc 2:70–72, 1994.

448. Muellner T, Funovics M, Nikolic A, et al: Patellar alignment evaluated by MRI. Acta Orthop Scand 69(5):489–492, 1998.

449. Sallay PI, Poggi J, Speer KP, et al: Acute dislocation of the patella. A correlative pathoanatomic study. Am J Sports Med 24:52–60, 1996.

450. Chatman AB, Hyams SP, Neel JM, et al: The patient-specific functional scale: measurement properties in patients with knee dysfunction. Physical Therapy 77:820–829, 1997.

451. Lucie RS, Wiedel JD, Messner DG: The acute pivot shift: clinical correlation. Am J Sports Med 12:189–191, 1984.

452. Rubinstein RA Jr, Shelbourne KD, McCarroll JR, et al: The accuracy of the clinical examination in the setting of posterior cruciate ligament injuries. Am J Sports Med 22:550–557, 1994.

453. Loos WC, Fox JM, Blazina ME, et al: Acute posterior cruciate ligament injuries. Am J Sports Med 9:86–92, 1981.

454. Moore HA, Larson RL: Posterior cruciate ligament injuries. Results of early surgical repair. Am J Sports Med 8:68–78, 1980.

455. Hughston JC, Andrews JR, Cross MJ, et al: Classification of knee ligament instabilities. Part II The lateral compartment. J Bone Joint Surg Am 58:173–179, 1976.

456. Clendenin MB, DeLee JC, Heckman JD: Interstitial tears of the posterior cruciate ligament of the knee. Orthopedics 3:764–772, 1980.

457. Greene CC, Edwards TB, Wade MR, et al: Reliability of the quadriceps angle measurement. Am J Knee Surg 14:97–103, 2001.

458. Fredericson M, Yoon K: Physical examination and patellofemoral pain syndrome. Am J Phys Med Rehabil 85:234–243, 2006.

459. Piva SR, Fitzgerald K, Irrgang JJ, et al: Reliability of measures of impairments asociated with patellofemoral pain syndrome. BMC Muscloskelet Disord 7:33, 2006.

460. Bremander AB, Peterson IF, Ross EM: Validation of the rheumatoid and arthritis outcome scores (RAOS) for the lower extremity. Health and Quality of Life Outcomes 1:1–11, 2003.

461. Augustsson J, Thomeé R, Linden C, et al: Single-leg hop testing following fatiguing exercise: reliabilty and biomechanical analysis. Scand J Med Sci Sports 16:111–120, 2006.

462. Kea J, Kramer J, Forwell L, et al: Hip abduction-adduction stretch and one-leg hop test: test-retest reliability and relationship to function in elite ice hockey players. J Orthop Sports Phys Ther 31(8):446–455, 2001.

463. Paterno MV, Greenberger HB: The test-retest reliability of a one legged hop for distance in young adults with and without ACL reconstruction. Isokinetics Exerc Sci 6:1–6, 1996.

464. Kramer JF, Nusca D, Fowler P, et al: Test-retest reliability of the one-leg hop test following ACL reconstruction. Clin J Sport Med 2:240–243, 1992.

465. Ageberg E, Zatterstrom R, Mortiz U: Stabiliometry and one leg hop test have high test-retest reliability. Scand J Med Sci Sports 8:198–202, 1998.

466. Birmingham TB: Test-retest reliability of lower extremity functional instability measures. Clin J Sports Med 10:264–268, 2000.

467. DiMattia MA, Livengood AL, Uhl TL, et al: What are the validity of the single-leg squat test and its relationship to hip-abduction strength? Sport Rehabil 14:108–123, 2005.

468. Shields RK, Enloe LJ, Evans RE, et al: Reliability, validity, and responsiveness of functional tests in patients with total joint replacement. Phys Ther 75:169–179, 1995.

469. Björklund K, Sköld C, Andersson L, et al: Reliability of a criterion-based test of athletes with knee injuries: where the physiotherapist and the patient independently and simultaneously assess the patient's performance. Knee Surg Sports Traumatol Arthrosc 14:165–175, 2006.

470. Björklund K, Andersson L, Dalén N: Validity and responsiveness of the test of athletes with knee injuries: the new criterion based functional performance test instrument. Knee Surg Sports Traumatol Arthrosc 17:435–445, 2009.

471. Gebhard F, Authenrieth M, Strecker W, et al: Ultrasound evaluation of gravity induced anterior drawer following anterior cruciate ligament lesion. Knee Surg Sports Traumatol Arthrosc 7(3):166–172, 1999.

472. McClure PW, Rothstein JM, Riddle DL: Intertester reliability of clinical judgements of medial knee ligament integrity. Phys Ther 69(4):268–275, 1989.

473. Garvin GJ, Munk PL, Vellet AD: Tears of the medial collateral ligament: magnetic resonance imaging findings and associated injuries. Can Assoc Radiol J 44:199–204, 1993.

SUGGESTED READINGS

Adams JC: Outline of orthopedics, London, 1968, E & S Livingstone.

Ahstrom JP: Reliability of history and physical examination in diagnosis of meniscus pathology. In Current practice in orthopedic surgery, vol 7, St Louis, 1977, Mosby.

Aichroth P, Freeman MAR, Smillie IS, et al: A knee function assessment chart. J Bone Joint Surg Br 60:308–309, 1978.

Amis AA: Anatomy and biomechanics of the posterior cruciate ligament. Sports Med Arthrosc Rev 7:225–234, 1999.

Ando T, Hirose H, Inoue M, et al: A new method using computed tomographic scan to measure the rectus femoris-patellar tendon Q-angle comparison with conventional method. Clin Orthop 289:213–219, 1993.

Andriacchi TP, Birac D: Functional testing in the anterior cruciate ligament-deficient knee. Clin Orthop 288:40–47, 1993.

Aprin H, Shapiro J, Gershwind M: Arthrography (plica views): a noninvasive method for diagnosis and prognosis of plica syndrome. Clin Orthop 183:90–95, 1984.

Arnold JA, Coker TP, Heaton LM, et al: Natural history of anterior cruciate tears. Am J Sports Med 7:305–313, 1979.

Back BR, Warren RF: Radiographic indicators of the anterior cruciate ligament injury. In Feagin JA, editor: The crucial ligaments, Edinburgh, 1988, Churchill Livingstone.

Bassett LW, Gold RH: Magnetic resonance imaging of the musculoskeletal system: an overview. Clin Orthop 244:17–28, 1989.

Bassett LW, Gold RH, Seeger LL: MRI atlas of the musculoskeletal system, London, 1989, Martin Dunitz.

Beetham WP, Polley HP, Slocumb CH, et al: Physical extremities of the joint, Philadelphia, 1965, WB Saunders.

Bigg-Wither G, Kelly P: Diagnostic imaging in musculoskeletal physiotherapy. In Refshauge K, Gass E, editors: Musculoskeletal physiotherapy: clinical science and practice, Oxford, 1995, Butterworth-Heinemann Ltd.

Booker JM, Thibodeau GA: Athletic injury assessment, St Louis, 1989, Mosby.

Brantigan OC, Voshell AF: The mechanics of the ligaments and menisci of the knee joint. J Bone Joint Surg 23:44–66, 1941.

Bryant JT, Cooke TD: A biomechanical function of the ACL: prevention of medial translation of the tibia. In Feagin JA, editor: The crucial ligaments, Edinburgh, 1988, Churchill Livingstone.

Bull AM, Andersen HN, Basso O, et al: Incidence and mechanism of the pivot shift—an in vitro study. Clin Orthop Relat Res 363:219–231, 1999.

Burk DL, Dalinka MK, Kinal E, et al: Meniscal and ganglion cysts of the knee: MR evaluation. Am J Roentgenol 150:331–336, 1988.

Cabaud HE, Slocum DB: The diagnosis of chronic anterolateral rotary instability of the knee. Am J Sports Med 5:99–104, 1977.

Cailliet R: Knee pain and disability, Philadelphia, 1973, FA Davis.

Clancy WG: Evaluation of acute knee injuries. In American Association of Orthopaedic Surgeons: Symposium on sports medicine: the knee, St Louis, 1985, Mosby.

Clarkson HM, Gilewich GB: Musculoskeletal assessment: joint range of motion and manual muscle strength, Baltimore, 1989, Williams & Wilkins.

Cole BJ, Harner CD: Degenerative arthritis of the knee in active patients: evaluation and management. J Am Acad Orthop Surg 7:389–402, 1999.

Collins HR: Anterolateral rotary instability. In American Association of Orthopaedic Surgeons: Symposium on the athlete's knee, St Louis, 1980, Mosby.

Conlan T, Garth WP, Lemons JE: Evaluation of the medial soft tissue restraints of the extensor mechanism of the knee. J Bone Joint Surg Am 75:682–693, 1993

Cooper DE: Tests for posterolateral instability of the knee in normal subjects: results of examination under anaesthesia. J Bone Joint Surg Am 73:30–36, 1991.

Crues JV, Ryu R, Morgan FW: Meniscal pathology: the expanding role of magnetic resonance imaging. Clin Orthop 252:80–87, 1990.

Cyriax J: Textbook of orthopaedic medicine, vol 1. Diagnosis of soft tissue lesions, London, 1975, Bailliere Tindall.

Danzig LA, Newell JD, Guerra J, et al: Osseous landmarks of the normal knee. Clin Orthop 156:201–206, 1981.

Davies GJ: Examining the knee. Phys Sportsmed 6:48–67, 1978.

De Haven KE, Collins HR: Diagnosis of internal derangement of the knee: the role of arthroscopy. J Bone Joint Surg Am 57:802–810, 1975.

Deutsch AL, Shellock FG, Mink JH: Imaging of the patellofemoral joint: emphasis on advanced techniques. In Fu FH, Stone DA, editors: Sports injuries: mechanisms, prevention, treatment, Baltimore, 1994, Williams & Wilkins.

Dietrini SD, LaPrade RL, Griffith CJ, et al: Radiographic identification of the primary posterolateral knee structures. Am J Sports Med 37:542–557, 2009.

Dontigny RL: Terminal extension exercises for the knee. Phys Ther 52:45–46, 1972.

Doppman JL: Baker's cyst and the normal gastrocnemiosemimembranosus bursa. Am J Roentgenol 94:646–652, 1965.

Dowd GS, Bentley G: Radiographic assessment of patellar instability and chondromalacia patellae. J Bone Joint Surg Br 68:297–300, 1986.

Ehrlich MG, Strain RE: Epiphyseal injuries about the knee. Orthop Clin North Am 10:91–103, 1979.

Ellison AE: The pathogenesis and treatment of anterolateral rotary instability. Clin Orthop 147:51–55, 1980.

Engle RP: Examination of the knee. In Engle RP, editor: Knee ligament rehabilitation, New York, 1991, Churchill Livingstone.

Evans RC: Illustrated essentials in orthopedic physical assessment, St Louis, 1994, Mosby.

Ewald FC: The knee society total knee arthroplasty roentgenographic evaluation and scoring system. Clin Orthop 248:9–12, 1989.

Feagin JA: Introduction: principles of diagnosis and treatment. In Feagin JA, editor: The crucial ligaments, Edinburgh, 1988, Churchill Livingstone.

Feagin JA, Cabaud HE, Curl WW: The anterior cruciate ligament: radiographic and clinical signs of successful and unsuccessful repairs. Clin Orthop 164:54–58, 1982.

Fetto JF, Marshall JL: The natural history and diagnosis of anterior cruciate ligament insufficiency. Clin Orthop 147:29–38, 1980.

Fleming BC, Beynnon BD, Johnson RJ: The use of knee laxity testers for the determination of anterior-posterior stability of the knee: pitfalls in practice. In Jackson DW, editor: The anterior cruciate ligament: current and future concepts, New York, 1993, Raven Press.

Fowler PJ: The classification and early diagnosis of knee joint instability. Clin Orthop 147:15–21, 1980.

Francis RS, Scott DE: Hypertrophy of the vastus medialis in knee extension. Phys Ther 54:1066–1070, 1974.

Frankel VH, Burstein AH, Brooks DB: Biomechanics of internal derangement of the knee. J Bone Joint Surg Am 53:945–962, 1971.

Franklin JL, Rosenberg TD, Paulos LE, et al: Radiographic assessment of instability of the knee due to rupture of the anterior cruciate ligament: a quadriceps contraction technique. J Bone Joint Surg Am 73:365–372, 1991.

Fu FH, Seel MJ, Berger RA: Patellofemoral biomechanics. In Fox JM, Del Pizzo W, editors: The patellofemoral joint, New York, 1993, McGraw-Hill.

Fulkerson JP: Awareness of the retinaculum in evaluating patellofemoral pain. Am J Sports Med 10:147–149, 1982.

Fulkerson JP: Evaluation of the peripatellar soft tissues and retinaculum in patients with patellofemoral pain. Clin Sports Med 8:197–202, 1989.

Fulkerson JP: Patellofemoral pain disorders: evaluation and management. J Am Acad Orthop Surg 2:124–132, 1994.

Gartland JJ: Fundamentals of orthopedics, Philadelphia, 1979, WB Saunders.

Gersoff WK, Clancy WG: Diagnosis of acute and chronic anterior cruciate ligament tears. Clin Sports Med 7:727–738, 1988.

Gillquist J: Diagnosis and classification of the instability of the knee joint. Semin Orthop 2:18–22, 1987.

Ginsburg JH, Ellsasser JC: Problem areas in the diagnosis and treatment of ligament injuries of the knee. Clin Orthop 132:201–205, 1978.

Goodfellow J, Hungerford DS, Woods C: Patellofemoral joint mechanics and pathology: chondromalacia patellae. J Bone Joint Surg Br 58:291–299, 1976.

Gough JV, Ladley G: An investigation into the effectiveness of various forms of quadriceps exercises. Physiotherapy 57:356–361, 1971.

Greenmill BJ: The importance of the medial quadriceps expansion in medial ligament injury. Can J Surg 10:312–317, 1967.

Griffin LY, Agel J, Albohm MJ, et al: Noncontact anterior cruciate ligament injuries: risk factors and prevention strategies. J Am Acad Orthop Surg 8:141–150, 2000.

Grood ES, Stowers SF, Noyes FR: Limits of movement in the human knee: effect of sectioning the posterior cruciate ligament and posterolateral structures. J Bone Joint Surg Am 70:88–97, 1988.

Gurtler RA, Stine R, Torg JS: Lachman test evaluated: quantification of a clinical observation. Clin Orthop 216:141–150, 1987.

Guzzanti V, Gigante A, DiLazzaro A, et al: Patellofemoral malalignment in adolescents: computerized tomographic assessment with and without quadriceps contraction. Am J Sports Med 22:55–60, 1994.

Hardy JR, Chimutengwende-Gordon M, Bakar I: Rupture of the quadriceps tendon—an association with a patellar spur. J Bone Joint Surg Br 87:1361–1363, 2005.

Hewett TE, Meyer GD, Ford KR: Anterior cruciate ligament injuries in female athletes. 1. mechanisms and risk factors. Am J Sports Med 34:299–311, 2006.

Heyerman WB, Hoyt WA: Anterolateral rotary instability associated with chronic anterior cruciate insufficiency. Clin Orthop Relat Res 134:144–148, 1978.

Hilyard A: Recent developments in the management of patellofemoral pain: the McConnell programme. Physiotherapy 76:559–565, 1990.

Hollinshead WH, Jenkins DB: Functional anatomy of the limbs and back, Philadelphia, 1981, WB Saunders.

Hoppenfeld S: Physical examination of the spine and extremities, New York, 1976, Appleton-Century-Crofts.

Hoppenfeld S: Physical examination of the knee joint by complaint. Orthop Clin North Am 10:3–20, 1979.

Hoskins W, Pollard H: The management of hamstring injury - part 1: issues in diagnosis. Manual Therapy 10:96–107, 2005.

Hughston JC, Bowden JA, Andrews JR, et al: Acute tears of the posterior cruciate ligament. J Bone Joint Surg Am 62:438–450, 1980.

Iobst CA, Stanitski CL: Acute knee injuries. Clin Sports Med 19:621–635, 2000.

Jackson JP: Internal derangement of the knee joint. Physiotherapy 52:229–232, 1966.

Jakob RP: Pathomechanical and clinical components of the pivot shift sign. Semin Orthop 2:9–17, 1987.

Jakob RP, Staubli HU, Deland JT: Grading the pivot shift: objective tests with implications for treatment. J Bone Joint Surg Am 69:294–299, 1987.

Jensen K: Manual laxity tests for anterior cruciate ligament injuries. J Orthop Sports Phys Ther 11:474–481, 1990.

Johnson TR, Steinbach LS: Essentials of musculoskeletal imaging, Rosemont, IL, 2004, American Academy of Orthopedic Surgeons.

Kapandji LA: The physiology of the joints, vol 2. Lower limb, New York, 1970, Churchill Livingstone.

Kennedy JC, Stewart R, Walker DM: Anterolateral rotary instability of the knee joint: an early analysis of the Ellison repair. J Bone Joint Surg Am 60:1031–1032, 1978.

Kursunoglu-Brahme S, Resnick D: Magnetic resonance imaging of the knee. Orthop Clin North Am 21:561–572, 1990.

LaPrade RF, Bollom TS, Wentorf FA, et al: Mechanical properties of the posterolateral structures of the knee. Am J Sports Med 33:1386–1391, 2005.

Larson RL: Clinical evaluation. In Larson RL, Grana WA, editors: The knee: form, function, pathology and treatment, Philadelphia, 1993, WB Saunders.

Lieb FJ, Perry J: Quadriceps function. J Bone Joint Surg Am 50:1535–1548, 1968.

Levangie PK, Norkin CC: Joint structure and function—a comprehensive analysis, Philadelphia, 2005. FA Davis.

Liu SH, Osti L, Dorey F, et al: Anterior cruciate ligament tear: a new diagnostic index on magnetic resonance imaging. Clin Orthop Relat Res 302:147–150, 1994.

Logan A: The knee: clinical applications, Gaithersburg, MD, 1994, Aspen Publishers.

Losee RE: Concepts of the pivot shift. Clin Orthop 172:45–51, 1983.

Losee RE: The pivot shift. In Feagin JA, editor: The crucial ligaments, Edinburgh, 1988, Churchill Livingstone.

Lucie RS, Wiedel JD, Messner DG: The acute pivot shift: clinical correlation. Am J Sports Med 12:189–191, 1984.

Macnicol MF: The problem knee: diagnosis and management in the younger patient, London, 1986, Wm Heinemann Medical Books.

Malek MM, Manjini RE: Patellofemoral pain syndrome: a comprehensive and conservative approach. J Orthop Sports Phys Ther 2:108–116, 1981.

Malone T, Kegerreis ST: Evaluation process. In Mangine RE, editor: Physical therapy of the knee, Edinburgh, 1988, Churchill Livingstone.

Mandelbaum BR, Browne JE, Fu F, et al: Articular cartilage lesions of the knee. Am J Sports Med 26:853–861, 1998.

Mandelbaum BR, Finerman GA, Reicher MA, et al: Magnetic resonance imaging as a tool for evaluation of traumatic knee injuries. Am J Sports Med 14:361–370, 1986.

Manner HM, Radler C, Ganger R, et al: Dysplasia of the cruciate ligaments: radiographic assessment and classification. J Bone Joint Surg Am 88:130–137, 2006.

Mayor D: Anatomical and functional aspects of the knee joint. Physiotherapy 52:224–228, 1966.

McLean SG, Neal RJ, Myers PT, et al: Knee joint kinematics during the sidestep cutting manoeuver: potential for injury in women. Med Sci Sports Exerc 31:959–968, 1999.

McRae R: Clinical orthopaedic examination, New York, 1976, Churchill Livingstone.

Meislin RJ: Managing collateral ligament tears of the knee. Phys Sportsmed 24:67–80, 1996.

Meister BR, Michael SP, Moyer RA, et al: Anatomy and kinematics of the lateral collateral ligament of the knee. Am J Sports Med 28:869–878, 2000.

Merchant AC: The lateral patellar compression syndrome. In Fu FH, Stone DA, editors: Sports injuries: mechanisms, prevention, treatment, Baltimore, 1994, Williams & Wilkins.

Meszler D, Manal TJ, Snyder-Mackler L: Disorders of the tibiofemoral joint—evaluation, diagnosis and intervention. Orthop Phys Ther Clin North Am 7:347–366, 1998.

Moller BN, Kadin S: Entrapment of the common peroneal nerve. Am J Sports Med 15:90–91, 1987.

Moran DJ, Floyd RT: The Lachman test: alternative techniques and applications for anterior cruciate ligament evaluation. Sports Med Update 5:3–5, 1990.

Muller W, Biedert R, Hefti F, et al: OAK knee evaluation: a new way to assess knee ligament injuries. Clin Orthop 232:37–50, 1988.

Myrer JW, Schulthies SS, Fellingham CW: Relative and absolute reliability of the KT-1000 arthrometer for injured knees. Am J Sports Med 24:104–108, 1992.

Nelson EW, LaPrade RF: The anterior intermeniscal ligament of the knee—an anatomic study. Am J Sport Med 28:74–76, 2000.

Neumann DA: Kinesiology of the musculoskeletal system—foundations for physical rehabilitation, St Louis, 2002, Mosby.

Norwood LA, Cross MJ: Anterior cruciate ligament: functional anatomy of its bundles in rotary instabilities. Am J Sports Med 7:23–26, 1979.

Norwood LA, Hughston JC: Combined anterolateral-anteromedial rotary instability of the knee. Clin Orthop 147:62–67, 1980.

Noyes FR, Grood ES: Diagnosis of knee ligament injuries: clinical concepts. In Feagin JA, editor: The crucial ligaments, Edinburgh, 1988, Churchill Livingstone.

Noyes FR, Grood ES, Butler DL: Clinical laxity tests and functional stability of the knee: biomechanical concepts. Clin Orthop 146:84–89, 1980.

Nunn KD, Mayhew JL: Comparison of three methods of assessing strength imbalances at the knee. J Orthop Sports Phys Ther 10:134–137, 1988.

Oberlander MA, Shalvoy RM, Hughston JC: The accuracy of the clinical knee examination documented by arthroscopy: a prospective study. Am J Sports Med 21:773–778, 1993.

O'Donoghue DH: Treatment of injuries to athletes, ed 4, Philadelphia, 1984, WB Saunders.

Ogata K, McCarthy JA, Dunlap J, et al: Pathomechanisms of posterior sag of the tibia in posterior cruciate deficient knees. Am J Sports Med 16:630–636, 1988.

Ombregt L, Bisschop P, ter Veer HJ, et al: A system of orthopedic medicine, London, 1995, WB Saunders.

Palmer ML, Epler M: Clinical assessment procedures in physical therapy, Philadelphia, 1990, JB Lippincott.

Patel D: Superior lateral-medial approach to arthroscopic meniscectomy. Orthop Clin North Am 13:299–305, 1982.

Percy EC, Strother RT: Patellalgia. Phys Sports Med 13:43–59, 1985.

Perry J: Function of quadriceps. J Can Physiother Assoc 24:130–132, 1972.

Pickett JC, Radin EL: Chondromalacia of the patella, Baltimore, 1983, Williams & Wilkins.

Pipkin G: Knee injuries: the role of the suprapatellar plica and suprapatellar bursa in simulating internal derangements. Clin Orthop 74:161–176, 1971.

Powers CM, Mortenson S, Nishimoto D, et al: Criterion-related validity of a clinical measurement to determine the medial/lateral component of patellar orientation. J Orthop Sports Phys Ther 29:372–377, 1999.

Pynsent P, Fairbank J, Carr A: Outcome measures in orthopedics, Oxford, 1993, Butterworth-Heinemann.

Reid DC: Functional anatomy and joint mobilization, Edmonton, 1980, University of Alberta Bookstore.

Reid DC: The myth, mystic and frustration of anterior knee pain. Clin J Sport Med 3:139–143, 1993.

Reid DC: Sports injury assessment and rehabilitation, New York, 1992, Churchill Livingstone.

Reider B, D'Agata SD: Factors predisposing to knee injury. In DeLee JC, Drez D, editors: Orthopedic sports medicine, Philadelphia, 1994, WB Saunders.

Reider B, Marshall JL, Koslin B, et al: The anterior aspect of the knee joint. J Bone Joint Surg Am 63:351–356, 1981.

Reilly BM: Practical strategies in outpatient medicine, Philadelphia, 1984, WB Saunders.

Renstrom P, Johnson RJ: Anatomy and biomechanics of the menisci. Clin Sports Med 9:523–538, 1990.

Resnick D, Kransdorf MJ: Bone and joint imaging, Philadelphia, 2005, Elsevier.

Ribn JA, Gross YJ, Harner CD, et al: The acutely dislocated knee: evaluation and management. J Am Acad Orthop Surg 12:334–346, 2004.

Robinson JR, Sanchez-Ballester J, Bull AM, et al: The posteromedial corner revisited: an anatomical description of the passive restraining structures of the medial aspect of the human knee. J Bone Joint Surg Br 86:674–681, 2004.

Rovere GD, Adair DM: Anterior cruciate-deficient knees: a review of the literature. Am J Sports Med 11:412–419, 1983.

Rubinstein RA, Shelbourne D, McCarroll JR, et al: The accuracy of the clinical examination in the setting of posterior cruciate ligament injuries. Am J Sports Med 22:550–557, 1994.

Rusche K, Mangine RE: Pathomechanics of injury to the patellofemoral and tibiofemoral joint. In Mangine RE, editor: Physical therapy of the knee, Edinburgh, 1988, Churchill Livingstone.

Sheehan FT, Drau JE: Human patellar tendon strain. Clin Orthop Relat Res 370:201–207, 2000.

Smillie IS: Diseases of the knee joint. Physiotherapy 70:144–150, 1984.

Solomon DH, Simel DL, Bates DW, et al: The rational clinical examination. Does this patient have a torn meniscus or ligament of the knee? Value of the physical examination. JAMA 286(13):1610–1620, 2001.

Stanitski CL: Patellofemoral mechanism. In Stanitski CL, DeLee JC, Drez D, editors: Pediatric and adolescent sports medicine, Philadelphia, 1994, WB Saunders.

Starkey C, Ryan J: Evaluation of orthopedic and athletic injuries, Philadelphia, 1996, FA Davis.

Swenson TM: Physical diagnosis of the multiple-ligament-injured knee. Clin Sports Med 19:415–423, 2000.

Tachdjian MO: Pediatric orthopedics, Philadelphia, 1972, WB Saunders.

Tegner Y, Lysholm J: Rating systems in the evaluation of knee ligament injuries. Clin Orthop 198:43–49, 1985.

Teitge RA, Faerber W, Des Madryl P, et al: Stress radiographs of the patellofemoral joint. J Bone Joint Surg Am 78:193–203, 1996.

Travell JG, Simons DG: Myofascial pain and dysfunction: the trigger point manual, Baltimore, 1983, Williams & Wilkins.

Tria AJ, Palumbo RC: Conservative treatment of patellofemoral pain. Semin Orthop 5:115–121, 1990.

Trickey EL: Injuries to the posterior cruciate ligament: diagnosis and treatment of early injuries and reconstruction of late instability. Clin Orthop 147:76–81, 1980.

Turner JS, Smillie IS: The effect of tibial torsion on the pathology of the knee. J Bone Joint Surg Br 63:396–398, 1981.

Wallace LA, Mangine RE, Malone TR: The knee. In Gould JA, editor: Orthopedic and sports physical therapy, St Louis, 1990, Mosby.

Walsh WM: Patellofemoral joint. In DeLee JC, Drez D, editors: Orthopedic sports medicine, Philadelphia, 1994, WB Saunders.

Warren LF, Marshall J: The supporting structures and layers on the medial side of the knee. J Bone Joint Surg Am 61:56–62, 1979

Warren LF, Marshall J, Girgis F: The prime static stabilizer of the medial side of the knee. J Bone Joint Surg Am 56:665–674, 1974.

Wechsler LR, Busis NA: Sports neurology. In Fu FH, Stone DA, editors: Sports injuries: mechanisms, prevention, treatment, Baltimore, 1994, Williams & Wilkins.

Weiss JR, Irrgang JJ, Sawhney R, et al: A functional assessment of anterior cruciate ligament deficiency in an acute and clinical setting. J Orthop Sports Phys Ther 11:372–373, 1990.

Weissman BNW, Sledge CB: Orthopedic radiology, Philadelphia, 1986, WB Saunders.

Welsh RP: Knee joint structure and function. Clin Orthop 147:7–14, 1980.

Wiles P, Sweetnam R: Essentials of orthopedics, London, 1965, J & A Churchill.

Wojtys EM, editor: The ACL deficient knee, Rosemont, IL, 1994, American Academy of Orthopedic Surgeons.

Woo SLY, Debski RE, Withrow JD, et al: Biomechanics of knee ligaments. Am J Sports Med 27:533–543, 1999.

Zachazewski JE, Magee DJ, Quillen WS: Athletic injuries and rehabilitation, Philadelphia, 1996, WB Saunders.

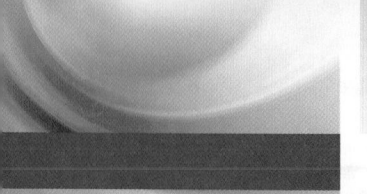

CHAPTER 13

Lower Leg, Ankle, and Foot

At least 80% of the general population has foot problems, but these problems can often be corrected by proper assessment, treatment, and, above all, care of the feet. Lesions of the ankle and foot can alter the mechanics of gait resulting in movement impairments and, as a result, cause stress on other lower limb joints, which in turn may lead to pathology in these joints.[1]

The foot and ankle combine flexibility with stability because of the many bones, their shapes, and their attachments. The lower leg, ankle, and foot have two principal functions: propulsion and support. For propulsion, they act like a flexible lever; for support, they act like a rigid structure that holds up the entire body.

Functions of the Foot

- Acts as a support base that provides the necessary stability for upright posture with minimal muscle effort
- Provides a mechanism for rotation of the tibia and fibula during the stance phase of gait
- Provides flexibility to adapt to uneven terrain
- Provides flexibility for absorption of shock
- Acts as a lever during push-off

Although the joints of the lower leg, ankle, and foot are discussed separately, they act as functional groups, not as isolated joints. As the terminal part of the lower kinetic chain, the lower leg, ankle, and foot have the ability to distribute and dissipate the different forces (e.g., compressive, shearing, rotary, tensile) acting on the body through contact with the ground.[2] This is especially evident during gait. In the foot, the movement occurring at each individual joint is minimal. However, when combined, there normally is sufficient range of motion (ROM) in all of the joints to allow functional mobility as well as functional stability. For ease of understanding, the joints of the foot are divided into three sections: hindfoot (rearfoot), midfoot, and forefoot.

APPLIED ANATOMY

Hindfoot (Rearfoot)

Tibiofibular Joint. The inferior (distal) tibiofibular joint is a fibrous or syndesmosis type of joint. It is supported by the anterior tibiofibular, posterior tibiofibular, and inferior transverse ligaments as well as the interosseous ligaments (Figure 13-1). The movements at this joint are minimal but allow a small amount of spread (1 to 2 mm) at the ankle joint during dorsiflexion. This same action allows the fibula to move up and down during dorsiflexion and plantar flexion. Dorsiflexion at the ankle joint causes the fibula to move superiorly, putting stress on both the inferior tibiofibular joint at the ankle and the superior tibiofibular joint at the knee. The fibula carries more of the axial load when it is dorsiflexed. On average, the fibula carries about 17% of the axial loading.[3] The joint is supplied by the deep peroneal and tibial nerves.

Talocrural (Ankle) Joint. The talocrural joint is a uniaxial, modified hinge, synovial joint located between the **talus,** the **medial malleolus** of the tibia, and the **lateral malleolus** of the fibula. The talus is shaped so that in dorsiflexion it is wedged between the malleoli, allowing little or no inversion or eversion at the ankle joint. The talus is approximately 2.4 mm (0.1 inch) wider anteriorly than posteriorly. The medial malleolus is shorter, extending halfway down the talus, whereas the lateral malleolus extends almost to the level of the subtalar joint. The joint is supplied by branches of the tibial and deep peroneal nerves.

The talocrural joint is designed for stability, especially in dorsiflexion. In plantar flexion, it is much more mobile. This joint is responsible for the anterior-posterior (dorsiflexion-plantar flexion) movement that occurs in the ankle-foot complex. Its close packed position is maximum dorsiflexion, and its capsular pattern is more a limitation of plantar flexion than of dorsiflexion. This joint is most stable in the dorsiflexed position. The resting position is 10° of plantar flexion, midway between maximum inversion and maximum eversion. The talocrural joint has one degree of freedom, and the movements possible at this joint are dorsiflexion and plantar flexion.

On the medial side of the joint, the major ligament is the **deltoid** or **medial collateral ligament,** which consists of four separate ligaments: the tibionavicular, tibiocalcanean, and posterior tibiotalar ligaments superficially, all of which resist talar abduction, and the anterior tibiotalar ligament, which lies deep to the other three ligaments and resists lateral translation and lateral rotation of the talus. On the lateral aspect, the talocrural joint is supported by the anterior talofibular ligament, which provides stability against excessive inversion of the talus; the posterior talofibular ligament, which resists ankle dorsiflexion, adduction ("tilt"), medial rotation, and medial translation of the talus; and the calcaneofibular ligament, which provides stability against maximum inversion at the ankle and subtalar joints. The anterior talofibular ligament is the ligament most commonly injured by a lateral ankle sprain, followed by the calcaneofibular ligament.

Subtalar (Talocalcanean) Joint. The subtalar joint is a synovial joint having three degrees of freedom and a close packed position of supination. Supporting the subtalar joint are the lateral talocalcanean and medial talocalcanean ligaments. In addition, the interosseous talocalcanean and cervical ligaments limit eversion.

The movements possible at the subtalar joint are gliding and rotation. With injury to the area (e.g., sprain, fracture), this joint and the talocrural joint often become

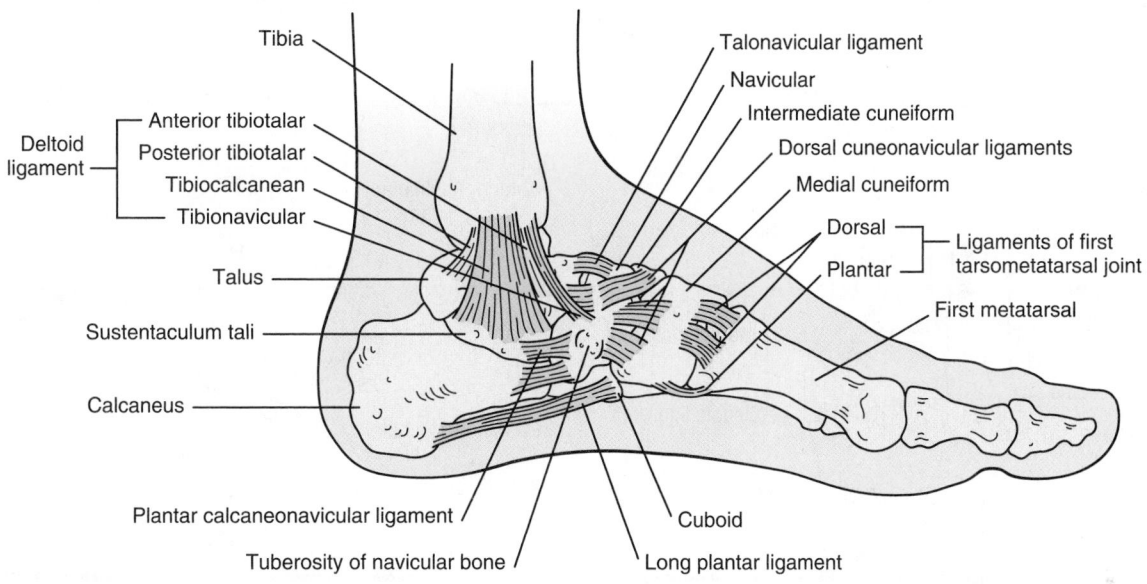

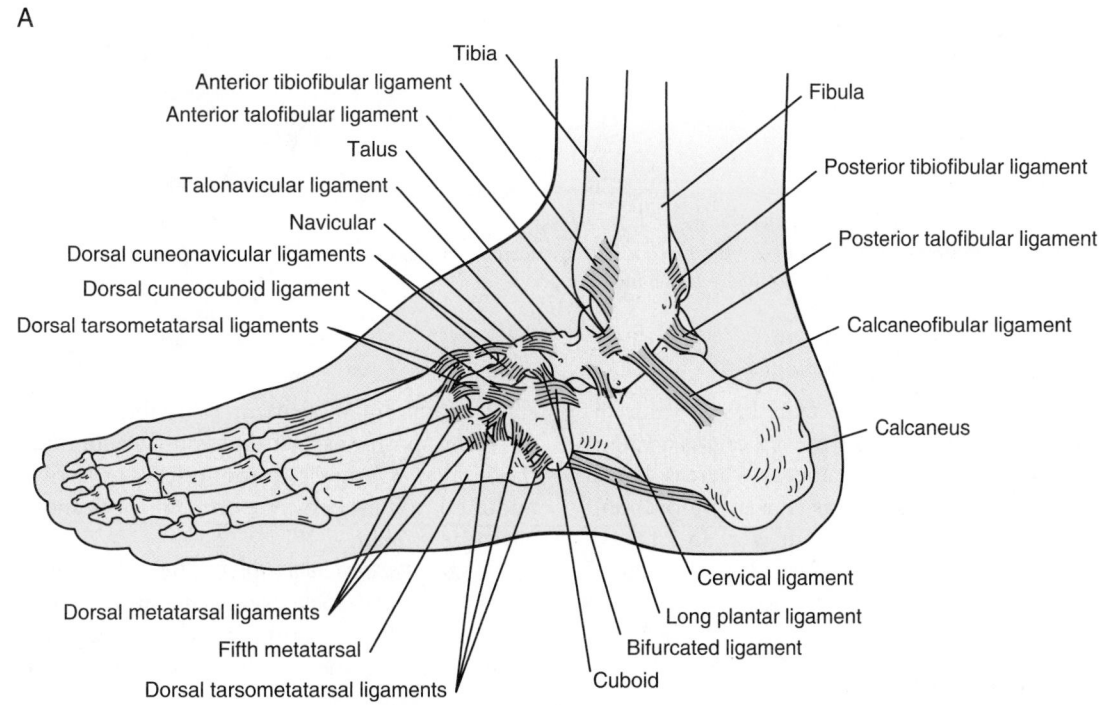

Figure 13-1 Ligaments of the hindfoot and midfoot. A, Medial view. **B,** Lateral view. *Continued*

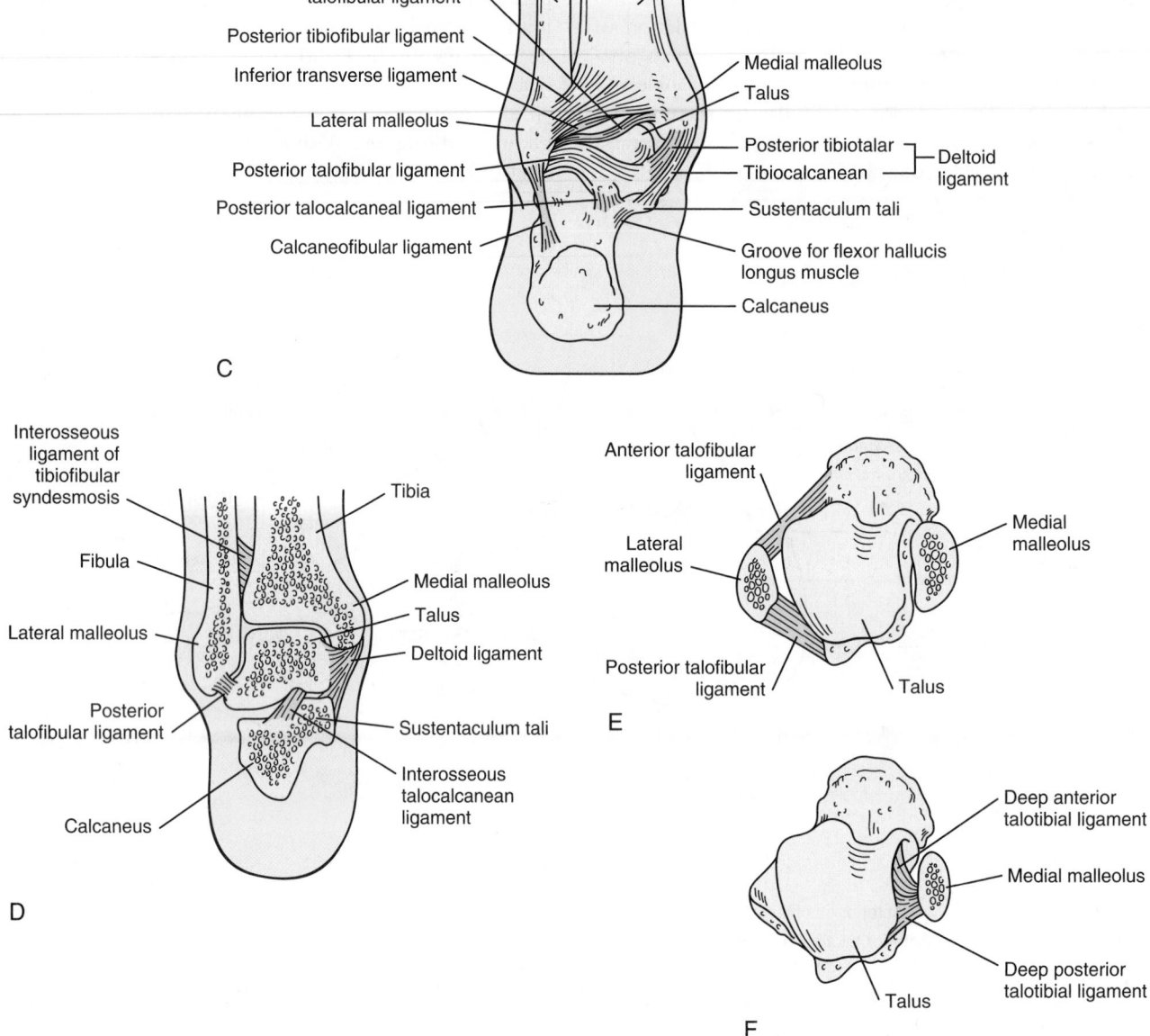

Figure 13-1, cont'd C, Posterior view. **D,** Coronal section through the left talocrural and talocalcanean joints. **E,** Superior view of ligaments on the lateral aspect. **F,** Superior view of deep deltoid ligament on the medial aspect.

hypomobile, partially because the talus has no muscles attaching to it. Medial rotation of the leg causes a valgus (outward) movement of the calcaneus, whereas lateral rotation of the leg produces a varus (inward) movement of the calcaneus. The axis of the joint is at an angle of 40° to 45° inclined vertically and 15° to 18° to the sagittal plane.

Midfoot (Midtarsal Joints)

In isolation, the midtarsal joints allow only a minimal amount of movement. Taken together, however, they

allow significant movement to enable the foot to adapt to many positions without putting undue stress on the joints. **Chopart joint** refers collectively to the midtarsal joints between the talus-calcaneus and the navicular-cuboid.

Talocalcaneonavicular Joint. The talocalcaneonavicular joint is a ball-and-socket synovial joint with 3° of freedom. Its close packed position is supination, and the dorsal talonavicular ligament, bifurcated ligament, and plantar calcaneonavicular (spring) ligament support the joint (see Figure 13-1; Figure 13-2). Movements possible at this joint are gliding and rotation.

Joints of the Hindfoot

TIBIOFIBULAR JOINT

Resting position:	Plantar flexion
Close packed position:	Maximum dorsiflexion
Capsular pattern:	Pain when joint is stressed

TALOCRURAL (ANKLE) JOINT

Resting position:	10° plantar flexion, midway between inversion and eversion
Close packed position:	Maximum dorsiflexion
Capsular pattern:	Plantar flexion, dorsiflexion

SUBTALAR JOINT

Resting position:	Midway between extremes of range of motion (ROM)
Close packed position:	Supination
Capsular pattern:	Limited ROM (varus, valgus)

Figure 13-2 Ligaments on plantar aspect of foot.

Cuneonavicular Joint. The cuneonavicular joint is a plane synovial joint with a close packed position of supination. The movements possible at this joint are slight gliding and rotation.

Cuboideonavicular Joint. The cuboideonavicular joint is fibrous, its close packed position being supination. The movements possible at this joint are slight gliding and rotation.

Intercuneiform Joints. The intercuneiform joints are plane synovial joints with a close packed position of supination. The movements possible at these joints are slight gliding and rotation.

Cuneocuboid Joint. The cuneocuboid joint is a plane synovial joint with a close packed position of supination. The movements of slight gliding and rotation are possible at this joint.

Calcaneocuboid Joint. The calcaneocuboid joint is saddle shaped with a close packed position of supination. Supporting this joint are the bifurcated ligament, the calcaneocuboid ligament, and the long plantar ligaments. The movement possible at this joint is gliding with conjunct rotation.

Joints of the Midfoot (Midtarsal Joints)

Resting position:	Midway between extremes of range of motion (ROM)
Close packed position:	Supination
Capsular pattern:	Dorsiflexion, plantar flexion, adduction, medial rotation

Forefoot

Tarsometatarsal Joints. The tarsometatarsal joints are plane synovial joints with a close packed position of supination. The movement possible at these joints is gliding. Taken together, these joints are referred to as **Lisfranc joint.**[4]

Intermetatarsal Joints. The four intermetatarsal joints are plane synovial joints with a close packed position of supination. The movement possible at these joints is gliding.

Metatarsophalangeal Joints. The five metatarsophalangeal joints are condyloid synovial joints with 2° of freedom. Their close packed position is full extension. Their capsular pattern is variable for the lateral four joints and more limitation of extension than flexion for the hallux (big toe); their resting position is 10° of extension. The movements possible at these joints are flexion, extension, abduction, and adduction.

Interphalangeal Joints. The interphalangeal joints are synovial hinge joints with 1° of freedom. The close packed position is full extension, and the capsular pattern is more limitation of flexion than of extension. The resting position of the distal and proximal interphalangeal joints is slight flexion. The movements possible at these joints are flexion and extension.

PATIENT HISTORY

It is important to take a detailed and complete history when assessing the lower leg, ankle, and foot. In addition to the questions listed under the "Patient History" section in Chapter 1 the examiner should obtain the following information from the patient:

1. *What is the patient's occupation?* Whether the patient stands a great deal and the types of surfaces on which

---

Joints of the Forefoot

TARSOMETATARSAL JOINTS

Resting position:	Midway between extremes of range of motion (ROM)
Close packed position:	Supination
Capsular pattern:	None

METATARSOPHALANGEAL JOINTS

Resting position:	10° extension
Close packed position:	Full extension
Capsular pattern:	Big toe: extension, flexion
	Second to fifth toe: variable

INTERPHALANGEAL JOINTS

Resting position:	Slight flexion
Close packed position:	Full extension
Capsular pattern:	Flexion, extension

---

injury, accompanied by a snapping and pain on the lateral aspect that rapidly diminishes, may indicate a tear of the peroneal retinaculum.[14] Taunton et al.[15] list some causes of overuse injuries in the lower limb.

Clinical Prediction Rule for Anterolateral Ankle Impingement[11]

Note: Five of six symptoms must be positive.
- Anterolateral ankle joint tenderness
- Anterolateral ankle joint swelling
- Pain on forced dorsiflexion
- Pain on affected side with single leg squat
- Pain with activities
- Absence of ankle instability

From Liu SH, Nuccion SL, Finerman G: Diagnosis of anterolateral ankle impingement: comparison between magnetic resonance imaging and clinical examination. Am J Sports Med 25:389–393, 1997.

---

the patient usually stands may have bearing on what is causing the problem.

2. *What was the mechanism of injury?* What was the position of the foot at the time of the injury? Ankle sprains occur most often when the foot is plantar flexed, inverted, and adducted, with injury to the anterior talofibular ligament, anterolateral capsule, and possibly the distal tibiofibular ligament.[5,6] This same mechanism can lead to peroneal tendon injury, a malleolar or talar dome fracture, and sinus tarsi syndrome.[7,8] Figure 13-3 outlines some of the common mechanisms of injury to the ankle. Table 13-1 outlines the **West Point Sprain Grading System** that can be used to determine the severity of ankle sprains.[9] With injury to the lateral ligaments, the structures (articular surfaces) may be damaged on the medial side owing to compression leading to medial as well as lateral pain.[10] In fact, if the lateral ligaments are completely torn and the capsule disrupted, medial pain may predominate. Anterolateral pain without a history of trauma may be the result of anterior impingement especially after injury to the anterior talofibular ligament. Lin et al.[11] developed a clinical prediction rule for ankle impingement (see the following box) that would preclude the need for magnetic resonance imaging (MRI). The impingement may be due to thickening of the joint capsule and/or bone spurs adjacent to the anterior talocrural joint.[12] Achilles tendinosis or paratenonitis often arises as the result of overuse, increased activity, or change in a high-stress training program. Osteochondral lesions most commonly occur with trauma and may accompany ankle sprains and fractures with symptoms being exacerbated by prolonged weight bearing or high impact activities.[13] A dorsiflexion

---

Causes of Overuse Injuries to the Lower Limb

- Prolonged training season
- Impact force of activity
- Training or competing on hard surfaces
- Change of training surface
- Downhill running
- Lack of flexibility
- Individual muscle weakness or poor reciprocal muscle strength
- Overstriding
- Poor posture
- High mileage or sudden change in mileage
- Too much, too soon
- Overtraining
- Anatomical factors (e.g., malalignment)
- Wrong type of footwear
- Road or sidewalk camber

---

3. *Did the patient notice a transient or fixed deformity of the foot or ankle at the time of injury?* Was there any transitory locking (e.g., loose body, muscle spasm)? An affirmative answer may indicate a fracture causing immediate swelling that decreased as it spread into the surrounding tissue.

4. *Was the patient able to continue the activity after the injury?* If so, the injury is probably not too severe, provided there is no loss of stability. Inability to bear weight, severe pain, and rapid swelling indicate a severe injury.[14] Walking is compatible with a second-degree sprain; pain with running usually indicates a first-degree injury.[16]

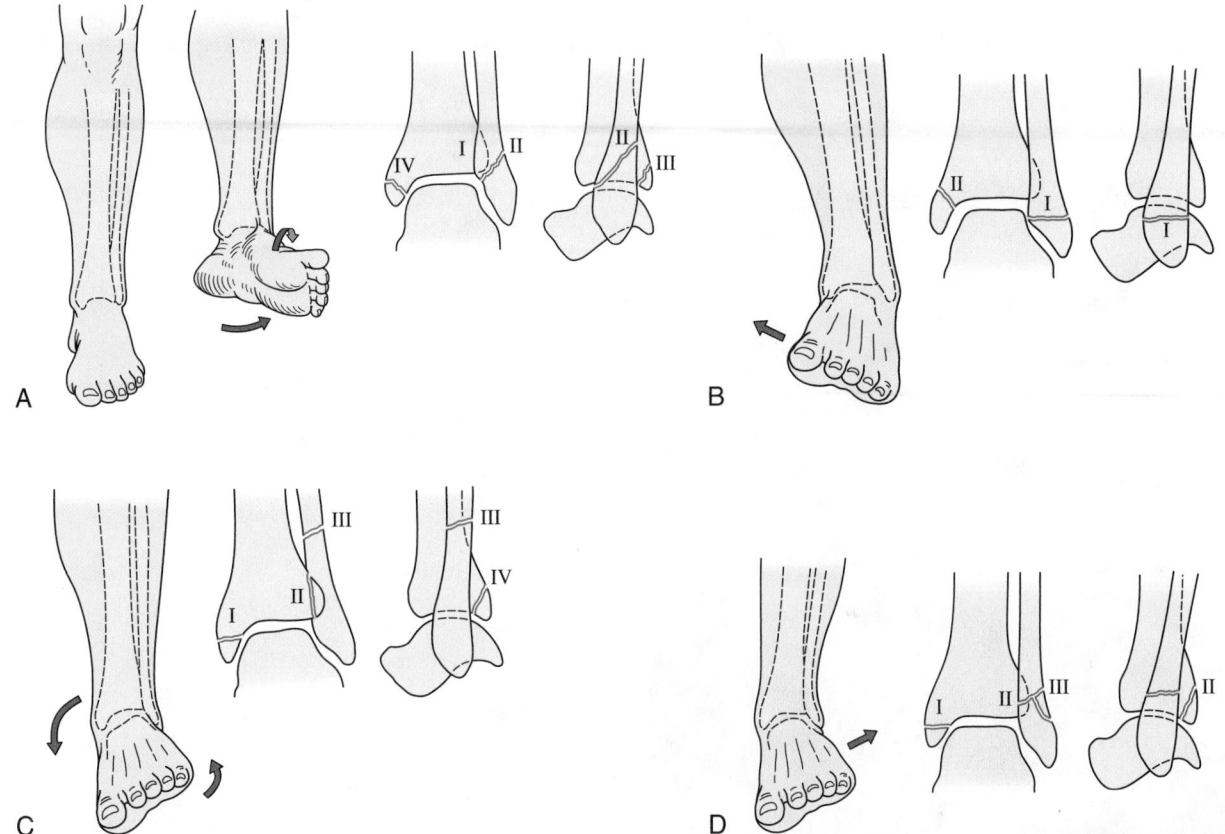

Figure 13-3 Ankle fracture injury mechanisms. A, Supination-lateral rotation injury. Lateral rotation forces applied to a supinated foot initially result in rupture of the anterior tibiofibular ligament (stage I). As the forces continue, a short oblique fracture of the distal portion of the fibula occurs (stage II). Stage III involves a fracture of the posterior aspect of the tibia. Stage IV is a fracture of the medial malleolus. **B,** Supination-adduction injury. Adduction forces applied to a supinated foot initially result in a traction or avulsion fracture of the distal portion of the fibula or rupture of the lateral ligaments (stage I). As forces continue, fracture of the medial malleolus or rupture of the deltoid ligament occurs (stage II). The fibular fracture is typically transverse, and that of the medial malleolus is oblique or nearly vertical. **C,** Pronation-lateral rotation injury. Forces of lateral rotation applied to a pronated foot initially result in rupture of the deltoid ligament or fracture of the medial malleolus (stage I). As forces continue, the anterior tibiofibular ligament is ruptured (stage II). A high fibular fracture (stage III) and fracture of the posterior tibial margin (stage IV) are the final stages in this mechanism of injury. **D,** Pronation-abduction injury. The first two stages of this injury are identical to those of the pronation-external rotation fracture complex. Stage III is a transverse supramalleolar fibular fracture that may be comminuted laterally. (Redrawn from Resnick D, Kransdorf MJ: Bone and joint imaging, Philadelphia, 2005, WB Saunders, pp. 867–868.)

TABLE 13-1

The West Point Ankle Sprain Grading System

Criterion	Grade I	Grade II	Grade III
Location of tenderness	Anterior talofibular ligament	Anterior talofibular ligament and calcaneofibular ligament	Anterior talofibular ligament, calcaneofibular ligament and posterior talofibular ligament
Edema and ecchymosis	Slight and local	Moderate and local	Significant and diffuse
Weight-bearing ability	Full or partial	Difficult without crutches	Impossible without significant pain
Ligament damage	Stretched	Partial tear	Complete tear
Instability	None	None or slight	Definite

From Dutton M: Dutton's orthopedic examination, evaluation and intervention, ed 3, New York, 2012, McGraw Hill. Data from Gerber JP, et al: Persistent disability associated with ankle sprains: a prospective examination of an athletic population. Foot Ankle Int 19:653–660, 1998.

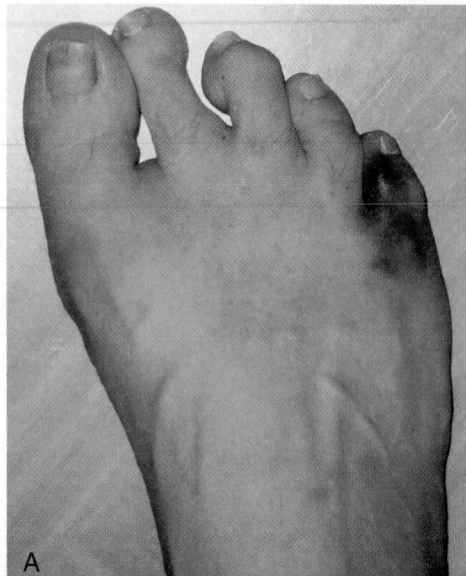

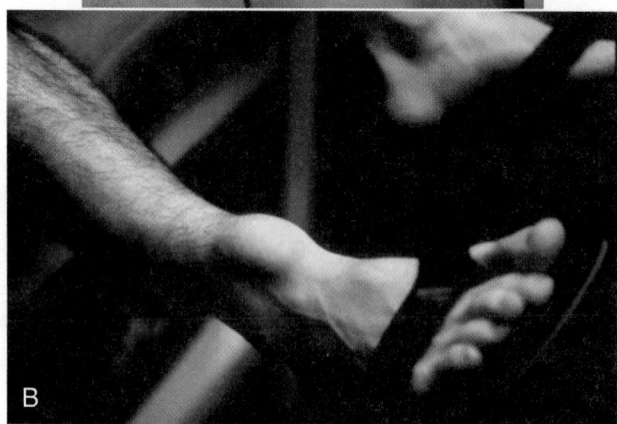

Figure 13-4 A, Ecchymosis following fracture of small toe. **B,** "Skate or lace bite." Swelling over extensor tendons.

Differential Diagnosis of Chronic Leg Pain in the Athlete

BONE PERIOSTEUM
- Medial tibial stress syndrome ("shin splints")*
- Stress fracture*

VASCULAR
- Popliteal artery entrapment syndrome
- Intermittent claudication

REFERRED PAIN
- Nerve entrapment
  - Peripheral
  - Spinal/radiculopathy
- Referred pain
  - Knee abnormality
  - Hip abnormality (especially in young patients)

MUSCLE/TENDON
- Chronic exertional compartment syndrome
- Muscle strains
- Tendinitis/tendinosis

NEOPLASM
INFECTION

Modified from Edwards PH, et al: A practical approach for the differential diagnosis of chronic leg pain in the athlete. Am J Sports Med 33:1244, 2005.

*These two conditions are commonly different stages of the same pathological continuum.

---

5. *Was there any swelling or bruising (ecchymosis)* (Figure 13-4, *A*)? *How quickly and where did it develop?* This question can elicit some idea of the type of swelling (e.g., blood, synovial, purulent) and whether it is intracapsular or extracapsular. Figure 13-4, *B*, shows "skate bite" in which there is swelling over the extensor tendons of the foot caused by irritation from doing up stiff ice skates too tight.

6. *Are symptoms improving, becoming worse, or staying the same?* It is important to know the type of onset (macrotrauma, microtrauma) and the duration and intensity of symptoms (acute, subacute, chronic). Edwards et al.[17] outlined some of the chronic causes of leg pain in athletes.

7. *What are the sites and boundaries of pain or abnormal sensation?* The examiner should note whether the pattern is one of a dermatome, a peripheral nerve, or another painful structure. If pain and other physical findings are "out of proportion" to what would normally be expected with injury especially in the rearfoot/talar region, a more diligent examination

including extra radiographic images of the talus and calcaneus may be necessary.[18]

8. *What is the patient's usual activity or pastime?* Answers to this question should give some idea of the stresses placed on the lower leg, ankle, and foot; how frequently they are applied; and whether the patient is suffering from a repetitive stress injury.

9. *Does activity make a difference?* Pain after activity suggests overuse. For example, with overuse injuries, pain initially comes on after the activity. As the injury progresses, pain or soreness is present at the beginning of the activity, and then it goes away during the activity only to return afterward. In later stages of the problem, the pain is constantly present. Pain during the activity suggests stress on the injured structure.

10. *Where is the pain? Does the patient indicate a specific location or area?* For example, with shin splints **(medial tibial stress syndrome)** or a compartment syndrome (acute or chronic type), the patient usually indicates a diffuse area.[19–22] With a stress fracture, the area of pain tends to be more specific. Anterolateral ankle impingement demonstrates anterolateral ankle joint tenderness, anterolateral ankle joint swelling (extracapsular), pain with force dorsiflexion and eversion, pain with single leg squat, pain with activities,

and possible absence of ankle instability.[11] Peroneal tendon problems show posterolateral pain and may be associated with lateral ankle instability.[23] Plantar fasciitis is the most common cause of heel pain on the antero-medial aspect of the heel.[24] It may be accompanied by a heel spur (see Figure 13-135, *C*), which is the result of the plantar fasciitis.

11. *Does walking on various terrains make a difference in regard to the foot problem?* If so, which terrains cause the most obvious problem? For example, walking on grass (an uneven surface) may bother the patient more than walking on a sidewalk (a relatively even surface), or the patient may find walking on a relatively soft surface (e.g., grass) easier than walking on a hard surface (e.g., cement). Prepared surfaces, such as sidewalks, roads, and playing fields, often have a camber to allow water runoff. This camber can cause problems in some cases of overuse.

12. *What types of shoes does the patient wear? What kind of heel do the shoes have? Are the shoes in good condition? Does the patient make use of orthoses? If so, are they still functional?* When an appointment is being made for an assessment, the patient should be told not to wear new shoes so that the examiner can use the shoes to determine the patient's usual shoe wear pattern. The examiner should also note whether the shoes offer proper support. The patient should bring any orthoses he or she is using to the assessment.

13. *Is there a history of previous injury, affliction or surgery?* For example, poliomyelitis may lead to a pes cavus. Systemic conditions, such as diabetes, gout, psoriasis, and collagen diseases, may manifest themselves first in the foot. If there was previous surgery, did the pain resolve following surgery? Is the pain the same as before surgery? Is it new pain?

14. For active people, especially runners or joggers, the following questions should also be considered[25]:
    a. *How long has the patient been running or jogging?*
    b. *On what type of terrain and surface does the patient train?*
    c. *In what types of workouts does the patient participate? Have the workouts changed lately? How many workouts are done per week? How far does the patient run per week?* (Joggers run approximately 2 to 30 km [1.2 to 18.6 miles] per week at a pace of 5 to 10 minutes/km, and sports runners run 30 to 65 km [18.6 to 40 miles] per week at a pace of 5 to 6 minutes/km. Long-distance runners run 60 to 180 km [37 to 112 miles] per week at a pace of 4 to 5 minutes/km. Elite runners run 100 to 270 km [62 to 168 miles] per week at a pace of 3.3 to 4 minutes/km.)
    d. *What types of warmup, stretching, and postexercise routines does the patient do?* The answers give the examiner some idea of whether the warmup and stretching activities are static or ballistic and whether these activities could be detrimental.
    e. *What types and styles of athletic shoes does the patient wear?* (The patient should have the shoes at the examination.) Are they "control" or "cushioning" shoes? People with a cavus foot are more likely to need a cushioning shoe, whereas those with a planus foot are more likely to need a control shoe. The examiner should be able to tell if the shoes fit properly.
    f. *Does the patient wear socks while training?* If so, what kind (e.g., cotton, wool, nylon), and how many pairs?
    g. *When was the patient's last race? How long was it? When is the patient's next race?* The answers give the examiner some idea of how long the problem has been present and how long it will be until maximum stress is again placed on the joints.

OBSERVATION

Observation of the foot is extensive. Because of the stresses the foot is subjected to and because it, like the hand, can project signs of systemic problems and disease, the examiner should carefully and meticulously inspect the foot.

When performing the observation, the examiner should remember to compare the weight-bearing (closed-chain) with the non–weight-bearing (open-chain) posture of the foot.[26] During open-chain motion, the talus is considered fixed; during closed-chain motion, the talus moves to help the foot and leg adapt to the terrain and to the stresses that are applied to the foot. Even though the calcaneus is touching a surface in closed-chain movement, for descriptive purposes, it is still considered to be moving. The weight-bearing stance of the foot shows how the body compensates for structural abnormalities (Figure 13-5). The non–weight-bearing posture shows functional and structural abilities without compensation (Figure 13-6). The observation includes looking at the patient from the front, from the side, and from behind in the weight-bearing (standing) position and from the front, from the side, and from behind in the sitting position with the legs and feet not bearing weight. The examiner should note the patient's willingness and ability to use the feet. The bony and soft-tissue contours of the foot should be normal, and any deviation should be noted. Often, painful callosities may be found over abnormal bony prominences. The examiner should note any scars or sinuses.

Weight-Bearing Position, Anterior View

With the patient in a standing position, the examiner should observe whether the patient's hips and trunk are in normal position. Excessive lateral rotation of the hip or rotation of the trunk away from the opposite hip

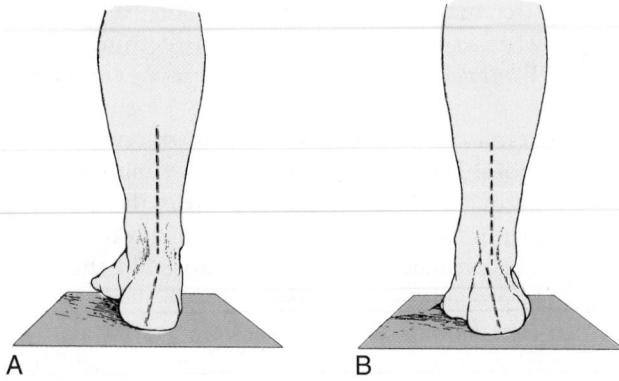

Figure 13-5 A, Closed-chain (weight-bearing) supination of the subtalar joint (right foot). Supination of the subtalar joint in the weight-bearing foot results in motion of both the calcaneus and the talus. The calcaneus moves in the frontal plane, and the talus moves in the transverse and sagittal planes. The calcaneus inverts, and the talus simultaneously abducts and dorsiflexes relative to the calcaneus. The leg follows the motion of the talus in the transverse plane and laterally rotates. The leg also follows the sagittal plane motion of the talus to some degree. The dorsiflexion motion of the talus on the calcaneus, therefore, tends to impart a slight extension motion to the knee. **B,** Closed-chain (weight-bearing) pronation of the subtalar joint (right foot). Pronation of the subtalar joint in the weight-bearing foot results in eversion of the calcaneus; the talus adducts and plantar flexes relative to the calcaneus. The leg follows the talus in a transverse plane and medially rotates. In a sagittal plane, the leg also moves to some extent with the talus. As the talus plantar flexes, the proximal aspect of the tibia moves forward to flex the knee slightly. (Redrawn from Root M, et al: Normal and abnormal function of the foot, Los Angeles, 1977, Clinical Biomechanics, p. 30.)

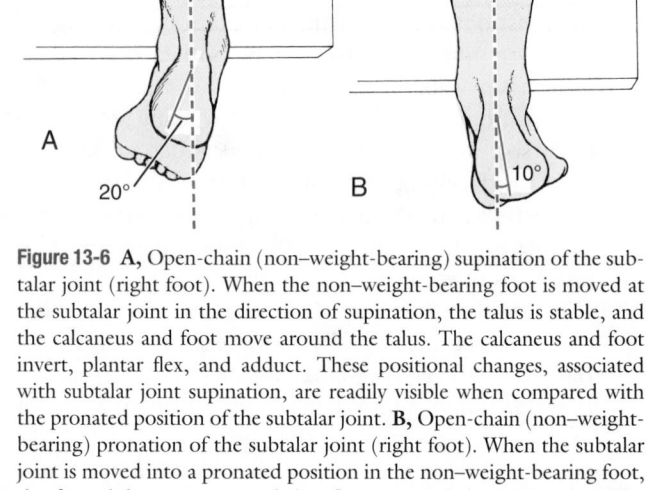

Figure 13-6 A, Open-chain (non–weight-bearing) supination of the subtalar joint (right foot). When the non–weight-bearing foot is moved at the subtalar joint in the direction of supination, the talus is stable, and the calcaneus and foot move around the talus. The calcaneus and foot invert, plantar flex, and adduct. These positional changes, associated with subtalar joint supination, are readily visible when compared with the pronated position of the subtalar joint. **B,** Open-chain (non–weight-bearing) pronation of the subtalar joint (right foot). When the subtalar joint is moved into a pronated position in the non–weight-bearing foot, the foot abducts, everts, and dorsiflexes around the stable talus. The positional variances can best be appreciated by comparing this illustration with the supinated position of the subtalar joint. (Redrawn from Root ML, et al: Normal and abnormal function of the foot, Los Angeles, 1977, Clinical Biomechanics, p. 29.)

elevates the medial longitudinal arch of the foot, whereas medial rotation of the hip or trunk rotation toward the opposite hip tends to flatten the arch (Figure 13-7). Medial rotation of the hip can also cause pigeon toes, which is a condition more commonly associated with medial tibial torsion or rotation. If the iliotibial band is tight, the tightness may cause eversion and lateral rotation of the foot.

The examiner should also look at the tibia to note any local or general bone swelling (Figure 13-8). Does the tibia have a normal shape, or is it bowed? Is there any torsional deformity? The medial malleolus usually lies anterior to the lateral malleolus. Pigeon toes, or toe-in deformity, result from a medial tibial torsion deformity; it does not constitute a foot deformity (Table 13-2).

Figure 13-9 shows the anterosuperior view of the feet in the weight-bearing stance. The examiner should note whether there is any asymmetry, malalignment (Table 13-3), or excessive supination or pronation of the foot. **Supination** of the foot involves inversion and outward rotation of the heel, adduction of the forefoot with inward rotation at the tarsometatarsal joints to maintain contact with the ground and outward rotation at the midtarsal joints, and plantar flexion at the subtalar joint and midtarsal joints so that the medial longitudinal arch is

accentuated (Figure 13-10, *A*). In addition, along with lateral rotation of the talus, there is lateral rotation of the leg in relation to the foot (Figure 13-11). Supination of the foot causes the proximal aspect of the tibia to move posteriorly. It is required during propulsion to give rigidity to the foot and requires less muscle work than pronation.

Pronation of the foot involves eversion and inward rotation of the heel, abduction of the forefoot with outward rotation at the tarsometatarsal joints and inward rotation at the midtarsal joints, and medial rotation of the talus causing medial rotation of the leg in relation to the foot, and dorsiflexion of the subtalar and midtarsal joints (Figure 13-12), resulting in a decrease in the medial longitudinal arch (Figure 13-10, *B*). This movement causes the proximal aspect of the tibia to move anteriorly. The pronated foot has greater subtalar motion than the supinated foot and requires more muscle work to maintain stance stability than the supinated foot. The foot is much more mobile in this position.

The definitions used in this chapter are the ones preferred by orthopedists and podiatrists. Anatomists and kinesiologists, such as Kapandji, refer to inversion as a combination of adduction and supination and to eversion as a combination of abduction and pronation.[27] Lipscomb

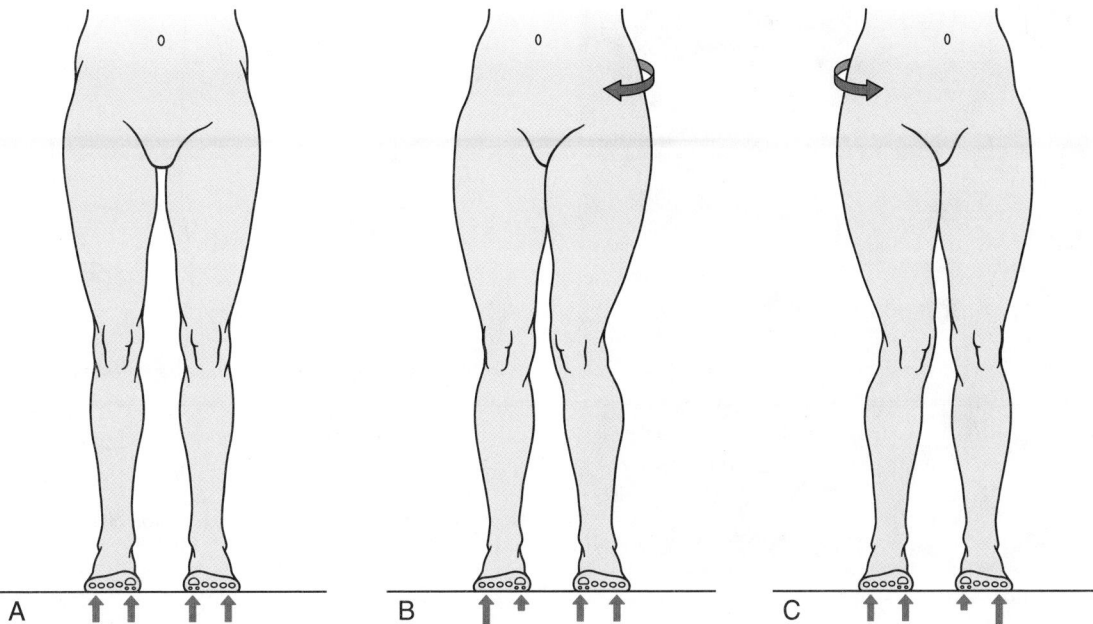

Figure 13-7 A, During static stance, ground reaction forces *(arrows)* directed upward against the plantar aspects of both feet maintain the transverse plane equilibrium and stability of the lower extremities and pelvis. Equal ground reaction forces are exerted on the lateral and medial plantar surfaces of both feet. **B,** When the trunk is rotated to the right, the right foot supinates and the left pronates. The right forefoot inverts from the ground; vertical ground reaction forces are greater against the lateral side of the forefoot *(large arrow)* and less against the medial side of the forefoot *(small arrow)*. The left forefoot remains flat on the ground, and vertical ground reaction forces are distributed evenly against the forefoot *(equal arrows)*. **C,** When the trunk is rotated to the left, ground reaction exerts unequal forces against the left forefoot and equal forces against the right forefoot. (Redrawn from Root ML, et al: Normal and abnormal function of the foot, Los Angeles, 1977, Clinical Biomechanics, p. 102.)

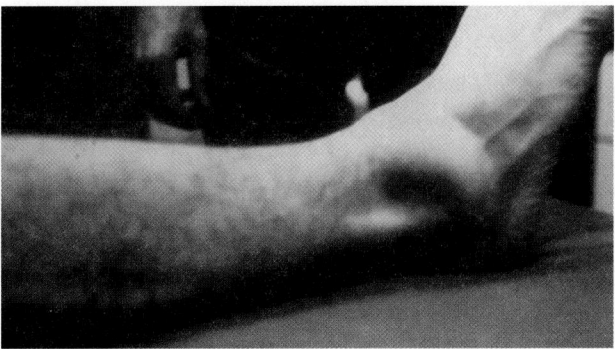

Figure 13-8 Swelling within the talocrural and subtalar joint capsule.

TABLE **13-2**

Causes of Toeing-In and Toeing-Out in Children

Level of Affection	Toe In	Toe Out
Feet-ankles	Pronated feet (protective toeing-in) Metatarsus varus Talipes varus and equinovarus	Pes valgus due to contracture of triceps surae muscle Talipes calcaneovalgus Congenital convex pes planovalgus
Leg-knee	Tibia vara (Blount disease) and developmental genu varum Abnormal medial tibial torsion Genu valgum—developmental (protective toeing-in to shift body center of gravity medially)	Lateral tibial torsion Congenital absence of hypoplasia of the fibula
Femur-hip	Abnormal femoral antetorsion Spasticity of medial rotators of hip (cerebral palsy)	Abnormal femoral retroversion Flaccid paralysis of medial rotators of hip
Acetabulum	Maldirected—facing anteriorly	Maldirected—facing posteriorly

From Tachdjian MO: Pediatric orthopedics, Philadelphia, 1990, WB Saunders, p. 2817.

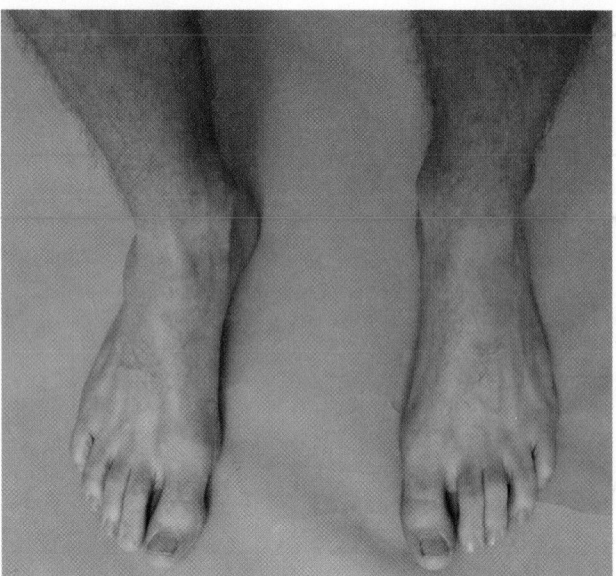

Figure 13-9 Anterosuperior view of the feet (weight-bearing position).

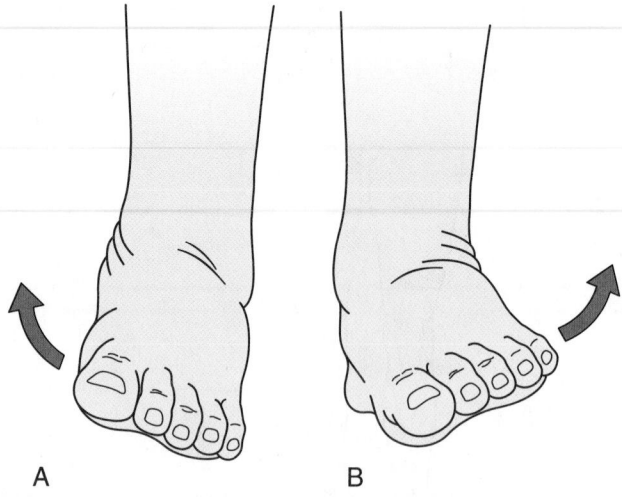

Figure 13-10 Supination (A) and pronation (B) of the (non–weight-bearing) foot.

TABLE **13-3**

Malalignment About the Foot and Ankle

Malalignment	Possible Correlated Motions or Postures	Possible Compensatory Motions or Postures
Ankle equinus		Hypermobile first ray Subtalar or midtarsal excessive pronation Hip or knee flexion Genu recurvation
Rearfoot varus Excessive subtalar supination (calcaneal varus)	Tibial; tibial and femoral; or tibial femoral, and pelvic lateral rotation	Excessive medial rotation along the lower quarter chain Hallux valgus Plantar flexed first ray Functional forefoot valgus Excessive or prolonged midtarsal pronation
Rearfoot valgus Excessive subtalar pronation (calcaneal valgus)	Tibial; tibial and femoral; or tibial, femoral, and pelvic medial rotation Hallux valgus	Excessive lateral rotation along the lower quarter chain Functional forefoot varus
Forefoot varus	Subtalar supination and related rotation along the lower quarter	Plantar flexed first ray Hallux valgus Excessive midtarsal or subtalar pronation or prolonged pronation Excessive tibial; tibial and femoral; or tibial, femoral, and pelvic medial rotation, or all with contralateral lumbar spine rotation
Forefoot valgus	Hallux valgus Subtalar pronation and related rotation along the lower quarter	Excessive midtarsal or subtalar supination Excessive tibial; tibial and femoral; or tibial, femoral, and pelvic lateral rotation, or all with ipsilateral lumbar spine rotation
Metatarsus adductus	Hallux valgus Medial tibial torsion Flatfoot Toeing-in	
Hallux valgus	Forefoot valgus Subtalar pronation and related rotation along the lower quarter	Excessive tibial; tibial and femoral; or tibial, femoral, and pelvic lateral rotation, or all with ipsilateral lumbar spine rotation

From Riegger-Krugh C, Keysor JJ: Skeletal malalignment of the lower quarter: correlated and compensatory motions and postures. J Orthop Sports Phys Ther 23:166, 1996.

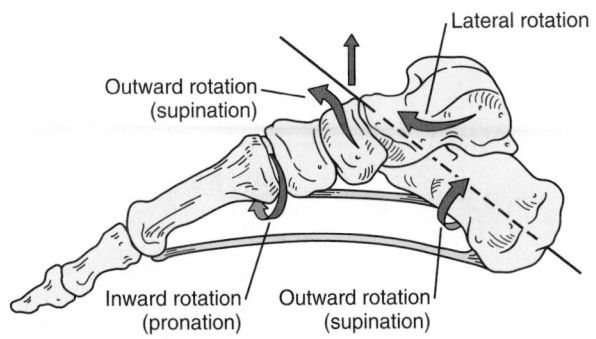

Figure 13-11 Supination of the foot produced by lateral rotation of the tibia. The rear foot and midfoot outwardly rotate (supinate) and the forefoot inwardly rotates (pronates) on the midfoot. As foot is plantar flexed, plantar fascia becomes tight along with ligaments to provide stable foot for push off. (Modified from Richardson JK, Iglarsh ZA, editors: Clinical orthopedic physical therapy, Philadelphia, 1994, WB Saunders, p. 513.)

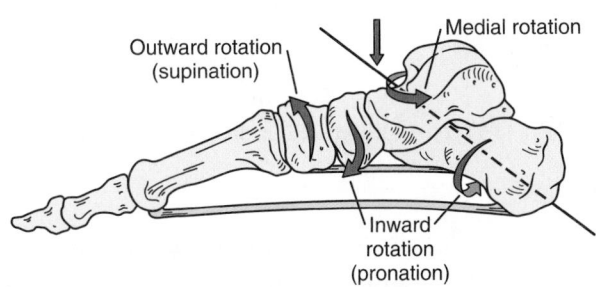

Figure 13-12 Pronation of the foot produced by medial rotation of the tibia. The rear foot and midfoot inwardly rotate (pronate) and the forefoot outwardly rotates (supinates) on the midfoot. Plantar fascia and plantar ligaments become taut as they absorb the ground reaction forces. (Modified from Richardson JK, Iglarsh ZA, editors: Clinical orthopedic physical therapy, Philadelphia, 1994, WB Saunders, p. 513.)

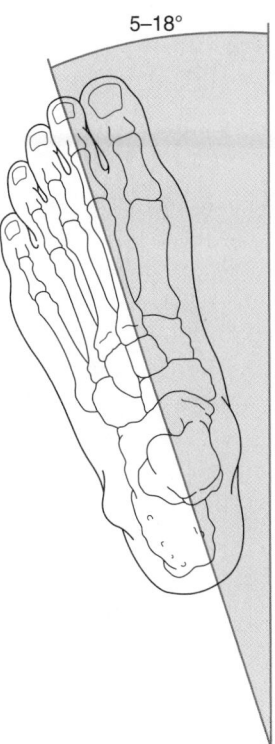

Figure 13-13 Fick angle.

and Ibrahim[28] and Williams and Warwick[29] have defined supination and pronation as opposite the terms just mentioned. Because of the confusion in terminology concerning the terms supination and pronation, readers of books and articles on the foot must be careful to discern exactly what each author means.

In the infant, the foot is normally pronated. As the child matures, the foot begins to supinate, accompanied by development of the medial longitudinal arch. The foot also appears to be more pronated in the infant because of the fat pad in the medial longitudinal arch.

The examiner should note how the patient stands and walks. Normally, in standing, 50% to 60% of the weight is taken on the heel and 40% to 50% is taken by the metatarsal heads. The foot assumes a slight toe-out position. This angle (the **Fick angle**) is approximately 12° to 18° from the sagittal axis of the body, developing from 5° in children (Figure 13-13).[30] Asymmetrical or excessive lateral rotation of the foot may be due to acetabular retroversion, femoral retrotorsion or femoral head neck abnormalities[31] (see Chapter 11). During movement, the foot is subjected to high loading, and pathology may

cause the gait to be altered. The cumulative force to which each foot is subjected during the day is the equivalent of 639 metric tons in a person who weighs approximately 90 kg, or the equivalent of walking 13 km per day.

Foot Loading During Gait

Walking:	1.2 times the body weight
Running:	2 times the body weight
Jumping (from height of 60 cm [2 feet]):	5 times the body weight

---

When weight-bearing, if the relation of the foot to the ankle is normal, all of the metatarsal bones bear weight, and all of the metatarsal heads lie in the same transverse plane. The forefoot and hindfoot should be parallel to each other and to the floor. The midtarsal joints are in maximum pronation, and the subtalar joint is in neutral position. The subtalar and talocrural joints should be parallel to the floor. Finally, the posterior bisection of the calcaneus and distal one third of the leg should form two vertical, parallel lines.[32]

If the examiner has noted any asymmetry in standing, the examiner should place the talus (or foot) in neutral (see the "Special Tests" section) to see if the asymmetry disappears. If the asymmetry is present in normal standing, it is a **functional asymmetry.** If it is still present when the foot is in neutral, it is also an **anatomical** or **structural**

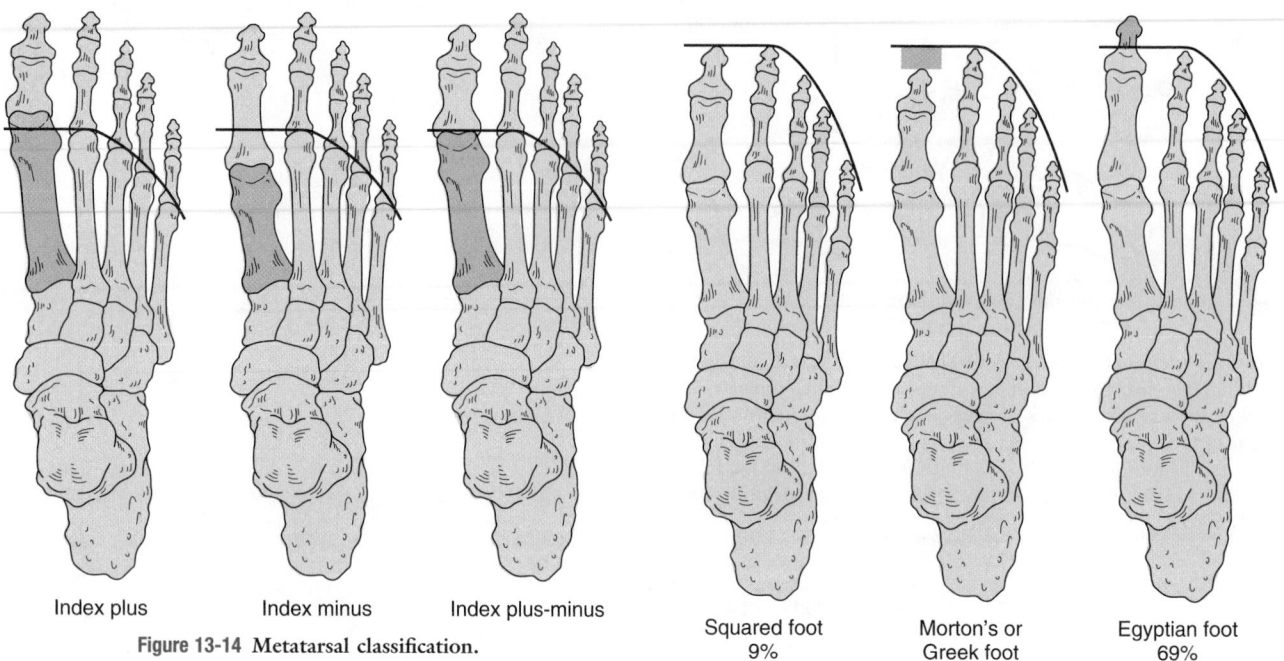

| Index plus | Index minus | Index plus-minus |

Figure 13-14 Metatarsal classification.

| Squared foot 9% | Morton's or Greek foot 22% | Egyptian foot 69% |

Figure 13-15 Types of feet seen in the general population.

asymmetry, in which case a structural deformity is probably causing the asymmetry. Leg-heel and forefoot-heel alignment (see the "Special Tests" section) may also be checked, especially if asymmetry is present.

The examiner should note whether the patient uses a cane or other walking aid. Use of a cane in the opposite hand diminishes the stress on the ankle joint and foot by approximately one third.

Any prominent bumps or exostoses should be noted, as should any splaying (widening) of the forefoot. Splaying of the forefoot and metatarsus primus varus is more evident in weight-bearing. There are three types of forefoot,[33] based on the length of the metatarsal bones (Figure 13-14):

1. **Index plus type:** The first metatarsal (1) is longer than the second (2), with the others (3, 4, and 5) of progressively decreasing lengths, so that $1 > 2 > 3 > 4 > 5$. This can result in an Egyptian type foot (Figure 13-15).
2. **Index plus-minus type:** The first metatarsal is equal in length to the second metatarsal, with the others progressively diminishing in length, so that $1 = 2 > 3 > 4 > 5$. This results in a squared type foot (see Figure 13-15).
3. **Index minus type:** The second metatarsal is longer than the first and third metatarsals. The fourth and fifth metatarsals are progressively shorter than the third, so that $1 < 2 > 3 > 4 > 5$. This results in a Morton's or Greek type foot (see Figure 13-15).

The examiner should note whether the toenails appear normal. Older individuals have more brittle nails. The examiner should look for warts, calluses, and corns. Warts are especially tender to the pinch (but not to direct pressure), but calluses are not. Plantar warts also tend to separate from the surrounding tissues, but calluses do not. Corns are similar to calluses but have a central nidus. They may be hard (on outside or upper aspect of toes) or soft (between toes) because of moisture.

Any swelling or pitting edema within the Achilles tendon, ankle, and foot should be noted (Figure 13-16). If there is any swelling, the examiner should note whether it is intracapsular or extracapsular. Swelling above the lateral malleolus may be related to a fibular fracture or disruption of the syndesmosis ("high" ankle sprain).[34,35] This injury takes a long time to heal and may involve the anterior and/or posterior tibiofibular ligament as well as the ligaments of the talocrural joint. Swelling posterior to the lateral malleolus may indicate peroneal retinacular injury. Lateral ankle sprains initially swell distal to the lateral malleolus, but swelling may spread into the foot if the capsule has been torn (Table 13-4).[14] The examiner should also check the patient's gait for the position of the foot at heel strike, at foot flat, and at toe off. The gait cycle is described in greater detail in Chapter 14.

Any vasomotor changes should be recorded, including loss of hair on the foot, toenail changes, osteoporosis as seen on radiographs, and possible differences in temperature between the limbs. Systemic diseases such as diabetes can also lead to foot problems as a result of altered sensation, which facilitates injury.

The examiner should look for any circulatory impairment or presence of varicose veins. Brick-red color or cyanosis when the limb is dependent is an indication of impairment. Does this condition change to rapid

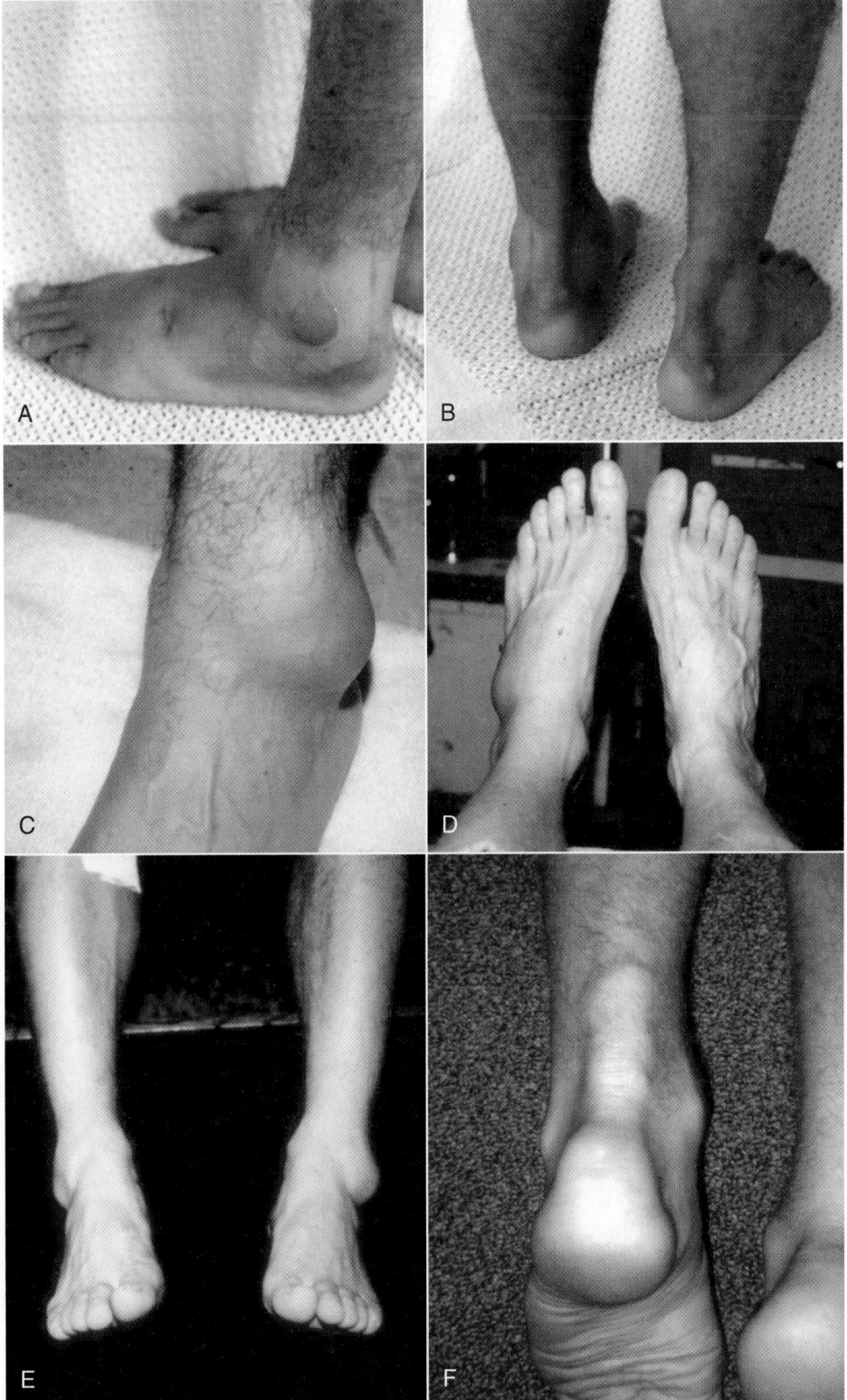

Figure 13-16 Ankle sprain. A, Note pattern of pitting edema on top of the left foot. **B,** The swelling is intracapsular, as indicated by swelling on both sides of the left Achilles tendon. **C,** Extracapsular swelling. **D,** Midtarsal swelling. **E,** Synovial thickening (not swelling) because of repeated ankle sprains. **F,** Achilles swelling.

TABLE **13-4**

Classification of Ankle Sprains

Severity	Pathology	Signs and Symptoms	Disability
Grade I (mild) stable	Mild stretch No instability Single ligament involved (usually anterior talofibular ligament)	No hemorrhage Minimal swelling Point tenderness No anterior drawer sign No varus laxity	No or little limp Minimal functional loss Difficulty hopping Recovery 8 days (range, 2 to 10)
Grade II (moderate) stable	Large spectrum of injury Mild to moderate instability Complete tearing of anterior talofibular ligament, or partial tearing of anterior talofibular plus calcaneofibular ligaments	Some hemorrhage Localized swelling (margins of Achilles tendon less defined) Anterior drawer sign may be present No varus laxity	Limp with walking Unable to toe raiase Unable to hop Unable to run Recovery 20 days (range, 10 to 30)
Grade III (severe) two-ligament, unstable	Significant instability Complete tear of anterior capsule, anterior talofibular and calcaneofibular ligaments	Diffuse swelling on both sides of Achilles tendon, early hemorrhage Possible tenderness medially and laterally Positive anterior drawer sign Positive varus laxity	Unable to bear weight fully Significant pain inhibition Initially almost complete loss of ROM Recovery 40 days (range, 30 to 90)

From Reid DC: Sports injury assessment and rehabilitation, New York, 1992, Churchill Livingstone, p. 226.
ROM, Range of motion.

blanching, or does it stay normal on elevation of the limbs? Change indicates circulatory impairment.

Weight-Bearing Position, Posterior View

From behind, the examiner compares the bulk of the calf muscles and notes any differences. Variation may be caused by peripheral nerve lesions, nerve root problems, or atrophy resulting from disuse after injury. The Achilles tendons on each side should be compared (see Figure 13-16, *F*). If a tendon appears to curve out (Figure 13-17), it may indicate a fallen medial longitudinal arch, resulting in a pes planus (flatfoot) condition **(Helbing sign).**[36]

The examiner observes the calcaneus for normality of shape and position. Runners often build up bone and a callus on the heel, producing a "pump bump" (**Haglund disease or deformity**) as a result of pressure on the heel (Figure 13-18).[37-39]

The malleoli are compared for positioning. Normally, the lateral malleolus extends farther distally than the medial malleolus; however, the medial malleolus extends farther anteriorly.

Weight-Bearing Position, Lateral View

With the side view, the examiner is primarily observing the longitudinal arches of the foot (Figure 13-19). The examiner should note whether the medial arch is higher than the lateral arch (as would be expected). Differences in the arches may often be determined by looking at the

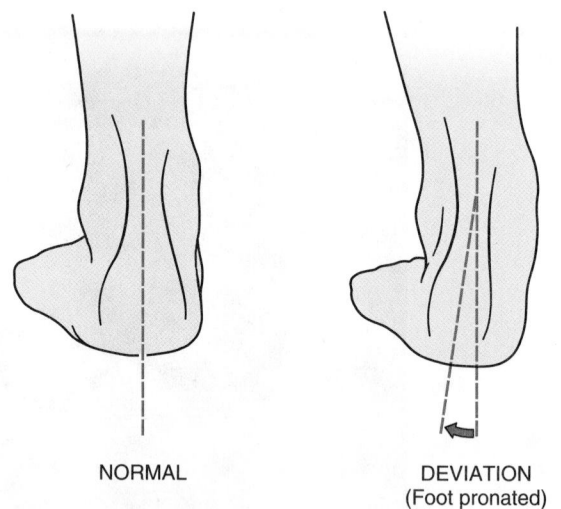

NORMAL   DEVIATION
(Foot pronated)

Figure 13-17 Normal and deviated Achilles tendon. The deviation is often seen with pes planus (flatfoot) and when the medial longitudinal arch is lower or has "dropped."

footprint patterns (Figure 13-20). The footprint pattern can be established by putting a light film of baby oil and then powder on the patient's foot and asking the patient to step down on a piece of colored paper.

The arches of the feet (Figure 13-21) are maintained by three mechanisms[40]: (1) wedging of the interlocking tarsal and metatarsal bones; (2) tightening of the ligaments on the plantar aspect of the foot; and (3) the

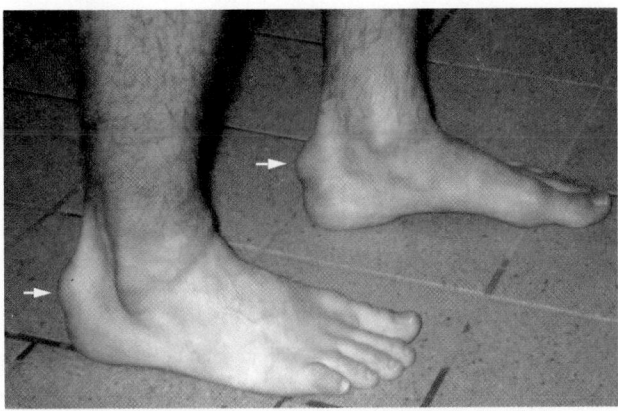

Figure 13-18 "Pump bumps" from tight ice skates.

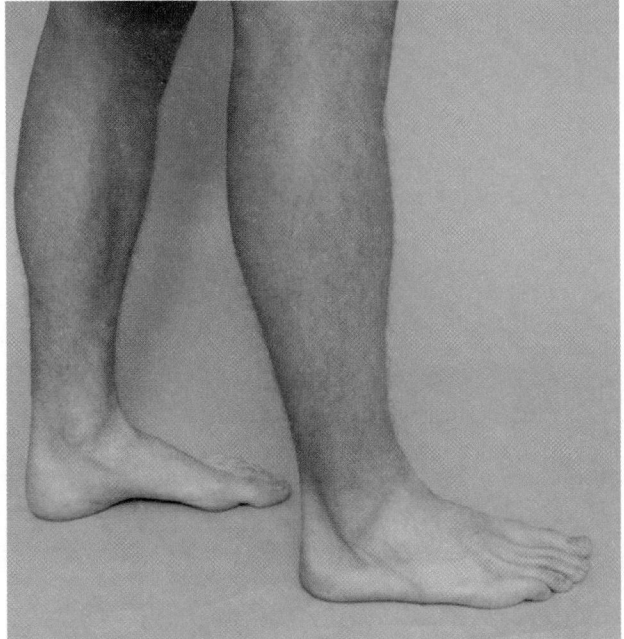

Figure 13-19 Lateral and medial views of the feet showing longitudinal arches.

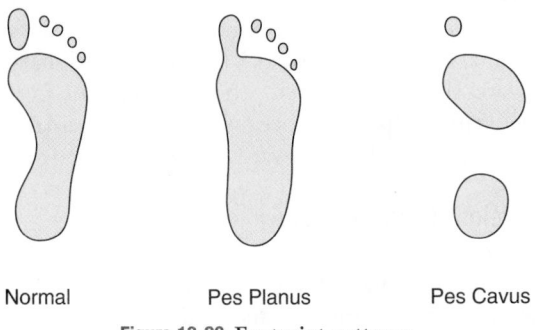

Normal   Pes Planus   Pes Cavus

Figure 13-20 Footprint patterns.

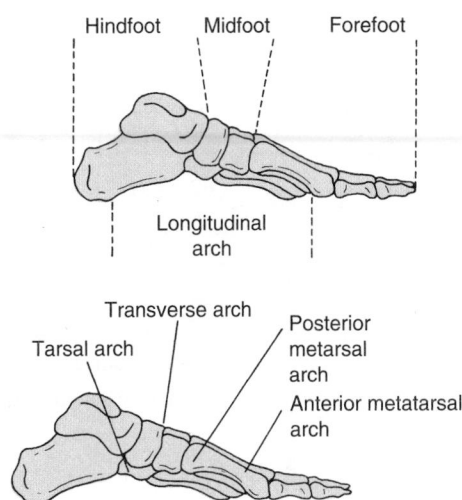

Hindfoot   Midfoot   Forefoot

Longitudinal arch

Transverse arch

Tarsal arch

Posterior metarsal arch

Anterior metatarsal arch

Figure 13-21 Divisions and arches of the foot (medial view).

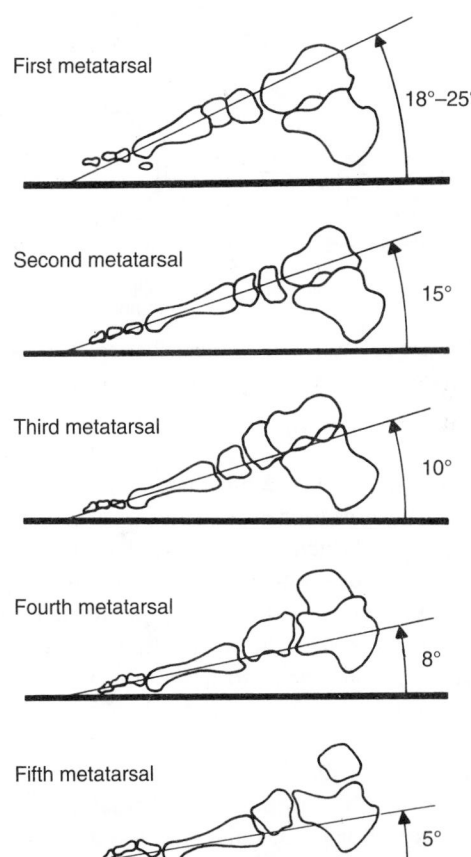

First metatarsal   18°–25°

Second metatarsal   15°

Third metatarsal   10°

Fourth metatarsal   8°

Fifth metatarsal   5°

Figure 13-22 Angle formed by each metatarsal with the floor. (Modified from Jahss MH: Disorders of the foot, Philadelphia, 1991, WB Saunders, p. 1231.)

intrinsic and extrinsic muscles of the foot and their tendons, which help to support the arches. The longitudinal arches form a cone as a result of the angle of the metatarsal bones in relation to the floor. With the medial longitudinal arch being more evident, this angle is greater on the medial side. The angle formed by each of the metatarsals with the floor is shown in Figure 13-22.

The **medial longitudinal arch** consists of the calcaneal tuberosity, the talus, the navicular, three cuneiforms, and the first, second, and third metatarsal bones (Figures

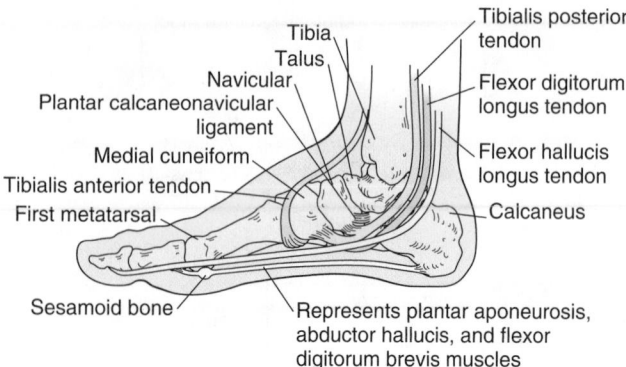

Figure 13-23 Supports of the medial longitudinal arch of the foot.

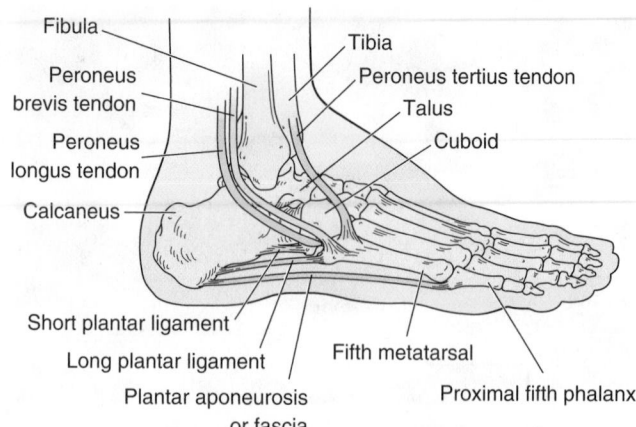

Figure 13-25 Supports of the lateral longitudinal arch of the foot: plantar aponeurosis (including the abductor digiti minimi and the flexor digitorum brevis IV and V); long plantar ligament; short plantar ligament.

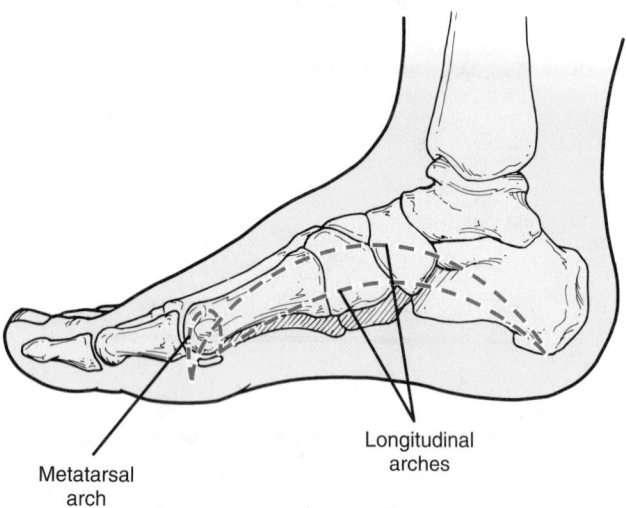

Figure 13-24 Arches of the foot (medial view).

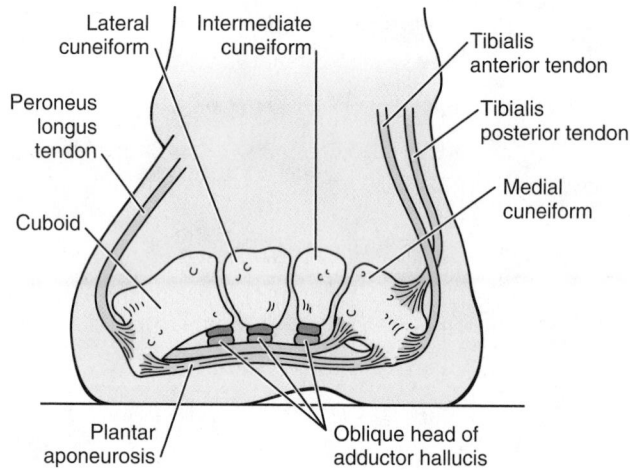

Figure 13-26 Supports of the transverse arch of the foot.

13-23 and 13-24). This arch is maintained by the tibialis anterior, tibialis posterior, flexor digitorum longus, flexor hallucis longus, abductor hallucis, and flexor digitorum brevis muscles; the plantar fascia or aponeurosis; and the plantar calcaneonavicular ligament. The plantar aponeurosis plays a major role during the stance and push-off phases of gait, which helps to distribute Achilles tendon forces under the forefoot to the metatarsal heads and phalanges.[41]

The calcaneus, cuboid, and fourth and fifth metatarsal bones make up the **lateral longitudinal arch** (Figure 13-25). This arch is more stable and less adjustable than the medial longitudinal arch. The arch is maintained by the peroneus longus, peroneus brevis, peroneus tertius, abductor digiti minimi, and flexor digitorum brevis muscles; the plantar fascia; the long plantar ligament; and the short plantar ligament.[40]

The **transverse arch** is maintained by the tibialis posterior, tibialis anterior, and peroneus longus muscles and the plantar fascia (Figure 13-26). This arch consists of the navicular, cuneiforms, cuboid, and metatarsal bones. The arch is sometimes divided into three parts: tarsal,

posterior metatarsal, and anterior metatarsal. A loss of the anterior metatarsal arch results in callus formation under the heads of the metatarsal bones (especially the second and third metatarsal heads). The metatarsophalangeal joints are slightly extended when the patient is in the normal standing position because the longitudinal arches of the foot curve down toward the toes.[40]

Non–Weight-Bearing Position

With the patient in a supine, non–weight-bearing position, the examiner should look for abnormalities, such as callosities, plantar warts, scars, and sinuses or pressure sores on the soles of the feet, as well as swelling, which is more prominent on the dorsum of the foot. In addition, by looking at the foot from anterior to posterior, as shown in Figure 13-27, the examiner can observe whether the patient has a "fallen" metatarsal arch. Normally, in the non–weight-bearing position, the arch is visible. If the arch falls, callosities are often found over the metatarsal

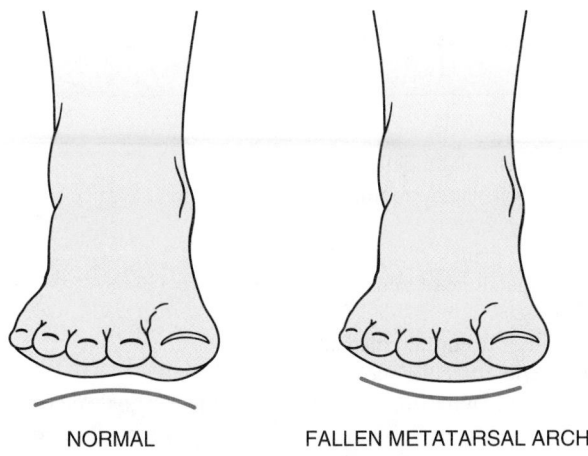

NORMAL   FALLEN METATARSAL ARCH

Figure 13-27 Fallen metatarsal arch.

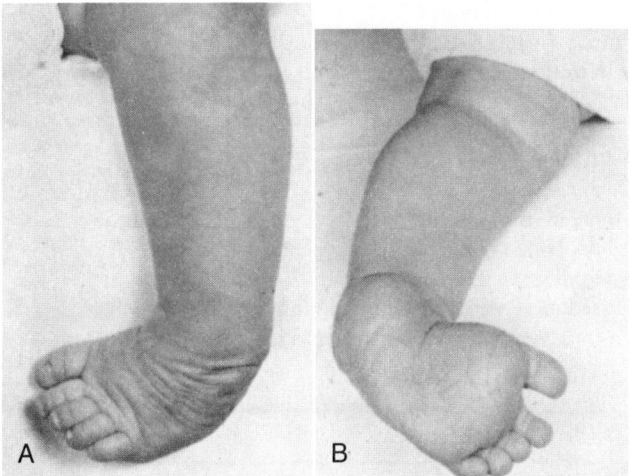

Figure 13-28 **Talipes equinovarus (clubfoot) in a child aged 4 months. A,** Anterior view. **B,** Posterior view. (From Klenerman L: The foot and its disorders, Boston, 1982, Blackwell Scientific, p. 64.)

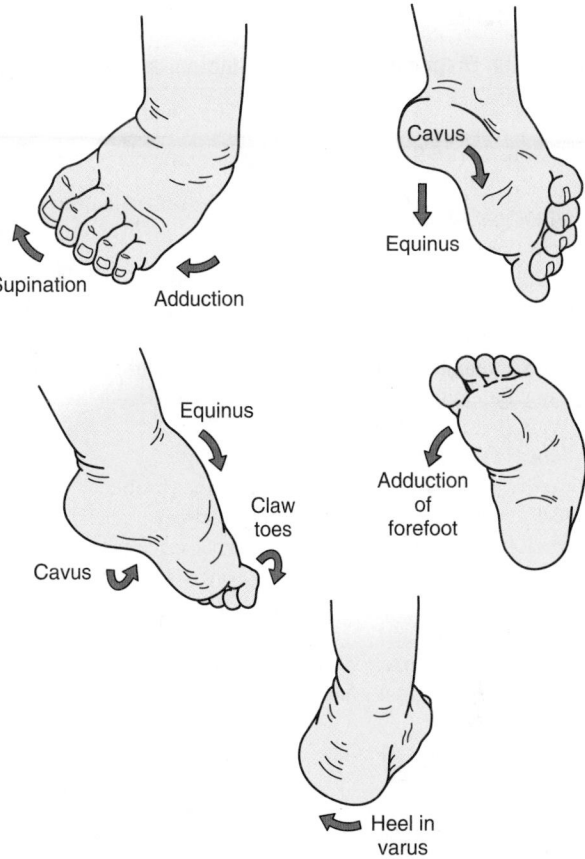

Figure 13-29 **Components of talipes equinovarus.**

heads. The arch may be reversed, or it may fall because of an equinus forefoot, pes cavus, rheumatoid arthritis, short heel cord, or hammertoes. Abnormal width of one ankle in relation to the other **(Keen sign)** may be caused by swelling, loss of integrity of the syndesmosis, or a malleolar fracture.

Young children should be assessed for clubfoot deformities, the most common of which is talipes equinovarus (Figures 13-28 and 13-29; Table 13-5). These types of deformities are often associated with other anomalies, such as spina bifida.

Common Deformities, Deviations, and Injuries

Bunionette (Tailor's Bunion). This deformity is characterized by prominence of the lateral aspect of the fifth toe metatarsal head (Figure 13-30).[42] If associated with hallux valgus, it results in a splayed foot. It is often associated with a pronated foot.

Claw Toes. A claw-toe deformity results in hyperextension of the metatarsophalangeal joints and flexion of the proximal and distal interphalangeal joints (Figure 13-31, *A*). Claw toes usually result from the defective actions of lumbrical and interosseus muscles that cause the toes to become functionless. This condition may be unilateral or bilateral and may be associated with pes cavus, fallen metatarsal arch, spina bifida, or other neurological problems.

Clubfoot. This congenital deformity is relatively common and can take many forms, the most common of which is **talipes equinovarus.** Its cause is unknown, but there are probably multifactorial genetic causes modified by environmental factors.[43] It sometimes coexists with other congenital deformities, such as spina bifida and cleft palate. The flexible form is easily treated, but the resistant type often requires surgery. On assessment, the ROM is limited and the foot has abnormal form (see Figure 13-29).

Crossover Toe. Crossover toe is the result of weakening of the lateral collateral ligament of the metatarsophalangeal joint and insufficiency of the plantar plate along with the pull of the extrinsic muscles resulting in medial deviation of the toe, most commonly in the second or third toe. It is often associated with hallux valgus.[44]

TABLE **13-5**

Differential Diagnosis of Postural Clubfoot and Talipes Equinovarus

	Postural Clubfoot	Talipes Equinovarus
Etiology	Intrauterine malposture	Primary germ plasm defect
		Defective cartilaginous anlage of the talus
Pathologic Anatomy		
Head and neck of talus	Normal	Medial and plantar tilt
	Declination angle of talus normal (150° to 155°)	Declination angle of talus decreased (115° to 135°)
Talocalcaneonavicular joint	Normal	Subluxed or dislocated medially and plantarward
Effect of manipulation in fetal specimens	Normal alignment of foot can be restored	Talocalcaneonavicular subluxation cannot be reduced unless ligaments connecting navicular to calcaneus, talus, and tibia are sectioned and posterior capsule and ligaments divided
Clinical Features		
Severity of deformity	Mild and flexible	Marked and rigid
Heel	Normal size	Small, drawn up
Relation between navicular and medial malleolus	Normal space between two bones; can insert finger	Navicular abuts medial malleolus: finger cannot be inserted between two bones
Lateral malleolus	Normal position	Posteriorly displaced with anterior part of talus very prominent in front of it
Skin creases on:		
Dorsolateral aspect of foot	Present; normal	Thin or absent
Medial and plantar aspects of foot	No furrowed skin	Furrowed skin
Posterior aspect of ankle	Normal	Deep crease
Calf and leg atrophy	None or very minimal	Moderate to marked
Treatment	Passive manipulation followed by retention by adhesive strapping, splint, or cast	Primary open reduction of talocalcaneonavicular joint often required; surgery is conservative
		Closed methods of reduction often unsuccessful
		Prolonged retentive apparatus essential
Prognosis	Excellent; result is normal foot	Poor with closed methods
		Prolonged cast immobilization results in smaller foot and atrophied leg

From Tachdjian MO: The child's foot, Philadelphia, 1985, WB Saunders, p. 163.

Curly Toe. A curly toe deformity involves a flexion deformity of both the proximal and distal interphalangeal joints with the metatarsophalangeal joint in neutral or flexion, often combined with rotation. It is the result of contracture of flexor digitorum brevis and longus tendons and is most commonly seen in the fifth toe in children.[44]

Equinus Deformity (Talipes Equinus). This deformity is characterized by limited dorsiflexion (less than 10°) at the talocrural joint, usually as a result of contracture of the gastrocnemius or soleus muscles or Achilles tendon. It may also be caused by structural bone deformity (primarily in the talus), trauma, or inflammatory disease. The deformity causes increased stress to the forefoot, which may lead to a rocker-bottom foot and excessive pronation at the subtalar joint. This deviation can contribute to conditions such as plantar fasciitis, metatarsalgia, heel spurs, and talonavicular pain.[25]

Exostosis (Bony Spur). Exostosis is an abnormal bony outgrowth extending from the surface of the bone (Figure 13-32). It is actually an increase in the bone mass at the site of an irritative lesion in response to overuse, trauma, or excessive pressure. The common areas of occurrence in the foot are on the dorsal aspect of the tarsometatarsal joint, the head of the fifth metatarsal bone, the calcaneus (where it is often called a pump bump or runner's bump), the insertion of the plantar fascia, and the superior aspect of the navicular bone. Most often these exostoses are the result of poorly fitting footwear that leads to undue pressure on the bone.

Forefoot Valgus. This structural midtarsal deviation involves eversion of the forefoot on the hindfoot when the subtalar joint is in the neutral position because the normal valgus tilt (35° to 45°) of the head and neck of the talus to its trochlea has been exceeded. With this deformity, during the weight-bearing phase of gait, the midtarsal joint is supinated so that the lateral aspect of the foot is brought into contact with the ground. Like hindfoot valgus, it contributes to decreasing the medial longitudinal arch and, therefore, clinically resembles a planus foot. The prolonged supination can contribute to

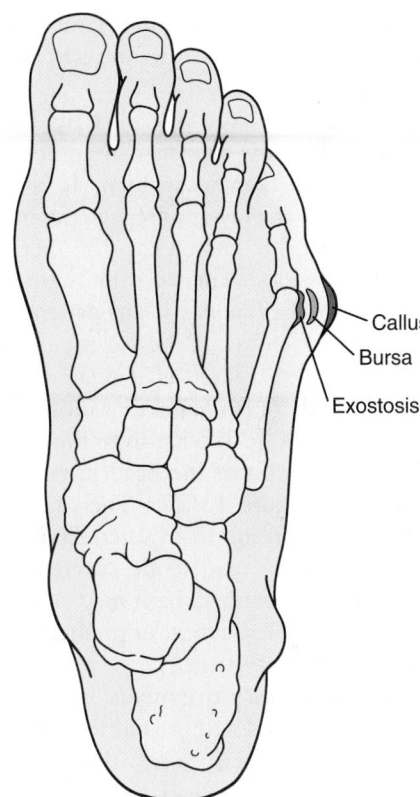

Figure 13-30 **A bunionette or tailor's bunion.**

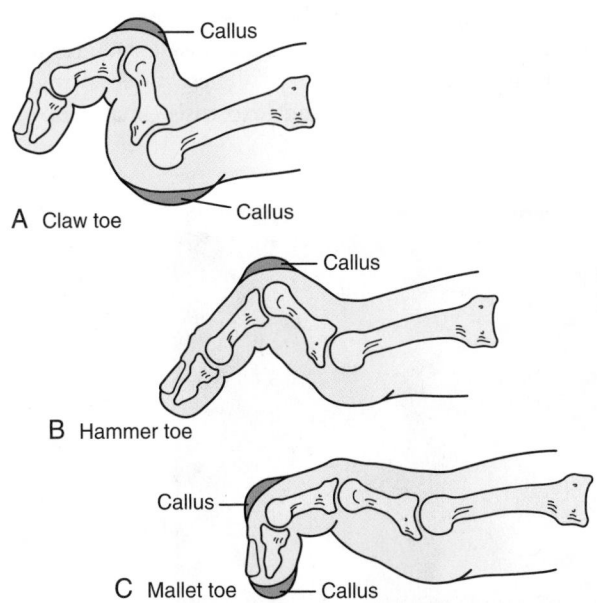

Figure 13-31 **Toe deformities. A,** Claw toe. Note that the proximal and distal interphalangeal joints are hyperflexed and the metatarsophalangeal joint is dorsally subluxated. **B,** Hammer toe. Note the flexion deformity of the proximal interphalangeal joints. The distal interphalangeal joint is in neutral position or slight flexion. **C,** Mallet toe. There is flexion contracture of the distal interphalangeal joint. The proximal interphalangeal and metatarsophalangeal joints are in neutral position.

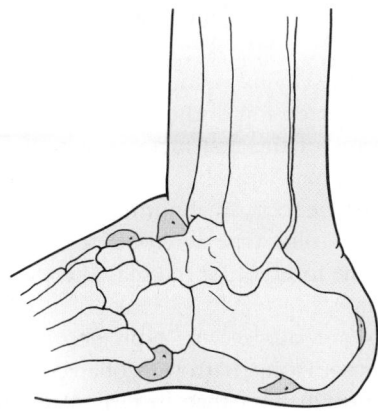

Figure 13-32 **Common areas of exostosis formation in the foot.**

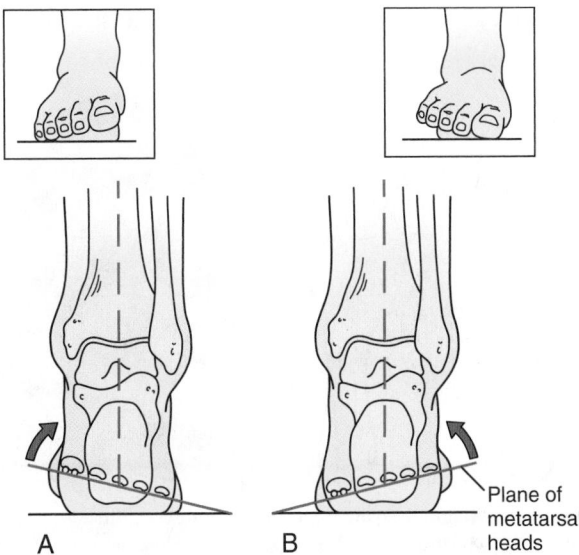

Figure 13-33 **Forefoot deformities (right foot). A,** Forefoot varus (metatarsal heads raised on medial side). **B,** Forefoot valgus (metatarsal heads raised on lateral side).

conditions such as lateral ankle sprains, iliotibial band syndrome, plantar fasciitis, anterior tarsal tunnel syndrome, toe deformities, sesamoiditis, and leg and thigh pain (Figure 13-33, *B*).[25,45]

Forefoot Varus. This structural midtarsal joint deviation involves inversion of the forefoot on the hindfoot when the subtalar joint is in the neutral position. It occurs because the normal valgus tilt (35° to 45°) of the head and neck of the talus to its trochlea has not been achieved.[25,45,46] Clinically, it contributes to decreasing the medial longitudinal arch and, therefore, resembles pes planus. With this deformity, during the weight-bearing phase of gait, the midtarsal joint is completely pronated in an attempt to bring the first metatarsal head in contact with the ground. The prolonged rotation that results can contribute to conditions, such as tibialis posterior paratenonitis, patellofemoral syndrome, toe deformities, ligamentous stress (medially), shin splints, plantar fasciitis, postural fatigue, and Morton's neuroma (Figure 13-33, *A*).

Hallux Rigidus. Hallux rigidus is a condition in which dorsiflexion or extension of the big toe is limited because of osteoarthritis of the first metatarsophalangeal joint.[47] Hallux rigidus may also be caused by an anatomical abnormality of the foot, an abnormally long first metatarsal bone (index plus type forefoot; see Figure 13-14), pronation of the forefoot, or trauma. There are two types: acute and chronic.

The acute, or adolescent, type occurs primarily in young people with long, narrow, pronated feet and occurs more frequently in boys than in girls. Pain and stiffness in the big toe come on quickly; the pain is described as constant, burning, throbbing, or aching. Tenderness may be palpated over the metatarsophalangeal joint, and the toe is initially held stiff because of muscle spasm. The first metatarsal head may be elevated, large, and tender. The weight distribution pattern in the gait is shown in Figure 13-34.

The second (chronic) type of hallux rigidus is much more common and occurs primarily in adults—again, in men more frequently than in women. It is frequently bilateral and is usually the result of repeated minor trauma resulting in osteoarthritic changes to the metatarsophalangeal joint of the big toe. The toe stiffens gradually, and the pain, once established, persists. The patient complains primarily of pain at the base of the big toe on walking.

Hallux Valgus. Hallux valgus is a relatively common condition in which there is medial deviation of the head of the first metatarsal bone in relation to the center of the body and lateral deviation of the head in relation to the center of the foot (Figure 13-35). The cause of hallux valgus is varied. It may result from a hereditary factor and is often familial. Women tend to be affected more than men. Trying to keep up with fashion may be a contributing factor if the patient wears tight or pointed shoes, tight stockings, or high-heeled shoes.[48]

As the metatarsal bones move medially, the base of the proximal phalanx is carried with it, and the phalanx pivots around the adductor hallucis muscle that inserts into it, causing the distal end as well as the distal phalanx to deviate laterally in relation to the center of the body. The long flexor and extensor muscles then have a bowstring effect as they are displaced to the lateral side of the joint, which can lead to increased stress on the proximal phalanx.[49]

A callus develops over the medial side of the head of the metatarsal bone, and the bursa becomes thickened and inflamed; excessive bone (exostosis) forms, resulting in a **bunion** (Figure 13-36).[15,50] These three changes—callus, thickened bursa, and exostosis—make up the

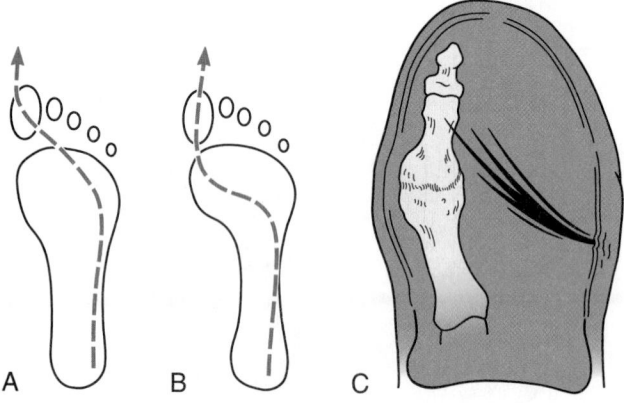

Figure 13-34 **Weight-bearing patterns in hallux rigidus. A,** Hallux rigidus gait pattern. **B,** Normal gait pattern. **C,** Shoe develops oblique creases with hallux rigidus. (**C,** Redrawn from Jahss MH: Disorders of the foot, Philadelphia, 1991, WB Saunders, p. 60.)

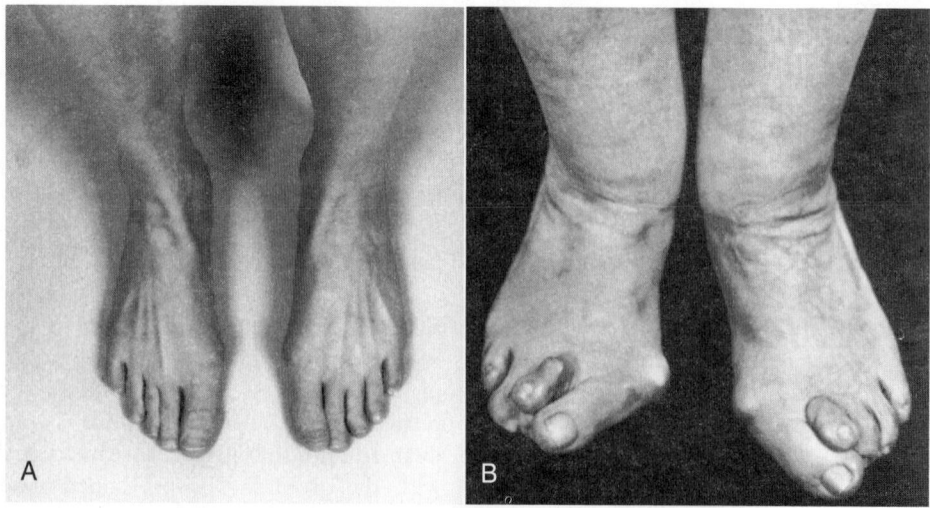

Figure 13-35 A, An example of congruous hallux valgus. **B,** Pathological hallux valgus with bilateral bunions and overlapped toes. Note how the deviating big toe (hallux) rotates and pushes under the second toe (crossover toe). (**B,** From Gartland JJ: Fundamentals of orthopedics, Philadelphia, 1987, WB Saunders, p. 401.)

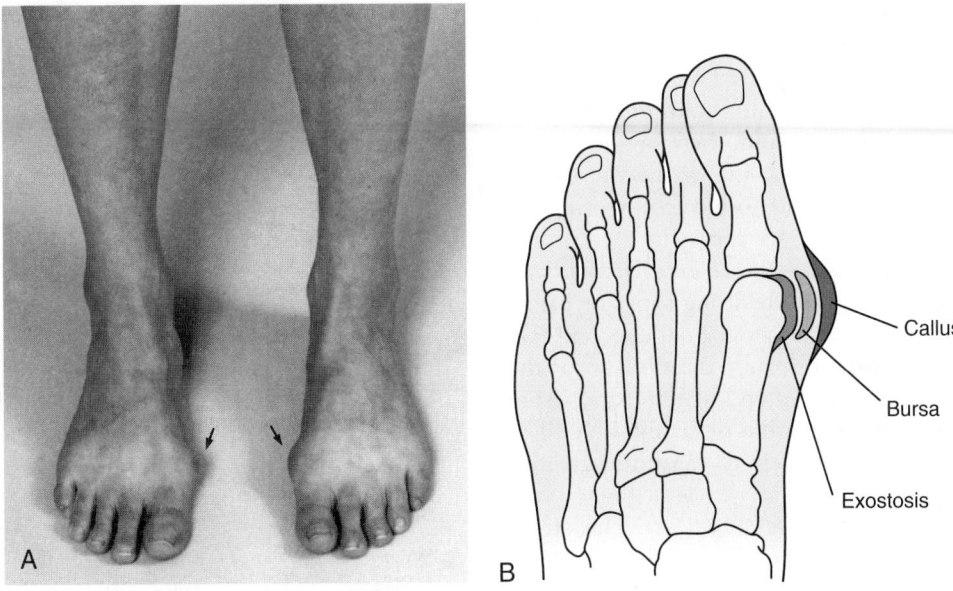

Figure 13-36 A, Bunions apparent on both feet. **B,** Schematic line drawing of a bunion.

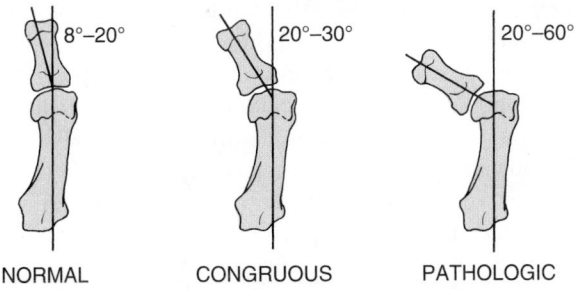

Figure 13-37 Metatarsophalangeal (hallux valgus) angle.

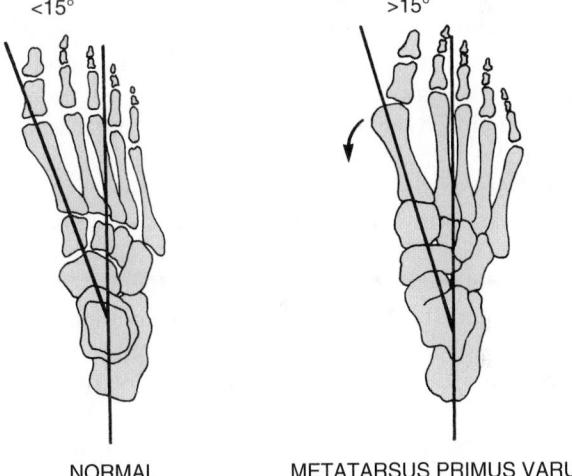

Figure 13-38 Normal foot and metatarsus primus varus. (Note increased intermetatarsal angle.)

bunion, a condition separate from hallux valgus, although it is the result of hallux valgus.

In normal persons, the **metatarsophalangeal angle** (the angle between the longitudinal axis of the metatarsal bone and the proximal phalanx) is 8° to 20° (Figure 13-37). This angle is increased to varying degrees in hallux valgus.

The first type (**congruous hallux valgus**) is a simple exaggeration of the normal relation of the metatarsal to the phalanx of the big toe. The deformity does not progress, and the valgus deformity is between 20° and 30°. The opposing joint surfaces are congruent. It requires little treatment, and often the biggest problem is cosmetic.

The second type (**pathological hallux valgus**) is a potentially progressive deformity, increasing from 20° to 60°. The joint surfaces are no longer congruent, and some may even go to subluxation. This type may occur in deviated (early) and subluxed (later) stages.

When looking at the foot, the examiner may find that there is a widening gap between the first and second metatarsal bones (increased **intermetatarsal angle**) and a lateral deflection of the phalanx at the metatarsophalangeal joint. The joint capsule lengthens on the medial

aspect and is contracted on the lateral aspect. The toes rotate on the long axis so that the toenail faces medially because of the pull of the adductor hallucis muscle. Sometimes, the big toe deviates so far that it lies over or under the second toe.

Of all hallux valgus cases, 80% are caused by **metatarsus primus varus,** in which the intermetatarsal or metatarsal angle is increased to more than 15° (Figure 13-38).[51,52] Metatarsus primus varus is an abduction deformity of the first metatarsal bone in relation to the tarsal and other metatarsal bones so that the medial border of the forefoot is curved. Normally, this angle is between 0° and 15°.

Hammer Toe. A hammer toe deformity consists of an extension contracture at the metatarsophalangeal joint and flexion contracture at the proximal interphalangeal joint; the distal interphalangeal joint may be flexed, straight, or hyperextended (Figure 13-31, *B*).[50,53] The interosseus muscles are unable to hold the proximal phalanx in the neutral position and, therefore, lose their flexion effect. This results in clawing of the toe by the long flexors and extensors leading to and accentuating the deformity. The causes of hammer toe include an imbalance of the synergic muscles, hereditary factors, and mechanical factors, such as poorly fitting shoes or hallux valgus. It is usually seen only in one toe—the second toe. Often, there is a callus or corn over the dorsum of the flexed joint. The condition is often asymptomatic, especially if the hammer toe is flexible or semiflexible. The rigid type of hammer toe is likely to cause the greatest problems.

Hindfoot Valgus (Subtalar or Rearfoot Valgus). This structural deformity involves eversion of the calcaneus when the subtalar joint is in the neutral position. The hindfoot is mobile, which may lead to excessive pronation and limited supination. It may result from genu valgum (knock knees) and may contribute to the appearance of a pes planus foot with the medial longitudinal arch appearing flattened. Because of the increased mobility, it is less likely to cause problems than hindfoot varus. It is often associated with tibia valgus (Figure 13-39, *B*) and has been associated with posterior tibial tendon insufficiency.[54]

Hindfoot Varus (Subtalar or Rearfoot Varus). This structural deviation involves inversion of the calcaneus when the subtalar joint is in the neutral position. The hindfoot is mildly rigid with calcaneal eversion; therefore, pronation is limited. It may contribute to the appearance of a pes cavus foot, making the medial longitudinal arch appear accentuated. It may be the result of tibia varus (genu varum), and, because of the extra subtalar pronation necessary at the beginning of stance, normal supination during early propulsion may be prevented. This deviation can contribute to conditions, such as retrocalcaneal exostosis (pump bumps), shin splints, plantar

fasciitis, hamstring strains, and knee and ankle pathology (Figure 13-39, *A*).[25]

Mallet Toe. Mallet toe is associated with a flexion deformity of the distal interphalangeal joint (Figure 13-31, *C*).[50,53] It can occur on any of the four lateral toes. Often, a corn or callus is present over the dorsum of the affected joint. The condition is usually asymptomatic. It is commonly seen with ill-fitting or poorly designed footwear.[42]

Metatarsus Adductus (Hooked Forefoot). This deformity is the most common foot deviation in children. It may be seen at birth but often is not noticed until the child begins to stand. The foot appears to be adducted and supinated (kidney shaped with medial deviation), and the hindfoot may or may not be in valgus.[55] It may be associated with hip dysplasia. Eighty-five to 90% of cases resolve spontaneously.[43]

Morton's (Atavistic or Grecian) Foot. With a Morton's foot, the second toe is longer than the first. The length difference may be due to different lengths of the metatarsals (see Figure 13-14). Increased stress is put on this longer toe, and the big toe tends to be hypomobile. There is often hypertrophy of the second metatarsal bone because more stress is put through the second toe. In fact, the second metatarsal can become as large as the first metatarsal. People with this deformity often have difficulty putting on tight-fitting footwear (e.g., skates, ski boots) or dancing (e.g., en pointe in ballet). The different types of feet and their proportional representations in the population are shown in Figure 13-15.

Morton's Metatarsalgia (Interdigital Neuroma). Morton's metatarsalgia (Morton's neuroma) refers to the formation of an interdigital neuroma as a result of injury to one of the digital nerves (Figure 13-40). Usually, it is the digital nerve between the third and fourth toes, so the examiner must take care to differentially diagnose the condition from a stress fracture of one of the metatarsals in the same area (**march fracture**). (A stress fracture will be more painful when the bone is palpated and a bone scan would be positive.) Title et al.[56] point out that if a Morton's neuroma is suspected, pressure palpation should be applied on the plantar aspect avoiding counter pressure on the dorsal aspect. Dorsal palpation pain is more likely to be associated with a stress fracture, metatarsophalangeal synovitis, or dorsal neuralgia. While walking or running, the patient is suddenly seized with an agonizing pain on the outer border of the forefoot. The pain is often intermittent, like a cramp, shooting up the side and to the tip of the affected toe or the adjacent two toes. Squeezing the metatarsal bones together elicits pain because of the pressure on the digital nerve. On palpation, pain is more likely to be between the bones rather than on the bone. The condition tends to occur more frequently in women than in men.

Pes Cavus ("Hollow Foot" or Rigid Foot). A pes cavus may be caused by a congenital problem; a neurological

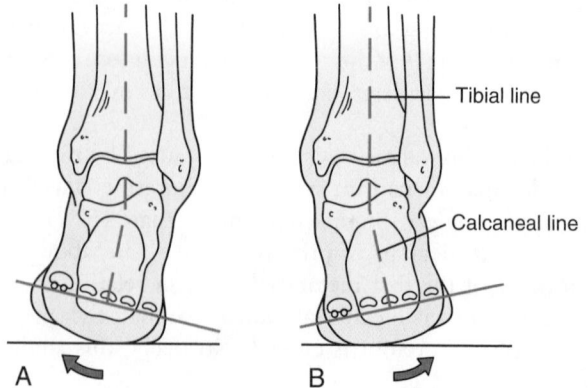

Figure 13-39 Hindfoot deformities (right foot). A, Hindfoot varus (heel appears inverted). **B,** Hindfoot valgus (heel appears everted).

problem, such as spina bifida, poliomyelitis, or Charcot-Marie-Tooth disease; talipes equinovarus; or muscle imbalance. There may also be a genetic factor, because it tends to run in families.

The longitudinal arches are accentuated (Figure 13-41), and the metatarsal heads are lower in relation to the hindfoot so that there is a dropping of the forefoot on the hindfoot at the tarsometatarsal joints (Figure 13-42). The soft tissues of the sole of the foot are abnormally short, which gives the foot a shortened appearance.

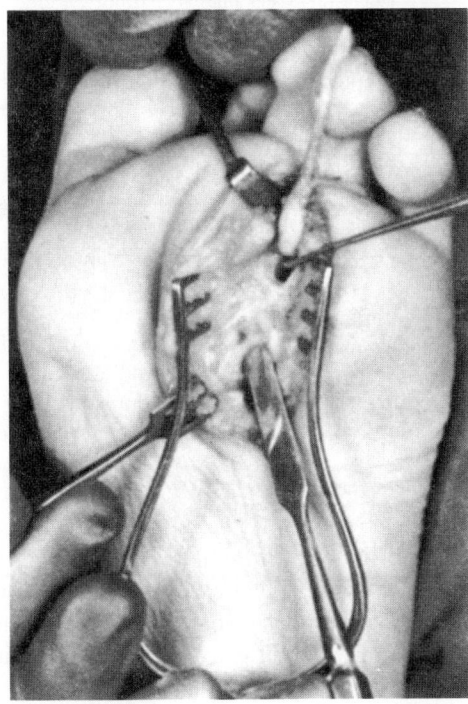

Figure 13-40 **The applied anatomy of Morton's metatarsalgia.** The interdigital nerve to the space between the third and fourth digits has been divided 2 cm above the neuroma and is reflected downward. The plantar digital vessels are shown entering the neuroma. The end of the flat dissector is on the upper margin of the transverse ligament. The end of the probe points to the intermetatarsophalangeal bursa. (From Klenerman L: The foot and its disorders, Boston, 1982, Blackwell Scientific, p. 143.)

If the deformity persists, the bones eventually alter their shape, perpetuating the deformity. The heel is normal, at least initially. Claw toes are often associated with the condition because of the dropping of the forefoot combined with the pull of the extensor tendons. The examiner often finds painful callosities beneath the metatarsal heads that are caused by the loss of the metatarsal arch and tenderness along the deformed toes. There is pain in the tarsal region after time because of osteoarthritic changes in these joints.

The longitudinal arches are high on both the medial and lateral aspects so that a lateral longitudinal arch occurs in some severe cases, and the forefoot is thickened and splayed (Table 13-6). The metatarsal heads are prominent on the sole of the foot, and the toes do not touch the ground, even on active or passive movement. This type of deformity leads to a rigid foot with little ability to absorb shock and adapt to stress. People with this deformity have difficulty doing repetitive stress activity (e.g., long-distance running, ballet) and require a cushioning shoe. In severe cases, the cavus foot is often associated with neurological disorders.[43]

Pes Planus (Flatfoot or Mobile Foot). Flatfoot may be congenital, or it may result from trauma, muscle weakness, ligament laxity, dropping of the talar head, paralysis, or a pronated foot. For example, a traumatic flatfoot may follow fracture of the calcaneus. It may also be caused by a postural deformity, such as medial rotation of the hips or medial tibial torsion. It is a relatively common foot deformity that often causes little or no problem. Therefore, the examiner should not necessarily assume that a flat, mobile foot needs to be treated. Because the foot is mobile, patients with flatfoot function well without treatment and often need only a control shoe to avoid problems in prolonged stress situations.

It must be remembered that all infants have flatfeet up to approximately 2 years of age. This appearance in part results from the fat pad in the longitudinal arch and in part from the incomplete formation of the arches. With pes planus, the medial longitudinal arch is reduced so that on standing its borders are close to or in contact with the

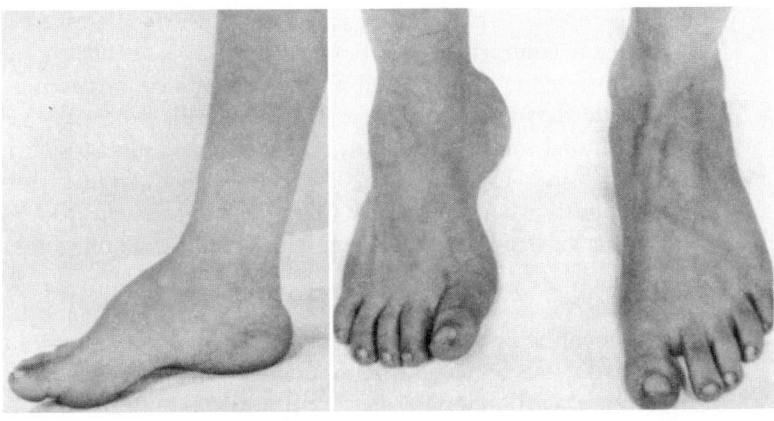

Figure 13-41 Pes cavus ("hollow foot"). Note the high medial longitudinal arch, early clawing of the big toe, and the heel in varus. (From Klenerman L: The foot and its disorders, Boston, 1982, Blackwell Scientific, p. 72.)

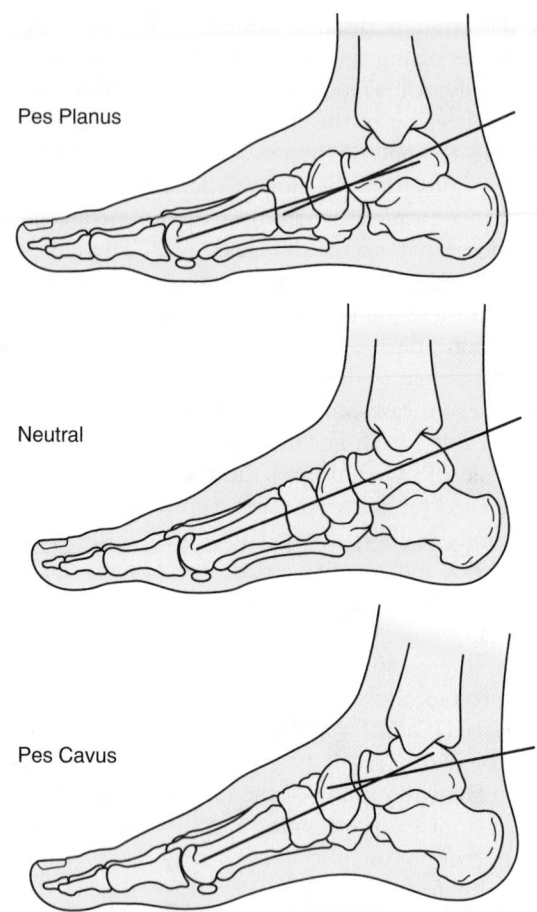

Pes Planus

Neutral

Pes Cavus

Figure 13-42 Talometatarsal angle used to define pes planus, neutral, and pes cavus foot types. (Redrawn from Jahss MH, editor: Disorders of the foot and ankle: medical and surgical management, ed 2, vol 1, Philadelphia, 1991, WB Saunders.)

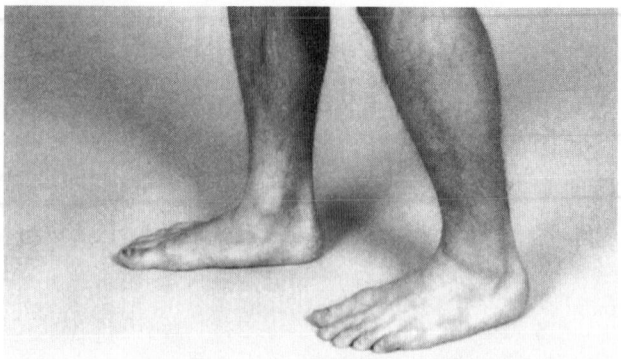

Figure 13-43 Pes planus (flatfoot).

TABLE **13-6**

Pes Cavus Classification

Classification	Features
1. Mild	Longitudinal arch appears high NWB
	Longitudinal arch almost normal WB
	Toes clawed NWB
	Toes may be normal WB
	May have hindfoot varus
2. Moderate	Longitudinal arch high NWB and WB
	Claw toes evident NWB and WB
	Calluses under prominent metatarsal heads
	Dorsiflexion may be limited
	Forefoot plantar flexed on hindfoot
3. Severe	Calcaneus cannot pronate past 5° varus
	Heel in varus, foot in valgus
	Decreased ROM in foot

NWB, Non–weight-bearing; *ROM,* range of motion; *WB,* weight-bearing.

TABLE **13-7**

Pes Planus Classification

Classification	Features
1. Mild	4° to 6° hindfoot valgus
	4° to 6° forefoot valgus
2. Moderate	6° to 10° hindfoot valgus
	6° to 10° forefoot varus
	Poor shock absorption at heel strike
3. Severe	10° to 15° hindfoot valgus
	8° to 10° forefoot varus
	Equinus deformity may be present

ground. This results from the hindfoot dropping in relation to the forefoot (see Figure 13-42). If the condition persists into adulthood, it may become a permanent structural deformity, leading to a defect or alteration of the tarsal bones and the talonavicular joints.

There are two types of flatfoot deformities. The first type (**rigid** or **congenital flatfoot**) is relatively rare. The calcaneus is found in a valgus position, whereas the midtarsal region is in pronation. The talus faces medially and downward, and the navicular is displaced dorsally and laterally on the talus. There are accompanying soft-tissue contractures and bony changes. The second type is **acquired** or **flexible flatfoot** (Figure 13-43). In this case, the deformity is similar to the rigid flatfoot, but the foot is mobile (Table 13-7); and there are few, if any, soft-tissue contractures and bony changes. It is usually caused by hereditary factors and is sometimes called a **hypermobile flatfoot.** Flexible flatfoot may result from tibial or femoral torsion, coxa vara, a defect in the subtalar joint, or injury to the posterior tibial tendon.[57] If the arch appears when the patient stands on tiptoes, the patient may have a mobile flatfoot. This type of flatfoot seldom needs treatment.

Plantar Flexed First Ray. This structural deformity occurs when the first ray (big toe) lies lower than the other four metatarsal bones so that the forefoot is everted when the metatarsal bones are aligned. If present congenitally, it is

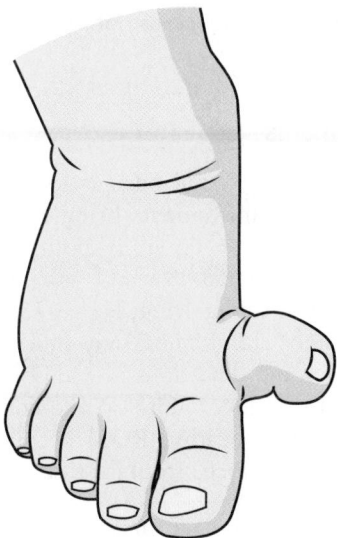

Figure 13-44 Polydactyly (extra digit). (These digits are commonly amputated early in life.)

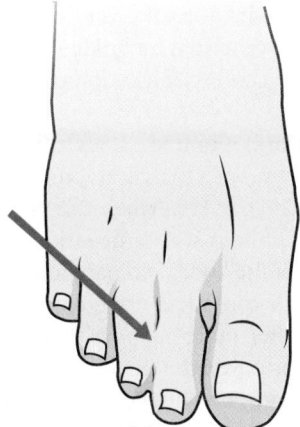

Figure 13-45 Syndactyly (webbing) of the second and third toe *(arrow).*

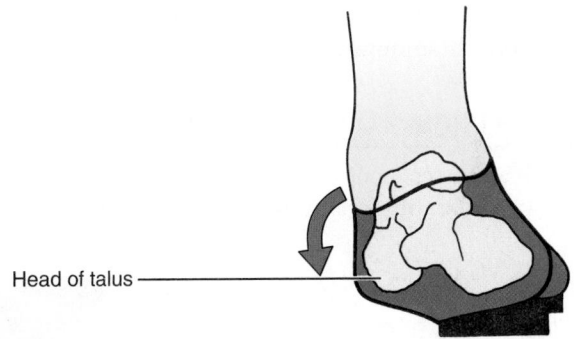

Head of talus

Figure 13-46 Pes planus (flatfoot) or calcaneus in valgus can lead to misshapen shoes. Note the prominence of the talar head.

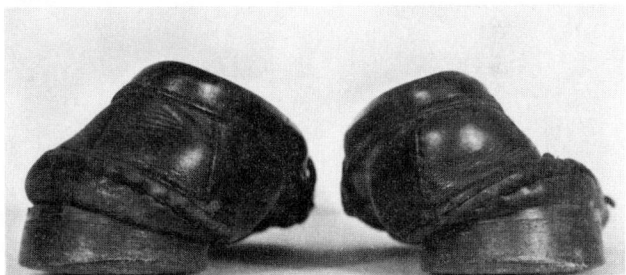

Figure 13-47 Misshapen shoes caused by severely pronated feet. (From Gartland JJ: Fundamentals of orthopedics, Philadelphia, 1987, WB Saunders, p. 398.)

indicative of a cavus foot. In its acquired form, it occurs as compensation for tibia varum (genu varum) with limited calcaneal eversion. This deformity can contribute to the same conditions seen with forefoot valgus.[25] The neutral position of the first ray is the position in which the first metatarsal head lies in the same transverse plane as the second through fourth metatarsal heads when they are maximally dorsiflexed.[58]

Polydactyly. This developmental anomaly is characterized by the presence of an extra digit or toe (Figure 13-44). It may be seen in isolation or with other anomalies, such as polydactyly of the hands and syndactyly (webbing) of the toes or hands (Figure 13-45). The primary concern with this anomaly is cosmesis.[59]

Rocker-Bottom Foot. In the rocker-bottom foot deformity, the forefoot is dorsiflexed on the hindfoot. This results in a "broken midfoot," so that the medial and longitudinal arches are absent and the foot appears to be bent the wrong way (i.e., convex to the floor instead of the normal concave).

Splay Foot. This deformity, which is broadening of the forefoot, is often caused by weakness of the intrinsic muscles and associated weakness of the intermetatarsal ligament and dropping of the anterior metatarsal arch.

Turf Toe. Turf toe is a hyperextension injury (sprain) combined with compressive loading to the metatarsophalangeal joint of the hallux. It can cause a significant functional disability, especially in sports, where the hallux is put under high loads. It is often related to the use of flexible footwear and artificial turf.[60–62]

Shoes

The examiner looks at the patient's shoes, both inside and outside, for weight-bearing and wear patterns (Figures 13-46 and 13-47). With the normal foot, the greatest wear on the shoe is beneath the ball of the foot and

slightly to the lateral side and the posterolateral aspect of the heel. If shoes are too small or too narrow, they may pinch the feet, causing deformities and affecting normal growth. If shoes are worn out, they offer little support. If shoes are stiff, they limit proper movement of the foot.

Platform-type or high-heeled shoes often cause painful knees, because the patient wearing these shoes usually walks with the knees flexed, which may increase the stress on the patella. Continuous wearing of high-heeled shoes may cause the calf muscles to contract and may lead to sore knees and a painful back, because the lumbar spine goes into increased lordotic posture to maintain the center of gravity in its normal position. In addition, these shoes increase the potential for ankle sprains and fractures because a raised center of gravity puts the wearer off balance.

High-heeled and pointed shoes often contribute to hallux valgus, bunions, march fractures, and Morton's metatarsalgia that may result because the toes are being pushed together. Shoes with a negative heel may lead to hyperextension of the knees and patellofemoral syndrome. High-cut or high-top shoes that cover the medial and lateral malleoli offer more support than low-cut shoes or those that do not cover the malleoli.

Excessive bulging on the medial side of the shoe suggests a valgus or everted foot, whereas excessive bulging on the lateral side suggests an inverted foot. Drop foot resulting from musculature weakness scuffs the toe of the shoe. Oblique forefoot creases in the shoe indicate possible hallux rigidus; absence of forefoot creases indicates no toe-off action during gait.

EXAMINATION

As with any assessment, the examiner must compare one side with the other and note any asymmetry. This comparison is necessary because of individual differences among normal people.

Active Movements

The first movements tested during the examination are active, with painful movements being tested last. These movements should be done in both weight-bearing (Figures 13-48 and 13-49) and non–weight-bearing (long leg sitting or supine lying; Figure 13-50) positions, and the examiner should note any differences because foot deformities and deviations in addition to decreased ROM can lead to injury.[63] Lindsjo and colleagues advocated testing weight-bearing ROM by putting the test foot on a 30-cm (12-inch) stool for ease of measurement and flexing the knee.[64]

Plantar Flexion

Plantar flexion of the ankle is approximately 50° (see Figure 13-50, *A*), and the patient's heel normally inverts when the movement is performed in weight bearing (Figure 13-51). If heel inversion does not occur, the foot is unstable, or there is tibialis posterior weakness or tightness.[37,65,66] The tibialis posterior muscle and tendon

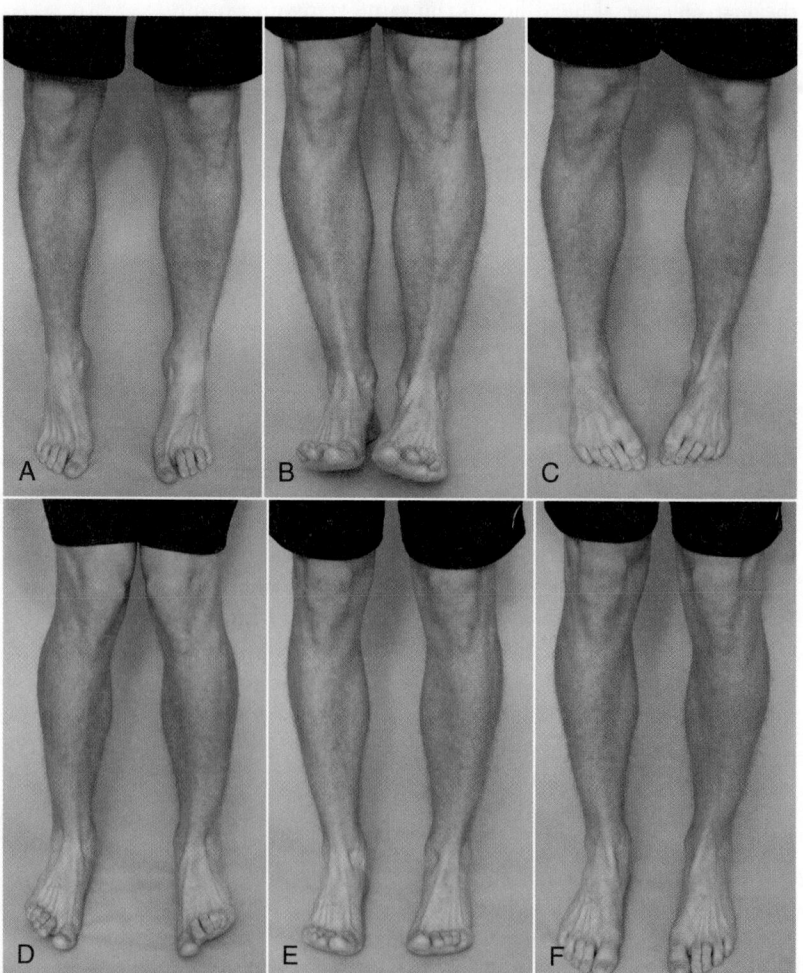

Figure 13-48 Active movements (weight-bearing posture). A, Plantar flexion. **B,** Dorsiflexion. **C,** Supination. **D,** Pronation. **E,** Toe extension. **F,** Toe flexion.

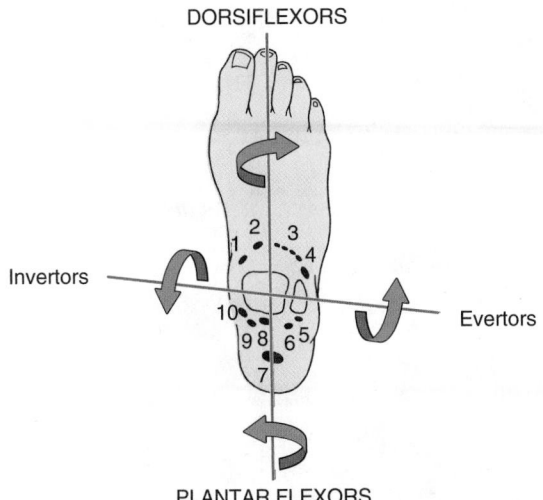

Figure 13-49 Motion diagram of the ankle. *1,* Tibialis anterior; *2,* extensor hallucis longus; *3,* extensor digitorum longus; *4,* peroneus tertius; *5,* peroneus brevis; *6,* peroneus longus; *7,* Achilles tendon (soleus and gastrocnemius); *8,* flexor hallucis longus; *9,* flexor digitorum longus; *10,* tibialis posterior.

Weight-Bearing Active Movements of the Lower Leg, Ankle, and Foot

- Plantar flexion (flexion), standing on the toes
- Dorsiflexion (extension), standing on the heels
- Supination, standing on the lateral edge of the foot
- Pronation, standing on the medial edge of the foot
- Toe extension
- Toe flexion
- Combined movements (if necessary)
- Sustained positions (if necessary)
- Repetitive movements (if necessary)

Non–Weight-Bearing Active Movements of the Lower Leg, Ankle, and Foot

- Plantar flexion (flexion), 50°
- Dorsiflexion (extension), 20°
- Supination, 45° to 60°
- Pronation, 15° to 30°
- Toe extension, lateral four toes (MTP, 40°; PIP, 0°; DIP, 30°) and great toe (MTP, 70°; IP, 0°)
- Toe flexion, lateral four toes (MTP, 40°; PIP, 35°; DIP, 60°) and great toe (MTP, 45°; IP, 90°)
- Toe abduction
- Toe adduction
- Combined movements (if necessary)
- Sustained positions (if necessary)
- Repetitive movements (if necessary)

DIP, Distal interphalangeal joint; *MTP,* metatarsophalangeal joint; *PIP,* proximal interphalangeal joint.

balance the pull of the peroneal muscles, protect the spring ligament, and invert and stabilize the hindfoot during toe off.[67] Pain in the spring ligament as well as the medial midfoot and hindfoot ligaments, hindfoot valgus, plantar flexed talar head, and forefoot abduction should lead the examiner to assessing the tibialis posterior for proper function.[37]

Dorsiflexion

Dorsiflexion of the ankle is usually 20° past the anatomical position (plantigrade), which is with the foot at 90° to the bones of the leg (see Figure 13-50, *B*). For normal locomotion, 10° of dorsiflexion and 20° to 25° of plantar flexion at the ankle are required. Functional dorsiflexion may be measured by the **ankle lunge test** ✓.[68,69] For this weight-bearing test, the patient is asked to place one foot perpendicular to a wall and lunge the same knee toward the wall (Figure 13-52, *A*). The foot is progressively moved away from the wall until the knee barely touches the wall and the foot remains flat on the floor. The distance from the wall to the big toe is measured (Figure 13-52, *B*). Both sides are compared. If desired, the angle of the tibial shaft to a vertical line can also be measured (Figure 13-53). Differences between sides may be due to a tight Achilles tendon or talocrural restriction.[70]

Supination and Pronation

Supination is 45° to 60° and pronation is 15° to 30°, although individuals vary (see Figure 13-50, *C* and *D*). It is more important to compare the movement with that of the patient's normal side (Figures 13-54 and 13-55). Supination combines the movements of inversion, adduction, and plantar flexion; pronation combines the movements of eversion, abduction, and dorsiflexion of the foot and ankle. As the patient does the movement, the examiner should watch for the possibility of subluxation of various tendons. The peroneal tendons are especially prone to subluxation, and their subluxation is evident on eversion (Figure 13-56). If tibialis anterior is weak, supination is affected. If the peronei are weak or the tendons sublux, pronation is affected.

Toe Extension and Flexion

Movement of the toes occurs at the metatarsophalangeal and proximal and distal interphalangeal joints (see Figure 13-50, *E* and *F*). Extension of the great toe occurs primarily at the metatarsophalangeal joint (70°); there is minimal or no extension at the interphalangeal joint. For the great toe, 45° flexion occurs at the metatarsophalangeal joint, and 90° occurs at the interphalangeal joint.

For the lateral four toes, extension occurs primarily at the metatarsophalangeal (40°) and distal interphalangeal joints (30°). Extension at the proximal interphalangeal joints is negligible. For the lateral four toes, 40° flexion occurs at the metatarsophalangeal joints, 35° occurs at

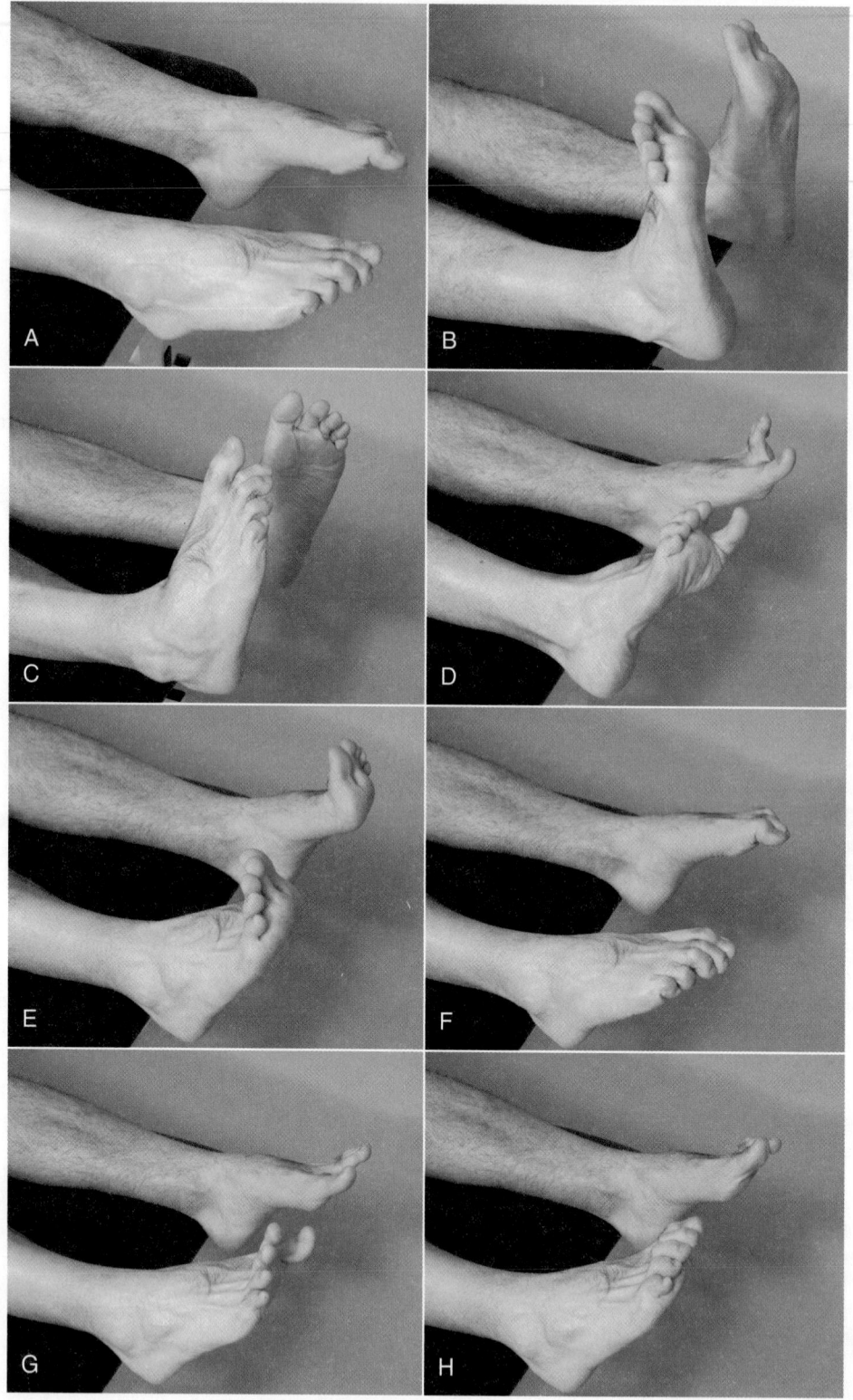

Figure 13-50 Active movements (non-weight-bearing posture). A, Plantar flexion. **B,** Dorsiflexion. **C,** Supination. **D,** Pronation. **E,** Toe extension. **F,** Toe flexion. **G,** Toe abduction. **H,** Toe adduction.

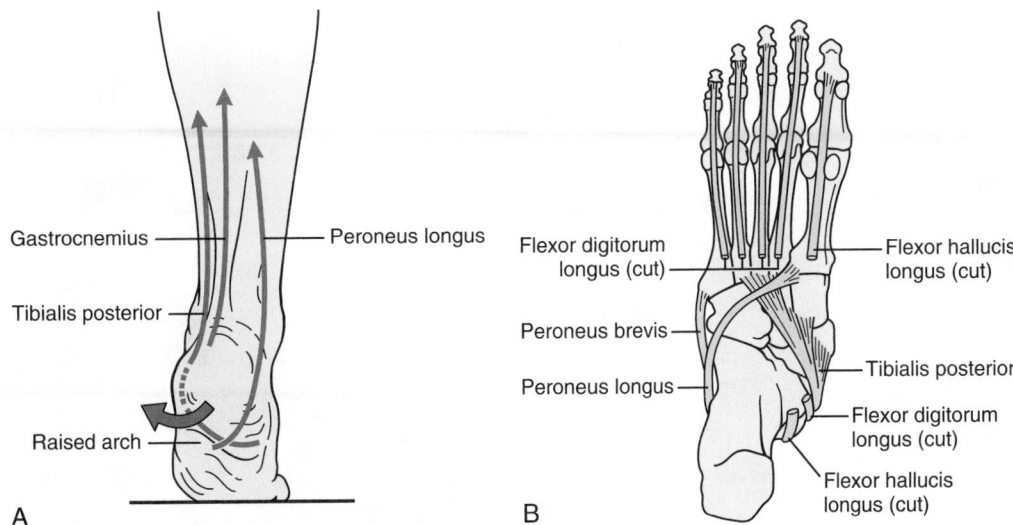

Gastrocnemius

Peroneus longus

Tibialis posterior

Raised arch

A

Flexor digitorum longus (cut)

Flexor hallucis longus (cut)

Peroneus brevis

Peroneus longus

Tibialis posterior

Flexor digitorum longus (cut)

Flexor hallucis longus (cut)

B

Figure 13-51 A, Inversion of heel while standing on toes (plantar flexion of ankle). Note that peroneus longus and tibialis posterior support the medial longitudinal and transverse arches. This motion is sometimes called "sickling" of the foot. **B,** Plantar view of the right foot shows the distal course of the tendons of the peroneus longus, peroneus brevis, and tibialis posterior. The tendons of the flexor digitorum longus and flexor hallucis longus are cut. Note the force couple relationship between the two peroneal muscles and tibialis posterior to control inversion and eversion along with the long flexors and extensors. (**B,** Redrawn from Neumann DA: Kinesiology of the musculoskeletal system: foundations for physical rehabilitation, St Louis, 2002, Mosby, p. 511.)

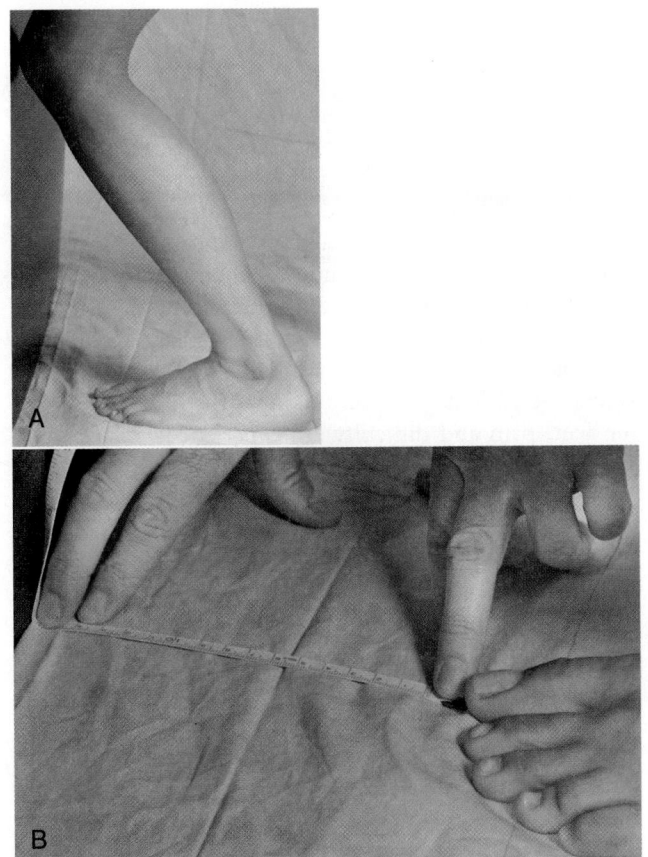

Figure 13-52 Ankle lunge test. A, Normal position: ankle fully dorsiflexed and knee against the wall. Note heel is firmly on floor. **B,** Measurement of the distance of the toes from the wall.

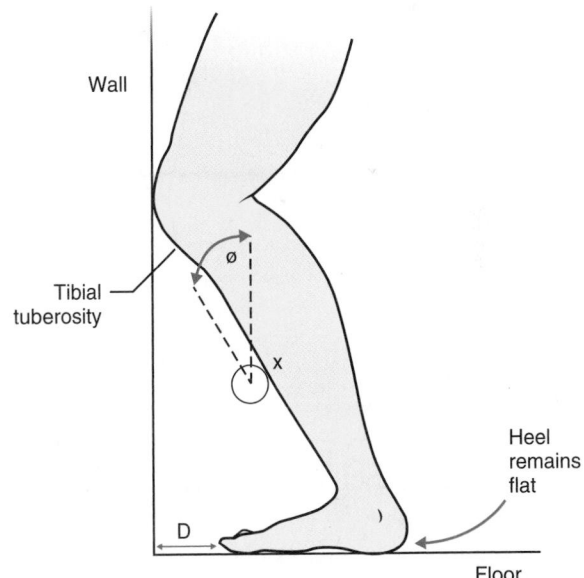

Wall

Tibial tuberosity

ø

x

Heel remains flat

D

Floor

Figure 13-53 Drawing depicting the two methods of measuring dorsiflexion lunge—distance from wall to big toe *(D)* and angle *(φ)* between line along anterior tibia *(x)* and vertical line.

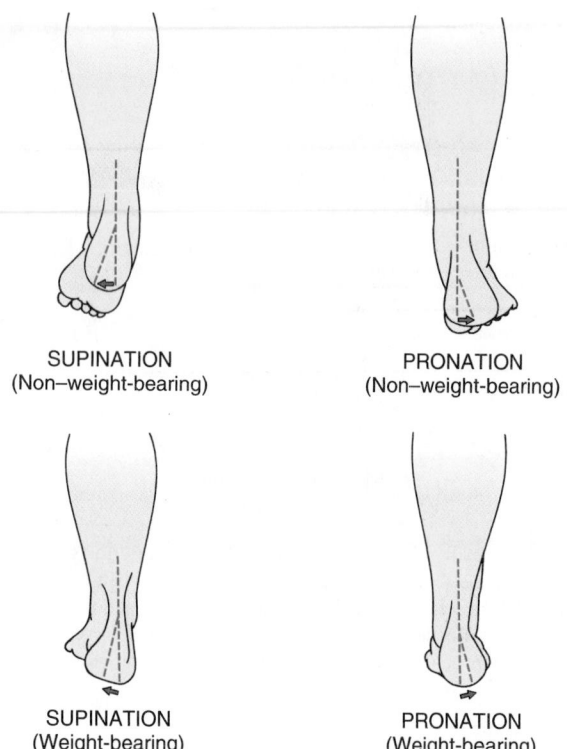

SUPINATION
(Non–weight-bearing)

PRONATION
(Non–weight-bearing)

SUPINATION
(Weight-bearing)

PRONATION
(Weight-bearing)

Figure 13-54 Supination and pronation of the foot in weight-bearing and non–weight-bearing postures (posterior views of the right limb).

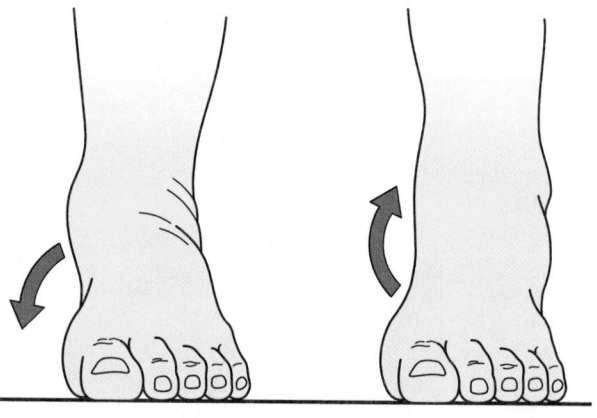

Foot in pronation

Foot in supination

Figure 13-55 Anterior view of the foot in pronation and supination (weight-bearing stance).

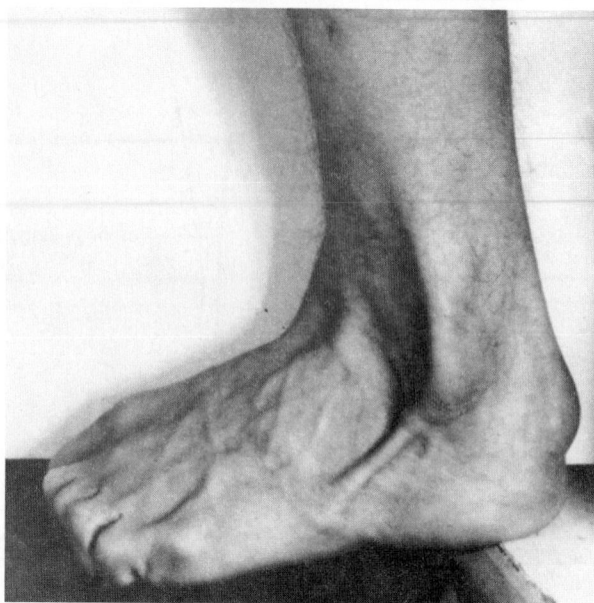

Figure 13-56 Habitual subluxation of the peroneal tendons. The peroneal tendons pass anterior to the retrofibular sulcus but not anterior to the distal fibula, in contradistinction to traumatic subluxation. (From Kelikian H, Kelikian AS: Disorders of the ankle, Philadelphia, 1985, WB Saunders, p. 765.)

the proximal interphalangeal joints, and 60° occurs at the distal interphalangeal joints.

Toe Abduction and Adduction

Abduction and adduction of the toes are measured with the second toe as midline. Although the ROM of abduction can be measured, this is not usually done. The common practice is to ask the patient to spread the toes and then bring them back together (see Figure 13-50, *G* and *H*). The amount and quality of movement are compared with those of the unaffected side.

If the history has indicated that weight-bearing or non–weight-bearing combined or repetitive movements or sustained postures result in symptoms, these movements should also be tested. The examiner should ask the patient to walk on the toes, heels, and outer and inner borders of the feet. These actions indicate the patient's muscle power and control and the functional ROM. With a third-degree strain (rupture) of the Achilles tendon, the patient is not able to walk on the toes. Lack of dorsiflexion makes it difficult for the patient to walk on the heels. When the patient walks on the inner or outer borders of the feet, pain and difficulty are experienced in the presence of a subtalar lesion.

The examiner should also check the efficiency of the toes. Are the toes straight and parallel? Is the patient able to flex, extend, adduct, and abduct the toes? The toes have a primarily ambulatory function, although, with training, they can develop a prehensile function. The toes extend the weight-bearing area forward and, by so doing, reduce the load on the metatarsal heads. The great toe also has a primary function of pushing off during gait.

When assessing the active movements, the examiner must remember that peripheral nerve injuries may alter the pattern of movement. For example, the common peroneal nerve may be injured, because it winds around the head of the fibula, resulting in altered nerve conduction to the peroneus longus and brevis muscles (superficial peroneal nerve) or the tibialis anterior, extensor digitorum longus, and extensor hallucis longus (deep peroneal nerve).[71] In such cases, the movements controlled by these muscles are altered. In addition, there are sensory changes that must be noted.

Passive Movements

The passive movements of the lower leg, ankle, and foot are performed with the patient in a non–weight-bearing position (Figure 13-57). As with other joints, if the active ROM is full, overpressure can be applied to test end feel during the active, non–weight-bearing movements to negate the need to do passive movements. Each

movement should be carefully checked, especially if deformities or asymmetries have been noticed during the observation. These deformities or asymmetries may cause problems in other areas of the lower kinetic chain. For example, limited dorsiflexion or tight heel cords may lead to anterior knee pain or ankle injuries.[72] Because the gastrocnemius is a two-joint muscle, dorsiflexion should be tested with the knee straight to test this muscles for tightness. Testing with the knee bent to 90°, isolates soleus. Stovitz and Coetzee recommended testing the Achilles tendon and its associated muscles with the

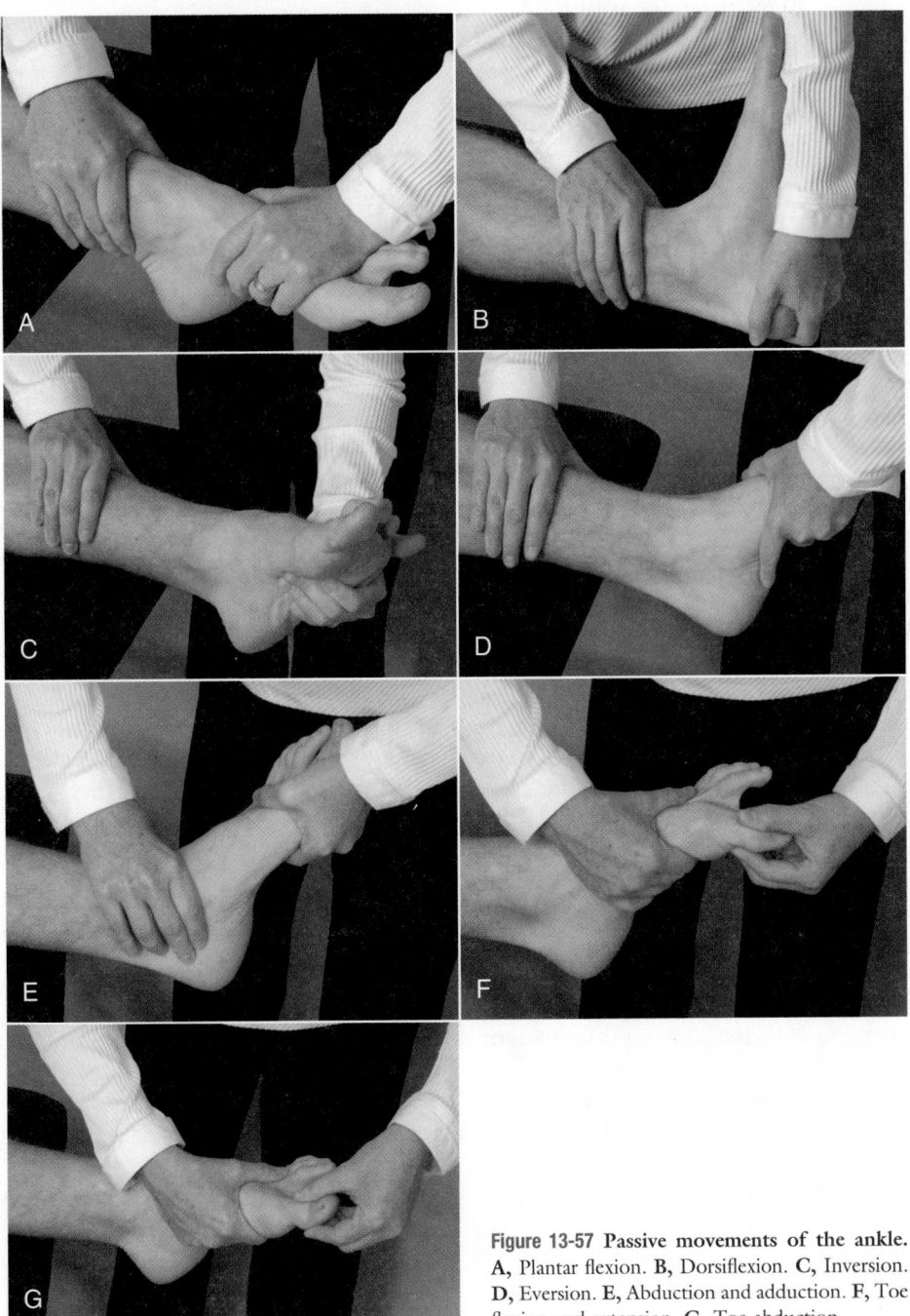

Figure 13-57 Passive movements of the ankle.
A, Plantar flexion. **B,** Dorsiflexion. **C,** Inversion.
D, Eversion. **E,** Abduction and adduction. **F,** Toe flexion and extension. **G,** Toe abduction.

subtalar joint in neutral with a lateral force applied to the talar neck to lock the foot during testing.[66] This eliminates calcaneal eversion or forefoot dorsiflexion from contributing to an apparent normal Achilles tendon. There is greater mobility and flexibility in the Achilles tendon in a baby or young child than there is in an adult. For example, in the newborn, the foot can readily be dorsiflexed passively so that the toes and dorsum of the foot touch the skin over the tibia. In the adult, however, dorsiflexion is limited to 20° more than plantigrade. If the patient can only attain plantigrade (90°), then the gastrocnemius or soleus is tight. If gastrocnemius is tight, the ankle ROM is limited with the knee extended. If soleus is tight, the ankle ROM is limited with the knee flexed. Conversely, increased ankle dorsiflexion (**Matles test ⚠**), compared to the other side, may indicate a torn achilles tendon, especially if combined with decreased plantar flexion strength.[73] If tibialis posterior is tight, supination of the foot is limited.

Passive Movements of the Lower Leg, Ankle, and Foot and Normal End Feel

- Plantar flexion at the talocrural joint (tissue stretch)
- Dorsiflexion at the talocrural joint (tissue stretch)
- Inversion at the subtalar joint (tissue stretch)
- Eversion of the subtalar joint (tissue stretch)
- Adduction at the midtarsal joints (tissue stretch)
- Abduction at the midtarsal joints (tissue stretch)
- Flexion of the toes (tissue stretch)
- Extension of the toes (tissue stretch)
- Adduction of the toes (tissue stretch)
- Abduction of the toes (tissue stretch)

Some movements may be tested in combination to more closely approximate what occurs functionally. For example, instead of testing plantar flexion, adduction, and inversion separately, supination, as a combined movement, may be tested. Similarly, pronation may be tested as a combined movement, instead of dorsiflexion, abduction, and eversion.

During passive movements of the ankle and foot, any capsular patterns should be noted. The capsular pattern of the talocrural joint is more limitation of plantar flexion than of dorsiflexion; the subtalar joint capsular pattern shows more limitation of varus range than of valgus ROM. The midtarsal joint capsular pattern is dorsiflexion most limited, followed by plantar flexion, adduction, and medial rotation. The first metatarsophalangeal joint has a capsular pattern in which extension is most limited, followed by flexion. The pattern for the second through fifth metatarsophalangeal joints is variable. The capsular pattern of the interphalangeal joints is flexion most limited, followed by extension.

Resisted Isometric Movements

The resisted isometric movements are performed to test the contractile tissue around the foot, ankle, and lower leg. The patient is in the sitting or supine lying position, and the patient's foot is placed in the anatomical position (plantigrade or 90°; Figure 13-58). Table 13-8 shows the muscles acting over the foot and ankle. Strength results may very depending on age and sex.[74]

Resisted Isometric Movements of the Lower Leg, Ankle, and Foot

- Knee flexion
- Plantar flexion
- Dorsiflexion
- Supination
- Pronation
- Toe extension
- Toe flexion

Dorsiflexion is sometimes tested with the patient's hip flexed to 45° and the knee flexed to 90°, as illustrated in Figure 13-58, *B*. Testing with the patient in this position enables the examiner to exert a greater isometric force. Resisted isometric knee flexion must be performed, because the triceps surae (gastrocnemius and soleus muscles together) act on the knee as well as on the ankle and foot.

If the history has indicated that eccentric, concentric, or econcentric muscle action has caused symptoms, these movements should also be tested, but only after the isometric tests have been completed.

Functional Assessment

If the patient is able to do the movements already described with little difficulty, functional tests may be performed to see whether these sequential activities produce pain or other symptoms. Full ROM is often not necessary for the patient to lead a functional life.

Functional Activities of the Lower Leg, Ankle, and Foot (in Sequential Order)

- Squatting (both ankles should dorsiflex symmetrically)
- Standing on toes (both ankles should plantar flex symmetrically)
- Squatting and bouncing at the end of a squat
- Standing on one foot at a time
- Standing on the toes, one foot at a time
- Going up and down stairs
- Walking on the toes
- Running straight ahead
- Running, twisting, and cutting
- Jumping
- Jumping and going into a full squat

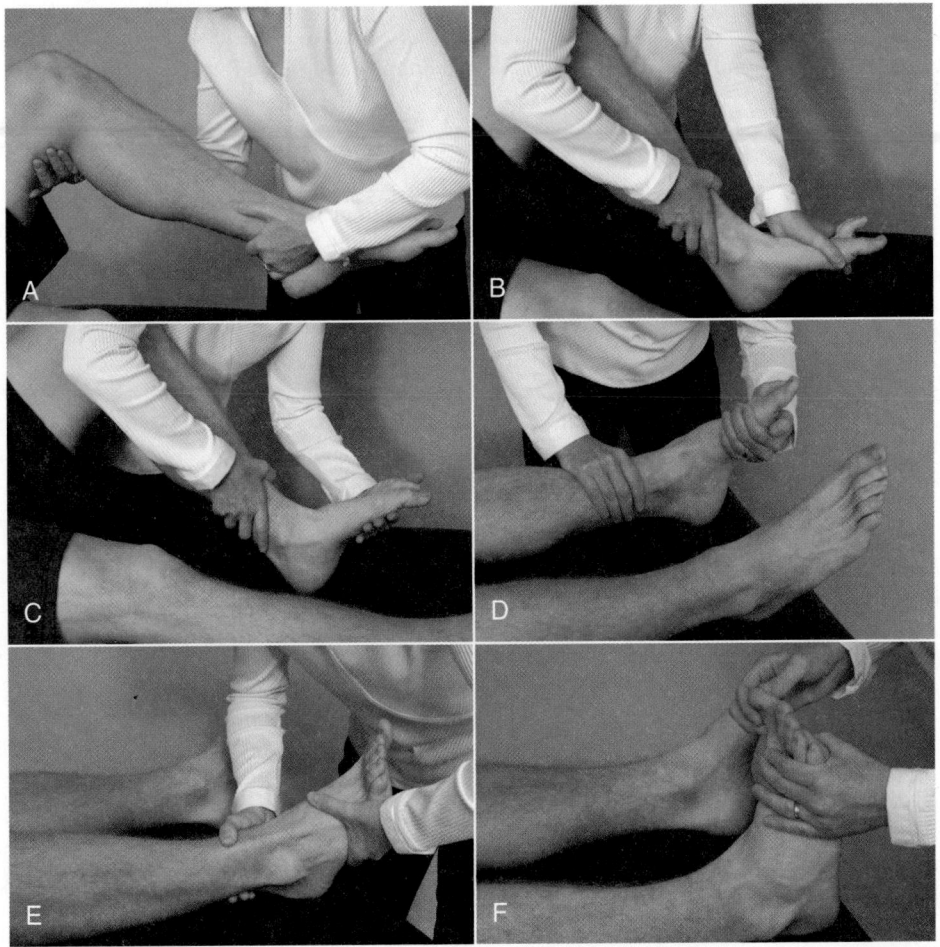

Figure 13-58 Resisted isometric movements of the lower leg, ankle, and foot. A, Knee flexion. **B,** Dorsiflexion. **C,** Plantar flexion. **D,** Supination. **E,** Pronation. **F,** Toe extension.

TABLE 13-8

Muscles of the Lower Limb, Ankle, and Foot: Their Actions, Nerve Supply, and Nerve Root Derivation (Peripheral Nerves)

Action	Muscles Acting	Nerve Supply	Nerve Root Derivation
Plantar flexion (flexion) of ankle	1. Gastocnemius*	Tibial	S1, S2
	2. Soleus*	Tibial	S1, S2
	3. Plantaris	Tibial	S1, S2
	4. Flexor digitorum longus	Tibial	S2, S3
	5. Peroneus longus	Superficial peroneal	L5, S1, S2
	6. Peroneus brevis	Superficial peroneal	L5, S1, S2
	7. Flexor hallucis longus	Tibial	S2, S3
	8. Tibialis posterior	Tibial	L4, L5
Dorsiflexion (extension) of ankle	1. Tibialis anterior	Deep peroneal	L4, L5
	2. Extensor digitorum longus	Deep peroneal	L5, S1
	3. Extensor hallucis longus	Deep peroneal	L5, S1
	4. Peroneus tertius	Deep peroneal	L5, S1
Inversion	1. Tibialis posterior	Tibial	L4, L5
	2. Flexor digitorum longus	Tibial	S2, S3
	3. Flexor hallucis longus	Tibial	S2, S3
	4. Tibialis anterior	Deep peroneal	L4, L5
	5. Extensor hallucis longus	Deep peroneal	L5, S1

Continued

TABLE **13-8**

Muscles of the Lower Limb, Ankle, and Foot: Their Actions, Nerve Supply, and Nerve Root Derivation (Peripheral Nerves)—cont'd

Action	Muscles Acting	Nerve Supply	Nerve Root Derivation
Eversion	1. Peroneus longus	Superficial peroneal	L5, S1, S2
	2. Peroneus brevis	Superficial peroneal	L5, S1, S2
	3. Peroneus tertius	Deep peroneal	L5, S1
	4. Extensor digitorum longus	Deep peroneal	L5, S1
Flexion of toes	1. Flexor digitorum longus	Tibial	S2, S3
	2. Flexor hallucis longus	Tibial	S2, S3
	3. Flexor digitorum brevis	Tibial (medial plantar branch)	S2, S3
	4. Flexor hallucis brevis	Tibial (medial plantar branch)	S2, S3
	5. Flexor accessorius (Quadratus plantae)	Tibial (lateral plantar branch)	S2, S3
	6. Interossei	Tibial (lateral plantar branch)	S2, S3
	7. Flexor digiti minimi brevis	Tibial (lateral plantar branch)	S2, S3
	8. Lumbricals (metatarsophalangeal joints)	Tibial (first by medial plantar branch; second through fourth by lateral plantar branch)	S2, S3
Extension of toes	1. Extensor digitorum longus	Deep peroneal	L5, S1
	2. Extensor hallucis longus	Deep peroneal	L5, S1
	3. Extensor digitorum brevis	Deep peroneal (lateral terminal branch)	S1, S2
	4. Lumbricals (interphalangeal joints)	Tibial (first by medial plantar branch; second through fourth by lateral plantar branch)	S2, S3
Abduction of toes	1. Abductor hallucis	Tibial (medial plantar branch)	S2, S3
	2. Abductor digiti minimi	Tibial (lateral plantar branch)	S2, S3
	3. Dorsal interossei	Tibial (lateral plantar branch)	S2, S3
Adduction of toes	4. Adductor hallucis	Tibial (lateral plantar branch)	S2, S3
	5. Plantar interossei	Tibial (lateral plantar branch)	S2, S3

*The gastrocnemius and soleus muscles are sometimes grouped together as the triceps surae muscles.

These activities, which are examples only, must be geared to the individual patient. Older patients should not be expected to do some of the activities unless they have been doing these or similar ones in the recent past (Table 13-9). Because the functional tests place a stress on the other lower limb joints (e.g., knee, hip, sacroiliac, lumbar joints), the examiner must ensure that these joints exhibit no pathology before all of the tests are completed. On the other hand, functional tests for other joints in the lower limb (e.g., hop test for the knee) may not be sensitive enough or deficits may be too small to test ankle function.[75,76] However, Wikstrom et al.[77] felt a modified hop test (jump test) was an effective way to determine functional ankle instability. Eechaute et al.[78] likewise, found a **multiple hop test** ⚠ (Figure 13-59) to be a reliable functional test. The test involves standing on two feet, jumping forward half the height of the patient's vertical jump and landing on one leg (good leg first).

Conditions, such as vascular intermittent claudication and anterior compartment syndrome, that occur within a specific time frame must also be considered in an assessment and when considering function.[79,80]

Balance and proprioception are tested by asking the patient to stand on the unaffected leg and then on the affected leg, first with the eyes open and then with

Range of Motion Necessary at the Foot and Ankle for Selected Locomotion Activities

Descending stairs:	Full dorsiflexion (20°)
Walking:	Dorsiflexion (10°); plantar flexion (20° to 25°)

the eyes closed. Any differences in balance time or difficulty in balancing give an idea of proprioceptive ability, especially differences that occurred when the patient's eyes were closed (Figure 13-60).[81]

Kaikkonen and colleagues[82] developed a numerical scoring system to evaluate functional outcome after ankle injury (Table 13-10). The **Ankle Joint Functional Assessment Tool (AJFAT)** (Figure 13-61), the **Foot and Ankle Ability Measure (FAAM)** (Figure 13-62), the **Foot and Ankle Outcome Score (FAOS)** (Figure 13-63), and the **Foot Functional Index (FFI)** (Figure 13-64),[12,83–87] which was developed for an elderly outpatient population, are two other functional tests. Other scales have been developed for specific pathologies (e.g., fractures, osteoarthritis) about the ankle or can be applied to injuries in any part of the lower limb (e.g., Lower Extremity Function Scale (LEF) scale; see Chapter 11).[88–98]

TABLE 13-9

Functional Testing of the Foot and Ankle

Starting Position	Action	Functional Test
Standing on one leg*	Lift toes and forefeet off ground (dorsiflexion)	10 to 15 Repetitions: Functional 5 to 9 Repetitions: Functionally fair 1 to 4 Repetitions: Functionally poor 0 Repetitions: Nonfunctional
Standing on one leg*	Lift heels off ground (plantar flexion)	10 to 15 Repetitions: Functional 5 to 9 Repetitions: Functionally fair 1 to 4 Repetitions: Functionally poor 0 Repetitions: Nonfunctional
Standing on one leg*	Lift lateral aspect of foot off ground (ankle eversion)	5 to 6 Repetitions: Functional 3 to 4 Repetitions: Functionally fair 1 to 2 Repetitions: Functionally poor 0 Repetitions: Nonfunctional
Standing on one leg*	Lift medial aspect of foot off ground (ankle inversion)	5 to 6 Repetitions: Functional 3 to 4 Repetitions: Functionally fair 1 to 2 Repetitions: Functionally poor 0 Repetitions: Nonfunctional
Seated	Pull small towel up under toes or pick up and release small object (i.e., pencil, marble, cottonball) (toe flexion)	10 to 15 Repetitions: Functional 5 to 9 Repetitions: Functionally fair 1 to 4 Repetitions: Functionally poor 0 Repetitions: Nonfunctional
Seated	Lift toes off ground (toe extension)	10 to 15 Repetitions: Functional 5 to 9 Repetitions: Functionally fair 1 to 4 Repetitions: Functionally poor 0 Repetitions: Nonfunctional

Data from Palmer ML, Epler M: Clinical assessment procedures in physical therapy, Philadelphia, 1990, JB Lippincott, pp. 308–310.
*Hand may hold something for balance only.

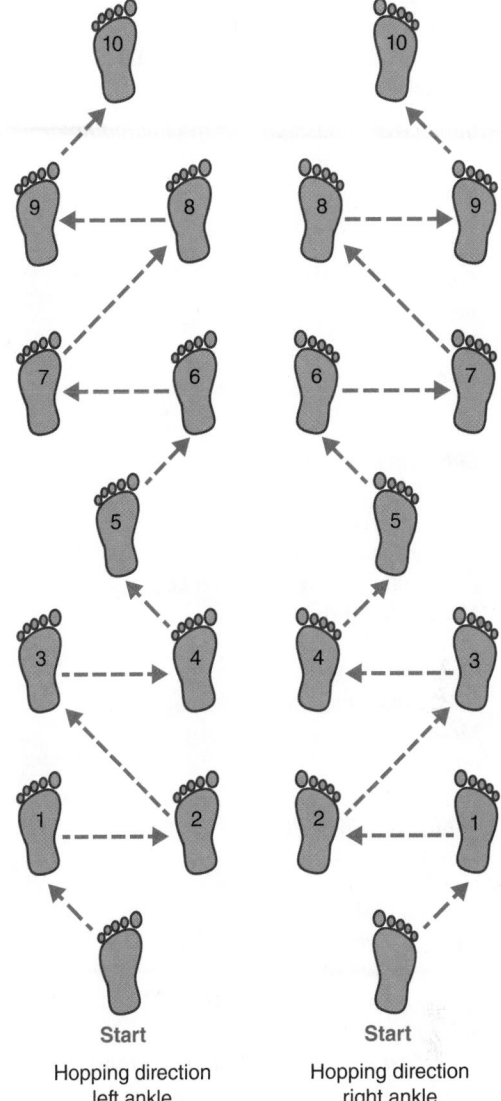

Figure 13-59 Multiple hop test. (Modified from Eechaute C, Vaes P, Duquet W: Functional performance deficits in patients with chronic ankle instability: validity of the multiple hop test. Clin J Sports Med 18:124–129, 2008.)

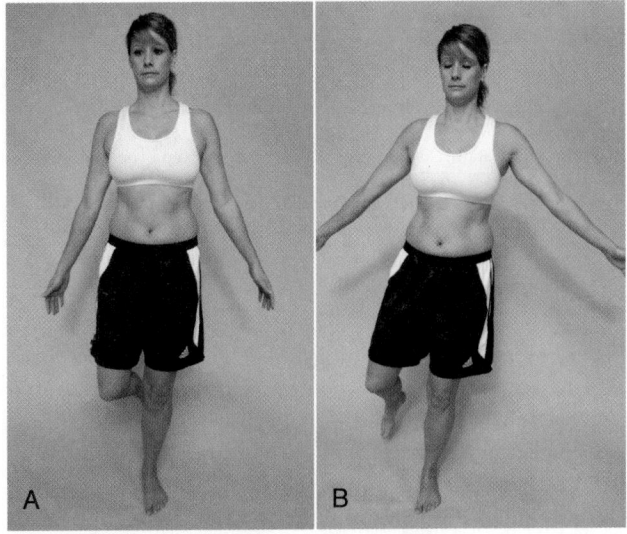

Figure 13-60 Balance and proprioception. A, One leg, with eyes open. **B,** One leg, with eyes closed.

TABLE **13-10**

Scoring Scale for Subjective and Functional Follow-Up Evaluation after Ankle Injury*

I	**Subjective Assessment of the Injured Ankle†**	
	No symptoms of any kind	15
	Mild symptoms	10
	Moderate symptoms	5
	Severe symptoms	0
II	**Can You Walk Normally?**	
	Yes	15
	No	0
III	**Can You Run Normally?**	
	Yes	10
	No	0
IV	**Climbing Down Stairs‡**	
	Less than 18 seconds	10
	18 to 20 seconds	5
	Longer than 20 seconds	0
V	**Rising on Heels with Injured Leg**	
	More than 40 times	10
	30 to 39 times	5
	Fewer than 30 times	0
VI	**Rising on Toes with Injured Leg**	
	More than 40 times	10
	30 to 39 times	5
	Fewer than 30 times	0
VII	**Single-Limbed Stance with Injured Leg§**	
	Longer than 55 seconds	10
	50 to 55 seconds	5
	Less than 50 seconds	0
VIII	**Laxity of the Ankle Joints (ADS)**	
	Stable (≤ 5 mm)	10
	Moderate instability (6 to 10 mm)	5
	Severe instability (> 10 mm)	0
IX	**Dorsiflexion Range of Motion, Injured Leg**	
	≥ 10°	10
	5° to 9°	5
	< 5°	0

From Kaikkonen A, et al: A performance test protocol and scoring scale for the evaluation of ankle injuries. Am J Sports Med 22:465, 1994.
ADS, Anterior drawer sign.
*Total: Excellent, 85–100; good, 70–80; fair, 55–65; poor, ≤ 50.
†Pain, swelling, stiffness, tenderness, or giving way during activity (mild, only one of these symptoms is present; moderate, two to three of these symptoms are present; severe, four or more of these symptoms are present).
‡Two levels of staircase (length, 12 m) with 44 steps (height, 13 cm; depth, 22 cm).
§On square beam (10 cm × 10 cm × 30 cm).

Special Tests

When assessing the lower leg, ankle, and foot, it is important to always assess the neutral position of the talus in both weight-bearing and non–weight-bearing situations. This will help the examiner to differentiate functional from structural deformities. Other tests that should be carried out include alignment, functional leg length, and tibial torsion tests. Of the other tests, only those that the examiner wishes to use as confirming tests need be performed. Special tests should never be used in isolation but can be used to confirm clinical findings.

For the reader who would like to review them, the reliability, validity, specificity, sensitivity, and odds ratios of some of the special tests used in the lower leg, ankle and foot are available on the Evolve website.

Tests for Neutral Position of the Talus

The neutral position of the talus is often referred to as the *neutral* or *balanced position* of the foot. This so-called neutral position is an ideal position that, in reality, is not commonly found in people in normal weight bearing.[26] For most patients, the subtalar joint is normally in slight valgus with the forefoot in slight varus and the calcaneus in slight valgus. The tibia is in slight varus,[99] so each joint slightly compensates for the adjacent one. The neutral position is used as a starting position to determine foot and leg deviations. When the subtalar joint is in neutral, calcaneal inversion is twice (2×) calcaneal eversion.[12,100] Functional asymmetry may occur in the lower limb in normal standing; the examiner should then put the talus in the neutral position to see whether the asymmetry remains. If it does, there is anatomical or structural asymmetry as well as functional asymmetry. If the asymmetry disappears, there is only functional asymmetry, which is often easier to treat.

⚠ *Neutral Position of the Talus (Prone—Non–Weight-Bearing Position).* The patient lies prone with the foot extended over the end of the examining table (Figure 13-65). The examiner grasps the patient's foot over the fourth and fifth metatarsal heads with the index finger and thumb of one hand. The examiner palpates both sides of the talus on the dorsum of the foot, using the thumb and index finger of the other hand. The examiner then passively and gently dorsiflexes the foot until resistance is felt (Figure 13-66). While maintaining the dorsiflexed position, the examiner moves the foot back and forth through an arc of supination (talar head bulges laterally) and pronation (talar head bulges medially). As the arc of movement is performed, there is a point in the arc at which the foot appears to fall off to one side or the other more easily. This point is the neutral, non–weight-bearing position of the subtalar joint.[32,46,58,101] This prone test position is best for determining the relation of the hindfoot to the leg.

⚠ *Neutral Position of the Talus (Supine—Non–Weight-Bearing Position).* The patient lies supine with the feet extending over the end of the examining table. The examiner grasps the patient's foot over the fourth and fifth metatarsal heads, using the thumb and index finger of one hand. The examiner palpates both sides of the head of the talus on the dorsum of the foot with the thumb and index finger of the other hand (Figure 13-67). The examiner then gently, passively dorsiflexes the foot until

1. How would you describe the level of pain you experience in your ankle?

___ (4) Much less than the other ankle
___ (3) Slightly less than the other ankle
___ (2) Equal in amount to the other ankle
___ (1) Slightly more than the other ankle
___ (0) Much more than the other ankle

2. How would you describe any swelling of your ankle?

___ (4) Much less than the other ankle
___ (3) Slightly less than the other ankle
___ (2) Equal in amount to the other ankle
___ (1) Slightly more than the other ankle
___ (0) Much more than the other ankle

3. How would you describe the ability of your ankle when walking on uneven surfaces?

___ (0) Much less than the other ankle
___ (1) Slightly less than the other ankle
___ (2) Equal in ability to the other ankle
___ (3) Slightly more than the other ankle
___ (4) Much more than the other ankle

4. How would you describe the overall feeling of stability of your ankle?

___ (0) Much less stable than the other ankle
___ (1) Slightly less stable than the other ankle
___ (2) Equal in stability to the other ankle
___ (3) Slightly more stable than the other ankle
___ (4) Much more stable than the other ankle

5. How would you describe the overall feeling of strength of your ankle?

___ (0) Much less strong than the other ankle
___ (1) Slightly less strong than the other ankle
___ (2) Equal in strength to the other ankle
___ (3) Slightly stronger than the other ankle
___ (4) Much stronger than the other ankle

6. How would you describe your ankle's ability when you descend stairs?

___ (0) Much less than the other ankle
___ (1) Slightly less than the other ankle
___ (2) Equal in amount to the other ankle
___ (3) Slightly more than the other ankle
___ (4) Much more than the other ankle

7. How would you describe your ankle's ability when you jog?

___ (0) Much less than the other ankle
___ (1) Slightly less than the other ankle
___ (2) Equal in amount to the other ankle
___ (3) Slightly more than the other ankle
___ (4) Much more than the other ankle

8. How would you describe your ankle's ability to "cut," or change direction, when running?

___ (0) Much less than the other ankle
___ (1) Slightly less than the other ankle
___ (2) Equal in amount to the other ankle
___ (3) Slightly more than the other ankle
___ (4) Much more than the other ankle

9. How would you describe the overall activity level of your ankle?

___ (0) Much less than the other ankle
___ (1) Slightly less than the other ankle
___ (2) Equal in amount to the other ankle
___ (3) Slightly more than the other ankle
___ (4) Much more than the other ankle

10. Which statement best describes your ability to sense your ankle beginning to "roll over"?

___ (0) Much later than the other ankle
___ (1) Slightly later than the other ankle
___ (2) At the same time as the other ankle
___ (3) Slightly sooner than the other ankle
___ (4) Much sooner than the other ankle

11. Compared with the other ankle, which statement best describes your ability to respond to your ankle beginning to "roll over"?

___ (0) Much later than the other ankle
___ (1) Slightly later than the other ankle
___ (2) At the same time as the other ankle
___ (3) Slightly sooner than the other ankle
___ (4) Much sooner than the other ankle

12. Following a typical incident of your ankle "rolling," which statement best describes the time required to return to activity?

___ (0) More than 2 days
___ (1) 1 to 2 days
___ (2) More than 1 hour and less than 1 day
___ (3) 15 minutes to 1 hour
___ (4) Almost immediately

Figure 13-61 Ankle Joint Functional Assessment Tool (AJFAT). (From Rozzi SL, Lephart SM, Sterner R, et al: Balance training for persons with functionally unstable ankles. J Orthop Sports Phys Ther 29:482, 1999.)

Key Tests Performed on the Lower Leg, Ankle, and Foot Depending on Suspected Pathology*

- *For determining the position of the talus:*
  - ❓ Navicular drop test
  - ⚠ Talar neutral position (non–weight-bearing) (supine and prone)
  - ⚠ Talar neutral position (weight-bearing)
- *For alignment:*
  - ⚠ Forefoot-heel alignment
  - ⚠ Leg-heel alignment
  - ⚠ Tibial torsion (prone)
  - ⚠ Tibial torsion (sitting)
  - ⚠ Tibial torsion (supine)
  - ⚠ "Too many toes" sign
- *For ligamentous instability:*
  - ✓ Anterior drawer test (supine and prone)
  - ⚠ Talar tilt

- *For joint instability (syndesmosis):*
  - ⚠ Cotton test
  - ✓ External rotation stress test
  - ⚠ Fibular translation test
  - ✓ Medial subtalar glide test
- *For third-degree strain (rupture):*
  - ⚠ Matles test
  - ⚠ Thompson's (Simmonds') test
- *For swelling:*
  - ⚠ Figure-eight measurement

*The author recommends these key tests be learned by the clinician to facilitate a diagnosis. See Chapter 1, p. 55, Key for Classifying Special Tests.

Foot and Ankle Ability Measure (FAAM)
Activities of Daily Living Subscale

Please answer every question with one response that most closely describes your condition within the past week.
If the activity in question is limited by something other than your foot or ankle, mark not applicable (N/A).

	No difficulty	Slight difficulty	Moderate difficulty	Extreme difficulty	Unable to do	N/A
Standing	☐	☐	☐	☐	☐	☐
Walking on even ground	☐	☐	☐	☐	☐	☐
Walking on even ground without shoes	☐	☐	☐	☐	☐	☐
Walking up hills	☐	☐	☐	☐	☐	☐
Walking down hills	☐	☐	☐	☐	☐	☐
Going up stairs	☐	☐	☐	☐	☐	☐
Going down stairs	☐	☐	☐	☐	☐	☐
Walking on uneven ground	☐	☐	☐	☐	☐	☐
Stepping up and down curbs	☐	☐	☐	☐	☐	☐
Squatting	☐	☐	☐	☐	☐	☐
Coming up on your toes	☐	☐	☐	☐	☐	☐
Walking initially	☐	☐	☐	☐	☐	☐
Walking 5 minutes or less	☐	☐	☐	☐	☐	☐
Walking approximately 10 minutes	☐	☐	☐	☐	☐	☐
Walking 15 minutes or greater	☐	☐	☐	☐	☐	☐

Because of your foot and ankle, how much difficulty do you have with:

	No difficulty at all	Slight difficulty	Moderate difficulty	Extreme difficulty	Unable to do	N/A
Home responsibilities	☐	☐	☐	☐	☐	☐
Activities of daily living	☐	☐	☐	☐	☐	☐
Personal care	☐	☐	☐	☐	☐	☐
Light to moderate work (standing, walking)	☐	☐	☐	☐	☐	☐
Heavy work (push/pulling, climbing, carrying)	☐	☐	☐	☐	☐	☐
Recreational activities	☐	☐	☐	☐	☐	☐

How would you rate your current level of function during your usual activities of daily living from 0 to 100 with 100 being your level of function prior to your foot or ankle problem and 0 being the inability to perform any of your usual daily activities?

☐ ☐ ☐ .0%

A

Foot and Ankle Ability Measure (FAAM)
Sports Subscale

Because of your foot and ankle, how much difficulty do you have with:

	No difficulty at all	Slight difficulty	Moderate difficulty	Extreme difficulty	Unable to do	N/A
Running	☐	☐	☐	☐	☐	☐
Jumping	☐	☐	☐	☐	☐	☐
Lunging	☐	☐	☐	☐	☐	☐
Starting and stopping quickly	☐	☐	☐	☐	☐	☐
Cutting/lateral movements	☐	☐	☐	☐	☐	☐
Low impact activities	☐	☐	☐	☐	☐	☐
Ability to perform activity with your normal technique	☐	☐	☐	☐	☐	☐
Ability to participate in your desired sport as long as you would like	☐	☐	☐	☐	☐	☐

How would you rate your current level of function during your sports related activities from 0 to 100 with 100 being your level of function prior to your foot or ankle problem and 0 being the inability to perform any of your usual daily activities?

☐ ☐ ☐ .0%

Overall, how would you rate your current level of function?

☐ Normal   ☐ Nearly normal   ☐ Abnormal   ☐ Severely abnormal

B

Figure 13-62 Foot and Ankle Ability Measure (FAAM). A, Activities of daily living subscale. **B,** Sports subscale. (From Martin RL, Irrgang JJ, Burdett RG, et al: Evidence of validity for the foot and ankle ability measure [FAAM]. Foot Ankle Int 26[11]:982–983, 2005.)

resistance is felt. While the examiner maintains the dorsiflexion, the foot is passively moved through an arc of supination (talar head bulges laterally) and pronation (talar head bulges medially). If the foot is positioned so that the talar head does not appear to bulge to either side, the subtalar joint will be in its neutral non–weight-bearing position.[32,46,58,101] This supine test position is best for determining the relation of the forefoot to the hindfoot.

⚠ *Neutral Position of the Talus (Weight-Bearing Position).* The patient stands with the feet in a relaxed standing position so that the base width and Fick angle are normal for the patient. Usually, only one foot is tested at a time. The examiner palpates the head of the talus on the dorsal aspect of the foot with the thumb and forefinger of one hand (Figure 13-68). The patient slowly rotates the trunk to the right and then to the left, which causes the tibia to medially and laterally rotate so that the

PAIN

P1. How often do you experience foot/ankle pain?   Never, Monthly, Weekly, Daily, Always
     What amount of pain have you experienced the
     last week during the following activities?

P2. Twisting/pivoting on your foot/ankle   None, Mild, Moderate, Severe, Extreme
P3. Straightening foot/ankle fully
P4. Bending foot/ankle fully
P5. Walking on flat surface
P6. Going up or down stairs
P7. At night while in bed
P8. Sitting or lying
P9. Standing upright

OTHER SYMPTOMS

S1. How severe is your foot/ankle stiffness after first   None, Mild, Moderate, Severe, Extreme
     wakening in the morning?
S2. How severe is your foot/ankle stiffness after
     sitting, lying, or resting later in the day?
Sy1. Do you have swelling in your foot/ankle?   Never, Rarely, Sometimes, Often, Always
Sy2. Do you feel grinding, hear clicking or any
     other type of noise when your foot/ankle moves?
Sy3. Does your foot/ankle catch or hang up when
     moving?
Sy4. Can you straighten your foot/ankle fully?   Always, Often, Sometimes, Rarely, Never
Sy5. Can you bend your foot/ankle fully?

ACTIVITIES OF DAILY LIVING

What difficulty have you experienced in the last week:

A1. Descending stairs   None, Mild, Moderate, Severe, Extreme
A2. Ascending stairs
A3. Rising from sitting
A4. Standing
A5. Bending to floor/pick up an object
A6. Walking on flat surface
A7. Getting in/out of car
A8. Going shopping
A9. Putting on socks/stockings
A10. Rising from bed
A11. Taking off socks/stockings
A12. Lying in bed (turning over, maintaining foot/ankle position)
A13. Getting in/out of bath
A14. Sitting
A15. Getting on/off toilet
A16. Heavy domestic duties (moving heavy boxes, scrubbing
     floors, etc.)
A17. Light domestic duties (cooking, dusting, etc.)

SPORT AND RECREATION FUNCTION

What difficulty have you experienced in the last week:

Sp1. Squatting   None, Mild, Moderate, Severe, Extreme
Sp2. Running
Sp3. Jumping
Sp4. Turning/twisting on your injured foot/ankle
Sp5. Kneeling

FOOT- AND ANKLE-RELATED QUALITY OF LIFE

Q1. How often are you aware of your foot/ankie problems?   Never, Monthly, Weekly, Daily, Always
Q2. Have you modified your life style to avoid potentially Not at all, Mildly, Moderately, Severly, Totally
     damaging activities to your foot/ankle?
Q3. Do you lack confidence in your ankle when doing activities? Not at all, Mildly, Moderately, Severly, Extremely
Q4. In general, how much difficulty do you have with your
     foot/ankle?   None, Mild, Moderate, Severe, Extreme

Figure 13-63 Foot and Ankle Outcome Score (FAOS). The 42 FAOS items arranged in the five subscales: 1) pain, 2) other symptoms, 3) activities of daily living, 4) sport and recreation function, and 5) foot- and ankle-related quality of life. The five answer options are given after each item. **In cases where several following items have identical answer options, the answer options are only given for the first item.** (Modified from Roos EM, Brandsson S, Karlsson J: Validation of the foot and ankle outcome scure for ankle ligament reconstruction. Foot Ankle Int 22[10]:790, 2001.)

A. Foot Pain Subscale
The line below each item represents the amount of pain you had during the past week performing an activity because of your foot condition. On the far left is "no pain," and on the far right is "worst pain imaginable." Place a vertical mark on the line to indicate how much pain you had performing each activity because of your feet during the past week. If you did not perform an activity during the past week, mark that item N/A.

How severe is your foot pain?

Foot pain at worst:
No pain _____ Worst pain imaginable

Foot pain in morning:
No pain _____ Worst pain imaginable

Pain walking barefoot:
No pain _____ Worst pain imaginable

Pain standing barefoot:
No pain _____ Worst pain imaginable

Pain walking with shoes:
No pain _____ Worst pain imaginable

Pain standing with shoes:
No pain _____ Worst pain imaginable

Pain walking with orthotics:
No pain _____ Worst pain imaginable

Pain standing with orthotics:
No pain _____ Worst pain imaginable

Foot pain end of day:
No pain _____ Worst pain imaginable

B. Foot Function Index Disability Subscale
The line below each item represents the amount of difficulty you had during the past week performing an activity because of your foot condition. On the far left is "no difficulty," and on the far right is "so difficult unable." Place a vertical mark on the line to indicate how much difficulty you had performing each activity because of your feet during the past week. If you did not perform an activity during the past week, mark that item N/A.

How much difficulty did you have?

Walking around the house:
No difficulty _____ So difficult, unable to do

Walking outside on uneven ground:
No difficulty _____ So difficult, unable to do

Walking four or more blocks:
No difficulty _____ So difficult, unable to do

Climbing stairs:
No difficulty _____ So difficult, unable to do

Descending stairs:
No difficulty _____ So difficult, unable to do

Standing on tip toe:
No difficulty _____ So difficult, unable to do

Getting out of a chair:
No difficulty _____ So difficult, unable to do

Climbing up or down curbs:
No difficulty _____ So difficult, unable to do

Walking fast or running:
No difficulty _____ So difficult, unable to do

Figure 13-64 Foot function index. (Data from Budiman-Mak E, Conrad KJ, Roach KE: The foot function index: a measure of foot pain and disability, J Clin Epidemiol 44:561–570, 1991.)

C. Activity Limitation Subscale
The line below each item represents the amount of activity that you were able to do during the past week relative to several questions.
On the far left is "no restriction," and on the far right is "no activity." Place a vertical mark on the line to indicate how much your foot enabled you to do during the past week in response to each of the questions. If a particular question does not apply, mark that item N/A.

Stayed inside all day because of feet:
No restriction _____ No activity

Stayed in bed all day because of feet:
No restriction _____ No activity

Limited activities because of feet:
No restriction _____ No activity

Used assistive device indoors:
No restriction _____ No activity

Used assistive device outdoors:
No restriction _____ No activity

Figure 13-64, cont'd

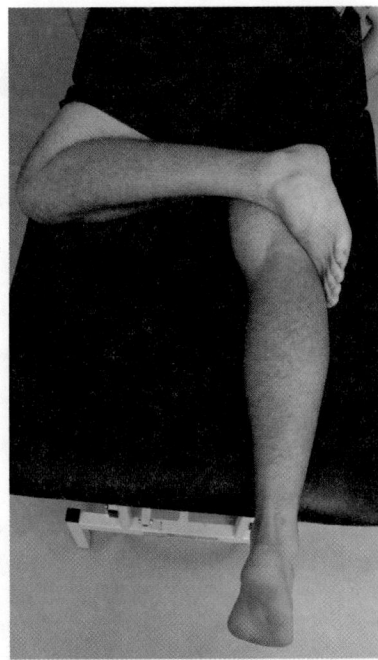

Figure 13-65 Prone lying with leg, which is not being assessed, in figure-4 position to allow easier assessment of the neutral position of the right subtalar joint.

talus supinates and pronates. If the foot is positioned so that the talar head does not appear to bulge to either side, then the subtalar joint will be in its neutral position in weight-bearing.[46] Mueller, et al.[102] described a progression of the neutral talus position in standing called the **navicular drop test** ❓ to quantify midfoot mobility and its effect on other parts of the kinetic chain.[103] Using a small rigid ruler, the examiner first measures the height of the navicular from the floor in the neutral talus position using the most prominent part of the navicular tuberosity and then measures the height of the navicular in normal relaxed standing (Figure 13-69, *A* and *B*). The difference is called the *navicular drop* and indicates the amount of

foot pronation or flattening of the medial longitudinal arch during standing (Figure 13-69, *C*).[103,104] Any measurement greater than 10 mm is considered abnormal. Experience in measuring is necessary to ensure reliable measures.[105] The test does not measure the amount of deformation that occurs with functional activities, such as walking or running.[106]

Tests for Alignment

Alignment tests are used to determine the relation of the leg to the hindfoot and the relation of the hindfoot to the forefoot.[107] These tests are used to differentiate functional from anatomical (structural) deformities or asymmetries.

❓ *Coleman Block Test.*[108] This test differentiates a hindfoot varus resulting from a forefoot valgus from a hindfoot varus resulting from a tight tibialis posterior. If the patient is found to have a hindfoot varus in standing, the examiner places a lift or block under the lateral side of the forefoot. If the hindfoot varus is corrected, it indicates the hindfoot is flexible and the hindfoot varus is due to a plantar flexed first ray or a valgus forefoot (Figure 13-70). If it does not correct, the tibialis posterior is tight.

⚠️ *Forefoot-Heel Alignment.* The patient lies supine with the feet extending over the end of the examining table. The examiner positions the subtalar joint in supine neutral position. While maintaining this position, the examiner pronates the midtarsal joints maximally and then observes the relation between the vertical axis of the heel and the plane of the second through fourth metatarsal heads (Figure 13-71). Normally, the plane is perpendicular to the vertical axis. If the medial side of the foot is raised, the patient has a forefoot varus; if the lateral side of the foot is raised, the patient has a forefoot valgus.[32,101]

⚠️ *Leg-Heel Alignment.* The patient lies in the prone position with the foot extending over the end of the examining table. The examiner places a mark over the

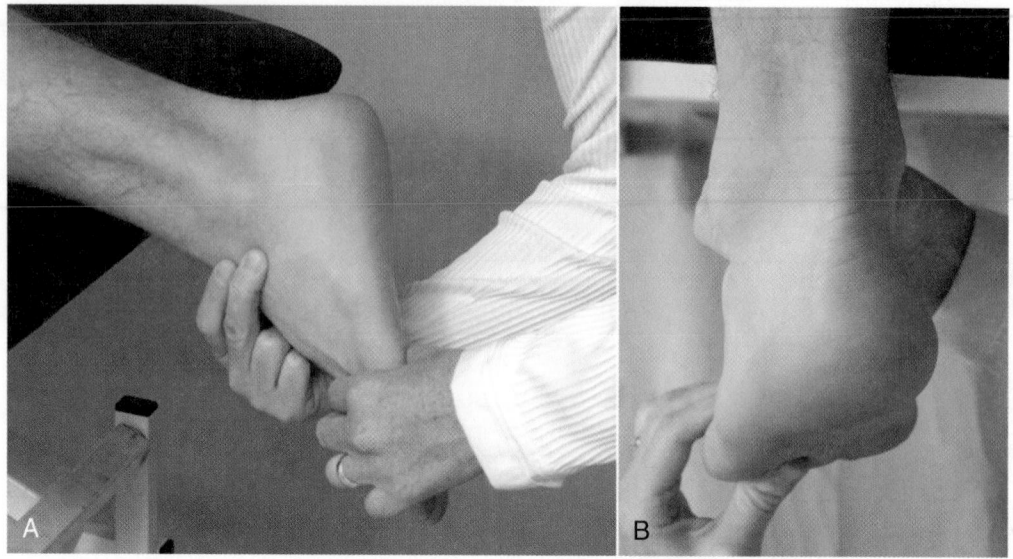

Figure 13-66 Determining the neutral position of the subtalar joints in the prone position. **A,** Side view. **B,** Superior view.

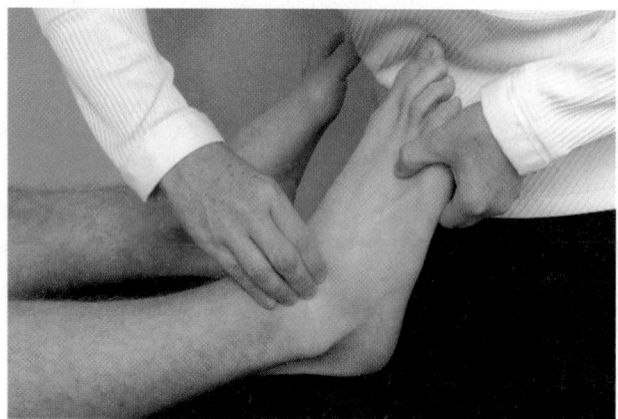

Figure 13-67 Determining the neutral position of the subtalar joint in supine position.

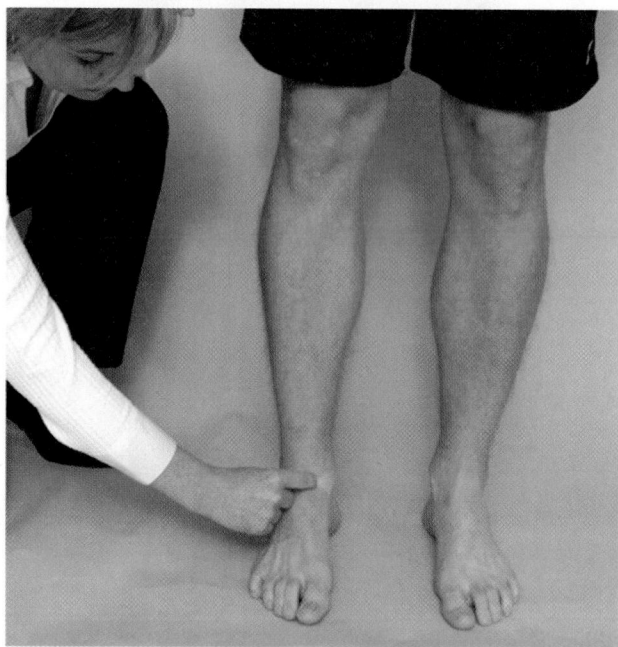

Figure 13-68 Determining the neutral position of the subtalar joint in standing (weight bearing).

midline of the calcaneus at the insertion of the Achilles tendon. The examiner makes a second mark approximately 1 cm distal to the first mark and as close to the midline of the calcaneus as possible. A **calcaneal line** is then made to join the two marks. Next, the examiner makes two marks on the lower third of the leg in the midline. These two marks are joined, forming the **tibial line,** which represents the longitudinal axis of the tibia. The examiner then places the subtalar joint in the prone neutral position. While the subtalar joint is held in neutral, the examiner looks at the two lines. If the lines are parallel or in slight varus (2° to 8°), the leg-to-heel alignment is considered normal.[101] If the heel is inverted, the patient has hindfoot varus; if the heel is everted, the patient has hindfoot valgus (Figure 13-72).

Tests for Tibial Torsion

When testing for tibial torsion, the examiner must realize that some lateral tibial torsion (13° to 18° in adults, less

in children) is normally present.[109] If tibial torsion is more than 18°, it is referred to as a *toe-out position.* If tibial torsion is less than 13°, it is referred to as a *toe-in position.* Excessive toeing-in is sometimes referred to as pigeon toes and may be caused by medial tibial torsion, medial femoral torsion, or excessive femoral anteversion (see Table 13-2).

    ▲ *Tibial Torsion (Prone).* The patient lies prone with the knee flexed to 90°. The examiner views from above the angle formed by the foot and thigh (Figure 13-73) after the subtalar joint has been placed in the neutral

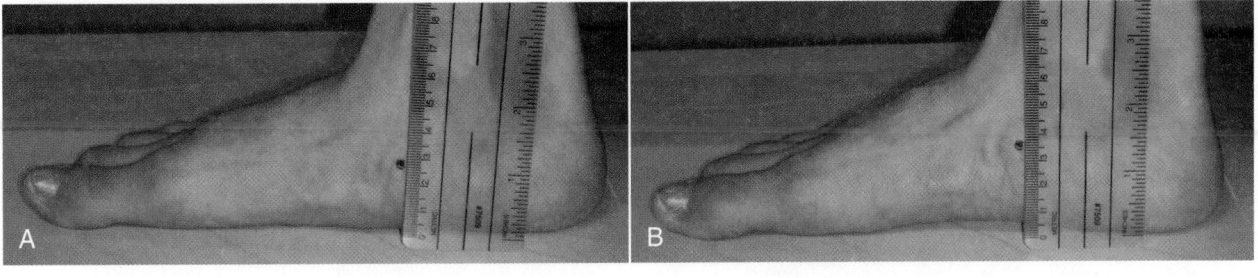

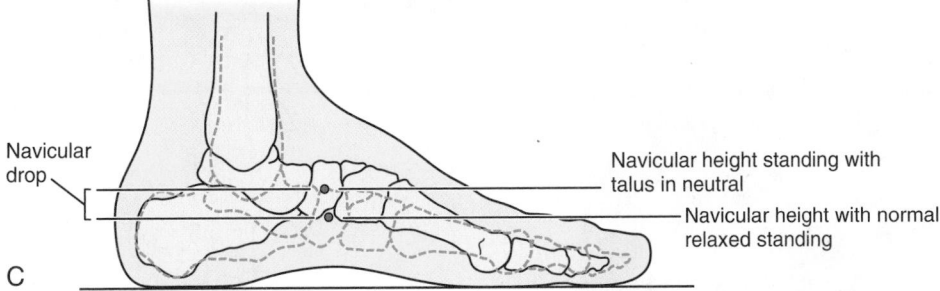

Figure 13-69 Navicular drop test. "Drop" is the difference in height between the navicular height in standing relaxed (**A**) and standing with talus in neutral (**B**). **C,** Illustration of two different foot positions required for navicular drop measurement.

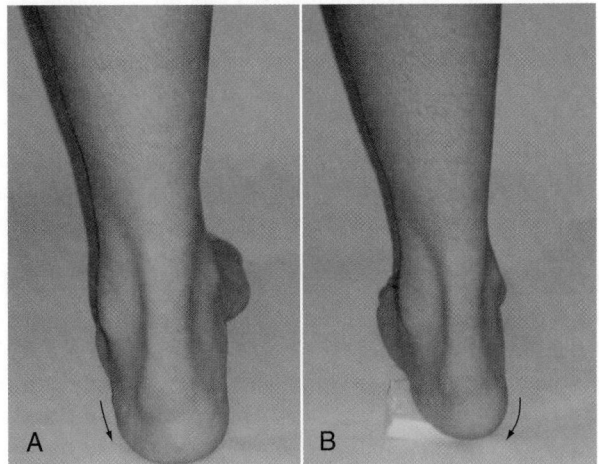

Figure 13-70 Coleman block test. A, On initial examination, the hindfoot is in varus. **B,** The patient stands with a book or block under the lateral side of the forefoot, and the hindfoot is reexamined. Heel varus correction indicates that the hindfoot deformity is flexible and that the varus position is secondary to the plantarflexed first ray, or valgus position of the forefoot.

position, noting the angle the foot makes with the tibia.[110] This method is most often used in children, because it is easier to observe the feet from above.

⚠ *Tibial Torsion (Sitting).* Tibial torsion is measured by having the patient sit with the knees flexed to 90° over the edge of the examining table (Figure 13-74). The examiner places the thumb of one hand over the apex of one malleolus and the index finger of the same hand over the apex of the other malleolus. Next, the examiner visualizes the axes of the knee and of the ankle. The lines are not normally parallel but instead form an angle of 12° to 18° owing to lateral rotation of the tibia.[25]

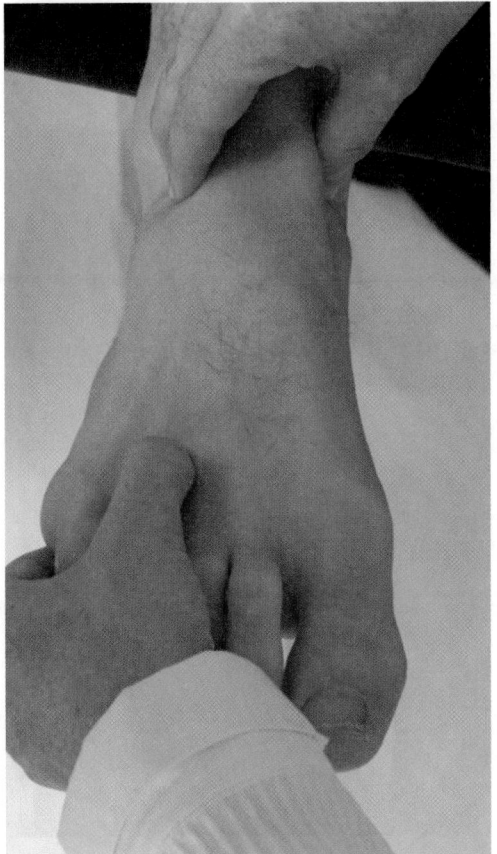

Figure 13-71 Alignment of forefoot and heel (superior view).

⚠ *Tibial Torsion (Supine).* The patient lies supine. The examiner ensures that the femoral condyle lies in the frontal plane (patella facing straight up). The examiner palpates the apex of both malleoli with one hand and draws a line on the heel representing a line joining the

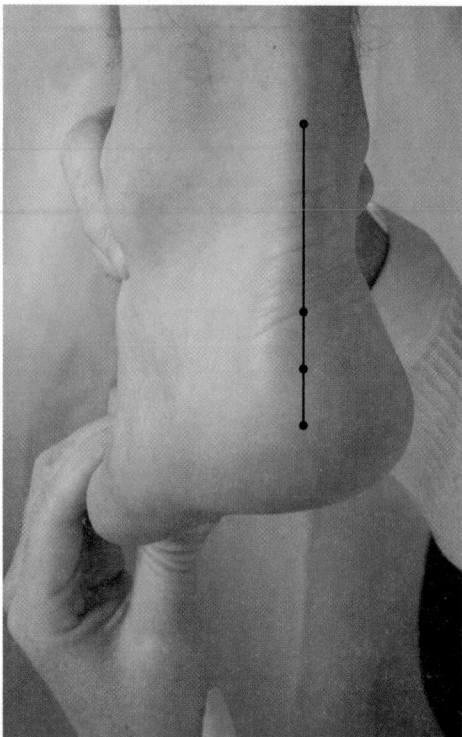

Figure 13-72 Alignment of leg and heel.

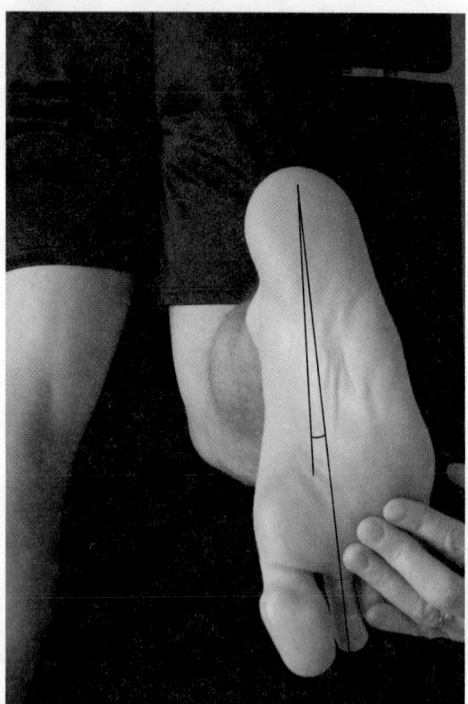

Figure 13-73 Measurement of tibial torsion in the prone position.

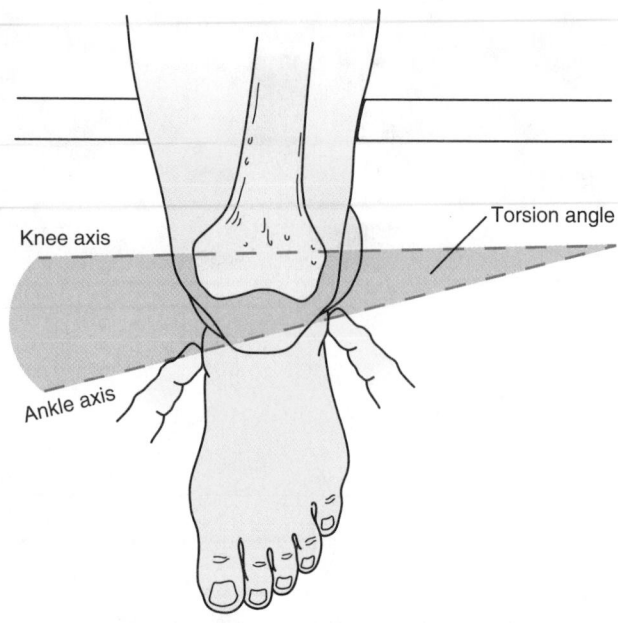

Figure 13-74 **Determination of tibial torsion in sitting (superior view).** The torsion angle (normal: 12° to 18°) determined by the intersection of the knee axis and the ankle axis. (Modified from Hunt GC, editor: Physical therapy of the foot and ankle, clinics in physical therapy, New York, 1988, Churchill Livingstone, p. 80.)

two apices. A second line is drawn on the heel parallel to the floor. The angle formed by the intersection of the two lines indicates the amount of lateral tibial torsion.

▲ *"Too Many Toes" Sign.* The patient stands in a normal relaxed position while the examiner views the patient from behind. If the heel is in valgus, the forefoot abducted, or the tibia laterally rotated more than normal (tibial torsion), the examiner can see more toes on the affected side than on the normal side (Figure 13-75).[111] Similarly, lateral femoral torsion could cause the "too many toes" test to be positive. If the talus is positioned in neutral and the calcaneus is in neutral, the "too many toes" sign means the forefoot is adducted on the rearfoot and may be seen with excessive pronation (hyperpronation).[66,112] Hyperpronation is often associated with metatarsalgia, plantar fasciitis, hallux valgus, and posterior tibial tendon pathology.[66]

Tests for Ligamentous Instability

✓ *Anterior Drawer Test of the Ankle.* This test is designed primarily to test for injuries to the anterior talofibular ligament, the most frequently injured ligament in the ankle.[113-115] The patient lies supine with the foot relaxed. The examiner stabilizes the tibia and fibula, holds the patient's foot in 20° of plantar flexion, and draws the talus forward in the ankle mortise (Figure 13-76).[116-119] Sometimes, a dimple appears over the area of the anterior talofibular ligament on anterior translation (**dimple** or **suction sign**) if pain and muscle spasm are minimal.[120-122] In the plantar-flexed position, the anterior talofibular ligament is perpendicular to the long axis of the tibia. By adding inversion, which gives an anterolateral stress, the examiner can increase the stress on the anterior talofibular ligament and the calcaneofibular ligament. A positive anterior drawer test may be obtained with a tear of only the anterior talofibular ligament, but anterior translation is greater if both ligaments are torn, especially if the foot is tested in dorsiflexion.[123] If straight anterior movement or translation occurs (Figure 13-77, *B*), the test indicates both medial and lateral ligament insufficiencies. This bilateral finding, which is often more evident in dorsiflexion, means that the superficial and deep deltoid ligaments, as well as the anterior talofibular ligament and anterolateral capsule, have been torn. If the tear is on only one side, only that side would translate forward. For example, with a lateral tear, the lateral side would translate forward, causing medial rotation of the talus and resulting in anterolateral rotary instability (Figure 13-77, *C*), which is increasingly evident with growing plantar flexion of the foot.[30,33,124-126]

Ideally, the knee should be placed in 90° of flexion to alleviate tension on the Achilles tendon. The test should be performed in plantar flexion and in dorsiflexion to test for straight and rotational instabilities.

The test may also be performed by stabilizing the foot and talus and pushing the tibia and fibula posteriorly on the talus (Figure 13-76, *B*). In this case, excessive posterior movement of the tibia and fibula on the talus indicates a positive test.

⚠ *Cotton Test (Lateral Stress Test).*[12,127,128] This test is used to assess for syndesmosis instability caused by separation of the tibia and fibula (diastasis). The two bones are normally held together by four ligaments (the tibiofibular

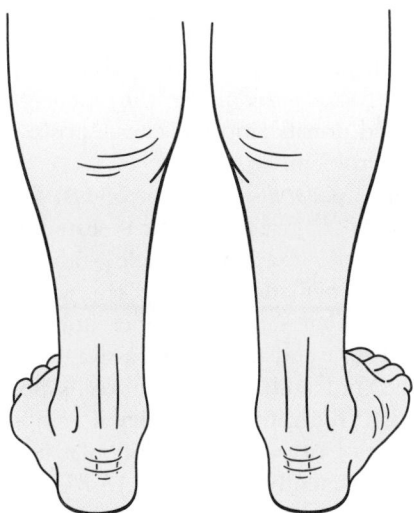

Figure 13-75 "Too-many-toes" sign signifying lateral foot or tibial rotation. Two-and-one-half toes shown on the left foot, four toes on the abnormal right foot. (Redrawn from Baxter DE, editor: The foot and ankle in sport, St Louis, 1995, Mosby, p. 45.)

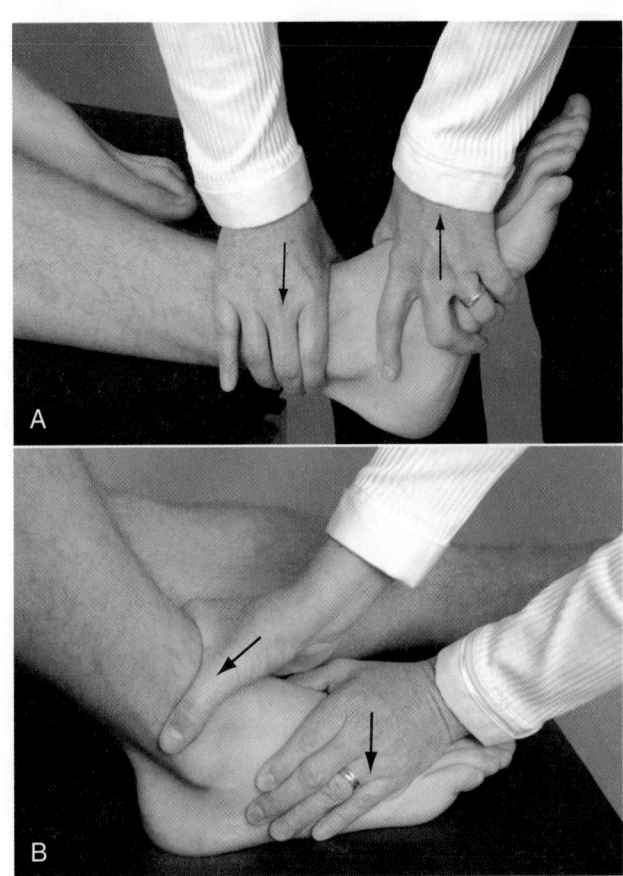

Figure 13-76 Anterior drawer test. **A,** Method 1—drawing the foot forward. **B,** Method 2—pushing the leg back.

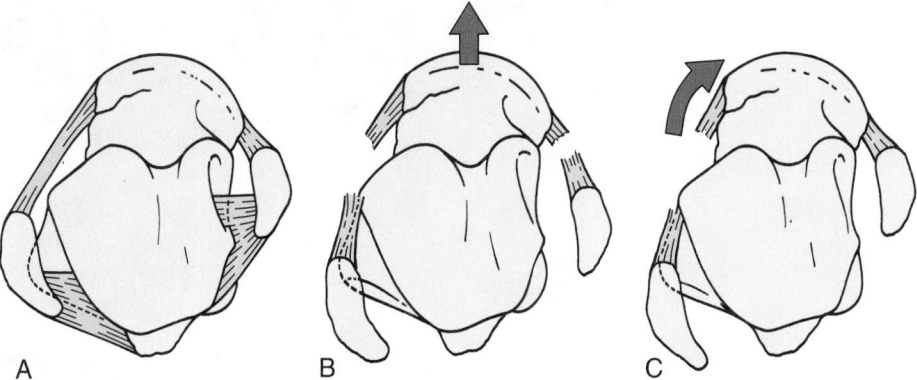

Figure 13-77 Anterior drawer test. **A,** Normal relation between talus and malleoli. **B,** Straight anterior translation (one-plane anterior instability). **C,** Lateral rotary translation (anterolateral rotary instability).

interosseous ligament, anteroinferior tibiofibular ligament, posteroinferior tibiofibular ligament, and transverse tibiofibular ligament).[129] The examiner stabilizes the distal tibia and fibula with one hand and applies a lateral translation force (not an eversion force) with the other hand to the foot.[12] Any lateral translation (more than 3 to 5 mm) or clunk indicates syndesmotic instability.[12,130] Stoffel, et al.[131] felt this test was better than the lateral rotation stress test for determining syndesmodic instability on stress x-ray. If the examiner applies a medial translation force, the test is called the **medial subtalar glide test** ☑.

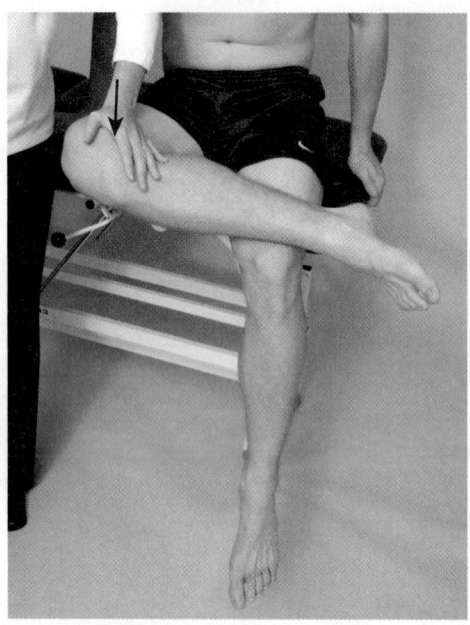

Figure 13-78 Crossed-leg test. The patient sits in a chair, with the injured leg resting across the knee of the uninjured leg. The examiner applies a gentle force on the medial knee of the injured leg.

? *Crossed Leg Test.*[132,133] The patient sits in a chair with the affected leg crossed over the opposite knee so the midpoint of the fibula is resting on the opposite knee (Figure 13-78). The examiner then applies a gentle force to the medial aspect of the knee of the injured leg. If the patient experiences pain in the area of the distal syndesmosis, it indicates a positive test.

? *Dorsiflexion Compression Test.*[132,134] While in bilateral weight-bearing, the patient is asked to move his or her ankle into extreme dorsiflexion (Figure 13-79, *A*). The patient is asked to note whether this maneuver is painful while the examiner notes the end ROM. The patient then assumes a normal standing position again. The examiner applies a compression force using two hands surrounding the malleoli of the injured leg. While this compression is maintained, the patient is asked to move into dorsiflexion again (Figure 13-79, *B*). A decrease in pain on dorsiflexion or an increase in dorsiflexion range indicates a positive test.

? *Dorsiflexion Maneuver.*[132,135,136] The patient sits on the edge of the table. The examiner stabilizes the patient's leg with one hand and with the other hand passively and forcefully dorsiflexes the foot by holding onto the heel and using the forearm to dorsiflex the foot (Figure 13-80). Pain on forced dorsiflexion indicates a positive test for a syndesmosis problem.

☑ *External (Lateral) Rotation Stress Test (Kleiger Test).*[115,122,127,132,134,137–139] The patient is seated with the leg hanging over the examining table with the knee at 90°. The examiner stabilizes the leg with one hand. With the other hand, the examiner holds the foot in plantigrade (90°) and applies a passive lateral rotation stress to the foot and ankle. The test is positive for a **syndesmosis ("high ankle") injury** if pain is produced over the anterior or posterior tibiofibular ligaments and the interosseous membrane (Figure 13-81). If the patient

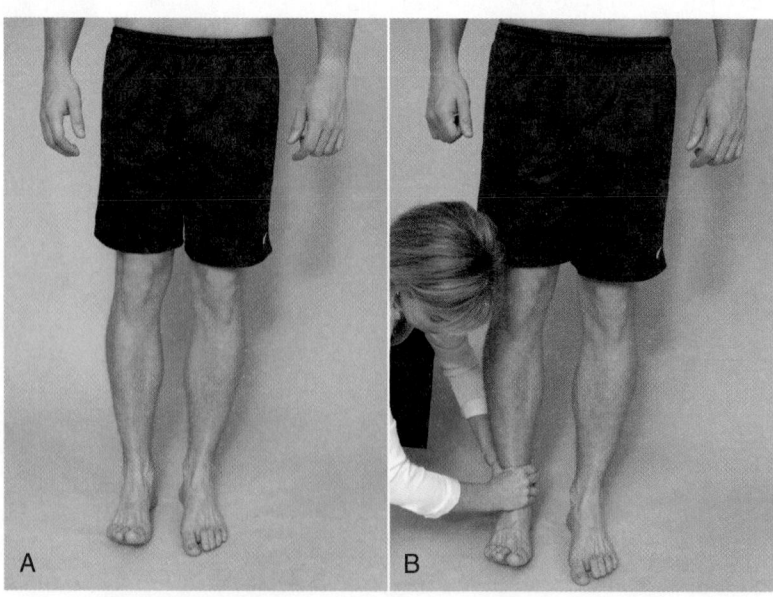

Figure 13-79 Dorsiflexion compression test. A, Step 1: Patient dorsiflexes feet while standing. **B,** Step 2: Patient dorsiflexes feet while examiner squeezes malleoli together.

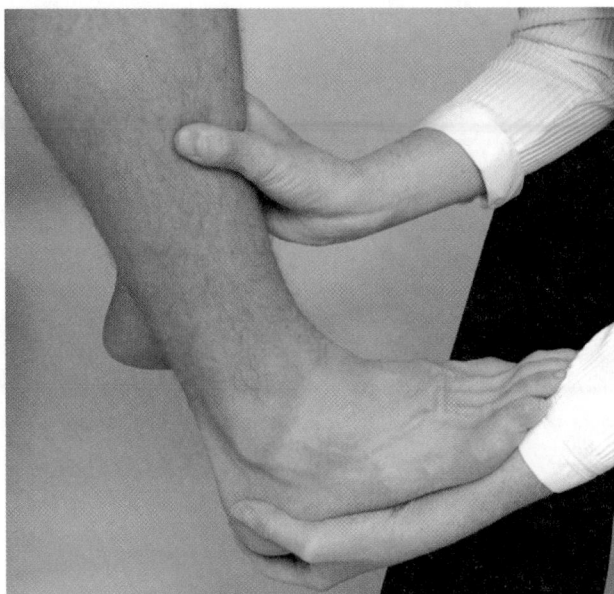

Figure 13-80 Dorsiflexion maneuver. The examiner stabilizes the leg with one hand and passively moves the foot toward dorsiflexion with the other hand using the forearm.

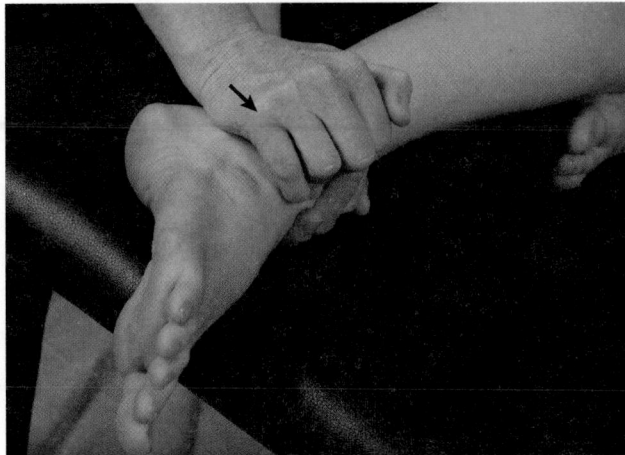

Figure 13-82 Fibular translation test showing anterior translation.

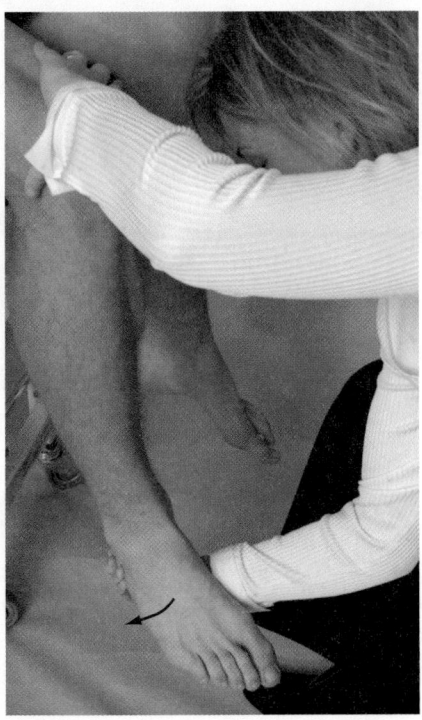

Figure 13-81 External rotation stress test.

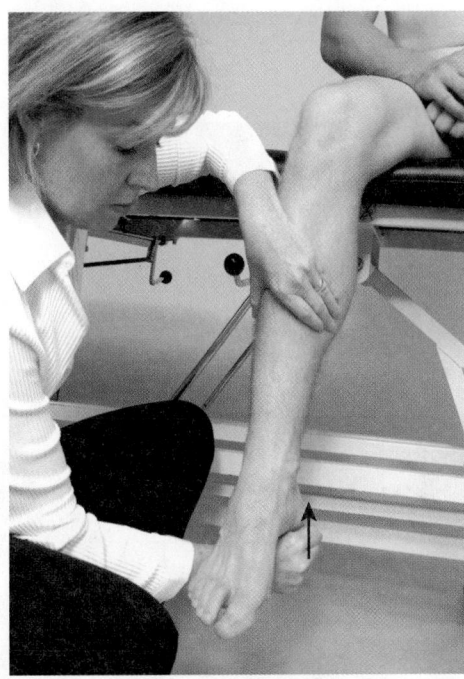

Figure 13-83 Heel thump test. The examiner holds the patient's leg with one hand and with the other hand applies a gentle but firm thump on the heel with the fist.

has pain medially and the examiner feels the talus displace from the medial malleolus, it may indicate a tear of the deltoid ligament. On a stress radiograph, if the medial clear space is increased (see Figure 13-129), it suggests rupture of the ligament (see the discussion in the Diagnostic Imaging section) if the lateral malleolus is intact.

Fibular Translation Test.[140,141] The patient is in sidelying. The examiner faces the foot to be examined from the front and stabilizes the tibia with one hand and translates the fibular malleolus anteriorly and posteriorly with the other hand (Figure 13-82). If pain occurs during the translation or if the movement is greater on the affected side, the test is considered positive for a syndesmosis injury.

Heel Thump Test.[132,142] The patient is in sitting or lying. The examiner uses one hand to stabilize the leg. With the other hand, the examiner applies a firm thump on the heel with the fist so that the force is applied to the center of the heel and in line with the long axis of the tibia (Figure 13-83). A positive test (i.e., pain) in the area of the ankle indicates a syndesmosis injury. Pain along the shaft of the tibia may indicate a stress fracture.

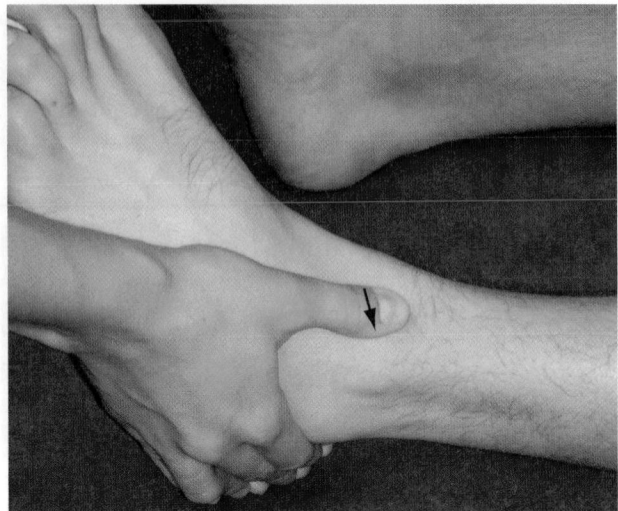

Figure 13-84 Point (palpation) test. The examiner applies pressure over the anterior aspect of the distal tibiofibular syndesmosis.

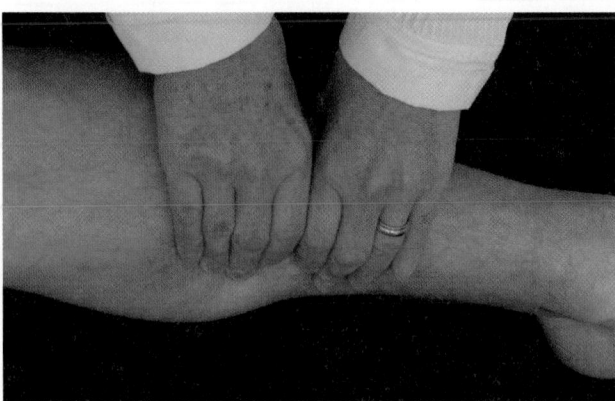

Figure 13-86 Squeeze test for stress fracture or ankle syndesmosis pathology.

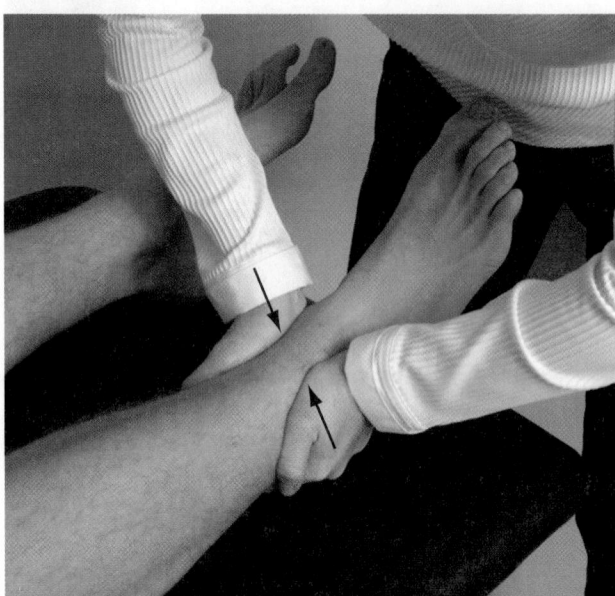

Figure 13-87 Distal tibiofibular compression test.

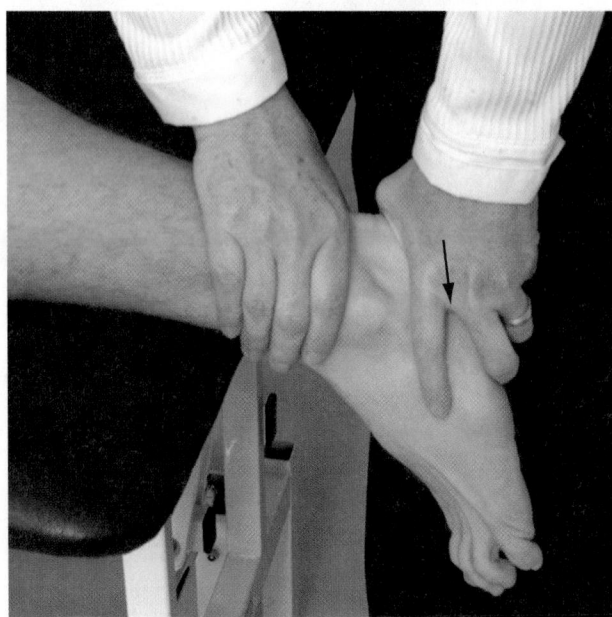

Figure 13-85 Prone anterior drawer test.

❓ Point (Palpation) Test.[35,132,134] The patient is positioned in sitting or supine. The examiner then applies a gradual pressure over the anteroinferior tibiofibular ligament (anterior aspect of the distal tibia fibular syndesmosis) using the index finger (Figure 13-84). Pain in the syndesmosis area indicates a positive test.

✓ Prone Anterior Drawer Test.[143] The patient lies prone with the feet extending over the end of the examining table. With one hand, the examiner pushes the heel steadily forward (Figure 13-85). Excessive anterior movement and a sucking in of the skin on both sides of the Achilles tendon indicate a positive sign. The test, like the

previous one, indicates ligamentous instability, primarily the anterior talofibular ligament.

❓ Squeeze Test of the Leg. The patient lies supine. The examiner grasps the lower leg at midcalf and squeezes the tibia and fibula together (Figure 13-86). The examiner then applies the same load at more distal locations moving toward the ankle. Pain in the lower leg may indicate a syndesmosis injury, provided that fracture, contusion, and compartment syndrome have been ruled out.[14,115,127,134,144,145] Brosky and associates called this test the **distal tibiofibular compression test** and applied the compression over the malleoli rather than the shaft of the tibia and fibula (Figure 13-87).[136] Nussbaum, et al.[137] reported that the "length of tenderness" above the lateral malleolus indicates severity.

⚠ Talar Tilt. The patient lies in the supine or side lying position with the foot relaxed (Figure 13-88).[30,146] The patient's gastrocnemius muscle may be relaxed by flexion

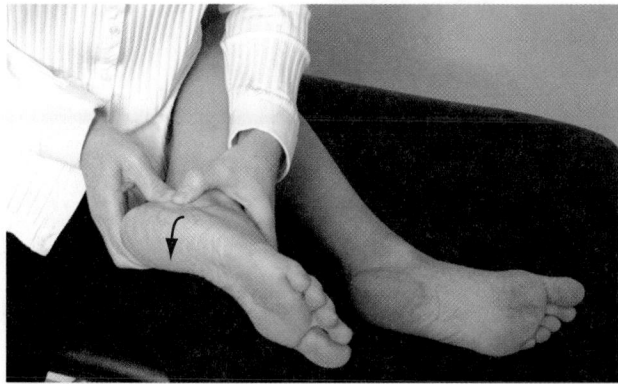

Figure 13-88 Talar tilt test.

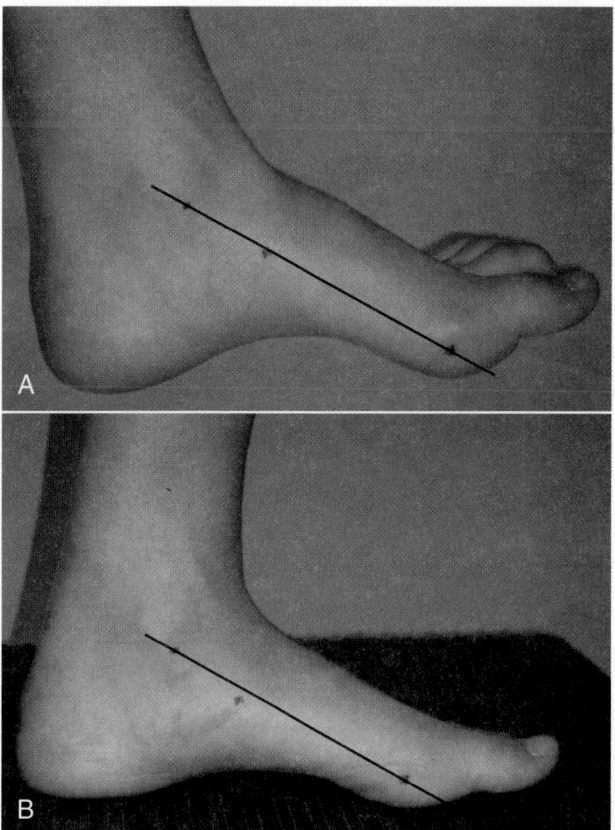

Figure 13-89 A, Feiss line in non–weight-bearing. Navicular is in normal position. **B,** Feiss line in weight-bearing. Navicular is slightly below line (within normal limits).

of the knee. This test is to determine whether the calcaneofibular ligament is torn.[114,123] The normal side is tested first for comparison. The foot is held in the anatomical (90°) position, which brings the calcaneofibular ligament perpendicular to the long axis of the talus. If the foot is plantar flexed, the anterior talofibular ligament is more likely to be tested (**inversion stress test**).[122] The talus is then tilted from side to side into inversion and eversion. Inversion tests the calcaneofibular ligament and, to some degree, the anterior talofibular ligament by increasing the stress on the ligament.[16] Eversion stresses the deltoid ligament, primarily the tibionavicular, tibiocalcaneal, and posterior tibiotalar ligaments. On a radiograph, the talar tilt may be measured by obtaining the angle between the distal aspect of the tibia and the proximal surface of the talus (see the discussion of stress radiographs in the Diagnostic Imaging section)

Other Tests

Buerger's Test. This test is designed to test the arterial blood supply to the lower limb.[36] The patient lies supine while the examiner elevates the patient's leg to 45° for at least 3 minutes. If the foot blanches or the prominent veins collapse shortly after elevation, the test is positive for poor arterial blood circulation. The examiner then asks the patient to sit with the legs dangling over the edge of the bed. If it takes 1 to 2 minutes for the limb color to be restored and the veins to fill and become prominent, the test is confirmed positive.

Duchenne Test.[36] The patient lies supine with the legs straight. The examiner pushes up on the head of the first metatarsal through the sole, pushing the foot into dorsiflexion. The test is positive for a lesion of the superficial peroneal nerve or a lesion of L4, L5, or S1 nerve root if, when the patient is asked to plantar flex the foot, the medial border dorsiflexes and offers no resistance while the lateral border plantar flexes.

Feiss Line.[32] The examiner marks the apex of the medial malleolus and the plantar aspect of the first metatarsophalangeal joint while the patient is not bearing weight. The examiner then palpates the navicular

tuberosity on the medial aspect of the foot, noting where it lies relative to a line joining the two previously made points. The patient then stands with the feet 8 to 15 cm (3 to 6 inches) apart. The two points are checked to ensure that they still represent the apex of the medial malleolus and the plantar aspect of the metatarsophalangeal joint. The navicular tubercle is again palpated (Figure 13-89). The navicular tubercle normally lies on or close to the line joining the two points. If the tubercle falls one third of the distance to the floor, it represents a first-degree flatfoot; if it falls two thirds of the distance, it represents a second-degree flatfoot; if it rests on the floor, it represents a third-degree flatfoot (see Figure 13-42, *A*).

Figure-Eight Ankle Measurement for Swelling.[147–150] The patient is positioned in long sitting with the ankle and lower leg beyond the end of the examining table with the ankle in plantigrade (90°). Rohner-Spengler, et al.[151] recommend placing the ankle in 20° plantar flexion (called **figure-of-eight-20**). Using a 6 mm (¼-inch) wide plastic tape measure, the examiner places the end of the tape measure on the tibialis anterior tendon, drawing the tape medially across the instep just distal to the navicular tuberosity. The tape is then pulled across the arch of the foot just proximal to the base of the fifth metatarsal,

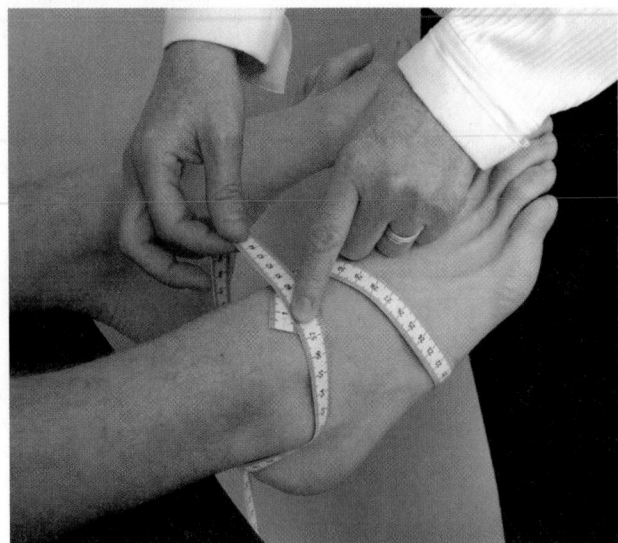

Figure 13-90 Figure-eight ankle measurement for swelling.

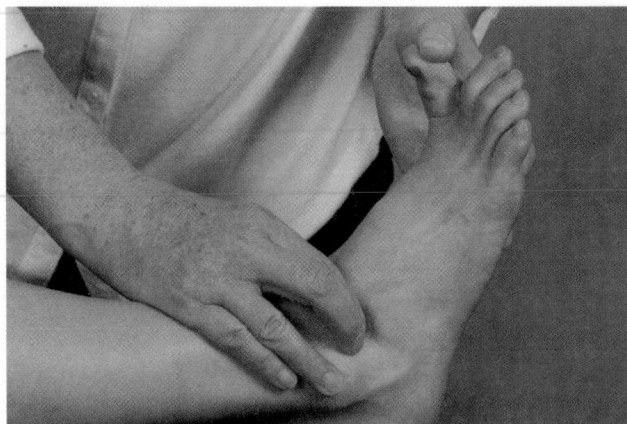

Figure 13-91 Functional hallux limitus test. Note the right hand of the examiner ensuring the foot is in the neutral position while the hallux is dorsiflexed or extended.

across the tibialis anterior tendon, and then around the ankle joint just distal to the tip of the medial malleolus, across the Achilles tendon, and just distal to the lateral malleolus, returning to the starting position (Figure 13-90). The measurement is repeated three times and an average taken.

⚠ *Functional Hallux Limitus Test.*[152,153] The patient lies supine with the leg supported on the bed. The examiner uses one hand to keep the subtalar joint in neutral while using the same hand to keep the first metatarsal in dorsiflexion. The examiner's other hand dorsiflexes the proximal phalanx of the hallux. If the first metatarsal plantar flexes when the toe is dorsiflexed, the test is considered positive for abnormal midtarsal joint function leading to abnormal midtarsal joint pronation during late midstance (Figure 13-91).

⚠ *Functional Leg Length.*[154] The patient stands in the normal relaxed stance (Figure 13-92). The examiner palpates the anterior superior iliac spines and then the posterior superior iliac spines and notes any differences. The examiner then positions the patient so that the patient's subtalar joints are in neutral position while weight bearing. The patient maintains this position with the toes straight ahead and the knees straight, and the examiner repalpates the anterior and the posterior superior iliac spines. If the previously noted differences remain, the pelvis and sacroiliac joints should be evaluated further. If the previously noted differences disappear, the examiner should suspect a functional leg length difference resulting from hip, knee, or ankle and foot problems—primarily, ankle and foot problems (Tables 13-11 and 13-12). The examiner must then determine what is causing the difference. For example, foot pronation is often seen with forefoot or hindfoot varus, tibial varus, tight muscles (e.g., calf, hamstrings, hip flexors), or weak muscles (e.g., ankle invertors, piriformis).

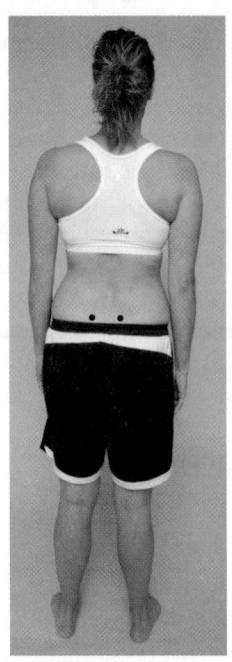

Figure 13-92 Functional leg length in standing position (subtalar joint in neutral). *Dots on back* indicate posterior superior iliac spines.

❓ *Hoffa's Test.* The patient lies prone with the feet extended over the edge of the examining table. The examiner palpates the Achilles tendon while the patient plantar flexes and dorsiflexes the foot. If one Achilles tendon (the injured one) feels less taut than the other one, the test is considered positive for a calcaneal fracture. Passive dorsiflexion on the affected side is also greater.

❓ *Homans Sign.* The patient's foot is passively dorsiflexed with the knee extended. Pain in the calf indicates a positive Homans sign for deep vein thrombophlebitis (Figure 13-93). Tenderness is also elicited on palpation of the calf. In addition to these findings, the examiner may find pallor and swelling in the leg and a loss of the dorsalis pedis pulse.

⚠ *Matles Test.*[155] The patient lies prone with the foot over the end of the examining table while the clinician stands near the end of the table. The patient is asked to actively flex the knee to 90° (Figure 13-94). During the motion, the examiner watches the foot. Normally, it will be slightly plantar flexed. If the foot falls into neutral or slight dorsiflexion, the test is positive for a 3° strain (rupture) of the Achilles tendon.

⚠ *Morton's Test.*[36] The patient lies supine. The examiner grasps the foot around the metatarsal heads and squeezes the heads together. Pain is a positive sign for stress fracture or neuroma.

❓ *Patla Tibialis Posterior Length Test.*[65] The patient is in prone lying with the knee flexed to 90° and the calcaneus held in eversion and the ankle in dorsiflexion with one hand (Figure 13-95). With the other hand, the examiner's thumb contacts the plantar surface of the bases of the second, third, and fourth metatarsals while the index and middle fingers contact the plantar surface of the navicular. The examiner then determines the end feel by pushing dorsally on the navicular and metatarsal heads. The end feel is compared with the normal side. A reproduction of the patient's symptoms indicates a positive test.

❓ *Swing Test for Posterior Tibiotalar Subluxation.*[156] The patient sits with feet dangling over the edge of the examining table (Figure 13-96). The examiner places the hands around the dorsum of the foot using the fingers to keep the feet parallel to the floor. With the thumbs, the examiner palpates the anterior portion of the talus. The examiner then passively plantar flexes and dorsiflexes the foot and compares the quality and degree of movement between feet, especially into dorsiflexion. Resistance to normal dorsiflexion in the injured ankle indicates a positive test for posterior tibiotalar subluxation.

⚠ *Test for Peroneal Tendon Dislocation.*[157] The patient is placed in prone on the examining table with the knee

TABLE 13-11

Functional Limb Length Difference

Joint	Functional Lengthening	Functional Shortening
Foot	Supination	Pronation
Knee	Extension	Flexion
Hip	Lowering	Lifting
	Extension	Flexion
	Lateral rotation	Medial rotation
Sacroiliac	Anterior rotation	Posterior rotation

Modified from Wallace LA: Lower quarter pain: mechanical evaluation and treatment. In Grieve GP, editor: Modern manual therapy of the vertebral column, Edinburgh, 1986, Churchill Livingstone, p. 467.

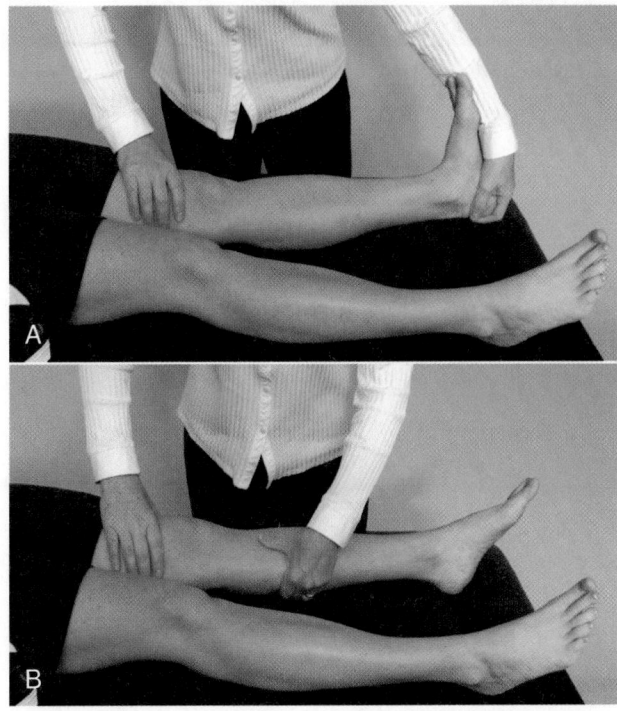

Figure 13-93 Homans sign for thrombophlebitis. **A,** Test. **B,** Palpation for tenderness in thrombophlebitis.

TABLE 13-12

Dynamic Limb Length Evaluation

Asymmetric Shoe Wear	Asymmetric Callus	Asymmetric Posture	Asymmetric Alignment or Movement
Shoe upper	Medial first distal interphalangeal	Foot	Toe-out
Heel counter	Medial first metatarsal	Ankle	Toe-grasp
Varus or valgus	Second and third metatarsal heads	Knee	Patellar alignment over foot
		Hip	Knee flexion
Shoe sole	Fourth and fifth metatarsal heads	Pelvis	Hip drop
Posterior lateral heel	Calcaneus		Propulsion
Posterior central heel	Lateral		
Posterior medial heel	Central		
	Medial		

Modified from Wallace LA: Limb length difference and back pain. In Grieve GP, editor: Modern manual therapy of the vertebral column, Edinburgh, 1986, Churchill Livingstone, p. 469.

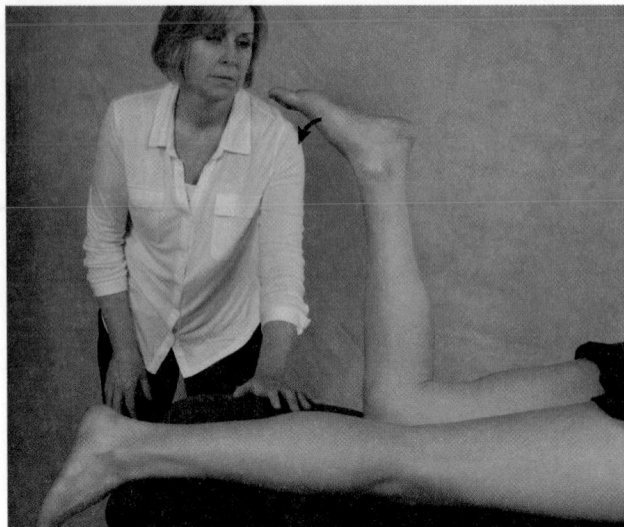

Figure 13-94 Matles test. Negative test is demonstrated. If the achilles tendon is ruptured, the foot would move into more dorsiflexion (*arrow*).

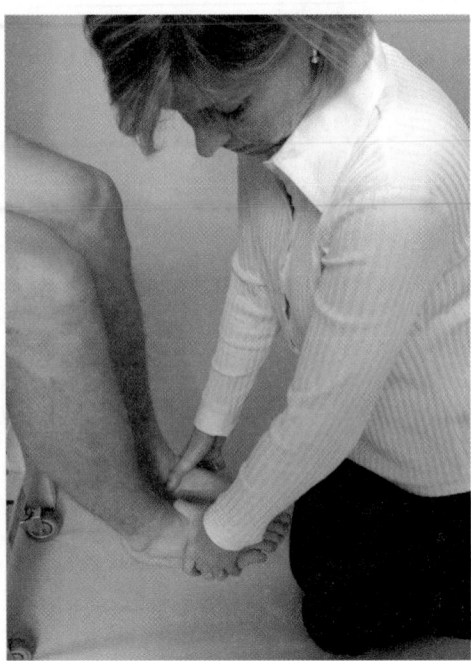

Figure 13-96 Swing test for posterior tibiotalar subluxation.

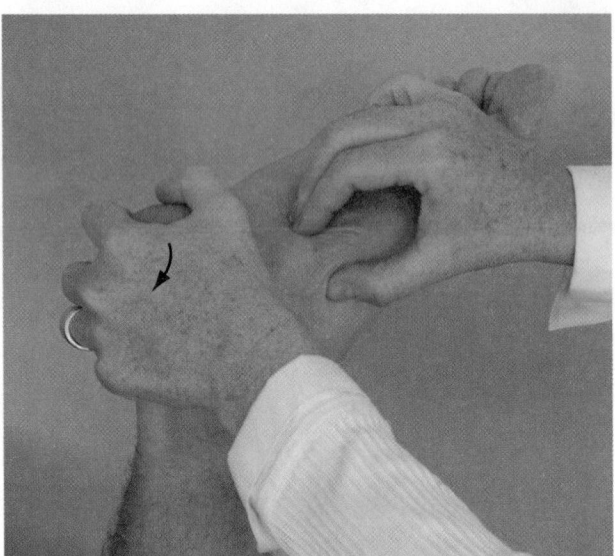

Figure 13-95 Patla tibialis posterior length test.

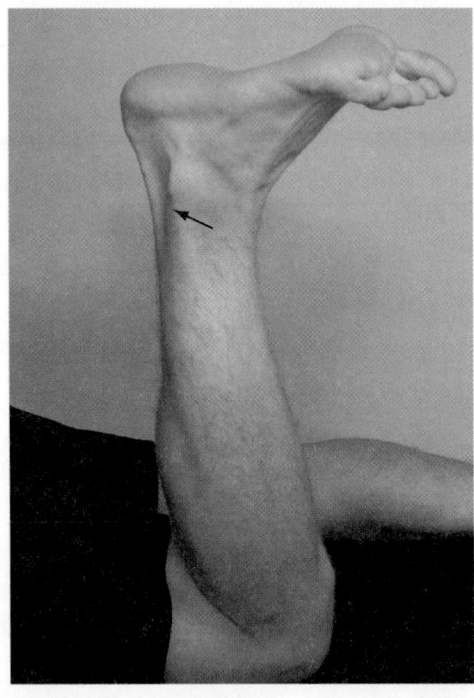

Figure 13-97 Test for peroneal tendon dislocation. Arrow indicates where to look for subluxing tendon.

flexed to 90°. The posterolateral region of the ankle is inspected for swelling. The patient is then asked to actively dorsiflex and plantar flex the ankle along with eversion against the examiner's resistance (Figure 13-97). If the tendon subluxes from behind the lateral malleolus, the test is positive.

▲ *Thompson's (Simmonds') Test (Sign for Achilles Tendon Rupture).* The patient lies prone or kneels on a chair with the feet over the edge of the table or chair (Figure 13-98). While the patient is relaxed, the examiner squeezes the calf muscles. The absence of plantar flexion when the muscle is squeezed indicates a positive test and a ruptured Achilles tendon (third-degree strain).[158-161] One should be careful not to assume that the Achilles tendon is not ruptured if the patient is able to plantar flex the foot while

not bearing weight. The long flexor muscles can perform this function in the non-weight-bearing stance even with a rupture of the Achilles tendon.

✓ *Tinel's Sign at the Ankle (Percussion Sign).* Tinel's sign may be elicited in two places around the ankle. The anterior tibial branch of the deep peroneal nerve may be percussed in front of the ankle (Figure 13-99, *A*). The

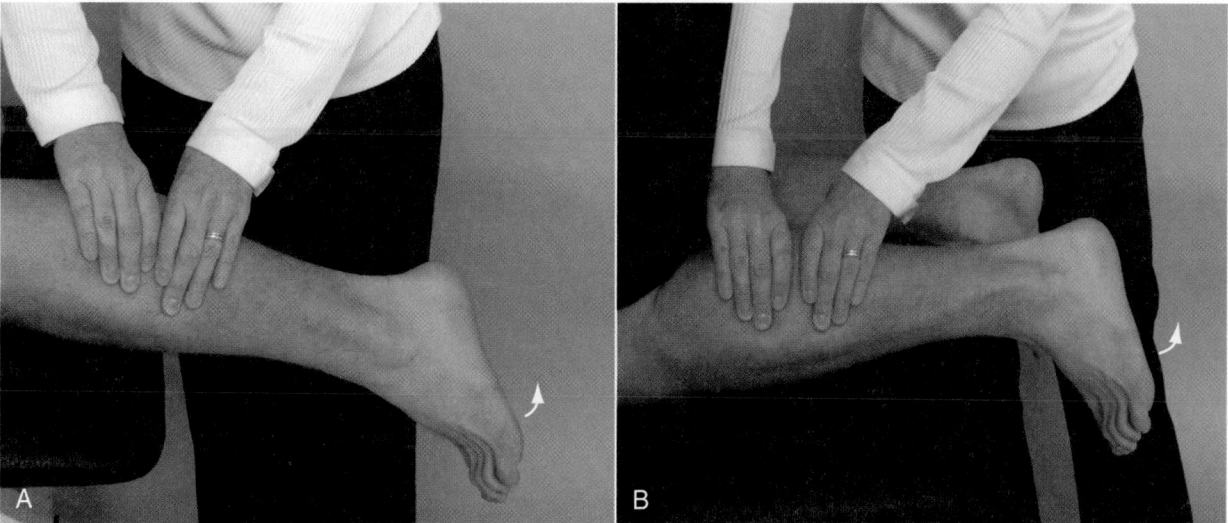

Figure 13-98 Thompson's test for Achilles tendon rupture. A, Prone lying position. **B,** Kneeling position. In each case, foot plantar flexes *(arrow)* if the test result is negative.

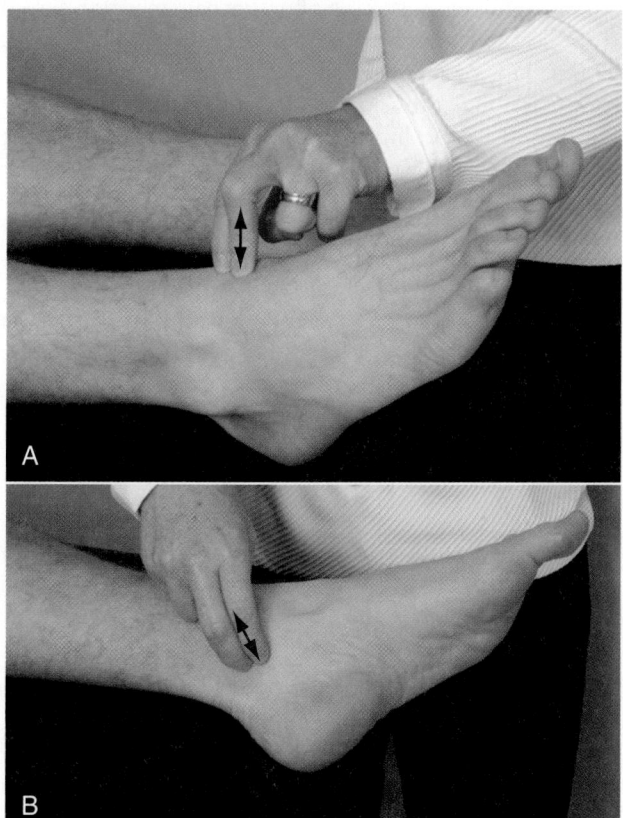

Figure 13-99 Tinel's sign. A, Anterior tibial branch of deep peroneal nerve. **B,** Posterior tibial nerve.

posterior tibial nerve may be percussed as it passes behind the medial malleolus (Figure 13-99, *B*). In both cases, tingling or paresthesia felt distally is a positive sign.

▲ *Windlass Test.*[153,162] The patient stands on a stool or chair with the foot positioned so that the metatarsal heads rest on the edge of the stool while the patient

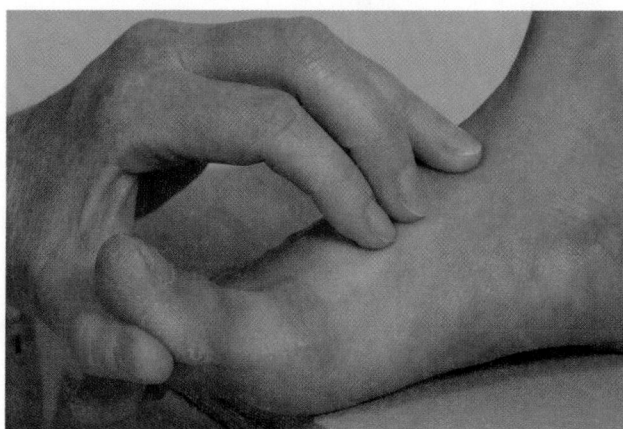

Figure 13-100 Windlass test.

maintains weight through the leg. The examiner then passively dorsiflexes the big toe (Figure 13-100). Pain or increased pain at the insertion of the plantar fascia (see Figure 13-25) indicates a positive test for plantar fasciitis. Lack of extension may indicate hallux rigidus.

Reflexes and Cutaneous Distribution

The examiner must be aware of the sensory distribution of the various peripheral nerves in the foot, especially the superficial peroneal, deep peroneal, and saphenous nerves, and the branches of the tibial nerve (sural, medial calcaneal, medial plantar, and lateral plantar; Figure 13-101).

The examiner must also differentiate between the peripheral nerve sensory distribution and the sensory nerve root distribution or dermatomes (Figure 13-102). Although dermatomes vary among individuals, their pattern is never identical to the peripheral nerve distribution, which tends to be more consistent among patients.

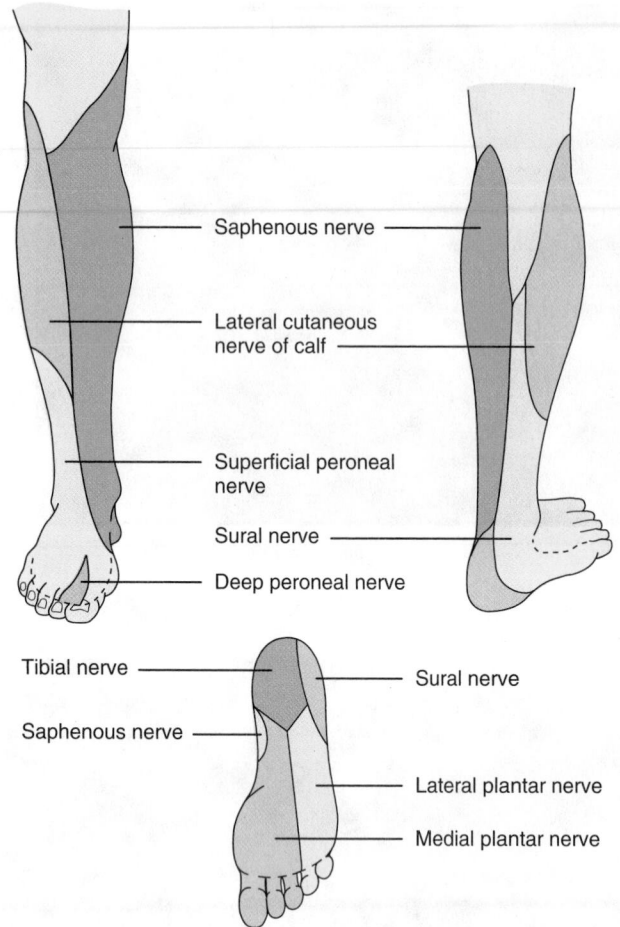

Figure 13-101 Peripheral nerve distribution in the lower leg, ankle, and foot.

The examiner should test the patient's sensation by running his or her hands over the anterior, lateral, medial, and posterior surfaces of the patient's leg below the knee, foot, and toes (sensation scanning examination). Any difference in sensation should be noted and can be mapped out in more detail with a pinwheel, pin, cotton batten, or brush.

The examiner must test the patient's reflexes. Commonly checked in this region are the Achilles reflex[163] (S1–S2; Figure 13-103) and the posterior tibial reflex (L4–L5; Figure 13-104). These reflexes may be affected by age and may be absent in older normal individuals.[163] The examiner may also wish to test for pyramidal tract (upper motor neuron) disease. There are various methods for testing the pathological reflexes, including the Babinski, Chaddock, Oppenheim, and Gordon reflexes (Figure 13-105). A positive sign in all of these tests is extension of the big toe. The Babinski reflex also causes fanning of the second through fifth toes. The most common and reliable test is the Babinski test.[164]

The examiner must remember that pain may be referred to the lower leg, ankle, or foot from the lumbar spine, sacrum, hip, or knee (Figure 13-106). Conversely, pain from a lesion in the lower leg, ankle, or foot may be transmitted to the hip or knee. Table 13-13 shows the muscles of the lower leg, ankle, and foot, and their patterns of pain referral.

Peripheral Nerve Injuries of the Lower Leg, Ankle, and Foot

Deep Peroneal Nerve (L4 to S2). The deep peroneal nerve, a branch of the common peroneal nerve, which is itself a

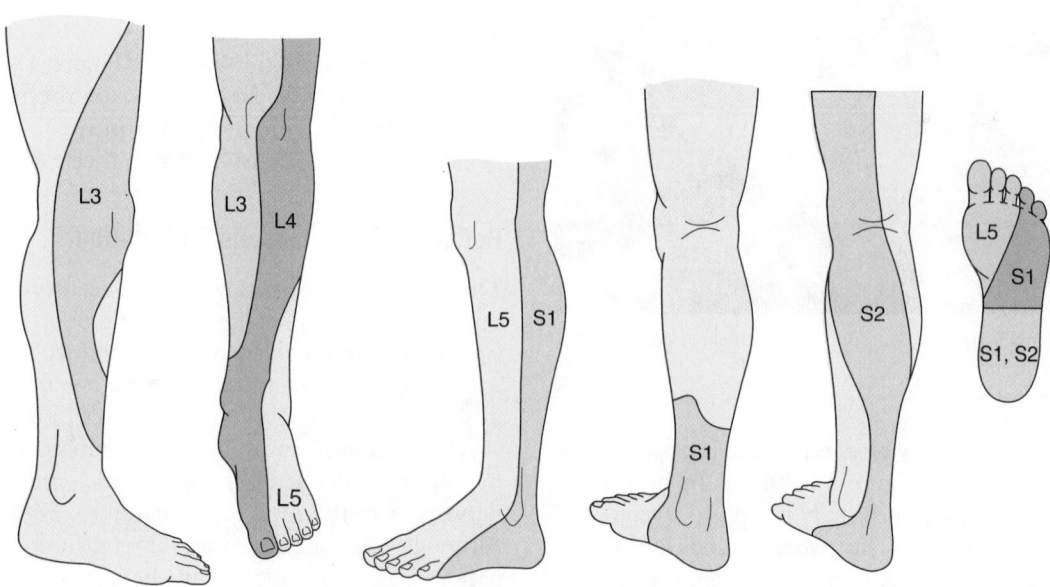

Figure 13-102 Dermatomes of the lower leg, ankle, and foot.

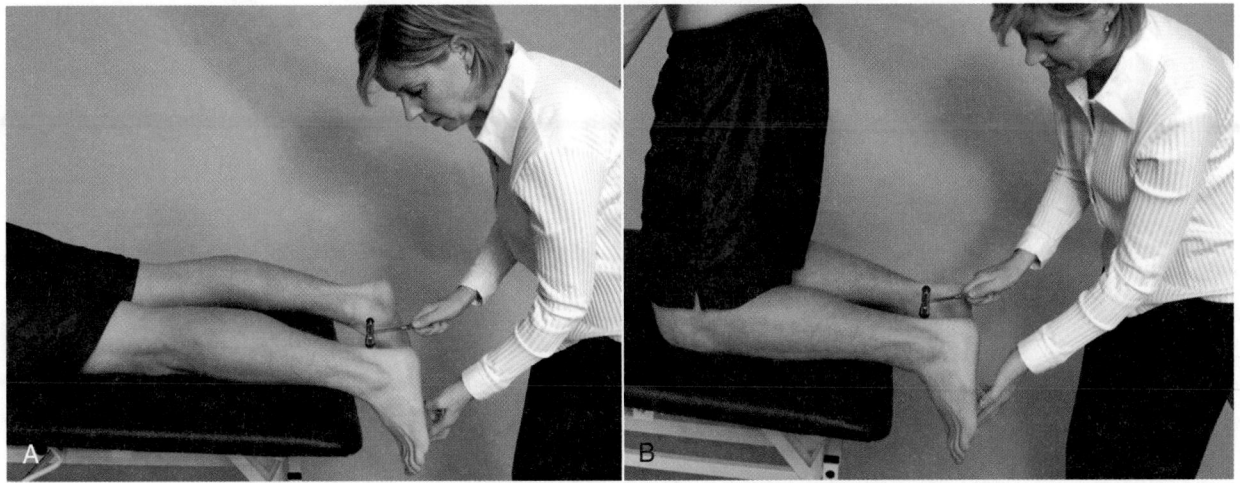

Figure 13-103 Test of Achilles reflex (S1–S2). **A,** Prone lying. **B,** Kneeling.

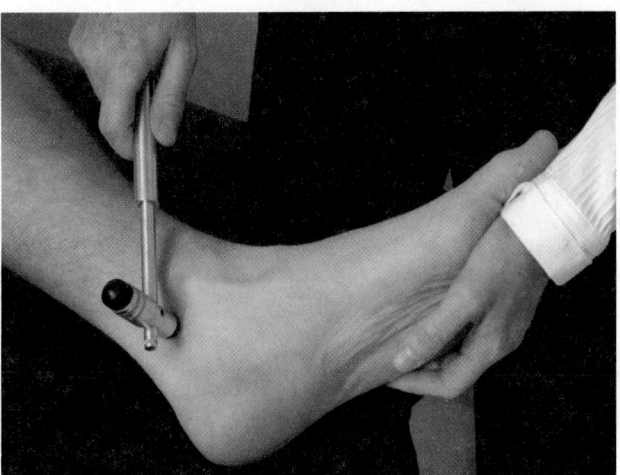

Figure 13-104 Tibialis posterior reflex.

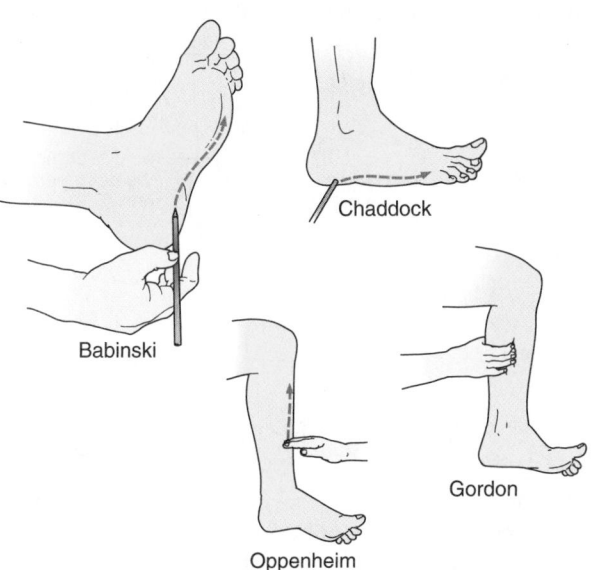

Figure 13-105 Pathological reflexes for pyramidal tract disease.

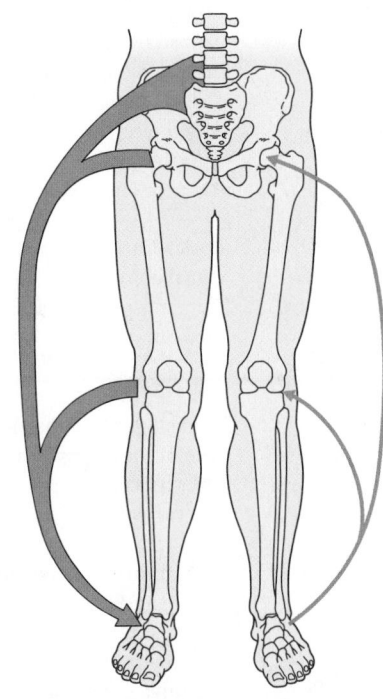

Figure 13-106 Pattern of referred pain to and from the ankle.

branch of the sciatic nerve (Figures 13-107 and 13-108), is most commonly injured (compressed) in **anterior compartment syndrome** in the leg, and where it passes under the extensor retinaculum (**anterior tarsal tunnel syndrome**).[110,165–171] Compression may be caused by trauma, tight shoelaces, a ganglion, or pes cavus.[167] Motor loss (Table 13-14) includes an inability to dorsiflex the foot (**drop foot**), which results in a high steppage gait and an inability to control ankle movement. Because the deep peroneal nerve is primarily motor, there is minimal sensory loss, but this loss can be aggravating, especially in anterior tarsal tunnel syndrome (see Figure 13-108). The sensory loss is a small triangular area between the first and second

TABLE **13-13**

Muscles of the Lower Leg, Ankle, and Foot and Referral of Pain

Muscle	Referral Pattern
Tibialis anterior	Anterior lower leg, medial dorsum of foot to hallux
Peroneus longus	Superolateral aspect of lower leg
Peroneus brevis	Lower lateral leg, over lateral malleolus and lateral aspect of foot
Peroneus tertius	Lower lateral leg, anterior to lateral malleolus and onto dorsum of foot, or behind lateral malleolus to lateral heel
Gastrocnemius	Behind knee, posterior leg to instep of foot
Soleus	Posterior leg to heel and sometimes to sole of foot
Plantaris	Posterior knee to upper half of posterior leg
Tibialis posterior	Posterior leg, Achilles tendon, heel, and sole of foot
Extensor digitorum longus	Anterolateral leg to dorsum of foot
Extensor hallucis longus	Anterior leg to dorsomedial foot
Flexor digitorum longus	Posteromedial leg, over medial malleolus, distal sole of foot
Flexor hallucis longus	Plantar aspect of hallux
Extensor digitorum brevis and extensor hallucis brevis	Dorsum of foot
Abductor hallucis	Medial heel and instep
Abductor digiti minimi	Sole of foot over fifth metatarsal
Flexor digitorum brevis	Over metatarsal head
Quadratus plantae (flexor accessorius)	Plantar aspect of heel
Adductor hallucis	Sole of foot over metatarsals
Flexor hallucis brevis	Dorsal and plantar aspect of first metatarsal and hallux
Interossei	Dorsum and plantar aspect of equivalent metatarsal and toe

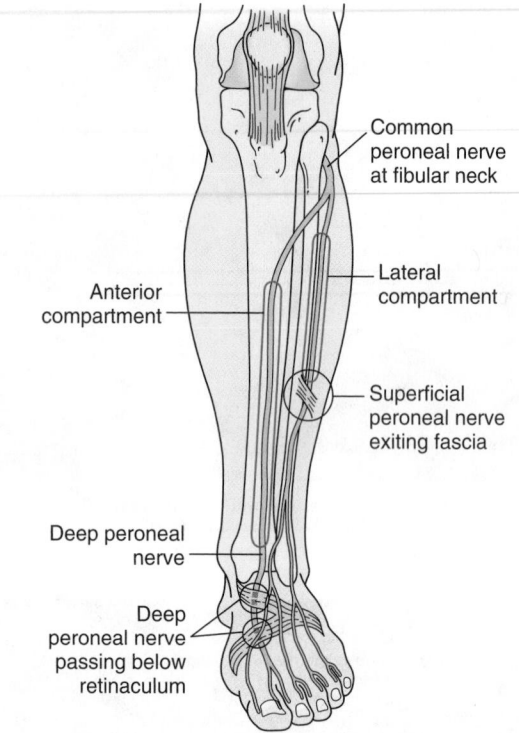

Figure 13-107 Superficial peroneal nerve travels in the lateral compartment of the leg and can be entrapped as it pierces the fascia 8 to 12 cm proximal to the tip of the lateral malleolus. The **deep peroneal nerve** can be compressed as it pierces the intermuscular septum to travel in the anterior compartment and under the retinaculum.

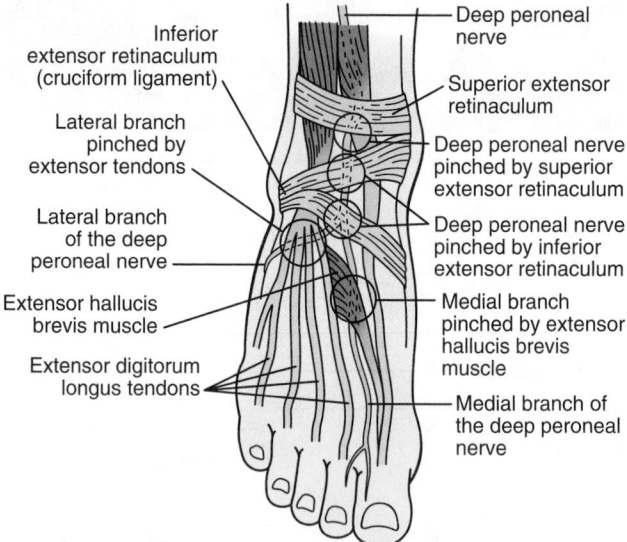

Figure 13-108 Compression of deep peroneal nerve by the extensor retinaculum or other structures.

toes. Pain is often accentuated by plantar flexion.[167] With the tunnel syndrome, muscle weakness is minimal (extensor digitorum brevis); there is burning pain between the first and second toes that is sometimes referred to the dorsum of the foot.

Superficial Peroneal Nerve (L4 to S2). Injuries to the superficial peroneal nerve, a branch of the common peroneal nerve (Figure 13-109; see Figure 13-107), are rare but they have been reported to be associated with lateral ankle (inversion) sprains causing stretching of the nerve, or the nerve may be entrapped as it pierces the deep fascia to become subcutaneous about 10 to 13 cm

(4 to 5 inches) above the lateral malleolus (Figure 13-110).[65,112,166,169,170,172–175] Motor loss with the high lesion near the head of the fibula is primarily loss of foot eversion and loss of ankle stability. With both lesions, the sensory loss is the same. The superficial peroneal nerve has a greater sensory role than the deep branch;

TABLE **13-14**

Peripheral Nerve Injuries (Neuropathy) of the Lower Leg, Ankle, and Foot

Nerve	Muscle Weakness	Sensory Alteration	Reflexes Affected
Deep peroneal nerve (L4 through S2)	Tibialis anterior Extensor digitorum longus Extensor digitorum brevis Extensor hallucis longus Peroneus tertius	Triangular area between the first and second toes	None
Superficial peroneal nerve (L4 through S2)	Peroneus longus Peroneus brevis	Lateral aspect of leg and dorsum of foot	None
Tibial nerve (L4 through S3)	Gastrocnemius Soleus Plantaris Tibialis posterior Flexor digitorum longus Flexor hallucis longus Flexor accessorius (quadratus plantae) Abductor digiti minimi Flexor digiti minimi Lumbricals Interossei Adductor hallucis Abductor hallucis Flexor digitorum brevis Flexor hallucis brevis	Sole of foot except medial border, plantar surface of toes	Achilles (S1–S2) Tibialis posterior (L4–L5)

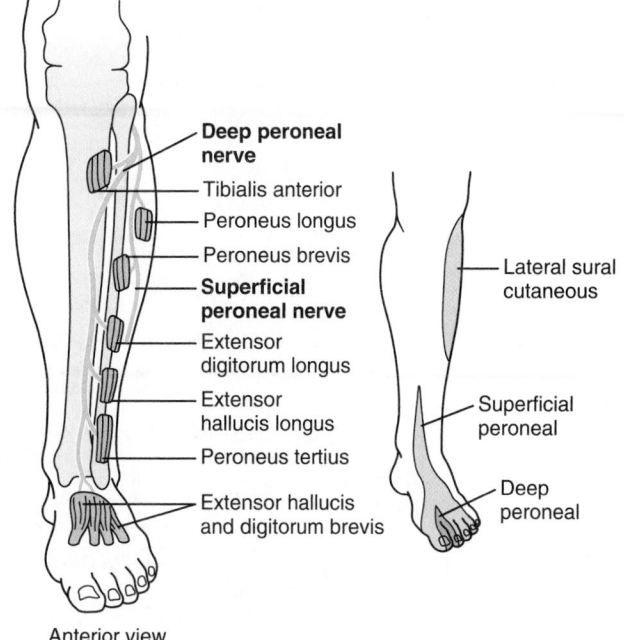

Anterior view

Figure 13-109 Common peroneal nerve and its branches, the superficial and deep peroneal nerves.

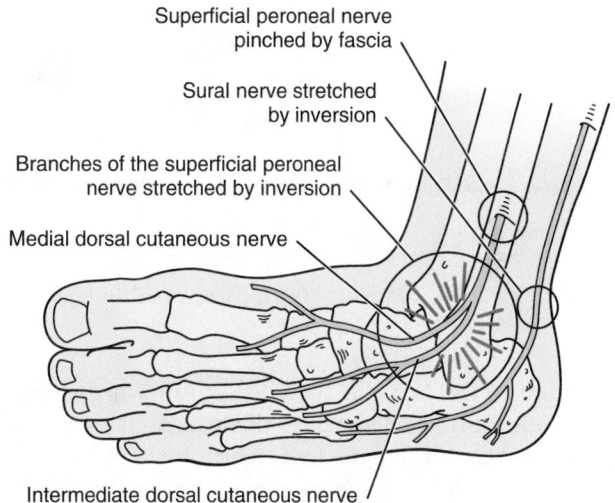

Figure 13-110 Stretching of the superficial peroneal nerve as a result of inversion of ankle.

it supplies the lateral side of the leg and dorsum of the foot (see Figure 13-109). This sensory alteration is often greater with activity. If the examiner plantar flexes and inverts the foot while applying pressure over the distal site, symptoms usually result.[176]

Pahor and Toppenberg reported that the slump test (see Chapter 9) combined with plantar flexion and inversion of the foot can be performed to rule out neurological injury to the nerve following lateral ankle sprains.[177]

Tibial Nerve (L4 to S3). The tibial nerve, a branch of the sciatic nerve (Figures 13-111 and 13-112), has a major role to play in the lower leg, ankle, and foot because it

supplies all the muscles in the posterior leg and on the sole of the foot. The nerve may be injured in the popliteal area at the knee from trauma (e.g., dislocation, blow) or from entrapment as it passes over the popliteus and under the soleus. **Popliteal entrapment** syndrome or injury may accompany an ankle sprain.[173] At the ankle, the nerve may be compressed as it passes through the tarsal tunnel, which is formed by the medial malleolus, calcaneus, and talus on one side and the deltoid ligament (primarily the tibiocalcanean ligament) on the other. This compression is referred to as **tarsal tunnel syndrome** (see Figure 13-112).[57,166,171,178,179]

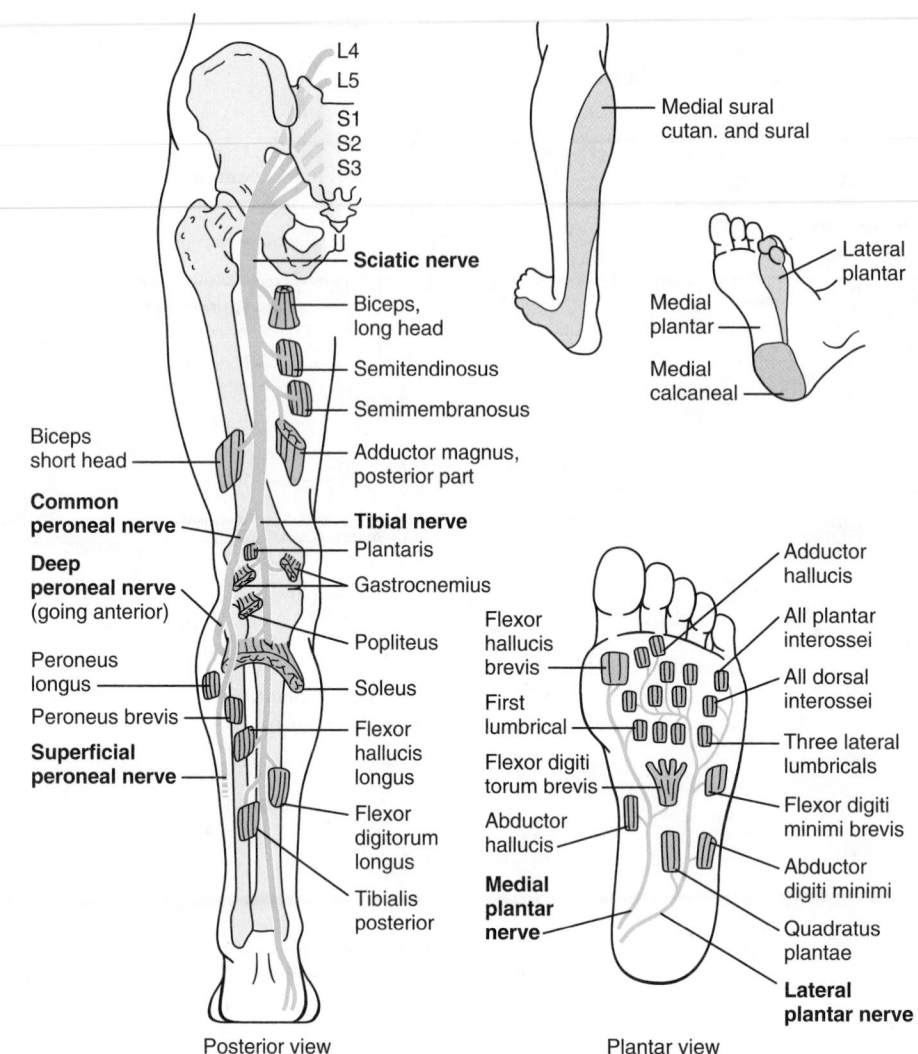

Posterior view

Plantar view

Figure 13-111 Distribution of the branches of the sciatic nerve with tibial nerve highlighted.

Injury to the nerve at the knee causes a major functional disability. Functionally, the patient is unable to plantar flex and invert the foot, which has a major effect on gait. In addition, the patient is unable to flex, abduct, or adduct the toes. Sensory loss involves primarily the sole of the foot, lateral surface of the heel, and plantar surfaces of the toes. With popliteal entrapment syndrome, the popliteal artery is often compressed with the nerve, leading to vascular symptoms (e.g., numbness, tingling, intermittent cramping, weakened dorsalis pedis pulse) and neurological signs.

Compression in the tarsal tunnel may be caused by swelling after trauma, a space-occupying lesion (e.g., ganglion), inflammation (e.g., paratenonitis), valgus deformity, or chronic inversion.[59,168–170,180–187] Sammarco and associates reported the possibility of **double crush injury** in the lower limb involving the sciatic nerve (L4 to S3) and one of its branches.[188] The examiner must always keep this possibility in mind when assessing for nerve pathology in the lower limb, especially in patients who

do not appear to be recovering. Pain and paresthesia into the sole of the foot are often present and are worse after long periods of standing or walking or at night.[166] The pain may be localized or may radiate over the medial side of the ankle distal to the medial malleolus. The condition is sometimes misdiagnosed as plantar fasciitis (Table 13-15).[189] In long-standing cases, motor weakness may become evident in the muscles of the sole of the foot that are supplied by the terminal branches of the tibial nerve (i.e., the medial and lateral plantar nerves).

The **sural nerve** (L5 to S2) is a sensory branch of the tibial nerve supplying the skin on the posterolateral aspect of the lower one third of the leg and the lateral aspect of the foot (Figure 13-113). Injury can result from a blow, trauma (e.g., fracture), or stretching (e.g., accompanying an ankle sprain).[59,112,169,187] Shooting pain and paresthesia in its sensory distribution are diagnostic signs.[166]

The **medial plantar nerve** (Figure 13-114), another branch of the tibial nerve that is found in the foot, may

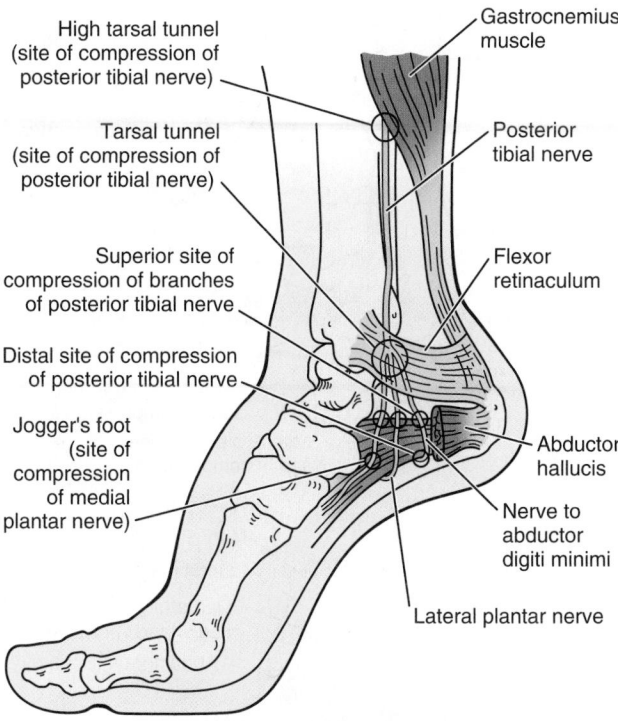

High tarsal tunnel
(site of compression of
posterior tibial nerve)

Gastrocnemius
muscle

Tarsal tunnel
(site of compression of
posterior tibial nerve)

Posterior
tibial nerve

Superior site of
compression of branches
of posterior tibial nerve

Flexor
retinaculum

Distal site of compression
of posterior tibial nerve

Jogger's foot
(site of
compression
of medial
plantar nerve)

Abductor
hallucis

Nerve to
abductor
digiti minimi

Lateral plantar nerve

Figure 13-112 Tarsal tunnel syndrome.

be entrapped in the longitudinal arch, causing aching in the arch, burning pain in the heel, and altered sensation in the sole of the foot behind the hallux. This condition is associated with hindfoot valgus and may be referred to as **jogger's foot.**[166,171,190,191]

Similarly, the **lateral plantar nerve** may be entrapped between the deep fascia of the abductor hallucis and the quadratus plantae (flexor accessorius) muscles (Figure 13-115).[166,192] The patient complains of chronic, dull, aching heel pain that is accentuated by walking and running. There is no complaint of numbness. The condition is accentuated by excessive foot pronation.[192]

The plantar digital nerves are branches of the tibial nerve. Injury to these nerves can result in a Morton's or interdigital neuroma[56] (see the "Morton's Metatarsalgia [Interdigital Neuroma]" section on p. 910).

Saphenous Nerve. This nerve is a sensory branch of the femoral nerve. If it is injured, sensation on the medial side of the leg and foot is affected.[193] More details are given in Chapter 12.

Joint Play Movements

The joint play movements (Figures 13-116 through 13-119) are performed with the patient in the supine or side lying position, depending on which movement is being performed. A comparison of movement between the normal or unaffected side and the injured side should be made.

TABLE 13-15

Differential Diagnosis of Plantar Fasciitis and Tarsal Tunnel Syndrome

	Plantar Fasciitis	Tarsal Tunnel Syndrome
Cause	Overuse	Trauma, space occupying lesion, inflammation, inversion, pronation, valgus deformity
Pain	Plantar aspect of foot, anterior calcaneus	Medial heel and medial longitudinal arch
	Worse with walking, running, and in the morning (sometimes improves with activity)	Worse with standing, walking, and at night
Electrodiagnosis	Normal	Prolonged motor and sensory latencies
Active movements	Full ROM	Full range of motion
Passive movements	Full ROM	May have pain on pronation
Resisted isometric movements	Normal	Weakness of foot intrinsics may be present
Sensory deficits	No	Possible
Reflexes	Normal	Normal

ROM, Range of motion.

Joint Play Movements of the Lower Leg, Ankle, and Foot

Talocrural (ankle joint)	Long-axis extension (traction) Anteroposterior glide
Subtalar joint	Talar rock Side tilt medially and laterally
Midtarsal joints	Anteroposterior glide Rotation
Tarsometatarsal joints	Anteroposterior glide Rotation
Metatarsophalangeal and interphalangeal joints	Long-axis extension (traction) Anteroposterior glide Lateral or side glide Rotation

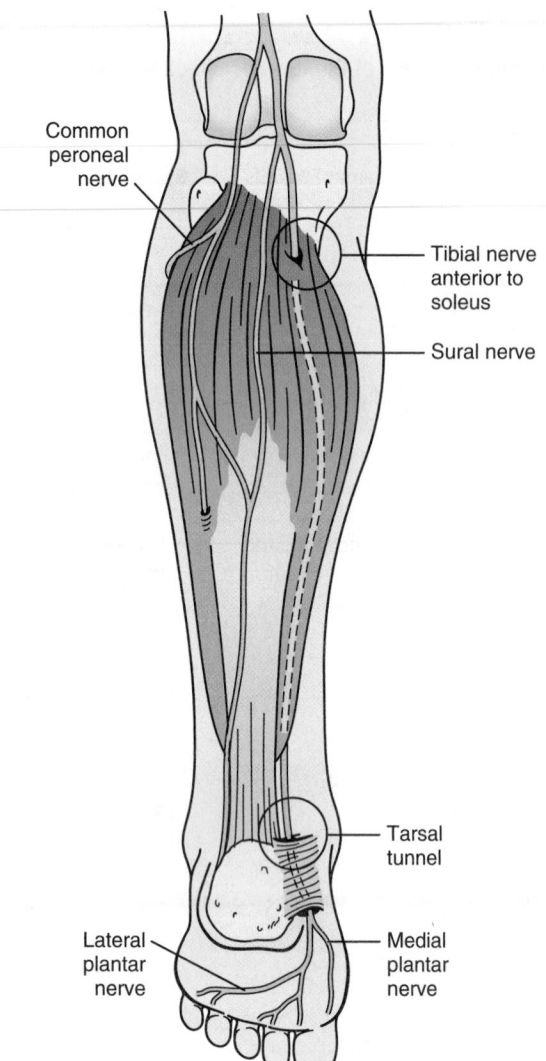

Figure 13-113 Sural nerve travels between the two heads of the gastrocnemius muscle and then becomes superficial in the distal third of the leg. The common peroneal nerve may become entrapped as it courses anteriorly between the fibular head and the peroneus longus. The tibial nerve may be entrapped as it passes through soleus and in the tarsal tunnel.

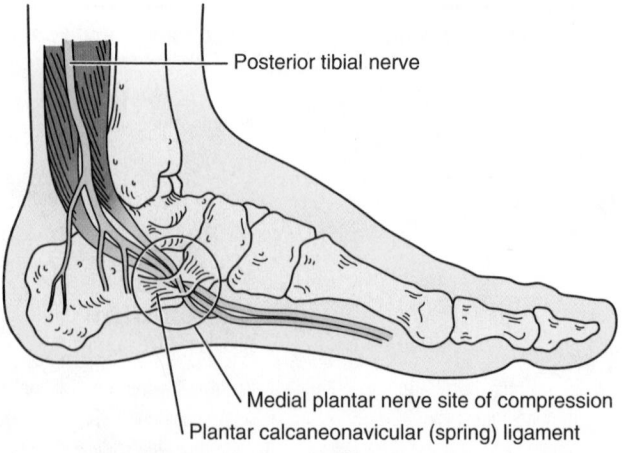

Figure 13-114 Jogger's foot (entrapment of the medial plantar nerve).

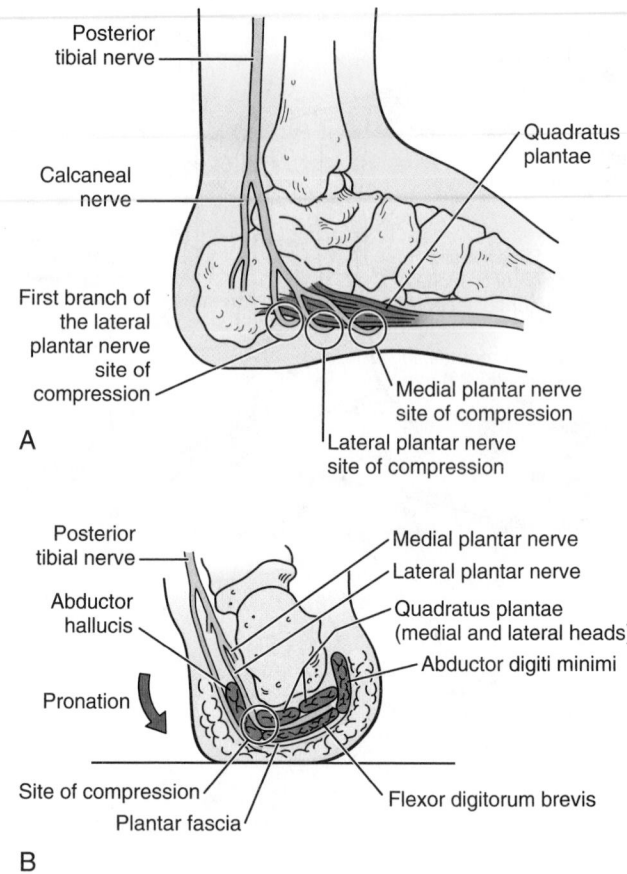

Figure 13-115 Entrapment of the lateral plantar nerve as it changes direction. A, Medial view. **B,** Posterior view.

Long-Axis Extension

Long-axis extension is performed by stabilizing the proximal segment and applying traction to the distal segment. For example, at the ankle, the examiner stabilizes the tibia and fibula by using a strap or just allowing the leg to relax. Both hands are then placed around the ankle, distal to the malleoli, and a longitudinal distractive force is applied. At the metatarsophalangeal and interphalangeal joints, the examiner stabilizes the metatarsal bone or proximal phalanx and applies a longitudinal distractive force to the proximal or distal phalanx, respectively.

Anteroposterior Glide

Anteroposterior glide at the ankle joint is performed by stabilizing the tibia and fibula and drawing the talus and foot forward. To test the posterior movement, the examiner pushes the talus and foot back on the tibia and fibula. There is a difference in the arc of movement between the two actions in tests of joint play. During the anterior movement, the foot should move in an arc into plantar flexion; during the posterior movement, the foot should move in an arc into dorsiflexion. Although similar to the anterior drawer test, the movements are not the same.

Anteroposterior glide at the midtarsal and tarsometatarsal joints is performed in a fashion similar to that used

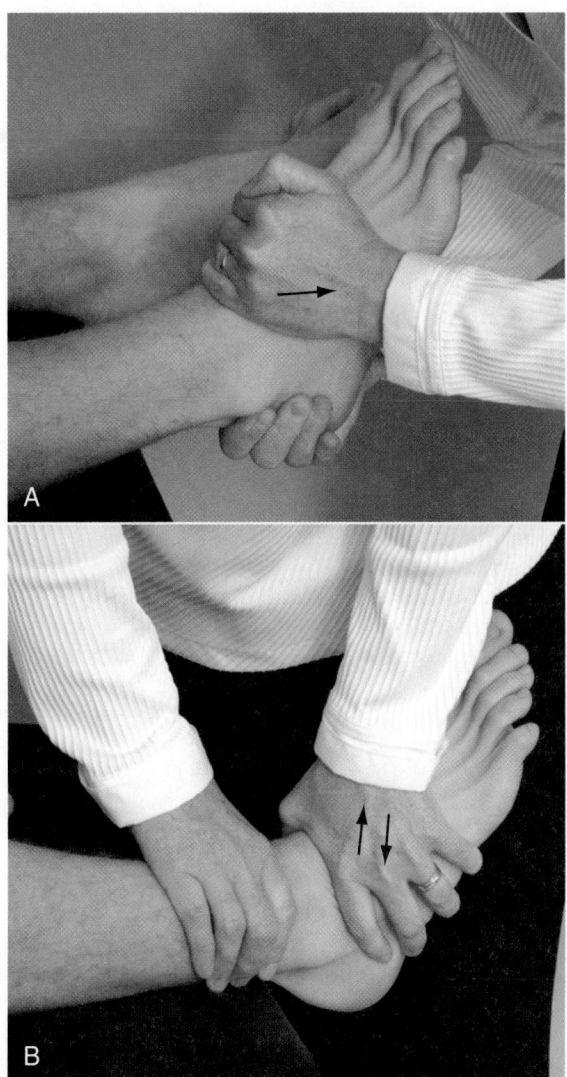

Figure 13-116 **Joint play movements at the talocrural joint.** **A,** Long-axis extension. **B,** Anteroposterior glide at the talocrural joint.

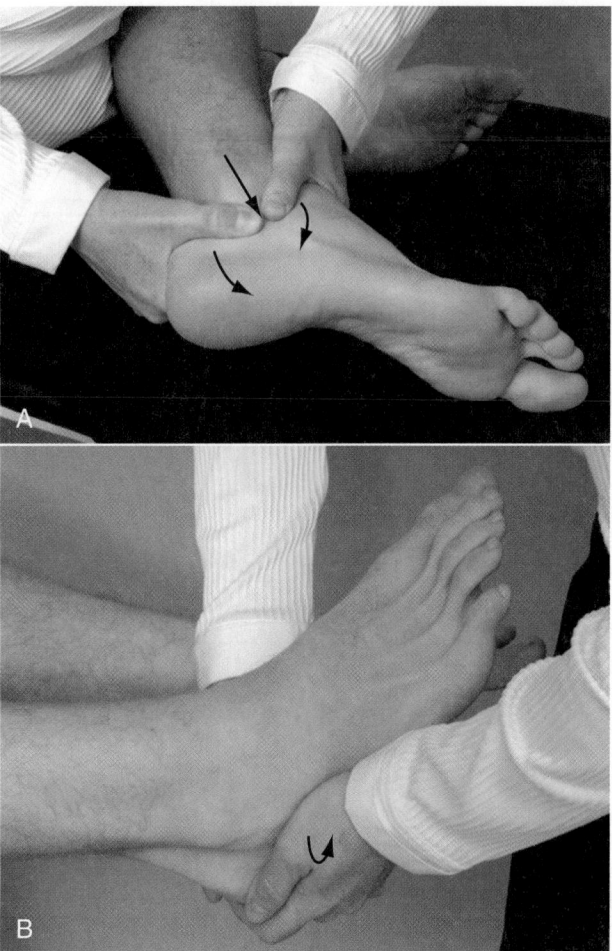

Figure 13-117 **Joint play movements at the subtalar joint.** **A,** Talar rock with slight traction applied. Talus is rocked anterior and posteriorly. **B,** Side tilt.

to test the carpal bones at the wrist. For the midtarsal joints, the examiner stabilizes the navicular, talus, and calcaneus with one hand by grasping the bones in the web space, thumb, and fingers. The other hand is placed around the distal row of tarsal bones (cuneiforms and cuboid). If the hands are positioned properly, they should touch each other, as in Figure 13-117. An anteroposterior gliding movement of the distal row of tarsal bones is applied while the proximal row of tarsal bones is stabilized. The examiner's hands are then moved distally so that the stabilizing hand rests over the distal row of tarsal bones and the mobilizing hand rests over the proximal aspect of the metatarsal bones. Again, the hands should be positioned so that they touch each other. An anteroposterior gliding movement of the metatarsal bones is applied while the distal row of tarsal bones is stabilized.

Anteroposterior glide of the metatarsophalangeal and interphalangeal joints is performed by stabilizing the proximal bone (metatarsal or phalanx) and moving the distal bone (phalanx) in an anteroposterior gliding motion in relation to the stabilized bone.

Talar Rock

Talar rock is the only joint play movement performed with the patient in the side lying position.[146] Both the hip and knee are flexed. The examiner sits with his or her back to the patient, as illustrated in Figure 13-117, *A,* and places both hands around the ankle just distal to the malleoli. A slight distractive force is applied to the ankle, and a rocking movement forward and backward (plantar flexion–dorsiflexion) is applied to the foot. Normally, the examiner should feel a clunk at the extreme of each movement. As with all joint play movements, the movement is compared with that of the unaffected side.

Side Tilt

Side tilt at the subtalar joint is performed by placing both hands around the calcaneus (see Figure 13-117, *B*). The wrists are flexed and extended, tilting the calcaneus

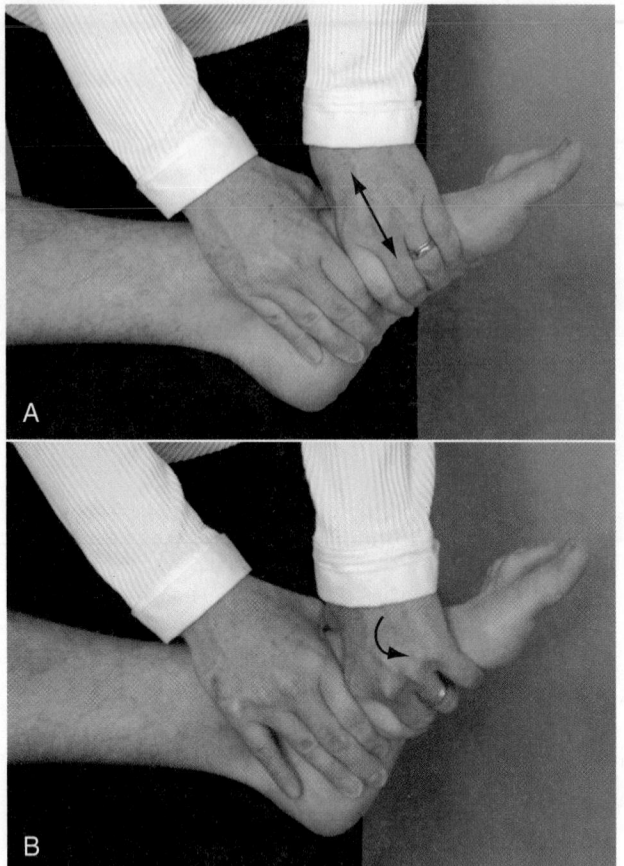

Figure 13-118 Joint play movements in the midtarsal and tarso-metatarsal joints. **A,** Anteroposterior glide. **B,** Rotation.

medially and laterally on the talus. The examiner keeps the patient's foot in the anatomical position while performing the movement. The movement is identical to that used to test the calcaneofibular ligament in the talar tilt test.

Rotation

Rotation at the midtarsal joints is performed in a similar fashion to the anteroposterior glide at these joints. The proximal row of tarsal bones (navicular, calcaneus, and talus) is stabilized, and the mobilizing hand is placed around the distal tarsal bones (cuneiforms and cuboid). The distal row of bones is then rotated on the proximal row of bones. Rotation at the tarsometatarsal joints is performed in a similar fashion. Rotation at the metatarsophalangeal and interphalangeal joints is performed by stabilizing the proximal bone with one hand, applying slight traction, and rotating the distal bone with the other hand.

Side Glide

Side glide at the metatarsophalangeal and interphalangeal joints is performed by stabilizing the proximal bone with one hand. The examiner then uses the other hand to apply slight traction to the distal bone and moves the distal bone

sideways (right and left) in relation to the stabilized bone without causing torsion motion at the joint.

Tests for Tarsal Bone Mobility

In addition to testing of the tarsal bones as a group, the bones should be tested individually, especially if symptoms resulted from group testing. The examiner may test these individual bones using whatever method is desired realizing that the amount of movement normally is minimal. An example of individual tarsal bone testing was put forward by Kaltenborn,[194] who advocates ten tests to determine the mobility of the tarsal bones.

Kaltenborn's Ten Tests for Tarsal Mobility

1. Fixate the second and third cuneiforms, and mobilize the second metatarsal bone.
2. Fixate the second and third cuneiform bones, and mobilize the third metatarsal bone.
3. Fixate the first cuneiform bone, and mobilize the first metatarsal bone.
4. Fixate the navicular bone, and mobilize the first, second, and third cuneiform bones.
5. Fixate the talus, and mobilize the navicular bone.
6. Fixate the cuboid bone, and mobilize the fourth and fifth metatarsal bones.
7. Fixate the navicular and third cuneiform bones, and mobilize the cuboid bone.
8. Fixate the calcaneus, and mobilize the cuboid bone.
9. Fixate the talus, and mobilize the calcaneus.
10. Fixate the talus, and mobilize the tibia and fibula.

Palpation

The examiner palpates for any swelling, noting whether it is intracapsular or extracapsular. Extracapsular swelling around the ankle is indicated by swelling on only one side of the Achilles tendon, whereas intracapsular swelling is indicated by swelling on both sides (see Figure 13-16). Pitting edema, if present, should be noted. If swelling is present at the end of the day and absent after a night of recumbency, venous insufficiency, caused by a weakening or insufficiency of the action of the muscle pump of the lower leg muscles, may be implied. Swelling in the ankle may persist for many weeks after injury as a result of this insufficiency.

The examiner should also notice the texture of the skin and nails. The skin of an ischemic foot shows a loss of hair and becomes thin and inelastic. In addition, the nails become coarse, thickened, and irregular. Many of the nail changes seen in the hand (see Chapter 7) in the presence of systemic disease are also seen in the foot. With poor circulation, the foot will also feel colder. The foot is palpated in the non-weight-bearing and long leg sitting or supine positions. The following structures, including the joints between them, should be palpated.

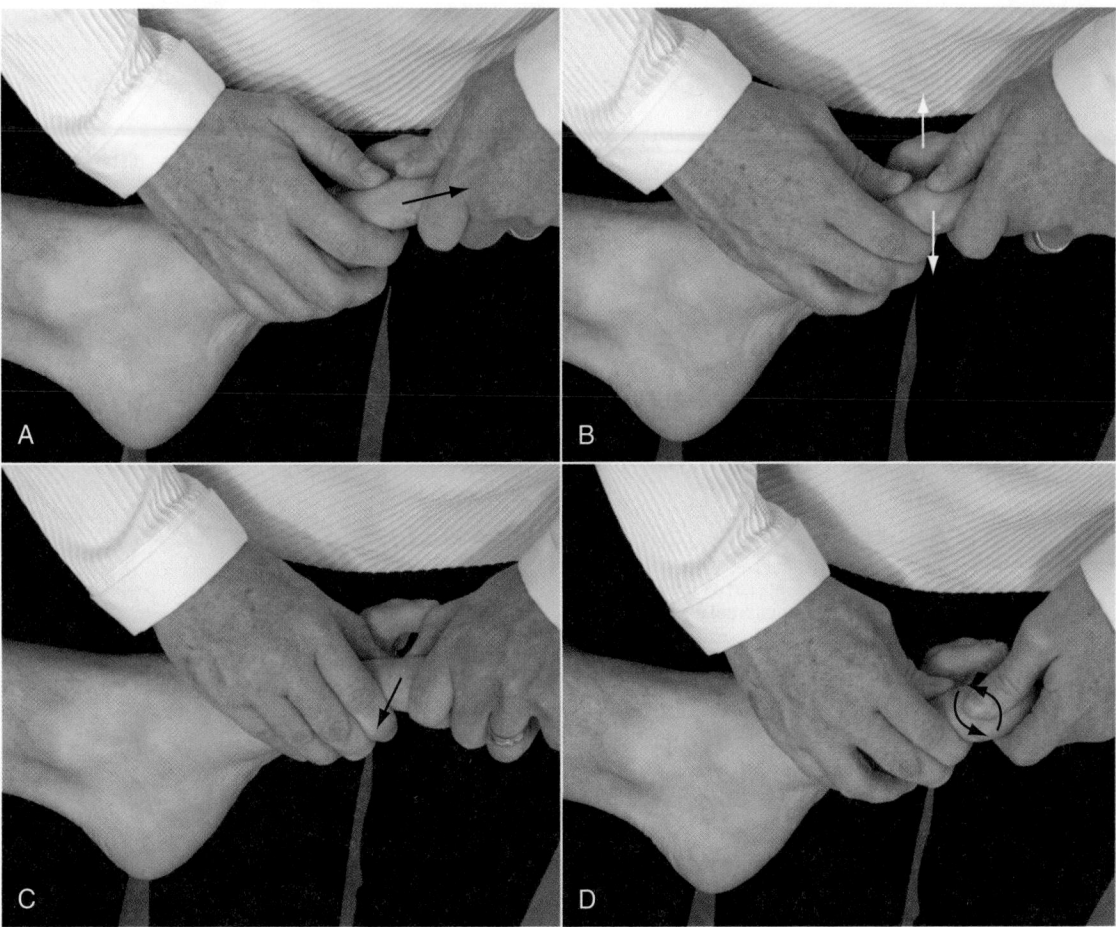

Figure 13-119 Joint play movements at the metatarsophalangeal and interphalangeal joints. A, Long-axis extension. **B,** Anteroposterior glide. **C,** Side glide. **D,** Rotation.

Palpation Anteriorly and Anteromedially

Toes and Metatarsal, Cuneiform, and Navicular Bones. Starting on the medial side, the great toe and its two phalanges are easily palpated. Moving proximally, the examiner comes to the first metatarsal bone (Figure 13-120). The head of the first metatarsal should be palpated carefully. On the medial aspect of the foot, the examiner palpates for any evidence of a bunion (exostosis, callus, and inflamed bursa), which is often associated with hallux valgus. On the plantar aspect, the two sesamoid bones just proximal to the head of the first metatarsal may be palpated.[195] The examiner then palpates the first metatarsal bone along its length to the first cuneiform bone and notes any tenderness, swelling, or signs of pathology. While moving proximally past the first cuneiform on its medial aspect, the examiner will feel a bony prominence, the tubercle of the navicular bone. The examiner then returns to the first cuneiform bone and moves laterally on the dorsal and plantar surface, palpating the second and third cuneiforms (Figure 13-121). Like the first cuneiform, the navicular and second and third cuneiform bones should be palpated on their dorsal and plantar aspects for

signs of pathology such as fracture, exostosis, or **Köhler's bone disease** (osteochondritis of the navicular bone).

Moving laterally, the examiner palpates the three phalanges of each of the lateral four toes. Each of the lateral four metatarsals is palpated proximally to check for conditions, such as **Freiberg disease** (osteochondrosis of the second metatarsal head). Under the heads of the second and third metatarsals on the plantar aspect, the examiner should feel for any evidence of a callus, which may indicate a fallen metatarsal arch. Care must be taken to palpate the base of the fifth metatarsal (styloid process) and adjacent cuboid bone for signs of pathology. Also, the lateral aspect of the head of the fifth metatarsal may demonstrate a bunion similar to that seen on the first toe; this is called a *tailor's bunion* (see Figure 13-30).

In addition to palpating the metatarsal bones, the examiner palpates between the bones for evidence of pathology (e.g., interdigital neuroma) as well as the intrinsic muscles of the foot.

Medial Malleolus, Medial Tarsal Bones, and Posterior Tibial Artery. The examiner stabilizes the patient's heel by holding the calcaneus with one hand and palpates the

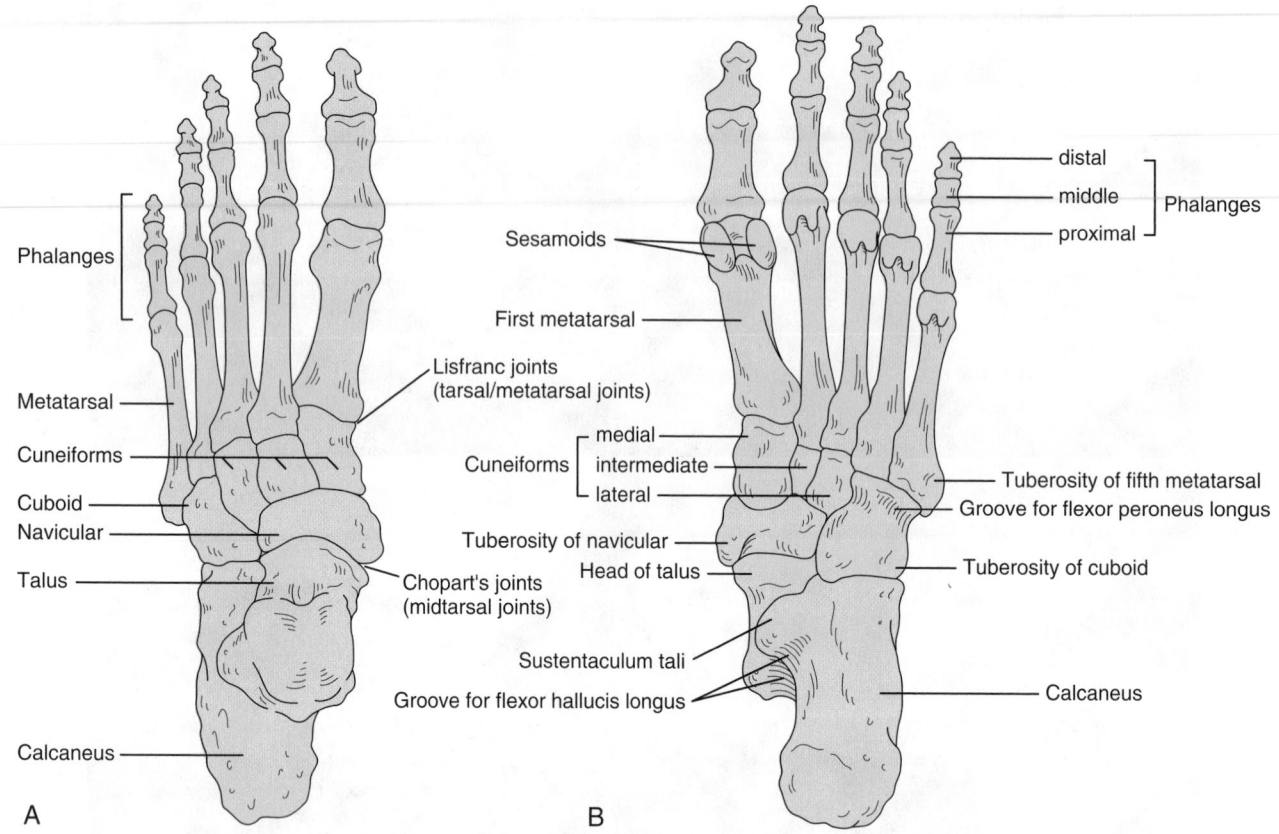

Figure 13-120 Bones of the ankle and foot. **A,** Dorsal view. **B,** Plantar view.

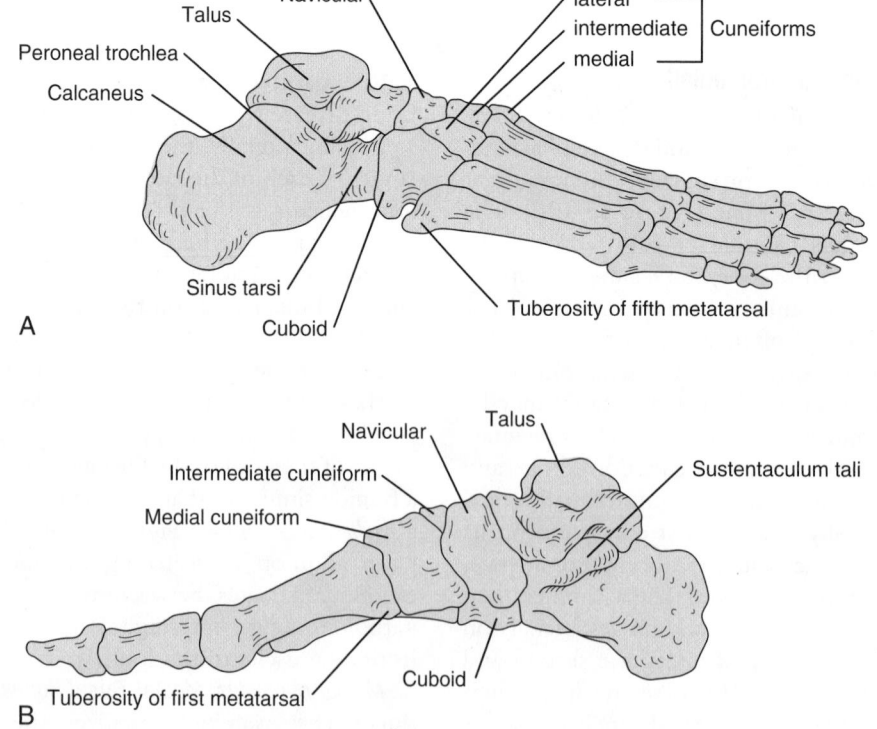

Figure 13-121 Bones of the foot from the lateral (A) and medial (B) sides.

distal edges of the medial malleolus for tenderness or swelling with the other hand. Moving from the distal extent of the medial malleolus along a line joining the navicular tubercle, the examiner moves along the talus until the head of the talus is reached. As the head of the talus is palpated, the examiner may evert and invert the foot, feeling the movement between the talar head and navicular bone. Eversion causes the talar head to become more prominent, as does pes planus. At the same time, the tibialis posterior tendon may be palpated where it inserts into the navicular and cuneiform bones. Rupture (third-degree strain) of this tendon leads to a valgus foot. The four ligaments that make up the deltoid ligament may also be palpated for signs of pathology.

Returning to the medial malleolus at its distal extent, the examiner moves further distally (approximately one finger width) until he or she feels another bony prominence, the sustentaculum tali of the calcaneus. This bony prominence is often small and difficult to palpate. Moving further posteriorly, the examiner palpates the medial aspect of the calcaneus for signs of pathology (e.g., sprain, fracture, tarsal tunnel syndrome). As the examiner moves to the plantar aspect of the calcaneus, the heel fat pad, intrinsic foot muscles, and plantar fascia are palpated for signs of pathology (e.g., heel bruise, plantar fasciitis, bone spur).

The examiner then returns to the medial malleolus and palpates along its posterior surface, noting the movement of the tibialis posterior and long flexor tendons (and checking for paratenonitis) during plantar flexion and dorsiflexion and noting any swelling or crepitus. At the same time, the posterior tibial artery, which supplies blood to 75% of the foot, may be palpated as it runs posterior to the medial malleolus. This pulse is often difficult to palpate in individuals with "plump" ankles and in the presence of edema or synovial thickening.

As the examiner moves proximally along the shaft of the tibia, he or she should feel for any tenderness or swelling (i.e., pitted edema) which may indicate the development of a medial tibial stress syndrome especially if palpating the posteromedial lower leg (Figure 13-122). This **shin palpation test** 🅐 causes pain in a positive test, or if there is pitting edema (**shin oedema test** 🅐) along the distal two thirds of the medial surface of the tibia, the test is positive.[196]

Anterior Tibia, Neck of Talus, and Dorsalis Pedis Artery. The examiner moves to the anterior aspect of the medial malleolus and follows its course laterally onto the distal end of the tibia. As the examiner moves distally, the fingers rest on the talus. If the ankle is then plantar flexed and dorsiflexed, the anterior aspect of the articular surface of the talus can be palpated for signs of pathology (e.g., osteochondritis dissecans, talar dome fracture). As the examiner moves further distally, the fingers can follow the course of the neck of the talus to the talar head. Moving distally from the tibia, the examiner should be able to

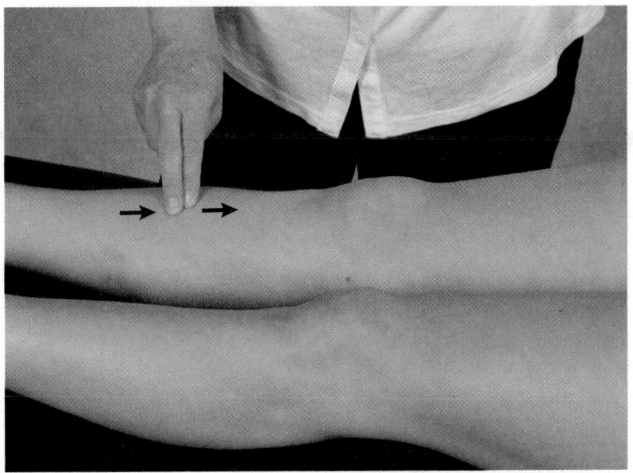

Figure 13-122 Shin palpation test.

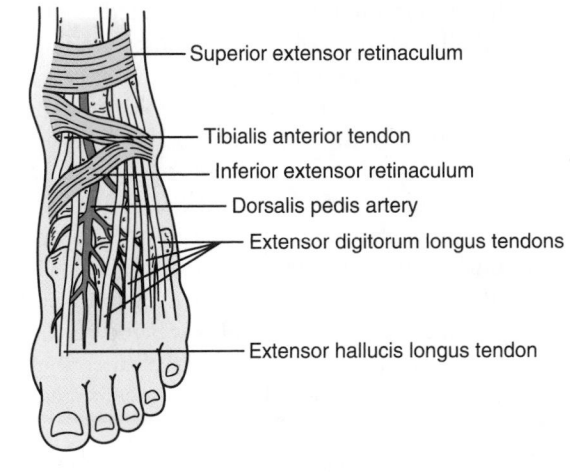

A

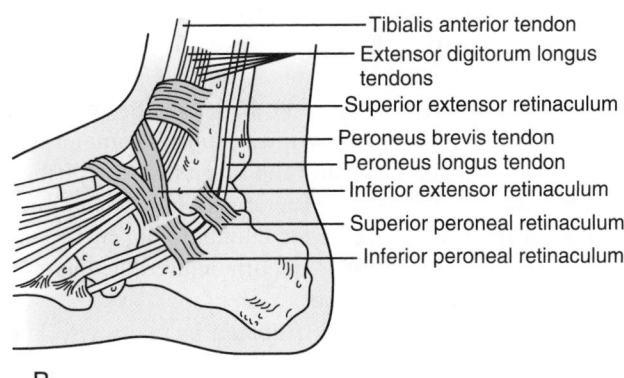

B

Figure 13-123 Retinaculum of the ankle. A, Anterior view. **B,** Lateral view.

palpate the long extensor tendons, the tibialis anterior tendon, and, with care, the extensor retinaculum (Figure 13-123). If the examiner moves further distally over the cuneiforms or between the first and second metatarsal bones, the dorsalis pedis pulse (branch of the anterior tibial artery) may be palpated. It may be found between the tendons of extensor digitorum longus and extensor hallucis longus over the junction of the first and second cuneiform bones. If an anterior compartment syndrome is suspected, this pulse should be palpated and compared with that of the opposite side. It should be remembered, however, that this pulse is normally absent in 10% of the population.

Palpation Anteriorly and Anterolaterally

Lateral Malleolus, Calcaneus, Sinus Tarsi, and Cuboid Bone. The lateral malleolus is palpated at the distal extent of the fibula. It should be noted that the lateral malleolus extends further distally and lies more posterior than the medial malleolus. The examiner then stabilizes the calcaneus with one hand and palpates with the other hand, as done previously. As the examiner moves distally from the lateral malleolus, the fingers lie along the lateral edge of the calcaneus, which is palpated with care. At the same time, the peroneal tendons can be palpated as they angle around the lateral malleolus to their insertion in the foot and up to their origin in the peroneal muscles of the leg. The peroneal retinaculum, which holds the peroneal tendons in place as they angle around the lateral malleolus, is also palpated for tenderness (see Figure 13-123). While palpating the retinaculum, the examiner should ask the patient to invert and evert the foot. If the peroneal retinaculum is torn, the peroneal tendons will often slip out of their groove or dislocate on eversion (see Figure 13-56). While the lateral malleolus is being palpated, the lateral ligaments (anterior talofibular, calcaneofibular, and posterior talofibular) should be palpated for tenderness and swelling (see Figure 13-1).

Returning to the lateral malleolus, the examiner palpates its anterior surface and then moves anteriorly to the extensor digitorum brevis muscle, the only muscle on the dorsum of the foot. By palpating carefully and deeply through the muscle, the examiner can feel a depression (the sinus tarsi) (Figure 13-124). If the fingers are left in the depression and the foot is inverted, the examiner will feel the neck of the talus, and the fingers will be pushed deeper into the depression. Tenderness in this area may indicate a sprain to the anterior talofibular ligament (see Figure 13-124), the most frequently injured ligament in the lower leg, ankle, and foot.

The cuboid bone may be palpated in two ways. The examiner may move further distally from the sinus tarsi (approximately one finger width) so that the fingers lie over the cuboid bone. Or the styloid process at the base of the fifth metatarsal bone may be palpated, and, as the examiner moves slightly proximally, the fingers lie over the cuboid bone. In either case, the cuboid should be palpated on its dorsal, lateral, and plantar surfaces for signs of pathology.

Inferior Tibiofibular Joint, Tibia, and Muscles of the Leg. Starting at the lateral malleolus and following its anterior border, the examiner should note any signs of pathology. The inferior tibiofibular joint is almost

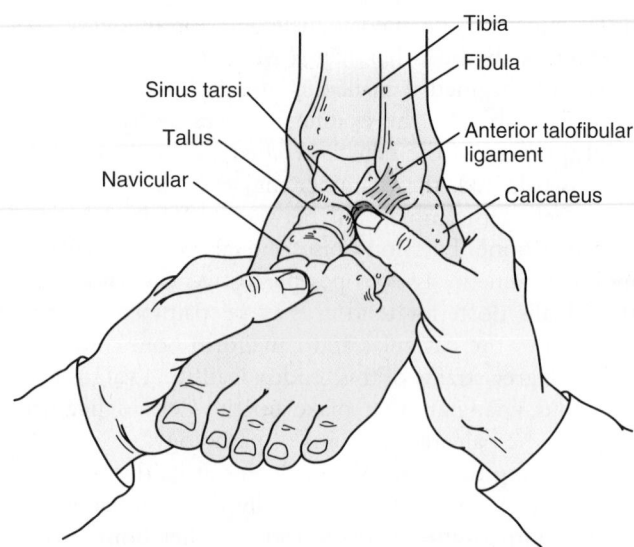

Figure 13-124 Palpation of the sinus tarsi and the anterior talofibular ligament.

impossible to feel; however, it lies between the tibia and fibula and just superior to the talus. The examiner then follows the shin, or crest, of the tibia superiorly, observing for signs of pathology (e.g., shin splints, anterior compartment syndrome, stress fracture). At the same time, the muscles of the lateral compartment (peronei) and anterior compartment (tibialis anterior and long extensors) should be carefully palpated for tenderness or swelling.

Palpation Posteriorly

The patient is then asked to lie in the prone position with the feet over the end of the examining table. The examiner palpates the following structures.

Calcaneus and Achilles Tendon. The examiner palpates the calcaneus and surrounding soft tissue for swelling (i.e., retrocalcaneal bursitis), exostosis (e.g., pump bump—Haglund deformity), or other signs of pathology. In children, care should be taken in palpating the calcaneal epiphysis for evidence of **Sever's disease** (calcaneal apophysitis; Figure 13-125). Moving proximally, the examiner palpates the Achilles tendon, noting any swelling or thickening (e.g., paratenonitis, retro-Achilles bursitis) or crepitation on movement. A palpable gap in the Achilles tendon may indicate a rupture of the tendon.[73] Any swelling caused by an intracapsular sprain of the ankle would also be evident posteriorly. Proximal to the Achilles tendon, the dome or superior surface of the calcaneus may also be palpated.

Posterior Compartment Muscles of the Leg. Moving further proximally, the examiner palpates the superficial (triceps surae) and deep posterior compartment muscles (tibialis posterior and long flexors) of the leg along their lengths for signs of pathology (e.g., strain, thrombosis).

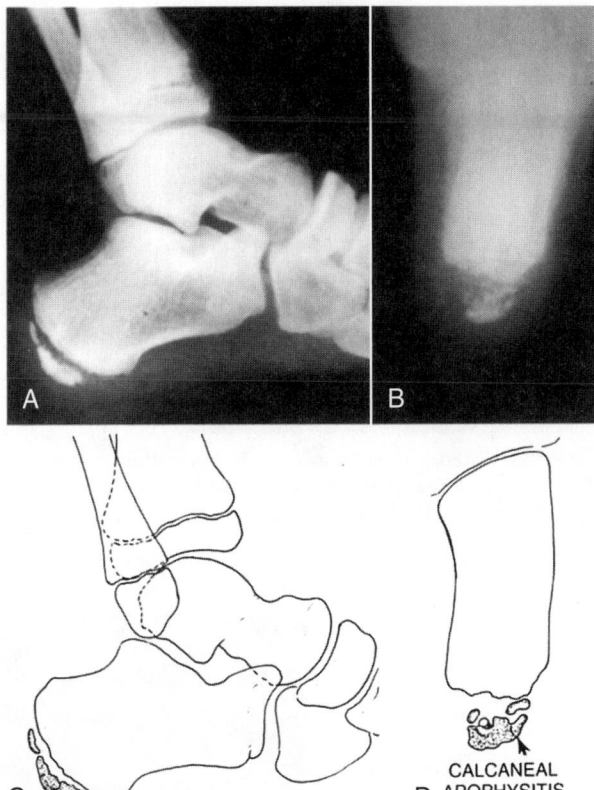

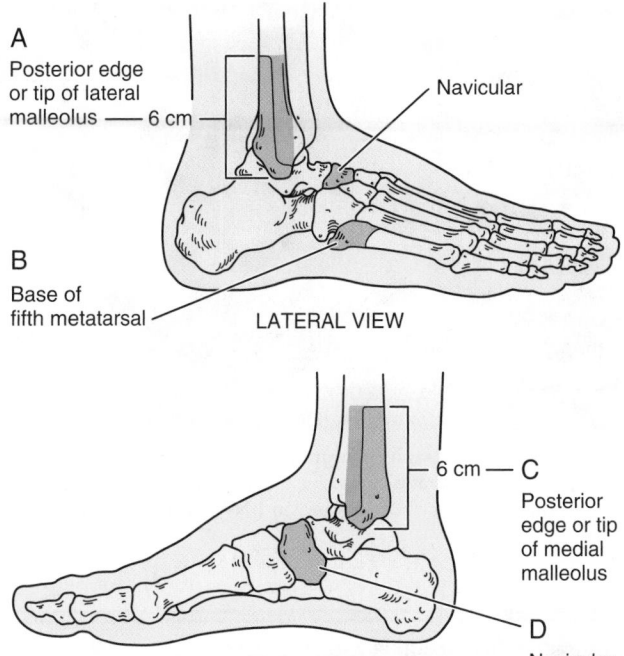

Figure 13-126 **Ottawa rules for ankle and foot radiographic series in ankle injury patients.** Radiographic series are needed only if there is bone tenderness at *A, B, C,* or *D;* inability to bear weight, and malleolar or midfoot pain. *Gray shaded areas* show Buffalo modification.

Figure 13-125 In **Sever's disease (calcaneal apophysitis),** there is fragmentation of the posterior apophysis off the calcaneus, causing achillodynia. **A,** Lateral roentgenogram of a 10-year-old boy with pain around the insertion of the Achilles tendon. **B,** Axial view of the calcaneus. **C** and **D,** Representations of films **A** and **B,** respectively. (From Kelikian H, Kelikian AS: Disorders of the ankle, Philadelphia, 1985, WB Saunders, p. 121.)

Diagnostic Imaging

Plain Film Radiography

When viewing any radiograph, the examiner should look for changes and differences between the right and left lower legs, ankles, and feet, such as osteoporosis or alterations in soft tissue, joint space, and alignment. Both weight-bearing and non–weight-bearing views should be taken. Routinely, anteroposterior, lateral, and mortise views are taken.[14,197,198] However, x-rays should not be used indiscriminately and findings should be considered in conjunction with other clinical signs and symptoms.[199] The following box shows common x-rays views taken of the lower leg, ankle, and foot.

Stiell and others have developed rules (**Ottawa ankle rules** ✓) for the proper use of x-rays after ankle or foot injuries (Figure 13-126).[200–205] Leddy and associates modified these rules with the Buffalo modification.[206] In addition to the Ottawa rules, the Buffalo modification includes the crest (midportion) of the malleolus, proximal to the ligament attachments (see Figure 13-126). Ottawa ankle rules do not apply to people under the age of 18, in the presence of multiple painful injury, head injury, intoxication, pregnancy, or neurological deficit.[122] Concern must

also be given for the mechanism of injury. For example, snowboarders commonly fracture the lateral process of the talus. Thus, a history of falling while snowboarding with tenderness below the lateral malleolus indicates the need for an x-ray.[67] To be viewed properly, individual radiographs must be made of the ankle, lower leg, or foot, and in some cases, all three to rule out injury proximal or distal to where the patient is complaining of pain.[14,32,207–210]

Common X-Ray Views of the Lower Leg, Ankle, and Foot Depending on Pathology

- Anteroposterior view of the leg and ankle (weight-bearing or non–weight-bearing) (Figure 13-131)
- Anteroposterior view of the foot/toes (routine) (Figure 13-132)
- Lateral view of the leg and ankle (see Figure 13-133)
- Mortise view (anteroposterior oblique) (routine—ankle) (see Figure 13-127, *B*)
- Anteroposterior view of the ankle (routine) (see Figure 13-127, *A*)
- Dorsoplanar view of the foot (see Figure 13-138)
- Medial 45° oblique view of the foot (non–weight-bearing) (see Figure 13-139)
- Stress (inversion) oblique view (see Figure 13-144)
- Anteroposterior lateral stress view (see Figure 13-146)
- Lateral view of foot/toes (see Figure 13-134)
- Medial oblique view of the ankle
- Lateral oblique view of the ankle
- Posterior tangential (subtalar)

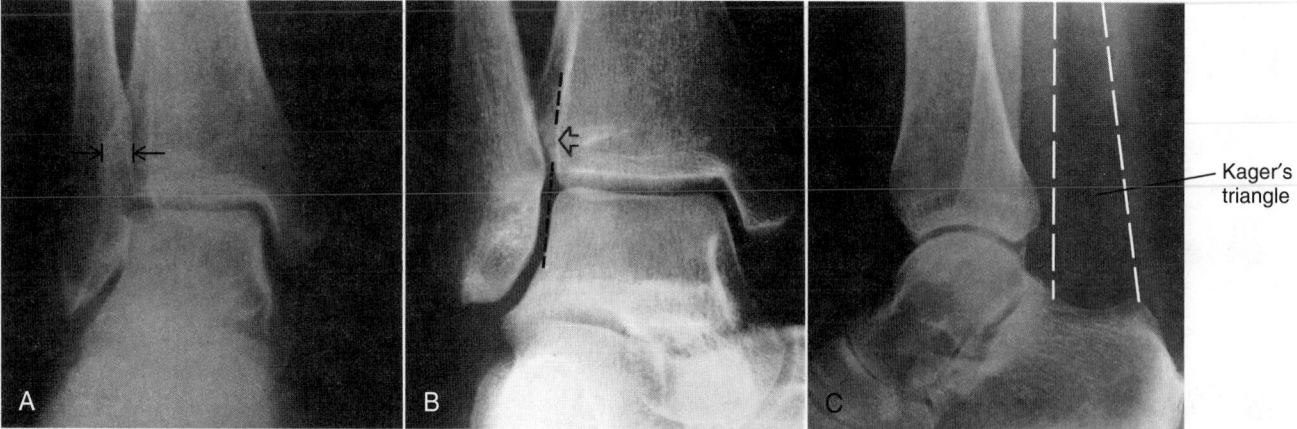

Figure 13-127 Radiographs of normal ankle. A, Anteroposterior view. Note tibiofibular overlap *(between arrows).* **B,** Internal oblique (mortise) view. *Arrow* demonstrates alignment of lateral talus with posterior cortex of tibia. **C,** Lateral view. Note the presence of Kager's triangle with an intact Achilles tendon. (From Weissman BNW, Sledge CB: Orthopedic radiology, Philadelphia, 1986, WB Saunders, pp. 590–591.)

Ottawa Rules for Ankle X-Rays (with Buffalo Modifications)

- Tenderness over lateral malleolus to 6 cm proximally
- Tenderness over medial malleolus to 6 cm proximally
- Tenderness over navicular
- Tenderness over base of fifth metatarsal

Anteroposterior View of the Ankle. The examiner notes the shape, position (whether the medial clear space is normal), and texture of the bones and determines whether there is any fractured or new subperiosteal bone (Figure 13-127). Figure 13-128 outlines the radiographic parameters of the ankle. The **medial clear space** is the space between the talus and medial malleolus (Figure 13-129). It is normally 2 to 3 mm wide, and values greater than this indicate a lateral talar shift with disruption of the ankle mortise (e.g., fibular fracture)[129,199] with disruption of the deltoid and tibiofibular ligaments[211] and, therefore, of the tibiofibular syndesmosis.[14,127,132,212] The **tibiofibular overlap** or **tibiofibular clear space** (see Figure 13-127, *A*) should be at least 6 mm, and greater than 1 mm in the mortise view although any alteration and related injury has been questioned.[129,211,213] In addition, the configuration, congruity, and inclination of the talar dome in relation to the tibial vault above it should be noted, because it may indicate an osteochondral lesion or osteochondritis dissecans (Figure 13-130).[30] If epiphyseal plates are present, the examiner should note whether they appear normal. Any increase or decrease in joint space, greater reduction of the tibial overlap, widening of the interosseus space, and greater visibility of the digital fossa should also be noted.

Mortise View of the Ankle. With this view, the ankle mortise and distal tibiofibular joint can be visualized (see

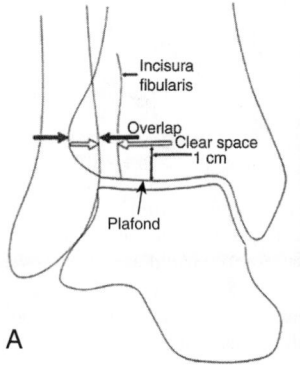
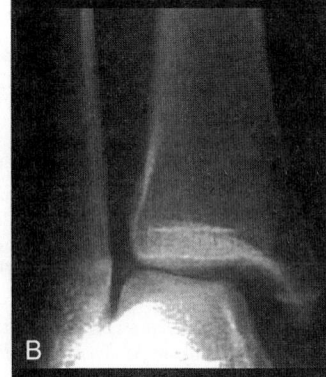

Figure 13-128 Ankle radiographic parameters. A, Normal syndesmotic relationships include a tibiofibular clear space *(open arrows),* 6 mm in both the anteroposterior (AP) and mortise views, as well as a tibiofibular overlap *(solid arrows)* > 6 mm or > 42% of the width of the fibula on the AP view, or > 1 mm on the mortise view. The overlap is measured 1 cm proximal to the plafond (ceiling of ankle joint or the articular surface of the distal end of the tibia). **B,** AP radiograph demonstrating a widened syndesmosis and increased medial clear space and no overlap. (**A** and **B,** From Stephen D: Ankle and foot injuries. In Kellam JF et al, editors: Orthopaedic knowledge update: trauma 2, p 210, Rosemont, IL, 2000, American Academy of Orthopaedic Surgeons).

Criteria for Syndesmosis Injury[32,214]

Medial clear space	> 4 mm
Tibiofibular overlap	< 2.1 mm ♀
	< 5.7 mm ♂
Clear space between fibula and peronea incisura of tibia	< 5.2 mm ♀
	< 6.5 mm ♂
Medial clear space	> Superior clear space

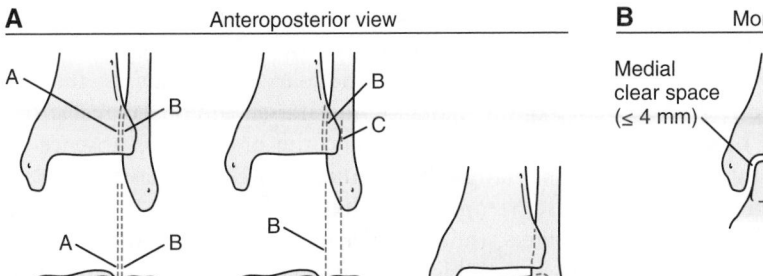

A Anteroposterior view

A
B

A
B

Clear space between
fibula and peroneal
incisura of the tibia
(≤ 5.2 mm in women,
≤ 6.5 mm in men)

B
C

B
C

Tibiofibular overlap
(≥ 2.1 mm in women,
≥ 5.7 mm in men)

Talar subluxation

B Mortise view

Medial
clear space
(≤ 4 mm)

Figure 13-129 Syndesmotic radiographic criteria. A finding outside any of these criteria indicates a syndesmosis injury. **A,** Anteroposterior view. **B,** Mortise view. *A,* Lateral border of posterior tibial malleolus; *B,* medial border of fibula; *C,* lateral border of anterior tibial tubercle.

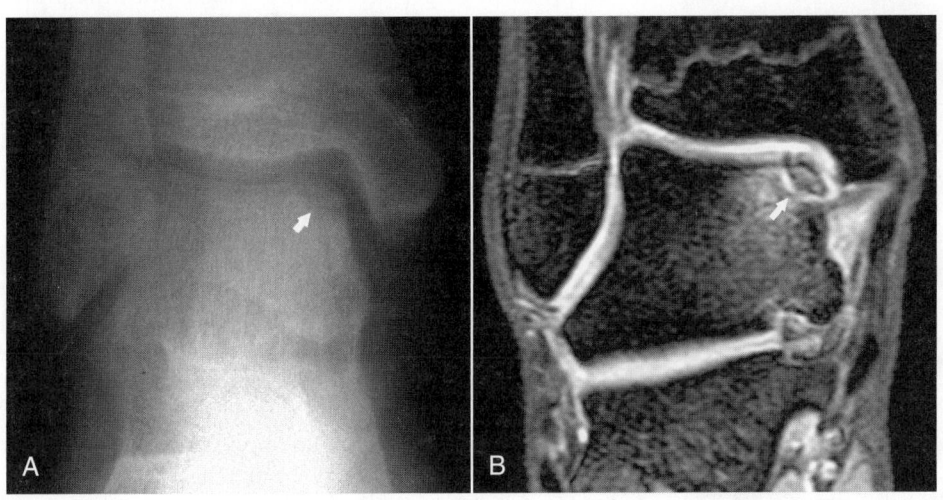

Figure 13-130 Osteochondritis dissecans of the talus: medial lesion. **A,** Note the lucent lesion of the medial talar dome *(arrow),* the site of an osteochondral fragment. **B,** Corresponding coronal, volume gradient (TR/TE, 28/7; flip angle, 25°) magnetic resonance (MR) image shows the nondisplaced fragment. (From Resnick D, Kransdorf MJ: Bone and joint imaging, Philadelphia, 2005, WB Saunders, p. 808.)

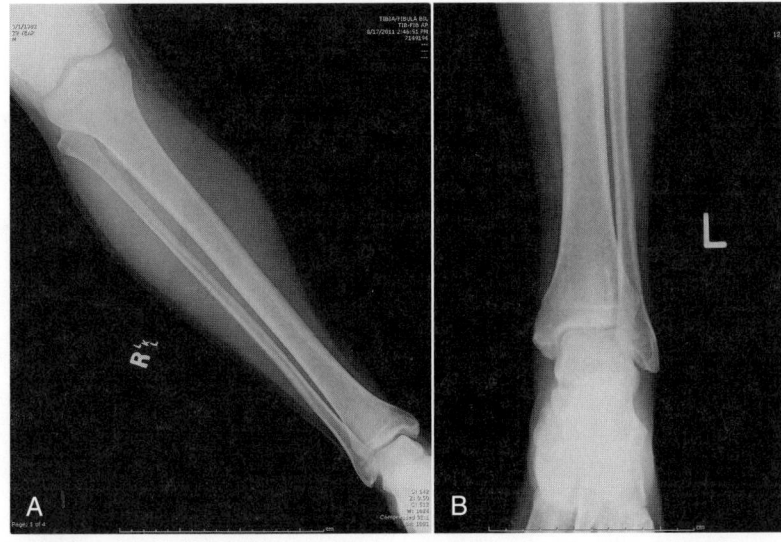

Figure 13-131 Radiographs of lower leg, ankle and foot. A, Anteroposterior view of the lower leg and ankle including the knee. **B,** Anteroposterior view of the lower leg, ankle, and foot.

Figure 13-127, *B*). To obtain this view, which is a modification of the anteroposterior view, the foot and leg are medially rotated 15° to 30°.

Lateral View of Leg, Ankle, and Foot. With this view, the examiner notes the shape, position, and texture of bones, including the tibial tubercle (Figures 13-133 and 13-134). Any fracture, new subperiosteal bone, or bone spurs should be noted (Figure 13-135). The examiner must note whether the epiphyseal lines are normal and whether there is any increase or decrease in joint space. Although this view clearly shows the talus and calcaneus, there is overlap of the midtarsal, metatarsal, and phalangeal structures. On the lateral x-ray, the presence or absence of **Kager's triangle** (see Figure 13-127, *C*) may be used to diagnose a ruptured Achilles tendon.[215] When viewing lateral films, the examiner must also be aware of Sever's disease and Köhler's disease (Figure 13-136). The presence of a Haglund deformity (abnormally enlarged posterosuperior aspect of calcaneus) or "pump bump" (abnormally large calcaneal protuberance as a result of retrocalcaneal bursitis and thickened Achilles tendon) can be determined by measuring parallel pitch lines (Figure 13-137).[37,38] Fowler and Phillip also used the posterior calcaneal angle to determine the same measurement (see Figure 13-137, *B*).[37,38,216]

Dorsoplanar View of the Foot. The dorsoplanar view is used primarily to project the forefoot. As with the previous views, the examiner should note the position, shape, and texture of the bones of the foot (Figure 13-138). The presence of a metatarsus primus varus or a condition, such as Köhler's disease, should be noted.

Medial Oblique View of the Foot. This view is often taken because it gives the clearest picture of the tarsal bones and joints and the metatarsal shafts and bases (Figures 13-139 to 13-141). The medial oblique view shows any pathology in the calcaneocuboid joint as well as the presence of a calcaneonavicular bar (Figures 13-142 and 13-143).

Stress Oblique View. The examiner should note whether there is a calcaneonavicular bar or abnormality of the calcaneus or navicular bones with this view (Figure 13-144).

Stress Film. The stress radiograph is used to compare the two ankles for integrity of the ligaments (Figures 13-145 and 13-146).[124,180,217–221] Anteroposterior views are most commonly used. With the application of an eversion or abduction stress, tilting of the talus by more than

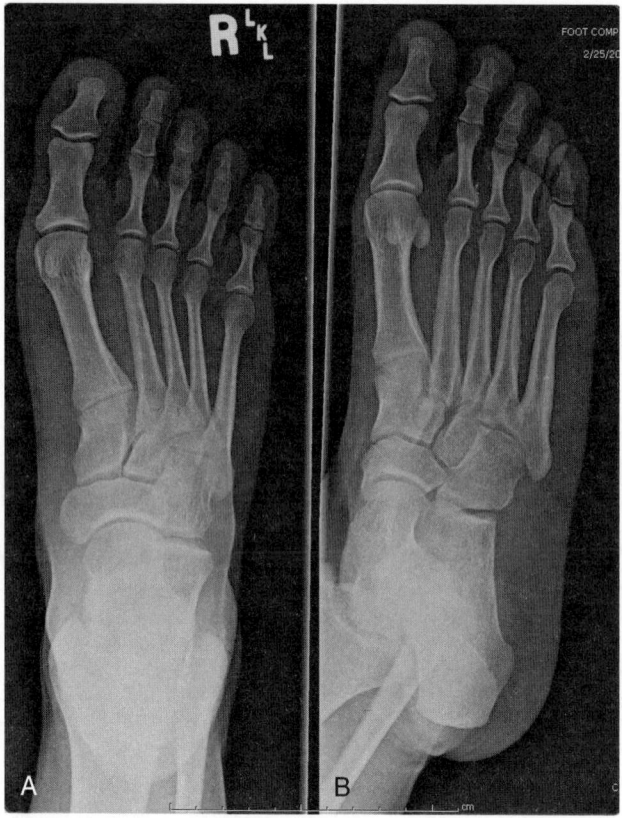

Figure 13-132 Anteroposterior (**A**) and oblique (**B**) views of the foot/toes.

Text continued on p. 965

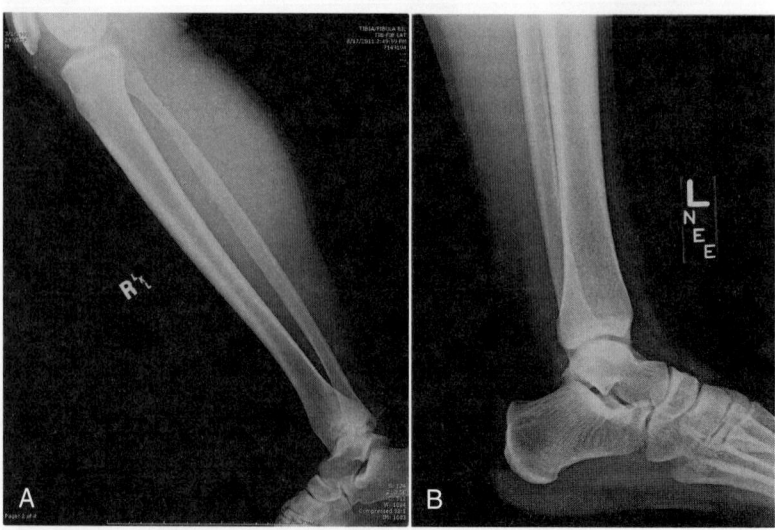

Figure 13-133 **A,** Lateral view of the leg and ankle including the knee. **B,** Lateral view of the leg and ankle including the foot.

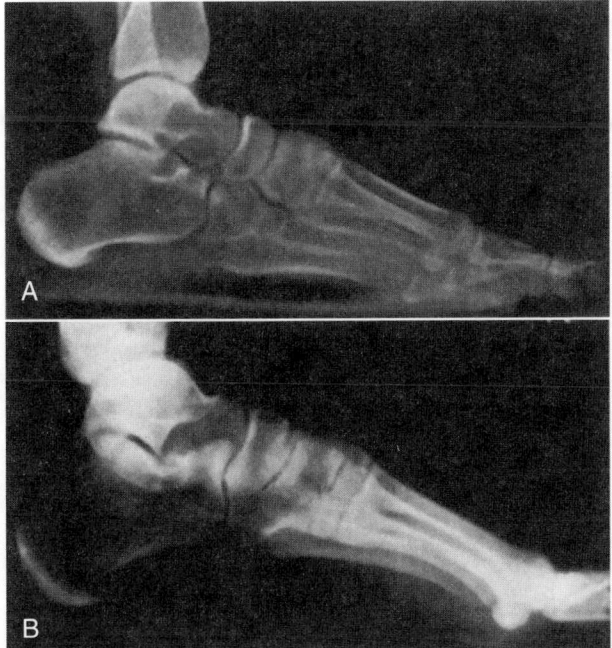

Figure 13-134 Lateral view of the foot. A, Weight-bearing posture. The soft-tissue pads are flattened beneath the heel and in the forepart of the foot, and the first metatarsal head is elevated by the sesamoids beneath it. **B,** Non–weight-bearing posture. The bony alignment and configuration are satisfactory, but the lack of resistance from the floor to the body weight permits variations, which make such views unsatisfactory for determining foot contours. (From Jahss MH: Disorders of the foot, Philadelphia, 1991, WB Saunders, pp. 68, 72.)

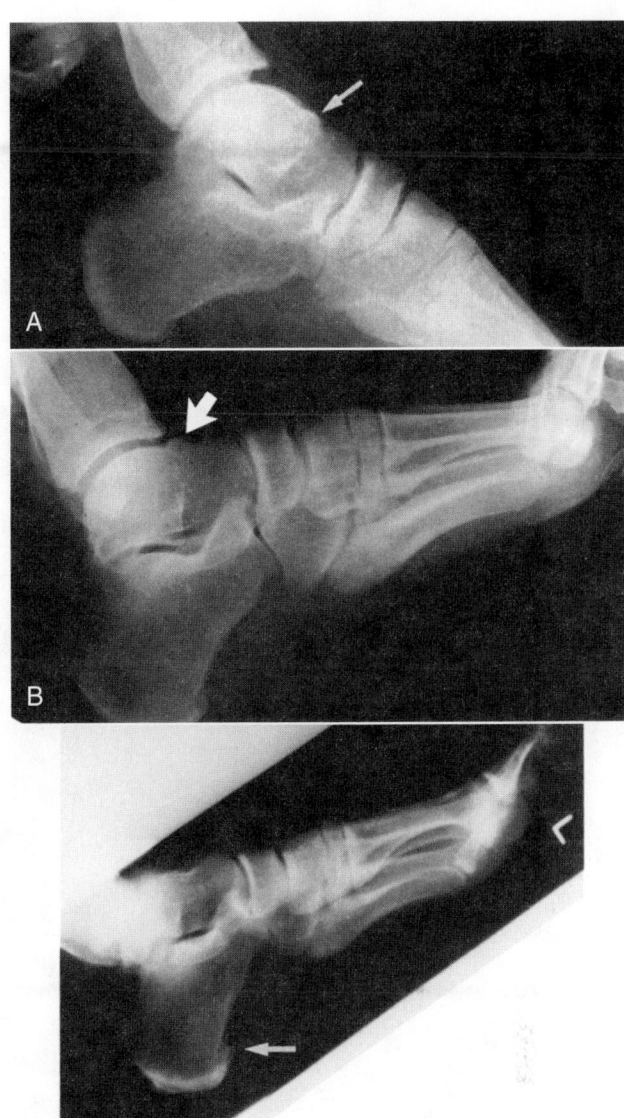

Figure 13-135 A, Talotibial spurs. **B,** Impingement occurs when foot is dorsiflexed. **C,** Heel spur. (**A** and **B,** From O'Donoghue DH: Treatment of injuries to athletes, ed 4, Philadelphia, 1984, WB Saunders, p. 627.)

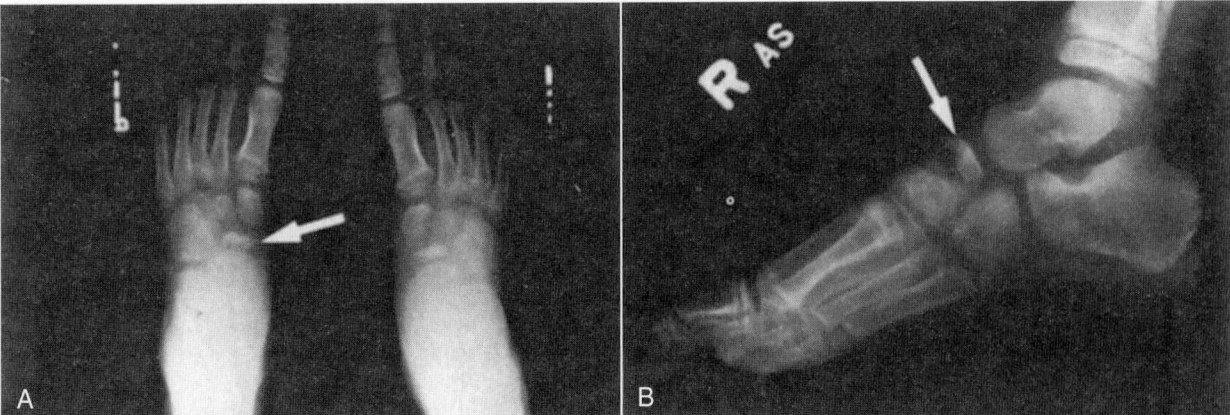

Figure 13-136 Radiographs of the foot. A, Bilateral involvement with condensation in the early stage of Köhler's disease. **B,** Same foot 2 years later shows restoration of contour on the way to completion. (From Jahss MH: Disorders of the foot, Philadelphia, 1991, WB Saunders, p. 608.)

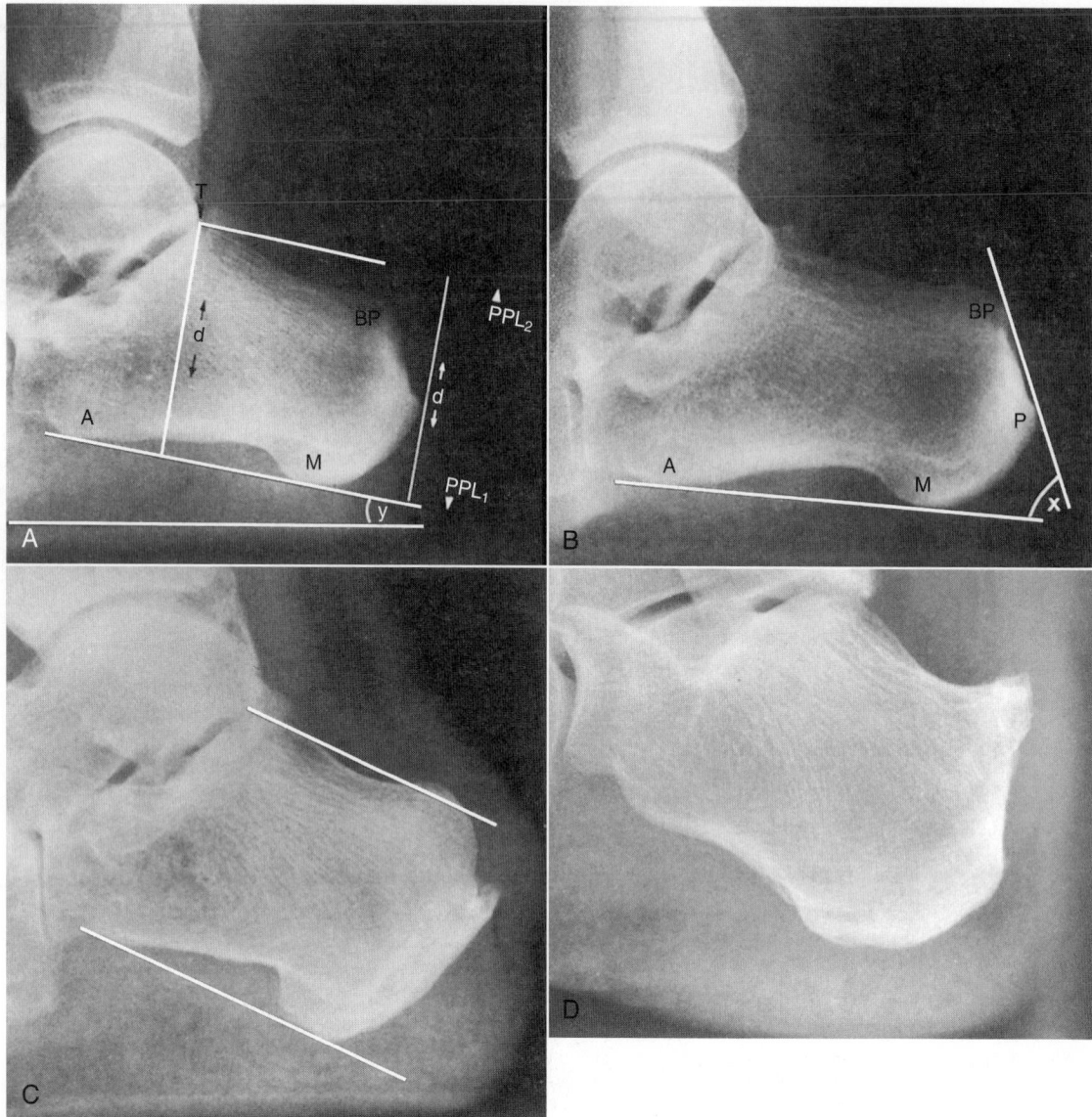

Figure 13-137 Quantitative evaluation of the shape and pitch of the os calcis. A, The parallel pitch lines *(PPL)* determine the prominence of the bursal projection *(BP)*. The lower PPL *(PPL₁)* is the base line, constructed as for the posterior calcaneal angle. A perpendicular *(d)* is constructed between the posterior lip of the talar articular facet *(T)* and the base line. The upper PPL *(PPL₂)* is drawn parallel to the base line at distance *d*. A bursal projection touching or below the PPL₂ is normal, not prominent, a −PPL. The pitch angle *(y)* is formed by the intersection of the base line *(PPL₁)* with the horizontal. **B,** The posterior calcaneal angle *(x)* of Fowler and Philip is that angle formed by the intersection of the base line tangent to the anterior tubercle A,[176] and the medial tuberosity *(M)* with the line tangent to the posterior surface of the bursal project *(BP)* and the posterior tuberosity *(P)*. **C,** Haglund syndrome is diagnosed on the lateral view of the heel by a +PPL; a cortically intact bursal projection; loss of the retrocalcaneal recess, indicating retrocalcaneal bursitis; thickening of the Achilles tendon, measuring over 9 mm at 2 cm above the bursal projection; loss of the sharp interface between the Achilles tendon and the pre-Achilles fat pad, indicating Achilles tendonitis; and convexity of the posterior soft tissues at the level of the Achilles tendon insertion, indicating superficial tendo Achilles bursitis. Clinically, this latter finding presents as a pump-bump. **D,** Patient with hypertrophic osteoarthritic spurring of the bursal projection. This bony projection displaces the Achilles tendon and adjacent soft tissues posteriorly and creates a pump-bump, which is prone to trauma if improper shoes are worn. Although this patient clinically had a pump-bump, it was produced by the posterior displacement of normal tissues at the level of a prominent bursal projection. (From Pavlov H, Heneghan MA, Hersh A, et al: The Haglund deformity: initial and differential diagnosis. Radiology 144:85–86, 1982.)

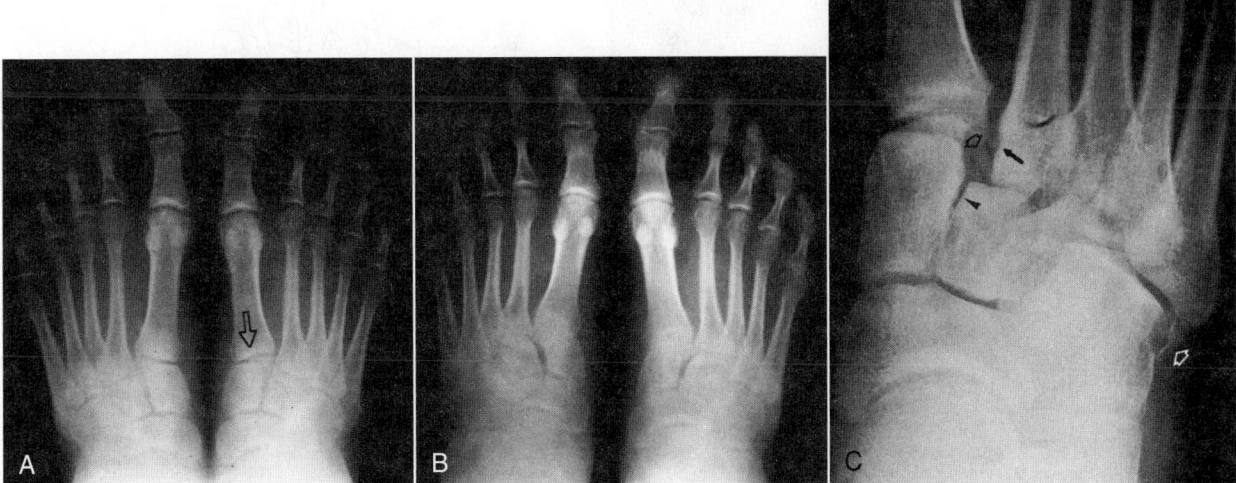

Figure 13-138 Dorsoplanar view of the foot. A, Weight-bearing posture. The cuneiform-first metatarsal joint is clearly shown *(arrow),* as are the transverse intertarsal joints, in contrast to the non–weight-bearing radiographs. **B,** Non–weight-bearing posture. The joint between the medial and middle cuneiforms is clearly shown; the other midtarsal joints are obscure. **C,** In this patient, note the subtle displacement of the second through fifth metatarsal bases. The medial edge of the second metatarsal base *(solid arrow)* is not aligned with the medial edge of the second cuneiform *(arrowhead).* Fractures of the base of the second metatarsal bone and cuboid are evident *(open arrows).* (**A** and **B,** From Jahss MH: Disorders of the foot, Philadelphia, 1991, WB Saunders, pp. 69, 71. **C,** From Resnick D, Kransdorf MJ: Bone and joint imaging, Philadelphia, 2005, WB Saunders, p. 873.)

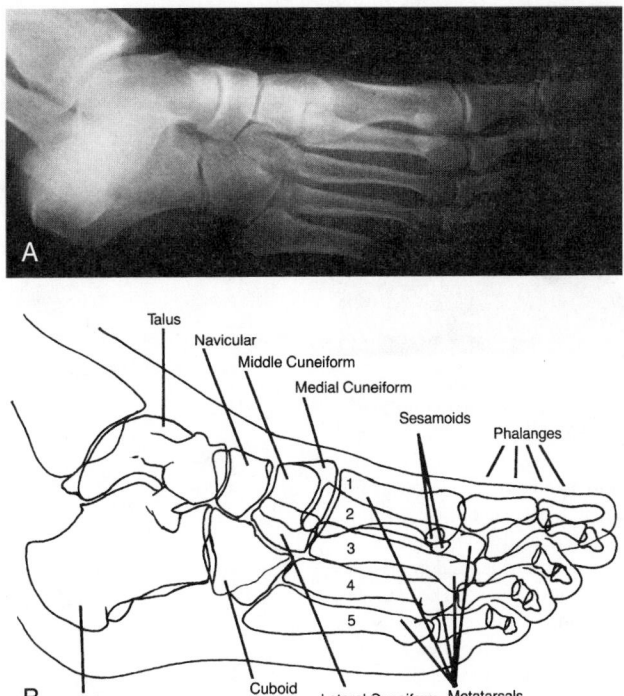

Figure 13-139 Medial oblique projection of the foot. A, Radiograph demonstrates the normal medial border alignment of the third and fourth metatarsophalangeal (MTP) joints. It also allows evaluation of the talonavicular and calcaneocuboid relationships. **B,** Anatomic drawing for correlation. (From Brotzman SB, Manske RC: Clinical orthopaedic rehabilitation: an evidence-based approach, ed 2, Philadelphia, 2003, Mosby.)

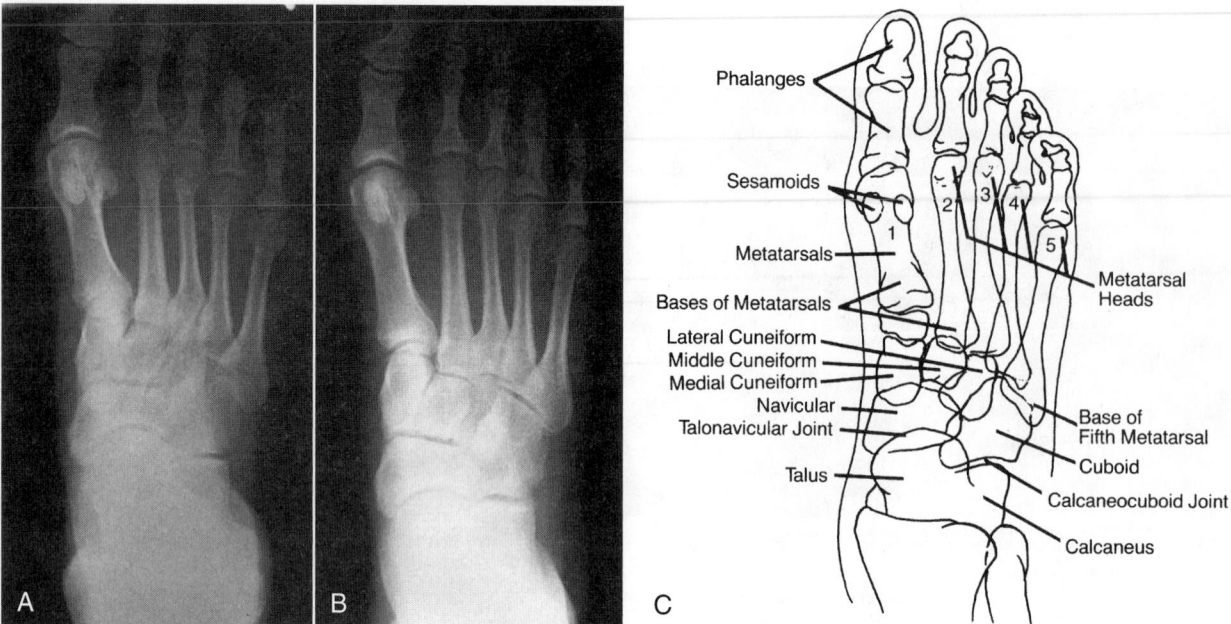

Figure 13-140 Anteroposterior projection of the foot. A, Perpendicular x-ray beam demonstrates the forefoot anatomy, particularly the phalanges and metatarsophalangeal (MTP) joints. Note the distal third and fourth metatarsal fractures. **B,** Angled x-ray beam provides improved detail of the midfoot anatomy, particularly illustrating the normal alignment of the lateral border of the first MTP joint and the medial border of the second MTP joint. **C,** Anatomic drawing for correlation. (From Brotzman SB, Manske RC: Clinical orthopaedic rehabilitation: an evidence-based approach, ed 2, Philadelphia, 2003, Mosby.)

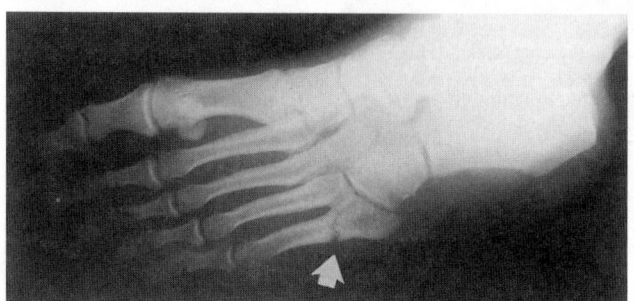

Figure 13-141 Fracture of the base of the fifth metatarsal. All fractures in this region have generally been referred to as "Jones fractures" after the original description put forth in 1902 by Sir Robert Jones, who personally sustained this fracture while dancing. Unfortunately, the persistence of this eponym has resulted in significant confusion in the management of these fractures, because at least two distinct fracture patterns occur at the base of the fifth metatarsal: avulsion fracture of the tuberosity at the attachment of the peroneus brevis, and transverse fracture of the proximal diaphysis, as shown here *(arrow)*. The management of these two types of fractures is distinctly different, because of the healing potential of the diaphyseal fracture is diminished and the rate of fibrous union or subsequent refracture is high. Inadequate initial treatment may contribute to nonunion or delayed union of the diaphyseal fracture, and thus this fracture must be distinguished from the less complicated, more proximal avulsion fracture. (From McKinnis LN: Fundamentals of musculoskeletal imaging, Philadelphia, 2005, FA Davis, p. 397.)

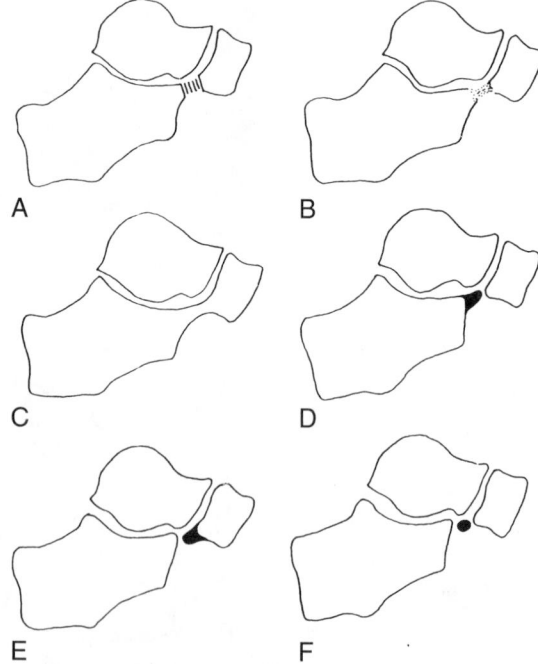

Figure 13-142 Diagrammatic representation of the types of union. A, Fibrous. **B,** Cartilaginous. **C,** Osseous. **D,** Prominent process on the calcaneus. **E,** Prominent process on the navicular. **F,** Separate calcaneonavicular ossicle (calcaneum secondarium). (From Klenerman L: The foot and its disorders, Boston, 1982, Blackwell Scientific, p. 336.)

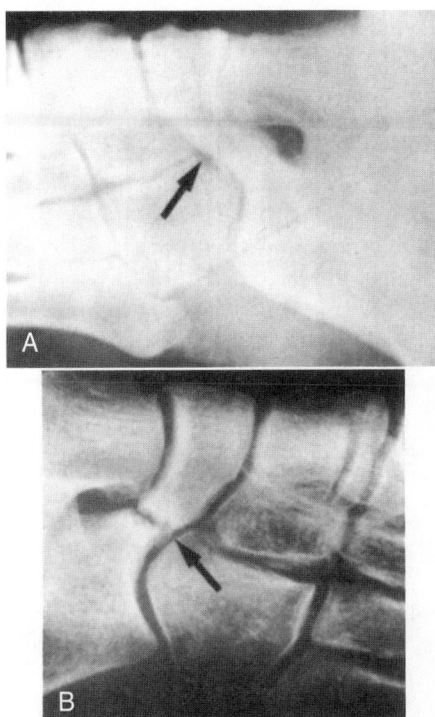

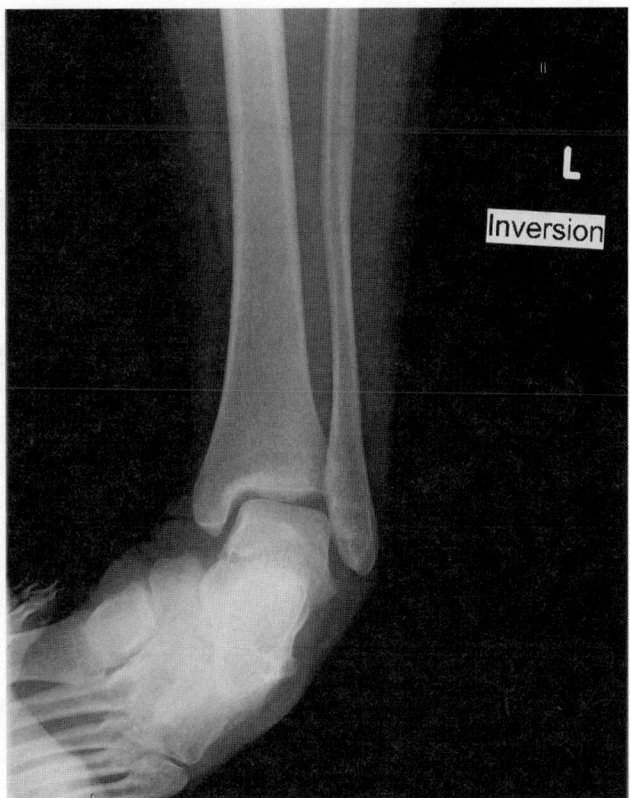

Figure 13-143 Calcaneonavicular coalition or bar. A, Total bony union, as well as bony breaks on the upper surfaces of the navicular and talus. The head of the talus may well be small. **B,** Fibrous or cartilaginous, rather than osseous, union between the bones is shown with osteoarthritic changes of the opposing bone surfaces and an enlarged navicular. (From Klenerman L: The foot and its disorders, Boston, 1982, Blackwell Scientific, p. 340.)

Figure 13-144 Ankle stress (inversion) view.

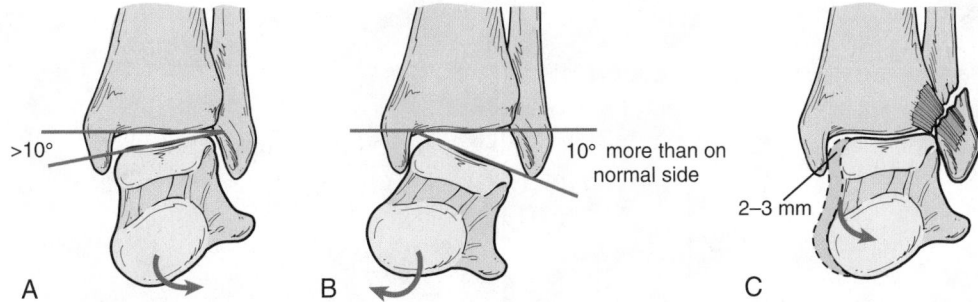

Figure 13-145 Positive findings on diagrammatic stress radiographs. A, Abduction stress. **B,** Adduction stress. **C,** Increased (2 to 3 mm) medial clear space (lateral rotary stress).

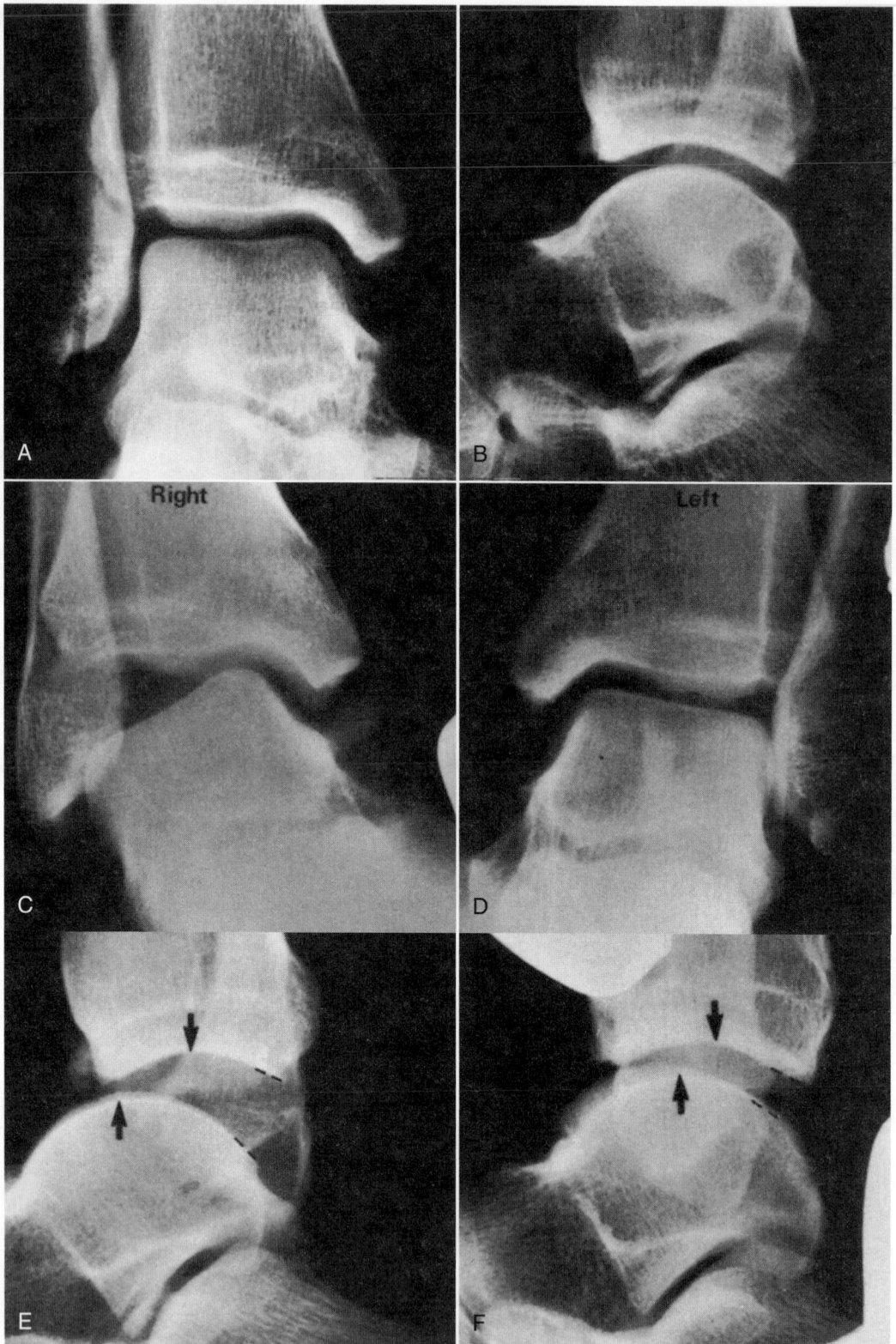

Figure 13-146 Abnormal stress views: anterior talofibular and calcaneofibular ligament tears. Anteroposterior (**A**) and lateral (**B**) views of the right ankle showing hypertrophic lipping from the anterior tibia and talus. The syndesmosis is slightly wide. Comparison varus stress views of the right (**C**) and left (**D**) ankles show abnormal talar tilt on the right, particularly when compared with the normal left side. This is diagnostic of an anterior talofibular ligament tear on the right, with or without a calcaneofibular ligament tear. The anterior drawer test is abnormal on the right (**E**) compared with the left (**F**). Comparison can be made by noting the anterior shift of the midtalus in relation to the midtibia *(arrows)* on each side, the loss of parallelism of the subchondral cortices on the right, or the marked widening of the posterior joint space *(lines)* on the abnormal as compared with the normal side. This is consistent with an anterior talofibular ligament tear on the right. (From Weissman BNW, Sledge CB: Orthopedic radiology, Philadelphia, 1986, WB Saunders, p. 600.)

10° is considered pathological.[222] An increase in the medial clear space (space between medial malleolus and talus) of more than 2 to 3 mm is considered pathological and usually indicates insufficiency of the deltoid ligament, especially the tibiotalar ligament. Instability may also be demonstrated by widening of the **syndesmosis** (the mortise between the tibia and fibula). An inversion or adduction stress causing 8° to 10° more movement on one ankle than the other is considered pathological and is indicative of torn lateral ligaments. If the talus has not moved, or if it is fixed but its distal end is unduly prominent, subtalar instability is suggested.

Measurements on Plain Radiographs. Plain radiographs may be used to measure different angles and axes. For example, Figure 13-147 shows the ankle joint axis, and Figure 13-148 shows the subtalar joint axis. Figures

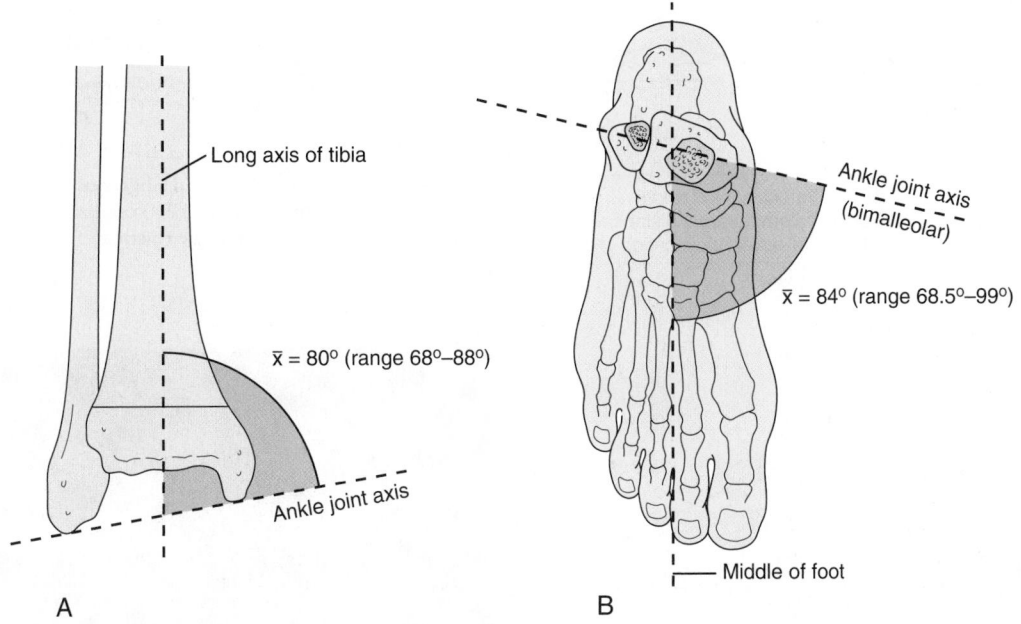

Figure 13-147 Orientation of the ankle joint axis. Mean values measure **(A)** 80° from a vertical reference and **(B)** 84° from the longitudinal reference of the foot. (Adapted from Hunt GC, editor: Physical therapy of the foot and ankle, New York, 1988, Churchill Livingstone; and Isman RE, Inman VT: Anthropometric studies of the human foot and ankle: technical report No. 58, San Francisco, 1968, University of California.)

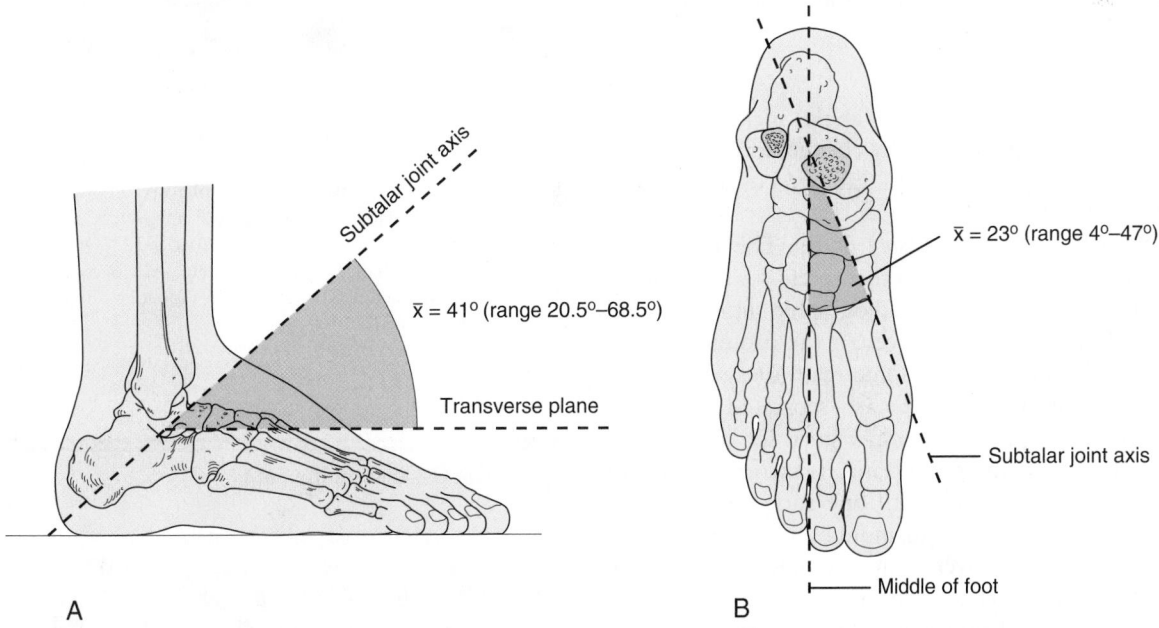

Figure 13-148 Orientation of the subtalar joint axis. Mean values measure **(A)** 41° from the transverse plane and **(B)** 23° medially from the longitudinal reference of the foot. (Adapted from GC Hunt, editor: Physical therapy of the foot and ankle, New York, 1988, Churchill Livingstone; and Isman RE, Inman VT: Anthropometric studies of the human foot and ankle: technical report no. 58, San Francisco, 1968, University of California.)

Normal Alignment

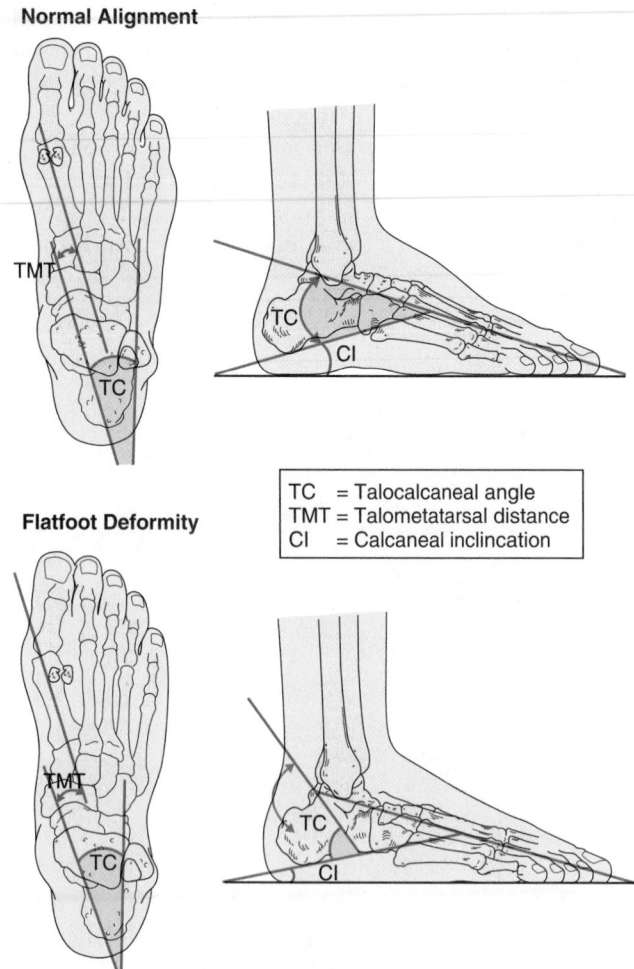

Flatfoot Deformity

TC	= Talocalcaneal angle
TMT	= Talometatarsal distance
CI	= Calcaneal inclincation

Figure 13-149 Drawing of normal and pathologic alignment of a pes planus in anteroposterior (AP) and lateral views. *CI,* Calcaneal inclination; *TC,* talocalcaneal angle; *TMT,* talometatarsal angle.

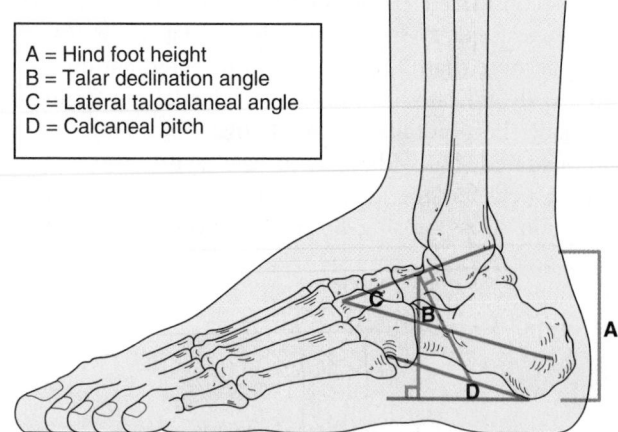

A = Hind foot height
B = Talar declination angle
C = Lateral talocalaneal angle
D = Calcaneal pitch

Figure 13-150 Drawing of normal alignment of a healthy foot in lateral weight-bearing view. *A,* Hindfoot height; *B,* talar declination angle; *C,* lateral talocalaneal angle (method 2); *D,* calcaneal pitch.

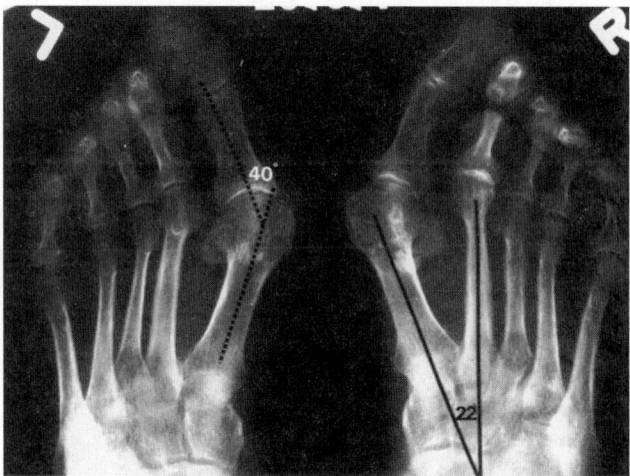

Figure 13-151 Measurement of hallux valgus deformity. On the left, the angle of intersection of the long axes of the proximal phalangeal and the first metatarsal shafts *(dotted lines)* is 40°. Normally, this angle is no greater than 10°. On the right, there is rotation of the great toe and lateral subluxation of the proximal phalanx, leaving about one half of the articular surface of the metacarpal uncovered. The angle of the first and second metatarsal shafts *(solid lines)* is 22°. On standing views, angles of greater than 10° indicate metatarsus primus varus. (From Weissman BNW, Sledge CB: Orthopedic radiology, Philadelphia, 1986, WB Saunders, p. 657.)

13-149 to 13-151 show various angles measured in the ankle and foot. These angles may change during development, so in some cases, serial radiographs may be of benefit.[223–225]

Abnormal Ossicles or Accessory Bones. The foot often exhibits abnormal ossicles, and their presence may lead to incorrect interpretation of radiographic films (Figure 13-152). These bones are pieces of the prominences of various tarsal bones that for some reason (e.g., fracture, secondary ossification center) are separated from the normal bone (e.g., os trigonum; Figure 13-153).[36,226] A sesamoid bone, on the other hand, is incorporated into the substance of a tendon with one surface articulating with the adjacent bones. A sesamoid bone moves with the tendon and is found over bony prominences or where the tendon makes a change in direction. In addition to the normal sesamoid bones under the big toe, sesamoid bones may also be found in the tendons of peroneus longus and tibialis posterior. Abnormal ossicles are more likely to occur in the foot than anywhere else in the body.

Common Ossicles in the Foot

- Os trigonum (separate posterior talar tubercle)
- Os tibiale externum (separate navicular tuberosity)
- Bipartite medial cuneiform (separated into upper and lower halves)
- Os vesalianum (separate tuberosity of the base of the fifth metatarsal)
- Os sustentaculi (separate part of the sustentaculum tali)
- Os supranaviculare (dorsum of the talonavicular joint)

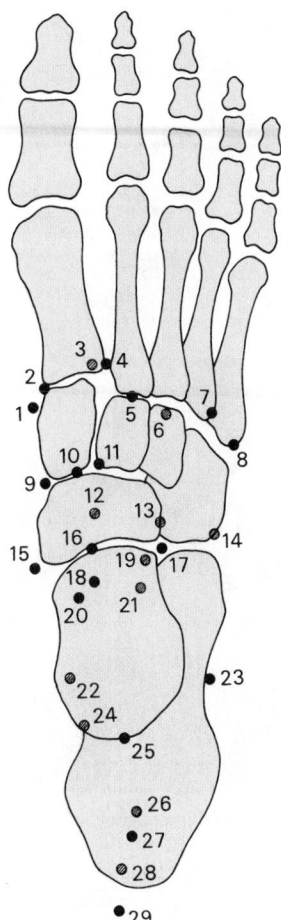

Figure 13-152 Accessory tarsal bones. *1,* Os sesamoideum tibialis anterior; *2,* os cuneometatarsale I tibiale; *3,* os cuneometatarsale I plantare; *4,* os intermetatarsale I; *5,* os cuneometatarsale II dorsale; *6,* os unci; *7,* os intermetatarsale IV; *8,* os vesalianum; *9,* os paracuneiforme; *10,* os naviculocuneiforme I dorsale; *11,* os intercuneiforme; *12,* os sesamoideum tibialis posterior (according to Trolle, this may be the same as *15*); *13,* os cuboideum secundarium; *14,* os peroneum; *15,* os tibiale (externum); *16,* os talonaviculare dorsale; *17,* os calcaneus secundarius; *18,* os supratalare; *19,* os trochleae; *20,* os talotibiale dorsale; *21,* os in sinu tarsi; *22,* os sustentaculi proprium; *23,* calcaneus accessorius; *24,* os talocalcaneare posterior; *25,* os trigonum; *26,* os aponeurosis plantaris; *27,* os supracalcaneum; *28,* os subcalcaneum; *29,* os tendinis Achilles. (Redrawn from Klenerman L: The foot and its disorders, Boston, 1982, Blackwell Scientific, p. 361.)

Films Showing Bone Development. Like the bones of the hand, the bones of the foot form within a certain time period (Figure 13-154). However, because the foot is subjected to greater forces and environmental effects than the hand, it is not usually used to determine skeletal age. X-rays of the foot often show the developing bone deformities seen in clubfoot (Figure 13-155). Although not all of the bones are present at birth, a series of films will show differences when compared with films of normal feet.

Arthrography

Arthrograms of the ankle are indicated whenever there is acute ligament injury, chronic ligament laxity, or

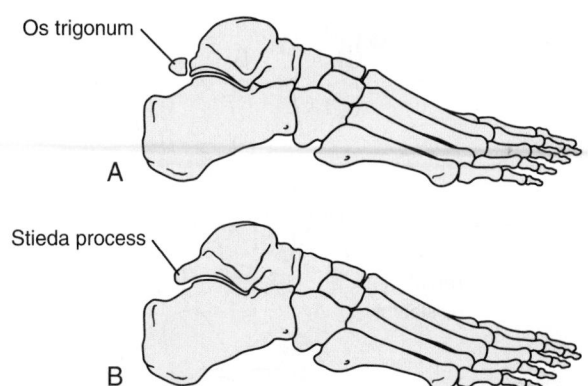

Figure 13-153 Lateral view of the ankle, showing the os trigonum (A) and Stieda's process (B). (Redrawn from Brodsky AE, Khalil MA: Talar compression syndrome. Foot Ankle 7:338–344, 1987.)

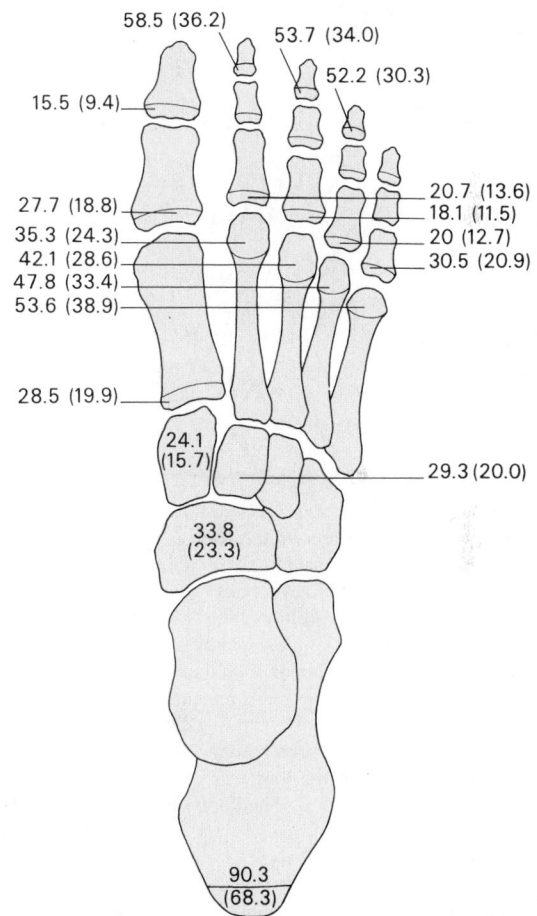

Figure 13-154 Anteroposterior diagram of the foot showing the times of appearance (in months) of the centers of ossification for boys (and for girls, in parentheses). (Redrawn from Hoerr NL, et al: Radiographic atlas of skeletal development of the foot and ankle, Springfield, IL, 1962, Charles C Thomas, with kind permission of Charles C Thomas, Springfield, IL.)

indications of loose body or osteochondritis dissecans (Figures 13-156 and 13-157).[14,30,227,228] Leakage of the contrast medium indicates tearing of the joint capsule or capsular ligaments. Normally, the talocrural joint admits only about 6 mL of contrast medium.

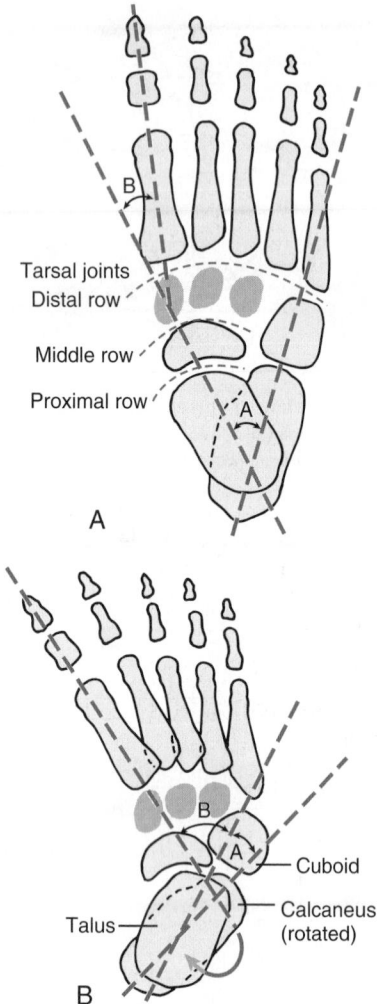

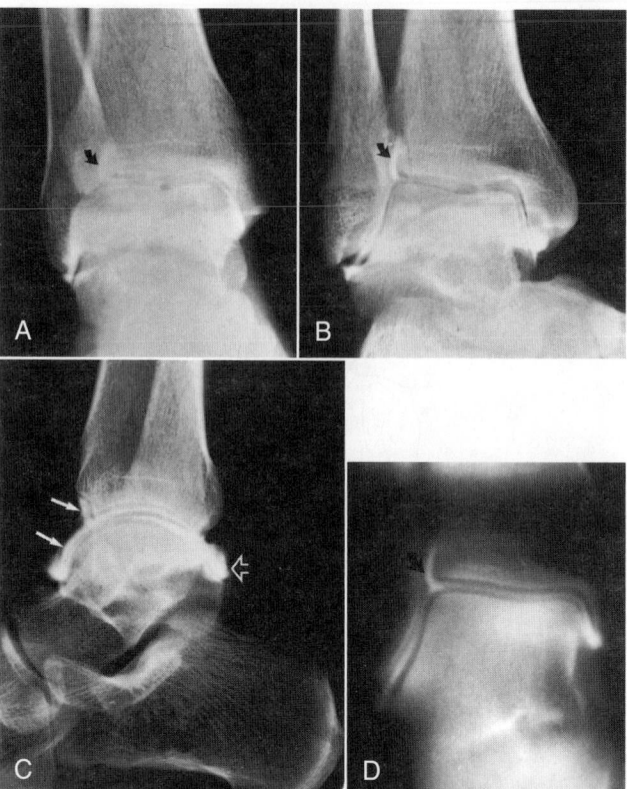

Figure 13-156 Normal positive-contrast ankle arthrogram. Antero-posterior **(A)**, internal oblique or mortise **B**, and lateral **C**, views and a tomogram **D**, in the internal oblique projection show contrast agent coating the articular surfaces and filling normally present anterior *(white arrows)*, posterior *(open arrow)*, and syndesmotic *(black arrows)* recesses. There is no extension of contrast medium into the soft tissue medially or laterally. (From Weissman BNW, Sledge CB: Orthopedic radiology, Philadelphia, 1986, WB Saunders, p. 596.)

Figure 13-155 Representations of the foot as seen on radiographs. A, Representation of the normal foot. The cuboid blocks medial movement of the foot at the middle row of tarsal joints because of its unique location. It alone occupies a position in both rows of tarsal joints. The talocalcaneal angle *(angle A)* is measured by drawing lines through the long axes of the talus and calcaneus. One should attempt to be as accurate as possible in making these measurements. The normal range for this measurement is 20° to 40° in the young child. The talus-first metatarsal angle *(angle B)* is measured by drawing lines through the long axis of the talus and along the long axis of the first metatarsal. The normal range is 0° to –20°. **B,** Hindfoot varus, as manifested by a decreased talocalcaneal angle *(angle A)*, and talonavicular subluxation, as manifested by a talocalcaneal angle of less than 15° and a talus-first metatarsal angle *(angle B)* of more than 15°. Talonavicular subluxation occurs through the medial movement of three bones, which move as a unit. The navicular, cuboid, and calcaneus move medially through the combined movements of medial translation and supination of the proximal tarsal bones, whereas the calcaneus inverts beneath the talus. (Redrawn from Simons GW: Analytical radiography and the progressive approach in talipes equinovarus. Orthop Clin North Am 9:189, 1978.)

Computed Tomography

Computed tomography scans are useful for determining the relation among the bones and for giving a view of the relation between bony and soft tissues (Figures 13-158 and 13-159).

Magnetic Resonance Imaging

MRI is an especially useful, although sometimes overused, technique for delineating bony and soft tissues around the ankle and foot (Figures 13-160 to 13-163).[11] MRI may be used to diagnose ruptured tendons (e.g., Achilles, peroneal), ligament tears (Figure 13-164), and fractures (e.g., stress fractures, osteochondral fractures, osteonecrosis).[229-238]

Bone Scans

Bone scans are used in the lower limb, ankle, and foot to diagnose stress fractures. Areas of high risk for stress fractures include the tibia (anterior diaphysis) (Figures 13-165 and 13-166), navicular, and proximal fifth metatarsal.[239]

Ultrasonography

This technique makes use of the ultrasonic waves to determine possible tissue injury. With an experienced operator, it may show injury to growth plates in the presence of a normal radiograph or prenatal pathology.[240,241]

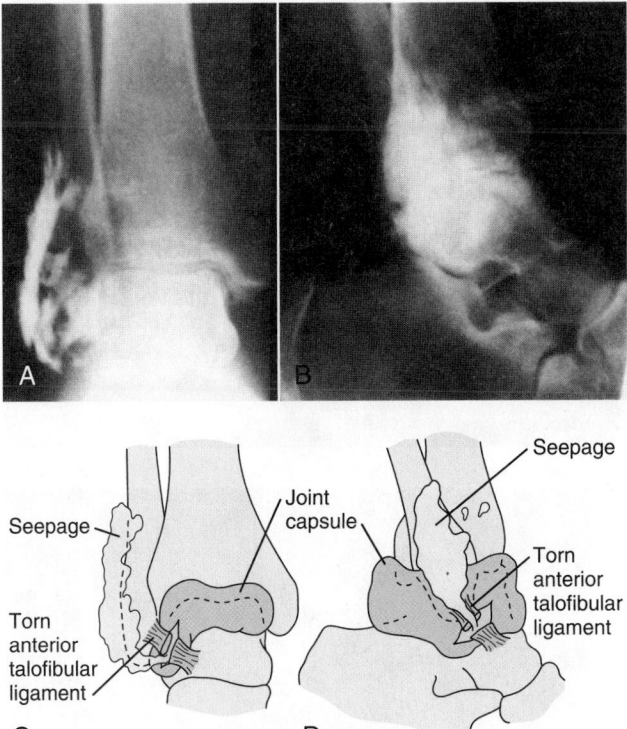

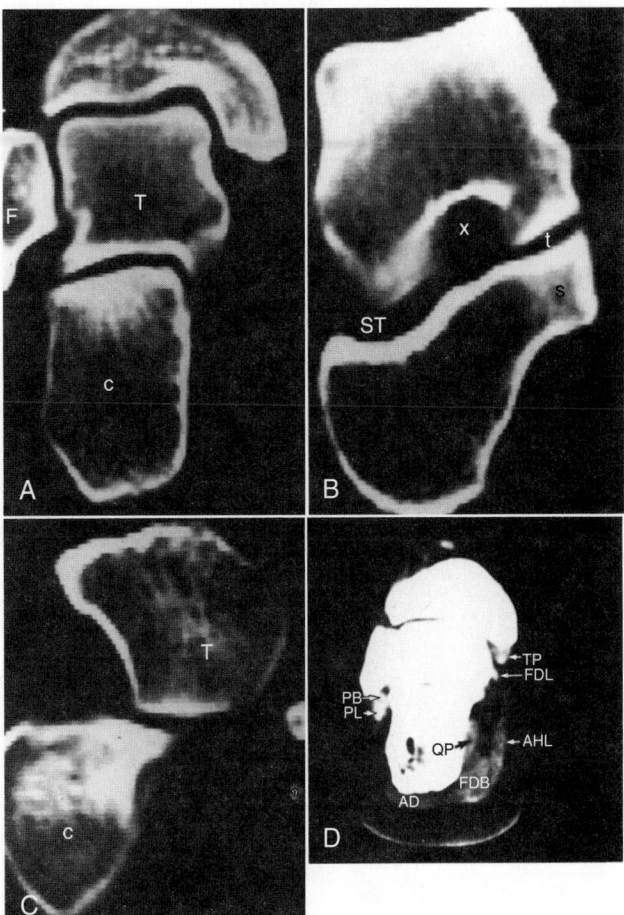

Figure 13-157 Contrast arthrography showing acute tear of the anterior tibiofibular ligament. A, Anteroposterior arthrogram of the right ankle 14 hours after the injury showing extravasation of contrast medium in front and around the lateral aspect of the fibula. **B,** Lateral view of the same. **C** and **D,** Illustrations of arthrograms **A** and **B,** respectively. (Modified from Kelikian H, Kelikian AS: Disorders of the ankle, Philadelphia, 1985, WB Saunders, p. 143.)

Figure 13-158 Normal anatomy of the ankle and foot as seen on computed tomography scans. A, Coronal section through the ankle and subtalar joint. *T,* Talus, *C,* calcaneus, *F,* fibula. **B,** Farther anteriorly, the sustentaculum tali *(S),* the site of insertion of the talocalcaneal ligament *(X),* the subtalar joint *(ST),* and the mid-talocalcaneonavicular joint *(t)* are shown. **C,** Anterior to the sustentaculum tali, the talus *(T)* and the calcaneus *(C),* are shown. **D,** The peroneus brevis *(PB),* peroneus longus *(PL),* posterior tibial *(TP),* and flexor digitorum longus *(FDL)* muscles are shown. *AD,* Abductor digiti quinti pedis; *AHL,* abductor hallucis longus, *FDB,* flexor digitorum brevis, *QP,* quadratus plantae. This scan is at the level of the posterior aspect of the sustentaculum tali. (From Weissman BNW, Sledge CB: Orthopedic radiology, Philadelphia, 1986, WB Saunders, p. 632.)

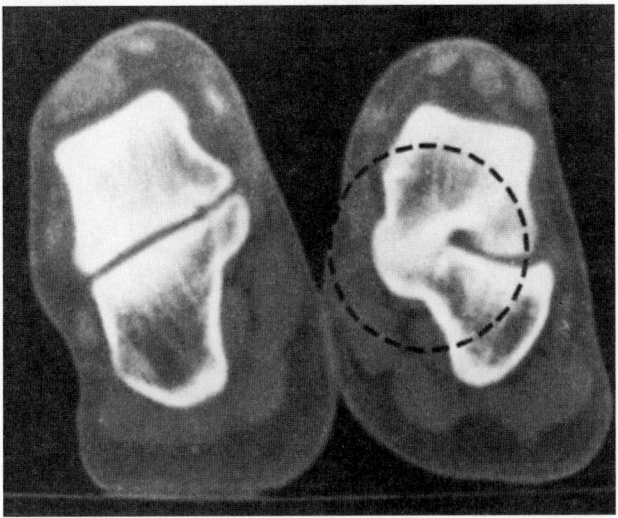

Figure 13-159 Coronal computed tomographic view showing talocalcaneal coalition on the right. (From Rettig AC, Shelbourne KD, Beltz HF, et al: Radiographic evaluation of foot and ankle injuries in the athlete. Clin Sports Med 6:914, 1987.)

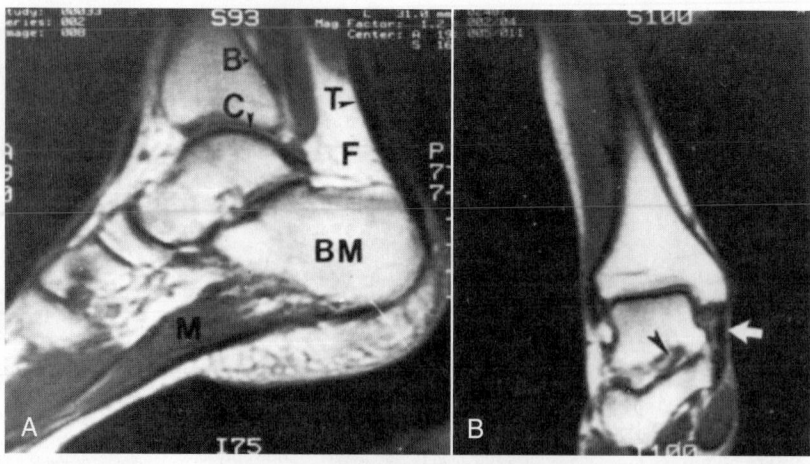

Figure 13-160 Sagittal and coronal magnetic resonance images of the ankle. A, Sagittal projection. Note the white bone marrow *(BM)* and subcutaneous fat *(F)*, black tendons *(T)* and ligaments, gray muscles *(M)* and articular cartilage *(C)*, and black cortical bone *(B)*. **B,** Coronal projection. Note the black appearance of the deltoid ligament *(white arrow)* and interosseous ligament *(black arrowhead)* between the talus and calcaneus. (From Kingston S: Magnetic resonance imaging of the ankle and foot. Clin Sports Med 7:19, 1988.)

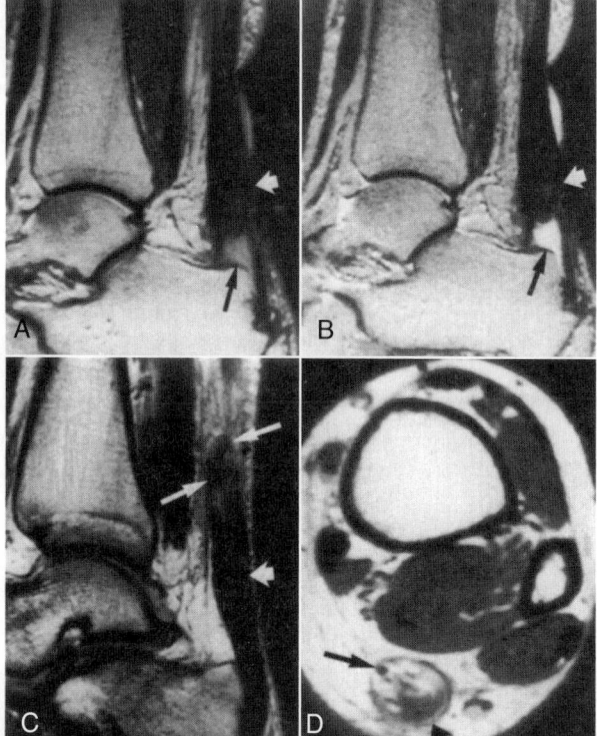

Figure 13-161 Magnetic resonance images showing partial Achilles tendon tear. Sagittal, proton-density **(A)** and T2-weighted magnetic resonance images **(B)** reveal a large tear at the Achilles insertion with intratendinous fluid *(long arrow)* and fraying and thickening of the distal tendon *(short arrow)*. **C,** Complete Achilles tendon tear. Sagittal, proton-density magnetic resonance (MR) image reveals disruption of the Achilles tendon *(long arrows)* and thickening of its distal portion *(short arrow)*. **D,** On an axial, T1-weighted MR image, only gray granulation tissue is shown within the paratenon *(short arrow)*. The intact plantaris tendon passes along the medial border of the paratenon *(long arrow)*. (From Kerr R, Forrester DM, Kingston S: Magnetic resonance imaging of foot and ankle trauma. Orthop Clin North Am 21:593, 1990.)

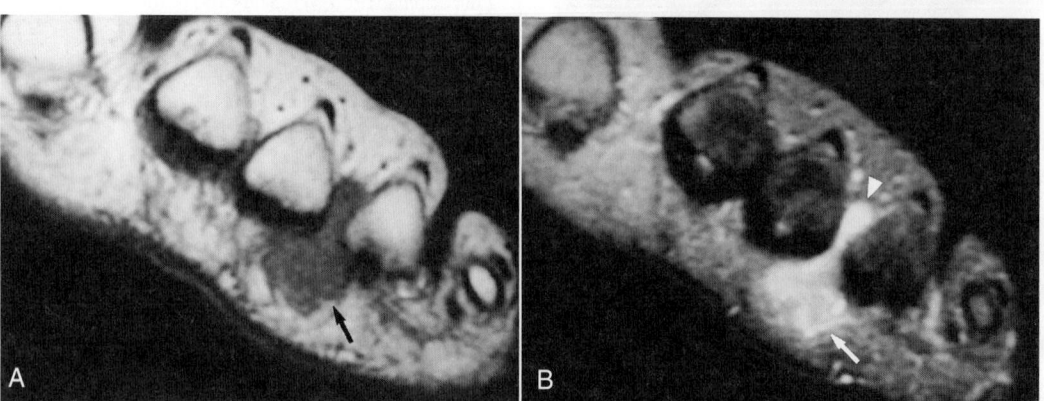

Figure 13-162 Morton's neuroma. A, Coronal T1-weighted (TR/TE, 600/20) spin echo magnetic resonance (MR) image shows a mass *(arrow)* of low signal intensity between the third and fourth metatarsal heads. **B,** This mass *(arrow)* has high signal intensity on a coronal fat-suppressed fast spin echo (TR/TE, 3500/50) MR image. A small amount of fluid may be present in the intermetatarsal bursa *(arrowhead)*. (From Resnick D, Kransdorf MJ: Bone and joint imaging, Philadelphia, 2005, WB Saunders, p. 1051.)

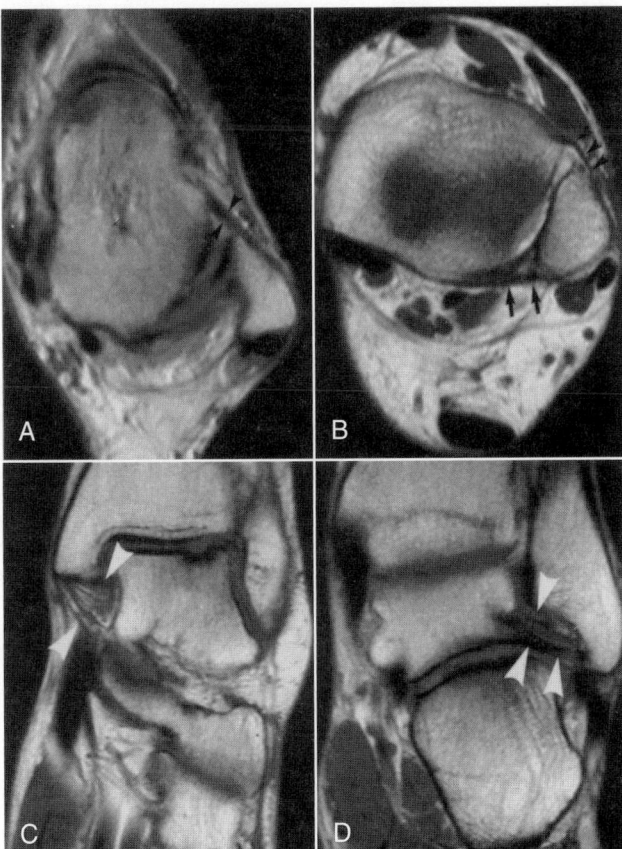

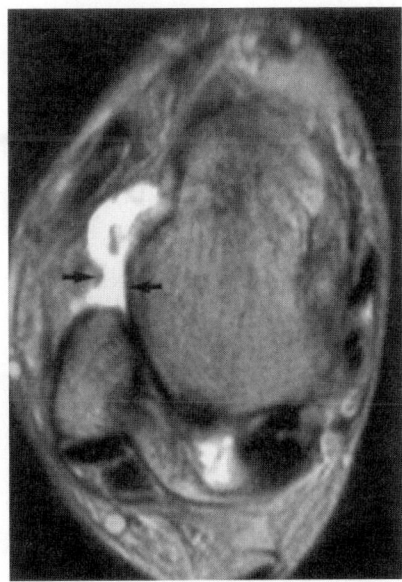

Figure 13-164 Chronic tear of the anterior talofibular ligament. This transaxial T2-weighted image demonstrates the absence of the anterior talofibular ligament, with high-signal-intensity fluid *(arrows)* filling the expected location of the ligament. (© 2001 American Academy of Orthopaedic Surgeons. Reprinted from the Journal of the American Academy of Orthopaedic Surgeons, vol 9[3], pp. 187–199, with permission.)

Figure 13-163 Appearance of normal ankle ligaments. A, The intact anterior talofibular ligament *(arrowheads)* is of low signal intensity on this T1-weighted transaxial image. Note the elliptical shape of the talus and the presence of the lateral malleolar fossa. **B,** Intact anterior *(arrowheads)* and posterior *(arrows)* tibiofibular ligaments are of uniform low signal intensity. The medial border of the lateral malleolus is flattened, indicating that this is the level of the tibiofibular ligaments. **C,** Intact tibiotalar component of the deltoid *(arrowheads)*. Note the osteochondral defect of the lateral talar dome. **D,** Posterior talofibular ligaments *(arrowheads)* on T1-weighted coronal image. The deltoid and posterior talofibular ligaments have a striated appearance rather than a homogeneous low-signal-intensity appearance like the anterior talofibular ligament. (© 2001 American Academy of Orthopaedic Surgeons. Reprinted from the Journal of the American Academy of Orthopaedic Surgeons, vol 9[3], pp. 187–199, with permission.)

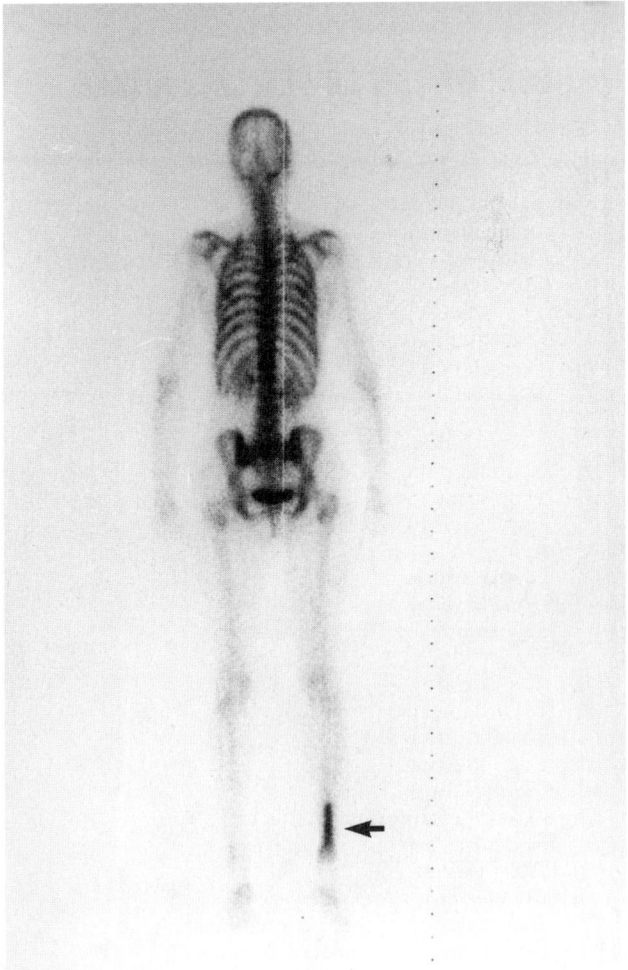

Figure 13-165 Bone scan of whole body. Arrow indicates area of increased isotope uptake ("hot spot") in the right tibia, which is consistent with a stress-related lesion.

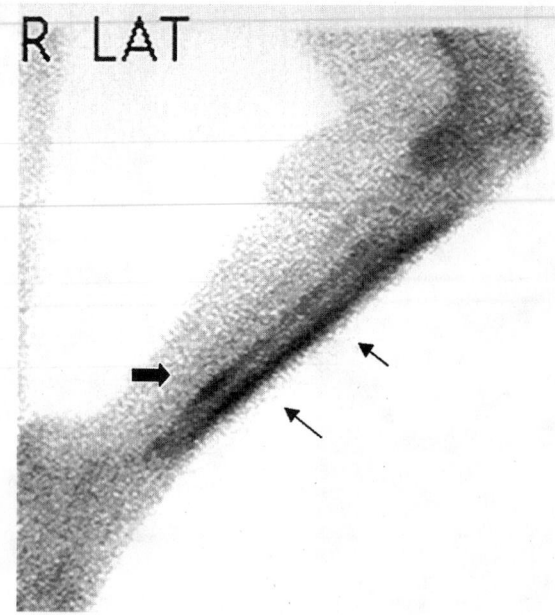

Figure 13-166 Stress fracture of the tibia and anterior shin splint. A short fusiform area of increased uptake in the posterior aspect of the distal shaft of the tibia represents a stress fracture *(large arrow)*. A long longitudinal area of increased uptake in the anterior aspect of the tibial shaft is consistent with a shin splint *(small arrows)*. (From Resnick D, Kransdorf MJ: Bone and joint imaging, Philadelphia, 2005, WB Saunders, p. 103.)

PRÉCIS OF THE LOWER LEG, ANKLE, AND FOOT ASSESSMENT*

History
Observation
Examination
   Active movements, weight-bearing (standing)
     Plantar flexion
     Dorsiflexion
     Supination
     Pronation
     Toe extension
     Toe flexion
   Functional assessment (standing)
   Special tests (standing)
     Neutral position of talus
     "Too many toes" sign
   Active movements, non-weight-bearing (sitting or supine lying)
     Plantar flexion
     Dorsiflexion
     Supination
     Pronation
     Toe extension
     Toe flexion
     Toe abduction
     Toe adduction
   Special tests (sitting)
     External rotation stress test
     Navicular drop test
     Tibial torsion
   Passive movements (supine lying)
     Plantar flexion at the talocrural (ankle) joint
     Dorsiflexion at the talocrural joint

     Inversion at the subtalar joint
     Eversion at the subtalar joint
     Adduction at the midtarsal joints
     Abduction at the midtarsal joints
     Flexion of the toes
     Extension of the toes
     Adduction of the toes
     Abduction of the toes
   Resisted isometric movements (supine lying)
     Knee flexion
     Plantar flexion
     Dorsiflexion
     Supination
     Pronation
     Toe extension
     Toe flexion
   Special tests (supine lying)
     Anterior drawer sign
     Figure-eight measurement of ankle
     Leg length
     Medial subtalar glide test
     Neutral position of talus
     Talar tilt
   Reflexes and cutaneous distribution (supine lying)
   Special tests (side lying)
     Fibular translation test
   Joint play movements (supine and side lying)
     Long-axis extension
     Anteroposterior glide
     Talar rock

PRÉCIS OF THE LOWER LEG, ANKLE, AND FOOT ASSESSMENT—cont'd

Side tilt
Rotation
Side glide
Tarsal bone mobility
Palpation (supine lying and prone lying)
Special tests (prone lying)
　Forefoot-heel alignment
　Leg-heel alignment

Matles test
Neutral position of talus
Tibial torsion
Thompson test
Diagnostic imaging

*The précis is shown in an order that limits the amount of moving that the patient has to do but ensures that all necessary structures are tested. It does not follow the order of the text. After any examination, the patient should be warned of the possibility that symptoms will exacerbate as a result of the assessment.

CASE STUDIES

When doing these case studies, the examiner should list the appropriate questions to be asked and why they are being asked, identify what to look for and why, and specify what things should be tested and why. Depending on the patient's answers (and the examiner should consider different responses), several possible causes of the patient's problem may become evident (examples are given in parentheses). A differential diagnosis chart should be made (see Table 13-16 as an example). The examiner can then decide how different diagnoses may affect the treatment plan.

1. A 38-year-old man ruptured his Achilles tendon 4 weeks earlier and had it surgically repaired. The cast has been removed. Describe your assessment plan for this patient.
2. A 24-year-old woman presents at your clinic with a painful left foot. There is no history of trauma; however, the pain has been present for approximately 6 years and has become worse in the past year. Describe your assessment plan for this patient (Morton's neuroma versus plantar fasciitis).
3. A 59-year-old man comes to you complaining of pain in his right calf and some numbness in his right foot. He also complains of some stiffness in his back. Describe your assessment plan for this patient (lumbar spondylosis versus tibial nerve palsy).
4. A 10-year-old boy recently had a triple arthrodesis for talipes equinovarus. The cast has now been removed. Describe your assessment plan for this patient.
5. A 16-year-old female volleyball player comes to you complaining of left ankle pain and difficulty walking after she stepped on another player's foot and went over on her ankle. The injury occurred 30 minutes earlier, and her ankle is swollen. Describe your assessment plan for this patient (malleolar fracture versus ligament sprain).
6. A 25-year-old woman tells you that she is training for a marathon but that every time she increases her mileage, her right foot hurts. Some time ago, someone told her she had a cavus foot. Describe your assessment plan for this patient.
7. Parents bring a 2-year-old boy to you and express concern that the child appears to have flat feet and "pigeon toes." Describe your assessment plan for this patient.
8. A 32-year-old woman comes to you complaining of ankle pain. She states that she sprained it 9 months earlier and thought it was better. However, she has now returned to training, and the ankle is bothering her. Describe your assessment plan for this patient (proprioceptive loss versus instability).

TABLE **13-16**

Differential Diagnosis of Lower Leg Compartment Syndrome

	Compartment Syndrome	Shin Splints*	Stress Fracture*	Tumor
Pain (type)	Severe cramping, diffuse pain, and tightness	Diffuse along medial two-thirds of tibial border	Deep, nagging localized with minimal radiation	Deep, nagging (bone) with some radiation
Pain with rest	Decreases or disappears	Decreases or disappears	Present, especially night pain	Present, often night pain
Pain with activity	Increases	Increases	Present (may increase)	Present
Pain with warm-up	May increase or become present	May disappear	Unilateral	Unaltered
Range of motion	Limited in acute phase	Limited	Normal	Normal
Onset	Gradual to sudden	Gradual	Gradual	?
Altered sensation	Sometimes	No	No	Sometimes
Muscle weakness or paralysis	Maybe	No	No	Not usually
Stretching	Increases pain	Increases pain	Minimal pain alteration	No increase in pain
Radiography	Normal	Normal	Early, negative; late, positive (?)	Usually positive
Bone scan	Negative	Periosteal uptake	Positive	Positive
Pulse	Affected sometimes	Normal	Normal	Normal
Palpation	Tender, tight compartment	Diffuse tenderness	Point tenderness	Point or diffuse tenderness
Cause	Muscle expansion	Overuse	Overuse	?
Duration and recovery	None without surgery	None without rest	Up to 3 months	None without treatment

From Magee DJ: Sports physiotherapy manual, Edmonton, 1988, University of Alberta Bookstore.
*These two conditions are different stages of tibial stress syndrome.

REFERENCES

1. Kangas J, Dankaerts W, Staes F: New approach to the diagnosis and classification of chronic foot and ankle disorders: identifying motor control and movement impairments. Manual Therapy 16:522–530, 2011.
2. Donatelli R: Abnormal biomechanics of the foot and ankle. J Orthop Sports Phys Ther 9:11–16, 1987.
3. Wang Q, Whittle M, Cunningham J, et al: Fibula and its ligaments in load transmission and ankle joint stability. Clin Orthop Relat Res 330:261–270, 1996.
4. Mantas JP: Lisfranc injuries in the athlete. Clin Sports Med 13:719–730, 1994.
5. Kleiger B: Mechanisms of ankle injury. Orthop Clin North Am 5:127–146, 1974.
6. Safran MR, Benedetti RS, Bartolozzi AR, et al: Lateral ankle sprains: a comprehensive review. Part 1: Etiology, pathoanatomy, histopathogenesis, and diagnosis. Med Sci Sports Exerc 31:S429–S437, 1999.
7. Klausner VB, McKeigue ME: The sinus tarsi syndrome: a cause of chronic ankle pain. Phys Sportsmed 28:75–80, 2000.
8. Heckman DS, Gluck GS, Pavekh SG: Tendon disorders of the foot and ankle. Part 1—peroneal tendon disorders. Am J Sports Med 37:614–625, 2009.
9. Gerber JP, Williams GN, Scoville CR, et al: Persistent disability associated with ankle sprains: a prospective examination of an athletic populations. Foot Ankle Int 19:653–660, 1998.
10. van Dijk CN, Bossuyt PM, Marti RK: Medial ankle pain after lateral ligament rupture. J Bone Joint Surg Br 78:562–567, 1996.
11. Liu SH, Nuccion SL, Finerman G: Diagnosis of anterolateral ankle impingement: comparison between magnetic resonance imaging and clinical examination. Am J Sports Med 25:389–393, 1997.
12. Dutton M: Dutton's orthopedic examination, evaluation and intervention, ed 3, New York, 2012, McGraw-Hill.
13. O'Loughlin PF, Heyworth BE, Kennedy JG: Current concepts in the diagnosis and treatment of osteochondral lesions of the ankle. Am J Sports Med 38:392–404, 2010.
14. Marder RA: Current methods for the evaluation of ankle ligament injuries. J Bone Joint Surg Am 76:1103–1111, 1994.
15. Taunton J, Smith C, Magee DJ: Leg, foot and ankle injuries. In Zachazewski JE, Magee DJ, Quillen WS, editors: Athletic injuries and rehabilitation, Philadelphia, 1996, WB Saunders.
16. Reid DC: Sports injury assessment and rehabilitation, New York, 1992, Churchill Livingstone.
17. Edwards PH, Wright ML, Hartman JF: A practical approach for the differential diagnosis of chronic leg pain in the athlete. Am J Sports Med 33:1241–1249, 2005.
18. Kou JX, Fortin PT: Commonly missed peritalar injuries. J Am Acad Orthop Surg 17:775–786, 2009.
19. Yates B, White S: The incidence and risk factors in the development of medial tibial stress syndrome among naval recruits. Am J Sports Med 32:772–780, 2004.
20. Gabisan GG, Gentile DR: Acute peroneal compartment syndrome following ankle inversion injury: a case report. Am J Sports Med 32:1059–1061, 2004.
21. van den Brand JG, Nelson T, Verleisdonk EJ, et al: The diagnostic value of intracompartmental pressure management, magnetic resonance imaging, and near-infrared spectroscopy in chronic exertional compartment syndrome: a prospective study of 50 patients. Am J Sports Med 33:699–704, 2005.
22. Gabisan GG, Gentile DR: Acute peroneal compartment syndrome following ankle inversion injury: a case report. Am J Sports Med 32:1059–1061, 2004.
23. Bonnin M, Tavernier T, Bouysset M: Split lesions of the peroneus brevis tendon in chronic ankle laxity. Am J Sports Med 25:699–703, 1997.
24. Neufeld SK, Cerrato R: Plantar fasciitis: evaluation and treatment. J Am Acad Orthop Surg 16:338–346, 2008.
25. Hunt GC, Brocato RS: Gait and foot pathomechanics. In Hunt GC, editor: Physical therapy of the foot and ankle: clinics in physical therapy, Edinburgh, 1988, Churchill Livingstone.
26. Lang LM, Volpe RG, Wernick J: Static biomechanical evaluation of the foot and lower limb: the podiatrist's perspective. Man Ther 2:58–66, 1997.
27. Kapandji IA: The physiology of the joints, vol 2: lower limb, New York, 1970, Churchill Livingstone.
28. Lipscomb AB, Ibrahim AA: Acute peroneal compartment syndrome in a well conditioned athlete: report of a case. Am J Sports Med 5:154–157, 1977.

29. Williams PL, Warwick R, editors: Gray's anatomy, ed 36, British, Philadelphia, 1980, WB Saunders.

30. Kelikian H, Kelikian AS: Disorders of the ankle, Philadelphia, 1985, WB Saunders

31. Sierra RJ, Trousdale RT, Ganz R, et al: Hip disease in the young active patient: evaluation and nonarthroplasty surgical options. J Am Acad Orthop Surg 16:689–703, 2008.

32. Palmer ML, Epler M: Clinical assessment procedures in physical therapy, Philadelphia, 1990, JB Lippincott.

33. Jahss MH: Disorders of the foot, Philadelphia, 1982, WB Saunders.

34. Smith AH, Bach BR: High ankle sprains: minimizing the frustration of a prolonged recovery. Phys Sportsmed 32(12):39–43, 2004.

35. Scranton PE: Isolated syndesmotic injuries: diastasis of the ankle in the athlete. Tech Foot Ankle Surg 1:88–90, 2002

36. Evans RC: Illustrated essentials in orthopedic physical assessment, St Louis, 1994, Mosby.

37. Mizel MS, Hecht PJ, Marymount JV, et al: Evaluation and treatment of chronic ankle pain. J Bone Joint Surg Am 86:622–632, 2004.

38. Pavlov H, Heneghan MA, Hersh A, et al: The Haglund deformity: initial and differential diagnosis. Radiology 144:83–88, 1982.

39. Meininger AK, Koh JL: Evaluation of the injured runner. Clin Sports Med 31:203–215, 2012.

40. Hamilton JJ, Ziemer LK: Functional anatomy of the human ankle and foot, American Association of Orthopaedic Surgeons, Symposium on the Foot and Ankle, St Louis, 1983, Mosby.

41. Erdemir A, Hamel AJ, Fauth AR, et al: Dynamic loading of the plantar aponeurosis in walking. J Bone Joint Surg Am 86:546–552, 2004.

42. Romash M: Deformities of the lesser toes and bunionette. In Lutter LD, Mizel MS, Pfeffer GB, editors: Orthopedic knowledge update: foot and ankle, Rosemont, IL, 1994, American Academy of Orthopaedic Surgeons.

43. Bowe JA: The pediatric foot. In Lutter LD, Mizel MS, Pfeffer GB, editors: Orthopedic knowledge update: foot and ankle, Rosemont, IL, 1994, American Academy of Orthopaedic Surgeons.

44. Shirzad K, Kiesau CD, deOrio JK, et al: Lesser toe deformities. J Am Acad Orthop Surg 19(8):505–514, 2011.

45. Brown LP, Yavorsky P: Locomotor biomechanics and pathomechanics: a review. J Orthop Sports Phys Ther 9:3–10, 1987.

46. McPoil TG, Brocato RS: The foot and ankle: biomechanical evaluation and treatment. In Gould JA, editor: Orthopedic and sports physical therapy, St Louis, 1990, Mosby.

47. McMaster MJ: The pathogenesis of the hallux rigidus. J Bone Joint Surg Br 60:82–87, 1978.

48. Pedowitz WJ: Deformities of the first ray. In Lutter LD, Mizel MS, Pfeffer GB, editors: Orthopedic knowledge update: foot and ankle, Rosemont, IL, 1994, American Academy of Orthopaedic Surgeons.

49. Yokoe K, Kameyama Y: Relationship between stress fractures of the proximal phalanx of the great toe and hallux valgus. Am J Sports Med 32:1032–1034, 2004.

50. Thompson GH: Bunions and deformities of the toes in children and adolescents. J Bone Joint Surg Am 77:1924–1936, 1995.

51. Durman DC: Metatarsus primus varus and hallux valgus. Arch Surg 74:128–135, 1957.

52. Price GFW: Metatarsus primus varus, including various clinicoradiologic features of the female foot. Clin Orthop 145:217–223, 1979.

53. Coughlin MJ: Conditions of the forefoot. In DeLee JC, Drez D, editors: Orthopedic sports medicine: principles and practice, Philadelphia, 1994, WB Saunders.

54. Beals TC, Pomeroy GC, Manoli A: Posterior tibial tendon insufficiency: diagnosis and treatment. J Am Acad Orthop Surg 7:112–118, 1999.

55. Churgay A: Diagnosis and treatment of pediatric foot deformities. Am Fam Physician 47:883–887, 1993.

56. Title CI, Schon LC: Morton neuroma: primary and secondary neurectomy. J Am Acad Orthop Surg 16:550–557, 2008.

57. Wukich DK, Tuason DA: Diagnosis and treatment of chronic ankle pain. J Bone Joint Surg Am 92:2002–2016, 2010.

58. Root ML, Orien WP, Weed JH: Normal and abnormal function of the foot, Los Angeles, 1977, Clinical Biomechanics.

59. Lian G: Nerve problems in the foot. In Lutter LD, Mizel MS, Pfeffer GB, editors: Orthopedic knowledge update: foot and ankle. Rosemont, IL, 1994, American Academy of Orthopaedic Surgeons.

60. Bowers KD, Martin RB: Turf toe: A shoe related football injury. Med Sci Sports Exerc 8:81–83, 1976.

61. Clanton TO, Ford JJ: Turf toe injury. Clin Sports Med 13:731–741, 1994.

62. Anderson RB, Hunt KJ, McCormick JJ: Management of common sports-related injuries about the foot and ankle. J Am Acad Orthop Surg 18:546–556, 2010.

63. Kaufman KR, Brodine SK, Schaffer RA, et al: The effect of foot structure and range of motion on musculoskeletal overuse injuries. Am J Sports Med 27:585–593, 1999.

64. Lindsjo U, Danckwardt-Lilliestrom G, Sahlstedt B: Measurement of the motion range in the loaded ankle. Clin Orthop 199:68–71, 1985.

65. Patla CE, Abbott JH: Tibialis posterior myofascial tightness as a source of heel pain: diagnosis and treatment. J Orthop Sports Phys Ther 30:624–632, 2000.

66. Stovitz SD, Coetzee JC: Hyperpronation and foot pain—steps toward pain-free feet. Phys Sportsmed 32(8):19–26, 2004.

67. McCrory P, Bladin C: Fractures of the lateral process of the talus: a clinical review: "snowboarder's ankle." Clin J Sports Med 6:124–128, 1996.

68. Bennell K, Talbot R, Wajswelner H, et al: Intra-rater and inter-rater reliability of a weight bearing lunge measure of ankle dorsiflexion. Austr J Physio 44:175–180, 1998.

69. Simondson D, Brock K, Cotton S: Reliability and smallest real difference of the ankle lunge test post ankle fracture. Manual Therapy 17:34–38, 2012.

70. Hoch MC, McKeon PO: Normative range of weight bearing lunge test performance asymmetry in healthy adults. Manual Therapy 16:516–519, 2011.

71. Hyslop GH: Injuries of the deep and superficial peroneal nerves complicating ankle sprain. Am J Surg 51:436–438, 1941.

72. Tabrizi P, McIntyre WM, Quesnel MB, et al: Limited dorsiflexion predisposes to injuries of the ankle in children. J Bone Joint Surg Br 82:1103–1106, 2000.

73. Chiodo CP, Glazebrook M, Bluman EM, et al: Diagnosis and treatment of acute achilles tendon rupture. J Am Acad Orthop Surg 18:503–510, 2010.

74. Jan MH, Chai AM, Lin YF, et al: Effects of age and sex on the results of an ankle plantar-flexor manual muscle test. Phys Ther 85:1078–1084, 2005.

75. Worrell TW, Booher LD, Hench KM: Closed kinetic chain assessment following inversion ankle sprain. J Sports Rehab 3:197–203, 1994.

76. Caffrey E, Docherty CL, Schrader J, et al: The ability of 4 single-limb hopping tests to detect functional performance deficits in individuals with functional ankle instability. J Orthop Sports Phys Ther 39:799–806, 2009.

77. Wikstrom EA, Tillman MD, Borsa PA: Detection of dynamic stability deficits in subjects with functional ankle instability. Med Sci Sports Exerc 37(2):169–175, 2005.

78. Eechaute C, Vaes P, Duquet W: Functional performance deficits in patients with chronic ankle instability: validity of the multiple hop test. Clin J Sports Med 18:124–129, 2008.

79. Mubarak S, Hargens A: Exertional compartment syndromes, American Association of Orthopaedic Surgeons, symposium on the foot and leg in running sports, St Louis, 1982, CV Mosby.

80. Reneman RS: The anterior and the lateral compartmental syndrome of the leg due to intensive use of muscles. Clin Orthop 113:69–80, 1975.

81. Freeman MAR, Dean MRE, Hanham IWF: The etiology and prevention of functional instability of the foot. J Bone Joint Surg Br 47:678–685, 1965.

82. Kaikkonen A, Kannus P, Jarvinen M: A performance test protocol and scoring scale for the evaluation of ankle injuries. Am J Sports Med 22:462–469, 1994.

83. Rozzi SL, Lephart SM, Scott M, et al: Balance training for persons with functionally unstable ankles. J Orthop Sports Phys Ther 29:478–486, 1999.

84. Martin RL, Irrgang JJ, Burdett RG, et al: Evidence of validity for the foot and ankle ability measure (FAAM). Foot Ankle Int 26:968–983, 2005.

85. Roos EM, Brandsson S, Karlsson J: Validation of the foot and ankle outcome score for ankle ligament reconstruction. Foot Ankle Int 22:788–794, 2001.

86. Budiman-Mak E, Conrad KJ, Roach KE: The foot function index: a measure of foot pain and disability. J Clin Epidemiol 44:561–570, 1991.

87. Martin RL, Irrgang JJ: A survey of self-reported outcome instruments for the foot and ankle. J Orthop Sports Phys Ther 37(2):72–84, 2007.

88. Seligson D, Gassman J, Pope M: Ankle instability: evaluation of the lateral ligaments. Am J Sports Med 8:39–42, 1980.

89. Hildebrand KA, Buckley RE, Mohtadi NG, et al: Functional outcome measures after displaced intra-articular calcaneal fractures. J Bone Joint Surg Br 75:119–123, 1996.

90. Merchant TC, Dietz FR: Long-term follow up after fractures of the tibial and fibular shafts. J Bone Joint Surg Am 71:599–606, 1989.

91. Olerud C, Molander H: A scoring scale for symptom evaluation after ankle fracture. Arch Orthop Trauma Surg 103:190–194, 1984.

92. Statford PW, Hart DL, Binkley JM, et al: Interpreting lower extremity functional status scores. Physiother Can 57:154–162, 2005.

93. Halasi T, Kynsburg A, Tallay A, et al: Development of a new activity score for the evaluation of ankle instability. Am J Sports Med 32:899–908, 2004.

94. Domsic RT, Saltzman CL: Ankle arthritis scale. Foot Ankle Int 19:466–471, 1998.

95. Andre M, Hagelberg S, Stenstrom CH: The juvenile arthritis foot disability index: development and evaluation of measurement properties. J Rheum 31:2488–2493, 2004.

96. Heffernan G, Knan F, Awan N, et al: A comparison of outcome scores in os calcis fractures. Irish J Med Sci 169:127–128, 2000.

97. Rowan K: The development and validation of a multidimensional measure of chronic foot pain: the Rowan foot pain assessment questionnaire. Foot Ankle Int 22:795–809, 2001.

98. Williams GN, Molloy JM, DeBerardino TM, et al: Evaluation of the sports ankle-rating system in

young, athletic individuals with acute lateral ankle sprains. Foot Ankle Int 24:274–282, 2003.

99. Astrom M, Arvidson T: Alignment and joint motion in the normal foot. J Orthop Sports Phys Ther 22:216–222, 1995.

100. Vaes PH, Duquet W, Casteleyn PP, et al: Static and dynamic roentgenographic analysis of ankle stability in braced and non-braced stable and functionally unstable ankle. Am J Sports Med 26:692–702, 1998.

101. Roy S, Irvin R: Sports medicine: prevention, evaluation, management and rehabilitation, Englewood Cliffs, NJ, 1983, Prentice-Hall.

102. Mueller MJ, Host JV, Norton BJ: Navicular drop as a composite measure of excessive pronation. J Am Pod Med Assoc 83:198–202, 1993.

103. Shrader JA, Poporich JM, Gracey GC, et al: Navicular drop measurement in people with rheumatoid arthritis: interrater and intrarater reliability. Phys Ther 85:656–664, 2005.

104. Loudon JK, Jenkins W, Loudon KL: The relationships between static posture and ACL injury in female athletes. J Orthop Sports Phys Ther 24:91–97, 1996.

105. Picciano AM, Rowlando MS, Worrell T: Reliability of open and closed kinetic chain subtalar joint neutral positions and navicular drop test. J Orthop Sports Phys Ther 18:553–558, 1993.

106. Dicharry JM, Franz JR, Croce UD, et al: Differences in static and dynamic movements in evaluation of talonavicular mobility in gait. J Orthop Sports Phys Ther 39:628–634, 2009.

107. Buchanan KR, Davis I: The relationship between the forefoot, midfoot, and rearfoot static alignment in pain-free individuals. J Orthop Sports Phys Ther 35:559–566, 2005.

108. Younger AS, Hansen ST: Adult cavovarus foot. J Am Acad Orthop Surg 13:302–315, 2005.

109. Staheli LT, Corbett M, Wyss C, et al: Lower extremity rotational problems in children: normal values to guide management. J Bone Joint Surg Am 67:39–47, 1985.

110. Staheli LT: Rotational problems of the lower extremities. Orthop Clin North Am 18:503–512, 1987.

111. Johnson KA: Posterior tibial tendon. In Baxter DE, editor: The foot and ankle in sport, St Louis, 1995, Mosby.

112. Pell RF, Khanuja HS, Cooley GR: Leg pain in the running athlete. J Am Acad Orthop Surg 12:396–404, 2004.

113. Lindstrand A: New aspects in the diagnosis of lateral ankle sprains. Orthop Clin North Am 7:247–249, 1976.

114. Hollis JM, Blasier RD, Flahiff CM: Simulated ankle ligamentous injury: change in ankle stability. Am J Sports Med 23:672–677, 1995.

115. Trojian TH, McKeag DB: Ankle sprains: expedient assessment and management. Phys Sportsmed 26(10):29–40, 1998.

116. Frost HM, Hanson CA: Technique for testing the drawer sign in the ankle. Clin Orthop 123:49–51, 1977.

117. Birrer RB, Cartwright TJ, Denton JR: Immediate diagnosis of ankle trauma. Phys Sportmed 22:95–102, 1994.

118. Tohyama H, Yasuda K, Ohkoshi Y, et al: Anterior drawer test for acute anterior talofibular ligament injuries of the ankle: how much load should be applied during the test? Am J Sports Med 31:226–232, 2003.

119. Parasher RK, Nagy DR, Em AL, et al: Clinical measurement of mechanical ankle instability. Manual Therapy 17:470–473, 2012.

120. Aradi AJ, Wong J, Walsh M: The dimple sign of a ruptured lateral ligament of the ankle: brief report. J Bone Joint Surg Br 70:327–328, 1988.

121. Davis PF, Trevino SG: Ankle injuries. In Baxter DE, editor: The foot and ankle in sport, St Louis, 1995, Mosby.

122. Hockenbury RT, Sammarco GJ: Evaluation and treatment of ankle sprains: clinical recommendations for a positive outcome. Phys Sportsmed 24(2):57–64, 2001.

123. Kjaersgaard-Andersen P, Frich LH, Madsen F, et al: Instability of the hindfoot after lesion of the lateral ankle ligaments: investigations of the anterior drawer and adduction maneuvers in autopsy specimens. Clin Orthop 266:170–179, 1991.

124. Colter JM: Lateral ligamentous injuries of the ankle. In Hamilton WC, editor: Traumatic disorders of the ankle, New York, 1984, Springer-Verlag.

125. Hamilton WC: Anatomy. In Hamilton WC, editor: Traumatic disorders of the ankle, New York, 1984, Springer-Verlag.

126. Rasmussen O, Tovberg-Jensen I: Anterolateral rotational instability in the ankle joint. Acta Orthop Scand 52:99–102, 1981.

127. Peng JR: Solving the dilemma of the high ankle sprain in the athlete. Sports Med Arthro Rev 8:316–325, 2000.

128. Cotton FJ: Fractures and fracture-dislocations, Philadelphia, 1910, WB Saunders.

129. Stiehl JB: Complex ankle fracture dislocations with syndesmotic diastasis. Ortho Rev 19:499–507, 1990.

130. Adamson C, Cymet T: Ankle sprains: evaluation, treatment, rehabilitation. Maryland Med J 46:530–537, 1997.

131. Stoffel K, Wysocki D, Baddour E, et al: Comparison of two intraoperative assessment methods for injuries to the ankle syndesmosis. J Bone Joint Surg Am 91:2646–2652, 2009.

132. Lin CF, Gross MT, Weinfeld P: Ankle syndesmosis injuries: anatomy, biomechanics, mechanism of injury, and clinical guidelines for diagnosis and intervention. J Orthop Sports Phys Ther 36:372–384, 2006.

133. Kiter E, Bukurt M: The crossed-leg test for examination of ankle syndesmosis injuries. Foot Ankle Int 26:187–188, 2005.

134. Alonso A, Khoury L, Adams R: Clinical tests for ankle syndesmosis injury: reliability and prediction of return to function. J Orthop Sports Phys Ther 27:276–284, 1998.

135. Taylor DC, Engelhardt DL, Bassett FH: Syndesmosis sprains of the ankle. The influence of heterotopic ossification. Am J Sports Med 20:146–150, 1992.

136. Brosky T, Nyland J, Nitz A, et al: The ankle ligaments: consideration of syndesmotic injury and implications for rehabilitation. J Orthop Sports Phys Ther 21:197–205, 1995.

137. Nussbaum ED, Hosea TM, Sieler SD, et al: Prospective evaluation of syndesmotic ankle sprains without diastasis. Am J Sports Med 29:31–35, 2001.

138. Boytim MJ, Fischer DA, Neuman L: Syndesmotic ankle sprains. Am J Sports Med 19:294–298, 1991.

139. Wright RW, Barile RJ, Surprenant DA, et al: Ankle syndesmosis sprains in national hockey league players. Am J Sports Med 32:1941–1945, 2004.

140. Beumer A, Swierstra BA, Mulder PG: Clinical diagnosis of syndesmotic ankle instability: evaluation of stress tests behind the curtain. Acta Orthop Scand 73:667–669, 2002.

141. Cook CE, Hegedus EJ: Orthopedic physical examination tests—an evidence based approach, Upper Saddle River, NJ, 2008, Prentice Hall/Pearson.

142. Lindenfeld T, Parikh S: Clinical tip: heel-thump test for syndesmotic ankle sprain. Foot Ankle Int 26:406–408, 2005.

143. Gungor T: A test for ankle instability: brief report. J Bone Joint Surg Br 70:487, 1988.

144. Hopkinson WJ, St Pierre P, Ryan JB, et al: Syndesmosis sprains of the ankle. Foot Ankle 10:325–330, 1990.

145. Norkus SA, Floyd RT: The anatomy and mechanisms of syndesmotic ankle sprains. J Athletic Train 36:68–73, 2001.

146. Mennell JM: Foot pain, Boston, 1969, Little, Brown.

147. Tatro-Adams D, McGann S, Carbone W: Reliability of the figure-of-eight method of ankle measurement. J Orthop Sports Phys Ther 22:161–163, 1995.

148. Petersen EJ, Irish SM, Lyons CL, et al: Reliability of water volumetry and the figure of eight method on subjects with ankle joint swelling. J Orthop Sports Phys Ther 29:609–615, 1999.

149. Mawdsley RH, Hoy DK, Erwin PM: Criterion-related validity of the figure of eight method of measuring ankle edema. J Orthop Sports Phys Ther 30:149–153, 2000.

150. Pugia ML, Middel CJ, Seward SW, et al: Comparison of acute swelling and function in subjects with lateral ankle injury. J Orthop Sports Phys Ther 31:384–388, 2001.

151. Rohner-Spengler M, Mannion AF, Babst R: Reliability and minimal detectable change for the figure-of-eight-20 method of measurement of ankle edema. J Orthop Sports Phys Ther 37:199–205, 2007.

152. Payne C, Chuter V, Miller K: Sensitivity and specificity of the functional hallux limitus test to predict foot function. J Am Podiatr Med Assoc 92:269–271, 2002.

153. Cleland JA, Koppenhaver S: Netter's orthopedic clinical examination—an evidence-based approach, ed 2, Philadelphia, 2011, Saunders/Elsevier.

154. Wallace LA: Limb length difference and back pain. In Grieve GP, editor: Modern manual therapy of the vertebral column, Edinburgh, 1986, Churchill Livingstone.

155. Maffulli N: The clinical diagnosis of subcutaneous tear of the achilles tendon. Am J Sports Med 26:266–270, 1998.

156. Blood SD: Treatment of the sprained ankle. J Am Osteopathic Assoc 79:680–692, 1980.

157. Safran MR, O'Malley D, Fu FH: Peroneal tendon subluxation in athletes: new exam technique, case reports and review. Med Sci Sports Exerc 31:S487–S496, 1999.

158. Thompson T, Doherty J: Spontaneous rupture of the tendon of Achilles: a new clinical diagnostic test. Anat Res 158:126–129, 1967.

159. Scott BW, Al-Chalabi A: How the Simmonds-Thompson test works. J Bone Joint Surg Br 74:314–315, 1992.

160. Simmonds FA: The diagnosis of a ruptured Achilles tendon. Practitioner 179:56–58, 1957.

161. Thompson TC: A test for rupture of the tendoachilles. Acta Orthop Scand 32:461–465, 1962.

162. Garceau DD, Bean D, Requejo SM, et al: The association between diagnosis of plantar fasciitis and Windlass test results. Foot Ankle Int 24:251–255, 2003.

163. Bowditch MG, Sanderson P, Livesey JP: The significance of an absent ankle reflex. J Bone Joint Surg Br 78:276–279, 1996.

164. Bassetti C: Babinski and Babinski's sign. Spine 20:2591–2594, 1995.

165. Chusid JG, McDonald JJ: Correlative neuroanatomy and functional neurology, Los Altos, CA, 1967, Lange Medical Publications.

166. Schon LC, Baxter DE: Neuropathies of the foot and ankle in athletes. Clin Sports Med 9:489–509, 1990.

167. Zengzhao L, Jiansheng Z, Li Z: Anterior tarsal tunnel syndrome. J Bone Joint Surg Br 73:470–473, 1991.

168. Pecina, MM, Krmpotic-Nemanic J, Markiewitz AD: Tunnel syndromes, Boca Raton, FL, 1991, CRC Press.

169. Wechsler LR, Busis NA: Sports neurology. In Fu FH, Stone DA, editors: Sports injuries: mechanisms, prevention, treatment, Baltimore, 1994, Williams & Wilkins.

170. Baxter DE: Functional nerve disorders. In Baxter DE, editor: The foot and ankle in sport, St Louis, 1995, Mosby.

171. Beskin JL: Nerve entrapment syndromes of the foot and ankle. J Am Acad Orthop Surg 5:261–269, 1997.

172. Sidey JD: Weak ankles: a study of common peroneal entrapment neuropathy. Br Med J 3:623–626, 1969.

173. Nitz AJ, Dobner JJ, Kersey D: Nerve injury and grades II and III ankle sprains. Am J Sports Med 13:177–182, 1985.

174. Kleinrensink GJ, Stoeckart R, Meulstee J, et al: Lowered motor conduction velocity of the peroneal nerve after inversion trauma. Med Sci Sports Exerc 26:877–883, 1994.

175. Schon LC, Clanton TO: Chronic leg pain. In Baxter DE, editor: The foot and ankle in sport, St Louis, 1995, Mosby.

176. Styf J: Entrapment of the superficial peroneal nerve: diagnosis and results of decompression. J Bone Joint Surg Br 71:131–135, 1989.

177. Pahor S, Toppenberg R: An investigation of neural tissue involvement in ankle inversion sprains. Man Ther 1:192–197, 1996.

178. Romani W, Perrin DH, Whiteley T: Tarsal tunnel syndrome: case study of a male collegiate athlete. J Sports Rehab 6:364–370, 1997.

179. Kinoshita M, Okuda R, Abe M: Tarsal tunnel syndrome and athletes. Am J Sports Med 34:1307–1312, 2006.

180. Kaplan, PE, Kernahan WT: Tarsal tunnel syndrome: an electrodiagnostic and surgical correlation. J Bone Joint Surg Am 63:96–99, 1981.

181. Massey EW, Plett AB: Neuropathy in joggers. Am J Sports Med 6:209–211, 1978.

182. Murphy PC, Baxter DE: Nerve entrapment of the foot and ankle in runners. Clin Sports Med 4:753–763, 1985.

183. Takakura Y, Kitada C, Sugimoto K, et al: Tarsal tunnel syndrome: causes and results of operative treatment. J Bone Joint Surg Br 73:125–128, 1991.

184. Stefko RM, Lauerman WC, Heckman JD: Tarsal tunnel syndrome caused by an unrecognized fracture of the posterior process of the talus (Cedell fracture). J Bone Joint Surg Am 76:116–118, 1994.

185. Trepman E: Tarsal tunnel syndrome following Achilles tendon injury in dancers: two cases. Clin J Sports Med 3:192–194, 1993.

186. Jackson DL, Haglund BL: Tarsal tunnel syndrome in runners. Sports Med 13:146–149, 1992.

187. Mann RA: Entrapment neuropathies of the foot. In DeLee JC, Drez D, editors: Orthopedic sports medicine: principles and practice, Philadelphia, 1994, WB Saunders.

188. Sammarco GJ, Chalk DE, Feibel JH: Tarsal tunnel syndrome and additional nerve lesions in the same limb. Foot Ankle 14:71–77, 1993.

189. Jackson DL, Haglund B: Tarsal tunnel syndrome in athletes: case reports and literature review. Am J Sports Med 19:61–65, 1991.

190. Rask MR: Medial plantar neuropraxia (jogger's foot): report of three cases. Clin Orthop 134:193–195, 1978.

191. Pfeffer GB: Plantar heel pain. In Baxter DE, editor: The foot and ankle in sport, St Louis, 1995, Mosby.

192. Johnson ER, Kirby K, Lieberman JS: Lateral plantar nerve entrapment: foot pain in the power lifter. Am J Sports Med 20:619–620, 1992.

193. House JA, Ahmed K: Entrapment neuropathy of the infrapatellar branch of the saphenous nerve. Am J Sports Med 5:217–224, 1977.

194. Kaltenborn FM: Mobilization of the extremity joints, Oslo, 1980, Olaf Norlis Bokhandel.

195. Richardson EG: Hallucal sesamoid pain: causes and surgical treatment. J Am Acad Orthop Surg 7:270–278, 1999.

196. Newman P, Adams R, Waddington G: Two simple clinical tests for predicting onset of medial tibial stress syndrome: shin palpation test and shin oedema test. Br J Sports Med 46:861–864, 2011.

197. Thordarson DB: Detecting and treating common foot and ankle fractures. Part 1: the ankle and hindfoot. Phys Sportsmed 24(9):29–38, 1996.

198. Thordarson DB: Detecting and treating common foot and ankle fractures. Part 2: the midfoot and forefoot. Phys Sportsmed 24(10):58–64, 1996.

199. Egol KA, Amirtharage M, Tejwani NC, et al: Ankle stress test for predicting the need for surgical fixation and isolated fibular fractures. J Bone Joint Surg Am 86:2393–2398, 2004.

200. Springer BA, Arceiro RA, Tenuta JJ, et al: A prospective study of modified Ottawa rules in a military population—interobserver agreement between physical therapists and orthopedic surgeons. Am J Sports Med 28:864–868, 2000.

201. Stiell IG, Greenberg GH, McKnight RD, et al: Decision rules for the use of radiography in acute ankle injuries: refinement and prospective validation. JAMA 269:1127–1132, 1993.

202. Stiell IG, McKnight RD, Greenberg GH, et al: Implementation of the Ottawa ankle rules. JAMA 271:827–832, 1994.

203. Stiell IG, Greenberg GH, McKnight RD, et al: A study to develop clinical decision rules for the use of radiography in acute ankle injuries. Ann Emerg Med 21:384–390, 1992.

204. Bachman LM, Kolb E, Koller MT, et al: Accuracy of Ottawa ankle rules to exclude fractures of the ankle and midfoot: systematic review. Br Med J 326:417–424, 2003.

205. Heyworth J: Ottawa ankle rules for the injured ankle. Br Med J 326:405–406, 2003.

206. Leddy JJ, Smolinski RJ, Lawrence J, et al: Prospective evaluation of the Ottawa ankle rules in a university sports medicine centre—with a modification to increase specificity for identifying malleolar fractures. Am J Sports Med 26:158–165, 1998.

207. Black H: Roentgenographic considerations. Am J Sports Med 5:238–240, 1977.

208. Hoffman JD: Radiography of the ankle. In Hamilton WC, editor: Traumatic disorders of the ankle, New York, 1984, Springer-Verlag.

209. Renton P, Stripp WJ: The radiology and radiography of the foot. In Klenerman L, editor: The foot and its disorders, ed 2, Boston, 1982, Blackwell Scientific.

210. Rettig AC, Shelbourne KD, Beltz HF, et al: Radiographic evaluation of foot and ankle injuries in the athlete. Clin Sports Med 6:905–919, 1987.

211. Nielson JH, Gardner MJ, Peterson MG, et al: Radiographic measurements do not predict syndesmotic injury in ankle fractures: an MRI study. Clin Orthop Relat Res 436:216–221, 2005.

212. Wuest TK: Injuries to the distal lower extremity syndesmosis. J Am Acad Orthop Surg 5:172–181, 1997.

213. Katcherian D: Soft-tissue injuries of the ankle. In Lutter LD, Mizel MS, Pfeffer GB, editors: Orthopedic knowledge update: foot and ankle, Rosemont, IL, 1994, American Academy of Orthopaedic Surgeons.

214. Beumer A, van Hemert WL, Niesing R, et al: Radiographic measurement of the distal tibiofibular syndesmosis has limited use. Clin Orthop Relat Res 423:227–234, 2004.

215. Cetti R, Andersen I: Roentgenographic diagnosis of ruptured Achilles tendon. Clin Orthop 286:215–221, 1993.

216. Fowler A, Philip JF: Abnormality of calcaneus as a cause of painful heel: its diagnosis and operative treatment. Br J Surg 32:494–498, 1945.

217. Rubin G, Witten M: The talar-tilt angle and the fibular collateral ligaments: a method for the determination of talar-tilt. J Bone Joint Surg Am 42:311–326, 1960.

218. Rijke AM, Jones B, Vierhout PA: Stress examination of traumatized lateral ligaments of the ankle. Clin Orthop 210:143–151, 1986.

219. Grace DL: Lateral ankle ligament injuries: inversion and anterior stress radiography. Clin Orthop 183:153–159, 1984.

220. Rijke AM: Lateral ankle sprains: graded stress radiography for accurate diagnosis. Phys Sportsmed 19:107–118, 1991.

221. Karlsson J, Bergsten T, Peterson L, et al: Radiographic evaluation of ankle joint stability. Clin J Sports Med 1:166–175, 1991.

222. Cox JS, Hewes TF: "Normal" talar tilt angle. Clin Orthop 140:37–41, 1979.

223. Vanderwilde R, Staheli LT, Chew DE, et al: Measurements on radiographs of the foot in normal infants and children. J Bone Joint Surg Am 70:407–415, 1988.

224. Banerjee R, Saltzman C, Anderson RB, et al: Management of calcaneal malunion. J Am Acad Orthop Surg 19:27–36, 2011.

225. Gluck GS, Heckman DS, Parekh SG: Tendon disorders of the foot and ankle. Part 3—the posterior tibial tendon. Am J Sports Med 38:2133–2144, 2010.

226. Klenerman L: Examination of the foot. In Klenerman L, editor: The foot and its disorders, ed 2, Boston, 1982, Blackwell Scientific.

227. Pavlov H: Ankle and subtalar arthrography. Clin Sports Med 1:47–49, 1982.

228. Raatikainen T, Putkanen M, Puranen J: Arthrography, clinical examination and stress radiograph in the diagnosis of acute injury to the lateral ligaments of the ankle. Am J Sports Med 20:2–6, 1992.

229. Kerr R, Forrester DM, Kingston S: Magnetic resonance imaging of foot and ankle trauma. Orthop Clin North Am 21:591–601, 1990.

230. Terk MR, Kwong PK: Magnetic resonance imaging of the foot and ankle. Clin Sports Med 13:883–908, 1994.

231. Rijke AM, Gietz HT, McCue FC, et al: Magnetic resonance imaging of injury to the lateral ankle ligaments. Am J Sports Med 21:528–534, 1993.

232. Verhaven EF, Shahabpour M, Handelberg FW, et al: The accuracy of three-dimensional magnetic resonance imaging in the diagnosis of ruptures of the lateral ligaments of the ligament. Am J Sports Med 19:583–587, 1991.

233. Haygood TM: Magnetic resonance imaging of the musculoskeletal system—the ankle. Clin Orthop Relat Res 336:318–336, 1997.

234. Patterson MJ, Cox WK: Peroneus longus tendon rupture as a cause of chronic lateral ankle pain. Clin Orthop Relat Res 365:163–166, 1999.

235. Stone JW: Osteochondral lesions of the talar dome. J Am Acad Orthop Surg 4:63–73, 1996.

236. Lazarus ML: Imaging of the foot and ankle in the injured athlete. Med Sci Sports Exerc 31:S412–S420, 1999.

237. Recht MP, Donley BG: Magnetic resonance imaging of the foot and ankle. J Am Acad Orthop Surg 9:187–199, 2001.

238. Bresler M, Mar W, Toman J: Diagnostic imaging in the evaluation of leg pain in athletes. Clin Sports Med 31:217–245, 2012.

239. Shindle MK, Endo Y, Warren RF, et al: Stress fractures about the tibia, foot and ankle. J Am Acad Orthop Surg 20(3):167–176, 2012.

240. Gleeson AP, Stuart MJ, Wilson B, et al: Ultrasound assessment and conservative management of inversion injuries of the ankle in children. J Bone Joint Surg Br 78:484–487, 1996.

241. Bar-On E, Mashiach R, Inbar O, et al: Prenatal ultrasound diagnosis of club foot: outcome and recommendations for counseling and followup. J Bone Joint Surg Br 87:990–993, 2005.

242. Brodovicz KG, McNaughton K, Uemura N, et al: Reliability and feasibility of methods to quantitatively assess peripheral edema. Clin Med Res 7:21–31, 2009.

243. Dennis RJ, Finch CF, Elliott BC, et al: The reliability of musculoskeletal screening tests used in cricket. Phys Ther Sport 9:25–33, 2008.

244. Menz HB, Tiedemann A, Kwan MM, et al: Reliability of clinical tests of foot and ankle characteristics in older people. J Am Podiatr Med Assoc 93(5): 380–387, 2003.

245. Martin RL, McPoil TG: Reliability of ankle goniometric measurements: a literature review. J Am Podiatr Med Assoc 95(6):564–572, 2005.

246. Greninger LO, Kark LA: The reliability of active ankle plantar flexion assessment. Clin Kinesiol 54(1):19–24, 2000.

247. Yildiz Y, Sekir U, Hazneci B, et al: Reliability of a functional test battery evaluating functionality, proprioception and strength of the ankle joint. Turk J Med Sci 1:115–123, 2009.

248. Spahn G: The ankle meter: an instrument for evaluation of anterior talar drawer in ankle sprain. Knee Surg Sports Traumatol Arthrosc 12:338–342, 2004.

249. Lohrer H, Nauck T, Arentz S, et al: Observer reliability in ankle and calcaneocuboid stress radiography. Am J Sports Med 36(6):1143–1149, 2008.

250. Phisitkul,P, Chaichankul C, Sripongsai R, et al: Accuracy of anterolateral drawer test in lateral ankle instability: a cadaveric study. Foot Ankle Int 30(7): 690–695, 2009.

251. Wilkin EG, Hunt A, Nightingale EJ, et al: Manual testing for ankle instability. Manual Therapy 17:593–596, 2012.

252. Dopcherty CL, Rybak-Webb K: Reliability of the anterior drawer and talar tilt tests using the ligmaster joint arthrometer. J Sport Rehabil 18:389–397, 2009.

253. Vela L, Tourville TW, Hertel J: Physical examination of acutely injured ankles: an evidence-based approach. Athletic Ther Today 8(5):13–19, 2003.

254. Menz HB, Munteanu SE: Validity of 3 clinical techniques for the measurement of static foot posture in older people. J Orthop Sports Phys Ther 35:479–486, 2005.

255. Friends J, Augustine E, Danoff J: A comparison of different assessment techniques for measuring foot and ankle volume in healthy adults. J Am Podiatr Med Assoc 98(2):85–94, 2008.

256. Eechaute C, Vaes P, Duquet W: The chronic ankle instability scale: clinimetric properties of a multidimensional, patient-assessed instrument. Phys Ther Sport 9:57–66, 2008.

257. Hiller CE, Refshauge KM, Bundy AC, et al: The Cumberland ankle instability tool: a report of validity and reliability testing. Arch Phys Med Rehabil 87:1235–1241, 2006.

258. Shambaugh P, Sclafani L, Fanselow AD: Reliability of the Derifeild-Thompson test for leg length inequality, and use of the test to demonstrate cervical adjusting efficacy. J Manip Physiol Ther 11(5):396–399, 1988.

259. Williams DS, McClay IS: Measurements used to characterize the foot and the medial longitudinal arch: reliability and validity. Physical Ther 80(9):864–871, 2000.

260. Kerkhoffs GM, Blankevoort L, Sierevelt LN, et al: Two ankle joint laxity testers: reliability and validity. Knee Surg Sports Traumatol Arthrosc 13:699–705, 2005.

261. Kim J, Hwang SK, Lee KT, et al: A simpler device for measuring the mobility of the first ray of the foot. Foot Ankle Int 29(2):213–218, 2008.

262. Weaver K, Price R, Czerniecki J, et al: Design and validation of an instrument package designed to increase the reliability of ankle range of motion measurements. J Rehabil Res Dev 38(5):471–475, 2001.

263. Meyer DC, Werner CM, Wyss T, et al: A mechanical equinometer to measure the range of motion of the ankle joint: interobserver and intraobserver reliability. Foot Ankle Int 27(3):202–205, 2006.

264. Hale SA, Hertel J: Reliability and sensitivity of the Foot and Ankle Disability Index in subjects with chronic ankle instability. J Athl Train 40:35–40, 2004.

265. Evans AM, Copper AW, Scharfbillig RW, et al: Reliability of the foot posture index and traditional measures of foot position. J Am Podiatr Med Assoc 93(3):203–213, 2003.

266. Redmond AC, Crosbie J, Ouvrier RA: Development and validation of a novel rating system for scoring standing foot posture: the foot posture index. Clin Biomech 21:89–98, 2006.

267. Jonson SR, Gross MT: Intraexaminer reliability, interexaminer reliability, and mean values for nine lower extremity skeletal measures in healthy naval midshipmen. J Orthop Sports Phys Ther 25(4):253–263, 1997.

268. Hubbard TJ, Kaminski TW, Vander Griend RA, et al: Quantitative assessment of mechanical laxity in the functional unstable ankle. Med Sci Sports Exerc 36(5):760–766, 2004.

269. Rose KJ, Burns J, Ryan MM, et al: Reliability of quantifying foot and ankle muscle strength in very young children. Muscle Nerve 37:626–631, 2008.

270. Kellin BM, McKeon PO, Gontkof LM, et al: Hand-held dynamometry: reliability of lower extremity muscle testing in healthy, physically active, young adults. J Sport Rehab 17:160–170, 2008.

271. Möller M, Lind K, Styf J, et al: The reliability of isokinetic testing of the ankle joint and a heel-raise test for endurance. Knee Surg Sports Traumatol Arthrosc 13:60–71, 2005.

272. Power CM, Maffucci R, Hampton S: Rearfoot posture in subjects with patellofemoral pain. J Orthop Sports Phys Ther 22(4):155–160, 1995.

273. Erichsen N, Lund H, Moller JO, et al: Inter-rater and intra-rater reliability of tests of translatoric movements and range of movements in the subtalar and talocrural joints. Adv Physiother 8:161–167, 2006.

274. Kwon OY, Tuttle LJ, Commean PK, et al: Reliability and validity of measures of hammer toe deformity angle and tibial torsion. The foot 19:149–155, 2009.

275. Van den Bekerom MPJ, Mutsaerts EL, Niek van Dijk C: Evaluation of the integrity of the deltoid ligament in supination external rotation ankle fractures: a systematic review. Arch Orthop Trauma Surg 129:227–235, 2009.

276. Cornwall MW, McPoil TG, Lebec M, et al: Reliability of the modified foot posture index. J Am Podiatr Med Assoc 98(1):7–13, 2008.

277. Glasoe WM, Getsoian S, Myers M, et al: Criterion-related validity of a clinical measure of dorsal first ray mobility. J Orthop Sports Phys Ther 35:589–593, 2005.

278. Gaebler C, Kukla C, Breitenseher MJ, et al: Diagnosis of lateral ankle ligament injuries: comparison between talar tilt, MRI and operative findings in 112 athletes. Acta Orthop Scand 68(3):286–290, 1997.

279. Picciano AM, Rowlands MS, Worrel T: Reliability of open and closed kinetic chain subtalar joint neutral positions and navicular drop test. J Orthop Sports Phys Ther 18(4):553–558, 1993.

280. Shultz SJ, Nguyen A, Windley TC, et al: Intratester and intertester reliability of clinical measures of lower extremity anatomic characteristics: implications for multicenter studies. Clin Sport Med 16(2):155–161, 2006.

281. Torbum L, Perry J, Gronley JK: Assessment of rearfoot motion: passive positioning, one-legged standing gait. Foot Ankle Int 19(10):688–693, 1998.

282. Smith-Oricchio K, Harris BA: Interrater reliability of subtalar neutral, calcaneal inversion and eversion. J Orthop Sports Phys Ther 12(1):10–15, 1990.

283. Elveru RA, Rothstein JM, Lamb RL: Goniometric reliability in a clinical setting: subtalar and ankle joint measurements. Phys Ther 68(5):672–677, 1988.

284. Sell KE, Verity TM, Worrell TW, et al: Two measurement techniques for assessing subtalar joint position: a reliability study. J Orthop Sports Phys Ther 19:162–167, 1994.

285. Yamamoto K, Miyata T, Onozuka A, et al: Plantar flexion as an alternative to treadmill exercise for evaluating patients with intermittent claudication. Eur J Vasc Endovasc Surg 33:325–329, 2007.

286. Pieper B, Templin TN, Birk TJ, et al: The standing heel-rise test: relation to chronic venous disorders and balance, gait, and walk time injection drug users. Ostomy Wound Manage 54(9):18–22, 24, 26–30, 2008.

287. Burns J, Redmond A, Ouvrier R, et al: Quantification of muscle strength and imbalance in neurogenic pes cavus, compared to health controls, using hand-held dynamometry. Foot Ankle Int 26(7):540–544, 2005.

SUGGESTED READINGS

American Academy of Orthopaedic Surgeons: Athletic training and sports medicine, Chicago, 1984, AAOS.

American Orthopedic Association: Manual of orthopaedic surgery, Chicago, 1972, AOA.

Anderson KJ, Lecocq JF, Lecocq EA: Recurrent anterior subluxation of the ankle joint: a report of two cases and an experimental study. J Bone Joint Surg Am 34:853–860, 1952.

Basmajian JV, Stecko G: The role of muscles in arch support of the foot. J Bone Joint Surg Am 45:1184–1190, 1964.

Baumann PA, Gallagher SP, Hamilton WG: Common foot, ankle and knee problems in professional dancers. Orthop Phys Ther Clin North Am 5:497–513, 1996.

Baumhauer JF, Alosa DM, Renstrom PA, et al: A prospective study of ankle injury risk factors. Am J Sports Med 23:564–570, 1995.

Beetham WP, Polley HF, Slocumb CH, et al: Physical examination of the joints, Philadelphia, 1965, WB Saunders.

Berridge FR, Bonnin JG: The radiographic examination of the ankle joint including arthrography. Surg Gynecol Obstet 79:383–389, 1944.

Best A, Giza E, Linklater J, et al: Posterior impingement of the ankle caused by anomalous muscles. J Bone Joint Surg Am 87:2075–2079, 2005.

Bigg-Wither G, Kelly P: Diagnostic imaging in musculoskeletal physiotherapy. In Refshauge K, Gass E, editors: Musculoskeletal physiotherapy, Oxford, 1995, Butterworth-Heinemann.

Bloedel PK, Hauger B: The effects of limb length discrepancy on subtalar joint kinematics during running. J Orthop Sports Phys Ther 22:60–64, 1995.

Bojsen-Moller F: Anatomy of the forefoot: normal and pathologic. Clin Orthop 142:10–18, 1979.

Bordelson RL: Heel pain. In DeLee JC, Drez D, editors: Orthopedic sports medicine: principles and practice, Philadelphia, 1994, WB Saunders.

Cailliet R: Foot and ankle pain, Philadelphia, 1968, FA Davis.

Campbell DG, Menz A, Isaacs J: Dynamic ankle ultrasonography: a new imaging technique for acute ankle ligament injuries. Am J Sports Med 22:855–858, 1994.

Campbell JW, Inman VT: Treatment of plantar fasciitis and calcaneal spurs with the UC-BL shoe insert. Clin Orthop 103:57–62, 1974.

Carroll NC, McMurtry R, Leete SF: The pathoanatomy of congenital clubfoot. Orthop Clin North Am 9:225–232, 1978.

Case WS: Ankle injuries. In Sanders B, editor: Sports physical therapy, Norwalk, CT, 1990, Appleton & Lange.

Catterall A: A method of assessment of the clubfoot deformity. Clin Orthop 264:48–53, 1991.

Cawthorn M, Cummings G, Walker JR, et al: Isokinetic measurement of joint inversion and evertor force in three positions of plantar flexion and dorsiflexion. J Orthop Sports Phys Ther 14:75–81, 1991.

Chen SC: Ankle injuries. In Helal B, King JB, Grange WJ, editors: Sports injuries: their treatment, London, 1986, Chapman & Hall Medical.

Chew JT, Tan SB, Sivathasan C, et al: Vascular assessment in the neuropathic diabetic foot. Clin Orthop 320:95–100, 1995.

Chiodo CP, Myerson MS: Developments and advances in the diagnosis and treatment of injuries to the tarsometatarsal joint. Orthop Clin North Am 32:11–20, 2001.

Clarkson HM, Gilewich GB: Musculoskeletal assessment: joint range of motion and manual muscle strength, Baltimore, 1989, Williams & Wilkins.

Clement DB, Taunton JE, Smart GW: Achilles tendinitis and peritendinitis: etiology and treatment. Am J Sports Med 12:179–184, 1984.

Close JR: Some applications of the functional anatomy of the ankle joint. J Bone Joint Surg Am 38:761–781, 1956.

Close JR, Inman VT, Poor PM, et al: The function of the subtalar joint. Clin Orthop 50:159–179, 1967.

Cohn SL, Taylor WC: Vascular problems of the lower extremity in athletes. Clin Sports Med 9:449–470, 1990.

Coleman SS, Chesnut WJ: A simple test for hindfoot flexibility in the cavovarus foot. Clin Orthop 123:60–62, 1977.

Cooper DL, Fair J: Managing the pronated foot. Phys Sportsmed 7:131, 1979.

Cox JS, Brand RL: Evaluation and treatment of lateral ankle sprains. Phys Sportsmed 5:51–55, 1977.

Cox PD: Isokinetic strength testing of the ankle: a review. J Orthop Sports Phys Ther 47:97–106, 1985.

Cyriax J: Textbook of orthopaedic medicine: diagnosis of soft tissue lesions, vol 1, ed 8, London, 1982, Balliere Tindall.

Dahle LK, Mueller M, Delitto A, et al: Visual assessment of foot type and relationship of foot type to lower extremity injury. J Orthop Sports Phys Ther 14:70–74, 1991.

DeBrunner HU: Orthopaedic diagnosis, London, 1970, E & S Livingstone.

DeCarlo MS, Talbot RW: Evaluation of ankle joint proprioception following injection of the anterior talofibular ligament. J Orthop Sports Phys Ther 8:70–76, 1986.

DeValentine S: Evaluation and treatment of ankle fractures. Clin Podiatr 2:325–348, 1985.

Donatto KC: Ankle fractures and syndesmosis injuries. Orthop Clin North Am 32:79–90, 2001.

Drecben S: Heel pain. In Lutter LD, Mizel MS, Pfeffer GB, editors: Orthopedic knowledge update: foot and ankle, Rosemont, IL, 1994, American Academy of Orthopaedic Surgeons.

Dreeben S, Thomas PB, Noble PC, et al: A new method for radiography of weight bearing metatarsal heads. Clin Orthop 224:260–267, 1987.

Ebbetts J: Manipulation of the foot. Physiotherapy 57:194–202, 1971.

Edgar MA: Hallux valgus and associated conditions. In Klenerman L, editor: The foot and its disorders, ed 2, Boston, 1982, Blackwell Scientific.

Engsberg JR: A new method for quantifying pronation in overpronating and normal runners. Med Sci Sports Exerc 28:299–304, 1996.

Faciszewski T, Burks RT, Manaster BJ: Subtle injuries of the Lisfranc joint. J Bone Joint Surg Am 72:1519–1522, 1990.

Fixsen JA: The foot in childhood. In Klenerman L, editor: The foot and its disorders, ed 2, Boston, 1982, Blackwell Scientific.

Forkin DM, Koczur C, Battle R, et al: Evaluation of kinesthetic deficits indicative of balance control in gymnasts with unilateral chronic ankle sprains. J Orthop Sports Phys Ther 23:245–250, 1996.

Fromherz WA: Examination. In Hunt GC, editor: Physical therapy of the foot and ankle: clinics in physical therapy, Edinburgh, 1988, Churchill Livingstone.

Garbalosa JC, Donatelli R, Wooden MJ: Dysfunction, evaluation and treatment of the foot and ankle. In Donatelli R, Wooden MJ, editors: Orthopedic physical therapy, Edinburgh, 1989, Churchill Livingstone.

Garrick JG: The injured ankle: a sports medicine nemesis. Sports Med Bull 10:8–10, 1975.

Gartland JJ: Fundamentals of orthopedics, Philadelphia, 1979, WB Saunders.

Giallonardo LM: Clinical evaluation of foot and ankle dysfunction. Phys Ther 68:1850–1856, 1988.

Gill LH: Plantar fasciitis: diagnosis and conservative management. J Am Acad Orthop Surg 5:109–117, 1997.

Grana WA: Chronic pain after ankle sprain: consider the differential diagnosis. Phys Sportsmed 23:67–79, 1995.

Gray GW: Chain reaction: successful strategies for closed chain testing and rehabilitation, Adrian, MI, 1989, Wynn Marketing.

Gregg JR, Das M: Foot and ankle problems in the preadolescent and adolescent athlete. Clin Sports Med 1:131–147, 1982.

Gutrecht JA, Espinosa RE, Dyck PJ: Early descriptions of common neurological signs. Mayo Clin Proc 43:807–814, 1968.

Ha'Eri GB, Fornasier VL, Schatzker J: Morton's neuroma: pathogenesis and ultrastructure. Clin Orthop 141:256–259, 1979.

Halpern JS: Lower extremity peripheral nerve assessment. J Emerg Med 15:333–337, 1989.

Hardy AE: Assessment of foot movement. J Bone Joint Surg Br 69:838–839, 1987.

Harter RA: Clinical rationale for closed kinetic chain activities in functional testing and rehabilitation of ankle pathologies. J Sports Med 5:13–24, 1996.

Hartsell HD: Isokinetics and muscle strength ratios of the ankle invertors/evertors: a pilot study. Isok Exerc Sci 4:116–121, 1994.

Helfet AJ, Gruebel-Lee DM: Disorders of the foot, Philadelphia, 1979, JB Lippincott.

Hertel J, Denegar CR, Monroe MM, et al: Talocrural and subtalar joint instability after lateral ankle sprain. Med Sci Sports Exerc 31:1501–1508, 1999.

Hlavac HF: The foot book: advice to athletes, Mountain View, CA, 1977, World.

Hoerr NL, Pyle SI, Francis CC: Radiographic atlas of skeletal development of the foot and ankle, Springfield, IL, 1962, Charles C Thomas.

Holden CEA: Compartmental syndromes following trauma. Clin Orthop 113:95–102, 1975.

Hollinshead WH, Jenkins DB: Functional anatomy of the limbs and back, Philadelphia, 1981, WB Saunders.

Hoppenfeld S: Physical examination of the spine and extremities, New York, 1976, Appleton-Century-Crofts.

Hutton WC, Stott JRR, Stokes IAF: The mechanics of the foot. In Klenerman L, editor: The foot and its disorders, ed 2, Boston, 1982, Blackwell Scientific.

Inman VT: The joints of the ankle, Baltimore, 1976, Williams & Wilkins.

Johanson NA, Liang MH, Daltroy L, et al: American Academy of Orthopedic Surgeons lower limb outcomes assessment instruments. J Bone Joint Surg Am 86:902–909, 2004.

Johnson TR, Steinbach LS: Essentials of musculoskeletal imaging, Rosemont, IL, 2004, American Academy of Orthopedic Surgeons.

Jones DC: Tendon disorders of the foot and ankle. J Am Acad Orthop Surg 1:87–94, 1993.

Judge RD, Zuidema GD, Fitzgerald FT: Clinical diagnosis: a physiological approach, Boston, 1982, Little, Brown.

Kaumeyer G, Malone T: Ankle injuries: anatomical and biomechanical considerations necessary for the development of an injury prevention program. J Orthop Sports Phys Ther 1:171–177, 1980.

Kerr R, Forrester DM, Kingston S: Magnetic resonance imaging of foot and ankle trauma. Orthop Clin North Am 21:591–601, 1990.

Kibler WB, Goldbert C, Chandler TJ: Functional biomechanical deficits in running athletes with plantar fasciitis. Am J Sports Med 19:66–71, 1991.

Kingston S: Magnetic resonance imaging of the ankle and foot. Clin Sports Med 7:15–28, 1988.

Kiruchi S, Hasue M, Watanabe M: Ischemic contracture in the lower limb. Clin Orthop 134:185–192, 1978.

Kitaoka HB, Luo ZP, An KN: Three-dimensional analysis of normal ankle and foot mobility. Am J Sports Med 25:238–242, 1997.

Kleiger B: The mechanism of ankle injuries. J Bone Joint Surg Am 38:59–70, 1956.

Klenerman L: Functional anatomy. In Klenerman L, editor: The foot and its disorders, ed 2, Boston, 1982, Blackwell Scientific.

Konradsen L, Ravn JB, Sorensen AI: Proprioception at the ankle: the effect of anaesthetic blockade of ligament receptors. J Bone Joint Surg Br 75:433–436, 1993.

Kopell HP, Thompson WA: Peripheral entrapment neuropathies of the lower extremity. N Engl J Med 262:56–60, 1960.

Kotwick JE: Biomechanics of the foot and ankle. Clin Sports Med 1:19–34, 1982.

Landeros O, Frost HM, Higgins CC: Post-traumatic anterior ankle instability. Clin Orthop 56:169–178, 1968.

Lassiter TE, Malone TR, Garrett WE: Injury to the lateral ligaments of the ankle. Orthop Clin North Am 20:629–640, 1989.

Lattanza L, Gray GW, Kantner RM: Closed vs open kinetic chain measurements of subtalar joint eversion: implications for clinical practice. J Orthop Sports Phys Ther 9:310–314, 1987.

Leach RE, James S, Wasilewski S: Achilles tendinitis. Am J Sports Med 9:93–98, 1981.

Liu SH, Jason WJ: Lateral ankle sprains and instability problems. Clin Sports Med 13:793–809, 1994.

MacConaill MA, Basmajian JV: Muscles and movements: a basis for human kinesiology, Baltimore, 1969, Williams & Wilkins.

Mack RP: Ankle injuries in athletics. Clin Sports Med 1:71–84, 1982.

Maitland GD: The peripheral joints: examination and recording guide, Adelaide, Australia, 1973, Virgo Press.

Malekafzali S, Wood MB: Tibial torsion: a simple clinical apparatus for its measurement and its application to a normal adult population. Clin Orthop 145:154–157, 1979.

Mann RA: Surgical implications of biomechanics of the foot and ankle. Clin Orthop 146:111–118, 1980.

Maquirriain J: Posterior ankle impingement syndrome. J Am Acad Orthop Surg 13:365–371, 2005.

Matsen FA: Compartment syndrome: a unified concept. Clin Orthop 113:8–14, 1975.

McGuine TA, Greene JJ, Best T, et al: Balance as a predictor of ankle injuries in high school basketball players. Clin J Sports Med 10:239–244, 2000.

McKinnis LN: Fundamentals of musculoskeletal imaging, Philadelphia, 2005, FA Davis.

McPoil TG, Hunt GC: Evaluation and management of foot and ankle disorders: present problems and future directions. J Orthop Sports Phys Ther 21:381–388, 1995.

McRae R: Clinical orthopaedic examination, New York, 1976, Churchill Livingstone.

Michelson JD, Varner KE, Checcone M: Diagnosing deltoid injury in ankle fractures: the gravity stress view. Clin Orthop Relat Res 37:178–182, 2001.

Milbauer DL, Patel S: Roentgenographic techniques. In Nicholas JA, Hershman EB, editors: The lower extremity and spine in sports medicine, vol 1, St Louis, 1986, Mosby.

Miller CM, Winter WG, Bucknell AL, et al: Injuries to the midtarsal joint and lesser tarsal bones. J Am Acad Orthop Surg 6:249–258, 1998.

Morris JM: Biomechanics of the foot and ankle. Clin Orthop 122:10–17, 1977.

Morton DJ: The human foot: its evolution, physiology and functional disorders, Cambridge, 1935, Cambridge University Press.

Mubarak SJ, Hargens AR: Compartment syndrome and Volkmann's contracture, Philadelphia, 1981, WB Saunders.

Nigg BM: The assessment of loads acting on the locomotor system in running and other sports activities. Semin Orthop 3:197–206, 1988.

Norfray JF, Schlachter L, Kernaham WT, et al: Early confirmation of stress fractures in joggers. JAMA 243:1647–1649, 1980.

O'Doherty D: The foot and ankle. In Pynsent P, Fairbank J, Carr A, editors: Outcome measures in orthopedics, Oxford, 1993, Butterworth-Heinemann.

O'Donoghue DH: Treatment of injuries to athletes, ed 4, Philadelphia, 1984, WB Saunders.

Ombregt L, Bisschop P, ter Veer HJ, et al: A system of orthopedic medicine, London, 1995, WB Saunders.

Omey ML, Micheli LJ: Foot and ankle problems in the young athlete. Med Sci Sports Exerc 31:S470–S486, 1999.

Parlasca R, Shoji H, D'Ambrosia RD: Effects of ligamentous injury on ankle and subtalar joints: a kinematic study. Clin Orthop 140:266–272, 1979.

Post M: Physical examination of the musculoskeletal system, Chicago, 1987, Year Book Medical.

Regan TP, Hughston JC: Chronic ankle "sprain" secondary to anomalous peroneal tendon. Clin Orthop 123:52–54, 1977.

Renstrom PA, Kannus P: Injuries of the foot and ankle. In DeLee JC, Drez D, editors: Orthopedic sports medicine: principles and practice, Philadelphia, 1994, WB Saunders.

Resnick D, Kransdorf MJ: Bone and joint imaging, Philadelphia, 2005, WB Saunders.

Richman JD, Barre PS: The plantar ecchymosis sign in fractures of the calcaneus. Clin Orthop 207:122–125, 1986.

Riddle DL: Foot and ankle. In Richardson JK, Iglarsh ZA, editors: Clinical orthopedic physical therapy, Philadelphia, 1994, WB Saunders.

Riegger-Krugh C, Keysor JJ: Skeletal malalignment of the lower quarter: correlated and compensatory motions and postures. J Orthop Sports Phys Ther 23:164–170, 1996.

Rockar PA: The subtalar joint: anatomy and joint motion. J Orthop Sports Phys Ther 21:361–372, 1995.

Root ML, Orien WP, Weed HJ: Normal and abnormal function of the foot, Los Angeles, 1977, Clinical Biomechanics.

Rorabeck CH, Macnab I: The pathophysiology of the anterior tibial compartment syndrome. Clin Orthop 113:52–57, 1975.

Rundle E: Foot and ankle. In Zuluaga M, et al, editors: Sports physiotherapy: applied science and practice, Melbourne, 1995, Churchill Livingstone.

Samuelson KM: Functional anatomy. In Hamilton WC, editor: Traumatic disorders of the ankle, New York, 1984, Springer-Verlag.

Scheller AD, Kasser JR, Quigley TB: Tendon injuries about the ankle. Orthop Clin North Am 11:801–811, 1980.

Shea MP, Manoli A: Recognizing talar dome lesions. Phys Sportsmed 21:109–120, 1993.

Sheehan G: Medical advice for runners, Mountain View, CA, 1978, World.

Sidey JD: Weak ankles: a study of common peroneal entrapment neuropathy. Br Med J 3:623–626, 1969.

Simons GW: Analytical radiography and the progressive approach in talipes equinovarus. Orthop Clin North Am 9:187–206, 1978.

Soma CA, Mandelbaum BR: Achilles tendon disorders. Clin Sports Med 13:811–823, 1994.

Spring JM, Hyatt GW: Treatment of sprained ankles. Gen Pract 36:78–94, 1967.

Staheli LT, Chew DE, Corbett M: The longitudinal arch. J Bone Joint Surg Am 69:426–428, 1987.

Stanish WD: Lower leg, foot and ankle injuries in young athletes. Clin Sports Med 14:651–668, 1995.

Starkey C, Ryan J: Evaluation of orthopedics and athletic injuries, Philadelphia, 1996, FA Davis.

Stricker PR, Spindler KP, Gautier KB: Prospective evaluation of history and physical examination: variables to determine radiography in acute ankle sprains. Clin J Sports Med 8:209–214, 1998.

Stuberg W, Temme J, Kaplan P, et al: Measurement of tibial torsion and thigh-foot angle using goniometry and computed tomography. Clin Orthop 272:208–212, 1991.

Subotnick SI: History and physical examination. In Subotnick SI, editor: Sports medicine of the lower extremity, Edinburgh, 1989, Churchill Livingstone.

Subotnick SI: Podiatric sports medicine, Mount Kisco, NY, 1975, Futura.

Subotnick SI: The running foot doctor, Mountain View, CA, 1977, World.

Sweetman R: Pes cavus. Physiotherapy 49:204–208, 1963.

Tatro-Adams D, McGann SF, Carbone W: Reliability of the figure of eight method of ankle measurement. J Orthop Sports Phys Ther 22:161–163, 1995.

Taylor DC, Bassett FH: Syndesmosis ankle sprains: diagnosing the injury and aiding recovery. Phys Sportsmed 21:39–46, 1993.

Testa VG, Capasso G, Maffulli N: Paresthesia of the anterior aspect of the ankle: an early sign of lumbar spinal disorders in sportsmen. Physiotherapy 75:205–206, 1989.

Thompson GH: Bunions and deformities of the toes in children and adolescents. J Bone Joint Surg Am 77:1924–1936, 1995.

Tomberlin JP, Saunders HD: Evaluation, treatment and prevention of musculoskeletal disorders, Chaska, MN, 1994, The Saunders Group.

Topp R, Mikesky A: Reliability of isometric and isokinetic evaluations of ankle dorsi/plantar strength among older adults. Isok Exerc Sci 4:157–163, 1994.

Travell JG, Simons DG: Myofascial pain and dysfunction: the trigger point manual (the lower extremities), Baltimore, 1992, Williams & Wilkins.

van Dijk CN, Lim LS, Bossuyt PM, et al: Physical examination is sufficient for diagnosis of sprained ankles. J Bone Joint Surg Br 78:958–962, 1966.

Vanderwilde RL, Stahei T, Chew DE, et al: Measurements on radiographs of the foot in normal infants and children. J Bone Joint Surg Am 70:407–415, 1988.

Wadsworth CT: Manual examination and treatment of the spine and extremities, Baltimore, 1988, Williams & Wilkins.

Walter NE, Wolf MD: Stress fractures in young athletes. Am J Sports Med 5:165–169, 1977.

Weissman BNW, Sledge CB: Orthopedic radiology, Philadelphia, 1986, WB Saunders.

Wilkerson GB, Nitz AJ: Dynamic ankle stability: mechanical and neuromuscular interrelationships. J Sports Rehab 3:43–57, 1994.

Williams A, Evans R, Shirley PD: Imaging of sports injuries, London, 1989, Bailliere Tindall.

Wilson RW, Gieck JH, Gansneder BM, et al: Reliability and responsiveness of disablement measures following acute ankle sprains among athletes. J Orthop Sports Phys Ther 27:348–355, 1998.

Yvars MF: Osteochondral fractures of the dome of the talus. Clin Orthop 114:185–191, 1976.

CHAPTER 14

Assessment of Gait

Walking is the simple act of falling forward and catching oneself. One foot is always in contact with the ground, and within a cycle, there are two periods of single-leg support and two periods of double-leg support. With running, there is a period of time during which neither foot is in contact with the ground, a period called "double float."

Winter[1] felt walking gait performs five main functions. First, it helps to support of the head, arms, and trunk by maintaining a semirigid lower limb. Second, it helps to maintain upright posture and balance. Third, it controls the foot to allow it to clear obstacles and enables gentle heel or toe landing through eccentric muscle action. Fourth, it generates mechanical energy by concentric muscle contraction to initiate, maintain, and, if desired, increase forward velocity. Finally, through eccentric action of the muscles, it provides shock absorption and stability and decreases forward velocity of the body.

The locomotion pattern tends to be variable and irregular until about the age of 7 years.[2] Several functional tasks are involved in gait, including forward progression, which is executed in a stepping movement in a wide range of rapid and comfortable walking speeds. Second, the body must be balanced alternately on one limb and then the other; this is accompanied by repeated adjustments of limb length. Finally, there is support of the upright body.

Gait assessment or analysis takes a great deal of time, practice, and technical skill combined with standardization for the clinician to develop the necessary skills.[3–5] Most gait analysis today is performed with force platforms to measure ground reaction forces, electromyography to measure muscle activity, and high-speed video motion analysis systems to measure movement. Discussion of these techniques, however, is beyond the scope of this book. This chapter gives only a brief overview of a complex task, assessment of normal and pathological gait; detailed assessment of gait is left to other authors.[6–15] The various terms commonly used to describe gait, the normal pattern of gait, the assessment of gait, and common abnormal gaits are reviewed.

DEFINITIONS[5–10]

Gait Cycle

The **gait cycle** is the time interval or sequence of motions occurring between two consecutive initial contacts of the same foot (Figure 14-1). It is synonymous with the stride length. For example, if heel strike is the initial contact, the gait cycle for the right leg is from one heel strike to the next heel strike on the same foot. The gait cycle is a description of what happens in one leg. The same sequence of events is repeated with the other leg, but it is 180° out of phase.[8] There are spatial descriptors of gait, such as stride length, step length and step width; time or temporal descriptors, such as cadence, stride time and step time; and, descriptors that involve time and space, such as walking speed.[16] Another spatial descriptor that is sometimes discussed with gait is foot angle (Fick angle; see Figure 14-14). Each of these descriptors can and should be very similar for both limbs. For example, osteoarthritis in one hip can change many of the descriptors and the examiner should watch for these changes. Simoneau[17] clearly described the terminology that applies to the gait cycle events (Figure 14-2). Table 14-1 demonstrates the periods or phases of the gait cycle, the function of each phase, and what is happening in the opposite limb.[8] The gait cycle consists of two phases for each foot: **stance phase,** which makes up 60% to 65% of the walking cycle, and **swing phase,** which makes up 35% to 40% of the walking cycle. In addition, there are two periods of double support and one period of single-leg stance during the gait cycle.

As the velocity of the cycle increases, the cycle length or stride length decreases. For example, in jogging, the gait cycle is 70% of the walking cycle, and in running, the gait cycle is 60% that of walking.[18] In addition, as the speed of movement increases, the function of the muscles changes somewhat, and their electromyographic activity may increase or decrease. Generally, gait velocity decreases with age.[19] Montero-Odasso et al.[20] found the gait velocity (less than 0.8 m/sec) could be used to determine mobility impairment in the elderly.

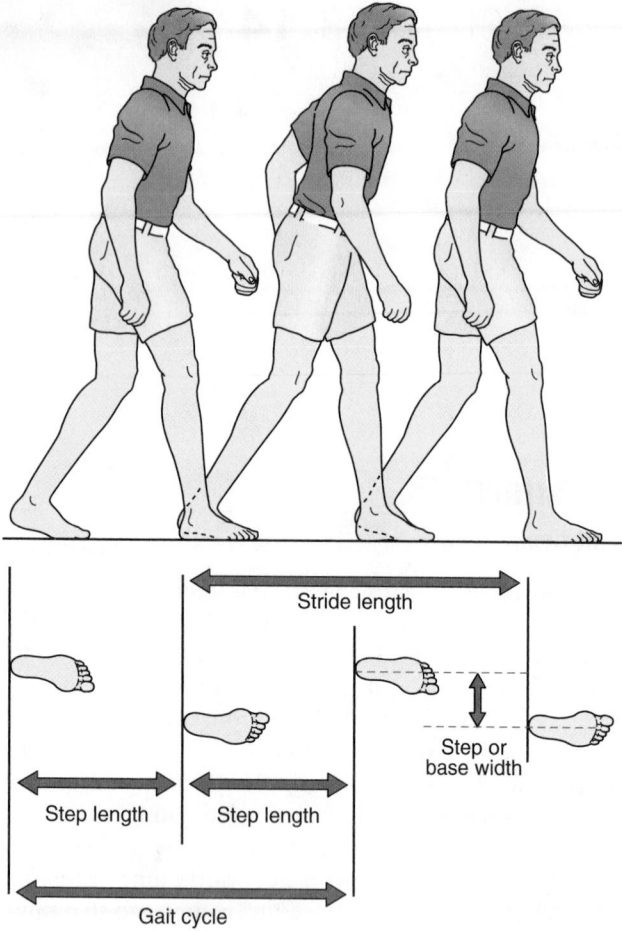

Figure 14-1 Gait cycle, stride length, and step length and width.

Stance Phase

The stance phase of gait occurs when the foot is on the ground and bearing weight (Figure 14-3). It allows the lower leg to support the weight of the body and, by so doing, acts as a shock absorber while allowing the body to advance over the supporting limb.[18] Normally, this phase makes up 60% of the gait cycle and consists of five subphases, or instants.

Stages (Instants) of Stance Phase

- Initial contact (heel strike)
- Load response (foot flat)
- Midstance (single-leg stance)
- Terminal stance (heel off)
- Preswing (toe off)

The **initial contact** instant is the **weight-loading** or **weight acceptance period** of the stance leg, which accounts for the first 10% of the gait cycle. During this period, one foot is coming off the floor while the other

foot is accepting body weight and absorbing the shock of initial contact. Because both feet are in contact with the floor, it is a period of **double support** or **double-leg stance.**

The **load response** and **midstance** instants consist of the **single support** or **single-leg stance,** which accounts for the next 40% of the gait cycle. During this period, one leg alone carries the body weight while the other leg goes through its swing phase. The stance leg must be able to hold the weight of the body, and the body must be able to balance on the one leg. In addition, lateral hip stability must be exhibited to maintain balance, and the tibia of the stance leg must advance over the stationary foot.

The **terminal stance** and **preswing** instants make up the **weight-unloading period,** which accounts for the next 10% of the gait cycle. During this period, the stance leg is unloading the body weight to the contralateral limb and preparing the leg for the swing phase. As with the first two instants, both feet are in contact, and so double support occurs for the second time during the gait cycle.

Swing Phase

The swing phase of gait occurs when the foot is not bearing weight and is moving forward (Figure 14-4). The swing phase allows the toes of the swing leg to clear the floor and allows for leg length adjustments. In addition, it allows the swing leg to advance forward. It makes up approximately 40% of the gait cycle and consists of three subphases.

Subphases (Instants) of Swing Phase

- Initial swing (acceleration)
- Midswing
- Terminal swing (deceleration)

Acceleration occurs when the foot is lifted off the floor. During normal gait, rapid knee flexion and ankle dorsiflexion occur to allow the swing limb to accelerate forward. In some pathological conditions, loss or alteration of knee flexion and ankle dorsiflexion leads to alterations in gait.

The **midswing** instant occurs when the swing leg is adjacent to the weight-bearing leg, which is in midstance.

During the final instant (**terminal swing** or **deceleration**), the swinging leg slows down in preparation for initial contact with the floor. With normal gait, active quadriceps and hamstring muscle actions are required. The quadriceps muscles control knee extension, and the hamstrings control the amount of hip flexion.

During running or with increased velocity, the stance phase decreases and a **float phase** or **double**

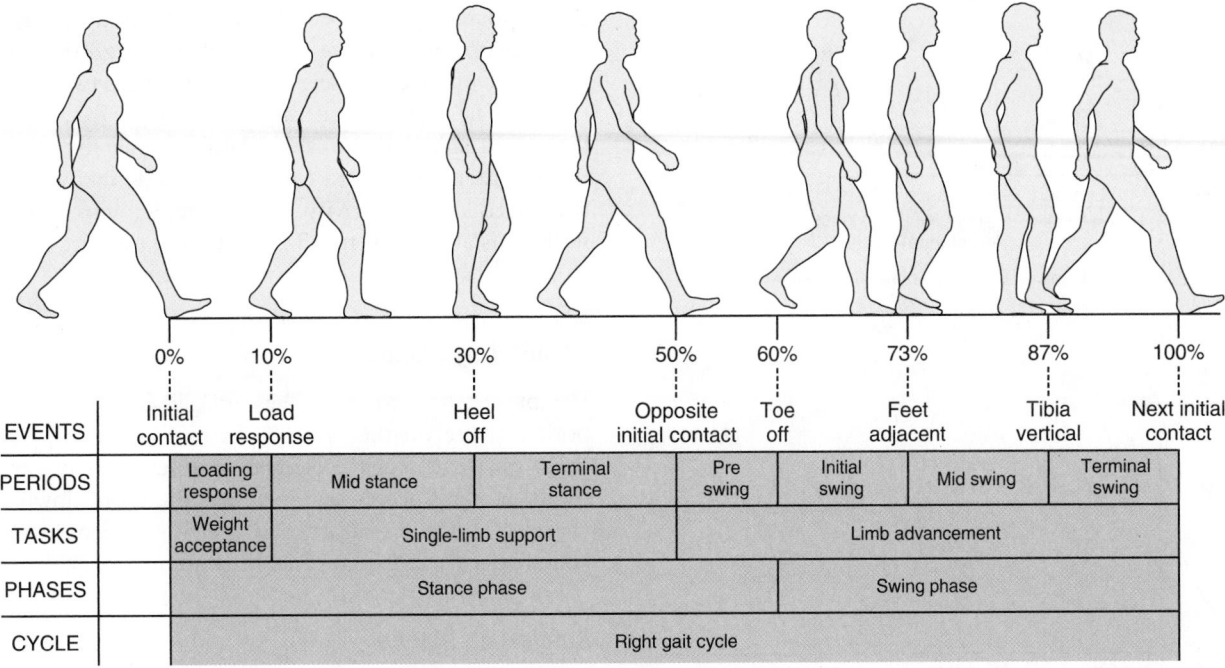

Figure 14-2 Terminology to describe the events of the gait cycle. *Initial contact* corresponds to the beginning of stance when the foot first contacts the ground at 0% of gait cycle. *Load response* occurs when the contralateral foot leaves the ground at 10% of gait cycle. *Heel off* corresponds to the heel lifting from the ground and occurs at approximately 30% of gait cycle. *Opposite initial contact* corresponds to the foot contact of the opposite limb, typically at 50% of gait cycle. *Toe off* occurs when the foot leaves the ground at 60% of gait cycle. *Feet adjacent* takes place when the foot of the swing leg is next to the foot of the stance leg at 73% of gait cycle. *Tibia vertical* corresponds to the tibia of the swing leg being oriented in the vertical direction at 87% of gait cycle. The final event is, again, initial contact, which in fact is the start of the next gait cycle. These eight events divide the gait cycle into seven periods. *Loading response*, between initial contact and opposite toe off, corresponds to the time when the weight is accepted by the lower extremity, initiating contact with the ground. *Midstance* is from opposite toe off to heel rise (10% to 30% of gait cycle). *Terminal stance* begins when the heel rises and ends when the contralateral lower extremity touches the ground, from 30% to 50% of gait cycle. *Preswing* takes place from foot contact of the contralateral limb to toe off of the ipsilateral foot, which is the time corresponding to the second double-limb support period of the gait cycle (50% to 60% of gait cycle). *Initial swing* is from toe off to feet adjacent, when the foot of the swing leg is next to the foot of the stance leg (60% to 73% of gait cycle). *Midswing* is from feet adjacent to when the tibia of the swing leg is vertical (73% to 87% of gait cycle). *Terminal swing* is from a vertical position of the tibia to immediately before heel contact (87% to 100% of the gait cycle). The first 10% of the gait cycle corresponds to a task of weight acceptance—when body mass is transferred from one lower extremity to the other. Single-limb support, from 10% to 50% of the gait cycle, bears the weight of the body as the opposite limb swings forward. The last 10% of stance phase and the entire swing phase advance the limb forward to a new location. (Modified from Simoneau GG: Kinesiology of walking. In Neumann DA, editor: Kinesiology of the musculoskeletal system: foundations of physical rehabilitation, ed 2, St Louis, 2010, Mosby, p. 636.)

TABLE **14-1**

Gait Cycle: Periods and Functions

Period	Percentage of Cycle	Function	Contralateral Limb
Initial double limb support	0 to 12	Loading, weight transfer	Unloading and preparing for swing (preswing)
Single limb support	12 to 50	Support of entire body weight: center of mass moving forward	Swing
Second double limb support	50 to 62	Unloading and preparing for swing (preswing)	Loading, weight transfer
Initial swing	62 to 75	Foot clearance	Single limb support
Midswing	75 to 85	Limb advances in front of body	Single limb support
Terminal swing	85 to 100	Limb deceleration, preparation for weight transfer	Single limb support

From Sutherland DH, et al: Kinematics of normal human walking. In Rose J, Gamble JG, editors: Human locomotion, Baltimore, 1994, Williams & Wilkins, p. 27.

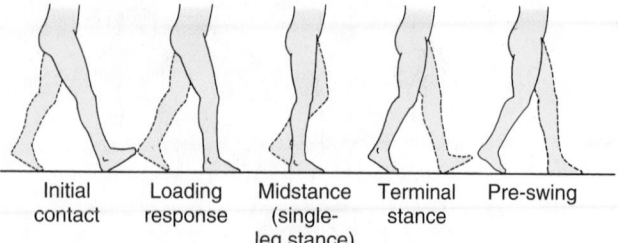

| Initial contact | Loading response | Midstance (single-leg stance) | Terminal stance | Pre-swing |

Figure 14-3 Stance phase of gait.

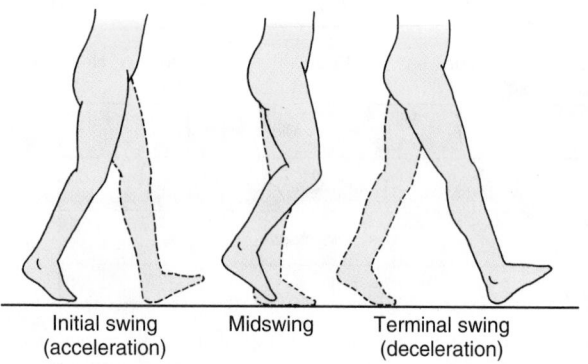

| Initial swing (acceleration) | Midswing | Terminal swing (deceleration) |

Figure 14-4 Swing phase of gait.

unsupported phase occurs while the double support phase disappears (Figure 14-5).[18,21] Although the single-leg stance phase decreases, the load increases two or three times.[22] The motion occurring at each of the joints (pelvis, hip, knee, ankle) is similar for walking and for running, but the required range of motion (ROM) increases with the speed of the activity. For example, hip flexion in walking is about 40° to 45°, whereas in running it is 60° to 75°.[23]

Double-Leg Stance

Double-leg stance is that phase of gait in which parts of both feet are on the ground. In normal gait, it occurs twice during the gait cycle and represents about 25% of the cycle. This percentage increases the more slowly one walks; it becomes shorter as walking speed increases (Figure 14-6) and disappears in running.

Single-Leg Stance

The single-leg stance phase of gait occurs when only one leg is on the ground; this occurs twice during the normal gait cycle and takes up approximately 30% of the cycle.

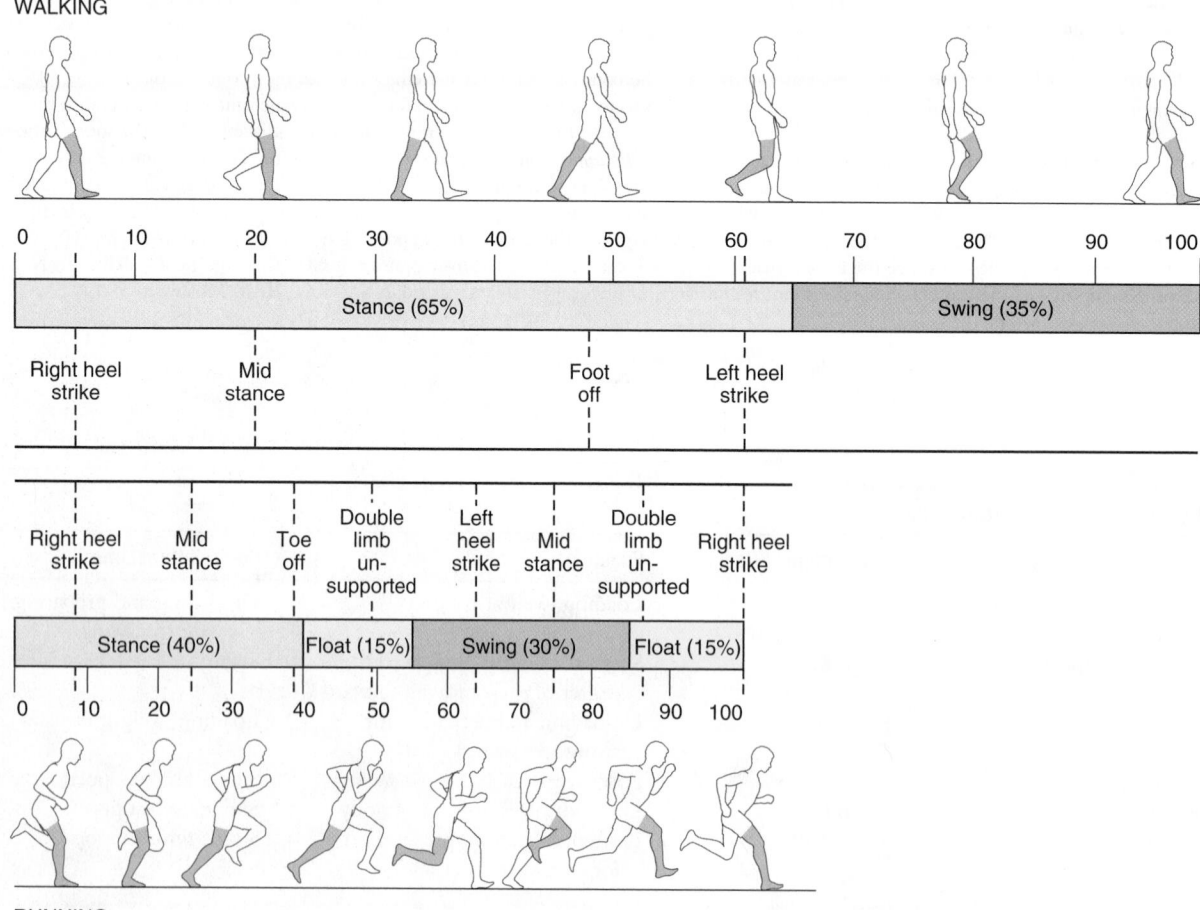

Figure 14-5 Comparison of the phases of the walking and running cycles.

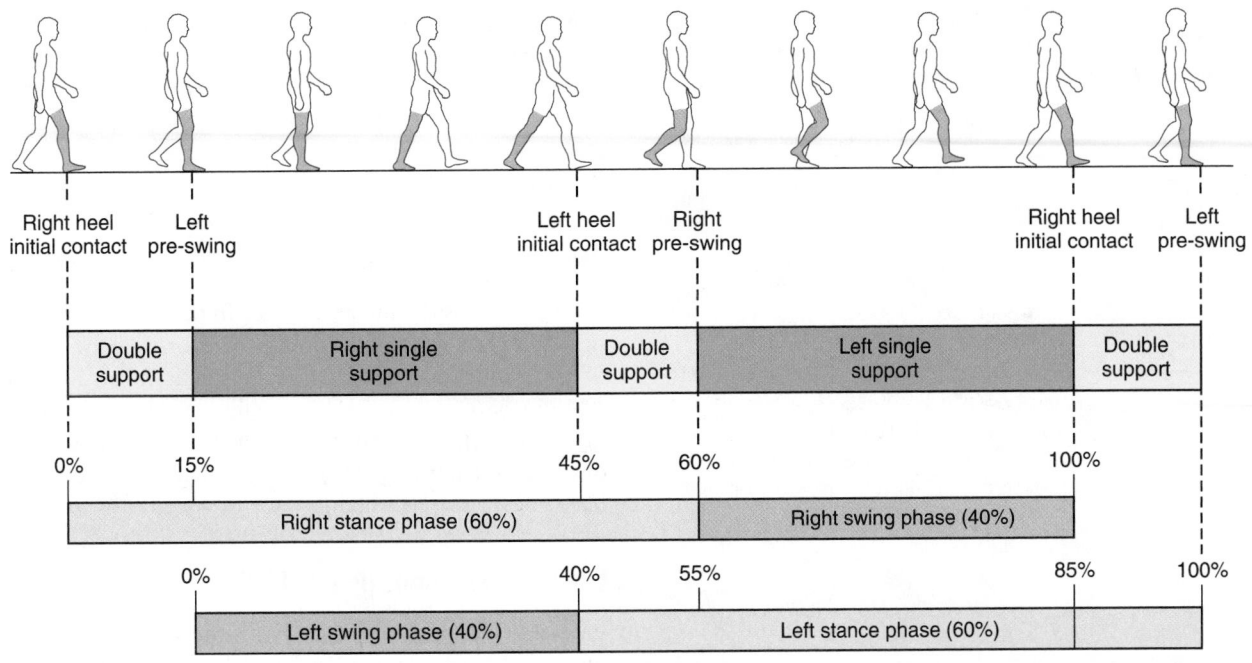

Figure 14-6 Time dimensions of the walking cycle. (Adapted from Inman VT, Ralston HJ, Todd F: Human walking, Baltimore, 1981, Williams & Wilkins, p. 26.)

NORMAL PARAMETERS OF GAIT[7–11,24]

The parameters that follow and their values are considered normal for a population between the ages of 8 and 45 years. It should be pointed out, however, that a relatively normal gait pattern is seen in persons as young as 3 years of age.[2] There are, however, differences between individuals of the same sex and between men and women.[25] For the majority of the population outside of these ages, there are alterations caused by neurological development, balance control, aging, changes in limb length, and maturation.[2] For example, with maturity, walking velocity and step length increase, and cadence decreases.[26] It is also important to evaluate gait on the basis of normal gait for someone the same age. This is especially true for children.

Base (Step) Width

The normal base width, which is the distance between the two feet, is 5 to 10 cm (2 to 4 inches; Figure 14-7). If the base is wider, the examiner may suspect some pathology (e.g., cerebellar or inner ear problems) that results in poor balance, a condition such as diabetes or peripheral neuropathy that may indicate a loss of sensation, or a musculoskeletal problem (e.g., tight hip abductors). In the first two cases, the patient tends to have a wider base to maintain balance. With increased speed, the base width normally decreases to zero, and in some cases, crossover

> **Gait Parameters That are Significantly Decreased in Women Compared with Men[24]**
>
> - Velocity
> - Stride and step length
> - Proportional distance of center of gravity from ground
> - Sagittal hip motion
> - Knee flexion in initial swing
> - Width of base of support
> - Vertical head excursion
> - Lateral head excursion
> - Shoulder sagittal motion
> - Elbow flexion

occurs, in which one foot lands where the other should and vice versa. Such **crossover** can lead to gait alterations and other problems.[27]

Step Length

Step length, or gait length, is the distance between successive contact points on opposite feet (see Figure 14-1). Normally, this distance is about 72 cm (28 inches) being relatively constant for each individual (i.e., step length is commonly related to preferred walking speed)[17,28] and should be equal for both legs. It varies with age and sex with children taking smaller steps than adults and females taking smaller steps than males.[22] Height also has an

Gait Descriptors or Parameters Which the Examiner Should Watch for When Observing Gait[16]

Stride:	The sequence of events between successive heel strikes of the same foot
Step:	The sequence of events between successive heel strikes of the opposite feet
Stride length:	The distance between two successive heel strikes of the same foot (average: 144 cm or 57 inches)
Step length:	The distance between successive heel strikes of two different feet (average: 72 cm or 28 inches)
Step or Base Width:	The lateral distance between the heel centers of two consecutive foot contacts (average: 8 to 10 cm or 3 to 4 inches)
Cadence (step rate):	Number of steps per minute (average: 90 to 120 steps/minute)
Stride time:	Time for a full gait cycle
Step time:	Time for completion of heel strike of right foot to heel strike of left foot
Walking or gait speed:*	Distance covered in a given amount of time (average: 1.4 m/second or 3 mph)

*All other values will vary depending on walking speed.

effect: a taller person takes larger steps. Step length tends to decrease with age, fatigue, pain, and disease. If step length is normal for both legs, the **rhythm of walking** is smooth. If there is pain in one limb, the patient attempts to take weight off that limb as quickly as possible, altering the rhythm.

Stride Length

Stride length is the linear distance in the plane of progression between successive points of foot-to-floor contact of the same foot. The stride length is normally about 144 cm (56 inches) and in reality is one gait cycle.[17] Stride length, like step length, decreases with age, pain, disease, and fatigue.[19,29] The age changes are often the result of decreased walking pace or speed.[29,30]

Lateral Pelvic Shift (Pelvic List)

Lateral pelvic shift, or pelvic list, is the side-to-side movement of the pelvis during walking. It is necessary to center the weight of the body over the stance leg for balance (Figure 14-8). The lateral pelvic shift is normally 2.5 to 5 cm (1 to 2 inches). It increases if the feet are farther

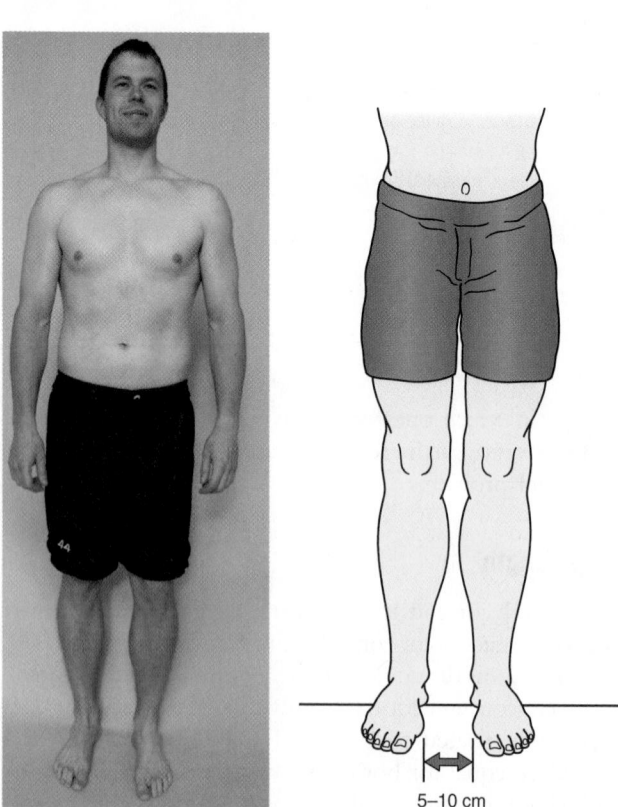

5–10 cm

Figure 14-7 Normal base or step width.

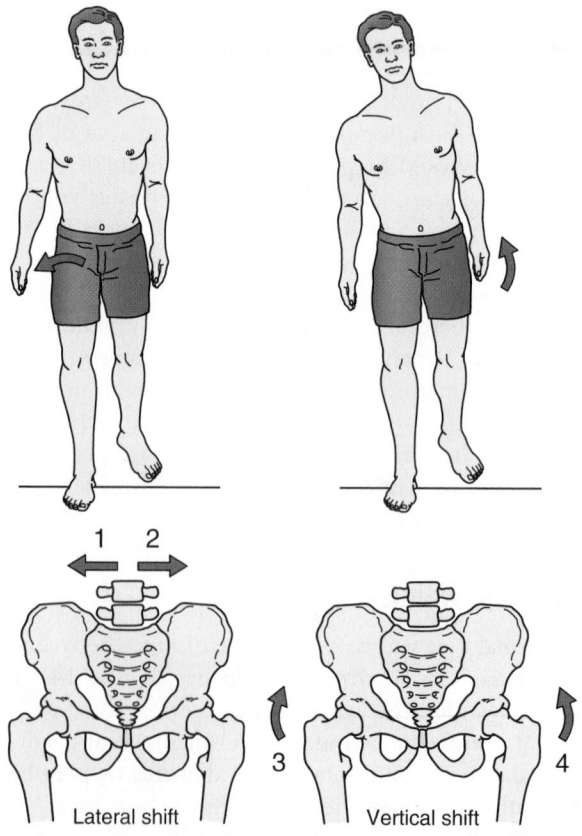

Lateral shift   Vertical shift

Figure 14-8 Pelvic shift. Numbers indicate that one lateral or vertical shift occurs and then the other; they do not occur at the same time. *1,* Right lateral shift; *2,* left lateral shift; *3,* right vertical shift; *4,* left vertical shift.

apart. The pelvic list causes relative adduction of the weight-bearing limb, facilitating the action of the hip adductors. If the abductor muscles are weak, a **Trendelenburg gait** results (see Figure 14-21).

Vertical Pelvic Shift

Vertical pelvic shift keeps the center of gravity from moving up and down more than 5 cm (2 inches) during normal gait. By means of a vertical pelvic shift, the high point occurs during midstance and the low point during initial contact; the height of these points may increase during the swing phase if the knee is fused or does not bend because of protective spasm or swelling. The head is never higher during normal gait than it is when the person is standing on both feet. Therefore, if a person can stand in an opening, he or she should be able to move through the opening without hitting the head.[7] On the swing phase, the hip is lower on the swing side, and the patient must flex the knee and dorsiflex the foot to clear the toe. This action shortens the extremity length at midstance and decreases the center of gravity rise.

Pelvic Rotation

Pelvic rotation is necessary to lessen the angle of the femur with the floor, and, in so doing, it lengthens the femur (Figure 14-9). The rotation decreases the amplitude of displacement along the path traveled by the center of gravity and thereby decreases the center-of-gravity dip. There is a total of 8° pelvic rotation with 4° forward on the swing leg and 4° posteriorly on the stance leg. To maintain balance, the thorax rotates in the opposite direction. When the pelvis rotates clockwise, the thorax rotates counterclockwise, and vice versa. These concurrent rotations provide counter-rotation forces and help regulate the speed of walking.

In the lower limb, rotation is evident at each joint (Figure 14-10). The farther the joint is from the trunk, the greater the amount of rotation. For example, rotation in the tibia is three times greater than rotation in the pelvis.[7]

Center of Gravity

Normally, in the standing position, the center of gravity is 5 cm (2 inches) anterior to the second sacral vertebra; it tends to be slightly higher in men than in women because men tend to have a greater body mass in the shoulder area. The vertical and horizontal displacements of the center of gravity describe a figure-eight, occupying a 5-cm (2-inch) square within the pelvis during walking. The vertical displacement, which describes a smooth sinusoidal curve during walking, can be observed from the side. The patient's head descends during weight-loading and weight-unloading periods and rises during single-leg stance.

Normal Cadence

The normal cadence is between 90 and 120 steps per minute which varies, in part, because of the height of the individual.[31-34] The cadence of women is usually six to nine steps per minute higher than that of men.[33] With age, the cadence decreases. Figure 14-11, *A*, illustrates the cadence of normal gait from heel strike to toe off showing the changing weight distribution. With pathology or deformity (e.g., a cavus foot [Figure 14-11, *B*]), this weight-bearing pattern may be altered. As the pace of walking increases, the stride width increases, and the toeing-out angle decreases. Gait speed is about 1.4 m/sec (3 mph).[17]

NORMAL PATTERN OF GAIT[6-11,17,31,35,36]

Stance Phase

As previously mentioned, there are five instants involved during the stance phase of gait. These are now described in order of occurrence. This phase is the **closed kinetic chain** phase of gait. The action occurring at the various joints causes a chain reaction because of the stresses put on the joints and supporting structures with weight-bearing. The foot becomes the fixed stable segment, and

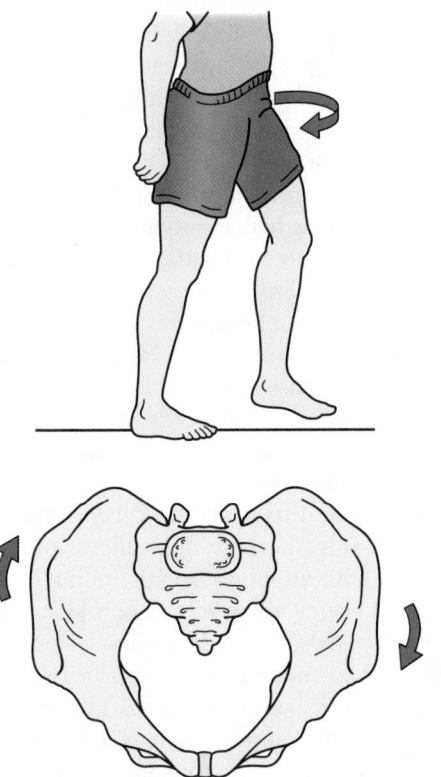

Figure 14-9 Pelvic rotation. Left forward pelvic rotation is illustrated.

Lower extremity kinematics (horizontal plane)

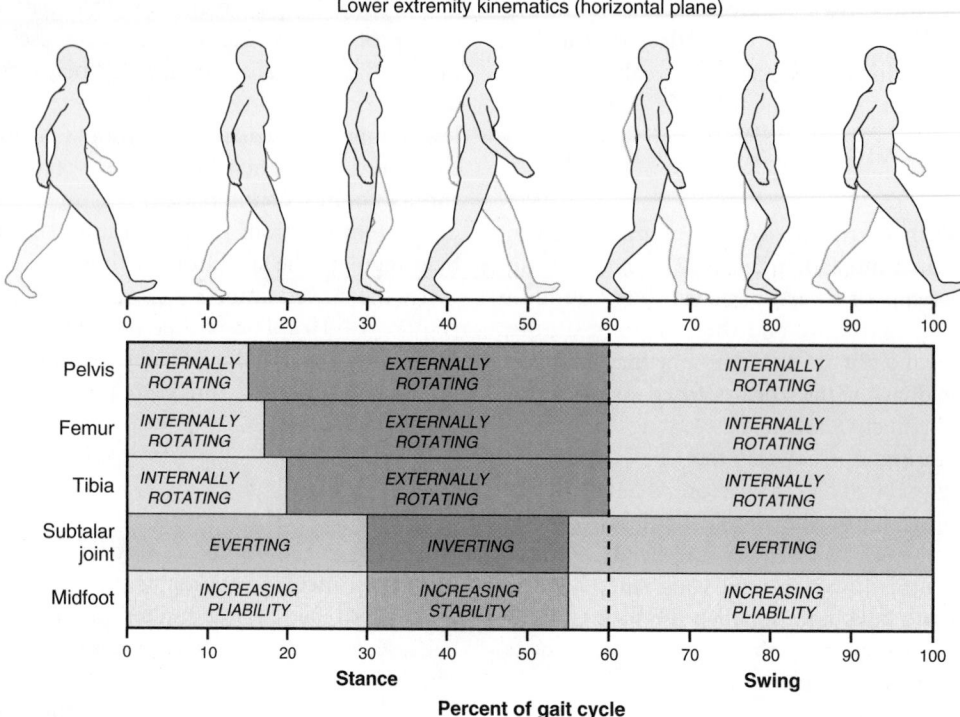

Figure 14-10 Horizontal plane rotation of the major bones of the lower extremity and subtalar joint during walking. The graph shows the direction of rotation, which is not necessarily the same as the absolute joint position. (From Simoneau GG: Kinesiology of walking. In Neumann DA: Kinesiology of the musculoskeletal system: foundations of physical rehabilitation, ed 2, St Louis, 2010, Mosby, p. 647.)

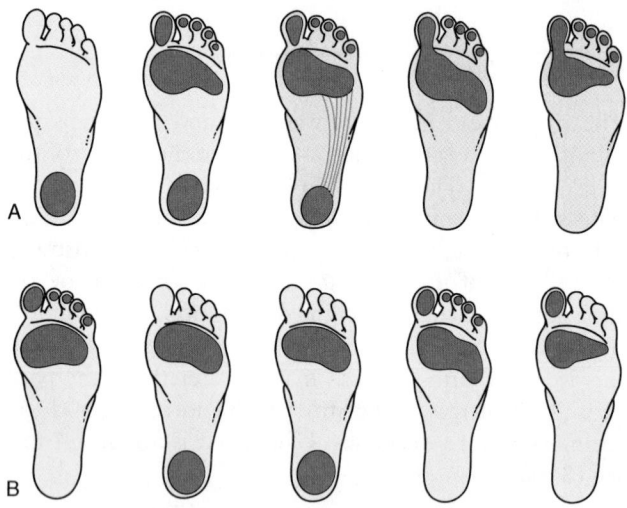

Figure 14-11 The cadence of gait. A, Normal foot. **B,** Cavus foot. (From Viladot A: Patologia del Antepié, Barcelona, 1975, Ediciones Toray, SA.)

alterations occur from the foot up with the joints of the foot adapting first, followed by those of the ankle, knee, hip, pelvis, spine, and finally the upper limb, which acts as a counterbalance to movement in the lower limb.[37] The relations between the joints are constantly changing. Table 14-2 summarizes the movement at the hip, knee, ankle, and foot during the stance phase.[38]

Initial Contact (Heel Strike)

Initial contact occurs when the limb first strikes the ground. Normally, this occurs when the heel strikes and the limb is being prepared to take weight. During the initial contact, the pelvis is level and medially rotated on the side of initial contact, whereas the trunk is aligned between the two lower limbs. The hip is flexed 30° to 49° and is medially rotated; the knee is slightly flexed or extended; the tibia is laterally rotated; the ankle is at 90° with the foot supinated; and the hindfoot is everted. At this instant, there is little force going through the limb.

If pain occurs in the heel at this time, it may be caused by a heel spur, bone bruise, heel fat-pad bruise, or bursitis. This pain may cause increased flexion of the knee with early plantar flexion to relieve the stress or pressure on the painful tissues. If the knee is weak, the patient may extend the knee by using the hand or may hit the heel hard on the ground to whip the knee into extension. A patient may do this because of weakness of the muscles (e.g., reflex inhibition, poliomyelitis, an internal derangement of the knee, a nerve root lesion [L2, L3, or L4], femoral neuropathy). In the past, this instant was referred to as "heel strike;" however, with some pathological gaits, heel strike may not be the first instant. Instead, the toes, the forefoot, or the entire foot may initially contact the ground. If the dorsiflexor muscles are weak, the foot drops, slaps, or flops down. The weakness may be caused

TABLE **14-2**

Summary of Joint Motions at the Hip, Knee, Tibia, Foot, and Ankle During the Stance Phase of Normal Gait

Hip

Phase	KINEMATIC MOTION	KINETIC MOTION	
	Hip	External Forces	Internal Forces
Heel strike	20° to 40° of hip flexion moving toward extension; slight adduction and lateral rotation	Reaction force in front of joint; flexion moment moving toward extension; forward pelvic rotation	Gluteus maximus and hamstrings working eccentrically to resist flexion moment; erector spinae working eccentrically to resist forward bend
Foot flat	Hip moving into extension, adduction, medial rotation	Flexion moment	Gluteus maximus and hamstrings contracting concentrically to bring hip into extension; erector spinae resisting trunk flexion
Midstance	Moving through neutral position; pelvis rotating posteriorly	Reaction force posterior to hip joint; extension moment	Iliopsoas working eccentrically to resist extension; gluteus medius contracting in reverse action to stabilize opposite pelvis; iliopsoas activity continuing
Heel off	10° to 15° extension of hip abduction, lateral rotation	Extension moment decreasing after double-limb support begins	
Toe off	Moving toward 10° extension, abduction, lateral rotation	Decrease of extension moment	Adductor magnus working eccentrically to control or stabilize pelvis; iliopsoas activity continuing

Knee and Tibia

Phase	KINEMATIC MOTION		KINETIC MOTION	
	Knee	Tibia	External Forces	Internal Forces
Heel strike	In full extension before heel contact; flexing as heel strikes floor	Slight lateral rotation	Rapidly increasing reaction forces behind knee joint causing flexion moment	Quadriceps femoris contracting eccentrically to control rapid knee flexion and to prevent buckling
Foot flat	In 20° flexion moving toward extension	Medial rotation	Flexion moment	After foot is flat, quadriceps femoris activity becoming concentric to bring femur over tibia
Midstance	In 15° flexion moving toward extension	Neutral	Maximum flexion moment	Quadriceps femoris activity decreasing; gastrocnemius working eccentrically to control excessive knee extension
Heel off	In 4° flexion moving toward extension	Lateral rotation	Reaction forces moving anterior to joint; extension moment	Gastrocnemius beginning to work concentrically to start knee flexion
Toe off	Moving from near full extension to 40° flexion	Lateral rotation	Reaction forces moving posterior to joint as knee flexes; flexion moment	Quadriceps femoris contracting eccentrically

Continued

TABLE **14-2**

Summary of Joint Motions at the Hip, Knee, Tibia, Foot, and Ankle During the Stance Phase of Normal Gait—cont'd

Foot and Ankle

Phase	KINEMATIC MOTION		KINETIC MOTION	
	Foot	Ankle	External Forces	Internal Forces
Heel strike	Supination (rigid) at heel contact	Moving into plantar flexion	Reaction forces behind joint axis; plantar flexion moment at heel strike	Dorsiflexors (tibialis anterior, extensor digitorum longus, and extensor hallucis longus) contracting eccentrically to slow plantar flexion
Foot flat	Pronation, adapting to support surface	Plantar flexion to dorsiflexion over a fixed foot	Maximum plantar flexion moment; reaction forces beginning to shift anterior, producing a dorsiflexion moment	Dorsiflexion activity decreasing; tibialis posterior, flexor hallucis longus, and flexor digitorum longus working eccentrically to control pronation
Midstance	Neutral	3° of dorsiflexion	Slight dorsiflexion moment	Plantar flexor muscles (gastrocsoleus and peroneal muscles), activated to control dorsiflexion of the tibia and fibula over a fixed foot, contracting eccentrically
Heel off	Supination as foot becomes rigid for push-off	15° dorsiflexion toward plantar flexion	Maximal dorsiflexion moment	Plantar flexor muscles beginning to contract concentrically to prepare for push-off
Toe off	Supination	20° plantar flexion	Dorsiflexion moment	Plantar flexor muscles at peak activity but becoming inactive as foot leaves ground

Modified from Giallonardo LM: Gait. In Myers RS, editor: Saunders manual of physical therapy practice, Philadelphia, 1995, WB Saunders, pp. 1108–1109.

by a peroneal neuropathy or nerve root lesion (L4). A knee flexion contracture or spasticity may cause the same alteration.

Load Response (Weight Acceptance or Foot Flat)

Load response is a critical event in that the person subconsciously decides whether the limb is able to bear the weight of the body. The trunk is aligned with the stance leg. The pelvis drops slightly on the swing leg side and medially rotates on the same side. The flexed and laterally rotated hip moves into extension, and the knee flexes 15° to 25°. The tibia is medially rotated and begins to move forward over the fixed foot as the body swings over the foot. The ankle is plantar flexed, and the hindfoot is inverted. The foot moves into pronation, because this position unlocks the foot and enables it to adapt to different terrains and postures. The forefoot is pronated, unlocking the subtalar and metatarsal joints to enable them to absorb the shock more effectively, and the plantar aspect is in contact with the floor.

Abnormal responses include excessive or no knee motion as a result of weak quadriceps, plantar flexor contractures, or spasticity.[9]

Midstance (Single-Leg Support)

The midstance instant is a period of stationary foot support. Normally, the weight of the foot is evenly distributed over the entire foot. The trunk is aligned over the stance leg, and the pelvis shows a slight drop to the swing leg side.

During this stage, there is maximum extension of the hip (10° to 15°) with lateral rotation, and the greatest force is on the hip. Painful hip, knee, or ankle conditions cause this phase to be shortened as the patient hurries through the phase to decrease the pain. If the gluteus medius (L5 nerve root) is weak, Trendelenburg sign is present. The knee flexes, and the ankle is locked at 5° to 8° of dorsiflexion, rolling forward on the forefoot (roll-off). The foot is in contact with the floor; the forefoot is pronated, and the hindfoot is inverted. This instant is a critical event for the ankle. If pain is elicited during this period, the phase is shortened and the heel may lift off early. This pain is commonly caused by conditions such as arthritis, rigid pes planus, fallen metatarsal or longitudinal arches, plantar fasciitis, or Morton metatarsalgia. Therefore, pathology at the hip, ankle, or knee can modify the gait in this phase.

Terminal Stance (Heel Off)

In the final stages, the trunk is initially aligned over the lower limbs and moves toward the stance leg. The pelvis is initially level and posteriorly rotated and then dips to the swing leg side, remaining posteriorly rotated. The heel is in neutral and slight medial rotation; the knee is extended with the tibia laterally rotated. At the ankle, plantar flexion occurs as the critical event. This action helps to smooth the pathway of the center of gravity. The forefoot is initially in contact with the floor, and then the weight on the foot moves forward with plantar flexion so that only the big toe is in contact with the floor. At the same time, the forefoot moves from inversion to eversion.

Preswing (Toe Off)

The preswing phase is the acceleration phase as the toe pushes the leg forward. The trunk remains erect, the pelvis remains posteriorly rotated, and the hip is extended and slightly medially rotated. The knee flexes to 30° to 35° (critical event), and the ankle is plantar flexed. Because the center of gravity is anterior to the hip, the hip can be accelerated forward in initial swing.

If pain is elicited during this instant, it may be caused by a hallux rigidus, turf toe, or any other pathology involving the great toe (hallux), especially the metatarsophalangeal joint of the hallux. With injury to the joint, the patient is unable to push off on the medial aspect of the foot; instead, the patient pushes off on the lateral aspect of the foot to compensate for the painful metatarsophalangeal joint or, in some cases, a painful metatarsal arch resulting from increased pressure on the metatarsal heads. If the plantar flexors are weak (e.g., S1–S2 nerve root pathology), push-off may be absent. During this phase, the foot pronates so that there is a rigid base for better push-off.

During walking, a cane can be used to decrease the load on the limb. Lyu and associates[39] have shown that using a cane in the contralateral upper limb, if the cane tip touches the ground at the same time as the heel, can reduce the force at heel strike by 34%, by 25% at midstance, and about 30% at toe off.

Swing Phase

The swing phase of gait involves the lower limb in an **open kinetic chain;** the foot is not fixed on the ground, and the stresses on the limb are therefore less and easier to dissipate. During this phase, alterations occur from the spine down through the pelvis, hip, ankle, and foot. The pelvis and hip provide the most stability in the lower limb during the non–weight-bearing phase. Table 14-3 summarizes the motions occurring in the lower limb during the swing phase.

The three instants composing the swing phase of gait are now described in order of occurrence.

Initial Swing

During the first subphase of acceleration (Figure 14-12), flexion and medial rotation of the hip and flexion of the knee occur. The pelvis medially rotates and dips to the swing leg side. The trunk is aligned with the stance leg. In addition, the ankle continues to plantar flex. The foot is not in contact with the floor. The forefoot continues supinating, and the hindfoot continues everting. The dorsiflexor muscles of the ankle contract to allow the foot to clear the ground, and the knee exhibits its maximum

TABLE **14-3**

Summary of Joint Motion and Forces During Swing Phase: Acceleration to Midswing and Midswing to Deceleration

Joint	ACCELERATION TO MIDSWING		MIDSWING TO DECELERATION	
	Kinematic Motion	Kinetic Motion	Kinematic Motion	Kinetic Motion
Hip	Slight flexion (0° to 15°) moving to 30° flexion and lateral rotation to neutral	Hip flexors working concentrically to bring limb through; contralateral gluteus medius concentrically contracting to maintain pelvis position	Continued flexion at about 30° to 40°	Gluteus maximus contracting eccentrically to slow hip flexion
Knee	30° to 60° knee flexion and lateral rotation of tibia moving toward neutral	Hamstrings concentrically contracting	Moving to near full extension and slight lateral tibial rotation	Quadriceps femoris contracting concentrically and hamstrings contracting eccentrically
Ankle and foot	20° dorsiflexion and slight pronation	Dorsiflexors contracting concentrically	Ankle in neutral; foot in slight supination	Dorsiflexors contracting isometrically

From Giallonardo LM: Gait. In Myers RS, editor: Saunders manual of physical therapy practice, Philadelphia, 1995, WB Saunders, p. 1110.

RANGE OF MOTION SUMMARY

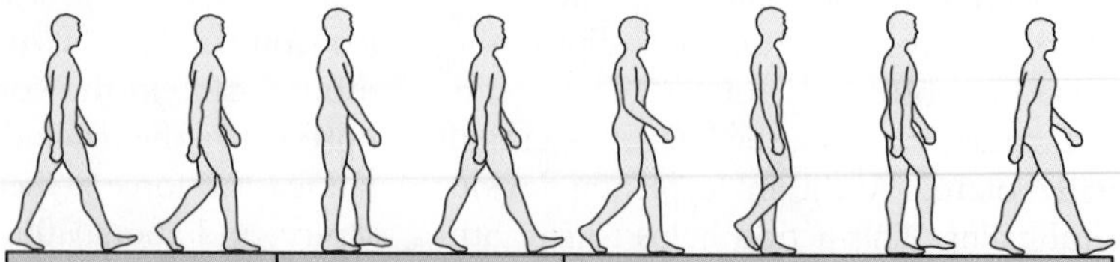

	Weight Acceptance		Single Limb Support		Swing Limb Advancement			
Reference Limb	IC	LR	MSt	TSt	PSw	ISw	MSw	TSw
Opposite Limb	PSw	PSw	ISw/MSw	TSw	IC/LR	MSt	MSt	TSt
TRUNK	Erect ➝							
PELVIS	5° Fwd Rotation	5° Fwd Rotation	0°	5° Bkwd Rotation	5° Bkwd Rotation	5° Bkwd Rotation	0°	5° Fwd Rotation
HIP	25° Flex	25° Flex	0°	20° Apparent Hyperext	0°	15° Flex	25° Flex	25° Flex
KNEE	0°	15° Flex	0°	0°	40° Flex	60° Flex	25° Flex	0°
ANKLE	0°	10° Plantar Flex	5° Dorsiflex	10° Dorsiflex	20° Plantar flex	10° Plantar flex	0°	0°
TOES	0°	0°	0°	30° MTP Ext	60° MTP Ext	0°	0°	0°

Figure 14-12 **Normal range of motion (ROM) during gait cycle.** *IC,* Initial contact; *ISw,* initial swing; *LR,* load response; *MSt,* midstance; *MSw,* midswing; *PSw,* preswing; *TSt,* terminal stance; *TSw,* terminal swing. (Copyright 1991 LAREI, Rancho Los Amigos Medical Center, Downey, CA 90242; from The Pathokinesiology Service and The Physical Therapy Department, Rancho Los Amigos Medical Center: Observational Gait Analysis. Downey, CA, Los Amigos Research and Educational Institute, Inc., 1996, p. 30.)

flexion during gait of about 60°. If the quadriceps muscles are weak, the trunk muscles thrust the pelvis forward to provide forward momentum to the leg.

Midswing

During the midswing instant, the hip continues to flex and medially rotate, and the knee continues to flex. The

ankle is in the anatomical or plantigrade position (90°) for the first 25% of the stance phase to permit the foot and midtarsal joints to unlock so that the foot can adapt to uneven terrain when it begins weight-bearing. The forefoot is supinated, and the hindfoot is everted. The pelvis and trunk are in the same position as during the previous stage. If the ankle dorsiflexor muscles are weak (e.g., drop foot), the patient demonstrates a **step-page gait** (see Figure 14-27). In such a gait, the hip flexes excessively so that the toes can clear the ground.

Terminal Swing (Deceleration)

During the final subphase, the hip continues to flex and medially rotate, and the knee reaches its maximum extension. At the ankle, dorsiflexion has occurred. The forefoot is supinated, and the hindfoot is everted. The trunk and pelvis maintain the same position as before. The hamstring muscles contract during the terminal phase to slow the swing; if the hamstrings are weak (e.g., S1–S2 nerve root lesion), heel strike may be excessively harsh to lock the knee in extension.

Joint Motion During Normal Gait

Although there is a tendency to talk about gait as action around joints, the examiner must not forget that muscles play a significant role in what happens at the joints. Table 14-4 illustrates the actions of some of the muscles used during gait.[40]

Hip. The function of the hip is to extend the leg during the stance phase and flex the leg during the swing phase. The ligaments of the hip help to stabilize it in extension. The hip extensors help to initiate movement, as do the hip flexors; both groups of muscles work phasically.[41] The hip flexors (primarily the iliopsoas muscle) contract to slow extension; the hip extensors (primarily the hamstring muscles) contract to slow flexion. In this way, they work eccentrically. The abductor muscles provide stability during single-leg support, a critical event for the hip.[41]

If there is loss of movement of the hip, the compensatory mechanisms are increased mobility of the knee on the same side and increased mobility of the contralateral hip. In addition, the lumbar spine shows increased mobility.

Knee. When the knee is in flexion during the first three instants of the stance phase of gait, it acts as a shock absorber. Painful knees are not able to do this. One of the critical events of the knee is extension. The functions of the knee during gait are to bear weight, absorb shock, extend the stride length, and allow the foot to move through its swing. The quadriceps muscles use only 4% to 5% of their maximum voluntary contraction to extend the knee, but in so doing, they help to control weight acceptance. The hamstring muscles flex the knee and slow the leg in the swing phase, working eccentrically.

If the knee has a flexion deformity, the hip is flexed and, therefore, loses its extension power, which is a critical event for the hip. Pathological conditions, such as patellofemoral syndrome, also cause deviations from normal gait. For example, patients with patellofemoral syndrome show less knee flexion during the single-leg stance phase, combined with lateral femoral rotation during the swing phase.[42] On heel strike to foot flat, the femur then medially rotates, and if this compensating medial rotation is too great, it causes excessive pronation, which then stresses the medial aspect of the patellofemoral joint.

Gastrocnemius and Soleus. The gastrocnemius and soleus muscles are important in gait. They use 85% of their maximum voluntary contraction during normal walking. These muscles help to restrain the body's forward

TABLE 14-4

Muscle Actions During Gait Cycle

Phase of Gait	Mechanical Goals	Active Muscle Groups	Examples
Stance Phase			
Initial contact	Position foot, begin deceleration	Ankle dorsiflexors, hip extensors, knee flexors	Anterior tibialis, gluteus maximus, hamstrings
Loading response	Accept weight, stabilize pelvis, decelerate mass	Knee extensors, hip abductors, ankle plantar flexors	Vasti, gluteus medius, gastrocnemius, soleus
Midstance	Stabilize knee, preserve momentum	Ankle plantar flexors (isometric)	Gastrocnemius, soleus
Terminal stance	Accelerate mass	Ankle plantar flexors (concentric)	Gastrocnemius, soleus
Swing Phase			
Preswing	Prepare for swing	Hip flexors	Iliopsoas, rectus femoris
Initial swing	Clear foot, vary cadence	Ankle dorsiflexors, hip flexors	Tibialis anterior, iliopsoas, rectus femoris
Midswing	Clear foot	Ankle dorsiflexors	Tibialis anterior
Terminal swing	Decelerate shank, decelerate leg, position foot, prepare for contact	Knee flexors, hip extensors, ankle dorsiflexors, knee extensors	Hamstrings, gluteus maximus, tibialis anterior, vasti

From Rab GT: Muscle. In Rose J, Gamble JG, editors: Human locomotion, Baltimore, 1994, Williams & Wilkins, p. 113.

momentum during forward movement. They also contribute to knee and ankle stability, restrain forward rotation of the tibia on the talus during the stance phase, and minimize the vertical pelvic shift, thereby conserving energy.[43] To accomplish these functions during gait, the triceps surae work eccentrically and concentrically.

Foot and Ankle. The foot and ankle play major roles in gait in that the various joints allow the foot to accommodate to the ground. The joints of the foot and ankle work interdependently during normal gait. When the heel contacts the ground, the lower limb becomes a closed kinetic chain, and movements and stresses must be absorbed by the structures of the lower limb.

When looking at the ankle, the examiner should observe immediate plantar flexion at initial contact. Loss of this plantar flexion (e.g., tibial nerve neuropathy) results in an inability to transfer weight to the anterior foot, increased ankle dorsiflexion, and increased knee flexion. In addition, the duration of single-leg stance on the affected side decreases, and the step length on the opposite side decreases. Furthermore, quadriceps action at the knee increases because of the lack of knee stability caused by the loss of the triceps surae with the end result being that walking velocity decreases.[43] The foot then dorsiflexes through midstance or single-leg stance, with maximum dorsiflexion being reached just before heel off. The examiner should note whether there is sufficient plantar flexion during push-off.

OVERVIEW AND PATIENT HISTORY

The assessment of a patient's gait should be included in any assessment of the lower limb. The examiner must keep in mind that the posture of the head, neck, thorax, and lumbar spine can affect gait even if no pathology is evident in the lower limb. The examiner must be able to identify the action of each body segment and note any deviation from normal during the individual phases of gait. For this reason, it is important to understand the normal parameters of gait and the mechanism of gait as it occurs. With this knowledge, the ways in which the gait is altered under pathological conditions can be better understood.

Musculoskeletal pathology tends to modify gait because of muscle weakness, pain, or altered ROM, so the examiner should watch closely for these factors when observing gait. Many patients can adapt automatically to these changes, provided they have normal sensation and can develop selective control.[9] Patients with upper motor neuron lesions have greater alterations and cannot easily adapt because, in addition to the musculoskeletal problems, they also present with spasticity, control problems, and sensory disturbances.[9] It is important that the examiner read the patient's chart and take a history from the patient regarding any disease or injury, past or present, that may be causing gait problems.

OBSERVATION

The examiner should first perform a general overview of the patient's posture, looking for any asymmetry, and then observe the patient's gait, looking at stride length, step frequency, time of swing, speed of walking, and duration of the complete walking cycle. This is normally done with the patient in shorts, wearing no shoes or socks. If gait is observed wearing shoes, the same shoes should be used for each test.[44] A steady gait pattern is usually established within three steps; it is initiated by the body's becoming unbalanced so that the patient can lift one foot off the ground to take the first step.[45] After this overview is completed, the examiner can look at specific parts of the gait in terms of phases and what happens at each joint during these phases.

Because gait constantly changes as one stops and starts, hurries, dawdles, and walks with others, it is important to remember whether the movements the patient is capable of are normal and whether the speeds, phases, strides, and durations of the cycles occur in normal combinations. In addition to observing walking at a normal speed, the patient's slow and fast gait speeds should be examined to see whether these changes affect the gait. The examiner must watch the upper limbs and trunk, as well as the lumbar spine, pelvis, hips, knees, feet, and ankles during these changes. Female patients should be in a bra and briefs, and male patients should be in shorts. The patient should walk barefoot. In this way, the motions of the toes, feet, legs, pelvis, trunk, and upper limbs can properly be observed.

The examiner should ask the patient to walk in the usual manner, using any aids necessary (e.g., parallel bars, crutches, walker, canes). While the patient is walking, the examiner makes an initial general observation of any obvious limp or deformity.

The examiner should observe the gait from the front, from behind, and from the side, in each instance observing from proximal to distal and watching the pelvis and lumbar spine down to the ankle and foot as well as from the foot up. For example, in the swing phase (open kinetic chain) movement starts proximally and moves distally. In the stance phase (closed kinetic chain), movement is reversed, starting in the foot and moving proximally. The examiner should observe the movements in the trunk and upper limbs, which normally are in the opposite direction to those of the lower limbs. This method provides a sequential, thorough manner of assessment. Rancho Los Amigos Medical Center has developed a useful gait analysis chart (Figure 14-13). By using the chart during observation, the examiner can determine deviations and their effect on gait in an easily used and easily retained method of recording. The dark gray boxes indicate what normally should occur; the lighter gray and white boxes indicate minor and major deviations from the normal, respectively. Minor deviations imply that the functional task of walking

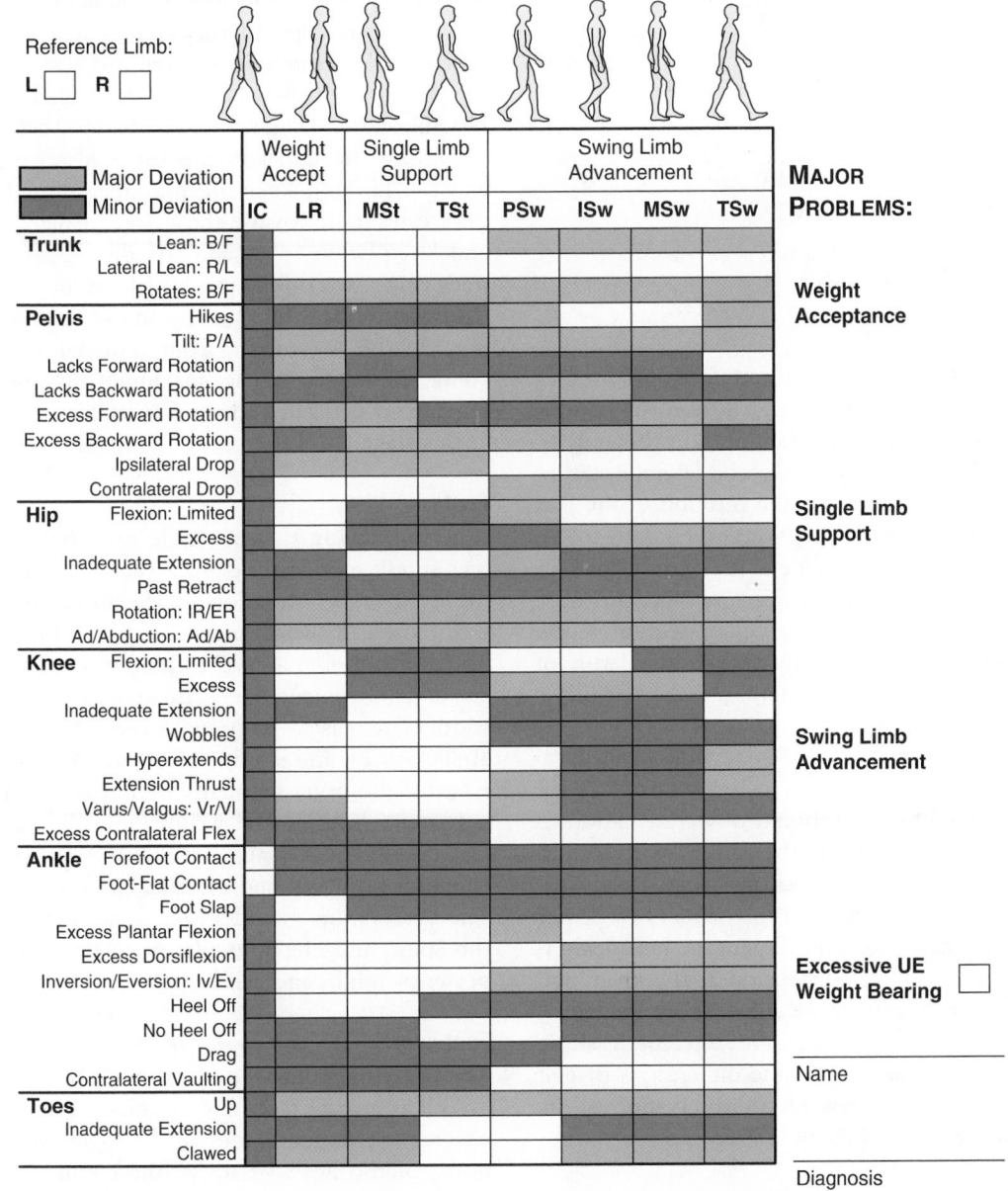

Gait Analysis: Full Body

Rancho Los Amigos Medical Center
Physical Therapy Department

Figure 14-13 **Gait analysis of the full body.** (Copyright 1996 LAREI, Rancho Los Amigos Medical Center, Downey, CA 90242; from the Pathokinesiology Service and the Physical Therapy Department, Rancho Los Amigos Medical Center: Observational Gait Analysis. Downey, CA, Los Amigos Research and Educational Institute, Inc., 1996, p. 64.)

is not affected. Major deviations imply that the mechanics of walking are affected adversely.[46]

Anterior View

When observing from the front as the patient walks, the examiner should note whether any lateral tilt of the pelvis occurs, whether there is any sideways swaying of the trunk, whether the pelvis rotates on a horizontal plane, whether the trunk and upper extremity rotate in the opposite direction to the pelvis, and whether reciprocal arm swing is present. Usually, the trunk and upper extremity rotation is approximately 180° out of phase with the pelvis—that is, as the pelvis and lower limb rotate one way, the trunk and upper limb rotate in the opposite direction. This action helps provide a balancing effect and smoothes the forward progression of the body. The examiner may also note movements at the hip (rotation and abduction-adduction), knee (rotation and

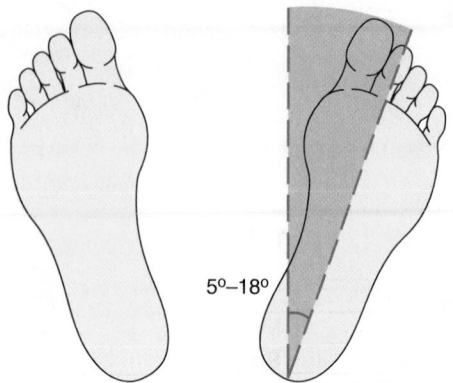

Figure 14-14　During stance and gait, the toes angle out 5° to 18° (Fick angle).

abduction-adduction), and ankle and foot (amount of toe-out and toe-in, dorsiflexion-plantar flexion, supination-pronation). The examiner should note any bowing of the femur or the tibia, any medial or lateral rotation of the hips, femur, or tibia, and the position of the feet as the patient goes through the gait cycle (Figure 14-14). This view is best used to examine the weight-loading period of the gait cycle. The examiner should also note whether there is any abduction or circumduction of the swing leg, whether there is atrophy of the musculature of the anterior thigh and leg, and whether the base width is normal.

Lateral View

From the side, the examiner should observe rotation of the shoulder and thorax during the gait cycle, as well as reciprocal arm swing. Spinal posture (e.g., lordosis), pelvic rotation, and movements in the joints of the lower limbs should be noted. These movements include flexion-extension at the hip, flexion-extension at the knee, and dorsiflexion-plantar flexion at the ankle. From the lateral aspect, the examiner may also observe step length, stride length, cadence, and the other time dimensions of gait (see Figure 14-6).[36] This view allows observation of the interactions between the walking surface and the various body parts.

The examiner must remember that there may be some compensation by the lumbar spine for limitation of movement in the hip. The patient should be observed to determine whether there is sufficient knee extension at initial contact, followed almost immediately by slight flexion until the foot makes contact with the floor; whether there is control of the slightly flexed knee during load response and midstance; and whether there is sufficient flexion during preswing and initial swing. Also, any hyperextension of the knee during the gait cycle should be noted. Finally, the examiner should note whether there is coordination of movement among the hip, knee, and ankle; even or uneven gait length; and even or uneven duration of steps.

As the patient moves from initial contact to loading response, the foot flexes immediately, and the knee flexes until the foot is flat on the floor. During this period, the hip is also flexed. During midstance, the ankle dorsiflexes as the body pivots in an arc over the stationary foot. At the same time, the hip and knee extend, lengthening the leg. As the patient moves from terminal stance to preswing, the ankle plantar flexes to raise the heel, and the hip and knee flex as the weight is transferred to the opposite leg.

During the initial swing, the ankle is plantar flexed, and the hip and knee are maximally flexed. As the leg progresses to midswing, the ankle dorsiflexes, and the hip and knee begin to extend. As the patient moves from midswing to terminal swing, the ankle remains in the neutral position while the hip and knee continue extending. As the leg moves from terminal swing to initial contact, the knee reaches maximum extension; the ankle remains in neutral, and no further hip extension occurs at this stage.

Posterior View

When observing the gait cycle from behind, the examiner should notice the same structures that were viewed from the front. Rotation of the shoulders and thorax, reciprocal arm swing, and pelvic list and rotation may be noted posteriorly, as well as hip, knee, ankle, and subtalar joint movement. Heel rise and base of support (base width) are easier to view posteriorly. Any abnormal abduction or adduction movements or lateral displacement of the body segments should be noted. This view is best to examine the weight-unloading period of the gait cycle. The examiner can note whether heel rise is equal for both feet and whether the heels turn in or out. The observation should also include lateral movement of the spine and the musculature of the back, buttocks, posterior thigh, and calf.

Footwear

The patient should be asked to walk in normal footwear as well as in bare feet. The examiner should take time to observe the patient's footwear and observe any wearing down of the heels or socks, the condition of the shoe uppers, creases, and so on. The feet should also be examined for callus formations, blisters, corns, and bunions. Different shoes can modify a patient's gait and the amount of energy necessary to perform gait. For example, high-heeled shoes alter movement, especially at the knee and ankle, which in turn increases the vertical loading.[47]

EXAMINATION

Most gait assessment involves observation. However, the examiner should take time, especially if he or she notices altered gait, to measure muscle strength (active and resisted movement) and range of movement (active and passive movement) at each joint involved in the gait cycle.

The parameters of gait (see normal parameters of gait) may also be measured to see if there are differences between the left and right gait cycles.[48,49] Leg length discrepancies (see Chapter 11 for leg length measurement) may also affect gait. Children tend to have better compensation mechanisms for leg length discrepancies than do adults.[50] Table 9-7 gives functional causes of leg length differences. Tables 11-10, 12-2, and 13-3 outline malalignments that may also affect gait.

Locomotion Scores

In addition to the detailed assessment of gait, locomotion scales or grading systems have been developed that include subjective and objective scores, which are combined for a total score. Figure 14-15 is a locomotion scoring scale that was developed for rheumatoid arthritis.[51] Figure 14-16 shows the modified Gait Abnormality Scale (GARS-M)

for elderly people who may be at high risk to falling.[52-54] In addition to including all aspects of locomotion, it gives an overall estimation of functional disability for patients with rheumatoid arthritis. Wolf and associates reported on the Emory Functional Ambulation Profile and established its reliability and validity.[55,56] The profile measures different tasks and surfaces for stroke patients and can differentiate between those suffering from a stroke and normals. The profile does time trials and measures such things as a 5-meter (16.4 feet) walk on bare floor and carpeted floor, an "up and go" task, negotiating an obstacle course, and stair climbing. The **Walking Safety Scale** (Grille d'évaluation de la sécurité à la marche [GEM]) is a scale developed to measure walking ability and safety.[16,57] It is a functional scale divided into basic level (walking short distances in different directions), advanced level (walking and doing other activities or walking on different surfaces), and outdoor activities, and can test patients with

---

Detailed and Total Locomotion Score in Chronic Arthritis

UPPER EXTREMITIES

A.   Subjective score (max. 100 points)

1. **Pain (max. 33 points)**
   33 None at ordinary activity ___
   25 Mild, inconstant, unilaterally, not interfering with normal activity
   17 Mild bilateral or moderate unilateral, constant use of analgesics
   10 Moderate pain despite large doses of analgesics, affecting activity
   5   Severe pain despite large doses of analgesics, affecting activity
   0   Severe bilateral, unable to work and use walking supports, prevents physical activity

2–4. **Pain score reduction** ___
   – 10% Unilateral hand pain
   – 25% Bilateral hand pain
   – 25% Severe pain from both lower extremities or neck
   Sum: ___

ABILITY (max. 67 points)

Degree of disability

General (max. 20 points)	None	Mild	Moderate	Severe or unable	
5–6. Manage work, household routines, shopping, child care (min. 3 of 4)	8☐	6☐	3☐	0☐	R 5 / L 6
7–8. ADL (home and kitchen chore, personal care, dressing, etc.)	7☐	5☐	2☐	0☐	R 7 / L 8
9–10. Drive a car or use public transportation	5☐		2☐	0☐	R 9 / L 10

Special (max. 47 points)					
11–12. Feeding (hold knife, cup, open milk pack)	10☐	7☐	4☐	0☐	R 11 / L 12
13–14. Carry 3 kg burden	5☐		2☐	0☐	R 13 / L 14
15–18. Use telephone	5☐		2☐	0☐	R 15 / L 16
17–18. Comb hair, brush teeth, shave	5☐		2☐	0☐	R 17 / L 18
19–20. Wash the axillas	5☐		2☐	0☐	R 19 / L 20
21–22. Reach things over shoulder level	5☐		2☐	0☐	R 21 / L 22
23–24. Use of walking support(s)	12☐	7☐	4☐	0☐	R 23 / L 24

Sum: right ___ left ___ Both (R/2 + L/2) ___

SUBJECTIVE SCORE: (pain: ___, ability: ___) _____

B.   Objective score—physical signs (max. 100 points)

		Right	Left
Shoulder (max. 35 points)			
25–26. Flexion:	>90° = 10p, 45-90° = 5 p, <45° = 0p	☐25	☐26
27–28. Extension:	>20° = 5p, 0-20° = 3p, 0° = 0p	☐27	☐28
29–30. Abduction:	>90° = 10p, 45-90° = 5p, <45° = 0p	☐29	☐30
31–32. Medial rot.:	>15° = 5p, <15° = 0p	☐31	☐32
33–34. Lateral rot.:	>10° = 5p, <10° = 0p	☐33	☐34
Elbow (max. 35 points)			
35–36. Flexion (from 90°):	>120° = 10p, 100-120° = 7p, 90-100° = 4p, 0° = 0p	☐35	☐36
37–38. Extension defect:	0-30° = 10p, 30-60° = 7p, 60-90° = 4p, 90° = 0p	☐37	☐38
39–40. Deformity: none + stable = 5p, rigid deformity = 2p, laxid = 0p		☐39	☐40
41–42. Varus-valgus: <5° = 10p, 5-10° = 7p stressed varus-valgus >15° = 3p, >25° = 0p		☐41	☐42
Wrist (max. 15 points)			
43–44. Deformity (rigid, laxid): none = 15p, mild = 10p, moderate = 5p, severe = 0p		☐43	☐44
Hand (max. 15 points)			
45–46. Deformity (rigid, laxid): none = 15p, mild = 10p, moderate = 5p, severe = 0p		☐45	☐46

Sum: right ___ left ___ Both (R/2 + L/2) ___

OBJECTIVE SCORE: ___   SUBJ. + OBJ. SCORE: ☐ (a)
                                  (upper extremities)

Figure 14-15 Locomotion scoring scale. (Modified from Larsson SE, Jonsson B: Locomotion score in rheumatoid arthritis. Acta Orthop Scand 60:272, 1989. © Munksgaard International Publishers, Ltd., Copenhagen, Denmark.)

Continued

Detailed and Total Locomotion Score in Chronic Arthritis—(Cont'd)

LOWER EXTREMITIES

C. Subjective score (max. 100 points)

47. **Pain (max. 44 points)** ___
    44 None at ordinary activity
    40 Slight, occasional ache or awareness of pain, not influencing activity
    30 Mild bilateral or moderate unilateral, may take analgesics
    20 Moderate, affecting ordinary activities and work, consistent use of analgesics.
    10 Severe pain in spite of optimal medication
    0 Severe, preventing most of activity or patient bedridden

48–50. **Pain score reduction** ___
    −25% Moderate or severe pain from more than one ipsilateral joint
    −50% Moderate or severe pain from more than one contralateral joint
    −10% Severe pain from upper extremities or neck

                                            Sum: ___

    ABILITY (max. 56 points)

Walk (max. 36 points)

51.	Limp:	none = 12p, slight = 8p, moderate = 5p, severe = 0p	☐
52.	Support:	none = 12p, cane for long walks = 8p, cane most of time = 5p one crutch or can't use = 3p, two canes = 2p two crutches or can't walk = 0p	☐
53.	Distance:	unlimited = 12p, >400m = 8p, <400m = 5p indoors only = 2p, bed or chair = 0p	☐

Special (max. 20 points)

54.	Climb stairs:	without difficulty = 6p with difficulty or by using banister = 3p with great difficulty or unable = 0p	☐
55.	Shoes and socks:	without difficulty = 6p, with difficulty = 3p, unable = 0p	☐
56.	Sitting:	without difficulty = 6p, only short time or on high chair = 3p, unable to use any chair = 0p	☐

| 57. | Transportation: | can use public transportation = 2p, unable = 0p | ☐ |

Sum: pain: ___, ability: ___ (walk: ___, special: ___)

                            SUBJECTIVE SCORE: ___

D.   Objective score—physical signs (max. 100 points)

		Right	**Left**
Hip (max. 35 points)			
58–59. Flexion:	>90° = 10p, 60–90° = 5p, <60° = 0p	☐58	☐59
60–61. Extension defect:	0-10° = 10p, 10–30° = 5p, >30° = 0p	☐60	☐61
62–63. Abduction/adduction:	>10° = 10p, −10–10° = 5p, <−10° = 0p	☐62	☐63
64–65. Rotation:	>0° = 5p, 0° = 0p	☐64	☐65
Knee (max. 35 points)			
66–67. Flexion:	>100° = 10p, 80–100° = 8p, 60–80° = 5p	☐66	☐67
68–69. Extension defect:	0° = 10p, 0–10° = 8p, 10–20° = 5p 20-30° = 2p, >30° = 0p	☐68	☐69
70–71. Varus-valgus:	<7° = 10p, 7–15° = 8p stressed v/v 15–30° = 5p, >30° = 0p	☐70	☐71
72–73. Deformity:	none + stable = 5p, rigid = 2p, laxid = 0p	☐72	☐73
Ankle (max. 15 points)			
74–75. Deformity (rigid, laxid): none = 15p, mild = 10p, moderate = 5p, severe = 0p		☐74	☐75
Feet (max. 15 points)			
76–77. Deformity (rigid, laxid): None = 15p, mild = 10p, moderate = 5p, severe = 0p		☐76	☐77

        SUM: right: ___ left: ___ Both (R/2 + L/2): ___

OBJECTIVE SCORE: ___   **SUBJ. + OBJ. SCORE:** ☐ **(b)**
                                      (lower extremities)

                           TOTAL LOCOMOTION SCORE: (a + b) ___

Figure 14-15, cont'd

MODIFIED GAIT ABNORMALITY RATING SCALE (GARS-M)

NAME _____ NO. _____ VISIT _____ DATE _____

1. VARIABILITY – A MEASURE OF INCONSISTENCY AND ARRHYTHMICITY OF STEPPING AND OF ARM MOVEMENTS

    0 = fluid and predictably paced limb movements
    1 = occasional interruptions (changes in velocity), approximately 25% of time
    2 = unpredictability of rhythm approximately 25%–75% of time
    3 = random timing of limb movements

2. GUARDEDNESS – HESITANCY, SLOWNESS, DIMINISHED PROPULSION, AND LACK OF COMMITMENT IN STEPPING AND ARM SWING

    0 = good forward momentum and lack of apprehension in propulsion
    1 = center of gravity of head, arms, and trunk (HAT) projects only slightly in front of push-off, but still good arm-leg coordination
    2 = HAT held over anterior aspect of foot, and some moderate loss of smooth reciprocation
    3 = HAT held over rear aspect of stance-phase foot, and great tentativity in stepping

3. STAGGERING – SUDDEN AND UNEXPECTED LATERALLY DIRECTED PARTIAL LOSSES OF BALANCE

    0 = no losses of balance to side
    1 = a single lurch to side
    2 = two lurches to side
    3 = three or more lurches to side

4. FOOT CONTACT – THE DEGREE TO WHICH THE HEEL STRIKES THE GROUND BEFORE THE FOREFOOT

    0 = very obvious angle of impact of heel on ground
    1 = barely visible contact of heel before forefoot
    2 = entire foot lands flat on ground
    3 = anterior aspect of foot strikes ground before heel

5. HIP ROM – THE DEGREE OF LOSS OF HIP RANGE OF MOTION SEEN DURING A GAIT CYCLE

    0 = obvious angulation of thigh backward during double support (10 degrees)
    1 = just barely visible angulation backward from vertical
    2 = thigh in line with vertical projection from ground
    3 = thigh angled forward from vertical at maximum posterior excursion

6. SHOULDER EXTENSION – A MEASURE OF THE DECREASE OF SHOULDER ROM

    0 = clearly seen movement of upper arm anterior (15 degrees) and posterior (20 degrees) to vertical axis of trunk
    1 = shoulder flexes slightly anterior to vertical axis
    2 = shoulder comes only to vertical axis, or slightly posterior to it during flexion
    3 = shoulder stays well behind vertical axis during entire excursion

7. ARM-HEEL STRIKE SYNCHRONY – THE EXTENT TO WHICH THE CONTRALATERAL MOVEMENTS OF AN ARM AND LEG ARE OUT OF PHASE

    0 = good temporal conjunction of arm and contralateral leg at apex of shoulder and hip excursions all of the time
    1 = arm and leg slightly out of phase 25% of the time
    2 = arm and leg moderately out of phase 25%–50% of the time
    3 = little or no temporal coherence of arm and leg

ROM = range of motion.

Figure 14-16 Modified Gait Abnormality Rating Scale (GARS-M). (From Dutton M: Orthopedic examination, evaluation and intervention, New York, 2004, McGraw-Hill, p. 389.)

TABLE **14-5**

Walking Items for Each Sub-Scale of the Walking Safety Scale

Sub-Scale	Items
Sub-scale A: Basic level	A1: Stand up from a chair (or wheelchair) and walk 10 m A2: Walk 1 m, then turn 180° and walk 1 m A3: Walk 2 m and turn the head to the right A4: Walk 2 m and turn the head to the left AS: Walk 2 m and stop abruptly A6: Walk backward 1 m A7: Walk sideways 1 m to the right A8: Walk sideways 1 m to the left A9: Walk 1 m, make an S around 2 chairs, and walk 1 m A10: Walk 1 m and sit down on the chair (or wheelchair)
Sub-scale B: Advanced level	B1: Walk 1 m and then sit on a chair without armrests B2: Get up from a chair without armrests and walk 1 m B3: Walk 1 m, go over a doorsill, and then walk 1 m B4: Walk 1 m, pick up a shoe, and walk 1 m B5: Walk 1 m and open then close a door B6: On carpet, walk 5 m B7: On carpet, walk 1 m then turn 180° and walk 1 m B8: On carpet, walk backward 1 m B9: On carpet, walk 1 m sideways to the right B10: On carpet, walk 1 m sideways to the left B11: On carpet, walk 1 m, make an S around 2 chairs, and walk 1 m B12: Walk 1 m, climb stairs, and walk 1 m B13: Walk 1 m, descend stairs, and walk 1 m
Sub-scale C: Pre-test for outdoor walking	Cl: Walk 1 m and step up onto a platform 15 cm high C2: Step down from a platform 15 cm high and walk 1 m C3: On mat, walk 2 m C4: On mat, walk 1 m then turn 180° and walk 1 m C5: On mat, walk 1 m and stop abruptly C6: On mat, walk backward 1 m C7: Walk 3 m up an incline C8: Walk 3 m down an incline C9: Walk 1 m, climb stairs, and walk 1 m C10: Walk 1 m, descend stairs, and walk 1 m

From Kaegi C, et al: Development of a walking safety scale for older adults. Part 1: content validity of the GEM scale. Physiother Can 60:264–273, 2008.

walking aids. It is a scale that has patient input (perception and safety) and examiner (rater) input. Table 14-5 shows the walking items for each subscale. The **modified Gait Efficacy Scale (mGES)** (Figure 14-17) was designed to measure walking confidence in older adults during everyday activities.[58] Other functional tests include the **Get Up and Go Test,**[59] the **Functional Ambulatory Classification Scale,**[60,61] **Figure-of-8 Walk Test,**[62] **Functional Gait Assessment,**[63] and the **Performance Oriented Balance and Mobility Assessment (POMA).**[64]

Compensatory Mechanisms

The examiner must try to determine the primary cause of gait faults and the compensatory factors used to maintain an energy-saving gait. The patient tries to use the most energy-saving gait possible.[65] Speed of walking can also

modify many of the normal parameters of gait.[66] Therefore, not only the gait pattern but also the speed of the activity and its effects must be noted. This type of assessment allows the examiner to set appropriate goals and plan a logical approach to treatment.

ABNORMAL GAIT

Gait deviations can occur for three reasons. First, they may occur because of pathology or injury in the specific joint (Table 14-6). Second, they may occur as compensations for injury or pathology in other joints on the same or ipsilateral side. Finally, they may occur as compensations for injury or pathology on the opposite or contralateral limb (Table 14-7).[17] Some of the more common gait abnormalities are discussed next, but this list is by no means inclusive.

The Modified Gait Efficacy Scale (mGES)

1. How much confidence do you have that you would be able to safely walk on a level surface such as a hardwood floor?

1	2	3	4	5	6	7	8	9	10

No Confidence   Complete Confidence

2. How much confidence do you have that you would be able to safely walk on grass?

1	2	3	4	5	6	7	8	9	10

No Confidence   Complete Confidence

3. How much confidence do you have that you would be able to safely walk over an obstacle in your path?

1	2	3	4	5	6	7	8	9	10

No Confidence   Complete Confidence

4. How much confidence do you have that you would be able to safely step down from a curb?

1	2	3	4	5	6	7	8	9	10

No Confidence   Complete Confidence

5. How much confidence do you have that you would be able to safely step up onto a curb?

1	2	3	4	5	6	7	8	9	10

No Confidence   Complete Confidence

6. How much confidence do you have that you would be able to safely walk up stairs if you are holding on to a railing?

1	2	3	4	5	6	7	8	9	10

No Confidence   Complete Confidence

7. How much confidence do you have that you would be able to safely walk down stairs if you are holding on to a railing?

1	2	3	4	5	6	7	8	9	10

No Confidence   Complete Confidence

8. How much confidence do you have that you would be able to safely walk up stairs if you are NOT holding on to a railing?

1	2	3	4	5	6	7	8	9	10

No Confidence   Complete Confidence

9. How much confidence do you have that you would be able to safely walk down stairs if you are NOT holding on to a railing?

1	2	3	4	5	6	7	8	9	10

No Confidence   Complete Confidence

10. How much confidence do you have that you would be able to safely walk a long distance such as ½ mile?

1	2	3	4	5	6	7	8	9	10

No Confidence   Complete Confidence

Figure 14-17 Modified Gait Efficacy Scale (mGES). (From Newell AM, et al: The modified gait efficacy scale: establishing the psychometric properties in older adults. Physical Therapy 92:327–328, 2012.)

TABLE **14-6**

Gait Deviations Secondary to Specific Impairments[*†]

Gait Deviations at the Hip/Pelvis/Trunk Secondary to Specific Hip/Pelvis/Trunk Impairments

Observed Gait Deviation at the Hip/Pelvis/Trunk	Likely Impairment	Selected Pathologic Precursors	Mechanical Rationale and/or Associated Compensations
Backward trunk lean during **loading response**	Weak hip extensors	Paralysis of poliomyelitis	This action moves the line of gravity of the trunk behind the hip and reduces the need for hip extension torque
Lateral trunk lean toward the **stance** leg; since this movement compensates for a weakness, it is often called "compensated" Trendelenburg gait and is referred to as a waddling gait if bilateral	Marked weakness of the hip abductors	Guillain-Barré or poliomyelitis	Shifting the trunk over the supporting limb reduces the demand on the hip abductors
	Hip pain	Arthritis	Shifting the trunk over the supporting lower extremity reduces compressive joint forces associated with the action of hip abductors
Excessive downward drop of the contralateral pelvis during **stance** (referred to as positive Trendelenburg sign if present during single-limb standing)	Mild weakness of the gluteus medius of the stance leg	Guillain-Barré or poliomyelitis	Although the Trendelenburg sign may be seen in single-limb standing, a compensated Trendelenburg gait is often seen in severe weakness of the hip abductors
Forward bending of the trunk during **mid and terminal stance**, as the hip is moved over the foot	Hip flexion contracture	Hip osteoarthritis	Forward trunk lean is used to compensate for lack of hip extension; an alternate adaptation could be excessive lumbar lordosis
	Hip pain	Hip osteoarthritis	Keeping the hip at 30° of flexion minimizes intraarticular pressure
Excessive lumbar lordosis in **terminal stance**	Hip flexion contracture	Arthritis	Lack of hip extension in terminal stance is compensated for by increased lordosis
Trunk lurches backward and toward the unaffected stance leg from **heel off to mid swing**	Hip flexor weakness	L2–L3 nerve compression	Hip flexion is passively generated by a backward movement of the trunk
Posterior tilt of the pelvis during **initial swing**	Hip flexor weakness	L2–L3 nerve compression	Abdominals are used during initial swing to advance the swing leg
Hip circumduction: semicircle movement of the hip during **swing**—combining hip flexion, hip abduction and forward rotation of the pelvis	Hip flexor weakness	L2–L3 nerve compression	Semicircular movement combining hip flexion, hip abduction, and forward rotation of the pelvis

TABLE **14-6**

Gait Deviations Secondary to Specific Impairments—cont'd

Gait Deviations at the Knee Secondary to Specific Knee Impairments

Observed Gait Deviation at the Knee	Likely Impairment	Selected Pathologic Precursors	Mechanical Rationale and/or Associated Compensations
Rapid extension of the knee (knee extensor thrust) immediately after **initial contact**	Spasticity of the quadriceps	Upper motor neuron lesion	Depending on the status of the posterior structures of the knee, may occur with or without knee hyperextension
Knee remains extended during the **loading response,** but there is no extensor thrust	Weak quadriceps	Femoral nerve palsy, L3–L4 compression neuropathy	Knee remains fully extended throughout stance; an associated anterior trunk lean in the early part of stance moves the line of gravity of the trunk, slightly anterior to the axis of rotation of the knee; this keeps the knee extended without action of the knee extensors; this gait deviation may lead to an excessive stretching of the posterior capsule of the knee and eventual knee hyperextension (genu recurvatum) during stance
	Knee pain	Arthritis	Knee is kept in extension to reduce the need for quadriceps activity and associated compressive forces; it may be accompanied by an antalgic gait pattern characterized by a reduced stance time and shorter step length
Genu recurvatum (hyperextension) during **stance**	Knee extensor weakness (see the two previously described gait deviations above)	Poliomyelitis	Secondary to progressive stretching of the posterior capsule of the knee
Varus thrust during **stance**	Laxity of the posterior and lateral ligamentous joint structures of the knee	Traumatic injury or progressive laxity	Rapid varus deviation of the knee during midstance, typically accompanied by knee hyperextension
Flexed position of the knee during **stance** and lack of knee extension in **terminal swing**	Knee flexion contracture > 10° (genu flexum) Hamstring overactivity (spasticity)	Upper motor neuron lesion	Associated increase in hip flexion and ankle dorsiflexion during stance
	Knee pain and joint effusion	Trauma or arthritis	Knee is kept in flexion since this is the position of lowest intraarticular pressure
Reduced or absent knee flexion during **swing**	Spasticity of knee extensors Knee extension contracture	Upper motor neuron lesion Immobilization (cast, brace) or surgical fusion	Compensatory hip hiking and/or hip circumduction could be noted

Continued

TABLE **14-6**

Gait Deviations Secondary to Specific Impairments—cont'd

Gait Deviations at the Ankle/Foot Secondary to Specific Ankle/Foot Impairments

Observed Gait Deviation at the Ankle/Foot	Likely Impairment	Selected Pathologic Precursors	Mechanical Rationale and/or Associated Compensations
"Foot slap": rapid ankle plantar flexion occurs following **heel contact;** the name foot slap is derived from the characteristic noise made by the forefoot hitting the ground	Mild weakness of ankle dorsiflexors	Common peroneal nerve palsy and distal peripheral neuropathy	Ankle dorsiflexors have sufficient strength to dorsiflex the ankle during swing but not enough to control ankle plantar flexion after heel contact; no other gait deviations
"Foot flat": Entire plantar aspect of the foot touches the ground at **initial contact,**‡ followed by normal, passive ankle dorsiflexion during the rest of stance	Marked weakness of ankle dorsiflexors	Common peroneal nerve palsy and distal peripheral neuropathy	Sufficient strength of the dorsiflexors to partially, but not completely, dorsiflex the ankle during swing; normal dorsiflexion occurs during stance as long as the ankle has normal ROM; no other gait deviations
Initial contact with the ground is made by the forefoot followed by the heel region; normal passive ankle dorsiflexion occurs during stance	Severe weakness of ankle dorsiflexors	Common peroneal nerve palsy and distal peripheral neuropathy	No active ankle dorsiflexion is possible during swing; normal dorsiflexion occurs during stance as long as the ankle has normal ROM; likely requires excessive knee and hip flexion during swing to avoid catching toes on the ground
Initial contact is made with the forefoot, but the heel never makes contact with the ground during stance	Heel pain Plantar flexion contracture (pes equinus deformity) or spasticity of ankle plantar flexors	Calcaneal fracture, plantar fasciitis Upper motor neuron lesion/cerebral palsy, CVA	Purposeful strategy to avoid weight bearing on the heel To maintain the weight over the foot, the knee and hip are kept in flexion throughout stance, leading to a "crouched gait"; requires short steps
Initial contact is made with the forefoot, and the heel is brought to the ground by a posterior displacement of the tibia **at midstance**	Plantar flexion contracture (pes equinus deformity) or spasticity of ankle plantar flexors	Upper motor neuron lesion (cerebral palsy, CVA) Ankle fusion in a plantar flexed position	Knee hyperextension occurs during stance owing to the inability of the tibia to move forward over the foot; hip flexion and excessive forward trunk lean during terminal stance occur to shift the weight of the body over the foot
Premature elevation of the heel in **midstance or terminal stance**	Lack of ankle dorsiflexion	Congenital or acquired muscular tightness of ankle plantar flexors	Characteristic bouncing gait pattern

TABLE **14-6**

Gait Deviations Secondary to Specific Impairments—cont'd

Gait Deviations at the Ankle/Foot Secondary to Specific Ankle/Foot Impairments

Observed Gait Deviation at the Ankle/Foot	Likely Impairment	Selected Pathologic Precursors	Mechanical Rationale and/or Associated Compensations
Heel remains in contact with the ground late in **terminal stance**	Weakness or flaccid paralysis of plantar flexors with or without a fixed dorsiflexed position of the ankle (pes calcaneus deformity)	Peripheral or central nervous system disorders Excessive surgical lengthening of the Achilles tendon	Excessive ankle dorsiflexion results in prolonged heel contact, reduced push off, and a shorter step length
Supinated foot position and weight bearing on the lateral aspect of the foot during **stance**	Pes cavus deformity	Congenital structural deformity	A high medial longitudinal arch is noted with reduced midfoot mobility throughout swing and stance
Excessive foot pronation occurs during **stance** with failure of the foot to supinate in mid stance; normal medial longitudinal arch noted during swing	Rearfoot varus and/or forefoot varus	Congenital or acquired structural deformity	Excessive foot pronation and associated flattening of the medial longitudinal arch may be accompanied by a general medial rotation of the lower extremity during stance
Excessive foot pronation with weight bearing on the medial portion of the foot during **stance;** the medial longitudinal arch remains absent during **swing**	Weakness (paralysis) of ankle invertors Pes planus deformity	Upper motor neuron lesion Congenital structural deformity	An overall excessive medial rotation of the lower extremity during stance is possible
Excessive inversion and plantar flexion of the foot and ankle occur during **swing** and at **initial contact**	Pes equinovarus due to spasticity of the plantar flexors and invertors	Upper motor neuron lesion (cerebral palsy, CVA)	Contact with the ground is made with the lateral border of the forefoot; weight-bearing on the lateral border of the foot during stance
Ankle remains plantar flexed during **swing** and can be associated with dragging of the toes, typically called *drop foot*	Weakness of dorsiflexors and/or pes equinus deformity	Common peroneal nerve palsy	Hip hiking, hip circumduction, or excessive hip and knee flexion of the swing leg or vaulting of the stance leg may be noted to lift the toes off the ground and prevent the toes from dragging during swing

From Simoneau GG: Kinesiology of walking. In Neumann DA, editor: Kinesiology of the musculoskeletal system—foundations of physical rehabilitation, ed 2, St Louis, 2010, Mosby, pp. 665, 666, 668.
CVA, Cerebrovascular accident; *ROM,* range of motion.
*An impairment is a loss or an abnormality in physiologic, psychologic, or anatomic structure or function.
†Note: Terms in **boldface** indicate when in the gait cycle the gait deviation is expressed.
‡Initial contact is often used instead of heel contact to reflect the fact that with many gait deviations the heel is not the section of the foot that makes initial contact with the ground.

TABLE **14-7**

Gait Deviations as a Compensation for a Lower Extremity Impairment*

Gait Deviations Seen at the Hip/Pelvis/Trunk as a Compensation for an Impairment of the Ipsilateral Ankle, Ipsilateral Knee, or Contralateral Lower Extremity

Observed Gait Deviation at the Hip/Pelvis/Trunk	Likely Impairment	Mechanical Rationale
Forward bending of the trunk during the **loading response**	Weak quadriceps	Trunk is brought forward to move the line of gravity anterior to the axis of rotation of the knee, thereby reducing the need for knee extensors
Forward bending of the trunk during **mid and terminal stance**	Pes equinus deformity	Lack of ankle dorsiflexion during stance results in knee hyperextension and forward trunk lean to move the weight of the body over the stance foot
Excessive hip and knee flexion during **swing**	Often due to lack of ankle dorsiflexion of the swing leg; may also be due to a functionally or anatomically short contralateral stance leg	Used to clear the toes of the swing leg
Hip circumduction during **swing**	Lack of shortening of the swing leg secondary to reduced hip flexion, reduced knee flexion, and/or lack of ankle dorsiflexion	Used to lift the foot of the swing leg off the ground and provide toe clearance
Hip hiking (elevation of the ipsilateral pelvis during **swing**)	Lack of shortening of the swing leg secondary to reduced hip flexion, reduced knee flexion, and/or lack of ankle dorsiflexion Functionally or anatomically short stance leg	Used to lift the foot of the swing leg off the ground and provide toe clearance
Excessive backward horizontal rotation of the pelvis on the side of the stance leg in **terminal stance**	Ankle plantar flexor weakness	Ankle plantar flexor weakness leads to prolonged heel contact and lack of push off; an increased pelvic horizontal rotation is used to lengthen the limb and maintain adequate step length

Gait Deviations Seen at the Knee as a Compensation for an Impairment of the Ipsilateral Ankle, Ipsilateral Hip, or Contralateral Lower Extremity

Observed Gait Deviation at the Knee	Likely Impairment	Mechanical Rationale
Knee is kept in flexion during **stance** despite the knee having normal ROM on examination	Impairments at the ankle or the hip, including a pes calcaneus deformity, plantar flexor weakness, and hip flexion contracture	Exaggerated ankle dorsiflexion or hip flexion during stance forces the knee in a flexed position; the contralateral (healthy) swing leg shows exaggerated hip and knee flexion to clear the toes owing to the functionally shorter stance leg
Hyperextension of the knee (genu recurvatum) from **initial contact to pre swing**	Ankle plantar flexion contracture (pes equinus deformity) or spasticity of ankle plantar flexors	Knee must hyperextend to compensate for the lack of forward displacement of the tibia during midstance
Antalgic gait	Painful stance leg	This is characterized by a shorter step length and stance time on the side of the painful lower extremity; it may be accompanied by ipsilateral trunk lean, if hip pain, contralateral trunk lean occurs with knee and foot pain
Excessive knee flexion in **swing**	Lack of ankle dorsiflexion of the swing leg or a short stance leg	Strategy to increase toe clearance of the swing leg and is typically accompanied by increased hip flexion

TABLE **14-7**

Gait Deviations as a Compensation for a Lower Extremity Impairment—cont'd

Gait Deviations Seen at the Ankle and Foot as a Compensation for an Impairment of the Ipsilateral Ankle, Ipsilateral Hip, or Contralateral Lower Extremity

Observed Gait Deviation at the Ankle/Foot	Likely Impairment	Mechanical Rationale
Vaulting: compensatory mechanism demonstrated by exaggerated ankle plantar flexion during **midstance;** leads to excessive vertical movement of the body	Any impairment of the contralateral lower extremity that reduces hip flexion, knee flexion, or ankle dorsiflexion during swing	Strategy used to allow the foot of a functionally long, contralateral lower extremity to clear the ground during swing
Excessive foot angle during **stance** that is called *toeing-out*	Retroversion of the neck of the femur or tight hip lateral rotators	Foot is in excessive toeing-out due to excessive lateral rotation of the lower extremity
Reduction of the normal foot ankle during **stance** that is called *toeing-in*	Excessive femoral anteversion or spasticity of the hip adductors and/or hip medial rotators	General medial rotation of the lower extremity

From Simoneau GG: Kinesiology of walking. In Neumann DA: Kinesiology of the musculoskeletal system—foundations of physical rehabilitation, ed 2, St Louis, 2010, Mosby, pp. 665–670.
ROM, Range of motion.
*Note: Terms in boldface indicate when in the gait cycle the gait deviation is expressed.

Antalgic (Painful) Gait

The antalgic or painful gait is self-protective and is the result of injury to the pelvis, hip, knee, ankle, or foot. The stance phase on the affected leg is shorter than that on the nonaffected leg, because the patient attempts to remove weight from the affected leg as quickly as possible; therefore, the amount of time on each leg should be noted. The swing phase of the uninvolved leg is decreased. The result is a shorter step length on the uninvolved side, decreased walking velocity, and decreased cadence.[36] In addition, the painful region is often supported by one hand, if it is within reach, and the other arm, acting as a counterbalance, is outstretched. If a painful hip is causing the problem, the patient also shifts the body weight over the painful hip. This shift decreases the pull of the abductor muscles, which decreases the pressure on the femoral head from more than two times the body weight to approximately body weight, owing to vertical instead of angular placement of the load over the hip. Flynn and Widmann have outlined some of the causes of a painful limp in children[67] (Table 14-8).

Arthrogenic (Stiff Hip or Knee) Gait

The arthrogenic gait results from stiffness, laxity, or deformity, and it may be painful or pain free. If the knee or hip is fused or the knee has recently been removed from a cylinder cast, the pelvis must be elevated by exaggerated plantar flexion of the opposite ankle and circumduction of the stiff leg (**circumducted gait**) to provide

toe clearance. The patient with this gait lifts the entire leg higher than normal to clear the ground because of a stiff hip or knee (Figure 14-18). The arc of movement helps to decrease the elevation needed to clear the affected leg. Because of the loss of flexibility in the hip, knee, or both, the gait lengths are different for the two legs. When the stiff limb is bearing weight, the gait length is usually smaller.

Ataxic Gait

If the patient has poor sensation or lacks muscle coordination, there is a tendency toward poor balance and a broad base (Figure 14-19). The gait of a person with cerebellar ataxia includes a lurch or stagger, and all movements are exaggerated. The feet of an individual with sensory ataxia slap the ground, because they cannot be felt. The patient also watches the feet while walking. The resulting gait is irregular, jerky, and weaving.

Contracture Gaits

Joints of the lower limb may exhibit contracture if immobilization has been prolonged or pathology to the joint has not been properly cared for. Hip flexion contracture often results in increased lumbar lordosis and extension of the trunk combined with knee flexion to get the foot on the ground. With a knee flexion contracture, the patient demonstrates excessive ankle dorsiflexion from late swing phase to early stance phase on the uninvolved

TABLE **14-8**

Differential Diagnosis of Antalgic Gait

Less than 4 Years	4 to 10 Years	More than 10 Years
• Toddler's fracture (tibia or foot) • Osteomyelitis, septic arthritis, discitis • Arthritis (juvenile rheumatoid arthritis, Lyme disease) • Discoid lateral meniscus • Foreign body in the foot • Benign or malignant tumor	• Fracture (especially physeal) • Osteomyelitis, septic arthritis, discitis • Legg-Calvé-Perthes disease • Transient synovitis • Osteochondritis dissecans (knee or ankle) • Discoid lateral meniscus • Sever apophysitis (calcaneus) • Accessory tarsal navicular • Foreign body in the foot • Arthritis (junveile rheumatoid arthritis, Lyme disease) • Benign or malignant tumor	• Stress fracture (femur, tibia, foot, pars interarticularis) • Osteomyelitis, septic arthritis, discitis • Slipped capital femoral epiphysis • Osgood-Schlatter disease or Sinding-Larsen-Johanssen syndrome • Osteochondritis dissecans (knee or ankle) • Chondromalacia patellae • Arthritis (Lyme disease, gonococcal) • Accessory tarsal navicular • Tarsal coalition • Benign or malignant tumor

© 2001 American Academy of Orthopaedic Surgeons. Reprinted from the Journal of the American Academy of Orthopaedic Surgeons, vol 9(2), pp. 89–98.

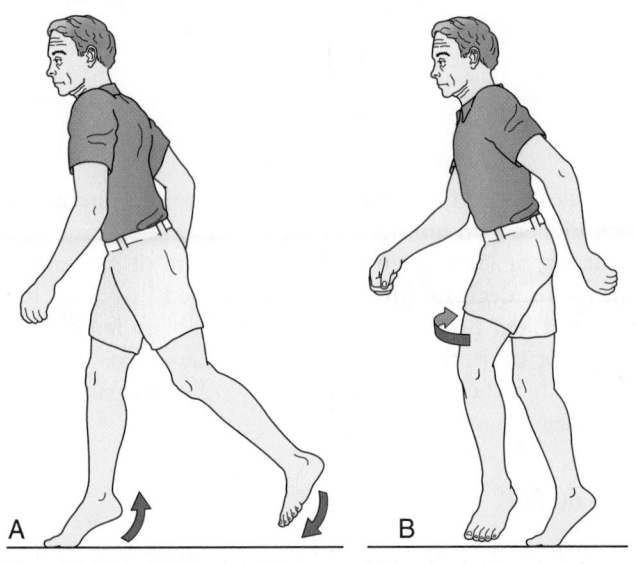

Figure 14-18 Arthrogenic (stiff knee or hip) gait. A, Excessive plantar flexion. **B,** Circumduction.

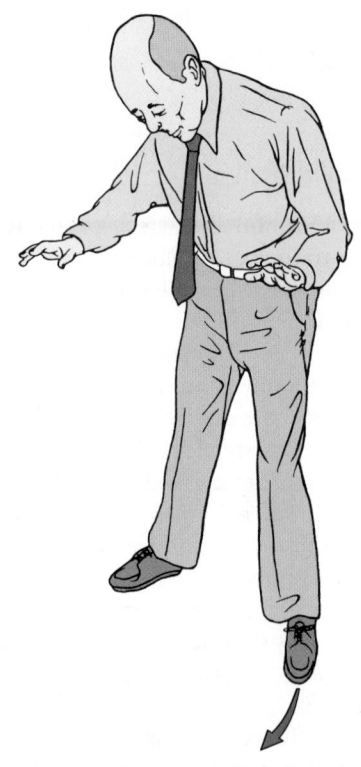

Figure 14-19 Ataxic gait. (Redrawn from Judge RD. Zuidema GD, Fitzgerald FT: Clinical diagnosis: a physiological approach, Boston, 1982, Little, Brown, p. 438.)

leg and early heel rise on the involved side in terminal stance. Plantar flexion contracture at the ankle results in knee hyperextension (midstance of affected leg) and forward bending of the trunk with hip flexion (midstance to terminal stance of affected leg). Heel rise on the affected leg also occurs earlier.[36]

Equinus Gait (Toe Walking)

This childhood gait is seen with talipes equinovarus (club foot) (Table 14-9). Weight-bearing is primarily on the dorsolateral or lateral edge of the foot, depending on the degree of deformity. The weight-bearing phase on the affected limb is decreased, and a limp is present. The

pelvis and femur are laterally rotated to partially compensate for tibial and foot medial rotation.[2]

Gluteus Maximus Gait

If the gluteus maximus muscle, which is a primary hip extensor, is weak, the patient thrusts the thorax

TABLE **14-9**

Differential Diagnosis of a Nonantalgic Limp

Equinus Gait (Toe-Walking)	Trendelenburg Gait	Circumduction Gait/Vaulting Gait	Steppage Gait
• Idiopathic tight Achilles tendon • Clubfoot (residual or untreated) • Cerebral palsy • Limb-length discrepancy	• Legg-Calvé-Perthes disease • Developmental dysplasia of the hip • Slipped capital femoral epiphysis • Muscular dystrophy • Hemiplegic cerebral palsy • Weak gluteus medius	• Limb-length discrepancy • Cerebral palsy • Any cause of ankle or knee stiffness	• Cerebral palsy • Myelodysplasia • Charcot-Marie-Tooth disease • Friedreich ataxia • Tibial nerve palsy

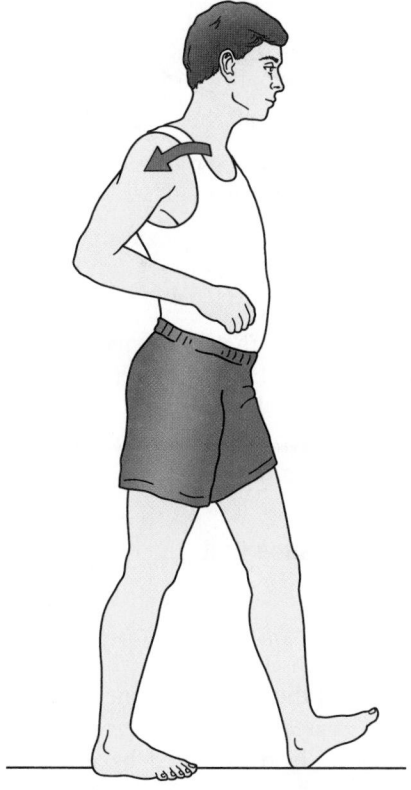

Figure 14-20 Gluteus maximus gait.

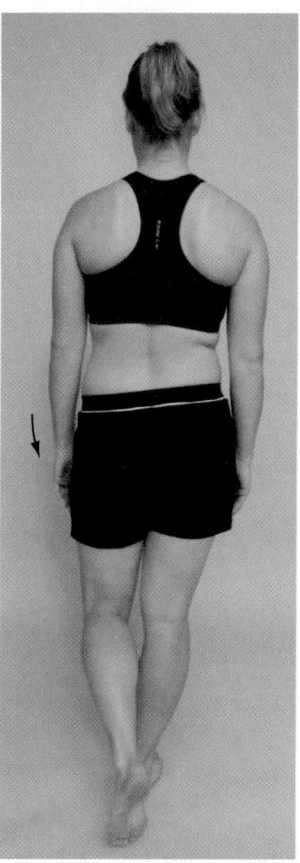

Figure 14-21 Gluteus medius (Trendelenburg) gait.

posteriorly at initial contact (heel strike) to maintain hip extension of the stance leg. The resulting gait involves a characteristic backward lurch of the trunk (Figure 14-20).

Gluteus Medius (Trendelenburg) Gait

If the hip abductor muscles (gluteus medius and minimus) are weak, the stabilizing effect of these muscles during stance phase is lost, and the patient exhibits an excessive lateral list in which the thorax is thrust laterally to keep the center of gravity over the stance leg (Figure 14-21). A positive Trendelenburg sign is also exhibited (i.e., the contralateral side droops because the ipsilateral hip

abductors do not stabilize or prevent the droop). If there is bilateral weakness of the gluteus medius muscles, the gait shows accentuated side-to-side movement, resulting in a wobbling gait or "chorus girl swing." This gait may also be seen in patients with congenital dislocation of the hip and coxa vara (see Table 14-9).

Hemiplegic or Hemiparetic Gait

The patient with hemiplegic or hemiparetic gait swings the paraplegic leg outward and ahead in a circle

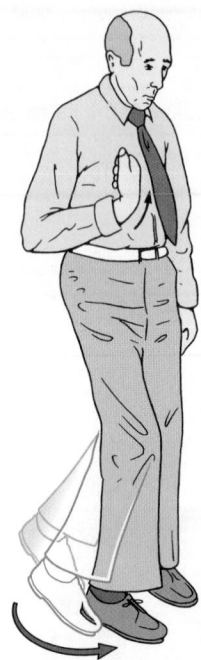

Figure 14-22 Hemiplegic (hemiparetic) gait. (Redrawn from Judge RD, Zuidema GD, Fitzgerald FT: Clinical diagnosis: a physiological approach, Boston, 1982, Little, Brown, p. 438.)

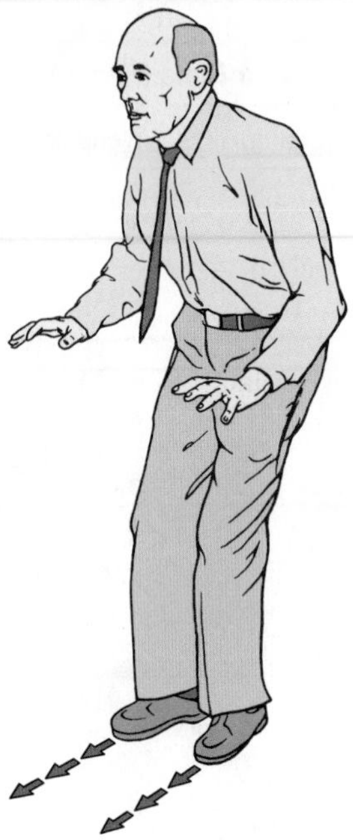

Figure 14-23 Parkinsonian gait. (Redrawn from Judge RD, Zuidema GD, Fitzgerald FT: Clinical diagnosis: a physiological approach, Boston, 1982, Little, Brown, p. 496.)

(circumduction) or pushes it ahead (Figure 14-22). In addition, the affected upper limb is carried across the trunk for balance. This is sometimes referred to as a **neurogenic** or **flaccid gait.**

Parkinsonian Gait

The neck, trunk, and knees of a patient with parkinsonian gait are flexed. The gait is characterized by shuffling or short rapid steps (marche à petits pas) at times. The arms are held stiffly and do not have their normal associative movement (Figure 14-23). During the gait, the patient may lean forward and walk progressively faster as though unable to stop (**festination**).[68]

Plantar Flexor Gait

If the plantar flexor muscles are unable to perform their function, ankle and knee stability are greatly affected. Loss of the plantar flexors results in decrease or absence of push-off. The stance phase is less, and there is a shorter step length on the unaffected side.[36]

Psoatic Limp

The psoatic limp is seen in patients with conditions affecting the hip, such as Legg-Calvé-Perthes disease. The patient demonstrates a difficulty in swing-through, and the limp may be accompanied by exaggerated trunk and pelvic movement.[36] The limp may be caused by weakness or reflex inhibition of the psoas major muscle. Classic manifestations of this limp are lateral rotation, flexion, and adduction of the hip (Figure 14-24). The patient exaggerates movement of the pelvis and trunk to help move the thigh into flexion.

Quadriceps Avoidance Gait

If the quadriceps muscles have been injured (e.g., femoral nerve neuropathy, reflex inhibition, trauma—3°strain), the patient compensates in the trunk and lower leg. Forward flexion of the trunk combined with strong ankle plantar flexion causes the knee to extend (hyperextend). The knee may be held extended by using the iliotibial band. If the trunk, hip flexors, and ankle muscles cannot perform this movement, the patient may use a hand to extend the knee.[36]

Scissors Gait

This gait is the result of spastic paralysis of the hip adductor muscles, which causes the knees to be drawn together so that the legs can be swung forward only with great effort (Figure 14-25). This is seen in spastic paraplegics and may be referred to as a neurogenic or **spastic gait.**

Short Leg Gait

If one leg is shorter than the other or there is a deformity in one of the bones of the leg, the patient may

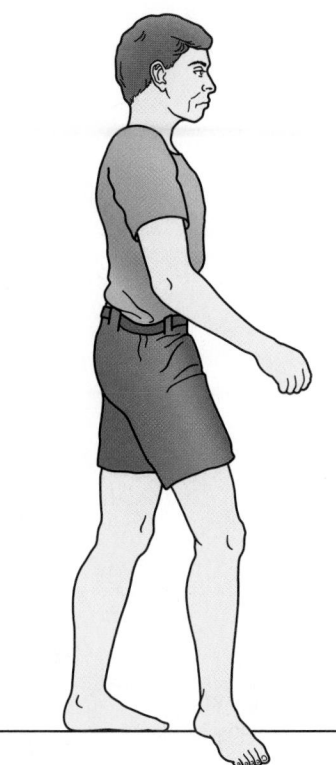

Figure 14-24 Psoatic limp. Note lateral rotation, flexion, and abduction of affected hip.

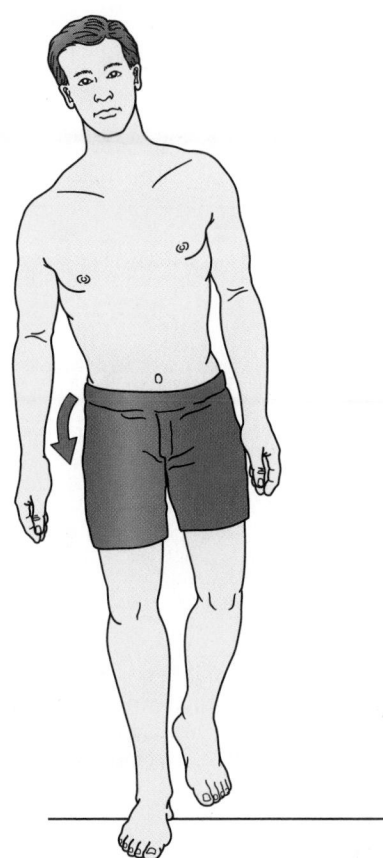

Figure 14-26 Short leg gait.

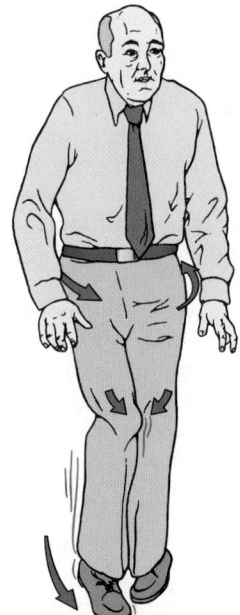

Figure 14-25 Scissors gait. (Redrawn from Judge RD, Zuidema GD, Fitzgerald FT: Clinical diagnosis: a physiological approach, Boston, 1982, Little, Brown, p. 439.)

demonstrate a lateral shift to the affected side, and the pelvis tilts down on the affected side, creating a limp (Figure 14-26). The patient may also supinate the foot on the affected side to try to "lengthen" the limb. The joints of the unaffected limb may demonstrate exaggerated flexion, or hip hiking may occur during the swing phase to allow the foot to clear the ground.[36] The weight-bearing period may be the same for the two legs. How a patient adapts for leg length difference has wide variability.[69,70] With proper footwear, the gait may appear normal. This gait may also be termed *painless osteogenic gait*.

Steppage or Drop Foot Gait

The patient with a steppage gait has weak or paralyzed dorsiflexor muscles, resulting in a drop foot. To compensate and avoid dragging the toes against the ground, the patient lifts the knee higher than normal (Figure 14-27). At initial contact, the foot slaps on the ground because of loss of control of the dorsiflexor muscles resulting from injury to the muscles, their peripheral nerve supply, or the nerve roots supplying the muscles (see Table 14-9).[71]

Table 14-10 lists common gait pathologies that can modify gait and the phase in which the deviation occurs.[38]

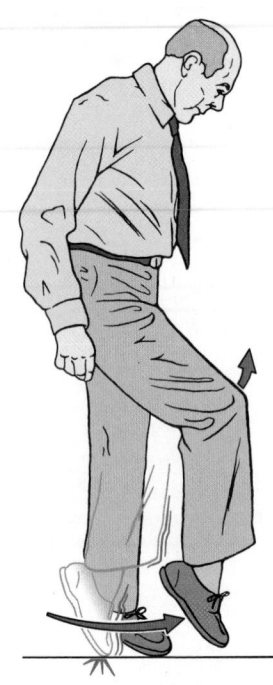

Figure 14-27 Steppage or drop foot gait. (Redrawn from Judge RD, Zuidema GD, Fitzgerald FT: Clinical diagnosis: a physiological approach, Boston, 1982, Little, Brown, p. 438.)

TABLE **14-10**

Common Gait Pathologies

Deviation	Phase	Cause
Excessive foot pronation	Midstance through toe off	Compensated forefoot or rearfoot varus deformity; uncompensated forefoot valgus deformity; pes planus; decreased ankle dorsiflexion; increased tibial varum; long limb; uncompensated medial rotation of tibia or femur; weak tibialis posterior
Excessive foot supination	Heel strike through midstance	Compensated forefoot valgus deformity; pes cavus; short limb, uncompensated lateral rotation of tibia or femur; limited calcaneal eversion; plantar flexed first ray; upper motor neuron muscle balance
Excessive calcaneal eversion	Initial contact through midstance	Excessive tibia vara; forefoot varus; tibialis posterior weakness; excessive lower extremity medial rotation (due to muscle imbalances, femoral anteversion)
Excessive varus	Heel strike to toe off	Contracture; overactivity of muscles on medial aspect of foot
Excessive valgus	Heel strike to toe off	Weak invertors; foot hypermobility
Bouncing or exaggerated plantar flexion	Midstance through toe off	Heel cord contracture; increased tone of gastrocnemius and soleus
Excessive dorsiflexion	Heel strike to toe off	Compensation for knee flexion contracture; inadequate plantar flexor strength; adaptive shortening of dorsiflexors; increased muscle tone of dorsiflexors; pes calcaneus deformity
Insufficient push-off	Midstance through toe off	Gastrocnemius and soleus weakness; Achilles tendon rupture; metatarsalgia; hallux rigidus

TABLE **14-10**

Common Gait Pathologies—cont'd

Deviation	Phase	Cause
Foot slap	Heel strike to foot flat	Dorsiflexor weakness; lack of lower limb sensation
Steppage gait (exaggerated hip and knee flexion to clear foot)	Acceleration through deceleration	Dorsiflexor weakness or paralysis; functional leg length discrepancy
Excessive knee flexion	Heel strike through toe off	Hamstring contracture; decreased ROM in ankle dorsiflexion; plantar flexor muscle weakness; lengthened limb; hip flexion contracture
Excessive knee extension/ inadequate knee flexion	Heel strike to foot flat, and swing	Pain; anterior trunk deviation/bending; weakness of quadriceps, hyperextension is a compensation and places body weight vector anterior to knee; spasticity of the quadriceps, noted more during the loading response and during initial swing intervals; joint deformity
Genu recurvatum (knee hyperextension)	Heel strike through midstance	Quadriceps femoris weak or short; compensated hamstring weakness; Achilles tendon contracture; habit
Abnormal internal hip rotation ("toe-in" gait)		Adaptive shortening of iliotibial band; weakness of hip lateral rotators; femoral anteversion; adaptive shortening of hip medial rotators
Abnormal external hip rotation ("toe-out" gait)		Adaptive shortening of hip lateral rotators; femoral retroversion; weakness of hip medial rotators
Increased hip adduction (scissors gait)	Heel strike to toe off	Spasticity or contracture of ipsilateral hip adductors; ipsilateral hip adductor weakness; coxa vara
Decreased hip swing through (psoatic limp)		Legg-Calvé-Perthes disease; weakness or reflex inhibition of psoas major muscle; pain
Excessive medial or lateral femur rotation (femoral torsion)	Heel strike through toe off	Medial or lateral hamstrings tight, respectively; opposite muscle group weakness; anteversion or retroversion, respectively
Increased base of support (> 4 inches/10 cm)	Heel strike through toe off	Abductor muscle contracture; instability; genu valgum; leg length discrepancy; fear of losing balance
Decreased base of support (< 2 inches/5 cm)	Heel strike through toe off	Adductor muscle contracture; genu varum
Circumduction	Acceleration through deceleration	Increased limb length; abductor muscle shortening or overuse; stiff hip or knee
Hip hiking	Acceleration through deceleration	Increased limb length; hamstring weakness; inadequate hip or knee flexion or ankle dorsiflexion; quadratus lumborum shortening
Vaulting (ground clearance of swinging leg is increased if subject goes up on toes of stance period leg)	Foot flat to toe off	Functional leg-length discrepancy; vaulting occurs on shorter limb side
Inadequate hip flexion	Acceleration through heel strike	Hip flexor muscle weakness; hip extensor muscle shortening; increased limb length; hip joint arthrosis
Inadequate hip extension (causes trunk forward bending, increased lordosis)	Midstance through toe off	Hip flexion contracture; hip extensor muscle weakness; iliotibial band contracture; hip flexor spasticity; pain
Increased lumbar lordosis	Foot flat to toe off	Inability to extend hip; hip flexion contracture or hip ankylosis
Excessive trunk back bending (gluteus maximus gait)	Heel strike through midstance	Hip extensor or flexor muscle weakness; hip pain; decreased ROM of knee

Continued

TABLE **14-10**

Common Gait Pathologies—cont'd

Deviation	Phase	Cause
Excessive trunk forward bending	Deceleration through midstance	Quadriceps femoris and gluteus maximus weakness; decreased ankle dorsiflexion; hip flexion contracture
Excessive trunk lateral flexion (compensated Trendelenburg gait)	Foot flat through heel off	Gluteus medius weakness; hip pain; unequal leg length; hip pathology; wide base
Pelvic drop	Foot flat through heel off	Contralateral gluteus medius weakness; adaptive shortening of quadratus lumborum; contralateral hip adductor spasticity
Excessive pelvic rotation	Heel strike to toe off	Adaptively shortened/spasticity of hip flexors on same side; limited hip joint flexion
Slower cadence than expected for person's age		Generalized weakness; pain; joint motion restrictions; poor voluntary motor control
Shorter stance phase on involved side and decreased swing phase on uninvolved side (shorter stride length on uninvolved side, decrease lateral sway over involved stance limb, decrease in cadence, decrease in velocity, use of assistive device)		Antalgic gait resulting from painful injury to lower limb and pelvic region
Stance phase longer on one side		Pain; lack of trunk and pelvic rotation; weakness of lower limb muscles; restrictions in lower limb joints; poor muscle control; increased muscle tone

Adapted from Giallonardo LM: Gait. In Myers RS, editor: Saunders manual of physical therapy practice, Philadelphia, 1995, WB Saunders, p. 1112; and Dutton M: Orthopedic examination, evaluation and intervention, New York, 2004, McGraw-Hill.
ROM, Range of motion.

REFERENCES

1. Winter DA: Biomechanics of normal and pathological gait: implications for understanding human locomotor control. J Motor Behav 21:337–355, 1989.
2. Sutherland DH, Valencia F: Pediatric gait: Normal and abnormal development. In Drennan JC, editor: The child's foot and ankle, New York, 1992, Raven Press.
3. Eastlack ME, Arvidson J, Snyder-Mackler L, et al: Interrater reliability of videotaped observational gait-analysis assessments. Phys Ther 71:465–472, 1991.
4. Martin PE, Heise GD, Morgan DW: Interrelationships between mechanical power, energy transfers, and walking and running economy. Med Sci Sports Exerc 25:508–515, 1993.
5. Wall JC, Kirtley C: Strategies for clinical gait assessment. Orthop Phys Ther Clin North Am 10:35–37, 2001.
6. Bowker JH, Hall CB: Normal human gait. In Atlas of orthotics: biomechanical principles and applications, St Louis, 1975, Mosby.
7. Inman VT, Ralston HJ, Todd F: Human locomotion. In Rose J, Gamble JG, editors: Human locomotion, Baltimore, 1994, Williams & Wilkins.
8. Sutherland DH, Kaufman KR, Moitoza JR: Kinematics of normal human walking. In Rose J, Gamble JG, editors: Human locomotion, Baltimore, 1994, Williams & Wilkins.

9. Adams JM, Perry J: Gait analysis: Clinical applications. In Rose J, Gamble JG, editors: Human locomotion, Baltimore, 1994, Williams & Wilkins.
10. Koerner IB: Normal human locomotion and the gait of the amputee, Edmonton, 1979, University of Alberta Bookstore.
11. Koerner I: Observation of human gait [videotapes], Health Sciences Audiovisual Education, 1984, University of Alberta.
12. Perry J: Gait analysis: normal and pathological function, Thorofare, NJ, 1994, Slack.
13. Olsson EC: Methods of studying gait. In Smidt GL, editor: Gait in rehabilitation, New York, 1990, Churchill Livingstone.
14. Shiavi R: Electromyographic patterns in normal adult locomotion. In Smidt GL, editor: Gait in rehabilitation, New York, 1990, Churchill Livingstone.
15. Kuo AD, Donelan JM: Dynamic principles of gait and their clinical implications. Physical Therapy 90:157–176, 2010.
16. Boudreau HR, Kaegi C, Rousseau J, editors: Grille d'évaluation de la securité à la marche (GEM), Ottawa 2002, Bibliothèque nationale du Canada.
17. Simoneau GG: Kinesiology of walking. In Neumann DA, editor: Kinesiology of the musculoskeletal

system: foundations of physical rehabilitation, ed 2, St Louis, 2010, Mosby.
18. Adelaar RS: The practical biomechanics of running. Am J Sports Med 14:497–500, 1986.
19. Larish DD, Martin PE, Mungiole M: Characteristic patterns of gait in the healthy old. Ann NY Acad Sci 515:18–32, 1988.
20. Montero-Odasso M, Magee M, Varela C, et al: Gait velocity in senior people: an easy test for detecting mobility impairment in community elderly. J Nutr Health Aging 8(5):340–343, 2004.
21. Mann RA, Moran GT, Dougherty SE: Comparative electromyography of the lower extremity in jogging, running, and sprinting. Am J Sports Med 14:501–510, 1986.
22. Barry-Greb TL, Harrison AL: Posture, gait and functional abilities of the adolescent, pregnant, and elderly female. Orthop Phys Ther Clin North Am 5:1–21, 1996.
23. Biden E, O'Conner J, Collins JJ: Gait analysis. In Daniel D, Akeson W, O'Conner J, editors: Knee ligaments: structure, function, injury and repair, New York, 1990, Raven Press.
24. Hoppenfeld S: Physical examination of the spine and extremities, New York, 1976, Appleton-Century-Crofts.

25. Barry-Greb TL, Harrison AL: Posture, gait, and functional abilities of the adolescent, pregnant and elderly female. Orthop Phys Ther Clin North Am 5:1–21, 1996.

26. Sutherland DH, Olshen R, Cooper L, et al: The development of mature gait. J Bone Joint Surg Am 62:336–353, 1980.

27. Subotnick SI: Variations in angles of gait in running. Phys Sportsmed 7:110–114, 1979.

28. Sekiya N, Nagasaki H, Ito H, et al: Optimal walking in terms of variability in step length. J Orthop Sports Phys Ther 26:266–272, 1997.

29. Ostrosky KM, Van Swearingen JM, Burdett RG, et al: A comparison of gait characteristics in young and old subjects. Phys Ther 74:637–646, 1994.

30. Waters RL, Hislop HJ, Perry J, et al: Comparative cost of walking in young and old adults. J Orthop Res 1:73–76, 1983.

31. Levangie PK, Norkin CC: Joint structure and function: a comprehensive analysis, Philadelphia, 2005, FA Davis.

32. Nuber GW: Biomechanics of the foot and ankle during gait. Clin Sports Med 7:1–13, 1988.

33. Rodgers MM: Dynamic foot mechanics. J Orthop Sports Phys Ther 21:306–316, 1995.

34. Rowe DA, Welk GJ, Heil DP, et al: Stride rate recommendations for moderate intensity walking. Med Sci Sports Exerc 43:312–318, 2011.

35. Perry J, Hislop HJ: The mechanics of walking: a clinical interpretation. In Perry J, Hislop HJ, editors: Principles of lower-extremity bracing, New York, 1970, American Physical Therapy Association.

36. Epler M: Gait. In Richardson JK, Iglarsh ZA, editors: Clinical orthopedic physical therapy, Philadelphia, 1994, WB Saunders.

37. Krebs DE, Wong D, Jevsevar D, et al: Trunk kinematics during locomotor activities. Phys Ther 72:505–514, 1992.

38. Giallonardo LM: Gait. In Myers RS, editor: Saunders manual of physical therapy practice, Philadelphia, 1995, WB Saunders.

39. Lyu SR, Ogata K, Hoshiko I: Effects of a cane on floor reaction force and centre of force during gait. Clin Orthop Relat Res 375:313–319, 2000.

40. Rab GT: Muscle. In Rose J, Gamble JG, editors: Human locomotion, Baltimore, 1994, Williams & Wilkins.

41. Krebs DE, Robbins CE, Lavine L, et al: Hip biomechanics during gait. J Orthop Sports Phys Ther 28:51–59, 1998.

42. Dillon PZ, Updyke WF, Allen WC: Gait analysis with reference to chondromalacia patella. J Orthop Sports Phys Ther 5:127–131, 1983.

43. Sutherland DH, Cooper L, Daniel D: The role of the ankle plantar flexors in normal walking. J Bone Joint Surg Am 62:354–363, 1980.

44. Arnadottir SA, Mereer VS: Effects of footwear on measurements of balance and gait in women between the ages of 65 and 93 years. Phys Ther 80:17–27, 2000.

45. Mann RA, Hagy JL, White V, et al: The initiation of gait. J Bone Joint Surg Am 61:232–239, 1979.

46. The Pathokinesiology Service and the Physical Therapy Department, Rancho Los Amigos Medical Center: Observational gait analysis, Downey, CA, 1996, Los Amigos Research and Educational Institute.

47. Ebbeling CJ, Hamill J, Crussemeyer JA: Lower extremity mechanics and energy cost of walking on high-heeled shoes. J Orthop Sports Phys Ther 19:190–196, 1994.

48. Coutts F: Gait analysis in the therapeutic environment. Man Ther 4:2–10, 1999.

49. Wall JC, Devlin J, Khirchof R, et al: Measurement of step widths and step lengths: a comparison of measurements made directly from a grid with those made from a video recording. J Orthop Sports Phys Ther 30:410–417, 2000.

50. Song KM, Halliday SE, Little DG: The effect of limb-length discrepancy on gait. J Bone Joint Surg Am 79:1690–1698, 1997.

51. Larsson SE, Jonsson B: Locomotion score in rheumatoid arthritis. Acta Orthop Scand 60:271–277, 1989.

52. Dutton M: Dutton's orthopedic examination, evaluation and intervention, ed 3, New York, 2012, McGraw-Hill.

53. Van Swearingen JM, Paschal KA, Bonino P, et al: The modified Gait Abnormality Rating Scale for recognizing the risk of recurrent falls in community-dwelling elderly adults. Phys Ther 76:994–1002, 1996.

54. Wolfson L, Whipple R, Amerman P, et al: Gait assessment in the elderly: a gait abnormality rating scale and its relation to falls. J Gerontol 45:M12–M19, 1990.

55. Wolf SL: A method of quantifying ambulatory activities. Phys Ther 59:767–768, 1979.

56. Wolf SL, Catlin PA, Gage K, et al: Establishing the reliability and validity of measurements of walking time using the Emory functional ambulation profile. Phys Ther 79:1122–1133, 1999.

57. Kaegi C, Boudreau R, Rousseau J, et al: Development of a walking safety scale for older adults. Part 1: content validity of the GEM scale. Physiother Can 60:264–273, 2008.

58. Newell AM, Van Swearingen JM, Hile E, et al: The modified gait efficacy scale: establishing the psychometric properties in older adults. Physical Therapy 92:318–328, 2012.

59. Matheis A, Nayak US, Isaacs B: Balance in elderly patients: the "get-up and go" test. Arch Phys Med Rehabil 67:387–389, 1986.

60. Holden MK, Gill KM, Magliozzi MR, et al: Clinical gait assessment in the neurologically impaired: reliability and meaningfulness. Phys Ther 64:35–40, 1984.

61. Holden MK, Gill KM, Magliozzi MR: Gait assessment for neurologically impaired patients: standards for outcome assessment. Phys Ther 66:1530–1539, 1986.

62. Hess RJ, Brach JS, Piva SR, et al: Walking skill can be assessed in older adults: validity of the Figure-of-8 Walk Test. Physical Therapy 90:89–99, 2010.

63. Wrisley DM, Kumar NA: Functional gait assessment: concurrent, discriminative and predictive validity in community-dwelling older adults. Physical Therapy 90:761–775, 2010.

64. Tinetti ME: Performance-oriented assessment of mobility problems in elderly patients. J Am Geriatr Soc 34:119–126, 1986.

65. Gleim GW, Stachenfeld NS, Nicholas JA: The influence of flexibility on the economy of walking and jogging. J Orthop Res 8:814–823, 1990.

66. Murray MP, Mollinger LA, Gardner GM, et al: Kinematic and EMG patterns during slow, free, and fast walking. J Orthop Res 2:272–280, 1984.

67. Flynn JM, Widmann RF: The limping child: evaluation and diagnosis. J Am Acad Orthop Surg 9:89–98, 2001.

68. Scandalis TA, Bosak A, Berliner JC, et al: Resistance training and gait function in patients with Parkinson's disease. Am J Phys Med Rehabil 80:38–43, 2001.

69. Kaufman KR, Miller LS, Sutherland DH: Gait asymmetry in patients with limb-length inequality. J Ped Orthop 16:144–150, 1996.

70. Song KM, Halliday SE, Little DG: The effect of limb-length discrepancy on gait. J Bone Joint Surg Am 79:1690–1698, 1997.

71. Morag E, Hurwitz DE, Andriacchi TP, et al: Abnormalities in muscle function during gait in relation to the level of lumbar disc herniation. Spine 25:829–833, 2000.

SUGGESTED READINGS

Andriacchi TP, Andersson GB, Fermier RW, et al: A study of lower-limb mechanics during stair climbing. J Bone Joint Surg Am 62:749–757, 1980.

Brown LP, Yavorsky P: Locomotor biomechanics and pathomechanics: a review. J Orthop Sports Phys Ther 9:3–10, 1987.

Burdett RG, Skrinar GS, Simon SR: Comparison of mechanical work and metabolic energy consumption during normal gait. J Orthop Res 1:63–72, 1983.

Chodera JD: Analysis of gait from footprints. Physiotherapy 60:179–181, 1974.

Cook TM, Farrell KP, Carey IA, et al: Effects of restricted knee flexion and walking speed on the vertical ground reaction force during gait. J Orthop Sports Phys Ther 25:236–244, 1997.

Crowinschield RD, Brand RA, Johnson RC: The effects of walking velocity and age on hip kinematics and kinetics. Clin Orthop 132:140–144, 1978.

Eberhart HD, Inman VT, Bresler B: Principal elements in human locomotion. In Klopsteg PE, Wilson PD, editors: Human limbs and their substitutes, New York, 1954, McGraw-Hill.

Engel GM, Staheli LT: The natural history of torsion and other factors influencing gait in childhood. Clin Orthop 99:12–17, 1974.

Finley FR, Cody KA, Finizie RV: Locomotion patterns in elderly women. Arch Phys Med Rehabil 50:140–146, 1969.

Gage JR, Ounpuu S: Gait analysis in clinical practice. Semin Orthop 4:72–87, 1989.

Garbalosa JC, Donatelli R, Wooden MJ: Dysfunction, evaluation and treatment of the foot and ankle. In Donatelli R, Wooden MJ, editors: Orthopedic physical therapy, Edinburgh, 1989, Churchill Livingstone.

Gaudet G, Goodman R, Landry M, et al: Measurement of step length and step width: a comparison of videotape and direct measurements. Physiother Can 42:12–15, 1990.

Gilbert JA, Maxwell GM, McElhaney JH, et al: A system to measure the forces and moments at the knee and hip during level walking. J Orthop Res 2:281–288, 1984.

Gray GW: Chain reaction successful strategies for closed chain testing and rehabilitation, Adrian, MI, 1989, Wynn Marketing.

Grieve DW: The assessment of gait. Physiotherapy 55:452–460, 1969.

Grieve DW: Timing and placement of the feet. Semin Orthop 4:130–134, 1989.

Gruebel-Lee DM: Disorders of hip, Philadelphia, 1983, JB Lippincott.

Herzog W, Conway PJ: Gait analysis of sacroiliac joint patients. J Manip Physiol Ther 17:124–127, 1994.

Hreljac A: Preferred and energetically optimal gait transition speeds in human locomotion. Med Sci Sports Exerc 25:1158–1162, 1993.

Inman VT: Functional aspects of the abductor muscles of the hip. J Bone Joint Surg 29:607–619, 1947.

Inman VT: The joints of the ankle, Baltimore, 1976, Williams & Wilkins.

Inman VT: Human locomotion: the classic. Clin Orthop 288:3–9, 1993.

Judge RD, Zuidema GD, Fitzgerald FT: Clinical diagnosis: a physiological approach, Boston, 1982, Little, Brown.

Kadaba, MP, Ramakrishnan HK, Wootten ME: Measurement of lower extremity kinematics during level walking. J Orthop Res 8:383–392, 1990.

Kadaba MP, Ramarkrishnan HK, Wootten ME, et al: Repeatability of kinematic, kinetic, and electromyographic data in normal adult gait. J Orthop Res 7:849–860, 1989.

Katoh Y, Chao EY, Laughman RK, et al: Biomechanical analysis of foot function during gait and clinical applications. Clin Orthop 177:23–33, 1983.

Kay RM, Dennis S, Rothlefson S, et al: The effect of preoperative gait analysis on orthopedic decision making. Clin Orthop Relat Res 372:217–222, 2000.

Krebs DE, Robbins CE, Lavine L, et al: Hip biomechanics during gait. J Orthop Sports Phys Ther 28:51–59, 1998.

Law HT: Introduction: techniques for the measurement of parameters related to human locomotion and their clinical applications. Semin Orthop 4:65–71, 1989.

Lee D: Instability of the sacroiliac joint and the consequences to gait. J Man Manip Ther 4:22–29, 1996.

Lehmann JF: Push off and propulsion of the body in normal and abnormal gait. Clin Orthop 288:97–108, 1993.

Macleod J: Clinical examination, New York, 1976, Churchill Livingstone.

Mann RA, Hagy JL: The function of the toes in walking, jogging, and running. [correction: *155*:293]. Clin Orthop 142:24–29, 1979.

McCulloch MU, Brunt D, Van der Linden D: The effect of foot orthotics and gait velocity on lower limb kinematics and temporal events of stance. J Orthop Sports Phys Ther 17:2–10, 1993.

McPoil TG, Cornwall MW: Applied sports biomechanics in rehabilitation: running. In Zachazewski JE, Magee DJ, Quillen WS, editors: Athletic injuries and rehabilitation, Philadelphia, 1996, WB Saunders.

Minetti AE, Capelli C, Zamparo P, et al: Effects of stride frequency on mechanical power and energy expenditure of walking. Med Sci Sports Exerc 27:1194–1202, 1995.

Murray MP: Gait as a total pattern of movement. Am J Phys Med 46:290–333, 1967.

Murray MP, Drought AB, Kory RC: Walking patterns of normal men. J Bone Joint Surg Am 46:335–360, 1964.

Murray MP, Gore DR, Clarkson BH: Walking patterns of patients with unilateral pain due to osteoarthritis and avascular necrosis. J Bone Joint Surg Am 53:259–274, 1971.

Olsson E: Gait analysis in orthopedics. Semin Orthop 4:111–119, 1989.

Perry J: Anatomy and biomechanics of the hindfoot. Clin Orthop 177:9–15, 1983.

Perry J: Pathological gait. In Atlas of orthotics: biomechanical principles and applications, St Louis, 1975, Mosby.

Perry J, Hislop H: Principles of lower extremity bracing, Washington, DC, 1967, American Physical Therapy Association.

Root ML, Orien WP, Weed JH: Normal and abnormal function of the foot, Los Angeles, 1977, Clinical Biomechanics.

Saunders JBM, Inman VT, Eberhart HO: The major determinants in normal and pathological gait. J Bone Joint Surg Am 35:543–558, 1953.

Schwab GH, Moynes DR, Jobe FW, et al: Lower extremity electromyographic analysis of running gait. Clin Orthop 176:166–170, 1983.

Simon SR, Mann RA, Hagy JL, et al: Role of the posterior calf muscles in a normal gait. J Bone Joint Surg Am 60:465–472, 1978.

Skinner S: Development of gait. In Rose J, Gamble JG, editors: Human locomotion, Baltimore, 1994, Williams & Wilkins.

Smidt GL: Gait assessment and training in clinical practice. In Smidt GL, editor: Gait in rehabilitation, New York, 1990, Churchill Livingstone.

Thurston AJ, Harris JD: Normal kinematics of the lumbar spine and pelvis. Spine 8:199–205, 1983.

Tiberio D, Gray GW: Kinematics and kinetics during gait. In Donatelli R, Wooden MJ, editors: Orthopedic physical therapy, Edinburgh, 1989, Churchill Livingstone.

Todd, FN, Lamoreux LW, Skinner SR, et al: Variations in the gait of normal children. J Bone Joint Surg Am 71:196–204, 1989.

Tomaro J, Burdett RG: The effects of foot orthotics on the EMG activity of selected leg muscles during gait. J Orthop Sports Phys Ther 17:532–536, 1993.

Tomberlin JP, Saunders HD: Evaluation, treatment and prevention of musculoskeletal disorders, Chaska, MN, 1994, Saunders Group.

Veicsteinas A, Aghemo P, Mrgaria R, et al: Energy cost of walking with lesions of the foot. J Bone Joint Surg Am 61:1073–1076, 1979.

Wadsworth CT: Manual examination and treatment of the spine and extremities, Baltimore, 1988, Williams & Wilkins.

Winter DA: Energy assessment in pathological gait. Physiother Can 30:183–191, 1978.

Wooten ME, Kadaba MP, Cochran GV: Dynamic electromyography: I. numerical representation using principal component analysis. J Orthop Res 8:247–258, 1990.

Wooten ME, Kadaba MP, Cochran GV: Dynamic electromyography: II. normal patterns during gait. J Orthop Res 8:259–265, 1990.

Wright DG, Desai SM, Henderson WH: Action of the subtalar and ankle joint complex during the stance phase of walking. J Bone Joint Surg Am 46:361–382, 1964.

Wyatt MP: Gait in children. In Smidt GL, editor: Gait in rehabilitation, New York, 1990, Churchill Livingstone.

CHAPTER 15

Assessment of Posture

POSTURAL DEVELOPMENT

Through evolution, human beings have assumed an upright erect or bipedal posture. The advantage of an erect posture is that it enables the hands to be free and the eyes to be farther from the ground so that the individual can see farther ahead. The disadvantages include an increased strain on the spine and lower limbs and comparative difficulties in respiration and transport of the blood to the brain.

Posture, which is the relative disposition of the body at any one moment, is a composite of the positions of the different joints of the body at that time. The position of each joint has an effect on the position of the other joints. Classically, ideal static postural alignment (viewed from the side) is defined as a straight line (line of gravity) that passes through the earlobe, the bodies of the cervical vertebrae, the tip of the shoulder, midway through the thorax, through the bodies of the lumbar vertebrae, slightly posterior to the hip joint, slightly anterior to the axis of the knee joint, and just anterior to the lateral malleolus (Figure 15-1).[1] **Correct posture** is the position in which minimum stress is applied to each joint. Upright posture is the normal standing posture for humans. Although upright posture allows one to see farther and provides freedom to move the arms, it does have disadvantages. It places greater stress on the lower limbs, pelvis, and spine; reduces stability; and increases the work of the heart.[2] If the upright posture is correct, minimal muscle activity is needed to maintain the position.

Any static position that increases the stress to the joints may be called **faulty posture.** If a person has strong, flexible muscles, faulty postures may not affect the joints because he or she has the ability to change position readily so that the stresses do not become excessive. If the joints are stiff (hypomobile) or too mobile (hypermobile), or the muscles are weak, shortened, or lengthened, however, the posture cannot be easily altered to the correct alignment, and the result can be some form of pathology. The pathology may be the result of the cumulative effect of repeated small stresses (microtrauma) over a long period of time or of constant abnormal stresses (macrotrauma) over a short period of time. These chronic stresses can result in the same problems that are seen when a sudden (acute) severe stress is applied to the body. The abnormal

stresses cause excessive wearing of the articular surfaces of joints and produce osteophytes and traction spurs, which represent the body's attempt to alter its structure to accommodate these repeated stresses. The soft tissue (e.g., muscles, ligaments) may become weakened, stretched, or traumatized by the increased stress. Thus postural deviations do not always cause symptoms, but over time, they may do so.[3] The application of an acute stress on the chronic stress may exacerbate the problem and produce the signs and symptoms that initially prompt the patient to seek aid.

At birth, the entire spine is concave forward, or flexed (Figure 15-2). Curves of the spine found at birth are called **primary curves.** The curves that retain this position, those of the thoracic spine and sacrum, are therefore classified as primary curves of the spine. As the child grows (Figure 15-3), **secondary curves** appear and are convex forward, or extended. At about the age of 3 months, when the child begins to lift the head, the cervical spine becomes convex forward, producing the cervical lordosis. In the lumbar spine, the secondary curve develops slightly later (6 to 8 months), when the child begins to sit up and walk. In old age, the secondary curves again begin to disappear as the spine starts to return to a flexed position as the result of disc degeneration, ligamentous calcification, osteoporosis, and vertebral wedging.

In the child, the center of gravity is at the level of the twelfth thoracic vertebra. As the child grows older, the center of gravity drops, eventually reaching the level of the second sacral vertebra in adults (slightly higher in males). The child stands with a wide base to maintain balance, and the knees are flexed. The knees are slightly bowed (genu varum) until about 18 months of age. The child then becomes slightly knock kneed (genu valgum) until the age of 3 years. By the age of 6 years, the legs should naturally straighten (Figure 15-4). The lumbar spine in the child has an exaggerated lumbar curve, or excessive lordosis. This accentuated curve is caused by the presence of large abdominal contents, weakness of the abdominal musculature, and the small pelvis characteristic of children at this age.

Initially, a child is flatfooted, or appears to be, as the result of the minimal development of the medial longitudinal arch and the fat pad that is found in the arch. As the child grows, the fat pad slowly decreases in size,

ANATOMIC LANDMARKS

SURFACE LANDMARKS

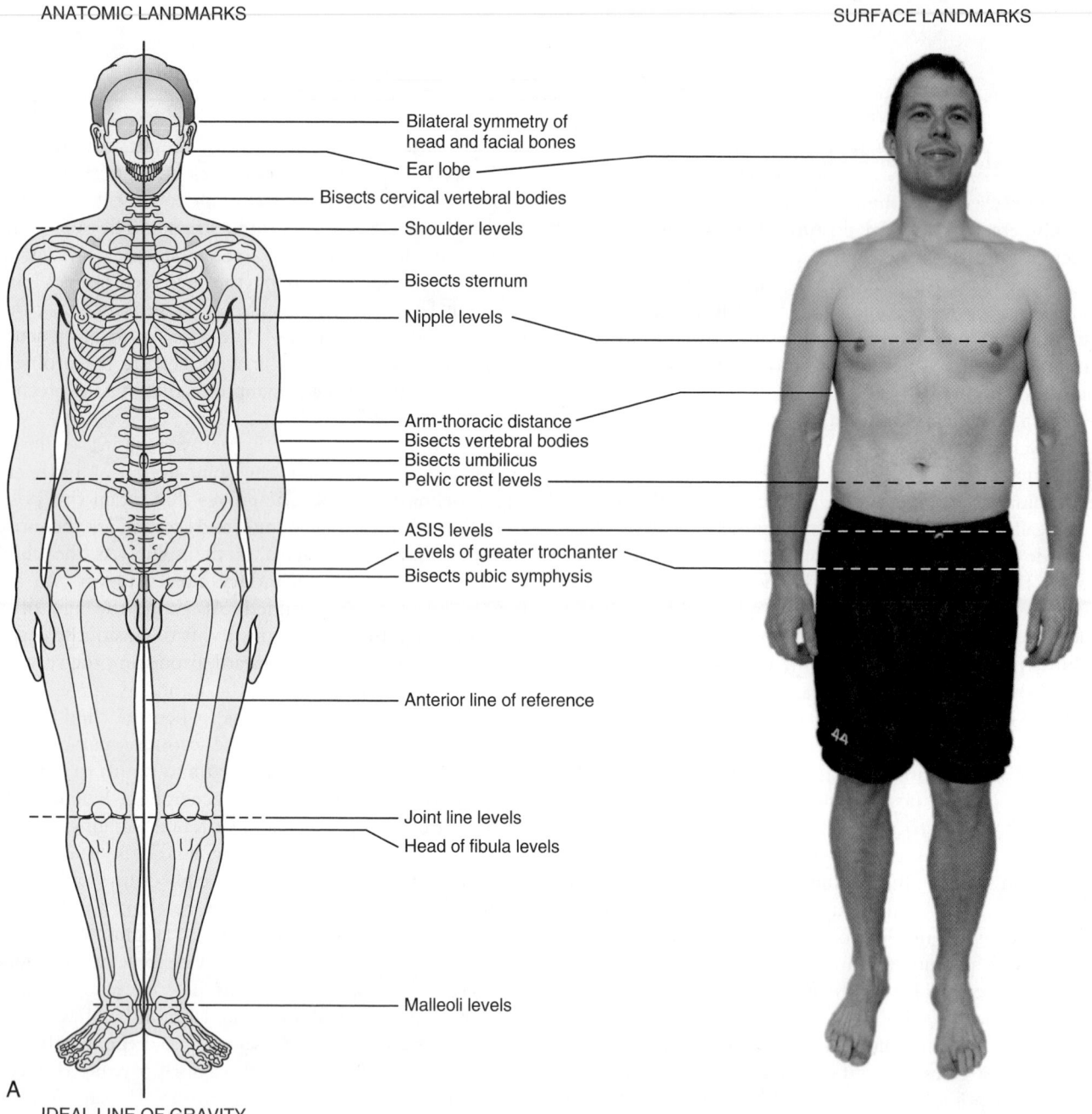

- Bilateral symmetry of head and facial bones
- Ear lobe
- Bisects cervical vertebral bodies
- Shoulder levels
- Bisects sternum
- Nipple levels
- Arm-thoracic distance
- Bisects vertebral bodies
- Bisects umbilicus
- Pelvic crest levels
- ASIS levels
- Levels of greater trochanter
- Bisects pubic symphysis
- Anterior line of reference
- Joint line levels
- Head of fibula levels
- Malleoli levels

A

IDEAL LINE OF GRAVITY

Figure 15-1 Ideal postural alignment. A, Front view. On a typical patient note the difference in shoulder height and nipple height and apparent arm length difference, arm-thorax difference, and difference in out-toeing.

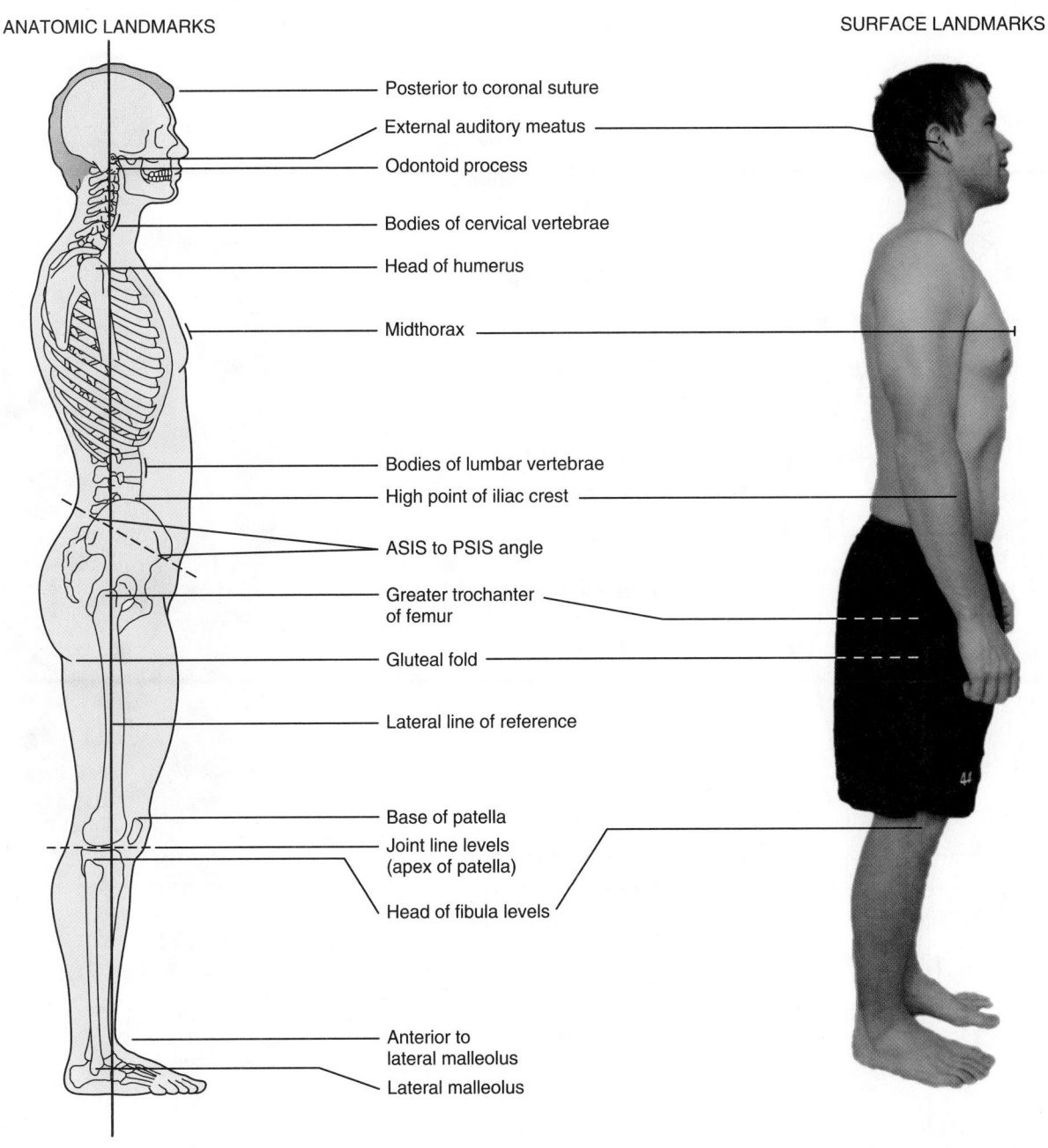

ANATOMIC LANDMARKS

SURFACE LANDMARKS

Posterior to coronal suture

External auditory meatus

Odontoid process

Bodies of cervical vertebrae

Head of humerus

Midthorax

Bodies of lumbar vertebrae

High point of iliac crest

ASIS to PSIS angle

Greater trochanter
of femur

Gluteal fold

Lateral line of reference

Base of patella

Joint line levels
(apex of patella)

Head of fibula levels

Anterior to
lateral malleolus

Lateral malleolus

B

IDEAL LINE OF GRAVITY

Figure 15-1, cont'd B, Side view. Typical patient with good lateral alignment.

Continued

ANATOMIC LANDMARKS

SURFACE LANDMARKS

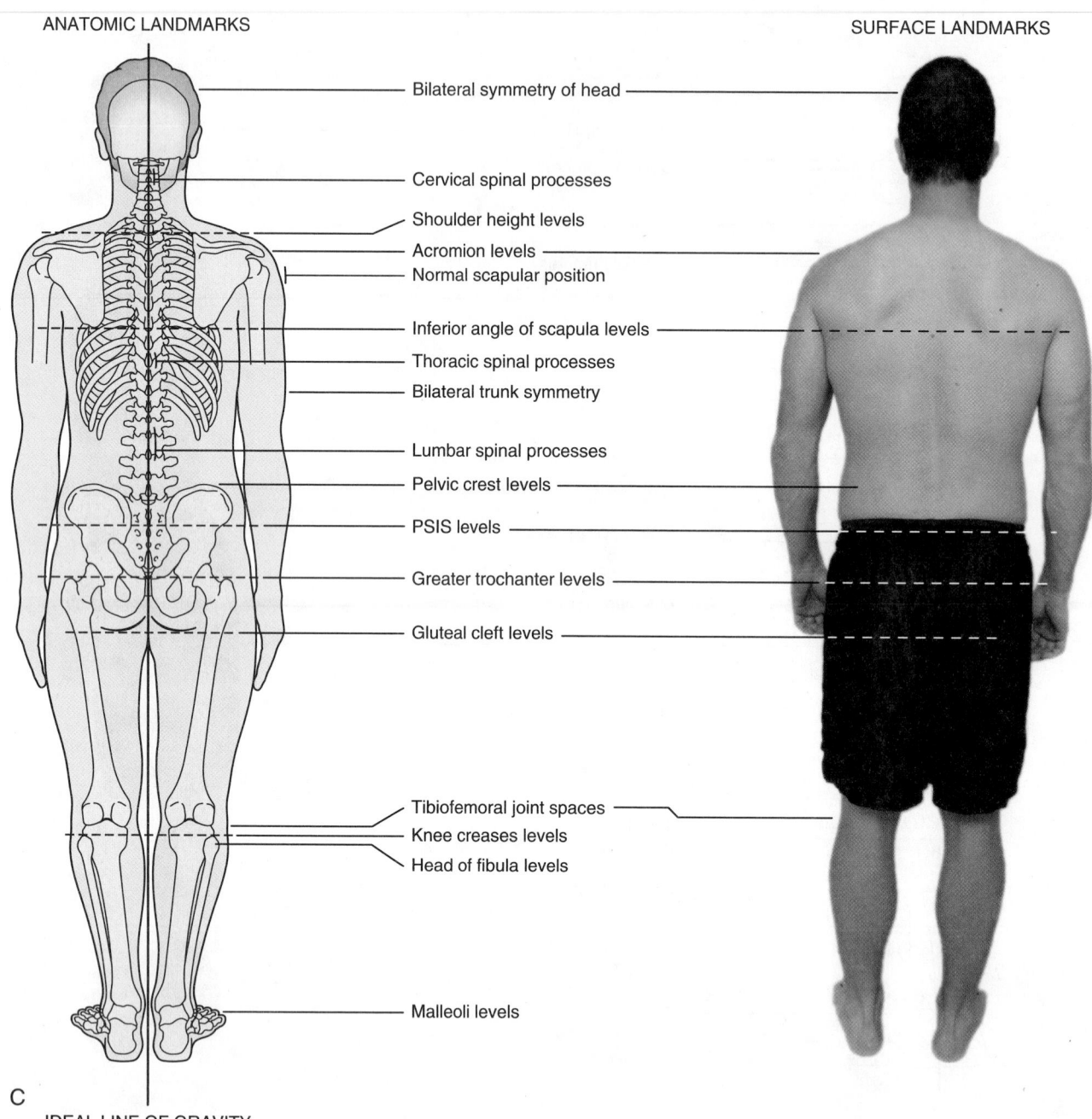

- Bilateral symmetry of head
- Cervical spinal processes
- Shoulder height levels
- Acromion levels
- Normal scapular position
- Inferior angle of scapula levels
- Thoracic spinal processes
- Bilateral trunk symmetry
- Lumbar spinal processes
- Pelvic crest levels
- PSIS levels
- Greater trochanter levels
- Gluteal cleft levels
- Tibiofemoral joint spaces
- Knee creases levels
- Head of fibula levels
- Malleoli levels

C

IDEAL LINE OF GRAVITY

Figure 15-1, cont'd C, Back view. On a typical patient note the difference in shoulder slope, shoulder height, height of inferior scapular angles, and rotation of arms. In this view, also note straight Achilles tendons.

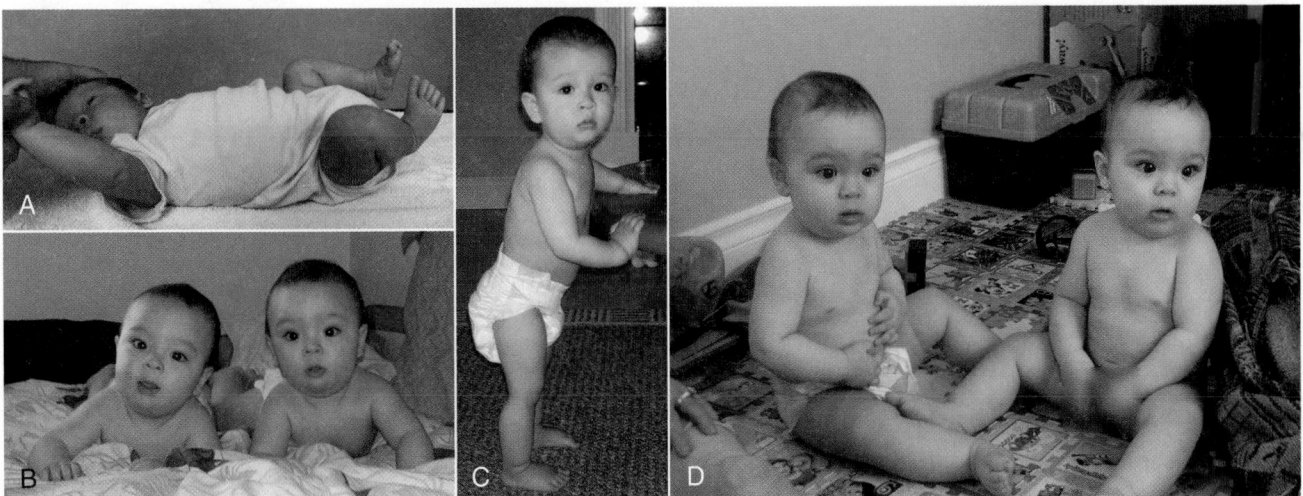

Figure 15-2 Postural development. A, Flexed posture in a newborn. **B,** Development of secondary cervical curve. **C,** Development of secondary lumbar curve. **D,** Sitting posture.

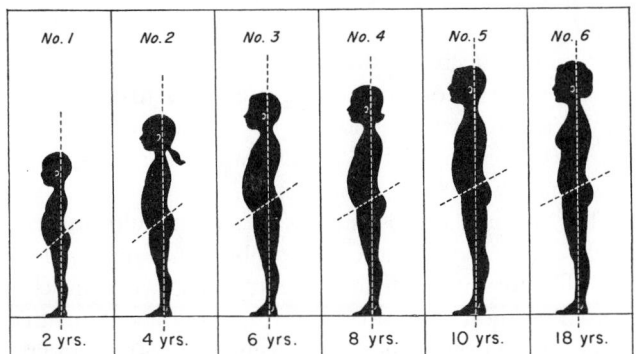

Figure 15-3 Postural changes with age. Apparent kyphosis at 6 and 8 years is caused by scapular winging. (From McMorris RO: Faulty postures. Pediatr Clin North Am 8:214, 1961.)

Newborn—
moderate genu varum

6 months—
minimal genu varum

1 year, 7 months—
legs straight

2 years, 6 months—
physiological
genu valgum

Protective toeing-in

4 to 6 years—
legs straight with
normal
toeing-out

Figure 15-4 Physiological evolution of lower-limb alignment at various ages in infancy and childhood. (Redrawn from Tachdjian MO: Pediatric orthopedics, Philadelphia, 1972, WB Saunders, p. 1463.)

making the medial arch more evident. In addition, as the foot develops and the muscles strengthen, the arches of the feet develop normally and become more evident.

During adolescence, posture changes because of hormonal influence with the onset of puberty and musculoskeletal growth. Human beings go through two growth spurts, one when they are very young and a more obvious one when they are in adolescence. This second growth spurt lasts 2.5 to 4 years.[4] During this period, growth is accompanied by sexual maturation. Females develop quicker and sooner than males. Females enter puberty between 8 and 14 years of age, and puberty lasts about 3 years. Males enter puberty between 9.5 and 16 years of age, and it lasts up to 5 years.[2] It is during this period that body differences arise between males and females with males tending toward longer leg and arm length, wider shoulders, smaller hip width, and greater overall skeletal size and height than females. Because of the rapid growth spurt, individuals, especially males, may appear ungainly, and poor postural habits and changes are more likely to occur at this age.

Factors Affecting Posture

Several anatomical features may affect correct posture. These features may be enhanced or cause additional problems when combined with pathological or congenital states, such as Klippel-Feil syndrome, Scheuermann disease (juvenile kyphosis), scoliosis, or disc disease.

Anatomical Factors Affecting Correct Posture

- Bony contours (e.g., hemivertebra)
- Laxity of ligamentous structures
- Fascial and musculotendinous tightness (e.g., tensor fasciae latae, pectorals, hip flexors)
- Muscle tonus (e.g., gluteus maximus, abdominals, erector spinae)
- Pelvic angle (normal is 30°)
- Joint position and mobility
- Neurogenic outflow and inflow

Causes of Poor Posture

There are many examples of poor posture (Figure 15-5). Some of the causes are postural (positional), and some are structural.

Postural (Positional) Factors

The most common postural problem is poor postural habit; that is, for whatever reason, the patient does not maintain a correct posture. This type of posture is often seen in the person who stands or sits for long periods and begins to slouch. Maintenance of correct posture requires muscles that are strong, flexible, and easily adaptable to environmental change. These muscles must continually work against gravity and in harmony with one another to maintain an upright posture.

Another cause of poor postural habits, especially in children, is not wanting to appear taller than one's peers. If a child has an early, rapid growth spurt there may be a tendency to slouch so as not to "stand out" and appear different. Such a spurt may also result in the unequal growth of the various structures, and this may lead to altered posture; for example, the growth of muscle may not keep up with the growth of bone. This process is sometimes evident in adolescents with tight hamstrings.

Muscle imbalance and muscle contracture are other causes of poor posture. For example, a tight iliopsoas muscle increases the lumbar lordosis in the lumbar spine.

Pain may also cause poor posture. Pressure on a nerve root in the lumbar spine can lead to pain in the back and result in a scoliosis as the body unconsciously adopts a posture that decreases the pain.

Respiratory conditions (e.g., emphysema), general weakness, excess weight, loss of proprioception, or muscle spasm (as seen in cerebral palsy or with trauma, as examples) may also lead to poor posture.

The majority of postural nonstructural faults are relatively easy to correct after the problem has been identified. The treatment involves strengthening weak muscles, stretching tight structures, and teaching the patient that it is his or her responsibility to maintain a correct upright posture in standing, sitting, and other activities of daily living (ADLs).

Structural Factors

Structural deformities that are the result of congenital anomalies, developmental problems, trauma, or disease may cause an alteration of posture. For example, a significant difference in leg length or an anomaly of the spine, such as a hemivertebra, may alter the posture.

Structural deformities involve mainly changes in bone and therefore are not easily correctable without surgery. However, patients often can be relieved of symptoms by proper postural care instruction.

COMMON SPINAL DEFORMITIES

Lordosis

Lordosis is an anterior curvature of the spine (Figure 15-6).[5-9] Pathologically, it is an exaggeration of the normal curves found in the cervical and lumbar spines. Causes of increased lordosis include (1) postural or functional deformity; (2) lax muscles, especially the abdominal muscles, in combination with tight muscles, especially

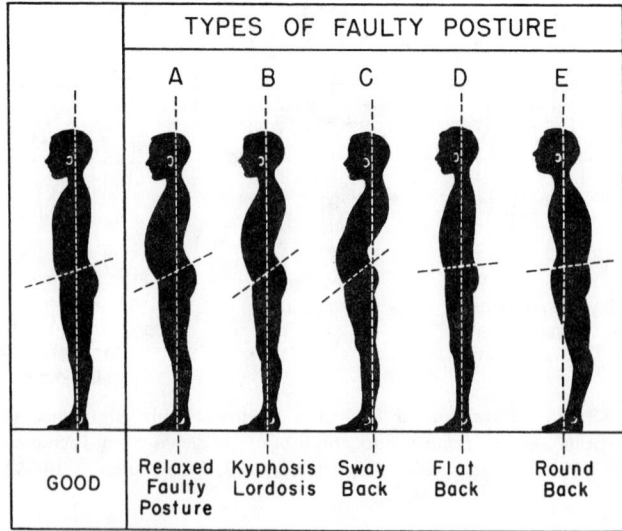

Figure 15-5 Examples of faulty posture. (From McMorris RO: Faulty postures. Pediatr Clin North Am 8:217, 1961.)

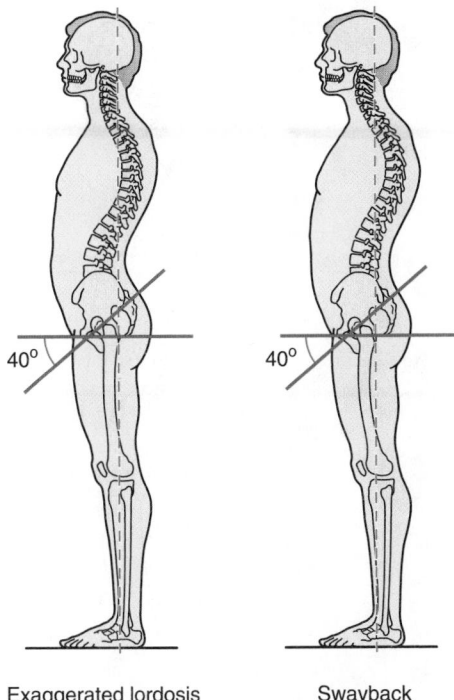

40°   40°

Exaggerated lordosis   Swayback

Figure 15-6 Examples of lordosis.

TABLE **15-1**

Changes Associated with Pathological Lordosis

Body segment alignment	Pelvis is anteriorly tilted with lordosis increased
	Knees are hyperextended
	Ankle joints slightly plantar flexed
Muscles commonly elongated and weak	Anterior abdominals
	Small muscles of lumbar spine (multifidus, rotators)
	Lower and middle trapezius
	Hamstrings may lengthen initially or shorten to compensate where posture has been present for some time
	Rhomboids (?)
	Upper (thoracic and cervical) erector spinae
	Hyoid muscles
Muscles commonly short and strong	Lumbar erector spinae
	Hip flexors
	Upper trapezius
	Pectoralis major and minor
	Levator scapulae
	Sternocleidomastoid
	Scalenes
	Suboccipital muscles
Joints commonly affected	Lumbar spine
	Pelvic joints
	Hip joints
	Thoracic spine
	Scapulothoracic joints
	Glenohumeral joints
	Cervical spine
	Atlanto-occipital joints
	Temporomandibular joints

Adapted from Kendall FP, McCreary EK: Muscles: testing and function, Baltimore, 1983, Williams & Wilkins; Giallonardo LM: Posture. In Myers RS, editor: Saunders manual of physical therapy practice, Philadelphia, 1995, WB Saunders.

hip flexors or lumbar extensors (Table 15-1); (3) a heavy abdomen, resulting from excess weight or pregnancy; (4) compensatory mechanisms that result from another deformity, such as kyphosis (Figure 15-7); (5) tight and commonly strong muscles (see Table 15-1); (6) spondylolisthesis; (7) congenital problems, such as bilateral congenital dislocation of the hip; (8) failure of segmentation of the neural arch of a facet joint segment; or (9) fashion (e.g., wearing high-heeled shoes). There are two types of exaggerated lordosis, pathological lordosis and swayback deformity.

Pathological Lordosis. In the patient with pathological lordosis, one may often observe sagging shoulders (scapulae are protracted and arms are medially rotated), medial rotation of the legs, and poking forward of the head so that it is in front of the center of gravity (Figure 15-8). This posture is adopted in an attempt to keep the center of gravity where it should be. Deviation in one part of the body often leads to deviation in another part of the body in an attempt to maintain the correct center of gravity and the correct visual plane. This type of exaggerated lordosis is the most common postural deviation seen.

The pelvic angle, normally approximately 30°, is increased with lordosis. With excessive or pathological lordosis, there is an increase in the pelvic angle to approximately 40°, accompanied by a mobile spine and an anterior pelvic tilt. Exaggerated lumbar lordosis is usually accompanied by weakness of the deep lumbar extensors and tightness of the hip flexors and tensor fasciae latae combined with weak abdominals (see Table 15-1).[10]

Swayback Deformity. With a swayback deformity, there is increased pelvic inclination to approximately 40°, and the thoracolumbar spine exhibits a kyphosis (Figure 15-9). A swayback deformity results in the spine's bending back rather sharply at the lumbosacral angle. With this postural deformity, the entire pelvis shifts anteriorly, causing the hips to move into extension. To maintain the center of gravity in its normal position, the thoracic spine flexes on the lumbar spine. The result is an increase in the lumbar and thoracic curves. Such a deformity may be associated with tightness of the hip extensors, lower lumbar extensors, and upper abdominals, along with weakness of the hip flexors, lower abdominals, and lower thoracic extensors (Table 15-2).[1]

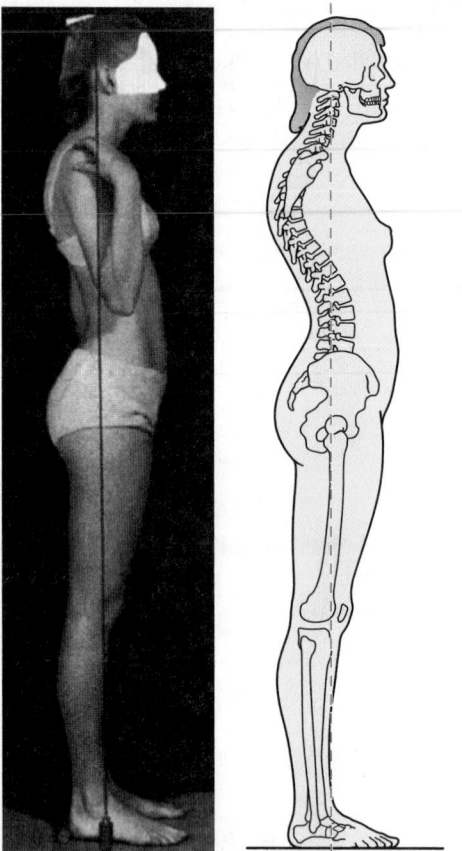

Figure 15-7 Faulty posture illustrating exaggerated lordosis and kyphosis. (From Kendall FP, McCreary EK: Muscles: testing and function, Baltimore, 1983, Williams & Wilkins, p. 281.)

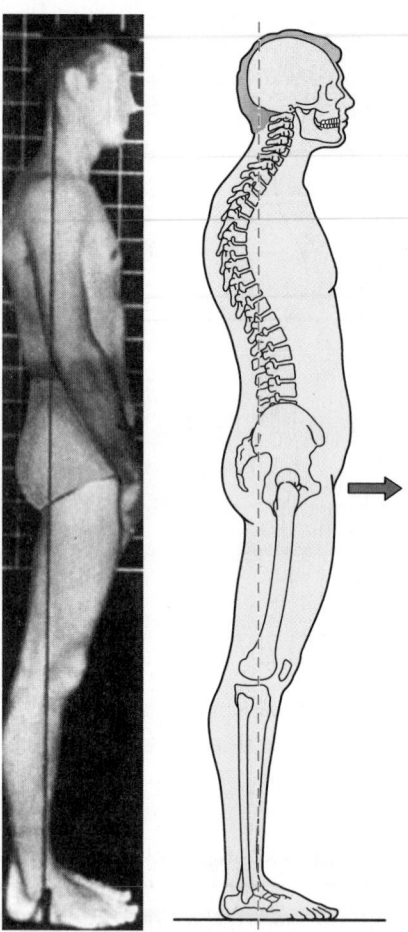

Figure 15-9 Faulty posture illustrating a swayback. (From Kendall FP, McCreary EK: Muscles: testing and function, Baltimore, 1983, Williams & Wilkins, p. 284.)

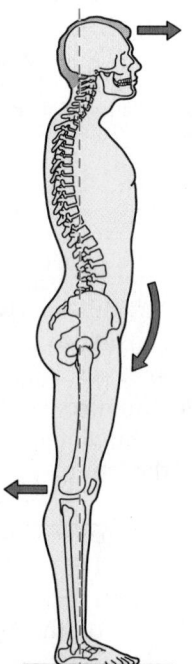

Figure 15-8 Pathological lordosis with compensatory forward head posture.

Kyphosis

Kyphosis is a posterior curvature of the spine (Figures 15-10 and 15-11).[7,9,11-15] Pathologically, it is an exaggeration of the normal curve found in the thoracic spine. There are several causes of kyphosis, including tuberculosis, vertebral compression fractures, Scheuermann disease, ankylosing spondylitis, senile osteoporosis, tumors, compensation in conjunction with lordosis, and congenital anomalies.[11] The congenital anomalies include a partial segmental defect, as seen in osseous metaplasia, or centrum hypoplasia and aplasia.[14,16,17] In addition, paralysis may lead to a kyphosis because of the loss of muscle action needed to maintain the correct posture combined with the forces of gravity.

Pathological conditions, such as Scheuermann vertebral osteochondritis, may also result in a structural kyphosis (Figure 15-12). In this condition, inflammation of the bone and cartilage occurs around the ring epiphysis of the vertebral body. The condition often leads to an anterior wedging of the vertebra. It is a growth disorder that affects approximately 10% of the population, and in most

TABLE **15-2**

Changes Associated with Swayback

Body segment alignment	Long kyphosis with pelvis the most anterior body segment, hip joint moves forwards of posture line (thoracic spine mobile to compensate) Lower lumbar area flattens Pelvis neutral or in posterior tilt Hip and knee joints hyperextended Where subject stands predominantly on one leg, pelvis is tilted down to non-favored side Favored leg appears longer in standing only
Muscles commonly elongated and weak	One joint hip flexors External obliques Lower thoracic extensors Lower abdominals Neck flexors Where one leg is favored, gluteus medius (especially posterior fibers) on favored side
Muscles commonly short and strong	Hamstrings Hip extensors Upper fibers of internal obliques Internal intercostals Low back musculature short but not strong Where one leg is favored, tensor fascia lata is strong and iliotibial band is tight on favored side
Joints commonly affected	Lumbar spine Pelvic joints Thoracic spine Hip joints Thoracic spine Scapulothoracic joints Glenohumeral joints Cervical spine Atlanto-occipital joints Temporomandibular joints

Adapted from Kendall FP, McCreary EK: Muscles: testing and function, Baltimore, 1983, Williams & Wilkins; Giallonardo LM: Posture. In Myers RS, editor: Saunders manual of physical therapy practice, Philadelphia, 1995, WB Saunders.

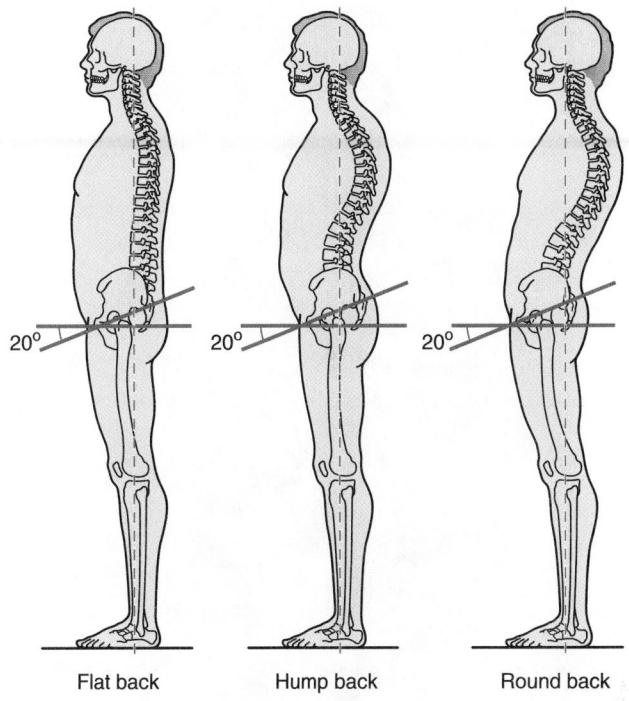

Flat back   Hump back   Round back

Figure 15-10 Examples of kyphosis.

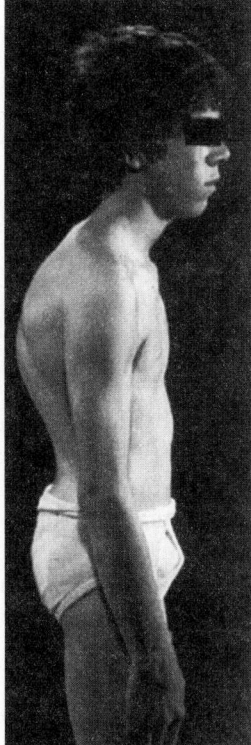

Figure 15-11 Faulty posture illustrating thoracic kyphosis. (From Moe JH, Bradford DS, Winter RB, et al: Scoliosis and other spinal deformities, Philadelphia, 1978, WB Saunders, p. 152.)

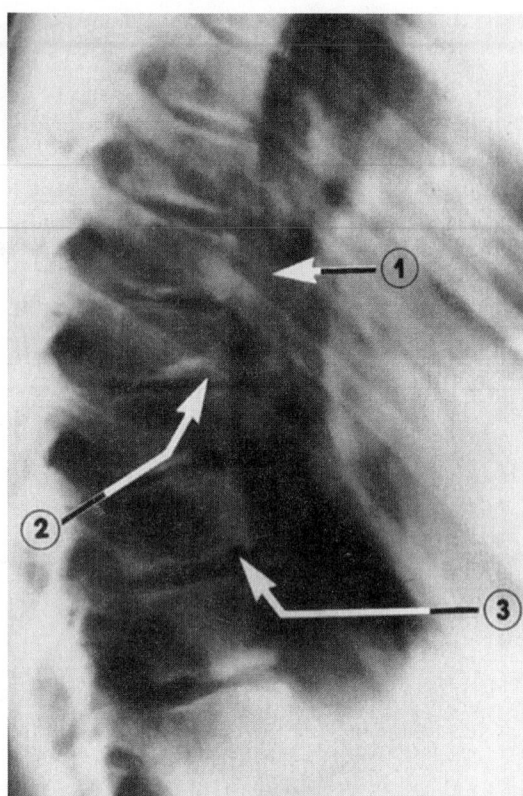

Figure 15-12 A classic x-ray appearance of the spine in a patient with Scheuermann disease. Note the wedged vertebra *(1)*, Schmorl nodules *(2)*, and marked irregularity of the vertebral end plates *(3)*. (From Moe JH, Bradford DS, Winter RB, et al: Scoliosis and other spinal deformities, Philadelphia, 1978, WB Saunders, p. 332.)

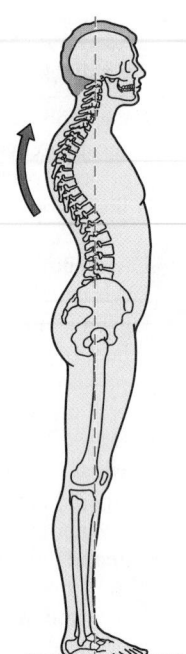

Figure 15-13 Round back form of kyphosis.

cases several vertebrae are affected. The most common area for the disease to occur is between T10 and L2.

The four types of kyphosis are round back, humpback, flat back, and dowager's hump.

Round Back. The patient with a round back has a long, rounded curve with decreased pelvic inclination (less than 30°) and thoracolumbar kyphosis. The patient often presents with the trunk flexed forward and a decreased lumbar curve (Figure 15-13). On examination, there are tight hip extensors and trunk flexors with weak hip flexors and lumbar extensors (Table 15-3).

Humpback or Gibbus. With humpback, there is a localized, sharp posterior angulation in the thoracic spine (Figure 15-14). This is commonly a structural deformity as the result of a fracture or pathology.

Flat Back. A patient with flat back has decreased pelvic inclination to 20° and a mobile lumbar spine (Figure 15-15). Table 15-4 outlines the structures affected.

Dowager's Hump. Dowager's hump is often seen in older patients, especially women. The deformity commonly is caused by osteoporosis, in which the thoracic vertebral bodies begin to degenerate and wedge in an anterior direction, resulting in a kyphosis (Figure 15-16).

TABLE **15-3**

Changes Associated with a Round Back Form of Kyphosis

Body segment alignment	Head held forward with cervical spine hyperextended
	Scapulae may be protracted
	Increased thoracic kyphosis
	Hips flexed, knees hyperextended
	Head is usually most anteriorly placed body segment
Muscles commonly elongated and weak	Neck flexors
	Upper erector spinae
	External obliques
	If scapulae are protracted, middle and lower trapezius
	Thoracic erector spinae
	Rhomboids
Muscles commonly short and strong	Neck extensors
	Hip flexors
	If scapulae are protracted, serratus anterior, pectoralis major and/ or minor, upper trapezius, levator scapulae
	Upper abdominal muscles
	Intercostales
Joints commonly affected	Thoracic spine
	Scapulothoracic joints
	Glenohumeral joints

Adapted from Kendall FP, McCreary EK: Muscles: testing and function, Baltimore, 1983, Williams & Wilkins; Giallonardo LM: Posture. In Myers RS, editor: Saunders manual of physical therapy practice, Philadelphia, 1995, WB Saunders.

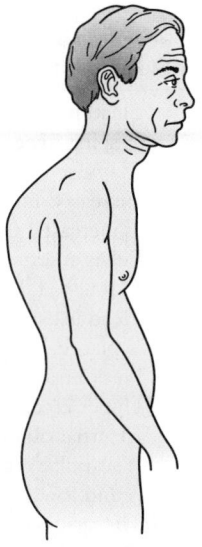

Figure 15-14 Humpback or gibbus deformity.

TABLE **15-4**

Changes Associated with a Flat Back Form of Kyphosis

Body segment alignment	Loss of lordosis with pelvis in posterior tilt Hip and knee joints hyperextended Forward head posture with increased flexion to upper thoracic spine
Muscles commonly elongated and weak	One joint hip flexors Lumbar extensors Local stabilizers (multifidus, rotatores) Scapular protractors (?) Anterior intercostals
Muscles commonly short and strong	Hamstrings Abdominals may be strong with back muscles slightly elongated Hip extensors Scapular retractors (?) Thoracic erector spinae
Joints commonly affected	Lumbar spine Pelvic joints Scapulothoracic joints (?) Thoracic spine (?) Cervical spine (?)

Adapted from Kendall FP, McCreary EK: Muscles: testing and function, Baltimore, 1983, Williams & Wilkins; Giallonardo LM: Posture. In Myers RS, editor: Saunders manual of physical therapy practice, Philadelphia, 1995, WB Saunders.

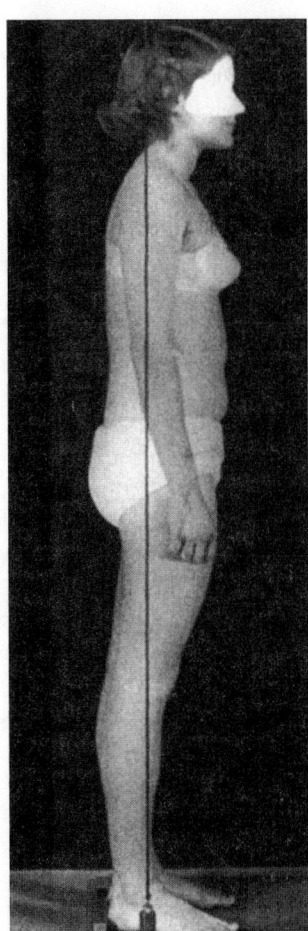 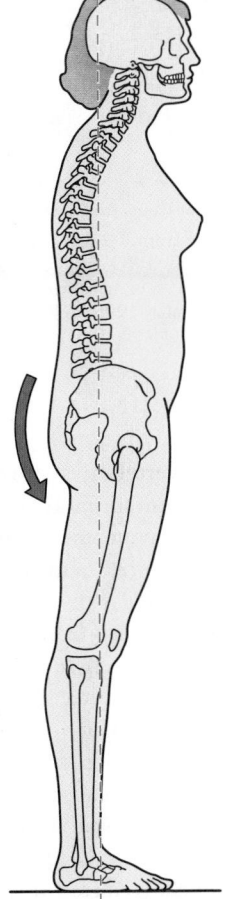

Figure 15-15 Faulty posture illustrating flat back. (From Kendall FP, McCreary EK: Muscles: testing and function, Baltimore, 1983, Williams & Wilkins, p. 285.)

Kypholordotic Posture. In some cases, both the thoracic and lumbar spine may be affected. Figure 15-17 and Table 15-5 outline the changes seen with this posture.

Scoliosis

Scoliosis is a lateral curvature of the spine.[11,13,18-24] This type of deformity is often the most visible spinal deformity, especially in its severe forms. The most famous example of scoliosis is the "hunchback of Notre Dame." In the cervical spine, a scoliosis is called a **torticollis.** There are several types of scoliosis, some of which are nonstructural (Figure 15-18) and some of which are structural. **Nonstructural** or **functional scoliosis** may be caused by postural problems, hysteria, nerve root irritation, inflammation, or compensation caused by leg length discrepancy or contracture (in the lumbar spine) (Table 15-6).[23] **Structural scoliosis** primarily involves bony deformity, which may be congenital or acquired, or excessive muscle weakness, as seen in a person with long-term quadriplegia. This type of scoliosis may be caused by

AGE   20   75

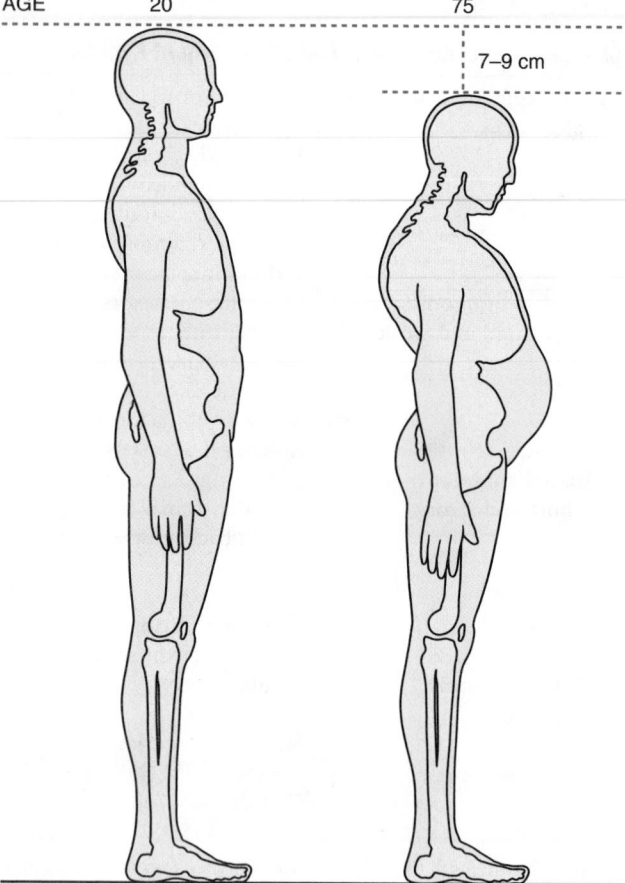

7–9 cm

Figure 15-16 Loss of height resulting from osteoporosis leading to dowager's hump. Note the flexed head and protruding abdomen, which occur partially to maintain the center of gravity in its normal position.

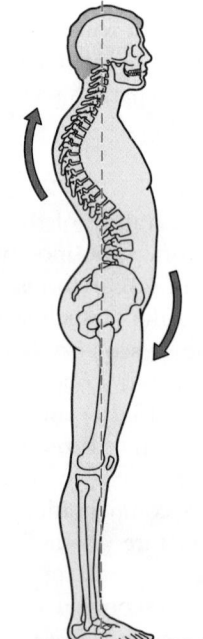

Figure 15-17 Kypholordotic posture.

TABLE **15-5**

Changes Associated with Kypholordotic Posture

Body segment alignment	Head held forward with cervical spine hyperextended Scapulae may be protracted Increased lumbar lordosis, and increased thoracic kyphosis Pelvis anteriorly tilted Hip flexed, knee hyperextended Head is usually most anteriorly placed body segment
Muscles commonly elongated and weak	Neck flexors Upper erector spinae External obliques If scapulae are protracted, middle and lower trapezius Thoracic erector spinae Middle and lower trapezius Rhomboids
Muscles commonly short and strong	Neck extensors Hip flexors If scapulae are protracted, serratus anterior, pectoralis major and/or minor, upper trapezius Intercostales
Joints commonly affected	Thoracic spine Lumbar spine Scapulothoracic joints Glenohumeral joints

Adapted from Kendall FP, McCreary EK: Muscles: testing and function, Baltimore, 1983, Williams & Wilkins; Giallonardo LM: Posture. In Myers RS, editor: Saunders manual of physical therapy practice, Philadelphia, 1995, WB Saunders.

wedge vertebra, hemivertebra (Figure 15-19), or failure of segmentation. It may be idiopathic (genetic) (Figure 15-20); neuromuscular, resulting from an upper or lower motor neuron lesion; or myopathic, resulting from muscular disease; or it may be caused by arthrogryposis, resulting from persistent joint contracture,[17] or by conditions such as neurofibromatosis, mesenchymal disorders, or trauma. It may accompany infection, tumors, and inflammatory conditions that result in bone destruction. Torticollis may occur because of neuromuscular problems, because of congenital problems (abnormal sternocleidomastoid muscle), or in conjunction with malocclusion of the temporomandibular joints or with ear problems (referred to the cervical spine).

With structural scoliosis, the patient lacks normal flexibility, and side bending becomes asymmetrical. This type of scoliosis may be progressive, and the curve does not disappear on forward flexion. It is most commonly seen in the thoracic or thoracolumbar spine. With nonstructural scoliosis, there is no bony deformity; this type of

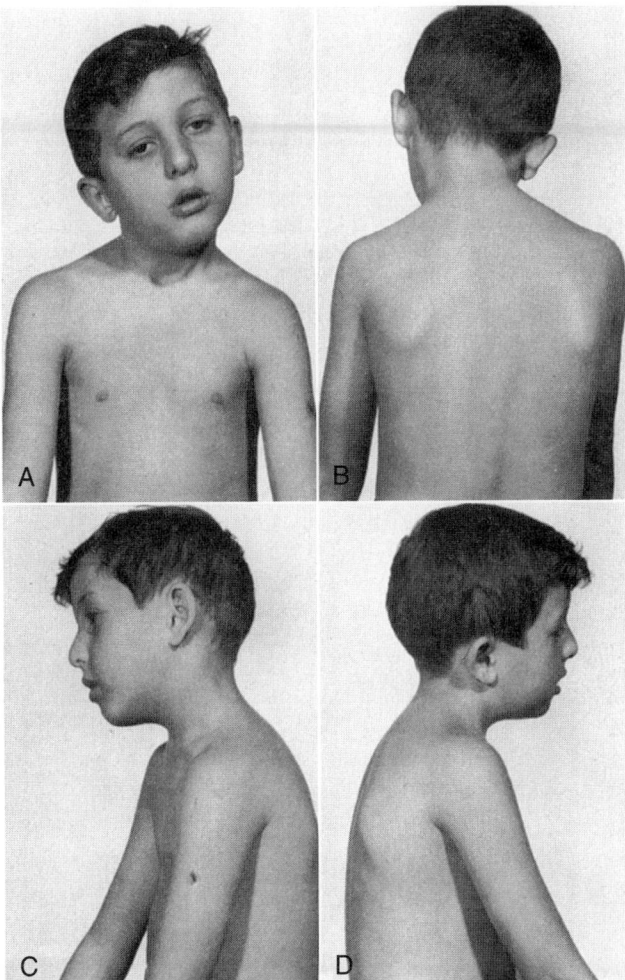

Figure 15-18 Congenital muscular torticollis on the right in a 10-year-old boy. Note the contracted sternocleidomastoid muscle. (From Tachdjian MO: Pediatric orthopedics, Philadelphia, 1972, WB Saunders, p. 74.)

TABLE 15-6

Changes Associated with Postural Scoliosis

Body segment alignment	Spine curves to left or right
	May have single or double curve or one main curve and one or two compensatory curves
	Ribs may protrude on one side and be depressed (paravertebral valley) on the other side ("hump and hollow" on forward flexion because of vertebral rotation)
	May have short leg—pelvis tilted laterally—concave side high
	Shoulder/scapula may drop on concavity side of curve
Muscles commonly elongated and weak	Muscles on the convex side
	Hip abductor muscles on concave side
	Foot pronator muscles on the long side
Muscles commonly short and strong	Muscles on concave side
	Hip adductors on convex side
	Foot supinators on short side
Joints commonly affected	Lumbar spine
	Thoracic spine
	Pelvic joints
	Hip joints
	Foot joints
	Scapulothoracic joints
	Glenohumeral joints
	Cervical spine (torticollis)
	Atlanto-occipital joints
	Temporomandibular joints

Adapted from Kendall FP, McCreary EK: Muscles: testing and function, Baltimore, 1983, Williams & Wilkins; Giallonardo LM: Posture. In Myers RS, editor: Saunders manual of physical therapy practice, Philadelphia, 1995, WB Saunders.

scoliosis is not progressive. The spine shows segmental limitation, and side bending is usually symmetrical. The nonstructural scoliotic curve disappears on forward flexion. This type of scoliosis is usually found in the cervical, lumbar, or thoracolumbar area.

Idiopathic scoliosis accounts for 75% to 85% of all cases of structural scoliosis. The vertebral bodies rotate into the convexity of the curve with the spinous processes going toward the concavity of the curve. There is a fixed rotational prominence on the convex side, which is best seen on forward flexion from the skyline view. This prominence is sometimes called a "razorback spine." The disc spaces are narrowed on the concave side and widened on the convex side. There is distortion of the vertebral body, and vital capacity is considerably lowered if the lateral curvature exceeds 60°; compression and malposition of the organs within the rib cage also occur. Examples of scoliotic curves are shown in Figure 15-21.

PATIENT HISTORY

As with any history, the examiner must ensure that the information obtained is as complete as possible. By listening to the patient, the examiner can often comprehend the problem. The information should include a history of the problem, the patient's general condition and health, and family history. If a child is being examined, the examiner must also obtain prenatal and postnatal histories, including the health of or injuries experienced by the mother during pregnancy, any complications during pregnancy or delivery, and drugs taken by the mother during that period, especially during the first trimester, which is the period when most of the congenital anomalies develop.

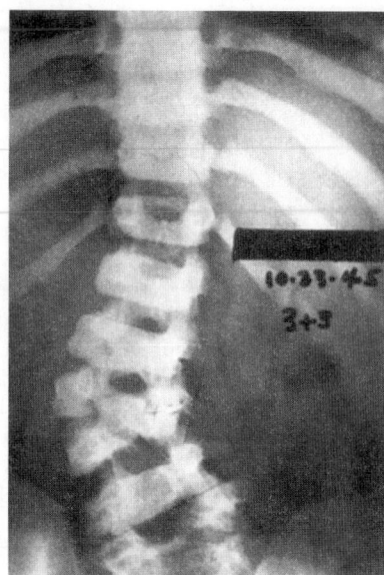

Figure 15-19 Scoliosis caused by hemivertebra. (From Moe JH, Bradford DS, Winter RB, et al: Scoliosis and other spinal deformities, Philadelphia, 1978, WB Saunders, p. 134.)

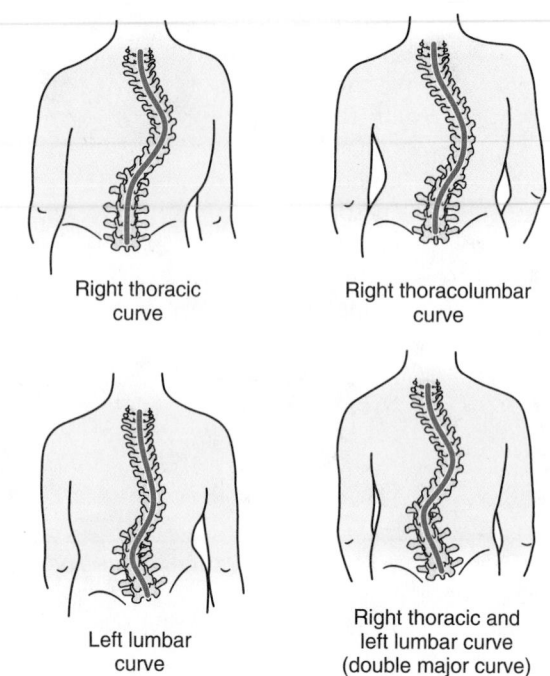

Right thoracic curve

Right thoracolumbar curve

Left lumbar curve

Right thoracic and left lumbar curve (double major curve)

Figure 15-21 Examples of scoliosis curve patterns.

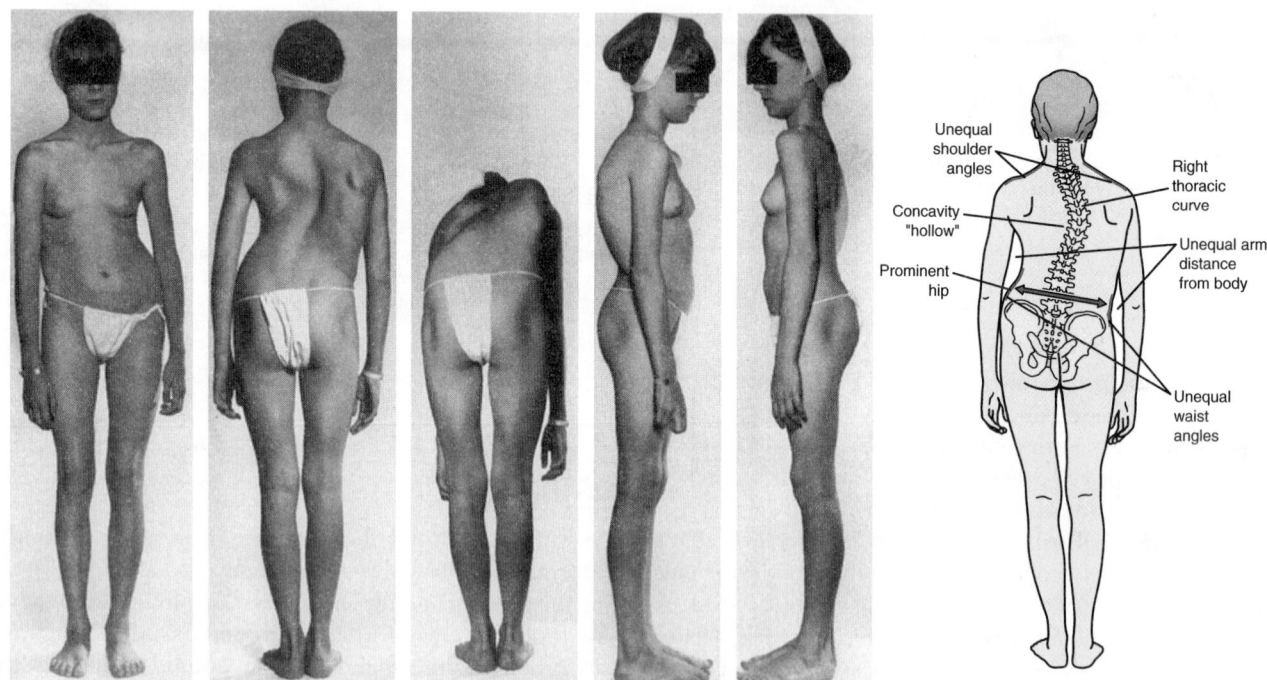

Figure 15-20 Idiopathic structural right thoracic scoliosis. Line drawing shows prominent features of scoliosis. (Photographs from Tachdjian MO: Pediatric orthopedics, Philadelphia, 1972, WB Saunders, p. 1200.)

It should be remembered that it is unusual for a patient to present with just a postural problem. It is the symptoms produced by the pathology that is causing the postural abnormality that initiate the consultation. The examiner therefore must be cognizant of various underlying pathological conditions when assessing posture.

The following questions should be asked:

1. *Was there any history of injury?* If so, what was the mechanism of injury? For example, lifting often causes lower spine problems, which may lead to altered posture.
2. *If there is a history of injury, had the patient experienced any back injury or pain previously?* If so, what caused that injury or pain? Was it a specific posture, sustained posture, or caused by repetitive movements? If so, what were the postures and/or movements?
3. *Are there any postures (e.g., standing with one foot on low stool, sitting with legs crossed) that give the patient relief or increase the patient's symptoms?*[25] The examiner can later test these postures to help determine the problem.
4. *Does the family have any history of back problems or other special problems?* Conditions, such as hemivertebra, scoliosis, and Klippel-Feil syndrome, may be congenital.
5. *Has the patient had any previous illnesses, surgery, or severe injuries?*
6. *Is there a history of any other conditions, such as connective tissue diseases, that have a high incidence of associated spinal problems?*
7. *Does footwear make a difference to the patient's posture or symptoms?* For example, high-heeled shoes often lead to excessive lordosis.[26]
8. *How old is the patient?* Many spinal problems begin in childhood or are the result of degeneration in the aged population.
9. *In the child, has there been a growth spurt?* If so, when did it begin? Growth spurts often lead to tight muscles and altered posture.
10. *For females, when did menarche begin?* Does back pain appear to be associated with menses? Menarche indicates the point at which approximately two thirds of the female adolescent growth spurt has been completed.
11. *For males, has there been a voice change?* If so, when? This question also gives an indication of maturity or onset of puberty.
12. *If a deformity is present, is it progressive or stationary?*
13. *Does the patient experience any neurological symptoms (e.g., a "pins and needles" feeling or numbness)?*
14. *What is the nature, extent, type, and duration of the pain?*
15. *What positions or activities increase the pain or discomfort?*

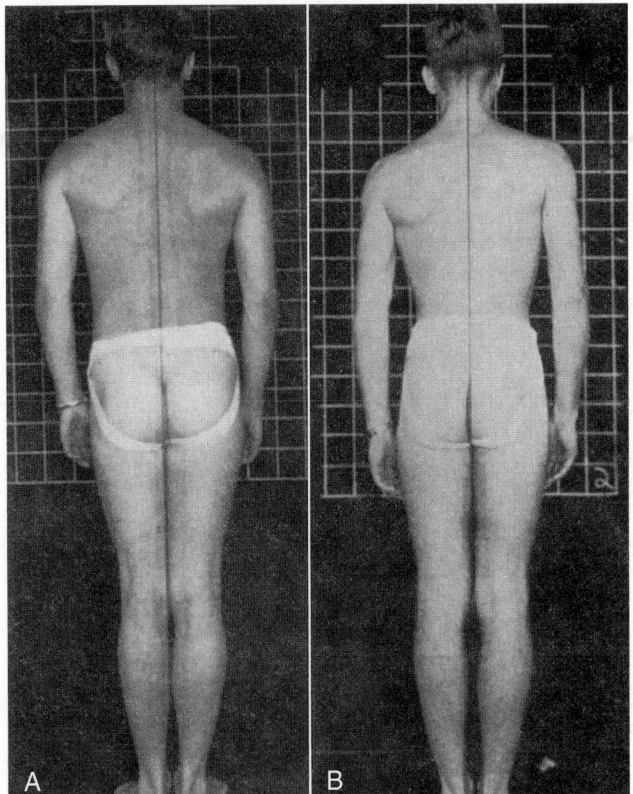

Figure 15-22 Effect of handedness on posture. A, Right hand dominant. **B,** Left hand dominant. (From Kendall FP, McCreary EK: Muscles: testing and function, Baltimore, 1983, Williams & Wilkins, p. 294.)

16. *What positions or activities decrease the pain or discomfort?*
17. *For children, is there difficulty in fitting clothes?* For example, with scoliosis, the hem of a dress is usually uneven because of the spinal curvature.
18. *Does the patient have any difficulty breathing?* Structural deformities, such as idiopathic scoliosis, can lead to breathing problems in severe cases.
19. *Which hand is the dominant one?* Often, the dominant side shows a lower shoulder with the hip slightly deviated to that side (Figure 15-22). The spine may deviate slightly to the opposite side, and the opposite foot is slightly more pronated.[7] The gluteus medius on the dominant side may also be weaker.
20. *Has there been any previous treatment?* If so, what was it? Was it successful?

OBSERVATION

Observation is the primary method of assessing posture and should be included in every assessment, looking for asymmetrical changes that may contribute to or be the result of faulty posture. The following sections outline static posture, which forms the basis of dynamic posture (e.g., walking, running, lifting, throwing).[2]

To assess posture correctly, the patient must be adequately undressed. Male patients should be in shorts, and female patients should be in a bra and shorts. Ideally, the patient should not wear shoes or stockings. However, if the patient uses walking aids, braces, collars, or orthotics, they should be noted and may be used after the patient has been assessed in the "natural" state to determine the effect of the appliances.

The patient should be examined in the habitual, relaxed posture that is usually adopted. Often, it takes some time for the patient to adopt the usual posture because of tenseness, uneasiness, or uncertainty.

In the standing and sitting positions, the assessment is the same as the observation for the upper and lower limb scanning examinations of the cervical and lumbar spines. Assessment of posture should be carried out with the patient in the standing, sitting, and lying (supine and prone) positions. After the patient has been examined in these positions, the examiner may decide to include other habitual, sustained, or repetitive postures assumed by the patient to see whether these postures increase or alter symptoms. The patient may also be assessed wearing different footwear to determine their effects on the posture and symptoms.

When observing a patient for abnormalities in posture, the examiner looks for asymmetry as a possible indication of what may be causing the postural fault (Figure 15-23). Some asymmetry between left and right sides is normal. The examiner must be able to differentiate normal deviations from asymmetry caused by pathology. Functional asymmetries usually refer to changes in alignment that occur with changes in posture. For example, nonstructural scoliosis may be present in standing because of a short leg but disappear on forward flexion. Anatomical or structural asymmetries are due to structural changes (e.g., idiopathic scoliosis).

As the examiner is watching for asymmetry, he or she should also note potential causes of asymmetry. For example, the examiner should always watch for the presence of muscle wasting, soft tissue or bony swelling or enlargement, scars, and skin changes that may indicate present or past pathology.

Standing

The examiner should first determine the patient's body type (Figure 15-24).[25] The three body types are **ectomorphic,** mesomorphic, and endomorphic. The ectomorph is a person who has a thin body build characterized by a relative prominence of structures developed from the embryonic ectoderm. The **mesomorph** has a muscular or sturdy body build characterized by relative prominence of structures developed by the embryonic mesoderm. The **endomorph** has a heavy or fat body build characterized by relative prominence of structures developed from the embryonic endoderm.

Body Types

- Ectomorph
- Mesomorph
- Endomorph

In addition to body type, the examiner should note the emotional attitude of the patient. Is the patient tense, bored, or lethargic? Does the patient appear to be healthy, emaciated, or overweight? Answers to these questions can help the examiner determine how much must be done to correct any problems. For example, if the patient is lethargic, it may take longer to correct the problem than if he or she appears truly interested in correcting the problem. The examiner must remember that posture is in many ways an expression of one's personality, sense of well-being, and self-esteem.

Anterior View

When observing the patient from the front (Table 15-7; see Figure 15-1, *A*), the examiner should note whether the following conditions hold true:

1. The head is straight on the shoulders (in midline). The examiner should note whether the head is habitually tilted to one side or rotated (e.g., torticollis) (Figure 15-25). The cause of altered head position must be established. For example, it may be the result of weak muscles, trauma, a hearing loss, temporomandibular joint problems, or the wearing of bifocal glasses.

2. The posture of the jaw is normal. In the resting position, normal jaw posture is when the lips are gently pressed together, the teeth are slightly apart (freeway space), and the tip of the tongue is behind the upper teeth in the roof of the mouth. This position maintains the mandible in a good posture (i.e., slight negative pressure in the mouth reduces the work of the muscles). It also enables respiration through the nose and diaphragmatic breathing.

3. The tip of the nose is in line with the manubrium sternum, xiphisternum, and umbilicus. This line is the **anterior line of reference** used to divide the body into right and left halves (see Figure 15-1, *A*). If the umbilicus is used as a reference point, the examiner should remember that the umbilicus is almost always slightly off center.

4. The upper trapezius neck line is equal on both sides. The muscle bulk of the trapezius muscles should be equal, and the slope of the muscles should be approximately equal. Because the dominant arm usually shows greater laxity by being slightly lower, the slope on the dominant side may be slightly greater.

5. The shoulders are level. In most cases, the dominant side is slightly lower.

POSTURE EVALUATION

NAME: AGE: SEX: HEIGHT: WEIGHT: DATE:

Body type: Ectomorph / Mesomorph / Endomorph / Slight Build / Medium Build / Heavy Build

Uncorrected Standing A   Corrected (Talus in Neutral) Standing B   Postural Deformity Corrected C

ANTERIOR VIEW	Comments:	
Head (aligned, forward, flexed, extended)		
Mandible (resting position, retracted)		
Shoulders (level, uneven)		
Rib cage (symmetric, asymmetric)		
Scoliosis (left, right, lumbar, thoracic, cervical)		
Pelvis (level, anterior/posterior tilt)		
Hips (coxa vara, coxa valga, anteversion, retroversion)		
Femurs (alignment, torsion)		
Knees (level, genu varum, genu valgum)		
Patellar position		
Tibias (alignment, torsions)		
Ankles (inversion, eversion)		
Rearfoot/forefoot alignment		
Feet (pes cavus, pes planus, supination/pronation)		
Toes (alignment, deformities)		
Leg length		
LATERAL VIEW	**Comments:**	
Head (forward, flexed/extended)		
Mandible (resting, protracted/retracted)		
Scapulae (winging, elevation/depression)		
Thoracic kyphosis (increased/decreased)		
Lumbar lordosis (increased/decreased)		
Pelvis (anterior/posterior tilt)		
Knees (hyperextension/flexion)		
Feet (longitudinal arch)		
POSTERIOR VIEW	**Comments:**	
Head (alignment, tilt)		
Shoulders (level)		
Scapulae (bilateral symmetry)		
Spine C-1 to sacrum (rotations, deviations)		
Pelvis (level, tilt)		
Sacrum (level at base and inferior lateral angles)		
Hips (level, uneven)		
Knees (creases level/uneven)		
Leg (rearfoot alignment)		
Ankles (inversion/eversion)		
Calcaneal position (inverted/everted)		

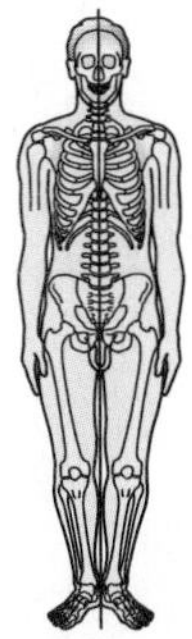

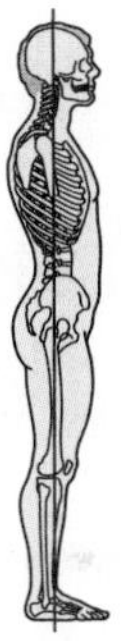

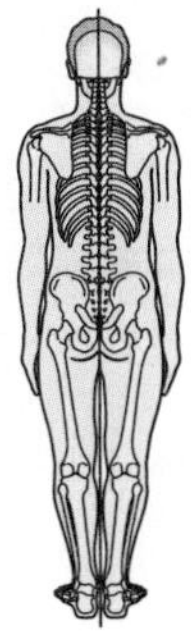

Pertinent Medical History:

Pertinent Radiographic Findings / Other Tests:

Figure 15-23 Example of standing posture evaluation form. Information is obtained by visual observation and palpation. (Modified from Richardson JK, Iglarsh ZA: Clinical orthopedic physical therapy, Philadelphia, 1994, WB Saunders.)

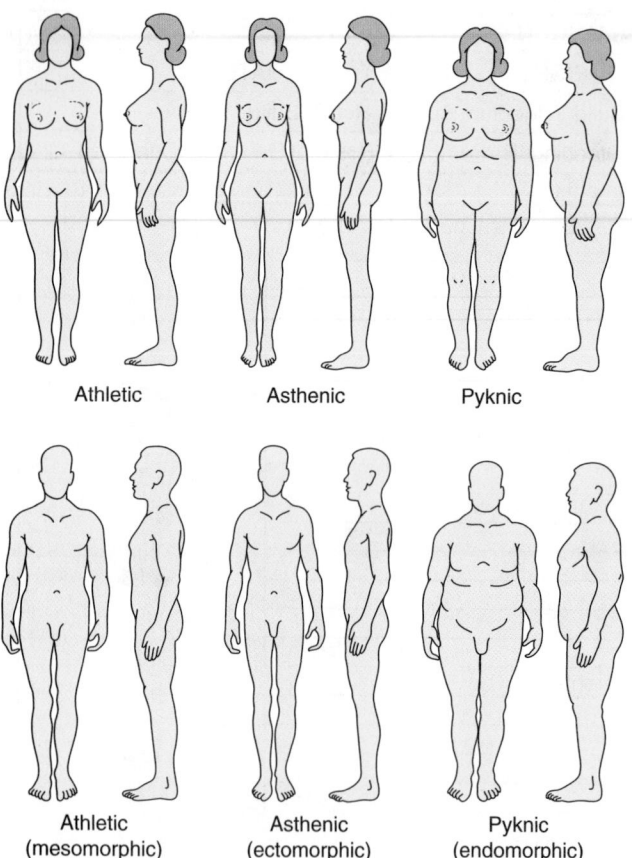

Athletic   Asthenic   Pyknic

Athletic
(mesomorphic)
Asthenic
(ectomorphic)
Pyknic
(endomorphic)

Figure 15-24 Male and female body types. (From Debrunner HU: Orthopedic diagnosis, London, 1970, E & S Livingstone, p. 86.)

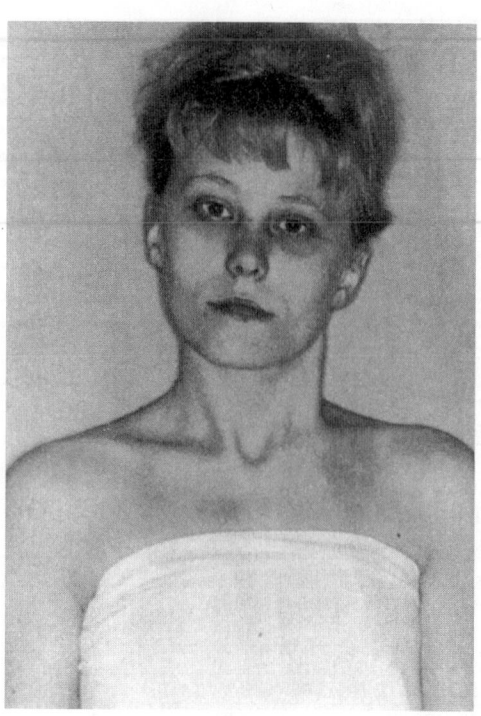

Figure 15-25 Congenital torticollis in 18-year-old girl. Note the asymmetry of the face. (From Tachdjian MO: Pediatric orthopedics, Philadelphia, 1972, WB Saunders, p. 68.)

TABLE **15-7**

Alignment in the Standing Posture: Anterior View

Body Segment	Line of Gravity Location	Observation
Head	Passes through middle of the forehead, nose and chin	Eyes and ears should be level and symmetrical
Neck/shoulders		Right and left angles between shoulders and neck should be symmetrical; clavicles also should be symmetrical
Chest	Passes through the middle of the xyphoid process	Ribs on each side should be symmetrical
Abdomen/hips	Passes through the umbilicus (navel)	Right and left waist angles should be symmetrical
Hips/pelvis	Passes on a line equidistant from the right and left ASISs; passes through the symphysis pubis	ASISs should be level
Knees	Passes between knees equidistant from medial femoral condyles	Patella should be symmetrical and facing straight ahead
Ankles/feet	Passes between ankles equidistant from the medial malleoli	Malleoli should be symmetrical, and feet should be parallel; toes should not be curled, overlapping, or deviated to one side

From Levangie PK, Norkin CC: Joint structures and function—a comprehensive analysis, Philadelphia, 2005, FA Davis, p. 498.
ASIS, Anterior superior iliac spine.

6. The clavicles and acromioclavicular joints are level and equal. They should be symmetrical; any deviation should be noted. Deviations may be caused by subluxations or dislocations of the acromioclavicular or sternoclavicular joints, fractures, or clavicular rotation.

7. There is no protrusion, depression, or lateralization of the sternum, ribs, or costal cartilage. If there are changes, they should be noted.

8. The waist angles are equal, and the arms are equidistant from the waist. If a scoliosis is present, one arm hangs closer to the body than the other arm. The examiner should also note whether the arms are equally rotated medially or laterally.

9. The carrying angles at each elbow are equal. Any deviation should be noted. The normal carrying angle varies from 5° to 15°.

10. The palms of both hands face the body in the relaxed standing position. Any differences should be noted and may give an indication of rotation in the upper limb.

11. The "high points" of the iliac crest are the same height on each side (Figure 15-26). With a scoliosis, the patient may feel that one hip is "higher" than the other. This apparent high pelvis results from the lateral shift of the trunk; the pelvis is usually level. The same condition can cause the patient to feel that one leg is shorter than the other.

12. The anterior superior iliac spines (ASISs) are level. If one ASIS is higher than the other, there is a possibility that one leg is shorter than the other or that the pelvis is rotated more or shifted up or down more on one side.

13. The pubic bones are level at the symphysis pubis. Any deviation should be noted.

14. The patellae of the knees point straight ahead. Sometimes the patellae face outward ("frog eyes" patellae) or inward ("squinting" patellae). The position of the patella may also be altered by torsion of the femoral neck (anteversion-retroversion), femoral shaft, or tibial shaft.

15. The knees are straight. The knees may be in genu varum or genu valgum. If the ankles are together and the knees are more than two finger-widths apart, the patient has some genu varum. If the knees are touching and the feet are apart, the patient has some genu valgum. Genu valgum is more likely to be seen in females. The examiner should note whether the deformity results from the femur, tibia, or both. In children, the knees go through a progression of being straight, going into genu varum (Figure 15-27), being straight, going into genu valgum (Figure 15-28), and finally being straight again during the first 6 years of life (see Figure 15-4).[13]

16. The heads of the fibulae are level.

17. The medial and lateral malleoli of the ankles are level. Normally, the medial malleoli are slightly anterior to the lateral malleoli, but the lateral malleoli extend farther distally.

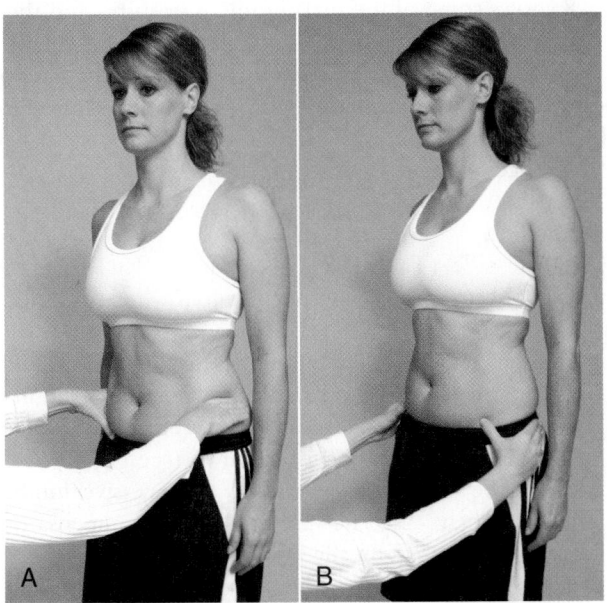

Figure 15-26 Viewing height equality. A, Iliac crests. **B,** Anterior superior iliac spines (ASISs).

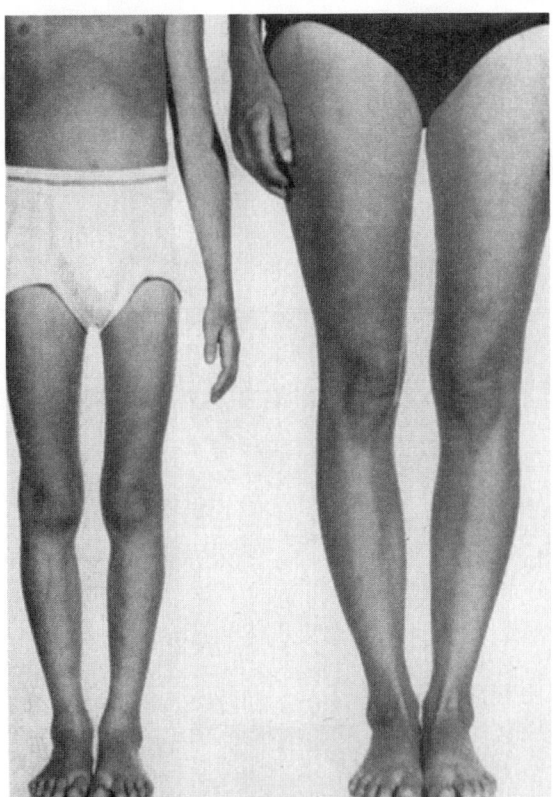

Figure 15-27 Bilateral genu varum in mother and son. Note the associated medial tibial torsion. (From Tachdjian MO: *Pediatric orthopedics,* Philadelphia, 1972, WB Saunders, p. 1462.)

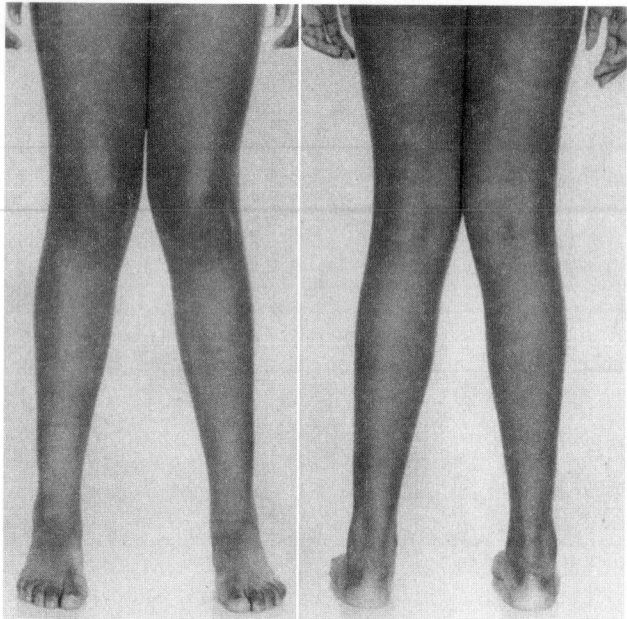

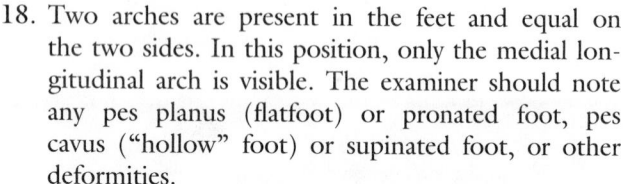

Figure 15-28 Bilateral genu valgum in an adolescent. (From Tachdjian MO: Pediatric orthopedics, Philadelphia, 1972, WB Saunders, p. 1467.)

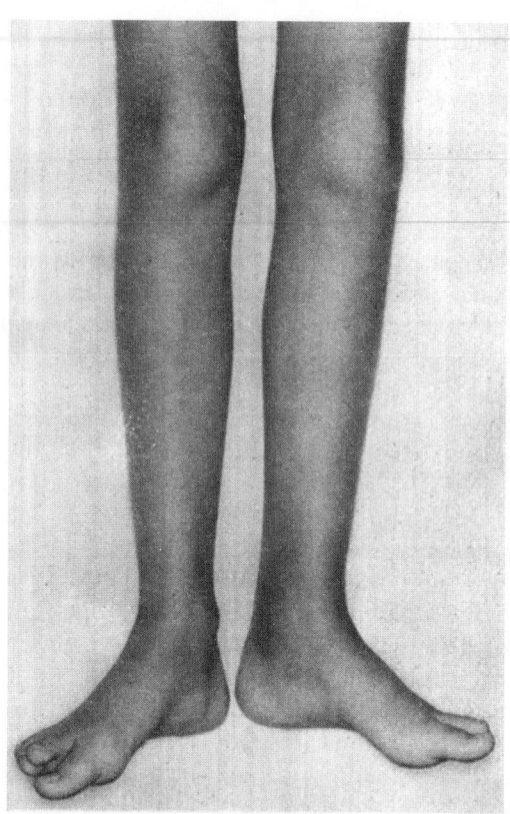

Figure 15-29 Exaggerated lateral tibial torsion. In stance, with the patellae facing straight forward, the feet point outward. (From Tachdjian MO: Pediatric orthopedics, Philadelphia, 1972, WB Saunders, p. 1461.)

18. Two arches are present in the feet and equal on the two sides. In this position, only the medial longitudinal arch is visible. The examiner should note any pes planus (flatfoot) or pronated foot, pes cavus ("hollow" foot) or supinated foot, or other deformities.

19. The feet angle out equally (this Fick angle is usually 5° to 18° [see Figure 14-14]; Figure 15-29). This finding means that the tibias are normally slightly laterally rotated (lateral tibial torsion). The presence of pigeon toes usually indicates medial rotation of the tibias (medial tibial torsion), especially if the patellae face straight ahead. If the patellae face inward (squinting patellae) in the presence of "pigeon toes" or outward, the problem may be in the femur (abnormal femoral torsion or hip retroversion-anteversion problems).

20. There is no bowing of bone. Any bowing may indicate diseases, such as osteomalacia or osteoporosis.

21. The bony and soft-tissue contours are equally symmetrical on the two halves of the body. Any indication of muscle wasting, muscle hypertrophy on one side, or bony asymmetry should be noted. Such a finding may indicate muscle or nerve pathology, or it may simply be related to the patient's job or recreational pursuits. For example, a rodeo bull rider will show hypertrophy of the muscles and bones on one side. (The arm that he uses to hang on!)

In addition, the patient's skin is observed for abnormalities, such as hairy patches (e.g., diastematomyelia), pigmented lesions (e.g., café au lait spots,

neurofibromatosis), subcutaneous tumors, and scars (e.g., Ehlers-Danlos syndrome), all of which may lead to or contribute to postural problems (Figure 15-30). Table 15-8 shows some of the malalignment postures and their effect.[2,13,27,28] Changes in one body segment cause changes in other segments as the body attempts to compensate or adjust for the malignment.[2] Compensatory postures are those that represent the body's attempt to normalize appearance or improve function.[2]

Lateral View

From the side (Table 15-9; see Figure 15-1, *B*), the examiner should note whether the following conditions hold true:

1. The earlobe is in line with the tip of the shoulder (acromion process) and the "high point" of the iliac crest. This line is the **lateral line of reference** dividing the body into front and back halves (see Figure 15-1, *B*). If the chin pokes forward, an excessive lumbar lordosis may also be present. This compensatory change is caused by the body's attempt to maintain the center of gravity in the normal position.

2. Each spinal segment has a normal curve (Figure 15-31). Large gluteus maximus muscles or excessive

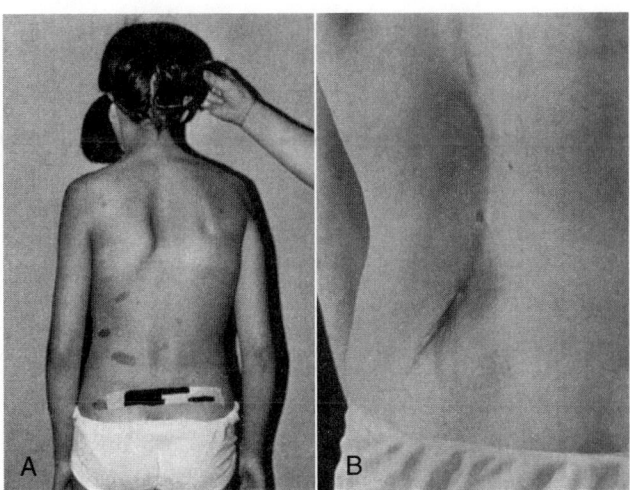

Figure 15-30 Abnormal skin markings. A, Café au lait areas of pigmentation seen in neurofibromatosis. **B,** Lumbar hair patch seen in diastematomyelia. (From Moe JH, Bradford DS, Winter RB, et al: Scoliosis and other spinal deformities, Philadelphia, 1978, WB Saunders, p. 20.)

fat may give the appearance of an exaggerated lordosis. The examiner should look at the spine in relation to the sacrum, not the gluteal muscles. Likewise, the scapulae may give the illusion of an increased kyphosis in the thoracic spine, especially if they are flat and the patient has rounded shoulders.

3. The shoulders are in proper alignment. If the shoulders droop forward (i.e., the scapulae protract), "rounded shoulders" are indicated. This improper alignment may be caused by habit or by tight pectoral muscles or weak scapular stabilizers.

4. The chest, abdominal, and back muscles have proper tone. Weakness or spasm of any of these muscles can lead to postural alterations.

5. There are no chest deformities, such as pectus carinatum (undue prominence of the sternum) or pectus excavatum (undue depression of the sternum).

6. The pelvic angle is normal (30°; Figure 15-32). The posterior superior iliac spine (PSIS) should be slightly higher than the ASIS.

TABLE 15-8

Malalignments Viewed Anteriorly[2,13,27,28]

Malalignment	Possible Correlated Motions or Postures	Possible Compensatory Motions or Postures
Torticollis	Rotation to same side limited Side flexion to opposite side limited	
Scoliosis	Side flexion to convex side limited Rotation to convex side limited Rib hump on convex side	
Lateral pelvic tilt (pelvic drop—right leg stance)	Right hip adduction Weak right abductors (positive Trendelenberg)	Right lumbar lateral flexion Tight left adductors
Lateral pelvic tilt (pelvic hitch—right leg stance)	Right hip abduction Weak left adductors	Left lumbar lateral flexion Tight right abductors
Forward rotation of one ilium on sacrum (right leg stance)	Right hip medial rotation Medial facing patella In-toeing Pronation of foot Long leg	Left lumbar rotation Scoliosis—concavity to left Knee flexion
Excessive anteversion	Toeing-in Subtalar pronation Lateral patellar subluxation Medial tibial torsion Medial femoral torsion	Lateral tibial torsion Lateral rotation at knee Lateral rotation of tibia, femur, and/or pelvis Lumbar rotation on same side
Excessive retroversion	Toeing-out Subtalar supination Lateral tibial torsion Lateral femoral torsion	Medial rotation at knee Medial rotation of tibia, femur, and/or pelvis Lumbar rotation on opposite side
Coxa vara	Pronated subtalar joint Medial rotation of leg Short ipsilateral leg Anterior pelvic rotation	Ipsilateral subtalar supination Contralateral subtalar pronation Ipsilateral plantar flexion Contralateral genu recurvatum Contralateral hip and/or knee flexion Ipsilateral posterior pelvic rotation and ipsilateral lumbar rotation

Continued

TABLE **15-8**

Malalignments Viewed Anteriorly—cont'd

Malalignment	Possible Correlated Motions or Postures	Possible Compensatory Motions or Postures
Coxa valga	Supinated subtalar joint Lateral rotation of leg Long ipsilateral leg Posterior pelvic tilt	Ipsilateral subtalar pronation Contralateral subtalar supination Contralateral plantar flexion Ipsilateral genu recurvatum Ipsilateral hip and/or knee flexion Ipsilateral anterior pelvic rotation and contralateral lumbar rotation
Medial femoral torsion	Excessive subtalar pronation In-toeing Medial facing or tilted patella ("squinting patella")	Excessive subtalar supination Functional forefoot valgus
Lateral femoral torsion	Excessive subtalar supination Out-toeing Lateral facing or tilted patella ("grasshopper eyes patella")	Excessive subtalar pronation Functional forefoot varus
Genu valgum	Pes planus Excessive subtalar pronation Lateral tibial torsion Lateral patellar subluxation Excessive hip adduction Ipsilateral hip excessive medial rotation Lumbar spine contralateral rotation	Forefoot varus Excessive subtalar supination to allow the lateral heel to contact the ground In-toeing to decrease lateral pelvic sway during gait Ipsilateral pelvic lateral rotation
Genu varum	Excessive lateral angulation of the tibia in the frontal plane; tibial varum Medial tibial torsion Ipsilateral hip lateral rotation Excessive hip abduction	Forefoot valgus Excessive subtalar pronation to allow the medial heel to contact the ground Ipsilateral pelvic medial rotation
Lateral tibial (malleolar) torsion	Out-toeing Excessive subtalar supination with related rotation along the lower quarter	Functional forefoot varus Excessive subtalar pronation with relaxed rotation along the lower quarter
Medial tibial (malleolar) torsion	In-toeing Metatarsus adductus Excessive subtalar pronation with related rotation along the lower quarter	Functional forefoot valgus Excessive subtalar supination with relaxed rotation along the lower quarter
Inadequate tibial retroflexion (bowing of the tibia)	Altered alignment of Achilles tendon causing altered associated joint motion	
Bowleg deformity of the tibia (tibial varum)	Medial tibial torsion	Forefoot valgus Excessive subtalar pronation
Ankle equinus		Hypermobile first ray Subtalar or midtarsal excessive pronation Hip or knee flexion Genu recurvation
Forefoot valgus	Hallux valgus Subtalar pronation and related rotation along the lower quarter	Excessive midtarsal or subtalar supination Excessive tibial; tibial and femoral; or tibial, femoral, and pelvic lateral rotation, or all with ipsilateral lumbar spine rotation
Metatarsus adductus	Hallus valgus Medial tibial torsion Flatfoot Toeing-in	
Hallus valgus	Forefoot valgus Subtalar pronation and related rotation along the lower quarter	Excessive tibial; tibial and femoral; or tibial, femoral, and pelvic lateral rotation, or all with ipsilateral lumbar spine rotation

TABLE **15-8**

Malalignments Viewed Anteriorly—cont'd

Malalignment	Possible Correlated Motions or Postures	Possible Compensatory Motions or Postures
In-toeing	Pronated foot Medial tibial torsion Metatarsus varus Talipes varus or equinovarus Tibia or genu varum Medial femoral torsion Excessive femoral anteversion Tight medial hip rotators Acetabular dysplasia (facing anteriorly)	
Out-toeing	Tight Achilles Talipes calcaneovalgus Convex pes planovarus Lateral tibial torsion Hypoplastic (absence) of fibula Lateral femoral torsion Abnormal femoral retroversion Tight lateral rotators Flaccid medial rotators Acetabular dysplasia (facing posteriorly)	
Rearfoot valgus (calcaneal eversion)	Tibial; tibial and femoral; or tibial, femoral, and pelvic rotation Hallux valgus	

TABLE **15-9**

Alignment in the Standing Posture: Side View

Joints	Line of Gravity	External Moment	Passive Opposing Forces	Active Opposing Forces
Atlanto-occipital	Anterior (anterior-to-transverse axis for flexion and extension)	Flexion	Ligamentum nuchae and alar ligaments; the tectorial, atlanto-axial, and posterior atlanto-occipital membranes	Rectus capitus posterior major and minor, semispinalis capitus and cervicis, splenius capitis and cervicis, and inferior and superior oblique muscles
Cervical	Posterior	Extension	Anterior longitudinal ligament, anterior anulus fibrosus fibers, and anterior zygapophyseal joint capsules	Anterior scalene, longus capitis and colli
Thoracic	Anterior	Flexion	Posterior longitudinal, supraspinous, and interspinous ligaments; posterior zygapophyseal joint capsules and posterior anulus fibrosus fibers	Ligamentum flavum, longissimus thoracis, iliocostalis thoracis, spinalis thoracis, and semispinalis thoracis
Lumbar	Posterior	Extension	Anterior longitudinal and iliolumbar ligaments, anterior fibers of the anulus fibrosus, and anterior zygapophyseal joint capsules	Rectus abdominis and external and internal oblique muscles
Sacroiliac joint	Anterior	Nutation	Sacrotuberous, sacrospinous, iliolumbar, and anterior sacroiliac ligaments	Transversus abdominis
Hip joint	Posterior	Extension	Iliofemoral ligament	Iliopsoas
Knee joint	Anterior	Extension	Posterior joint capsule	Hamstrings, gastrocnemius
Ankle joint	Anterior	Dorsiflexion		Soleus, gastrocnemius

From Levangie PK, Norkin CC: Joint structures and function—a comprehensive analysis, Philadelphia, 2005, FA Davis, p. 493.

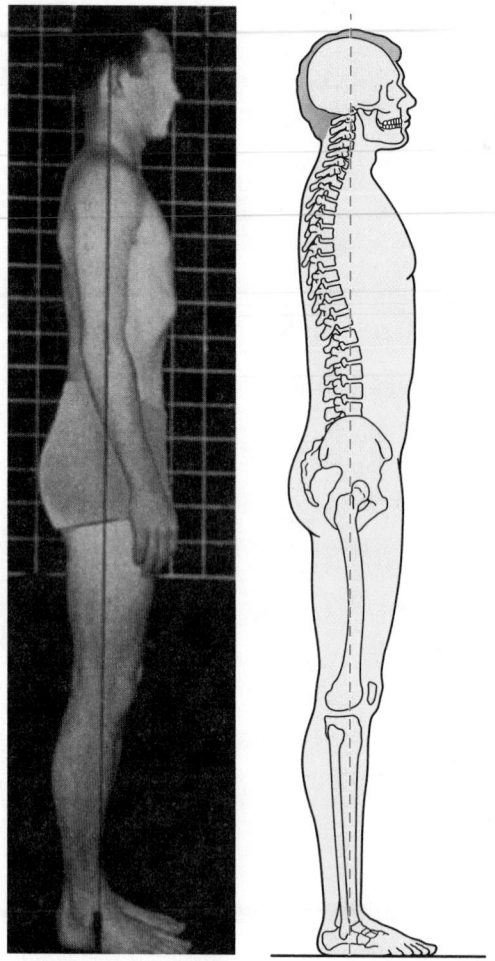

Figure 15-31 Correct postural alignment. (From Kendall FP, McCreary EK: Muscles: testing and function, Baltimore, 1983, Williams & Wilkins, p. 280.)

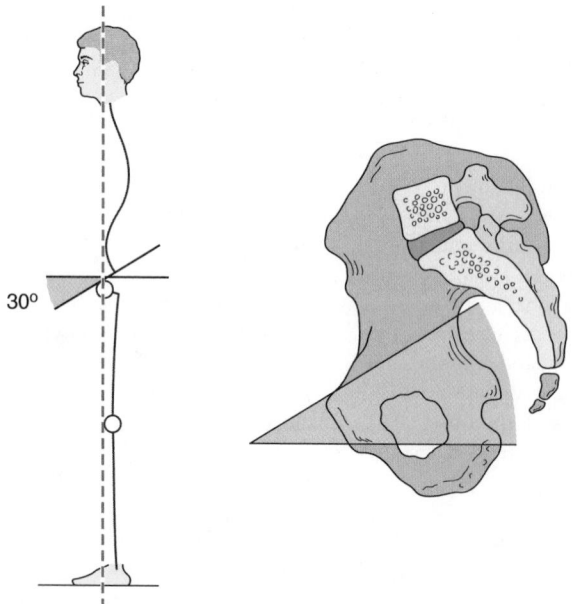

30°

Figure 15-32 Normal pelvic angle.

7. The knees are straight, flexed, or in recurvatum (hyperextended). Usually, in the normal standing position, the knees are slightly flexed (0° to 5°). Hyperextension of the knees may cause an increase in lordosis in the lumbar spine. Tight hamstrings or gastrocnemius muscles can also cause knee flexion.

Figure 15-33 illustrates normal posture and some of the abnormal deviations seen when viewing the patient from the side. Table 15-10 shows some of the malalignment postures and their effect.[2,27-29]

Posterior View

When viewing from behind (Table 15-11; see Figure 15-1, *C*), the examiner should note whether the following conditions hold true:

1. The shoulders are level, and the head is in midline. These findings should be compared with those from the anterior view.
2. The spines and inferior angles of the scapulae are level (Figure 15-34), and the medial borders of the scapulae are equidistant from the spine. If not, is there a rotational or winging deformity of one of the scapulae? Defects, such as Sprengel's deformity, should be noted (Figure 15-35).
3. The spine is straight or curved laterally, indicating scoliosis. A plumb line may be dropped from the spinous process of the seventh cervical vertebra (Figure 15-36).[30] Normally, the line passes through the gluteal cleft. This line is the **posterior line of reference** used to divide the body into right and left halves posteriorly (see Figure 15-1, *C*). The distance from the vertical string to the gluteal cleft can be measured. This distance is sometimes used as a measurement of spinal imbalance, and it is noted whether the deviation is to the left or right. If a torticollis or cervicothoracic scoliosis is present, the plumb line should be dropped from the occipital protuberance.[11]
4. The ribs protrude or are symmetrical on both sides.
5. The waist angles are level.
6. The arms are equidistant from the body and equally rotated.
7. The PSISs are level (Figure 15-37). If one is higher than the other, one leg may be shorter or rotation of the pelvis may be present. The examiner should note how the PSISs relate to the ASISs. If the ASIS on one side and the PSIS on the other side are higher, there is a torsion deformity (anterior or posterior) at the sacroiliac joint. If the ASIS and PSIS on one side are higher than the ASIS and PSIS on the other side, there may be an up-slip at the sacroiliac joint on the high side.
8. The gluteal folds are level. Muscle weakness, nerve root problems, or nerve palsy may lead to asymmetry.

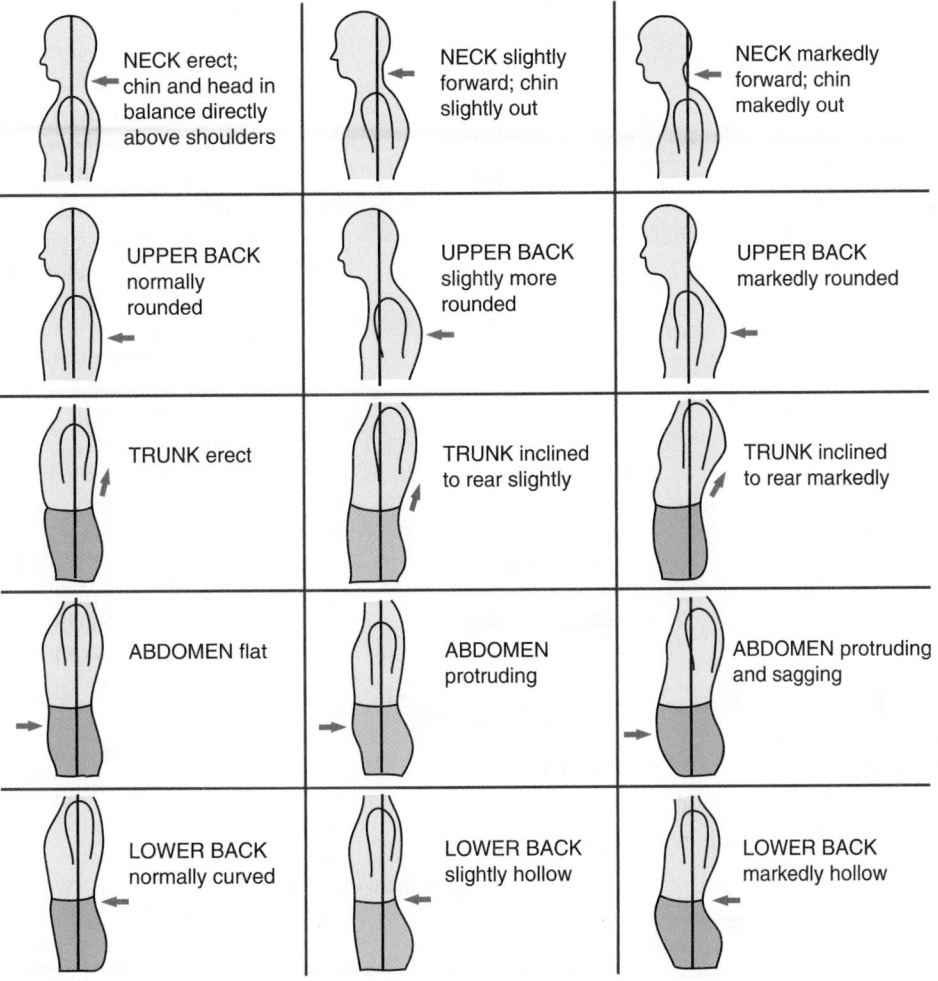

Figure 15-33 Postural deviations obvious from the side view. (Redrawn from Reedco Research, Auburn, NY.)

TABLE **15-10**

Malalignments Viewed Laterally[2,27-29]

Malalignment	Possible Correlated Motions or Postures	Possible Compensatory Motions or Postures
Forward head posture	Extension of cervical spine Protracted scapula	Increased kyphosis in thoracic spine Increased lordosis in lumbar spine Medially rotated humerus
Round back	Extension of cervical spine Protracted scapula	Forward head posture Hips flexed Knees extended
Flat back	Posterior pelvic tilt	Hips extended Knees extended Forward head posture
Swayback	Pelvic neutral or posterior tilt	Pelvis slides anterior Kyphosis Hips extended Knees extended
Pathological lordosis	Pelvis anteriorly tilted Tight hip flexors	Knees extended Ankles plantar flexed

Continued

TABLE **15-10**

Malalignments Viewed Laterally—cont'd

Malalignment	Possible Correlated Motions or Postures	Possible Compensatory Motions or Postures
Anterior pelvic tilt	Hip flexion (tight hip flexors)	Lumbar extension (increased lordosis) Hyperextended knees Poking chin (cervical extension) Rounded shoulders (protracted scapula) Thoracic kyphosis Ankles plantar flexed
Posterior pelvic tilt	Hip extension	Lumbar flexion (flat back) Hips extended Knees extended Forward head posture
Backward rotation of one ilium on sacrum (right leg stance)	Right hip lateral rotation Lateral facing patella Out-toeing Supination of foot Short leg	Right lumbar rotation Scoliosis—concavity to right Knee extension
Genu recurvatum	Ankle plantar flexion Excessive anterior pelvic tilt	Posterior pelvic tilt Flexed trunk posture Excessive thoracic kyphosis
Excessive tibial retroversion (posterior slant of tibial plateaus)	Genu recurvatum	
Inadequate tibial retrotorsion (posterior deflection of proximal tibia due to hamstrings pull)	Flexed knee posture	
Rearfoot valgus (calcaneal eversion)	Forward pelvic tilt (bilateral) Lateral pelvic tilt (unilateral)	

TABLE **15-11**

Alignment in the Standing Posture: Posterior View

Body Segment	Line of Gravity Location	Observation
Head	Passes through middle of head	Head should be straight with no lateral tilting; angles between shoulders and neck should be equal
Arms		Arms should hang naturally so that the palms of the hands are facing the sides of the body
Shoulders/spine	Passes along vertebral column in a straight line, which should bisect the back into two symmetrical halves	Scapulae should lie flat against the rib cage, be equidistant from the line of gravity and be separated by about 4 inches in the adult
Hips/pelvis	Passes through gluteal cleft of buttocks and should be equidistant from PSISs	The PSISs should be level; the gluteal folds should be level and symmetrical
Knees	Passes between knees equidistant from medial joint aspects	Look to see that the knees are level
Ankles/feet	Passes between ankles equidistant from the medial malleoli	The heel cords should be vertical and the malleoli should be level and symmetrical

From Levangie PK, Norkin CC: Joint structures and function—a comprehensive analysis, Philadelphia, 2005, FA Davis, p. 499.
PSIS, Posterior superior iliac spine.

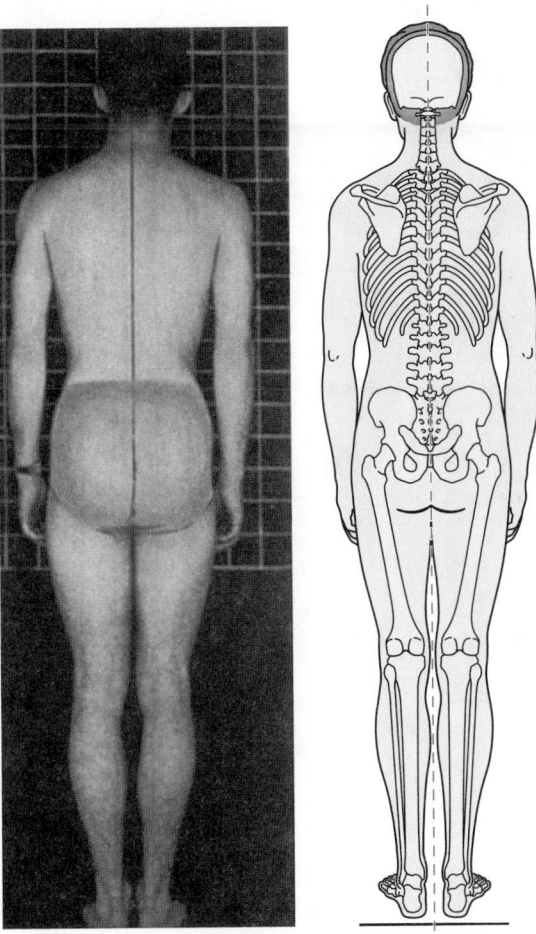

Figure 15-34 Correct postural alignment. (From Kendall FP, McCreary EK: Muscles: testing and function, Baltimore, 1983, Williams & Wilkins, p. 290.)

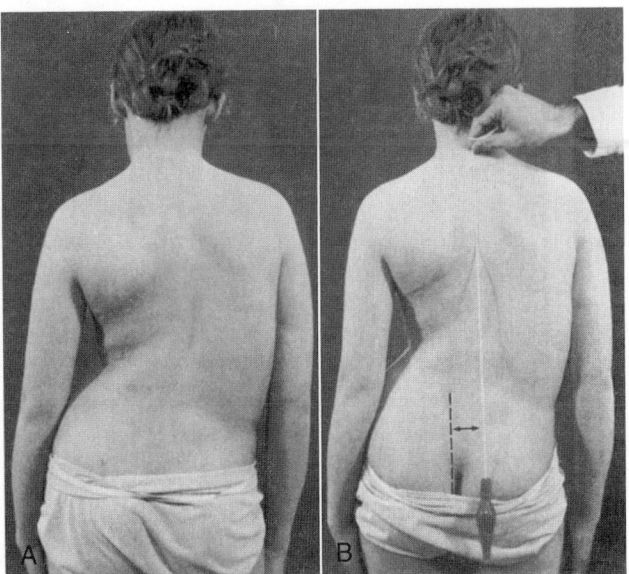

Figure 15-36 The patient is viewed from the back to evaluate the spine deformity. A, A typical right thoracic curve is shown. The left shoulder is lower, and the right scapula more prominent. Note the decreased distance between the right arm and the thorax with the shift of the thorax to the right. The left iliac crest appears higher, but this is caused by the shift of the thorax with fullness on the right and elimination of the waistline. The high hip is thus only apparent, not real. **B,** Plumb line dropped from the prominent vertebra of C7 (vertebra prominens) measures the decompensation of the upper thorax over the pelvis. The distance from the vertical plumb line to the gluteal cleft is measured in centimeters and is recorded, noting the direction of fall from the occipital protuberance (inion). (From Moe JH, Bradford DS, Winter RB, et al: Scoliosis and other spinal deformities, Philadelphia, 1978, WB Saunders, p. 14.)

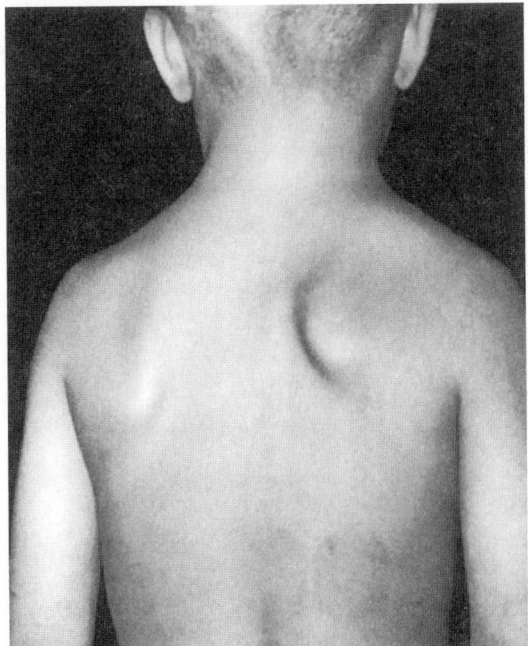

Figure 15-35 Sprengel's deformity. Note the small, high scapula on the right. (From Tachdjian MO: Pediatric orthopedics, Philadelphia, 1972, WB Saunders, p. 82.)

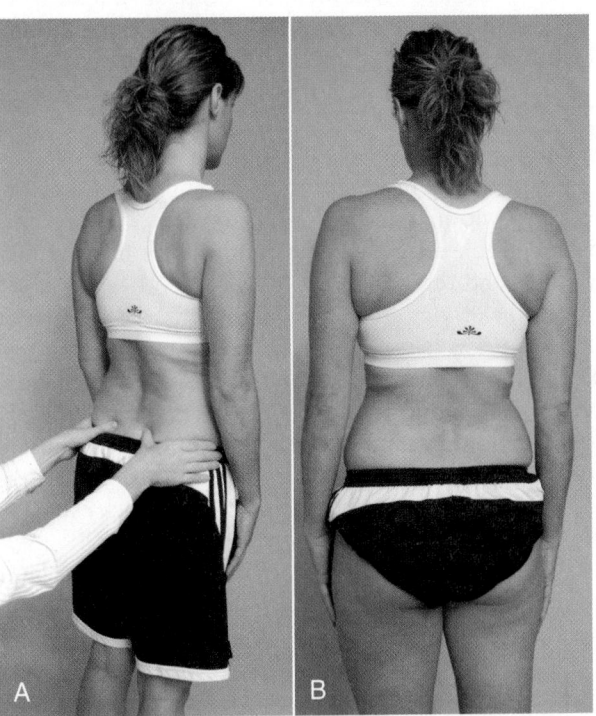

Figure 15-37 Viewing height equality. A, Posterior superior iliac spines (PSISs). **B,** Gluteal folds.

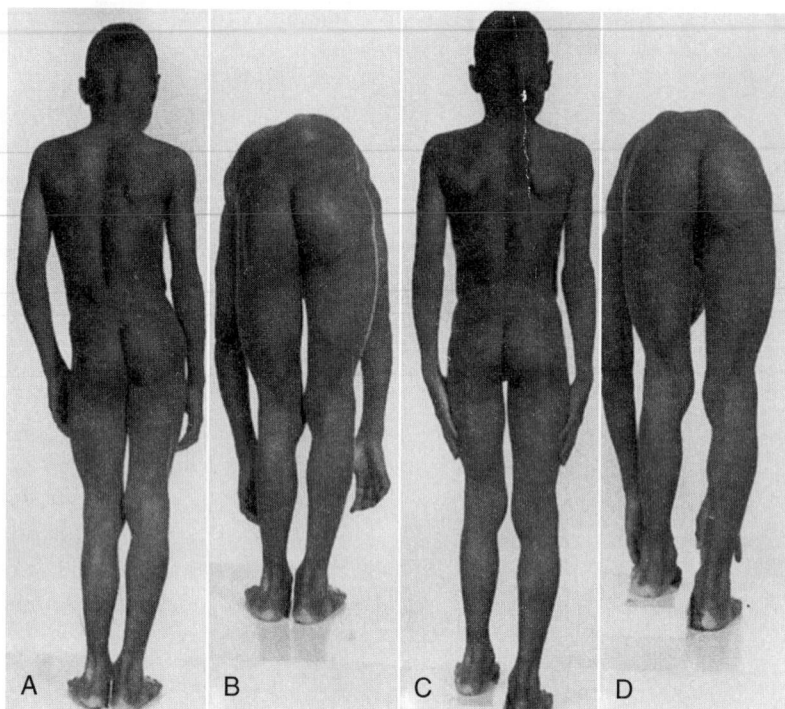

Figure 15-38 A and **B,** Functional scoliosis resulting from short leg. **C** and **D,** The spinal position with short leg is corrected. (From Tachdjian MO: Pediatric orthopedics, Philadelphia, 1972, WB Saunders, p. 1192.)

9. The knee joints are level. If they are not, it may indicate that one leg is shorter than the other (Figure 15-38).
10. Both of the Achilles tendons descend straight to the calcanei. If the tendons angle out, it may indicate a flatfoot deformity (pes planus).
11. The heels are straight or are angled in (rear-foot varus) or out (rear-foot valgus).
12. Bowing of femur or tibia is present or absent.

Figure 15-39 illustrates the normal posture and some of the abnormal deviations seen when viewing from behind. Table 15-12 highlights some of the malalignment postures and their effect.[2,13,27,28]

When viewing posture, the examiner should remember that the pelvis is usually the key to proper back posture. The normal pelvic angle is 30°, and the pelvis is held or balanced in this position by muscles. For the pelvis to "sit properly" on the femur, the following muscles must be strong, supple (mobile), and balanced: abdominals, hip flexors, hip extensors, superficial and deep back extensors, hip rotators, and hip abductors and adductors.

If the height of the patient is measured, especially in a child, the focal height of the child may be estimated by the use of a chart, such as the one shown in Table 15-13.[31]

After the standing posture has been assessed, the examiner may decide to assess some additional postures (e.g., positional, sustained, or repetitive), especially if the patient

has stated in the history that these different positions have caused problems or symptoms.

Forward Flexion

Having completed the assessment of normal standing, the examiner asks the patient to flex forward at the hips with the fingertips of both hands together so that the arms drop vertically (Figure 15-40). The feet should be together, and both knees should be straight. Any alteration from this posture will cause the spine to rotate, giving a false view.

From this position, using the anterior and posterior skyline views, the examiner can note the following:
1. Whether there is any asymmetry of the rib cage (e.g., rib hump); if a hump is present, a level and tape measure may be used to obtain the perpendicular distance between the hump and hollow (Figure 15-41)[11]
2. Whether there is any asymmetry in the spinal musculature
3. Whether a pathological kyphosis is present
4. Whether lumbar spine straightens or flexes as it normally should
5. Whether there is any restriction to forward bending, such as spondylolisthesis or tight hamstrings (Figures 15-42 and 15-43)

If, in the history, the patient said that sustained forward flexion caused symptoms, the examiner should ask the

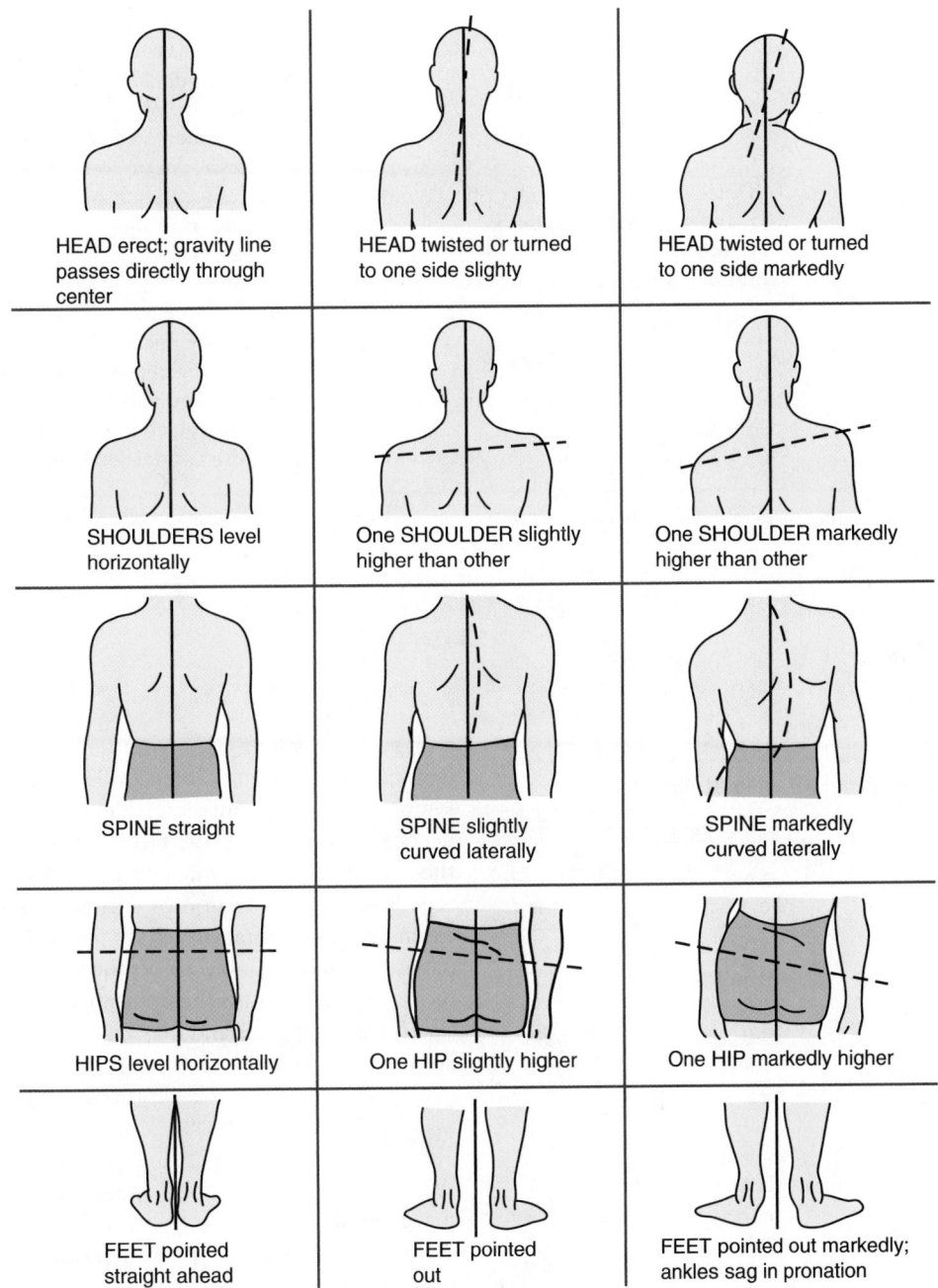

Figure 15-39 Postural deviations obvious from the posterior view. (Redrawn from Reedco Research, Auburn, NY.)

TABLE **15-12**

Malalignments Viewed Posteriorly*[2,13,27,28]

Malalignment	Possible Correlated Motions or Postures	Possible Compensatory Motions or Postures
Scoliosis	Side flexion to convex side limited Rotation to convex side limited Rib hump on convex side	
Rearfoot varus Excessive subtalar supination (calcaneal varus)	Tibial; tibial and femoral; or tibial, femoral, and pelvic lateral rotation	Excessive medial rotation along the lower quarter chain Hallux valgus Plantar flexed first ray Functional forefoot valgus Excessive or prolonged midtarsal pronation
Rearfoot valgus Excessive subtalar pronation (calcaneal valgus)	Tibial; tibial and femoral; or tibial, femoral, and pelvic medial rotation Hallus valgus	Excessive lateral rotation along the lower quarter chain Functional forefoot varus
Forefoot varus	Subtalar supination and related rotation along the lower quarter	Plantar flexed first ray Hallux valgus Excessive midtarsal or subtalar pronation or prolonged pronation Excessive tibial; tibial and femoral; or tibial, femoral, and pelvic medial rotation, or all with contralateral lumbar spine rotation

*Many of the posterior malalignments are also seen anteriorly.

TABLE **15-13**

Percentage of Mature Height Attained at Different Ages

Chronological Age (Years)	PERCENTAGE OF EVENTUAL HEIGHT	
	Boys	Girls
1	42.2	44.7
2	49.5	52.8
3	53.8	57.0
4	58.0	61.8
5	61.8	66.2
6	65.2	70.3
7	69.0	74.0
8	72.0	77.5
9	75.0	80.7
10	78.0	84.4
11	81.1	88.4
12	84.2	92.9
13	87.3	96.5
14	91.5	98.3
15	96.1	99.1
16	98.3	99.6
17	99.3	100.0
18	99.8	100.0

From Bayley N: The accurate prediction of growth and adult height. Mod Probl Pediatr 7:234–255, 1954.

patient to assume the symptom-causing posture and maintain it for 15 to 30 seconds to determine whether symptoms arise or increase. Flexion has been found to decrease the stress on the facet joints, but it can increase the pressure in the nucleus pulposus.[32,33] Likewise, if repetitive forward flexion or combined movements (e.g., extension and rotation) have caused symptoms, the patient should be asked to do the repetitive or combined movements. Loading the spine by lifting an object may also cause symptoms and may be investigated if symptoms are not too great.

Sitting

With the patient seated on a stool so that the feet are on the ground and the back is unsupported, the examiner looks at the patient's posture (Figure 15-44). Sitting without a back support causes the patient to support his or her own posture and increases the amount of muscle activity needed to maintain the posture.[32] This observation is carried out, as in the standing position, from the front, back, and side. If any anteroposterior or lateral deviations of the spine are observed, the examiner should recall whether they were present when the patient was examined while standing. It should be noted whether the spinal curves increase or decrease when the patient is in

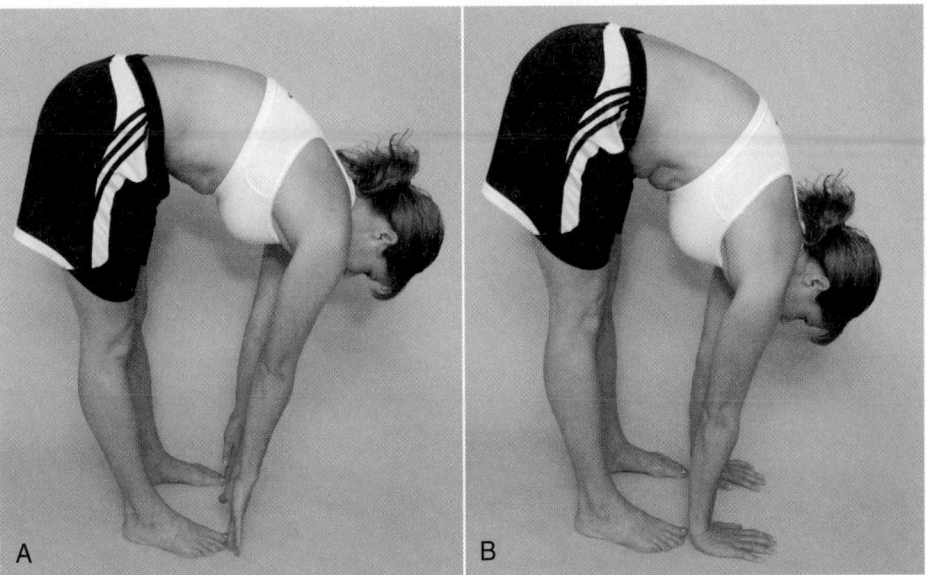

Figure 15-40 Posture in forward flexion. A, Normal range of motion. Note reversal of lumbar curve. **B,** Excessive range of motion caused by excessive hip mobility.

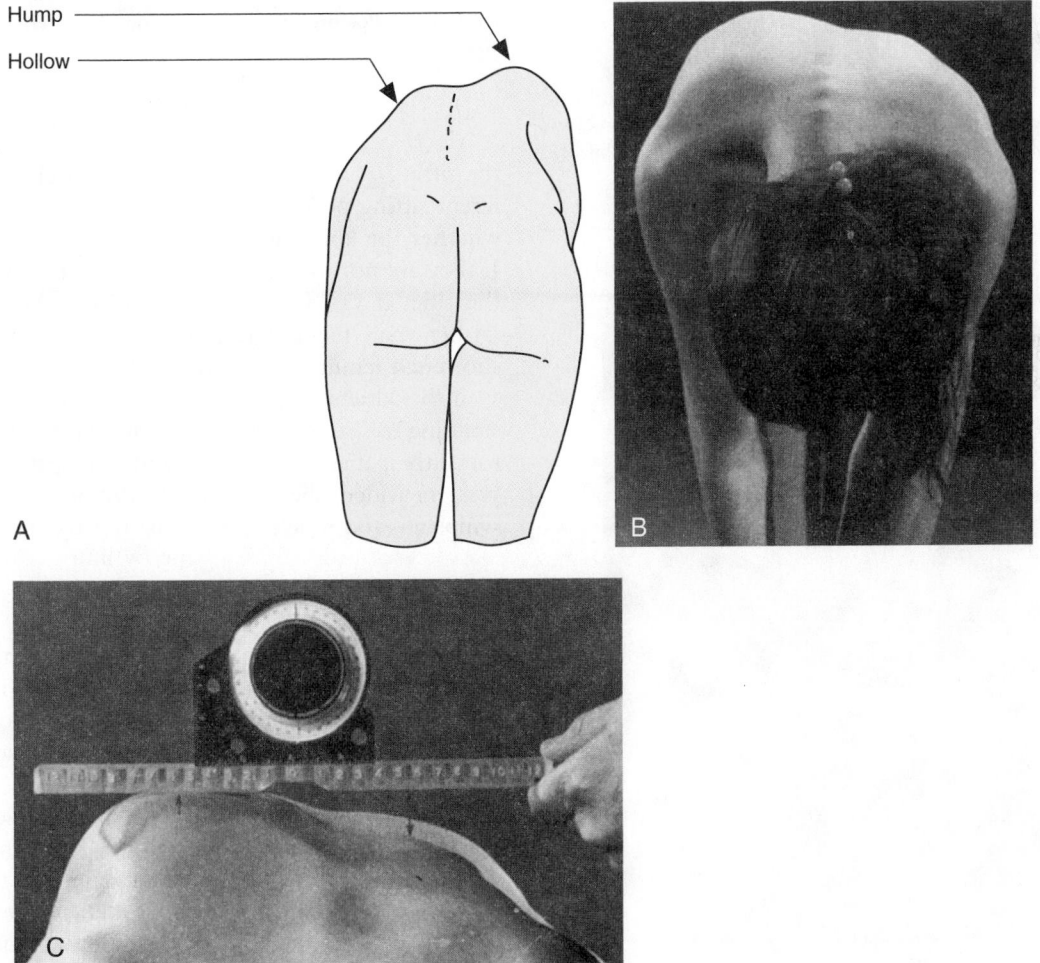

Hump

Hollow

Figure 15-41 Rib hump in forward-bending test. A, Posterior view. **B,** Anterior view. The two sides are compared. Note the presence of a right thoracic prominence. **C,** Measurement of the prominence. The spirit level is positioned with the zero mark over the palpable spinous process in the area of maximal prominence. The level is made horizontal, and the distance to the apex of the deformity (5 to 6 cm) noted. The perpendicular distance from the level to the hollow is measured at the same distance from the midline. A 2.4-cm right thoracic prominence is shown. (From Moe JH, Bradford DS, Winter RB, et al: Scoliosis and other spinal deformities, Philadelphia, 1978, WB Saunders, p. 17.)

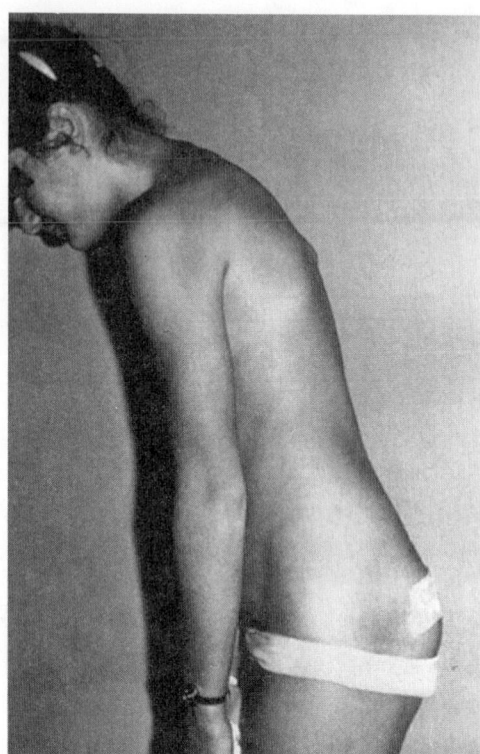

Figure 15-42 Abnormal forward bending resulting from tight hamstrings in a patient with spondylolisthesis. (From Moe JH, Bradford DS, Winter RB, et al: Scoliosis and other spinal deformities, Philadelphia, 1978, WB Saunders, p. 19.)

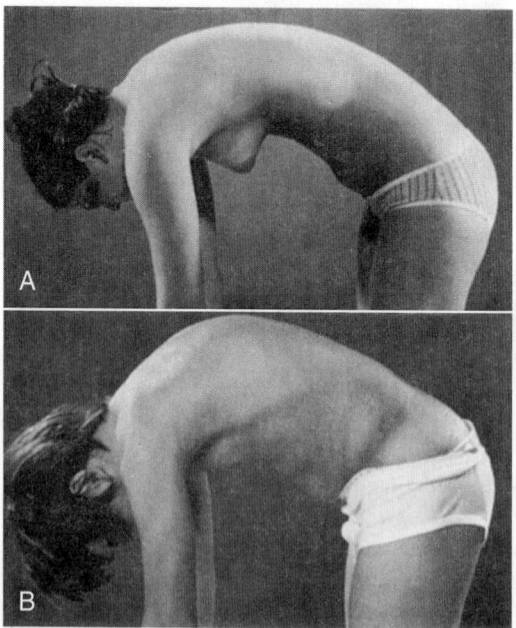

Figure 15-43 Forward-bending position for viewing kyphosis (lateral view). A, Normal thoracic roundness is demonstrated with a gentle curve to the whole spine. **B,** An area of increased bending is seen in the thoracic spine, indicating structural changes, in a patient with Scheuermann disease. (From Moe JH, Bradford DS, Winter RB, et al: Scoliosis and other spinal deformities, Philadelphia, 1978, WB Saunders, p. 18.)

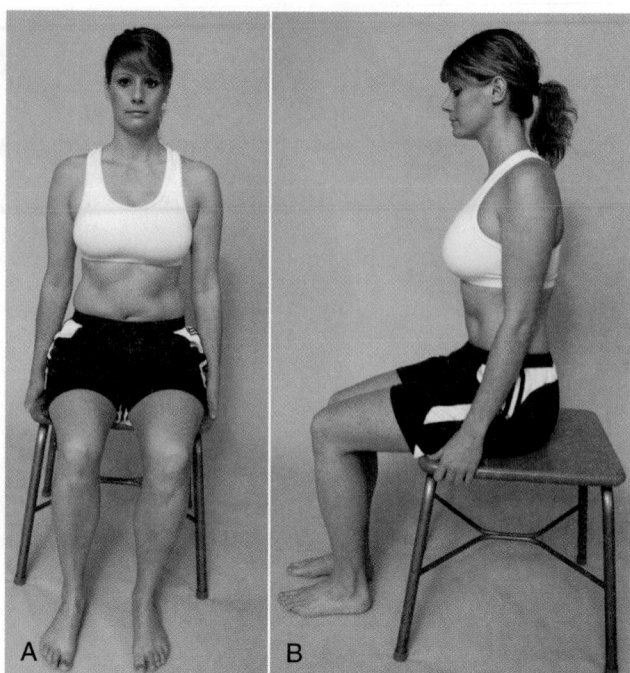

Figure 15-44 Posture in sitting position. A, Anterior view. **B,** Side view.

the sitting position and how the curves change with different sitting postures.[34] From the front, it can be noted whether the knees are the same distance from the floor. If they are not, this may indicate a shortened tibia. From the side, it can be noted whether one knee protrudes farther than the other. If it does, this may indicate a shortened femur on the other side.

If the patient has stated in the history that going from standing to sitting or sitting to standing resulted in symptoms, the patient should be asked to repeat these maneuvers, provided the movements do not exacerbate the symptoms too much.

Supine Lying

With the patient in the supine-lying position, the examiner notes the position of the head and cervical spine as well as the shoulder girdle. The chest area is observed for any protrusion (e.g., pectus carinatum) or sunken areas (e.g., pectus excavatum).

The abdominal musculature should be observed to see whether it is strong or flabby, and the waist angles should be noted to see whether they are equal. As in the standing position, the ASISs should be viewed to see if they are level. Any extension in the lumbar spine should be noted. In addition, it should be noted whether bending the knees helps to decrease the lumbar curve; if it does, it may indicate tight hip flexors. The lower limbs should descend parallel from the pelvis. If they do not, or if they cannot be aligned parallel and at right angles to a line joining the

ASISs, it may indicate an abduction or adduction contracture at the hip.

If, in the history, the patient has complained of symptoms on arising from supine lying or from going into the supine position, the examiner should ask the patient to repeat these movements, provided they do not exacerbate the symptoms.

Prone Lying

With the patient lying prone, the examiner notes the position of the head, neck, and shoulder girdle, as previously described. The head should be positioned so that it is not rotated, side flexed, or extended. Any condition, such as Sprengel's deformity or rib hump, should be noted, as should any spinal deviations. The examiner should determine whether the PSISs are level and should ensure that the musculature of the buttocks, posterior thighs, and calves is normal (Figure 15-45).

As with supine lying, if assuming the position or recovering from the position causes symptoms, the patient should be asked to repeat these movements, as long as symptoms are not made worse.

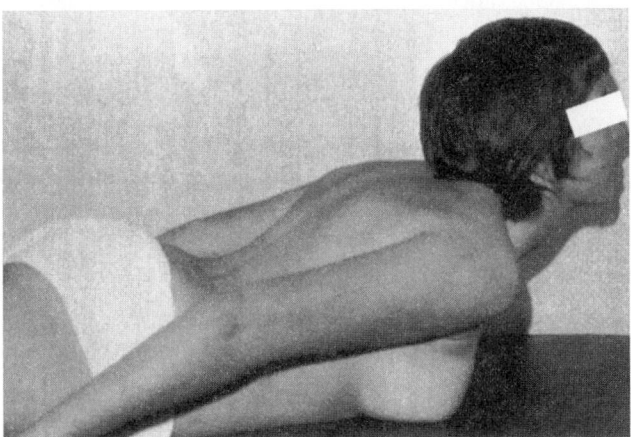

Figure 15-45 Structural kyphosis does not disappear on extension. (From Moe JH, Bradford DS, Winter RB, et al: Scoliosis and other spinal deformities, Philadelphia, 1978, WB Saunders, p. 339.)

EXAMINATION

Assessment of posture primarily involves history and observation. If, on completing the history and observation, the examiner believes that a direct examination is necessary, the procedures outlined in this text for the various areas of the body should be followed. In addition, there are postural alignment measures, such as the Flexicurve ruler and other measures that may be used to record postural alignments and changes.[35] With every postural assessment, however, the examiner should perform two tests: the leg length measurement[36-39] and the slump test.

Leg Length Measurement. The patient lies supine with the pelvis set square or "balanced" on the legs (i.e., the legs at an angle of 90° to a line joining the ASISs). The legs should be 15 to 20 cm (6 to 8 inches) apart and parallel to each other (Figure 15-46). The examiner then places one end of the tape measure against the distal aspect of the ASIS, holding it firmly against the bone. The index finger of the other hand is placed immediately distal to the medial or lateral malleolus and pushed against it. The thumbnail is brought down against the tip of the index fingers so that the tape measure is pinched between them. A reading is taken where the thumb and finger pinch together. A slight difference, up to 1.0 to 1.5 cm (0.4 to 0.6 inch), is considered normal but can still be relevant if pathology is present. Further information on measurement of true leg length may be found in Chapter 11.

Slump Test. The patient is seated on the edge of the examining table with the legs supported, the hips in neutral position (i.e., no rotation or abduction-adduction), and the hands behind the back (see Figure 9-62). The examination is performed in several steps. First, the patient is asked to "slump" the back into thoracic and lumbar flexion. The examiner maintains the patient's chin in the neutral position to prevent neck and head flexion. The examiner then uses one arm to apply overpressure across the shoulders to maintain flexion of the thoracic and lumbar spines. While this position is held, the patient

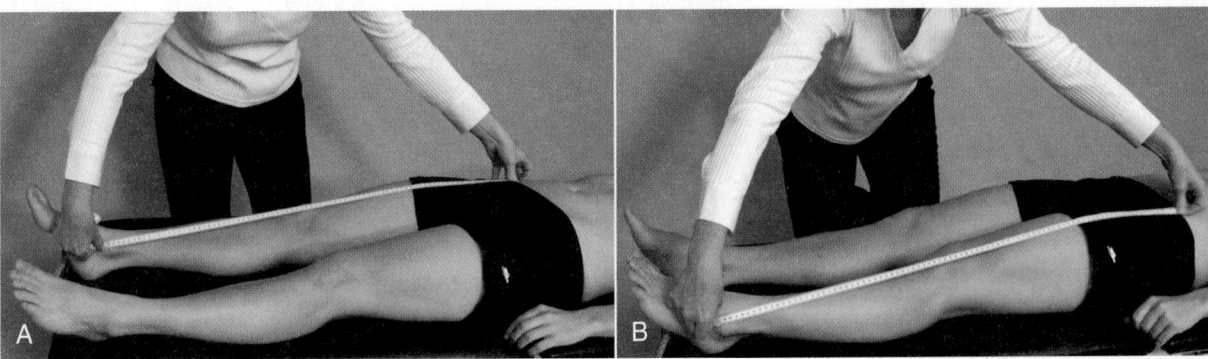

Figure 15-46 Measuring leg length. A, To medial malleolus. **B,** To lateral malleolus.

is asked to actively flex the cervical spine and head as far as possible (i.e., chin to chest). The examiner then applies overpressure to maintain flexion of all three parts of the spine (cervical, thoracic, lumbar), using the hand of the same arm to maintain overpressure in the cervical spine. With the other hand, the examiner then holds the patient's foot in maximum dorsiflexion. While the examiner holds these positions, the patient is asked to actively straighten the knee as much as possible. The test is repeated with the other leg and then with both legs at the same time. If the patient is unable to fully extend the knee because of pain, the examiner releases the overpressure to the cervical spine and the patient actively extends the neck. If the knee extends farther, the symptoms decrease with neck extension, or the positioning of the patient increases the patient's symptoms, then the test is considered positive for increased tension in the neuromeningeal tract.[40–42] Further information on the slump test may be found in Chapter 9.

Additional Tests. Other tests may also be performed based on what the examiner has observed. For example, if the hip flexors appear tight, the Thomas test should be performed (see Chapter 11). Refer to Table 15-14 for a detailed presentation of good and faulty posture.

TABLE **15-14**

Good and Faulty Posture: Summary Chart

Good Posture	Part	Faulty Posture
Head is held erect in a position of good balance.	Head	Chin up too high. Head protruding forward. Head tilted or rotated to one side.
Arms hang relaxed at the sides with palms of the hands facing toward the body. Elbows are slightly bent, so forearms hang slightly forward. Shoulders are level, and neither one is more forward or backward than the other when seen from the side. Scapulae lie flat against the rib cage. They are neither too close together nor too wide apart. In adults, a separation of approximately 10 cm (4 inches) is average.	Arms and shoulders	Holding the arms stiffly in any position forward, backward, or out from the body. Arms turned so that palms of hands face backward. One shoulder higher than the other. Both shoulders hiked up. One or both shoulders drooping forward or sloping. Shoulders rotated either clockwise or counterclockwise. Scapulae pulled back too hard. Scapulae too far apart. Scapulae too prominent, standing out from the rib cage ("winged scapulae").
A good position of the chest is one in which it is slightly up and slightly forward (while the back remains in good alignment). The chest appears to be in a position about halfway between that of a full inspiration and a forced expiration.	Chest	Depressed, or "hollow-chest," position. Lifted and held up too high, brought about by arching the back. Ribs more prominent on one side than on the other. Lower ribs flaring out or protruding.
In young children up to about the age of 10, the abdomen normally protrudes somewhat. In older children and adults, it should be flat.	Abdomen	Entire abdomen protrudes. Lower part of the abdomen protrudes while the upper part is pulled in.
The front of the pelvis and the thighs are in a straight line. The buttocks are not prominent in back but instead slope slightly downward. The spine has four natural curves. In the neck and lower back, the curve is forward, and in the upper back and lowest part of the spine (sacral region), it is backward. The sacral curve is a fixed curve, whereas the other three are flexible.	Spine and pelvis (side view)	The low back arches forward too much (lordosis). The pelvis tilts forward too much. The front of the thigh forms an angle with the pelvis when this tilt is present. The normal forward curve in the low back has straightened out. The pelvis tips backward, and there is a slightly backward slant to the line of the pelvis in relation to the front of the hips (flat back). Increased backward curve in the upper back (kyphosis or round upper back). Increased forward curve in the neck. Almost always accompanied by round upper back and seen as a forward head. Lateral curve of the spine (scoliosis); toward one side (C-curve), toward both sides (S-curve).

TABLE **15-14**

Good and Faulty Posture: Summary Chart—cont'd

Good Posture	Part	Faulty Posture
Ideally, the body weight is borne evenly on both feet, and the hips are level. One side is not more prominent than the other as seen from front or back, nor is one hip more forward or backward than the other as seen from the side. The spine does not curve to the left or the right side. (A slight deviation to the left in right-handed individuals and to the right in left-handed individuals should not be considered abnormal. Also, because a tendency toward a slightly low right shoulder and slightly high right hip is frequently found in right-handed people, and vice versa for left-handed, such deviations should not be considered abnormal.)	Hips, pelvis, and spine (back view)	One hip is higher than the other (lateral pelvic tilt). Sometimes it is not really much higher but appears so because a sideways sway of the body has made it more prominent. (Tailors and dressmakers often notice a lateral tilt because the hemline of skirts or length of trousers must be adjusted to the difference.) The hips are rotated so that one is farther forward than the other (clockwise or counterclockwise rotation).
Legs are straight up and down. Patellae face straight ahead when feet are in good position. Looking at the knees from the side, the knees are straight (i.e., neither bent forward nor "locked" backward).	Knees and legs	Knees touch when feet are apart (genu valgum). Knees are apart when feet touch (genu varum). Knee curves slightly backward (hyperextended knee) (genu recurvatum). Knee bends slightly forward, that is, it is not as straight as it should be (flexed knee). Patellae face slightly toward each other (medially rotated femurs). Patellae face slightly outward (laterally rotated femurs).
In standing, the longitudinal arch has the shape of a half dome. Barefoot or in shoes without heels, the feet toe-out slightly. In shoes with heels, the feet are parallel. In walking with or without heels, the feet are parallel, and the weight is transferred from the heel along the outer border to the ball of the foot. In running, the feet are parallel or toe-in slightly. The weight is on the balls of the feet and toes because the heels do not come in contact with the ground	Foot	Low longitudinal arch or flatfoot. Low metatarsal arch, usually indicated by calluses under the ball of the foot. Weight borne on the inner side of the foot (pronation). "Ankle rolls in." Weight borne on the outer border of the foot (supination). "Ankle rolls out." Toeing-out while walking or while standing in shoes with heels ("outflared" or "slue-footed"). Toeing-in while walking or standing ("pigeon-toed").
Toes should be straight, that is, neither curled downward nor bent upward. They should extend forward in line with the foot and not be squeezed together or overlap.	Toes	Toes bend up at the first joint and down at middle and end joints so that the weight rests on the tips of the toes (hammer toes). This fault is often associated with wearing shoes that are too short. Big toe slants inward toward the midline of the foot (hallus valgus). This fault is often associated with wearing shoes that are too narrow and pointed at the toes.

Modified from Kendall FP, McCreary EK: Muscles: testing and function, Baltimore, 1983, Williams & Wilkins.

PRÉCIS OF THE POSTURAL ASSESSMENT*

History
Observation
   Standing (front, side, behind)
   Forward flexion (front, side, behind)
   Sitting (front, side, behind)
   Supine lying
   Prone lying

Examination
   Leg length measurement
   Slump test
Examination of specific joints (see appropriate chapter)

*As with any assessment, the patient must be warned that there may be some discomfort after the examination and that this discomfort is normal. Discomfort after any assessment should decrease within 24 hours. The examiner must keep in mind that several joints may be affected at the same time, either as the result of or as the cause of faulty posture. Therefore the examination of posture may be an extensive one, with observation both of the posture in general and of several specific joints in detail.

REFERENCES

1. Kisner C, Colby LA: Therapeutic exercise: foundations and techniques, Philadelphia, 1985, FA Davis.
2. Levangie PK, Norkin CC: Joint structures and function—a comprehensive analysis, Philadelphia, 2005, WB Saunders.
3. Griegel-Morris P, Larson K, Mueller-Klaus K, et al: Incidence of common postural abnormalities in the cervical, shoulder, and thoracic regions and their association with pain in two age groups of healthy subjects. Phys Ther 72:425–430, 1992.
4. Barry-Greb TL, Harrison AL: Posture, gait, and functional abilities of the adolescent, pregnant, and elderly female. Orthop Phys Ther Clin North Am 5:1–21, 1996.
5. Fahrni WH: Backache: assessment and treatment, Vancouver, Canada, 1976, Musquean Publishers.
6. Finneson BE: Low back pain, Philadelphia, 1981, JB Lippincott.
7. Kendall FP, McCreary EK: Muscles: testing and function, Baltimore, 1983, Williams & Wilkins.
8. McKenzie RA: The lumbar spine: mechanical diagnosis and therapy, Waikanae, New Zealand, 1981, Spinal Publications.
9. Wiles P, Sweetnam R: Essentials of orthopaedics, London, 1965, J & A Churchill.
10. Porterfield JA, DeRosa C: Mechanical low back pain: perspectives in functional anatomy, Philadelphia, 1991, WB Saunders.
11. Moe JH, Bradford DS, Winter RB, et al: Scoliosis and other spinal deformities, Philadelphia, 1978, WB Saunders.
12. McMorris RO: Faulty postures. Pediatr Clin North Am 8:213–224, 1961.
13. Tachdjian MO: Pediatric orthopedics, Philadelphia, 1972, WB Saunders.
14. Tsou PM: Embryology and congenital kyphosis. Clin Orthop 128:18–25, 1977.
15. White AA, Panjabi MM, Thomas CC: The clinical biomechanics of kyphotic deformities. Clin Orthop 128:8–17, 1977.
16. Hensinger RN: Kyphosis secondary to skeletal dysplasias and metabolic disease. Clin Orthop 128: 113–128, 1977.
17. Tsou PM, Yau A, Hodgson AR: Embryogenesis and prenatal development of congenital vertebral anomalies and their classification. Clin Orthop 152:211–231, 1980.
18. Cailliet R: Scoliosis: diagnosis and management, Philadelphia, 1975, FA Davis.
19. Figueiredo UM, Mames JIP: Juvenile idiopathic scoliosis. J Bone Joint Surg Br 63:61–66, 1981.
20. Goldstein LA, Waugh TR: Classification and terminology of scoliosis. Clin Orthop 93:10–22, 1973.
21. James JIP: The etiology of scoliosis. J Bone Joint Surg Br 52:410–419, 1970.
22. White AA: Kinematics of the normal spine as related to scoliosis. J Biomech 4:405–411, 1971.
23. Papaioannou T, Stokes I, Kenwright J: Scoliosis associated with limb length inequality. J Bone Joint Surg Am 64:59–62, 1982.
24. Debrunner HU: Orthopaedic diagnosis, London, 1970, E & S Livingstone.
25. Dolan P, Adams MA, Hutton WC: Commonly adopted postures and their effect on the lumbar spine. Spine 13:197–201, 1988.
26. Opila KA, Wagner SS, Schiowitz S, et al: Postural alignment in barefoot and high-heeled stance. Spine 13:542–547, 1988.
27. Giallonardo LM: Posture. In Myers RS, editor: Saunders manual of physical therapy practice, Philadelphia, 1995, WB Saunders.
28. Riegger-Krugh C, Keysor JJ: Skeletal malalignment of the lower quarter: correlated and compensatory motions and postures. J Orthop Sports Phys Ther 23:164–170, 1996.
29. Pinto RZ, Souza TR, Trede RG, et al: Bilateral and unilateral increases in calcaneal eversion affect pelvic alignment in standing position. Manual Therapy 13:513–519, 2008.
30. McLean IP, Gillan MG, Ross JC, et al: A comparison of methods for measuring trunk list—a simple plumb line is best. Spine 21:1667–1670, 1996.
31. Bayley N: The accurate prediction of growth and adult height. Mod Probl Pediatr 7:234–255, 1954.
32. Adams MA, Hutton WC: The effect of posture on the lumbar spine. J Bone Joint Surg Br 67:625–629, 1985.
33. Adams MA, Hutton WC: The effect of posture on the role of the apophyseal joints in resulting intervertebral compressive forces. J Bone Joint Surg Br 62:358–362, 1980.
34. Black KM, McClure P, Polansky M: The influence of different sitting positions on cervical and lumbar posture. Spine 21:65–70, 1996.
35. Arnold CM, Beatty B, Harrison EL, et al: The reliability of five clinical postural alignment measures for women with osteoporosis. Physiother Can 52:286–294, 2000.
36. Clarke GR: Unequal leg length: an accurate method of detection and some clinical results. Rheumat Phys Med 11:385–390, 1972.
37. Fisk JW, Baigent ML: Clinical and radiological assessment of leg length. NZ Med J 81:477–480, 1975.
38. Nichols PJR, Bailey NTJ: The accuracy of measuring leg-length differences. Br Med J 2:1247–1248, 1955.
39. Woerman AL, Binder-Macleod SA: Leg-length discrepancy assessment: accuracy and precision in five clinical methods of evaluation. J Orthop Sports Phys Ther 5:230–239, 1984.
40. Maitland GD: The slump test: examination and treatment. Aust J Physiother 31:215–219, 1985.
41. Philip K, Lew P, Matyas TA: The inter-therapist reliability of the slump test. Aust J Physiother 35:89–94, 1989.
42. Butler DS: Mobilisation of the nervous system, Melbourne, 1991, Churchill Livingstone.

SUGGESTED READINGS

Anderson BJG, Ortengon R, Nachemson Al, et al: The sitting posture: an electromyographic and discometric study. Orthop Clin North Am 6:105–120, 1975.

Cailliet R: Nerve and arm pain, Philadelphia, 1964, FA Davis.

Cartas O, Nordin M, Frankel VH, et al: Quantification of trunk muscle performance in standing, semistanding, and sitting postures in healthy men. Spine 18:603–609, 1993.

Cyriax J: Textbook of orthopaedic medicine, vol 1. Diagnosis of soft tissue lesions, London, 1982, Bailliere Tindall.

Dieck GS, Kelsey JL, Goel VK, et al: An epidemiological study of the relationship between postural asymmetry in the teen years and subsequent back and neck pain. Spine 10:872–877, 1985.

During J, Goudfrooij H, Keessen W, et al: Towards standards for posture—postural characteristics of the lower back system in normal and pathological conditions. Spine 10:83–87, 1985.

Fischer P: Clinical measurement and significance of leg length and iliac crest height discrepancies. J Man Manip Ther 5:57–60, 1997.

Itoi E: Roentgenographic analysis of posture in spinal osteoporotics. Spine 16:750–756, 1991.

Kapandji IA: The physiology of the joints, vol 2. The trunk and vertebral column, New York, 1974, Churchill Livingstone.

Kappler R: Postural balance and motion patterns. J Am Osteopath Assoc 81:598–606, 1982.

Littler WA: Cardiorespiratory failure and scoliosis. Physiotherapy 60:69–70, 1974.

MacDougall JD, Wenger HA, Green HJ: Physiological testing of the elite athlete, Ottawa, 1982, Canadian Association of Sports Sciences.

Matthews DK: Measurement in physical education, Philadelphia, 1973, WB Saunders.

McKinnis DL: The posture-movement dynamic. In Richardson JK, Iglarsh ZA, editors: Clinical orthopedic physical therapy, Philadelphia, 1994, WB Saunders.

Mellin G, Poussa M: Spinal mobility and posture in 8- to 16-year-old children. J Orthop Res 10:211–216, 1992.

Mennell J: Back pain: diagnosis and treatment using manipulative techniques, Boston, 1960, Little, Brown.

Murray MP, Seireg A, Scholz RC: Centre of gravity, center of pressure and supportive forces during human activities. J Appl Physiol 23:831–838, 1967.

Nashner LM: Sensory, neuromuscular and biomechanical contributions to human balance. In Duncan PW, editor: Balance: proceedings of the American Physical Therapy Association Forum, Alexandria, VA, 1990, American Physical Therapy Association.

Opila KA: Gender and somatotype differences in postural alignment: response to high-heeled shoes and simulated weight gain. Clin Biomech 3:145–152, 1988.

Pacelli LC: Straight talk on posture. Phys Sportsmed 19:124–127, 1991.

Portnoy H, Morin F: Electromyographic study of postural muscles in various positions and movements. Am J Physiol 186:122–126, 1956.

Richardson JK, Iglarsh ZA: Clinical orthopedic physical therapy, Philadelphia, 1994, WB Saunders.

Riemann BL, Caggiano NA, Lephart SM: Examination of a clinical method of assessing postural control during a functional performance task. J Sports Rehab 8:171–183, 1999.

Rothman RH, Simeone FA: The spine, Philadelphia, 1982, WB Saunders.

Torell G, Nordwall A, Nachemson A: The changing pattern of scoliosis treatment due to effective screening. J Bone Joint Surg Am 63:337–341, 1981.

Tsai L, Wredmark T: Spinal posture, sagittal mobility and subjective rating of back problems in former female elite gymnasts. Spine 18:872–875, 1993.

Vakos JP, Nitz AJ, Threlkeld AJ, et al: Electromyographic activity of selected trunk and hip muscles during a squat lift. Spine 19:687–695, 1994.

Walker ML, Rothstein JM, Finucane SD, et al: Relationships between lumbar lordosis, pelvic tilt, and abdominal muscle performance. Phys Ther 67:512–516, 1987.

Williams MM, Hawley JA, McKenzie RA, et al: A comparison of the effects of two sitting postures on back and referred pain. Spine 16:1185–1191, 1991.

Wolfson LI, Whipple R, Amerman P, et al: Stressing the postural response: a quantitative method for testing balance. J Am Geriatr Soc 34:845–850, 1986.

Woollacott M: Postural control mechanisms in the young and old. In Duncan PW, editor: Balance: proceedings of the American Physical Therapy Association Forum, Alexandria, VA, 1990, American Physical Therapy Association.

CHAPTER **16**

Assessment of the Amputee

An amputation is defined as the removal of part or all of a limb or some other outgrowth of the body. If fingers and partial non-mutilating hand injuries are excluded, lower-limb amputations are much more frequent than upper-limb amputations.[1] However, upper-limb amputations cause greater functional loss because the upper limbs are used more functionally and in many more diverse ways. There is also a greater functional sensory loss when an upper limb is involved. In addition, the upper-limb amputation causes a more obvious disfigurement and alteration of body image, which affects the actions and reactions of both the amputee and those with whom he or she interacts.[1,2] Amputations are considered to be a treatment of last resort when other methods, such as revascularization or reattachment, have failed or are not considered suitable treatment options.[2-5] Assessment of the amputee patient may involve assessing a patient before the amputation or after the amputation has taken place. In the first instance, the assessment is primarily carried out by one or more physicians deciding whether there is a need for such a procedure and then deciding the level at which the amputation should occur. In some cases, indexes or scores[6-19] may be used although some[20] have questioned their usefulness in the final outcome, especially in the case of trauma.

There are several indications for amputations.[21] The most common are trauma caused by compound fractures, blood vessel rupture, stab or gunshot injuries, compression injuries, severe burns, or cold injuries;[22] and vascular disease as the result of systemic problems, such as diabetes, arteriosclerosis, embolism, venous insufficiency, or peripheral vascular disease often aggravated by cigarette smoking.[23] About 75% of amputations in older patients fall within this second category.[24] The presence of suspected vascular disease may include more than the physical examination when considering whether to amputate. These other tests include blood tests, chest x-rays, electrocardiography, Doppler studies, arteriography, venograms, thermography, and transcutaneous PO_2 readings.[22] When trauma is the cause, the aim of the amputation is to restore maximum length with good soft-tissue covering.[22] In addition, amputations may be performed because of infections, tumors (both benign and more commonly, malignant types), neurological disorders (e.g., an anaesthetic limb from, for example, a complete plexus

avulsion[25]), congenital deformity (e.g., partial or total absence of a limb), and amputations for cosmetic reasons (e.g., extra digit).[25-28] Younger people tend to experience more congenital, malignancy, and trauma-related amputations, whereas older people experience multiple pathophysiological mechanisms, as previously mentioned.

Causes of Amputation

- Trauma
- Vascular disease
- Infection
- Tumors
- Neurological disorders
- Congenital deformity

The examiner who has the opportunity to do a preoperative physical assessment of the patient who has been scheduled for an amputation should take the time to determine the patient's available muscle strength, range of motion (ROM), and functional mobility **bilaterally** to provide a baseline for future comparison if necessary. The size and position of any abnormal tissue degeneration or potential pressure areas should be recorded accurately, and functional levels should be assessed and recorded. If at all possible in this preoperative period, the patient should be given some instruction in bed mobility, as well as climbing in and out of bed with or without support. In addition, the examiner should ensure that the patient knows how to provide suitable care for pressure areas and preserve joint mobility to prevent any contractures from forming. If a lower-limb amputation is anticipated, the patient should be taught to use ambulatory aids such as crutches or wheelchair so that he or she can maintain as much mobility as possible after the amputation.

LEVELS OF AMPUTATION

Amputation surgery, whether performed to the upper limb or the lower limb, can occur at various levels (Figures 16-1 and 16-2).[29] For the most part, this chapter deals with assessment of the lower-limb amputee primarily, because these amputations are more common. However,

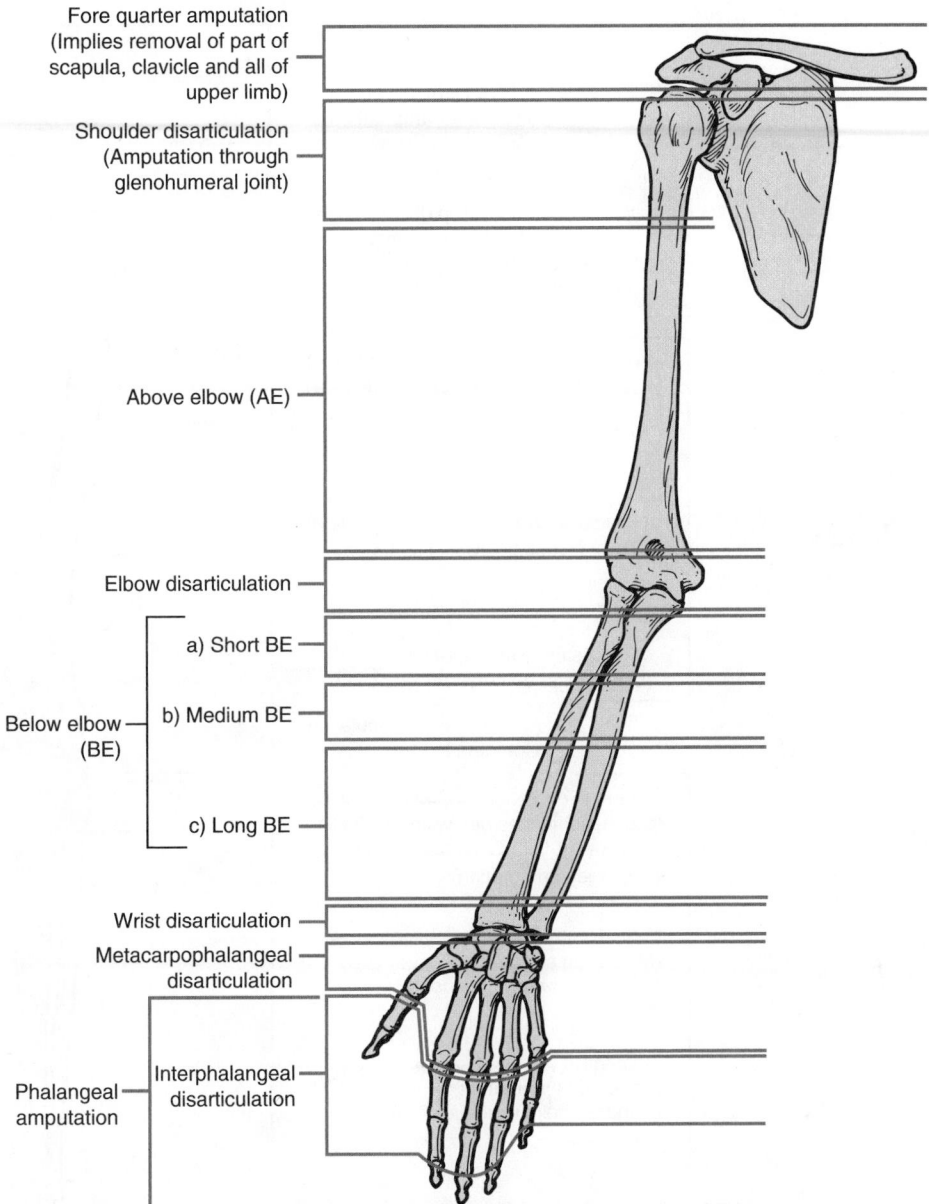

Fore quarter amputation
(Implies removal of part of
scapula, clavicle and all of
upper limb)

Shoulder disarticulation
(Amputation through
glenohumeral joint)

Above elbow (AE)

Elbow disarticulation

a) Short BE

Below elbow
(BE)
b) Medium BE

c) Long BE

Wrist disarticulation

Metacarpophalangeal
disarticulation

Phalangeal
amputation
Interphalangeal
disarticulation

Figure 16-1 Common levels of amputation—upper limb.

functional loss is usually greater for upper-limb amputees. Thus upper-limb amputee assessment deals much more with different functional demands than lower-limb assessment. Figure 16-3 shows the percentage impairment caused by an upper-limb amputation.[30]

Amputation surgery may be one of two types—open or closed. Open, or primary, amputation is used in cases of infection in which the wound is left open after the amputated part is removed to allow clearance of infection. It requires a second procedure to close the wound. More commonly, a closed amputation is performed. This procedure is used when tissue viability is as normal as possible. At the time of the amputation, the skin flaps are closed, as is the wound. Commonly, the skin flaps are closed on the posterior and distal aspect of the stump because adhesions are less likely and an incision line is further from the bone, but other methods are also sometimes used.[31] The goal of amputation surgery is to create a dynamically-balanced residual limb with good motor control and sensation.[32] The patient will need a well-healed, well-shaped residual stump with the greatest functional length possible in the limb.[32] The higher the level of the amputation, the greater the handicap.[25] In the lower limb, immediate prosthetic fitting helps facilitate early mobilization with more normal gait patterns.[26] Amputation should be considered to be a reconstructive procedure leaving the patient with the best of possible alternatives.[33]

The second opportunity where the amputee patient may be assessed is following the surgery. This is more

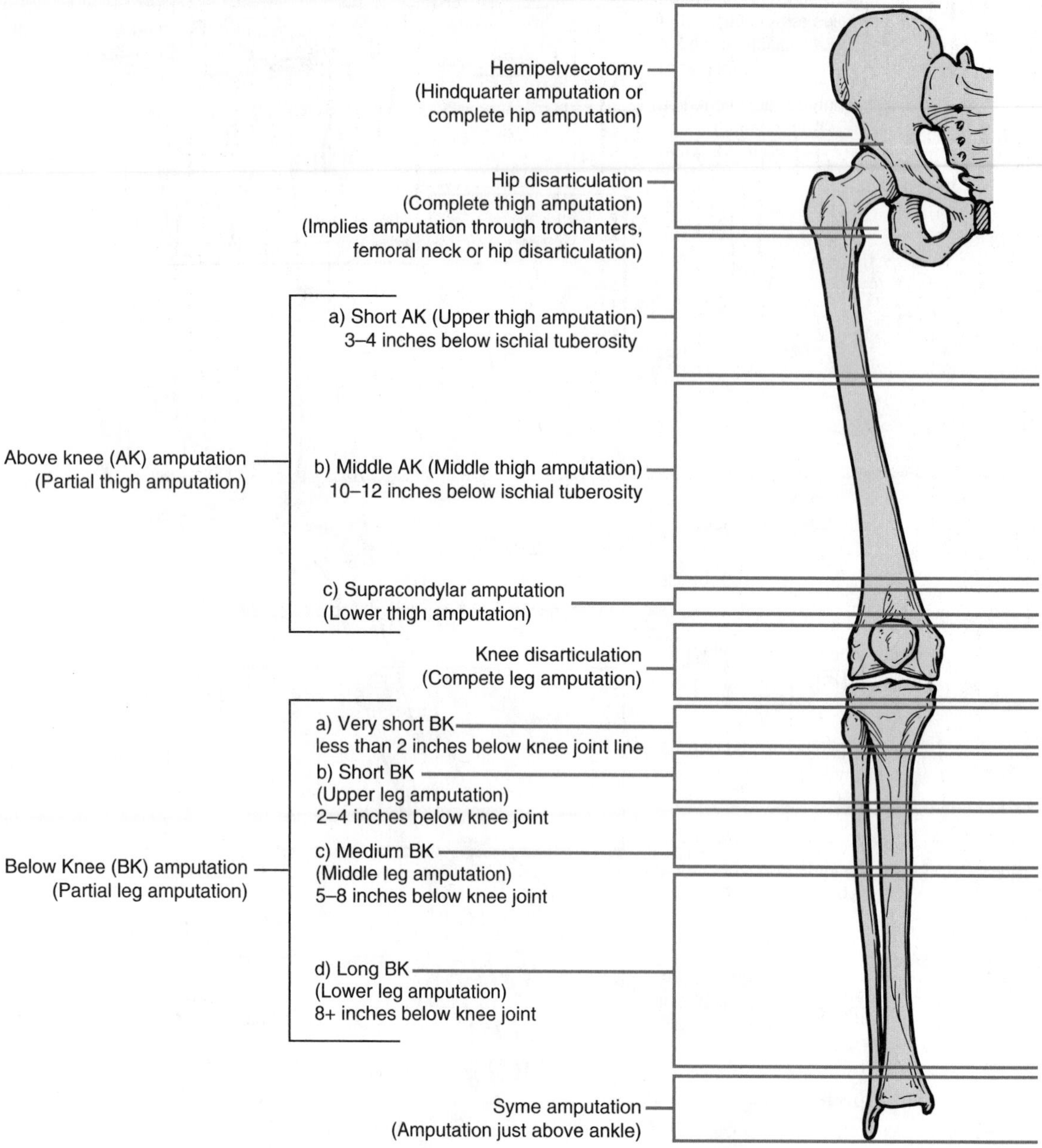

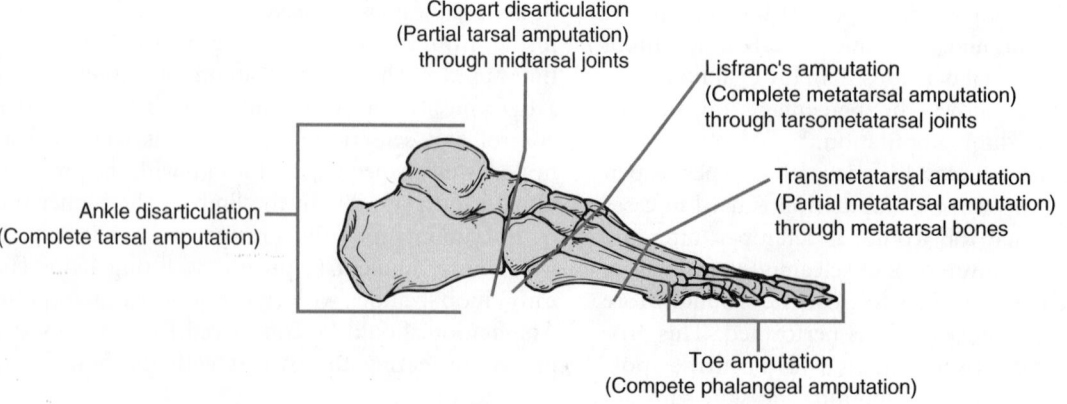

Hemipelvecotomy
(Hindquarter amputation or
complete hip amputation)

Hip disarticulation
(Complete thigh amputation)
(Implies amputation through trochanters,
femoral neck or hip disarticulation)

Above knee (AK) amputation
(Partial thigh amputation)

a) Short AK (Upper thigh amputation)
3–4 inches below ischial tuberosity

b) Middle AK (Middle thigh amputation)
10–12 inches below ischial tuberosity

c) Supracondylar amputation
(Lower thigh amputation)

Knee disarticulation
(Compete leg amputation)

Below Knee (BK) amputation
(Partial leg amputation)

a) Very short BK
less than 2 inches below knee joint line

b) Short BK
(Upper leg amputation)
2–4 inches below knee joint

c) Medium BK
(Middle leg amputation)
5–8 inches below knee joint

d) Long BK
(Lower leg amputation)
8+ inches below knee joint

Syme amputation
(Amputation just above ankle)

Chopart disarticulation
(Partial tarsal amputation)
through midtarsal joints

Lisfranc's amputation
(Complete metatarsal amputation)
through tarsometatarsal joints

Transmetatarsal amputation
(Partial metatarsal amputation)
through metatarsal bones

Ankle disarticulation
(Complete tarsal amputation)

Toe amputation
(Compete phalangeal amputation)

Figure 16-2 Common levels of amputation—lower limb.

history (which may include information on alcohol or drug abuse), current stressors (including recent losses), pain tolerance, previous association with patients who have disabilities, and compliance with medical treatments.[24] In addition, information on family structure and possible support groups, including family and friends, must be discussed. Issues such as marital status, sexual history, family roles including familial support, strengths, and problems should be ascertained, because they can impact greatly the outcome and how the patient ultimately functions as an amputee.[35,36]

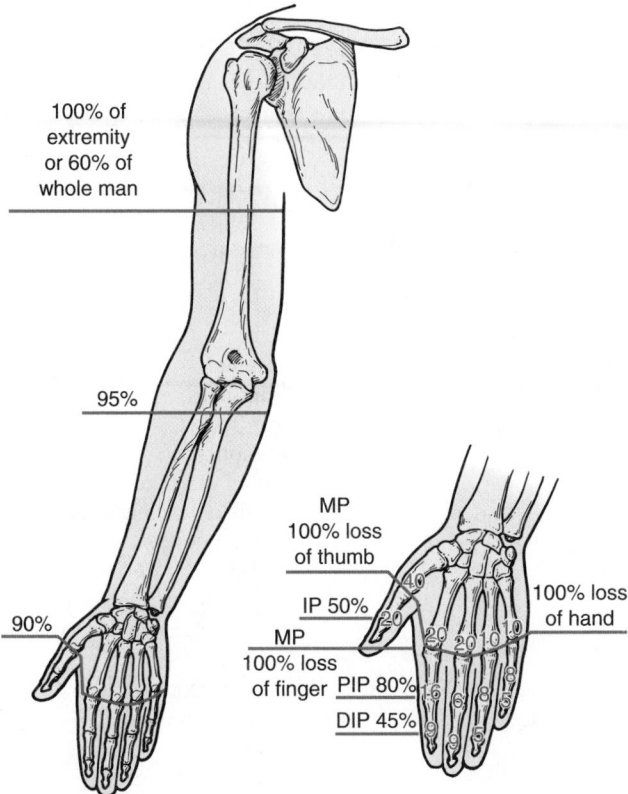

Figure 16-3 Amputation impairment. Percentage of impairments related to whole body, extremity, hand, or digit. *DIP,* Distal interphalangeal; *IP,* interphalangeal; *MP,* metacarpophalangeal; *PIP,* proximal interphalangeal. (Redrawn from Swanson AB, de Groot Swanson G, Goran-Hagert C: Evaluation of hand function. In Hunter JM, Schneider LH, Mackin EJ, et al, editors: Rehabilitation of the hand, St Louis, 1990, Mosby, p. 119.)

likely to be done by the physician or other health care professionals. In this case, the aim of the assessment is primarily to determine what functional deficits the patient has, to assess the fitting of the prosthesis, and to watch for complications. A good assessment enables the clinician to assist the patient in understanding and dealing with the specific physical and social limitations that the amputation has brought to his or her pattern of life.[34] This second scenario is described in the remainder of this chapter.

PATIENT HISTORY[34]

As with any assessment, the initial part of the examination will include the patient's history as it relates to the amputation, its cause, and any related factors. When doing the assessment of the amputee, it is important to determine the patient's past medical, surgical, preoperative ambulatory, and functional status for both upper and lower limbs, and preoperative symptoms. As part of this "past history," the examiner must develop some understanding of the patient's recreational activities, past psychiatric

Pertinent Information in Patient Assessment[24]

RELEVANT PATIENT INFORMATION
- Educational level
- Occupational history
- Avocational activities
- Psychiatric history, alcohol and drug use, problems with the law (It is important to have objective corroboration from the family.)
- Current stressors, including recent losses
- Any pain sensitivity or tolerance
- Previous associations with patients having disabilities
- Compliance with medical treatment; obstacles to compliance

FAMILY STRUCTURE
- Marital adjustment
- Sexual history
- Family roles; strengths and problem areas
- Health of others

THE PATIENT'S PERSPECTIVE
- Current mood
- Anxieties and ideas associated with them
- What the patient imagines his or her future to be (that is, how the disability will change lifestyle, social relations, vocational future); self-concept
- The degree to which self-esteem is related to physique and physical skills
- Comfort in meeting a psychiatrist or psychologist
- How the patient thinks the adjustment is going
- The most pressing immediate concern
- The patient's understanding of the cause and probable course of disability
- How much the patient wants to know about the treatment as it progresses; how the patient prefers having a medical update

The examiner must determine and develop an understanding for any patient anxieties, why they are present, whether these anxieties can be dealt with by the examiner or if other health care specialists need to be involved, what the patient imagines his or her future to be, and how the disability will change his or her lifestyle, social relations, vocational future, and self-concept (Table 16-1). All these

TABLE **16-1**

Patient Motivational and General Problems

Problem	Cause	Findings	Solution
Discouraged patient	Performance does not equal expectations	Does not wear prosthesis Complaints not related to physical findings	Sympathetic explanation of reasonable realistic goals Training
Failure to maintain good prosthetic habits	Lack of training New situations Poor motivation	Hip or knee flexion contracture Pressure sores Poor socket fit Abnormal gait patterns	Retraining Sympathetic encouragement
Poor hygiene	Poor motivation	Dermatitis Abscess formation Hidradenitis (inflammation of sweat glands)	Wash limb Clean socks Clean socket Antibiotics Surgical drainage
Rest pain	Phantom pain/sensation	Pain in missing segment of limb	Provide distracting sensation (a) Wrapping (b) Temperature changes (c) Activity with prosthesis (d) Transcutaneous nerve stimulation
	Neuroma Ischemia	Positive Tinel sign Crampy pain aggravated by activity	Excise neuroma Unweight limb Stop smoking Revise amputation

Modified from Smith AG: Common problems of lower extremity amputees. Orthop Clin North Am 13:576, 1982.

factors must be considered if the examiner hopes to have a successful outcome to treatment.

For the present medical history, the following questions should be asked:

1. *What is the patient's occupation?* Does the patient have any concerns about returning to his or her job? If so, what are the patient's future occupational plans? Is any vocational guidance or training required?

2. *What is the patient's present medical status?* For example, what was the reason for the amputation? Any systemic disease, such as diabetes, cardiovascular or respiratory problems, arthritic joints, and lifestyle factors, has a bearing on successful treatment outcomes. Systemic disease or trauma may prolong the healing process, and the speed of recovery may be delayed.

3. *How long ago did the amputation occur?* In recent amputations, the initial concern is the healing of the stump and the prevention of complications. If the amputation surgery was a revision procedure, why was the revision necessary? Was the problem one of poor tissue viability, or was the procedure performed to enable the patient to obtain better functional results?

4. *If the amputation occurred some time ago (3 to 6 months or longer), has the patient experienced any complications over that period, such as tissue breakdown, ulcer formation, or blisters?*

5. *If the patient has a prosthesis, what does the patient think about the prosthesis, its fit, and its function?* How long has the prosthesis been worn? (Years? Months?) How long is the prosthesis worn each day? Is it worn every day? Is the suspension adequate? Are there any skin abrasions? Inadequacies in these areas will lead to patient frustration, to disappointment, and, ultimately, to the patient becoming discouraged about using the prosthesis and, in fact, may come to the state where the patient does not want to wear the prosthesis. If the prosthesis is uncomfortable or excessively noisy, it is unlikely the patient will use it, or if it is used, it is unlikely the patient will use it properly. In the case of a lower-limb prosthesis, the patient may refuse to bear weight on the prosthesis. Cosmesis is another problem that is often of concern for amputees, especially for women, and when the amputation is in the upper limb the extremity is sometimes not covered with clothing. The examiner must differentiate between the discomfort of using something new and the discomfort caused by a specific prosthetic fault. In some cases, a prosthesis evaluation questionnaire (PEQ)[37] may be useful (Figure 16-4).

6. *Has the patient been looking after the stump properly, ensuring proper limb and sock hygiene?* Failure to do so easily leads to complications, such as skin breakdown, infection, and ulcers (see Table 16-1).[32] The

Sample Items in the 10 Prosthesis Evaluation Questionnaire

(Respondents are asked to rate the item over the past 4 weeks.)

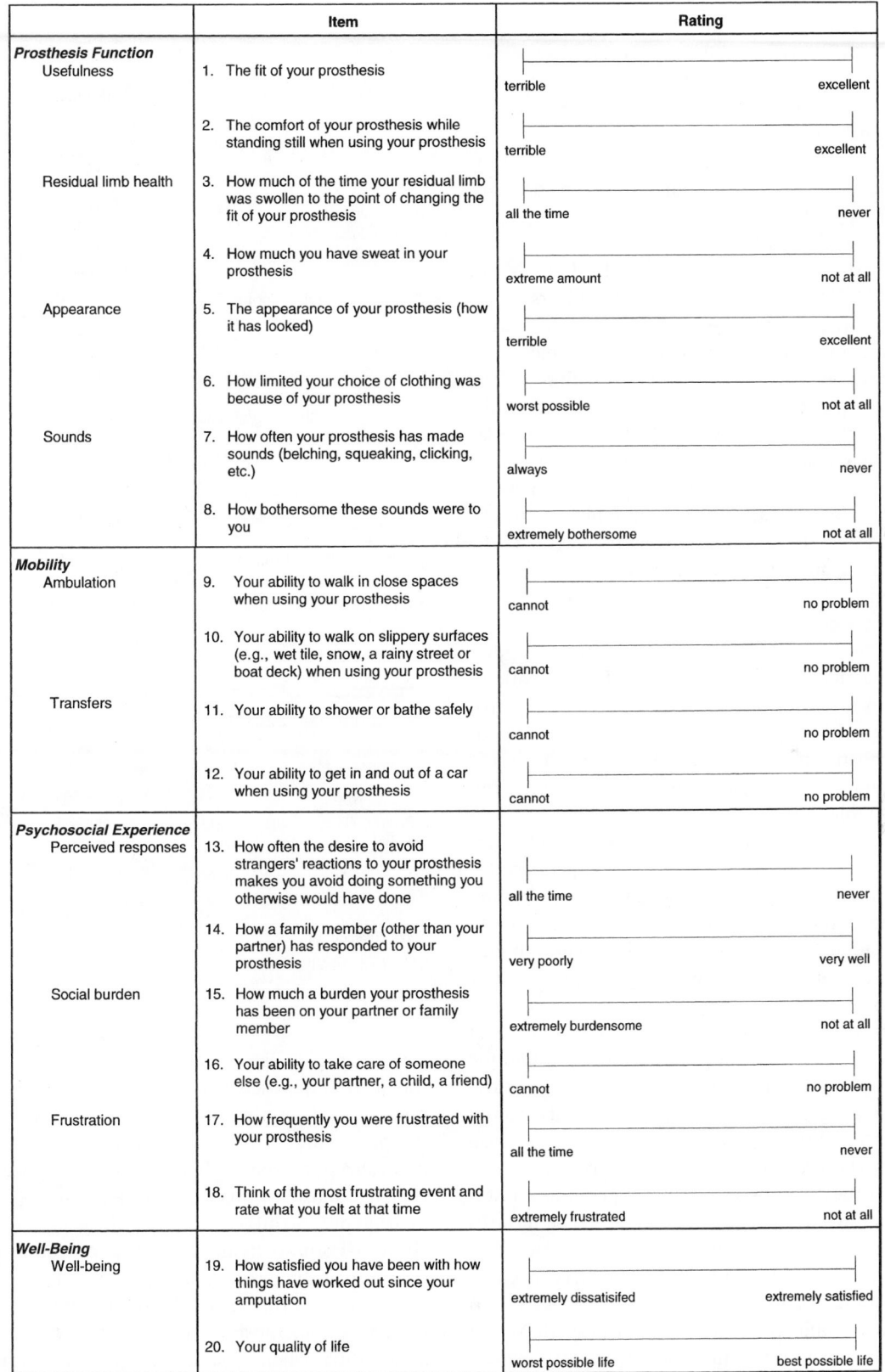

Figure 16-4 Sample items in the ten prosthesis evaluation questionnaire (PEQ) scales. (Modified from Legro MW, Reiber GD, Smith DG, et al: Prosthetic evaluation questionnaire for persons with lower limb amputations: assessing prosthesis-related quality of life. Arch Phys Med Rehabil 79:934, 1998.)

remaining stump should be washed with care using mild soap. The stump sock should be changed and cleaned regularly, and the prosthesis socket should also be cleaned regularly with mild soap and water.[32]

7. *Does the patient have any pain or abnormal sensation?* Where is the pain or abnormal sensation? Is the pain intermittent or constant? What is the intensity of the pain (a visual analogue scale may be used—see Figure 1-4)? Where is the pain? What type of pain or abnormal sensation is it? **Phantom sensation** is an abnormal feeling the patient has for the limb, but the patient feels the sensation as being in the amputated part of the limb even though that part of the limb is not there.[22,38–40] This sensation is an almost universal consequence of limb amputation.[41,42] It may take numerous forms, including the feeling that someone is touching the amputated limb, pressure being applied to the missing body part, cold, wetness, itching, tickle, pain, or fatigue. The intensity of these sensations may vary and may change over time. The sensations commonly have different meaning to different people. Phantom sensations are more commonly felt in the distal part of the excised extremity, because the distal part of an extremity tends to be more richly innervated.[38]

Phantom pain is described as a painful sensation perceived in the missing body part in the case of an amputation, in the paralyzed part of a spinal cord injury patient, or following a nerve root avulsion in the case of a neurological injury.[22,38–41] Eighty percent of amputees experience some phantom pain sometime during the injury healing process. Phantom pain is relatively common, but it is unpredictable in terms of predisposing factors, severity, frequency, duration or character, aggravation by internal or external stimuli, or type of pain experienced.[38] Phantom pain is more likely to be seen in the upper-limb amputee than in the lower-limb amputee, and it tends to be more prolonged in the upper limb. Some patients report that the pain is of very high intensity, which may be evoked by some external or internal stimuli, whereas others report a dull, continuous aching or burning that does not seem to be episodic. Many amputees describe the pain as being knifelike, burning, sticking, shooting, prickling, throbbing, cramplike, squeezing, "like something trying to pull my leg off," or some type of electrical phenomenon (Figure 16-5).[39,41] Phantom pain generally begins within the first postsurgical week, commonly stabilizes after a few months, but may occur several months or years after the amputation. It seems to decrease in frequency, duration, and severity during the first 6 months. Most commonly, phantom pain persisting beyond 6 months is very difficult to treat and usually does not change in character after that time. Some people, however, report that the intensity of pain changes with time. Prolonged healing or other complications, such as fractures, may cause phantom pain to persist for longer periods.

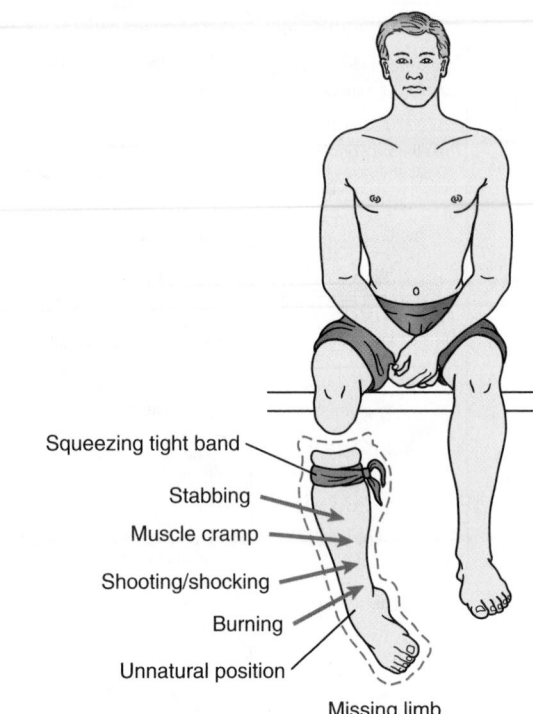

Figure 16-5 Phantom limb pain. Some of the typical painful feelings that seem to stem from the missing limb. (Redrawn from Sherman RA: Stump and phantom limb pain. Neurol Clin 7:250, 1989.)

Phantom Pain Sensations[39]	
• Knifelike*†	• Throbbing
• Sticking*	• Pressing
• Shooting	• Cramplike
• Prickling	• Sawing
• Burning†	• Dull
• Squeezing†	

*More common early
†More common after 6 months

Stump pain is pain arising from the residual part of the body as opposed to phantom pain, which is felt in the missing part of the body.[22,38,39,41,42] It is commonly a sharp, sticking, or pressure feeling that, although diffuse, is localized to the end of the stump.[39] Stump pain is usually the result of six primary etiologies—prosthogenic, neurogenic, arthrogenic, sympathogenic, referred, and abnormal stump tissues.[38] The most common cause of stump pain is prosthogenic, which implies improper fitting of the prosthesis. The second type of stump pain is neurogenic, most commonly from the formation of a neuroma where the nerve was cut during surgery. Neuroma pain is usually characterized by sharp, shooting pain that can be evoked by light tapping over the neuroma (Tinel sign). Third, stump pain may be arthrogenic or coming from an adjacent joint or surrounding tissues, usually as a result of changing stresses to the tissues or because sufficient time has not been allowed for the tissues to adapt to the new stresses being applied to them. For example, back pain is initially a common finding in above-knee (AK) amputees.[42] Fourth, stump pain may be sympathogenic or associated with the sympathetic nerve system. This pain is sometimes called *causalgia, reflex sympathetic dystrophy,* or, as some people now call it, *sympathetically maintained pain.* Fifth, the pain may be referred. Non-radicular referred pain can come from the joints, muscles, or myofascial conditions. Last, abnormal tissue, such as bony exostosis, heterotrophic ossification, adherent scar, or sepsis (infection), can lead to pain in the remaining stump. Virtually every amputee experiences stump pain after amputation. Stump pain is a normal result of major surgery. However, it is frequently a shock to those patients who are not warned to expect it.[41] Stump pain is usually severe immediately after amputation and subsides quickly with healing. It tends to be more evident in patients who have nondecreasing phantom pain.[39] About 80% of amputees have functionally significant episodes of phantom or stump pain every year and may have almost constant, very low level, stump and phantom pain that they define as being over the threshold of nonpainful sensation.[41]

There is no evidence that phantom pain or stump pain is caused by psychological disorders although stress and psychological disturbances can exacerbate the pain.[41] They are both considered to be physiological phenomena.

OBSERVATION[34]

Following surgery, the examiner will observe the stump for any swelling and whether healing is occurring properly. The condition of the skin as well as the presence of joint contractures, especially if the amputation is close to a joint (e.g., below-knee [BK] amputation), should be noted. The amputee should be observed both without the prosthesis and while wearing the prosthesis. Generally, the lower-limb amputee is observed in three positions while wearing the prosthesis: standing, sitting, and walking.

To begin the observation of the amputee, the examiner first looks at the remaining good limb, noting sensation, pulses, temperature, and skin condition. The examiner takes time to observe the remaining limb that will have to take a greater functional role and often greater stresses because of the amputation to the other limb. If it is a lower-limb amputation, the remaining limb will have to take a greater load during gait. Are the skin and nails normal, or are trophic changes evident? Are there any sores or open areas? These changes may indicate circulatory impairment. What are the color and temperature of the remaining limb? Do they fall within normal

limits? Are the pulses (e.g., femoral, tibial, dorsalis pedis) normal? Does the limb exhibit any deformity or swelling? Will the remaining limb be able to take the additional stress?

The examiner notes whether the patient is wearing the prosthesis or not. If the patient has the prosthesis on, then observation of the patient functioning with the prosthesis is first done with the patient standing, walking, and sitting. If the patient is not wearing the prosthesis, the examiner spends the initial period checking the stump and its condition, noting whether the wound is healing properly or whether there are any signs of drainage or weeping from the wound or evidence of tissue breakdown.[32] If the stump is covered with an elastic wrap or shrinker to assist in decreasing swelling, the examiner should note how it is applied, whether it fits smoothly or contains wrinkles, and whether the application is effective in reducing swelling. The examiner can then ask the patient to remove the wrap. At this stage, the examiner can ask the patient to demonstrate how he or she applies the wrap (if the patient does it himself or herself), or this may be left until later.

With the wrap off, the examiner then inspects the stump, noting its shape. The stump may be classed as cylindrical, conical, bony, bulbous, or edematous. The examiner looks for signs of unusual patterns of swelling (an indication the wrap has been applied incorrectly) (Figure 16-6); causes of residual limb edema (Figure 16-7); presence of skin abrasions, skin breakdown, or blisters (all of which may indicate poor prosthesis fit); or presence of infection (Table 16-2).[32] The examiner should note whether the scar is healing normally and whether the sutures have been removed or some remain. The scar may be classed as non-tender, sensitive, invaginated, well-healed, open, or adherent. The location of the scar and

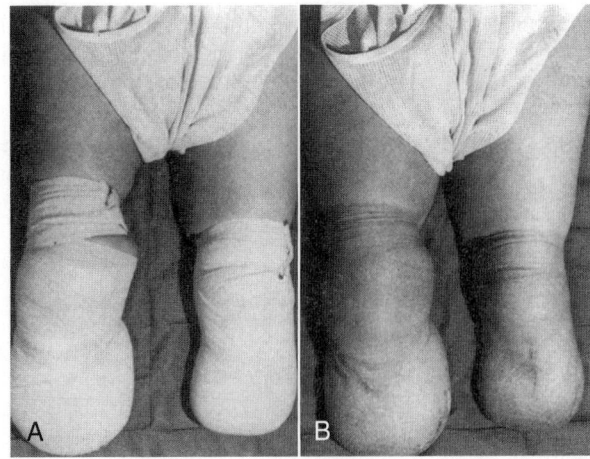

Figure 16-6 The effect of bad bandaging. A, An incorrectly applied bandage. **B,** The uneven residual limb contour produced by the incorrectly applied bandage. (From Engstrom B, Van de Ven C: Therapy for amputees, Edinburgh, 1999, Churchill Livingstone, p. 53.)

whether it will affect the fitting of the prosthesis should be noted. Any "dog ears" to the suture, which may interfere with the prosthesis, should also be noted. The mobility of the scar and tension of the skin and its mobility, especially over the distal end of the stump, should be observed. In addition, the color and temperature of the stump should be noted. Any potential weight-bearing areas (e.g., ischial tuberosity–AK amputation; patellar tendon–BK amputation) should also be inspected because these tissues will receive greater stress with the use of a

prosthesis. The condition of the remaining joints and their supporting musculature (e.g., atrophied, fleshy, strong) should be noted.

If the patient has a prosthesis, the prosthesis is then inspected (Table 16-3). The examiner should note the socket type, the material used to construct it, and the type of suspension. The general workmanship of the prosthesis and whether it is satisfactory should be noted. The examiner should inspect the trim lines, the rivets, and other fastenings to see if they are neat and secure. Joint covers should shield mechanical joint heads to prevent damage to clothing. There should be no scratches or rough areas on the prosthesis. Plastic lamination should be uniform without appreciable missed areas.

Next, provided the patient is at the stage where the prosthesis has been fitted (in some cases, especially in the lower limb, the prosthesis may be fitted right after surgery; in other cases, the prosthesis is fitted after tissue healing is ensured), the patient is asked to put the prosthesis on while the examiner determines whether the patient can correctly and easily do this independently or only with help.

For the lower-limb amputee, once the prosthesis is fitted, the patient is first observed in standing position. As with the patient who is not an amputee, posture of the patient is assessed (see Chapter 15) and the examiner must determine if any deviations are structural or due to the prosthesis. In addition, the examiner notes the following:

1. Does the patient appear to be comfortable while standing, especially with the heels no more than 15 cm (6 inches) apart as seen in normal standing?

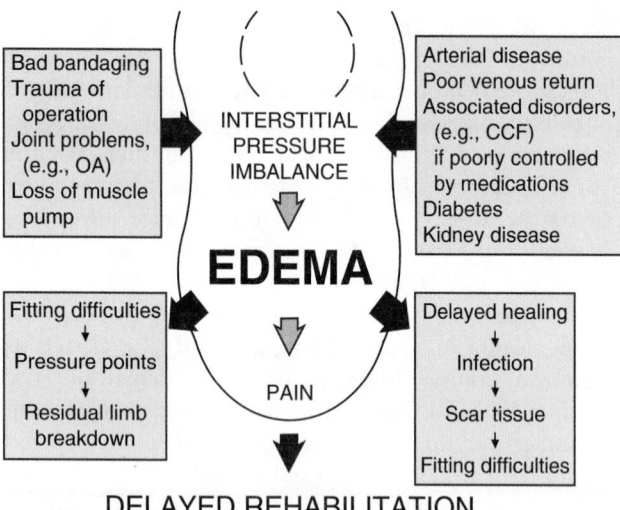

Figure 16-7 Causes of residual limb edema. (From Engstrom B, Van de Ven C: Therapy for amputees, Edinburgh, 1999, Churchill Livingstone, p. 52.)

TABLE **16-2**

Amputation Problems

Problem	Cause	Findings	Solution
Limb shrinkage	Normal shrinkage with activity Weight loss	Limb too deep in socket Pressure areas on bony prominences Pressure on end of amputation Limb too short	Add stump socks Modify liners in socket New socket or prosthesis
Limb swelling	Edema Weight gain Failure to continue limb wrapping in recent amputee Failure to wear prosthesis for prolonged period without wrapping	Limb not fitting into socket Pressure on bony prominences Choking on end of stump Limb too long	Treat medical cause of edema Diet control Training in proper limb wrapping Socket relief Remove stump socks Wear stump shrinker
Joint contracture	Failure of preprosthetic training Lack of patient cooperation Patient does not wear prosthesis	Limb short Heel of prosthesis off floor Unstable gait Excessive knee and hip flexion when prosthesis off	Sympathetic encouragement Training Temporary prosthesis that is adjustable as contracture decreases

Modified from Smith AG: Common problems of lower extremity amputees. Orthop Clin North Am 13:570, 1982.

TABLE **16-3**

Problems Related to the Prosthesis

Problem	Cause	Findings	Solution
Improper socket fit	Improper fabrication	Same as for limb swelling or shrinkage shortly after Delivery	Socket relief New socket
Improper prosthetic alignment	Improper fabrication Patient changes height of shoe heel Joint contracture	Limb too long or too short with good socket fit Heel or toe off the floor Gait abnormalities Pressure areas on limb	Realign prosthesis Heel pads in shoe or shoes with original heel height Training to correct contracture
Inadequate suspension	Improper fabrication of suspension	Pistoning of limb in socket Insecurity on weight bearing Abrasions Gait abnormality that is similar to findings when prosthesis is too long Prosthesis incorrectly rotated Restriction of joint motion	Readjust suspension

Modified from Smith AG: Common problems of lower extremity amputees. Orthop Clin North Am 13:574, 1982.

2. Is the patient able to "balance" on the prosthesis when standing on two legs or when weight shifting between the two legs? At the same time, the examiner should note whether the anteroposterior alignment of the prosthesis is satisfactory so that the patient does not feel the knee is unstable or that the knee is being forced backward, in the case of a BK amputee. Also, the clinician should note whether the mediolateral alignment is satisfactory with the foot flat on the floor. There should be no uncomfortable pressure on the lateral or medial brim of the socket.

3. Is the prosthesis of correct length? When the patient rises on the prosthesis, is there any piston action of the stump in the prosthesis? Normally, there should be very little movement. Are the anterior, medial, and lateral walls of the prosthesis of adequate height? Do the medial and lateral walls of the stump contact the prosthesis in the correct places so that there is no weight on the end of the prosthesis? In the case of a joint disarticulation, weight-bearing through the end of the stump may be allowed, at least partially.

4. Are the size, contours, and colors of the prosthesis approximately the same as those of the sound limb? Are the "joints" similarly placed to the normal limb? The prosthesis should be inspected from the front, back, and side to check this. The patient should be asked if he or she is satisfied with the appearance of the prosthesis.

5. Is the suspension, if present, adequate and fully supporting the prosthesis during weight-bearing? Is the suspension adjustable if necessary?[43]

6. Does the patient consider the prosthesis satisfactory? This question will help to ensure that any items that may have been overlooked will be brought to the attention of the clinical team.

Next, the patient is observed seated while wearing the prosthesis. The examiner notes the following:

1. Can the patient sit comfortably with minimal bunching of the soft tissue around the prosthesis?

2. Does the socket remain securely on the stump? Is the patient able to sit comfortably with minimum functioning of the soft tissues around the prosthesis? Are the soft tissues and bony prominences free from excessive pressure? Does the prosthesis remain in good alignment?

The third phase of lower-limb amputee observation is to view the patient walking while wearing the prosthesis. During walking, the examiner should watch for hip or knee instability or abnormal gait. During this phase, the examiner observes the following:

1. Is the patient's performance and walking on a level surface satisfactory? Any gait deviation that requires attention should be noted. Gait deviations include an abducted or adducted gait, lateral trunk bending, circumduction, medial or lateral whip of the prosthesis, foot rotation on heel strike, uneven heel rise, foot slap, uneven step length, and vaulting. Also, the stump may be oversensitive and/or painful. A very short stump may fail to provide a sufficient lever arm for the pelvis. Finally, an abnormal gait pattern may develop because of a habitual pattern of movement.[22,44] A prosthesis aligned in abduction may cause a wide base gait resulting in this abnormal gait pattern. Amputee balance may be difficult if an adduction contracture is present. An abducted gait is characterized by a very wide base with the prosthesis held away from the midline at all

times. If the prosthesis is the cause of the abducted gait, it may be that the prosthesis is too large or that too much abduction may have been built into the prosthesis. A high medial wall may cause the amputee to hold the prosthesis away to avoid pressure on the pubic ramus. The pelvic band may be positioned too far away from the patient's body. This defective gait may also be caused by an abduction contracture or a poor habitual pattern of gait.[22,44]

Lateral bending of the trunk is characterized by excessive bending laterally, generally toward the prosthetic side, from the midline. If the prosthesis is the cause, it may be that it is too short or has an improperly shaped lateral wall that fails to provide adequate support for the femur. A high medial wall may cause the amputee to lean away to minimize the discomfort.

A circumduction gait is a swinging of the prosthesis laterally in a wide arc during the swing phase of gait. This defect may be due to the prosthesis being too long or the prosthesis having too much alignment stability or friction in the knee, making it difficult to bend the knee during the swing-through phase of gait. The amputee may have an abduction contracture of the stump or may lack confidence in flexing the prosthetic knee because of muscle weakness, or the amputee may fear stubbing the toe. Finally, this abnormal gait pattern may be the result of a habitually incorrect gait pattern.[22,44]

Medial or lateral whips are observed best when the patient walks away from the observer. A medial whip is present when the heel travels medially on initial flexion at the beginning of the swing phase, whereas a lateral whip exists with the heel moving laterally. If whipping occurs, then it is the fault of the prosthesis. Lateral whips are commonly seen from excessive medial rotation of the prosthetic knee. A medial whip may result from excessive lateral rotation of the knee. The socket may fit too tightly, thus reflecting stump rotation. Excessive valgus in the prosthetic knee may contribute to this defect. Also, a badly aligned toe break in the conventional foot may cause twisting at toe-off. Faulty walking habits by the amputee may also result in whips.[22,44]

Rotation of the prosthetic foot on heel strike is due to too much resistance to plantar flexion caused by the plantar flexor bumper or heel wedge.[22,44] If too much toe-out has been built into the prosthesis or if the socket fits too loosely, it may also cause a similar gait fault. If the amputee has poor stump muscle control or extends the stump too vigorously at heel strike, the same gait fault can occur.

If the amputee exhibits uneven arm swing, the altered gait may be due to poor balance, fear or insecurity, or a poor habitual pattern.

A long prosthetic step is seen when the amputee takes a longer step with the prosthesis than with the normal leg. If the prosthesis is at fault, it is usually due to insufficient initial flexion in the socket where a stump flexion contracture is present.[22,44]

Foot slap is a too rapid descent of the anterior portion of the prosthetic foot. It is commonly the result of plantar flexion resistance in the prosthesis being too soft, or the amputee may be driving the prosthesis into the walking surface too forcefully to ensure extension of the knee.[22,44]

Uneven heel rise is characterized by the prosthetic heel rising too much or too rapidly when the knee is flexed at the beginning of the swing phase. If the prosthesis is at fault, the knee joint may have insufficient friction, and there may be an inadequate extension aid. The amputee may also be using more power than necessary to force the knee into flexion.[22,44]

Uneven timing is characterized by steps of unequal duration or length, usually by a very short stance phase on the prosthetic side. An improperly fitting socket may cause pain and a desire to shorten the stance phase on the prosthetic side. A weak extension aid or insufficient friction in the prosthetic knee can cause excessive heel rise and thus result in uneven timing because of a prolonged swing-through. Alignment stability may also be a factor if the knee buckles too easily. In addition, the amputee may have weak muscles in the stump and may not have developed good balance. Fear and insecurity may also contribute to this defect.[22,44]

Terminal swing impact is characterized by rapid forward movement of the shin piece allowing the knee to reach maximum extension with too much force before heel strike. If the prosthesis has insufficient knee friction or the knee extension aid is too strong, this gait fault may be seen. In addition, the amputee may be trying to assure himself or herself that the knee is in full extension by deliberately and forcefully extending the stump.[22,44]

The amputee who feels unstable at the prosthetic knee may develop a feeling of instability that could lead to the danger of falling. In this case, the prosthetic knee joint may be too far ahead of the thigh, knee, ankle (TKA) line and insufficient initial flexion may have been built into the socket. Plantar flexion resistance may also be too great, causing the knee to buckle at heel strike. Failure to limit dorsiflexion can lead to incomplete knee control. Also, the amputee may have weak hip extensor muscles or a severe hip flexion contracture leading to instability.[22,44]

Drop-off at the end of stance phase is characterized by a downward movement of the trunk as the body moves forward over the prosthesis. The prosthesis is at fault if there is inadequate limitation of dorsiflexion of the prosthetic foot. The keel of a solid ankle cushion heel (SACH)-type foot may be too short, or the toe break of the conventional foot may be too far posterior. The socket may have been placed too far anterior in relation to the foot.[22,44]

Excessive trunk extension during the stance phase in which the amputee creates an active lumbar lordosis may also be seen in some amputees. If the prosthesis is at fault, it may be due to an improperly shaped posterior wall causing forward rotation of the pelvis to avoid full weight bearing on the ischium. It may also be due to insufficient initial flexion being built into the socket. In addition, the amputee may demonstrate hip flexor tightness or weakness of the hip extensors and may be attempting to substitute with the lumbar erector spinae muscles. Weak abdominal muscles contribute to this defect. The deviation may be due to a habitual pattern with the patient moving his or her shoulders backward in an effort to obtain better balance.[22,44]

Vaulting is characterized by rising on the toe of the normal foot to permit the amputee to swing the prosthesis through with little or no knee flexion. If the prosthesis is the cause, it may be too long or there may be inadequate socket suspension. Excessive alignment stability or some limitation of knee flexion, such as a knee lock or strong extension aid, may lead to altered gait. Vaulting is a fairly frequent habitual pattern that amputees develop. The amputee may also have fear of stubbing the toe, which could lead to this abnormal gait, or there may be some stump discomfort.[22,44]

The reader is referred to Lusardi, et al.[44] and Engerstrom and Van de Ven[22] for further information on prosthetic gait. Normally, gait deviations observed in BK amputees are fewer and less noticeable than in AK amputees.

2. Is the patient able to go up and down inclines and stairs satisfactorily? Is the patient able to kneel, bend down, and get up from kneeling?
3. Are the socket and suspension systems comfortable?
4. Does the prosthesis function quietly? Any noises coming from the prosthesis should be noted and the source of the noise determined. Occasionally, hissing may be heard as air enters and escapes from the socket as the amputee walks. This is associated with the piston action caused by inadequate suspension and poor socket fit or poor congruence between the socket and liner.[32,43]

After checking the gait while wearing the prosthesis, the prosthesis should be removed to check the patient's stump for tissue stress from the gait activity. At this stage, the examiner observes the following:

1. Does the patient's stump appear to be free of abrasions, discolorations, or excessive perspiration when the prosthesis is removed? Pressure discolorations and redness because of the prosthesis should normally disappear within 10 to 15 minutes. If they persist, then the causes of the irritation or pressure should be determined.

2. Is weight bearing distributed over the proper areas of the stump? For example, for a BK amputation with weight bearing on the patellar tendon, the medial-tibial flare, lateral distal, and posteroproximal aspects of the stump should bear weight. An indication of the weight-bearing area sometimes may be obtained by noting the imprint of the stump sock on the skin of the stump. To determine the concentration and location of the distal pressure, it may be desirable to insert a piece of modeling clay in the bottom of the socket. Flattening of the clay will indicate distal contact.

EXAMINATION

Before the examination, the examiner should read the operative report to determine which muscles have been cut or how they have been stabilized along with the amputation since this gives the examiner some idea of the muscles available to move the limb and prosthesis and to provide stability during functional movement.

Measurements Related to Amputation

The examiner should note the length and circumference of the stump as well as scar length. Methods of measuring for prosthesis fitting are shown in the accompanying forms (Figures 16-8 and 16-9). Other measurements include the following:

1. Amputation type: short (10% to 33% of sound side length); medium (34% to 67% of sound side length); long (68% to 100% of sound side length)
2. Ulcer measurements (if present) and descriptions

Active Movements

When assessing the amputee, the examiner must determine the ability (strength and endurance) of the muscles to move the remaining joints in the remaining stump and the range of active motion available in those joints. Ideally, ROM at the remaining joints should be close to normal but may be affected by contractures or scarring. This is especially true for the hip and knee in lower-limb amputees. The ROM available helps determine the patient's ability to move and control the prosthesis as well as whether the muscles are able to control the available ROM and provide stability when the patient is in the prosthesis. In addition, the strength, endurance, and ROM of the opposite good limb must be assessed, because greater stress will be placed on this limb, especially in the lower-limb amputee. In the case of an upper-limb amputee, if it has been the dominant limb that has experienced the amputation, the other limb will become the dominant limb of necessity, and new skills will have to be learned by that limb. In either case, a thorough assessment of the functional status of the remaining whole limb will be necessary, in addition to the examination of the

UPPER-EXTREMITY PROSTHETIC MEASUREMENTS

Name of Patient_____ Phone_____ Date_____

Address_____ City_____ State/Zip_____

Male ☐   Female ☐   Date of Birth_____ Height_____ Weight_____

Type of Prosthesis_____ Right_____ Left_____

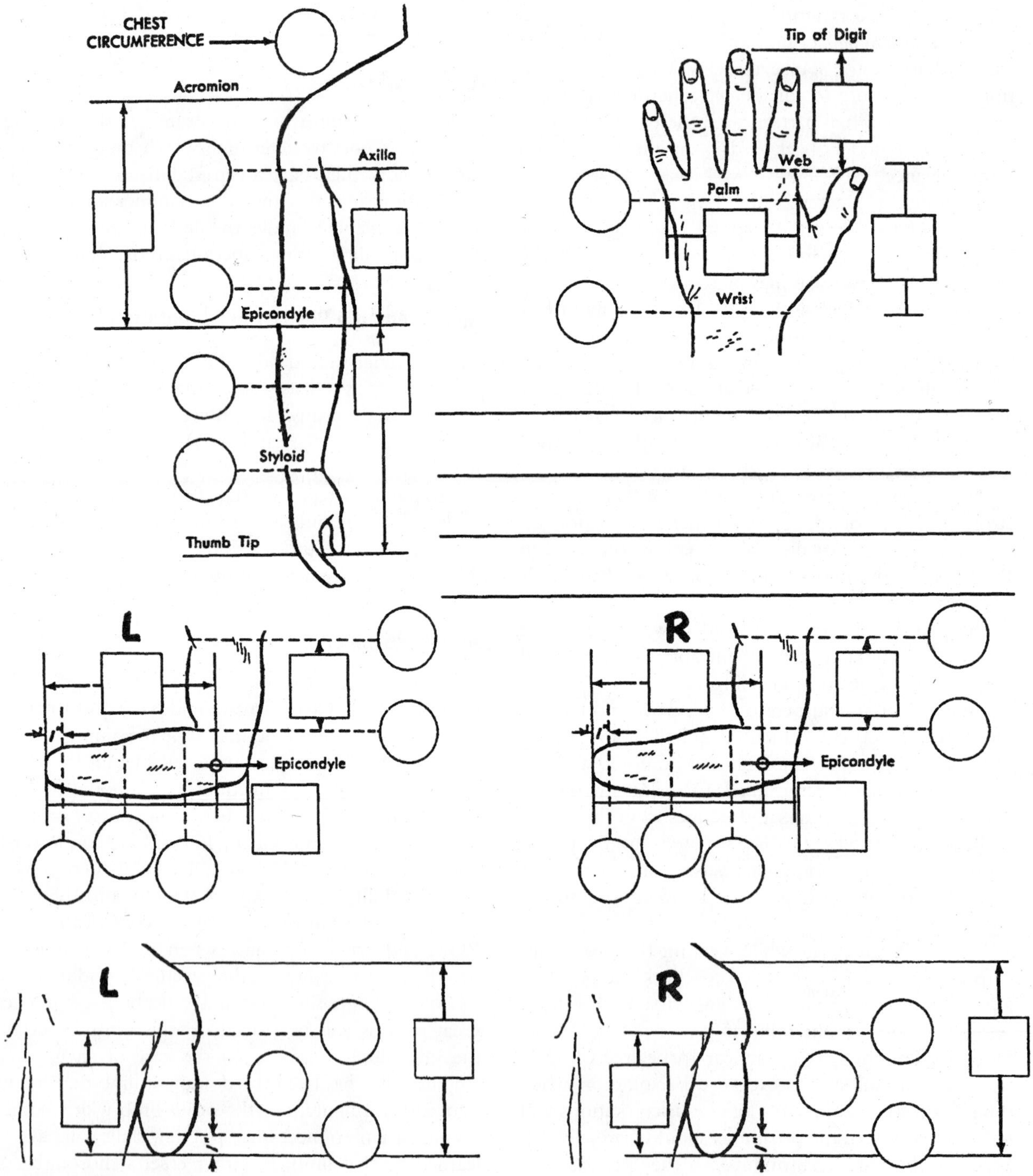

Figure 16-8 Upper-extremity prosthetic measurements. (Permission granted by the American Orthotic and Prosthetic Association, Alexandria, VA.)

LOWER-EXTREMITY PROSTHETIC MEASUREMENTS

Name of Patient _____ Phone _____ Date _____

Address _____ City _____ State_____

Age _____ Height _____ Weight _____

Type Prosthesis _____ Right _____ Left _____

Shoe Furnished:　One ☐　Both ☐　None ☐

Shoe Lace Opening:　Top ☐　Bottom ☐

Extra Light-Weight Limb: ☐

Extra Strong Limb: ☐

KB or BK Knee Joints: Size _____ Style _____

Angle Joint:　　Size _____ Style _____

KB or BK Thigh Lacing:

　　　Eyelets ☐　Hooks ☐　Both ☐

Thigh Lacer Height:_____

Shoulder Loop Size: _____

Waist Belt Size: _____

Color: Caucasian ☐　Negroid ☐

　Light Brown ☐　Medium ☐　Dark Brown ☐

Check Strap: Lace ☐　Leather Strap ☐

Measured by: _____

Shop Alterations

Lengthen Thigh _____ In. Shorten Thigh _____ In.

Lengthen Shin _____ In. Shorten Shin _____ In.

KB or BK Lace Opening: Top _____ In. Bottom _____ In.

Set BK Lacer on Joints:

　　　Higher _____ In.　Bottom _____ In.

Outside BK Joint Head:

　　　Set In _____ In.　Set Out _____ In.

Inside BK Joint Head:

　　　Set In _____ In.　Set Out _____ In.

Fit Foot In Shoe: Tight ☐ Loose ☐ Medium ☐

Make Heel Cushion: Soft ☐ Medium ☐ Firm ☐

Special Changes: _____

_____

Fitted By: _____

Finished BK Limb, Knee Center to Floor:_____ In.

Finished AK Limb, Ischium to Floor: _____ In.

Weight of Finished Limb: _____ lbs. _____ oz.

Finish of Limb: Plastic Laminate ☐

　　　　　　Rawhide Enamel ☐

Special Features : _____

_____

_____

Date Completed: _____

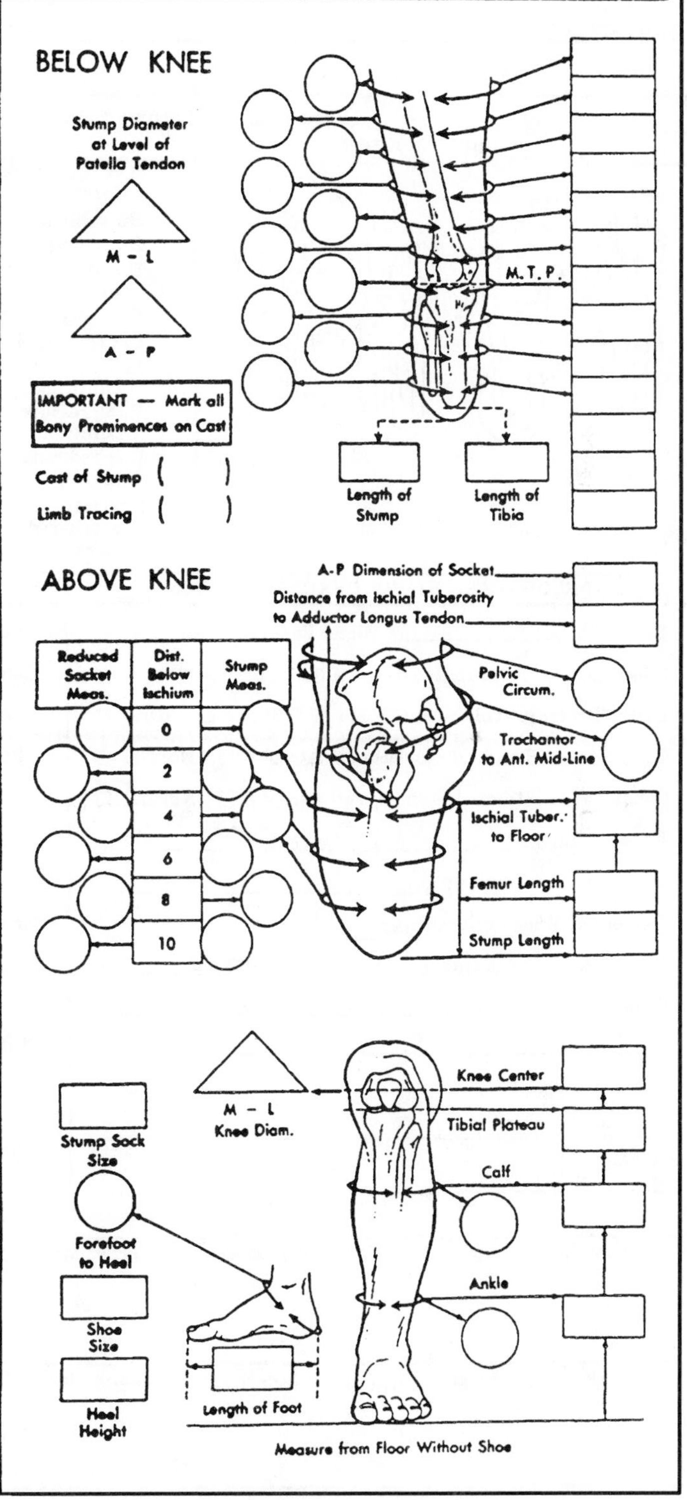

BELOW KNEE

Stump Diameter at Level of Patella Tendon

M – L

A – P

IMPORTANT — Mark all Bony Prominences on Cast

Cast of Stump ( )

Limb Tracing ( )

M.T.P.

Length of Stump

Length of Tibia

ABOVE KNEE

A-P Dimension of Socket_____

Distance from Ischial Tuberosity to Adductor Longus Tendon_____

Reduced Socket Meas.	Dist. Below Ischium	Stump Meas.
	0	
	2	
	4	
	6	
	8	
	10	

Pelvic Circum.

Trochanter to Ant. Mid-Line

Ischial Tuber. to Floor

Femur Length

Stump Length

M – L Knee Diam.

Stump Sock Size

Forefoot to Heel

Shoe Size

Heel Height

Knee Center

Tibial Plateau

Calf

Ankle

Length of Foot

Measure from Floor Without Shoe

A

Figure 16-9 A, Lower-extremity prosthetic measurements. (Medial tibial plateau *(MTP)*, the anatomical landmark of reference for establishing prosthetic build height and for starting circumferential measurements on the transtibial amputated residual limb.)　　　*Continued*

LOWER-EXTREMITY PROSTHETIC INFORMATION

Name of Patient _____

Site of Amputation _____ Right _____ Left _____

Clinic _____ Physician _____

(Show Location of Stump Details, Identify with Code Letters)

BELOW KNEE

Anterior   Posterior   Medial   Lateral

A = abrasion
B = boil or skin infection
Bu = bursa
Bs = bone spur
D = discoloration
E = edema
I = irritation
M = muscle bunching
P = pressure point
R = redundant tissue
S = scar
T = trigger point

ABOVE KNEE

Anterior   Posterior   Medial   Lateral

BELOW-KNEE STUMP CHARACTERISTICS

Stump Shape: _____ Distal Padding: _____

Subcutaneous Tissue: Heavy ☐ Light ☐

Distal Pressure Tolerance: None ☐ Slight ☐ Good ☐

Condition of Thigh Musculature: Atrophy ☐ Normal ☐

Condition of Stump Musculature: Atrophy ☐ Normal ☐

Knee Stability: _____

Range of Knee Motion: _____

Degrees of Knee Contracture: _____

Condition of Cut Bones: Tibia _____ Fibula _____

Remarks: _____

_____

_____

_____

ABOVE-KNEE STUMP CHARACTERISTICS

Stump Musculature	Soft	Average	Hard
General			
Hamstring Group			
Gluteal Group			
Rectus Femorus			
Adductor Longus			

Subcutaneous Tissue: Heavy ☐ Light ☐

Ischium: Toughened ☐ Pressure Sensitive ☐

    Muscle Padding _____ Prominent _____

Previous Ischial Bearing: Yes ☐ No ☐

Stump Lateral Convex   Concave
    Contour: Out ☐   Flat ☐   In ☐
Degree of Contracture: Hip Flexion _____°
                        Abduction _____°

Stump Adduction _____° Remarks: _____

Prescription for Prosthesis

3 Foot Comp. Model	5 Knee Comp. Model	Socket Materials	Type of Symes	6 Hip-Joint Model Type
4 Ankle Comp. Model	Type of Socket	Shank Materials	Hip Disartic. Type	Type of Suspension

B

Figure 16-9, cont'd B, Lower-extremity prosthetic information. (Permission granted by the American Orthotic and Prosthetic Association, Alexandria, VA.)

amputated limb. The active movements performed would be the same as those listed for the individual joints in other chapters in this book.

Passive Movements

Passive movements of the amputated limb and remaining normal limb are necessary to ensure the necessary ROM is available and to prevent contractures or to restore ROM after contractures occur. For example, BK amputees are prone to hip flexion and knee flexion contractures, especially if the amputee spends long periods sitting in bed or in a wheelchair. The passive movements performed would be the same as those listed for the individual joints in other chapters in this book. Passive movements give the examiner an understanding of the end feel present so that if contractures occur, proper stretching treatment can be instituted. If laxity or instability is present, the patient can be instructed in proper stabilization exercises.

Resisted Isometric Movements

Resisted isometric movements should be performed on the muscles of the amputated limb as well as the remaining normal limb to ensure the patient has the strength and endurance (or exercise tolerance) that will enable the patient to use a prosthesis.[45] Resisted movements of all muscles of the remaining joints on both the amputated limb and the remaining limb must be tested. These resisted movements would be the same as those listed for the individual joints in other chapters in this book. In lower-limb amputations, the muscles of the hip and knee are especially important to check. In the upper limb, the muscles of the shoulder, which play a significant role in positioning the prosthesis, must be assessed. Such testing enables the examiner to develop an exercise program to ensure maximum functionality of the patient.

Functional Assessment

For the amputee, functional assessment, for example, the Rivermead Mobility Index (RMI),[46] takes primary importance, so the examiner must determine the amputee's level of function and independence both with and without a prosthesis. This assessment may involve the care of the remaining stump, ability to put on and take off the prosthetic device, and determining the patient's anticipated level of activity and whether this activity level can be realistically met given the patient's handicap.

For the lower-limb amputee, the examiner should determine the following:
1. The patient's gait and endurance when walking and whether external support (crutches, cane) is necessary. Tests such as the 6- and 10-minute walk test, timed "up and go" test (TUG test), L-test for functional mobility, the modified Emory Functional Ambulation Profile, and the Amputee Mobility Predictor are outcomes that have been found to be both reliable and valid for amputees.[47]
2. The patient's bed mobility. That is, can the patient move easily in bed, or does he or she require assistance? Can the patient roll over, move from lying to sitting, or lie prone?
3. The patient's ability to transfer from sitting to standing and from bed to wheelchair.
4. The patient's ability to balance in sitting and standing (e.g., the Activities Specific Balance Confidence Scale[47]).
5. The patient's ability to get up from and down to different types of chairs.
6. The patient's ability to use aids (e.g., crutches, walker) for gait training. Can the patient manage a wheelchair?
7. The patient's ability to go up and down stairs and ramps and ability to move in confined spaces.
8. The patient's ability to get up from and down to the floor, as well as his or her ability to kneel, pick objects up from the floor, and do similar activities.

For the upper-limb amputee, the examiner should determine the following:
1. Whether the amputated part is from the dominant or nondominant limb
2. The patient's ability to perform functions of activities of daily living (ADLs) and instrumental activities of daily living (IADLs) (see Table 1-25)

Sensation Testing

The sensitivity of the stump must be tested to ensure normal sensation. Commonly, hypersensitive areas may be present that have to be desensitized. At the opposite extreme, some areas may have no sensation and require protection. In any case, sensation testing of the stump should involve, at a minimum, hot and cold sensation and light touch.

Psychological Testing

If necessary, psychological testing may be performed.[1,48] Some people have little difficulty adapting to the idea of losing a limb, whereas others have great difficulty accepting the fact that they have lost a limb. This acceptance may be related to how the patient lost the limb (trauma [suddenly] or from long-term problems, such as peripheral vascular disease), how active and independent the patient was before the amputation, or the patient's age (generally, children adapt much better to amputation and a prosthesis than adults). Sometimes, a psychological screening test, such as the Minnesota Multiphasic Personality Inventory (MMPI), may be used to determine the presence of depression, situational anxiety, and possible hysterical reaction to limb loss.[41]

Palpation

The examiner must take time during the examination to palpate the remaining stump of the limb. When palpating, the examiner is looking for normal mobility of the remaining tissues or any tissues that are adherent that may be amenable to treatment, any tissue tenderness, state of the overlying skin, tissue tension and texture, and any differences in tissue thickness, especially in "wear areas" where pressure is applied by the prosthesis. The uninvolved side should also be palpated for comparison.

Diagnostic Imaging

Although diagnostic imaging is not commonly a prerequisite for amputation surgery, especially in trauma cases, it may be used to evaluate the amputated stump. In this case, the examiner would be looking for the following:
1. The level of amputation to determine whether end weight bearing is possible; for example, a joint disarticulation is more likely to allow end weight bearing.
2. The presence of deformity, bony spurs, or loose fragments.
3. The size and shape, especially of the end bone of the amputation.

PRÉCIS OF THE AMPUTEE ASSESSMENT*

History
Observation (with and without prosthesis on)
   Standing (front, side, behind)
   Sitting (front, side, behind)
   Walking (front, side, behind) (watch for gait faults in
     lower-limb amputees)
   Stump examination
   Prosthesis examination
Examination
   Stump measurements
   Active movements

Passive movements
Resisted isometric movements
Functional assessment
Sensation testing
Psychological testing
Palpation
Diagnostic imaging

*As with any assessment, the patient must be warned that there may be some discomfort after the examination and that this discomfort is normal. Discomfort after any assessment should decrease within 24 hours.

REFERENCES

1. Beasley RW: General considerations in managing upper limb amputations. Orthop Clin North Am 12:743–749, 1981.
2. Beasley RW: Surgery of hand and finger amputations. Orthop Clin North Am 12:763–803, 1981.
3. Zhong-Wei C, Meyer VE, Kleinert HE, et al: Present indications and contraindications for replantation as reflected by long-term functional results. Orthop Clin North Am 12:849–870, 1981.
4. Jaeger SH, Tsai TM, Kleinert HE: Upper extremity replantation in children. Orthop Clin North Am 12:897–907, 1981.
5. Burton RI: Problems in the evaluation of results from replantation surgery. Orthop Clin North Am 12:909–913, 1981.
6. Slauterback JR, Britton C, Moneim MS, et al: Mangled extremity severity score: an accurate guide to treatment of the severely injured upper extremity. J Orthop Trauma 8:282–285, 1994.
7. O'Toole DM, Goldberg RT, Ryan B: Functional changes in vascular amputee patients: evaluation by Barthel Index, PULSES Profile and ESCROW Scale. Arch Phys Med Rehabil 66:508–511, 1985.
8. Spence VA, McCollum PT, Walker WF, et al: Assessment of tissue viability in relation to the selection of amputation level. Prosthet Orthot Int 8:67–75, 1984.
9. McCollum PT, Spence VA, Walker WF: Amputation for peripheral vascular disease: the case for level selection. Br J Surg 75:1193–1195, 1988.

10. Johansen K, Daines M, Howey T, et al: Objective criteria accurately predict amputation following lower extremity trauma. J Trauma 30:568–573, 1990.
11. Gregory RT, Gould RJ, Peclet M, et al: The mangled extremity syndrome (M.E.S.): a severity grading system for multisystem injury of the extremity. J Trauma 25:1147–1150, 1985.
12. Lange RH, Bach AW, Hansen ST, et al: Open tibial fractures with associated vascular injuries: prognosis for limb salvage. J Trauma 25:203–208, 1985.
13. Howe HR, Poole GV, Hansen KJ, et al: Salvage of lower extremities following combined orthopedic and vascular trauma—a predictive salvage index. Am Surg 53:205–208, 1987.
14. Fairs SL, Ham RO, Conway BA, et al: Limb perfusion in the lower limb amputee—a comparative study using a laser Doppler flowmeter and a transcutaneous oxygen electrode. Prosthet Orthot Int 11:80–84, 1987.
15. McCollum PT, Spence VA, Walker WF: Circumferential skin blood flow measurements in the ischemic limb. Br J Surg 72:310–312, 1985.
16. Helfet DL, Howey T, Sanders R, et al: Limb salvage versus amputation—preliminary results of the mangled extremity severity score. Clin Orthop Relat Res 256:80–86, 1990.
17. Johansen K, Daines M, Howey T, et al: Objective criteria accurately predict amputation following lower extremity trauma. J Trauma 30:568–573, 1990.

18. Gregory RT, Gould RJ, Peclet M, et al: The mangled extremity syndrome (MES): a severity grading system for multisystem injury of the extremity. J Trauma 25:1147–1150, 1985.
19. Howe HR, Poole GV, Hansen KJ, et al: Salvage of lower extremities following combined orthopedic and vascular trauma—a predictive salvage index. Am Surg 53:205–208, 1987.
20. Bonanni F, Rhodes M, Lucke JF: The futility of predictive scoring of mangled lower extremities. J Trauma 34:99–104, 1993.
21. Gottschalk F: Transfemoral amputation—biomechanics and surgery. Clin Orthop Relat Res 361:15–22, 1999.
22. Engerstrom B, Van de Ven C: Therapy for amputee, Edinburgh, 1999, Churchill Livingstone.
23. Lind J, Kramhoft M, Bodtker S: The influence of smoking on complications after primary amputation of the lower extremity. Clin Orthop Relat Res 267:211–217, 1991.
24. Fitzpatrick MC: The psychologic assessment and psychosocial recovery of the patient with an amputation. Clin Orthop Relat Res 361:98–107, 1999.
25. Baumgartner RF: The surgery of arm and forearm amputations. Orthop Clin North Am 12:805–817, 1981.
26. Pandian G, Kowalske K: Daily functioning of patients with an amputated lower extremity. Clin Orthop Relat Res 361:91–97, 1999.

27. Aitken GT, Frantz CH: The child amputee. Clin Orthop Relat Res 148:3–8, 1980.
28. Lamb DW, Scott H: Management of congenital and acquired amputation in children. Orthop Clin North Am 12:977–994, 1981.
29. Kay HW, Newman JD: Relative incidence of new amputations. Orthotics and Prosthetics 29:3–16, 1975.
30. Swanson AB, de Groot Swanson G, Goran-Hagert C: Evaluation of hand function. In Hunter JM, Schneider LH, Mackin EJ, et al, editors: Rehabilitation of the hand, St Louis, 1990, Mosby.
31. Smith DG, Fergason JR: Transtibial amputations. Clin Orthop Relat Res 361:108–115, 1999.
32. Smith AG: Common problems of lower extremity amputees. Orthop Clin North Am 13:569–578, 1982.
33. Beasley RW, de Bese GM: Upper limb amputations and prostheses. Orthop Clin North Am 17:395–405, 1986.
34. Postgraduate Medical School—Prosthetics and Orthotics: Lower limb prosthetics, New York, 1988, New York University Medical Centre.
35. High RM, McDowell DE, Savrin RA: A critical review of amputation in vascular patients. J Vasc Surg 1:653–655, 1984.
36. Helm P, Engel T, Holm A, et al: Function after lower limb amputation. Acta Orthop Scand 57:154–157, 1986.
37. Legro MW, Reiber GD, Smith DG, et al: Prosthetic evaluation questionnaire for persons with lower limb amputations: assessing prosthesis-related quality of life. Arch Phys Med Rehabil 79:931–938, 1998.
38. Davis RW: Phantom sensation, phantom pain and stump pain. Arch Phys Med Rehabil 74:79–91, 1993.
39. Jensen TS, Krebs B, Nielsen J, et al: Phantom limb, phantom pain and stump pain in amputees during the first six months following limb amputation. Pain 17:243–256, 1983.
40. Omer GE: Nerve, neuroma, and pain problems related to upper limb amputations. Orthop Clin North Am 12:751–762, 1981.
41. Sherman RA: Stump and phantom limb pain. Neurol Clin 7:249–264, 1989.
42. Smith DG, Ehde DM, Legro MW, et al: Phantom limb, residual limb and back pain after lower extrem-ity amputations. Clin Orthop Relat Res 361: 29–38, 1999.
43. Kapp S: Suspension systems for prostheses. Clin Orthop Relat Res 361:55–62, 1999.
44. Lusardi MM, Berke GM, Psonak R: Prosthetic gait. Orthop Phys Ther Clin North Am 10:77–116, 2001.
45. Cruts HE, de Vries J, Zilvold G, et al: Lower extremity amputees with peripheral vascular disease: graded exercise testing and results of prosthetic training. Arch Phys Med Rehabil 68:14–19, 1987.
46. Franchignoni F, Brunelli S, Orlandini D, et al: Is the Rivermead Mobility Index a suitable outcome measure in lower limb amputees? A psychometric validation study. J Rehabil Med 35:141–144, 2001.
47. Stevens P, Fross N, Kapp S: Clinically relevant outcome measures in orthotics and prosthetics. Advancing orthotic and prosthetic care through knowledge. Am Acad Orthotists Prosthetists 5(1):1–14, 2009.
48. Pinzux MS, Graham G, Osterman H: Psychologic testing in amputation rehabilitation. Clin Orthop Relat Res 229:236–240, 1988.

SUGGESTED READINGS

Ashley RK, Vallier GT, Skinner SR: Gait analysis in pediatric lower extremity amputees. Orthop Rev 21:745–749, 1992.
Boulas HJ: Amputations of the fingers and hand: indications for replantation. J Am Acad Orthop Surg 6:100–105, 1998.
Burgess EM, Romano RL, Zettl JH: The management of lower extremity amputations, Washington, DC, 1969, US Government Printing Office.
Dowd GS: Predicting stump healing following amputation for peripheral vascular disease using the transcutaneous oxygen monitor. Ann R Coll Surg Engl 68:31–35, 1986.
Fletcher GF, Lloyd A, Waling JF, et al: Exercise testing in patients with musculoskeletal handicaps. Arch Phys Med Rehabil 69:123–127, 1988.
Frantz CH, Aitken GT: Management of the juvenile amputee. Clin Orthop Relat Res 14:30–49, 1959.
Ham R, Regan JM, Roberts VC: Evaluation of introducing the team approach to the care of the amputee: the Dulewich study. Prosthet Orthot Int 11:25–30, 1987.
Helm P, Engel T, Holm A, et al: Function after lower limb amputation. Acta Orthop Scand 57:154–157, 1986.
High RM, McDowell DE, Savrin RA: A critical review of amputation in vascular patients. J Vasc Surg 1:653–655, 1984.
Hume MC, Gellman H, McKellop H, et al: Functional range of motion of the joints of the hand. J Hand Surg Am 15:240–243, 1990.
Koerner I: Re-evaluation of amputee training. 1. Pre-prosthetic training. Physiother Can 16:79–85, 1964.
Koerner I: The gait of the amputee. Physiother Can 19:321–329, 1967.
Koerner IB: The phantom limb phenomenon in amputee training. Physiother Can 21:90–100, 1969.
Koerner IB: Rehabilitation of the lower extremity amputee, Edmonton, 1972, University of Alberta Printing Services.
Krouskop TA, Dougherty D, Yalcinkaya MI, et al: Measuring the shape and volume of an above-knee stump. Prosthet Orthot Int 12:136–142, 1988.
Lange RH, Bach AW, Hansen ST, et al: Open tibial fractures with associated vascular injuries: prognosis for limb salvage. J Trauma 25:203–208, 1985.
McCollum PT, Spence VA, Walker WF: Amputation for peripheral vascular disease: the case of level selection. Br J Surg 75:1193–1195, 1988.
Mitchell JW, Gailey RS, Bowker JH: New developments in recreational prostheses and adaptive devices for the amputee. Clin Orthop Relat Res 256:64–75, 1990.
O'Toole DM, Goldberg RT, Ryan B: Functional changes in vascular amputee patients: evaluation by Barthel index, PULSES profile, and ESCROW scale. Arch Phys Med Rehabil 66:508–511, 1985.
Pillet J: The aesthetic hand prosthesis. Orthop Clin North Am 12:961–969, 1981.
Radcliffe CW: Functional considerations in the fitting of above knee prostheses. Artif Limbs 2:40, 1955.
Shurr DG, Cook TM: Prosthetics and orthotics, Norwalk, Conn, 1990, Appleton & Lange.
Spence VA, McCollum PT, Walker WF, et al: Assessment of tissue viability in relation to the selection of amputation level. Prosthet Orthot Int 8:67–75, 1984.
Summers GD, Morrison JD, Cochrane GM: Foot loading characteristics of amputees and normal subjects. Prosthet Orthot Int 11:33–39, 1987.
Torburn L, Schweiger GP, Perry J, et al: Below-knee amputee gait in stair ambulation—a comparison of stride characteristics using five different prosthetic feet. Clin Orthop Relat Res 308:185–192, 1994.
Van Wirdum P: A new explanation of phantom symptoms. Psychiatry Neurol Neurochir 66:306–313, 1963.
Wilson AB: Limb prosthetics—1970. Artif Limbs 14:1–52, 1970.
Winter DA, Sienko SE: Biomechanics of below-knee amputee gait. J Biomech 21:361–367, 1988.

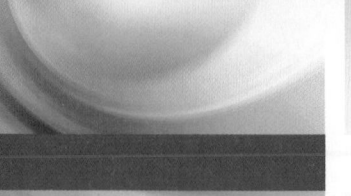

CHAPTER 17

Primary Care Assessment

Although it would be ideal for a family physician who is familiar with the patient's and the family's history to perform a primary care assessment because he or she would more likely be aware of any congenital or developmental problems, the patient's immunization status, and any recent injuries or illnesses and therefore could provide continuity of care,[1-3] many people today do not have a family physician. As health care changes occur, more and more health care professionals are becoming involved in assessment of patients who come to them as first-level providers of medical care. This may involve nurse practitioners, physician assistants, and other health care providers, as well as physicians in primary care facilities, physical therapists with direct access in private practice, clinicians in sole-charge facilities, and sports therapists working and traveling with teams.[4-8] Thus it becomes important for clinicians to be able to evaluate and recognize the potential for health care problems, including systemic disease as a disease entity itself or a disease masquerading as neuromuscular dysfunction, that must be referred to the appropriate health professional.[9,10] Primary care assessment is a form of triage in which the clinician decides whether the patient's problem or problems fall within his or her scope of practice or should be referred to other health care professionals.[11-15]

In many ways, a primary care assessment is similar to a preparticipation examination used in sports because both assessments are used to clear patients of having certain problems that could affect activity and also to provide a mechanism in which problems can be referred to the appropriate health care professional.[16-22] This process involves an understanding of disease as well as an ability to distinguish what system may be affected through a detailed history, observation and examination, and an understanding of different levels of reporting ability of the patient.[9,23] It also requires the clinician to understand his or her limitations, the scope of practice of his or her chosen profession, and why the patient has come to see the clinician. For example, what is the patient's complaint? Is it related to how the patient feels? Is it related to his or her occupation? Is it related to a certain population, age, or gender?[18,24,25]

If the patient has symptoms, several questions should be asked that relate to the symptoms[26]:
1. Where is the symptom, and does it radiate?
2. What does the symptom feel like?
3. How bad is the symptom?
4. Where does (did) the symptom start?
5. How long does the symptom last?
6. How often does the symptom occur?
7. What brings the symptom on?
8. What makes the symptom better or worse?
9. Are there other symptoms associated with it?

Once these questions, and the ones discussed under the different systems as outlined later in the chapter, are answered, the examiner can decide to treat the patient or refer on to another health care professional, usually a physician. Goodman and Snyder[27] clearly outline cases in which referral to a physician is necessary (Table 17-1). This chapter is not meant to be all inclusive of conditions and systems that may need referral. Complete systems assessment is left to other sources.[26,27]

McKeag[28] has outlined five specific populations in which special areas of possible concern should be included in an examination. In the prepubescent patient (6 to 10 years of age), assessments should include examination for congenital abnormalities that may not have been diagnosed previously. In the pubescent patient (11 to 15 years of age), the examination should include an evaluation of physical maturity and good health practices. The postpubescent or young adult group (16 to 30 years of age) has the widest variety of skills, levels, and motivation. For this group, the history of previous injuries and any sport-specific or activity-specific problems is particularly important. For the adult population (30 to 65 years of age), injury prevention (e.g., overuse), previous injury patterns, health concerns, and conditioning should be included in the examination. The final group consists of elderly patients (65 years of age or older), who require an examination based on individual requirements, because many of these people take up exercising or increased physical activity after a medical illness.[20] Age-related changes and their possible consequences are outlined in Table 17-2.

TABLE **17-1**

Physician Referral

Immediate Medical Attention	Patient with anginal pain not relieved in 20 minutes
	Patient with angina who has nausea, vomiting, profuse sweating
	Diabetic patient demonstrating signs of confusion, lethargy, or changes in mental alertness and function
	Patient with bowel/bladder incontinence and/or saddle anesthesia secondary to cauda equine lesion
	Patient in anaphylactic shock
Medical Attention Necessary	***General Systemic***
	Unknown cause
	Lack of significant objective neuromusculoskeletal signs and symptoms
	Lack of expected progress with physical therapy treatment
	Development of constitutional symptoms or associated signs and symptoms over the course of treatment
	Discovery of significant PMH unknown to physician
	Changes in health status that persist 7 to 10 days beyond expected time period
	Patient who is jaundiced and has not been diagnosed or treated
	Changes in size, shape, tenderness and consistency of lymph nodes in more than one area, which persist more than 4 weeks; painless, enlarged lymph nodes
	For Women
	Low back, hip, pelvic, groin, or sacroiliac symptoms without known etiology and in the presence of constitutional symptoms
	Symptoms correlated with menses
	Any spontaneous uterine bleeding after menopause
	For pregnant women: Vaginal bleeding, elevated blood pressure, increased Braxton-Hicks contractions during exercise
	Vital Signs (Report These Findings)
	Persistent rise or fall of blood pressure
	Blood pressure evaluation in any woman taking birth control pills (should be closely monitored by her physician)
	Pulse amplitude that fades with inspiration and strengthens with expiration
	Pulse increase over 20 BPM lasting more than 3 minutes after rest or changing position
	Difference between systolic and diastolic measurements of more than 4 mm Hg in pulse pressure
	Persistent low-grade (or higher) fever, especially associated with constitutional symptoms, most commonly sweats
	Cardiac
	Angina at rest
	Anginal pain not relieved in 20 minutes
	More than three sublingual nitroglycerin tablets required to gain relief
	Nitroglycerin does not relieve anginal pain
	Rest does not relieve angina
	Angina continues to increase in intensity after stimulus (e.g., cold, stress, exertion) has been eliminated
	Changes in pattern of angina
	Abnormally severe chest pain
	Patient has nausea, vomiting
	Anginal pain radiates to jaw/left arm
	Upper back feels abnormally cool, sweaty, or moist to touch
	Patient has any doubts about his or her condition

Continued

TABLE **17-1**

Physician Referral—cont'd

Cancer

Early warning sign(s) of cancer: seven early warning signs plus two additional signs pertinent to the physical therapy examination: proximal muscle weakness and change in deep tendon reflexes

All soft tissue lumps that persist or grow, whether painful or painless

Any women presenting with chest, breast, axillary, or shoulder pain of unknown etiology, especially in the presence of a positive medical history (self or family) of cancer

Bone pain, especially on weight-bearing, that persists more than 1 week and is worse at night

Pulmonary

Shoulder pain that is aggravated by supine positioning

Shoulder, chest (thorax) pain that subsides with autosplinting (lying on the painful side)

For the patient with asthma: Signs of asthma or bronchial activity during exercise

Genitourinary

Abnormal urinary constituents (e.g., change in color, odor, amount, flow of urine)

Any amount of blood in urine

Musculoskeletal

Symptoms that seem out of proportion to the injury, or symptoms persisting beyond the expected time for the nature of the injury

Severe or chronic back pain accompanied by constitutional symptoms, especially fever

Precautions/ Contraindications to Therapy	Uncontrolled chronic heart failure or pulmonary edema Active myocarditis Resting heart rate > 120 or 130 BPM* Resting systolic rate > 180 to 200 BPM* Resting diastolic rate > 105 to 110 BPM* Moderate dizziness, near-syncope Marked dyspnea Unusual fatigue Unsteadiness Loss of palpable pulse Postoperative posterior calf pain For the patient with diabetes: Chronically unstable blood sugar levels must be stabilized (normal: 80 to 120 mg/dL; "safe": 100 to 250 mg/dL)

From Goodman CC, Snyder TE: Differential diagnosis in physical therapy, Philadelphia, 1995, WB Saunders, pp. 18–20.

BPM, Beats per minute; *PMH,* past medical history.

*Unexplained or poorly tolerated by patient

TABLE **17-2**

Selected Age-Related Changes and Their Consequences

Organ/System	Age-Related Physiologic Change*	Consequence of Age-Related Physiologic Change	Disease, Not Age
General	↑ Body fat	↑ Volume of distribution for fat-soluble drugs	Obesity
	↓ Total body water	↓ Volume of distribution for water-soluble drugs	Anorexia
Eyes/Ears	Presbyopia	↓ Accommodation	Blindness
	Lens opacification	↑ Susceptibility to glare	Deafness
	↓ High-frequency acuity	Difficulty discriminating words if background noise is present	

TABLE **17-2**

Selected Age-Related Changes and Their Consequences—cont'd

Organ/System	Age-Related Physiologic Change*	Consequence of Age-Related Physiologic Change	Disease, Not Age
Endocrine	Impaired glucose tolerance	↑ Glucose level in response to acute illness	Diabetes mellitus
	↓ Thyroxine clearance (and production)	↓ T_4 dose required in hypothyroidism	Thyroid dysfunction
	↑ ADH, ↓ renin, and ↓ aldosterone	—	↓ NA^+, ↑ K^+
	↓ Testosterone	—	Impotence
	↓ Vitamin D absorption and activation	Osteopenia	Osteoporosis Osteomalacia
Respiratory	↓ Lung elasticity and ↑ chest wall stiffness	Ventilation/perfusion mismatch and ↓ pO_2	Dyspnea Hypoxia
Cardiovascular	↓ Arterial compliance and ↑ systolic BP → LVH	Hypotensive response to ↑ HR, volume depletion, or loss of atrial contraction	Syncope
	↓ β-adrenergic responsiveness	↓ Cardiac output and HR response to stress	Heart failure
	↓ Baroreceptor sensitivity and ↓ SA node automaticity	Impaired blood pressure response to standing, volume depletion	Heart block
Gastrointestinal	↓ Hepatic function	Delayed metabolism of some drugs	Cirrhosis
	↓ Gastric acidity	↓ Ca^+ absorption on empty stomach	Osteoporosis Vitamin B_{12} deficiency
	↓ Colonic motility	Constipation	Fecal impaction
	↓ Anorectal function	—	Fecal incontinence
Hematologic/ Immune system	↓ Bone marrow reserve (?)	—	Anemia
	↓ T-cell function	False-negative PPD response	—
	↑ Autoantibodies	False-positive rheumatoid factor, antinuclear antibody	Autoimmune disease
Renal	↓ Glomerular filtration rate	Impaired excretion of some drugs	↑ Serum creatinine
	↓ Urine concentration/ dilution (see also Endocrine)	Delayed response to salt or fluid restriction or overload; nocturia	↑↓ Na^+
Genitourinary	Vaginal/urethral mucosal atrophy	Dyspareunia Bacteriuria	Symptomatic urinary tract infection
	Prostate enlargement	↑ Residual urine volume	Urinary incontinence Urinary retention
Musculoskeletal	↓ Lean body mass, muscle	—	Functional impairment
	↓ Bone density	Osteopenia	Hip fracture
Nervous system	Brain atrophy	Benign senescent forgetfulness	Dementia Delirium
	↓ Brain catechol synthesis	—	Depression
	↓ Brain dopaminergic synthesis	Stiffer gait	Parkinson disease
	↓ Righting reflexes	↑ Body sway	Falls
	↓ Stage 4 sleep	Early wakening, insomnia	Sleep apnea

From Resnick NM: Geriatric medicine. In Isselbacher KJ, et al, editors: Harrison's principles of internal medicine, ed 13, New York, 1994, McGraw-Hill.

ADH, Antidiuretic hormone; *BP,* blood pressure; *HR,* heart rate; *LVH,* left ventricular hypertrophy; *PPD,* purified protein derivative, *SA,* sinoatrial; *T4,* thyroxine.

The table displays selected changes that occur normally with age and their physiologic consequences. Changes due to disease rather than to age are listed in the last column.

*Changes generally observed in healthy elderly subjects free of symptoms and detectable disease in the organ system studied. The changes are usually important only when the system is stressed or other factors are added (e.g., drugs, disease, or environmental challenge); they rarely result in symptoms otherwise.

A primary care assessment may vary from a minimal medical examination or physical to rule out possible systemic problems to a very extensive examination involving laboratory tests, stress testing, profiling, x-rays, and other special protocols.[29] History, as well as a physical examination, plays a major role.[30–32] If the patient is going to be asked to do strenuous activity as part of his or her treatment program, various systems (e.g., heart, lungs) must be cleared to ensure the patient is capable of doing the activity.[33]

Characteristics of Systemic Symptoms

- No known cause or unknown etiology
- Gradual onset with progressive, cyclical course (worse/better/worse)
- Persist beyond expected time for that condition
- Constant
- Intense
- Bilateral symptoms (e.g., edema, nail bed changes, clubbing, numbness or tingling, weakness, skin pigmentation changes, or rash)
- Unrelieved by rest or change in position
- If relieved by rest or positional change, over time even these relieving factors no longer reduce symptoms
- Do not fit the expected mechanical or neuromusculoskeletal pattern; symptoms are out of proportion to the injury
- Symptoms cannot be altered (provoked, reproduced, alleviated, eliminated, aggravated) during examination
- Constitutional symptoms, especially fever and night sweats
- Disproportionate pain relief with aspirin (red flag for bone cancer)
- Night pain
- Pain described as knifelike, boring, deep, colicky, deep aching
- Pattern of pain coming and going like spasms

From Goodman CC, Snyder TE: Differential diagnosis in physical therapy, Philadelphia, 1995, WB Saunders, p. 16.

OBJECTIVES OF THE EVALUATION

Primary care evaluations have many useful purposes.[1,9,29,34,35] However, the examiner must remember that the primary purpose of the examination is to determine the patient's health problem and to either treat the patient or refer him or her to the appropriate health care professional.[1,9] As part of the examination, the examiner can establish **baseline values** for the patient. These may be compared with normal "textbook" values or used to determine change in the future. In other words, the assessment should not consist of simple "yes/no" questions. Instead, it must be very thorough to establish proper baseline levels.

The primary care assessment is used to determine the health status of the patient. It also helps to prevent injuries through identification of any abnormalities, physical inadequacies, or poor conditioning that may put the

---

Objectives of Primary Care Assessment

- Determine if disease is present
- Uncover pre-existing conditions
- Determine unsuspected correctable conditions
- Determine health status
- Prevent injuries
- Avoid misinterpretation of findings
- Establish baseline values
- Act as a screening process
- Foster good health practices
- Develop rapport with the patient
- Establish guidelines
- Develop a musculoskeletal profile
- Counsel the patient
- Classify the patient
- Meet legal and insurance requirements
- Determine if referral is necessary

---

patient at risk.[36] The examination may identify previously unsuspected conditions that are amenable to correction or that preclude participation in the desired activity. Similarly, the evaluation helps to avoid misinterpretation of findings that appear to be new but existed previously. For this reason, a review of previous health records, if possible, is also part of the primary care assessment.

The primary care assessment is also worthwhile to ensure that treatments have been carried out previously and that conditions previously diagnosed have been properly cared for. In this way, it acts as a screening process to ensure that treatment of potentially serious medical and surgical conditions has taken place. It also helps to rule out potentially serious or threatening conditions that may temporarily preclude the patient from participation in work or recreational activities. For example, with infectious mononucleosis, contact sports may be precluded for a time, because the patient's spleen is enlarged and is more easily injured or ruptured.

The assessment also gives the clinician an opportunity to foster good health practices and to promote optimum health and fitness. The assessment enables the health care provider to give proper health guidance and to determine the general state of health of the patient.

The assessment also gives the examiner a chance to develop a rapport with the patient. The examiner can learn what motivates the patient and, at the same time, help establish the patient's confidence in the health care staff. The examination may also be used to establish guidelines for the patient and health care team on questions of health, safety, and care. In addition, it provides an opportunity to counsel the patient.

PRIMARY CARE HISTORY

For a primary care assessment, the history plays a predominant role to ensure that questions related to the various systems are asked. A complete history can usually identify 60% to 75% of the problems affecting a patient.[22,29,37] For the young person or the patient with communication problems, both the patient and his or her parent or guardian should provide the history to ensure completeness. The rest of the assessment proceeds from the information determined in the history. The history provides details regarding health problems and injuries and enables the examiner to focus on any abnormalities that it brings out.[29] Generally, the history is completed by the patient's answering questions in a yes/no format (see Appendix 17-1 on the Evolve website for a generic primary care assessment questionnaire). Using such a format decreases the chance of the patient forgetting something.[23] The "yes" answers then are investigated further in other parts of the assessment (see Appendix 17-2 on the Evolve website). It is important, however, that the "no" answers also be checked for accuracy. Ideally, oral histories, in which the health care professional asks the questions, are more accurate; but usually, because of time constraints, this is not possible. The history should include the patient's medical history as well as the family's medical history to rule out any congenital, hereditary, or injury problems. It is important that a complete health history be obtained, because the patient may leave out or hide information that may preclude the patient from taking part in a desired activity or because of possible secondary gain.[37]

Some general questions can be asked initially, and these can be used to cross-reference questions asked in specific areas of assessment:[29]

1. *Have you ever been a patient in a hospital, emergency room, or clinic?*
2. *Have you ever seen a physician for an injury or illness?*
3. *Have you ever had x-rays?*
4. *Have you ever had an operation?*
5. *Are you presently taking any medication or pills?*
6. *Do you have any allergies (to medications, insects, food, or other things)?*
7. *When was your last vaccination? What was the vaccination for?*
8. *Have you ever been unable to work or participate in exercise or sports?*
9. *Have you ever experienced chest pain, dyspnea, or syncope during work, exercise, or activity?*
10. *Have you ever had a seizure?*
11. *Have you ever been told you had high blood pressure?*
12. *Have you ever been told you had high cholesterol?*
13. *Do you have trouble breathing or do you cough during or after activity?*

These general questions cover wide areas, and the specific parts of the assessment should corroborate the answers given to these general questions. In addition, the examiner must consider the effect of psychosocial issues on both the patient and his or her reported symptoms. Haggman et al.[38] believed two questions were useful to screen for symptoms of depression:

1. *During the past month, have you often been bothered by feeling down, depressed, or hopeless?*
2. *During the past month, have you been bothered by little interest or pleasure in doing things?*

If the answer to both questions is yes, further psychological investigation may be warranted.[39,40] Waddell and Main[40] talked about illness behavior, a normal and reasonable behavior, which is what people do and say to communicate that they are ill. The examiner should always keep in mind the role psychosocial issues may have in anyone seeking primary care help.

The following assessment sections outline questions pertaining to specific body systems that may lead to further examination or testing and possible concerns or issues that must be dealt with if the patient is going to take part in a particular activity. The examiner may want to cover all of the systems or only those that appear pertinent to the problem.

EXAMINATION

The medical examination must be not only thorough but also applicable to the job, activity, exercise, or sport to which the person hopes to return or take part in. Health care professionals should always be alert for concealment, denial, or invention of problems on the part of the patient.

Parts of Primary Care Examination

- History
- Vital signs
  - Temperature
  - Blood pressure
  - Heart rate
  - Weight
- Head and face examination
- Neurological examination and convulsive disorders
- Musculoskeletal examination
- Cardiovascular examination
- Pulmonary examination
- Urogenital examination
- Gastrointestinal examination
- Dermatological examination
- Examination for heat illness
- Laboratory tests
- Physical fitness profile
  - Body composition
  - Maturity index
  - Flexibility
  - Strength, endurance, and power
  - Agility, balance, and reaction time
  - Cardiovascular fitness

Vital Signs

The initial part of the examination is performed to establish the patient's baseline physiological parameters and vital signs (see Chapter 1, Table 1-7), including pulse or heart rate, respiratory rate, blood pressure (systolic and diastolic), weight, and temperature (normal: 98.4°F [37°C], range: 96.5°F [35.8°C] to 99.4°F [37.4°C]). This part of the examination may be performed by any health care professional who has knowledge or an understanding of the techniques, and it is part of any primary care examination.[41,42]

Table 1-8 (see Chapter 1) outlines guidelines for blood pressure measurement.[43] High blood pressure values should be checked several times at 15- to 30-minute intervals with the patient resting in between to determine whether a high reading is accurate or is being caused by anxiety ("white coat syndrome") or some similar reason. If three consecutive readings are high, the patient is said to have high blood pressure (hypertension) (see Chapter 1, Table 1-9). If the readings remain high, further investigation may be warranted.[1,43,44] Table 17-3 outlines the risk factors of hypertension.

Complications of Hypertension

- Cardiovascular disease
- Heart failure
- Left ventricular hypertrophy
- Stroke
- Intracerebral hemorrhage
- Chronic renal insufficiency
- Renal disease

TABLE **17-3**

Risk Factors of Hypertension

Primary	Secondary
• One or both parent with hypertension • Increased salt intake • Excessive alcohol consumption • Obesity • Race (Black individuals are more commonly affected.) • Personality traits (tense, hostile) • Smoking • Diabetes • Physical inactivity • Cholesterol > 6.5 mmol/L or low-density lipoprotein cholesterol > 4.0 mmol/L	• Renal disease • Oral contraceptives • Cushing syndrome • Sleep apnea syndrome • Endocrine (thyroid, parathyroid conditions) • Coarctation of aorta • Renovascular disease • Adrenal cortex dysfunction

The following examination sections may be part of the primary care examination, but this will depend on what has been found from taking the history and vital signs. Only those sections that the examiner feels are relevant or are areas of concern would normally be investigated.

General Medical Problems

There are general systemic problems that the examiner must always keep in mind when doing an assessment. Some of the general medical (systemic) questions include the following[13,27,45]:

1. Have you ever been diagnosed with a systemic disease (e.g., diabetes)?
2. Have you ever been diagnosed with a progressive disease (e.g., muscular dystrophy, multiple sclerosis)?
3. Have you ever been told you have cancer?
4. Have you ever had anything similar to what you have now? How often?
5. Where exactly is your pain? What is the quality, frequency, and pattern of the pain?[46] What have you tried to do to alleviate the pain? On a scale of 1 (no pain) to 10 (pain is bad as it could possibly get), how would you rate your pain level?
6. Do you have any other symptoms?
7. Have you ever had any infections? How were they treated?
8. Do you have unexplained fatigue?
9. Have you ever had any unexplained weakness?
10. Do you bruise easily?

The presence of systemic disease (e.g., diabetes) does not rule out work or activity, but the examiner must ensure that there is either good control by the use of medication or that the disease will not cause undue risk to the patient or his or her well-being. It must also be determined whether the extent or intensity of the activity the patient has to do poses a significant threat to the patient's physical condition.[47] The examiner also has to be concerned about problems, such as acute infection and malignancy, and progressive diseases, such as multiple sclerosis.

Acute illnesses tend to be self-limiting and usually require only that the patient temporarily withdraw from work or activity, often to prevent spread to others.[29] Dehydration is made worse by febrile illness, which could, in certain circumstances, lead to heat disorders.

Head and Face

Eye Examination

Visual acuity is usually examined with the use of a Snellen or common eye chart. Peripheral vision and depth perception may also be tested. Questions related to the eye examination include the following[29,48]:

1. Have you had any problems with vision or your eyes?
2. Have you ever injured your eyes?

3. Do you wear glasses, contact lenses, or protective eyewear?
4. Are you color-blind?
5. Do you have a peripheral vision problem?
6. Have you ever used medications for an eye problem?
7. Have you ever had an eye infection?

Any abnormalities found or positive answers may require further examination. Uncorrected vision of less than 20/40 should be checked further.[34] Visual loss of 20/50 means that the patient can read at 20 feet what the average person can read at 50 feet. The health care professional should watch for problems that may preclude work, preclude participation in the chosen activity or sport, or affect the safety of the patient. Vision in only one eye results in lack of depth perception, which can be detrimental in certain activities. Patients with sight in only one eye should work at specific jobs or participate in physical activities only if they have an understanding of the dangers of participating and accept the risks. Such patients should not work or participate in sports for which there is no adequate eye protection.

Examples of Eye Conditions or Signs and Symptoms Requiring Further Examination

- Sudden vision loss
- Visual loss greater than 20/40
- Vision in one eye only
- Severe myopia
- Retinal detachment
- Retinal tear
- Corneal abrasion
- Iritis
- Conjunctivitis
- Proptosis (protrusion) of eye

If the patient wears glasses, the health care professional should ensure that the lenses are plastic, polycarbonate, or heat-treated (safety) glass to prevent them from shattering during work or activity.

Myopia, or nearsightedness, should be noted on the chart; such patients are more likely to suffer retinal degeneration, which increases the possibility of retinal detachment. Patients who have had a retinal detachment are sometimes excluded from contact sports or high-exertion jobs. People who have a retinal tear should be allowed to do strenuous activities only if cleared by a physician or specialist, and they should have a qualifying letter allowing them to return to work.

Pupil size should also be evaluated. In some patients, the pupils are of obvious different sizes (**anisocoria**). This difference should be noted in case the patient has to be evaluated for a head injury at a later date.[49] Assessment of the eyes is shown in Chapter 2.

Dental Examination

Questions to be asked concerning the patient's dental record include the following[48]:
1. When did you last see a dentist?
2. Have you ever had any problems with your teeth or gums?
3. Have you ever had any teeth knocked out, damaged, or extracted?
4. Do you wear a mouth guard?
5. Do you smoke or chew tobacco?
6. Have you ever had an injury to your face or jaws?

When looking for dental problems, which is usually done by a dentist, it is important to determine how many teeth the patient has and the last time he or she saw a dentist.

Ear Examination

Questions to be asked concerning the patient's ear problems include the following:
1. Do you have any problems with hearing?
2. Do you have an earache? (What was the onset? How long is the duration?)
3. Is the earache associated with a cold, flu, or trauma?
4. Is there pain in the ear?
5. Is there any discharge from the ear?

Ear problems are commonly referred to a physician or an ear, nose, and throat specialist. Assessment of the ear is shown in Chapter 2.

Nose Examination

Questions to be asked concerning the patient's nose problems include the following:
1. What is the problem with your nose?
2. Can you breathe through the nose?
3. Do you have any discharge from the nose (e.g., blood, mucus)?
4. Do you use any medication through your nose (nose drops, nasal spray)?
5. Are both nostrils affected?

Assessment of the nose is shown in Chapter 2. Nose problems other than colds are commonly referred to a physician.

Neurological Examination and Convulsive Disorders (Including Head Injury)

The neurological examination is very important, especially in contact or collision activities or when there is a suspected head injury. Some of the more common questions asked in the neurological examination include the following[13,29]:
1. Have you ever been knocked out or been unconscious?
2. Have you ever had a head injury?
3. Have you had or do you have frequent or severe headaches?

4. Have you ever had a stinger or burner?
5. Have you ever had a time when one or more of your limbs went numb or "to sleep" during activity?
6. Have you ever fainted (syncope)?
7. Have you ever had a paralyzed limb?
8. Have you ever lost feeling or muscular control of your arms or legs?
9. Have you ever had a seizure?
10. Have you ever been in a motor vehicle accident or fallen and hit your head?

A positive answer to any of these questions could have a significant impact on what the patient is allowed to do and whether the patient is allowed to return to work or participate in contact or collision activities.

In the neurological examination, the examiner may assess the status of a head injury (see Chapter 2), perform a cranial nerve assessment (see Chapter 2) and sensation scan, and evaluate the different reflexes (see Chapter 1) if problems are suspected. The examiner must check for concussions and nerve palsies. Any positive neurological signs and symptoms uncovered in the examination, such as recurrent concussions or nerve palsies, should preclude strenuous activity until investigated further by a specialist before clearance to return to previous activities is given.

Examples of Neurological Conditions or Signs and Symptoms Requiring Further Examination

- More than one concussion
- Post-concussion syndrome
- Any history of head injury
- Expanding intracranial lesion
- Any history of seizure
- Neurological symptoms of undetermined cause
- Any history of stinger, burner, or neurapraxia
- Persistent weakness, numbness, or arm or leg pain
- Any history of transient quadriplegia
- Upper motor neuron symptoms
- Any history of nerve palsy

With convulsive disorders, the examiner needs to know the frequency of the episodes; how or whether control of the convulsions has been achieved; the use of routine medication; any circumstances that activate the convulsions; and whether the patient understands the disorder, its hazards, and its predisposing factors. Patients with epilepsy should be discouraged from activities, such as skiing, scuba diving, parachuting, and climbing, because of their inherent dangers.[29] If the activity involves water sports (e.g., swimming alone, scuba diving), auto racing, or any activity in which recurrent head trauma or unexpected falls may cause serious injury (e.g., mountain climbing, working at heights), then the patient with convulsive disorders should be discouraged from doing these activities. Patients whose activities should be restricted include those who experience daily or weekly seizures, those who display bizarre forms of psychomotor epilepsy, and those whose postconvalescent state is prolonged or typically includes marked abnormal behavior. It is important to understand whether the medication taken can maintain good control of the patient's condition, not only in everyday situations but also in stress situations. For example, hyperventilation may precipitate an epileptic seizure, and seizures tend to occur after exercise, not during the event. In addition, it is important to know whether the extent or intensity of the participation poses a significant threat to the patient's physical condition.

Musculoskeletal Examination

Like the neurological examination discussed previously, the musculoskeletal examination is often a very important part of an evaluation. Questions in the history related to this examination include the following[31,50–54]:

1. Have you ever pulled (strained) or hurt a muscle?
2. Have you ever torn (sprained) or stretched a ligament?
3. Have you ever subluxated or dislocated a joint or had a bone come out of joint?
4. Have you ever broken (fractured) a bone?
5. Have any of your joints ever swollen?
6. Have you ever had pain in the muscles or joints at work or during or after activity, exercise, or sports (Table 17-4)?
7. Have you ever had regular prolonged (more than 30 minutes) morning stiffness?

TABLE **17-4**

Comparison of Systemic and Musculoskeletal Joint Pain

Systemic	Musculoskeletal
• Awakens at night	• Decreases with rest
• Deep aching, throbbing	• Sharp
• Reduced by pressure	• Ceases when stressful action is stopped
• Constant or waves/spasm	
• Jaundice	• Associated signs and symptoms
• Migratory arthralgias	• Usually none
• Skin rash	• Trigger points may be accompanied by nausea, sweating
• Fatigue	
• Weight loss	
• Low-grade fever	
• Muscular weakness	
• Cyclic, progressive symptoms	
• History of infection (hepatitis, streptococcosis, mononucleosis, measles)	

From Goodman CC, Snyder TE: Differential diagnosis in physical therapy, Philadelphia, 1995, WB Saunders, p. 526.

8. Have you ever had any rashes, eye infections, diarrhea associated with joint pains, and/or swelling?
9. Have you ever had any proximal weakness, excessive cramping, or muscle fasciculations?

A positive response to any of these questions requires further investigation.

The musculoskeletal examination begins with observation of the patient's posture (see Chapter 15), looking for any asymmetry. Asymmetry, combined with the history, may lead the examiner to do a detailed assessment of a specific joint (see Chapters 3 to 13). If no problems are noted, the examiner can do a quick **upper and lower scanning** or **screening examination** to check for potential problems and abnormal movement (e.g., hypomobility, hypermobility, capsular patterns, weakness, abnormal movement patterns, cheating movements).[41,55]

Upper and Lower Scanning Examination

- Cervical spine: flexion, extension, side flexion, rotation
- Shoulder shrug (resistance may be added)
- Shoulder: elevation through abduction, forward flexion and the plane of the scapula; medial and lateral rotation (resistance may be added)
- Elbow: flexion, extension, supination, pronation
- Wrist: flexion, extension, radial, and ulnar deviation
- Fingers and thumb: open hands wide, make a tight fist
- Thoracic and lumbar spine: flexion (touch toes, knees straight—watch for spine versus hip movement), extension, side flexion, rotation
- Tighten quadriceps (quadriceps strength, symmetry)
- Test hamstring tightness
- Hip, knee, ankle, and foot: squat and bounce, heel-toe walking

---

If any deviation, weakness, or abnormality is found, or if the patient has reported a previous injury to a joint, a more detailed examination may be performed to assess active movements, passive movements, resisted isometric movements, special tests, functional tests, reflexes, sensation, myotomes, joint play, and palpation of that joint or associated joints.

When looking for musculoskeletal problems, it is important to consider whether the patient's job or what he or she wants to do will exacerbate an existing disease or injury, increase an existing deformity, or cause further bone or joint damage. When looking for musculoskeletal problems, the examiner may look at the patient's flexibility, strength, and endurance, as well as static and dynamic stability. Spinal instability (especially instability of the cervical or lumbar spine) or spondylolisthesis may preclude the patient from taking part in some activities. Maturation may also have to be considered when dealing with patients who are still growing, as may previous injuries, congenital problems, and growth abnormalities.

Examples of Musculoskeletal Conditions or Signs and Symptoms Requiring Further Examination

- Joint or spinal instability (static and dynamic)
- Joint swelling
- Unhealed muscle or ligament injury (especially 3° or if avulsion suspected)
- Possible fractures or dislocations/subluxations
- Unhealed or healing fracture
- Degenerative diseases
- Inflammatory diseases
- Unusual hypermobility or hypomobility
- Muscle weakness
- Growth or maturation disorders
- Repetitive stress disorders
- Myopathy
- Metabolic disease

Cardiovascular Examination

The cardiovascular examination should be performed in a quiet area because of the need to auscultate. In this part of the evaluation, the examiner looks for subtle but significant cardiac abnormalities to reduce the incidence of unexpected sudden death in sports or similar incidences at work.[2,32,56-61] In some cases, electrocardiograms (ECGs) or stress ECGs may be appropriate.[62] More than 90% of sudden deaths in exercise and sports among participants younger than 30 years of age involve the cardiovascular system.

The following questions should be asked in the history concerning the cardiovascular system[9,13,27,29]:

1. Have you ever had a heart attack?
2. Do you have a pacemaker or other device to assist your heart?
3. Have you ever had heart surgery?
4. Have you ever had frequent heartburn?
5. Have you ever experienced dizziness, fainting, or passing out during or after activity, exercise, or sports?
6. Have you ever experienced chest pain, tightness, crushing sensation, squeezing, or pressure in the chest at work or during or after activity, exercise, or sports (Table 17-5 and 17-6)?
7. When working or doing an activity, exercise, or sport, do you tire more quickly than others doing the same things?
8. Have you ever had high blood pressure?
9. Has your heart ever "raced" or skipped beats?
10. Have you ever been told you have a heart murmur?
11. Has anyone in your family ever had or died from heart problems?
12. Has anyone in your family died suddenly before the age of 50 years?
13. Have you had a severe viral infection (myocarditis, mononucleosis) within the last month?

14. Has a physician denied or restricted your participation in any activity for any heart problems?
15. Do your ankles and/or legs swell?[63]

If the answer to any of these questions is yes, the examiner must consider the possibility of cardiomyopathy, conduction abnormalities, arrhythmias, valvular problems, coronary artery defects, and lung or related problems.[64] If cardiovascular problems are suspected, the examiner may organize further tests (e.g., ECG, treadmill stress tests, laboratory tests)[65] to detect cardiac abnormalities.

TABLE 17-5

Causes of Chest Pain

Systemic Causes	Neuromuscular Causes
<ul><li>Pulmonary<ul><li>Pulmonary embolism</li><li>Spontaneous pneumothorax</li><li>Pulmonary hypertension</li><li>Cor pulmonale</li><li>Pleurisy with pneumonia</li></ul></li><li>Cardiac<ul><li>Myocardial ischemia (angina)</li><li>Pericarditis</li><li>Myocardial infarct</li><li>Dissecting aortic aneurysm</li></ul></li><li>Epigastric/Upper GI<ul><li>Esophagitis</li><li>Upper GI index</li></ul></li><li>Breast<ul><li>Breast tumor</li><li>Abscess</li><li>Mastitis</li><li>Lactation problems</li><li>Mastodynia</li><li>Trigger point</li></ul></li><li>Other<ul><li>Rheumatic diseases</li><li>Anxiety</li></ul></li></ul>	<ul><li>Tietze syndrome</li><li>Costochondritis</li><li>Hypersensitive xiphoid</li><li>Slipping rib syndrome</li><li>Trigger points</li><li>Myalgia</li><li>Rib fracture</li><li>Cervical spine disorders</li><li>Neurologic<ul><li>Thoracic outlet syndrome</li><li>Neuritis</li><li>Shingles (herpes zoster)</li><li>Dorsal nerve root irritation</li></ul></li></ul>

From Goodman CC, Snyder TE: Differential diagnosis in physical therapy, Philadelphia, 1995, WB Saunders, p. 532.
GI, Gastrointestinal.

TABLE 17-6

Characteristics of Cardiac Chest Pain

Angina	Myocardial Infarct	Mitral Valve Prolapse	Pericarditis
<ul><li>1 to 5 minutes</li><li>Moderate intensity</li><li>Tightness, chest discomfort</li><li>Subsides with rest or nitroglycerin</li><li>Pain related to tone of arteries (spasm)</li></ul>	<ul><li>30 minutes to hours</li><li>Severe (can be painless)</li><li>Crushing pain; intolerable (can be painless)</li><li>Unrelieved by rest or nitroglycerin</li><li>Pain related to heart ischemia</li></ul>	<ul><li>Hours</li><li>Rarely severe</li><li>May be asymptomatic; unlike angina in quality or quantity</li><li>Unrelieved by rest or nitroglycerin</li><li>Mechanism of pain unknown</li></ul>	<ul><li>Hours to days</li><li>Varies; mild to severe</li><li>Asymptomatic; varies; can mimic MI</li><li>Relieved by keeling on all fours, leaning forward, or sitting upright</li><li>Pain related to inflammatory process</li></ul>

From Goodman CC, Snyder TE: Differential diagnosis in physical therapy, Philadelphia, 1995, WB Saunders, p. 94.
MI, Myocardial infarct.

Examples of Cardiovascular Conditions or Signs and Symptoms Requiring Further Examination

- Chest pain
- Dizziness with activity or vertigo
- Irregular heartbeat (rate, rhythm)
- Hypertension (labile or organic)
- Heart murmur
- Family history of heart problems
- Hypertrophic cardiomegaly
- Conduction abnormalities
- Arrhythmias
- Myocarditis
- Valvular problems
- Aortic coarctation
- Marfan syndrome
- Enlarged (athlete's) heart
- Atherosclerotic disease (positive ankle-arm index [AAI])
- Mitral insufficiency
- Anemia
- Enlarged spleen
- Unexplained fatigue

When looking for cardiovascular problems, the examiner should be alert for the following unusual or abnormal findings:

1. Heart rate faster than 120 beats/min or inappropriate tachycardia for a specific activity
2. Arrhythmias or irregular beats[66]
3. Midsystolic clicks, indicating a leaky valve or mitral valve prolapse
4. Murmurs that are grade 3 or louder

The loudness of **systolic murmurs** is graded from 1 to 6 with grade 1 being a very faint murmur requiring concentration to be heard. A grade 2 murmur is a faint murmur but one that is heard immediately after the stethoscope is placed on the chest. Grade 3 is an intermediate murmur louder than grade 2. Most human dynamically significant murmurs are at least grade 3. Grade 4 is a loud murmur, frequently associated with palpable sensation, known as a thrill. A grade 5 murmur is a very loud murmur still requiring at least the edge of the stethoscope to remain in contact with the chest. The grade 6 murmur is a murmur audible with the stethoscope just breaking contact with the chest.[67] **Diastolic murmurs** are graded from 1 to 4, 1 representing the faintest and 4 the loudest murmur. A benign functional murmur or systemic mitral valve prolapse does not preclude exercise or sports but must be evaluated on an individual basis.

The examiner must be aware of congenital heart abnormalities, such as aortic coarctation (stenosis of the artery), which may be revealed by a difference in the femoral and brachial pulses. In such a case, strenuous activity is contraindicated. As another example, 90% of patients with Marfan syndrome (an autosomal dominant condition) have cardiac abnormalities. The examiner must be aware of atrial septal defects (an abnormal communication between the chambers of the heart), dextrocardia (the heart is moved within the thoracic cavity), and paroxysmal auricular tachycardia (an abnormal increase in heartbeat for short periods). Patients with these conditions should be cleared by a specialist before any strenuous activity because of the possibility of fainting in a stressful situation. The examiner must also be aware of heart enlargement (athlete's heart). This condition does not necessarily preclude activity but should be investigated further if found. If any of these abnormalities have been surgically corrected, they should be evaluated by a specialist on an individual basis to determine whether the patient can take part in the proposed activity.

Hypertrophic cardiomyopathy is the most common cause of sudden death in athletes, followed by aortic rupture associated with Marfan syndrome, congenital coronary artery anomalies, and atherosclerotic coronary artery disease.[29,68] If any of these conditions is present, strenuous activity is precluded.

Other cardiovascular problems include thromboembolic disease, pulse irregularities, valvular problems (such as, mitral insufficiency or mitral valve prolapse), and abnormally high blood pressure (hypertension). Systolic pressure of 140 mm Hg on repeated measurements is considered abnormal (see Chapter 1, Table 1-9).[58] Also, patients with labile hypertension (an unstable condition of free and rapid change in tension) or organic hypertension caused by structural problems should be investigated further. These patients should have a complete comprehensive coronary risk factor work-up. Mild hypertension does not preclude strenuous activity, but this slight abnormality should be noted and evaluated on an individual basis.[29] When taking blood pressure, a proper cuff size must be used to ensure an accurate reading. If the initial reading is high, the reading should be repeated two or three times after the patient has been lying supine for 20 to 30 minutes. Only if the blood pressure is elevated after the third reading should the patient be considered hypertensive.

Detecting Cardiac Risks in Examinations: Key Physical Findings of Cardiac Evaluation by Physician

Heart rate faster than 120 beats/min
- If repeated tests on second occasion are high, suggest monitoring and recording of pulse at home by a trained parent or nurse friend.
- Pulse recovery tests after jumping or hopping exercises are useless routines except for multiple extrasystoles or arrhythmias.

Multiple extrasystoles or arrhythmias. Check after jumping or hopping 20 times to ascertain if arrhythmias appear or disappear.

Resting blood pressure higher than 130/80 mm Hg for students aged 6 to 11 years, 140/90 mm Hg for students aged 12 to 18 years.
- For validity, be certain that the pressure cuff covers at least two thirds of the upper arm, from elbow to shoulder (adult cuff = 30 × 13 cm; pediatric cuff = 22 × 10 cm; obese cuff = 39 × 15 cm).
- If high, repeat test three times and take average.

All systolic murmurs grade 3 to 6 or louder at any location; all diastolic murmurs of any intensity at any location; or any continuous murmur. Heart should be auscultated at four chest locations:
- Pulmonic area (second intercostal space at left sternal border)
- Aortic area (second intercostal space at right sternal border)
- Tricuspid area (fourth intercostal space at left sternal border)
- Mitral area (fourth intercostal space at left midclavicular line)

Routinely palpate femoral and brachial pulses. Note if absent or if large discrepancy exists between them.

Modified from Schell NB: Cardiac evaluation of school sports participants: guidelines approved by the Medical Society of New York. NY State J Med 78:942–943, 1978.

Detecting Cardiac Risks in Examinations: Key Historical Facts Obtained from Students, Parents, and School Health Records

- Cyanotic heart disease early in life
- Murmur early in life based on anatomical diagnosis of left-to-right shunt or pulmonic or aortic stenosis
- Rheumatic heart disease
- Fainting spells (syncope)
- Chest or abdominal pains (not otherwise diagnosed)
- Dyspnea on exertion
- Cardiac surgery
- Enlarged heart
- Cardiac rhythm disturbances
- Familial heart disease* or rhythm disturbances
- Functional or innocent murmur of 4 or more years' duration

Modified from Schell NB: Cardiac evaluation of school sports participants: guidelines approved by the Medical Society of New York. NY State J Med 78:942–943, 1978.

*Hypertension, early stroke (before 50 years), or early coronary (before 50 years) in close relatives.

Another condition the examiner should be aware of is anemia. If anemia is suspected, the level of hemoglobin (the oxygen-carrying pigment in human blood) is tested. Anemia is more likely to be seen in women during menstruation, and sickle cell anemia is more common in black individuals. In some cases, anemia is caused by an increase in blood volume, which decreases the concentration of red blood cells. In this case, the individual has normal red blood cells but appears to be anemic.

If cardiovascular or cardiopulmonary disease is suspected, an exercise stress test is often recommended.[34,69] Figure 17-1 outlines a flowchart for considerations before doing such a test. Twenty to thirty-five percent of those with heart disease have a normal stress test, so it is important to remember that any stress test is only valid to the load at which the heart has been stressed when doing the test. Forty-five percent of runners older than 40 years of age have irregular results on ECGs. Further, different types of activity (e.g., static or dynamic) lead to different stresses on the heart.

The ankle-arm index (AAI) may also be used to screen for atherosclerotic (cardiovascular) disease.[70,71] This is the ratio of the ankle to arm systolic pressure when measured using a Doppler ultrasound device.[70] The lower the AAI, the greater the risk of disease.[71]

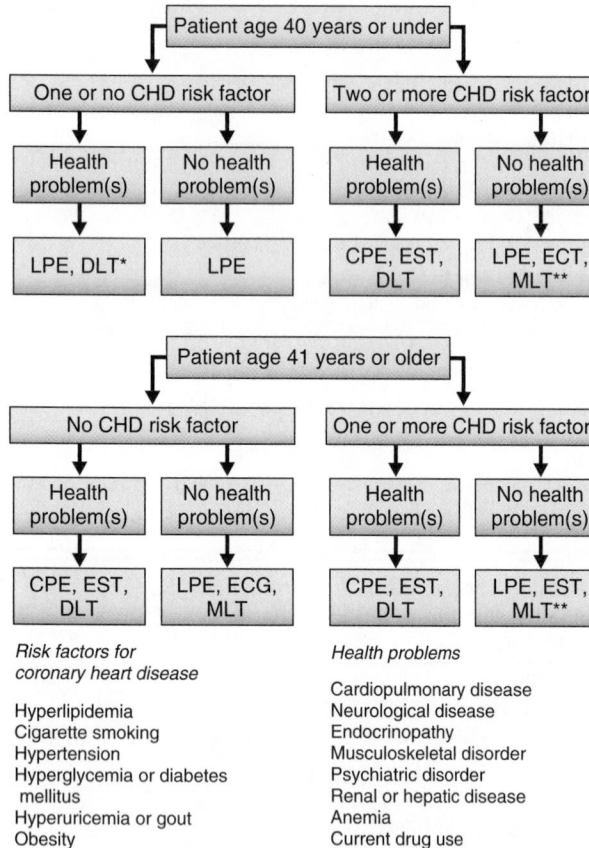

Risk factors for
coronary heart disease

Hyperlipidemia
Cigarette smoking
Hypertension
Hyperglycemia or diabetes
mellitus
Hyperuricemia or gout
Obesity

Health problems

Cardiopulmonary disease
Neurological disease
Endocrinopathy
Musculoskeletal disorder
Psychiatric disorder
Renal or hepatic disease
Anemia
Current drug use
Other acute or chronic disease

* Exercise stress testing is recommended if patient has cardiopulmonary disease.

** Diagnostic laboratory testing is indicated if CDH risk factors include hyperlipidemia, hyperglycemia, or hyperuricemia.

Figure 17-1 Pre-exercise evaluation flow sheet. *CDH,* Coronary heart disease; *CPE,* comprehensive physical examination; *DLT,* diagnostic laboratory testing; *ECG,* resting electrocardiogram; *EST,* exercise stress test; *LPE,* limited physical examination; *MLT,* minimal laboratory testing. (Redrawn from Taylor RB: Pre-exercise evaluation: which procedures are really needed? Consultant, April 1983, pp. 94–101.)

Contraindications to Exercise Testing

- Physical inability to walk on the treadmill
- Unstable angina or new resting ECG changes
- Acute pericarditis, myocarditis, endocarditis
- Uncompensated CHF, S3 gallop, rales
- Severe aortic stenosis
- Hypertrophic cardiomyopathy
- Known LMCA or equivalent stenoses
- Uncooperative patient
- Other serious medical problem or problems

From Cavell RM: The exercise treadmill test for diagnosis and prognosis of coronary artery disease. J La State Med Soc 147:198, 1995.

CHF, Congestive heart failure; *ECG,* electrocardiogram; *LMCA,* left main coronary artery.

Common Causes of False-Positive Exercise Tests

- Congenital and valvular heart disease
- Digoxin
- Electrolyte abnormalities
- Non-fasting state
- Pre-excitation syndromes, WPW
- Bundle branch block
- Mitral valve prolapse
- Left ventricular hypertrophy
- Hyperventilation

From Cavell RM: The exercise treadmill test for diagnosis and prognosis of coronary artery disease. J La State Med Soc 147:198, 1995.

WPW, Wolff-Parkinson-White syndrome.

Indications for Termination of the Exercise Test

- Patient's request
- Achievement of maximum effort
- Appearance of serious arrhythmia, multiform PVCs, triplets, rapid SVT
- Fall in systolic BP in the face of increasing workload
- Progressive anginal pain
- CNS symptoms, dizziness, ataxia
- Signs of poor perfusion, pallor, cyanosis, cool extremities
- More than 0.3 mV of horizontal or down-sloping SVT depression
- Technical loss of monitoring ability

From Cavell RM: The exercise treadmill test for diagnosis and prognosis of coronary artery disease. J La State Med Soc 147:198, 1995.

BP, Blood pressure; *CNS,* central nervous system; *PVC,* premature ventricular contraction; *SVT,* supraventricular tachycardia.

Pulmonary Examination

The pulmonary examination is often done in conjunction with the cardiovascular examination in a quiet area. Questions related to the pulmonary system may include the following[13,27,32]:

1. Have you ever had trouble breathing?
2. Have you ever had a pulmonary disease?
3. Do you use any breathing aids?
4. Have you ever had a chest x-ray? When?
5. Have you ever experienced long periods of intermittent coughing?
6. Do you cough anything up? Have you had a recent productive cough (e.g., sputum, blood, what color?)?
7. Have you ever experienced coughing at work or during or after activity, exercise, or sports?
8. Have you ever experienced shortness of breath or wheezing at work or during or after activity, exercise, or sports?
9. Is your breathlessness related to anything (e.g., exercise, pollen, emotion)?
10. Do you have asthma? If so, how do you treat it?
11. Have you ever broken your nose?
12. Do you suffer from chronic sinus irritation or a runny nose?

Examples of Pulmonary Conditions or Signs and Symptoms Requiring Further Examination

- Abnormal coughing
- Abnormal shortness of breath
- Abnormal breath sounds (e.g., wheezing, rhonchi, rales)
- Asthma (uncontrolled or exertional)
- Exercise-induced bronchospasm
- Pulmonary insufficiency
- Severe allergies
- Nasal deviation or occlusion
- Chronic sinusitis

The examiner auscultates for clear breath sounds and watches for symmetrical diaphragm excursion.[29] Any required controlling medications should be noted and recorded. The ears, nose, and mouth may also be checked during this examination. If abnormalities are found, appropriate lung function tests or arterial blood gases may be ordered (Table 17-7).[72] If there is concern about an active disease process, a chest x-ray may be in order.

Respiratory problems, such as tuberculosis, uncontrolled asthma, exertional asthma, exercise-induced bronchospasm, pulmonary insufficiency resulting from a collapsed lung, or bronchial asthma, should be checked and discussed with the patient.[34,73,74]

TABLE 17-7

Arterial Blood Gas Values

Normal Values	
pH	7.35 to 7.45
pCO₂ (partial pressure of carbon dioxide)	35 to 45 mm Hg
HCO₃ (bicarbonate ion)	22 to 26 mEq/L
pO₂ (partial pressure of oxygen)	80 to 100 mm Hg
O₂ saturation (oxygen saturation)	95% to 100%

Critical Values	
pH	< 7.25 or > 7.45
pCO₂	< 20 or > 60 mm Hg
HCO₃	< 15 or > 40 mEq/L
pO₂	< 40 mm Hg
O₂ saturation	< 75%

From Goodman CC, Snyder TE: Differential diagnosis in physical therapy, Philadelphia, 1995, WB Saunders, p. 151. Adapted from Pagana D, Pagana T: Mosby's diagnostic and laboratory test reference, St Louis, 1992, Mosby-Year Book, p. 104.

Gastrointestinal Examination

The gastrointestinal examination involves evaluation of the digestive system, eating habits, and nutrition. Some of the questions that may be asked include the following[13,27,78]:

1. Do you have a problem with bowel movements (e.g., diarrhea, constipation)?
2. Do you have any problems chewing or swallowing food?
3. Have you been vomiting lately?
4. Do you have any pain related to eating?
5. Do your stools appear normal?
6. Do you feel you eat regularly and have a well-balanced diet?
7. Are there certain food groups you will not eat?
8. Have you ever been on a diet?
9. Do you view yourself as too thin, too fat, or just right?
10. Have you ever tried to control your weight? If so, how?
11. Have you ever had excessive heartburn or indigestion?
12. Have you had any heartburn or dyspepsia after using anti-inflammatory medications?

A positive answer to any of these questions requires further investigation.

The examiner should palpate the abdomen for masses or organomegaly.[1] The examiner has to ensure that there is no inflammation of the liver (hepatitis, enlarged liver) or enlarged spleen, especially if the patient is involved in contact sports.

In some cases, it is advisable to check the patient's nutritional status, especially if there appears to be a tendency toward eating disorders, such as anorexia or

---

Examples of Gastrointestinal Conditions or Signs and Symptoms Requiring Further Examination

- Organomegaly (e.g., enlarged liver, spleen)
- Anorexia
- Bulimia
- Female athlete triad (anorexia/bulimia, amenorrhea, osteoporosis)
- Ulcers
- Blood in stools

Examples of Urogenital Conditions or Signs and Symptoms Requiring Further Examination

- Hernia (femoral, inguinal, abdominal, sports)
- Absent or undescended testicle
- Lump in testicle
- One kidney or diseased kidney
- Albuminuria
- Hemoglobinuria
- Nephroptosis
- Hematuria
- Exercise amenorrhea
- Diabetes
- Sexually transmitted diseases

---

bulimia.[79] This is best done by having the patient record his or her food intake for at least 3 days and having the record analyzed by a nutritionist, who can then calculate dietary intake in relation to the activity level of the patient. It also provides an opportunity to determine what supplements the patient is using, in case they contain banned substances.

Urogenital Examination

Depending on whether the patient is male or female, the examination is modified to meet the individual needs. For example, females may be asked about their menstrual history (e.g., when did menses begin? when was the last period? are there any abnormalities?) or about gynecological problems. Males may be given a genital examination looking for abnormalities, hernias, or absence of a testicle.[29] Common history questions asked in the urogenital examination (males and females) include the following:

1. Have you ever had any problems with your kidneys or bladder?
2. Has there been a change in the number of times you urinate daily?
3. When you urinate, do you have trouble starting, continuing, or stopping?
4. Have you ever been treated for venereal disease?
5. Is your urine clear?
6. Have you ever been diagnosed as having sugar, albumin, or blood in your urine?
7. Have you felt any bulges in your groin, testicle, or abdomen?
8. Have you felt a painless hard mass in your testicle (testicular cancer screen)?
9. Have you had any urethral discharge or dysuria?

The examiner should check for hernias, kidney problems, albuminuria (excessive protein in the urine), and venereal disease if a problem of the urogenital system is suspected.[75] Generally, patients with one kidney should be warned of the danger of contact sports, especially if the kidney is abnormally positioned or is diseased.[76] In males, the examiner should be aware of an undescended or atrophied testicle or testicular torsion. A urinalysis should be performed if diabetes or kidney disease is suspected. These conditions do not preclude activity,

exercise, or sports, but they may be amenable to treatment, and the patient must be made aware of potential dangers caused by these conditions.

Dehydration, athletic pseudonephritis, hemoglobinuria, nephroptosis, and hematuria are all possible problems of the urogenital system. For females in sports, it is important to determine whether they have a regular period and menstrual pattern because of concern about exercise amenorrhea and its relation to bone density and osteoporosis.[34,77]

Dermatological Examination

The primary care assessment may involve examination for any developing skin conditions and those that may be amenable to treatment. Generally, the questions that relate to the dermatological examination would be the following[13]:

1. Have you had any problems with acne?
2. Have you had any problems with rashes or itching, especially in areas covered by clothes, equipment, or footwear?
3. Do you have a history of fungal infections?

The answers to such questions give the examiner some idea of skin conditions, most of which are easily dealt with by treatment.

Examples of Dermatological Conditions or Signs and Symptoms Requiring Further Examination

- Severe acne
- Dermatitis (e.g., contact, clothes)
- Herpes (e.g., simplex, gladiatorum)
- Fungal infection (tinea capitis or corporis)
- Boils
- Warts
- Impetigo
- Molluscum contagiosum
- Psoriasis

The examiner must ensure that the patient with dermatological problems has them under control, because many of these conditions are contagious, including bacterial, fungal, or viral infections (such as, herpes simplex, herpes gladiatorum, boils, impetigo, or warts), and contact dermatitis.

Examination for Heat (Hyperthermic) Disorders

Examination for heat disorders should be included if the patient's work, activity, exercise, or sport has involved working or activity where there is high temperature, high humidity, or a combination of the two (e.g., moderate temperature and high humidity) or where a heat injury is suspected.[80–85] These are often the conditions that lead to heat disorders. Questions in the history related to heat disorders may include the following:

1. Have you ever experienced a heat disorder?
2. Have you ever had muscle cramps?
3. Have you ever participated in an activity, exercise, or sport in a high-temperature, high-humidity environment?
4. Have you ever passed out or become dizzy in the heat?
5. Have you been on medication, or do you drink a lot of caffeinated beverages or use stimulants?
6. Have you recently lost a considerable amount of weight in a short time?

Examples of Heat Disorders or Heat-Related Signs and Symptoms Requiring Further Examination

- Heat exhaustion
- Heat stroke
- Excessive muscle cramps in heat
- Excessive dehydration

Intake of antihistamines or excessive caffeine, as well as lack of fluid and/or metabolites, can increase the risk of heat disorders. If a patient has a history of heat-related disorders, the condition should be thoroughly investigated because it could lead to life-threatening situations.

Examination for Cold (Hypothermic) Disorders

Examination for hypothermia should be included if the patient's work, activity, exercise, or sport involves working or activity where there are low temperatures (below freezing), a significant wind chill factor, high humidity (or patient wearing wet clothes), or a combination of the three.[83,85–91] Any of these may lead to environmental factors, such as acute (immersion), chronic (exposure), or urban hypothermia. Questions in the history related to hypothermic (cold) disorders may include the following:

1. Have you ever frozen your ears, toes, or fingers?
2. How long have you been in the cold? (Note: This could be in a cold building, not just outside.)
3. Were you working or participating in an activity, exercise, or sport in low-temperature, windy conditions and/or a humid environment?
4. Have you been in poor health in the last 6 months?
5. Have you been eating well?
6. Have you consumed any drugs or alcohol in the last 24 hours?
7. Do you smoke?

Factors That Increase Susceptibility to Cold

- General: Infancy, advanced age, malnutrition, exhaustion
- Drug use: Alcohol, sedatives, meperidine, clonidine, neuroleptic agents
- Endocrine system: Hypoglycemia, hypothyroidism, adrenal insufficiency, diabetes
- Cardiovascular system: Peripheral vascular disease, nicotine use
- Neurological system: Peripheral neuropathy, spinal cord damage, autonomic neuropathy, hypothalamic disease
- Trauma: Falls (head or spinal injury), fracture causing immobility
- Infection: Sepsis (diaphoresis, hypothalamic dysfunction)

From Biem J, et al: Out of the cold: management of hypothermia and frostbite. Can Med J 168:306, 2003.

Questions 4 to 7 are asked because of their effect on the circulation and neurological systems. Often the patient experiencing hypothermia is shivering, is apathetic and lethargic, and may demonstrate an inability to perform simple meaningful tasks.

LABORATORY TESTS

Laboratory tests are often included in a primary care assessment. If the examiner suspects problems for which laboratory tests can be diagnostic, then they should be ordered. For example, if heart disease is suspected or an older population is being examined, serum cholesterol, triglyceride, or high-density lipoprotein tests may be ordered (Tables 17-8 to 17-11).

The incidence of iron deficiency anemia in postmenarche female athletes is as high as 15%. Plasma ferritin may be used to measure iron status. In males, anemia may occur during a growth spurt, with inadequate diet, or with a peptic ulcer. Hemoglobin is often checked if sickle cell anemia (common in black people) is suspected. The prepubertal level of hemoglobin is about 11.5 g/dL of blood, and the postpubertal value is 14.5 g/dL of blood for males and 12.0 g/dL or higher for females.

TABLE **17-8**

Blood Cholesterol Levels

Age (Years)	Values (mg/dL)
< 25	125 to 200
25 to 40	140 to 225
40 to 50	160 to 245
50 to 65	170 to 265
> 65	< 265

From Goodman CC, Snyder TE: Differential diagnosis in physical therapy, Philadelphia, 1995, WB Saunders, p. 134.

TABLE **17-9**

Triglyceride Levels

Age (Years)	Value (mg/dL)
Female Adult	
20 to 29	10 to 100
30 to 39	10 to 110
40 to 49	10 to 122
50 to 59	10 to 134
> 59	10 to 147
Female Child	
1 to 19	10 to 121
Male Adult	
20 to 29	10 to 157
30 to 39	10 to 182
40 to 49	10 to 193
50 to 59	10 to 197
> 59	10 to 199
Male Child	
1 to 19	10 to 103

From Chernecky C, et al: Laboratory tests and diagnostic procedures, Philadelphia, 1993, WB Saunders, p. 932.

TABLE **17-10**

Serum Electrolyte Levels

Test	Normal Values
Serum potassium	3.5 to 5.3 mEq/L
Serum sodium	136 to 145 mEq/L
Serum calcium	8.2 to 10.2 mg/dL (4.5 to 5.5 mEq/L)
Serum magnesium	1.8 to 3 mg/dL (1.5 to 2.5 mEq/L)

Adapted from Chernecky C, et al: Laboratory tests and diagnostic procedures, Philadelphia, 1993, WB Saunders.

TABLE **17-11**

Urine Analysis (Urinalysis)

	Test	Normal Result
General measurements	Color	Yellow-amber
	Turbidity	Clear
	pH	4.6 to 8.0
	Specific gravity	1.01 to 1.025
Other components	Glucose	Negative
	Ketones	Negative
	Blood	Negative
	Protein	Negative
	Bilirubin	Negative
Sediment	RBCs	Negative
	WBCs	Negative
	Casts	Occasional
	Mucous threads	Occasional
	Crystals	Occasional

From Goodman CC, Snyder TE: Differential diagnosis in physical therapy, Philadelphia, 1995, WB Saunders, p. 258. Normal values are taken from Kee J: Laboratory and diagnostic tests with nursing implications, ed 3, Norwalk, CT, 1991, Appleton & Lange. *RBCs,* Red blood cells; *WBCs,* white blood cells.

Common Laboratory Tests

- Hematocrit
- Urinalysis
- Blood chemistry (glucose, creatine, electrolytes)
- Fasting lipid profile
- Electrocardiogram

DIAGNOSTIC IMAGING

Diagnostic imaging may also be part of a primary care assessment but should not be used indiscriminately.[92] For the most part, diagnostic imaging should be used following set guidelines and to confirm a clinical diagnosis. The type of imaging depends on the information sought. More detailed information on diagnostic imaging may be found in Chapter 1 and other more detailed references.[93-95]

PHYSICAL FITNESS PROFILE (FUNCTIONAL ASSESSMENT)

In some cases, it may be important for the examiner to establish a physical fitness profile for the patient to determine if he or she can meet the stresses of work or sports or to determine his or her functional level.[96] Basically, profiling is the gathering of information about the physical attributes of the participant.[97] Such profiling helps to determine whether the person possesses the attributes, skills, and abilities necessary for a job or participation in various activities and to meet the demands of the job or activity, and it should be geared to the specific job, activity, exercise, or sport (Table 17-12).[97–103] It should be designed to stress the body so that any weakness or pathology that exists will be apparent. In this way, it may be used as a **screening device** to prevent injury.[97,104] The profile also provides a **baseline** in the event of injury or to demonstrate the need for, or effect of, conditioning necessary to do the job or take part in the activity. A physical fitness profile can involve many parameters or aspects, including strength, endurance, flexibility, cardiovascular fitness, and maturation. To be effective, the program or test must exhibit several characteristics.[105]

Movement Patterns of Functional Movement Screen[107–109]

- Deep squat (bilateral, functional and symmetrical mobility)
- Hurdle step* (stride mechanics)
- In-line lunge* (lower limb stability and flexibility)
- Shoulder mobility* (including scapular stabilization)
- Active straight leg raise* (hamstring flexibility and pelvic stability)
- Trunk stability push up (trunk stabilization with upper extremity motion)
- Rotary stability* (multiplane trunk stability with upper and lower extremity motion)

*Test both left and right sides.

Characteristics of Physical Fitness Profile

- The variables being tested must be relevant to the job, activity, exercise, or sport
- The test must be reliable and valid
- Test protocols must be as specific to the job, activity, exercise, or sport as possible
- The test must be standardized and controlled
- The rights of the patient and confidentiality must be respected
- Testing may be repeated at regular intervals if the purpose is to show effectiveness of a training program
- Results must be conveyed to the patient in a meaningful way that the patient can understand

---

Functional Movement Screen (FMS).[106–108] This screen was developed by Move2Perform® to determine if individuals had poor movement patterns or pre-existing movement impairments. The functional movement screen consists of seven movement tests for balance, mobility and stability. Each test is scored from 0 (unable to do) to 3 (able to do with no compensatory movement or no pain). If scores are different between sides, there is an imbalance. Kiesel et al[106,107] showed that if an individual's FMS score was 14 or less, the probability of serious injury occurring in the future increased from 15% to 51%. The same company has developed the **"Y Balance Test" (Star Excursion Balance Test)** using an excursion balance, which is used to measure upper and lower limb control and balance. These values can be used to determine when a patient is ready to return to activity especially for the active individual.[110–114]

Strength

Strength is one of the attributes that is commonly examined in a physical fitness profile. The way in which the examiner determines strength depends on the job, activity, exercise, or sport; the equipment available; and the demands of the activity. It has been reported that strength

declines 1% per year after the age of 30 years.[115] The strength measures may involve isometric, isotonic, or isokinetic testing; functional activities; lifting of free weights; or, in some cases, simply a hand grip test.[116,117] In some cases, it may involve muscle fiber typing. If a general indication of strength is desired, a hand grip is relatively easy, and standard tests can be used (see Chapter 7). For the elderly population, plantar flexor, hip abductor, and hip extensor strengths are important to test.[118] Functional strength tests are often used, because they are easy and provide comparable results.[1] However, the examiner should make these tests as job or activity specific as possible.

Examples of Functional Strength Tests

- Bench press, leg press
- Sit-ups
- Push-ups
- Pull-ups
- Grip strength

More sophisticated methods may be used, especially if the patient has a history of injury to specific muscles or joints (see the sections on functional testing in Chapters 3 to 13). Isokinetic testing (i.e., Cybex, KinCom, Biodex) is more likely to be used to test specific joints, looking for potential discrepancies between left and right sides, agonist versus antagonist, and differences in strength and endurance. However, it is important to realize that many of these tests are not usually done in functional job- or activity-specific positions or ways.

Power

Power is the ability to move a weight over a distance. This weight may be an object or the human body. Depending

TABLE 17-12

Used to Determine Athletic Fitness for Specific Sports*

	Speed	Strength	Muscle Endurance	Power	Quickness and Agility	Reaction Time	Flexibility	Cardiorespiratory Endurance	Balance	Anaerobic Endurance	Body Composition	Kinesthetic Perception
Football	X	X	—	X	X	X	X		X	X	X	X
Basketball	X	—	X	X	X	—	X	X	X	X	X	X
Baseball	X	—	—	X	—	X	X	—	—	X	—	—
Track and field												
Sprinters	X	X	—	X	—	X	X	—	—	X	X	—
Thrower	—	X	—	X	X	—	X	—	X	X	X	X
Jumpers	X	X	—	X	—	—	X	—	X	X	X	X
Distance	—	—	X	—	—	—	X	X	—	—	X	—
Volleyball	—	—	X	X	X	X	X	—	X	X	X	X
Soccer	X	—	X	—	X	X	X	X	X	—	X	X
Rodeo	—	X	—	X	X	X	X	—	X	—	—	X
Tennis	—	—	X	X	X	X	X	—	—	X	X	X
Golf	—	—	X	—	—	—	X	X	X	—	X	X
Skiing	—	X	X	X	—	—	X	X	X	—	X	X
Wrestling	—	X	X	X	X	—	X	X	X	—	X	X
Gymnastics	X	X	X	X	X	—	X	—	X	—	X	X

From Bridgman R: A coach's guide to testing for athletic attributes. National Strength Conditioning Assoc J 13:35, 1991.

*X denotes areas of physical fitness that are most needed in each sport.

Test examples:

Speed: 20-, 40-, 100-yard dashes
Strength: 1 repetition max
Muscle endurance: 225-lb or 285-lb bench test, sit-up, pull-up, dip, push-up
Power: Vertical jump, standing broad jump, two-hand medicine ball put
Agility: 20-yard shuttle run, Semo agility test, T-test
Reaction time: Dekan Auto Performance Analyzer
Flexibility: Sit and reach test, shoulder rotation test
Cardiorespiratory endurance: 1.5-mile run, 12-minute run
Balance: Nelson balance test
Anaerobic endurance: Margaria-Kalamen leg power test, 40-yard repeated sprint test
Body composition: Skinfold measurements
Kinesthetic perception: Distance perception jump

on the job, activity, exercise, or sport, power may be included as part of the physical fitness profile. As with all profile parameters, power measurements should be related to the job, activity, exercise, or sport in which the patient will be participating.

Examples of Power Activities

- Throwing a medicine ball (equivalent to weight the patient would throw on the job)
- Lifting a weight and placing it at a higher level
- Stair climbing or running
- Walking up and down stairs
- Bending and lifting
- Jump for height (vertical jump test)
- Two-legged hop
- Single-leg hop for distance

Flexibility and Range of Motion

Flexibility is a very important consideration when profiling a patient for a specific job or activity.[119,120] In some cases, less flexibility is better than too much, but in some activities, excessive flexibility (laxity) is necessary to succeed. Therefore flexibility testing must be specific to the job or activity in which the patient wishes to take part, or it may be position specific. For example, in running activities, lower limb flexibility (especially hip flexors, hamstrings, rectus femoris, iliotibial band, and gastrocnemius) is of greatest importance, whereas in swimming, upper limb flexibility (especially shoulder abduction and medial and lateral rotation) is more important, as it is with jobs involving a large amount of overhead work. In some activities, such as ballet, gymnastics, and synchronized swimming, overall flexibility is essential. In baseball, pitchers often require greater shoulder, hip, and trunk flexibility than other players.[18] Flexibility may be measured with the use of devices, such as a goniometer, Flexometer, or tape measure.[120]

When considering range of motion (ROM), the examiner must realize that hypermobility or laxity in one joint or in one direction of joint movement does not necessarily mean hypermobility in all joints or in all directions. Similarly, normal ROM charts are often not valid when dealing with persons who, by virtue of their job or activities (e.g., ballet, gymnastics, synchronized swimming), are hypermobile. Values that are considered normal for these types of activities would be considered hypermobile or abnormal for the general population. It is also important to realize that hypermobility (laxity) and hypomobility are not necessarily pathological states. In pathological states, hypermobility may lead to instability and is usually the result of the individual being unable to control movement in the available ROM (through strength,

---

Determinants of Range of Motion[121]

- Shape of the bone and cartilage
- Muscle power and tone
- Muscle bulk
- Ligaments and joint capsule laxity
- Extensibility of the skin and subcutaneous tissue
- Race (Indians are more flexible than Blacks, who are more flexible than Caucasians)
- Gender (women are more flexible than men)
- Age (ROM decreases with age)
- Genetic makeup
- The dominant limb tends to be less mobile (decreased ROM) than the nondominant limb
- Day to day stresses on joints

ROM, Range of motion.

---

endurance, passive stabilizers, and neurological input) (see Chapter 1). The ROM available may be the result of genetic makeup or the stresses placed on individual joints. Tight-jointed people tend to be more susceptible to muscle strains, nerve pinch syndromes, and overstress paratenonitis. Hypermobile, or loose-jointed, people are more susceptible to ligament sprains, chronic back pain, disc prolapse, spondylolisthesis, pes planus, joint effusion, and paratenonitis caused by lack of control of the joint. In the hypermobile individual, if strength and endurance are not at the appropriate level to support the joints, the joints are often unstable or are subjected to potentially injuring loads.

Various criteria can be used to determine a patient's generalized joint laxity. However, the points previously mentioned must be kept in mind when looking at these generalized values. Carter and Wilkinson[122] have developed a five-point system. The patient who meets all criteria is said to exhibit general joint hypermobility. Beighton and Horan developed a 9-point system (see Chapter 1, p. 34), which is a modification of Carter and Wilkinson's criteria.[123,124] In this case, the patient who scores 4 or more is said to exhibit general joint hypermobility.

Carter and Wilkinson's Criteria for Generalized Joint Laxity (Hypermobility)[122]

- Passive apposition of the thumb to the flexor aspect of the forearm
- Passive hyperextension of the fingers so they lie parallel with the extensor aspect of the forearm
- Ability to hyperextend elbows at least 10°
- Ability to hyperextend knees at least 10°
- Excessive passive dorsiflexion of the ankle and eversion of the foot

Nicholas[125] established criteria for determining whether a patient is tight jointed (hypomobile). It should be realized, however, that under these criteria, the majority of the North American population today would be classified as hypomobile!

Nicholas's Criteria for Hypomobility[125]

- Patient is unable to touch the floor with the palms, bending at the knees with the waist straight
- Patient is unable to sit comfortably in the lotus position
- Patient demonstrates less than 20° hyperextension at the knees when lying prone with the legs hanging over the end of the table
- Patient is unable to position the feet at 180° while standing with the knees flexed at 15° to 30°
- Patient has no upper limb laxity on shoulder flexion, elbow hyperextension, or forearm hypersupination

---

It is important to understand the principles of hypermobility and hypomobility. A person who is hypermobile must avoid further stretching and support the joint through strengthening (concentric and eccentric exercise) and endurance programs. The patient must be taught proper positioning, and if there are hypermobile joints, there are probably hypomobile joints nearby that need to be mobilized. It is essential to make sure that these patients have improved strength, endurance, muscular speed of reaction, and balanced activities to help support the hypermobile joints.

The person who is hypomobile may be treated by mobilization or manipulation of the affected joint in the direction of tightness. Tight supporting structures also must be stretched, and active exercises must be given to maintain the restored ROM. It is important with these patients to retrain their kinesthetic sense so that they can maintain and control the acquired ROM.

Speed

Speed is often considered an important component of a physical fitness profile, depending on the job, activity, exercise, or sport. It is a function of distance covered per unit of time.[1]

Examples of Functional Speed Tests

- Timed moving things from one station to another
- Time to assemble "something"
- Timed 40-yard (40-m) run or walk
- Timed 100-yard (100-m) run or walk
- Timed 440-yard (400-m) run or walk

Cardiovascular Fitness and Endurance

Because almost every activity involves stresses on the heart and vascular system, it is important to know the level of the stresses produced and whether the cardiovascular system can respond to these stresses. Aerobic fitness has been reported to decline 9% per decade for sedentary adults after the age of 25 years.[126] Therefore the cardiovascular system must be evaluated to determine how it responds to these or equivalent loads.[127,128]

Many methods can be used to determine cardiovascular (aerobic) fitness, but the method chosen should be related to the specific job, activity, or population.[129,130] As an example, ice hockey players who are tested on a bicycle may show very good cardiovascular fitness; however, when they get on the ice and skate, their cardiovascular fitness may not be as evident, because they are being tested in a different type of activity.

Examples of Common Endurance Tests

- Harvard step test
- 12-minute walk-run
- 1.5-mile (2.4-km) run
- Submaximal ergometer test
- Treadmill test

The Harvard step test is one of the most common general cardiovascular fitness tests done for a physical fitness profile. It is relatively simple, is easy to set up, and takes a minimal amount of time to do. To set up the test, an 18-inch platform is used. The patient is instructed to step with both feet onto the platform at a rate of about 30 times per minute (a metronome is used for cadence). The patient is made to step for 3.5 minutes at a pace of 2 seconds per step and then sprint as fast as possible for 30 seconds (total time: 4 minutes). The patient then immediately sits down in a chair and relaxes for 3 minutes while the pulse is determined. The pulse is taken at 30, 60, 120, and 180 seconds after the exercise. The index formula for the pulse is as follows:

$$Index = \frac{Duration\ of\ exercise(in\ sec) \times 100}{2 \times the\ sum\ of\ any\ three\ pulse\ counts}$$

The higher the index, the better the person's fitness. If the index is less than 65, the patient is not ready for high-level activity. Cooper[131,132] developed an indirect method for measuring fitness using a 12-minute walk-run test. From the distance covered in 12 minutes, he developed tables for men and women that showed the patient's fitness category. He later went on to use a similar method for activities such as swimming and cycling, thus making the testing more activity specific. For older

TABLE 17-13

How to Administer the Kasch Pulse-Recovery Test

1. Measure pulse at rest
2. Ask the patient to step up and down (with both feet) a 12-inch step 24 times per minute for 3 minutes
3. Measure pulse 1 minute after the test
4. Determine patient's fitness level on the following scale:

Fitness Level	POST-EXERCISE BEATS/MINUTE	
	Age 56 to 65 Years	Age 66+ Years
Men		
Excellent	72 to 82	72 to 86
Good	89 to 97	89 to 95
Above average	98 to 101	97 to 102
Average	105 to 111	104 to 113
Below average	113 to 118	114 to 119
Poor	122 to 128	122 to 128
Very poor	131 to 150	133 to 152
Women		
Excellent	74 to 92	73 to 86
Good	97 to 103	93 to 100
Above average	106 to 111	104 to 114
Average	113 to 117	117 to 121
Below average	119 to 127	123 to 127
Poor	129 to 136	129 to 134
Very poor	142 to 151	135 to 151

From Kligman EW, et al: Recommending exercise to healthy older adults—the preparticipation evaluation and exercise prescription. Phys Sportsmed 27(11):49, 1999. Reproduced with permission of McGraw-Hill, Inc.

individuals, the **Kasch Pulse-Recovery Test**[20,133] can be used (Table 17-13).

Other, more detailed aerobic and anaerobic tests may be performed, including a respiratory quotient test (direct method), the Astrand nomogram (indirect method), the Sjostrad PWC$_{170}$ test (indirect method), and the Yo-Yo tests (see later discussion).[134]

Although not commonly done except in high-level sports, maximum tests are necessary to get the most complete diagnostic data on a patient's response to exercise. This is important, because half of the heart abnormalities are missed if the test stops at 85% of predicted maximum heart rate, which the simplest tests tend to do.[135] Even if a maximum test is performed, 10% to 15% of the normal population may show an abnormal response.[135] It must be remembered that cardiovascular tests clear the subject only up to the heart rate at which he or she has been tested. In most cases, maximum testing is not done, but if a person is showing abnormalities, such a test may be performed as a second diagnostic procedure. These tests must, however, be performed under very controlled conditions, where there are proper facilities to handle cardiac emergencies.

Although anaerobic fitness is not directly related to the cardiovascular system, it is tested through its effects on the cardiovascular system. If the patient's job, activity, exercise, or sport is primarily anaerobic, consideration must be given to including this measurement as part of the profile.[136] Anaerobic tests can be divided into short-term tests (10 seconds or less), intermediate-term tests (20 to 50 seconds), and long-term anaerobic tests (60 to 120 seconds). Probably the most common anaerobic test used today in a laboratory or clinic setting is the 30-second Wingate test.[137]

Agility, Balance, and Reaction Time

For activities requiring agility, balance, and reaction time, the physical fitness profile should include these items. Balance testing is especially important in the elderly population.[118] O'Brien[118] advocated the Sharpened Romberg test, functional reach test, timed get-up-and-go test (see Chapter 11), and Tinetti assessment tool for balance and gait. The functional reach test involves the patient reaching forward as far as possible without falling forward or taking a step while the examiner measures a horizontal for distance. The Tinetti assessment tool has two parts. One part measures static and dynamic sitting and standing balance (Table 17-14), whereas the second part assesses gait (Table 17-15).[138] Ideally, testing should be related to the specific activity. Agility is defined as the ability to change directions rapidly when moving at a high rate of speed.[1] Agility and balance tests are often measured by time or accuracy (e.g., correct two out of three).[1,139]

Maturation and Growth

Maturation assessment is a method of determining how far a patient has progressed toward physical maturity. It also helps to identify periods of rapid growth.[137,140,141] This is especially important where there is a possibility that there will be stress applied to the growth plate, which is commonly the "weak link" in traumatic injury. That is,

Agility and Balance Tests

- Carioca
- Run-and-cut drills
- Back-pedal and throw at stationary or moving target
- Kick at stationary or moving target (different distances)
- One-arm spin
- Shuttle drills
- Pivoting drills
- Blocking drills
- Figure-eight running
- Front-to-back and side-to-side hops
- Sidestep tests
- Beam-walking tests

Sharpened Romberg Test[115,118]

1. With eyes open, stand with feet together for 10 seconds
2. Repeat step 1 with eyes closed
3. With eyes open, place one foot halfway in front of the other for 10 seconds
4. Repeat step 3 with eyes closed
5. With eyes open, place one foot directly in front of the other for 10 seconds
6. Repeat step 5 with eyes closed

during a rapid growth spurt period, the growth plate is weaker and more susceptible to injury than the ligaments and/or capsule. Maturation profiling should not be used to push children into specific activities unless chosen by the child, and it should not be used to exclude a child unless documented evidence demonstrates unacceptable risk for the child.[142] In adolescents, growth patterns can have an effect on participation in activities, exercise, and sports and may affect injury patterns. For example, a growth spurt for a gymnast may adversely affect balance and flexibility. Pubertal growth accounts for 20% to 25% of final adult height, and pubertal weight gain accounts for 50% of ideal adult weight.[78]

TABLE **17-14**

Performance-Oriented Assessment of Balance*

Maneuver	RESPONSE		
	Normal	Adaptive	Abnormal
Sitting balance	Steady, stable	Holds onto chair to keep upright	Leans, slides down in chair
Arising from chair	Able to arise in a single movement without using arms	Uses arms (on chair or walking aid) to pull or push up, and/or moves forward in chair before attempting to arise	Multiple attempts required or unable without human assistance
Immediate standing balance (first 3 to 5 seconds)	Steady without holding onto walking aid or other object for support	Steady, but uses walking aid or other object for support	Any sign of unsteadiness†
Standing balance	Steady, able to stand with feet together without holding object for support	Steady, but cannot put feet together	Any sign of unsteadiness regardless of stance or holds onto object
Balance with eyes closed (with feet as close together as possible)	Steady without holding onto any object with feet together	Steady with feet apart	Any sign of unsteadiness or needs to hold onto an object
Turning balance (360°)	No grabbing or staggering; no need to hold onto any objects; steps are continuous (turn is a flowing movement)	Steps are discontinuous (patient puts one foot completely on floor before raising other foot)	Any sign of unsteadiness or holds onto an object
Nudge on sternum (patient standing with feet as close together as possible, examiner pushes with light even pressure over sternum three times; reflects ability to withstand displacement)	Steady, able to withstand pressure	Needs to move feet, but able to maintain balance	Begins to fall, or examiner has to help maintain balance
Neck turning (patient asked to turn head side to side and look up while standing with feet as close together as possible)	Able to turn head at least half way side to side and be able to bend head back to look at ceiling; no staggering, grabbing, symptoms or lightheadedness, unsteadiness, or pain	Decreased ability to turn side to side to extend neck, but no staggering, grabbing, symptoms of lightheadedness, unsteadiness, or pain	Any sign of unsteadiness or symptoms when turning head or extending neck
One leg standing balance	Able to stand on one leg for 5 seconds without holding object for support		Unable

TABLE **17-14**

Performance-Oriented Assessment of Balance—cont'd

Maneuver	RESPONSE		
	Normal	Adaptive	Abnormal
Back extension (ask patient to lean back as far as possible, without holding onto object if possible)	Good extension without holding object or staggering	Tries to extend, but decreased ROM (compared with other patients of same age) or needs to hold object to attempt extension	Will not attempt or no extension seen or staggers
Reaching up (have patient attempt to remove an object from a shelf high enough to require stretching or standing on toes)	Able to take down object without needing to hold onto other object for support and without becoming unsteady	Able to get object but needs to steady self by holding on to something for support	Unable or unsteady
Bending down (patient is asked to pick up small objects, such as pen, from the floor)	Able to bend down and pick up the object and is able to get up easily in single attempt without needing to pull self up with arms	Able to get object and get upright in single attempt but needs to pull self up with arms or hold onto something for support	Unable to bend down or unable to get upright after bending down or takes multiple attempts to upright
Sitting down	Able to sit down in one smoother movement	Needs to use arms to guide self into chair or not a smooth movement	Falls into chair, misjudges distances (lands off center)

From Tinetti ME: Performance oriented assessment of mobility problems in elderly patients. J Am Geriatr Soc 34(2):119–126, 1986.
ROM, Range of motion.
*The patient begins this assessment seated in a hard, straight-backed, armless chair.
†Unsteadiness defined as grabbing at objects for support, staggering, moving feet, or more than minimal trunk sway.

TABLE **17-15**

Performance-Oriented Assessment of Gait*

Components†	OBSERVATION	
	Normal	Abnormal
Initiation of gait (patient asked to begin walking down hallway)	Begins walking immediately without observable hesitation; initiation of gait is single, smooth motion	Hesitates; multiple attempts; initiation of gait not a smooth motion
Step height (begin observing after first few steps: observe one foot, then the other; observe from side)	Swing foot completely clears floor but by no more than 1 to 2 inches	Swing foot is not completely raised off floor (may hear scraping) or is raised too high (> 1 to 2 inches)‡
Step length (observe distance between two steps of stance foot and heel of swing foot; observe from side; do not judge first few or last few steps; observe one side at a time)	At least the length of individual's foot between the stance toe and swing heel (step length usually longer but foot length provides basis for observation)	Step length less than described under normal‡
Step symmetry (observe the middle part of the patch not the first or last steps; observe from side; observe distance between heel of each swing foot and toe of each stance foot)	Step length same or nearly same on both sides for most step cycles	Step length varies between sides or patient advances with same foot with every step
Step continuity	Begins raising heel of one foot (toe off) as heel of other foot touches the floor (heel strike); no breaks or stops in stride; step lengths equal over most cycles	Places entire foot (heel and toe) on floor before beginning to raise other foot; or stops completely between steps; or step length varies over cycles‡

Continued

TABLE **17-15**

Performance-Oriented Assessment of Gait—cont'd

Components[†]	OBSERVATION	
	Normal	Abnormal
Path deviation (observe from behind; observe one foot over several strides; observe in relation to line on floor [e.g., tiles] if possible; difficult to assess if patient uses a walker)	Foot follows close to straight line as patient advances	Foot deviates from side to side or toward one direction[§]
Trunk stability (observe from behind; side to side motion of trunk may be a normal gait pattern, need to differentiate this from instability)	Trunk does not sway; knees or back are not flexed; arms are not abducted in effort to maintain stability	Any of preceding features present[§]
Walk stance (observe from behind)	Feet should almost touch as one passes other	Feet apart with stepping**
Turning while walking	No staggering; turning continuous with walking; and steps are continuous while turning	Staggers; stops before initiating turn; or steps are discontinuous

From Tinetti ME: Performance oriented assessment of mobility problems in elderly patients. J Am Geriatr Soc 34(2):119–126, 1986.
*The patient stands with examiner at end of obstacle-free hallway. Patient uses usual walking aid. Examiner then asks patient to walk down hallway at his or her usual pace. Examiner observes one component of gait at a time (analogous to heart examination). For some components, the examiner walks behind the patient; for other components, the examiner walks next to patient. May require several trips to complete.
[†]Also ask patient to walk at a "more rapid than usual" pace and observe whether any walking aid is used correctly.
[‡]Abnormal gait finding may reflect a primary neurologic or musculoskeletal problem directly related to the finding or reflect a compensatory maneuver for other, more remote problem.
[§]Abnormality may be corrected by walking aid (such as, cane); observe with and without walking aid if possible.
**Abnormal finding is a usually compensatory maneuver rather than a primary problem.

Skeletal development is usually measured by wrist x-rays, using the *Radiographic Atlas of Skeletal Development of the Wrist and Hand,* by W.W. Greulich and S.U. Pyle,[143] for interpretation.

The most common method of measuring maturation in males and females is the Tanner scale.[28,137,144] The five stages of the Tanner scale are based on pictorial standards of genitalia and pubic hair for males and breast development and pubic hair for females (Figures 17-2 to 17-4 and Table 17-16). Some people have recommended that collision sports not be allowed for boys until they reach level 5 of development. For females, onset of menstruation is another suitable index of maturity and maturation.

Body Composition and Anthropometry

Body composition profiling is designed to provide a relatively detailed analysis of an individual's muscle, fat, and bone mass.[141,145] Anthropometry may be used to determine the individual's body type (mesomorphic, endomorphic, ectomorphic) to see whether he or she is properly suited for the desired activity, exercise, sport, or position played in a sport.

Anthropometry also involves body fat measurements, such as skinfold measurements or underwater weighing.[146] Of the two, skinfold measurement is more common, because it is easier and faster. Seven skinfold sites are most commonly used (Figure 17-5), although some people believe that measurement at three sites is sufficient (i.e., a different three for males and females).[146] Most males should fall below 12% to 15% body fat. Endurance athletes (e.g., distance runners, gymnasts, wrestlers) are often below 7%. Football, baseball, and soccer players average 10% to 12%.[147] No one should be below 5% body fat. Generally, if the percentage of body fat is greater than the upper normal limit of 14% for males and 17% for females, the patient should be put on a weight loss program or weight training to increase lean body mass; but again, this depends on the activity in which the patient wishes to participate.

Other methods of body composition measurement include girth measurements, bone diameter measurements, ultrasound measurement, and arm radiograph measurements.[145]

TESTS FOR RETURN TO ACTIVITY FOLLOWING INJURY

Tests for return to activity should attempt to replicate the activity the patient is returning to. They should be functional, while testing such parameters as strength, endurance, flexibility, and proprioception to decrease the

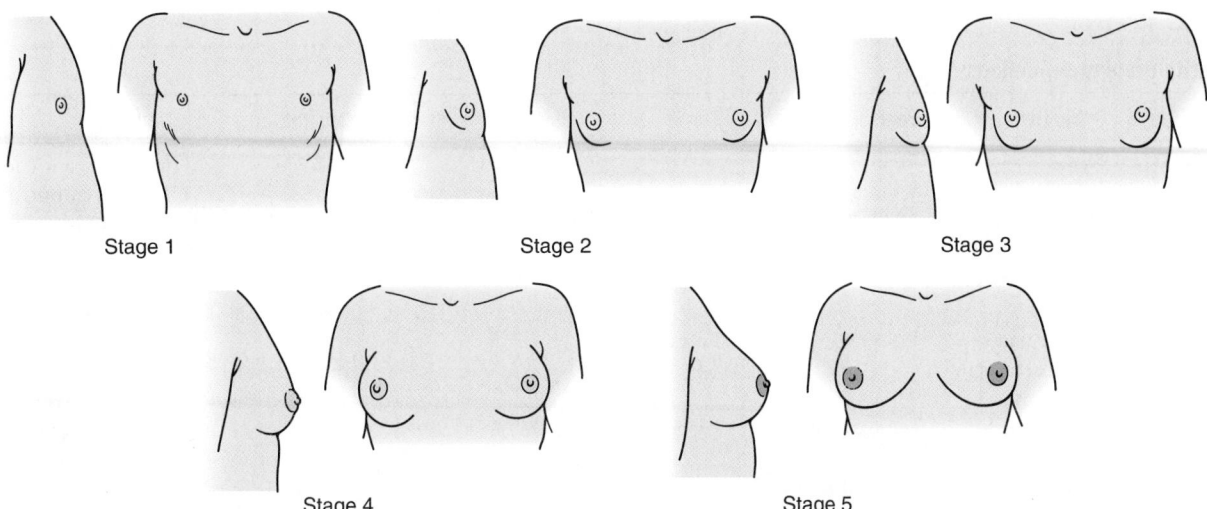

Figure 17-2 Breast development in girls. The development of the mammae can be divided into five stages. In stage 1, only the nipple is raised above the level of the breast (as in the child). In stage 2, the budding stage, there is bud-shaped elevation of the areola. On palpation, a fairly hard button can be felt that is disc or cherry shaped. The areola is increased in diameter, and the surrounding area is slightly elevated. In stage 3, there is further elevation of the mammae; the areolar diameter is further increased, and the shape of mammae is visibly feminine. In stage 4, fat deposits increase, and the areola forms a secondary elevation above that of the breast. This secondary mound occurs in approximately half of all girls and in some cases persists in adulthood. In stage 5, the adult stage, the areola usually subsides to the level of the breast and is strongly pigmented. (Redrawn from Halpern B, Blackburn T, Incremona B, et al: Preparticipation sports physicals. In Zachazewski JE, Magee DJ, Quillen WS, editors: Athletic injuries and rehabilitation, Philadelphia, 1996, WB Saunders, p. 855.)

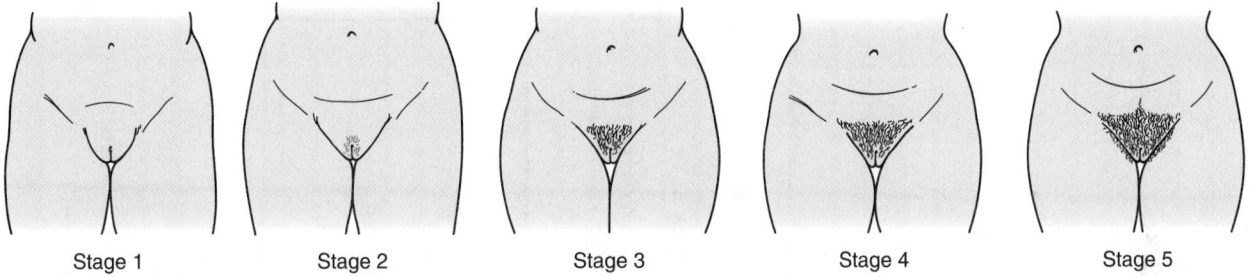

Figure 17-3 Pubic hair development in females. In the development of pubic hair, five stages can be distinguished. In stage 1, there is no growth of pubic hair. In stage 2, initial, scarcely pigmented hair is present, especially along the labia. In stage 3, sparse dark, visibly pigmented, curly pubic hair is present on the labia. In stage 4, hair that is adult in type but not in extent is present. In stage 5, there is lateral spreading (type and spread of hair are adult). (Redrawn from Halpern B, Blackburn T, Incremona B, et al: Preparticipation sports physicals. In Zachazewski JE, Magee DJ, Quillen WS, editors: Athletic injuries and rehabilitation, Philadelphia, 1996, WB Saunders, p. 855.)

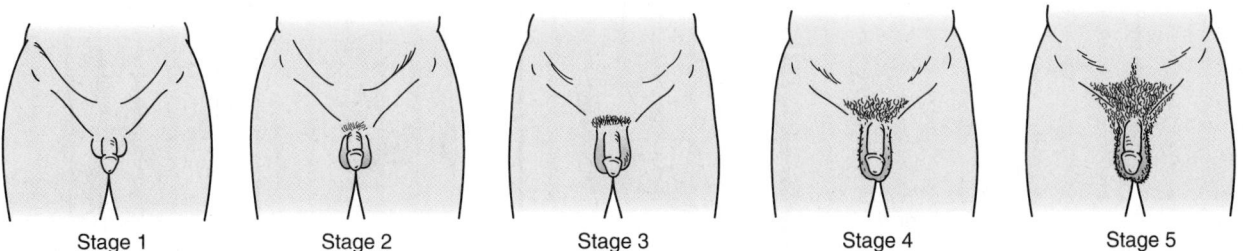

Figure 17-4 Genital and pubic hair development in males. The development of external genitalia and pubic hair can be divided into five stages. In stage 1, the testes, scrotum, and penis are the same size and shape as in the young child, and there is no growth of pubic hair (hair in pubic area is no different from that on the rest of the abdomen). In stage 2, there is enlargement of the scrotum and testes. The skin of the scrotum becomes redder, thinner, and wrinkled. The penis has not grown (or just slightly so). Pubic hair is slightly pigmented. In stage 3, there is enlargement of the penis, especially in length, further enlargement of testes, and descent of scrotum. Dark, definitely pigmented, curly pubic hair is present around the base of penis. In stage 4, there is continued enlargement of the penis and sculpturing of the glans with increased pigmentation of the scrotum. This stage is sometimes best described as not quite adult. Pubic hair is definitely adult in type but not in extent (no further than the inguinal fold). In stage 5, the adult stage, the scrotum is ample, and the penis reaches almost to the bottom of the scrotum. Pubic hair spreads to the medial surface of the thighs but not upward. In 80% of men, hair spreads along the linea alba. (Redrawn from Halpern B, Blackburn T, Incremona B, et al: Preparticipation sports physicals. In Zachazewski JE, Magee DJ, Quillen WS, editors: Athletic injuries and rehabilitation, Philadelphia, 1996, WB Saunders, p. 855.)

TABLE **17-16**

Maturity Staging Guidelines

Boys' Stage	Pubic Hair	Penis	Testis	Girls' Stage	Pubic Hair	Breasts
1	None	Preadolescent (infantile)	—	1	Preadolescent (none)	Preadolescent (no germinal button)
2	Slight, long, slight pigmentation	Slight enlargement	Enlarged scrotum, pink slight rugae	2	Sparse, lightly pigmented, straight medial border of labia	Breast and papilla elevated as small mound; areolar diameter increased
3	Darker, starts to curl, small amount	Longer	Larger	3	Darker, beginning to curl, increased	Breast and areola enlarged; no contour separation
4	Coarse, curly, adult type, but less quantity	Increase in glans size and breadth of penis	Larger, darker scrotum	4	Coarse, curly, abundant, but less than adult	Areola and papilla form secondary mound
5	Adult, spread to inner thighs	Adult	Adult	5	Adult female triangle and spread to medial surface	Mature, nipple projects, areola part of general breast contour

From Tanner JM: Growth and adolescence. Oxford, England, 1962, Blackwell Scientific.

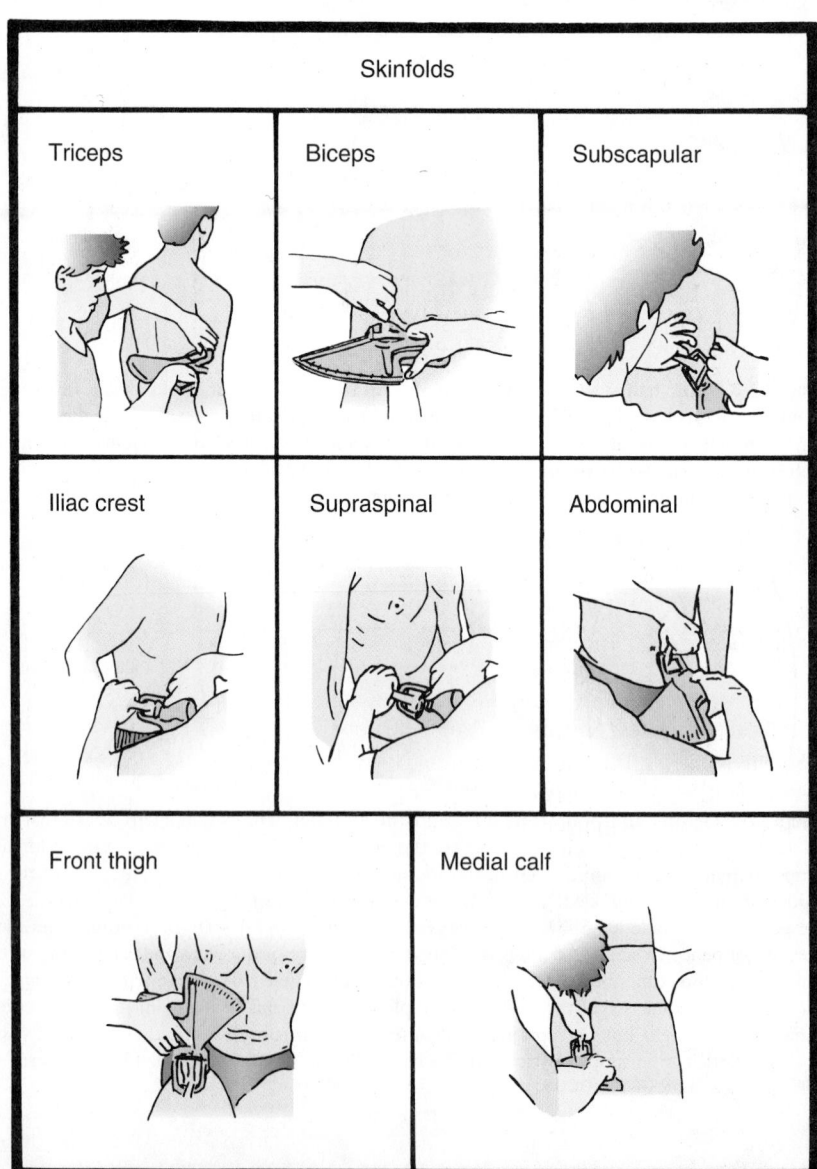

Figure 17-5 Skinfold sites for measuring body fat. (Reprinted, by permission, from Ross WD, Marfell-Jones MJ: Kinanthropometry. In Mac-Dougal JD, Wenger HA, Green HJ, editors: Physiological testing of the high performance athlete, ed 2, Champaign, IL, 1991, Human Kinetics, p. 238.)

chance of the patient being reinjured. The tests are more commonly used for individuals returning to sport activities but could be modified to test the functional level of a patient. For people who are less active, different timing or load tests could be used. For more sedentary people, numerical rating scales or walking tests (see Chapter 11 for examples) could be used. The following tests are simply examples of functional tests that may be used to test a patient for return to activity.

Forward Step Down Test.[148] This test is used to determine eccentric muscle strength for lowering the body to the ground. If a force plate is used, a vertical impact score that is greater on the affected side indicates loss of motor control coinciding with knee extensor weakness. The patient is asked to step down from an 8 inch (20 cm) step. As the patient does so, the examiner should watch for such things as contralateral hip drop, ipsilateral hip hike, increased knee valgus, and increased plantar flexion (reaching), which may indicate imbalances or weaknesses.

Yo-Yo Endurance Test (Also Called the Beep, Bleep, Progressive Shuttle Run, and the Leger Shuttle Run).[148,149] This is a "field" test used to evaluate physical capacity and basic fitness involving the lower limb. For the test, two markers (pylons) are placed 20 m (66 feet) apart and an audio CD or metronome is used to control the speed that is regularly increased over time (i.e., a "beep" occurs at set intervals when the individual should be at the marker) until the patient can no longer maintain a specific speed (Figure 17-6, *A*). The test involves running continuously between two points that are 20 m apart while the interval between successive beeps decreases, forcing the individual to increase velocity over the test until he or she can no longer keep synchronized with the beep; that is, the individual reaches each pylon at a beep, runs around pylon, and starts to return to go back the other way. The recording normally is structured with twenty-three "levels" with the time to complete each interval varying from 68 to 61 seconds (to complete 20 meters). The highest level attained before failing to keep up is recorded as the score of the test. Test results are the distance covered and can be related to the specific activity the individual wants to return to. The test usually takes 5 to 15 minutes to complete.

Yo-Yo Intermittent Endurance Test.[148] This test is set up as described earlier, but the patient does intermittent intense exercise repeatedly (Figure 17-6, *B*). This too can be geared to the specific activity the patient is returning to. The test lasts 10 to 20 minutes doing 5- to 18-second intervals interspersed with 5-second rest periods. It evaluates the patient's ability to perform repeated activity intervals over time. It is a test of the aerobic system and is a good test for sports, such as tennis, soccer, hockey, basketball.

Yo-Yo Intermittent Recovery Test (Yo-Yo 1R2 Test).[148] This test is set up as described earlier and lasts 2 to 15 minutes,

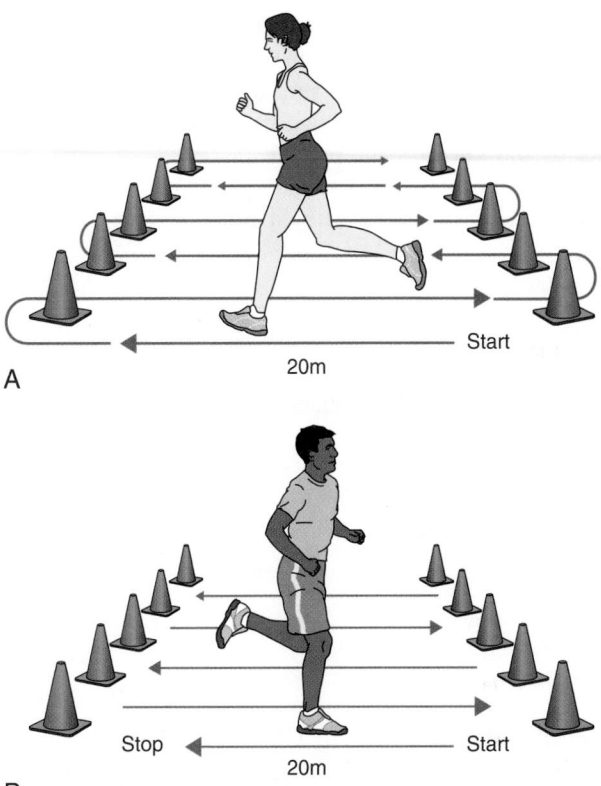

Figure 17-6 A, Beep or Yo-Yo test. The individual times the run so that he or she arrives at the pylon at the beep, runs around pylon, and runs back to the other pylon repeating the process until he or she no longer keeps up with the beep. **B,** Beep or Yo-Yo intermittent test. The individual times the runs so that he or she arrives at the pylon at the beep and has a 5-second rest period before running back to the other pylon repeating the process until he or she no longer keeps up with the beep. The time to complete the interval is decreased as the test progresses while the rest period remains the same.

and it determines the ability of the patient to recover after intense exercise. It is designed to test the anaerobic system. Between each exercise bout (5 to 15 seconds), there is a 10-second pause. The number of repetitions is measured and can be equated to the activity repetitions the individual will do when returning to his or her specific activity. It is a good test for sports, such as football, soccer, and hockey.

SPORTS PARTICIPATION

For any primary care evaluation, the physician is the final arbitrator. Any decision as to whether someone should be allowed to work or participate in an activity or as to the patient's functional level must be based on accurate diagnosis of the condition, knowledge of the disease process for the condition, knowledge of the job or sport, knowledge of the physical needs of the patient and the activity, and direct evaluation of the individual.[96] The examiner must also keep in mind the rights of handicapped people and the limits of informed consent. Although standards are often given for participation, in the end, the examiner must make his or her final decision on an individual basis, being primarily concerned with the health and safety of the patient.

Any individual with a solitary paired organ, such as an eye, kidney, or testicle, should not take part in contact sports, especially if the organ is abnormal. Children should be channeled into noncontact sports. High-caliber or older athletes know the rules and should make their own decision. Table 17-17 lists conditions that are contraindications to specific sports, and the level of these activities can be extrapolated to the physical stresses of everyday jobs.[3,28]

TABLE **17-17**

Conditions Commonly Disqualifying an Individual from Participation in Sports

Conditions	TYPE OF SPORT			
	Collision*	Contact†	Noncontact‡	Others§
Eyes				
Absence of one eye	??	??	—	—
Congenital glaucoma	X	X	—	—
Retinal detachment	X	X	—	—
Severe myopia	?	?	—	—
Musculoskeletal				
Acute inflammatory conditions	X	X	X	X
Spinal instability	X	X	?	?
Congenital or growth abnormalities that are incompatible with demands of sport	X	X	X	—
Chronic or unhealed conditions (unless cleared by physician)	X	X	X	X
Neurological				
Uncontrolled convulsive disorder	X	X	X	?
Controlled convulsive disorder	?	?	?	?
Repeated concussions	X	X	—	—
Serious head trauma	X	X	—	—
Previous head surgery	X	X	—	—
Transient quadriplegia (unless cleared by physician)	X	X	—	—
Cardiovascular				
Acute infection	X	X	X	X
Cardiomegaly	X	X	X	X
Enlarged spleen	X	X	—	—
Hemorrhage (bleeding) disorders	X	X	X	—
Heart abnormalities (unless cleared by cardiologist)	X	X	X	X
Organic hypertension	X	X	X	X
Previous heart surgery (unless cleared by cardiologist)	X	X	X	X
Pulmonary				
Acute infection	X	X	X	X
Pulmonary insufficiency	X	X	X	X
Uncontrolled asthma (unless cleared by pulmonary physician)	X	X	X	X
Urogenital				
Absence of one kidney	??	??	—	—
Acute infection	X	X	X	X
Enlarged liver	X	X	—	—
Hernia (inguinal or femoral, unless cleared by physician)	X	X	X	—
Renal disease	X	X	X	X
Absent or undescended testicle (unless cleared by physician)	??	??	—	—

TABLE **17-17**

Conditions Commonly Disqualifying an Individual from Participation in Sports—cont'd

Conditions	TYPE OF SPORT			
	Collision*	Contact†	Noncontact‡	Others§
Gastrointestinal				
Jaundice		X	X	X
Dermatological				
Acute infection (e.g., boils, herpes simplex, impetigo)	X	X	?	?
General or Systemic Disease				
Acute systemic infection or illness	?	?	?	?
Uncontrolled diabetes	X	X	X	X
Physical immaturity (relative to level of competition)	X	X	—	—

Adapted from the Committee on Medical Aspects of Sports: Medical evaluation of the athlete: a guide, American Medical Association, ©1966.
*Examples include boxing, football, hockey (ice and field), rugby.
†Examples include baseball, basketball, lacrosse, martial arts, rodeo, soccer, volleyball, wrestling.
‡Examples include dance, rowing, skiing, squash, swimming, tennis, track^h cross-country.
§Examples include archery, bowling, golf, shooting, track and field events.
?, Depends on individual case and clearance by physician; ??, athlete may compete if athlete knows risks and informed consent form is completed (protective equipment may be necessary); X, participation prohibited; —, participation permitted.

REFERENCES

1. Sanders B, Nemeth WC: Preparticipation physical examination. J Orthop Sports Phys Ther 23:144–163, 1996.
2. American Academy of Orthopaedic Surgeons: Athletic training and sports medicine, Rosemont, IL, 1991, The Academy.
3. Harvey J: The preparticipation examination of the child athlete. Clin Sports Med 1:353–369, 1982.
4. Clyne ME, Forlenza M: Consumer-focused preadmission testing: a paradigm shift. J Nurs Care Qual 11(3):9–15, 1997.
5. Daker-White G, Carr AJ, Harvey I, et al: A randomized controlled trial: shifting boundaries of doctors and physiotherapists in orthopedic outpatient departments. J Epidemiol Community Health 53:643–650, 1999.
6. Hattam P, Smeatham A: Evaluation of an orthopedic screening service in primary care. Clin Perform Qual Health Care 7:121–124, 1999.
7. Breen A, Carr E, Mann E, et al: Acute back pain management in primary care: a qualitative pilot study of the feasibility of a nurse-led service in general practice. J Nurs Manage 12:201–209, 2004.
8. Moore JH, Goss DL, Baxter RE, et al: Clinical diagnostic accuracy and magnetic resonance imaging of patients referred by physical therapists, orthopedic surgeons and nonorthopedic providers. J Orthop Sports Phys Ther 35:67–71, 2005.
9. International Olympic Committee: Lausanne recommendations: sudden cardiovascular death in sports—preparticipation screening, 2004, The Committee.
10. Hall K, Zalman B: Evaluation and management of apparent life-threatening events in children. Am Fam Physician 71:2301–2308, 2005.
11. Harrington JT, Dopf CA, Chalgren CS: Implementing guidelines for interdisciplinary care of low back pain: a critical role for pre-appointment management of specialty referrals. Jt Comm J Qual Improv 27:651–663, 2001.
12. Lynch JR, Gardner GC, Parsons RR: Musculoskeletal workload vs. musculoskeletal clinical confidence among primary care physicians in rural practice. Am J Orthop 34:487–492, 2005.
13. Eathorne SW: Medical problems in a sports medicine setting. Med Clin North Am 78:479–503, 1994.
14. Vlek JF, Vierhout WP, Knottnerus JA, et al: A randomized controlled trial of joint consultations with general practitioners and cardiologists in primary care. Br J Gen Pract 53:108–112, 2003.
15. Moore MN: Orthopedic pitfalls in emergency medicine. South Med J 81:371–378, 1988.
16. Superko HR, Bernauer E, Voss J: Effects of a mandatory health screening and physical maintenance program for law enforcement officers. Phys Sportsmed 16:99–109, 1988.
17. Binda C: Precamp physical exams: their value may be greater than you think. Phys Sportsmed 17:167–169, 1989.
18. Gurry M, Pappas A, Michaels J, et al: A comprehensive preseason fitness evaluation for professional baseball players. Phys Sportsmed 13:63–74, 1985.
19. Metzel JD: The adolescent preparticipation physical examination—is it helpful? Clin Sports Med 19:577–592, 2000.
20. Kligman EW, Hewitt MJ, Crowell DL: Recommending exercise to healthy older adults – the preparticipation evaluation and exercise prescription. Phys Sportsmed 27(11):42–62, 1999.
21. Glover DW, Maron DJ, Matheson GO: The preparticipation physical examination—steps toward consensus and uniformity. Phys Sportsmed 27:29–34, 1999.
22. Peltz JE, Haskell WL, Matheson GO: A comprehensive and cost-effective preparticipation exam implemented on the world wide web. Med Sci Sports Exerc 31:1727–1740, 1999.
23. Scheitel SM, Boland BJ, Wollan PC, et al: Patient-physician agreement about medical diagnoses and cardiovascular risk factors in the ambulatory general medical examination. Mayo Clin Proc 71:1131–1137, 1996.
24. Tanji TL: The preparticipation exam: special concerns for the Special Olympics. Phys Sportsmed 19:61–68, 1991.
25. Hudson PB: Preparticipation screening of Special Olympics athletes. Phys Sportsmed 16:97–104, 1988.
26. Bickley LS: Bates' guide to physical examination and history taking, Philadelphia, 1999, Lippincott, Williams & Wilkins.
27. Goodman CC, Snyder TE: Differential diagnosis in physical therapy, Philadelphia, 1995, WB Saunders.
28. McKeag DB: Preparticipation screening of the potential athlete. Clin Sports Med 8:373–397, 1989.
29. Hunter SC: Preparticipation physical examination. In Griffin LY, editor: Orthopedic knowledge update: sports medicine, Rosemont, IL, 1994, American Academy of Orthopaedic Surgeons.
30. Woolf AD: History and physical examination. Best Pract Res Clin Rheum 17:381–402, 2003.
31. Yazici Y, Gibofsky A: A diagnostic approach to musculoskeletal pain. Office Rheum 2(2):1–10, 1999.
32. Cayley WE: Diagnosing the cause of chest pain. Am Fam Physician 72:2012–2021, 2005.
33. Committee on Sports Medicine: Recommendations for participation in competitive sports. Pediatrics 81:737–739, 1988.
34. Stanley K: Preparticipation evaluation of the young athlete. In Stanitski CL, DeLee JC, Drez D, editors: Pediatric and adolescent sports medicine, Philadelphia, 1994, WB Saunders.
35. Smilkstein G: Health evaluation of high school athletes. Phys Sportsmed 9:73–80, 1981.
36. Heidt RS, Sweeterman LM, Carlonas RL, et al: Avoidance of soccer injuries with preseason conditioning. Am J Sports Med 28:659–662, 2000.

37. Carek PJ, Futrell M, Hueston WJ: The preparticipation physical examination history: who has the correct answers? Clin J Sports Med 9:124–128, 1999.

38. Haggman S, Maher CG, Refshauge KM: Screening for symptoms of depression by physical therapists managing low back pain. Phys Ther 84:1157–1166, 2004.

39. Grotle M, Brox JI, Veierod MB, et al: Clinical course and prognostic factors in acute low back pain: patients consulting primary care for the first time. Spine 30(8):976–982, 2005.

40. Waddell G, Main CJ: Illness behavior. In Waddell G, editor: The back pain revolution, New York, 1998, Churchill Livingstone.

41. Farnell S, Maxwell L, Tan S, et al: Temperature measurement: comparison of non-invasive methods used in adult critical care. J Clin Nurs 14:632–639, 2005.

42. Carroll M: An evaluation of temperature measurement. Nurs Standard 14:39–43, 2000.

43. Kaplan NM, Deveraux RB, Miller HS: Systemic hyperextension. Med Sci Sports Exerc 26:S268–S270, 1994.

44. Zabetakis PM: Profiling the hypertensive patient in sports. Clin Sports Med 3:137–152, 1984.

45. Staats PS, Argoff CE, Brewer R, et al: Neuropathic pain: incorporating new consensus guidelines into the reality of clinical practice. Adv Stud Med 4:S550–S566, 2004.

46. Potter RG, Jones JM: The evolution of chronic pain among patients with musculoskeletal problems: a pilot study in primary care. Br J Gen Pract 42:462–464, 1992.

47. Nelson MA: The child athlete with chronic disease. In Stanitski CL, DeLee JC, Drez D, editors: Pediatric and adolescent sports medicine, Philadelphia, 1994, WB Saunders.

48. Bonci CM, Ryan R: Preparticipation screening in intercollegiate athletics: postgraduate advances in sports medicine, Philadelphia, 1988, University of Pennsylvania Medical School and Forum Medicum.

49. Halpern B, Blackburn T, Incremona B, et al: Preparticipation sports physicals. In Zachazewski JE, Magee DJ, Quillen WS, editors: Athletic injuries and rehabilitation, Philadelphia, 1996, WB Saunders.

50. Wall EJ: Practical primary pediatric orthopedics. Nurs Clin North Am 35:95–113, 2000.

51. Barth WF: Office evaluation of the patient with musculoskeletal complaints. Am J Med 102(suppl 1A): 3S–10S, 1997.

52. Calkins E: Rheumatic diseases in the elderly—finding a way through the maze. Prim Care 9:181–195, 1982.

53. Davis AE: Primary care management of chronic musculoskeletal pain. Nurse Pract 21:74–82, 1996.

54. Pimentel L: Orthopedic trauma: office management of major joint injury. Med Clin North Am 90:355–382, 2006.

55. Gomez JE, Landry GL, Bernhardt DT: Critical evaluation of the 2-minute orthopedic screening examination. Am J Dis Child 147:1109–1113, 1993.

56. Strong WB, Steed D: Cardiovascular evaluation of the young athlete. Pediatr Clin North Am 29:1325–1339, 1982.

57. Huston TP, Puffer JC, Rodney WM: The athletic heart syndrome. N Engl J Med 313:24–32, 1985.

58. McGrew CA: Clinical implications of the AHA preparticipation cardiovascular screening guidelines. Athletic Ther Today 5:52–56, 2000.

59. Fuller CM: Cost effectiveness analysis of screening of high school athletes for risk of sudden cardiac death. Med Sci Sports Exerc 32:887–890, 2000.

60. Maron BJ, Pollac DC, Kaplan JA, et al: Blunt impact to the chest leading to sudden death from cardiac arrest during sports activities. N Engl J Med 333:337–342, 1995.

61. Potera C: AHA Panel outlines sudden death screening standards. Phys Sportsmed 24(10):27–28, 1996.

62. Fuller CM, McNulty CM, Spring DA, et al: Prospective screening of 5,615 high school athletes for risk of sudden cardiac death. Med Sci Sports Exerc 29:1131–1138, 1997.

63. Blankfield RP, Finkelhor RS, Alexander JJ, et al: Etiology and diagnosis of bilateral leg edema in primary care. Am J Med 105:192–197, 1998.

64. Salem DN, Isner JM: Cardiac screening in athletes. Orthop Clin North Am 11:687–695, 1980.

65. Keffer JH: The cardiac profile and proposed practice guidelines for acute ischemic heart disease. Am J Clin Pathol 107:398–409, 1997.

66. Heger JJ: Ventricular arrhythmias: guidelines for primary care management. J Indiana St Med Assoc 76:819–822, 1983.

67. Pflieger KL, Strong WB: Screening for heart murmurs: what's normal and what's not. Phys Sportsmed 20:71–81, 1992.

68. Braden DS, Strong WB: Preparticipation screening for sudden cardiac death in high school and college athletes. Phys Sportsmed 16:128–144, 1988.

69. Cavell RM: The exercise treadmill test for diagnosis and prognosis of coronary artery disease. J La State Med Soc 147:197–201, 1995.

70. Shinozaki T, Hasegawa T, Yano E: Ankle-arm index as an indicator of atherosclerosis: its application as a screening method. J Clin Epidemiol 51:1263–1269, 1998.

71. Newman AB, Siscovick DS, Manolio TA, et al: Atherosclerosis: ankle-arm index as a marker of atherosclerosis in the cardiovascular health study. Circulation 88:837–845, 1993.

72. Belman MJ, King RR: Pulmonary profiling in exercise. Clin Sports Med 3:119–136, 1984.

73. Ross RG: The prevalence of reversible airway obstruction in professional football players. Med Sci Sports Exerc 32:1985–1989, 2000.

74. Rundell KW, Wilber RL, Szmedra L, et al: Exercise-induced asthma screening of elite athletes: field versus laboratory exercise challenge. Med Sci Sports Exerc 32:309–316, 2000.

75. Khosla RK: Detecting sexually transmitted disease—a new role for urinalysis in the preparticipation exam? Phys Sportsmed 23(1):77–80, 1995.

76. Dorsen PJ: Should athletes with one eye, kidney or testicle play contact sports? Phys Sportsmed 14:130–138, 1986.

77. Lombardo JA: Preparticipation physical evaluation. Prim Care 11:3–21, 1984.

78. Johnson MD: Tailoring the preparticipation exam to female athletes. Phys Sportsmed 20:61–72, 1992.

79. Slavin JL: Assessing athletes' nutritional status: making it part of the sports medicine physical. Phys Sportsmed 19:79–94, 1991.

80. American Academy of Pediatrics: Climatic heat stress and the exercising child. Phys Sportsmed 11:155–159, 1983.

81. Henry C: Heatstroke. Crit Care Update 30–35, 1983.

82. American College of Sports Medicine Position Statement: Prevention of heat injuries during distance running. Am J Sports Med 3:194–196, 1975.

83. Bota DP, Ferreira FL, Melot C, et al: Body temperature alterations in the critically ill. Intensive Care Med 30:811–816, 2004.

84. Poumadere M, Mays C, LeMer S, et al: The 2003 heat wave in France: dangerous climate change here and now. Risk Anal 25:1483–1494, 2005.

85. Moran DS: Potential applications of heat and cold stress indices to sporting events. Sports Med 31:909–917, 2001.

86. Claremont AD: Taking winter in stride requires proper attire. Phys Sportsmed 4:65–68, 1976.

87. Nelson WE, Gieck JH, Kolb P: Treatment and prevention of hypothermia and frostbite. Athletic Training 330–332, 1983.

88. Roach JJ: Coping with killing cold. Phys Sportsmed 3(6):35–39, 1975.

89. Sherry E, Richards D: Hypothermia among resort skiers: 19 cases from the Snowy Mountains. Med J Aust 144:457–461, 1986.

90. Biem J, Koehnecke N, Classen D, et al: Out of the cold: management of hypothermia and frostbite. Can Med J 168:305–311, 2003.

91. Mallet ML: Pathophysiology of accidental hypothermia. Q J Med 95:775–785, 2002.

92. Twomey P: Making the best use of a radiology department: an example of implementation of a referral guideline within a primary care organization. Qual Prim Care 11:53–59, 2003.

93. McKinnis LN: Fundamentals of musculoskeletal imaging, Philadelphia, 2005, FA Davis.

94. Johnson TR, Steinbach LS: Essentials of musculoskeletal imaging, Rosemont, IL, 2004, American Academy of Orthopedic Surgeons.

95. Resnick D, Kransdorf MJ: Bone and joint imaging, Philadelphia, 2005, Elsevier.

96. O'Brien K: Getting around: a simple office workup to assess patient function. Geriatrics 49(7):38–42, 1994.

97. Nicholas JA: The value of sports profiling. Clin Sports Med 3:3–10, 1984.

98. Feinstein RA, Soileau EJ, Daniel WA: A national survey of preparticipation physical examination requirements. Phys Sportsmed 16:51–59, 1988.

99. Marino M: Profiling swimmers. Clin Sports Med 3:211–229, 1984.

100. Sapega AA, Minkoff J, Valsamis M, et al: Musculoskeletal performance testing and profiling of elite competitive fencers. Clin Sports Med 3:231–244, 1984.

101. Bridgman R: A coach's guide to testing for athletic attributes. National Strength Conditioning Assoc J 13:34–37, 1991.

102. Gleim GW: The profiling of professional football players. Clin Sports Med 3:185–197, 1984.

103. Skinner JS: Exercise testing and exercise prescription for special cases: theoretical basis and clinical application, Philadelphia, 1993, Lea & Febiger.

104. Hershman E: The profile for prevention of musculoskeletal injury. Clin Sports Med 3:65–84, 1984.

105. MacDougal JD, Wenger HA: The purpose of physiological testing. In MacDougal JD, Wenger HA, Green HJ, editors: Physiological testing of the high performance athlete, Champaign, IL, 1991, Human Kinetics.

106. Kiesel K, Plisky PJ, Voight ML: Can serious injury in professional football be predicted by a preseason functional movement screen? North Am J Sports Phys Ther 2:147–158, 2007.

107. Kiesel K, Plisky PJ, Butler R: Functional movement test scores improve following a standardized off-season intervention program in professional football players. Scand J Med Sci Sports 21:287–292, 2011.

108. Teyhen DS, Schaffer SW, Lorenson CA, et al: The functional movement screen: a reliability study. J Orthop Sports Phys Ther 42:530–540, 2012.

109. Kiesel K, Plisky PJ, Voight ML: Can serious injury in professional football be predicted by a preseason functional movement screen? North Am J Sports Phys Ther 2:147–158, 2007.

110. Gribble PA, Hertel J, Denegar CR: Chronic ankle instability and fatigue create proximal joint alterations during performance of the Star Excursion Balance. Int J Sports Med 28:236–242, 2007.

111. Hale SA, Hertel J, Olmsted-Kramer LC: The effect of a 4-week comprehensive rehabilitation program on postural control and lower extremity function in individuals with chronic ankle instability. J Orthop Sports Phys Ther 37:303–311, 2007.

112. Herrington L, Hatcher J, Hatcher A, et al: A comparison of Star Excursion Balance Test reach distances between ACL deficient patients and asymptomatic controls. Knee 16:49–52, 2009.

113. Plisky PJ, Rauh M, Kaminski T, et al: Star Excursion Balance Test as a predictor of lower extremity injury in high school basketball players. J Orthop Sports Phys Ther 30:911–919, 2006.

114. Kiesel KB, Plisky PJ, Kersey P: Functional movement test score as a predictor of time-loss during a professional football team's preseason. Med Sci Sports Exerc 40(5)Suppl:S234, 2008.

115. Guccione AA: Geriatric physical therapy, St Louis, 1993, Mosby.

116. Marino M, Gleim GW: Muscle strength and fiber typing. Clin Sports Med 3:85–100, 1984.

117. Sale DG: Testing strength and power. In MacDougal JD, Wenger HA, Green HJ, editors: Physiological testing of the high performance athlete, Champaign, IL, 1991, Human Kinetics.

118. O'Brien K: Getting around: a simple office workup to assess patient function. Geriatrics 49:38–40, 1994.

119. Corbin CB: Flexibility. Clin Sports Med 3:101–117, 1994.

120. Hubley-Kozey CL: Testing flexibility. In MacDougal JD, Wenger HA, Green HJ, editors: Physiological testing of the high performance athlete, Champaign, IL, 1991, Human Kinetics.

121. Kibler WB, Chandler TJ, Uhl T, et al: A musculoskeletal approach to the preparticipation physical examination: preventing injury and improving performance. Am J Sports Med 17:525–531, 1989.

122. Carter C, Wilkinson J: Persistent joint laxity and congenital dislocation of the hip. J Bone Joint Surg Br 46:40–45, 1969.

123. Remvig L, Jensen DV, Ward RC: Are diagnostic criteria for general hypermobility and benign joint hypermobility syndrome based on reproducible and valid tests? A review of the literature. J Rheumatol 34(4):798–803, 2007.

124. Juul-Kristensen B, Rogind H, Jensen DV, et al: Inter-examiner reproducibility of tests and criteria for generalized joint hypermobility and benign joint hypermobility syndrome. Rheumatology 46:1835–1841, 2007.

125. Nicholas JA: Risk factors, sports medicine and the orthopedic system: an overview. J Sports Med 3:243–259, 1975.

126. American College of Sports Medicine: Recommended quantity and quality of exercise for developing and maintaining cardio-respiratory and muscular fitness in healthy adult. J Cardiopulmon Rehab 10:235–245, 1990.

127. Squires RW, Bove AA: Cardiovascular profiling. Clin Sports Med 3:11–29, 1984.

128. Morrison CA, Norenberg RG: Using the exercise test to create the exercise prescription. Prim Care 28:137–158, 2001.

129. Wasserman K, Hansen JE, Sue DY, et al: Principles of exercise testing and interpretation, Philadelphia, 1994, Lea & Febiger.

130. Thoden JS: Testing aerobic power. In MacDougal JD, Wenger HA, Green HJ, editors: Physiological testing of the high performance athlete, Champaign, IL, 1991, Human Kinetics.

131. Cooper KH: The new aerobics, New York, 1970, Bantam Books.

132. Cooper KM: A means of assessing maximal oxygen intake. JAMA 203:201–204, 1968.

133. Kasch FW, Phillips WH, Ross WD, et al: A comparison of maximal oxygen uptake by treadmill and step test procedures. J Appl Physiol 21:1387–1388, 1966.

134. Astrand PD, Rodahl K: Textbook of work physiology, Toronto, 1977, McGraw-Hill.

135. Kowal DM, Daniels WL: Recommendations for the screening of military personnel over 35 years of age for physical training programs. Am J Sports Med 7:186–190, 1979.

136. Bouchard C, Taylor AW, Simoneau JA, et al: Testing anaerobic power and capacity. In MacDougal JD, Wenger HA, Green HJ, editors: Physiological testing of the high performance athlete, Champaign, IL, 1991, Human Kinetics.

137. Caine DJ, Broekhoff J: Maturity assessment: a viable preventive measure against physical and psychological insult to the young athlete. Phys Sportsmed 15:67–80, 1987.

138. Tinetti ME: Performance oriented assessment of mobility problems in elderly patients. J Am Geriatr Soc 43:119–126, 1986.

139. Tippett SR, Voight ML: Functional progressions for sports rehabilitation, Champaign, IL, 1995, Human Kinetics.

140. Whieldon D: Maturity sorting: new balance for young athletes. Phys Sportsmed 6:127–132, 1978.

141. Ross WD, Marfell-Jones MJ: Kinanthropometry. In MacDougal JD, Wenger HA, Green HJ, editors: Physiological testing of the high performance athlete, Champaign, IL, 1991, Human Kinetics.

142. Goldberg B, Boiardo R: Profiling children for sports participation. Clin Sports Med 3:153–169, 1984.

143. Greulich WW, Pyle SU: Radiographic atlas of skeletal development of the wrist and hand, Stanford, CA, 1959, Stanford University Press.

144. Tanner JM: Growth and adolescence, Oxford, England, 1962, Blackwell Scientific.

145. Katch FI, Katch VL: The body composition profile: techniques of measurement and applications. Clin Sports Med 3:31–63, 1984.

146. Jackson AS, Pollock ML: Practical assessment of body composition. Phys Sportsmed 13:772–790, 1985.

147. Coleman AE: Skinfold estimates of body fat in major league baseball players. Phys Sportsmed 9:77–82, 1981.

148. Cates W, Cavanaugh J: Advances in rehabilitation and performance testing. Clin Sports Med 28:63–76, 2009.

149. Léger L, Lambert J: A maximal multistage 20m shuttle run test to predict VO$_2$ max. Eur J Appl Physiol 49:1–5, 1982.

150. Stratford PW, Spadoni GF: Assessing improvement in patients who report small limitations in functional status on conditions-specific measures. Physiother Can 57:234–239, 2005.

SUGGESTED READINGS

Abdenour TE, Weir NJ: Medical assessment of the prospective student athlete. Athletic Training 122–123, 1986.

Anderson BD: Office orthopedics for primary-care diagnosis and treatment, Philadelphia, 1995, WB Saunders.

Armstrong C: Preseason medical examinations and an injury recording profile. Can Athl Ther Assoc J 13–14, 1981.

Boissonnault WG, Bass C: Medical screening examination: not optional for physical therapists. J Orthop Sports Phys Ther 14:241–242, 1991.

Brown RT: Targeting teen health problems: maximizing the preparticipation exam. Phys Sportsmed 21:77–80, 1993.

Cahill BR, Griffith EH: Effect of preseason conditioning on the incidence and severity of high school football knee injuries. Am J Sports Med 6:180–184, 1978.

Cheitlen MD, Douglas PS, Parmley WW: Acquired valvular heart disease. Med Sci Sports Exerc 26:S254–S260, 1994.

Clement JD, Graves RA, Lane RM, et al: Minimum standards of physical fitness required of candidates for collision sports at the University of Maine. J Maine Med Assoc 58:121–123, 1967.

Cottone J: Preparticipation physical examinations. Athletic Ther Today 4:55–60, 1999.

Dyment PG: New guidelines for sports participation. Phys Sportsmed 16:45–46, 1988.

Eggart JS, Leigh D, Vargamini G: Preseason athletic physical examination. In Gould JA, editor: Orthopedic and sports physical therapy, St Louis, 1990, Mosby.

Feinstein RA, Colvin E, Oh MK: Echocardiographic screening as part of a preparticipation examination. Clin J Sports Med 3:149–152, 1993.

Feiring DC, Derscheid GL: The role of preseason conditioning in preventing athletic injuries. Clin Sports Med 8:361–372, 1989.

Gettman LR, Storer TW, Ward RD: Fitness changes in professional football players during preseason conditioning. Phys Sportsmed 15:92–101, 1987.

Goldberg B, Saraniti A, Witman P, et al: Preparticipation sports assessment: an objective evaluation. Pediatrics 66:736–745, 1980.

Gomolak C: Problems in matching young athletes: baby fat, peach fuzz, muscle and mustache. Phys Sportsmed 3:96–98, 1975.

Graham TP, Bricker JT, James FW, et al: Congenital heart disease. Med Sci Sports Exerc 26:S246–S253, 1994.

Hutter AM: Cardiovascular abnormalities in the athlete: the role of the physician. Med Sci Sports Exerc 26:S227–S229, 1994.

Lin LY: Scuba divers with disabilities, challenges, medical protocols, and ethics. Phys Sportsmed 15:224–235, 1987.

Linder CW, DuRant RH, Seklecki RM, et al: Preparticipation health screening of young athletes: results of 1268 examinations. Am J Sports Med 9:187–193, 1981.

Maron BJ, Isner JM, McKenna WJ: Hypertrophic cardiomyelopathy myocarditis and other myopericardial diseases and mitral valve prolapse. Med Sci Sports Exerc 26:S261–S267, 1994.

Minkoff J: Evaluating parameters of a professional hockey team. Am J Sports Med 10:285–292, 1982.

Mitchell JH, Blomquist G, Haskell WL, et al: Classification of sports. J Am Coll Cardiol 6:1198–1199, 1985.

Mitten MJ: Athletic participation with a contagious blood-borne disease. Clin J Sports Med 5:153–154, 1995.

Moore M: Preparticipation exams: Just "a lick and a promise"? Phys Sportsmed 10:113–116, 1982.

Round Table: The office examination of the athlete. Phys Sportsmed 4:86–105, 1976.

Savastano AA: Physical basis for restriction of participation in sports. J Maine Med Assoc 55:146–148, 1964.

Shephard RJ, Thomas S, Weller I: The Canadian home fitness test: 1991 update. Sports Med 11:358–366, 1991.

Sterner TG, Burke EJ: Body fat assessment: a comparison of visual estimation and skinfold techniques. Phys Sportsmed 14:101–107, 1986.

Taunton JE, Clement DB: The medical care of the elite athlete. Medicine North Am 84–90, 1987.

Thompson PD, Klocke FJ, Levine BD, et al: Coronary artery disease. Med Sci Sports Exerc 26:S271–S275, 1994.

Vincent GM: Sudden death in a young athlete. Phys Sportsmed 26:59–62, 1998.

Weidenbener EJ, Krauss MD, Waller BF, et al: Incorporation of screening echocardiography in the preparticipation exam. Clin J Sports Med 5:86–89, 1995.

Weistart JC: Legal consequences of standard setting for competitive athletes with cardiovascular abnormalities. J Am Coll Cardiol 6:1191–1197, 1985.

Zipes DP, Garson A: Arrhythmias. Med Sci Sports Exerc 26:S276–S283, 1994.

CHAPTER 18

Emergency Sports Assessment

This chapter will enable the health care professional to immediately assess a patient before applying first aid or transportation to the hospital. This assessment should be divided into two parts. The first part concerns the primary evaluation or survey, which usually takes place at the location in which the patient is found to ensure that life-threatening situations are handled immediately. The second part of the assessment is performed when the examiner has more time and the patient is not under immediate threat of death or permanent disability.

PRE-EVENT PREPARATION

Before any sporting event, the examiner should establish and practice **emergency protocols** and review sideline preparedness.[1-3] This preparation includes designating personnel for specific tasks and establishing emergency vehicle routes and entrances. The examiner and the assistants should know the location of additional medical assistance, emergency equipment (e.g., spinal board, neck supports, sandbags, stretchers, blankets, emergency first-aid kit), and a telephone. The equipment must be compatible with the needs, size, and age of the athletes, and with the equipment of other health care professionals. Near the telephone, the examiner should post emergency telephone numbers (e.g., ambulance, physician, dentist), identify the name and address of the sports facility, specify the entrance to be used, and note any obvious landmarks, because the person making the emergency call may forget information or give inappropriate information when under stress (Figure 18-1). Included in the preparation is a communication plan for on-field or at-site injuries. This plan may involve pre-established hand signals (e.g., crossed arms may mean "send a physician out," whereas a hand on top of one's head may signify "send ambulance or emergency medical services [EMS] personnel") or walkie-talkies to communicate with other professionals working on the sideline.[4]

The examiner should take the time to give the facility a **safety check** by looking for potential hazards. Visiting teams should also be informed of emergency protocols. In addition, emergency situations and protocols must be practiced repeatedly to ensure that proper care will be given in an emergency.

Emergency Protocol

- Designated personnel
- Emergency vehicle access routes
- Location of emergency equipment
- Location of telephone
- Communication plan

PRIMARY ASSESSMENT

After an injury occurs, the examiner must first take control of the situation and ensure that no additional harm comes to the patient. The primary survey, which takes 30 seconds to 2 minutes with the maximum on-scene time being 10 minutes, is carried out with little or no movement of the patient.[5] It is used to determine whether injuries are life threatening, the severity of injury, and how the patient can be moved. With severe injuries, the longer the assessment takes, the higher the mortality rate is likely to be. If, at any time, the examiner finds that a major injury has occurred (Table 18-1), he or she may terminate the assessment process and ensure the patient receives higher levels of care by calling for the ambulance or EMS. The examiner is designated as the **charge person,** or person in control. The examiner takes control by not allowing the patient to be moved until some type of assessment is made, the spine is supported as much as possible, and, if required, assistance is obtained.

Emergency Evaluation

- Airway evaluation (A):	5 to 7 seconds
- Ventilation check (B):	5 to 8 seconds
- Circulation/heart rate (C):	20 to 30 seconds
- Blood loss:	20 to 30 seconds
- Neurological injury:	10 to 20 seconds
TOTAL TIME:	60 to 95 seconds

For the primary emergency assessment, the examiner should call at least one person to provide immediate assistance, relay messages, and obtain additional help, if

<table>
<tr><td>

Emergency Telephone Numbers

Ambulance _____ Fire/Inhalator _____

Acute Care Hospital (who will receive your athletes)

_____

Emergency Protocol

When you call the ambulance, state:

1. Your name

2. "There has been a suspected _____
   (*insert injury*)

   at _____ (*location*).

   Please send an ambulance to _____
   (*designated meeting spot*)

   I will meet the ambulance there."

3. Ask the estimated time of arrival (ETA).

4. Give them your phone number.

5. DO NOT HANG UP UNTIL THE OTHER PARTY DOES!

Note: If this information cannot be kept by the telephone it should be kept in your first-aid kit with a quarter ($0.25) in case you need to phone the ambulance from a pay phone.

Ambulance Route

Draw a map of the ambulance route to your facility and the designated meeting location.

</td></tr>
</table>

Figure 18-1 Telephone emergency protocol (to be put near emergency telephones or taped to mobile phone). (Modified from Sports Physiotherapy Division Newsletter, Canadian Physiotherapy Association, July/August 1991, p. 3.)

TABLE **18-1**

Priorities in the Management of Injuries: Beware of Injury to the Cervical Spine!

Highest Priority
1. Respiratory and cardiovascular impairment: Facial, neck, and chest injuries
2. Hemorrhage: External, severe

High Priority
3. Retroperitoneal injuries: Shock, hemorrhage
4. Intraperitoneal injuries: Shock, hemorrhage
5. Craniocerebral spinal cord injuries: Open or closed, observation
6. Severe burns: Extensive soft-tissue wounds

Low Priority
7. Lower genitourinary tract: Hemorrhage, extravasation
8. Peripheral vascular, nerve, locomotor injuries: Open or closed
9. Facial and neck injuries: Except priorities 1 and 2
10. Cold exposure

Special
11. Fractures, dislocations: Splinting
12. Tetanus prophylaxis

From Steichen FM: The emergency management of the severely injured. J Trauma 12:787, 1972.

▼ **Emergency Telephone Information**

- Caller's name
- Number of telephone being used
- Type of emergency
- Degree of urgency
- Exact location of facility
- Emergency vehicle access route
- Estimated time of arrival
- Best entrance

---

necessary. This person is designated the **call person,** and he or she should know the location of the closest telephone (a cell phone would be ideal) and what telephone numbers to call in specific emergencies. This information can be posted on or by the telephone (see Figure 18-1). When telephoning, the call person should state the caller's name, the number of the telephone being used, the exact emergency (type of injury), the degree of urgency, and the exact location of the facility; ask for an estimated time of arrival; and explain the location of the best entrance to the facility for responding emergency personnel. Other individuals (as many as six or seven) may be called as necessary to act as transporters or help move the patient.

While performing the initial assessment, the examiner must keep in mind that six situations can immediately threaten the life of a patient: airway obstruction, respiratory failure, cardiac arrest, severe heat injury, head (craniocerebral) injury, and cervical spine injury.[6] It is for these situations, along with severe bleeding, that the examiner must be most prepared, because they are the most common emergency life-threatening situations. Only practice can ensure proper care in an emergency.

Initially, the examiner **stabilizes and immobilizes** the patient's head and cervical spine in case the patient has suffered a cervical spine injury (Figure 18-2).[7] If the patient has suffered trauma above the clavicles, he or she should be considered to have suffered a spinal injury to the cervical spine until proven otherwise.[8] Simultaneously, the examiner **talks to the patient.** If the patient replies in a normal voice and gives logical answers to questions, the examiner can assume that the airway is

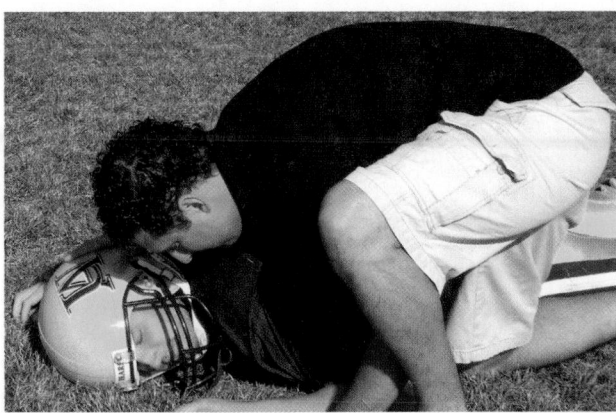

Figure 18-2 Stabilization of the patient's head and neck before initial assessment.

Life-Threatening Emergency Situations

- Airway obstruction
- Respiratory failure
- Cardiac arrest
- Severe heat/cold injury
- Head (craniocerebral) injury
- Cervical spine injury
- Severe bleeding

patent and the brain is receiving adequate perfusion. The examiner asks the patient what happened to determine how the injury occurred (mechanism of injury). The patient is asked to describe the symptoms (e.g., pain, numbness) and how severe he or she thinks the injury is. The examiner then explains what he or she is going to do and reassures the patient.[9] If the patient is unable to speak or is unconscious, the examiner must ask witnesses what happened. If the patient is unconscious ("collapsed athlete"), the examiner must work with the assumption that a neck (cervical spine) injury has occurred until proven otherwise.[10]

Emergency On-Field Procedures

- Stabilize head and spine (Do not move patient.)
- Talk to patient and determine level of consciousness
- Move patient only if in respiratory or cardiac distress
- Check or establish airway
- Check heartbeat
- Check for bleeding, shock, cerebrospinal fluid
- Check pupils
- Check for spinal cord injury (Neural Watch)
- Position the patient
- Check for head injury
- Assess for heat injury
- Assess movement

While the examiner is talking to the patient, he or she should be observing whether the patient moves, is still, or is having a seizure. If the patient moves, it means he or she is at least partially conscious, has no apparent neurological dysfunction, and has some cardiopulmonary function. If the patient is still, it means he or she is unconscious, has some neurological dysfunction, or has some other major system failure. A seizure indicates neurological, systemic, or psychological dysfunction. The examiner should also observe the position of the patient (e.g., normal, deformity) and look for altered joint alignment (e.g., fracture, dislocation), swelling, or discoloration.[4] In case there is a spinal cord injury, the patient should be left in the original position until the nature and severity of the injury have been determined, except in cases of respiratory or cardiac distress. If the athlete is suspected of having a head injury and is mobile, the examiner can use a **Pocket Concussion Recognition Tool™** (Figure 18-3) on the sideline to determine if a concussion has occurred.[11] A rapid assessment of the **brain and spinal cord** can be accomplished by asking the patient to do simple movements, such as sticking out the tongue[12] (see the "Assessment for Spinal Cord Injury" section, presented later). If a concussion is suspected, the procedures in the following box should be followed.[13]

On-Field or Sideline Evaluation of Acute Concussion

When a player shows *any* features of a concussion (see Table 2-7):

A. The player should be evaluated by a physician or other licensed health care provider on-site using standard emergency management principles and particular attention should be given to excluding a cervical spine injury.

B. The appropriate disposition of the player must be determined by the treating health care provider in a timely manner. If no health care provider is available, the player should be safely removed from practice or play and urgent referral to a physician arranged.

C. Once the first aid issues are addressed, an assessment of the concussive injury should be made using the SCAT3 (see Figure 2-11) or other sideline assessment tools.

D. The player should not be left alone following the injury and serial monitoring for deterioration is essential over the initial few hours following injury.

E. A player with diagnosed concussion should not be allowed to return to play on the day of injury.

From McCrory P, Meeuwisse WH, Aubry M, et al: Consensus statement on concussion in sport: the 4th International Conference on Concussion in Sport held in Zurich, November 2012. Br J Sports Med 47:250–258, 2013.
SCAT3, Sideline Concussion Assessment Tool—3rd edition.

Level of Consciousness

The examiner must quickly determine whether the patient is conscious. At no time during the initial assessment should ammonia inhalants be used to arouse the patient. Inhalants should be used only after the examiner is

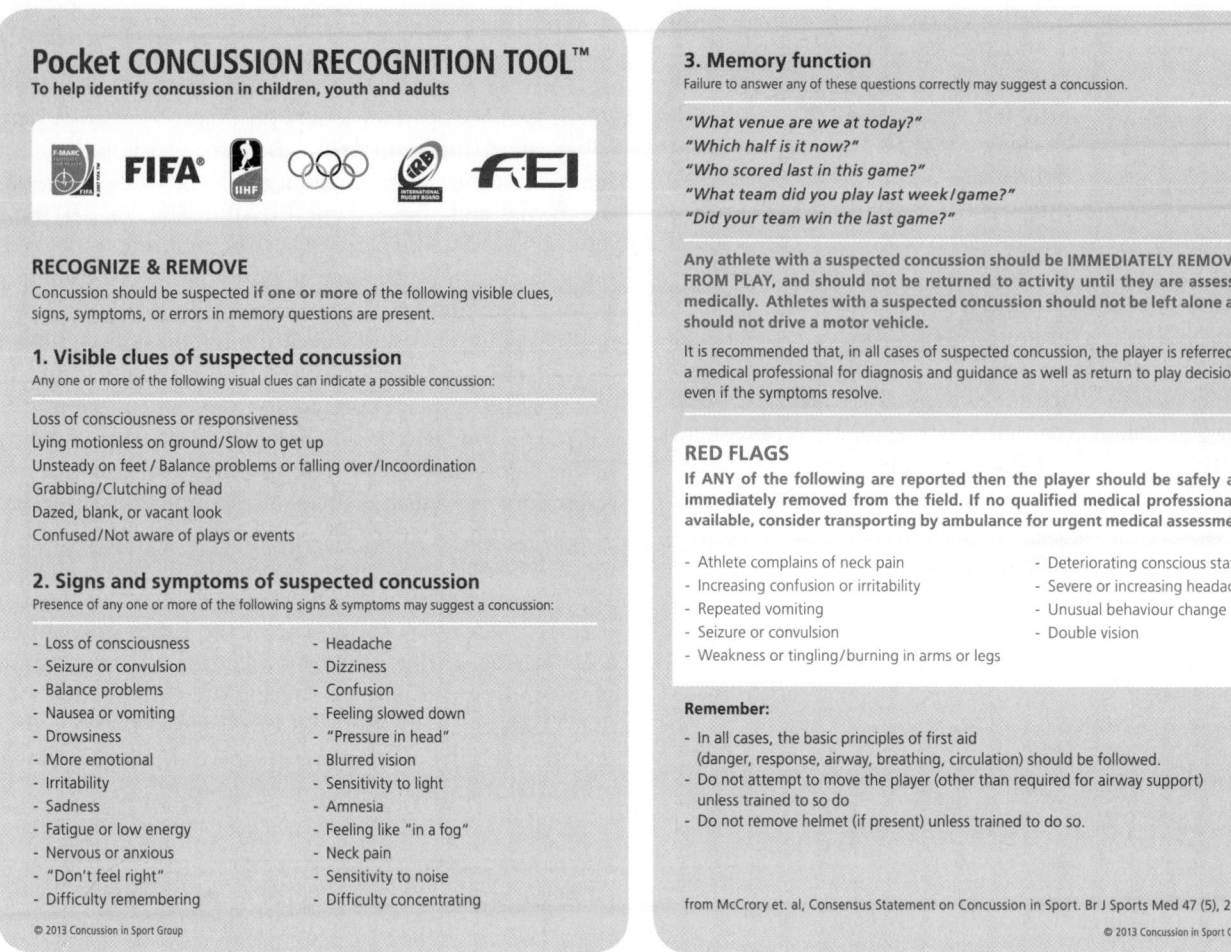

Pocket CONCUSSION RECOGNITION TOOL™
To help identify concussion in children, youth and adults

RECOGNIZE & REMOVE
Concussion should be suspected if one or more of the following visible clues, signs, symptoms, or errors in memory questions are present.

1. Visible clues of suspected concussion
Any one or more of the following visual clues can indicate a possible concussion:

Loss of consciousness or responsiveness
Lying motionless on ground/Slow to get up
Unsteady on feet / Balance problems or falling over/Incoordination
Grabbing/Clutching of head
Dazed, blank, or vacant look
Confused/Not aware of plays or events

2. Signs and symptoms of suspected concussion
Presence of any one or more of the following signs & symptoms may suggest a concussion:

- Loss of consciousness
- Seizure or convulsion
- Balance problems
- Nausea or vomiting
- Drowsiness
- More emotional
- Irritability
- Sadness
- Fatigue or low energy
- Nervous or anxious
- "Don't feel right"
- Difficulty remembering

- Headache
- Dizziness
- Confusion
- Feeling slowed down
- "Pressure in head"
- Blurred vision
- Sensitivity to light
- Amnesia
- Feeling like "in a fog"
- Neck pain
- Sensitivity to noise
- Difficulty concentrating

© 2013 Concussion in Sport Group

3. Memory function
Failure to answer any of these questions correctly may suggest a concussion.

"What venue are we at today?"
"Which half is it now?"
"Who scored last in this game?"
"What team did you play last week/game?"
"Did your team win the last game?"

Any athlete with a suspected concussion should be IMMEDIATELY REMOVED FROM PLAY, and should not be returned to activity until they are assessed medically. Athletes with a suspected concussion should not be left alone and should not drive a motor vehicle.

It is recommended that, in all cases of suspected concussion, the player is referred to a medical professional for diagnosis and guidance as well as return to play decisions, even if the symptoms resolve.

RED FLAGS
If ANY of the following are reported then the player should be safely and immediately removed from the field. If no qualified medical professional is available, consider transporting by ambulance for urgent medical assessment:

- Athlete complains of neck pain
- Increasing confusion or irritability
- Repeated vomiting
- Seizure or convulsion
- Weakness or tingling/burning in arms or legs

- Deteriorating conscious state
- Severe or increasing headache
- Unusual behaviour change
- Double vision

Remember:
- In all cases, the basic principles of first aid (danger, response, airway, breathing, circulation) should be followed.
- Do not attempt to move the player (other than required for airway support) unless trained to so do
- Do not remove helmet (if present) unless trained to do so.

from McCrory et. al, Consensus Statement on Concussion in Sport. Br J Sports Med 47 (5), 2013

© 2013 Concussion in Sport Group

Figure 18-3 Pocket Concussion Recognition Tool. (©2013 Concussion in Sport Group. From McCrory, Meeuwisse WH, Aubry M, et al: Consensus statement on concussion in sport: the 4th International Conference on Concussion in Sport held in Zurich, November 2012. Br J Sports Med 47[5]:267, 2013.)

absolutely sure there is no spinal injury, because the fumes may cause a reflex head jerk, complicating the possible neck injury.[8] At this early stage, the examiner simply determines whether the patient is alert (fully conscious), confused (drowsy), in delirium, in obtundation (dulled sensations, especially pain and touch), in a stupor, or in a coma. A patient is classified as **alert** if he or she is able to carry on an appropriate conversation with no delays and is aware of time, place, and identity. See Chapter 2 for an explanation of the levels of consciousness.

The examiner determines the level of consciousness or arousal by talking to the patient, not by moving the patient. This stage is sometimes referred to as the "shake and shout" stage, in which the examiner tries to arouse the unconscious individual by gentle shaking (without allowing movement of the head and neck) and by shouting into each ear. If the patient does not respond to this verbal stimulus, the examiner can, at least initially, assume that the patient is unconscious or not fully conscious and proceed under that assumption. Further neurological assessment is left until the examiner is sure that the patient

has a patent airway, is breathing normally, and has a heartbeat. If the patient is conscious, the examiner should reassure the patient that help has arrived. The patient should be informed of what the examiner is doing and proposes to do in terms of examining and moving the patient. Regardless of the patient's state of consciousness, he or she should not move or be moved until the examination has been completed.

On the sideline, the examiner can perform a **Sideline Concussion Assessment Tool—3rd edition (SCAT3) exam** (see Chapter 2) and begin a **Neural Watch** to provide serial monitoring (see later discussion) for the possibility of an increasingly severe head injury (i.e., progressive deterioration of signs and symptoms). In addition, balance testing may be performed using the **Balance Error Scoring System (BESS).**[14] This is a quantifiable low technology test that uses only a stopwatch and a piece of medium density foam. The athlete is asked to do three different stances (double, single and tandem) twice on two different surfaces (the ground and the foam) (see Figure 2-37) for a total of six trials. The athlete begins in the required stance with the hands on the iliac crests and, while standing quiet and motionless, is asked to close both eyes for 20 seconds. During the single leg stance, the athlete stands on the non-dominant foot and is asked to hold the opposite non–weight-bearing limb in 20° to 30° of hip flexion and 40° to 50° of knee flexion. For tandem stance, the non-dominant foot is placed behind the dominant foot. If the athlete is losing his or her balance, he or she can make any necessary adjustments and returns to the test position as quickly as possible. The athlete is scored by adding one error point for each committed error (see Table 2-22). If the athlete cannot maintain the desired stance for at least 5 seconds of the 20 second test period, the athlete has failed the test. The maximum error score for normal athletes is 10.

Indications That Athlete Should Be Referred to an Emergency Facility

- Worsening headache
- Very drowsy or cannot be easily awakened
- Cannot recognize people or places
- Develops significant nausea or vomiting
- Behaves unusually, more confused or irritable
- Develops seizures
- Weakness or numbness in the arms or legs
- Slurred speech or unsteadiness of gait

Modified from Putukian M, Raftery M, Guskiewicz K, et al: Onfield assessment of concussion in the adult athlete. Br J Sports Med 47:285–288, 2013.

Establishing the Airway

While waiting for assistance, the examiner can immediately begin to check for abnormal or arrested breathing, abnormal or arrested pulse, internal and external bleeding, and shock. This initial assessment is called the **airway, breathing, and circulation (ABCs)** of cardiopulmonary resuscitation (CPR). New guidelines also include the use of automated defibrillators if required.[15] The first priority is to maintain an adequate airway, normal ventilation, and hemodynamic stability (see Table 18-1).[16,17] Also, obvious bleeding should be controlled by compression.

While the cervical spine is protected and immobilized, the examiner quickly assesses the airway for patency by looking, listening, and feeling for spontaneous respirations.[5,8] Respirations can be determined by watching for movement of the chest, feeling the breath on the examiner's cheek, or hearing the air move in and out (Figure 18-4). The normal resting ranges of respirations are 10 to 25 breaths per minute for adults and 20 to 25 breaths per minute for children. An athlete or someone who has been exerting before injury may show a higher rate. If a patient is not breathing and has no heartbeat, clinical death occurs between 0 and 4 minutes (Figure 18-5). If breathing and heartbeat are not restored within 4 to 6

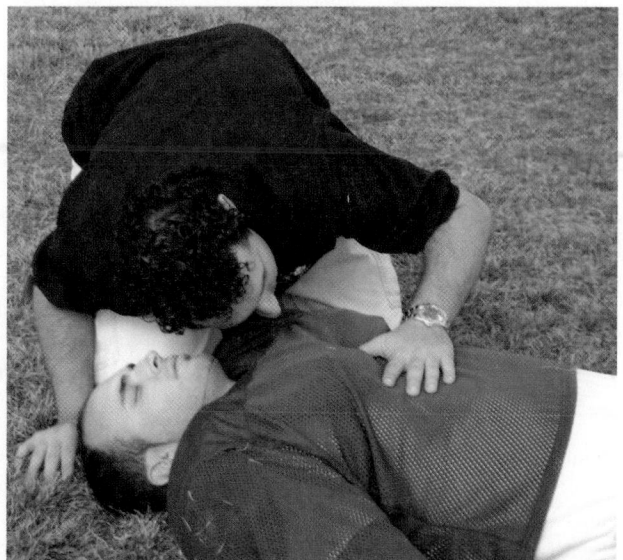

Figure 18-4 Examiner positioning to determine respiration of the patient. The examiner can feel the breath on the cheek, hear the breath, and watch the chest move.

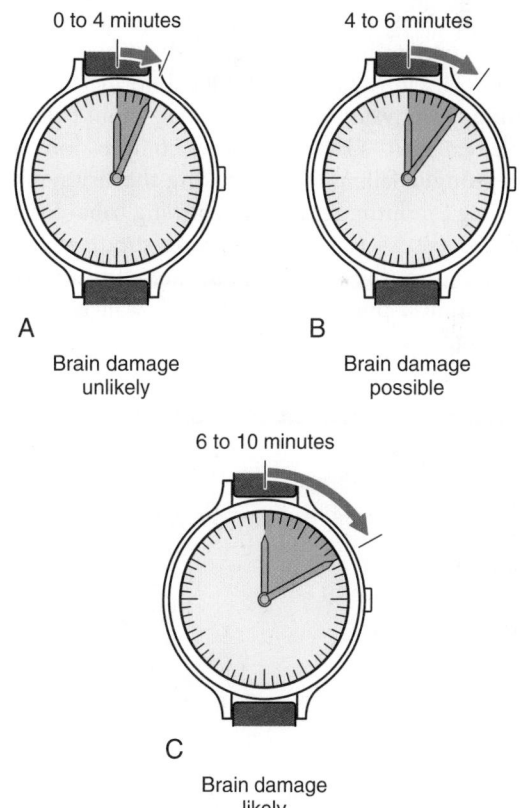

Figure 18-5 If the brain is deprived of oxygen for 4 to 6 minutes, brain damage is possible. After 6 minutes, brain damage is extremely likely.

minutes, brain damage is probable. If there is no breathing and no heartbeat for 6 to 10 minutes, biological death occurs, and brain damage is likely.[18]

If the patient is breathing without difficulty, the rate and rhythm of the respirations and their characteristics

TABLE **18-2**

Abnormal Breathing Patterns

Term	Description	Location of Possible Neurological Lesions
Hyperpnea	Abnormal increase in the depth and rate of the respiratory movements	
Apnea	Periods of non-breathing	Pons
Ataxic breathing (Biot respiration)	Irregular breathing pattern, with deep and shallow breaths occurring randomly	Medulla
Hyperventilation	Prolonged, rapid hyperpnea, resulting in decreased carbon dioxide blood levels	Midbrain, pons
Cheyne-Stokes respirations	Periods of hyperpnea regularly alternating with periods of apnea, characterized by regular acceleration and deceleration in depth	Cerebrum, cerebellum, midbrain, pons
Cluster breathing	Breaths follow each other in disorderly sequence with irregular pauses between them	Pons, medulla

Adapted from Hickey JV: The clinical practice of neurological and neurosurgical nursing, Philadelphia, 1986, JB Lippincott, p. 138.

should be noted. Cheyne-Stokes and ataxic respirations are often associated with head injuries.[19] Table 18-2 indicates some of the abnormal breathing patterns that may occur in a patient in an emergency situation.

If the conscious patient exhibits abnormal or arrested breathing (asphyxia), the examiner should look for possible causes.[20] Causes include compression of the trachea; tongue falling back, blocking the airway; foreign bodies (e.g., mouthguard, gum, chewing tobacco); swelling of the tissues (e.g., anaphylactic shock after a bee sting); fluid in the air passages; presence of harmful gases or fumes; pulmonary and chest wall trauma; and suffocation.[20,21]

Causes of Asphyxia

- Compression of trachea
- Tongue blocking airway
- Foreign bodies
- Tissue swelling
- Fluid in air passages
- Harmful gases or fumes
- Suffocation

Falling back of the tongue is the most common cause of airway obstruction after a sport injury, especially in the unconscious patient. Normally, the tone of the tongue muscles ensures airway patency. However, the unconscious person, especially one in the supine position, loses muscle tone and the tongue falls back, potentially leading to an obstruction. If the tongue is the cause of obstruction, the examiner can simply pull the chin forward in a **chin lift** or **jaw thrust maneuver** to restore the airway, being careful to keep movement of the cervical spine to

a minimum. The chin lift maneuver is less likely to compromise the cervical spine.[22,23] Either maneuver pulls the retropharyngeal musculature forward, thus opening the airway.[20]

If the examiner can see an object obstructing the airway, an oral screw and tongue forceps can be used to remove the object. The mouth should be held open with the oral screw or something similar, and the examiner can use a finger to sweep the mouth clear of debris (e.g., broken teeth, dentures, mouthguard, chewing gum, tobacco). If the jaw is not held open and blocked from closing, the examiner should put fingers in the patient's mouth only with caution. If the cause of the blockage is something other than the tongue (e.g., foreign body), the patient, if conscious, should be asked to cough. If this does not expel the object, the Heimlich maneuver should be performed until the patient expels the object. If the patient loses consciousness, he or she should be placed supine and ventilation attempted. If it is unsuccessful, six to ten subdiaphragmatic abdominal thrusts are applied. This sequence of ventilation and subdiaphragmatic abdominal thrusts is repeated until a physician or EMS personnel arrive to perform a laryngoscopy.[24] Other causes of asphyxia may be treated by epinephrine (anaphylaxis) or intubation.[24] If the examiner is concerned about maintaining a patent airway, an oropharyngeal airway may be used. As a last resort, a wide-bore needle (18-gauge or larger) may be inserted into the trachea to ensure an airway.[20]

If the patient is not breathing, artificial ventilation (mouth-to-mouth resuscitation) must be initiated immediately, by using the breathing portion of the CPR techniques or by using a similar artificial breathing method.

If the patient is conscious but obviously in respiratory or cardiac distress, the examiner must deal with the presenting situation immediately (Table 18-3). If the patient

TABLE **18-3**

Airway Obstruction

Conscious Athlete	Unconscious Athlete
1. If patient is breathing or coughing, leave him/her alone but continue to watch 2. If no air is going in and out of lungs, administer four abdominal thrusts (Heimlich maneuver); some people also administer four back blows 3. Repeat until patient can breathe independently or patient becomes unconscious	1. Perform head tilt if no cervical spine injury is suspected 2. If no response, try to ventilate 3. If no success, reposition head and try to ventilate again 4. If unsuccessful, follow with four abdominal thrusts (Heimlich maneuver); some people also administer four back blows 5. Perform a quick sweep of the mouth 6. If unsuccessful, repeat steps 1 through 5 until there is no longer obstruction, or qualified help arrives; a tracheotomy may follow if obstruction continues

Adapted from American Academy of Orthopaedic Surgeons: Athletic training and sports medicine, Park Ridge, IL, 1984, AAOS, p. 454.

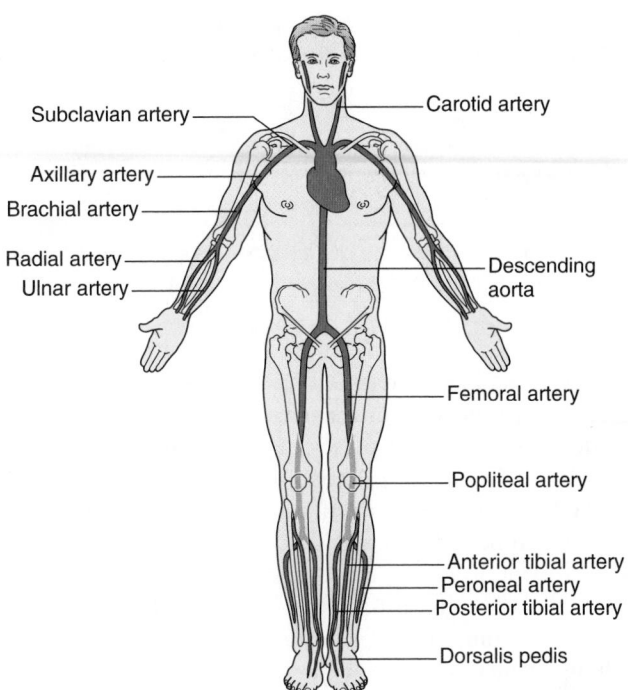

Figure 18-6 Major arteries in the body. Pressure applied to any of the arteries (pressure points) can decrease bleeding if applied proximal to the bleeding.

does not have a patent airway, an airway must be established, as has been described. If the patient is moving in an attempt to get air into the lungs, the examiner may assume that a severe cervical injury is less likely to have occurred. However, movement of the head in relation to the cervical spine should be kept to a minimum. Keeping in mind the possibility of a cervical injury, the examiner should position the patient so that airway clearance and resuscitation can easily be accomplished. This change in position must be performed carefully to ensure that movement of the cervical spine is kept to a minimum. If the patient is reasonably comfortable in the side-lying or prone position and there is no problem with cardiac function or breathing, it is not necessary to move the patient to the supine position.

After the airway has been established, whether by the use of an airway device, by proper head or jaw positioning, by the use of tongue forceps, or by a tracheotomy, the examiner must ensure that the airway is maintained and that the patient continues breathing. If respiration is not spontaneous, assisted ventilation (e.g., mouth-to-mouth, bagging) should be instituted. Ventilation can be compromised by a flail chest or pneumothorax (tension or open).[8,21] Endotracheal intubation is necessary if nasopharangeal bleeding, laryngeal trauma, secretions, or aspirations prevent maintenance of an adequate airway or

end-ventilation.[16,20,25] Transtracheal ventilation is the treatment of choice for patients with breathing problems caused by brain, cervical spine, or maxillofacial injuries. An endotracheal tube may cause straining and venous hypertension, leading to increased brain edema, and extension of the head and neck to open upper airways may aggravate cervical spine injuries. Also, hemorrhage in maxillofacial injuries prevents the effective use of a breathing mask and does not allow adequate visualization.[17]

Establishing Circulation

While the examiner is determining whether breathing is normal, the patient's circulation should be checked for 10 or 15 seconds using the carotid (preferred), brachial, radial, or femoral pulse (Figure 18-6). For a sedentary adult, the normal heart rate is 60 to 90 beats per minute. For children, the rate is 80 to 100 beats per minute. In the highly trained athlete of either sex, the rate may be as low as 40 beats per minute. With activity, the heart rate will be above these levels, and the examiner should take this fact into account when taking the pulse. Depending on the type and level of the individual's activity, the heart rate for a fit person should decrease to slightly above normal values *within 5 minutes*. The examiner should note whether the pulse is absent, rapid and rebounding, or weak and diminishing.

The pulse is most often checked at the carotid artery, because this artery is large and easy to locate. Therefore,

Rapid Assessment Criteria for Circulation

1. Skin color
2. Carotid pulse palpable (systolic blood pressure, ≥ 60 mm Hg)
3. Femoral pulse palpable (systolic blood pressure, ≥ 70 mm Hg)
4. Radial pulse palpable (systolic blood pressure, ≥ 80 mm Hg)

Modified from Driscoll P, Skinner D: Initial assessment and management: I. Primary survey. Br Med J 300:1266, 1990.

the examiner has less chance of missing the pulse and does not have to move from the area of the patient's head to perform palpation. If a pulse cannot be detected, it should be assumed that the patient does not have a heartbeat, and CPR should be initiated using either manual methods or an automated external defibrillator. The use of the defibrillator increases the chance of survival in cardiac arrest.[26] Although cardiac arrest is rare in athletes, sudden death or commotio cordis resulting from low-impact blunt trauma is always a possibility in sports.[27] When the pulse is assessed, the examiner should estimate its rate, strength, and rhythm to obtain an indication of the cardiac output. Circulatory sufficiency may also be determined by squeezing the nail bed or hypothenar eminence. **Capillary refill** is delayed if the pink color does not return to the nail bed or hypothenar eminence within 2 seconds after release of the pressure.[28] Squeezing the hypothenar eminence is a better indicator if the patient is hypothermic.

The pulse may also be used to determine the patient's blood pressure. If a carotid pulse can be palpated, systolic blood pressure is 60 mm Hg or higher. If the femoral pulse is palpable, systolic blood pressure is 70 mm Hg or higher. If the radial pulse can be palpated, the systolic blood pressure is 80 mm Hg or higher.[12,19,28] Like heart rate, blood pressure should drop to almost normal levels within 5 minutes following termination of exercise.

A **weak** or **rapid pulse** usually indicates shock, heat exhaustion, hypoglycemia, fainting, or hyperventilation. A **slowing pulse** is sometimes seen when there is a large increase in intracranial pressure, which usually indicates a severe lower brain stem compression.[29] A pulse that is **rebounding and rapid** is often the result of hypertension, fright, heat stroke, or hyperglycemia.

If the pulse rate is beginning to weaken, the patient may be going into **shock** (Figure 18-7). Shock is characterized by signs and symptoms that occur when the cardiac output is insufficient to fill the arterial tree and the blood is under insufficient pressure to provide organs and tissues with adequate blood flow. It should be noted, however, that patients who maintain pink skin, especially in the face and extremities, are seldom hypovolemic after injury. If the skin of the face or extremities turns ash-gray or white, this usually indicates blood loss of at least 30%.[8] Common types of shock and their causes are shown in

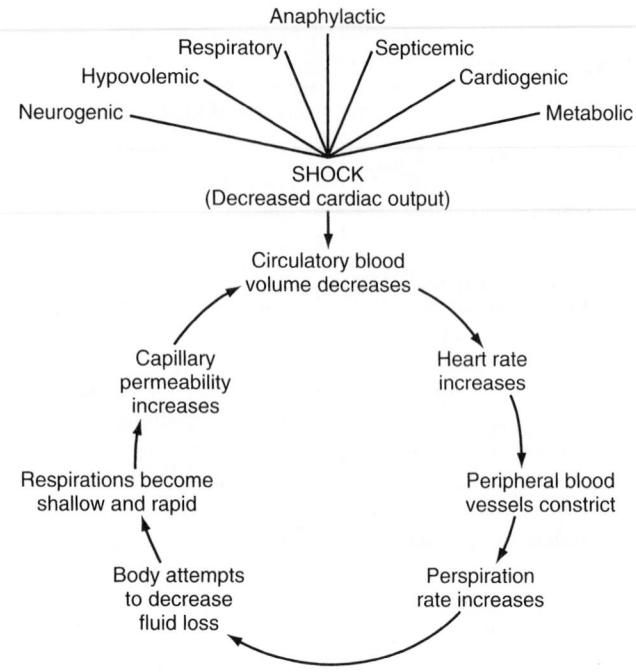

Figure 18-7 The shock cycle.

TABLE **18-4**

Types of Shock and Their Causes

Type	Cause
Hemorrhagic (hypovolemic)	Blood loss
Respiratory	Inadequate blood supply
Neurogenic	Loss of vascular control by nervous system
Psychogenic	Common fainting
Cardiogenic	Insufficient pumping of blood by the heart
Septic	Severe infection and blood vessel damage
Anaphylactic	Allergic reaction
Metabolic	Loss of body fluid

Table 18-4. A patient going into shock becomes restless and anxious. The pulse slowly becomes weak and rapid, and the skin becomes cold and wet, often clammy. Sweating may be profuse, and the face is initially pale and later cyanotic (blue) around the mouth. Respirations may be shallow, labored, rapid, or possibly irregular and gasping, especially if a chest injury has occurred. The eyes usually become dull and lusterless, and the pupils become increasingly dilated. The patient may complain of thirst and feel nauseated or vomit. If shock develops quickly, the patient may lose consciousness. To prevent or delay the onset of shock, the examiner may cover the patient, elevate the patient's legs, or attempt to eliminate the cause of the problem.

Circulatory collapse in trauma patients is caused primarily by blood loss from vascular damage or fracture, or

Signs and Symptoms of Shock

- Increased and weak heart rate
- Cold, clammy, pale skin
- Increased and shallow respiratory rate
- Profuse sweating
- Increased thirst
- Restlessness and anxiousness
- Altered level of consciousness
- Dilated pupils
- Nausea or vomiting

TABLE **18-5**

Bleeding Characteristics and Their Source

Source	Bleeding Characteristics
Artery	Bright red, sputting or pulsating flow
Vein	Dark red, steady flow
Capillary	Slow, even flow
Lungs	Bright red, frothy
Stomach	"Coffee grounds" vomitus
Upper bowel	Tarry black stools
Kidneys	Smoky, red urine
Bladder	Red urine, difficulty urinating
Abdomen	Blood not visible; abdominal rigidity, pain, difficulty breathing

hypovolemic shock, but the examiner must remember that shock in trauma may also be caused by tension pneumothorax, central nervous system injury, or pericardial tamponade (heart compression resulting from blood in the pericardium)—all emergency conditions that require physician intervention.[30] By the time hypovolemic shock becomes evident, blood loss may be as high as 20% to 25%. The normal range of blood pressure is 100 to 120 mm Hg for systolic pressure and 60 to 80 mm Hg for diastolic pressure. With shock, the blood pressure gradually decreases. If the blood pressure can be measured, it is best to assume that shock is developing in any injured adult whose systolic blood pressure is 100 mm Hg or less.

If the examiner is caring for a dark-skinned person, it may be difficult to determine from observation whether the patient is going into shock. A healthy person with dark skin usually has a red undertone and shows a healthy pink color in the nail beds, lips, and mucous membranes of the mouth and tongue. A dark-skinned patient in shock, however, has a gray cast to the skin around the nose and mouth, especially if experiencing respiratory shock. The mucous membranes of the mouth and tongue, the lips, and the nail beds have a blue tinge. If the shock is caused by hypovolemia, the mucous membranes of the mouth and tongue will not be blue; rather they will have a pale, graying, waxy pallor.[31]

If no pulse is present, then the cardiac portion of CPR techniques should be initiated. Sports equipment (such as, shoulder pads or rib pads) should be removed, at least anteriorly, to give the examiner clear access to the anterior chest wall. CPR provides only approximately 25% of normal cardiac output, so it is imperative that it is performed properly by knowledgeable persons.[32] CPR is maintained until the patient recovers or EMS personnel arrive. If a cervical spine injury is suspected, CPR must be done with care, because compression to the heart can cause repeated flexion-extension of the cervical spine.[17]

Assessment for Bleeding, Fluid Loss, and Shock

The examiner should look for any signs of external bleeding or hemorrhage (Table 18-5). The types of wounds in

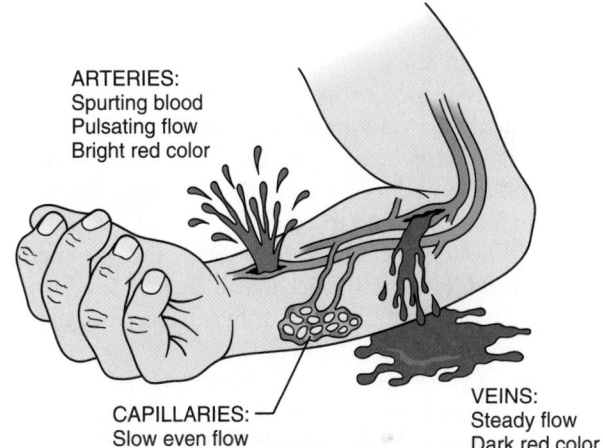

Figure 18-8 Bleeding characteristics.

ARTERIES:
Spurting blood
Pulsating flow
Bright red color

CAPILLARIES:
Slow even flow

VEINS:
Steady flow
Dark red color

which external bleeding or hemorrhage may be seen are incisions, which are clean cuts, or lacerations that have jagged edges. A contusion may produce internal bleeding, whereas a puncture or abrasion may also show bleeding or oozing on the surface. Major traumatic injuries, such as fractures (e.g., pelvis, femur), can cause a great deal of internal bleeding. Of the five types of wounds, the puncture wound is probably the most difficult to treat, because it has the highest probability of infection. The examiner should watch for bleeding from the lungs, the stomach, the upper bowel, the lower bowel, the kidneys, or the bladder. If the liver, spleen, or kidney is injured, serious internal bleeding may result; the blood will not be visible because it is contained within the abdominal cavity. In this case, the patient may experience abdominal rigidity, pain, and difficulty breathing (pressure on diaphragm).

When inspecting a bleeding structure, the examiner should note the type of vessel affected. For example, an artery spurts blood, whereas a vein provides an even flow. Capillaries tend to ooze bright blood (Figure 18-8).[18] Because arterial bleeding is of greatest concern, the examiner must be aware of the pressure points in the body (see Figure 18-6) so that he or she will know where to apply proper treatment. The examiner chooses the pressure point closest to the area of bleeding and applies pressure to the artery to slow or stop the bleeding. Tourniquets should be used only with extreme caution and in selected instances (e.g., accidental amputation of a limb, very severe bleeding from a major artery, or the need to apply CPR with no assistance available) and then only with enough pressure to stop bleeding. If a tourniquet is used, the time of tourniquet application should be noted carefully to prevent unnecessary tissue damage. Hemodynamic stability is best maintained by applying direct pressure to an open wound, keeping the patient in a recumbent position, and minimizing the number of times the patient is moved.[16]

If signs and symptoms of shock are present but visible bleeding is minimal, the examiner should suspect hidden bleeding within the abdomen, chest, or extremities.[19,33] If bleeding is suspected in the abdomen, the examiner should palpate the abdominal wall for shape and distention. To check for bleeding in the chest or extremities, the examiner should look for deformities (e.g., fractures). The fingers may be used to percuss the chest area, noting any loss of hollow sounds, to help locate the presence of fluid or blood. Hyporesonance may indicate a solid organ or the presence of fluid or blood; hyperresonance usually indicates air- or gas-filled spaces.[19]

After the ABCs systems have been assessed and controlled, the examiner can proceed to the remainder of the primary assessment. The examiner should check the ears and nose for the presence of cerebrospinal fluid. If blood or cerebrospinal fluid leaks from the ear, this may indicate a skull fracture. The examiner should incline the head toward the affected side to facilitate drainage, unless a cervical injury is suspected. The examiner can place a gauze pad over the patient's ear or nose where the bleeding is occurring to collect the fluid on the gauze (Figure 18-9). The examiner should look for an orange halo forming on the pad (see Figure 2-42). The halo is cerebrospinal fluid, the presence of which is a good indication of a skull fracture.[34]

Pupil Check

The examiner checks the pupils for shape and for response to light by using a penlight or by covering the eye with one hand and then taking it away. The pupil normally reacts to the intensity of light or focal distance. The pupils dilate in a dark environment or with a long focal distance, and they constrict in a light environment or with a short focal distance. Normally, the pupils are equally or almost equally dilated (diameter range, 2 to 6 mm; mean of 3.5 mm), but injury to the central nervous system (e.g., head injury) may cause the pupils to dilate unevenly. Some people normally have unequal pupil sizes, and the

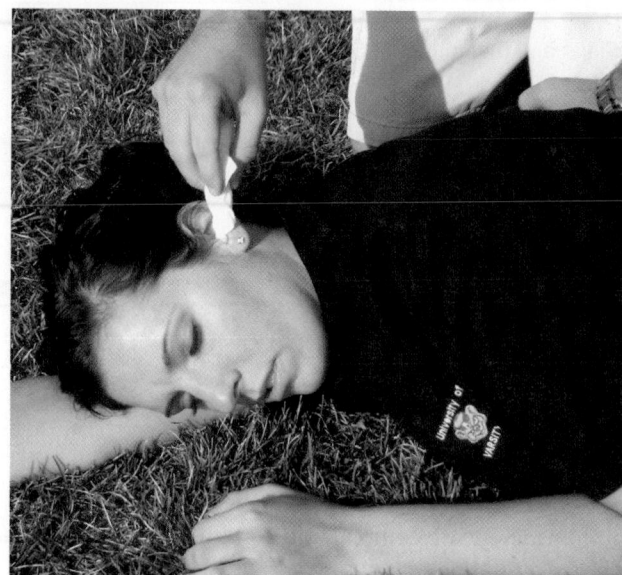

Figure 18-9 Checking the ear for blood or cerebrospinal fluid.

health care professional must be aware of this possibility. In a fully conscious, alert person who has sustained a blow near the eye, a dilated, fixed pupil is most likely the result of trauma to the short ciliary nerves of that eye rather than the result of third cranial nerve compression caused by brain herniation.[16] Drugs may also affect the pupillary size. For example, opiate drugs cause pinpoint pupils, whereas amphetamines may cause dilated pupils.[19]

To test pupil reaction, the examiner holds one hand over one eye and then moves the hand away quickly, or shines the light from a penlight into the eye, and observes the pupil's reaction when the light is shone on the eye (normal reaction: constriction) or when the light source is removed (normal reaction: dilation). The examiner tests the other eye in a similar fashion and compares the results. The **pupillary reaction** is classified as brisk (normal), sluggish, nonreactive, or fixed. An ovoid or slightly oval pupil or a fixed and dilated pupil indicates increasing intracranial pressure.[19] If both pupils are midsize, midposition, and nonreactive, midbrain damage is usually indicated. The fixation and dilation of both pupils is a terminal sign of anoxia and ischemia to the brain.[19,35]

Assessment for Spinal Cord Injury

Spinal cord injuries can have catastrophic and irreversible neurologic consequences, so early recognition of the problem is essential.[36] If the athlete walks off the field before notifying the medical staff of a potential neck injury, he or she should be examined using a regular cervical assessment (see Chapter 3). If the player appears to have or communicates a neck injury on the field or is unconscious, then a neck or head injury should be assumed, and he or she is treated as indicated below. The cervical assessment is modified so as much of the examination as possible is done without moving the athlete. After examination, the athlete is immobilized and transported to a medical facility.[37]

An upper spinal cord injury should be suspected, at least initially, if the patient has neck pain; the patient's head position is asymmetric or abnormal; the patient is having respiratory difficulty, especially if the chest is not moving (absence of abdominal or diaphragmatic breathing); the patient is demonstrating priapism (erection of the penis); or the patient is unconscious after a fall or other contact activity. Other indications of neurological injuries in the conscious patient include numbness, tingling, or burning, especially below the clavicles; muscle weakness; twitching; or paralysis of the arms or legs, especially bilaterally (flaccid paralysis).[19]

The examiner may ask the patient to stick out the tongue, wiggle the toes, move the feet or arms, or squeeze the examiner's fingers.[12] This quick test provides a rapid assessment of the brain and spinal cord by showing whether the patient can follow instructions and can do the activity.

If the patient is unconscious (Table 18-6), the examiner should reassess the level of unconsciousness if

Situations in Which Cervical Spine Injury Must Be Suspected Until Proven Otherwise

- Neck pain or stiffness
- Cervical muscle spasm
- Asymmetric or abnormal head position
- Respiratory difficulty (chest not moving)
- Priapism
- Unconsciousness
- Numbness, tingling, or burning
- Muscle weakness or paralysis
- Loss of bowel or bladder control

possible and treat the patient as though a spinal injury has occurred. In the unconscious patient, the examiner should watch for spontaneous limb movement, especially after the application of a painful stimulus, because movement indicates that the patient is less likely to have suffered a severe cervical injury.[19] In addition, the examiner should look for tonic posturing that indicates a severe head injury. The **fencing response** may occur at the time of impact with one limb extending and the other flexing regardless of position or gravity (Figure 18-10).[38]

TABLE 18-6

Some Common Causes of Unconsciousness in Patients

Category	Problem	Cause	Pathophysiology	Management
General	Loss of consciousness	Injury or disease	Shock, head injury, other injuries, diabetes, arteriosclerosis	Need for CPR, triage
Disease	Diabetic coma	Hyperglycemia and acidosis	Inadequate use of sugar, acidosis	Complex treatment for acidosis
	Insulin shock	Hypoglycemia	Excess insulin	Sugar
	Myocardial infarct	Damaged myocardium	Insufficient cardiac output	Oxygen, CPR, transport
	Stroke	Damaged brain	Loss of arterial supply to brain or hemorrhage within brain	Support, gentle transport
Injury	Hemorrhagic shock	Bleeding	Hypovolemia	Control external bleeding, recognize internal bleeding, CPR, transport
	Respiratory shock	Insufficient oxygen	Paralysis, chest damage, airway obstruction	Clear airway, supplemental oxygen, CPR, transport
	Anaphylactic shock	Acute contact with agent to which patient is sensitive	Allergic reaction	Intramuscular epinephrine, support, CPR, transport
	Cerebral contusion, concussion, or hematoma	Blunt head injury	Bleeding into or around brain, concussive effect	Airway, supplemental oxygen, CPR, careful monitoring, transport
Emotions	Psychogenic shock	Emotional reaction	Sudden drop in cerebral blood flow	Place supine, make comfortable, observe for injuries

Continued

TABLE **18-6**

Some Common Causes of Unconsciousness in Patients—cont'd

Category	Problem	Cause	Pathophysiology	Management
Environment	Heatstroke	Excessive heat, inability to sweat	Brain damage from heat	Immediate cooling, support, CPR, transport
	Electric shock	Contact with electric current	Cardiac abnormalities, fibrillation	CPR, transport; do not treat until current controlled
	Systemic hypothermia	Prolonged exposure to cold	Diminished cerebral function, cardiac arrhythmias	CPR, rapid transport, warming at hospital
	Drowning	Oxygen, carbon dioxide, breath holding, water	Cerebral damage	CPR, transport
	Air embolism	Intravascular air	Obstruction to arterial blood flow by nitrogen bubbles	CPR, recompression
	Decompression sickness ("bends")	Intravascular nitrogen	Obstruction to arterial blood flow by nitrogen bubbles	CPR, recompression
Injected or ingested agents	Alcohol	Excess intake	Cerebral depression	Support, CPR, transport
	Drugs	Excess intake	Cerebral depression	Support, CPR, transport (bring drug)
	Plant poisons	Contact, ingestion	Direct cerebral or other toxic effect	Support, recognition, CPR, identify plant, local wound care, transport
	Animal poisons	Contact, ingestion, injection	Direct cerebral or other toxic effect	Recognition, support, CPR, identify agent, local wound care, transport
Neurological	Epilepsy	Brain injury, scar, genetic predisposition, disease	Excitable focus of motor activity in brain	Support, protect patient, transport in status epilepticus

From the American Academy of Orthopaedic Surgeons: Athletic training and sports medicine, ed 2, Park Ridge, IL, 1991, AAOS, pp. 618–619. *CPR,* Cardiopulmonary resuscitation.

Decerebrate rigidity is evidenced by all four extremities being in extension. With **decorticate rigidity,** the lower limbs are in extension and the upper limbs are in flexion (see Figure 2-33).

Assessment for Head Injury (Neural Watch)

The patient's level of consciousness is then reassessed. The examiner should now institute a Neural Watch (Figure 18-11) or a similar observation scheme to note any changes in the patient over time. The Neural Watch should initially be performed **every 5 to 15 minutes,** because it also facilitates monitoring of the patient's vital signs.[19] After the patient has stabilized, Neural Watch recordings may be made **every 15 to 30 minutes.**[29] If possible, reassessment by the same examiner allows the detection of subtle changes.

The examination should include an evaluation of the patient's facial expression; a determination of the patient's orientation to time, place, and person; and the presence of both posttraumatic amnesia and retrograde amnesia.

Signs and symptoms that demand emergency action in a patient who has sustained a blow to the head are increased headache, nausea and vomiting, inequality of pupils, disorientation, progressive or sudden impairment of consciousness, gradual increase in blood pressure, and diminution of pulse rate.

Emergency Signs and Symptoms of Head Injury

- Increased headache
- Nausea and vomiting
- Inequality of pupils
- Disorientation
- Altered level of consciousness
- Increased blood pressure
- Decreased pulse rate
- Decreased reaction to pain
- Decreased or altered values on Neural Watch chart or GCS

GCS, Glasgow Coma Scale.

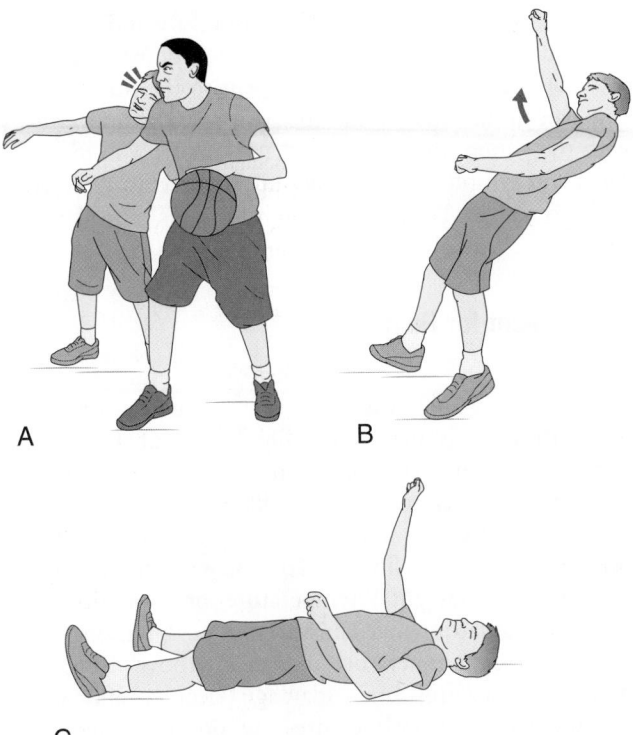

Figure 18-10 The fencing response during a knockout. A, Athlete receives a blow to the head. **B,** After the traumatic blow to the head, the unconscious athlete immediately exhibits extension in one arm and contralateral flexion while falling to the ground. **C,** During prostration, the rigidity of the extended and flexed arms is retained for several seconds as flaccidity gradually returns.[38]

Neural Watch Chart

Unit		Time 1 ( )	Time 2 ( )	Time 3 ( )
I. Vital signs	Blood pressure Pulse Respirations Temperature			
II. Conscious and	Oriented Disoriented Restless Combative			
	Unconscious			
III. Speech	Clear Rambling Garbled None			
IV. Will awaken to	Name Shaking Light pain Strong pain			
V. Nonverbal reaction to pain	Appropriate Inappropriate "Decerebrate" None			
VI. Pupils	Size on right Size on left Reacts on right Reacts on left			
VII. Ability to move	Right arm Left arm Right leg Left leg			
VIII. Sensation	Right side (normal/abnormal) Left side (normal/abnormal) Dermatome affected (specify) Peripheral nerve affected (specify)			

Figure 18-11 Neural Watch chart. (Modified from American Academy of Orthopaedic Surgeons: Athletic training and sports medicine, Park Ridge, IL, 1984, AAOS, p. 399.)

Reaction to pain and the level of consciousness can be determined by the use of physical and verbal stimuli. If there is no cervical injury, the verbal stimuli may include calling the patient's name and shaking and shouting at the patient. Physical stimuli (see Figure 2-32) include squeezing the Achilles tendon, squeezing the trapezius muscle, squeezing the soft tissue between the patient's thumb and index finger, squeezing an object (pen or pencil) between the patient's fingers, squeezing a fingertip, or applying a knuckle to the sternum. (This must be done with caution because it may cause bruising.) In comatose patients, a motor response to a painful stimulus to an extremity may indicate intact pain appreciation from that site, especially if it is accompanied by a more remote response, such as a grimace or a change in respiration or pulse.[16]

The level of consciousness can best be determined with the use of the **Glasgow Coma Scale (GCS)** (see Table 2-20).[39-41] The sooner the patient is tested with the scale, the better, because the initial assessment can be used as a baseline for improvement or deterioration in the patient. The GCS is often used in conjunction with the Neural Watch. For a description of the test, see Chapter 2.

Deterioration of consciousness may result from many conditions, such as increased intracranial pressure caused by an expanding intracranial lesion, hypoxia (which can aggravate cerebral edema and increase the intracranial pressure), epilepsy, meningitis, or fat embolism. The examiner should always look for signs of expanding intracranial lesions (see Chapter 2), especially if the patient is conscious. These lesions are emergency conditions that must be attended to immediately because of their potentially high mortality rate (up to 50%).

If the patient experiences loss of consciousness or appears to have disturbed senses, is seeing stars or colors, is dizzy, or has auditory hallucinations or a severe headache, the patient should not be left alone or allowed to return to activity (Table 18-7). In addition, nausea, vomiting, lethargy, increasing blood pressure, disturbed sensation of smell, or a diminished pulse should lead the

TABLE 18-7

Indications for Immediate Removal from Activity

Area of Injury	Indications for Immediate Removal from Activity
Eye	Blunt trauma, visual difficulty, pain, laceration, obvious deformity
Head	Loss of consciousness, disturbed sensorium, stars or colors being seen, dizziness, auditory hallucinations, nausea, vomiting, lethargy, severe headache, rising blood pressure, disturbed smell, diminishing pulse, amnesia, hyperirritability, large contusion, open wounds, unequal pupils, leakage of cerebrospinal fluid or blood from ears or nose, numbness of one side of body
Spine	Obvious deformity, restricted motion, weakness of extremity, pain on movement, localized tenderness, numbness of extremity (pinched nerve), paresthesias
Extremities	Obvious deformity, crepitus, loss of range of motion, loss of sensation, effusion, pain on use, unstable joint, open wounds, significant tenderness, significant swelling
Abdomen	Dizziness or syncope, nausea, persisting pallor, vomiting, history of infectious mononucleosis, abnormal thirst, muscle guarding, localized tenderness, shoulder pain, distension, rapid pulse, clamminess and sweating

Reprinted by permission from the New York State Journal of Medicine, copyright by the Medical Society of the State of New York
Adapted from Greensher J, Mofenson HC, Merlis NJ: First aid for school athletic emergencies. NY State J Med 79:1058, 1979.

examiner to the same conclusion. Amnesia, hyperirritability, an open wound, unequal pupils, or leaking of cerebrospinal fluid or blood from the ears or nose also indicates an emergency condition. Numbness on one side of the body or a large contusion in the head area should likewise lead the examiner to handle the patient with care. If the frontal area of the brain is affected, the patient may experience lapses of memory, personality changes, or impairment of judgment. If the temporal lobe has been affected, the patient may experience feelings of unreality, déjà vu, or hallucinations involving odors, sounds, or visual disturbances, such as macropsia (seeing objects as larger than they really are) or micropsia. The literature indicates that head injury depends not only on the magnitude and direction of impact and the structural features and physical reactions of the skull but also on the state of the head/brain at the moment of impact.[6,42,43]

If the patient has received a head injury and has been checked by a physician and it has been determined that it is not necessary to send the patient to the hospital, the clinician should ensure that the patient and whoever lives with the patient understands what to look for in terms of signs and symptoms that may indicate increasing severity of head injury. Figure 2-34 demonstrates typical home health care guidelines.

Assessment for Heat Injury

If the examiner suspects a heat-type injury with no cervical injury, only heat exhaustion and heat stroke need be considered as life-threatening.[10,44] **Heat fatigue** or exhaustion occurs when a person is exposed to high environmental temperature or humidity and perspires excessively without salt or fluid replacement. **Heat stroke** can occur when a non-acclimatized person is suddenly exposed to high environmental temperature or humidity. The thermal regulatory mechanism fails, perspiration stops, and the body temperature increases. Above 42°C oral body temperature, brain damage occurs, and death follows if emergency measures are not instituted. The diagnostic keys in this situation are the **high body temperature** and the **absence of sweating.** Initial signs of heat injury include muscle cramps, excessive fatigue or weakness, loss of coordination, decreased reaction time, headache, decreased comprehension, dizziness, and nausea and vomiting.

Signs of Heat Injury

- Muscle cramps
- Excessive fatigue or weakness
- Loss of coordination
- Headache
- Decreased comprehension
- Dizziness
- Nausea and vomiting
- Decreased reaction time

The body temperature varies according to the site at which the measurement is taken. The oral body temperature is 37°C (98.6°F). Taken in the armpit or axilla, the temperature is 36.4°C to 36.7°C (97.5°F to 98.1°F), and in the rectum, it is 37.3°C to 37.6°C (99.1°F to 99.7°F).

The examiner may palpate the skin to get some idea of the external temperature of the body and possible pathology (Table 18-8). Hot and dry skin is often caused by heat stroke, high fever, or hyperglycemia. Cold and clammy skin is caused by hypoglycemia, shock, fainting, or hyperventilation. Cool and moist skin is often caused by heat exhaustion, whereas cool and dry skin is caused by exposure to cold.

Skin color can also play a significant role. Pallor, or whitish skin, indicates circulatory disturbance or decreased circulation and is most often associated with trauma and shock. Cyanosis, or a blue tint to the skin, indicates respiratory distress, as does a gray tint. Redness indicates an increase in blood flow as a result of fever, heat stroke, or exercise.

Assessment for Movement

While doing the initial assessment, the examiner should also be considering how the patient will be moved and immobilized (e.g., self-ambulation, stretcher, spinal board) depending on the severity of the injury, and

TABLE 18-8

Skin Changes and Their Cause

Skin Change	Cause
Hot and dry	Heat stroke, high fever, hyperglycemia
Cold and clammy	Fainting, hypoglycemia, hyperventilation, shock
Cool and moist	Heat exhaustion
Cool and dry	Cold
White pallor	Decreased circulation
Cyanosis (blue pallor)	Respiratory distress
Red pallor	Fever, heat stroke, inflammation, exercise

whether the patient can move him or herself or can move only with assistance.[45]

If the patient has not already done so, the examiner asks the patient to move the limbs to reassess for a cervical spine injury and look for major trauma (e.g., fracture, dislocation, third-degree strain, third-degree sprain). At the same time, the examiner may palpate the areas of potential injury, noting any pain, abnormal bone or joint alignment, swelling, hypersensitive or hyposensitive areas, or palpable defect (third-degree strain).[4] If movement is relatively normal, the examiner quickly checks the myotomes of the upper or lower body for any possible motor involvement or motor impairment. Changes in limb power may be caused by a contractile tissue injury, a neurological injury, or an expanding intracranial lesion, which will be displayed as progressive weakness in the contralateral arm or leg.[29] Decreased limb power can also be caused by reflex inhibition as a result of previously unrecognized limb injury. In these cases, contractions are weak and painful. These types of injuries are placed in the low-priority group (see Table 18-1) because they represent a threat to the limb rather than to the life of the patient.[17]

Positioning the Patient

Normally, a patient is left in the position in which he or she is found until the primary assessment is completed. However, if the patient is having difficulty breathing or there is no pulse, the patient must be positioned to do CPR. If the conscious patient is prone and in respiratory difficulty, the examiner, with assistance, should **log-roll** the patient (Figure 18-12) onto a spinal board so that an

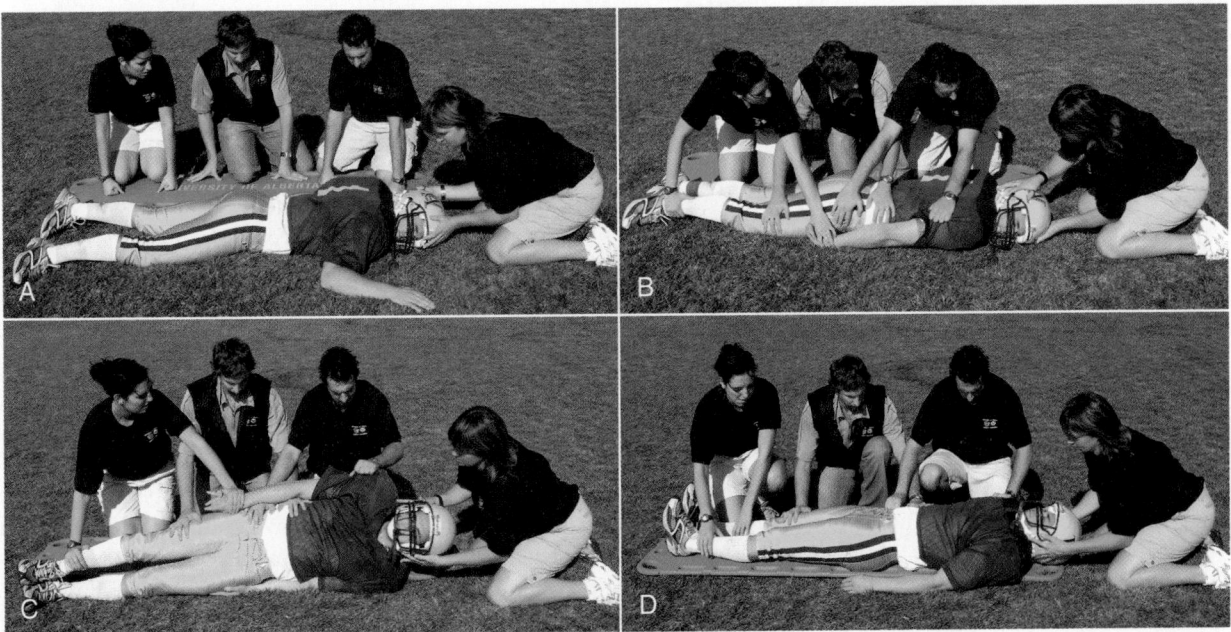

Figure 18-12 Moving a patient to the supine position after injury. Note that the head and neck are stabilized throughout the movement. **A,** Patient prone, examiner stabilizes head and gives instruction to helpers. **B through D,** Patient is log-rolled onto spinal board.

attempt can be made to restore the airway. During any movement of the patient, the examiner should apply traction of about 4.5 kg (10 lbs) to the cervical spine to maintain stability. The patient should be reassured that others are going to carefully move the patient while he or she remains still. Before any movement is attempted, the patient and those who are going to assist the examiner should know what the examiner plans to do and what their jobs are. This requires *frequent practicing of emergency procedures.* The sequence of movement and positioning of the extremities and body of the patient should be thought out beforehand so that everyone is aware of what is going to happen and in what order. The proper procedure for moving the patient should be practiced often to ensure competency.

To roll the patient, at least three assistants are needed. There should be two-way communication between the examiner and the patient at all times to continually evaluate the patient's comfort level and neurological signs. The assistants should place the spinal board beside the patient and then kneel beside the spinal board and patient (see Figure 18-12, *A*). They should reach over the patient and hold the patient's shoulder, hip, and knees (see Figure 18-12, *B*). On command from the examiner, the assistants roll the patient toward them while the examiner stabilizes the head (see Figure 18-12, *C*) until the patient is lying supine on the spinal board (see Figure 18-12, *D*). Only rolling—not lifting—should occur. With the patient in the supine position, proper CPR techniques may be applied, or the patient may be transported. The patient may also be covered with a blanket to provide warmth.

If a spinal injury is suspected and the conscious patient is in the prone position but has no difficulty breathing, the patient is log-rolled halfway toward the assistants while another assistant slides the spinal board as close as possible to the patient's side. The patient is then rolled directly onto the spinal board in the prone position. Similarly, if a spinal injury is suspected and the patient is in the supine position and breathing normally, the patient is rolled toward the assistants while another assistant slides the spinal board under the patient as far as possible. The patient is then rolled back onto the spinal board in the supine position. If a spinal injury is suspected and the patient is in side lying, the patient is log-rolled directly onto the spinal board and into the supine position. In each of these cases, the examiner controls the head, applies traction, and instructs the assistants. The patient's head is then stabilized and immobilized with sandbags, a head immobilizer, or triangular bandages, and the patient is strapped to the spinal board with restraining belts. If a collar is used to stabilize the spine, it must do so during movement as well as when the patient is stationary; it must not hinder access to the carotid pulse, airway, or performance of CPR; it must be easy to assemble and apply; it must be adaptable to patients of all ages and sizes; and it must allow radiological examination without

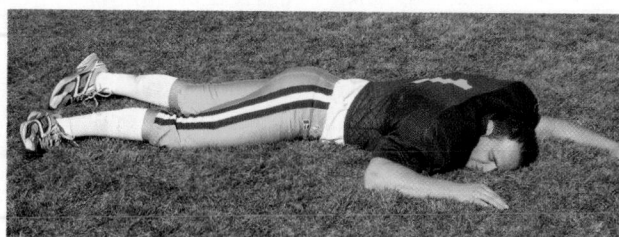

Figure 18-13 Recovery position.

removal.[46,47] Any major injury (such as, a head injury, a spinal injury, or a fracture) requires appropriate handling, slow and deliberate management, and proper transportation to provide a satisfactory outcome. These techniques must be practiced repeatedly.

If possible and if time permits, especially if the assistants are not used to working together, a simulated roll and transport using an uninjured person should be attempted before moving the patient to ensure that all involved know what they are doing in terms of patient positioning, movement sequence, and specific handling (e.g., head, hands, feet) so that any transfer or movement of the patient is effective and organized.

During the emergency assessment, if the patient is nauseated, is vomiting, or has fluid draining from the mouth, and provided breathing and circulation are normal, the patient should be placed in the **recovery position** (Figure 18-13) as long as there is no suspicion of a spinal injury. This side lying position enables the patient to be continually monitored (ABCs) and allows the examiner to easily observe any change in condition while waiting for emergency personnel. The patient's head should be positioned to keep the airway open and to allow drainage from the throat and mouth. If the blood flow to the heart and brain has diminished, circulation can be improved by elevating the lower limbs, provided that the position change can be accomplished without causing further pain or breathing problems or aggravating an injury. If the patient has breathing difficulties or a chest injury or has experienced a heart attack or stroke, it may be desirable to lower blood pressure in the injured parts by elevating the upper part of the body slightly, if the position change can be accomplished without causing further pain or breathing problems.

If the patient is unconscious and the cardiac and circulatory functions are not compromised, the patient should be left in the original position until consciousness is regained. However, if the patient is unconscious and lying supine, the examiner should always watch for the possibility that the patient may "swallow" the tongue and obstruct the airway. Also, an unconscious patient loses the cough reflex, and if vomiting or bleeding occurs, vomitus, mucus, or blood may enter and obstruct the airway. Therefore, the examiner may elect to put the patient in the recovery position.

If the patient is unconscious and in respiratory or cardiac distress, the examiner must quickly assess the patient and attempt to restore respiratory and cardiac function. This patient is then treated the same as the conscious patient.

If the patient's spine is twisted or flexed and the patient is reasonably comfortable, the patient should be stabilized in that position until a spinal injury is ruled out. If there has been a loss of breathing or cardiac function, the examiner must carefully correct the deformity, place the patient in the supine lying position, and perform the appropriate measures to deal with the problem.

If a cervical spine injury has occurred to a child of 7 years of age or younger, the examiner should realize that in these children, the head is normally larger in proportion to the rest of the body. If the child is positioned on a spinal board without modification, the neck will be forced into some flexion. To alleviate this problem, the spinal board should have a cutout for the head, or a pad for the chest or rest of the body should be added to elevate it in relation to the head.[48]

If the patient is in the water and unconscious, he or she must be reached as quickly as possible. The rescuer should not jump into the water, because this action creates waves that may rock the victim's head and could cause severe consequences if a neck injury has occurred. The examiner should approach the patient head-on and place an extended arm down the middle of the patient's back with the patient's head in the examiner's axilla. The examiner then grasps the patient's biceps with the forearm around the patient's forehead, slowly lifts the arm, and turns the patient face up. The examiner's forearm locks the patient's head in the examiner's axilla during the turn. Once the patient is supine, both of the examiner's arms support the patient's head and spine in the water. An assistant then slides the spinal board under the patient in the water and blocks the patient's head with towels. The patient is next strapped to the spinal board with restraining straps and is lifted out of the water.[49] If a spinal board is not available and a cervical injury is suspected, the patient should be supported in the water until emergency personnel arrive.

In some sports (e.g., ice hockey, lacrosse, motor car or motorcycle racing, football), the athletes wear helmets. Whether the helmet should be removed to institute emergency procedures is a controversial issue and often depends on the type of training (EMS versus sports therapy) and experience of the health care professional.[2,45,50-53] Generally, if the patient is unconscious, the helmet should not be removed unless the examiner is absolutely certain that there has not been a neck injury. In the patient who wears both helmet and shoulder pads, both should be left on the patient, because they help to maintain the cervical sagittal alignment close to normal. Ideally, the helmet and shoulder pads should be removed in a controlled setting, such as the emergency department.[2,54,55] Helmets should be removed only if the facemask or visor interferes with adequate ventilation;[54,56] if the facemask interferes with the clinician's ability to restore an adequate airway;[54,56] if the helmet is so loose that it does not provide adequate immobilization of the head when secured to the spinal board;[54,56] if life-threatening hemorrhage under the helmet cannot be controlled;[54,56] if, in children, the helmet is too large and causes flexion of the neck when used as part of the immobilization;[48,54,56] or if it is necessary to defibrillate the patient. In the last case, the shoulder pads must be removed, so the helmet should be removed to maintain spinal position.[4] If the patient is in respiratory distress, facemasks can usually be easily removed with the use of an X-Acto knife or similar device to release the restraining straps while holding the mask in place.

If, for whatever reason, the decision is made to remove the headgear, the neck and head must be held as rigid as possible. Therefore, at least two people are needed: one to stabilize the head and neck and one to remove the facemask. One person, usually the assistant, first applies in-line traction is to the helmet to ensure initial stability. A second person, usually the examiner, then stands at the side of the patient and employs in-line traction by applying a traction force through the patient's chin and occiput. The assistant stops applying traction and, if the helmet is a football helmet, first removes the cheek pads by sliding a flat object (e.g., scissors handle) between the cheek pad and helmet, twisting the object to cause the pads to unsnap. After the pads are removed, the assistant applies bilateral expansion to the helmet so that the ears are cleared as the helmet is removed.[4] After the helmet has been removed, the assistant reapplies in-line traction from the head, and the examiner then releases the traction and continues the primary examination.[43] If desired, the examiner may apply a cervical collar, such as the Stifneck collar, but this should be done with caution because cervical collars do not completely eliminate movement in the cervical spine.[57]

If the helmet is removed and the patient is wearing shoulder pads, the person holding the head must ensure that the head does not fall back into extension, and a modification must be made to the spinal board. The shoulder pads should be removed only if it is impossible to do this or if defibrillation is necessary.

If the patient is conscious and there appears to be no cervical injury or other severe injury, the patient may be moved to another area for a more appropriate and complete secondary assessment. If the injury is in the upper limb and the injured part is immobilized, the patient may first be moved from a supine to a sitting or kneeling position, then from sitting or kneeling to supported standing, to unsupported standing, and finally the person may walk off the field. During these changes in position, the examiner or assistants are positioned to provide support and assistance if the patient feels dizzy or unsteady. If the injury is in the lower limb, the athlete may be helped off the field by teammates, stretcher, or cart. Spinal injuries require greater care and the use of a spinal board and cervical collar with support. Again, assistance may be required, and everyone, including the patient and assistants, should be aware of the movement sequence before it is attempted.

Movement Sequence to Remove Conscious, Mobile Athlete from Field of Play

Supine lying
↓
Sitting (supported)
↓
Kneeling (supported, 4 point → 2 point)
↓
Standing (supported)
↓
Standing (unsupported)
↓
Walk off field (assistance ready)

Injury Severity

During the primary assessment, the examiner must use some method of determining the severity of injury. There are several scales that may be used to test the severity of injury or to triage the patient, including the Galveston Orientation and Amnesia Test,[58] which tests for posttraumatic amnesia; the Abbreviated Injury Scale;[59] the Injury Severity Score;[59-61] the Trauma Score;[62] the Triage Index;[63,64] the Circulation, Respiration, Abdomen, Motor, and Speech (CRAMS) Scale;[65,66] and the Trauma Index.[67] Of these, the Trauma Score illustrates the ease of scoring (Figure 18-14) and the survival probabilities (Table 18-9) that can be expected in trauma patients. This tool provides a dynamic score that monitors changes in the patient's condition and is useful in making triage decisions. The CRAMS scale illustrates a similar scoring pattern (Table 18-10).

SECONDARY ASSESSMENT

The examiner can proceed to the secondary assessment if the patient is conscious, is able to respond by talking coherently, shows minimal or no distress in terms of breathing, and displays normal circulation. However, the examiner must keep in mind that the patient may still have suffered a catastrophic injury (e.g., cervical spine injury) that, although not life-threatening at the present time, could lead to significant problems. For the most part, the secondary survey is predicated on the patient's being clinically stable.[8]

If the patient is conscious, the examiner must constantly reassure the patient to reduce potential anxieties. By the time the secondary assessment begins, the examiner should have eliminated any possible life-threatening situations and can then complete the injury assessment. In the case of a sudden injury, the examiner should remember that the patient has had no time to prepare psychologically or practically for the injury. Therefore, the injury can represent a sudden and frightening change in the patient's physical state. Other concerns experienced by the patient may be related to the patient's job, financial situation, family, or prognosis, and these concerns, suddenly magnified, may affect the patient's behavior, especially in later secondary or "sideline" assessments.

The secondary assessment is a head-to-toe rapid physical examination[68] and can be performed after the examiner has ascertained that there is no threat to the patient's life. The patient must be conscious for the examiner to perform the secondary assessment properly. The secondary survey involves a complete body survey to detect other injuries that may cause serious complications or lead to a patient's not being allowed to return to activity. The patient should be instructed not to move unless requested by the examiner, who should also explain to the patient what is being done while the examination is being performed. It is important to maintain communication with the patient throughout the examination. During this time, the examiner is testing for possible spinal injuries, fractures, dislocations, or soft-tissue injuries. Care must be taken that injuries are not missed.[69]

Musculoskeletal Injuries Commonly Missed during Emergency Assessment[69]

- Closed tendon injuries of the hand
- Carpal bone injuries
- Occult elbow fractures
- Femoral neck fractures
- Posterior shoulder dislocations
- Epiphyseal plate injuries
- Pubic ramus fractures
- Patellar tendon rupture
- Lisfranc (tarsometatarsal) fractures
- Compartment syndromes

While performing the secondary assessment, the examiner is considering whether the patient should be allowed to return to activity. The examiner must decide whether further evaluation is required on-site or whether the patient should be taken to some other venue (e.g., training room, hospital). In addition, the examiner should keep in mind that home monitoring may be necessary and

Trauma Score

Trauma Score	Value	Points	Score
A. Respiratory rate	10–24	4	
Number of respirations in 15 sec, multiply by four	25–35	3	
	>35	2	
	<10	1	
	0	0	A. _____
B. Respiratory effort	Normal	1	
Shallow—markedly decreased chest movement or air exchange	Shallow or retractive	0	
Retractive—use of accessory muscles or intercostal retraction			B. _____
C. Systolic blood pressure	>90	4	C. _____
Systolic cuff pressure—either arm; auscultate or palpate	70–90	3	
	50–69	2	
	<50	1	
No carotid pulse	0	0	
D. Capillary refill			
Normal—forehead, lip mucosa or nail bed color refill in 2 sec	Normal	2	
Delay—more than 2 sec of capillary refill	Delayed	1	
None—no capillary refill	None	0	D. _____

E. Glasgow Coma Scale (GCS)

Total GCS Points	Score
14–15	5
11–13	4
8–10	3
5–7	2
3–4	1	E. _____

1. Eye opening
   - Spontaneous _____ 4
   - To voice _____ 3
   - To pain _____ 2
   - None _____ 1

2. Verbal response
   - Oriented _____ 5
   - Confused _____ 4
   - Inappropriate words _____ 3
   - Incomprehensible words _____ 2
   - None _____ 1

3. Motor response
   - Obeys command _____ 6
   - Purposeful movement (pain) _____ 5
   - Withdraw (pain) _____ 4
   - Flexion (pain) _____ 3
   - Extension (pain) _____ 2
   - None _____ 1

Trauma Score
(Total points A + B + C + D + E): _____

Total GCS points (1 + 2 + 3) _____

Figure 18-14 Trauma score (see Table 18-9 for survival rate based on trauma score). (From Champion HR, Sacco WJ, Carnazzo AJ, et al: Trauma score. Crit Care Med 9:673, 1981.)

therefore should determine whether a responsible person is at home to watch for changing signs and symptoms in the patient (see Figure 2-34).

When progressing to the secondary assessment, the examiner must continue to do the Neural Watch or the GCS and watch for signs of an expanding intracranial lesion or other complications. Advanced cerebral edema may further reduce the perfusion of an already damaged hemisphere of the brain, and compression of the descending motor tracts may decrease limb power. Also, the patient's level of consciousness can reveal a deficit previously overshadowed by other evidence of severe brain injury.

During the secondary assessment, there is time to carry out a more thorough assessment for head injury or perform other tests in addition to the Neural Watch and GCS. The patient's abilities to assimilate information and

Emergency Care Levels of Decision

1. Is the injury life-threatening?
2. What care (first aid) must be given on-site or "on the field"?
3. Can and should the patient be moved?
4. If the patient is to be moved, what is the best way to do it?
5. What steps are to be taken before the patient is moved? Spinal board? Splinting? Instruction?
6. If the patient is to be moved, where to? Sidelines? Locker room? Training room? Hospital?
7. How is the patient to be transported? Ambulance? Parent's vehicle?
8. If the injury is not severe enough to require transportation to the hospital, what protocols are to be followed for return to activity?
9. If the patient is not allowed to return to activity, what protocols are to be followed?

Adapted from Haines A: Principles of emergency care. Athletic J 26:66–67, 1984.

TABLE 18-9

Trauma Score and Probability of Survival Based on the Score

Trauma Score	Probability
16	0.99
15	0.98
14	0.95
13	0.91
12	0.83
11	0.71
10	0.55
9	0.37
8	0.22
7	0.12
6	0.07
5	0.04
4	0.02
3	0.01
2	0.00
1	0.00

From Champion HR, Sacco WJ, Carnazzo AJ, et al: Trauma score. Crit Care Med 9:674, 1981.

TABLE 18-10

CRAMS Scale

Circulation
2: Normal capillary refill and BP over 100 mm Hg systolic
1: Delayed capillary refill or BP 85 to 99 systolic
0: No capillary refill or BP less than 85 systolic   ____

Respiration
2: Normal
1: Abnormal (labored, shallow, or rate over 35)
0: Absent   ____

Abdomen
2: Abdomen and thorax not tender
1: Abdomen or thorax tender
0: Abdomen rigid, thorax flail, or deep penetrating injury to either abdomen or thorax   ____

Motor
2: Normal (obeys commands)
1: Responds only to pain—no posturing
0: Posturing or no response   ____

Speech
2: Normal (oriented)
1: Confused or inappropriate
0: No sounds or unintelligible sounds
(Score of 6 or less indicate referral to trauma center should be initiated)

TOTAL   ____

From Hawkins ML, Treat RE, Mansberger AR: Trauma victims: Field triage guidelines. South Med J 80:564, 1987. Reprinted by permission from the Southern Medical Journal.
BP, Blood pressure; *CRAMS*, circulation, respiration, abdomen, motor, and speech.

act with split-second timing are more likely to be impaired after a concussion than are strength and endurance. If a head injury is suspected, it is important to determine the patient's reasoning and processing ability (see Chapter 2).

The examiner also checks coordination or motor neurological function.[70] When testing for proper neurological function, the examiner should palpate the neck and back for any pain or tenderness.[71] There are a number of tests for eye-hand coordination (see Chapter 2). Balance and motor coordination can be tested by determining whether the patient can maintain balance through unsupported standing, the Romberg test, standing with eyes closed, being pushed from side to side, balancing on one leg, or normal walking. Motor neurological function is tested by checking the patient's grip strength or the various myotomes.

Eye coordination and peripheral vision can be checked by asking the patient to follow the examiner's fingers up and down, side to side, diagonally, and in circles, noting any wandering eye movements. To test visual disturbance, the patient is asked to read or observe something from a short distance (e.g., eye chart, how many fingers the examiner is holding up). To test for vision at distance, the patient can be asked to read the score clock, as an example.

After brain function has been tested, the remainder of the secondary assessment is similar to the "clearing," or scanning, assessments performed for the cervical or lumbar spine. The examiner clears the different areas of the body so that a detailed assessment of the specifically injured joints or structures can be performed. At this stage, the assessment follows the same basic protocol as in the detailed assessment of specific joints—that is, a more detailed history of the injury is taken, the patient is observed for obvious or potential problems, and the entire body is quickly scanned for injury. This is followed by a detailed examination of the specifically injured structures, including active, passive, and resisted isometric movements, special tests, testing of reflexes and cutaneous sensory distribution, joint play movement tests (if applicable), and, finally, palpation and other diagnostic tests, such as imaging and laboratory tests (see Chapters 3 to 13).

Because the examiner is one of the first persons to talk to the patient, the examiner will probably obtain the most accurate history. Simple non-leading questions should be asked, and information should be clarified in an attempt to find out what happened and what injury or injuries the patient believes have occurred. Appropriate questions related to specific joints or areas of the body can be found elsewhere in this text. The patient often can provide the examiner with the diagnosis if the examiner listens carefully. After the patient has been thoroughly questioned, others who witnessed the accident or injury may also be questioned to complete the history. Informed conversation with other persons sometimes helps the examiner to detect abnormal behavior that may not be noticed initially. If the patient has a previous medical file, it may also prove beneficial to review the contents for information regarding preexisting conditions, previous trauma, and medications.

While obtaining the patient's history, the examiner continues to observe the patient and notes levels of consciousness, developing symptoms, pain patterns, and altered functional abilities. In addition, the examiner should carefully watch for developing signs and symptoms of an expanding intracranial lesion by noting changes in facial expression, the pupils, and the level of consciousness and by performing the Neural Watch and GCS several times. The basic observation is the same as that performed during joint assessment and includes observation of bony and soft-tissue contours, scars, deformities, the ability to move, and body alignment.

The next part of the secondary assessment is the scanning examination, in which the examiner quickly scans the entire body through observation, by asking the patient to make particular movements (depending on where the suspected injury has occurred), and by testing myotomes, dermatomes, and reflexes. During this phase, the examiner should explain what is being done and why, not only to reassure the patient but also to ensure cooperation and relaxation. This part of the examination may be done without removing the patient's clothes, although it is better to do so because clothing may obstruct the view of the injured area. However, if the examination is being performed in the presence of other people, clothing removal should be left to a later time, or the patient should be moved to a more appropriate location. If the clothes need to be removed, the patient should be warned, especially if in a public place, and every effort should be made to maintain the patient's dignity.

After the specific area or areas of injury have been narrowed down through the scanning examination, the examiner can perform a detailed assessment of the appropriate parts of the body, as specified in other chapters. Failure to perform a proper examination may lead to a missed assessment and more problems than originally anticipated.

The patient must be immediately sent to a hospital or trauma center if at any time during the primary or secondary evaluation the following signs are exhibited: pupillary or extraocular movement abnormality, facial or extremity weakness, amnesia, confusion or lethargy, sensory or cranial nerve abnormality, positive Babinski sign, deep tendon reflex asymmetry, or posttraumatic seizures.[35,72] Proper care for the patient must always be uppermost in the mind of the examiner.

Signs Indicating Need for Immediate Transport to Hospital

- Abnormal pupil or extraocular movement
- Increasing facial or extremity weakness or flaccid paralysis
- Amnesia, confusion, or lethargy
- Sensory or cranial nerve abnormality
- Decreasing value in GCS
- Positive Babinski sign
- Deep tendon reflex asymmetry
- Posttraumatic seizures
  GCS, Glasgow Coma Scale.

After the assessment has been completed and the patient has been stabilized, has returned to competition, or has been referred for further medical care by ambulance, the examiner should be sure to document what happened and the subsequent care that was given, noting any potential difficulties. These notes, if taken at the sideline, should be transferred to the patient's medical record as soon as possible.

PRÉCIS OF THE EMERGENCY SPORTS ASSESSMENT

The sequence to be followed for assessment of acute injury is shown in Figure 18-15 on next page.

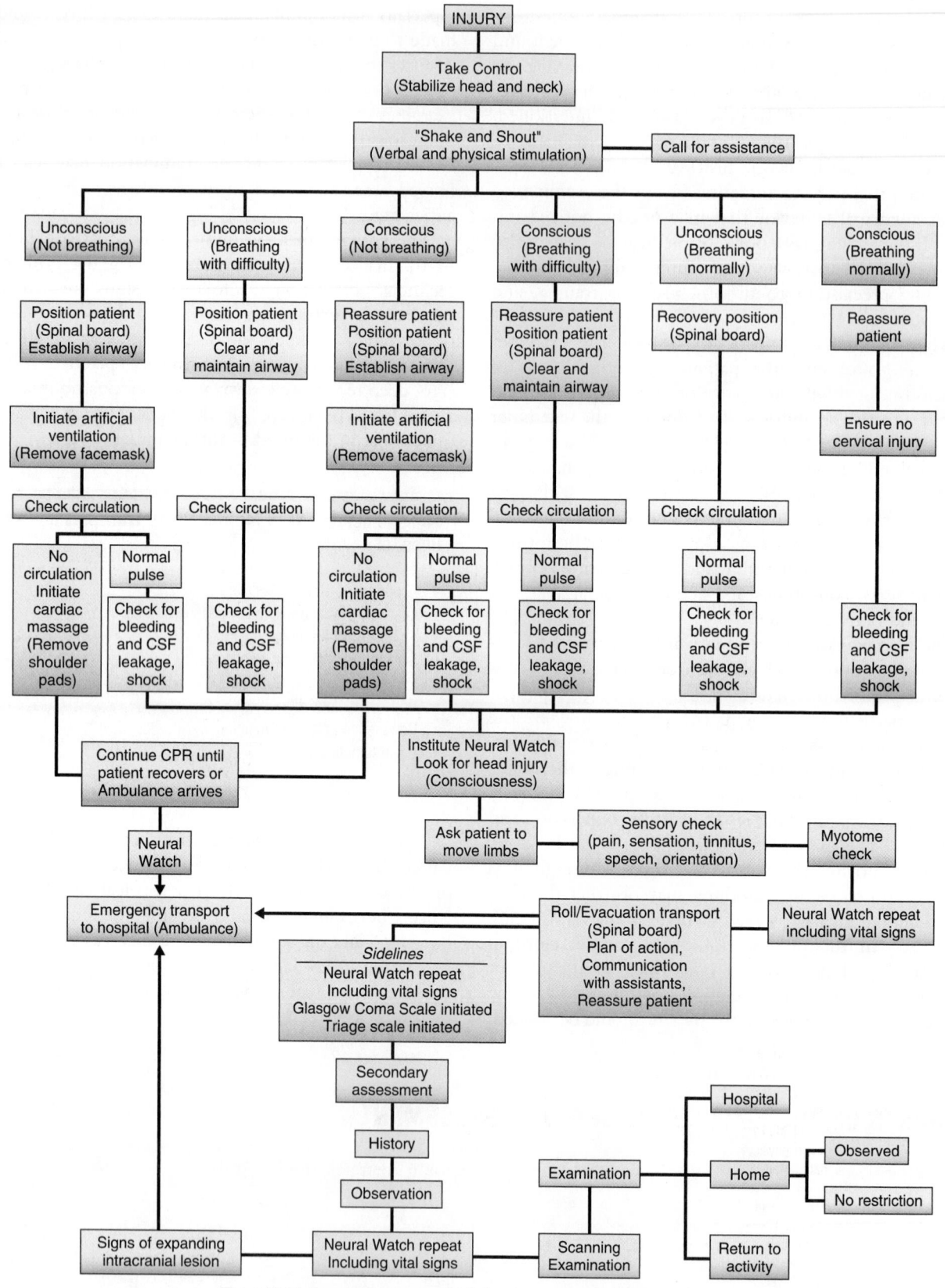

Figure 18-15 Assessment sequence following acute head/neck injury.

CASE STUDIES

When reviewing or practicing these case studies, the examiner should outline the necessary protocol for dealing with the situations described. The examiner can develop different scenarios depending on the degree of severity of the injury. These scenarios, including assessment and movement of the patient, should be practiced often so that the examiner is fully aware of what to do and how to handle emergency situations.

1. A diver misjudges his take-off from the 10-m board, hits his head on the concrete platform, and falls unconscious into the pool, displaying decorticate rigidity as he falls. Describe your emergency protocol for this patient.

2. During a squash game, a player is struck near the eye by her opponent's squash racquet. Describe your emergency protocol for this patient.

3. A 22-year-old professional basketball player is under his own net and suddenly collapses and lapses into unconsciousness during a game. Describe your emergency protocol for this patient.

4. During a race on a hot, humid day, a 10,000-m runner collapses on the track during the event and lies motionless. Describe your emergency protocol for this patient.

5. During a baseball game, a batter is hit on the chest by a pitched ball and collapses at home plate. Describe your emergency protocol for this patient.

6. A defensive back tackles a runner and makes the tackle but does not move when the other players get up, even though he is conscious. He is having difficulty breathing. Describe your emergency protocol for this patient.

7. A rugby player hits his head during a collapsing scrum. He is knocked unconscious, is not breathing, and has no pulse. Describe your emergency protocol for this patient.

8. A hockey player receives a deep cut to the neck when another player's skate accidentally cuts him. He is bleeding profusely. Describe your emergency protocol for this patient.

9. A gymnast on the balance beam misses her dismount and lands on her head, neck, and shoulders and is knocked unconscious. Describe your emergency protocol for this patient.

10. A wrestler is thrown to the mat near the end of the first round. He lands hard on the side of his face with his neck twisted. He is lying prone and unconscious. Describe your emergency protocol for this patient.

11. While playing soccer, an athlete is stung by a bee and develops anaphylactic shock. Describe your emergency protocol for this patient.

12. A hockey player is "checked" into the boards from behind. He falls to the ice and has difficulty breathing; he had been chewing gum. Describe your emergency protocol for this patient.

REFERENCES

1. Kleiner DM, Almquist JL, Bailes J, et al: Player down: step by step guidelines for the injured athlete. Sports Med Update 16:34–38, 2001.
2. Banerjee R, Palumbo MA, Fadale PD: Catastrophic cervical spine injuries in the collision sport athlete: part 2—principles of emergency care. Am J Sports Med 32:1760–1764, 2004.
3. Herring SA, Kibler WB, Putukian M, et al: Sideline preparedness for the team physician: a consensus statement—2012 update. Med Sci Sports Exerc 44:2442–2445, 2012.
4. Starkey C, Ryan J: Evaluation of orthopedics and athletic injuries, Philadelphia, 1996, FA Davis.
5. Beaver BM: Care of the multiple trauma victim: the first hour. Nurs Clin North Am 25:11–21, 1990.
6. Torg JS, Quedenfeld TC, Newell W: When the athlete's life is threatened. Phys Sportsmed 3:54–60, 1975.
7. Fourré, M: On-site management of cervical spine injuries. Phys Sportsmed 19:53–56, 1991.
8. Dick BH, Anderson JM: Emergency care of the injured athlete. In Zachazewski JE, Magee DJ, Quillen WS,

editors: Athletic injuries and rehabilitation, Philadelphia, 1996, WB Saunders.
9. Allman FL, Crow RW: On-field evaluation of sports injuries. In Griffin LY, editors: Orthopedic knowledge update: sports medicine, Rosemont, IL, 1994, American Academy of Orthopaedic Surgeons.
10. Blue JG, Pecci MA: The collapsed athlete. Ortho Clin North Am 33:471–478, 2002.
11. McCrory P, Meeuwisse W, Johnson K, et al: Consensus statement on concussion in sport, 3rd International Conference on Concussion in Sport held in Zurich, November 2008. Clin J Sports Med 19:185–200, 2009.
12. Driscoll P, Skinner D: Initial assessment and management: I. Primary survey. Br Med J 300:1265–1266, 1990.
13. McCrory P, Meeuwisse WH, Aubry M, et al: Consensus statement on concussion in sport: the 4th International Conference on Concussion in Sport held in Zurich, November 2012. Br J Sports Med 47:250–258, 2013.

14. Guskiewicz KM: Balance assessment in the management of sport-related concussion. Clin Sports Med 30:89–102, 2011
15. Rubin A, Araujo D: Advanced cardiac life support. Phys Sportsmed 28(8):29–35, 1995.
16. Hugenholtz H, Richard MT: The on-site management of athletes with head injuries. Phys Sportsmed 11:71–78, 1983.
17. Steichen FM: The emergency management of the severely injured. J Trauma 12:786–790, 1972.
18. American Academy of Orthopaedic Surgeons: Emergency care and transportation of the sick and injured, Chicago, 1981, AAOS.
19. Ward R: Emergency nursing priorities of the head injured patient. AXON 11:9–12, 1989.
20. Veenema KR, Swenson J: Laryngeal trauma: Securing the airway on the field. Phys Sportsmed 28(8):71–75, 1995.
21. Erickson SM, Rich BS: Pulmonary and chest wall emergencies: on-site treatment of potentially fatal conditions. Phys Sportsmed 23:95–104, 1995.

22. Hochbaum SR: Emergency airway management. Emerg Med Clin North Am 4:411–425, 1986.

23. Vegso JJ, Lehman RC: Field evaluation and management of head and neck injuries. Clin Sports Med 6:1–15, 1987.

24. Profera LM, Paris P: Managing airway obstruction. Phys Sportsmed 19:35–40, 1991.

25. Stackhouse T: On-site management of nasal injuries. Phys Sportsmed 26(8):69–74, 1998.

26. Rubin A, Roberts WO: Automated external defibrillators: selection and use. Phys Sportsmed 28(3):112–114, 2000.

27. Vincent GM, McPeak H: Commotio cordis: a deadly consequence of chest trauma. Phys Sportsmed 28(11):31–39, 2000.

28. Keitz JE: Emergent assessment of the multiple trauma patient. Orthop Nurs 8:29–32, 1989.

29. Hayward R: Management of acute head injuries, Oxford, 1980, Blackwell Scientific.

30. Erickson SM, Rich BS: Pulmonary and chest wall emergencies: on-site treatment of potentially fatal conditions. Phys Sportsmed 23:95–104, 1995.

31. Hafen BQ, Karren KJ: First aid and emergency care skills manual, Englewood, CA, 1982, Morton.

32. Jackson RE, Freeman SB: Hemodynamics of cardiac massage. Emerg Med Clin North Am 1:501–513, 1983.

33. Rose CC: Radiologic triage of the multiply-injured patient. Emerg Med Clin North Am 3:425–436, 1985.

34. Booher JM, Thibodeau GA: Athletic injury assessment, St Louis, 1989, Mosby.

35. Mahoney BD, Ruiz E: Acute resuscitation of the patient with head and spinal cord injuries. Emerg Med Clin North Am 1:583–594, 1983.

36. Schouten R, Albert T, Kwan BK: The spine-injured patient: initial assessment and emergency treatment. J Am Acad Orthop Surg 20:336–346, 2012.

37. Kepler CK, Vaccaro AR: Injuries and abnormalities of the cervical spine and return to play criteria. Clin Sports Med 31:499–508, 2012.

38. Hosseini AH, Lifshitz J: Brain injury forces of moderate magnitude elicit the fencing response. Med Sci Sports Exerc 41:1687–1697, 2009.

39. Teasdale G, Jennett B: Assessment of coma and impaired consciousness: practical scale. Lancet 2:81–83, 1974.

40. Menegazzi JJ, Davis EA, Sucov AN, et al: Reliability of the Glasgow Coma Scale when used by emergency physicians and paramedics. J Trauma 34:46–48, 1993.

41. Durand P, Adamson CJ: On the field management of athletic head injuries. J Am Acad Orthop Surg 12:191–195, 2004.

42. Gerberich SG, Priest JD, Grafft J, et al: Injuries to the brain and spinal cord: assessment, emergency care and prevention. Minnesota Med, 691–696, 1982.

43. Vegso JJ, Bryant MH, Torg JS: Field evaluation of head and neck injuries. In Torg JS, editor: Athletic injuries to the head, neck and face, Philadelphia, 1982, Lea & Febiger.

44. Casey EB: Heat emergencies. Athletic Ther Today 11:44–45, 2006.

45. Haight RR, Shiple BJ: Sideline evaluation of neck pain: when it is time for transport? Phys Sportsmed 29(3):45–62, 2001.

46. Karbi OA, Caspari DA, Tator CH: Extrication, immobilization and radiologic investigation of patients with cervical spine injuries. Can Med Assoc J 139:617–621, 1988.

47. Chandler DR, Nemejc C, Adkins RH, et al: Emergency cervical spine immobilization. Ann Emerg Med 21:1185–1188, 1992.

48. Herzenberg JE, Hensinger RN, Dedrick DK, et al: Emergency transport and positioning of young children who have an injury of the cervical spine. J Bone Joint Surg Am 71:15–22, 1989.

49. Richards RN: Rescuing the spine-injured diver. Phys Sportsmed 3:67–71, 1975.

50. Patel MN, Rund DA: Emergency removal of football helmets. Phys Sportsmed 22:57–59, 1994.

51. Waninger KN: On-field management of potential cervical spine injury in helmeted football players: leave the helmet on! Clin J Sports Med 8:124–129, 1998.

52. Peris MD, Donaldson WF, Towers J, et al: Helmet and shoulder pad removal in suspected cervical spine injury: human control model. Spine 27:995–999, 2002.

53. Waninger KN: Management of the helmeted athlete with suspected cervical spine injury. Am J Sports Med 32:1331–1350, 2004.

54. Zachazewski JE, Geissler G, Hangen D: Traumatic injuries to the cervical spine. In Zachazewski JE, Magee DJ, Quillen WS, editors: Athletic injuries and rehabilitation, Philadelphia, 1996, WB Saunders.

55. Veenema K, Greenwald R, Kamali M, et al: The initial lateral cervical spine film for the athlete with a suspected neck injury: helmet and shoulder pads on or off? Clin J Sports Med 12:123–126, 2002.

56. Heckman JD: Emergency care and transport of the sick and injured, Rosemont, IL, 1993, American Academy of Orthopaedic Surgeons.

57. Aprahamian C, Thompson BM, Finger WA, et al: Experimental cervical spine injury model: evaluation of airway management and splinting techniques. Ann Emerg Med 13:584–587, 1984.

58. Davidoff G, Jakubowski M, Thomas D, et al: The spectrum of closed-head injuries in facial trauma victims: incidence and impact. Ann Emerg Med 17:27–30, 1988.

59. Baker SP, O'Neill B, Haddon W, et al: The injury severity score: a method for describing patients with multiple injuries and evaluating emergency care. J Trauma 14:187–196, 1974.

60. Baker SP, O'Neill B: The injury severity score: an update. J Trauma 16:882–885, 1976.

61. Greenspan L, McLellan BA, Greig H: Abbreviated injury scale and injury severity score: a scoring chart. J Trauma 25:60–64, 1985.

62. Champion HR, Sacco WJ, Carnazzo AJ, et al: Trauma score. Crit Care Med 9:672–676, 1981.

63. Champion HR, Sacco WJ, Hannon DS, et al: Assessment of injury severity: the triage index. Crit Care Med 8:201–208, 1980.

64. Lindsey D: Teaching the initial management of major multiple system trauma. J Trauma 20:160–162, 1980.

65. Hawkins ML, Treat RC, Mansberger AR: Trauma victims: field triage guidelines. South Med J 80:562–565, 1987.

66. Clemmer TP, Orme JF, Thomas F, et al: Prospective evaluation of the CRAMS scale for triaging major trauma. J Trauma 25:188–191, 1985.

67. Kirkpatrick JR, Youmans RL: Trauma index: an aid in the evaluation of injury victims. J Trauma 11:711–714, 1971.

68. Hugenholtz H, Richard MT: Return to athletic competition following concussion. Can Med Assoc J 127:827–829, 1982.

69. Moore MN: Orthopedic pitfalls in emergency medicine. Southern Med J 81:371–378, 1988.

70. Guskiewitz KM: Assessment of postural stability following sport-related concussion. Curr Sports Med Rep 2:24–30, 2003.

71. Topel JL: Examination of the comotose patient. In Weiner WJ, Goetz C, editors: Neurology for the non-neurologist, Philadelphia, 1989, JB Lippincott.

72. Jones RK: Assessment of minimal head injuries: indications for in-hospital care. Surg Neurol 2:101–104, 1974.

SUGGESTED READINGS

Adelman DC, Spector SL: Acute respiratory emergencies in emergency treatment of the injured athlete. Clin Sports Med 8:71–79, 1989.

American Academy of Orthopaedic Surgeons: Athletic training and sports medicine, Park Ridge, IL, 1984, AAOS.

Andrews J: Difficult diagnoses in blunt thoracoabdominal trauma. J Emerg Nurs 15:399–404, 1989.

Arnheim DD: Modern principles of athletic training, St Louis, 1985, Mosby.

Axe MJ: Limb-threatening injuries in sport. Clin Sports Med 8:101–109, 1989.

Bailes JE, Maroon JC: Management of cervical spine injuries in athletes. Clin Sports Med 8:43–58, 1989.

Baker JH: The first aid management of spinal cord injury. Semin Orthop 4:2–14, 1989.

Bernardo LM, Comway A, Bove M: The ABC method of emotional assessment and intervention: a new approach in pediatric emergency care. J Emerg Nurs 16:70–76, 1990.

Blanchard BM, Castaldi CR: Injuries in youth hockey: on-ice emergency care. Phys Sportsmed 19:54–71, 1991.

Brennan FH: Recurrent epitaxis in a college athlete. Clin J Sports Med 9:239–240, 1999.

Brukner P, Khan K: Sporting emergencies. In Zuluaga M, Briggs C, Carlisle J, editors: Sports physiotherapy: applied science and practice, Melbourne, Australia, 1995, Churchill Livingstone.

Cantwell JD: Automatic external defibrillators in the sports arena: the right place, the right time. Phys Sportsmed 26(12):33–34, 1998.

Champion HR, Sacco WJ, Lepper RL, et al: An anatomic index of injury severity. J Trauma 20:197–202, 1980.

Coady C, Stanish WD: Emergencies in sports: the young athlete. Clin Sports Med 7:625–640, 1988.

Dailey RH: Acute upper airway obstruction. Emerg Med Clin North Am 1:261–277, 1983.

Davies GJ, Anast CY: The fractured femur: acute emergency care treatment. J Orthop Sports Phys Ther 1:53–58, 1979.

De Podesta M: A practical and effective approach in dealing with emergency situations. Can Athletic Ther Assoc J 9:5–8, 1982.

Diamond DL: Sports-related abdominal trauma. Clin Sports Med 8:91–99, 1989.

Fahey TD: Athletic training: principles and practice, Palo Alto, CA, 1986, Mayfield.

Frazier JE: Acute cardiac emergencies in the injured athlete. Clin Sports Med 8:81–90, 1989.

Gausche M, Henderson DP, Seidel JS: Vital signs as part of the prehospital assessment of the pediatric patient: a survey of paramedics. Ann Emerg Med 19:173–178, 1990.

Greensher J, Mofenson HC, Merlis NJ: First aid for school athletic emergencies. NY State J Med 79:1058–1062, 1979.

Haines A: Principles of emergency care. Athletic J 26:8–10, 1984.

Halpern JS: Clinical notebook: lower extremity peripheral nerve assessment. J Emerg Nurs 15:333–337, 1989.

Halpern JS: Clinical notebook: upper extremity peripheral nerve assessment. J Emerg Nurs 15:261–265, 1989.

Hawkins ML, Treat RC, Mansberger AR: The trauma score: a simple method to evaluate quality of care. Am Surg 54:204–206, 1988.

Heckman JD: Fractures: emergency care and complications. Clin Symposia 43(3):1–32, 1992.

Hickey JV: The clinical practice of neurological and neurosurgical nursing, Philadelphia, 1986, JB Lippincott.

Jacobs LM, Sinclair A, Beisner A, et al: Prehospital advanced life support: benefits in trauma. J Trauma 24:8–13, 1984.

Kane G, Engelhardt R, Celentino R, et al: Empirical development and evaluation of prehospital trauma triage instruments. J Trauma 25:482–489, 1985.

Levin HS, O'Donnell VM, Grossman RG: The Galveston orientation and amnesia test (GOAT): a practical scale to assess cognition after head injury. J Nerv Ment Dis 167:675–684, 1979.

Long SE, Reid SE, Sweeney HJ, et al: Removing football helmets safely. Phys Sportsmed 8:119, 1980.

Lowery DW: Soft tissue trauma of the head and neck. Phys Sportsmed 19:21–24, 1991.

Martinez R: Catastrophies at sporting events: a team physician's pivotal role. Phys Sportsmed 19:42–44, 1991.

McKnight W: Understanding the patient in emergency. Can Nurse 20–23, 1976.

Meislin HW, Iserson KV, Kaback KR, et al: Airway trauma. Emerg Med Clin North Am 1:295–312, 1983.

Moore S: Airway maintenance: A primary consideration in the unconscious athlete. Athletic Training, 48–49, 1981.

Patterson D: Legal aspects of athletic injuries to the head and cervical spine. Clin J Sports Med 6:197–210, 1987.

Putukian M, Raftery M, Guskiewicz K, et al: Onfield assessment of concussion in the adult athlete. Br J Sports Med 47:285–288, 2013.

Round Table: Guidelines to help you in giving on-field care. Phys Sportsmed 3:51–63, 1975.

Roy S, Irvin R: Sports medicine: prevention, evaluation, management, and rehabilitation, Englewood Cliffs, NJ, 1983, Prentice Hall.

Ryan AJ: On-field diagnosis of head injuries. Phys Sportsmed 4:82–84, 1976.

San Diego Sports Medicine Center: Athletic injury disaster plan San Diego, Valhalla High School, 1987.

Schneider RC: The treatment of the athlete with neck, cervical spine and cervical cord trauma. In Schneider RC, Kennedy JC, Plant ML, editors: Sports injuries: mechanisms, prevention and treatment, Baltimore, 1985, Williams & Wilkins.

Schneider RC, Kiss FC: First aid and diagnosis: the treatment of head injuries. In Schneider RC, editor: Head and neck injuries in football, Baltimore, 1973, Williams & Wilkins.

Shatney CH: Initial resuscitation and assessment of patients with multisystem blunt trauma. South Med J 81:501–506, 1988.

Shires GT: Initial management of the severely injured patient. JAMA 213:1872–1878, 1970.

Stuart MJ: On-field examination and care: an emergency checklist. Phys Sportsmed 26(11):51–55, 1998.

Swaine BR, Sullivan SJ: Reliability of the scores for the finger-to-nose test in adults with traumatic brain injury. Phys Ther 73:71–78, 1993.

Teasdale G, Jennett B: Assessment of coma and impaired consciousness: a practical scale. Lancet 2:81–83, 1974.

Torg JS: Management guidelines for athletic injuries to the cervical spine. Clin Sports Med 6:53–60, 1987.

Waecherle JF: Planning for emergencies. Phys Sportsmed 19:35–38, 1991.

Walters BC, McNeill I: Improving the record of patient assessment in the trauma room. J Trauma 30:398–409, 1990.

Warren WL, Bailes JE: On the field management of athletic head and neck injuries. In Cantu RC, editor: Neurologic athletic head and spine injuries, Philadelphia, 2000, WB Saunders.

Watkins RG, Dillin WM: Cervical spine and spinal cord injuries. In Fu FH, Stone DA, editors: Sports injuries: mechanisms, prevention, treatment, Baltimore, 1994, Williams & Wilkins.

Weigelt JA: Initial management of the trauma patient. Crit Care Clin 2:705–716, 1986.

Werman HA, Nelson RN, Campbell JE, et al: Basic trauma life support. Ann Emerg Med 16:1240–1243, 1987.

West JG, Murdock MA, Baldwin LC, et al: A method for evaluating field triage criteria. J Trauma 26:655–659, 1986.

Wilberger JE, Maroon JC: Head injuries in athletes. Clin Sports Med 8:1–9, 1989.

Yarnell PR, Lynch S: The "ding": amnesic states in football trauma. Neurology 23:196–197, 1973.

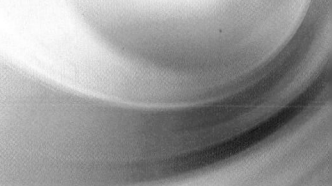

Index

Page numbers followed by "f" indicate figures, "t" indicate tables, and "b" indicate boxes.